BASIC NURSING

A PSYCHOPHYSIOLOGIC APPROACH

KAREN CREASON SORENSEN, R.N., B.S., M.N.

Formerly, Lecturer in Nursing, University of Washington;
Formerly, Instructor of Nursing, Highline College;
Formerly, Nurse Clinical Specialist, University Hospital and
Firland Sanatorium, Seattle, Washington

JOAN LUCKMANN, R.N., B.S., M.A.

Formerly, Instructor of Nursing, University of Washington,
Highline College, Seattle, Oakland City College, and
Providence Hospital College of Nursing, Oakland, California

W. B. SAUNDERS COMPANY
PHILADELPHIA • LONDON • TORONTO

W. B. Saunders Company: West Washington Square
Philadelphia, PA 19105

1 St. Anne's Road
Eastbourne, East Sussex BN21 3UN, England

1 Goldthorne Avenue
Toronto, Ontario M8Z 5T9, Canada

BASIC NURSING: A Psychophysiologic Approach   ISBN 0-7216-8498-X

Last digit is the print number: 9   8   7   6

CONTRIBUTORS, REVISERS AND REVIEWERS

ROSEMARIAN BERNI, R.N., M.N.
Associate Professor, Department of Rehabilitation Medicine, School of Medicine, University of Washington, Seattle; Adjunct Associate Professor, Department of Physiological Nursing, School of Nursing, University of Washington, Seattle; Rehabilitation Nurse Specialist, Department of Rehabilitation, University of Washington Hospitals and Clinics, Seattle

MARY X. BRITTEN, R.N., Ed.D.
Assistant Professor of Nursing, School of Nursing, State University of New York at Binghamton

MARGARET AULD BRUYA, R.N., M.N.
Doctoral Candidate, Boston University, Boston, Mass.; Associate Professor, Intercollegiate Center for Nursing Education, Spokane, Washington; Formerly Associate Professor, University of Oregon Health Sciences Center, Portland

JAMES BUSH, R.N., M.N.
Assistant Professor, School of Nursing, University of Washington, Seattle

MARY A. CHELGREN, R.N., Ph.D.
Formerly Assistant Professor of Nursing, Goshen College, Goshen, Ind.; Assistant Professor of Nursing, Berea College, Berea, Ky.; Pre-doctoral Lecturer, University of Washington, Seattle. Presently Consultant in Cardio-Pulmonary Care

ROSEMARY J. CRAIG, B.S., R.N., C.R.T.T., R.R.T.
Clinical Associate, Department of Physiologic Nursing, School of Nursing, University of Washington, Seattle; Technical Director, Respiratory Therapy Department, Swedish Hospital Medical Center, Seattle

MARYLIN JANE DODD, R.N., B.Sc.N., M.N.
Doctoral applicant, Wayne State University, Detroit

JAMES C. HANKEN, J.D.
Lecturer, Seattle University; Partner, Lenihan, Ivers and McAteer, Seattle

TY HONGLADAROM, M.D.
Attending Physician, Physical Medicine and Rehabilitation, Mason Clinic, Virginia Mason Hospital, Seattle

BARBARA S. INNES, R.N., M.S.
Associate Professor, Seattle Pacific University, Seattle

DOLLY M. ITO, R.N., D.N.Sc.
Professor of Nursing, School of Nursing, Seattle University, Seattle

CAROLYN MUELLER JARVIS, R.N., M.S.N.
Assistant Professor, School of Nursing, University of Missouri, Columbia, Missouri

LINDA A. KENT, R.N., M.N.
Coordinator, Division of Staff Development, Department of Nursing Services, University Hospital, University of Washington, Seattle

CAROLYN ANN LIVINGSTON, R.N., B.S.N., M.N.
Doctoral Candidate at the Institute for Advanced Study of Human Sexuality, San Francisco

MARGARET MARY McMAHON, R.N., B.S.N., CCRN
Project Director, Washington EDNA Education Programs; Consultant to Washington State Emergency Medical Services

RUTH McCORKLE, R.N., Ph.D.
Assistant Professor, Community Health Care Systems Department, School of Nursing, University of Washington, Seattle

DORIS I. MILLER, Ph.D.
Associate Professor of Physical Education, University of Washington, Seattle

MAUREEN B. NILAND, R.N., M.S.
Formerly Assistant Professor, School of Nursing, University of Washington, Seattle; Presently Nursing Program Chief, Ambulatory Care, Seattle Veterans Administration Hospital, Seattle

GEORGE R. NOCK, B.A., J.D.
Professor of Law, School of Law, University of Puget Sound, Tacoma

MARGARET HELEN PARKINSON, R.N., R.M.N., Dip. N., B.Soc.Sc., M.N.
Formerly Nurse Instructor, School of Nursing, Auckland Technical Institute, Auckland, New Zealand

WANDA ROBERTS, R.N., B.S.N., M.N.
Instructor, School of Nursing, Seattle University, Seattle

SARAH J. SANFORD, R.N., M.A.
Instructor, School of Health Sciences, Seattle Pacific University, Seattle

JEAN SAXON, R.N., M.N., Ph.B.
Formerly Assistant Professor, School of Nursing, University of Washington, Seattle

HELENE A. STITH, R.N., B.S.N., C.R.N.A.
Coordinator of Blood Services, University Hospital, Seattle

MARTHA L. TYLER, R.N., M.N., R.R.T.
Assistant Professor of Nursing, School of Nursing, University of Washington, Seattle; Adjunct Assistant Professor of Medicine, School of Medicine, University of Washington; Respiratory Nurse Specialist, Respiratory Disease Division, Harborview Medical Center, Seattle

ALMA MILLER WARE, R.N., M.N.
Assistant Professor, School of Nursing, University of Washington, Seattle; Consultant, Veterans Administration Hospital, American Lake, Tacoma, Washington

BONNIE S. WORTHINGTON, Ph.D.
Associate Professor, School of Nutrition Sciences and Textiles, University of Washington, Seattle; Chief Nutritionist, Child Development and Mental Retardation Center, University of Washington, Seattle

JOYCE V. ZERWEKH, R.N., M.A.
Formerly Assistant Professor of Nursing, Pacific Lutheran University; Presently Home Health Coordinator, Group Health Cooperative of Puget Sound

PREFACE

Dear Reader,

Once again we are privileged to prepare a textbook for the increasingly complex and important nursing profession. The publication of *Basic Nursing: A Psychophysiologic Approach* represents the fulfillment of a long-term plan to jointly publish books containing fundamental nursing content and specialized medical-surgical nursing content. Now we have *Basic Nursing*, which can be used in conjunction with or independently from our other book, *Medical-Surgical Nursing: A Psychophysiologic Approach.*

Over the years we have noted large overlaps in some content areas between introductory nursing and medical-surgical nursing texts. Overlaps, with unnecessary repetition, consume reader time and book space—crucial factors in a dynamic profession with a rapidly expanding knowledge base. We have carefully divided content between *Basic Nursing* and the second edition of our *Medical-Surgical Nursing* text to avoid unnecessary duplication and yet provide important content bridges, for example, in areas such as nursing process, fluid-electrolyte balance and imbalances, and caring for a person experiencing pain.

Basic Nursing has been designed as a text for students of nursing in any professional program and as a reference book for all nurses. Additionally, anyone—professional or nonprofessional—who wishes to understand the circumstances and events surrounding human problems of a health-illness nature may find it interesting reading.

We are dedicated to a psychophysiologic approach and have consistently used it throughout the text. We combine a systems approach with a conceptual model, believing that both frameworks have a place in providing clarity and meaning to the presentation of knowledge basic to nursing.

While it is difficult to "step outside" of one's own culture, we have gone to considerable effort to broaden the scope of *Basic Nursing* beyond the United States. We believe this book is appropriate for international use.

By the time you finish studying this text, it can be expected that you will:

▶Have a firm grasp of nursing and medical terminology.

▶Be able to discuss and utilize key concepts currently underlying nursing practice, e.g., stress, adaptation, homeostasis, scientific method of problem solving, nursing process, changing roles of nurses, the therapeutic nurse-patient relationship, introductory physical and psychosocial assessment, patient rights, patient-family education, illness prevention and principles of rehabilitation.

▶Be ready to apply the knowledge gained from your reading to actual nursing practice in clinical areas.

▶Effectively utilize steps of the nursing process in diagnosing and solving patients' problems and meeting patients' needs.

▶Be acquainted with certain frequently performed basic nursing procedures and the scientific rationale underlying procedural steps.

▶Be prepared to help patients and their significant others learn basic information they need to maintain their physical and psychologic health.

▶Be prepared to explore more advanced areas of nursing study (e.g., medical-surgical nursing, psychosocial nursing, maternal-child health nursing) using the concepts of basic nursing in this text as a foundation.

Basic Nursing is divided into ten units. In *Unit I* we consider unifying concepts underlying nursing practice. We describe human bonds that unite people everywhere: the healthy self and the self in illness; the therapeutic nurse-patient relationship, and nurses' growing and changing roles within modern society. In *Unit II* basic concepts of stress, adaptation, and homeostasis are considered. We also discuss changing definitions and patterns of health and disease, evolving theories of disease causation, and changing concepts of health care. The existence of the ill is investigated in detail in *Unit III*. This section describes anxieties and worries patients may feel, recognizing the need for health care, psycho-behavioral reactions to illness, disorganized behavior and thought processes that accompany illness, disturbances of body image, and the sick and impaired roles.

Unit IV is in some ways the heart of this book. In this unit we develop those vital practical concepts that excellent nurses use every day as they work with patients, e.g., the scientific method; the nursing process (assessment, diagnosis, care planning, care plan implementation and evaluation); principles of diagnosis, therapy, and rehabilitation; and methods of charting and reporting on patient status. In *Unit V* we consider the age-old problems of ethics and legalities within the nursing profession as well as the more current topic of patients' rights. *Unit VI* explores the subject of biomechanics in nursing. In that unit you will discover that biomechanics—a subject that combines basics of anatomy and physiology with statics and dynamics—is the application of the principles of mechanics to the study of living organisms. Providing patients with food and fluids is the topic of *Unit VII*. This section discusses basic concepts of good nutrition, the factors that influence a person's diet, assessment of a patient's nutritional status, nutritional considerations for various ages, special diets, and feeding methods. In addition, we present an overview of the complex subject of fluid and electrolyte balance and imbalance. *Unit VIII,* titled "Basic Clinical Considerations," includes discussion of the safe and therapeutic patient environment, providing rest and sleep, patient hygiene, monitoring vital signs, urinary and bowel elimination, medication administration, minimizing problems arising from immobility, and providing pain relief. A number of fundamental procedures are presented in this unit, e.g., giving a bed bath, administering oral and topical medications. *Unit IX,* "Advanced Clinical Considerations," delves into more complex nursing concepts and procedures, e.g., cardiopulmonary resuscitation, respiratory therapy, sterile technique, injection of medications, blood administration. Finally, *Unit X* considers the special nursing care needs of persons requiring isolation, ill children, ill elderly persons, and grieving and terminally ill people.

The concepts, principles, practices, and procedures described in these ten units build upon each other from chapter to chapter—some progressing from simpler to more complex material. Terms are defined within the context of each chapter. Each unit is written from a holistic and humanitarian viewpoint and therefore focuses primarily on the whole experience of a person under stress.

This book contains many learning aids that will make your hours of study both profitable and interesting. As you read through this text, note the study devices and use them to speed and enliven your learning. An *overview* of each chapter sets the stage for learning. Be certain to read it carefully before proceeding further into the chapter. *Study guides* also precede chapter content. These guides frequently identify concepts that may be new to you and contain vocabulary lists as well as thought-provoking questions and suggested activities.

Nursing is a vast and complex subject. Therefore, we have used special format devices to emphasize key information throughout this text. For example, *boxes* and *arrows* identify points of special importance. Many drawings, tables, and photographs are included to enhance clarity and readability.

Metric measurements and *apothecary equivalents* are stated as appropriate throughout the text. Careful *documentation,* frequent *cross-referencing,* and extensive *bibliographies* are presented to help you obtain additional information. Specific *examples* illustrate theoretical concepts. Also, we have utilized *patient histories* to help you remember that nursing theory always centers around people.

Thirty-six *nursing procedures* are described, giving a practical emphasis to the book. The procedure format is clear and concise. Significant concepts of patient-family education and patient preparation (psychologic and physical) are included.

While we acknowledge and support the view that nursing is much more than a set of tasks (procedures), we also realize that eventually principles must be translated into activities. Nurses performing technical activities must be skilled and knowledgeable. Such competence matters a lot to a patient! Thus, selected step-by-step procedures are provided to help the beginning nursing student obtain skills in the technical aspects of nursing practice. The rationale and principles supporting each step are detailed to enable the experienced nurse to adapt performance of the procedures in response to the inevitable variations in circumstances surrounding nursing practice. The procedures present *one* way of doing a task—the rationale/discussion provides a safe basis for other possible approaches to the same activity. Procedures are included for those who find them helpful; however, the text of the book is not dependent upon them.

Throughout the preparation of *Basic Nursing* painstaking attention has been given to accuracy and detail. It is recognized, however, that opinions vary and changes occur concerning "appropriate" nursing practice. The reader is thus advised to review current literature (including journals and drug and other product information sheets and brochures) and to participate in additional educational activities. Of course, textbook writing usually presents generalized information; in practice an individual patient's needs must always be assessed and individualized care planned accordingly.

The conscientious practice of nursing requires investigation of sound conceptual frameworks; thoughtful application of knowledge through the sensitive, yet incisive implementation of the nursing process; a willingness to embark upon a life course of study, and a dedication to the constant improvement of patient care. A truly professional person constantly searches for knowledge and delights in its application. This may be especially true when such application can prevent or reduce suffering.

We found again, in the preparation of *Basic Nursing*, that the most exciting part of finding new knowledge is sharing it with others. It is, thus, with a sense of excitement that we place this book in your hands.

KAREN CREASON SORENSEN

JOAN LUCKMANN

ACKNOWLEDGMENTS

We wish to express our thanks to the many experts who have contributed to the preparation of *Basic Nursing*. Our contributing authors and revisers are listed on a separate page. Special thanks are due to Jean Saxon for the various procedures that she developed and for her consultation services. The vast number of original illustrations for this work were skillfully prepared by Marjorie Domenowske. We are deeply indebted to Margaret Parkinson for her valuable contributions as author and consultant and for her careful review of proof. Of course the staff of the W. B. Saunders Company has contributed to the publication of our book. We particularly express our gratitude to Helen L. Dietz for assisting with the publication of this book and to Ilze Rader for her extremely thorough editing. Finally we thank all of the individuals and firms whose literature we have used in researching and writing this text.

KAREN CREASON SORENSEN
JOAN LUCKMANN

CONTENTS

CONTENTS

UNIT IX   ADVANCED CLINICAL CONSIDERATIONS

UNIT X   CARING FOR PERSONS WITH SPECIAL NEEDS

LIST OF PROCEDURES

UNIFYING CONCEPTS BASIC TO NURSING PRACTICE

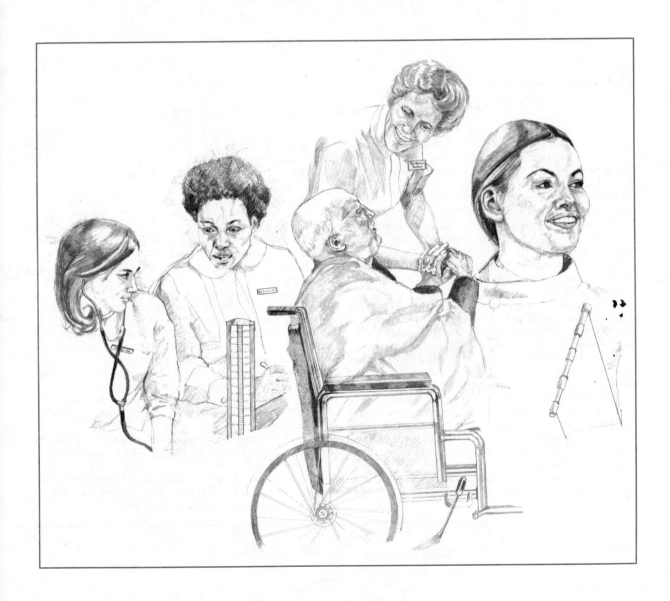

CHAPTER 1

HUMAN BONDS

...man is not only a biological organism but also a psychological actor, a member of a society and a bearer of culture. He is a biological organism with vital processes that are characteristic of life or of living matter. He is a psychological actor in that he feels, acts, and engages in such activities as thinking, learning, talking, and perceiving. He is a member of a society in that he not only occupies a status, both ascribed and achieved, but he also enacts one or more roles through interaction with others. He is a bearer of culture in that he carries the beliefs, values, customs, and mores from generation to generation. All of these facets of man must be understood singularly and jointly, for it is their combined effect that guides and determines man's total behavior.

R. WU[25]

INTRODUCTION AND STUDY GUIDE

The purpose of this chapter is to discuss those human bonds that you, as a person, share with all other people—and thus, with patients. Despite individual differences in age, appearance, personality and social background, nurses and patients have in common many basic characteristics, behaviors and needs, and they face many of the same problems and stresses. A fundamental knowledge of "man" and an understanding of the commonalities as well as the differences between people enable the nurse to give intelligent empathic care to patients from divergent cultures, life-styles and backgrounds.

In Chapter 1, then, we consider man's basic characteristics and needs, since in order to understand a patient's needs we must first be knowledgeable about people in general. More specifically, we discuss the following: (a) the hospital as a human world in microcosm, (b) man as a biologic and social being, (c) man as a natural system, (d) man's basic needs, and (e) man's universal experiences.

While some of the terms and concepts discussed in Chapter 1 will be familiar to you, many of the words and ideas may be new. Therefore, we suggest that you use the following study guide to make your reading more meaningful:

As you study this chapter, strive to learn the general meaning of the following terms:

cell

internal milieu
external environment
stress
adaptation
systems theory
goal
need

As you read this chapter, attempt to answer the following general questions:

1. What biologic characteristics do all living organisms share?

2. What common characteristics, experiences, problems and needs do all human beings share?

3. In what way does anthropologist Clyde Kluckhohn attempt to reconcile the conflict between the uniqueness of each individual versus the universality of human needs and problems?

4. What is a "system" and in what ways can the "systems approach" be used to study mankind?

5. Using the systems approach, how is "man" defined? Describe the hierarchy of natural systems constituting "man."

6. How does Maslow describe human needs? In what way does Maslow arrange human needs within a hierarchical system?

7. What are man's universal experiences? How does an appreciation of universal human experiences aid nurses in caring for patients?

THE HOSPITAL: A HUMAN WORLD IN MICROCOSM

Anyone who works in a hospital soon realizes that a hospital is a miniature world in itself, populated by people with special problems. One finds in the hospital environment numerous personality types, cultural varieties and endless human problems similar to those found in the larger world outside. But because patients are people *undergoing stress*, the hospital environment is one in which certain elements are exaggerated more than they are in the community at large. The hospital environment is intense, filled with strange odors, frightening sounds and sudden tragedy; it is a place in which the extremes of infancy and old age, birth and death, anesthesia and chronic pain come together.

Within the hospital, as well as in the outside community, a knowledge of human bonds helps nurses give compassionate care to persons of different ages, cultures, races, religions and ethnic backgrounds. Indeed, this knowledge enables the nurse to bring order and meaning into her work with patients despite the tremendous range of human variability that exists in any patient community. As an example of the variety of personalities and the multitude of individual problems that nurses face daily, consider the following situation.

Today you have been assigned to care for four women occupying a four-bed ward. Both the head nurse and your instructor have briefed you concerning these patients, and now you are entering the room to survey the situation.

In one bed lies Mrs. Kowalski, an obese, jaundiced, Polish woman about 55 years of age. Mrs. Kowalski has terminal cancer that has metastasized, or spread, throughout her body. Before becoming so ill, she had been an obstetric nurse in this hospital. Consequently, she knows many doctors and nurses from different wards who come almost daily to visit and comfort her. One reason for their devotion is that she herself had assisted with the delivery of some of their children. You look carefully at her, now that she is sleeping, and you note that she breathes deeply and slowly. She has recently been given an injection of morphine sulfate, which she must receive frequently to subdue her constant pain. The head nurse has told you that Mrs. Kowalski is very bitter about her illness. She feels resentful toward all whom she has served—her children, her grandchildren, her patients. She views her life as one of sacrifice for others, which forced her to give up her own pleasures and happiness. Now she feels that her attitude toward life was a mistake and that she should have devoted more time to her own pleasure. Mrs. Kowalski has always wanted to travel—to see this country, to see Europe, to see the world—and now she knows that she never will.

In bed two lies Rita Rolands. An anxious young girl of 16, Rita is a high school dropout as well as a habitual drug user. A few days ago Rita overdosed with amphetamines and was brought into the emergency room in a state bordering on psychosis. Today, Rita is being seen by a psychiatrist for a preliminary assessment of her mental condition and psychosocial background. According to her social worker, Rita will be discharged later today to foster parents. Apparently, Rita's parents feel that their daughter is incorrigible, and thus, they have asked the court to place Rita in a foster home.

Mrs. Arethra Jones, an obese black woman, gazes pleasantly at you from bed three. She has suffered for many years from diabetes mellitus (a problem of faulty sugar metabolism), complicated by severe arteriosclerosis, a condition known to the public as "hardening of the arteries." Mrs. Jones is the mother of four children, all of whom are devoted to her and visit her almost daily, bringing their own spouses and children whenever possible. Mrs. Jones has worked much of her life in hospitals as a vocational nurse. Consequently she sympathizes with the nursing staff almost as much as they sympathize with her. Although she has been a diabetic for many years, she has never really accepted the limitations imposed by her condition in regard to diet and activities. Now, as a result of some severe dietary indiscretions, she is in the hospital, worried every minute about her finances, her younger children and her home.

Finally, you turn to Miss Claire Hopkins, an aging woman, propped up on pillows. She looks tired and faintly apprehensive, and she seems to breathe with difficulty. Miss Hopkins has severe congestive heart failure; in other words, her heart is failing to pump blood adequately through her lungs and throughout her body. You give Miss Hopkins the oxygen prescribed for her, and when she feels better, she begins to talk to you. You find that she can't recall what she ate yesterday, or what she did, but she can remember the world of her youth with brilliant acuity. In her younger days Miss Hopkins was a secretary. In the evenings, she tells you, she attended night classes in many different fields—anthropology, history, art, civics. This kept her life from being too lonely. But as she grew older and her vision failed, she found that she could no longer read as she once had. Thus, she tended to remain alone in her room for long periods, going over and over in her mind the fascinating things she had learned in school. This is how she passes time, even here in the hospital. In talking to her, you find that Miss Hopkins has the memory changes seen with age. You note that she is strangely distant and preoccupied, as if the world in which she lives has no link or connection with yours. You wonder about this woman, her life, her knowledge, her loneliness and her increasing isolation.

Now, with initial rounds made, you walk out the door and down the hall to the nurses' desk. You realize that within a few minutes you must pull together a plan of care that will give to each patient the emotional support, the instruction and guidance, and the physical care that she uniquely needs—a plan that will help each patient to obtain, if not optimum health, at least a diminution of her suffering.

You consider the many problems that face you. You wonder how you should respond to Mrs. Kowalski's feelings about her disease, to her disappointment in her life. How should you interpret her pain—is it a completely physical phenomenon or does it have a mental component? What are her feelings about death? Does she think a great deal about it and is she afraid? Equally important, how can you, an inexperienced nurse, be empathic with this patient when you yourself have never known the pain of cancer, the fear of impending death, or the despair of a life ending before its time?

You think next of Rita Rolands. This teenage girl may be only a few years younger than you and yet her life experiences have been radically different from yours. Will you, a serious student, be able to empathize with a person who has dropped out of school to lose and abuse herself in the world of drugs?

Then, there's Mrs. Jones. How can you approach her with instructions concerning a disease that she has lived with for so many years? Except for her hospital experience, what do you have in common with this patient if she is of a different race than you are; when she has four children and you are not even married?

When you consider Miss Hopkins, you feel an even greater gap—a gap in age, a gap in life experience. You, who are probably young, healthy and active, must work and communicate effectively with a woman who is aging, physically very ill and emotionally isolated. What can you do with these problems?

Given this situation, there are three possible approaches that you can take: First, you can plan to care for these patients on a purely mechanical, technical level, ignoring all the intricate, painful and delicate human problems that arise. That is, you can make sure that Mrs. Kowalski receives her injections for pain, that Mrs. Jones is given instruction booklets concerning diabetes, that Rita Rolands is discharged properly, and that Miss Hopkins is given oxygen when necessary, as well as any medications that have been ordered. At the same time, you close your eyes and ears and ignore, as much as possible, Mrs. Kowalski's fears and bitterness, Rita Rolands' need for guidance and reassurance as to her basic worth, Mrs. Jones' basic misconceptions about her diabetes, and Miss Hopkins' pathetic attempts to establish contact with another person. As a result, you will "do your job" without either taxing yourself intellectually or investing yourself emotionally. A comfortable illusion of patient care will be created without any really thorough care ever being given. Unfortunately, this form of mechanized nursing practice is not uncommon.

Second, you can approach this group of patients in a helter-skelter fashion, recognizing that patient problems do indeed exist but being unable to organize and understand the mass of signs, symptoms, clues and responses that these problems create. Unlike the mechanically oriented nurse, you do not ignore the differences between patients, nor the many subtle details inherent in every human situation. Instead, you tend to think mainly in terms of differences and details without ever relating these details to each other or to any larger frame of reference. With this approach, you may feel that Mrs. Kowalski's bitterness over her illness, Rita Rolands' rejection of parental and societal values, Mrs. Jones' rejection of her illness, and Miss Hopkins' rejection of the real world are responses totally isolated from one another. Furthermore, you fail to see any interlinking threads between these four people and their problems, and yourself and your problems. Naturally, you come to feel frustrated and overwhelmed. To plan care with this attitude is like attempting to write a play without a plot, to create characters who act and react without basic human motivations. The end result, for both plan and play, is an unintelligible jumble of action without any unity or purpose.

Finally, you can approach nursing care with an appreciation of the diversity of human life and personality, but without losing sight of the basic similarities that unite all people, patients and nurses. These similarities, consequently, make planning care easier. You recognize that Mrs. Kowalski, Rita Rolands, Mrs. Jones, Miss Hopkins and yourself are first of all *people;* consequently, you all share certain basic human experiences. Furthermore, you all share the same basic human needs, some of which are satisfied and some of which are not. You all are being acted upon by stresses arising either within the environment or within yourselves. Each of you is attempting to adapt as well as you can to these stresses in the hope of reaching some sort of balance or equilibrium, both psychologically and physiologically. However, you tend to *differ* from one another in that some of you are meeting the challenges and stresses inherent in life more successfully than others, and some of you have more stresses at this period in your individual lives than others.

In conclusion, if we view this ward with its four patients as a sample of the hospital population, and the hospital as a sample of the general population, then it is obvious that we must begin our study of patients by studying people. It has been pointed out by Martin and Prange that "nursing needs a better conceptualization of . . . the human phenomena with which it deals."[16] They continue by citing Galdston, who said about medicine:

Medicine is founded on, pursues, and cultivates the knowledge and understanding of man as a living creature whose being is framed by a world of many and varied realities. Medicine is not only a body of knowledge and skills which aims at benefiting man but also an understanding of the nature of the universe, and of man's position in it.[9]

In sum, nursing and medicine are concerned with total man, not a part of man. We strive for a holistic view of man, and begin by thinking of the broad science of man. We care for people, not facts or theories or principles. With this concept in mind, we shall now turn to a general discussion of man both as a biologic being and as a thinking, feeling person, living in a complex social environment.

MAN AS A BIOLOGIC AND SOCIAL BEING*

Man As a Living Organism. Western man, with characteristic egotism, likes to consider himself as being unique and thus totally dif-

---

*In this book, we use the term "man" to represent both men and women, and the words "she" and "her" to refer to both male and female nurses. We have employed these designations, despite their sexist connotations, simply for convenience because they are less cumbersome than such constructs as "he/she" and "him/her."

ferent from "lower" life forms. The humiliating truth is that we have *much* in common with any cat, dog, fish, snail, gutter rat, or even the tiny amoeba. We share, with these and with all other living organisms, the struggle for life—for a continued existence in a changing environment. All of us, then, from the complex organism called man to the one-celled amoeba, share the following biologic properties:

1. All living material, in its many forms, is chemically composed of carbon, hydrogen, oxygen, nitrogen, sulfur, phosphorus, calcium, iron, potassium and magnesium. Sodium and chlorine, as well as smaller amounts of manganese, copper and iodine, are typically present also. These chemicals interact within the *protoplasm,* a viscous colloidal substance that constitutes the physical basis of living organisms.

2. With rare exceptions, *the protoplasm of living organisms is organized into cells.* We define a *cell* as a unit of life. A dynamic, highly organized structure, the cell is actively involved in the processes of growth and reproduction. Even those few organisms that appear to be noncellular (e.g., the virus) still contain the same basic substances found in ordinary cells. Thus, despite the great variety of living things that surround us, all life can be reduced ultimately to the same vital components. Furthermore, all life today can be traced back to certain ancient and primitive cells that must have evolved at least 2 billion years ago.

3. In all living organisms, *respiration* is vital to the formation, maintenance and eventual breakdown of the cells that form them.

4. *All organisms have an internal environment as distinguished from the exterior world or environment surrounding them.* This "internal milieu" is created by an encapsulating membrane, which serves to protect the organism from the atmosphere external to it. The maintenance of the internal milieu is absolutely essential for life. Some of its major functions are to (a) help the organism adjust to changes in the external environment, (b) reduce the intrusion of noxious substances that could disturb the function of the organism, and (c) maintain a continuously open system for the exchange of vital substances between the internal and external environments. It is obvious that any breakdown or disruption of this internal milieu could be fatal to the organism.

5. All living things seem to pass through a

definite life cycle. The processes of birth, growth and development, maturation and reproduction, decline and death surround us everywhere in nature. In man, as in other organisms, the regulation of these processes is primarily determined by *genes,* which are the units of heredity.

6. As implied above, all living things have the ability to *reproduce,* resulting in the continuation of their species.

7. All living things are characterized by *physiologic and behavioral rhythms;* these rhythms are apparently initiated and controlled within all organisms by internal timers called *biologic clocks.* Examples of biologic rhythms include the menstrual cycle in women, sleep-awake cycles, seasonal migrations of birds, daily fluctuations in body temperature and daily cell division rhythms.[24]

8. All organisms, if they are to survive and reproduce, must have *the capacity to adapt themselves internally to changes in the external environment.* This ability enables the organism to escape harm, to minimize injury, to cope with stress and to restore internal balance once this balance is lost. Hans Selye, an authority on stress, has written that "adaptability is probably the most distinctive characteristic of life."[23] Indeed, Selye goes so far as to equate adaptability with life and the loss of adaptability with death.

Thus, we and our patients share with all other living organisms a similar chemical structure. We and all other living things depend for life upon respiration, the maintenance of an internal milieu, the ability to grow and reproduce and, finally, the ability to adapt to changing environmental conditions. Man's health can be upset if any of these vital functions are disturbed.

If these are the properties that man shares with other organisms, what then are the properties that are common to human beings and set them apart from other organisms?

Man As a Social Being. Basically, people everywhere are alike. On the other hand, we realize from personal experience that there is nothing quite so variable and seemingly unpredictable as individual human actions and reactions. This conflict between the variability of individual human beings and the universality of human nature has fascinated scholars for centuries. Over the years, scientists, artists, philosophers and physicians have attempted to solve and resolve the basic contradictions inherent in man's personality.

In a profession such as nursing, we see these contradictions daily. Almost all our patients experience pain, but some cry, some react with bitterness, some are stoical. Almost all patients experience fear and apprehension—but some hide it behind a smile, some bury it in resignation, and others express it in anger. What is the basis for these different reactions to the same experience? Anthropologist Clyde Kluckhohn[13] attempted to summarize the essence of this enigma with elegant simplicity when he wrote that "Every man is in certain respects (a) like all other men, (b) like some other men, and (c) like no other man."

Let's break this statement down and examine it for a moment as it applies to nursing. We will begin with the last statement.

> *Every man is in certain respects like no other man.*

While we readily recognize our own individuality, we often find it difficult to realize the uniqueness of others. We tend to want to "group" others in our minds; at the same time we want others to recognize our special qualities and *not* group us. It is a fact, however, that every patient we care for *is* an individual; there is no other patient and no other person in the world exactly like him.

Our patients vary from each other for two main reasons: (1) they have inherited particular characteristics from their parents or earlier ancestors, and (2) they each come from a different environmental background (social, physical, psychologic and economic). Each of our patients has grown up under different circumstances and has experienced dissimilar stresses, traumas and triumphs. These experiences have been critical in shaping their unique personalities. Also, the distinct manner in which they view themselves and their relationship to the world around them contributes to their individuality. Past experience plays a significant role in determining how a patient will face a diagnosis and accept a regimen of treatment. Consequently it is possible for many patients to suffer from exactly the same disease, and yet for each to react so differently to the diagnosis that many divergent approaches are required in giving care.

For example, let us consider an actual situation involving two male patients, both of whom were very ill with coronary heart disease. One patient was a postman: he was a timid, small, fearful person who never took chances and avoided changes in his life as much as possible. The other patient was an attractive airline pilot, accustomed to a life of travel, glamor and danger. His whole self-image revolved around himself as *the* man of action. Both patients were faced with the real possibility of sudden death from a heart attack. To prevent another attack, it was imperative that they rest, change their diet, take prescribed medications and, in general, follow prescribed treatment. The shy postman, terrified of dying, accepted without question the restrictions placed upon him. The pilot, on the other hand, refused to drastically change his life or his diet. He rejected the thought that he should modify his activities. For this man, the possibility of dying was easier to accept than even a temporary dependence on other people.

Both these patients, interestingly enough, had the same doctor. This physician wisely realized that the classic rules of treatment expressed in textbooks often must be modified when applied to real people. Whereas a routine treatment program could be followed with the postman, it would not be successful with the pilot. The doctor accepted this fact and did not force the pilot into a way of life that would have destroyed him psychologically. Instead, he compromised with the patient's need for independence by allowing him as much freedom as possible and by placing as few restrictions on him as necessary. As a result, the pilot did relax and rest, and eventually he left the hospital, as did the postman. If the doctor had failed to consider individual differences and had rigidly adhered to a "routine program" of care, this patient's anxiety and anger over his restrictions might have precipitated a fatal heart attack or he might have become despondent and committed suicide.

This example illustrates that while two patients may face the same problem, the same solution may not be applicable. Consequently, the skilled practitioner is not rigid in approaching patient care. What the book says about treatment should be weighed along with what the patient says about himself. Good care results only when both factors are carefully evaluated. Patients know themselves better than we know them, although they may sometimes be incapable of making sound judgments about what is in their best interest.

> *Every man is in certain respects like some other men.*

Nursing care is complicated by the fact that we must consider our patients not only as individuals but also as members of various groups. The ward situation described earlier in this chapter provides a good example of the various group affiliations that patients are likely to have. For example, Mrs. Kowalski is Polish. She belongs to a distinct ethnic group, which may in turn affect her attitudes about diet, disease, hospitalization and other matters. In this same room we have one black patient and three white patients. Although these patients share many things in common, there are certain cultural differences that must be considered in planning care.

Furthermore, not only do we have differing ethnic, racial, and economic groups present on this ward, but there are also different age and occupational groups. An elderly woman like Miss Hopkins cannot be approached in the same manner as a young girl of 16 like Rita Rolands. Consequently, we need to be well informed as to the general characteristics of the aged as compared to the characteristics of the adolescent and young adult. Two of the women, Mrs. Kowalski and Mrs. Jones, have worked in hospitals, and that gives them a common bond with each other and with you, the nurse. It is possible that because of their experience, they will have to be approached somewhat differently from the person who has never worked in a hospital setting. Perhaps the two who have worked in a hospital are more anxious about being patients than the other two; perhaps this is not the situation at all. These possibilities must be considered and evaluated. Also, Mrs. Kowalski and Mrs. Jones share the common bond of parenthood. Together they can discuss the trials and tribulations of child rearing, no matter how divergent their social and economic situations. Finally, all the women in this ward belong to the group, patient, as compared to the group of nurses, doctors and technicians who surround them as staff members. The bond that patients feel toward each other is often extremely strong, especially among those with chronic illnesses.

As a nurse, the more knowledge you have about different groupings of people—age, racial, ethnic, occupational and religious—the more comprehensive and intelligent your care will be.

> *Every man is in certain respects like all other men.*

Patients and nurses have their individual differences and their group differences. But, basically, we all belong to the same species, and consequently, we all have similar biologic characteristics. We all experience certain universal problems and share certain universal needs. It is this universality of need and experience that gives us a common stage upon which to act and interact with our patients. It is this mutuality, the sense of being part of humanity, that allows us to be empathic and to understand, to some degree at least, another human being.

MAN AS A NATURAL SYSTEM

Scientists and philosophers are always searching for unifying concepts with which to correlate the biologic, social, individual and cultural dimensions of "man" and of human life. One way to integrate these various facets into a unified whole is to use the *systems approach.*

Systems theory,* which has been growing in popularity over the past two decades, can be applied to any structure in the universe from a planet to a subatomic particle.

> *In essence, a* system *(which can be natural or manmade) is "a relatively stable whole" composed of various components which are integrated and coordinated in their activities by a communications network.*[1]

The activities of a system are always directed toward particular ends—states, or *goals.* For a system to attain a goal, it must interact continuously and adaptively with its environment; also, its various components must interact correctly together.

Highly complex systems (e.g., our solar system) are characterized by components (e.g., the various planets). Each component, in turn, is a natural system in its own right as well as part of a greater system. Also, each component can itself be broken down into smaller and simpler systems, thus forming a *hierarchy of systems* ranging from the complex to the simple. Thus, one can visualize life as a vast system, as does Potter, who writes: "Life is characterized by the exquisite organization of living organisms, whether they are single cells or human beings

consisting of millions upon millions of individual cells combined into a fabulous cybernetic system."[22]

Using the systems approach, an individual human being is defined as a *natural system within a hierarchy of natural systems,* which range from the biosphere to subatomic particles (see Fig. 1–1).[4] Note in Figure 1–1 that the part of the hierarchy that is labeled "Person" corresponds to each individual man, woman, or child, with all of his memories, needs and aspirations. Note, too, that the various behaviors and experiences which make up the person can also be broken down into sublevels extending hierarchically through

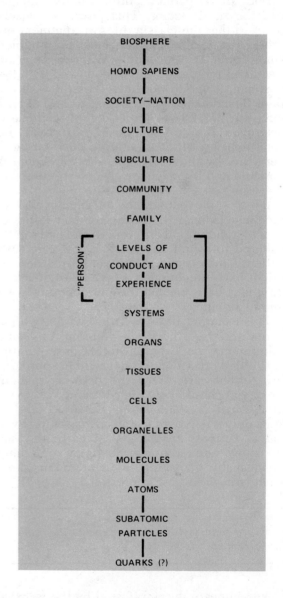

Figure 1–1. Hierarchy of natural systems constituting "man." (Taken from Brody, H.: The systems view of man: Implications for medicine, science and ethics. *Perspectives in Biology and Medicine,* Autumn 1973, p. 74.)

---

*Throughout this text we will be mentioning systems theory as it applies to health and disease, systems of health care, and the nursing process.

time from infancy to old age. Thus "man," like other natural systems, is four-dimensional, existing in both space and time.

Like all other systems, man is *goal-oriented.* That is, all his activities and behaviors are directed toward the achievement of certain end states, e.g., the satisfaction of basic needs for food, oxygen, safety, love, and acceptance by a group. Thus, goals may be biologic, cultural or social. Different individuals, societies and cultures may have different goals as a result of divergent needs and expectations. Moreover, one's goals may vary at different stages in one's life. Nevertheless, everyone has certain fundamental needs which he must strive to satisfy and toward which his behavior is directed. These needs which are basic to people everywhere will be considered next.

MAN'S BASIC NEEDS

Man has many needs, some of which are more vital than others. Physiologists, biologists and psychologists have worked out many ways of grouping needs, and the following scheme represents one such classification. According to Maslow,[12] there is a hierarchy of motivated needs, ranging from the most basic to the most sophisticated (see Fig. 1–2). In his scheme, there are the following six levels:

1. Survival needs: food, air, water, temperature, elimination, rest, pain avoidance
2. Stimulation needs: sex, activity, exploration, manipulation, novelty
3. Safety and security needs: safety, security, protection
4. Love needs: love, belonging, closeness
5. Esteem needs: esteem of others, self-esteem
6. Self-actualization: the process of making maximum use of one's abilities and potential

Maslow has made a number of assumptions about human needs. In his book *Motivation and Personality* Maslow points out that basic needs are arranged within a hierarchy on the "basis of relative potency"; i.e. if a person is starving, he is, at that moment, more concerned with finding food than he is with writing a poem or story. However, once this individual has eaten, he may then feel a need to write about his experience of starving. Thus, the need that has the *greatest potency* at the time is the need that will be satisfied first. Maslow also states that while the lower needs (e.g., the physiologic needs) *must* be satisfied if life is to continue, the higher needs also have survival value—a fact which is sometimes forgotten by doctors and nurses. In this context Maslow states:

Living at the higher need level means greater biological efficiency, greater longevity, less disease, better sleep, appetite, etc. The psychosomatic re-

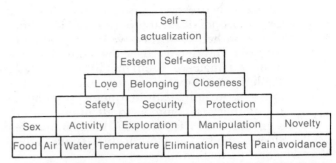

Figure 1–2. Maslow's hierarchy of needs, as adapted by Kalish. (From Kalish, R. A.: *The Psychology of Human Behavior.* Belmont, CA, Wadsworth Publishing Co., 1966.)

searchers prove again and again that anxiety, fear, lack of love, domination, etc. tend to encourage undesirable physical as well as undesirable psychological results. Higher need gratifications have survival value and growth value as well.[17]

When we consider the area of human needs in relationship to patients, it is obvious that (1) patients, as people, have the same basic needs as the nurse, (2) the patient cannot satisfy many of his needs because of physical or mental incapacity or illness, and (3) it is the nurse's task to help the patient to gratify his needs realistically within the confines of his illness and hos-

TABLE 1–1. THE COMPONENTS OF BASIC NURSING CARE

1. Helping patient with respiration
2. Helping patient with eating and drinking
3. Helping patient with elimination
4. Helping patient to maintain desirable posture in walking, sitting, and lying and to move from one position to another
5. Helping patient to rest and to sleep
6. Helping patient with selection of clothing and with dressing and undressing
7. Helping patient to maintain body temperature within normal range
8. Helping patient to keep body clean and well groomed and to protect integument
9. Helping patient to avoid dangers in the environment and protecting others from any potential danger from the patient such as infection or violence
10. Helping patient to communicate with others to express his needs and feelings
11. Helping patient to practice his religion or to conform to his concepts of right and wrong
12. Helping patient with work or productive occupation
13. Helping patient with provision for recreational activities
14. Helping patient to learn

Source: Henderson, V.: *I.C.N. Basic Principles of Nursing Care.* London, International Council of Nurses House, 1960.

pitalization, preserving as much independence for him as possible, and permitting his dependence on her as necessary. In her pamphlet, Virginia Henderson lists the components of basic nursing care. From this list (presented in Table 1–1), it is evident that the basic role of the nurse is to help patients meet those human needs that are common to all human beings, e.g., the needs for oxygen, food, fluids, rest, sleep, safety, communication with others, work, recreation.

Clearly, some needs require constant gratification, whereas the attainment of other needs can be postponed. For example, we cannot live for long without air, but sexual activity can be postponed indefinitely. However, it must be recognized that although the gratification of needs can be postponed or modified for varying periods of time, *the needs are still present.*

Sensitivity to patients and intelligent nursing care depend upon a recognition of the entire gamut of human needs. Certainly we cannot ignore the patient's survival and protection needs. If he is cyanotic (skin has a bluish hue), he may need oxygen; if he is in pain, he may need medication or a position change; if he is unconscious or delirious, he needs the protection of side rails on his bed.

On the other hand, the needs for love, stimulation and esteem, although not so obvious, are equally important. For example, consider the case of the airline pilot with severe heart disease. His need for self-esteem, which involved the preservation of his masculine, daring self-image, was actually as great, if not greater, than his survival needs. Furthermore, patients on bed rest are known to deteriorate (mentally and physically) if their needs for mental stimulation and physical movement are not met. Even under the most aseptic hospital conditions, children have failed to grow and have even died because of lack of affection and love.

In sum, patients, like ourselves, want to do more than just exist. Too frequently in nursing care only the survival needs are considered. Patients want to live as completely as possible; they desire and need a certain amount of novelty, love and esteem in their lives. They should not be denied self-actualization.

MAN'S UNIVERSAL EXPERIENCES

Because of the universality of human needs, it follows that there are also certain universal human experiences and problems. For example, people everywhere experience a sense of the passage of time, memories of the past, and an awareness of the future. Throughout the world, in tribal communities as well as in cities, men and women develop and sustain relationships with others in their society. In addition, all human beings undergo the biologic and developmental changes involved in aging. The emotions of joy and sorrow, and the realities of birth, disease, pain and death are always a part of man's existence. The fundamental experience of stress and the struggle to adapt to change is a continuous and ultimately exhausting aspect of everyone's life.

Nurses share with all humans these universal experiences as well as the drive to satisfy basic needs. The recognition of human bonds and common interests should help us to feel empathy with the patients in our care. In Chapter 2 we will further explore how the nurse can use her knowledge of human beings and human bonds to form truly therapeutic relationships with her patients—relationships that provide patients with support, help and warmth and the nurse with a feeling of satisfaction and personal growth.

BIBLIOGRAPHY

1. Aakster, C. W.: Psycho-social stress and health disturbances. *Social Science in Medicine*, 8:77, Feb. 1974.
2. Arnold, H. M.: I-Thou. *American Journal of Nursing*, 70:2554, Dec. 1970.
3. Aspy, V. H.: Are patients people? *Nursing Times*, 68:690, June 1, 1972.
4. Brody, H.: The systems view of man: Implications for medicine, science, and ethics. *Perspectives in Biology and Medicine*, 17:71, Autumn 1973.
5. Cybernetic man, *J.A.M.A., 210*:1752, 1969.
6. Dubos, R.: *Man Adapting.* New Haven, Yale University Press, 1965.
7. Dubos, R.: *Man, Medicine, and Environment.* New York, Encyclopedia Britannica, 1968.
8. Fletcher, J.: Medicine and the nature of man. *Science, Medicine, and Man*, 50:93, 1973.
9. Galdston, I. (ed.): *Beyond the Germ Theory.* New York, Health Education Council, 1954.
10. Guyton, A. C.: *Textbook of Medical Physiology*, 5th ed. Philadelphia, W. B. Saunders Co., 1976.
11. Henderson, V.: *I. C. N. Basic Principles of Nursing Care.* London, I. C. N. House, 1960.
12. Kalish, R. A.: *The Psychology of Human Behavior.* Belmont, CA, Wadsworth Publishing Co., 1966.
13. Kluckhohn, C., and Murray, H.: Personality formation: The determinants. *In* Kluckhohn, C., and Murray, A. (eds.): *Personality in Nature, Society, and Culture.* New York, Alfred A. Knopf, 1959.
14. Libby, W. F.: Man's place in the physical world. *Health Physics*, 17:531, Oct. 1969.
15. Man in his world. *Lancet*, 2:27, July 1972.
16. Martin, H. W., and Prange, A. J.: Human adaptation—a conceptual approach to understanding patients. *Canadian Nurse*, 58:234, March 1962.
17. Maslow, A. H.: *Motivation and Personality*, 2nd ed. New York, Harper & Row, 1970.

18. Mathwig, G. M.: Living, open systems, reciprocal adaptation and the life process. *Nursing Research, 18:*523, Nov.-Dec. 1969.

19. Murdock, G. P.: The common denominator of cultures. *In* Linton, R. (ed.): *The Science of Man in the World Crisis.* New York, Columbia University Press, 1945.

20. Norris, C. M.: Delusions that trap nurses. *Nursing Outlook, 21:*18, January 17, 1973.

21. Pierce, L. M.: A patient model. *American Journal of Nursing, 69:*1700, Aug. 1969.

22. Potter, V. R.: Probabilistic aspects of the human cybernetic machine. *Perspectives in Biology and Medicine,* p. 165, Winter 1974.

23. Selye, H.: *Stress without Distress.* Philadelphia, J. B. Lippincott, 1974.

24. Volpe, P.: *Man, Nature, and Society: An Introduction to Biology.* Dubuque, W. C. Brown Co., 1975.

25. Wu, R.: *Behavior and Illness.* Englewood Cliffs, NJ, Prentice-Hall, 1973.

CHAPTER 2

THE SELF IN
HEALTH AND ILLNESS

INTRODUCTION AND STUDY GUIDE

The three main topics discussed in this chapter are (1) psychologic homeostasis, (2) the healthy self and (3) the self in illness. Adaptation and homeostasis are discussed more fully in Unit II. Here we wish to offer an introduction to the concepts of mental and emotional balance and imbalance. Psychologic defense mechanisms are reviewed in Chapter 11.

We wish to emphasize that while we use such terms as "mental," "psyche," "emotional," and "psychologic," or "physical," "soma," "somatic," and "physiologic," it is not actually possible to dichotomize (separate) man into such entities. These terms have filtered down from the time in history when it was incorrectly believed that a separation did exist between mind and body.

A true understanding of illness and the ill person is based upon the knowledge that the mind does not exist separately from the body, and vice versa. This point is intentionally emphasized repeatedly because it is imperative that a nurse realize that:

> *Every ill person is experiencing* both *physiologic and psychologic imbalances. Physiologic imbalance creates an emotional disequilibrium, and emotional imbalance causes physiologic disturbances.*

As you read this chapter you may wish to clarify in your thinking the following terms and concepts:
introspection
dichotomize
consciousness
self-actualization
self-perception
autonomy
"public self"
"private self"
existence
alienation
self-knowledge
subjectivity
objectivity
values
self-image
self-deception
motivations
self-acceptance
self-rejection

When you have completed studying this chapter, try to discuss in general, in your own words, the following:
1. Components of the healthy self
2. Why it is difficult to gain self-understanding
3. Ways of meeting the needs of the normal self in illness
4. How self-understanding can help a nurse in giving patient care

THE HEALTHY SELF

It is easier to sail many thousand miles through cold and storm and cannibals . . . than it is to explore the private sea, the Atlantic and Pacific Ocean of one's being alone.

Henry David Thoreau—*Walden*

It is only through subjective reflection that we can explore what we mean by the "self." We have no conceptual definition of the self to begin with because no definition has been universally accepted. Descriptions of what the self is like invite disagreement, for we each tend to describe *the* self in terms of how we think about *our* self. It is possible, however, to pull together some generalizations about the healthy, normal self (see Table 2–1).

1. *The healthy, adjusted self is not entirely*

TABLE 2–1. SOME CHARACTERISTICS OF THE "SELF"

1. The healthy, adjusted self is not entirely free from emotional conflicts or symptoms of illness.
2. Ample energy and a drive toward self-actualization characterize the healthy self.
   a. Some of the values and goals of life that people seek vary from culture to culture.
   b. Individuals vary in their ability to become aware of deeper levels of the self and to gain insight or self-awareness.
   c. The self is simultaneously composed of sameness and change.
3. The healthy self has a sense of personal integration or of a coherent wholeness.
4. The healthy self strives to maintain some autonomy and therefore it is not necessarily of a socially conformist nature.
5. Owing to the unique consciousness of man, the self is capable of introspection and is aware of time.
6. The self is composed of a "public self" and a "private self."
7. Even though individual "selves" are isolated from one another, it is possible to form bonds with others.
8. The self is largely determined by and recognized from the values that it assumes.
9. The concept of oneself is founded upon perceptions of oneself; at times we perceive ourselves differently from the way others perceive us.
10. Each self is individual and unique from all others.

free from emotional conflicts or symptoms of illness. A certain amount of illness, imbalance, or conflict is a natural aspect of life. The healthy self is able to live with and resolve conflicts rather than be overwhelmed or immobilized by them. Stress and conflict will produce some mental disequilibrium, even in the healthy self, and therefore some of the symptoms of mental illness may appear.

2. *Ample energy and a drive toward self-actualization characterize the healthy self.* It takes energy to resolve conflicts. The well-adjusted individual is able to cope with his life's problems without depleting his supply of energy. He thus has ample energy to be productive in life and to enjoy the pleasures that are available to him. This means that it is possible for him to achieve a fairly high level of self-actualization, personally and with others.

a. *Some of the values and goals of life that people seek vary from culture to culture.* In addition, variation is found among personal goals and values. These are determined in part by an individual's personal constitutional endowment and also by his life experience. In spite of this diversity of cultural and personal goals, people everywhere strive toward self-actualization as fully as their cultural and personal situations permit. They strive to fulfill their potentials, to grow and to achieve as much as they can. None of this is possible without encountering conflict. The healthy individual attempts to learn from his conflicts so

that he may achieve a higher level of self-actualization.

b. *Individuals vary in their ability to become aware of deeper levels of the self and to gain insight or self-awareness.* Although many people recognize the *need* for self-awareness, too few work to attain it.

Avoiding responsibility and decision through avoiding inner resources and powers, we evade the challenge to be what we are or can be. We are truly adrift, like a ship in irons.[20]

Even for those who do work to attain it, complete self-awareness is impossible.

c. *The self is simultaneously composed of sameness and change.* We remain the same person, recognizable to ourselves and to others, even though we change and grow physically and psychologically.

I was a moment ago; I am part of the past. Yet it is I who now am, who then was. Though I passed with time, I did persist.[37]

It is through this quality of persistence that we are able to remain ourselves while undergoing change. The fact that we remain the same and yet change in a nebulous manner makes it difficult to track the elusive self, much less to understand it.

3. *The healthy self has a sense of personal integration or of a coherent wholeness.* As individuals we must come to know ourselves, to develop a feeling and sense about the person we are. This involves reaching a consciousness of ourselves, our values, and our life directions. It further means forming our own values, thoughts, and opinions by choice from the complex variety of ideas and ways of life that surround us. In order to do this, life's contradictions and inconsistencies must be considered.

All this introspection about oneself, one's behavior, and the values of the outer world (that which is outside the self) is carried out in an attempt to achieve some inner sense of order and meaning for life. We cannot live with too great a sense of disorder. We need to feel related to our world and to have a relatedness within ourselves. We must feel that we are not impulsive and erratic, lacking direction in our lives and buffeted by fate. It is important to feel able to predict, to some extent, what the world is like—to know it and to understand it. We must have a similar sense about ourselves and our self-concepts. If one hopes to know the world and himself, he must be prepared to look realistically and as objectively as possible at what he finds. This process is not easy, as Kierkegaard has demonstrated:

> To venture causes anxiety, but not to venture is to lose one's self. . . And to venture in the highest sense is precisely to become conscious of one's self.

4. *The healthy self strives to maintain some autonomy and therefore it is not necessarily of a social conformist nature.* Although we want to know what others are like, and wish to conform and be like them to some extent, the healthy individual also wants to maintain his own individuality. The strong self strives toward the idea of maintaining a sense of its own uniqueness or authentic being. However, by nature we are also social beings, and so, in addition to wanting autonomy, the self also seeks involvement with the world and with others.

5. *Owing to the unique consciousness of man, the self is capable of introspection and is aware of time.*

> What presumably began as some barely living jelly much like protoplasm which still fills the cells of our bodies is now Man the Maker and Man the Thinker. Because something we call Mind has emerged from that merely mechanical ability to react, which is the most primitive characteristic of life, Man has taken control of his own destiny, to at least some limited extent, instead of leaving it in the hands of whatever mysterious power first created life. He can send capsules . . . far out into the measureless space which surrounds the globe to which he was once confined. What is much more remarkable and perhaps more fateful is that he can also wonder and speculate about his origins, his destiny and the meaning of his existence.
>
> Joseph Wood Krutch
> (Introduction to Eiseley[7])

Man has developed a unique consciousness. Loren Eiseley[7] writes that man evolved into something the world had never seen before—a "dream animal." Unlike the rest of the animal world, man escaped the eternal present into a knowledge of past and future.

Thus, it is possible for men to think of their lives in ways that animals cannot: imagining tomorrow, remembering yesterday, and dreaming about how things might be. This consciousness favors men above other animals, but it also carries with it burdens and responsibilities. Just as a man can imagine future good times and dream his future dreams, he can also imagine terror, suffering, and death. Through his unique consciousness, a man can become

morbidly preoccupied with the past or the future to the point of becoming mentally ill. Or he can become so introspective that he shuts out the rest of the world.

The self is not "found," it is "achieved" through introspection. Many people speak of finding themselves as if, quite by accident, they had stumbled upon something lost. The self is ever-present, although it may be present behind a variety of masks; it is ever-evolving, ever-becoming; it is evanescent and appears as reflections of its parts. What it represents, at any given time, is the life achievement of the individual. We do not lose our old self, we outgrow it and achieve something more.

It is through the baffling ability for introspection that a man can know his consciousness. Man, unlike other animals, can perceive himself in the act of perceiving. That is, we can see ourselves seeing ourselves. We can question ourselves and what our existence is all about.

The healthy self uses introspection for growth and better self-understanding, striving for maximum achievement. Man's introspection generally serves to guide him in the direction best for him. Because he can transcend time, he can learn from the past and, to some extent, plan for the future. Thus, he can use the present creatively in a conscious, constructive effort for self-actualization.

Man is in the unique position of being aware of time's passage and also of living in knowledge of his fate. However, the healthy individual is able to use this knowledge constructively. Through developing a consciousness of the present, and by realizing that the present is all that he has, he can strive to make his time more meaningful. It is not the quantity of time that is important, but rather the quality of it. In discussing "Man, Transcender of Time," Rollo May states:

> It is by no means as easy as it may look to live in the immediate present. For it requires a high degree of awareness of one's self as an experiencing "I." . . . But the more awareness one has—that is, the more he experiences himself as the acting, directing agent in what he is doing—the more alive he will be and the more responsive to the present moment. Like self-awareness itself, this experiencing of the quality of the present can be cultivated.[27]

6. *The self is composed of a public self and a private self.* Karl Marx among others has called our attention to the division of man into a "public" and "private" person. We all know that our public self is often not quite the same as our real or private self since we may feign or disguise our real self in public. We also know that as individuals we are isolated from others in the sense that we can never become another person

and no one can become us. We can present a part of ourselves to the world or to others, but we cannot give our self-perception to others.

The newborn baby is not aware of himself as existing separately from his environment or from others. It is as we grow that we learn of the distances between ourselves and the world around us.

As man becomes aware of himself as apart from his environment and as separate from his fellow men, the original oneness of life with its matrix is lost.[38]

Because of the existence of a public and private self we have a consciousness of ourselves as separate from other people, i.e., a feeling of otherness. A part of this feeling is the realization that we exist alone. This separateness of the self makes one feel helpless and insignificant. We are not referring here to an absence of any religious unification, but rather to the fact that we are all our separate selves.

The healthy self is able to accept the division between the public and private self and the alienation from others. For the healthy self, the public self and the private self are fairly similar. Also, the sense of alienation and isolation from others is balanced by those life experiences that can be shared with others. These shared experiences become bonds that unite men in their experience, e.g., in the areas of religion, culture, family, groups, and roles. Thus, even though we are isolated and see things from our own viewpoint, we can communicate with others. However, if we hope to communicate as accurately as possible and to establish bonds we must carefully explore our private self. As Eiseley wrote: "Men see differently. I can best report from my own wilderness. The important thing is that each man possess such a wilderness and that he consider what marvels are to be observed there."[7]

7. *Even though individual "selves" are isolated from one another, it is possible to form bonds with others.* Communication and self-knowledge are the tools with which we subjectively work to leave the isolation of our own experience and form bonds with others. In doing this we attempt to look at our own experience and to relate it to the experience of others, and then we turn the question around and look at the experience of others and try to relate it to our own. How are the experiences similar? How do they differ? Why do they differ? We constantly work to sharpen our awareness of our self and of others and to reduce our prejudices and biases. We try to sharpen the blunt tool of subjectivity. We look at the limitations of the tool and we consider its assets.

An ability to communicate with others is essential to the life of a healthy self. Communi-

cation is a bond with others; it is our means of feeling less like separate planets pursuing our individual orbits, and more like a united galaxy. The great philosopher Karl Jaspers repeatedly emphasized the necessity of communication. He wrote: "The thesis of my philosophizing is this: The individual cannot become human by himself. Self-being is only real in communication with another self-being. Alone, I sink into gloomy isolation—only in community with others can I be revealed in the act of mutual discovery."[17]

8. *The self is largely determined by and recognized from the values that it assumes.** Ultimately the search for oneself is the responsibility of onself. Others cannot do this for us because we are isolated from them and live in a state of alienation. The self that we choose to be results to a large extent from our choice of values. In discussing values, Wheelis has discussed how alone we are in making our choices: "[The alienated person] is thrown back on his own resources, becomes himself the referent of meaning and value."[38] Wheelis continues to point out that in the end we decide for ourselves the values by which we will live; they are a matter of choice. From all the possible variety of values that we *might* embrace, we select those by which we *will* live. We choose some values that we believe are "better than" others. Our values may or may not conform to those that predominantly surround us. Perhaps our values are valid and perhaps they are not; at times values transcend the evidence of proof for them at hand.

Our identity is ultimately founded upon the values that we assume, because our values determine our goals and our goals define our identity. Often our values change through life. Our values are *not* what we say, but rather are what we do, because "values cannot function as values unless they are held as such. A value which is forgotten or ignored is, empirically, not a value."[38]

9. *The concept of oneself is founded upon perceptions of oneself; at times we perceive ourselves differently from the way others perceive us.* As early as the 1700's, David Hume

---

*Certain philosophers believe that man does not determine what his own self will become, but rather that his self is determined for him by his heredity and environment. Today self-determination and free choice of values in life are being increasingly accepted by philosophers and psychologists.

was aware of the fact that we see ourselves in terms of perceptions. When he wrote on "Personal Identity" he stated:

> For my part, when I enter most intimately into what I call *myself,* I always stumble on some particular perception or other, of heat or cold, light or shade, love or hatred, pain or pleasure. I never can catch *myself* at any time without a perception, and never can observe anything but the perception.[12]

We perceive ourselves, or think of ourselves, in many different ways. In part, we think of ourselves in terms of our feelings, abilities, and actions. Our perceptions evoke feelings about ourselves, and *our feelings about ourselves are usually intense.* This fact is easily verified from one's own experience. We know how easily our feelings may be hurt or how insecure we may feel if our self-image is threatened. We know self-disappointment as well as dreams of fulfillment. Surprisingly enough, however, we usually know very little about what we actually *are* like! *One's feelings about oneself (or one's self-concept) may correspond with the truth or reality or they may not.* In addition, *our behavior nearly always appears more consistent to us than it does to others who observe it.* We all tend to see what we want to see.

We may not be as we think we are. This fact of self-deception often goes unrecognized. When it is discovered, we may find that we are in truth a part of what we had denied that we were. This realization means that, unknown to us, we possess attributes that we have despised or disliked in others. We may also have qualities that we admire in others but do not realize that we also possess. If some of my ideas about myself are inaccurate, it may mean such diverse things as these: I may describe myself as friendly, while others say I am hard to get to know; or I may think I don't do well in some activity, whereas others may think I excel.

Self-knowledge will help one to obtain a more realistic view of himself over a period of time. It will enable one to better understand how he presents himself to others and to see those incongruities that may exist between how he appears to others and how he appears to himself. Such insight is essential, for regardless of the accuracy of one's self-concept, it greatly influences how others react to us and how we behave toward others.

Let us now look at some of the reasons why it is difficult to perceive oneself accurately or to gain self-understanding. *First* of all, the process is difficult because self-understanding involves attempting to understand our own unconscious psychologic defenses* and unconscious motivations. Thus, our vision is often distorted. *Second,* we may find it too psychologically painful to *believe* facts about ourselves which do not support our own "good" self-image. If we are incapable of looking at aspects of ourselves that displease us, then we cannot hope to look honestly at ourselves. *Third,* because the process of self-understanding is psychologically painful and uncomfortable, we often prefer focusing our attention on the behavior of *others.* This is a hazard inherent in nursing and in other occupations that require some "understanding" of others.

We must realize that self-understanding *precedes the ability to begin to understand others.*

Because we never completely understand ourselves or others, the process becomes one continous attempt at self-knowledge while engaged in trying to understand others.

A *fourth* factor that makes self-knowledge difficult to achieve is that some people may lack the intelligence, and thus the knowledge, that is necessary to penetrate the complex self with its hidden and disguised motivations and experiences. Language skills, vocabulary, memory, and foresightedness are closely related to intelligence and vary from person to person. In part, then, the self we can become is determined by our vocabulary and verbal ability because thinking requires the use of concepts, and our concepts are most often verbal. Therefore, the more concepts an individual can build and consider (in terms of his vocabulary), the better able he is to think. Individuals also vary in their ability to think in abstractions, e.g., mathematics and philosophy. Consequently they have difficulty in thinking about the self, or the mind, because the self is an abstraction.

Self-knowledge will help one to obtain a more realistic view of himself and to achieve a balance of *self-acceptance* and *self-rejection.* This means that the individual is able to maintain a kind of psychologic homeostasis or equilibrium about his self-concept. An individual who *completely* accepts himself "as is" cannot reach his full potential, for he does not grow. On the other hand, a person who is overly harsh

---

*These defenses are briefly discussed on pp. 000 to 000.

or rejecting of himself suffers a crippling imbalance. It is the ability to change, evolve, and be flexible, then, that facilitates growth through self-knowledge. Flexibility thus makes healthy psychologic adaptation possible.

Because we are not bound to a static existence, change is possible and is our human privilege. As life progresses, change occurs. Some changes are beyond man's control (e.g., physical aging); other changes can be made voluntarily (e.g., behavior). Fortunately, awareness of oneself can lead to growth or productive change in behavior and insights. An individual is, thus, not bound to always act as he acts today.

10. *Each self is individual and unique from all others.* Although this fact increases the difficulties of knowing one another (because we cannot predict what individuals are like in advance of knowing them), it does make life the interesting experience that it is.

How can we best describe *why* each individual is unique? We can think of every organism and each part of every organism as consisting of the interaction of at least three factors: *time, heredity* and *environment.* Each of these factors is indispensable for life. Time is the life-span in which to grow and develop. Growth and development are guided by the blueprint of heredity, which controls the selection and use of materials, and by the environment. Each individual or oganism embodies a unique combination of these factors. Another way of viewing the development of the self-concept (identity) is to consider it as evolving in a flowing manner from the interaction of *biologic, social* and *experiential* forces. The interaction of these forces is depicted in Figure 2–1.

We can read about man for just so long. And then, if we really want to strive to understand people, we must meet the people themselves. The nurse is in a unique position to do this. She meets people most often during periods of crisis or intense experience in their lives. These are times when pretense is reduced to a minimum and the true self appears more clearly. Such times call for wisdom.

THE SELF IN ILLNESS

How does all this information about the self relate to nursing? We shall now see.

1. *Healthy, adjusted individuals are not entirely free from emotional conflicts or symptoms of illness.* This statement can orient the nurse to the fact that conflict and illness are often "normal" life experiences. Since the nurse will often care for patients who are *not* healthy and adjusted, it will be helpful if she can view imbalances in their proper perspective. She needs to recognize those imbalances that are temporary, and view them as temporary, and she also must recognize those imbalances that are permanent and accept the fact that they cannot be reversed. In *both* situations, a nurse must look for and develop the strengths that her patients have as well as recognize and prevent a deepening of impairments.

> *A nurse's concept of health, adjustment, and balance is as important as her concept of illness, maladjustment, and imbalance.*

The nurse must also strive for an awareness of her own emotional conflicts so that she does not project these upon persons in her care and upon her coworkers.

2. *Ample energy and a drive toward self-actualization characterize the healthy self.* A lack of energy is a general characteristic of physical and mental illness. The *body* is often weak and fatigued when combating physical stresses and illness; the *mind* is likewise weary, and people lack energy when they are experiencing mental stress and anxiety. When one is ill, however, the drive toward self-actualization is not necessarily absent. The

Figure 2–1. A model for the development of identity. (From Donovan, M. I., and Pierce, S. G.: *Cancer Care Nursing.* New York, Appleton Century Crofts, 1976, p. 205.)

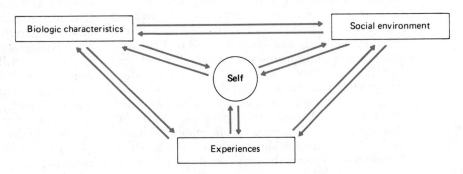

nurse's responsibility then becomes one of helping ill individuals to continue to fulfill their potentials, and to grow and achieve as much as they can within the limitations imposed by their illness. People can grow and learn *from* periods of stress and *within* such periods. They do not usually become emotionally and psychologically immobilized and cease being themselves merely because they are ill.

The nurse also can learn from periods of stress that she herself experiences, and she can strive to become aware of the many possibilities for self-actualization in her personal and professional life.

3. *A sense of personal integration or a coherent wholeness about oneself is essential for healthy functioning.* An individual who is ill needs a sense of order and personal integration as much as a healthy individual. The nurse can help to keep order in the patient's universe by preparing him as best she can for what will be happening to him. She can do this in small ways, for it is mainly in small ways that we all order our lives. For example, she can tell the newly admitted patient what the general routine of the hospital is. The nurse can tell a patient *what* she will be doing for him when she is assigned to care for him and *when* she will do these things. She can allow the patient to order some of his time by making some decisions *with* him about when they should do something. For example, would he like his bath early this morning or later? When would be the best time to take him to a telephone so he can phone home?

People who are ill may become confused or disoriented so that they lose the important sense of personal integration. When this occurs the nurse can help to reorient the patient by telling him where he is, what time it is, what day it is, who she is, and so forth.

4. *The healthy self strives to maintain some autonomy, and therefore mentally healthy individuals are not necessarily social conformists.* Even when ill and hospitalized, the individual needs to maintain a sense of his own uniqueness and autonomy. Many of the daily "problems" that nurses encounter center around this fact. Individuals do not like to conform to enforced ways of behaving (and neither do nurses). Autonomy expresses itself in thousands of different preferences. These preferences come to the nurse as innumerable requests—requests that express the wish to be treated differently from the "rest of the group." Basically such requests are for recognition of individuality. No one wants to be thought of as a part of a nameless, faceless group in which individuals cease to exist. No one wants to be thought of as a "gallbladder" or "room 214." Patients fear that they may be thought of in this kind of depersonalized manner.

The requests directed to the nurse, then, are serious; they are important to the self-concept of the patient even though they may seem minute and unimportant to the point of being "picky." The bids for autonomy may sound like this: "This meat is overcooked. I like mine rare." "I don't want a spread on my bed." "I don't care if it isn't visiting hours, I'm expecting company." "I want to wear my own pajamas." "I don't like ice water, I want a cup of warm water." "My roommate wants the window up, but I want it down." "I want a scrambled egg, not a boiled one." "I simply *cannot* use a bedpan." And so, the nurse must mediate between the necessity for some conformity as a part of group living and the equally important necessity for some autonomy.

5. *Owing to the unique consciousness of man, the self is capable of introspection and is aware of time.* Let us first look at his introspective nature. Illness is often a time of great uncertainty and, thus, a time of deep introspection. Because man is (as Eiseley says) a "dream animal," because he is capable of introspection and of projecting his thoughts forward and backward in time, he will dream, muse, rejoice, fret, and worry in the presence of the nurse. Often a patient needs, and wants, to think out loud and to talk with those around him. This is perfectly natural. What is unnatural for the patient is that those around him, at this time of crisis or concern for him, are not his familiar friends and family. He must talk with strangers about concerns that are often deeply personal.

Through introspection a man comes to know his inner feelings. Through his communications *we* can come to know his feelings and concerns. Consequently nursing requires skills in communication. It is necessary that a nurse help people to feel comfortable with her. This requires sensitivity to *both* verbal and nonverbal communication—the nurse's own as well as that of others. Furthermore, a nurse must be able to talk with people from extremely divergent backgrounds. The ability to speak simply and slowly will greatly enhance clarity of communication. The nurse should attempt to speak to patients without using complicated terms and the jargon of her profession.

Let us now turn to a consideration of the relation of the self to time. It is not time in and of itself that is important, but the *quality* and *meaning* of time for the patient and the nurse.

Because we can determine to a large extent what the quality of our time will be, the nurse can create a *quality* in the time she spends with patients. A conscious awareness of this ability can greatly influence the quality of nursing time spent with all patients.

It does not matter whether a nurse will be with a patient for one minute or eight hours, she will determine the quality of her relations with the patient (e.g., her pleasantness) and thus will determine the quality of that time. No one but the nurse herself determines how much she will consciously *give* to the time she spends with a patient. She can grudgingly merely "put in time," or she can spend time with the patient helpfully and creatively.

Let us look at another aspect of time. The present is all that any of us has. Although the past and future are important to us, we live only in the present. Occasionally people (both patients and nurses) view illness and hospitalization as a time *away* from life—that is, as if the patient's life were suspended in time and would begin again when he is well or out of the hospital. This negation of the present needs to be guarded against, for it is the present that is truly meaningful.

The nurse can help the patient to be a constructive agent of his time. One of the commonest examples of negation of the present is seen in the attitude that nurses often convey in their care of terminal patients. Because his future life appears brief, the nurse often overlooks the importance of the present for the patient. These patients need more than others perhaps the comfort, warmth, and security that any of us want. They still want the *quality of their present life to be meaningful*. The dying are still living, only the dead are dead. And the dying live in the present time, as they have always lived, and as we all live.

6. *The self is composed of a public self and a private self.* Both patient and nurse have public and private selves. We often "fool" with our own and are "fooled" by others' public selves. Occasionally we are brought to the realization that we really didn't know someone at all in terms of his private self; all we saw was the public self. Let us see how "Richard Cory" was known:

Whenever Richard Cory went down town,
We people on the pavement looked at him:
He was a gentleman from sole to crown,
Clean favored, and imperially slim.
And he was always quietly arrayed,
And he was always human when he talked;
But still he fluttered pulses when he said,
"Good morning," and he glittered when he walked.

And he was rich—yes, richer than a king,
And admirably schooled in every grace:

In fine, we thought that he was everything
To make us wish that we were in his place.

So we worked and waited for the light
And went without the meat, and cursed the bread;
And Richard Cory, one calm summer night
Went home and put a bullet through his head.

E. A. Robinson[31]

Just as you may not appear to others as you think you appear, so your patients may not appear to you as they think they do. A patient may think he appears calm when, in fact, he looks very apprehensive. Or a patient may think he doesn't seem irritable, when he actually is very short-tempered. He may think you know that he feels faint as he stands by the bed, when you really can't tell this, and so on. A doctor may think he appears calm, when he actually looks very pressured and acts tense. You may think you don't appear hurried to your patient, but you make him feel rushed.

The nurse must strive to see both her public self and her private self. She will also need to try to distinguish between the public and private selves of her patients. Just as she understands that her own public behavior does not always express her private feelings, so she must understand the same thing concerning the behavior of patients. As she must become skilled in verbal communication, so she must develop sensitivity and awareness to nonverbal communication so that she can see glimpses of the veiled private self behind the public mask.

The private self is isolated and alienated from other selves. Understanding these feelings that *all men* have, the nurse can empathize with those who are feeling lonely, isolated, and alienated in their illness. Illness, misfortune, and suffering make people realize strongly how separate from other people they really are. *They* are in pain, *they* face death, *they* are frightened, but the world goes on. And no one can assume the pain, death, or fear of others. The nurse, however, can reduce the feelings of isolation by her skilled, comforting presence and by her willingness to allow the patient to talk with her about his life situation. She can work to alleviate pain and to reduce fears. She can strive to reduce the differences between the public and private self.

7. *Even though individual "selves" are isolated from one another, it is possible to form bonds with others.* Although our interpretation of the feelings and behavior of others is largely subjective, we can manage to find common

bonds with other people. We all must work within the limitations of subjectivity. Thus, when a patient says, "I'm miserable and full of pain," or "The doctor told me this morning I have cancer," the nurse cannot factually say, "I know how you feel." The nurse can, however, draw on her own experience. She can look for common bonds of experience with which she can attempt to understand the feelings of other persons as she talks with them, observes them, and attempts to be "with" them. To use a phrase of Loomis, we hope the nurse and patient can, in the purest sense, "resonate together."

To "resonate" with another human being is to know that when you speak you are heard by him. The echoes that reverberate to you in his voice are rich with the sounds of your own concern. Similarly, your own voice, echoing back to him, has been affected by what you have heard him say and what you felt that he believed.[20]

The nurse who is capable of this level of communication is a nurse who is a *student of man*. She understands his isolation from others and his bonds with them. She studies human experience as carefully as she studies anatomy and physiology. Such a nurse is an "idea person" as well as a "fact person." It has been pointed out that

nursing needs a better conceptualization of its own functions and the human phenomena with which it deals. This path to better ways and techniques will be opened by ideas, not by discrete, poorly related principles to be slavishly followed as techniques.[24]

If we deal with separate facts we fail to see the relationships between them; if we think only of separate people we fail to recognize that there are bonds that unite them. A factual approach to nursing is oriented toward objects as instruments for health (e.g., medications, hypodermics, dressings) rather than people. On the other hand, the nurse who works with "ideas" recognizes that consciousness, subjectivity, and communication are instruments for health and that she *herself* is an instrument that can be therapeutically applied . . . or denied.

8. *The self is largely determined by and recognized from the values that it assumes.* A nurse's value system will greatly influence her nursing practice. It may not influence how she talks about her nursing practice, but it will be directly reflected in the actual practice itself. A nurse may say that she values and respects individual differences, but the manner in which she treats individuals with differences will ultimately show what her values really are. As we have said previously, values are not values unless they are held as such and are the basis for action.

A nurse must be able to tolerate ideas and values that are foreign to her. Eiseley has said, "On the world island we are all castaways so that what is seen by one may often be obscure to another."[7] It is the task of the nurse to try to understand the obscure; it is her privilege to come to know differing visions of life on this "world island."

9. *The concept of oneself is founded upon perceptions of himself; however, at times we perceive ourselves differently from the way others perceive us.* How fragile one's self-concept is! How easily it is influenced or damaged! Every time a nurse speaks of a patient, she is speaking of a self. Her challenge becomes one of seeing how honestly, how accurately, and how fairly she can refer to that self. In attempting to describe a patient, she must invest as much effort in that description as she would in her own self-description. If others see us differently from our own self-perception, and we see them differently from theirs, we must evaluate ourselves and others cautiously.

How do others describe you? Do they do it partially in terms of themselves and their needs? In part they do, and you too describe others partially in terms of yourself. The beginning, then, is self-knowledge. Your feelings and perceptions about yourself will serve as your "antenna," your baseline for understanding others.

10. *Each self is individual and unique from all others.* Realizing this, the nurse can *expect* and enjoy the differences in patients whom she meets. She will not personally like all those she meets, but she can find that one of nursing's most rewarding aspects is the fact that she will meet so many different people. An appreciation of individuality and a conscious effort to allow it to flourish as much as possible can contribute greatly to patient care.

SIGNIFICANT OTHERS

Interaction with "significant others" (i.e., persons who play significant parts in the life of an individual) is highly important in the development of one's self. Significant others may include such persons as friends, peers and teachers, as well as family members. Family groups are typically categorized into (a) the *nuclear family* and (b) the *extended family*. Robinson (drawing on the work of Kincaid) summarizes family living as follows:

The family may be perceived of as a cohesive group, consisting of the original dyad—a male and a female, and their offspring. This total unit is the nuclear family. The extended family includes aunts, uncles, cousins, and other related persons. In the contemporary world, groups differing from the traditional model are observed. Homosexual marriages occur; single adults form family units with adopted children. There is some experimentation with group marriage, communal life, and the rearing of children within those structures. All of these types of relationships have in common the principal's desires for intimacy and sharing. The evolving units remain together for reasons of biological, sociological, psychological and economic need.[32]

BIBLIOGRAPHY

1. Bakker, C. B., and Bakker-Rabdou, M. K.: *No Trespassing*. San Francisco, Chandler and Sharp Publishers, 1973.
2. Braden, W.: *The Private Sea*. Chicago, Quadrangle Books, 1967.
3. Brammer, L.: *The Helping Relationship: Process and Skills*. Englewood Cliffs, NJ, Prentice-Hall, 1973.
4. Brill, N. Q.: The importance of understanding yourself. *In* Mereness, D. (ed.): *Psychiatric Nursing*, Vol. I. Dubuque, Iowa, W. C. Brown Co., 1966.
5. Combs, A. W., Avila, D. L., and Purkey, W. W.: *Helping Relationships: Basic Concepts for the Helping Professions*. Boston, Allyn & Bacon, 1971.
6. Dubos, R.: *Man Adapting*. New Haven, Yale University Press, 1965.
7. Eiseley, L.: *The Immense Journey*. New York, Time-Life, Inc., Time Reading Program, 1962.
8. Engel, G. L.: *Psychological Development in Health and Disease*. Philadelphia, W. B. Saunders Co., 1962.
9. Erb, E. D., and Hooker, D.: *The Psychology of the Emerging Self*. Philadelphia, F. A. Davis Co., 1967.
10. Francis, G. M.: How do I feel about myself? *American Journal of Nursing*, 67:1244, June 1967.
11. Goffman, E.: *The Presentation of Self in Everyday Life*. Garden City, NY, Doubleday Anchor Books, 1959.
12. Hume, D.: Personal identity. *In* Hammer, L. Z. (ed.): *Value and Man*. New York, McGraw-Hill Book Co., 1966.
13. Johnson, D.: *Reaching Out*. Englewood Cliffs, NJ, Prentice-Hall, 1972.
14. Jourard, S. M.: *Disclosing Man to Himself*. Princeton, NJ, D. Van Nostrand Co., 1968.
15. Jourard, S. (ed.): *To Be or Not to Be*. Gainesville, University of Florida Press, 1967.
16. Jourard, S.: *The Transparent Self*. Princeton, NJ, D. Van Nostrand Co., 1964.
17. Levi, A. W.: Existentialism and the alienation of man. *In* Lee, E., and Mandelbaum, M. (eds.): *Phenomenology and Existentialism*. Baltimore, The Johns Hopkins Press, 1967.
18. Levine, M. E.: Holistic nursing. *Nursing Clinics of North America*, 6:253, June 1971.
19. Lewis, J. A.: Reflections on self. *American Journal of Nursing*, 60:828, June 1960.
20. Loomis, E. A., Jr.: *The Self in Pilgrimage*. New York, Harper & Row, 1960.
21. Lucia, S. P.: The psyche of man and his illness. *Medical Times*, 99:140, Aug. 1971.
22. Lyon, H.: *Learning to Feel—Feeling to Learn*. Columbus, Ohio, Charles E. Merrill Publishing Co., 1971.
23. Lyons, S. M. L.: The creative use of self in human relations. *AORN*, 5:47, Feb. 1967.
24. Martin, H. W., and Prange, A. J.: Human adaptation: a conceptual approach to understanding patients. *The Canadian Nurse*, 58:234, March 1962.
25. Maslow, A. H.: *Motivation and Personality*. New York, Harper & Row, 1954.
26. Maslow, A. H.: *Toward a Psychology of Being*. Princeton, NJ, D. Van Nostrand Co., 1962.
27. May, R.: *Man's Search for Himself*. New York, W. W. Norton and Co., 1953.
28. Mayeroff, M.: *On Caring*. New York, Harper & Row, 1971.
29. Menninger, K., Mayman, M., and Pruyser, P.: *The Vital Balance: The Life Process in Mental Health and Illness*. New York, Viking Press, 1963.
30. Purtilo, R.: *Health Professional/Patient Interaction*, 2nd ed. Philadelphia, W. B. Saunders Co., 1978.
31. Robinson, E. A.: "Richard Cory." *In* Saunders, G., and Nelson, J. (eds.): *Chief Modern Poets of England and America*, 3rd ed. New York, The Macmillan Co., 1943.
32. Robinson, L.: *Liaison Nursing: Psychological Approach to Patient Care*. Philadelphia, F. A. Davis Co., 1974.
33. Rogers, C.: *On Becoming a Person*. Boston, Houghton Mifflin Co., 1961.
34. Romey, W.: *Risk-Trust-Love*. Columbus, Ohio, Charles E. Merrill Publishing Co., 1972.
35. Stevens, L. F.: Understanding ourselves. *American Journal of Nursing*, 57:1022, Aug. 1957.
36. Watts, A. W.: *Psychotherapy East and West*. New York, Ballantine Books, 1961.
37. Weiss, P.: *Reality*. Carbondale, IL, Southern Illinois University Press, 1967.
38. Weelis, A.: *The Quest for Identity*. New York, W. W. Norton and Co., 1958.

CHAPTER 3

THERAPEUTIC NURSE-PATIENT RELATIONSHIP

By Margaret Helen Parkinson, R.N., R.M.N., Dip.N., B.Soc.Sc., M.N.

The word is a mighty power—it can end fear, abolish pain, instil joy, increase pity.

GORGIAS

OVERVIEW AND STUDY GUIDE

Overview

This chapter (a) presents principles basic to a therapeutic or helpful nurse-patient relationship; (b) examines the nature of helping, relationships and communication; and (c) describes in detail the essential characteristics of helping people and the skills involved in communicating such helpfulness to other people.

Material presented in this chapter is essential to good nursing practice. However, it is not easy to internalize and put into practice. A nurse will fall short of the ideals discussed many times. What is important, however, is that she is aware of their significance and be committed to developing them within herself throughout her professional life.

Study Guide

Material presented in this chapter is absolutely basic to excellent nursing practice. It is among the most difficult to learn, although this may not appear to be true on first reading. You will need to do more than simply remember the material in a cognitive way. You will need to be involved in affective learning as well. This means you need not only to understand the depth of meaning contained in the concepts but also to examine your attitudes, values and behaviors to see that they are consistent with concepts central to a therapeutic nurse-patient relationship. You probably will study this chapter many times before you will feel that you are beginning to understand the meanings it contains.

To help you with this task we suggest you periodically undertake the following tasks.

1. Make a list of the characteristics you believe to be basic to all human beings. Test this list against your own behavior toward other people. Take each item on your list and ask yourself the question: "How does my behavior toward other people show that I really believe this?"

2. Examine your motives for seeking to become a nurse. Ask yourself the question: "What satisfactions do I get from caring for people who need nursing care?"

3. In your own words, write a paragraph describing what you believe nursing to be. Compare your description with the description given in this chapter. Examine your own nursing behavior and ask yourself the question: "How does my behavior within the nurse-patient relationship illustrate what I believe to be true of the nurse-patient relationship?"

4. Make a list of the ways you care about yourself in physical, emotional and intellectual ways. Set goals for ways you plan to care for yourself more. Evaluate your movement toward these goals in 2 weeks.

5. Make periodic process recordings of your interactions with patients and their families and evaluate them for genuineness, nonpossessive warmth, accurate empathy, concreteness in communication, immediacy in communication and sensitive confrontation. Set goals and make plans to improve your skills in communicating each of these characteristics.

6. Make periodic process recordings of your interactions with patients and their families. From

these, identify any ways you blocked their communication.

7. Set up regular "role-play sessions" with another nursing student or friend to practice the skills described in this chapter. It is sometimes helpful to have a third person observe the role play and give you objective feedback on your behavior. Audio or video tape recordings can also give helpful feedback. Note that it is not always necessary to discuss "problems" in role play. Any conversation topic will do to help you identify the ways you both facilitate and block communication.

8. *Be gentle with yourself. It takes a long time and a lot of patience to learn how to be really helpful to another person.*

Objectives of this chapter: by studying this material, you will

1. Understand the basic characteristics common to all helping professionals.

2. Appreciate the interdependence of both expressive and instrumental roles in nursing.

3. Be willing to give attention to your own personal growth in physical, emotional and intellectual realms.

4. Examine your own behavior within the nurse-patient relationship to assess your functioning in genuineness, nonpossessive warmth, accurate empathy, concreteness in communication, immediacy in communication and sensitive confrontation.

5. Develop skills in the art of listening.

6. Become aware of the continual need to reevaluate your professional practice within the nurse-patient relationship.

INTRODUCTION

So you have decided to study nursing! You probably have a number of thoughts and fantasies about the things you will be required to do as a nurse. Maybe you imagine yourself giving injections and skillfully manipulating intravenous infusion equipment. Sometimes you may see yourself caring for a patient as he regains consciousness following surgery, or maybe caring for a patient as his heart beat and blood pressure are mechanically monitored or feeding a newborn child or skillfully helping an elderly person use walking aids. Perhaps you see yourself discussing a disease process with a physician and carefully carrying out his orders concerning treatment. You will certainly do all these things, and more, when you become a nurse, but there is more to nursing than tasks and techniques.

In Chapter 1 it was pointed out that a successful nurse both understands and applies scientific principles in order to practice nursing care with technical skill and that a nurse clearly communicates with a variety of patients in an empathic, warm and honest manner.

> *For excellence in nursing care both scientifically based technical skill and genuine empathic understanding in communication are essential.*

The above two functions are the basis of a nurse's role. We may call the first function the nurse's instrumental role and the second her expressive role.

We can define an *instrumental role* as a set of behaviors that are "directly related to moving a system toward its goal."[30] For example, consider Janet Martin who at age 14 is admitted to the hospital to have an appendectomy for acute appendicitis. As the nurse shaves and prepares the skin over the operation area, withholds food and fluid for several hours before surgery and carefully administers the prescribed premedication, she is carrying out instrumental functions. The more skillfully the nurse performs such tasks, the greater is her

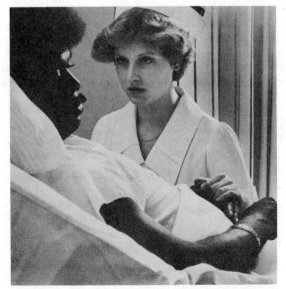

Figure 3-1. The therapeutic use of self. (From Krovisky, E. W., Mitch and me: cancer patients with the same prognosis. *RN, 40*:60, Jan. 1977.)

contribution to helping Janet (in this case, "the system") reach a goal of restored health.

An *expressive role*, on the other hand, can be defined as behaviors that are "related to maintaining motivational equilibrium in the individual."[30] Let us consider Janet Martin again. Suppose this is the first time she has ever been in a hospital but she has heard unpleasant stories about what happens to people who have operations. She is a quiet person and hesitates to speak, let alone to ask questions. The excellent nurse would make sure she always explained what was going to happen to Janet *before* it happened. Such a nurse may also spend time with Janet even when there was not a task to perform. She may say something like: "I imagine having an operation may seem rather scary to you. I'd like to listen to you if you want to talk about the things that may be worrying you." Such a nurse is likely to win Janet's trust and thus enable Janet to express her fears.

The above nursing actions are ways by which Janet's anxieties may be reduced to help her to go to her operation in a state of relative peace and balance of "equilibrium." Janet would then be more able to use her energy (i.e., be motivated) to do the things she needed to do to move toward health. Energy would not be dissipated by unnecessary anxieties. The nurse who works well in this way is carrying out expressive functions.

Instrumental and expressive functions complement each other. *No matter how efficiently a nurse performs instrumental tasks, their effectiveness will be reduced if she does not practice expressive roles in a sensitive and caring way.*

In many ways instrumental tasks are easier to learn than the skills necessary for expressive functions because instrumental tasks are often concrete and precise. The purpose of this chapter is to help you develop the more difficult skills and attitudes essential to a facilitative expressive nursing role.

NURSING IS A WAY OF HELPING

Many people who present themselves to a nursing school as prospective students state that they want to become a nurse so that they can "help people." Maybe you decided to become a nurse for the same reason. This is a commendable purpose, and to become excellent nurses we need to understand what "helping people" means.

The American College Dictionary defines the verb "to help" as "(1) to cooperate effectively with a person, (2) to furnish aid to, contribute strength or means to, assist in doing, (3) to succor, save, (4) to relieve (someone) in need, sickness, pain, or distress."[5] Being helpful, then, is doing something that is seen as relevant, positive and useful by some other person or persons.

"Help" could be summarized as all the behaviors of a person (helper) that assist another person (helpee) to more comfortably engage in a productive and enjoyable life.

Everybody is both a "helper" and a "helpee" at different times in their lives. A mother can be a helper to her child; a child can be a helper to his mother; friends can be helpers to each other; teachers can be helpers to students; doctors, dentists and other health professionals can be helpers to patients. In fact, anyone can be a helper to anyone else. What particular kinds of useful things do nurses do when they are being helpers to patients?

Many people think of nurses as helping people who are sick in *hospitals*. In fact, there was a time when this was the only thing nurses were trained to do. Today, however, many nurses do not practice in hospitals, and their clients are not always defined as "sick." Some nurses work in the *community* in areas such as (a) public health in clients' homes; (b) occupational health in factories and other places of work; (c) mental health in clinics such as community mental health centers; and (d) private practices as nurse-therapists with various specializations. It has become important then, to identify commonalities in nursing practice whether inside or outside a hospital.

Nursing leaders have suggested that there is a unique function common to all nurses wherever they practice. Henderson defines this function as follows:

The unique function of the nurse is to assist the individual, sick or well, in the performance of those activities contributing to health or its recovery (or to a peaceful death) that he would perform unaided if he had the necessary strength, will or knowledge. And to do this in such a way as to help him gain independence as rapidly as possible.[23]

A nurse, then, is a person who helps someone else in meeting his basic human needs when, for a period of time, he cannot meet them for himself. (See Chapter 1 for a description of basic human needs.) Human beings are normally able to arrange for the meeting of their own needs without help. However, sometimes individuals may need help because their strength, will or knowledge is insufficient. In such circumstances a nurse, by using the nursing process, helps patients to identify unmet needs, plans ways of having those needs satisfied and evaluates the effectiveness of the plans. (Nursing process is discussed in Chapter 17.)

> *The skillful nurse's actions encourage independence rather than dependence on others. Appropriate dependence is, of course, comfortably facilitated.*

Sometimes a nurse *does things for a patient,* but the excellent nurse always allows and encourages a patient to *do things for himself,* as soon as he is able.

For example, suppose you are responsible for Ms. Thompson, who has been admitted to the hospital unconscious, in a diabetic coma. (A diabetic coma is a state of unconsciousness brought about in diabetic persons by excess sugar in the blood.) Let us consider this patient's physiologic need to eat and drink adequately. While in this state of total dependence Ms. Thompson is unable to do anything to meet this need for herself. Nourishment and fluids are thus provided, probably by intravenous infusion. Once she has regained consciousness, Ms. Thompson gradually regains the strength to eat the meals delivered to her from the dietary department. The excellent nurse provides opportunities for Ms. Thompson to learn the special dietary considerations necessary for diabetic control. Also, through her relationship with Ms. Thompson, the nurse makes it comfortable for the patient to discuss her illness experience. Efforts are made to identify and discuss aspects of diabetes that Ms. Thompson does not understand, including any concerns she has about developing appropriate dietary patterns in her own home. In this way Ms. Thompson and the nurse work together to find solutions to the problems that may exist. Ms. Thompson could then return to her home with the necessary strength, will and knowledge to enable her to eat and drink more healthily than she had before hospitalization.

This example illustrates the way in which the excellent nurse modifies her interventions to facilitate a patient's return to maximal independence. Nursing interventions vary as a patient moves from positions of dependence to independence. You will observe that the nurse in this example used both instrumental and expressive roles.

NURSING TAKES PLACE WITHIN INTERPERSONAL RELATIONSHIPS

It will be clear from the previous discussion that the kind of "helping" called "nursing" involves interaction between at least two persons. This is rather simplistic, however. Nursing is more an interaction between two systems, i.e., the patient or "helpee system" and the "health or helper system."

The *patient,* a helpee system, includes the individual seeking help and those individuals within the patient's personal social matrix, i.e., his "significant others." (The helpee is sometimes referred to as the "client.") The composition of this system varies with each patient but most commonly includes a patient's family and friends.

The *health or helper system* includes the individual nurse interacting with a patient and with the whole organizational matrix of persons making up the institution within which the interaction take place. This institution may be a hospital or some other community health service.

It is important to remember then that whenever a nurse and a patient interact, there is more to the interaction than simply the meeting of two people. The nurse and the patient each bring with them (1) their *personal experiences,* e.g., individual emotions, knowledge, perceptions and attitudes; (2) their *specific health-oriented experiences,* e.g., their connections and experiences with illness, wellness and with the health care system; and (3) their general life experiences and associations (see Fig. 3–2). In other words, both the nurse and the patient bring to the nurse-patient relationship a "life history," which influences their perceptions and expectations of each other and affects the processes between them. Figure 3–2 illustrates the coming together of a patient and a nurse system. It shows the relationship between personal experiences, specific health-oriented experiences and general life experiences for both the patient and the nurse. Figure 3–2 indicates interactions occurring within and between the patient and the nurse system. It also shows the "functional focus" (i.e., where action takes place) of nursing as the interface

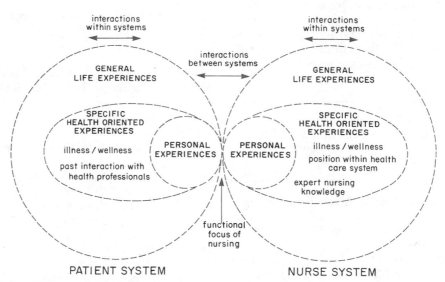

Figure 3–2. Factors influencing the nurse-patient relationship. Both the patient and the nurse bring the effects of past experiences to their interactions with each other. (See text for full discussion.)

between the nurse and the patient, i.e., the point at which they are meeting face to face. It is this interaction that constitutes the nurse-patient relationship. King expresses these concepts in the following way:

> . . . a nurse-patient relationship is viewed as a functional closeness between two individuals, usually strangers, who bring to the nursing situation their individual expectations, goals, needs and values.[36]

We need to look rather carefully at the meanings and consequences of the concept of a "relationship" if it is the "functional focus" of nursing. *The Random House Dictionary* defines a "relationship" as (1) a connection, association or involvement, (2) an emotional or other connection between people.[69] Jourard uses the term "interpersonal behavior" for relationship and defines it as "any and all behavior which a person undertakes in the presence of others."[32]

There are always consequences from the interpersonal behavior that occurs within relationships. These consequences can be positive or negative (i.e., can have "good" or "bad" consequences) for the persons involved in the relationship. The relationship between a nurse and a patient occurs at a time of vulnerability for the patient—a time when he is susceptible to failure in meeting his basic human needs. Encounters with a nurse would therefore be of some significance, either toward patient well-being

or deterioration. A nurse has a responsibility, then, to facilitate the kind of relationship that is most likely to have constructive or positive consequences for the patient rather than negative or deteriorative consequences for him.

The nurse-patient relationship is not a casual connection. It is established purposefully, maintained deliberately, and ended carefully in relation to the particular health needs of the patient. The nurse is most often in the position of "power" in a nurse-patient relationship. This means her behaviors either can allow healthful growth to take place or can accentuate differences between the patient and nurse systems so that tension increases.

While a nurse can get great satisfaction from her work, the helpful nurse does not allow her personal needs to take precedence over the needs of the patient. The helpful nurse is a "real person" within the nurse-patient relationship. However, the focus of the interactions is directed toward patient need. Saunders has expressed this concept in the following way:

> Whenever and wherever the nursing function is performed, there are always present two indispensable components, the patient and the nurse—one needing, one giving.[60]

The fact that the patient's needs are central to the nurse-patient relationship differentiates this relationship from other interpersonal relationships, e.g., casual interpersonal relationships. As well as the personal factors arising from her personal experiences, specific health-oriented experiences and general life experiences, the nurse brings to the nurse-patient relationship her professional nursing knowledge and skills. It is this combination that allows a nurse to enter into a *professional* helping relationship. Brammer sees the professional helping relationship as an equation that adds the personality of the helper to his helping skills, producing growth-facilitating conditions that lead to specific outcomes for the helper.

The nurse, then, brings herself and her acquired nursing skills (expressive and instrumental) to the nurse-patient relationship. These factors, combined with the problem-solving potential of the patient can lead to the improved functioning of the patient.

PHASES OF A RELATIONSHIP

Self-limiting relationships, such as the nurse-patient relationship, have fairly clear, although overlapping, phases (see Fig. 3–3). Certain things commonly occur in each phase, and certain nurse behaviors are appropriate to each phase.

Phase 1, or the *initiation phase*, begins as soon as the nurse and the patient meet. This is when the nurse and the patient get to know each other. The important task of the initiation phase is to *build trust*. During this time the patient will *test* the nurse to see just how much he can trust her. Testing may be done through actions or words, but it will usually be disguised. A patient may use his call bell for no apparent reason other than to find out how quickly the nurse responds to it. A patient will watch the nurse's behavior carefully to see how much he can rely on her physically and emotionally.

During the initiation phase the nurse commonly seeks out information about the patient. During this time a nursing history is taken and a nursing care plan begun. The growth-facilitating conditions of genuineness, nonpossessive warmth and accurate empathy are most important during this phase (see pp. 31–34). They contribute to the building of trust.

Phase 2, or the *working phase*, commences when trust has been established. This is when *patient problems can be worked on successfully*. The action-oriented conditions of helping—concreteness in communication, immediacy in communication and sensitive confrontation—may be used at this time (see pp. 34–35). Growth-facilitating conditions are continued. The action-oriented conditions are too threatening until trust has been established.

Phase 3, or the *termination phase*, is the time to *say good-bye*. Whenever possible, this should be begun long before the final moments of the nurse-patient relationship. The nurse and the patient should talk with each other about the time when they will no longer be interacting together. The relationship may end because the patient is "discharged" from the nurse's care or because the nurse no longer has the patient assigned to her.

A nurse-patient relationship should never end without the completion of *unfinished business*. The good and bad times of the whole relationship should be discussed by the nurse and the patient. The growth-facilitating conditions of genuineness, nonpossessive warmth and accurate empathy are most important at the termination phase. New material should not be introduced if it cannot be completed.

The shapes used in Figure 3–3 illustrate the interconnections between the three phases. The phases overlap, but each phase has a time of prime emphasis.

The three phases extend over the entire relationship. They also exist on a smaller scale at each interaction. Pause in your reading for a few moments and recall the ways you have experienced these phases in your relationships with patients.

THE NURSE AS A HELPER

We have shown that a nurse is a professional helper who usually practices within the health

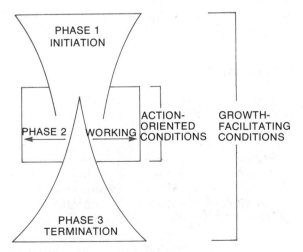

Figure 3–3. The phases of a relationship.

care system. A nurse's unique function is concerned with assisting people to meet their basic human needs when, for some reason or another, they are unable to meet their needs for themselves. She does much of her work by involving herself in interpersonal relationships with patients and with members of a patient's social network. The basic purpose of these interpersonal relationships is solving problems concerning unmet or inadequately met patient needs.

The *nurse herself* is a very important factor in this helping process. It is she who has most control in setting the tone and pace of the process within the relationship. Interpersonal relationships of any kind require constant and honest work. The quality of a relationship depends on the abilities of both parties to put as much energy into the relationship as possible.

> *An excellent or truly helpful nurse is a person who cares about and accepts herself. Only such a person is free to care about others.*

A nurse, then, has an obligation to keep herself healthy in physical, emotional and intellectual realms. We will discuss in a little more detail the ways a nurse may choose to do this.

Physical Realm

The professional nurse attends to her own physical health. She makes sure her own basic physiologic needs are met satisfactorily. For example, she eats well, maintaining a weight appropriate to her height and body build. The person who is either too fat or too thin is not taking care of himself/herself physically. The physically healthy nurse eats a diet balanced in essential nutrients and finds pleasure in the social components of eating. Also, the nurse attending to her own physical health makes certain she gets adequate exercise from activities she finds personally enjoyable and satisfying. Exercise is kept in balance with obtaining adequate rest. In other words, the excellent nurse strives to meet her basic physiologic needs in a balanced and health-producing way. She does not tolerate a "mediocre" physical existence.

The excellent nurse pays attention to symptoms that may indicate illness, seeking

appropriate consultation. Additionally, she has a regular physical examination and rests whenever she develops symptoms of a cold, influenza or fatigue.

The nurse who is functioning at a high level in the physical realm is aware of her own body. For example, she knows what she looks like physically and she enjoys that. The "healthy" nurse is aware of her own common physiologic reactions to stressful situations, i.e., physical symptoms she tends to develop when stressed. By having an awareness of these patterns, she can strive to change either herself or her environment in ways that will reduce relievable stresses.

For example, as nursing student Ms. Smith becomes increasingly aware of herself and her own physiologic reactions, she discovers that she is inclined to eat excessively when her anxiety levels rise. She observes that such overeating makes her feel uncomfortable and angry with herself. Knowing this about herself, Ms. Smith tries to make certain modifications in her life when times of increased stress are anticipated. For instance, when examination times approach, Ms. Smith (a) makes sure she does not have large quantities of high-calorie foods in her cupboards; (b) consciously strives to eat regular, adequate meals; (c) keeps a brief food diary, listing everything she eats; (d) tries to increase her intake of water in an attempt to avoid between-meal snacking; and (e) prepares a snack plate of pieces of fresh vegetables.

The means that Ms. Smith uses to eliminate uncontrolled eating at examination times are based on her knowledge about herself and the behaviors that are satisfying to her. In this way, Ms. Smith becomes more and more in control of herself and her physiologic processes.

The excellent nurse in the physical realm is the one who (a) takes care of herself physically; (b) likes and enjoys her own body; and (c) uses her knowledge about healthy ways to meet basic physiologic needs to her own advantage.

Emotional Realm

It is very important that a nurse have a satisfactory and healthy emotional life. *If a nurse is not aware of her own feelings and typical emotional reactions, it is likely that unresolved emotional energy will interfere with her nurse-patient relationships.* When a nurse lacks such self-awareness, tensions originating in her private life may find ventilation in interactions with patients in ways that are far from helpful.

For example, nursing student Ms. Smith may have had a very difficult relationship with her mother. Suppose her mother developed strong patterns of controlling her daughter's life in ways that Ms. Smith found unpleasant, yet was unable to counteract. Under these circumstances Ms. Smith is likely to experience anger toward her mother which she may not be aware of, let alone express. It may happen, then, that whenever Ms. Smith cares for a woman resembling her mother (in appearance or behavior) the unresolved anger enters into the relationship. In order to establish satisfactory nurse-patient relationships it would thus be important for Ms. Smith to clarify her relationship with her mother and become aware of the influence of this relationship. Ms. Smith's feelings toward her mother (avoidance, anger) could then be appropriately resolved instead of being transferred inappropriately to a nursing situation.

If a nurse is to be an effective helper, it is therefore important that she develop ways of measuring self-awareness of her feelings and reactions. There are a number of ways a nurse may choose to help herself do this. For example, she may keep a personal "feelings" and "experiences" journal, i.e., a diary recording her reactions toward daily life events. Or the nurse may join some kind of awareness or growth group. In some cases a nurse may choose one-to-one psychotherapy as a way of increasing her own self-awareness. If a nurse chooses a group or psychotherapy approach, she is well advised to make inquiries about the nature and purpose of the experience and the qualifications and experiences of the facilitator or therapist. This will help her to obtain the kind of experience she really wants.

A nurse also takes care of her own emotional realm when she maintains satisfactory relationships within her own social sphere. This involves clarifying her family relationships so that she knows her position within that system as an adult. It also involves building satisfying reciprocal friendships and developing a comfortable life-style of her own. It is sometimes useful for a nurse to periodically assess her personal social support system. The nurse needs resource persons available to her own personal support outside the nursing situation. It is not appropriate to use nurse-patient relationships for this purpose. You may wish to diagram your own personal support system. Figure 3–4 shows an example of a diagrammatic representation of a social support system. The length of connecting lines indicates the degree of closeness experienced between the two persons involved. Such a diagram will change over time, and periodic review of a social support system can help the nurse assess her interpersonal patterns.

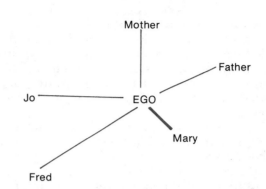

Figure 3–4. Representation of a social support system.

Many nursing students are young persons, experiencing the last phases of the adolescent life stage. This is the time when sexual factors are becoming clarified in interpersonal relationships. It can be important for the nurse to become aware of his or her sexual orientation at this time and the mode of sexual interaction that is most comfortable within the developing life-style. Again, it is not appropriate for the nurse to do this within nurse-patient relationships.

As a nurse works to maintain herself at a high level of emotional functioning she becomes more and more able to take responsibility for herself and her own actions and choices. Such a nurse finds that she blames other people less frequently for her circumstances and experiences. She gradually learns that she alone creates her own happiness and peace, and she becomes less likely to criticize other people for not producing such feelings for her.

In summary, the excellent nurse attends to her own emotional life. She works to increase her own self-awareness. She develops and maintains facilitative and satisfying private interpersonal relationships. And she seeks to take responsibility for herself and her own behavior.

Intellectual Realm

Nursing is a profession based on a body of knowledge derived from the physical, social and behavioral sciences. A truly professional nurse always seeks to maintain a high intellectual standing in areas pertaining to her work. She does this not only during her basic educational experiences but also throughout her entire professional life. The excellent nurse takes advantage of educational opportunities that will increase her knowledge and skills, thus improving her professional competency. She also pursues personal research, gaining individual knowledge through reading and discussion.

The professional nurse may also maintain interest in learning about areas not specifically related to nursing, e.g., crafts and literature. These activities not only increase her own pleasure but also help her remain an interesting person as well as a competent nurse.

In summary, if a nurse is to be an excellent or really helpful nurse, she not only cares about patients but also cares about herself. In fact, she cannot care about patients satisfactorily unless she first likes and cares about herself. It is not easy to really care about oneself. In the Judeo-Christian culture it has often been viewed as more worthy to care about others and to ignore one's own needs and growth. We are now beginning to see that caring for others and caring for oneself go together. Carkhuff has said:

> If the helper is not committed to his own physical, emotional, and intellectual development, he cannot enable another to find fulfillment in any or all of these realms of functioning.[10]

Attending to one's own personal development in physical, emotional and intellectual realms, then, is both a private and a professional responsibility.

THE NECESSARY CHARACTERISTICS OF HELPING PERSONS

Nursing is one of the professions that help people in their lifelong task of growing toward self-actualization and of thus finding increasingly effective ways of interacting with personal and nonpersonal aspects of the environment. (See Chapter 1 for a discussion on self-actualization.) The most helpful nurse is concerned with *all* aspects of the patients she cares for. She cares about the "total person." The nurse, along with all other helping professionals, must know the ways in which such comprehensive caring can be communicated to others.

This section will consider the factors involved in creating a therapeutic environment; the general characteristics of helping persons;

the specific facilitative characteristics of genuineness, nonpossessive warmth and accurate empathy; and the specific action-oriented characteristics of concreteness in communication, immediacy in communication and sensitive confrontation.

Creating a Therapeutic Environment

Creating a therapeutic environment means providing circumstances within which a person can feel comfortable and can work toward health when this is possible. This involves consideration of physical comfort and psychosocial comfort. The excellent or really helpful nurse makes sure that her patient is able to have his basic physiologic needs met. For example, she will make sure that he can breathe normally, that he can get relaxing rest and sleep, that he is able to get the kind of dietary nutrients he needs and that he can eliminate his bodily wastes with ease and without embarrassment. Furthermore, the excellent nurse does not "assume" that *she* knows the best ways for the patient to have these needs met. Rather she discusses each need with her patient. Through these discussions, the nurse finds out ways in which the patient has habitually most adequately met his physiologic needs and she does all that is possible to enable him to continue to meet his needs in similar ways. The nurse commonly uses a nursing history to gather such information and uses the nursing process to find solutions to any problems that arise. (See Chapter 17 for a discussion on nursing histories and the nursing process.) Let us consider the following example:

Ms. Smith is the nurse taking care of Mr. Jones, a 24-year-old man confined to bed with an orthopedic splint on his leg to provide healing of a fractured femur. Ms. Smith learns that Mr. Jones has difficulty in having bowel movements while in bed. Ms. Smith would not be creating a therapeutic environment if she merely told Mr. Jones that he "must have" a bowel movement every day in order to maintain health and that he must sit on a bedpan at 9 AM everyday—because that is the time that pans are given—until his bowels move. Such an approach is unlikely to be successful.

Ms. Smith would do better to sit down near Mr. Jones and in privacy discuss his normal bowel habits with him. She would probably ask questions about how many bowel movements he normally had during a week's time, the time of day his bowel movement usually occurred, the usual consistency of his feces (e.g., liquid, soft, hard) and what he was in the practice of doing when constipation or diarrhea occurred. She would also encourage Mr. Jones to discuss the things that made it particularly difficult for him to have normal bowel movements in his present circumstances. Ms. Smith may find that

Mr. Jones usually ate a bran cereal for breakfast and that he believes this helped him to maintain comfortable regular bowel movements. Or she may discover that the curtains around Mr. Jones' bed did not close properly, causing him acute embarrassment. Possibly she would learn that the window curtains were never drawn by Mr. Jones' bed while he was on the bedpan and that he felt tense because of outsiders walking past. There are probably many other things Mr. Jones would be able to tell Ms. Smith if she listened carefully.

Having gathered such information, Ms. Smith and Mr. Jones can then proceed to discuss ways of eliminating each of these problems and they can make plans that are appropriate for Mr. Jones, Ms. Smith, the health team and other persons involved (e.g., family members). Mr. Jones would thus be more likely to overcome his problem of constipation. By approaching patient concerns and patient problems in the above described way, Ms. Smith creates an environment that is therapeutic and she facilitates satisfactory problem solving.

It can be observed that the nurse in this example was not merely focusing on the patient's physical need for elimination but was also concerned with his psychosocial needs. She was concerned about privacy, for example. She also showed the patient that she was interested in his feelings and considered his ideas and life patterns important.

Sometimes psychosocial needs are even more primary than in the example of Mr. Jones:

Ms. White, a 63-year-old woman, is in the early stages of recovery from a heart attack. She persistently rings her call bell every half hour with apparently trivial requests. Such behavior can make a nurse become so irritated that she is tempted to ignore Ms. White's calls and deny her such requests. However, if the nurse is actively creating a therapeutic environment, she would be more likely to discuss the situation with Ms. White. She may sit down and say something like, "I notice that you are using your call bell a lot, Ms. White, and often you do not seem to want whatever it is you ask for. I want to help you but I do not seem to be doing that very well. Would you help me to know what you need?" If she listens carefully and does not make Ms. White feel she has been reprimanded, the nurse may discover that Ms. White is very frightened that she will have another heart attack while she is alone in her room. By discussing this together, Ms. White and the nurse could find ways of helping Ms. White feel less isolated and more cared about. As part of the plan, the nurse may explain to Ms. White that it is not necessary to make requests in order to have the nurse stop by. The nurse may promise that she and other staff members will look in frequently without being called. The nurse then coordinates her plan with other staff members.

In the two examples concerning Mr. Jones and Ms. White, it can be seen that the outcomes depended very much on the nurse. In each case

the nurse could have made the situation worse if by her manner and her words the patients had felt "put down" and "foolish" and if they had sensed that the nurse didn't really care about their concerns. If this had happened, the patients would have been unable to discuss their personal concerns openly, and a helpful solution would not have been reached. The helpful nurse is thus the kind of person who allows patients to feel comfortable, accepted and worthwhile.

The Necessary Conditions of Helping

We have already discussed the fact that *all helping occurs through the medium of interpersonal relationships.* It is now relevant to ask how we can conduct our professional relationships so that the helping process can be most effective. In other words, how can a nurse behave toward her patients in ways that are most likely to be helpful to them?

MAIN TYPES OF HELPFUL CHARACTERISTICS

Several researchers have suggested that there are two main types of helpful characteristics: (1) *facilitative characteristics,* i.e., conditions that create an emotional environment in which a person feels comfortable and safe in communicating; and (2) *action-oriented characteristics,* i.e., conditions that assist a person to move toward his goals. The facilitative characteristics used by a helper are
   a. Genuineness
   b. Nonpossessive warmth
   c. Accurate empathy
The action-oriented characteristics used by a helper are
   a. Concreteness in communication
   b. Immediacy in communication
   c. Sensitive confrontation
Let us look at each of the six conditions of helping and consider their application to nursing.

Facilitative Characteristics

Genuineness. Rogers maintained that *if a helper is not genuine, all else he does will be a waste of time.*[57] In fact, a helper who is not genuine is very threatening to a helpee. This is detrimental because a threatened person must use a lot of energy in defending himself and thus has very little energy left for working toward wellness.

> *Genuineness is considered to be the most basic of the helping conditions.*

Words that are sometimes used instead of "genuineness" include "authenticity," "congruence" and "realness." Regardless of the word used, the concept has been described by Rogers in the following way:

[the helper] . . . is what he *is*, when in the relationship with his client he is genuine and without "front" or façade, openly being the feelings and attitudes which at that moment are flowing in him. . . . By this we mean that the feelings the therapist is experiencing are available to him, available to his awareness, and he is able to live these feelings, be them, and able to communicate them if appropriate.[57]

This concept means that a *helper needs to be aware of his own changing feelings.* He must have a high enough level of self-knowledge and be comfortable enough with who he is so that he does not block out his own feelings from himself. For example, he does not deny unacceptable feelings in himself. Next, *the helper must have enough skill to be able to put his feelings into words in such a way that they are not condemning of the other person.* In addition to that, *the helper must have the judgment to allow him to decide when it is appropriate to express his feelings and when it is not.*

It is difficult to be genuine. Rogers has something to say about this difficulty. "No one fully achieves this condition [of genuineness], yet the more the therapist is able to listen acceptantly to what is going on within himself, and the more he is able to be the complexity of his feelings, without fear, the higher the degree of his congruence."[57]

Let us take some examples from a nursing context to illustrate ways a nurse can be genuine in nurse-patient relationships and the judgment she most appropriately makes when deciding when to communicate her feelings and when not to.

The nurse, Ms. Smith, is taking care of a young man, Bob Aspey, in a rehabilitation unit. He became a paraplegic several months ago and is now trying to come to terms with life in a wheelchair. Ms. Smith is gradually getting the feeling that Bob is becoming romantically interested in her and she is uncomfortable with that. One morning, while she is working with Bob, he says, "We could really have a great life together, you and I. If I wasn't in this wheelchair I think I would ask you to marry me." Ms. Smith could laugh at Bob and say "Come on now, Bob, don't be silly." Such a response would not be helpful to either Bob or Ms. Smith, since it does not acknowledge the real feelings of either of them.

A more genuine response might be, "Bob, I have the feeling that you are wishing we could become close friends in a romantic kind of way. I find I am uncomfortable with this and I would like to clarify it with you." Such a response would be likely to facilitate a more direct discussion about Bob's attraction to Ms. Smith and his frustration at the prospect of being confined to his wheelchair for the rest of his life. Through conversation Ms. Smith may be able to convey to Bob the ways in which she likes him even though she is not romantically interested in him.

Ms. Smith may also find that she has some angry feelings toward Bob—feelings she suspects may come from a private relationship she has with another person who persuaded her to take responsibility for him in a possessive kind of way. These feelings do not really relate to Bob, so it would not be appropriate to burden him with the details of that situation. However, Ms. Smith should not try to ignore those feelings because they would inevitably be communicated to Bob in nonverbal ways. It would be better for her to discuss that situation with someone she trusted in her own social network. In this way she can remain congruent to Bob while allowing his needs to take precedence over hers in that particular nurse-patient relationship.

Let us consider another example of genuineness in a nurse.

Ms. Smith is working as a public health nurse and is visiting Ms. Blogs and her newborn baby. When Ms. Smith calls at the house she feels that Ms. Blogs is reluctant to let her come into the house or to see the baby. Ms. Smith explains carefully who she is, but she still has the feeling that Ms. Blogs does not want her to come in. An unhelpful response from Ms. Smith in terms of genuineness might be, "Come now, Ms. Blogs, I am here to help you. You must let me see your baby if I am to do that." This response is directive in that it tells the client what she "must do." Such a response would probably make Ms. Blogs feel more defensive and more reluctant to let Ms. Smith into the house. A more genuine response would be, "Ms. Blogs, I have the feeling that you are a bit nervous about me. I am wondering if there is something I am doing that is upsetting to you?" Such a response reflects Ms. Smith's real feelings and is more likely to lead to understanding between her and her client.

It can be seen that genuineness requires "self-disclosing" statements. These are not easy statements to make, and many people confuse them with accusing statements about another person. (The reader is referred to the section on self-disclosure later in the chapter.)

Nonpossessive Warmth. Nonpossessive

warmth is another condition necessary for the creation of an emotional environment in which a person can grow toward "wellness."

> *A helper must be able to communicate genuine caring and warmth to another person in ways that are nonjudgmental and unconditional.*

Other words sometimes used for "nonpossessive warmth" are "unconditional positive regard," "respect for the other" and "prizing the other." These terms all mean that a helper believes in the basic goodness of another and cares about him regardless of what he feels and does. This does not mean that the helper approves of or agrees with everything another feels or does. Rather, *the helper neither "approves" nor "disapproves" but "accepts."* He encourages the other to express his feelings rather than act them out, and he continues to communicate feelings of caring in whatever he says or does.

The following examples illustrate ways a nurse can show high levels of nonpossessive warmth in nurse-patient relationships.

Ms. Smith is this time taking care of Ms. Grey, who is in the terminal stages of metastatic carcinoma. In other words, the patient is dying of cancer that has spread from one place in her body to other places. Ms. Grey appears very withdrawn and depressed one morning, rejecting everything Ms. Smith tries to do for her. Ms. Smith would not be expressing nonpossessive warmth if she were to stand at the end of the bed and say: "Come now, Ms. Grey, you are really being very difficult this morning. Your husband will be disappointed in you." It would be an equally nonhelpful response if she were to ignore the patient's behavior and say: "I am going to give you a bed bath now" and then proceed to mechanically wash Ms. Grey. Ms. Grey may end up being clean but she is unlikely to feel any more comfortable or feel understood and truly "cared for."

Ms. Smith may respond at a higher level of nonpossessive warmth if she accepts that Ms. Grey is behaving in the only way she can at that moment. The nurse may then say warmly, "I can see that you are feeling miserable this morning, Ms. Grey. Do you want to talk about it?" Ms. Grey may or may not want to talk. However, regardless of what Ms. Grey wants, Ms. Smith is most helpful if she does not reject Ms. Grey. Ms. Smith is helpful when she shows, by her words and actions, that she cares about and respects Ms. Grey's feelings rather than trying to "snap her out" of her withdrawal and depression.

Whenever a nurse hears herself doing or saying things that mean, "You should not be feeling what you are feeling" or "I like you sometimes but not at others," then she can know that she is not truly indicating nonpossessive warmth. A nurse needs to maintain a high level of self-awareness in order to know just how nonjudgmental she is really being. In other words, as previously emphasized, the helpful nurse frequently identifies and assesses her feelings and behaviors.

Nonpossessive warmth is often communicated to others in *nonverbal ways.* Facial expression, tone of voice, body posture and gesture can make the difference between a warm and a cold message. Pause in your reading for a few moments and practice a series of facial expressions, voice tones, body postures and gestures that you think convey warmth. Then practice another series that you think convey coldness. Compare the two. The feedback of another person would be helpful to you. A mirror, audio tape or video tape may also help you.

Warmth is usually conveyed by

▶ maintaining eye contact

▶ soft but clearly audible voice volume

▶ a gentle but not condescending voice tone

▶ words in common usage rather than technical jargon

▶ body position that brings your face at the same level as the patient's face

▶ body position about 3 or 4 feet away from the patient

▶ listening more than talking

▶ occasional gentle touching of the patient's hand or shoulder (A nurse should be sensitive to a patient's nonverbal response to touch and should not use touch to the extent that it appears to make a patient uncomfortable.)

Accurate Empathy.   Accurate empathy is the third condition necessary for the creation of an environment in which a person can grow toward wellness. Other terms sometimes used for accurate empathy are "empathic understanding," "active listening" and "creative listening." Communicating accurate empathy is particularly difficult and requires continuous practice by a helper.

> Accurate empathy *means that the helper is always striving to understand exactly what the other is feeling and experiencing. It does not mean that the helper feels or experiences those feelings himself (this is sympathy) but rather that he accepts and understands what the other person is feeling.*

A helper seeks to understand another person's experiences and feelings by observing the other's verbal and nonverbal behavior. A helper then verbally "checks out" or validates his perceptions (i.e., what he *thinks* the helpee is feeling and experiencing) with the helpee. He puts into words his ideas about what he thinks the helpee is feeling or experiencing and talks with the helpee to find out if he has understood the helpee's situation accurately. These activities require considerable communication skills. The reader is referred to the later section on communication, particularly those discussing reflection, paraphrasing, clarifying and summarizing (see pp. 42–43). A person is often helped considerably if he feels another person understands him or is at least trying very hard to understand him.

The following example presents a nurse practicing accurate empathy on a high level within a nurse-patient relationship.

Ms. Smith has been caring for Mr. Elliot while he is hospitalized to receive care during a regressive episode of multiple sclerosis (a degenerative condition of the nervous system). Ms. Smith observes the patient's wife, Mrs. Elliot, sitting alone at the end of the hospital hallway. Ms. Smith approaches Mrs. Elliot quietly, make eye contact with her and sits down beside her. The following conversation takes place.
Ms. Smith: "Good morning, Mrs. Elliot. You are looking rather thoughtful today" (putting into words her assessment of Mrs. Elliot's appearance).
Mrs. Elliot: "Oh, good morning. Well, I've just been visiting my husband. He seems to be getting a lot worse to me."
Ms. Smith: "Would you like to talk about it for a while? I can imagine it would be very difficult to feel your husband is getting worse."
Mrs. Elliot: "Yes, it really is difficult. There doesn't seem to be anyone I can turn to for help."
Ms. Smith: I can appreciate that it could be a very lonely time for you right now."

Such a conversation could go on for quite a few minutes if Ms. Smith continued to convey her attempts to understand. On the other hand, Ms. Smith would quickly put an end to any helpful conversation if, for example, she tried to talk Mrs. Elliot "out of" her feelings. An untherapeutic, unhelpful remark could be, "Oh, surely it's not as bad as all that. How can I cheer you up a little bit?" Here the nurse's remarks minimize and deny the real feelings of Mrs. Elliot, possibly causing Mrs. Elliot to feel embarrassed for feeling as she does. Undoubtedly Mrs. Elliot would be reluctant to try again to have a meaningful, honest conversation with Ms. Smith.

Ms. Smith would also be unhelpful to Mrs. Elliot if she made a response like, "Well, we are all doing our best to make him most comfortable. Why don't you go home and get some rest. I'm sure you'll feel better in the morning." Such a response suggests to Mrs. Elliot that she can forget or "push back" her feelings by resting. This response also closes off discussion of Mrs. Elliot's concerns and sounds as if this nurse is defensive about Mr. Elliot's care. Mrs. Elliot would be unlikely to feel that Ms. Smith understood her feelings at all.

Ms. Smith is helpful by (a) carefully focusing on Mrs. Elliot's verbal and nonverbal messages; and (b) continuing to give back to Mrs. Elliot messages (verbal and nonverbal) that show that she cares about Mrs. Elliot and wants to understand Mrs. Elliot's feelings and experiences. In this way the nurse practices accurate empathy.

To briefly summarize, we have been discussing the *facilitative characteristics* (genuineness, nonpossessive warmth and accurate empathy) used by a helper. You will recall that facilitative conditions create an emotional environment in which a person feels comfortable and safe in communicating.

Action-Oriented Characteristics

The action-oriented characteristics (concreteness in communication, immediacy in communication and sensitive confrontation) will be discussed in somewhat less detail, since the beginning nurse will probably want to concentrate on developing the facilitative characteristics. The action-oriented skills, while important, may be learned once the facilitative skills are firmly established.

Concreteness in Communication. A person is helped when he is encouraged to express his concerns in specific and personal terms. The most helpful nurse, then, is willing to clearly and explicitly discuss personal issues of a patient's situation rather than dealing only with generalized and vague topics. For example, Ms. Smith would probably be providing opportunity for concreteness when she makes such comments as: "Can you give me some examples?" "Does that problem apply to you personally?" "Tell me how that situation applies to you and your family now." Ms. Smith would be avoiding concreteness in communication (thus, being less helpful) if she makes statements such as: "Everyone feels like that." "Yes, that is often the way things are."

Immediacy in Communication. The most effective helper does not avoid discussion about the dynamics (interaction) occurring within the helper-helpee relationship itself. Such a helper knows that the therapeutic relationship is itself a reality that is influential in the helpee's life. A nurse, then, will initiate and encourage acknowledgment of any emotional content occurring between her and a patient. For example, suppose Ms. Smith has a patient who refuses to cooperate with her in any way, yet other nurses seem to be able to work with this patient quite successfully. Ms. Smith could avoid such a patient as much as possible and try to ignore the tension between them. However, she would be functioning at a higher level of immediacy if she approached the patient and said something like, "Mr. Jones, I am concerned about the tension that seems to exist between us. I am finding it difficult to find ways of helping you. Could we talk about that a little bit?"

Sensitive Confrontation. Many people confuse the concept of "confrontation" as meaning "attack." This is a misconception. *Sensitive confrontation is the nonjudgmental pointing out of discrepancies* in a helpee's behavior. If used well, it can be of considerable help but it should be used carefully. Sensitive confrontation should never be used in the initial (early) phases of a therapeutic relationship before trust has been established.

Sensitive confrontation is seen most clearly in a psychiatric nursing context but may be appropriate in other areas as well. For example, suppose Ms. Smith has been taking care of John Brown over several weeks. He is a young man who is recovering from a fractured femur (i.e., a break in the long bone of the thigh). John talks a lot about wanting to get well and return to work. Yet he refuses to do any of the exercises necessary to build up the strength in his muscles. Ms. Smith may helpfully use sensitive confrontation by pointing out this inconsistency to him. "John, I am a little confused. You talk a lot about wanting to be able to return to your normal life, yet you aren't doing any of the exercises that would help this to happen. Can you talk to me about that?"

Summary

We have considered six characteristics found by research to be important to the helping process. They are divided into two main groups: (1) the facilitative characteristics of genuineness, nonpossessive warmth and accurate empathy and (2) the action-oriented characteristics of concreteness in communication, immediacy of communication and sensitive confrontation. Helpful professionals, including nurses, must work on developing these characteristics throughout their professional lives. They are difficult to develop and maintain. Students of nursing should be diligent in their attempts to develop them in themselves but should not become disheartened if they do not always manage to function at the highest levels. Be gentle with yourself!

The reader will recognize that *the six conditions of helping are not used in isolation.* The most helpful nurse uses all three facilitative conditions simultaneously.

▶ She behaves as a real human being toward patients (genuineness).

▶ She allows the patient to be himself and to express any thoughts and feelings he is experiencing (nonpossessive warmth). Obviously, she does not simply accept behaviors that threaten her personal safety. She encourages verbal expression rather than acting-out behavior.

▶ She accepts the patient in a nonjudgmental way (nonpossessive warmth).

▶ She attempts at all times to understand exactly what a patient is telling her by his behavior and his words (accurate empathy).

The most helpful nurse uses the action-oriented conditions from time to time once the nurse-patient relationship has progressed beyond the initiation phase.

▶ She encourages her patient to be specific.

▶ She attends to any interpersonal processes occurring within the therapuetic relationship.

▶ She sensitively points out discrepancies in the patient's behavior.

Appropriate Confidentiality

If the conditions of helping are present within a nurse-patient relationship, it is likely that the patient will share information, feelings and experiences that are personally significant to him. The nurse, then, learns some things that are important and maybe private to the patient and has the responsibility of handling them gently and sensitively.

The nurse may, of course, use the knowledge she has about the patient to improve the quality of his nursing care. She may make changes in the nursing care plan in the light of this knowledge. The nurse would also discuss with the patient any issues she feels important to share with other professionals.

The nurse never shares information about the patient with anyone who is not involved with the care of the patient, however. In other words, she does not gossip with her friends; she does not talk about patients while riding home on the bus; she does not betray a patient's confidence in her. Such behavior breaks professional confidentiality and is unethical.

HELPING RELATIONSHIPS REQUIRE EFFECTIVE COMMUNICATION

Having identified and described the necessary characteristics of helping persons, we must emphasize that simply "knowing" what they are is not enough. To be really helpful a nurse must be able to communicate such characteristics to her patients. This section considers (a) the concept of communication; (b) verbal and nonverbal elements of communication; (c) the levels at which communication occurs; and (d) some common blocks to effective communication.

Communication

Smith, Bealer and Sim define communication in the following way:

Communication is the process through which a set of meanings embodied in a message is conveyed to a person or persons in such a way that the meanings received are equivalent to those which the initiator(s) of the message intended.[65]

Communication occurs, then, when meaning is transmitted from one person to another. Communication is most effective when the meaning the sender intended to send is the meaning received.

There is more to be considered than just sending and receiving messages. Person A may have a message that he wishes to send to Person B:

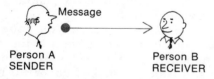

Perfect communication has occurred if the exact message person A intended to send is the one person B received:

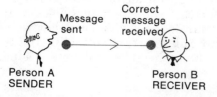

This does not always occur, however. Many times the message is distorted or changed in some way. We may illustrate such change or distortion by a change in the shape of the "message":

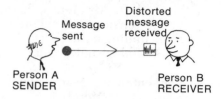

Distortion of Messages

Various personal and environmental factors may contribute to the distortion or change of messages.

Personal Factors. Factors relating to the internal processes of either Person A or Person B may impede the clear, accurate transmission of a message. Examples of such factors are as follows:

▶ *Emotional factors*, e.g., anger, anxiety, excitement, resentment, antagonism, grief

▶ *Physical factors*, e.g., tiredness, illness, speech defects, deafness, pain

▶ *Intellectual factors*, e.g., differing intellectual abilities, language use, knowledge levels

▶ *Social factors*, e.g., differences in culture, language, socioeconomic class, race, ethnic groups, professional status

Such factors may narrow the perceptual field of one or both of the persons involved in the communication process. Thus, messages sent from one person to the other may be distorted or changed.

Environmental Factors. Factors relating to the physical and social circumstances in which the communication takes place may "get in the way" of the message. Examples of such environmental factors are:

▶ *Physical factors*, e.g., environmental noise, lack of privacy, uncomfortable accommodations

▶ *Social factors*, e.g., presence of other people, expecting the presence of other people.

Such factors may increase tension or discomfort between the two persons attempting to communicate with each other. Environmental factors thus contribute to the distortion or change of messages sent from one person to another.

Ross Transactional Communication Model. Ross[58] has developed a model to illustrate

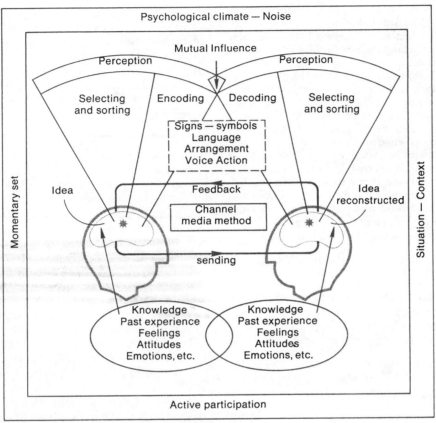

Figure 3–5. Ross Transactional Communication Model. (From Ross, R. S.: *Speech Communication: Fundamentals and Practice,* 3rd ed. Englewood Cliffs, NJ: Prentice-Hall, 1974, p. 15.)

in another way the factors involved in the communication process (see Fig. 3–5). The Ross transactional communication model illustrates factors that can bring about discrepancies between the idea (message sent) and the idea reconstructed (message received). Study Figure 3–5 carefully. It contains a lot of useful information.

Nurse-Patient Communication

A nurse needs to be aware of factors that can distort messages. Obviously, they affect nurse-patient communication as well as the nurse's communication with others, e.g., staff members. Keeping these factors in mind, the skillful nurse makes every effort to *prevent* communication difficulties and to *reduce* communication difficulties as they arise.

It is important for a nurse to be aware of personal factors that may be operating *within*

herself and to deal with such factors outside nurse-patient relationships. By making genuine statements about herself and her own feelings, a nurse can reduce interpersonal tensions that may arise between herself and the patient.

It is also important for a nurse to recognize personal factors that may be operating *within the patient.* The nurse can strive to reduce the potential communication distorting effects of such factors by carefully using the skills involved in accurate empathy.

Additionally, the skillful nurse takes particular notice of the *environment* surrounding the communication process. She makes every attempt to reduce distracting factors such as disturbing noises and lack of privacy.

Let us look at a situation in which a nurse does not attend to the above-mentioned factors.

Suppose our nurse Ms. Smith is preparing Ms. Frank for abdominal surgery. She goes to Ms. Frank's room and gives her all the information she considers necessary and leaves, feeling she has done a good job. What Ms. Smith does not realize however is that Ms. Frank has some hearing loss. Also, Ms. Frank has been waiting for her surgery for 6 weeks and is very anxious about it. Ms. Frank is tired and worried about "home." She has six children at home with her husband, and she spent days getting their clothes and food ready for the time she will be in the hospital. Further, Ms. Frank has difficulty communicating with authority figures and is thus unlikely to question anything Ms. Smith said. Ms. Smith herself has an important examination the next day and is worrying about that. She has made similar explanations to patients many times before and has ceased thinking carefully about what she should say. All these factors would make it unlikely that the messages Ms. Smith thought she had sent Ms. Frank were in fact the messages Ms. Frank received.

Ms. Smith could have done much better if she had:

▶ Acknowledged to herself that she was under stress because of the impending examination and so needed to take extra care when communicating with others.

▶ Spent some moments initiating a comfortable relationship with Ms. Frank before attempting the explanation.

▶ Made herself aware of Ms. Frank's hearing loss by consulting the patient's nursing history and then made deliberate efforts to speak clearly and slowly while directly facing Ms. Frank.

▶ Remembered that Ms. Frank will have some perceptual narrowing due to anxiety and so talked slowly and calmly.

▶ Carefully communicated nonpossessive warmth to help Ms. Frank feel important and accepted and to reduce the patient's anxiety of the nurse as an authority figure.

▶ "Checked out" (i.e., sought validation about) Ms. Frank's understanding of the explanations to ensure that an accurate message had indeed been received.

Verbal and Nonverbal Communication

We have seen that communication involves both the verbalization of a message and a number of nonspoken events and circumstances.

Verbal communication involves use of the spoken or written word and is dependent on *language*. "Language" is really the code used to convey a message from one person to another. To be effective, a code must be clearly and exactly understood by *both* the sender and the receiver. It is simple for a nurse to discover whether another person uses the same language system (e.g., English, French, Spanish) as herself. However, it is not so simple to determine whether another person attaches the same *meanings* to the same words. Additional difficulties can arise if a nurse uses technical words and abbreviations that are familiar to her but are unfamiliar to the patient or a family member.

> *A nurse must always seek "feedback," or validation, of her message from a patient to make sure that the message sent by the nurse is the same message received by the patient.*

The unspoken events and circumstances that accompany and affect communication are called nonverbal communication and include facial expression; body posture; tone, pitch and volume of voice; gait; gesture; touch; and eye contact. This very powerful component of the communication process can alter the meaning of verbal communication considerably. This truth is conveyed in the proverb, "What you do speaks so loudly that I cannot hear what you say."

Consider, for example, the different shades of meaning that can be given to the phrase "We were expecting you" by changing the tone of voice or the emphasis on various words. Or think of the differences in meaning of "I'm to be your nurse today," depending on whether it is said as the nurse (a) hurries out of the patient's room; (b) stands restlessly reading her watch at the end of the patient's bed; or (c) sits down or stands beside the patient, looking at the patient in a relaxed, friendly manner.

The truly helpful nurse pays attention to the nonverbal messages she receives from patients along with their verbal messages. Such a nurse "checks out" any inconsistencies she notices between the verbal and nonverbal messages. For example, "You say you don't mind staying in the hospital a few more days, yet you look worried as you say that." *Nonverbal messages are often much closer to the truth than verbal messages* because nonverbal communication is much more difficult to cover up or distort. However, nonverbal messages are not clear messages. It is thus important to encourage a patient to express significant nonverbal messages in verbal terms when possible. This is best done by gentle use of the skills that communicate accurate empathy.

A nurse needs to become particularly skilled at identifying the nonverbal signs of anxiety, as this is an emotion experienced commonly by patients. Behavioral clues to anxiety include quick and agitated movements; tenseness of muscles; trembling of extremities; rapid speech; increased talking or severely reduced talking; irritability and the making of seemingly "trivial" demands; inability to concentrate; and excessive smoking or other repetitious behaviors. The excellent nurse notices such behavioral clues and encourages the patient to discuss his anxieties, although he may find this difficult. This expression is facilitated by the nurse using skills that communicate genuineness, nonpossessive warmth and accurate empathy.

Levels of Communication

The kind of communication between a nurse and her patients can be of an intimate and personal nature. Any discussion about one's feelings is very personal and is not usually done with strangers or persons outside one's close circle of friends and relatives. Yet, we have seen that to be really helpful, a nurse must appropriately share her own feelings with a patient and encourage him to share his feelings with her. Because this can be threatening, a safe interpersonal environment must be created. It is then possible to share feelings more comfortably. Let us now look at the levels of communication that exist and the factors that influence the level used at any particular time.

Powell[53] has suggested that there are five levels of communication: (1) cliché conversation; (2) reporting facts; (3) sharing personal ideas and judgments; (4) sharing feelings; and (5) peak communication. The differences between these levels are a consequence of the extent to which a person is willing to share his real feelings.

Levels of Communication[53]

Peak communication	
Sharing feelings	Communication progresses upward as a consequence of trust
Sharing personal ideas and judgments	
Reporting facts	
Cliché conversation	

The level with least sharing of feelings is *cliché conversation*. At this level people exchange the pleasantries of superficial social interaction: "How are you?" "I'm just fine thanks." "It's a nice day today." These kinds of conversations are familiar to everyone. To a certain extent such conversation helps us feel "safe," as it does not require any thought and eliminates the unexpected. A nurse may usefully employ cliché conversation briefly at the beginning of an interaction with a patient in an attempt to establish trust. However, the skillful nurse quickly attempts to encourage a patient to communicate with her at a more meaningful level. It is especially important not to ask the patient "How are you?" in a cliché tone of voice. To do so would indicate to the patient a lack of interest in how he *really* is feeling.

The second level of communication, *reporting facts,* is objective and does not reveal very much about the persons involved in the interaction. A nurse may allow a patient to speak at this level if it seems he has a need to; however, she would be careful not to suggest by her behavior anything that would stop him from sharing more of himself.

The third level of communication is the *sharing of personal ideas and judgments*. When a person begins to talk at this level, some trust has been developed in the relationship, since some sharing of self is taking place. At such a level, for example, a patient may tell a nurse his opinions regarding his treatment. The helpful nurse is careful not to communicate messages of disapproval or ridicule to a patient who is communicating in this way. Such messages would be likely to stop the patient from sharing and cause him to talk at more superficial and uninvolved levels.

When a person communicates at the fourth level he is *sharing feelings*. He is telling another person his beliefs and reactions to past and present events. Such sharing is helpful and healthy and is most easily done in an environment of interpersonal trust and security. A nurse can help build such trust and security with a patient by (a) being a real person herself (genuineness); (b) caring warmly for the patient (nonpossessive warmth); and (c) attempting to understand him accurately (accurate empathy).

The fifth level of communication is that of *peak communication,* or a sense of "oneness." This is achieved by few and even then for only short periods of time. It will occasionally occur spontaneously if level four has been reached.

All five levels of communication may occur within the nurse-patient relationship at one time or another. It is important to allow a patient to communicate at the level that is most comfortable for him and not to force him into a higher level before he is ready. A nurse needs to continually assess her own communication patterns, however, to make sure she is not keeping the communication between herself and her patients at an unnecessarily superficial level by her own behavior.

Blocks to Effective Communication

The nature of the nurse-patient relationship is to a large degree dependent on the quality of communication, which is influenced by the behavior of both the nurse and the patient. It is the professional responsibility of the nurse, however, to make sure that there is nothing in her behavior that prevents a patient from communicating at a personal level when he wants to and has a need to. Sometimes a nurse may block deeper communication without being aware of it. Her intentions may be to allow the patient to discuss whatever he wants; however, by some simple remark she may stop him from doing so, leaving the patient feeling lonely and misunderstood. A nurse thus needs to be aware of the kinds of remarks that can block effective communication.

Hewitt and Pesznecker[25] have reported five major categories of remarks that are likely to block effective communication.* When a nurse understands the nature of each of these categories she can work to eliminate them from her communication patterns with patients and so facilitate more effective communication. Also, the informed nurse will be more likely to communicate the characteristics of a helping person that have been identified and described earlier in this chapter.

The five categories of remarks that block effective conversation are as follows:[25]

1. Changing the subject.
2. Stating one's own opinions and ideas about the patient and his situation.
3. False or inappropriate reassurance.
4. Jumping to conclusions or offering solutions to the problem.

---

*This classification is based on an original system developed by Joan Bachand: "Problematic Verbal Patterns of Student Nurses in Initial Interviews with Psychiatric Patients: A Tool and Its Application," Newark, NJ, Rutgers University, 1959 (unpublished master's thesis).

5. Inappropriate use of medical facts or nursing knowledge.

Changing the Subject. A nurse may stop a patient from discussing a topic of importance to him either by *directly changing the subject* or by *shifting the focus of the conversation* by responding to an insignificant aspect of the patient's comment.

For example, in the following conversation, note how Ms. Smith directly changes the subject away from what Mr. Armstrong says.

Ms. Smith: "Good morning, Mr. Armstrong, how are you today?"

Mr. Armstrong (slow, depressed speech): "Oh, I'm all right, I guess, except I'm beginning to wonder if I'll ever get well enough to leave the hospital."

Ms. Smith: "Well, it's time to take your bath now."

By this remark, Mr. Armstrong would get the message that Ms. Smith was either unable or unwilling to discuss his feelings of concern about his recovery. The patient may not risk talking about his feelings again. Thus, his feelings of depression and anxiety would not be relieved. Notice also that Ms. Smith opened the conversation by asking "How are you?" in a cliché sense. She did not focus on the patient's response to this question.

Stating One's Own Opinions. This kind of response usually has a "moralizing tone" and communicates to the patient that he ought not be feeling what he is feeling and that his thoughts and opinions are inappropriate or wrong. Consider the following example:

Ms. Smith: "Good morning, Mr. Armstrong, how are you today?"

Mr. Armstrong (slow, depressed speech): "Oh, I'm all right I guess, except I'm beginning to wonder if I'll ever get well enough to leave the hospital."

Ms. Smith: "Oh, I'm sure you will, Mr. Armstrong. You shouldn't feel that way."

By this remark Mr. Armstrong would probably feel foolish and "put down." He may feel that Ms. Smith did not understand him at all, and he may not attempt to discuss his concerns with her again.

False or Inappropriate Reassurance. In an attempt to help a patient "cheer up," a nurse may make quick, trite remarks. Such comments are easy to offer but are rarely appropriate or reassuring.

Ms. Smith: "Good morning, Mr. Armstrong, how are you today?"

Mr. Armstrong (slow, depressed speech): "Oh, I'm all right I guess, except I'm beginning to wonder if I'll ever get well enough to leave the hospital."

Ms. Smith: "Oh, yes you will, Mr. Armstrong. Things are brighter than that. You'll have a clean bill of health before you know it."

Again, Mr. Armstrong would probably be unable to express his anxieties and fears, as he might feel that Ms. Smith could not or did not want to try to understand his real feelings.

Jumping to Conclusions or Offering Solutions to the Problem. It is often tempting to offer solutions to a patient's problems too quickly. When this is done there is a danger of responding to only a part (perhaps an insignificant part) of the patient's concern. People very rarely express their real concerns in the first few sentences. Often they need time to "think out loud"—to express their anxieties and discover for themselves what is really troubling them. Commonly, "solutions" from other people are not needed as much as an opportunity to talk with others about concerns. Notice in the following example how Ms. Smith "jumps to conclusions" about Mr. Armstrong's thoughts and how she then "offers a solution" to what she thinks is the problem.

Ms. Smith: "Good morning, Mr. Armstrong, how are you today?"

Mr. Armstrong (slow, depressed speech): "Oh, I'm all right I guess, except I'm beginning to wonder if I'll ever get well enough to leave the hospital."

Ms. Smith: "Now, I think you are worrying about that laboratory test your doctor has ordered for you today. You think that means you are more seriously ill than you really are. You just need to forget about that and everything will be all right."

Mr. Armstrong may not have been worrying about the laboratory test at all. In this interaction, Ms. Smith did not take the time to find out what Mr. Armstrong really meant by his remarks. Instead, Ms. Smith jumped to her own conclusion about his concerns, and she offered premature, unhelpful solutions. Such remarks by the nurse could not only introduce new concerns to the patient but also block expression of the patient's initial concerns. No doubt Mr. Armstrong was left feeling isolated with his problems and misunderstood.

Inappropriate Use of Medical Facts or Nursing Knowledge. A nurse may offer facts to a patient *too quickly,* i.e., *before* she has really found out what facts, if any, he is looking for. Information given too quickly can cut off a patient's expression of feeling.

Ms. Smith: "Good morning, Mr. Armstrong. How are you today?"

Mr. Armstrong (slow, depressed speech): "Oh, I'm all right I guess, except I'm beginning to wonder if I'll ever get well enough to leave the hospital."

Ms. Smith: "Well, I'm not sure that is true. Your doctor is very pleased with your progress. Your blood pressure is almost back to normal, those tablets you are taking are the best possible treatment you can have for your condition."

While the facts Ms. Smith offered might be accurate, offering them so soon in a conversation would most likely do little more than stop Mr. Armstrong from talking about his concerns and clarifying what they are. Mr. Armstrong has a need to be listened to by a nurse who is making a real effort to understand him. A more helpful response to Mr. Armstrong's

concerns that he would never leave the hospital would be:

"You are looking very concerned, Mr. Armstrong. I can appreciate that a long hospitalization would worry you. Can we talk about that for a while?"

Such a remark is more likely to help Mr. Armstrong feel that the nurse really wanted to listen to him. He would thus be more likely to express his feelings and so gain some comfort and relief from his fears.

It is easy to block a patient's communication of feelings quite unintentionally. If a nurse becomes aware that she has done this, she may be able to correct her mistake by making a genuine statement to the patient about what has happened. For example, after any of the blocking statements Ms. Smith made, she could try to repair any damage by saying, "Mr. Armstrong, I think you were starting to tell me of a real worry you have and I cut you off by answering you too quickly. I'm sorry I did that. I really would like to listen to you and try to understand if you feel you could talk about it now."

Interpersonal communication is a very sensitive process; however, as indicated above, mistakes are not irreversible. A nurse need not fear making a mistake, but it would be a serious error if a nurse didn't care about her communication and thus didn't work to develop helpful communication patterns with patients and coworkers. As with other skills, communication skills develop with awareness, practice and performance evaluation.

SKILLS THAT FACILITATE COMMUNICATION

To be really helpful, a nurse continually develops her skills of effective communication. There are a number of fairly specific techniques that can be learned, practiced and used within therapeutic relationships. When properly used, these techniques facilitate a smooth, two-way communication flow between a helper and a helpee. It must be remembered, however, that techniques are never helpful in themselves. Communication techniques may actually be perceived as threatening and destructive if they are not accompanied by the helpful characteristics described earlier in this chapter.

The communication skills described here are the more common ones: listening, problem solving and self-disclosure. These skills are all aimed at increasing the levels of two-way understanding between a helper and helpee by encouraging the helpee to talk. This encouragement is given so that change can occur for the helpee in a goal-directed manner.

Listening Skills

There is more to listening than simply hearing the words of another. In addition to hearing the words it is important to consider tone of voice, fluency of speech, choice of language, facial expressions, body posture and body movements. Listening involves attending to the "whole person" and trying to understand the "total message" the individual is trying to relate. The words are only part of this total message. In sum, listening involves attending to verbal and nonverbal communication.

We will look at the specific listening skills of attending, perception checking and reflecting. Specific examples of each skill are given in a nursing context.

Attending. Attending is the way of giving a person the comfortable, warm feeling of having the total attention of another person. Ivey[27] and others have identified four components of successful attending. The first component is *eye contact*. If eye contact is maintained at a comfortable distance for both nurse and patient (usually not less than 3 feet), the patient will feel attended to.

The second component of attending is *posture*. The interested nurse may sit in a comfortable, relaxed position, facing the patient and leaning a little toward the patient.

The third component of attending is *gesture*. The nurse conveys nonverbal messages to the patient through her gestures. If she shifts around in her chair and looks at her watch repeatedly, the patient will probably receive (nonverbally) the message that the nurse is in a hurry, has no time to talk and is thinking about other things. It is extremely important for helpers to be aware of their individual common gestures and the kinds of nonverbal messages these "typical" gestures give to others. It is especially important to become aware of gestures used when feeling stressed, e.g., pressured by time, fearful, anxious. Some gestures can be helpful to the attending process, e.g., gestures that are natural, relaxed and congruent to the whole interaction.

The fourth component of attending is *verbal behavior*. A nurse shows attention by offering a few verbal comments relating to the topic the patient is presenting. Such comments are made without changing the subject or interrupting the patient.

If a patient feels he has a nurse's attention, he will be encouraged to talk and express his feelings in more detail. Brammer[8] offers the following list as a summary of guidelines for effective attending behavior:

▶ Establish contact through looking at the helpee when he talks.

▶ Maintain a natural, relaxed posture that indicates your interest.

▶ Use natural gestures that communicate your intended messages.

▶ Use verbal statements that relate to the helpee's statements without introducing interruptions, questions or new topics.

Perception Checking. Perception checking is a way of getting and giving feedback. A helper may listen very carefully and observe nonverbal behavior and then check his perceptions by asking the helpee if what he (helper) understands about what he has seen or heard is correct. This checking may be done in a number of ways.

One way of checking perceptions is by *paraphrasing*. Paraphrasing involves restating the helpee's message in different words. For example, a patient may tell a nurse about numerous visits he has made to doctors about a pain problem and how he felt about the limited help he considered he received. The nurse may paraphrase the patient's comments by saying: "You've really been bothered by this pain for a long time and it doesn't seem as though any of the doctors you have seen have been able to help you."

Another way of perception checking is by *clarifying*. This involves trying to get more specific information from messages that seem vague and confused to the listener. A nurse may seek clarification by making the following kinds of statements: (a) "I don't quite understand. Are you telling me that . . ." (b) "Do you mean that . . ." (c) "It sounds like you are saying that . . ."

> *Whenever perception checking is done the nurse must always pause to allow the patient to correct, modify or confirm her understandings. Perception checking skills lead to the establishment of accurate empathy.*

Reflecting. Reflecting involves saying back to the helpee or demonstrating to him what he communicated (verbally and nonverbally) so that the helpee can re-evaluate his communication. Reflecting allows the helpee to (a) know that the helper is trying to understand and (b) have a clarifying experience by hearing and seeing himself in someone else. Consider the following examples of reflections by one nursing student, Ms. Smith.

Example 1

Mr. George: "I feel so bad today, nurse. I have no energy at all. I think it would be better if I was no longer here."

Ms. Smith: "This is really a hard day for you today, Mr. George, and you are wondering if you have enough strength to keep going."

Example 2

Ms. White: "The doctor tells me I have cancer in my stomach. I wonder if that means I am going to die."

Ms. Smith: "You are not sure what it means when the doctor says 'cancer.' You don't know if that means he can cure you or not."

Again, a nurse should always pause after making a reflective statement to allow the patient to tell her if she has correctly understood the patient's communication. Reflecting also helps create accurate empathy.

Problem-Solving Communication Skills

There are some communication skills that are concerned more specifically with problem solving. We consider here the following common problem-solving communication skills: (a) information seeking; (b) focusing; (c) summarizing; and (d) informing.

Information Seeking. The first step in the nursing process is the collection of information (see Chap. 17). It is on the basis of collected information that a nurse makes her nursing assessment and diagnosis and consequently develops a plan for nursing action. If the information collected is not accurate, then the consequent assessment and plan will be less than helpful. It is therefore important to collect accurate information. This activity is facilitated by asking questions in such a way that the patient feels comfortable in responding in his own way.

Open-ended questions are usually most appropriate. Such questions are asked in such a way that they do not imply the answer. For example, "Would you tell me how today has been for you, Mr. Brown?" is an open-ended question. "You have been much better today, Mr. Brown, haven't you?" is *not* an open-ended question. Open-ended questions require more than a "yes" or "no" answer and encourage the person to give more detail. Here are two more examples of open-ended questions: "Could you tell me about the circumstances that brought you into hospital?" "Can we talk a bit about how you are managing to prepare your baby's special diet at home?"

A nurse is unlikely to get the information she requires if her mode of questioning conveys judgment, condescension or preconceived answers.

Focusing. Anxious people often have difficulty identifying the concerns that are central for them and may thus tend to "wander" in their communication. Focusing is a way of helping a person keep to the point, e.g., helping to direct the comments of an anxious person. A nurse should not use the focusing technique too early in an interaction. If she does, she may unintentionally "focus" the patient on an issue that is not really important to him. Examples of focusing statements are as follows: "You mentioned that you are having difficulty getting your son to go to school. Would you like to talk about that for a little bit?" "You were talking about the pain you had in your chest and we got away from that a bit. Is there anything more you would like to tell me about that?"

Focusing can be helpful to a patient, but a nurse must always be aware that by doing this she may be taking the patient's communication in a direction he doesn't really want it to go.

Summarizing. It is often helpful for a person to hear a summary or concise overview of what he has been saying. Summarizing is a way of tying together, in one statement, several ideas and feelings. It can give a person a sense of movement in problem solving and help him to clarify the direction he is going in. Examples of summarizing statements may be: "Let's see, we've talked about several things in the last half hour. You told me about your mother's serious illness and how she reacted to it by withdrawing and feeling depressed. And you wondered if you might be reacting in ways similar to hers. Also, you started telling me that you are concerned about your daughter's health."

Summary statements can be very useful at the end of an interaction. They may also be appropriate during the course of a conversation if a number of themes or topics are being covered. If a nurse is involved in a series of conversations with a patient around a particular problem, it may be useful to summarize the material covered in previous sessions at the beginning of a new session. After a nurse uses a summarizing statement, she should pause to ask the patient if she has been accurate in her statements.

Informing.   There are times when a nurse has information that a patient needs and has a right to know. Common examples of such information include (a) the normal routines and practices at the health service the patient is involved in, e.g., hospital, clinic, community health agency; and (b) explanations of procedures and treatments the patient is involved in. Whenever a nurse gives information she should first make sure it is accurate. Also, the nurse should know if other members of the health team consider it appropriate to give the patient the information. The skillful nurse presents information in a clear simple manner without condescension, avoiding the use of technical and medical jargon. Also, the nurse pauses to give the patient an opportunity to ask questions or to seek clarification of what he has been told. It is sometimes helpful to give information in writing as well as verbally.

Self-Disclosure

This chapter has shown that the helpful nurse is one who encourages a patient to talk about himself. Jourard[32] has said that self-disclosure, or the sharing of oneself with others, is an indicator of personality health and at the same time is a way of increasing or improving personality health. Jourard has also shown through research that people are more likely to be self-disclosing to people who are sharing something of themselves as well. As Jourard[32] says, "Self-disclosure breeds self-disclosure." The concept of genuineness of self, already discussed, supports the principle that excellent or really helpful nurses are willing to share something of themselves with patients.

There are two types of self-disclosure. The first is the sharing of *biographical and personal historical information*. If a nurse shares this kind of information, she will tell of happenings in her past and private life. Some of this can be useful. For example, a nurse should always tell every patient her name and whether she is a nursing student or a registered nurse. Further information of this nature can be useful when appropriate if the nurse feels comfortable sharing it and if she is not doing so in an attempt to meet her own needs. As has been pointed out previously, the needs of the patient must always be primary in the nurse-patient relationship.

The second type of self-disclosure is the *sharing of oneself in the here and now*. This is a very important kind of self-disclosure for the helping process. It is this kind of self-disclosure that was predominantly described in the discussion on genuineness of self. The nurse who is "real" or "genuine" with her patients is willing to make self-disclosure statements about her feelings and reactions within the present relationship she is maintaining with her patients. This is not easy to do. It requires a lot of self-awareness and skill. The nurse needs to work hard to develop nonjudgmental and nonthreatening ways of sharing herself. When done well and appropriately, however, such self-disclosure is one of the most successful ways of being helpful to patients.

Use of Silence

Much of the material presented thus far has emphasized the verbal skills a nurse can use to facilitate communication. Verbal skills are important, but they are not the only way to be helpful to another person. Warm silences can be very comforting and useful to a patient. They give a patient time to think and time to "just be" in the company of someone who cares. A nurse need never feel that time must always be filled with speech.

Many nurses are not comfortable with silences, however, and they communicate this discomfort to patients. A conversation that could be therapeutic can be prematurely terminated because of the tension created by the nurse's discomfort.

You may find it useful to try to increase your self-awareness by examining your own reactions to silence. Try to answer the following questions:

► Do you feel it necessary to break silences when you are in a group?

► Are you usually the first to talk in a group?

► How do you feel when in the company of someone who does not talk very much?

► Do you find it necessary to fill silences with chatter?

It may be useful to discuss these questions with a group of nursing students. Others may be able to give you useful feedback about your behavior during silences.

If nurses do not become comfortable with

silences, they lose important opportunities to be therapeutic. An effective nurse is able to sit quietly with a patient and give him the space to think while the nurse communicates nonpossessive warmth with nonverbal messages. The nurse may even give the patient permission to be quiet by saying something like, "You don't need to talk if you don't want to. I'd like to stay here with you for a while though." Silence is an important therapeutic tool. Maybe it "lets the air" into a relationship.

THE PATIENT AND HIS SIGNIFICANT OTHERS

Very few people are completely isolated from other people. Most people live within a social matrix of people who are "significant" to them to a greater or lesser extent. Such significant people usually include a number of family members and friends. When an individual is ill, the illness not only affects the ill person himself but also places stress on the significant others in his life. His social roles alter and so do the reciprocal roles of the people with whom he lives and interacts. (The sick role is discussed in Chapter 13.)

A nurse needs to be aware of this phenomenon and be willing to enter into therapeutic relationships with the patient's family and friends. The material covered in this chapter is as important to the relationships a nurse has with a patient's significant others as it is to the nurse-patient relationship itself.

Therefore, the problem solving involved in the nursing process (see Chap. 17) must take into account the social matrix surrounding the patient. If this is not done, solutions reached may seem ideal for the patient but be totally inappropriate for the social milieu in which the patient lives.

EVALUATING SUCCESS IN THERAPEUTIC RELATIONSHIPS

The fifth step in the nursing process is the "evaluation of the plan" (see Chap. 17). It is particularly important to evaluate nursing action on the basis of purposes or goals, e.g., "Have I done what I intended to do?" Evaluation becomes the basis for further planning.

The excellent nurse undertakes frequent evalution of her interpersonal relationships with patients. A nurse can evaluate her behavior in terms of the six characteristics of a helping professional: (1) genuineness, (2) nonpossessive warmth, (3) accurate empathy, (4) concreteness in communication, (5) immediacy in communication, and (6) sensitive confrontation. This can be done generally, e.g., "How have I rated on the six characteristics of a helping professional in my overall behavior toward patients today?"

It is probably more useful to be somewhat more specific, however. A nurse's behavior can be evaluated more effectively if she makes periodic process recordings of interactions with patients. This can be done from memory or occasionally it may be possible to audio or video tape an interaction for the purposes of evaluation. These interactions can be reviewed by communication experts or skilled coworkers.

Nursing action can also be evaluated in terms of patient behavior: Aiken and Aiken[1] suggest that a patient's behavior is a consequence of a nurse's behavior. A nurse may thus try to evaluate her own effectiveness by looking at her patient's responses. To do this she might ask questions such as:

▶ Does the patient appear more physically comfortable?

▶ Did the patient talk about his feelings and reactions or did he talk only superficially?

▶ If the patient talked only superficially, did the nurse block his communication? If so, specifically how did the nurse block communication?

THE NURSE AS PART OF THE THERAPEUTIC TEAM

Nursing is not an individualistic professional practice. A nurse most often works with a nursing team and a wider medical and paramedical team. To a large extent the success of nursing care is dependent upon the successful working together of all members of the health team. This coordinated effort requires a considerable amount of energy on the part of all team members if it is to be done well.

Successful team work requires sharing of information and giving of support to each other. Many of the previously discussed important characteristics of a therapeutic relationship can be appropriately applied to the relationships a nurse has with colleagues as well as her relationships with patients. Health workers who are being genuine, nonpossessively warm and accurately empathic with each other are more likely to be able to offer an excellent service to patients than those who are not.

A nurse need never feel she is alone in her work. Instead, she may seek out other cooperative team members for support, feedback and consultation.

THE EXPRESSIVE ROLE OF THE NURSE DURING TECHNICAL PROCEDURES

Many chapters in this book present technical and scientific information that will help you carry out numerous instrumental procedures required by a therapeutic plan for a patient. Examples of such procedures are injection techniques, intravenous therapy, applications of heat and cold, the use of mechanical lifts. With practice and familiarity you will become very skilled and will consider such procedures uncomplicated. This will not be so for the patients you care for.

The nurse does well to anticipate that almost all patients will experience some degree of anxiety at requiring medical or nursing help. Anxiety will increase whenever a patient is required to undergo an unfamiliar technical procedure. Any experience that is not part of the everyday life of the individual is anxiety producing.

It is a nursing task to identify the origins of a patient's anxieties and to use an expressive role to promote comfort and relative freedom from fear. (See p. 24 for a description of expressive roles.) Throughout this book, descriptions are given of the kinds of anxieties patients often have when subjected to particular procedures. These and other concerns may be reduced if the nurse

▶ really understands the nature and reasons for the treatment and is able to communicate these to the patient and help him gain confidence and trust

▶ takes time to explain the procedure quietly and clearly both before and during the procedure

▶ recognizes that anxious people have a narrowed perceptual field and is therefore willing to repeat herself as many times as the patient needs

▶ encourages the patient to ask questions and answers them clearly, making sure the patient is satisfied with the answers each time

▶ makes sure the patient can get attention at any time during long procedures, i.e., that he has a call bell available and feels comfortable using it

▶ responds to patients' requests quickly and willingly

A patient may be concerned about some things other than those anticipated by the nurse, however. A nurse should never assume that she knows what a patient is concerned about until she has listened carefully to what the patient is saying both verbally and nonverbally. Most people require some encouragement to be able to identify and express fears and anxieties. The excellent nurse is able to provide encouragement with the use of genuineness, accurate empathy and nonpossessive warmth. Accurate empathy is probably the most important way of helping a patient cope with unfamiliar and fear-producing procedures. If a nurse uses this expressive skill well she will be able to

▶ identify the patient's fears accurately

▶ communicate appropriate reassuring information at the right time and the right level of sophistication

▶ assess the extent her reassurance has allayed anxieties and whether she must seek further means of promoting psychologic comfort for the patient

BIBLIOGRAPHY

1. Aiken, L., and Aiken, J. L.: A systematic approach to evaluation of interpersonal relationships. *American Journal of Nursing*, 73:863–867, May 1973.
2. Amacher, N. J.: Touch is a way of caring. *American Journal of Nursing*, 73:852–854, May 1973.
3. Avila, D. L., Combes, A. W., and Purkey, W. W.: *The Helping Relationship Source Book*. Boston, Allyn and Bacon, 1971.
4. Backscheider, J.: The use of self as the essence of clinical supervision in ambulatory patient care. *Nursing Clinics of North America*, 6:785–794, Dec. 1971.
5. Barnhart, C. L. (ed.): *The American College Dictionary*. New York, Random House, 1967.
6. Benjamin, A.: *The Helping Interview*, 2nd ed. Boston, Houghton Mifflin Co., 1969.
7. Bernstein, L., Bernstein, R., and Dana, R.: *Interviewing: A Guide for Health Professionals*. New York, Appleton-Century-Crofts, 1974.
8. Brammer, L. M.: *The Helping Relationship—Process and Skills*. Englewood Cliffs, NJ, Prentice-Hall, 1973.
9. Burnside, I. M.: Touching is talking. *American Journal of Nursing*, 73:2060–2063, Dec. 1973.
10. Carkhuff, R. R.: *Helping and Human Relations*, Vol. I. New York, Holt, Rinehart and Winston, 1969.
11. Carkhuff, R. R.: *Helping and Human Relations*, Vol. II. New York, Holt, Rinehart and Winston, 1969.

12. Combs, A. W., Avila, D. L., and Purkey, W. W.: *Helping Relationships: Basic Concepts for the Helping Professions.* Boston, Allyn & Bacon, 1971.

13. Costley, D. L.: Basis for effective communication. *Supervisor Nurse, 4*:16–22, Jan. 1972.

14. De Jean, S.: Empathy: A necessary ingredient of care. *American Journal of Nursing, 68*:559–560, March 1968.

15. Giammatteo, M. C.: Patient management and interpersonal relationships. *AORN Journal, 16*:71–73, July 1972.

16. Goldsborough, J.: Involvement. *American Journal of Nursing, 69*:66–68, Jan. 1969.

17. Goldsborough, J.: On becoming nonjudgmental. *American Journal of Nursing, 70*:2340–2344, Nov. 1970.

18. Haggerty, V. C.: Listening: an experiment in nursing. *Nursing Forum, 10*(4):382–391, 1971.

19. Hart, J. T., and Tomlinson, T. M.: *New Directions in Client Centered Therapy.* Boston, Houghton Mifflin Co., 1970.

20. Hein, E. C.: *Communication in Nursing Practice.* Boston, Little, Brown and Co., 1973.

21. Hein, E. C.: Listening. *Nursing 75,* pp. 93–102, March 1975.

22. Henderson, V.: Excellence in nursing. *American Journal of Nursing, 69*:2133–2137, Oct. 1969.

23. Henderson, V.: *The Nature of Nursing.* New York, The Macmillan Co., 1966.

24. Henderson, V.: The nature of nursing. *American Journal of Nursing, 64*:62–68, Aug. 1964.

25. Hewitt, H. E., and Pesznecker, B. L.: Blocks to communicating with patients. *American Journal of Nursing, 64*:101–103, July 1964.

26. Hornby, C.: The patient who needed a friend. *Canadian Nurse, 67*:37–39, Nov. 1971.

27. Ivey, A., et al.: Micro-counselling and attending behavior. *Journal of Counseling Psychology,* Vol. 15; monogr. suppl. 1–12.

28. Johnson, B.: The meaning of touch in nursing. *Nursing Outlook, 13*:59–60, Feb. 1965.

29. Johnson, D. W.: *Reaching Out.* Englewood Cliffs, NJ, Prentice-Hall, 1972.

30. Johnson, M., and Martin, H. W.: A sociological analysis of the nurse's role. *American Journal of Nursing, 58*:373–377, March 1958.

31. Jourard, S.: *Disclosing Man to Himself.* Princeton, D. Van Nostrand Co., 1968.

32. Jourard, S.: *The Transparent Self,* 2nd ed. New York, D. Van Nostrand Co., 1971.

33. Kalisch, B. J.: Strategies for developing nurse empathy. *Nursing Outlook, 19*:714–718, Nov. 1971.

34. Kalisch, B. J.: What is empathy? *American Journal of Nursing, 73*:1548–1552, Sept. 1973.

35. Kelly, D. N.: Do you mean what you think you mean?" *Supervisor Nurse, 1*:44–47, Oct. 1970.

36. King, I. M.: *Toward a Theory for Nursing.* New York, John Wiley and Sons, 1971.

37. Kron, T.: *Communication in Nursing,* 2nd ed. Philadelphia, W. B. Saunders Co., 1972.

38. Kron, T.: How we communicate nonverbally with patients. *The Canadian Nurse, 68*:21–23, Nov. 1972.

39. Lewis, Garland: *Nurse-Patient Communication.* Dubuque, Iowa, W. C. Brown Co., 1973.

40. Loesch, L. C., and Loesch, N. A.: What do you say after you say mm-hmm? *American Journal of Nursing, 75*:807–809, May 1975.

41. Luft, J.: *On Human Interaction.* Palo Alto, National Press Books, 1969.

42. Lundberg, G. A., Schrag, C. C., and Larsen, O. N.: Elements of communication. *In* Folta, J., and Deck, E. (eds.): *A Sociological Framework for Patient Care.* New York, John Wiley and Sons, 1966.

43. Mahoney, S. C.: *The Art of Helping People Effectively.* New York, Association Press, 1967.

44. Mansfield, E.: Empathy: concept and identified psychiatric nursing behavior. *Nursing Research, 22*:525–530, Nov.–Dec. 1973.

45. Mayeroff, Merton: *On Caring.* New York, Harper & Row, 1971.

46. Muecke, M. A.: Overcoming the language barrier. *Nursing Outlook, 18*:53–54, April 1970.

47. Naar, R.: Client-centered therapy: a theory of interpersonal relationships. *Mental Hygiene, 50*:146–149, 1966.

48. Naugle, E. H.: The difference caring makes. *American Journal of Nursing, 73*:1890–1891, Nov. 1973.

49. Parkhurst, R.: A bedside manner: do we have it? *Nursing Care, 6*:16–20, March 1973.

50. Peplau, H. E.: *Basic Principles of Patient Counselling,* 2nd ed. Philadelphia, Smith, Kline & French Laboratories, 1964.

51. Peplau, H. E.: Nurse-doctor relationships. *Nursing Forum, 5*(1):60–75, 1966.

52. Peters, N. J.: The X factor in nursing. *RN, 34*:39–43, July 1971.

53. Powell, J.: *Why Am I Afraid to Tell You Who I Am?* Chicago, Peacock Books, Argus Communication, 1969.

54. Rogers, C.: *Client Centered Therapy.* Boston, Houghton Mifflin Co., 1965.

55. Rogers, C.: The characteristics of a helping relationship. *Personnel and Guidance Journal, 37*:6–16, 1958.

56. Rogers, C.: The necessary and sufficient conditions of therapeutic personality change. *In* Ard, B. (ed.): *Counselling and Psychotherapy.* Palo Alto, Science and Behavior Books, 1966, pp. 126–141.

57. Rogers, C.: *On Becoming a Person.* Boston, Houghton Mifflin Co., 1961.

58. Ross, R. S.: *Speech Communication: Fundamentals and Practice,* 3rd ed. Englewood Cliffs, NJ, Prentice-Hall, 1974.

59. Ruesch, J.: *Therapeutic Communication.* New York, W. W. Norton and Co., 1961.

60. Saunders, L.: Permanence and change. *American Journal of Nursing, 58*:969–971, July 1958.

61. Saupe, R.: How do you feel, nurse? *American Journal of Nursing, 74*:1105, June 1974.

62. Schwartz, L. H., and Schwartz, J. L.: Transference: the hidden element in your relations with patients. *Nursing 73, 3*(10):37–41, 1973.

63. Skipper, J. K., Tagliasozzo, D. L., and Mauksch, H. O.: What communication means to patients. *American Journal of Nursing, 64*:101–103, April 1964.

64. Smiley, O. R., and Smiley, C. W.: Interviewing techniques for nurses. *Canadian Journal of Public Health, 65*:281–283, July–Aug. 1974.

65. Smith, J., Bealer, R., and Sim, F.: Communication and the consequences of communication. *Sociological Inquiry,* Winter 1962.

66. Stewart, J.: *Bridges Not Walls.* Reading, MA, Addison-Wesley Publishing Co., 1973.

67. Triplett, J. L.: Empathy is. . . . *Nursing Clinics of North America, 4*:673–681, Dec. 1969.

68. Truax, C. B.: Toward the effective use of interpersonal skills in psychiatric nursing. *Canadian Journal of Psychiatric Nursing, 13*:12–14, July–Aug. 1972.

69. Uraang, L., and Flexner, S. B. (eds.): *The Random House Dictionary of the English Language.* New York, Random House, 1969.

70. Van Dersal, W. R.: How to be a good communicator—and a better nurse. *Nursing 74, 4*:57–64, Dec. 1974.

71. Zderad, L. T.: Empathetic nursing. *Nursing Clinics of North America, 4*:655–662, Dec. 1969.

CHAPTER 4

TRADITIONAL AND EXPANDING ROLES OF NURSES

By Margaret Helen Parkinson, R.N., R.M.N., Dip.N., B.Soc.Sc., M.N.

INTRODUCTION AND STUDY GUIDE

What do nurses do? What should nurses be doing? Are there some things nurses should not be doing? What do nurses believe about themselves? What does the public expect of nurses? These are the kinds of questions concerning role and function that nurses are expected to consider throughout their professional lives. Self-examination is the responsibility of a profession that intends to remain relevant to the time and people it intends to serve.

It is unlikely (and inappropriate) that permanent answers will be found to such questions. If the nursing profession is to remain useful, it will modify its role and function in response to changes in the health needs of society. The profession that defines itself in unchanging terms is a dead (or, at best, dying) profession. A viable profession makes concrete plans for the present and creates the machinery for future adaptation and change. It does this not only within its own professional boundaries but also in cooperation with associated professions. It is important that professional reassessment keep pace with societal changes so that its service remains relevant.

This chapter is prepared to help you understand issues concerning present and future roles of the nursing profession. It presents material that enables you to enter constructively into ongoing debates about the roles and functions of nurses. The material includes consideration of (a) past, present and possible future nursing roles; (b) educational requirements and opportunities for nurses; (c) settings in which nurses work and the people they work with; (d) characteristics of a professional person and the setting of standards for nursing practice; (e) expectations the public has of nurses; (f) legal implications concerning nurses' roles; and (g) issues around sexism in nursing practice.

To more fully understand the content of this chapter, you may find it useful to follow the suggestions outlined in the following *study guide:*

1. Write out, in your own words, meanings of the following terms:

role
status
philosophy
interdisciplinary conflict
intradisciplinary conflict
intentional learning
incidental learning
basic nursing education
graduate nursing education
continuing education
inservice education
expanded nursing roles
nurse practitioner
nurse clinician
clinical nurse specialist
physician's assistant
patient advocate
professionalism
accountability

2. Read as many nursing philosophies as you can and identify the similarities and differences among them.

3. Write down ideas that form your own philosophy of nursing. Include your preconceptions of nursing before you entered nursing school. You may find it useful to repeatedly complete the sentence: I believe that nursing is . . . . Write your own definition of the unique function of the nurse.

4. Find out the structural arrangement of nursing services in each of the clinical areas you go to for clinical experience. Also find out methods of communication, delegation of authority and evaluation of nursing care that are used in each area.

5. Obtain a copy of the Nursing Practice Act appropriate to you. Then summarize legal requirements the act places on nurses.

Our *objectives* for this chapter are to enable you, by studying this material, to do the following:

1. Appreciate the ways historical and societal influences affect the practice of nursing today.

2. Understand the importance of philosophies of nursing and begin to develop your own.

3. Know the structural and functional machinery that operates within nursing.

4. Know the range of educational opportunities available to nurses at basic and higher levels.

5. Become aware of ways the nursing role is currently expanding.

6. Appreciate the need to identify community needs in the planning of nursing services.

7. Perceive yourself as a beginning professional person.

THE MEANING OF ROLE

The word *role* is a term borrowed by social scientists from drama. In the theatrical context role refers to a person pretending to be someone else for the purposes of entertainment. It implies a certain deception. This is not the way the word "role" is used in the phrase "the nurse's role."

"Role" is the term applied to human behavior, based on the fact that human beings behave in certain relatively predictable patterns. *Role is a descriptive word for relatively predictable behavorial patterns.* The nursing role, then, refers to all behaviors that are considered appropriate for a nurse.

HISTORICAL INFLUENCES ON THE NURSE'S ROLE

A knowledge and appreciation of history are important for an understanding of the present. The way in which nursing roles are enacted today is a consequence of how these roles were enacted in the past. Similarly, the way present-day nurses enact their roles will influence the development of future nursing roles. We are connected with the past and the future by invisible yet strong bonds.

Some major trends that have influenced nursing roles are identified in this section.

Historical Images of the Nurse

Traditionally, the nurse has been seen as an uneducated woman taking care of the sick, disabled, young, elderly and dying. She was the sickroom attendant. While parts of this traditional view are still true, it does not adequately describe the current role of the professional nurse.

Since Florence Nightingale established the first nursing school in the mid-19th century, nursing has developed in both depth and breadth. This has not been an easy development, however, and some historical images continue to inhibit progress. Uprichard[109] identifies three historically traditional images that still influence the nursing profession:

The Folk Image. The folk image of the nurse as "mother" arises from the original use of the word "nurse" to mean to suckle the young. This

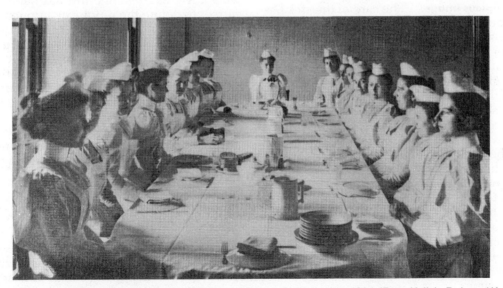

Figure 4–1. Nurses at dinner, Jefferson Medical College Hospital, Philadelphia, 1894. (From Kalish, B. J., and Kalish, P. A.: Slaves, servants, or saints? *Nursing Forum, 14*(3):222, 1975.)

The Role of a Nurse in 1887*

The following directives were given to floor nurses by a hospital in 1887.

In addition to caring for your 50 patients, each nurse will follow these regulations:

1. Daily sweep and mop the floors of your ward, dust the patient's furniture and window sills.

2. Maintain an even temperature in your ward by bringing in a scuttle of coal for the day's business.

3. Light is important to observe the patient's condition. Therefore, each day fill kerosene lamps, clean chimneys, and trim wicks. Wash the windows once a week.

4. The nurse's notes are important in aiding the physician's work. Make your pens carefully; you may whittle nibs to your individual taste.

5. Each nurse on day duty will report every day at 7 a.m. and leave at 8 p.m., except on the Sabbath on which day you will be off from 12 to 2 p.m.

6. Graduate nurses in good standing with the director of nurses will be given an evening off each week for courting purposes or two evenings a week if you go regularly to church.

7. Any nurse who smokes, uses liquor in any form, gets her hair done at a beauty shop, or frequents dance halls will give the director of nurses good reason to suspect her worth, intentions and integrity.

---

meaning quickly broadened to that of caring for the sick and the aged. Such care was provided by simple methods passed on from one person to another. The folk image, which is still held today, is an emotional view of the nurse as "mother: gentle, kind, always available, nurturing life by natural means, wise but not learned."[109]

The Religious Image.   The care of the sick has always been seen as a Christian duty in Western civilization. In the past the church viewed caring for the sick as important for the salvation of the soul of the care giver. Over the centuries, this religious image reinforced the characteristics of the folk image, since it suggested that nursing should be done for love and required no formal learning. It added other notions, among which were the beliefs that a nurse should be "celibate, cloistered, unworldly and strictly disciplined."[109]

The Servant Image.   This image arose during the 16th to the 19th centuries—the dark ages in nursing history. During this time illness was seen as a punishment for sin, and the care, if any, given to the sick was far from charitable. Any nursing that was available generally was given by ill-paid, ignorant and sometimes immoral women.

---

*Reprinted from *Nursing Forum,* 10(1):31, 1971.

Traces of the three traditional images are still seen. Views of nurses as mothers, saints, or sometimes lower socioeconomic class servants remain in the minds of the public and sometimes even in the minds of nurses themselves. Such images present obstacles to the development of professional nurses as educated, well-paid, respected and independent practitioners.

THE PRESENT—A TIME OF CLARIFICATION

Significant progress in the last hundred years has taken nurses from a position of unskilled laborers to that of well-educated members of the professional health team. Along with these changes has been the tremendous development in medical and scientific knowledge. Changing societal values have also had an influence, e.g., the development of humanitarian principles stating that every human being has a right to the best available health care. Nursing has established its place in professional health teams offering such care. An important question is not whether nursing has a function in the health care team but rather exactly what that function should be.

The major influence upon nursing's development over the last century has been advancement in medical knowledge. Until quite recently nurses have been taught by doctors instead of nurses, and their actions essentially were directed by doctors according to the medical regimen planned for the patient. However, over the last few decades nurses have been considering whether the role of a "doctor's assistant" is the appropriate primary role for the nurse. A great deal of effort has been made by nurses to define the unique or autonomous role of the nurse. *The role that is the center of the nursing profession is called the unique or primary role of the nurse.* Nursing literature is teeming with material concerning the independent, interdependent and dependent roles of nurses in light of societal needs and the roles of other health professionals. Various philosophies of nursing have been developed in an attempt to give clarification to this important issue. We will look briefly at a few of these philosophies.

PHILOSOPHIES OF NURSING

A philosophy may be defined as a set of beliefs and attitudes that direct the behavior of individuals in the achievement of goals. Every nurse has a philosophy or a set of beliefs upon which she bases her action. Such philosophies are not always consciously recognized, however. The following are brief descriptions of two nurses' attempts to make their philosophies of nursing explicit and able to be communicated to others.

The Philosophy of Nursing of Virginia Henderson

Henderson[46] sees nursing as being appropriately involved in three areas directed toward *assisting* the patient. These areas are

▶ Helping a patient carry out the therapeutic plan initiated by the doctor.

▶ Helping and receiving help from other members of the health team to plan and carry out a total program of care for a patient. This program may be directed toward improvement of health, recovery from illness or support in death

▶ Providing basic nursing care.

Henderson sees providing basic nursing care as the *unique function of the nurse*. This is the area over which the nurse has authority and the area in which the nurse should be legally responsible. Basic nursing care (the unique function of the nurse) is concerned with helping a patient meet his basic human needs until he can meet them for himself without assistance.

Definition of Nursing

The unique function of the nurse is to assist the individual sick or well, in the performance of those activities contributing to health or its recovery (or to a peaceful death) that he would perform unaided if he had the necessary strength, will or knowledge. And to do this in such a way as to help him gain independence as rapidly as possible. This aspect of her work, this part of her function, she initiates and controls; of this she is master.

—Virginia Henderson[46]

Henderson identifies 14 activities, or basic needs, that a nurse may help a patient perform. A patient may be unable to perform such activities for himself for a time because of his age, temperament, social or cultural status, physical or intellectual capacity or particular pathologic state. The nurse helps him with such activities until he is able to perform them for himself unaided.

Components of basic nursing consist of assisting the patient with these functions or providing conditions that will enable him to do the following:[46]

▶ Breathe normally

▶ Eat and drink adequately

▶ Eliminate by all avenues of elimination

▶ Move and maintain a desirable posture (walking, sitting, lying and changing from one position to another)

▶ Sleep and rest

▶ Select suitable clothing; dress and undress

▶ Maintain body temperature within normal range by adjusting clothing and modifying the environment

▶ Keep the body clean and well groomed and protect the integument

▶ Avoid dangers in the environment and avoid injuring others

▶ Communicate with others in expressing emotions, needs, fears, etc.

▶ Worship according to his faith

▶ Work at something that provides a sense of accomplishment

▶ Play or participate in various forms of recreation

▶ Learn, discover, or satisfy the curiosity that leads to "normal" development and health

The Philosophy of Nursing of Frances Reiter Kreuter

Reiter Kreuter sees nursing as a service for the care of the sick, the prevention of illness and the promotion of health, "a portion of which is carried out under medical authority."[55] Nursing practice comprises the following components:[55]

▶ *Providing nursing care.*

▶ *Coordinating* nursing care with the care provided by medical and allied professionals.

▶ *Planning for continuity* of patient care in home, school, industry, clinic or hospital with other nurses.

▶ *Evaluating* total patient care with members of allied health professions.

▶ *Directing* the family and the nursing auxiliary as they give nursing care.

Reiter Kreuter considers nursing care to be the component of nursing practice that is the primary function of the nurse and the area over which the nurse should have complete control.[88]

Definition of Nursing Care

. . . acting and interacting with the patient through physical and personal contact for his welfare, and intervening in his behalf between him and those stresses in the physical environment and in the social climate that impinge upon him.

—Frances Reiter Kreuter[55]

Reiter Kreuter clarifies her definition of nursing care by differentiating it from the care offered by other helping professions in terms of nursing ministrations. The purpose of nursing care is to minister to the basic human needs of the patient.

The Ministrations of Nursing Care

. . . doing for a person that which he would do for himself but is unable to do for a time or for all times; performing these nursing measures for personal and mental hygiene as he would if he were able. The basic ministrations in nursing care are comforting measures that contribute to the sense of well-being—being there and seeing him, bathing, feeding, toileting, dressing, listening to him, moving and sheltering him, and feeling his feelings. To comfort is an object of care.[55]

Philosophies of nursing help us clarify central purposes of the nursing role. The reader is encouraged to examine the wide range of philosophies available in nursing literature and the definitions of nursing they include. A range of definitions written by nurses is presented below. Read each carefully and try to rewrite each in your own words. Also, try to identify similarities and differences between the definitions.

Some Other Definitions of Nursing

Florence Nightingale. ". . . what nursing has to do . . . is to put the patient in the best condition for nature to act upon him."[77]

Imogene King. "Nursing is a process of ac-

tion, reaction, interaction, and transaction, whereby nurses assist individuals of any age and socioeconomic group to meet their basic needs in performing activities of daily living and to cope with health and illness at some particular point in the life cycle."[54]

Hildegard Peplau. "Nursing is a significant therapeutic, interpersonal process. . . . It functions cooperatively with other human processes that make health possible for individuals in communities. In specific situations in which a professional health team offers health services, nurses participate in the organization of conditions that facilitate natural ongoing tendencies in human organisms. Nursing is an educative instrument, a maturing force, that aims to promote forward movement of personality in the direction of creative, constructive, productive, personal, and community living."[83]

Martha Rogers. "Nursing aims to assist people in achieving their maximum health potential. Maintenance and promotion of health, prevention of disease, nursing diagnosis, intervention, and rehabilitation encompass the scope of nursing's goals. Nursing is concerned with people—all people—well and sick, rich and poor, young and old. The arenas of nursing's services extend into all areas where there are people: at home, at school, at work, at play; in hospital, nursing home, and clinic; on this planet and now moving into outer space."[91]

Sister Madeleine Clemence Vaillot. "Nursing does not aim at restoring the patient's biologic integrity but at helping the patient to live as fully as possible. This may mean that the nurses assist the patient to carry out the prescribed medical regimen. But, beyond this, it can also mean that the goal of nursing is to help the patient reach out for a plentitude of being that is always possible, in spite of biologic limitations against which medicine is helpless."[110]

Some Conclusions about Philosophies of Nursing

While each philosophy and definition is expressed in a different way, some common ideas emerge. Nurses carry out a wide variety of functions. Some of the functions can be seen as "primary" to the nurse's role and others are "secondary" to the nurse's role.

Primary Functions. Primary functions are those functions specific to nursing. They make up the human caring service for which nursing exists. They are "care" functions rather than "cure" functions.

Secondary Functions. Secondary functions are those things a nurse does while assisting other health professionals with their primary functions. Secondary nursing functions are often related to cure and have to do with the disease and its treatment. It is appropriate for nurses to carry out secondary functions insofar as they do not mitigate against or interfere with their primary function.

Care-Cure Concept. Most nurses practice in situations in which, if a cooperative relationship has been developed between the nurse and other health professionals (especially the physician), care and cure functions can be coordinated for the benefit of the patient. Figure 4–2 shows a model of the care-cure concept relating to the primary and the secondary functions of physicians and nurses.

The physician has a primary function to "cure" and a secondary function to "care," which is best carried out in cooperation with the nurse. The nurse has a primary function to care and a secondary function to cure, which is carried out in cooperation with the physician. Curing is most effectively done within an environment of caring. It is the creation of such an environment that is the challenge of creative nursing. The National Commission for the Study of Nursing and Nursing Education of 1970 stated, "It may be that nursing, in particular, holds the key to maintenance of humane, individualistic concern for people and their health problems. And this capacity must be zealously enlarged."[75]

The Fifth Report of the World Health Organization Expert Committee on Nursing[116] states that complete health care should offer service in five stages of health and illness.

▶ *Health maintenance stage:* To help the individual achieve and maintain the highest level of health possible.

▶ *Increased risk stage:* To help the individual in a "pre-disease" stage to avoid the development of a health problem.

▶ *Early detection stage:* To identify the individual in the early stages of disease and prevent unnecessary suffering or death by early diagnosis and treatment.

▶ *Clinical stage:* To help the individual who is experiencing acute illness.

▶ *Rehabilitation stage:* To help the individual avoid disability resulting from disease or to achieve maximum potential within his disability or to support him as he faces death.

SETTINGS IN WHICH NURSES WORK

Hospitals

Nursing Structure. The largest concentration of health services is in the clinical stage. This concerns the treatment of people suffering from acute illness in a hospital setting. The majority of nurses work in this area.

Nursing services within hospitals have traditionally been arranged in a hierarchical system with authority coming from the Director of Nursing through nursing supervisors to the charge nurses or head nurses of hospital floors who direct nurse team leaders and staff nurses. Countries of British influence have a hierarchical structure similar to that of American hospitals, although different titles may be used.

Lower still on the hierarchy may be licensed practical nurses (State Enrolled Nurses in Britain), licensed vocational nurses and other nursing assistants. Nursing students may appear in the lower echelons of the hierarchy in hospitals that operate schools of nursing and therefore employ students to give some of the nursing care.

Twenty-four Hour Service. Nursing service operates on a 24-hour basis within a hospital. Nurses are often scheduled in shifts to cover three 8-hour periods. *Full-time* nurses are employed by hospitals for 40 hours a week. The work week usually consists of five 8-hour days,

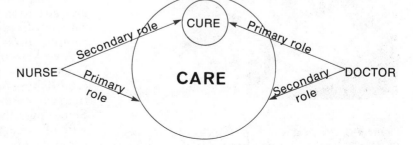

Figure 4–2. Showing the coordination of care and cure functions and the associated responsibilities of the nurse and the doctor.

but different combinations of hours may occur, e.g., four 10-hour days. *Part-time* nurses are sometimes employed by hospitals to routinely work less than 40 hours per week. *Temporary* nurses are employed by a nursing contracting service on a full-time or part-time basis. The contracting service makes nurses available to health services as they are required. Hospitals sometimes use a temporary nurse to cover gaps or emergencies in their routine staffing structure.

The 24-hour nature of hospital nursing has important consequences. As the only part of the health team that offers service on a continuous basis, nursing has the opportunity to be the coordinator of all patient services. This is a task entirely consistent with the nursing role as described earlier in this chapter. The entire 24 hours can never be covered by the same personnel, however, so careful and efficient systems of communication are established to ensure continuity of care.

Specialized Areas of Practice. Hospitals are usually divided into areas of specialized practice according to the variety of medical services offered. For example, such divisions may be made according to

▶ The patient's age—e.g., neonatal units, pediatric units, geriatric units

▶ The systems of the body—e.g., orthopedic units, cardiovascular units, neurologic units, urologic units, eye-ear-nose-throat (EENT) units

▶ Disease entities—e.g., alcoholism units, oncology (cancer) units, mental retardation units, psychiatric units

▶ Severity of the illness—e.g., intensive care units (ICU), progressive care units, self-care units

Nurses may develop an interest in particular areas of hospital care and through experience and education may become specialists in that area of nursing.

Community

Over recent decades emphasis has been given to the provision of health services outside the hospital setting. This has come partially from an increased awareness of the importance of health maintenance and illness prevention.

Public Health. Nurses work along with other health professionals within government departments of health. These nurses are called *public health nurses* or *community health nurses*. The primary emphasis of such work is on the promotion and maintenance of health within families. They work both in the family home and in community clinics.

Community Centers. The development of community health centers is of relatively recent origin. Examples of such centers are community mental health centers and planned parenthood clinics. Nurses, along with other health workers, function within such clinics to provide specialized services to individuals and families.

Occupational Health. Since a major part of adult life is spent within the work force, greater attention is being given to the health of workers. Nursing care is offered in this area by *industrial nurses* and *office nurses*.

School Health. Health centers are frequently established within educational institutions to give attention to the health of students. Nursing care is offered in such centers by *school or campus nurses*.

Private Practice. With the adoption of Private Practice Acts in some states, a few nurses are establishing private practices. This trend is particularly evident in the area of mental health. Sometimes these practices are in cooperation with physicians in medical practice. This is one example of an expanded nursing role and is discussed later in this chapter.

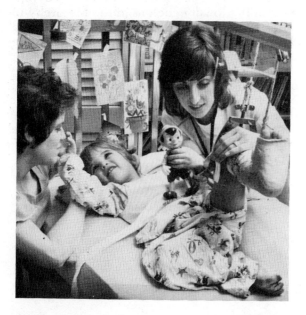

Figure 4–3. Nurse at work in pediatric setting. (Courtesy of Massachusetts General Hospital, Boston, Massachusetts.)

While there is an awareness of the need to create a health service for all stages on the health-illness continuum, it is still easy to place emphasis on the clinical stage. This is so even within the community services. (Careful observation may show that a "health center" may really be a "sickness center" in its function.) One of the reasons for this may be that the clinical stage is more identifiable and immediate than the other stages and that medical knowledge is greatest in the clinical area.

Since health services are frequently established from a therapeutic or medical model, it is possible for nurses functioning within them to lose sight of their primary nursing role. It is easy for them to become absorbed in the instrumental, delegated, medical care aspects of their responsibilities and neglect the more expressive nursing aspects.

The problem could be avoided in part by clear job descriptions. Every nurse should seek a job description from a prospective employer before taking a position. The nurse should be satisfied that the job description reflects the purpose of the service and that it gives scope for the practice of the primary nursing role.

PEOPLE WITH WHOM NURSES WORK

There is more to health care than one discipline can provide. The most effective health service thus comes from a team of health professionals, each bringing their individual expertise to the needs of the patient and his significant others in a cooperative way.

Ideally, each team member (a) communicates directly with the patient in formulating plans and (b) coordinates with other members of the team to ensure a cooperative approach consistent with the patient's needs.

In practice the team approach does not always work as it should. Interdisciplinary conflict (i.e., conflict between members of the total health team) can occur. Members may be distrustful of each other and may resent actions that appear to be an intrusion into the functions or territory once held by one profession alone. In the past the health team consisted simply of the doctor and his "nurse helper." The demands of the modern health service are greater than can be handled by this simple "partnership." Defensive behaviors of health team members impede patient care.

The efficiency of the health team depends upon the ability of team members to work together. This ability of team members to work together depends, in part, on the quality of the interpersonal relationships achieved in daily practice.

An understanding and appreciation of each other's primary role, a commitment to patient-centered care and an ability to communicate clearly with each other are important factors to the success of the health team.

Failure in any one factor will bring disorganization to patient care. Let us examine briefly the relationships between doctors and nurses as an example of the relationships within the health team and the origins of some potential interaction problems.

Nurse-Doctor Relationships

The doctor has traditionally been the head of the health team. This is still true in many areas of practice. Typically, some aspects of medical practice can legally be performed only by a doctor, e.g., prescribing drugs. Team work does not depend upon doing each other's jobs but rather on valuing the particular skills and functions of each.

There are several factors, however, that have tended to place doctors and nurses in different status positions, making communication and cooperation between them difficult. Hoekelman[47] identifies some of these factors:

▶ *Traditional sex roles.* Doctors are most often men, and nurses are most often women. The traditional male dominance can occur within the health team as much as anywhere else. As sexist attitudes toward women gradually become less prevalent, discrimination within the health team should diminish.

▶ *Differing educational preparation.* Doctors have tended to spend more time in educational preparation than nurses. This is becoming less true as the extent of nursing education increases. The effects of educational differences should diminish as both nurses and doctors come to appreciate the unique contribution each can make to patient care.

► *Economic differential.* On the whole, doctors have a greater earning power than nurses. Doctors earn more because men tend to earn more than women and because they often provide more vital specialized services. They are often the employers of nurses, and they hold a higher hierarchical position than nurses within the health system. Present trends indicate the beginnings of change in these areas.

► *Lack of understanding about roles.* Nurses often complain that doctors do not understand what nursing has to offer. This may not always be the fault of the doctor. Nurses sometimes behave from an internalized subordinate position. Nurses need to communicate their worth and abilities to others more clearly and confidently.

The Nursing Team

Rather than a group of identical people, a nursing team consists of persons with different personalities, educational preparation, interests, specialties and experiences. Although all team members are nurses, they have differences that can lead to intradisciplinary conflict (conflict between members of the same discipline).

The same factors that facilitate successful functioning within the health team facilitate successful functioning within the nursing team, i.e., an understanding and appreciation of each other's abilities and functions, a commitment to patient-centered care and an ability to communicate clearly with each other. Interpersonal relationships are very powerful. Nurses in positions of leadership would do well to remember that other members of the nursing team are people too!

THE PREPARATION OF NURSES FOR THEIR ROLE

Roles have to be learned. The learning of roles is called *socialization.* Socialization occurs in two ways: through *intentional learning* and through *incidental learning.*[94] A nurse is socialized intentionally through the formalized education experiences received in nursing schools and through continuing education. Incidental socialization occurs in more subtle ways. It involves the attitudes and beliefs a person develops about the nurse's role from personal contacts with the nursing profession both as a recipient and a deliverer of nursing care. The role modeling of professional nurses is a very powerful instrument in the process of socialization into the nursing role.

Intentional Learning

Basic Nursing Education. In the United States nursing students may study toward registered nurse (RN) qualification in one of three ways:

► Hospital-based school of nursing program

► Community college, Associate Degree (AD) program

► University baccalaureate degree program

Each of these programs offers educational preparation based on the physical and social sciences as well as clinical nursing instruction and experience in health facilities covering all stages of the health-illness continuum.

Persons who desire to be involved in nursing activities but who do not wish to become registered nurses may train as licensed practical nurses (LPN) or licensed vocational nurses (LVN) in various types of settings.

Higher Nursing Education. 1. GRADUATE EDUCATION. Registered nurses holding a baccalaureate degree in nursing may undertake graduate education at a master's and then a doctoral level. Master's programs in nursing involve a specialized nursing area such as psychosocial nursing, community health nursing, medical-surgical nursing, or administration. Doctoral degrees may be obtained in nursing or in other related fields, e.g., sociology, anthropology, or educational psychology.

2. CONTINUING EDUCATION. Every registered nurse has a responsibility to continue learning after graduating. Any educational opportunity available to a nurse beyond a basic program is part of continuing education.

3. INSERVICE EDUCATION. Inservice education refers to programs developed and offered by health service institutions for employees. They usually provide instruction around issues central to the nurse's function within her employment. Many hospitals and other health facilities employ inservice educators who are responsible for planning and implementing inservice education programs.

4. SPECIAL PROGRAMS. As the role of the nurse changes and expands, new and special educational programs are developed to prepare nurses to function in special ways. Examples of such programs are nurse practitioner programs

and clinical specialist programs. The role and preparation of nurses in these special programs is discussed later in this chapter.

Incidental Learning

The process of socialization into the nursing role is not confined to formal educational programs. It also occurs through the more casual interactions a person has within the health care system.

Nursing students develop some attitudes and beliefs about what nurses do and how they behave long before entry into a nursing school. Beliefs and attitudes may be developed through the presentation of nurses' roles in the mass media, e.g., books, newspapers, television and films. Contacts with nurses through childhood and family experiences also influence an individual's expectations of a nurse.

After entry into a nursing program a nursing student becomes socialized into a role through the incidental interactions she has with professional nurses and other nursing students both in the nursing school and in clinical settings. This kind of learning is often unconscious and unplanned. We can never be quite sure of the influences we are having on other people or of their influences upon us.

THE CHANGING ROLES OF THE NURSE

As far back as 1948 a nursing leader, Esther Lucille Brown,[14] advised nurses to view their functions as evolutionary and dynamic rather than static. Present-day nursing is in a period of change and adaptation. Terms such as the *expanded* or the *extended* role of the nurse are under much discussion. (We use the phrase "expanded role" to refer to any area in which the traditional role of the nurse is broadening.)

The Direction of Expanding Roles

In 1971 a report was published by the U.S. Department of Health, Education and Welfare committee that studied the extended (expanded) roles for nurses.[98] The committee saw the expanding roles of the nurse as being an important physician-nurse collaboration to meet the increasing health care needs of the public. The committee set up by the Secretary of Health, Education and Welfare identified areas of the expansion of a nurse's role in spheres of primary care, acute care and long-term care. Areas of expanded function included the following:

▶ Increased skills in assessment leading to medical and nursing diagnosis

▶ More formalized methods of history taking for both medical and nursing purposes

▶ Increased peer collaboration with physicians in the planning and implementation of medical intervention

▶ Increased responsibility for nurses in areas of health surveillance and health maintenance for individuals and families not classified as acutely ill.

Further education is required if nurses are to undertake functions not previously included within their role. Numerous educational opportunities are developing for this purpose both within university graduate degree programs and in other continuing education facilities. (Further information regarding these programs can be obtained through the American Nurses' Association, Inc., 2420 Pershing Road, Kansas City, Missouri 64108.)

Emerging Expanded Roles

At the present time many titles are being used to describe the areas of expansion in the nurse's role. We will discuss the three roles defined by the American Nurses' Association Congress for Nursing Practice in 1974.[2] The terms used by the American Nurses' Association broadly cover all the expanded roles presently evolving.

Nurse Practitioner. A nurse practitioner has "advanced skills in the assessment of the physical and psychosocial health-illness status of individuals, families or groups in a variety of settings through health and development history taking and physical examination."[2] A nurse practitioner is a registered nurse who develops further skills in assessment through formal programs of continuing education. Skills are developed in specialty areas such as family health and pediatric care. Other titles sometimes used for the nurse practitioner are *nurse associate, family nurse practitioner* (FNP) and *PRIMEX*.

Nurse Clinician. A nurse clinician has "well-developed competencies in utilizing a broad range of cues. These cues are used for prescribing and implementing both direct and indirect care and for articulating nursing therapies with other planned therapies. Nurse clinicians demonstrate expertise in nursing practice and insure ongoing development of expertise through clinical experience and continuing education."[2] A nurse clinician offers comprehensive nursing care in a specific specialty area. The minimal qualification for a nurse clinician is a baccalaureate degree in nursing.

Clinical Nurse Specialist.   The clinical nurse specialist usually holds a master's degree in a specific clinical area of nursing. Such clinical specialties include psychosocial nursing, psychiatric nursing, oncologic nursing, midwifery, emergency nursing, and geriatric nursing. Clinical nurse specialists are "primarily clinicians with a high degree of knowledge, skill and competence in a specialized area of nursing. These are made directly available to the public through the provision of nursing care to clients and indirectly available through guidance and planning of care with other nursing personnel."[2]

In Great Britain the term *clinical nurse consultant* is sometimes used instead of clinical nurse specialist. It should be noted that although the American Nurses' Association differentiates between the nurse clinician and the clinical nurse specialist, the terms are often used synonymously in practice.

The Physician's Assistant

The physician's assistant (PA) is a new member of the health team emerging in the United States. Such a person is often not a nurse. The physician's assistant is trained by doctors to help doctors with their work. Physician's assistants may function within a hospital or within the community and are associated with and work for the medical team.

Nurses As Managers

Management in nursing implies the "coordination and facilitation of the process of patient care."[80] Nurses have assumed management functions since Florence Nightingale systematized nursing services in the late 19th century. Nurses are involved in the management of nursing care by communication (a) with patients themselves, (b) within the nursing team and (c) within the wider health team. The higher the position of a nurse in the nursing hierarchy, the broader are the accompanying management responsibilities. The broader the management responsibilities become, the more the nurse is concerned with long-term goals.

Successful management requires successful *leadership,* as every manager depends upon the cooperation of a number of other people. One of the most important aspects of leadership is the facilitation of clear two-way communication. Nurses would do well to include the development of management and leadership skills in their continuing education activities.

Nurses As Researchers

The nursing process itself is based on the application of research principles. (Nursing process is discussed in Chap. 17.) To this extent, every nurse is a researcher. Some nurses, however, have undertaken more deliberate research roles in attempts to expand the body of nursing knowledge available for nursing practice.

Research is an essential component of graduate nursing degree programs. Some nurses with master's and doctoral degrees undertake nursing research as a full-time occupation. They most often work in university settings but also in institutions offering health services. The results of significant nursing research are published in professional journals and are eventually included in nursing textbooks. Nursing can advance in usefulness only if careful research is done and the information discovered is communicated to those actively involved in nursing practice.

Nurses As Teachers

Insofar as nurses are involved in helping people develop successful health practices and insofar as every nurse is involved in the incidental learning of colleagues, every nurse is a teacher. Some nurses choose to be involved in formal nursing education and hold positions as faculty members in schools of nursing or as inservice educators in health service institutions.

Teachers of nursing usually possess expertise in both nursing and teaching, and they combine both roles. They attempt to maintain their clinical skills and to facilitate the development of nursing skills in students.

Nurses As Authors

Nursing knowledge must be disseminated as widely as possible if nursing practice is to keep pace with the health needs of the community. Numerous professional journals selectively publish material concerning nursing issues. The quality of the journals depends upon the quality of the material submitted. Many institutions (particularly universities) encourage nurse faculty members to publish. It is a responsibility of nurses to attempt to publish any new knowledge they gain.

Nurses As Patient Advocates

An advocate is a person who speaks or acts for another person. As the resources and personnel involved in health service increase, there is an increasing need for someone who will take responsibility for explaining, interpreting, defending and protecting patients' rights. The primary orientation of nursing is toward human well-being. The nurse is most concerned with the ways a patient is experiencing what is happening to him. This may not always be the primary concern of other health workers. A nurse may need to speak for a patient at times when he cannot speak for himself. (Patient rights are discussed in Chap. 20.)

Patient advocacy goes beyond direct patient care. It includes involvement in decision-making procedures concerning health services at local, state and national levels. Whenever health-related issues are being debated, nurses should be represented to ensure that a humanitarian approach to total patient care is maintained.

THE NURSE AS A PROFESSIONAL

Is nursing a profession or not? Nursing literature contains argument around this question. On the whole, however, nurses see themselves as professional people who strive individually and collectively to fulfill the requirements of professionalism.

The Characteristics of Professions

Sociologists have identified a number of attributes that characterize professions. They include the following:

▶ Altruistic or service-based purposes

▶ Intellectual and educative basis for action

▶ Autonomy or self-regulation

A profession is an occupation primarily motivated toward service for others. It is dedicated to improvement in the quality of life. While a professional person does not expect to work without monetary remuneration, the availability of service comes before economic gain.

A profession is an occupation in which performance is based on scientific principles. It requires extensive educative preparation, and sets standards of minimal attainment before allowing individuals to practice. Such education takes place within a recognized and approved educational institution, e.g., a university or community college. Its members are expected to continue learning throughout their professional lives.

A profession claims an autonomy or independence in its functioning. It regulates and controls itself. A profession does this through an organization made up of its own members.

In many countries, including the United States, nursing has developed the characteristics of a profession to a high degree. Nursing exists for the service of others; rigorous educational commitment is required for the commencement and maintenance of practice; and self-regulation is seen as an ideal. Despite a traditional subservient status in the field of medicine, nursing has achieved considerable autonomy in administrative and managerial functions and is developing more autonomy in practice as the specific nursing role is more clearly defined.

Professional Organizations

All professions have developed professional organizations. The professional organization for nurses in the United States is the American Nurses' Association, which has a membership of about 200,000. The American Nurses' Association is one of the members of the international organization for nurses—the International Council of Nurses. The other national organization for nurses is the National League for Nursing, to which lay persons also belong. The professional organization in Canada is the Canadian Nurses' Association.

Professional organizations have dual functions. They work to maintain a high standard of service to the community and they work for the welfare of members. The first function is sometimes termed a *professional function* and the second a *unionized function*. Sometimes these two functions are in conflict, but it is generally

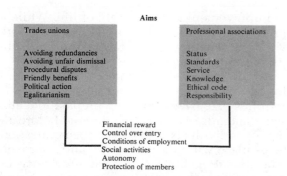

Figure 4–4. The usual aims of trade unions and professional associations and those aims common to both. (From McEvoy, P.: Unionisation or professionalisation. Which way for nurses? *Nursing Mirror, 141*:70–72, Nov. 20, 1975.)

seen as appropriate for both to be attempted by one organization in order to balance the relative priorities of each (see Fig. 4–4).

Professional nurses' organizations achieve their professional functions by such means as setting standards of practice, encouraging or requiring ongoing continuing education, establishing codes of ethics, publications, providing forums for the discussion and dissemination of knowledge through conventions and workshops. Professional nurses' organizations achieve their unionized functions by such means as collective bargaining, indemnity insurance, negotiations with employers and government, and welfare programs. Some nurses find the activities involved in the unionized functions difficult to accept, particularly if strike action is involved. Other nurses feel that quality in nursing care may not be possible unless nurses have satisfactory working conditions.

The Individual and Professionalism

The ultimate responsibility for professional practice lies with the individual nurse. A professional organization can provide (and at times enforce) opportunities for professionalism, but it is the individual nurse who must retain a commitment to patient care, maintain a high academic standard, take responsibility and be accountable for individual professional practice.

As the nursing profession develops its rights to autonomy and to control its own practice, it also increases its responsibilities to be concretely and systematically accountable for its own performance. Evaluation is a vital step in the nursing process. Each individual member of the nursing profession must take responsibility for maintaining high standards in individual practice. The profession as a whole also has this responsibility.

Being accountable in nursing service means providing systematic evidence to show that the level of care provided meets the "standards" that have been previously agreed upon as indicators of quality care.

Standards of Practice

Standards for nursing practice should be stated in clear objective and behavioral terms. In other words, they must be expressed in such a way that they can be used as concrete measures of actual nursing performance. Individual nursing service agencies frequently formulate a set of standards for their own institutions. The American Nurses' Association has committees developing both generic (general) and specific standards for various individual clinical areas, e.g., community health nursing, geriatric nursing, maternal and child health nursing, medical-surgical nursing, and psychiatric–mental health nursing. The eight generic standards of nursing practice published by the American Nurses' Association in 1973 and their implementation are discussed in Chapter 17.

Evaluation

Phaneuf and Wandelt[85] have identified three purposes served by the systematic evaluation of nursing care:

To account for the level of care provided.
To make comparisons (of different situations, settings or times)
—to determine the effects of changes made in care practices.
—to determine differences in care.
—to determine the extent to which objectives of a program have been attained.
To provide bases for planning for improvement.

Several methods of achieving sound evaluations are developing within nursing practice. Among them are the following:

Nursing Audit. A selection of patient charts are audited (formally examined) at regular intervals according to a predetermined set of criteria. Evidence of inadequate care is investigated and necessary changes are made.

Peer Review. Nurses are involved in evaluative discussions about their own performance with each other. One of the purposes is to reduce the defensive reaction that can be produced by evaluation from an external group.

Patient Audit. Patients are given the opportunity to offer their evaluations of the nursing care they received or are receiving. This is usually done through a questionnaire completed and returned by the patient, who may remain anonymous.

The reader is referred to Chapter 17 for further discussion of the evaluation of nursing practice.

PUBLIC EXPECTATIONS OF NURSING

There is very little reliable information about the public's expectations of nursing. This is unfortunate because if nurses are to offer a useful service, they need to know what the recipients of their care want and expect.

It seems likely, however, that the public in general holds images of nurses that are somewhat consistent with the traditional images described earlier in this chapter.

A study done by Tagliacozzo[105] showed that patients ideally want personalized care; friendly, kind and cheerful personal attributes in the nurse; and prompt and efficient services. These expectations are within the sphere of the nursing role. It would seem, however, that nurses need to seek more information from the public regarding their needs and expectations. It is only on the basis of knowledge of community need that nursing services can expand realistically.

LEGAL IMPLICATIONS FOR NURSING

Nurses function within legal boundaries. Every nurse must be aware of the legal requirements that determine her responsibilities in the country in which she practices. This involves knowledge of both *statutory law* and *common law* (see Chap. 19).

In the United States each state has a *Nursing Practice Act*. This legislation determines the educational and examination requirements for nurses, provides for licensure (or registration) of qualified practitioners, and describes the professional practice of nurses in broad terms.

Every nurse should be completely familiar with the contents of the Nursing Practice Act in her state.

As nurses accept more responsibility and accountability for their functions, the possibility of legal action against nurses increases. While it is not expected that a nurse will function outside the law or be negligent in the delivery of nursing care, it is wise for every nurse to be adequately covered by professional *liability insurance* (indemnity insurance).

NURSING AND SEXISM

Nursing has traditionally been a "women's occupation." Many of the issues facing women in their struggle for equal rights affect the nursing profession as a whole.

The Nurse and the Women's Movement

In spite of the fact that many of the obstacles to the development of nursing as a viable and autonomous profession stem from sexist issues, nurses have been surprisingly slow to become involved in activities of the women's movement. This is particularly surprising when it is remembered that some of nursing's greatest leaders (Florence Nightingale, Lavinia Dock, Lillian Ward and Margaret Sanger) were involved in some way with the demand for women's rights.

The issues facing nursing today are the same as those facing all women. In essence, they involve the struggle to emerge from rigid traditionalism that maintains stereotyped, ritualistic, subservient roles. The most effective nurse is the same as a most effective woman—a person who is forward thinking, able to make decisions and initiate change, and aware of and fulfilled in her perception of self. Nursing and the women's movement have much to offer each other.

Men in Nursing

Although increasing numbers of men are entering the nursing profession, they still compose a very small percentage of it. The central concepts of nursing—care, nurturing and support—are viewed by many as "female characteristics." Scientists have shown that this is not true genetically. Men are as capable of providing these services as are women.

Misconceptions are still prevalent, however. Male nurses are inclined to experience mistrust from people inside and outside nursing. It is difficult for some people to understand why a man should choose a so-called "female" occupation. Such attitudes are unfair to both men and women.

There is nothing within the nature of nursing that makes it more appropriate for one sex or the other. It is more important that those in the profession be committed to its purposes and functions. Nursing can only benefit from an increase of dedicated men into the profession. Nursing needs to be presented as a professional opportunity for both men and women.

NURSING AND THE FUTURE

What of the future? Some say that nursing will disappear because it is neglecting its primary role of care through direct humanitarian service. Others say that nursing will survive and flourish as a body of well-educated people able to adapt creatively to the needs of an advanced, changing society. All such discussion is, of course, speculation. No one really knows.

What is known, however, is that behaviors of the present-day nursing profession are determining the directions and priorities of the nurses of the future. What is also known is that knowledge is exploding at such a rate that the acquisition of facts is no longer sufficient to maintain a viable professional person. The abilities to think, to create, to seek out information, and to solve problems are much more important. The nurse of the future must be educated toward a process more than toward static content.

So long as human beings exist there will be a need for personal helping services that facilitate human actualization at times of vulnerability. Nursing has the potential to offer this kind of service. Whether it does or not will depend on the diligence with which it defines and practices its role in response to a changing society.

CONCLUSION

This chapter has presented material that will help you understand the issues affecting the profession you have entered—the nursing profession. The issues are changing issues, and you will need to work hard to keep up to date. One of the best ways to do this is through membership and participation in your professional organization. Welcome to the nursing profession! Your intelligent contribution is needed.

BIBLIOGRAPHY

1. Abdellah, F. G., et al.: *New Directions in Patient-Centered Nursing.* New York, The Macmillan Co., 1973.
2. American Nurses' Association Congress for Nursing Practice: "Definition: Nurse Practitioner, Nurse Clinician and Clinical Nurse Specialist." May 8, 1974.
3. American Nurses' Association: Establishing standards for nursing practice. *American Journal of Nursing,* 69:1458–1463, July 1969.
4. American Nurses' Association: Standards for organized nursing services. *American Journal of Nursing,* 65:76–79, March, 1965.
5. Andreoli, K. G.: A look at the physician's assistant. *American Journal of Nursing,* 73:658–661, April 1973.
6. Auld, M. E., and Birum, L. H. (eds.): *The Challenge of Nursing.* St. Louis, C. V. Mosby Co., 1973.
6a. Bandman, B., and Bandman, E.: Do nurses have rights? No! Yes! *American Journal of Nursing,* 78:84–86, Jan. 1978.
7. Bates, B.: Doctor and nurse: Changing roles and relations. *In* Reinhardt, A. M., and Quinn, M. D.: *Family-Centered Community Nursing.* St. Louis, C. V. Mosby Co., 1973.
8. Bates, B.: Twelve paradoxes: a message for nurse practitioners. *Nursing Outlook,* 22:686–688, Nov. 1974.
9. Beland, I. L.: Future directions. *In* Abdellah, F. G., et al.: *New Directions in Patient-Centered Nursing.* New York, The Macmillan Co., 1973.
10. Bell, C.: Competencies for "expanded role." *Supervisor Nurse,* 5:58–62, March 1974.
11. Biggs, B.: Nurse-clinician-practitioner-assistant-associate. *American Journal of Nursing,* 71:1936–1937, Oct. 1971.
12. Brand, K. L., and Glass, L. K.: Perils and parallels of women and nursing. *Nursing Forum,* 14(2):160–174, 1975.
13. Brodt, D. E.: Excellence or obsolescence: the choice for nursing. *Nursing Forum,* 9(1):19–26, 1976.
14. Brown, E. L.: *Nursing for the Future.* New York, Russell Sage Foundation, 1948.
15. Brown, E. L.: *Nursing Reconsidered: A Study of Change.* Part 1. Philadelphia, J. B. Lippincott Co., 1970.
16. Brown, E. L.: *Nursing Reconsidered: A Study of Change.* Part 2. Philadelphia, J. B. Lippincott Co., 1971.
17. Browning, M. H., and Lewis, E. P. (eds.): *The Expanded Role of the Nurse.* New York, The American Journal of Nursing Co., 1973.
18. Bullough, B.: Influences on role expansion. *American Journal of Nursing,* 76:1476–1481, Sept. 1976.
19. Bullough, B. (ed.): *The Law and the Expanding Nursing Role.* New York, Appleton-Century-Crofts, 1975.
20. Bullough, B., and Bullough, V. (eds.): *Issues in Nursing.* New York, Springer Publishing Co., 1966.
21. Bullough, B., and Bullough, V. (eds.): *New Directions for Nurses.* New York, Springer Publishing Co., 1971.

22. Castronovo, F.: The effective use of the clinical specialist. *Supervisor Nurse*, 6:48–56, May 1975.
23. Christman, L.: What the future holds for nursing. *Nursing Forum*, 9(1):12–18, 1970.
24. Christy, T. E.: New privileges . . . new challenges . . . new responsibilities. *Nursing '73*, 3:8–11, Nov. 1973.
25. Clemence, Sister M.: Existentialism: a philosophy of commitment. *American Journal of Nursing*, 66:500–505, March 1966.
26. Copp, L. A.: How to plan for an expanded nursing role. *RN*, 36:62–66, Nov. 1973.
27. Davis, M. Z., Krammer, M., and Strauss, A. L. (eds.): *Nurses in Practice: A Perspective on Work Environments*. St. Louis, C. V. Mosby Co., 1975.
28. Denton, J. A.: Attitudes toward alternative models of unions and professional associations. *Nursing Research*, 25:178–180, May–June 1976.
29. Donovan, H. M.: Toward a definition of nursing. *Supervisor Nurse*, 1:12–15, Oct. 1970.
30. Dougherty, M. C.: A cultural approach to the nurses' roles in health care planning. *Nursing Forum*, 11(3):311–322, 1972.
31. Driscoll, V.: Liberating nursing practice. *Nursing Outlook*, 20:24–27, Jan. 1972.
32. Dworkin, C.: Spotlight on the clinical nurse specialist. *The Canadian Nurse*, 69:40–42, Sept. 1973.
33. Epstein, C.: Breaking the barriers to communications on the health team. *Nursing '74*, 4:65–68, Sept. 1974.
34. Fagin, C.: Accountability. *Nursing Outlook*, 19:249–251, April 1971.
35. Fagin, C.: Professional nursing—the problems of women in microcosm. *Supervisor Nurse*, 2:62–68, Sept. 1971.
36. Ford, L. C.: Educating the health professions for high-quality care: nursing education. *Bulletin of the New York Academy of Medicine*, 52:93–104, Jan. 1976.
37. Georgopoulos, B. S., and Christman, L.: The clinical nurse specialist: a role model. *American Journal of Nursing*, 70:1030–1039, May 1970.
38. Godfrey, M.: Someone should represent nurses. *Nursing '76*, 6:73–85, June 1976.
38a. Gortner, S. R.: Strategies for Survival in the Practice World. *American Journal of Nursing*, 77:618–619, April 1977.
39. Grand, N. K.: Nightingaleism, employeeism and professional collectivism. *Nursing Forum*, 10(3):289–299, 1971.
40. Greenberg, E., and Levine, B.: Role strain in men nurses. *Nursing Forum*, 10(4):416–430, 1971.
41. Greenough, K.: Determining standards for nursing care. *American Journal of Nursing*, 68:2153–2157, Oct. 1968.
42. Gross, P. F.: The future of health care and nursing in the 1980's. *Australian Nurses' Journal*, 6:24–28, Oct. 1976.
42a. Gunderson, K., et al.: How to control professional frustration. *American Journal of Nursing*, 77:1180–1183, July 1977.
43. Heide, W. S.: Nursing and women's liberation—a parallel. *American Journal of Nursing*, 73:824–827, May 1973.
44. Henderson, V.: *Basic Principles of Nursing Care*. New York, International Council of Nurses, S. Karger, 1969.
45. Henderson, V.: Excellence in nursing. *American Journal of Nursing*, 69:2133–2137, Oct. 1969.
46. Henderson, V.: *The Nature of Nursing*. New York, The Macmillan Co., 1964.
47. Henderson, V.: The nature of nursing. *American Journal of Nursing*, 64:62–68, Aug. 1964.
48. Hoekelman, R. A.: Nurse-physician relationships. *American Journal of Nursing*, 75:1150–1152, July 1975.
49. Jacox, A.: Collective action and control of practice by professionals. *Nursing Forum*, 10(3):239–257, 1971.
50. Johnson, D.: Development of a theory: a requisite for nursing as a primary health profession. *Nursing Research*, 23:372–377, Sept.–Oct. 1974.
51. Johnson, M. M., and Martin, H. W.: A sociological analysis of the nurse role. *American Journal of Nursing*, 58:373–377, March 1958.
52. Judge, D.: The new nurse: a sense of duty and destiny. *Nursing Digest*, 3:20–24, Nov.–Dec. 1975.
53. Keller, N. S.: The nurse's role: is it expanding or shrinking? *Nursing Outlook*, 21:236–240, April 1973.
54. King, I. M.: *Toward a Theory for Nursing: General Concepts of Human Behavior*. New York, John Wiley & Sons, 1971.
55. Kreuter, F. R.: What is good nursing care? *Nursing Outlook*, 5:302–304, May 1957.
56. Lambertsen, E. C.: Perspective on the physician's assistant. *Nursing Outlook*, 20:32–36, Jan. 1972.
57. Levine, M. E.: *Renewal for Nursing*. Philadelphia, F. A. Davis Co., 1971.
58. Levine, M. E.: The pursuit of wholeness. *American Journal of Nursing*, 69:93–98, Jan. 1969.
59. Lewis, E. P. (ed.): *Changing Patterns of Nursing Practice*. New York, The American Journal of Nursing Co., 1971.
60. Lewis, E. P.: *The Clinical Nurse Specialist*. New York, The American Journal of Nursing Co., 1970.
61. Lewis, F. M.: The nurse as lackey: a sociological perspective. *Supervisor Nurse*, 7:24–27, April 1976.
62. Linn, L. S.: A survey of the "care-cure" attitudes of physicians, nurses, and their students. *Nursing Forum*, 14(2):145–159, 1975.
63. Little, D.: The nurse specialist. *American Journal of Nursing*, 67:552–556, March 1967.
64. Lysaught, J. P. (National Commission for the Study of Nursing and Nursing Education): *An Abstract for Action*. New York, McGraw-Hill Book Co., 1970.
65. Mauksch, H. O.: Nursing: churning for change. *In* Freeman, H. E., Levine, S., and Reeder, L. G. (eds.): *Handbook of Medical Sociology*, 2nd ed. Englewood Cliffs, NJ, Prentice-Hall, 1972.
66. Mauksch, H. O.: The nurse coordinator of patient care. *In* Skipper, J. K., and Leonard, R. C. (eds.): *Social Interaction and Patient Care*. Philadelphia, J. B. Lippincott Co., 1965.
67. Mauksch, H. O.: The organizational context of nursing practice. *In* Davis, F. E. (ed.): *The Nursing Profession*. New York, John Wiley & Sons, 1966.
68. Mauksch, I. G.: Attainment of control over professional practice. *Nursing Forum*, 10(3):232–238, 1971.
69. Marriner, A.: Continuing education in nursing. *Supervisor Nurse*, 6:20–28, June 1975.
70. McEvoy, P.: Unionisation or professionalisation. Which way for nurses? *Nursing Mirror*, 141:70–72, Nov. 20, 1975.
71. McFarland, M. B.: Adaptability in the nurse clinician. *Supervisor Nurse*, 14:23–29, Feb. 1973.
72. Meleis, A.: The clinical nurse specialist in community health nursing. *In* Bullough, B., and Bullough, V. (eds.): *New Directions for Nurses*. New York, Springer Publishing Co., 1971.
73. Mullane, M. K.: Nursing care and the political arena. *Nursing Outlook*, 23:699–701, Nov. 1975.
74. Mussallem, H. K.: The expanding role: where do we go from here? *The Canadian Nurse*, 67:31–34, Sept. 1971.

75. National Commission for the Study of Nursing and Nursing Education: Summary report and recommendations; *The American Journal of Nursing,* 70:279–294, Feb. 1970.

76. Nightingale, F.: *Florence Nightingale to Her Nurses.* London, Macmillan Co., 1914.

77. Nightingale, F.: *Notes on Nursing: What It Is and What It Is Not.* London, Gerald Duckworth and Company Ltd., 1970.

78. Nuckolls, K. B.: Who decides what the nurse can do? *Nursing Outlook,* 22:626–631, Oct. 1974.

79. O'Dell, M. L.: Physicians' perceptions of an extended role for the nurse. *Nursing Research,* 23:348–351, July–Aug. 1974.

80. Parkis, E. W.: The management role of the clinical specialist. Part 1. *Supervisor Nurse,* 5:44–51, Sept. 1974.

81. Parkis, E. W.: The management role of the clinical specialist. Part 2. *Supervisor Nurse,* 5:24–35, Oct. 1974.

81a. Partridge, K. B.: Nursing values in a changing society. *Nursing Outlook,* 26:356–360, June 1978.

82. Pearson, L. E.: The clinical specialist as role model or motivator? *Nursing Forum,* 11(1):71–77, 1972.

83. Peplau, H.: *Interpersonal Relations in Nursing.* New York, G. P. Putnam and Sons, 1952.

84. Peplau, H.: Nurses as a collectivity must take a stand. *American Journal of Nursing,* 70:2123–2124, Oct. 1970.

85. Phaneuf, M. C., and Wandelt, M. A.: Quality assurance in nursing. *Nursing Digest,* 4:32–35, Summer 1976.

86. Plawecki, J. A.: A viewpoint on the preparation of the clinical nurse specialist. *Supervisor Nurse,* 2:49–63, Jan. 1971.

87. Pluckhan, M. L.: Professional territoriality. *Nursing Forum,* 11(3):300–310, 1972.

88. Reiter, F.: The nurse clinician. *American Journal of Nursing,* 66:274–280, Feb. 1966.

89. Riehl, J. P., and McVay, J. W. (eds.): *The Clinical Nurse Specialist: Interpretations.* New York, Appleton-Century-Crofts, 1973.

90. Robinson, A. M.: Men in nursing: their career, goals and image are changing. *RN,* 36:36–41, Aug. 1973.

91. Rogers, M. E.: *An Introduction to the Theoretical Basis of Nursing.* Philadelphia, F. A. Davis Co., 1970.

92. Rogers, M. E.: Nursing: to be or not to be. *Nursing Outlook,* 20:42–46, Jan. 1972.

93. Rubin, C. F., Rinaldi, L. A., and Dietz, R. R.: Nursing audit—nurses evaluating nursing. *American Journal of Nursing,* 72:916–921, May 1972.

94. Sarbin, T. R.: Role theory. *In* Lindsay, G. (ed.): *Handbook of Social Psychology.* Reading, PA, Addison-Wesley, 1954.

94a. Schipani, C. C.: From the ideal to the real. *American Journal of Nursing,* 78:1034–1035.

95. Schlofeldt, R. M.: On the professional status of nursing. *Nursing Forum,* 13(1):16–31, 1974.

96. Schulman, S.: Basic functional roles in nursing: mother surrogate and healer. *In* Jaco, E. B. (ed.): *Patients, Physicians and Illness.* Glencoe, IL, Free Press, 1958.

97. Schoenmaker, A., and Radosevich, D. M.: Men nursing students: how they perceive their situation. *Nursing Outlook,* 24:298–303, May 1976.

98. Secretary of Health, Education and Welfare Committee to Study Extended Roles for Nurses: Extending the scope of nursing practice. *American Journal of Nursing,* 71:2346–2351, Dec. 1971.

99. Shaw, B. L.: The nurse–P.A.: one experiment that's working. *RN,* 34:44–47, June 1971.

100. Sheahan, Sister D.: The game of the name: nurse professional and nurse technician. *Nursing Outlook,* 20:440–444, July 1972.

101. Shockley, J. S.: Perspectives in femininity. Implications for nursing. *Nursing Digest,* 3:49–52, Nov.–Dec. 1975.

102. Silver, H. K., and McAtee, P. A.: Health care practice: an expanded profession for men and women. *American Journal of Nursing,* 72:78–80, Jan. 1972.

103. Snyder, D. J.: Role conflict is here to stay. *American Journal of Nursing,* 69:809–810, April 1969.

104. Stein, L. I.: The doctor-nurse game. *American Journal of Nursing,* 68:101–105, Jan. 1968.

105. Tagliacozzo, D.: The nurse from the patient's point of view. *In* Skipper, J. K., and Leonard, R. C. (eds.): *Social Interaction and Patient Care.* Philadelphia, J. B. Lippincott Co., 1965.

106. TenBrink, C. L.: The process of socialization into a new role: the professional nurse. *Nursing Forum,* 7(2):146–160, 1968.

107. Thomstad, B., et al.: Changing the rules of the doctor-nurse game. *Nursing Outlook,* 23:422–427, July 1975.

108. Torres, G.: Educators' perceptions of evolving nursing functions. *Nursing Outlook,* 22:184–187, March 1974.

109. Uprichard, M.: Ferment in nursing. *International Nursing Review,* 16(3):222–234, 1969.

110. Vaillot, Sister M. C.: Living and dying. Hope. The restoration of being. *American Journal of Nursing,* 7:268–273, Feb. 1970.

111. Vaughan, B. A.: Role fusion, diffusion and confusion. *Nursing Clinics of North America,* 8:703–713, Dec. 1973.

112. Wakeley, J.: The role of the nurse (UK). *Supervisor Nurse,* 3:12–15, Dec. 1972.

113. Walker, A. E.: PRIMEX—the family nurse practitioner program. *Nursing Outlook,* 20:28–31, Jan. 1972.

114. Walton, M. H.: Professional: cost and quality. *Nursing Clinics of North America,* 8:685–689, Dec. 1973.

115. Walsh, M. E.: On nursing's role in health care delivery. *Nursing Outlook,* 20:592–593, Sept. 1972.

115a. Winstead-Fry, P.: The need to differentiate a nursing self. *American Journal of Nursing,* 77:1452–1454, Sept. 1977.

116. World Health Organization Expert Committee on Nursing: Fifth Report. Geneva, World Health Organization, 1966.

117. Wright, E.: Registered nurses' opinions on an extended role concept. *Nursing Research,* 25:112–114, March–April 1976.

UNIT
II
BASIC CONCEPTS OF STRESS, HOMEOSTASIS, HEALTH AND ILLNESS

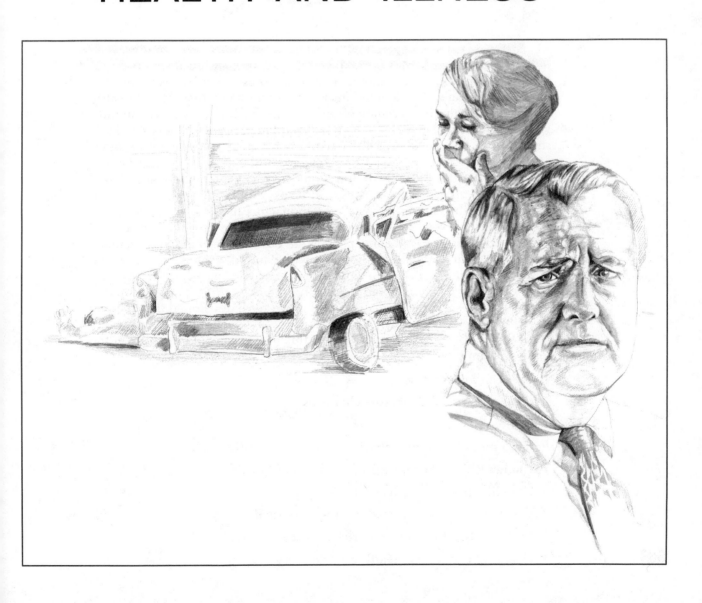

UNIT II

BASIC CONCEPTS OF STRESS, HOMEOSTASIS, HEALTH AND ILLNESS

To a scientist, stress is any action or situation that places special physical or psychological demands upon a person — anything that can unbalance his individual equilibrium. And while the physiological response to such demands is surprisingly uniform, the forms of stress are innumerable. A divorce is stressful — but so is a marriage. Getting fired is stressful — but so is a promotion. Stress may even be all but unconscious, like the noise of a city or the daily chore of driving a car. Perhaps the one incontestable statement that can be made about stress is that it belongs to everyone — to businessmen and professors, to mothers and their children, to factory workers, garbagemen and writers. A keyed-up feeling is part of the fabric of life.

OGDEN TANNER[142]

INTRODUCTION AND STUDY GUIDE

Adapting to stress, coping with crisis, maintaining homeostatic balance in an unstable world, preserving health and preventing disease are all basic goals of man. Furthermore, not only are these goals basic but they are also closely related to one another. For example, to be in a state of health, a person must also be in a state of relative equilibrium or balance; an individual's state of balance, in turn, depends upon his ability to adapt to life's stresses and to cope successfully with crises as they arise. On the other hand, disease states appear to be linked with states of homeostatic imbalance or disequilibrium. An individual enters a state of imbalance when he is unable to adapt to the "physical or psychological demands" placed upon him by the various stress-producing factors in his environment.

As you can see, stress and adaptation, balance and imbalance, and health and disease are all concepts that are basic to the health professional. The nurse who understands how people adapt adequately to stress, and how they normally maintain homeostatic balance, will have a basis for understanding *faulty* adaptation and the *breakdown of homeostasis* that occurs in illness. It is for this reason that we have developed the chapters describing these subjects in some detail.

As a brief overview, our object in this unit is to explore with you the following important topics:

▶ stress and adaptation

▶ crisis theory and coping mechanisms

▶ homeostatic mechanisms

▶ biorhythms and biofeedback

▶ changing concepts of health, disease and health care

▶ changing patterns of disease

▶ the significance of disease for the individual

▶ traditional and modern theories of disease causation

▶ changing patterns of health care delivery

Because this unit covers a large and complex subject area, it contains many terms, theories and concepts that may be new to you. The following guides may help you to gain the most from your reading.

Upon finishing this unit, you should be aware of the meaning of the following key terms:

health
disease
stress
strain
stressors
adaptation
  physiologic
  psychologic
  sociocultural
  technologic
crises
coping
defenses
crisis intervention
homeostatic mechanisms
negative feedback
positive feedback
feed forward
thermostat-like regulators

servomechanisms
deviation
overshoot
oscillations
  stable
  unstable
  damped
  runaway
biologic rhythms
circadian rhythms
chronobiology
rhythm synchronizers
endogenous clock theory
exogenous clock theory
biofeedback
community health care
comprehensive health care
primary care

You should be able to discuss generally the following theories of disease:

1. Theory of the body machine
2. Pathologic anatomic theories
3. Mind-body dichotomy
4. Germ theory
5. Cellular theory
6. Molecular theory
7. Multicausal theories

You should be able to discuss generally the following concepts:

1. Stress theory
2. Levels of adaptation
3. Characteristics of life crises
4. Basic characteristics of homeostatic mechanisms
5. Positive and negative feedback
6. Applications of the concept of homeostasis to patient care
7. Types of circadian rhythms in man
8. Basic techniques of biofeedback training
9. The changing definition of illness
10. The continuum of health and disease
11. Disease as a failure of adaptation
12. The false dichotomies of mind and body, mental and physical disease.
13. The antiquity of disease

14. Man's life expectancy
15. Shifting geographic disease patterns
16. Characteristics of modern theories of disease
17. Six emerging patterns of health care

Before our discussion begins, three important points need to be made. First, much of the subject matter presented in this unit is controversial and lies in the area of theory and speculation. Although a great deal has been written about man and his adaptive abilities, we actually *know* very little about ourselves. The precise ways in which we function and adapt— physically, mentally and emotionally—are only dimly understood. Thus, theories about human nature are subject to correction and change as man better comprehends the mystery of himself.

Second, although unifying concepts such as those of adaptation and homeostasis are helpful in integrating seemingly unrelated data, it would be a gross oversimplification to imply that knowledge of ourselves can ever be reduced to any one common denominator. Unifying concepts have value for nurses mainly because they serve as reference points from which we can gain a perspective on the complexities of our own behavior and that of our patients.

Third, we must caution you that even general information concerning health and disease is in a constant state of change and growth. Much of what was believed true yesterday has been discredited today. What seems to be true today may be virtually meaningless tomorrow. Thus, it is best to approach the study of theories of disease causation with an open mind and in an inquiring and critical spirit.

Let us now turn to Chapter 5 and our discussion of stress, adaptation and crisis.

CHAPTER 5

ADAPTING TO STRESS AND COPING WITH CRISIS

THE CONCEPT OF STRESS

Stress is a universal human experience that bridges personalities, cultures and time. As an old saying states: "To be alive is to be under stress."

Clearly, the concept of stress is very old. The ancients, who faced a brutal, uncompromising environment, must have recognized, however vaguely, that sense of being "under stress." Hans Selye, a world-renowned authority on stress, describes primitive man's concept of stress in this manner.

It must have occurred even to prehistoric man that the loss of vigor and the feeling of exhaustion that overcame him after hard labor, prolonged exposure to cold or heat, loss of blood, agonizing fear, or any kind of disease had something in common. He may not have been consciously aware of this similarity in his response to anything that was simply too much for him, but when the feeling came he must have realized instinctively that he had exceeded the limits of what he could reasonably handle—that, in other words, he had "had it."[126]

While the idea of stress has been alive throughout the ages, it was not until the 20th century that scientists attempted to crystallize this vague concept into precise scientific terminology. During the first part of this century, famous physicians such as William Osler and Walter Cannon began to talk and write about stress as a possible cause of illness. By the 1950's, Selye was linking stress with certain specific diseases, e.g., gastric and duodenal ulcers and high blood pressure. As it became increasingly evident that stress was an important factor in physical and mental disease, research was undertaken by authorities from a myriad of academic fields—medicine, biology, physiology, psychology, sociology and anthropology. As a result of widespread interest, tens of thousands of articles have been written and innumerable studies have been conducted on the causes of and responses to stress. Medical and nursing clinicians have become fascinated by the notion of applying stress theory to patient care. Currently, physicians and nurses are specifically trained to observe for the signs of stress in their patients and to consider the effects of stress upon their clients' physical and mental health.

Today the concept of stress is undergoing criticism as a result of the difficulties in defining stress and the almost impossible task of quantitatively measuring stress.[69, 107] Nevertheless, the stress concept, despite its limitations, still stands as an important cornerstone in the study of health and disease.

Attempting to Define Stress

Difficulties in Defining Stress. Stress is a very difficult concept to define in anything but general terms. Reasons for this difficulty are as follows:

▶ Stress is a *highly complex concept* that involves several dimensions, e.g., causes of stress, the nature of the stressor (physical injury, mental shock), the immediate physical, social and psychologic responses to stress, and the permanent or semipermanent physical and mental changes created by the stress experience.

▶ Stress has an *ambiguous nature*. It is often difficult to know whether stress is the *cause* or the *consequence* of certain events.

▶ The term stress is used by *different authorities* from different fields in divergent ways. A physiologist may describe stress through its physiologic correlates (e.g., an elevation of blood pressure), whereas a psychologist may define stress in terms of anxiety.

▶ Engineers and physicists also employ the terms "stress" and "strain" in relationship

69

to solid bodies; this further adds to the confusion. In physics and engineering, stress can be *quantitatively measured,* whereas in human relations, stress can only be described.

▶ The concept of stress has been *"popularized."* The term "stress" constantly arises in popular literature (e.g., women's magazines and newspaper articles), and it is frequently used in conversations of persons outside the sciences. Unfortunately, use of the word "stress" by lay persons has further obscured and confused its meaning.

Despite these difficulties, knowledgeable persons have attempted to define stress in relatively precise terms. We will now consider some of the more outstanding definitions and conceptions.

Definitions and Conceptions of Stress.   Originally a Latin derivative, the term "stress" has evolved through many definitions over the centuries.[69] During the 17th century "stress" was linked with "hardship, straits, adversity or affliction." By the 18th and 19th centuries, the meaning of stress had changed to mean "force, pressure, strain, or strong effort" that acts upon a person or an object. Hinkle states that this view of stress as a "force" had an impact on our modern definition of the term. He writes:

It [the 18th century definition of stress] then carried with it the connotation of an objects's [or person's] being acted upon by forces from without, resisting the distorting effects of these forces, attempting to maintain its integrity and trying to return to its original state. The word was taken over into science in this sense, and probably the scientific use of the term reinforced the popular usage.[69]

During the 19th century, the word "stress" was incorporated into the vocabularies of physicists and engineers. In physics, stress is defined as "the ratio of the internal force brought into play when a substance is distorted to the area over which the force acts." Engineers calculate stress in dynes per square centimeter.[69]

Throughout the 20th century, physicians, physiologists and biologists have attempted to define stress from physiologic, psychologic and sociologic points of view. Some of the most useful definitions and concepts of stress have been developed by Hans Selye, the late Harold Wolff, Basowitz, Scott, Howard, and Aakster.

Selye, a physician and endocrinologist, defines stress as follows:

Stress. In biology the nonspecific response of the body to any demand made upon it. For general orientation, it suffices to keep in mind that by stress the physician means the common results of exposure to any stimulus. For example, the bodily changes produced whether a person is exposed to nervous tension, physical injury, infection, cold, heat, X rays, or anything else are what we call stress.[126]

Selye further defines *nonspecific* response as "one which affects all or most parts of a system without selectivity." He also states, "A nonspecifically caused change is one which can be produced by many or all agents."[126] Thus, when Selye writes of the "nonspecific response of the body" to stimuli, he means that the *entire* body or the majority of its systems must try to adjust to any specific agent that places demands upon it.

For example, exposure to extreme heat or cold is a specific problem to which the body must respond and adjust by either shivering (in

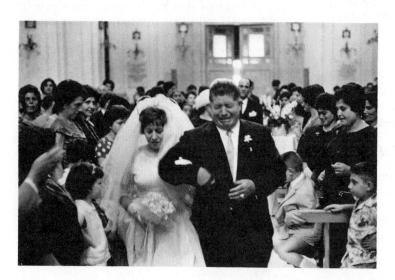

Figure 5–1. Joyful events can be stressful. An Italian father breaks down and cries uncontrollably while escorting his daughter to the altar on her wedding day. (From Paul Schutzer, *Life Magazine* © Time, Inc.)

the case of cold) or perspiring (in the case of heat). While the specific responses to them are different, heat and cold are nonetheless similar in that they *force the body to perform adaptive functions with the goal of returning the body to its previous state of balance.*

On an *emotional level,* the body also responds nonspecifically to joyful (pleasant but stressful) events and to unpleasant, traumatic (distressful) events. Selye emphasizes that it is a fallacy to believe that stress responses arise only during distressful events. For example, a person can be under as much stress at his wedding as he is at the funeral of a loved one (see Fig. 5–1). In both cases (one of joy and one of sorrow) the body's systems are responding as a whole (nonspecifically) to specific events.

According to Selye, the multiple and constant stresses to which one is exposed throughout life constitute the "wear and tear" on the body that produces the physical and psychologic signs of *aging.* While Selye once equated stress and aging as the same phenomenon, Selye currently believes that aging is the *result* of stress. Stress responses continue throughout life. The only time a person's body ceases to respond to life's challenges is when he dies. As Selye says: "Complete freedom from stress is death."

Another important viewpoint on stress was developed by the late Harold Wolff. Wolff's work in the laboratory and in clinical situations focused on the pathologic changes that can be produced by social and psychologic problems. He defined stress as "the internal or resisting force brought into action in part by external forces or loads."[107] He further stated, "Stress becomes the *interaction* between external environment and organism, with the past experience of the organism as a major factor."[107] Wolff believed that life stress was mediated through the nervous system.

Basowitz, another student of stress, developed the concept of stress in terms of *anxiety.* Based on his studies of army paratroopers during training, Basowitz defined stress as "the threat to the fulfillment of basic needs, the maintenance of regulated (homeostatic) functioning, and to growth and development."[107] Basowitz believed that the term "stress" applied to that "class of conditions" which evoke anxiety in the majority of people and force individuals to respond physically, psychologically and behaviorally. He proposed that responses to stress could be either adaptive (enabling the individual to adjust) or pathologic.

At a Symposium on Stress (1976), Jeanne Benoliel described stress in *sociologic terms.* She defined *social stress* as "a situation which places objective demands on an individual so as to overload his adaptive capacities."[14] As an example of social stress, Benoliel spoke of the nurse in the intensive care unit (ICU) who must cope daily with heavy work loads, exposure to death and dying, continuous contact with difficult situations, crowded work space and communication problems. To overcome these social stresses, the nurse must learn how to cope physically and mentally with her demanding work situation.

Aakster defines stress by using a systems approach. We stated in Chapter 1 that all systems are always directed toward a particular goal or *end state.* In order to reach its goals, a system must adjust to the various disequilibriums (imbalances) that arise within its environment. According to Aakster, "Forces which create such disequilibriums are termed stress."[1]

While all the definitions and viewpoints we have presented are helpful, they all have their limitations:

1. Each of these definitions appears to be geared to one particular discipline—sociology, psychology or physiology. None of the definitions adequately integrates concepts from each of the physiologic and behavioral sciences.

2. Many definers of stress tend to equate stress with distress and trauma and fail to recognize that stress may accompany pleasant experiences.

3. Some models of stress assume that if a situation is stressful for one person it will be stressful for everyone.

4. Certain definitions imply that the results of stress are always pathologic, and they ignore the beneficial aspects of stress: e.g., jogging is stressful but will result in body conditioning; mountain climbing is stressful, but for some people it is an exhilarating experience.

Stress: Sources and Responses

However we define stress, it is helpful to distinguish between sources of stress and responses to stress.

There are four *general sources* of stress. First, stress can arise from situations that are difficult, threatening or rapidly changing; in this context, stress can also result from a *pathologic* change in the body as a result of disease or injury. Second, stress can be the outcome of *normal living* when no injury or illness has occurred. Daily commuting, entertaining, and attending classes all can be considered mildly stressful yet normal activities of modern life. Third, stress can be the outcome of planned activities, or even therapies, and can be *curative*. For instance, competitive sports, though stressful, help us to work off certain emotions; electroconvulsive therapy (ECT), a stressful procedure, can relieve mental depression in some patients. Finally, stress can arise in anticipation of a stressful event. *Anticipatory stress* occurs frequently in daily life; for example, consider the anxiety a person feels prior to an important examination, a critical courtroom hearing, or a crucial or painful diagnostic test.

Important specific sources of stress are

▶ attacks by bacteria, viruses or parasites

▶ trauma (injury, burns, assaults, electric shock)

▶ inadequate food, warmth, protection

▶ disruptive social and family relationships

▶ conflicting social and cultural expectations

▶ basic needs (e.g., sexual desires) that must be denied because of social pressure

▶ imagined threats of injury (sources of stress do not have to be based in reality)

▶ changes in the internal physiology (e.g., puberty, menstruation, pregnancy, menopause)

▶ battle conditions (war)

▶ periods of unrelieved isolation

▶ natural disasters (earthquakes, floods)

▶ geographic relocation (change of residence, travel)

▶ hard competitive sports

Responses to stress are generally categorized into four general areas: (1) *physiologic* responses (e.g., changes in cardiovascular function, increased gastric secretion); (2) *behavioral* responses (increased reaction time, error increase, tremor, loss of sphincter control); (3) *subjective* responses (anxiety, depression, unresolved problems); (4) *psychologic* responses (use of various defense mechanisms* such as denial or repression of a stressful situa-

---

*Defense mechanisms are defined and discussed in Unit III, Chapter 11.

tion).[73, 107] The precise manner in which each individual responds to stressful situations is mediated by (a) his personality, (b) the manner in which he characteristically responds to stressful events (response repertoire) and (c) how he basically perceives his problem.[73]

Despite these individual differences in response to stress, social scientists have learned that all people

▶ experience deprivation, frustration and stress when needs are not satisfied

▶ tend to avoid stresses, such as injury, temperature extremes and pain

▶ react in similar ways to extreme stress

▶ tend to adapt to stress and to satisfy basic needs by deliberately modifying the environment (e.g., inventing clothing, housing, medicines)

▶ tend to seek a state of equilibrium in the face of environmental and internal stresses

Summary of Conclusions from Stress Studies

Stress has been studied in many settings: laboratories (using both animals and human beings), disaster situations, military training centers, battle situations, within primitive cultures, and in hospital wards and clinics. Some general conclusions drawn from stress studies are as follows:[107, 124, 142]

1. Stress is usually described as "a state of the total organism under extenuating circumstances rather than as an event in the environment"[107] (i.e., stress is generally perceived as a generalized response that develops within the individual rather than an upsetting event that acts upon the person).

2. A stress state can develop in response to a great variety of stimuli.

3. Different people respond to different stressors in a variety of ways.

4. The same person may develop a stress response in reaction to one critical situation but not to another critical situation.

5. The theory that there is *one* common physiologic stress reaction that develops in all persons in critical situations is subject to question.

6. The intensity and duration of the stress state in an individual is dependent upon the following subjective factors: past experiences, socialization patterns during childhood, and the meaning of the situation to the person.

7. A certain amount of stress is beneficial and too little stress can actually be harmful.

8. Stress is linked with some diseases; however, whether stress is a major causative factor in heart disease is debatable.

9. When people are subjected to severe stress they become accident prone.

10. Life in the country or suburbs is as stressful as life in the city. However, the stresses are of a different nature.

THE CONCEPT OF ADAPTATION

Adaptation is a universal characteristic of life and, thus, serves as a unifying concept for understanding human behavior. Biologists and behavioral scientists have shown that whenever a person encounters stress, from any source, he attempts to adapt to it. If adaptation is successful, the individual's balance is not disturbed or is restored. If adaptation is faulty, the individual becomes ill, and then, as a sick person, he must adapt to his illness. Thus, the concept of adaptation is of vital concern to nurses and physicians who daily cope with the adaptive changes that illness has forced upon patients.

The word "adapt" comes from the Latin word *adaptare,* meaning "to adjust." Thus, originally, adaptation simply meant adjustment. Today, *Dorland's Illustrated Medical Dictionary* defines adaptation as "the adjustment of an organism to its environment, or the process by which it enhances such fitness."

Since the process of adaptation is characteristic of all living things, adaptation has been a subject for intensive study in many disciplines, ranging from plant biology to psychiatry. The result is that the word "adaptation" can be considered from the standpoints of both biology and human behavior. In its most comprehensive sense, the concept of adaptation includes the whole range of protective adjustments from the simplest motor action to the most complex interaction between individuals or entire nations. It involves organisms that are as simple as the one-celled amoeba and those as complicated as man. As Selye aptly states:

The great capacity for adaptation is what makes life possible on all levels of complexity. It is the basis of homeostasis and of resistance to stress. . . . *Adaptability is probably the most distinctive characteristic of life.*[129]

In sum, adaptation is found at all levels of life; it is probably the one characteristic that separates living organisms from inanimate objects. At the human level, adaptation is more complicated than among less complex organisms. It involves more than a simple biologic process. Man does not just react to his environment as an insect would; instead, he *responds* to his environment with its multiple stresses. With body, intellect and emotion, man attempts to meet the challenges of life actively and aggressively.

Levels of Adaptation

We may consider human adaptation as functioning at the following four levels: (1) physiologic or biologic, (2) psychologic, (3) sociocultural, and (4) technologic. For purposes of convenience, we shall examine these levels separately. However, it is essential to remember that, in terms of human experience, these levels are fully interrelated.

The Physiologic Level. Adaptation in the biologic sense is defined by *Webster's New World Dictionary* as a "change in structure, function, or form that produces better adjustment of an animal or plant to its environment." Physiologic or biologic adaptation involves compensatory changes that occur within the body in response to either (1) increased or altered demands being made upon the body, or (2) stresses (either internal or environmental) that are impinging upon the body and threatening to destroy its physiologic balance.

For example, consider the increased demands made upon the body by jogging. Many of the people undertaking this form of exertion have led sedentary lives before beginning a jogging program. Consequently, they experience a considerable degree of physical stress during their first exercise sessions. They may feel exhausted; they may experience muscular soreness and aching; their hearts may beat quite rapidly in an effort to circulate a sufficient supply of blood to their muscles; their respirations may accelerate as a result of the additional amounts of oxygen needed. However, if these persons follow the recommended jogging schedule, increasing their efforts a little every day, they may eventually be able to jog quite a distance, at a moderate rate, without undue strain. Their muscles, hearts and lungs will have gradually increased in strength and functional efficiency in order to best *adapt* to the additional demands placed upon them.

Man's ability to adjust to extreme changes in temperature and to climatic variations provides another example of physiologic adaptation. For instance, if a person is suddenly exposed to extreme cold, he tends to shiver, to stamp his feet, to wave his arms, and to move about generally. This muscular activity helps to increase his body's heat production so that his body temperature remains normal despite the cold environment. On the other hand, individuals who live in cold climates for lengthy periods maintain the increased heat production necessary for survival by developing a higher rate of metabolism. Further, not only is heat production generally increased, but heat loss from the body is prevented by the development of protective mechanisms. For instance, sweating is reduced, the blood vessels that supply the skin tend to constrict more, and an insulating layer of subcutaneous fat develops as a result of an increased food intake. Because of these physiologic adaptations, and because of such technologic adaptations as specially designed clothing, heating and housing, explorers have been able to survive for considerable periods in extremely frigid environments in which they would normally perish. In contrast, the Eskimo, with a relatively simple technology, has developed genetic adaptations as a result of centuries of life in a frozen habitat. Consequently, these people have a short, thick body build with a heavy layer of subcutaneous fat. These physical attributes are most advantageous for life in cold climates.

The body's reaction to invading microorganisms serves as a further illustration of physiologic adaptation to stress. Man resists attacks by viruses and bacteria by developing an immunity to them. Briefly, immunity may be either inherited or acquired. When it is *inherited,* an individual is *naturally* resistant to certain organisms. When it is *acquired,* the individual develops immunity as a result of previous contact with an organism by either having a particular infectious disease and surviving it or being inoculated against that disease. His body, in this situation, *adapts* to the presence of disease through forming protective antibodies in his blood. He thus develops immunity for specific diseases.

As a final example, in the field of sensory physiology, adaptation is viewed as a decrease in the intensity of a sensation resulting from "steady state stimulation" or continuous responses. The olfactory sense provides a good example of sensory adaptation. We all know that when we come into contact with a noxious odor, we are immediately offended. However, if we remain in contact with this odor (steady state stimulation) and the odor remains constant, we become accustomed to it rather quickly; thus, there is a decrement in the inten-

sity of sensation until we are oblivious of its existence. In other words, we adapt.

The Psychologic Level. Psychologic adaptation involves adjustment to stress through the use of learning, perception, and conscious and unconscious processes, including the various psychologic defense mechanisms. This mode of adaptation is based primarily on complex neurochemical processes, many of which are as yet unexplained. It also involves our genetic endowment as well as the many associations, both pleasant and unpleasant, which arise from our past experiences.

At the psychologic level, David Mechanic defines adaptation as "the way in which a person deals with his situation and his feelings aroused by the situation."[103] Mechanic writes that adaptation is composed of the following two components:

1. *Coping:* how an individual handles his *situation.* Coping involves relieving stress by removing or attenuating the sources of stress.

2. *Defenses:* how an individual handles his *feelings* of anxiety, fear, discomfort, etc. about a situation.

Psychologic defenses are called into play when coping is impossible; e.g., when the person's anxiety level is too high. For example, picture typical college students during examinations—usually a very stressful time for students. To deal with the problem of examinations, one student called John may try *coping* measures to get through his exams; e.g., he makes arrangements to be absent from his part-time job that week, thereby gaining more time for study. In addition, he may forgo dates and social occasions during exams. In areas of his studies about which he is uncertain, he may arrange to talk with his instructor or with other students who are more knowledgeable. In these ways this student is handling a difficult situation by reducing stress as much as possible.

Another student, named Bill, might feel so immobilized by anxiety that he becomes totally unable to cope with exam week. Instead of coping he employs various inappropriate defense mechanisms in order to deal with his anxiety. For example, he may deny the significance of his examinations. Thus, he may tell himself: "I don't care what happens with these exams. It's a waste of time to go to college anyway." Or he may project his anxiety onto his instructors or college in the form of angry denunciations. He may think, "If that teacher was any good or really cared about his students, I wouldn't have to worry about this exam." Or "This is such a lousy school! How can they expect students to pass." In addition, this student may develop a cold or the flu on the day of a particularly feared exam, thus bypassing the whole horrible experience. As a result of these defenses, this student has diluted his anxiety but may have failed his exam. Thus, while adaptation is always *useful*, it does not always result in what is best for the *total* individual; i.e., *unhealthy adaptation* also occurs. In an attempt to respond to stress, an individual may adapt in a manner that *temporarily* may function to relieve his discomfort but ultimately may not be in his best interest.

As another example, a man who unconsciously wishes to be dependent on other people may develop an incapacitating illness. This allows him to be dependent without experiencing guilt feelings over his dependency. He does not feel guilty because he accepts the idea that sick people can be dependent. This is not, of course, the situation with all illnesses. It does serve, however, as an example of adaptation that ultimately proves harmful to the individual, but that meets his immediate need to reduce the stress that his dependent feelings create.

Moreover, some psychiatrists believe that certain neurotic behavior has protective value. For instance, suppose that an obese individual cannot control his eating and feels driven to eat all the time ("compulsive" overeating). This is neurotic behavior, assuming there is no physiologic imbalance. The resulting obesity may protect the individual from becoming involved in threatening sexual relationships. If this person diets and loses weight, he will consequently become more sexually attractive. Then he will have to either come to terms with the problems of sexuality or develop a new protective neurosis. As long as he remains obese he is protected by his neurotic overeating. Even though he may say he wishes he were not so heavy, his neurotic need for protection is greater than his drive to be more attractive physically.

This person's adaptation is protective to him and should not be tampered with by unskilled persons. It may be that even though his adaptation appears unsuccessful, it is the most successful adaptation that he can make. Obese individuals have been known to commit suicide when losing weight because they could not adapt to the new problems created. For them, obesity was a successful, life-sustaining adaptation.

The student is cautioned not to generalize from this example or apply it to all obese people. Neurotic problems vary from individual to individual and are identified only through skilled exploration. This example is presented merely to illustrate neurotic adaptation.

Protection of the psyche from overwhelming trauma is seen not only in the neurotic, but in the extreme behavior of the psychotic as well.

For instance, total withdrawal from the world serves to isolate the psychotic from an unbearable life experience; hallucinations may help him to recognize and control a threatening and chaotic existence. Thus, he is adapting to life in the only way he can at the time.

In summary, when we adapt psychologically to stress, we are attempting to protect ourselves so that we can continue to survive in life. Individuals adapt to stress in the best way they can at the time. Adaptive behavior may not always appear appropriate; however, it is always purposeful.

The Sociocultural Level. Adaptation at this level includes the various patterns of behavior by which people adjust to the society and the culture that surrounds them. More explicitly, sociocultural adaptation involves, first of all, the adjustment of an individual's actions and conduct to the norms, conventions, beliefs, and pressures of various groups. The family, professional societies, labor unions, social clubs, and sororities are but a few examples of the wide assortment of groups that demand our involvement and commitment. Second, adaptation at this level means adjustment of our behavior to the concepts, ideals, traditions and institutions that define a culture. Examples of cultural groups include racial groups, geographic groups (e.g., American, European) and certain religious groups.

As an illustration of sociocultural adaptation at the *group level*, consider your own experience as a student preparing for the profession of nursing. When you first entered your school of nursing, you were probably exposed, almost immediately, to a new set of ethics that you had to accept, to a new vocabulary that you had to learn, and to certain standards of performance that you had to achieve. All these demands perhaps seemed overwhelming at first. Furthermore, your first experiences with patients may have been overshadowed by a sense of uncertainty, nervousness, and even fear. But gradually, over a period of months, you begin to speak the medical language fluently, you come to believe in the values that you were taught, and you develop the confidence to function fairly efficiently in the nurse-patient relationship.

You may safely assume that the longer you remain in nursing, the more natural it will seem to you to be a nurse. This is because you, as an individual, will have adapted to the nursing profession. You will have become a bona fide member of the group. You may eventually become so well adapted to nursing that you will find it difficult to relate to other professional and social groups. This sense of exclusiveness is a common characteristic of professional societies, and one of the dangers of social adaptation. If this occurs, you will have adapted so exclusively to one group that you have lost your ability to adapt to others.

Adaptation at the *cultural level* can be exemplified in several ways. For instance, a cowboy who leaves the wilds of Wyoming to take up residence in Los Angeles must make many sweeping adjustments. He must adapt himself to urban sprawl, smog, roaring freeways, glaring lights, constant noise, numerous people, and the general turmoil of city life. He must adjust to crowding, competitive attitudes, emotional stresses, varying ideas and conventions, as well as to the multiple value systems found in a megalopolis.

The cowboy may at first feel awed and shocked by city life. He may even become emotionally disturbed by the changes in his own life-style which this new situation demands. However, if he remains in the city long enough he may gradually develop the appropriate attitudes, habits and behaviors. As a result, he will come to feel as at home in the heavily populated Los Angeles environment as he once did in the open country of Wyoming.

The process of cultural adaptation is also illustrated by the anthropologist who goes into the field to work with a group of primitive people, or by the Peace Corps worker who volunteers to serve in an underdeveloped country. Both anthropologists and Peace Corps workers often tell of the "cultural shock" that they experienced when they first came into contact with the customs and activities of the people with whom they were working. Gradually, however, the sense of shock subsided as they became acclimated to the situation. Indeed, these workers sometimes become so well adapted to the foreign culture that the eventual re-entry into the confines of their own culture proves difficult. Nurses may experience "cultural shock" as their nursing practice brings them into contact with various cultural groups.

In short, when we adapt to a group or to a culture, we modify and, in some instances, radically change our attitudes and behavior so that they merge with the norms, values, and institutions of the group or culture we are involved with. Of course, in order to adapt socially, we must also adapt psychologically, and in some instances, physiologically. For example, when the cowboy moved from Wyoming to Los Angeles, he was obliged to adapt psychologically to the emotional stresses inherent in city living, and physiologically to the air pollution characteristic of industrial areas.

The Technologic Level. Technologic adaptations are those scientific and industrial arts and innovations that man himself has created through the use of his cultural heritage. These adaptations have built for man an artificial world in place of the primitive pre-industrial world in which he once lived. Technology, an outgrowth of culture, has allowed us to modify and change our surrounding environment and to control many of the stresses that are part of that environment. Unfortunately, modern technology has also created certain new stresses to which man must adapt—for example, water, air, and noise pollution. On the whole, however, advances in science enable men to live longer with less discomfort than was ever before possible. Although we, as human animals, are still ruled by general biologic laws, we are more and more in control of our own destiny through industrial, scientific, and medical innovations.

Modern medicine, in particular, has evolved at a tremendous rate over the last decades. Because of medical science, man is adapting with greater success to the stresses of disease and injury, birth, and death than would have been believed possible in past centuries. For example, today medical technology eases population stresses through the use of contraceptives; emotional stresses through the use of tranquilizing drugs; the problems of infectious disease through the use of inoculations and sanitation; the dangers of childbirth through the development of better obstetric techniques; and the once fatal problems of heart and kidney failure through the use of transplants.

As a result of our technology, then, we are gaining a certain control over the universal problems of disease, pain, and death. The successes of medical science, however, have not been obtained without a price. Serious dilemmas (philosophic, ethical, and legal) have developed as a result of our technologic adaptations. These dilemmas are complex and far-reaching in their implications. These medical problems often have an effect on nursing practice, and they will be discussed as appropriate throughout the text.

CHARACTERISTICS OF ADAPTATION

All adaptive mechanisms (whether physiologic, psychologic, cultural or technologic) tend to have certain common characteristics. These characteristics can be summarized as follows:

1. *All adaptive mechanisms are attempts to maintain within the individual optimum physical and chemical conditions.* Thus, through the process of adaptation, those physiologic processes necessary to life can be carried on to best effect. The process of maintaining a fairly steady internal environment for the individual is called *homeostasis.* The concept of homeostasis is so important that it will be explained at length in the following chapter.

2. *Individuals always retain their own identity despite the use of adaptive mechanisms.* Thus, we are able to adapt to changing conditions without losing those characteristics of appearance and behavior that particularly distinguish us. For example, we, as individuals, may undergo tremendous stresses during certain periods of our lives. We may be forced to adapt to painful trauma and to upsetting changes. As a result, we may wrinkle, develop gray hair, and age visibly. Nevertheless, we are still recognizable as human beings in general, and as ourselves in particular. We still retain the gross appearance and general behavior patterns that have characterized us throughout our lives. In sum, we exhibit a certain stability in the midst of change.

3. *Adaptation is a dynamic and active process.* Individuals do not passively submit to environmental or internal stresses; for example, such *internal* stimuli as hunger and thirst result in our *actively* seeking release from these tensions through such actions as seeking food and water. When *external* stresses threaten us, we may run from them, or block them from our consciousness (for example, by fainting), or actively struggle against them. Moreover, to further protect ourselves from danger, we may intensify the action of those sensory receptors that are necessary for our survival. For instance, in a life-threatening situation, our hearing tends to become more acute and our vision sharper than it "normally" is. Vision sharpens because the pupil of the eye dilates when we are under extreme stress. Involved in all these protective adaptive actions are the sympathetic and parasympathetic nervous systems as well as certain circulatory, endocrine, and sensory mechanisms.

4. *When individuals adapt to change or to stress, they tend to adapt as total organisms.* In other words, adaptation does not occur exclusively at any one level of human experience. Rather, it tends to embrace all levels—the physiologic, the psychologic, the sociocultural, and perhaps even the technologic. When you became a nursing student, you had to adapt physiologically to the greater work load, to the long hours of study, and to the muscular stresses required for lifting and moving patients. Psychologically you had to adapt on an intellectual level to the new and different subject matter, and emotionally to the responsibilities and problems inherent in patient care. At the sociocultural level you had to adjust to the ethics and norms of the nursing profession and of hospital culture. Technologically it was necessary to familiarize yourself with equipment new to you.

5. *Adaptation, as a process, has its definite limitations.* Although adaptive mechanisms and behavior exploit the available potentialities of the individual, they must also operate within the limitations of that individual's hereditary make-up, physiologic constitution, intelligence, and emotional stability. As one scientist has written, "a cornered amoeba cannot escape by flying."[44] Likewise, a man cannot flap his arms and fly or remain submerged in water indefinitely. He must adapt within the confines of his nature or through technologic innovations.

6. *Adaptive responses are much more limited in number and scope at the physiologic level than they are at the social and psychologic levels.* For instance, our blood sugar, the oxygen content of our blood, and our internal temperature can fluctuate only within certain narrow limits and still be consistent with life. On the other hand, there are many possible adaptive solutions available to us in situations involving emotional or social crises. However, even in these circumstances the number of possible solutions is finite.

7. *Adaptation can be viewed in relationship to time.* The individual who has sufficient time can adapt more readily to stress than can the individual who must adapt quickly. For example, the body is able to adapt remarkably well to a *gradual* blood loss. Individuals with hemorrhoids, slowly bleeding peptic ulcers, or unsuspected gastrointestinal tract cancer may lose up to one-half of their total red blood cell volume *without* experiencing the usual symptoms of anemia. This is because the blood loss is occurring over a prolonged period of time. Under these conditions, the bone marrow is able to increase the production of erythrocytes sufficiently to compensate for the blood loss.

In contrast, the body tends to adapt much less readily to a *sudden,* rapid blood loss. Consequently, persons suffering from sudden hemorrhage due to any number of causes *do* tend to develop anemia, with such symptoms as asthenia (weakness), fatigue, and pallor. If the blood loss has been considerable (1000 ml. or more), it may take 2 months or longer for the body to compensate adequately. Moreover, patients with sudden rapid bleeding may develop signs of shock such as rapid pulse, lowered blood pressure, and restlessness. These signs develop in response to the sudden drop in circulating fluid volume that occurs with hemorrhage. If the body is unable to compensate quickly enough and appropriate medical measures are not taken swiftly, the shock may become irreversible and death may result. *Time* is, thus, an important aspect of adaptation.

8. *Adaptability varies from individual to individual.* Flexible individuals who are readily responsive to change, and who employ a wide range of compensatory mechanisms, are more adaptable than those persons lacking these qualities. Consequently they are more likely to survive stress and change than are rigid individuals.

Although open to many philosophical interpretations, Franz Kafka's story "The Hunger Artist" can be used to illustrate this principle as it applies to an individual life. "The Hunger Artist" centers around a man who practiced, for a livelihood, the highly specialized art of fasting. Living in a time when public fasting was popular, the Hunger Artist was very successful. He fasted while perched atop a pole or in other extreme situations. He was applauded and honored by people everywhere for his performances. Times changed, however, and people lost all interest in the art of fasting. The Hunger Artist, unfortunately, was unable to change with the times. Not only was he too old, but more important, he was too fanatically devoted to fasting to learn another profession. Fasting was the only thing he knew how to do well, and the only way of life he enjoyed. Finally, with no economic means left and deserted by everyone, the Hunger Artist joined a circus where he continued to pursue his art. There, in a cage, virtually unknown and almost completely neglected by the public he had once thrilled, the artist continued to fast day after day until finally he died in total obscurity. To sum up, the Hunger Artist had become extremely specialized and rigid in his response to the environment in which he lived. Consequently when that environment unexpectedly changed, he did not have the flexibility to change with it. As a result he could not adapt and he did not survive.

For the Hunger Artist, the ultimate price of an inability to adapt to change was death. For other individuals, the price of inadequate adaptation may be less drastic. Nevertheless, it may involve such serious problems as the development of mental illness, physical disease, or both.

Physical illness is not always the *result* of failure to adapt. Sometimes physical illnesses may *cause* problems in adaptation. Patients with an incapacitating disease such as a severe heart problem may be called upon suddenly to change their occupation and life-style. Like the Hunger Artist, these changes may be demanded of them at a time in their life when they are most set in their ways and least able to change. Unless these patients are given reassurance and guidance in planning the future, they may not be able to adapt to the new way in which they must live to survive.

9. *Adapation is a process that may make us, at the same time, less sensitive to some stimuli and more sensitive to other stimuli.* For example, when we attend a matinee on a sunny afternoon, entering a darkened theater from the outside, we are at first unable to see at all. Gradually, however, our eyes adapt to the dark and we are able to see fairly well. But while our eyes are becoming adjusted to the dark, they are becoming, at the same time, more sensitive to bright light. Consequently, by the time the show is over, we find that we can see very well inside the darkened theater, but when we go outside we are again temporarily blinded, this time by the light. In sum, exposure to darkness makes us more sensitive to light and vice versa.

10. Hans Selye suggests that *"an essential feature of adaptation is the delimitation of stress to the smallest area capable of meeting the requirements of the situation."*[129] As an example of the principle of delimitation, Selye discusses the inflammatory process.

Inflammation is a local reaction to injury characterized by heat, pain, redness and swelling. This injury may result from the invasion of viruses or bacteria. It may also be caused by irritants and allergens. Inflammation serves the purpose of barricading off infected or irritated areas of tissue from those areas that are healthy. This localization of infection allows white blood cells to deal more effectively with dangerous invading organisms. Localization also prevents a serious infection from spreading throughout the body by way of the blood vessels to cause septicemia (generalized blood poisoning). In sum, then, the inflammatory process is an adaptive mechanism that *limits* a stress to the area capable of dealing with it. This localization of stress spares the individual from widespread trauma.

11. *Adaptive responses may be adequate to meet stress or change and to re-establish homeostatic balance. However, adaptive mechanisms may also be inadequate, excessive, or inappropriate.*

To illustrate, inflammation can, in some instances, serve *adequately* as an adaptive function. By means of connective tissue barriers, inflammation can prevent dangerous organisms from spreading throughout the body. If the inflammatory response to infection is *inadequate*, however, the body may be overwhelmed by the invading organisms. On the other hand, an inflammatory process can be maladaptive because it is *excessive*. If, for example, the irritant to our tissues is *not* a dangerous microbe but a harmless pollen, then inflammation acts as an excessive and *inappropriate* adaptive mechanism. Inflammation, in this case, is not aiding the individual; instead it is creating unnecessary pathologic changes that do not serve any protective purpose.

12. *Even though adaptation helps individuals to adjust to stress and to maintain or establish homeostatic balance, adaptive mechanisms may, in themselves, be stressful.* For instance, inflammation is an adaptive mechanism that can prevent the spread of highly infectious organisms throughout the body. However, the inflammatory process is, in itself, stressful for the individual because it causes certain physiologic changes that result in the symptoms of heat, swelling, redness and pain. These symptoms are uncomfortable and, therefore, are stressful. In striving to achieve homeostatic balance, the individual may sometimes develop imbalances. These imbalances, in turn, will require the use of further compensatory adaptive mechanisms.

THE CONCEPT OF CRISIS

Key Definitions and Concepts

Unlike stress, which continuously permeates our daily lives from birth to death, a crisis is a sporadic phenomenon which punctuates our existence rarely but dramatically. Bircher attempts to define a crisis in general terms:

"What is a crisis?" It is a decisive moment or turning point, a situation in which turns of events and decisions determine whether the results will be for better, or for worse. A crisis is a challenge, an opportunity for learning and growth. It is a subjective experience in which old ways of doing things no longer assure success and survival.

A crisis demands change and reintegration at a level of mastery higher than that previously attained.

If adaptation and mastery are not achieved, the outcome tends to be progressive maladaptation.[19]

Gerald Caplan, an authority in crisis theory, concludes that a crisis develops "when a person faces an obstacle to important life goals, that is, for a time, insurmountable through the utilization of customary methods of problem-solving. A period of disorganization ensues, a period of upset, during which many abortive attempts at solution are made."[3, 33]

Obstacles to life goals which can produce the periods of disorganization and disturbance called crises are exemplified below:

▶ Sudden death of a family member

▶ Severe family discord

▶ Spouse or child abuse

▶ Serious automobile accident

▶ Loss of a limb

▶ Loss of a job with severe financial ramifications

▶ Rape or attempted rape

In each of the critical situations listed above, the individual has suffered an abrupt interruption in the normal routine of his life; i.e., he has experienced a serious upset in his equilibrium and has been thrown off balance. Furthermore, because such traumas as sudden death, limb loss and rape are not everyday events, the person typically has not developed problem-solving methods for dealing with these upsets. Thus, the individual is thrown from his normal "steady state" into a state of crisis or disorganization. During this chaotic period, the frantic individual typically tries to solve his problem through trial and error. If the individual survives the crisis either by solving his problem or by adapting to a non-solution, he may emerge a mentally healthier person who has emotionally "grown" because of his ordeal. On the other hand, the person who does *not* satisfactorily "work through" his dilemma will find it more difficult than ever to deal with future problems. Ultimately, the outcome or resolution of a crisis (for better or for worse) depends upon the individual's perception of his life and upon the resources (family, friends, psychiatrist, minister, etc.) available to him in his environment.

Thus, people in crisis need help of a special nature if they are to cope successfully with their problems. Long-term psychotherapy, which is often prescribed for the chronically stressed individual, is inappropriate for the person undergoing crisis. Patients in crisis need *immediate* counseling. The form of therapy recommended for these persons is called *crisis intervention*. According to Jacobson, crisis intervention may be defined as "activities designed to influence the course of crisis so that a more adaptive outcome will result including the ability to better cope with future crises."[76]

Characteristics of Life Crises

There are seven major characteristics of life crises:

▶ Crisis is a *universal* experience; crises develop among individuals in all races and at all socioeconomic levels.

▶ According to Frederick, all crises have a common element: *"difficulty with significant people* in our lives along with an insecure view of ourselves"[53] (italics added).

▶ A crisis, unlike chronic stress, is usually *time-limited;* it typically is resolved (hopefully successfully) within 4 to 6 weeks.

▶ Almost all crises develop in a *predictable fashion.*

Caplan outlines the *four developmental phases of crisis* as follows: (1) When a serious problem or threat develops, the individual (who has been in a state of relative equilibrium) becomes increasingly tense as he attempts to employ his usual problem-solving techniques. (2) The person grows more upset with each failure of his coping methods and enters a state of disequilibrium. (3) As tensions continue to build, the person mobilizes all possible internal and external resources in an attempt to restore equilibrium. At this stage, the problem may be reevaluated and attacked from a new angle, or the problem may be distorted and viewed as unsolvable. (4) If the problem is not resolved, the internal emotional pressures continue to build, and the individual falls into a state of disorganization and/or immobilization due to his severe anxiety and/or depression.[3, 34]

▶ People in crisis display typical psychologic and physiologic reactions.

Immediate reactions to a critical problem include fear, anxiety, anger, panic, the drive to act, and heightened tension. All these responses are of an *emergency nature;* thus they help a threatened individual or animal to "fight or flee." When a crisis *extends* over a period of time, a person develops the following responses: confusion, depression, immobilization and a breakdown of the ability to make decisions. These responses are *not* helpful, and in fact, prevent him from satisfactorily resolving his problem.

▶ Crises tend to occur in *cycles,* with one crisis following another.

For example, a man who has been involved in a serious automobile accident usually must be hospitalized. If hospitalization is extensive, he may lose his job at the very time he needs additional money to pay hospital bills. If he is married, his wife may be forced to work or moonlight on a second job, thereby leaving the children unattended. As a consequence, the children may develop serious behavioral problems at school and at home, and so forth. Thus, as the old saying goes, "troubles never come singly."

▶ People undergoing crisis are highly *susceptible to the influence of other persons* in their environment; thus these patients are usually quite responsive to crisis intervention techniques.

Coping with Potential Crises

Personal problems, no matter how serious, *do not* have to culminate in a crisis; crises are preventable. According to Aguilera, whether or not a person with a problem will go into crisis depends upon the following three balancing factors: (1) the individual's *perception of the problem* or event, (2) available *situational supports,* and (3) *coping mechanisms* (see Fig. 5–2).[3]

Note in Figure 5–2 that if a person undergoing a stressful event perceives his situation realistically and has adequate situational support (e.g., family or friends with whom he can discuss the problem) and adequate coping mechanisms (e.g., ways of reducing tension by expressing anger, frustration, etc.), he will resolve his problem, regain his balance and avert a crisis. On the other hand, if one or more balancing factors are missing, the problem will not be resolved, balance will not be regained, and a crisis will develop.

For example, consider the two students, John and Bill, whom we discussed earlier. As you recall, for John, exam week was a stressful event, but taking exams did not force him into a

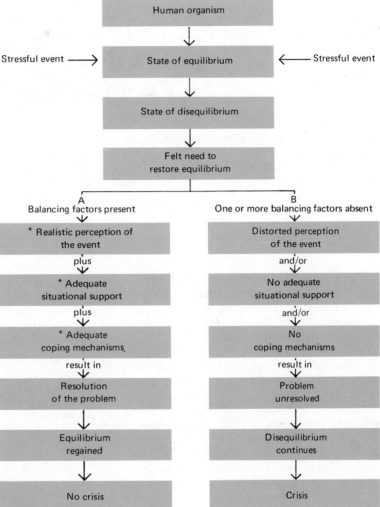

Figure 5–2. Paradigm: effect of balancing factors in a stressful event. (From Aguilera, D. C., et al.: *Crisis Intervention: Theory and Methodology.* St. Louis, The C. V. Mosby Co., 1970, p. 52.)

Human organism

Stressful event ⟶ State of equilibrium ⟵ Stressful event

State of disequilibrium

Felt need to restore equilibrium

A
Balancing factors present

B
One or more balancing factors absent

* Realistic perception of the event

plus

* Adequate situational support

plus

* Adequate coping mechanisms

result in

Resolution of the problem

Equilibrium regained

No crisis

Distorted perception of the event

and/or

No adequate situational support

and/or

No coping mechanisms

result in

Problem unresolved

Disequilibrium continues

Crisis

*Balancing factors.

state of crisis. A crisis was averted because John perceived his situation realistically, he had good situational supports (teachers, friends) and he used adequate coping mechanisms (sought help when needed, lessened pressures at work and in his social life). The other student, Bill, tended to see exam week in a distorted fashion, and exaggerated its importance to the point of being immobilized by anxiety. He did not use the situational supports available (friends, teachers); also, he utilized inappropriate defense mechanisms (denial, projection of hostility onto teachers, illness) instead of coping mechanisms. As a result, he felt increasingly disorganized and emotionally unbalanced and finally entered a state of crisis.

BIBLIOGRAPHY

The references for Chapters 5 to 7 will be found at the end of Unit II, p. 114.

CHAPTER 6

THE STRUGGLE TO MAINTAIN A STATE OF BALANCE

The process by which we living beings resist the general stream of corruption and decay is known as homeostasis. We can continue to live in the very special environment which we carry forward with us until we begin to decay more quickly than we can reconstitute ourselves.

NORBERT WEINER[157]

For generations scientists believed that constancy and stability were fundamental characteristics of life. Today, we recognize that the essence of life is change and instability. Thus, for a living organism to preserve its life it must be able to (1) adapt satisfactorily to change and (2) maintain internal stability in the face of a variable and stressful environment. The need to maintain some stability amid constant environmental changes has forced living organisms, over eons of time, to develop certain techniques for *automatically* maintaining balance despite constant threats to their equilibrium. Those self-regulatory techniques that preserve an organism's ability to adapt to stresses and yet to maintain its inner balance are called *homeostatic mechanisms*. A vital form of adaptations, homeostatic mechanisms operate at all levels of life, regulating biologic functioning and counteracting change and imbalance.

HISTORICAL PERSPECTIVES

Although the scientific study of homeostatic regulation is comparatively new, the concept of the need for physiologic balance has existed for centuries. Hippocrates, the father of medicine, conceived of health as the result of a balance or harmony between individuals and their environment. The French physiologist, Claude Bernard, around the middle of the 19th century, wrote of the *"milieu interne"* (internal milieu). He believed that life and health depended upon the constancy and stability of the circulat-ing fluids of the body. In 1939 Cannon created the term *homeostasis* from the Greek words *homoios*, meaning "like," and *stasis*, meaning "standing." In his classic text, *The Wisdom of the Body*, Cannon wrote:

The constant conditions which are maintained in the body might be termed *equilibria*. That word, however, has come to have fairly exact meaning as applied to relatively simple physio-chemical states, in closed systems, where known forces are balanced. The coordinated physiological processes which maintain most of the steady states in the organism are so complex and so peculiar to living things—involving as they may, the brain and nerves, the heart, lungs, kidneys and spleen, all working cooperatively—that I have suggested a special designation for these states, *homeostasis*. The word does not imply something set and immobile, a stagnation. It means a condition—a condition which may vary, but which is relatively constant.[32]

Cannon conceived of homeostasis as a type of *dynamic* equilibrium as opposed to a static condition. His use of the term "homeostasis" applied mainly to the self-regulation of such internal physiologic processes as the following:
body temperature
blood pressure
blood sugar concentration
water balance
electrolyte balance
muscle tone
blood oxygen level
blood carbon dioxide level
Norbert Weiner later expanded the concept of homeostasis and helped develop the science

of *cybernetics;* also, he introduced the concept of feedback. *Cybernetics* is defined as "the science of the processes of communication and control in the animal and in the machine." *Feedback* basically involves reinserting (or feeding back) into an organism or a machine the results of its past performance in order to control its present and future performance. Weiner wrote of feedback in relation to homeostasis in his book *Cybernetics.* He states:

A great group of cases in which some sort of feedback is not only exemplified in physiological phenomena but is absolutely essential for the continuation of life is found in what is known as homeostasis.

The conditions under which life, especially healthy life, can continue in the higher animals are quite narrow. A variation of one-half degree centigrade in the body temperature is generally a sign of illness, and a permanent variation of five degrees is scarcely consistent with life. The osmotic pressure of the blood and its hydrogen-ion concentration must be held within strict limits. . . . In short, our inner economy must contain an assembly of thermostats, automatic hydrogen-ion-concentration controls, governors, and the like, which would be adequate for a great chemical plant. These are what we know collectively as our homeostatic mechanism.[156]

Today the concept of homeostasis has far wider applications than simply to physiologic processes. Currently, homeostasis is being used to explain perceptual and cognitive processes, activities leading to the satisfaction of basic needs, instinctive reactions, and even intellectual and creative behavior. Also, the concept of feedback is being employed in developing biofeedback techniques for the control of various physiologic functions (discussed later in this chapter).

Moreover, homeostatic principles have been applied to such diversified fields as genetics; growth; human, plant and animal ecology; psychiatry; and engineering. In industry, the basic concept of homeostasis has been used in the creation of such self-regulating devices as automatic airplane pilots, missile guidance systems, computers and servomechanisms* for industrial automation. Although it is true that human technology has been able to produce very sophisticated self-regulating devices, these manmade mechanisms cannot begin to rival the biologic systems in complexity or in precision.

Thus, the concept of homeostasis has, in itself, adapted to changing environmental demands. Once thought of as simply the regulation of steady states in mammals, the term has now been expanded to include any self-regulating system aiding survival.

---

*This term is discussed on page 86.

BASIC CHARACTERISTICS OF HOMEOSTATIC MECHANISMS*

All homeostatic devices tend to be characterized by certain distinctive traits. In the following discussion of homeostatic mechanisms, these distinguishing characteristics are boxed.

> *Homeostatic devices are compensatory in nature.*

In other words, homeostatic devices help to counterbalance any variation from those conditions that are most normal and optimal for the individual. Adjustments in the pH and glucose levels of the blood, body fluid and electrolyte levels, and body temperature as well as the compensatory growth of tissues and proliferation of cells all provide examples of homeostatic *compensatory mechanisms.* Let us briefly discuss two of these examples: temperature regulation and compensatory growth.

Temperature Regulation.† As discussed earlier, a stable body temperature is vital for organisms that live in constantly changing climatic environments. For instance, normally body temperature registers at 37°C. (98.6°F.). If we walk from a warm house into icy weather, body temperature remains at 37°C. instead of dropping to the low temperature outdoors. This remarkable stability of our body temperature is the result of certain *compensatory mechanisms:* specifically, vasoconstriction of our peripheral arteries and arterioles; pilomotor action resulting in "goose flesh"; increased muscular activity; and shivering.

Conversely, if we walk from an airconditioned house out into a desert-like climate, our body temperature does not rise in response to this hot environment. Instead body temperature again tends to remain fairly steady at 37°C. This stability is the result of the action of certain other *compensatory mechanisms:* namely, an increased circulation of blood to the peripheral blood vessels; increased sweating, which leads to cooling; and an increase in thirst and water intake, which pre-

---

*For information concerning the characteristics of homeostasis, the authors have relied especially on the work of Thomas Overmire.[111]

†Temperature regulation is discussed in detail in Chapter 28.

vents dehydration. As a result of these mechanisms for stabilizing temperature, we are able to adapt to changing climates while still retaining our internal equilibrium.

Compensatory Growth. The proliferation of cells and the enlargement, or hypertrophy, of organs and tissues provide further illustrations of the compensatory nature of homeostasis. For example, red blood cell levels rise in response to increased demands for oxygen; muscles hypertrophy or enlarge when additional demands are made upon them by exercise or stress; and the spleen and lymphatic organs increase in size when the body is invaded by infectious organisms. Moreover, when an organ such as a kidney is severely damaged or removed, the remaining kidney increases in size so that it is able to do the work of both kidneys. Finally, if the heart, for any reason, should begin to fail as a circulatory pump, the left ventricle of the heart enlarges, or hypertrophies, in order to pump out more blood into the arteries, thus *compensating* for the breakdown in circulatory function.

In summary, homeostatic mechanisms preserve the integrity of the body by counterbalancing stress and compensating for change.

> *Homeostatic mechanisms are self-regulatory.*

In other words, homeostatic devices *automatically* attempt to correct any deviation from what is characteristically normal function for the individual. It is fortunate for us as human beings that this is so. As Cannon expressed it:

Without homeostatic devices we should be in constant danger of disaster, unless we were always on the alert to correct voluntarily what normally is corrected automatically. With homeostatic devices, however, that keep essential bodily processes steady, we as individuals are free from such slavery—free to enter into agreeable relations with our fellows, free to enjoy beautiful things, to explore and understand the wonders of the world about us, to develop new ideas and interests, and to work and play, untrammeled by anxieties concerning our bodily affairs.[32]

Homeostasis, then, provides us with the opportunity for a creative life rather than a bare existence continually centered around the problems of *consciously* adapting to changes, both large and small.

Of course, it is only the healthy individual who enjoys the privilege of a body that is essentially self-regulating. When severe illness strikes, physiologic homeostatic mechanisms tend to break down and to lose their automaticity. It is at this point that doctors, nurses and other medical personnel attempt to regulate those functions that are normally self-adjusting, using such technologic devices as intravenous fluids, hypothermia, and so forth.

> *Homeostatic systems tend to be negative feedback systems.*

The main objective of a homeostatic mechanism is to minimize the difference between how a system *should* behave ideally and how it *is* behaving in reality. *Feedback* is the mechanism that enables the system to sense to what degree it is deviating from the set norm and to make the necessary adjustments to correct the deviation.

There are two major types of feedback: *negative* feedback and *positive* feedback. *Almost all*

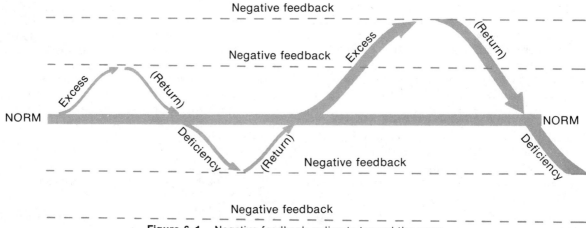

Figure 6–1. Negative feedback redirects toward the norm.

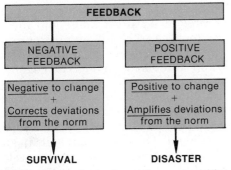

Figure 6–2. Comparison of negative and positive feedback mechanisms.

biologic systems are controlled by negative feedback rather than by positive feedback. This is because a *negative* feedback system always leads the organism *back* to a state that is optimum for it. In other words, it *negates* and attempts to correct any radical change from the norm either toward excess or toward a deficiency. This point is explained diagrammatically in Figure 6–1.

Positive feedback systems, on the other hand, tend to lead the organism consistently *away* from the normal state. The original error, rather than being corrected, is repeated again and again, thus compounding the problem. Consequently, death or some other disaster results unless, at some point, the positive feedback is corrected or controlled by negative feedback. The essential difference between the two systems is shown diagrammatically in Figure 6–2.

How Negative Feedback Works

As stated earlier, negative feedback controls almost all biologic systems. To comprehend how a system of negative feedback operates within the body, it is helpful to first use a mechanical or electrical *model* for purposes of explanation. (Models are frequently used to explain biologic phenomena.) A model in this sense can be defined as a replica of a relationship or group of events, used to clarify a complex phenomenon, and expressed in a mathematical form or by means of mechanical or electrical apparatus.

Although mechanical models can be helpful, they can also be misleading because they tend to *greatly oversimplify* the biologic activities and processes that they represent. Models serve only to provide us with a way of explaining complex phenomena; *they do not duplicate the physiologic phenomena themselves.* The ideas expressed by feedback mechanisms thus provide us with a way of thinking about the control of physiologic mechanisms, but they do not actually present distinct physiologic processes.

There are two major types of negative feedback mechanisms: *thermostat-like* mechanisms and *continually fluctuating* mechanisms. We shall first consider the thermostat-like regulator.

Thermostat-like Mechanisms. Thermostat-like regulators are distinguished by two features: First, these mechanisms operate by correcting deviations from a definite *predetermined goal* or "setting." Second, they operate intermittently rather than continuously, turning off and on as needed to correct errors. Thus, whenever an error is signaled, the system is triggered toward that activity which will return it to its normal range of function.

One obvious example of this type of regulator is the thermostat that controls the heating within homes. Let us say that you have set the thermostat at 22°C. (72°F.), but the temperature of the house itself registers only 18°C. (65°F.). A small deviation from the goal is allowable, but if the deviation becomes too great, the system is triggered into action. Once the heat turns on, the temperature in the house may increase to as much as 23 or 24°C. (74 or 75°F.), i.e., the deviation will now be in excess of the goal. One can readily detect the error of overheating by comparing the actual temperature of the house and the thermostat setting. The furnace will then shut off until the house again becomes too cool. If the system is working properly, the house will remain at approximately the same temperature indefinitely despite weather conditions outside.

A second example of "stat" regulation is the *temperature control system within the body.* In this case the thermostat that controls temperature stability is located within the hypothalamus, a vital structure found at the base of the brain. Operating by means of negative feedback, the thermostat control in the hypothalamus keeps the body temperature fairly steady at 37°C. (98.6°F.) despite environmental conditions. When a temperature elevation does occur, with resulting signs of fever, or when the temperature is subnormal, it is believed that the *goal* or *reference level* has been changed in some way. For instance, as we might accidentally set the thermostat within our homes incorrectly, the reference level within our hypothalamus may become altered by disease or accident. As a result, there is a corresponding alteration in body temperature.

A third illustration of "stat" control is the *regulation of food intake*. Physiologists now believe that there is an "appestat" (or appetite-regulating center), which is also located in the hypothalamus. This structure contains two groups of cells with different functions. One group of cells constitutes the "feeding center," which causes us to want to eat. The other group of cells makes up the "satiety center," which signals us to stop eating when we have consumed a sufficient amount of food. Physiologists suggest that appetite regulation is a typical negative feedback system. They theorize that such factors as blood sugar concentration, hormones, changes in fat reserve levels, and psychologic factors possibly provide the signals that activate the feedback system. Variables such as body structure, state of health, psychologic make-up, and activity determine the *goal*. Appetite acts as a type of *error signal* that "turns on" when the individual has not consumed sufficient food to meet his needs. The *response* is that the individual continues to eat until he becomes satiated. His appetite then "shuts off," until the sensor is again activated. Physiologists now postulate that if any component of the feedback system is not working properly, appetite does not "shut off" and the person, as a result, overeats; eventually, *obesity* develops.

The *control of blood sugar levels* provides a final illustration of thermostat-like regulation. The *normal limits* for blood glucose are from 80 to 100 mg./100 ml. If we eat a substantial breakfast, our blood sugar will rise very rapidly until it passes the upper limits of normal. At this point there is, of course, a discrepancy between the *normal* blood sugar range and the *actual* glucose level. As a result, an error is signaled, and the excess glucose is removed from the blood and stored in the liver as glycogen. As the day proceeds, however, we may, as a result of activity and metabolic demands, use up a large percentage of our circulating blood sugar. Consequently, the level of glucose may drop below 80 mg./100 ml. This, in turn, results in an *error signal,* and the glycogen that has been stored is reconverted to sugar. This reconversion, in turn, raises the blood glucose level till it is again within a safe and normal range.

Continually Fluctuating Mechanisms. A second type of negative feedback control system is the *continually fluctuating mechanism* (or *servomechanism*). This system differs from the "stat" type of regulator in two ways: First, the *goal* or reference point is *continually fluctuating*, and second, the *system is in continuous operation* rather than shutting off and on (see Fig. 6–3).

The control of hormonal levels within the body provides an illustration of this type of feedback. For example, let us consider the interrelationship between the adenohypophysis (anterior lobe of the pituitary gland) and the adrenal glands. The adenohypophysis secretes a hormone called adrenocorticotropic hormone (ACTH). When the ACTH level rises in the blood, the adrenal glands are stimulated to release hormones called glucocorticoids. However, when the blood level of glucocorticoids rises too high, the adenohypophysis is signaled by means of negative feedback to *inhibit* its release of ACTH. As a result, the blood level of ACTH drops and, consequently, so does the blood level of glucocorticoids. Eventually, the glucocorticoid level drops so low that again the adenohypophysis is stimulated to release ACTH which, in turn, raises the level of

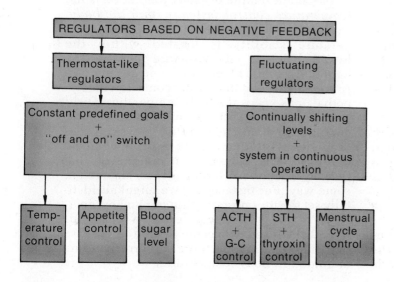

Figure 6–3. Types of regulators based on negative feedback.

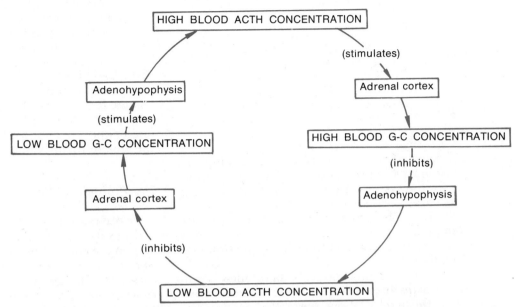

Figure 6–4. Control of ACTH secretion by the adenohypophysis—a feedback mechanism and also a homeostatic mechanism.

glucocorticoids, and so forth. This process is illustrated in Figure 6–4.

Similar examples of feedback controls that involve endocrine balance are found in the relationship between the adenohypophysis and the thyroid gland as well as in the complex hormonal control involved in the menstrual cycle.

> *The regulation of a single physiologic process may require the operation of multiple homeostatic negative feedback systems.*

In the examples given thus far, homeostatic regulation for a particular variable (temperature, appetite, etc.) has apparently been controlled by *one* negative feedback system. It is important, however, to realize that some variables (for example, blood pressure) may be under the control of *several* different feedback systems, which must *all* function so that they complement each other.

Deviation and Error

> *Some degree of deviation or error exists in all homeostatic systems.*

The concept of homeostatic balance essentially represents an ideal. Actually in every self-regulating system there is *always* some degree of deviation from what is optimum or normal for that system. As Overmire states, "Homeostatic regulators can never be expected to function perfectly, since control is achieved only through adjustment of error."[111]

When an error is signaled in a homeostatic system, several problems may result, including the following:

1. A considerable *time lag* may be present between the moment the error is discovered and the moment corrective action is started.

2. As a result of this time lag, the system may attempt to overcompensate for the error and what is called an *overshoot* will take place.

3. This overshoot, in itself, is an error. Consequently a new time lag and another overshoot in the *opposite** direction will then result.

4. These overshoots in opposite directions create fluctuations *(oscillations)*, or *hunting*, as the system attempts to correct itself and return to normal.

5. If the oscillations or overshoots *increase in magnitude,* then a condition of *unstable os-*

---

*Note the difference between overshoots and positive feedback. Positive feedback, as we said earlier, goes continually *out* from the norm. Overshoots move back and forth around the norm.

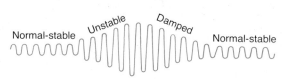

Figure 6–5. Types of oscillations.

cillations develops. This is a problem, and these unstable oscillations may result in disaster for the system. Another term for disaster, in this case, is *runaway.*

6. If, on the other hand, the oscillations are *damped,* or they *decrease in magnitude,* then the system can return to normal function (see Fig. 6–5).

Within the human body, homeostatic systems are *always* oscillating to some degree. However, these oscillations normally occur within *very narrow limits.* If the oscillations become too great, the continued existence of the individual is severely threatened.

As an example of oscillations in a negative feedback system, consider the control of arterial blood pressure. If, for some reason, arterial blood pressure begins to fall, an error is signaled. In response to this signal, and as a result of various physiologic mechanisms, the blood pressure will begin to rise. However, the effect of the mechanism activated by the error signal to raise the blood pressure will persist until the pressure increases not only to the point considered normal but *beyond* that point; the blood pressure then becomes too high, and another error is signaled. A new set of responses to this "too-high" error signal then acts to lower the blood pressure, but again, the effect of the activity will persist beyond the "normal" point, the blood pressure will become too low, and still another error will be signaled.

Under these conditions, the blood pressure continues to *oscillate* or *overshoot* between high and low extremes. If the oscillations become too wild and unstable, the system may be driven to disaster. Fortunately, however, oscillations within the human body are readily *damped;* i.e., they decrease in size as a result of various compensatory physiologic reactions. Consequently, unstable blood pressure oscillations will most likely be damped. This means that the blood pressure either will return to the reading that preceded the upset or will become readjusted at a different reading.

To summarize, some overshoots are un-avoidable in any homeostatic system, because all homeostatic systems are continually adjusting to new strains and new disturbances. Adjustment of homeostatic mechanisms is the result of various compensatory reactions that develop in response to change or stress. If a homeostatic system is not too badly disturbed by a stressor, it will very likely return to its former status. However, if a system is severely disturbed, it may either break down entirely or go on to a completely new "steady state," a change that may not be reversible. In the latter case, the system *will* stabilize, but it will no longer operate at the same level as it did prior to the severe disturbance.

The Problem of Positive Feedback

Positive feedback develops when a product of the system exerts a stimulating effect on a key step in the control mechanism, causing the output or responses of the system to *increase continuously.* In other words, there is a continuous *reinforcing of the original error,* resulting in a *runaway* of the system. When this happens, negative feedback mechanisms break down; positive feedback causes an uncontrolled, constantly increasing deviation from the norm; and a vicious circle results, leading to *disaster and death* for the individual (see Fig. 6–6).

As an example of the dangers of positive feedback, consider the patient suffering from a sudden severe hemorrhage. As a result of blood loss, this person first experiences a severe drop in arterial blood pressure. The drop in blood pressure diminishes the flow of blood to the heart muscle, and as a result the heart beat is greatly weakened. This weakness, in turn, leads to even less blood being pumped to the arterial system. Consequently, the blood pressure drops still lower and even less blood is returned to the heart. As a result, the heart beat is further weakened, and so on. This vicious circle, unless stopped, will be repeated until finally the patient dies.

If, on the other hand, the patient receives medical and nursing care before his blood loss becomes too great, his body's negative feedback mechanisms will continue to operate. As a result, compensatory mechanisms involving blood pressure, the arterial system, and the heart beat will overbalance the positive feedback. A vicious circle will not occur, and the patient will live.

This example illustrates how valuable a knowledge of feedback can be to the nurse. Although the theory of homeostasis is initially somewhat complex, once the student familiarizes herself with it she will see daily implications for its use in nursing care.

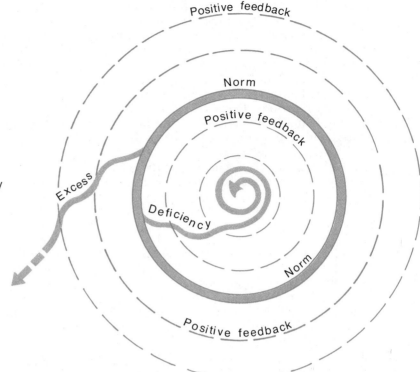

Figure 6–6. Positive feedback constantly leads away from the norm.

The Concept of Feedforward

Functioning organisms, in their struggle to maintain equilibrium, utilize not only feedback processes but "feedforward" processes as well. As we have seen, *feedback processes* are *goal-directed* and *self-correcting* in nature. Correction of error principally depends upon information that is gathered from the environment and is fed back into the machine or organism. On the other hand, *feedforward processes* are *predetermined* and *automatic* patterns of response to certain stimuli. Feedforward controls are either *genetic* in nature (e.g., protective neuromuscular reflexes such as pulling one's hand away from a hot stove) or they have been established by repetitive training of the organism over time. Organisms combine both feedback and feedforward mechanisms for smooth functioning.[123]

LIMITATIONS OF HOMEOSTATIC SYSTEMS

It is essential to recognize that self-regulating homeostatic mechanisms, however complex and sophisticated, have definite limitations. Extreme stress, reduction in adaptive energy, or damage to any part of the system will lead to either of the following consequences: (1) a *continued* but *inadequate* performance of the mechanism, leading eventually to an *overdriven system*, or (2) the complete *breakdown of negative feedback control*, leading rapidly to disaster and death.

A breakdown in a homeostatic mechanism which may lead to an overdriven system and the possibility of eventual death can be illustrated by again considering the regulation of blood sugar in the body. You will recall that in our discussion of normal blood sugar regulation, we stated that blood sugar must remain within certain clearly defined limits. We also stated that if the blood sugar exceeds these limits, glucose is then converted to glycogen and stored in the liver to be reconverted to glucose as needed. However, the smooth operation of this homeostatic mechanism depends upon a pancreatic hormone called *insulin*.

When an insulin *deficiency* exists, two things happen. First, sugar is not oxidized and utilized properly, and second, excess glucose cannot be converted to glycogen. These pathologic changes result in the individual's excreting large amounts of excess sugar in the urine. The abnormal excretion of sugar, in turn, leads to such compensatory mechanisms as a "craving for sweets," an increased urinary output, thirst, and so forth. This person (who has developed the condition of *diabetes mellitus*) can survive for a while by means of these inadequate compensatory reactions. However, if his condition is not eventually diagnosed so that he can be treated with a proper diet and with insulin, his system will become overdriven. As a result, he will suffer irreparable damage to his body organs, and without treatment he will eventually die.

The second limitation of homeostatic systems (more rapid breakdown of negative feedback control) is exemplified by the hemorrhaging patient who continues to lose blood rapidly. At first, this patient's peripheral blood vessels will constrict, his blood pressure will oscillate for a while, and his heart, though weak, will beat very rapidly in order to compensate for the blood loss. Eventually, however, if this patient continues to bleed, negative feedback will totally break down. The patient's blood pressure will fall precipitously; his heart beat will become very weak and then will stop entirely; his respirations will cease; and he will expire. The final evidence, then, that homeostatic mechanisms have limitations, and can fail, is death.

HOMEOSTASIS: THEORETICAL AND CLINICAL CONSIDERATIONS

Some of the most exciting scientific advances made in recent years are based upon the concepts of: (a) homeostatic balance; (b) the rhythmic oscillating quality of living things; and (c) feedback control of physiologic and behavioral processes. We will discuss two important new areas of research which have arisen from these concepts and which carry vital implications for the health and welfare of people now and in the future. The first area is concerned with the biologic rhythms that regulate both the body and behavior. The second section discusses the relatively new area of biofeedback theory and training.

Biologic Rhythms (Chronobiology)

THE RHYTHMIC NATURE OF LIVING SYSTEMS

Most scientists agree that living organisms, in order to adapt to a changing environment, have evolved as *oscillating* systems that fluctuate in a rhythmic fashion.[122] Clearly, living things at all levels of the plant and animal kingdoms are controlled by daily physiologic and behavioral rhythms, e.g., activity-inactivity cycles, sleep-wakefulness cycles, changes in body temperature. Rhythmic cycles appear to be initiated and sustained within the organism by innate internal timers called *biologic clocks*. The recently developed science of biologic clocks and their effects on living systems is named *chronobiology* (based on the Greek word *chronos*, meaning "time").

Biologic clocks play a vital role in regulating both the physiology and the social lives of all animals. The basic function of these clocks is to help the organism to adjust constantly to its surrounding physical environment (e.g., rhythmic change in light and/or barometric pressure) as well as to changes in social routines (e.g., bird migrations, jet travel, changes in work shifts).

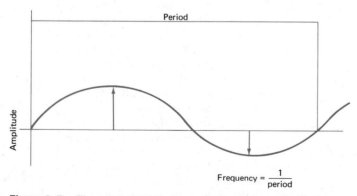

Figure 6–7. The relationship between the period, amplitude, and frequency of a cycle. (From Luce, G. G.: *Body Time: Physiological Rhythms and Social Stress.* New York, Bantam Books, 1973, p. 29.)

TABLE 6–1. BASIC TERMS USED IN DESCRIBING RHYTHMS

TERM	DEFINITION
Cycle	An event which repeats itself at predictable intervals, e.g., the menstrual cycle
Period	The interval of time it takes for a cycle to repeat itself, e.g., around 24 hours, 1 month
Frequency	The number of times a cycle repeats itself within a time interval, e.g., the menstrual cycle occurs at a frequency of approximately once every 28 days
Amplitude	The largeness, fullness or extent of a rhythm; e.g., the daily variance in degrees of an individual's body temperature (temperature variance may range from as little as 1.5 to 2.1 degrees)

The various clocks that operate within the body are set to regulate rhythmic cycles of various periods of time, frequencies and amplitudes. For definitions and an illustration of these terms, see Table 6–1 and Figure 6–7.

There are several types of rhythmic cycles. One set of rhythms are called *circadian rhythms.* The word circadian was derived from the Latin words *circa* (around) and *dies* (day). Thus, a circadian rhythm is a cycle which occurs at intervals of *around 24 hours*—i.e., the rhythm is slightly longer or shorter than 24 hours.

Cycles occurring at intervals that are *shorter* than 24 hours are called *ultradian* rhythms. For instance, the nerve action potential has a period of 1 millisecond. Brain wave rhythms and certain enzyme rhythms are also extremely rapid, occurring in microseconds.

At the other end of the scale, rhythms with *longer* cycles than circadian rhythms are called *infradian* rhythms. One example of an infradian rhythm is the menstrual cycle, which occurs in women every 28 days or so. Certain rhythms of migration and hibernation have a period of a year. Some scientists now believe that the whole process of aging may be basically an extended rhythm.[17]

While our various physiologic rhythms adhere to basic time schedules, the period and amplitude of each rhythm varies somewhat from individual to individual. For instance, one woman may have her menstrual period every 24 days and she may experience a heavy menstrual flow. Another woman's menstrual period may appear every 32 days and her menstrual flow may be light.

The importance of biologic rhythms to the smooth functioning of our daily lives has only recently been recognized. In the next section, we will briefly consider some of the most basic rhythms, their interrelationships, and their possible origins. Because a patient's circadian rhythms should be an important factor in planning his daily care, we will focus primarily upon this type of rhythm.

CIRCADIAN RHYTHMS IN MAN

There are many different circadian rhythms that regulate our physiologic functioning, rest and activity schedules, health, and susceptibility to disease. Some of the most important rhythms (from the standpoint of planning patient care) are as follows:

Sleep-Wakefulness Rhythms. Most living organisms experience alternating periods of relative activity and inactivity—sleep and wakefulness. These contrasting states reflect the catabolic and anabolic phases that underlie the

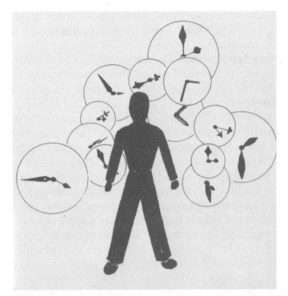

Figure 6–8. Daily rhythms. (From Ward, R. R.: *The Living Clocks.* New York, New American Library—Mentor Books, 1971, p. 325.)

rhythm of proper metabolic function.[46] During *catabolic* periods (wakefulness), food compounds are broken down into simpler compounds and energy is expended. During the *anabolic* state (sleep), more complex compounds (hormones, protoplasm) are synthesized from simpler compounds; and repair, renewal and growth of the organism are fostered. Sleep-wakefulness patterns have apparently arisen from a family and social life that developed on the basis of light/darkness, night/day alterations. Also, sleep-wakefulness patterns seem to arise from neural and endocrine mechanisms. When sleep-wakefulness rhythms are disrupted (as is often the case on a hospital ward), the waking mood of the individual suffers, and psychomotor performance deteriorates. Apparently, disruption of an established sleep-wakefulness rhythm has a more detrimental effect on the individual than does a decrease in the total number of hours of sleep.[17, 42, 86]

Performance Rhythms. The ability to perform tasks requiring muscular coordination, mental acuity, strength, timing and vigilance is greater at certain times within a 24-hour period than at other times.[97] For example, the athlete who performs skillfully in the ballpark at 3 o'clock in the afternoon would find it difficult, if not impossible, to give the same performance at 3 o'clock in the morning! Also, his viewers might find it difficult to cheer very enthusiastically at such an hour.

Body Temperature Rhythms. * The body temperature of human beings alternately rises and drops by approximately 2 degrees over each 24-hour period. This cycle occurs daily despite the individual's life-style, sleeping and activity patterns, and eating habits. Note in Figure 6–9 that body temperature begins to drop at night, is lowest upon waking, gradually rises during the morning, levels off somewhat in the afternoon and then drops again in the evening. This small change of around 2 degrees in temperature has an important effect on metabolic and physiologic functions as well as upon performance levels. For example, "morning people" (individuals who function best early in the day) experience an earlier rise in body temperature than do "night people" (individuals who function most efficiently late in the day). The biologic clock that controls the circadian rhythm of body temperature may possibly be located in the hypothalamus.[150]

---

*The circadian rhythm associated with body temperature is also discussed in Chapter 28.

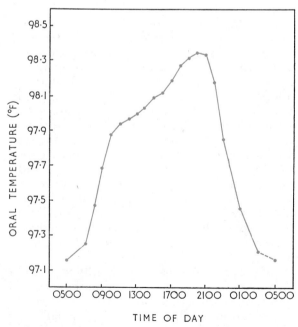

Figure 6–9. Rhythm of oral temperature in a group of 70 males. (From Colquhoun, W. P. (ed.): *Biological Rhythms and Human Performance.* New York, Academic Press, 1971.)

Hormone and Enzyme Rhythms. The concentration of adrenocortical hormones (released by the adrenal cortex) in the serum may vary more than fourfold over a 24-hour period; this same variance is true for many enzymes of the liver and serum. The level of adrenocortical hormone secretion appears to be correlated with (a) an individual's state of *alertness* and *wakefulness* and (b) *body temperature* rhythms. Thus, the level of hormones of the adrenal cortex rises early in the morning while we normally sleep, peaks around the time we typically awaken in the morning, and then drops to a low point by late evening when we usually feel fatigued. Note that this cycle is similar to the cyclic changes in body temperature mentioned above.

Levels of adrenocortical hormones are also inversely related to *taste* and *smell* sensitivity. Thus, when circulating levels of these hormones fall at the end of a day, the individual's senses of taste and smell sharpen, and consequently his appreciation of food increases. This fact may explain why most of us enjoy a hearty evening meal and spurn the substantial breakfast advocated by many nutritionists.[150]

Urine Flow. Urine is secreted in a circadian rhythm with urine output being greatest in the morning and at midday and least during the night. This rhythmic pattern holds true even when the individual is drinking fluids around the clock. Moreover, the excretion of *sodium* and *potassium* in the urine follows a circadian rhythm, with the greatest amount of these electrolytes being excreted around midday and during the afternoon[97] (see also Chap. 24).

Cell Division Rhythms. The rate of replacement of tissue cells roughly approximates the rate of cell damage and erosion. However, cell division is more rapid during certain hours of a 24-hour period than at others. For example, the division of skin cells, which require constant replacement, occurs primarily during our deepest hours of sleep—roughly between midnight and 4 AM. It is possible that this nightly period of cellular renewal is one of the outstanding functions of sleep.[97, 122]

RHYTHM SYNCHRONIZERS

The two major sets of factors that help to synchronize an individual's internal circadian rhythms with the world around him are (1) environmental factors arising from the earth's rotation on its axis and (2) social factors.

Environmental factors include such predictable phenomena as sunrise, sunset and moonrise. It is in response to these physical clues of alternating light and darkness that we set our watches and develop our sleep and activity schedules. While environmental clues do not govern our circadian rhythms, they can reset the timing of our rhythm. For example, if a person flies to a country halfway around the world, he will have to adjust to a new pattern of light and darkness, and thus his internal rhythms will reset themselves to synchronize with the clock time in the new country.

Social factors include the hours of jobs (the shift we work), classes, family routines and social events. For human beings, social and work routines are apparently more powerful synchronizers than are environmental factors. On the other hand, the rhythms of birds and animals are more tuned to light-darkness alterations than to social factors.

THE ORIGIN OF CIRCADIAN RHYTHMS

What is the fundamental nature of circadian rhythms? Where do they originate? How are they controlled and what factors control them? To these questions there are as yet no answers. However, scientists have advanced two opposing theories, each of which purports to explain rhythmic phenomena. These theories are the endogenous-clock hypothesis and the exogenous-clock hypothesis.

The *endogenous-clock theory* primarily advocated by Colin Pittendrigh, states that body rhythms are generated and controlled by *independent internal timepieces* (i.e., biologic clocks), which are located *within* the organism. Furthermore, even though these pacemakers are influenced by external clues from the environment, they *do not* depend on these clues for their operation. For example, an organism's circadian rhythms persist even under laboratory conditions in which periods of light and dark and humidity and temperature settings are carefully controlled. This hypothesis, then, compares the biologic clock to "a self-winding wristwatch with a built-in timer."[150]

On the other hand, the *exogenous clock theory,* advocated by Dr. F. A. Brown, proposes that our circadian rhythms are dependent for their operation upon *geophysical forces external* to the organism; e.g., electrostatic, electromagnetic, magnetic and gravitational fields and cosmic rays. Thus, in this viewpoint, a biologic clock can be compared to an electric clock that must be plugged into an electrical outlet to function. Because of the impossibility of isolating the particular geophysical forces responsible for each body rhythm, Brown's theory (sometimes called the "cosmic theory") is difficult to prove or disprove.[150]

THE DISRUPTION OF CIRCADIAN RHYTHMS

Physiologic rhythms can be disrupted by (1) physiologic and emotional changes and (2) time changes. The *physiologic* and *emotional* changes that disrupt biologic rhythms are as follows:

▶ Physical or mental illness; e.g., high fevers, manic-depressive psychosis

▶ Drugs and toxins; e.g., barbiturates

▶ Immobilization and isolation; e.g., patients who are immobilized, placed in isolation because of a communicable disease, or treated in intensive care units may experience serious disturbances of body rhythms similar to those affecting astronauts in space. Concerning this problem, Edelstein quotes Stevens: "Some patient-care environments, to some extent perhaps of necessity, partake of the essence of the space capsule mockup. Immobility, painful monotony, aberrant schedule—all might conspire to be stressors of an already tenuous physiologic adaptation."[42]

The *time changes* that demand a readjustment or resetting of circadian rhythms include the following:

▶ Jet travel: Flight across time zones produces a group of symptoms sometimes labeled "jet fatigue" or "jet lag" (i.e., irritability, extreme sense of tiredness, inability to sleep at the appropriate time). Adjustment to radical time changes due to jet flight occurs at the rate of approximately one hour per day.[150]

▶ Changing work shifts: Rotating work shifts also upset circadian rhythms by forcing workers to adjust to new eating, sleeping and social patterns.[50]

▶ Daylight-saving time: This yearly time change requires some behavioral and physiologic adjustment because one rises and retires an hour earlier than usual and eats at slightly earlier times.

▶ Institutionalization or hospitalization: When an individual is admitted to a hospital, jail or military setting, he is forced to fit into a rigid new time schedule over which he has little control. In a hospital, for example, times for meals, sleeping, and socializing are typically dictated by institutional rules rather than by the desires of individual patients. Thus, patients are forced to accommodate their physiologic rhythms to a new temporal environment at the very time they are undergoing stress due to illness.

Individuals vary in their rate of adjustment to rapid time changes. Some persons adapt rapidly, others slowly, and others not at all. Also, our biologic rhythms themselves adjust to time changes at different rates. For example, some cardiovascular rhythms adjust to a new time schedule within a few days. On the other hand, readjustment of adrenal hormonal secretions may require up to 2 weeks.[97]

Everyone who must adjust to rapid temporal changes undergoes some stress in the process. Occasionally stress may be so great that the various biologic rhythms become disassociated from one another and illness results.

CLINICAL APPLICATIONS OF CHRONOBIOLOGIC PRINCIPLES

The application of chronobiologic principles to patient care is still in its early stages. However, in the future, our growing knowledge of biologic rhythms will probably be employed in a number of practical ways.

First of all, the study of circadian rhythms can lead to a greater understanding of the *nature of disease.* For example, some researchers believe that susceptibility to disease-causing bacteria, toxins, drugs, and alcohol may be greater at certain times of day.[42, 150] Other researchers are attempting to relate the cause of some cancerous growths to the disruption of cell division rhythms. Curt Richter, professor emeritus of psychobiology at the Johns Hopkins Medical School, has studied the cyclical nature of certain physical and mental disorders since 1919. He has found that peptic ulcer, migraine headache and epilepsy tend to be periodic disorders. Emotional disorders that seem to recur periodically include elation, stupor, excitement, manic depression and paranoia.[97] With the progress of medical research, it may someday be possible to link *all* diseases to the desynchronization of the body's rhythmic cycles and to loss of precision in biologic timing.

Second, knowledge of circadian rhythms could be used to revolutionize *diagnostic testing* in the laboratory. Currently, most diagnostic test results are inaccurate because the technicians who develop such tests and analyze the data fail to acknowledge that each patient is a *biochemically different entity* at different times during each 24-hour period owing to biologic cycles. For example, the majority of specimens for laboratory tests are collected in the morning rather than at different times over a 24-hour period. Then the patient's test results are compared with *standard* laboratory normal values, which have typically been established without consideration of man's daily physiologic fluctuation. As a result, the patient's blood and urine data are inaccurate and incomplete.[122] Medical laboratories of the future will undoubtedly assess the effects of rhythmic cycles on such factors as blood, urine, and electrolyte levels in determining their results.

Determination of circadian rhythms could also be useful in the *treatment of disease.* For instance, there may be an optimum time of the day for an individual to undergo surgery or to receive x-ray treatment. Also, proper timing is undoubtedly an important but neglected area in *drug administration.* Rodin's studies, for example, have shown that a dose of barbiturates that would be safe in the evening may have dangerously potent effects if taken in the morning.[97] Thus, the patient-consumer should know at what time a particular drug will have its greatest impact on his body and at what time its toxicity is at its highest. But as Ward points out: "Who has ever seen a warning label on a prescription bottle that reads *"Not* to be taken between 10:00 PM and 8 AM"? In the future, drug companies may be required to publish this type of vital information.

Finally, an understanding of circadian rhythms may eventually be used to *prevent disease.* It is possible that some day each person will be identified not only by his thumb print and voice print but by a time print. An individual's time print would show the variety and range of his rhythmic cycles as well as the factors that act to disrupt them. Health practitioners could then use time prints to predict when a patient would be particularly vulnerable to a disorder, thereby averting a serious, crippling, or deadly illness.

Biofeedback Training

Biofeedback training utilizes the concept of feedback to help individuals monitor and control their automatic physiologic functions (e.g., blood pressure, heart rate), with the result that these functions are maintained at a desirable level. Biofeedback is a new and evolving scientific concept which is still in its early stages of development.

BASIC CONSIDERATIONS

Until recently, biologists have traditionally divided physiologic functions into two distinct groups:

1. *Voluntary functions* are governed by the

conscious mind, e.g., motor skills and speech.

2. *Involuntary biologic functions* (sometimes called *visceral* functions) are governed by the autonomic nervous system and operate *automatically* without the individual's conscious awareness or control, e.g., temperature regulation, brain wave activity, control of cardiovascular function.

However, within the last decade, the concept of feedback has been applied with considerable success to the behavioral regulation of the so-called "involuntary" biologic functions—thus, the term *biofeedback*. As a result, the rigid dichotomy which has always existed between voluntary and involuntary physiologic functions is gradually breaking down. Indeed, scientists now believe that with biofeedback training, man may learn to beneficially control responses, e.g., blood pressure, that were once termed uncontrollable.

TECHNIQUES OF BIOFEEDBACK TRAINING

Biofeedback training is a scientifically planned program that trains selected subjects to control one or more of their "involuntary" functions. What essentially is involved in a training program which can teach an individual to regulate his blood pressure at will, speed or slow his heart rate, alter brain waves, tense or relax "involuntary" muscles, and raise or lower skin temperature?

In essence, biofeedback training involves (a) attaching the subject to complex electronic monitoring equipment; (b) monitoring a particular physiologic function (e.g., the subject's heart beat); (c) "feeding back" selected information about that function (e.g., increases or decreases in heart rate) to the subject by pictures, sounds, etc.; and (d) rewarding him for successfully learning to partially control that function.

To understand the mechanisms of biofeedback more fully, examine Figure 6–10, which contains a diagram of a generalized biofeedback circuit. Note that a generalized feedback circuit is composed of the following:[22]

a. The *subject* or patient who is learning to control a visceral function, e.g., heart rate, blood pressure, brain waves

b. The *physiologic monitor*, which picks up the minute electrical signals produced by muscle activity, brain wave activity, etc., e.g., the electrocardiogram (ECG) used to measure the electrical activity of the heart, the electroencephalogram (EEC) used to measure brain electrical patterns, and the electromyogram (EMG) used to measure tonic (contracted) muscle discharge

c. The *physiologic amplifier,* which en-

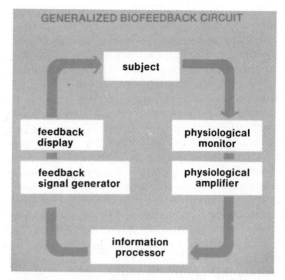

Figure 6–10. Generalized biofeedback circuit. (From Breeden, S. A., and Kondo, C.: Using biofeedback. *American Journal of Nursing, 75*:2010, Nov. 1973.)

larges the minute electrical signals, thereby making them easier to perceive

d. The *information processor,* which selects the significant data to be presented to the subject, e.g., an increase or decrease in heart rate per minute above or below a predetermined rate

e. The *feedback signal generator,* which changes the significant feedback data from the processor into a form the subject can use to assess and modify his physiologic responses, e.g., a beeping sound to indicate a change in heart rate or a pretty picture to indicate that the subject has lowered his blood pressure

f. The *feedback display,* which transmits the signal (e.g., headphones, a projection screen)

While biofeedback training seems novel, it is nevertheless similar to the conscious learning techniques we employ every day. For instance, biofeedback training resembles the trial-and-error learning approach one uses to master driving a car or playing a game of tennis. While learning to play tennis, the novice must continuously gather information about his own actions, his opponent's level of skill, the height of the net, the layout of the court, etc. The player then uses this information to modify his performance. At first the beginning player may have great difficulty hitting the ball properly and scoring points, but with practice and by using trial-and-error tactics, he eventually learns to play the game. Thus, both in conscious trial-and-error learning and in biofeedback training, one uses *information* to modify and improve performance. However, conscious learning differs from biofeedback training in that the information for modifying *voluntary* functions is easily available to the learner. For example, the tennis player can readily gather information concerning his performance both through his senses and from the critical comments of his instructor. On the other hand, the person who attempts to control involuntary functions (outside the laboratory) lacks the essential information he must have to modify a biologic function. As Neal Miller, a pioneer in biofeedback, points out: it is as difficult to modify a physiologic function without biofeedback training as it is "to learn to play tennis at night with the lights off."[79]

Fortunately, today research in biofeedback training is shedding light on the conscious control of visceral functions and malfunctions (e.g., the correction of an irregular heart beat). In the next section, we will briefly consider some of the important studies in the clinical uses of biofeedback.

BIOFEEDBACK RESEARCH AND CLINICAL APPLICATIONS

Some fascinating studies in biofeedback research and application have been conducted in the following areas: (a) yoga techniques of self-control, (b) control of cardiovascular symptoms, and (c) alleviation of conditions associated with abnormal muscle tension.

Yoga Techniques. While the notion of biofeedback training is new, the conscious control of visceral functions has been practiced for centuries by the Eastern yogis. Recently, scientists have begun to seriously study and analyze some of the yoga methods of body self-control. In 1970, at the Menninger Clinic in Topeka, Kansas, Green (a psychologist) studied, under laboratory conditions, the remarkable physiologic feats of an Indian yogi, Swami Rama.[63, 79] The Swami demonstrated his ability to (a) breathe at a rate of one to two breaths per minute without discomfort; (b) stop his heart from pumping blood for 17 seconds; (c) create a 10-degree difference in the skin temperature of different areas of his palm by dilating one of the two arteries supplying his palm while simultaneously constricting the second artery; and (d) consciously produce alpha, beta and delta brain

waves. It had taken the Swami 40 years to achieve this level of self-control. Concerning Swami Rama's accomplishments, Green writes:

The importance of Swami Rama's demonstrations did not lie in the performances themselves but in their implications. I do not intend to practice stopping my heart or to try to teach anyone else according to Swami's instructions, but the fact that *it can be done* is of major scientific importance. Aside from supporting the psychophysiological theory previously discussed, it more importantly gives us additional reason to believe that *training programs are feasible for the establishment and maintenance of psychosomatic health.* If every young student knew by the time he finished his first biology class, in grade school, that the body responds to self generated psychological inputs, that blood flow and heart behavior, as well as a host of other body processes, can be influenced at will, it would change prevailing ideas about both physical and mental health. It would then be quite clear and understandable that we are *individually responsible to a large extent for our state of health or disease.*

Control of Cardiovascular Symptoms. The control of heart disease and hypertension—both major health problems in the United States—has been another field for exploration by scientists in biofeedback. In 1970, Weiss and Engel attempted to train eight patients with cardiac disease to control their heart rates.[79] In this classic study, colored lights were used to notify the patients of their progress: a green light indicated that the patient's heart was beating too slowly, a red light indicated too rapid a rate, and a yellow light indicated a normal beat. By using this system, all the patients learned to control their heart rates to some extent, and five succeeded in regulating their heart rate to a significant degree. According to the researchers, these patients probably learned to stabilize their heart rates by controlling the sympathetic and vagal stimulation to the heart muscle. Exactly how patients learned to modify neural stimulation to the heart is not clear. However, the subjects reported using mental images to force changes in their heart rates, e.g., thinking about an argument or running down a dark street (for speeding the heart) or swinging leisurely in the park (for slowing the heart).[79, 80, 131]

Since Weiss and Engel did their pioneering research, other scientists have attempted to use biofeedback methods to modify cardiovascular responses. While results of research have been promising, it remains questionable whether biofeedback techniques, used alone, can cure or even significantly help patients with cardiovascular diseases.[22]

Control of Abnormal Muscle Tension and Its Effects.[22, 80, 131] One of the most favorable areas of biofeedback research involves the treatment of patients suffering from severe muscle tension due to anxiety. For example, electromyographic biofeedback has been successfully used in the treatment of persons with *tension headache.** Tension headaches are apparently caused by the sustained habitual contraction of muscles in the head and neck—particularly the frontalis muscle. Patients with incapacitating tension headaches have been taught to consciously relax their frontalis muscle with EMG biofeedback techniques. First EMG electrodes, which measure muscle tension, are placed over the frontalis muscle. Feedback concerning frontalis muscle tension is then given to the patient in the form of tones or clicking noises. High-pitched tones or rapid clicking sounds indicate increased muscle tension, while low-pitched tones or fewer clicks indicate that the muscle is relaxing. By using this feedback, patients learn just how tense the frontalis muscle is and how to consciously relax this muscle, thereby preventing headaches.

Patients with *lower back pain* due to chronic torso muscle tension have also responded well to biofeedback techniques. In one study, 80 per cent of the patients who received EMG biofeedback training for 1 month reported a substantial lessening of chronic pain and were able to return to their normal activities.[139]

Finally, biofeedback training for deep muscle relaxation has been helpful in the relief of *insomnia* due to anxiety and muscle tension.

Other Clinical Applications. Biofeedback training is also being tried in a more limited way to treat the following conditions:

▶ *Neuromuscular disorders* such as paralysis and muscle spasticity

▶ *Epilepsy*, which is caused by a disturbance in the electrical activity of the brain and characterized by seizures

▶ *Phobias*, which are mental disorders characterized by the extreme fear of or aversion to certain conditions (high places), objects (elevators) or persons

THE ROLE OF THE PATIENT IN BIOFEEDBACK TRAINING

For biofeedback training to be successful, the patient must play an extremely active role in his treatment program. Unlike other forms of therapy in which the patient may be passive (e.g., undergoing surgery, receiving medications) the patient in a biofeedback program is almost completely responsible for his own progress. Thus, the successful patient is highly

*You will recall that an electromyogram (EMG) measures tonic (contracted) muscle discharge.

motivated and intelligent; furthermore, the patient must be willing to travel regularly to the laboratory, to tolerate the application of electrodes, and to practice the techniques he has learned for months to years—by which time the novelty has worn off.

Given these patient requirements, some researchers question whether biofeedback training can ever be used among large segments of the population or whether it will be limited to the more affluent and educated persons. Shapiro states that perhaps the use of home feedback devices marketed on a national scale and supervised by physicians will make it possible for more people to use biofeedback training techniques.[130]

EVALUATING BIOFEEDBACK TRAINING

It has been difficult for scientists and physiologists to evaluate the role of biofeedback in patient care. For one reason, biofeedback training is a relatively new science and treatment method. Second, the studies that have been performed are often inconclusive because of the small number of subjects or uncontrolled laboratory conditions. Third, patient responses are difficult to evaluate. There is always the question: are patients responding to the biofeedback training itself or are they simply responding to the attention they receive as subjects in a scientific experiment? Finally, biofeedback training is an area that, in unscrupulous hands, can easily lead to commercial exploitation of the unwary consumer. For these reasons, researchers have tended to view biofeedback research with caution.

Nonetheless, many scientists believe that biofeedback training is essentially beneficial. Biofeedback training has definitely helped to relieve the symptoms of patients with psychosomatic illness (e.g., tension headache) without the use of potentially dangerous drugs. Moreover, not only does this training help to lessen symptoms, but it also appears to modify the underlying cause of the illness. Furthermore, biofeedback training may help to prevent diseases in the future. For example, researchers Budzynski and Stoyva have been attempting to teach subjects to voluntarily slow their metabolic processes. This ability could be used by trained individuals to retard biologic or mental breakdown during periods of great stress.[79] Finally, biofeedback research may enable us to better understand the relationship between mind and body and the extent to which the control of the body by the mind is possible.

HOMEOSTASIS AS A UNIFYING CONCEPT

In summary, the concept of homeostasis has added a new and vital dimension to our comprehension of life processes. Knowledge of homeostatic mechanisms has contributed greatly to the study of (1) physiology, (2) health and disease, and (3) the general dynamics of living.

The field of physiology has benefited from the concept of homeostasis in at least three ways. First, the idea of homeostasis has brought a *sense of order and of unity* into the study of physiologic processes. Body changes and adjustments that formerly had seemed to conflict with each other can now be better understood as adaptive manifestations of homeostasis and as functions related to the *total* needs of the individual. Second, the concept of homeostasis has demonstrated the *interdependence of the body's systems.* For example, the circulatory, endocrine and nervous systems are no longer conceived of as isolated units, operating independently of each other. Instead, they are now considered as part of a functioning whole, working together to enable the individual to survive emergencies and everyday stresses. Third, homeostasis has enabled us to see physiology as a *dynamic process* of continuous self-regulation and self-adjustment. Consequently, we can better understand the many fluctuations and oscillations that occur constantly within the body. In the light of these factors, it is not surprising that many scientists conceive of homeostasis as the single most important concept in physiology.

Further, our appreciation of *health* and *disease* has been greatly expanded by the concept of homeostasis. A knowledge of basic homeostatic mechanisms has enabled persons in the health care fields to meet their responsibilities in a more logical and intelligent way. A brief summary of principles, based on the concept of homeostasis, that have implications for patient care follows:

▶ The body adapts to stress and defends itself against radical changes by means of self-regulating homeostatic systems.

▶ Living things adapt to changes in their physical and social environment with the aid of internal timers called biological clocks.

▶ Self-regulating systems can break down as a result of extreme stress, a reduction in energy, or·damage to a part of the system.

▶ Biologic rhythms can be upset by numerous factors including toxins, drugs, and time changes; disturbances in rhythmic cycles can result in illness.

▶ Self-regulating systems that break down to any degree may elicit responses that are inadequate, inappropriate, unstable or maladaptive.

▶ Homeostatic systems can destroy themselves through the continuous repetition of error, thereby leading to a vicious circle.

▶ Medical and nursing intervention, if *appropriate and timely,* can aid the body in returning to homeostatic balance—either to approximately the same level of balance or to a new "steady state," which may be irreversible but is still functional.

▶ Patients can be trained with biofeedback techniques to regulate physiologic processes such as blood pressure and heart rate. Biofeedback training holds great implications for the future physical and mental health of mankind.

Finally, we can see that every aspect of life involves successful and unsuccessful attempts at developing and maintaining equilibrium. The process of living, then, on any level, from cellular operations to community interactions, from the moment of birth to the hour of death, can be better appreciated when approached from the standpoint of homeostatic balance.

BIBLIOGRAPHY

The references for Chapters 5 to 7 will be found at the end of Unit II, p. 114.

CHAPTER 7

CHANGING CONCEPTS OF HEALTH, DISEASE AND HEALTH CARE

INTRODUCTION

Rene Dubos once wrote: "Life is an adventure where nothing is static . . . complete and lasting freedom from disease is but a dream."[40] A dream or not, people still long to be free from pain, to experience the joy of a healthy body and mind, to prolong their existence on earth, to live in harmony with their environment, and to lead productive lives. To promote this dream, endless hours and millions of dollars have been spent on medical research; schools have developed throughout the world for the training of health practitioners; and health care services have expanded to the point that health is currently the number one industry of the United States. Yet, despite these advances, our dream of mental and physical health for all people everywhere has remained just that—a dream. Nevertheless, despite obstacles and setbacks, mankind continues to combat the problems of disease.

As we all know, the relative presence or absence of disease is both a personal and a societal problem. It is a *personal* problem because an individual's ability to work, to be productive, to love and to play are all related to how he feels and functions, both mentally and physically.

It is a *societal* problem because the illness of one person can adversely affect other people; e.g., the sick individual's family and/or fellow workers. Moreover, if the disease or injury is serious or disabling, a person may be forced to depend upon his family or society (the taxpayers, workmen's compensation, church organizations) for financial support and physical care. In addition, some diseases may spread from one person to another, possibly disrupting the social order; the great influenza, small pox and plague epidemics of the past immobilized entire populations.

To offset these problems, a variety of social institutions have developed over the centuries. Laws have been passed to control disease and its spread and to fight environmental pollution. Public health services have developed to control sanitation and to prevent and treat communicable diseases. Private insurance and government programs have been created to finance health care services. In addition, philosophers and clerics have attempted to explain disease and death to their followers and have offered comfort to those afflicted. Writers and artists have endeavored to depict human suffering as well as its powerful consequences; doctors and nurses have sought to diagnose and to treat disease and to alleviate suffering.

Because of the universal nature of disease, and its far-reaching personal and social consequences, thoughtful individuals have always asked questions about disease. Some of the most important questions are: What is disease and *why* does disease exist? What is health in relation to disease? What effect does disease have upon the individual and upon the society in which he lives? To what extent do the pressures exerted by society upon an individual cause disease? What can be done to alleviate disease, or at least to minimize its consequences? How can health care services best be delivered to all people regardless of their geographic location, race or economic status?

A basic purpose of this unit is to explore these questions, all of which are central to the medical and nursing professions. Again, as in preceding chapters, much of the information imparted is of a theoretical and speculative nature. Man is only beginning to learn about himself as a total entity—a physical, intellectual, emotional, social being—struggling to adapt to a challenging environment. We are only beginning to study the broad concepts of health and disease in a manner that is holistic and yet precise.

HEALTH, DISEASE AND HEALTH CARE: EVOLVING AND EXPANDING CONCEPTS

Health and disease are not static conditions. Rather, they are vital concepts that are variable in their meaning and are subject to the same continuous processes of evaluation and change as is man himself. In recent years, largely because of expanded medical and nursing research, our view of health and disease has changed in at least four major ways:

1. Broader and more inclusive definitions and viewpoints of health and disease
2. Awareness of changes in disease patterns and distribution
3. Changes in our concepts of disease causation
4. Changes in our pattern of health care delivery

Health and Disease: Changing Definitions and Viewpoints

In the not so distant past, disease was often defined as "an absence of health," and health was defined as "an absence of disease"—definitions that obviously led nowhere. Some authorities saw disease and health as states of physical discomfort or well-being; unfortunately, such rigid, narrow viewpoints totally disregarded the emotional and social pressures that affect us all.

Today, the experts are continuing to argue and disagree over exactly what constitutes health as opposed to disease. In her article "To Your Health—Whatever That May Mean," Siegel lists some of the problems involved in defining and understanding the concept of health—difficulties which are equally applicable to the defining of disease:[133]

▶ It is a value judgment.

▶ It is a subjective state.

▶ It is an abstraction which cannot be measured in objective terms.

▶ It is a spectrum with the distinction between health and illness often almost imperceptible except for certain acute illnesses.

▶ It is a relative concept.

▶ It is culturally determined.

Despite such obstacles, individuals and groups have continued to develop a number of definitions for health and disease. Let us first consider *health.*

One of the most widely accepted current definitions of health is stated in the Constitution of the World Health Organization (WHO) signed in 1946. This definition reads:

> *Health is a state of complete physical, mental, and social well-being and not merely the absence of disease or infirmity.*

The WHO definition of health has been both praised and criticized for its all-inclusive nature. On the one hand, the WHO definition excels because it includes the psychologic and social aspects of health as well as the physical. This definition thus avoids the error of traditional definitions that rigidly dichotomize mind, body and society (see later in this chapter). The WHO definition therefore places the concept of health into the broad context of human life. On the other hand, critics point out that the WHO definition is imprecise and unrealistic. Callahan, in his interesting article on the WHO definition, takes particular issue with the word "complete." He writes:

. . . it is doubtful that there ever was, or ever will be more than a transient state of "complete physical, mental, or social wellbeing" for individuals or societies; that's just not the way life is or could be.

Callahan then goes on to cite the major danger which the WHO definition of health fosters:

The demands which the word "complete" entail set the stage for the worst false consciousness of all: the demand that life deliver perfection. Practically speaking, this demand has led in the field of health to a constant escalation of expectation and requirement, never ending, never satisfied.[31]

A second definition of health which is growing in popularity is the *"systems" definition of health.* To quickly review Chapter 1, recall that man (according to systems theory) is defined as a hierarchy of natural systems. The system "man," like other systems, is goal-oriented and its various components are integrated and coordinated by means of signals transmitted through feedback loops. Therefore, "health," according to systems theory, is that "state of harmonious and dynamic equilibrium that characterizes a properly functioning hierarchy of natural systems."[24]

Like health, *disease* can be viewed as a *broad comprehensive concept*. For example, Engel broadly defines disease as follows:

> *Disease corresponds to failures or disturbances in the growth, development, functions, and adjustments of the organism as a whole or of any of its systems.*[44]

Thus, Engel implies that disease is not something that a person *has* and that is imposed upon him from the outside world; rather, it is a failure of the *total* individual to grow, function and adapt successfully to life's stresses.

The *systems definition of disease* revolves around the concept of *system and subsystem breakdown*. Brody identifies the concept of disease with "the disruption of the hierarchical system . . . [which] is generally precipitated by some disruptive force or perturbation from the external environment . . . using 'external' in the broad sense and remembering that what is external to one cell in a tissue may be internal to the tissue, and so on."[24]

Gerson and Skipper distinguish between (a) disease, (b) illness, and (c) sickness. According to their concept, *disease* is a pathologic state ("biologic dimension"), *illness* is the manner in which the patient interprets the pathologic states ("perceptive dimension") and *sickness* is the response of the patient to his perception of the pathologic state ("action dimension"). These three dimensions (biologic, perceptual and action) are separate steps in the *health action process*. For the individual, the perceptual dimension is the important aspect of the disease process, while the action dimension is most important to the society in which the person lives.[58]

Other definitions of health and disease have been advanced by various schools of thought, including physiologic, epidemiologic, ecologic, sociologic, and consumer viewpoints. These various definitions are briefly summarized and contrasted in Table 7–1.

As you study Table 7–1, note that these definitions can be broad or narrow, the distinctions between health and disease can be "hard" or "soft" (i.e., blurred) and the definitions may mainly focus on the individual or upon the society or species as a whole. Also note that it is almost impossible to understand the concept of health except in relation to disease and vice versa.[137]

While it is difficult to define health and disease precisely, it is even more difficult to apply the concepts of health and disease to *people*. For example, consider the following individuals; which of them are sick and which are well?

▶ An American business executive has experienced two relatively severe heart attacks, yet he continues to function satisfactorily on the job.

▶ A young housewife suffers every month from nervousness and instability due to premenstrual tension.

TABLE 7–1.   DEFINITIONS OF HEALTH AND DISEASE

VIEWPOINT	HEALTH	DISEASE
Physical or biologic view	"Health is a state of physical well-being."[30]	"In a biologic perspective the term 'disease' designates a medical concept whose meaning or intention involves an abnormality in function and/or structure of any part, process, or system of the body."[49]
Epidemiologic view	Health is a state in which the host has remained *resistant* to pathogenic agents in his environment (see discussion of the infection chain, Chap. 25)	Disease is a state resulting from the *susceptibility* of the host to pathogenic agents in his environment.
Ecologic view	"Health is the product of a harmonized relationship between man and his ecology."[118]	Disease is the product of a nonadaptive maladjusted relationship between man and his ecology.
Sociologic view	Health is *conformity* to that physical and/or behavioral state that is considered normal (or modal in statistical terms) within a particular group.	Disease is *deviancy* from that physical and/or behavioral state which is considered normal within a particular group.
Consumer viewpoint	"Health is . . . a commodity, an investment" which can to some degree be purchased.[133]	Disease is an abnormal condition that can be treated, controlled, and possibly cured through the purchase of health care services.

▶ A middle-aged hard-working engineer suffers from an aortic aneurysm but does not know it. This condition is often symptomless but is nevertheless life-threatening.

▶ A ballet dancer, though physically strong and lithe, tends, when taxed by work, to lose her sense of reality to the point of hallucinating.

▶ A college student occasionally escapes the realities and painful aspects of his life by using marijuana, a practice approved by his peer group.

▶ A lower class slum-dweller and his large family of 13 all suffer from infected teeth, a condition that he and other members of the lower class accept as "normal."

▶ A young boy of Tristan da Cunha, an island in the South Atlantic, is a powerful swimmer and mountain climber even though he suffers from worm infestations, a condition he ignores because it is so common on his island.

▶ A Los Angeles salesman suffers from congested lungs and weeping eyes on smoggy days, a condition to which he has become accustomed.

Who is sick and who is well? Or are all these people sick to some degree and healthy to some degree? How does each of these individuals define sickness and health? Do their definitions differ markedly from doctors' or nurses' definitions?

It is almost certain that each of these people will view disease and health in terms of their meaning to himself and his group. Thus, they may define disease in terms of whether or not they can continue to work, produce or study; whether signs and symptoms are present or absent; whether a state of discomfort is short or prolonged; whether a problem is physical, mental or social. Their definitions of health and disease will vary according to their peer groups, their cultural setting, their geographic location and their social class.

As you can see from the above, both professionals and laymen view health and disease in broad terms. Our conceptions of health and disease have expanded over the past decades in the following ways:

1. We view health and disease as *relative* concepts and not as separate absolutes. All living things are diseased to some extent; they progressively undergo aging, and eventually die. Thus, it is important to consider health and disease as a *continuum,* or graduated scale, with excellent health at one extreme and death at the other. To illustrate, the individuals just described each occupy a certain position on this disease-health continuum, somewhere in between the two extremes. Moreover, their positions vary from year to year, day to day, hour to hour, depending upon their life situation. For example, the housewife with premenstrual tension will experience symptoms only at a certain time of the month; the ballerina hallucinates only when severely overtaxed physically. These women, then, are to some degree continually shifting up and down the continuum in response to various internal and environmental stresses.

2. We realize today that each person has his *own* unique definitions of health and disease. These personal definitions are based upon the individual's own life experience, which includes his cultural and social background and geographic setting. Thus, a man from Los Angeles might regard a worm infestation as a sign of illness, but will ignore the potentially dangerous physical discomforts stemming from a smoggy and polluted environment. On the other hand, a native of Tristan da Cunha would probably acknowledge himself as ill on a smoggy day in Los Angeles, but is able to ignore his worm infestation since it is common to his culture.

3. Disease today is defined not just as a morbid pathologic process within the body, but rather as a *failure of adaptation to the internal or external environment—a homeostatic imbalance that ultimately affects the total individual.* For example, the housewife with premenstrual tension may become so irritable with her husband and children every month that her marriage and consequently her life become severely disrupted.

4. Finally, disease is now defined as including both the mental and physical aspects of illness; physical and mental diseases cannot be rigidly placed into separate categories. Thus, Harold Wolff cautions: "It is unprofitable to establish a separate category of illness to be defined as psychosomatic or to separate sharply—as regards genesis—psychiatric, medical, and surgical diseases."[159a]

To sum up, health and disease are now viewed as two sides of the same coin, a coin that is set in motion by unseen forces and that spins so rapidly that it is difficult to clearly distinguish one side of the coin from the other. As Romano states:

Health and disease are not static entities, but are phases of life, dependent at any time on the balance maintained by devices, genetically and experimentally determined, intent on fulfilling needs and adapting to and mastering stresses as they may arise from within the organism or from without.[120]

Shifting Patterns of Health and Disease

Disease has always existed; in an infinite variety of ways it has manifested itself throughout man's history. However, within the United States over the last 80 years, the statistical picture of life expectancy and disease patterns for Americans has greatly altered owing to (a) the remarkable medical and public health advances made during the 20th century and (b) greater longevity for Americans coupled with increased social and environmental stresses. More precisely, since 1900, the following four changes in our total health patterns have evolved:

1. *A decline in the death rate.* Note in Figure 7–1 that the death rate for the United States population declined significantly between 1900 and 1950—the years during which some of the major battles against infectious diseases were won.

2. *Life expectancy has significantly increased.* Today, people live considerably longer than did their forefathers. For example, it is thought that only 10 per cent of prehistoric men lived past the age of 40, and only one-half of them lived past 20. The Greek citizens of the classical era lived only slightly longer than did their primitive predecessors, while the average Egyptian of 2000 years ago lived only 22 years. As a result of some improvement in life-style, a man born in the Middle Ages could expect to live to be around 35. However, it was not until the 19th century, in the United States and England, that life expectancy increased to any appreciable degree. In 1900, as a result of improvements both in sanitation and in the control of some infectious diseases, a male at birth could expect to live to the age of 47.3 years.

Today, because of our more sophisticated medical knowledge and practices, an American has a life expectancy of 71.9 years—a tremendous increase in length of life as compared with the past.[136]

3. *Infectious diseases have greatly declined in prevalence.* Until the early 1920's infectious maladies such as smallpox, pneumonia, influenza, and tuberculosis were major killers. Today, only 6 Americans out of 100 will die of an infectious disease whereas in 1901, 36 persons out of every 100 died from an infectious process.[60] Unfortunately, as you see in Figure 7–2, the decline of infectious disease has been coupled with a dramatic rise in the prevalence of chronic disorders such as heart disease, the degenerative diseases associated with aging, and disorders resulting from environmental pollution.

4. *Chronic diseases rank as the major causes of death and disability today.* The three leading causes of death are heart disease, cancer and cerebrovascular accidents. Glazier points out that since 1900 heart disease has increased by 268 per cent and cancer by 240 per cent. Furthermore, these chronic disorders not only kill, but also disable their typically middle-aged and elderly victims. Thus Glazier writes:

The death rates tell only part of the story, since the chronic diseases also afflict large numbers of the living for long periods of time. According to estimates made in 1968, heart and circulatory disorders afflicted 26.2 million people in the U. S., mental and emotional disorders 20 million and arthritis and rheumatic diseases 16 million. The inescapable legacy of improved health in early and middle life is the increased prevalence of these less tractable forms of disease and disability in middle and later life.[60]

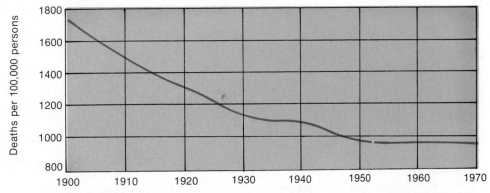

Figure 7–1. Decline in the death rate in the United States from 1900 to 1970. (Modified from Glazier, W. H.: The task of medicine. *Scientific American, 228*:13, April 1973.)

On an international scale, there have evolved, during the 20th century, distinctive differences in geographic disease patterns between the underdeveloped, overpopulated countries and the technologically developed countries of the Western world. In underdeveloped nations of the world, overcrowding, malnutrition, and poverty are common and consequently so are diseases and early death. For example, the life expectancy in India from 1951 to 1960 was 41.89 years for men and 40.55 years for women; from 1970 to 1975, life expectancy in Bolivia was 45.7 years for men and 47.9 years for women. Compare these statistics to the life expectancy at birth in the United States which is currently 71.9 years (68.2 years for men and 75.9 years for women). In Venezuela in 1974, the infant mortality rate was 53.6 deaths per 1000 live births. In the United States the infant mortality rate in that same year was 16.7 deaths per 1000 live births.[136, 161]

From these statistics you can infer that the United States, by means of technologic advances, has partially eradicated such problems as starvation, severe overcrowding, and infection. Through the development and use of public health measures (e.g., chlorination of water, vaccines, and antibiotics), through the enforcing of pure food and drug laws, and by means of health education, the people in this country have been spared many of the infectious and depleting conditions common to non-Western countries. Life in America has been substantially enriched and improved, at least for the more affluent classes.

On the other hand, the statistics shown in Figure 7–2 demonstrate that Americans are by no means disease-free. We have simply exchanged one pattern of disease for another. The chronic diseases that plague modern Americans may strike more slowly and more insidiously than the infectious diseases, but they are just as painful, frightening and deadly. Americans may live longer lives than their less wealthy and sophisticated neighbors, but they suffer no less.

Changes in Theories of Causation of Disease

What factors ultimately cause disease? This question remains one of the great mysteries facing man—a mystery demanding solution.

Like all things mysterious, the question of disease causation has given rise to many theories over the centuries, some of which are still, in part, acceptable today. As a student of nursing, it is useful for you to have some idea of the changes in these theories. The changes in viewpoint have powerfully affected the philosophy of the medical and nursing fields—and consequently the goals of patient care. Let us first study the transition from the traditional theories of disease causation to the more modern theories of illness. Then, in the light of these transitional changes, let us examine more closely the current view of disease.

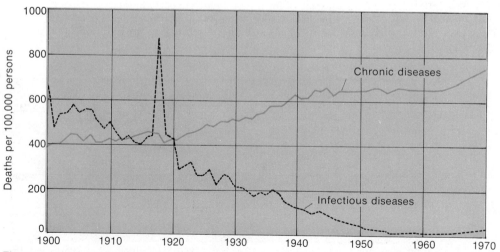

Figure 7–2. Changing role of infectious diseases and chronic diseases as causes of death in the United States between 1900–1970. (Modified from Glazier, W. H.: The task of medicine, *Scientific American*, 228:13, April 1973.)

To study a mysterious object and to understand its many facets, it is usually necessary to take that object apart and examine its separate components. This is precisely what scientists and doctors, in the past, have done to human beings. In their effort to comprehend man, they have taken him apart, torn him away from his natural environment, divorced his mind from his body, fragmented even his physical being—dissecting system from system, organ from organ, and tissue from tissue. In the final analysis, science has reduced man to a molecular, even atomic level, so that he is no longer a whole and living being but rather a mechanized, dehumanized abstraction. Moreover, scientists in the past not only have split man into particles but have neglected to reunite him. Thus, until recently, man has been left in a sadly disjointed state, being appreciated as a group of parts rather than as a total entity.

It is not surprising, then, that traditional theories of human disease causation also tended toward a fragmentation of man, concentrating upon a single dimension of a patient's self, but never upon his whole being. Many of these traditional and limited theories of disease continue to influence modern medicine and nursing, creating a fragmentation in our patient care. Let us now briefly examine some of these older concepts that continue to influence us and the newer theories that are replacing them.

1. One early theory of disease causation viewed the *human body as a machine, and disease as the result of a defective part*. This old way of considering disease is sometimes termed the *pathologic-anatomic concept*.[90] The basis for the theory originated with Descartes, a 17th century French philosopher who envisioned man as a well-functioning "body machine." Doctors, searching for ways to cope with disease processes, believed they saw in Descartes's mechanistic theories a solution to the problem of sickness. They reasoned that if disease was caused by a malfunctioning of the machine or by a defective part, then the cure for disease was simply to repair or remove the defective part or parts. Thus, the rationale for surgery as treatment is actually based upon Descartes's ideas, as are many other medical procedures.

Today newer theories have expanded upon this limited concept. For example, we now consider disease as *a failure in the growth, development, or adjustment of the organism as a whole rather than a part*. Moreover, we currently recognize the interrelationships which exist between the mind and the body as well as the total person and his environment. In sum, we see disease as more than a physiologic, pathologic process; instead we view it as a process that is intimately linked with the individual's total life experience.

2. A second traditional theory of disease is that *the disease process tends to be localized, affecting a single organ or system*.[159] This view of sickness, like the concept of the "body machine," is based upon the pathologic-anatomic concept of disease. It, too, tends to oversimplify highly complex phenomena. Advocates of this view stressed the importance of one individual organ or system in the study of disease because they noted that generally a single organ appeared pathologically altered. The effects that one diseased organ have upon the total body went undetected.

Today we recognize that *the body organs and the body systems are not separate entities but are closely interrelated* by means of the nervous, circulatory, and endocrine systems. Increasingly we realize that although disease may indeed affect one particular organ or system, the manifestations and consequences of that disease affect the entire body as well as the psyche of the individual. It is unfortunate that in spite of our present advanced medical knowledge, remnants of the outmoded "organ-centered" way of thinking still remain.

3. A third way of viewing disease in the past has centered around *the mind-body dichotomy*. Advocates of this obsolete point of view saw the mind and body as separate from each other; consequently they believed that no relationship existed between the intellectual-emotional component of man and bodily disease.

This dualistic theory, like the body machine theory, has dominated medical thinking since the days of Descartes. For centuries it has prevented nurses and physicians from developing a holistic view of disease. Only recently has science begun to conceive of man as a *total unit with body and mind integrated*. We realize today that every system of the body is capable of responding to psychologic pressures. The modern nurse recognizes that (1) certain diseases coincide with periods of emotional or mental stress in a patient's life, and (2) "purely" physical problems and disabilities such as a broken leg or arm can result in serious mental disturbance.

4. A fourth traditional view of disease causa-

tion is that *illness is the result of a single etiologic agent or cause.* Single-factor theories of disease causation have been popular in medicine because, like the preceding outdated concepts, these theories have tended to simplify the problems of diagnosis, treatment, and prevention. Doctors reasoned that if there was a single cause for disease, and that cause could be discovered and controlled, then disease could be eradicated.[44]

Medical history abounds with examples of single-factor theories. For instance, the body's chemistry was once regarded as the key to health and disease. Old medical writings emphasized that a proper balance of the four "humors" of the body—phlegm, blood, black bile, and yellow bile—guaranteed good physical health. Even a person's temperament was supposedly affected by the humors. For example, a phlegmatic man (a man with too much phlegm) was lazy; a sanguine person (from the Latin word *sanguis*, meaning "blood") was hearty and sensual; too much black bile made a person melancholy, whereas too much yellow bile made him violent.

With the advent of Pasteur's *germ theory,* modern medicine was born. But even this theory, heralded by many scientists as the last word in disease causation, fell short. At first, physicians were hopeful that by simply identifying and killing dangerous microorganisms, disease could be eradicated forever. But we realize today that such a simple solution is not possible. Infectious diseases continue to exist despite the fact that many pathogenic organisms have been identified, vaccines and antibiotics have been developed, and public health and sanitation measures have been improved. Moreover, the germ theory, while partially solving the problem of infectious disease, is not applicable to the widespread pattern of noninfectious chronic disease which so drastically affects modern civilization.

Despite the failure of the germ theory to explain all disease, doctors have continued to search for the single causative agent behind many illnesses. Indeed, the tradition of the single-factor theory still flourishes to some extent in modern medicine. The "concept of the biochemical defect" provides one example of a contemporary single-factor theory.[44] The supporters of this concept hypothesize that defective enzymes or impaired biochemical systems cause disease. This viewpoint, to some degree, neglects emotional and environmental factors in disease causation, and instead stresses chemical and molecular factors.

Even in the field of psychiatry, single-factor theories are prevalent. For example, certain psychiatrists try to explain mental disease solely in terms of the person's early childhood. Other psychiatrists have concentrated upon thwarting of the sexual drive as the major problem in mental disease. More recently, some have theorized that biochemical changes are the cause of mental disturbance.

In sum, a wide variety of single-factor theories of disease have evolved over time. Although these theories help to explain certain aspects of disease, no single-factor theory has been shown to answer the *whole* question of disease causation. Even individual diseases do not seem to have a single cause or a single remedy. This discovery is slowly having an impact on modern medicine. As Selye points out:

The principal endeavor of medicine in general is beginning to change. It is no longer the search for specific pathogens and for specific remedies with which to eradicate them. We always used to accept as a self-evident fact that each well-characterized disease must have its own specific cause. This tenet is self-evident no longer. It becomes increasingly more manifest that an agent does or does not produce disease, depending upon a variety of conditions.[128]

Only a *multicausal theory* of sickness, then, which takes into account all possible factors and predisposing conditions, can complete the puzzle of disease causation from which so many pieces are still missing.

5. A fifth traditional belief is that *the agents that cause disease are always external to man;* they are never a part of him. Since primitive times, man has tried to externalize and project away from himself those things that he considers evil or "bad." As Engel has said:

The mechanism of projecting to the outside what is felt or experienced as uncomfortable, painful, or dangerous is universal in every human being and is characteristic of one phase of the psychological development of every child. So too is the idea that what is felt as bad or painful inside got there from the outside.[44]

Men consider disease to be painful, evil and dangerous. It is not surprising, then, that people have thought of disease as an "invader" that enters a person's body from the outside world. This notion of disease is very old, dating back to primitive man, who viewed the world as a magical place filled with devils, charms and spells.

In modern society, we too often view sickness as something apart from ourselves. Examples of this attitude are common in our everyday speech. We say we are "invaded" by microbes, "contaminated" by infectious material, we "breathe in" pollen and allergens, we "ingest" foods that sicken us, we "catch" colds, are "driven" by our primitive instincts, and we are corrupted by our vices. When we visit a physician, we want him to "rid us" of our disease with medicines and treatment. We want the surgeon to "cut out" the organ that has become diseased or the cells that have become cancerous. When mentally disturbed, we visit a psychiatrist who lets us "talk out" our feelings and objectify our fears. In sum, man, both primitive and modern, has tried to externalize disease by reducing it to a "bad thing" that has its own independent existence apart from the sufferer.

This objective way of thinking about disease is psychologically comforting to both patient and doctor. If we can project the cause of a disease outside ourselves, we can then put it under a microscope, study it, fight it, and cure it. However, this point of view can dangerously simplify the approach to nursing care. Nurses will feel no need to understand patients if they believe that what has caused disease is an external factor rather than an internal problem. Such nurses will believe their task ends with the giving of medications and the performance of procedures.

Conversely, the belief that disease is caused by some factor that is an intimate part of ourselves is psychologically disquieting. For then the enemy that causes us so much sickness, pain, and discomfort is no longer external to us—it is within us and *a part of us.* With such a view, the cause of illness cannot be exorcised like a devil or exterminated like a microbe. It becomes necessary for doctors and nurses to study *the patient himself* as well as the disease if they want to effect a cure.

Modern medical theorists are taking as much cognizance of the "enemy within" as they are of those disease-producing factors that exist in the external world. Consequently many broad questions are being asked today. Why, for example, when three people are exposed to the tuberculosis bacillus, does only one of the three develop tuberculosis? And why, since all of us are exposed to many different infectious microorganisms, does this one person develop tuberculosis and not some other infectious disease? Is it something in the person that predisposes him to tuberculosis or is it something in the *environment?* Or is it the result of some peculiar interrelationship between the two?

Such questions must be answered. However, the external-factor theory alone does not offer the solution. In recent years, science has been looking more carefully at man himself and at the way in which he *responds internally* to external stressors and invaders. Medicine has shifted its emphasis from the study of environmental factors to the study of man's internal

milieu and his adaptive processes. As Stewart Wolf points out:

> Newer concepts of disease hold that illness and incapacity arise from efforts on the part of the body to deal with adverse forces in the environment more frequently than they do from the direct effect or intrinsic nature of the adverse stimulus itself. In a sense, disease is a reaction to rather than an effect of noxious forces.[159]

Thus, for the final answer to disease causation we must look to the individual man himself as well as to the external world surrounding him.

COMPARISON OF TRADITIONAL AND MODERN THEORIES OF DISEASE CAUSATION

Traditional theories of disease causation are usually anatomically oriented and they tend to support etiologic concepts of illness that are rigid, narrow, and mechanistic.

Modern theories of disease differ from traditional theories in at least four ways: (1) Modern theories are based upon the *total man* rather than upon bodily processes. (2) They are more *unified* and less fragmented. The interrelationships between the various organs, between mind and body, and between the total man and his environment are increasingly being recognized. (3) Current theories consider man's unique *response* to disease as well as the disease itself. (4) Finally, the etiology of disease tends to be multicausal in scope rather than unicausal.

Changing Patterns of Health Care Delivery

Over the past 50 years, methods of delivering health care services have changed greatly in this country and throughout the world. In this section we will briefly consider (1) the attitudes, trends and concepts which have brought about change; (2) new and evolving patterns of health care; (3) the different methods for financing health care; (4) the strengths and weaknesses of our current methods for delivering health services; and (5) emerging priorities in the health care fields.

TRENDS, ATTITUDES AND CONCEPTS AFFECTING HEALTH CARE DELIVERY

A number of new and developing trends, attitudes and concepts have evoked radical changes in our current American philosophy of health care delivery. The most important of these trends and attitudes (some of which we have discussed earlier in this chapter) can be summarized as follows:

▶ Recognition of the patient as a *total person* who has not only physical needs, but emotional, intellectual, and social needs as well.

▶ Emergence of the patient as a *health consumer* who should have a voice in the policies and therapies that affect his physical and emotional well-being.

▶ Development of the theory that disease is *multicausal* in origin and that therapy must be directed toward a patient's emotional and social problems as well as toward treatment of physical malfunctions and disabilities.

▶ Shifts in the *incidence* of diseases as exemplified by a *decrease* in acute and infectious disease and an *increase* in (a) chronic illnesses (heart disease, arthritis); (b) the degenerative disorders associated with aging; (c) illnesses which are essentially "man made" (arising from smoking and environmental pollution); and (d) nervous and mental disorders which now rank as the fourth most prevalent chronic health problem.[60, 134]

▶ *Population shifts* characterized by (a) an increasing worldwide population; (b) increased life expectancy, which results in increased numbers of old people who require extensive health services; and (c) increased movement of persons from sparsely populated areas to urban and suburban centers.

▶ Increase in *social problems* such as divorce, unemployment, alcoholism, drug addiction, venereal disease, behavioral disorders, poverty, and isolation of elderly and chronically ill.

▶ Increase in *scientific knowledge* in the physical, social and medical sciences coupled with a tremendous growth in *biomedical technology* (e.g., the use of computers, patient monitoring devices).

▶ Shift from a disease-oriented philosophy of therapy to a *comprehensive philosophy* of health care oriented toward the promotion of health, the prevention and treatment of disease, and rehabilitation of the patient following accident or illness.

There are at least six emerging patterns of health care which have evolved from the concepts summarized above. Let us consider each briefly.

Community Health Care.   With the increase in long-term chronic disorders and the decrease in acute diseases, the care of patients has increasingly shifted *from the hospital to the community*. As Battistella points out:

> In point of fact, in the course of a year, only about 10% of the population at risk are admitted to a hospital, and only about 1% are admitted to a teaching hospital. By far the bulk of care is provided by practitioners in ambulatory settings for largely routine, and, by prevailing medical standards, prosaic conditions.[11]

Thus, the majority of patients today are being treated in clinics, outpatient departments of hospitals, neighborhood health centers, doctor's offices, and at home under the supervision of visiting nurses or public health nurses.

The "back to the community" policy has also radically affected the care of psychiatric patients. Over the last 10 years, patients with mental disorders have been discharged from the wards of psychiatric hospitals into the community where they are supervised in day-care hospitals, transitional half-way houses, and aftercare clinics. This important change in the care of psychiatric patients, in part, developed in response to the following policies stated in 1961 by the Joint Commission on Mental Illness and Health.

> We must enable the patient to maintain himself in the community in a normal manner by 1) saving the patient from the debilitating effects of institutionalization as much as possible; 2) returning the patient home to community life as soon as possible after a hospitalization; and (3) thereafter maintaining him in the community as long as possible.[134]

Unfortunately, this program has resulted in increased isolation and loneliness for many patients as well as rising readmission rates for many psychiatric hospitals.

Nevertheless, community-based health care for patients of all types is a reality with which the health fields are attempting to cope. One positive out-growth of the "return to the community" movement has been the development of the fields of *community medicine* and *community nursing*. Increasingly, departments of Social Medicine, Community Medicine, and Family and Community Nursing are being created within hospitals and medical and nursing schools. These departments primarily train health practitioners to help patients to physically and emotionally cope with their daily lives within the community.[29] With the rise of community health services has come an increased emphasis on comprehensive health care.

Comprehensive Health Care. The modern health practitioner is being taught to view comprehensive health care as the ideal form of health care delivery as opposed to outmoded disease-oriented systems of care. In essence, comprehensive health care is composed of the following four components:

1. *Health promotion* involves such activities as (a) education of the public in regard to health practices and good nutrition; (b) development of physical education and activity programs, as well as mental health counseling services; and (c) environmental controls such as the designation of "no-smoking areas" and anti-pollution laws.

2. *Disease prevention* can be exemplified by (a) *public health programs* for administration of immunizations against smallpox, poliomyelitis, etc. and the control of disease-carrying insects and rodents; (b) *screening programs* for early identification of hereditary and chronic disorders (e.g., sickle-cell anemia, hypertension); (c) the *enforcement of safe working conditions* in order to prevent accidents; (d) *prenatal care* for pregnant women designed to alleviate the complications of pregnancy and childbirth; (e) *school health programs* for the detection of nutritional, visual, hearing and dental problems in children; (f) increased emphasis in the "media" on cancer detection, e.g., women are instructed to have a yearly "Pap" smear* and to examine their breasts monthly for lumps in order to ensure early treatment of cancer should it develop; (g) outpatient clinics where individuals who suspect they have *venereal disease* can be examined; and (h) educational programs which give information concerning the signs of *alcoholism* and *drug addiction* as well as naming community resources to which addicted individuals can turn for help.

3. *Diagnosis and treatment of disease* is increasingly characterized by the use of sophisticated technological devices; e.g., clinical laboratory data systems, multiphasic screening centers, the use of computers in diagnosis, continuous monitoring devices for patients in surgery, intensive care units, and coronary care units; biofeedback machines for teaching patients new and healthier behavioral and physiologic responses (see Chap. 6); and automated classification, storage and retrieval systems for patient records and medical research data.

4. *Rehabilitation* involves, in its broadest sense, the restoration of the physically or emotionally disabled person to the highest level of physical and mental health possible for that individual. Rehabilitation is an integral part of the patient's total plan of care which should be commenced upon the health practitioner's initial contact with the patient. Some major rehabilitative goals are as follows: (a) protecting the patient from further disability; (b) strengthening and supporting the patient in the use of his remaining abilities; (c) assisting the patient to adapt physically, psychologically and socially to permanent disabilities. Rehabilitation will be discussed in Chapter 16.

The Health Care Team. The demands of patient care today are so heavy and so varied that no one health professional is equipped to deal with all of them. Thus, the growing complexity of comprehensive health care has triggered the development of *health care teams*. Typically, a health care team such as one might find in a large hospital or clinic is composed of a physician, nurse, social worker, physical therapist, occupational therapist, respiratory therapist, and psychologist or psychiatrist. Sometimes the team also utilizes a public health nurse who functions as a liaison worker between the hospital and the patient's home and community environment. In the ideal health team, no one person is seen as *the* leader of the group. Instead each health professional is respected as an authority in his field and as an individual with a unique contribution to make to the patient's health and welfare.

Primary Care. What is modern primary nursing? Let's consider Hegyvary's comprehensive definition:

Primary nursing is a form of organization that aims to overcome weaknesses in team and functional organizations by establishing nursing responsibility and accountability for specific patients. The central concept in primary nursing is that the *nursing care of a specific patient is under the continuous guidance of one nurse from admission through discharge....* In essence, the primary nurse is responsible for the total nursing process* with that patient during the period of hospitalization.[68]

The modern primary nurse resembles the private duty nurse of the past in that she pro-

---

*The "Pap smear," or Papanicolaou test, is a simple cytologic examination used primarily to detect cancer of the uterus and cervix. This test was named for its originator Dr. Papanicolaou.

*The nursing process is discussed in Chapter 17.

vides *continuous* patient-centered care to patients throughout their hospitalization. The primary nurse differs from the private duty nurse in that she does *not* provide 24-hour care to the patient *herself.* Instead, she is responsible for *developing* and *supervising* the patient's plan of care around the clock. Ideally, the primary nurse performs the following activities.[43]

► Collects data concerning the patient's present problems and past history

► Assesses the patient's problems and strengths upon admission

► Assists the patient in developing short- and long-range goals

► Devises an individualized plan for giving the patient 24-hour nursing care

► Sets up learning situations for the patient and his family

► Cooperates with other team members in planning the patient's care

► Evaluates the patient's progress

► Is available for consultation in event of an emergency or the development of unforeseen patient problems

► Prepares the patient for discharge and arranges for home or clinic care as necessary

In sum, the primary nurse is the individual who is responsible for coordinating a patient's total diagnostic, therapeutic and rehabilitative program from inception to completion—from admission to discharge.

Increased Patient-Consumer Involvement.* Until very recently, patients were often treated like dependent children by those in charge of their care. Indeed the "ideal patient" was an individual who seldom complained about his care (no matter how poorly he was treated), rarely asked questions or demanded answers, acted as a willing "guinea pig" in therapeutic experiments, smilingly underwent humiliating physical and psychologic examinations during staff rounds, and above all else, never criticized his physician, nurse or hospital facility. In other words, the patient was a person without rights or privileges; he truly had no voice in his own

*The rights of the patient-consumer are discussed in detail in Chapter 20.

affairs. Patients were expected to do as they were told and to be grateful for any help received. Today, the patient has finally emerged as a consumer of health services who has a *right* to good care and who is due the respect and privacy that should be accorded any human being.

The battle for patients' rights has been in the making for decades. However, only recently has the concept of the patient as a *consumer* had an impact on patient care. The shift of power from the health professional to the health consumer has been brought about by a number of factors. For example, health consumers are more knowledgeable today about health care and medical services. Popular magazines and television shows have enabled the modern layman to become far more sophisticated about his physical and mental health needs than were his predecessors. Also, consumers are beginning to organize politically and to demand representation on policy-making boards that deal with health care. Currently consumers are participating in planning neighborhood health centers, clinics and community hospitals.[88] In addition, hospitals and health practitioners are at last beginning to recognize the rights of consumers. In 1973 the American Hospital Association approved "A Patient's Bill of Rights" (see Chap. 20), and the American Medical Association officially recognized the right of patients to state grievances concerning their care. As a result, many hospitals today have health practitioners who act as "patient advocates" as well as grievance boards with whom patients can register complaints.

Nevertheless, while the patient-consumer has come a long way in terms of promoting his own welfare, he clearly has a long way to go before he receives the care to which he is entitled.

Increased Government Involvement in Health Care. Government at the local, state and national level is playing a greater and greater role in health care service delivery within the United States. As you will read in the next section, the government has become particularly involved in the financing of both health care and medical research.

CHANGING PATTERNS OF HEALTH CARE FINANCING

Health care has become the largest industry in the United States. The costs of health care are high and still rising at both the personal level and the national level.[60]

At the *personal* level, yearly health care expenditures per person rose from $79 in 1950 to $324 in 1970—a 310 per cent increase! In 1971, the average American spent $358 on health care while individuals over 65 spent over $1200 on medical services.[21]

On the national level, health care expenditures increased from 4 billion dollars in 1940 to between 50 and 75 billion dollars in 1971. Some statisticians estimate that with the current trend, expenditures may mount to as high as 200 billion dollars in 1980.[60] This trend reflects the steady rise in the cost of living in this country, sharp increases in the price of physician's fees, hospitalization, medications, etc.; the enormous expenditures for medical and educational research; and the fact that consumers are purchasing more health services.

How is money raised for the purchase and delivery of health services? Throughout the world, there are six major methods for financing health care: individual personal payment, charity, industry, voluntary insurance, social insurance, and general revenues (taxation).* While one method of financing may be more popular in one nation than another, all six methods are used to some degree throughout the world. Let us consider each method briefly.

Individual Personal Payment. The time-honored system for obtaining and financing health care is for the consumer to select a particular practitioner (doctor, dentist, nurse) and pay him a fee for services received. The personal fee-for-service method still predominates in the United States (especially in the purchase of ambulatory services, dental care, and drugs), while other nations such as the U.S.S.R. and Great Britain rely heavily on public funding. However, in the United States, the sharply rising cost of health services is forcing Americans to depend increasingly on voluntary insurance, social insurance, and public funding for paying their health care bills. Our substantial population of the poor and the aged is relying more and more on government-sponsored health services because, on their low, often fixed, incomes, they cannot afford current physician and hospital fees.

Charity. In the past, the sick poor were largely dependent upon charitable (often church-administered) institutions for health care. In the modern world, donations, contributions and bequests (money willed to a charitable cause) play a relatively minor role in financing health care. Within the United States, charity provides less than 5 per cent of the monies needed for health financing. Charitable funds are typically used for hospital endowments, medical research, and construction of health care facilities. Examples of organizations that have made important charitable contributions include the Rockefeller Foundation, the March of Dimes and the United Fund.

Industrial Health Care. The medical care of workers by private industries is not a predominant method of health financing anywhere in the world. However, some private industries—for example, British and American oil companies and the Firestone Rubber Company in Saudi Arabia—continue to finance health care for their employees. The developing countries of Latin America, Asia and Africa still rely (to a degree) on doctors, nurses, dentists, etc. employed by industries (frequently owned by North American or European corporations) to meet workers' health needs as well as to provide health education and environmental sanitation. Nevertheless, there is a worldwide trend to gradually replace health care financing by industries with funds raised through voluntary and social insurance.

Voluntary Insurance. Historically, voluntary insurance was an important method for financing health care; during the 18th and 19th centuries in Europe various occupational groups, benefit societies and sickness funds provided monies for contributors who became ill or were injured. On the other hand, few people in the United States before 1930 had voluntary insurance. Today, however, at least 85 per cent of persons in the United States carry some form of private insurance to help pay medical expenses. The tremendous upsurge in the use of private insurance was inspired by the spiraling cost of medical services and by the threat of socialized medicine.

Voluntary insurance has been primarily promoted by hospital and medical associations and by commercial insurance companies. Insurance coverage may be purchased either by individuals or by groups. For example, many businesses and industries offer insurance coverage to their employees; in some cases the employers may pay a percentage of the employee's costs.

Basically there are two types of voluntary insurance: indemnity insurance plans and pre-paid insurance plans, which are also called health maintenance organizations (HMO's).

Indemnity insurance compensates the insurance holder (within the limits of his policy) should he require visits to his physician, surgery, or hospitalization. This type of insurance is offered to individuals and to groups by such insurance companies as Blue Cross and

---

*In writing this section, the author relied extensively on the article by M. I. Roemer entitled "Health Care Financing and Delivery Around the World."[119]

Blue Shield. Cost of indemnity insurance for the policy holder depends upon his age, state of health, history of past disorders, the amount and type of coverage, deductibility of certain expenses, etc. Indemnity insurance has *not* altered the traditional fee-for-service method in which health services are delivered in this country—i.e., the health consumer still contacts a practitioner or hospital of his choice and then the practitioner receives a fee for services rendered from the patient's insurance company.

Pre-paid insurance or *HMO's,* on the other hand, have *departed* from the traditional method of health delivery. A health maintenance organization is typically composed of hospital and clinic facilities that are staffed by health practitioners (physicians with various specialized backgrounds, nurses, etc.) salaried by the plan for their services. Thus the policy holder of a pre-paid insurance plan has a more limited group of physicians and facilities to select from than does the holder of indemnity insurance—a deficiency of this system. On the positive side, HMO's are far more geared to health maintenance and the prevention of disease than are indemnity plans, which typically render no benefits unless the holder is seriously ill or injured. Classic and successful

examples of pre-paid plans include Health Insurance Plan of Greater New York, Kaiser-Permanente Health Plan in California and the Group Health Cooperative of Puget Sound, Washington. Despite the advantages offered, pre-paid plans have attracted only about 6 per cent of insured persons.

While the development of private voluntary insurance has provided a large percentage of the populace with a realistic means for financing their medical services, this form of coverage has failed to meet the health needs of the poor, the aged, and the rural populace. As a result, mandatory social insurance (i.e., social security programs) have arisen in the United States and throughout the world.

Social Insurance. In most countries, social insurance is supported to varying degrees by government taxation. In the United States, the federal government has played a vital role in the development of social insurance. The most important step was taken in 1965 when the following two amendments of the Social Security Act were passed: (1) Title XVIII (Medicare) and (2) Title XIX (Medicaid). *Medicare* provides hospital care and other health services to the aged; it is financed through federally collected Social Security taxes. *Medicaid* provides health services to the poor; participation in this program is voluntary. Note in Figure 7–3 the extent to which these federal programs have changed the pattern of payment for medical services during the years from 1960 to 1970. Although social insurance, like voluntary insurance, has changed the pattern of payment for care, it clearly has *not* changed the basic system for health care service delivery. The health consumer still contacts the practitioner of his choice and the practitioner then receives a fee for his services—in this case, from the federal government rather than from the patient or an insurance company.

Even though there have been problems in the administration of Medicare and Medicaid, these programs have benefited large numbers of the aged and poor. All in all, social insurance seems to be more advantageous than other forms of health financing. As Roemer states:

In general, social insurance is believed to have the advantage of fiscal stability, in contrast to other methods of financing medical care. It is not subject to the uncertainties of legislative appropriation, nor to the ups and downs of charity or voluntary enrollment. At the same time, most of the laws give a voice to workers and employers in the administration of the program. And in most countries, the social insurance fund need not fear invasion by other government ministries; it is reserved for benefits to the insured.[119]

Government Taxation (General Revenues). Throughout the world, taxes are used to

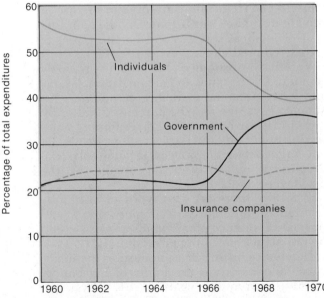

Figure 7–3. Changes in the pattern of payment for medical care. (Modified from Glazier, W. H.: The Task of Medicine. *Scientific American, 228*:13, April 1973.)

help finance health care services; within the United States, federal, state, and local taxes support a variety of health programs, e.g., (a) programs for *special groups* such as the elderly, the indigent, veterans, merchant seamen, native Americans; (b) programs to treat *patients with certain diseases* such as psychiatric disorders, crippling disabilities, venereal disease; (c) *public health* programs for disease prevention and environmental control; and (d) *research* and *educational* programs.

While tax revenues play an increasingly important role in supporting health care in the United States, other countries rely almost exclusively on taxation. Roemer believes that these countries fall into three distinct groups:

▶ Countries such as New Zealand, Great Britain and Chile where the social insurance system evolved into a government institution completely supported by general revenues

▶ Developing countries in Africa and Asia where large masses of poor people depend upon government financing for health services

▶ Socialist countries such as the U.S.S.R. where public health services are the predominant channel for health care delivery

Noting the worldwide trends toward government involvement in health care delivery, Roemer writes in summary:

On the whole, one can observe throughout the world—in its capitalist-parliamentary, its socialist, and its developing sectors alike—a clear trend toward increasing collectivization of health care financing. With this has evolved an increasing organization of resources designed to enhance both the efficiency and the effectiveness of medical care delivery.[119]

THE CRISIS IN HEALTH CARE

The current system of health care in the United States is said to be in a state of crisis. Despite vital growth in medical technology, outstanding educational programs for health practitioners, advances in medical research, plentiful funds for health care, and government-sponsored programs for the aged and poor (Medicare and Medicaid), the system is undergoing tremendous criticism from both health consumers and health professionals. One writer states the basic problem strongly:

The problem, as I see it, is the serious gap between available health resources—ways in which health resources are organized and distributed—and expectations and needs of consumers. The existing organizations of health resources are totally ineffective for vast portions of our society. They

work neither quantitatively nor qualitatively. In other words, comprehensive health care is a myth![61]

According to its critics, the crisis in health care has developed for several reasons.

Medical domination is one of the major causes of the breakdown in delivery of comprehensive medical services. Medical domination, or "imperialism" (in Gorman's terms), is based on the tradition that the physician is the ultimate expert on all matters pertaining to health and disease and is thus consistently seen as the most powerful member of hospital staffs. This myopic view of the physician has alienated other health professionals and has intimidated consumers. It has also resulted in an emphasis on *medical* technology and research rather than on general health care. As a result, there has been a disproportionate allocation of government funds into medical research, technology and medical schools rather than into projects that would improve the quality of health care services for consumers.[61, 84]

Fragmentation of health service is another cause of the current crisis. Fragmentation has basically evolved from the overspecialization of physicians (90 per cent of medical school graduates are trained as specialists); the demise of the family practitioner; the multiplicity of federal, state and local programs of health care; the lack of interest in integrating these health programs; and the development of dual programs of care to service the poor versus the well-to-do. Fragmentation has resulted in a decrease in primary care and a lack of comprehensive health care.[29, 67] Consumers today experience little continuity of service from hospitals, physicians and nurses.

A third cause of the crisis is the teaching by some medical schools of an *antiquated disease model*. As we stated earlier, the treatment of infectious and acute disorders was at one time the top priority of health professionals. Today, the picture has changed, and chronic disorders as well as social and mental problems have emerged as the dominant disease models. Unfortunately many schools still emphasize the care of acute disease to the exclusion of degenerative and environmental disorders. The result is a system of health care which is built to meet the needs of the consumer 50 years ago but fails to adequately help the modern patient. In Battistella's words:

. . .while there is an abundant, if not excessive, supply of highly sophisticated and costly services available for the treatment of serious and esoteric acute illnesses, there is a shortage of personnel and services for the treatment of more commonplace nondramatic illnesses associated with primary care and the care of the chronically ill and handicapped.[11]

Rising medical costs constitute a fourth problem. Zerwekh reported in 1972 that, "In the last five years the costs of health care have risen five times faster than the cost of living. . . ."[162] *Costs are soaring* in response to our growing technology, our use of sophisticated equipment, and the unnecessary duplication and overlap of medical and hospital services. And yet, even though huge sums of money are being poured into the business of health care, the health needs of whole segments of our population still remain unmet.

> Inequities in the delivery of health care services and the demand for equality for consumers are probably the roots of the crisis in health care.[60, 61]

Despite our advanced technology and economic assets, the aged, the poor, and minorities are not receiving proper care. Below, Swan asks a vital question and employs some frightening statistics concerning inequities in health services in the United States.

Why, then, in spite of these advantages, does our country rank fourteenth among the industrialized nations of the world in infant mortality—the gauge by which a country's health standards are measured? This poor showing is due mainly to the high morbidity and mortality figures among the poor, especially the black poor. For example, infant mortality among black babies is twice that of the white babies, the maternal mortality three times as high, the tuberculosis rate seven times as high, and the life expectancy seven years less. From conception, the poor run a greater risk of disease because we know that a high percentage of women whose babies are delivered in municipal hospitals have had no prenatal care at all.[140]

The *uneven geographic distribution of physicians* in the United States creates further inequities in the delivery of health services. The majority of physicians (and especially specialists) are located in the metropolitan areas while rural areas suffer from a definite shortage of specialists.

The problems of medical domination, fragmentation of services, decreases in primary care, and spiraling costs coupled with inequities in the delivery of health care services must be met if we are to resolve the crisis in health care. We will now briefly present some of the goals and priorities that have recently evolved in an attempt to combat the growing crisis.

EMERGING PRIORITIES IN HEALTH CARE

The major health care goals today as envisioned by health professionals and consumers alike are as follows:

▶ Improvement of the care of the poor, the aged, and minority populations

▶ Greater access to health care facilities for the disadvantaged and for persons who live in sparsely populated areas of the country

▶ Greater emphasis by medical schools, federally funded programs, etc. on the prevention and treatment of the chronic and degenerative diseases as well as those disorders arising from environmental pollution

▶ The promotion of the primary care concept with an emphasis on continuity of care for the consumer from his first contact with the health care system until he is rehabilitated

▶ Maximal recognition of the need to reduce the current epidemics of alcoholism, venereal disease, drug addiction, malnutrition, mental illness, and social isolation of the elderly and chronically ill

▶ Improved and more communicative relationships between health professionals and consumers

▶ Advanced programs for educating individuals in the area of primary care, e.g., family nurse practitioners, general medical practitioners

Whether or not these goals will be met depends to a large extent on government funding and on current and future legislative rulings. Realization of these goals also depends upon the commitment of each individual health practitioner (doctor, nurse, technician, student) to the concepts of primary comprehensive health care and to the ideal that good health care is the basic right of every person regardless of age, race, cultural background or economic circumstances.

BIBLIOGRAPHY: UNIT II

1. Aakster, C. W.: Psycho-social stress and health disturbances. *Social Science and Medicine*, 8:77, Feb. 1974.
2. Abdellah, F. G.: A national health strategy for the delivery of long term health care: implications for nursing. *Nursing Digest*, 4:15, Winter 1976.
3. Aguilera, D., et al.: *Crisis Intervention: Theory and Methodology.* St. Louis, C. V. Mosby Co., 1970.

4. Anderson, O. W., and Andersen, R. M.: Patterns of use of health services, *In* Freeman, H. E., et al. (eds.): *Handbook of Medical Sociology,* 2nd ed. Englewood Cliffs, NJ, Prentice Hall, 1972, p. 386.

5. Andreoli, K. G.: The ambulatory health care system. *Nursing Digest,* 5:16, Spring 1977.

6. Arnold, M.: *Administering Health Services: Issues and Perspectives.* New York, Aldine-Atherton, 1971.

7. Auld, M. E., and Birum, L. H.: *The Challenge of Nursing: A Book of Readings.* St. Louis, C. V. Mosby Co., 1973.

8. Barach, A. L.: Homeostasis: a physiologic and psychologic function in man. *Perspectives in Biology and Medicine,* 17:522, Summer 1974.

9. Barnett, G. O., and Robbins, A.: Information technology and manpower productivity. *Journal of the American Medical Association,* 209:546, 1969.

10. Bassler, S. F.: The origins and development of biological rhythms. *Nursing Clinics of North America,* 11:575, Dec. 1976.

11. Battistella, R. M.: The right to adequate health care. *Nursing Digest,* Jan.–Feb. 1976.

12. Bell, U. R., and Schwartz, G. E.: Voluntary control and reactivity of human heart rate. *Psychophysiology,* 12:399, 1975.

13. Bell, J. M.: Stressful life events and coping methods in mental-illness and wellness behaviors. *Nursing Research,* March–April, 1977.

14. Benoliel, J. Q.: "Staff Responses to Stress," a presentation given at the *Symposium on Stress* in Seattle, Washington, March 31 and April 1, 1976. Presentation sponsored by the Puget Sound Chapter of the American Association of Critical-Care Nurses.

15. Benson, H.: *The Relaxation Response.* New York, William Morrow, 1975.

16. Benson, H.: Your innate asset for combating stress. *Nursing Digest,* May–June, 1975, p. 38.

17. Berger, R. J.: Bioenergetic functions of sleep and activity rhythms and their possible relevance to aging. *Federation Proceedings,* 34:97, Jan. 1975.

18. Berliner, B. S.: Nursing a patient in crisis. *American Journal of Nursing,* 70:2154, Oct. 1970.

19. Bircher, A. U.: Mankind in crisis: an application of clinical process to population-environment. *Nursing Forum,* 11:1, 1972.

20. Birley, J. L.: Stress and disease. *Journal of Psychosomatic Reasearch,* 16:235, Aug. 1972.

21. Boyce, T., and Michael, M., III.: Nine assumptions of western medicine. *Man and Medicine,* 1:311, Summer 1976.

22. Breeden, S. A., and Kondo, C.: Using biofeedback. *American Journal of Nursing,* 75:2010, Nov. 1973.

23. Brock, J. F.: Nature, nurture and stress in health and disease. *Lancet,* 1:701, April 1, 1972.

24. Brody, H.: The systems view of man: implications for medicine, science, and ethics. *Perspectives in Biology and Medicine,* 17:71, Autumn 1973.

25. Brower, H. T. F., and Baker, B. J.: Using the adaptation model in a practitioner curriculum. *Nursing Outlook,* 24:686, Nov. 1976.

26. Brown, B. B.: *Stress and the Art of Biofeedback.* New York, Harper & Row, Publishers, 1977.

27. Brown, F. A., et al.: *The Biological Clocks: Two Views.* New York, Academic Press, 1970.

28. Bruhn, J. G.: The diagnosis of normality. *Texas Reports on Biology and Medicine,* 32:241, Spring 1974.

29. Burns, E. M.: Critical issues in social health policies: today and tomorrow. *Man and Medicine,* 1:205, Spring 1976.

30. Busse, E. W., and Pfeiffer, E.: *Behavior and Adaptation in Late Life.* Boston, Little, Brown & Co., 1970.

31. Callahan, D.: The WHO definition of "Health." *Center Studies,* 1:77, 1973.

32. Cannon, W. B.: *The Wisdom of the Body.* New York, W. W. Norton & Co., 1939.

33. Caplan, G.: *An Approach to Community Mental Health.* New York, Grune & Stratton, Inc., 1961.

34. Caplan, G.: *Principles of Preventative Psychiatry.* New York, Basic Books, Inc. 1964.

35. Carter, P.: "Crisis Intervention," a presentation given at the *Symposium on Stress,* in Seattle, Washington, March 31 and April 1, 1976. Presentation sponsored by the Puget Sound Chapter of the American Association of Critical-Care Nurses.

36. Conroy, R., and Mills, J. M.: *Human Circadian Rhythms.* Baltimore, The Williams & Wilkins Co., 1971.

37. Dreitzel, H. P.: Introduction. *In The Social Organization of Health.* New York, The Macmillan Co., 1971.

38. Dubos, R.: *Man Adapting.* New Haven, Yale University Press, 1965.

39. Dubos, R.: *Man, Medicine, and Environment.* New York, Encyclopedia Britannica, Inc., 1968.

40. Dubos, R.: *Mirage of Health, Utopias, Progress and Biological Change.* Garden City, NY, Doubleday and Co., 1959.

41. Dubos, R., and Pines, M.: *Health and Disease.* Life Science Library. New York, Time-Life Inc., 1965.

42. Edelstein, R. R. G.: The time factor in relation to illness as a fertile nursing research area: review of the literature. *Nursing Research,* 21:72, Jan.–Feb. 1972.

43. Elpern, E. H.: Structural and organizational supports for primary nursing. *Nursing Clinics of North America,* 12:205, June 1977.

44. Engel, G. L.: A unified concept of health and disease. *Perspectives in Biology and Medicine,* 3:459, Spring 1960.

45. Engel, G. L.: Homeostasis, behavioral adjustment, and the concept of health and disease. *In* Grinker, R. S. (ed.): *Mid-Century Psychiatry,* Springfield, IL, Charles C Thomas, Publisher, 1953.

46. Engel, G. L., and Schmale, A. H.: Conservation-withdrawal: a primary process for oganismic homeostasis. *CIBA Foundation Symposium,* 8:57, 1972.

47. Engelhardt, H., Jr.: Explanatory models in medicine: facts, theories, and values. *Texas Reports on Biology and Medicine,* 12:225, Spring 1974.

48. Fabrega, H.: Concepts of disease: logical features and social implications. *Perspectives in Biology and Medicine,* 15:583, Summer 1972.

49. Fabrega, H.: *Disease and Social Behavior: An Interdisciplinary Perspective.* Cambridge, MA, M.I.T. Press, 1974.

50. Felton, G.: Body rhythm effects on rotating work shifts. *Nursing Digest,* Jan.–Feb. 1976, p. 29.

51. Fletcher, S.: Medicine and the nature of man. *Science, Medicine, and Man,* 1:93, Dec. 1973.

52. Fox, F. W.: Nature, nurture and stress. *Lancet,* 2:183, July 22, 1972.

53. Frederick, C. J.: The role of the nurse in crisis intervention and suicide prevention. *Journal of Psy-*

chiatry and Neurology and Mental Health Services, Jan.–Feb. 1973, pp. 70–81.

54. Freeman, H. E., et al.: *Handbook of Medical Sociology,* 2nd ed. Englewood Cliffs, NJ, Prentice-Hall, 1972.
55. Fried, C.: An analysis of "equality" and "rights" in medical care. *Nursing Digest, 5:*68, Spring 1977.
56. Fuchs, V.: The economics of health care in the 70's. *Hospitals J.A.H.A., 44:*66, Jan. 1970.
57. Galdston, I. (ed.): *Beyond the Germ Theory: the Roles of Deprivation and Stress in Health and Disease.* New York, Health Education Council, 1954.
58. Gerson, L. W., and Skipper, J. K., Jr.: A conceptual model for the study of the health action process. *Canadian Journal of Public Health, 63:*477, Nov.–Dec. 1972.
59. Glasser, M. A.: What price health care? *Nursing Digest, 4:*48, Winter 1976.
60. Glazier, W. H.: The task of medicine. *Scientific American, 228:*13, April 1973.
61. Gorman, M.: Societal constraints to comprehensive health care. *Nursing Forum, 12:*175, 1973.
62. Graham, S., and Reeder, L. G.: Social factors in the chronic illnesses. *In* Freeman, H. E., et al.: *Handbook of Medical Sociology,* 2nd ed. Englewood Cliffs, NJ, Prentice-Hall, 1972.
63. Green, E.: Biofeedback for mind-body-self regulation: healing and creativity. *In* Barber, T. X., et al. (eds.): *Biofeedback and Self-Control, 1972.*
64. Gunderson, E. K., and Rahe, R. H. (eds.): *Life Stress and Illness.* Springfield, IL, Charles C Thomas, Publishers, 1974.
65. Halberg, F.: Biological rhythms. *Advances in Experimental Medicine and Biology, 54:*1, 1975.
66. Halpern, H. A.: Crisis theory: a definitional study. *Community Mental Health Journal, 9:*342, Winter 1973.
67. Haynes, M. A.: Planning unifying health care. *Hospitals J.A.H.A., 44:*67, March 16, 1970.
68. Hegyvary, S. T.: Foundations of primary nursing. *Nursing Clinics of North America, 12:*187, June 1977.
69. Hinkle, L. E., Jr.: The concept of "Stress in the biological and social sciences." *Science, Medicine, and Man, 1:*31, April 1973.
70. Hinkle, L. E.: Normal stress in normal experience. *In* Galdson, J. (ed.): *Beyond the Germ Theory.* New York, Health Education Council, 1954.
71. Hitchcock, J. M.: Crisis intervention. *American Journal of Nursing, 73:*1388, Aug. 1973.
72. Horowitz, M. J.: *Stress Response Syndromes.* New York, Jason Aronson, 1976.
73. House, J. S.: Occupational stress and coronary heart disease: a review and theoretical integration. *Journal of Health and Social Behavior, 15:*12, March 1974.
74. Hoyman, H.: Models of human nature and their impact on health education. *Nursing Digest, 3:*37, Sept.–Oct. 1975.
75. Hyndman, B. W.: The role of rhythms in homeostasis. *Kybernetik, 15:*227, July 1974.
76. Jacobson, G., et al.: Generic and individual approaches to crisis intervention. *American Journal of Public Health, 58:*339, 1968.
77. Jamann, J. S.: Health is a function of ecology. *American Journal of Nursing, 71:*5, May 1971.
78. Joint Commission on Mental Illness and Health: *Ac-*

tion for Mental Health. Final Report. New York, Basic Books, 1961.
79. Jonas, G.: Mind over muscle. *In Nature/Science Annual.* New York, Time-Life Books, 1973.
80. Jonas, G.: *Visceral Learning: Toward a Science of Self Control.* New York, Cornerstone Library, 1974.
81. Katz, A. H.: The social causes of disease. *In* Dreitzel, H. P. (ed.): *The Social Organization of Health.* New York, The Macmillan Co., 1971, p. 3.
82. Kiely, W. F.: Coping with severe illness. *Advances in Psychosomatic Medicine, 8:*105, 1972.
83. King, L. S.: Causation: a problem in medical philosophy. *Clio Medica, 10:*95, 1975.
84. Kisch, A. I.: Planning for a sensible health care system. *Nursing Outlook, 20:*641, Oct. 1972.
85. Kleinman, A. M.: Toward a comparative study of medical systems: an integrated approach to the study of the relationship of medicine and culture. *Science, Medicine, and Man, 1:*55, April 1973.
86. Kleitman, N.: *Sleep and Wakefulness.* Chicago, University of Chicago Press, 1963.
87. Koppman, J. W., et al.: Voluntary regulation of temporal artery diameter by migraine patients. *Headache, 14:*133, 1974.
88. Kramer, M.: The consumer's influence on health care. *Nursing Outlook, 20:*574, Sept. 1972.
89. Kuenzi, S. H., and Fenton, M. V.: Crisis intervention in acute care areas. *American Journal of Nursing, 75:*830, May 1975.
90. Kuiper, F. C.: A few notes on the disease concept. *Psychiatria, Neurologia, Neurochirurgia, 70:*187, May–June 1967.
91. Lanuza, D. M.: Circadian rhythms of mental efficiency and performance. *Nursing Clinics of North America, 11:*583, Dec. 1976.
92. Lesparre, M.: Interview: the federal role in health. *Hospitals, J.A.H.A., 47:*45, Sept. 16, 1973.
93. Leventhal, H.: Changing attitudes and habits to reduce risk factors in chronic disease. *American Journal of Cardiology, 31:*571, May 1973.
94. Levine, M. E.: Holistic nursing. *Nursing Clinics of North America, 6:*253, June 1971.
95. Levine, S., and Scotch, N. A.: *Social Stress.* Chicago, Aldine Publishing Co., 1970.
96. Lipkin, M.: *The Care of Patients: Concepts and Tactics.* New York, Oxford University Press, 1974.
97. Luce, G. G.: *Body Time: Physiological Rhythms and Social Stress.* New York, Bantam Books, 1973.
98. Man in his world. *Lancet, 2:*27, July 1972.
99. Martin, H. W., and Prange, A. J.: Human adaptation—a conceptual approach to understanding patients. *Canadian Nurse, 58:*234, March 1962.
100. Maslow, A. H.: *Motivation and Personality,* 2nd ed. New York, Harper & Row, 1970.
101. McInnes, W. J.: Three dimensional health care. *Supervisor Nurse, 3:*17–23, July 1972.
102. McQuade, W., and Aikman, A.: *Stress.* New York, E. P. Dutton & Co., 1974.
103. Mechanic, D.: Health and illness in technological societies. *Center Studies, 1:*7–18, 1973.
104. Miller, N.: Learning of glandular and visceral responses. *In* Barber, T. X., et al. (eds.): *Biofeedback and Self Control, 1972.* Chicago, Aldine Publishing Co., 1973, p. 90.
105. Mitchell, C. E.: Identifying the hazard: the key to crisis intervention. *American Journal of Nursing, 77:*1194, July 1977.
106. Morley, W. E., et al.: Crisis: paradigms of intervention. *Journal of Psychiatric Nursing, 5:*537, 1967.
107. Moss, G. E.: *Illness, Immunity and Social Interaction.* New York, John Wiley & Sons, 1973.
108. Nenner, V. C., et al.: Primary nursing. *Supervisor Nurse, 8:*14, May 1977.
109. O'Dell, M. L.: Human biorhythmology: implications for nursing practice. *Nursing Forum, 14:*43, 1975.

110. Oelbaum, C. H.: Hallmarks of adult wellness. *American Journal of Nursing*, 74:1623, Sept. 1974.
111. Overmire, T. G.: *Homeostatic Regulation.* American Institute of Biological Sciences, Biological Sciences Curriculum Study, Pamphlet 9, Sept. 1963.
112. Parsons, T.: *The Social System.* Glencoe, IL, The Free Press, 1951.
113. Patel, C.: 12 month follow-up of yoga and biofeedback in the management of hypertension. *Lancet*, 27:62, 1975.
114. Peason, B. D.: Nursing implications of "What Price Health Care?" by M. A. Glasser. *Nursing Digest*, 4:51, Winter 1976.
115. Penfield, W.: *The Mystery of the Mind.* Princeton, Princeton University Press, 1975.
116. Potter, V. R.: Probabilistic aspects of the human cybernetic machine. *Perspectives in Biology and Medicine*, 17:164, Winter 1974.
117. Raskin, M., et al.: Chronic anxiety treated by feedback-induced muscle relaxation. *Archives of General Psychiatry*, 28:263, Feb. 1973.
118. Reverby, S.: A perspective on the root causes of illness. *American Journal of Public Health*, 62:1040, Aug. 1972.
119. Roemer, M. I.: Health care financing and delivery around the world. *American Journal of Nursing*, 71:1158, June 1971.
120. Romano, J.: *Adaptation.* Ithaca, NY, Cornell University Press, 1949.
121. Roy, C.: Adaptation: A conceptual framework for nursing. *Nursing Outlook*, 18:42, March 1970.
121a. Roy, C.: Comment: the Roy adaptation model. *Nursing Outlook*, 24:690, Nov. 1976.
122. Scheving, L., and Pauly, J.: Circadian rhythms: some examples and comments on clinical application. *Chronobiologia*, 1:3, Jan.–March 1974.
123. Schmitt, O. H.: Chronobiophysics. *Chronobiologia*, 1:28, Jan.–Feb. 1974.
124. Scott, R., and Howard, A.: Models of stress. *In* Levine, S., and Scotch, N. (eds.): *Social Stress.* Chicago, Aldine Publishing Co., 1970.
125. Sedgwick, P.: Illness—mental and otherwise. *Center Studies*, 1:19, 1973.
126. Selye, H.: *Stress without Distress.* Philadelphia, J. B. Lippincott Co., 1974.
127. Selye, H.: *The Physiology and Pathology of Exposure to Stress: A Treatise Based on the Concepts of the General Adaptation Syndrome and the Diseases of Adaptation.* Montreal, Acta, 1950.
128. Selye, H.: The physiopathology of stress. *Postgraduate Medicine*, Vol. 25, June 1959.
129. Selye, H.: *The Stress of Life.* New York, McGraw-Hill Book Co., 1956.
130. Shapiro, D.: Preface. *In* Barber, T. X., et al. (eds.): *Biofeedback and Self-Control, 1972.* Chicago, Aldine Publishing Co., 1973, p. v.
131. Shapiro, D., and Schwartz, G. E.: Biofeedback and visceral learning: clinical applications. *In* Barber, T. X., et al. (eds.): *Biofeedback and Self-Control, 1972.* Chicago, Aldine Publishing Co., 1973, p. 477.
132. Sheldon, A.: Toward a general theory of disease and medical care. *Science, Medicine and Man*, 1:237, Dec. 1974.
133. Siegel, H.: To your health—whatever that may mean. *Nursing Forum*, 12:280, 1973.
134. Slavensky, A. T., et al.: Back to the community: a dubious blessing. *Nursing Outlook*, 24:370, June 1976.
135. Smolensky, M. H., and Reinberg, A.: The chronotherapy of corticosteroids: practical application of chronobiologic findings to nursing. *Nursing Clinics of North America*, 11:609, Dec. 1976.
136. *Statistical Abstracts 1974:* United States Department of Commerce, Bureau of the Census, 1974.
137. Steinfels, P.: The concept of health: an introduction. *The Hasting's Center Studies*, 1:3, 1973.
138. Stephens, G. J.: Periodicity in mood, affect, and instinctual behavior. *Nursing Clinics of North America*, 11:595, Dec. 1976.
139. Sterman, L. T.: Clinical biofeedback. *American Journal of Nursing*, 75:2006, Nov. 1975.
140. Swan, L. F.: Group approach to medical care. *Nursing Outlook*, 18:56, Jan. 1970.
141. Swanson, B. E.: The politics of health. *In* Freeman, H., et al. (eds.): *Handbook of Medical Sociology*, 2nd ed. Englewood Cliffs, NJ, Prentice-Hall, 1972, p. 435.
142. Tanner, O.: *Stress: Time-Life Library of Human Behavior.* New York, Time-Life Books, 1976.
143. Taylor, F. K.: A logical analysis of the medicopsychological concept of disease. *Psychological Medicine*, 1:356, 1971.
144. Timiras, P. S.: Decline in homeostatic regulation. *In Developmental Physiology and Aging.* New York, Macmillan, 1972, p. 546.
145. Timiras, P. S.: Aging of homeostatic control system. *Federation Proceedings*, 34:81, Jan. 1975.
146. Tom, C. K.: Nursing assessment of biological rhythms. *Nursing Clinics of North America*, 11:621, Dec. 1976.
147. Tom, C. K., and Lanuza, D. M. (eds.): Introduction: symposium on biological rhythms. *Nursing Clinics of North America*, 11:569, Dec. 1976.
148. Torrey, H. B.: Adaptation as a process. *Scientific Monthly*, Dec. 1915.
149. Twaddle, A. C.: Illness and deviance. *Social Science and Medicine*, 7:751, Oct. 1973.
150. Volpe, P.: *Man, Nature, and Society: An Introduction to Biology.* Dubuque, William C. Brown Co., 1975.
151. Wadsworth, M.: Health and sickness: the choice of treatment. *Nursing Digest*, Sept.–Oct. 1975.
152. Wagner, P.: Testing the adaptation model in practice. *Nursing Outlook*, 24:682, Nov. 1976.
153. Ward, R. R.: *The Living Clocks.* New York, New American Library–Mentor Books, 1971.
154. Weiss, J. M.: Psychological factors in stress and disease. *Scientific American*, 226:104, June 1972.
155. Wender, P. H.: Vicious and virtuous circles: the role of deviation amplifying feedback in the origin and perpetuation of behavior. *Psychiatry*, 31:309, Nov. 1968.
156. Wiener, N.: *Cybernetics*, 2nd ed. Cambridge, MA, Massachusetts Institute of Technology Press, 1961.
157. Wiener, N.: *The Human Use of Human Beings: Cybernetics Society*, Garden City, NY, Doubleday Co., 1956.
158. Williams, J.: Hart, E., and Sechrist, W. (eds.): *Dynamics of Wellness.* Belmont, CA, Wadsworth Publishing Co., 1970.
159. Wolf, S.: Disease as a way of life. *Perspectives in Biology and Medicine*, 4:288, Spring 1961.
159a. Wolff, H. G.: A concept of disease in man. *Psychosomatic Medicine*, 24:25, Jan.–Feb. 1962.
160. Wolff, H. G.: *Stress and Disease*, 2nd ed. Springfield, IL, Charles C Thomas, Publisher, 1968.
161. *World Health Organization (WHO) Demographic Year Book 1975:* Department of Economic and Social Affairs, United Nations Statistical Office, 1975.
162. Zerwekh, J. M.: The health-care nightmare. *Nursing Forum*, 11:336, 1972.
163. Zola, I. K.: The concept of trouble and sources of medical assistance. *Social Science and Medicine*, 6:673, 1972.

UNIT
III

UNDERSTANDING THE EXISTENCE OF THE ILL

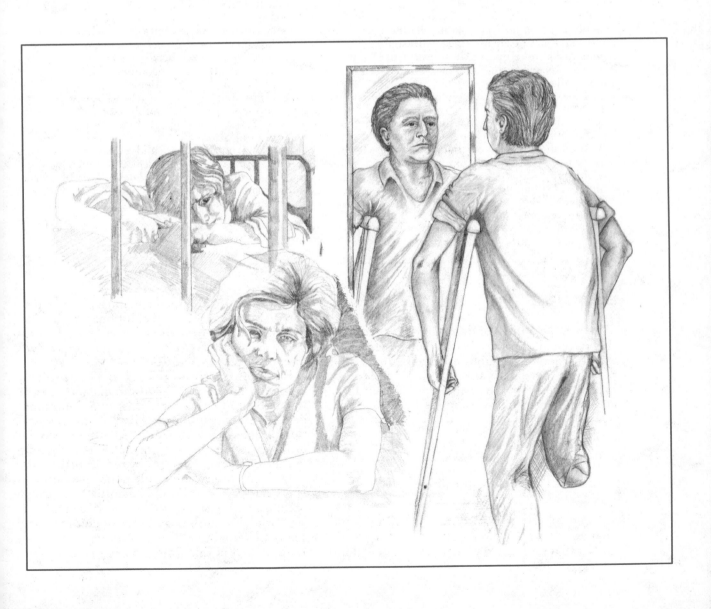

CHAPTER 8

ANXIETY . . . THE MOTIVATING EMOTION

INTRODUCTION AND STUDY GUIDE

This chapter opens with a brief general discussion of emotions. The nature of anxiety is next reviewed, e.g., causes of anxiety, communication of anxiety, levels of anxiety. In the final section of this chapter physiologic and psychologic responses to anxiety are considered, mental defense mechanisms are defined, and examples in nursing are presented. These mechanisms are referred to in subsequent chapters.

As you proceed to study this chapter, the following study guide may be helpful:

1. Identify the three levels on which emotions exist.

2. Define anxiety and distinguish between anxiety and fear.

3. Identify three factors that influence whether anxiety is helpful or harmful.

4. Identify situations in your own experience which made you feel anxious.

5. Identify your physical and mental feelings when you are anxious.

6. Try to recall your behaviors the last time you experienced a fairly high level of anxiety.

7. Consider how patient teaching is affected if the patient is highly anxious and identify other ways patient care might be affected if a patient's anxiety level is high (this would be a suitable topic for group discussion).

8. In your own words state the functions and general characteristics of mental defense mechanisms.

9. Provide your own examples of

rationalization	compensation
projection	denial
repression	reaction formation
suppression	sublimation
regression	displacement
identification	

As you give patient care and work with coworkers try to be aware of the presence of anxiety in yourself and these other people. Whenever suitable, make appropriate interventions to reduce high levels of unproductive anxiety.

EMOTIONS

In order to understand the concept of anxiety it is necessary first to examine some basic facts about emotions. Emotions are feelings that prompt a person to observable action or to internal mental and physiologic changes. They are thus crucial in the adaptive process.

> *Physiologic changes take place within the body when emotional states occur, and it is known that specific patterns of physiologic change are related to specific emotions.*

Some physiologic activities that undergo changes as a result of emotional states are (1) brain waves, (2) the electrical resistance of the skin surface, (3) heart rate, (4) muscular tension, and (5) breathing rate. All emotions may be said to exist on three levels: (1) a neuroendocrine level; (2) a motor-visceral level; and (3) a level of conscious awareness.

Emotions motivate behavior. The resultant behavior may be impulsive and maladaptive, or it may be appropriate and adaptive. Emotional development is influenced by both the maturation process and learning. Emotions can be aroused by projecting oneself ahead in time (anticipating the future) or by recalling the past.

In the mature adult a wide range of emotional behavior is possible. One familiar emotional state is *anxiety*. Since the concept of anxiety is essential for understanding psychic life and many physiologic disorders, let us turn our attention to it at this time.

Anxiety may be considered to be essentially a human experience, since it is associated with the capacity for delayed reaction, choice of action, self-reflection of motivation, and projection of the self into the future. Thus, anxiety can be present only in humans, who have evolved a form of self-reflective consciousness. Because anxiety is an emotion, it is not directly observable. Instead, the physiologic and behavioral *results* of anxiety can be observed.

We are said to be living in the "age of anxiety." Anxious feelings are familiar to us; however, these feelings are not unique to our period in history. Anxiety has always been a part of human existence because it is the result of frustrations and conflicts that occur with life. Of the variety of unpleasant emotions that are the end product of conflict and frustration, anxiety is the most outstanding.

Anxiety can be described as apprehension, dread, foreboding, or uneasiness that is related to an *unidentifiable* source of anticipated danger. *"Anxiety" and "fear" are not the same, because with fear the source of danger is recognized and can be identified* (see Table 8–1). Generally when we feel anxious we are aware of feeling uncomfortable; indeed, at times we may experience intense discomfort. Such feelings are usually an admixture of both physical and mental states: (1) we are aware of a feeling of nervousness or mental uneasiness; (2) we also experience a variety of physiologic states that are disturbing. The results of such unpleasant feelings are a variety of manifestations of anxiety, for example, a quavering voice. Uncomfortable as we may be when anxious, we generally cannot identify exactly what it is that causes us to feel as we do. It is precisely because we cannot readily recognize its source that anxiety can become so disturbing. Usually we are unable to tolerate anxious feelings for a sustained period of time. As further discussion will demonstrate, we attempt to terminate anxiety in many different ways.

Even though anxiety may be uncomfortable to experience, it is, nevertheless, an essential life ingredient. Anxiety can be thought of as being helpful or harmful, depending on the following: (1) its degree of intensity, (2) its appropriateness, and (3) its duration.

> *An appropriate degree of anxiety serves a useful integrative purpose.*

Unless we are mildly anxious as students, for example, we tend to lack appropriate motivation to study and learn. Excessive anxiety, on the other hand, may have a disintegrative effect because it can immobilize an individual or lead to panic states in which appropriate goal-directed behavior is not possible. However, when anxiety is absent, in apathy for example, goal-directed behavior is also impossible. In nursing, one is often faced with the critical issue of how best to manage an apathetic patient. It is not uncommon to witness the death of patients who lack the will to live and thus become apathetic and die, even though their presenting illness need not have been fatal. Such events are further testimony to the fact that we cannot separate the mental and physical states—the one pervades the other and they are mutually interactive.

> *In addition to the degree of anxiety present, we must consider its appropriateness and duration.*

It is appropriate and expected that individuals experience anxiety in certain situations and not in others. Also, the expected duration of anxiety will vary with the situation itself and with the individual's perception of it. Ultimately, of course, we find that the same situation may prove to be anxiety-provoking for one person but not for another. Such matters of individual perception vary greatly, depending upon an individual's learning and degree of maturation.

As Figure 8–1 indicates, perception contributes greatly to the production of anxiety. The emotional state of anxiety makes its appearance during infancy. Usually the first behavioral signs of anxiety appear at about 7 or 8 months of age. Did the picture on the left make you feel "anxious" when you first noticed it? Can you identify why it made you feel "anxious"?

Anxiety forces change. It is the piston-like driving force in the dynamics of all human ad-

TABLE 8–1.   ANXIETY VS. FEAR

ANXIETY	FEAR
Unknown threat	Recognizable threat
Internal threat	External threat
Related to the future	Immediate
Vague in character	Definite in character
Consequence of psychologic conflict	Not a consequence of psychologic conflict

Source: Eiland, D. C., Jr.: The chronically anxious patient. *American Family Physician*, 9:157, Feb. 1974.

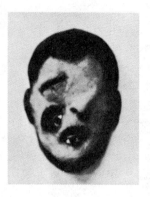
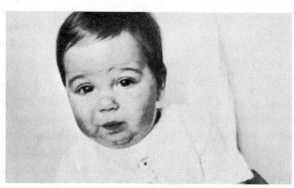

Figure 8–1. Perceptual distortion and anxiety. Violation of perceptual expectancies makes the baby of about eight months express anxiety when he sees the distorted mask at left. At an earlier period, before he learned what the human face is supposed to look like, he might have smiled at the mask. (From Kagan, J., and Havemann, E.: *Psychology: An Introduction.* New York, Harcourt Brace and World, 1968.)

justment. The important factor is the *direction* of the change, for anxiety can produce both constructive and destructive change. An individual can grow through the changes that anxiety forces or he can be destroyed by them. Sustained anxiety clearly can produce mental and physical illness if the individual's adaptive pattern is unhealthy for him.

> *Anxiety is our life partner; either we can strive to recognize its presence and use it constructively, or we can succumb to it.*

What Causes Anxiety?

A countless variety of situations involving frustration, conflict, and stress cause anxiety and are familiar to us all. We all have incentives or are motivated toward certain goals in life for a variety of reasons. However, life experience shows us that we do not always reach the goals we seek. Obstacles to goal satisfaction may be either external or internal. When our goal-directed behavior is thwarted or interfered with, we experience frustration. Frustration produces feelings of anxiety within us; these feelings are also produced by conflicting motives that force us to make choices.

Whether or not an event is perceived as anxiety-producing is an individual matter. Generally we may say that *situations of frustration, conflict, or stress that threaten the* *physical or mental security of an individual produce anxiety.* Certainly the major anxiety-producing conditions that the nurse will encounter are illness and death. Threats to physical existence can be recognized more easily than threats to one's mental self-concept. It is possible to see clearly an uncontrolled infection producing bodily changes that are life-threatening, but it is more difficult to identify the threats to the patient's mental self-image that such an illness produces.

Illness is both physically and mentally taxing. The skilled nurse recognizes that illness produces anxious feelings in patients; she also tries to be sensitive to the individual anxieties that patients experience when illness interferes with their unique self-expectations and needs.

Anxiety Is Communicated

Both verbally and nonverbally we receive messages that tell us when other people are anxious. An individual's voice may shake or break; his words may convey anxiety; his manner of speaking may change from his usual pattern to one that is more rapid or slow; the pitch of his voice may change. A tense posture, nervous movements, "wide-eyed" appearance, and perspiration are a few nonverbal clues to anxiety. Anxious feelings can be communicated from one person to another. One anxious patient in a ward can make the other patients anxious; the anxious nurse communicates her anxiety to patients and coworkers.

It is important that the nurse understand the ways in which anxiety is believed to affect such important processes as learning, perception, awareness and thinking. Because the nurse daily works with anxious people, she can help to meet their needs better if she can understand what their mental experiences are like. As always, she can learn best from her own experience.

Peplau[31] and Francis and Munjas[15] help us conceptualize anxiety by placing degrees of anxiety on a continuum, ranging from ataraxy to panic (see Fig. 8–2). Briefly summarized, the levels on this continuum are as follows:[15]

▶ *Ataraxy:* An uncommon state characterized by the absence of anxiety or the presence of anxiety which is so minimal in degree that it does not affect the individual in terms of desires or motivations. (*Note:* drugs given for the purpose of reducing anxiety levels are called "ataractics.")

▶ *Well-being:* That state, which typically follows satisfying experiences, in which the individual feels relaxed, comfortable and happy. In this state of minimal anxiety the individual is not very alert. This level of anxiety is believed to be healing.

▶ *Mild anxiety:* This attentive, gentle level of anxiety is useful and is experienced by most productive, healthy persons.

▶ *Moderate anxiety:* This intermediate, tempered level of anxiety can take on the qualities of either mild or severe anxiety, being neither restrained nor excessive. At its lower levels, moderate anxiety can heighten one's productivities and abilities; at its higher levels, it can narrow perception in such a way that the individual is unaware of peripheral activities.

▶ *Severe anxiety:* This painful, harsh level of anxiety is not useful and hence should be reduced through appropriate interventions. Severe anxiety consumes most of the individual's energy, inhibiting his physiologic powers of restoration. The person in severe anxiety may be aware of his overwhelming anxiety or he may be unaware of it and dissociate himself from the anxiety.

▶ *Panic:* This frightening, violent, disintegrating, overpowering level of anxiety causes the individual to lose control of himself. This level of anxiety is not frequently encountered; however, when it does occur it is critical—perhaps a matter of life or death. Panic, the most severe state of psychologic disequilibrium, cannot be endured for very long. Prompt intervention is required. The individual in panic cannot perceive, make decisions, remember, or control his affect (emotional feeling or tone) or his motor activities.

Mild anxiety is an asset to successful adaptation in life. When we are mildly anxious we are alerted in such a manner that we can "take in" more than usual and thus our perception becomes keener, and we are in a state that is conducive to learning. A mild state of anxiety may thus help a nurse to function effectively; it may also help a patient to learn or to understand what the nurse or doctor may be attempting to tell him.

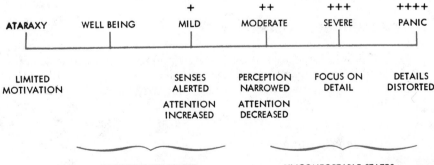

Figure 8–2. Anxiety continuum. (From Francis, G. M., and Munjas, B.: *Promoting Psychological Comfort.* Dubuque, Iowa, W. C. Brown Co., 1968, p. 22.)

Adapted from H. E. Peplau, *Interpersonal Relations in Nursing*, page 126. © G. P. Putnam's Sons, 1952.

As the level of anxiety increases, however, we lose our ability to function effectively over a period of time. When anxiety mounts we become less able to consider a situation in its entirety; our perceptual field is reduced so that we perceive only part of a situation. In situations of *extreme anxiety (panic)* we may find that we "blow up" one area of concern out of all proportion and are unable to comprehend the total situation. Panic also may produce a state of mind in which our attention is greatly scattered and we are unable to maintain any goal-directed activity. Heightened anxiety thus tends to produce confusion and becomes maladaptive. Perceptual distortions of time, space, people, and the meaning of events also occur. Such distortions impede learning because they interfere with our ability to relate one item to another, to recall, or to concentrate generally.

> *As a patient's level of anxiety increases he will become increasingly unable to understand clearly what is happening to him and what is expected of him.*

Thus, if a patient's level of anxiety is excessively high, it will interfere with effective patient teaching. Because the extremely anxious person easily misunderstands what is said to him, communication with him should be clear and directions brief. Repeating statements is frequently helpful, as anxious persons tend to forget easily. Nonverbal motions may aid in clarifying communication at such times. The anxious person needs an opportunity to discuss his feelings with a calm person.

RESPONSES TO ANXIETY

Anxiety produces physiologic (somatic) responses and psychologic responses simultaneously; our awareness of these responses varies.

Physiologic Responses

In response to anxiety the body alerts itself in preparation to "fight or flee." When we are anxious we can feel our heart beat faster (tachycardia) or "flutter" (palpitate); we may breathe rapidly (hyperventilate) or experience

TABLE 8–2. COMMON PHYSIOLOGIC EFFECTS OF ANXIETY

EFFECTS THAT MAY BE CONSCIOUSLY FELT	EFFECTS THAT CANNOT BE CONSCIOUSLY FELT
Heart beats faster or flutters	Blood pressure rises
Difficult or rapid breathing	Blood temporarily removed from gastrointestinal tract and made available to muscles
Frequent yawning; dry mouth	Liver releases sugar
Chest pain	Adrenal glands produce epinephrine
Anorexia, nausea, vomiting, abdominal cramps, diarrhea, gas pains, "butterflies"	Peristaltic activity is reduced
Flushing, excessive perspiration, "cold sweats," shifts in body temperature	Pupils dilate
Urgency to urinate, frequent urination	
Dysmenorrhea, frigidity	
Impotence	
Aching muscles and joints	
Arthralgia, arthritis	
Backache, headache, wryneck	

difficulty in breathing (embarrassed respirations); perhaps we yawn a lot or feel chest pain. Some other physiologic effects of anxiety that we may consciously experience are anorexia, nausea, vomiting, abdominal cramps or diarrhea. We may feel flushed or perspire excessively. Some individuals experience an urgency to urinate or may need to urinate more frequently. Anxiety can produce dysmenorrhea and frigidity in women; men may experience impotence. The musculoskeletal response may be manifested as aching muscles or joints and complaints of arthralgia or arthritis. Backache, headache or wryneck also may be attributable to anxiety. These are all physiologic results of anxiety that we may consciously be aware of and thus *feel*.

Other changes in body function occur that are *not* within our conscious awareness. For example, in order to force more blood into the muscles, the blood pressure is maintained or elevated. Moreover, blood is made available to the muscles by means of its temporary removal from the gastrointestinal tract. Also, the liver releases sugar, the adrenals produce epinephrine, and peristaltic activity is reduced. The pupils dilate so that we can "see more" and thus be ready to respond to emergencies. In general, the cardiovascular system is stimulated and the gastrointestinal system is inhibited. Table 8–2 presents a summary of some common physiologic effects of anxiety (see also Fig. 8–3).

As individuals each of us tends to experience anxiety differently: one person may experience mainly gastrointestinal symptoms while another may most commonly notice cardiovascular symptoms. If the anxiety is short-lived, that is, successfully dealt with, these psychic and physiologic effects do no harm. However, it can be seen clearly that sustained or chronic anxiety will eventually take its toll of the body by keeping it in an abnormal state.

Although these are some of the typical major responses to anxiety, the nurse is cautioned not to assume automatically that anxiety is the sole basis for these symptoms or bodily responses. For example, anxiety may or may not be a contributing factor in the etiology of headache. Only a precise diagnostic work-up can demonstrate the specific etiology of such symptoms in a given patient. Furthermore, if anxiety should prove to be a significant factor, the nurse must remember that the symptom is out of the patient's conscious control. The pain

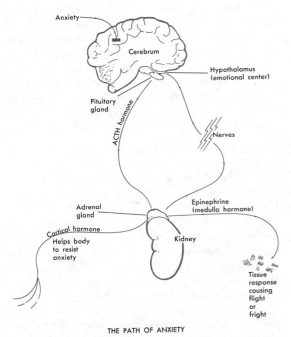

THE PATH OF ANXIETY

Figure 8–3. Anxiety reaches the cerebrum and stimulates both the pituitary gland and the hypothalamus. This action results in two responses: (1) the pituitary gland excretes the ACTH hormone, which in turn stimulates the cortex of the adrenal gland, which then produces the cortical hormone to help the body resist anxiety; and (2) the hypothalamus sends out stimuli along the autonomic nervous system to the medulla of the adrenal gland, which then produces epinephrine and prepares the tissues for the fight or flight response. (From Saxton, D. F., and Haring, P. W.: *Care of Patients with Emotional Problems,* 2nd ed. St. Louis, The C. V. Mosby Co., 1975, p. 22.)

experienced from headache caused by anxiety may be as intense as that of a headache resulting from brain tumor.

The physiologic responses to anxiety that we have been discussing may exist in varying degrees or levels, depending upon the intensity of the anxiety. The greater the anxiety, the more extreme the physiologic response tends to be. These physiologic responses to anxiety are of obvious interest to the nurse, as she studies the body in health as well as in conditions in which physiologic changes are disease-producing.

Psychologic and Behavioral Responses to Anxiety

Anxiety tends to motivate us to behaviors and attitudes that we hope will reduce the anxiety and the resultant discomfort that it produces. As individuals we each tend to develop our own patterns of reacting to the frustrations, conflicts and anxious feelings that are a part of life. Much of our personality actually consists of our individual manner of dealing with anxiety.

MENTAL DEFENSE MECHANISMS

There are many different ways of classifying reactions to anxiety. Although our individual responses are all unique to some extent, there are broad common patterns of reacting that have been identified and named "defense mechanisms," "basic adjustive techniques" or "adaptive mental mechanisms." These are mental processes and behavior that serve the important function of protecting our self-esteem by defending us against excessive anxiety.

Adequate self-esteem and self-respect are necessary for healthy function. We all use certain types of behavior, especially in stressful situations, in attempts to maintain and improve our self-concept. All of us more or less regularly encounter anxiety-producing situations through which we feel our "self" threatened. Defense mechanisms comprise those habits that we have developed for defending our self-regard and at times enhancing it. The self is protected, by means of defense mechanisms, not only from the threats that may present themselves in our external environment (i.e., from other people and from situations in which we find ourselves) but also from the dangers that arise from within ourselves (i.e., from our own impulses or affects).

Defense mechanisms have several general characteristics: First, they defend the self and protect it from injury by bolstering self-esteem or through self-enhancement. Second, defense mechanisms are not used deliberately, but rather they are unconscious, or at least partly so. Defense mechanisms also tend to have in common the quality of self-deception; that is, they operate by (1) masking or disguising our true motives or (2) denying the existence within ourselves of impulses, actions or memories that might be anxiety-provoking to us. Adaptive mental mechanisms thus protect us from anxiety by distorting (1) perception, (2) memory, (3) action, (4) motivation, and (5) thinking or by completely blocking out some psychologic process.

Defense mechanisms are essential for healthy adaptation. Like anxiety, defense mechanisms can contribute in a positive sense to an individual's developing life or they can, through overuse or their failure when needed, lead to a disruptive, unhappy life pattern.

Defense mechanisms usually are studied in detail in courses in psychology and psychiatry. We include here a brief outline of some common defense mechanisms to facilitate the transfer of psychologic theory into patient care (see Table 8–3).

We can understand more clearly the fears and concerns of patients if we can identify when they use adaptive mechanisms and what their behavioral adaptive patterns are. Let us briefly summarize some major points concerning defense mechanisms and look at some nursing implications:

▶ Defensive behavior often evokes, in others, feelings of retaliation or retreat. The nurse who reacts to anxious patients in this manner (because she does not recognize their anxiety and understand it) may intensify a patient's anxiety rather than reduce it. Furthermore, the nurse should examine her own defensive behavior and recognize that such behavior, on her part, can create problems for her with patients and coworkers.

▶ While it is possible to describe defense mechanisms and resultant behavior, we often cannot identify or understand the specific needs that make the person rely on the mechanisms he is using. Therefore, the nurse should not tamper with a patient's system of defenses; rather, she should recog-

nize the behavior as being defensive in nature and as serving the function of protecting the individual from anxiety. While a patient's behavior may seem maladaptive to her (because of the defenses used), it may be that the patient's defenses are serving adaptive purposes for him at the time. Without them his anxiety might be overwhelming.

▶ Defense mechanisms are not "abnormal" or "bad." They are used daily by everyone as a means of adaptation to life. They are helpful and necessary because they reduce anxiety and help us to retain emotional equilibrium. However, psychopathology or psychologic maladaptation can occur when (1) certain defense mechanisms are overused, and the individual becomes overly dependent on their usage; or (2) they fail to protect the individual as they once did. A nurse needs extensive education and experience before she can identify when the use of defense mechanisms is pathologic in degree. Patient behavior that she feels is maladaptive should be discussed with the attending physician.

▶ Defensive behavior, like all behavior, may be thought of as existing on a continuum or in various degrees. The classification of behavior into defense mechanisms is an arbitrary procedure and it would be unfortunate if it resulted in the stereotyping or labeling of individuals. There are no clear borderlines between various types of defensive behavior. Often when an individual reacts to a stressful situation, his behavior is a combination of several mechanisms.

▶ Defense mechanisms normally function to help to conserve emotional energy. Healthy living should be a process of expedient use of energy—both physical and mental. An individual whose self-esteem is chronically low or who lacks self-respect (consciously or unconsciously) may utilize so much energy through overuse of defense mechanisms (in an attempt at self-justification) that he has little energy available for use in constructive self-realization. This may be the situation with a person experiencing an illness. Illness produces frustrations, conflicts and anxiety. In trying to ward off anxiety and retain a satisfactory self-concept, a patient may overuse certain mechanisms, thus taxing his mental energy and flexibility. Also, he may find that certain mechanisms that helped him to adapt when he was well fail him in illness. Recognizing that illness and hospitalization are stressful experiences, the nurse should *expect* that patients may react to their situation with some exaggerated use

TABLE 8–3. DEFENSE MECHANISMS AND THEIR USAGE

DEFENSE MECHANISM	DESCRIPTION	EXAMPLES IN NURSING CARE
Rationalization	Assigning logical reasons or plausible excuses for what we have done impulsively or for motives that we do not wish to acknowledge; serves to maintain self-respect and prevents feelings of guilt	A patient is extremely rude and demanding; he thinks to himself that it is all right for him to behave this way because he is sick; he thus excuses his behavior
Projection	Attributing to others exaggerated amounts of undesirable qualities that we have but do not wish to recognize in ourselves	The rude, demanding patient may not recognize his behavior; instead he thinks the nurse is behaving in this way, thus projecting his feelings onto her; actually her behavior is misinterpreted by him, as she has not been rude or demanding
Repression	Involuntarily forgetting about unacceptable ideas, impulses or events; serve to protect us from being constantly aware of anxiety-producing situations	A patient had a sudden strong urge to defecate and was incontinent before the nurse could help her onto the bedpan; the patient was extremely embarrassed by the situation; a month later she had totally forgotten about the incident and did not remember it again
Suppression	Consciously putting unacceptable ideas, impulses or events out of mind; the material can readily be recalled	A patient has been told by her physician that she needs to undergo surgery; this thought is upsetting to her; she leaves the doctor's office and says to herself, "I won't think about it now; I'll do some shopping instead"
Regression	Returning to an earlier level of emotional adjustment; an unconscious process	A patient is usually quite self-sufficient when he is feeling well; however, with his illness he becomes somewhat more dependent than his physical condition necessitates; thus, he returns to an earlier level of dependency
Identification	Unconsciously adopting the personality characteristics of another individual whom the subject admires—the opposite of projection; not consciously trying to be like someone else	Two patients with multiple sclerosis share a room in the hospital for several weeks; one admires the other very much and over a period of time her attitude toward her illness becomes similar to that of the friend she admires A nurse's professional, kind attitude with patients is unconsciously adopted by other members of the staff who admire her
Compensation	A conscious or unconscious attempt to overcome real or imagined inferiorities	A patient paralyzed from the waist down works hard to develop the muscles in his trunk and arms to compensate for his inability to use his legs
Denial	Unconsciously refusing to acknowledge to oneself a known fact that is uncomfortable to accept; not consciously lying to oneself	A patient is proved to have cancer and is told the diagnosis by his physician; the patient does not consciously admit to himself that he has cancer; he denies the diagnosis
Reaction formation	A forbidden motive or behavior is denied, and the individual develops behavior displaying the opposite motive	A patient is fearful of surgery but instead of appearing fearful he acts unconcerned and nonchalant about it; he jokes about surgery and says, "There's nothing to it. I don't know why some guys are such babies about going"
Sublimation	The "socialization of energy" by diverting unacceptable impulses into socially accepted behavior	A patient is angry because he was hit by a car, injured and is hospitalized for several weeks; he is missing work and his wife is home taking care of their three young children by herself; he directs his "angry energy" into pounding designs into leather and selling the purses, wallets, etc.; he sends home the small amount of money he makes and thus has a sense of contributing to his home and family
Displacement	Emotion or behavior is redirected from the original object or person to a more acceptable substitute object	A patient hopes to go home but is told by his doctor that he probably cannot be discharged for some time; the patient is angry at what the doctor says but doesn't want to appear angry at the doctor; the rest of the day he is short-tempered with the nurses; he thus displaces his anger from the doctor to the nurses

of their defense patterns and with mental fatigue and irritability.

▶ When we say that a certain type of behavior serves as a defense mechanism we are speaking theoretically. Behavior that is classified as functioning as a defense mechanism in one situation may not be used as a defense mechanism in another situation. Whether or not the behavior is used defensively depends upon the individual's motivation and whether the behavior has distorted his sense of reality.

BIBLIOGRAPHY

1. Aasterud, M.: Defenses against anxiety in the nurse-patient relationship. *Nursing Forum, 1*:35, Summer 1962.
2. Appley, M., and Turnbull, R.: *Psychological Stress.* New York, Appleton-Century-Crofts, 1965.
3. Basowitz, H.: *Anxiety and Stress: An Interdisciplinary Study of a Life Situation.* New York, Blakiston Division, McGraw-Hill Book Co., 1955.
4. Boulette, T. R.: Anxiety and the nurse. *P.N., 17*:28, Aug. 1967.
5. Burd, S. F., and Marshall, M. A. (eds.): *Some Clinical Approaches to Psychiatric Nursing.* New York, The Macmillan Co., 1963.
6. Burkhardt, M.: Response to anxiety. *American Journal of Nursing, 69*:2153, Oct. 1969.
7. Cattell, R. B.: The nature and measurement of anxiety. *Scientific American,* Vol. 96, March 1963.
7a. Chernus, J.: Finding clues to anxiety. *Consultant, 14*:74–75, March 1974.
8. Cleland, V. S.: Effects of stress on thinking. *American Journal of Nursing, 67*:108, Jan. 1967.
9. Cloudsley, T., and Leonard, J.: *Animal Conflict and Adaptation.* Chester Springs, PA, Dufour Editions, 1965.
10. Cofer, C., and Appley, M.: *Motivation: Theory and Research.* New York, John Wiley & Sons, 1964.
11. Drage, E. M.: Recall of panic episodes. *American Journal of Nursing, 68*:1254, June 1968.
12. Dumas, R., and Leonard, R.: The effect of nursing on the incidence of postoperative vomiting. *Nursing Research, 12*:12, 1963.
13. Durand, M.: The nurse and the anxious patient. Paper presented at the Institute "Anxiety, Depression and Suicide," sponsored by University of Washington School of Nursing, February 10, 1966.
14. Eiland, D. C., Jr.: The chronically anxious patient. *American Family Physician, 9*:156, Feb. 1974.
15. Francis, G. M., and Munjas, B.: *Promoting Psychological Comfort.* Dubuque, Iowa, W. C. Brown Co., 1968.
16. Freud, S.: *The Problem of Anxiety.* New York, W. W. Norton, 1966.
17. Fromm-Reichmann, F.: Psychiatric aspects of anxiety. *In* Stein, M., Vidich, A. J., and White, D. M. (eds.): *Identity and Anxiety.* Glencoe, IL, The Free Press, 1960.
18. Glasrud, C. A. (ed.): *The Age of Anxiety.* Boston, Houghton Mifflin Co., 1960.
19. Gregg, D.: Anxiety, a factor in nursing care. *American Journal of Nursing, 52*:1363, Nov. 1952.
20. Gregg, D.: Reassurance. *American Journal of Nursing, 55*:171, Feb. 1955.
21. Hinkle, L. E., Jr.: Normal stress in normal experience. *In* Galdston, I. (ed.): *Beyond the Germ Theory.* New York, New York Academy of Medicine, 1954.
22. Hughes, J. M.: Anxiety. *Nursing Mirror, 132*:17, March 12, 1971.
23. Kalkman, M. E.: Recognizing emotional problems. *American Journal of Nursing, 68*:536, March 1968.
24. King, J. M.: Denial. *American Journal of Nursing, 66*:1010, May 1966.
24a. Lagina, S. M.: A computer program to diagnose anxiety levels. *Nursing Research, 20*:484, Nov.–Dec. 1971.
25. Mangili, G., et al.: Steroid control of the central nervous system and control of ACTH secretion. *In* Weiner, N., and Schade, J. P. (eds.): *Progress in Biocybernetics.* New York, American Elsevier Co., 1964.
26. May, R.: Centrality of the problems of anxiety in our day. *In* Stein, M., Vidich, A. J., and White, D. J. (eds.): *Identity and Anxiety.* Glencoe, IL, The Free Press of Glencoe, 1960.
27. Meares, A.: *The Management of the Anxious Patient.* Philadelphia, W. B. Saunders Co., 1963.
28. Neyland, M. P.: Anxiety. *American Journal of Nursing, 62*:110, May 1962.
29. Oskendorf, M.: Emotional responses of patients to physical illness. *ANA Clinical Sessions,* p. 145, 1966.
30. Parley, K.: How to balance your tensions. *American Journal of Nursing, 67*:2099, Oct. 1967.
31. Peplau, H. E.: *Interpersonal Relations in Nursing.* New York, G. P. Putnam's Sons, 1952.
32. Powers, M. E., and Storlie, F.: The apprehensive patient. *American Journal of Nursing, 67*:58, 1972.
33. Robinson, L.: *Liaison Nursing: Psychological Approach to Patient Care.* Philadelphia, F. A. Davis Co., 1974.
34. Robinson, L.: *Psychological Aspects of the Care of Hospitalized Patients,* 2nd ed. Philadelphia, F. A. Davis Co., 1972.
35. Sartain, A., et al.: *Psychology: Understanding Human Behavior,* 2nd ed. New York, McGraw-Hill Book Co., 1962.
36. Sheafer, D. W.: The symptom complex of anxiety: its interplay with fear. *Medical Insight, 3*:16, April 1971.
37. Smerdon, A. C.: The development of tension. *Occupational Health, 19*:15, Jan–Feb. 1967.
38. Stine, J. J.: Anxiety—a factor in somatic symptoms. *American Journal of Psychiatry, 127*:1099, Feb. 1971.
39. Sullivan, H. S.: The meaning of anxiety in psychiatry and in life. *Psychiatry, 11*:1, Feb, 1948.
40. Tarnower, W.: Psychological needs of the hospitalized patient. *Nursing Outlook, 13*:28, 1965.
41. Townsend, R. E., House, J. F., and Addario, D.: A comparison of biofeedback-mediated relaxation and group therapy in the treatment of chronic anxiety. *American Journal of Psychiatry, 132*:6, June 1975.
42. Williams, J. G.: Systematic management of the anxious patient. *American Family Physician, 15*:124–129, Feb. 1977.

CHAPTER 9

ILLNESS: A "NORMAL" STATE OF EXISTENCE

Illness is a universal phenomenon that is experienced by people in all societies. It has been with us since the beginning of time. Like birth, death, work, and play, illness is an accepted part of our lives. It is talked about, heard about, and "seen" in all segments of society, and yet its definition and its very nature remain elusive.[4]

INTRODUCTION AND STUDY GUIDE

In illness, one's "normal" state of existence or life pattern is altered. The nature of this alteration is as varied as the individual lives of those who are ill. In order to help patients most effectively and most compassionately, the skillful nurse attempts to comprehend how the state of illness is being experienced by each patient in her care. This chapter and several following chapters review some common experiences associated with illness and the existence of the ill. Because there are many possible interpretations of the meanings of illness and the experience of illness, our discussions are limited to those that we believe are representative or "typical."

This chapter considers illness as a "normal" state of existence (we are not referring here to serious, critical or terminal illness) and reviews some typical experiences we have probably all had with minor illnesses. Because of the shared nature of

illness it is possible for a nurse to reflect on her own experiences with illness and thus better understand how others who are ill may feel. As the chapter progresses, therefore, the reader is asked to devote some time to thinking carefully about his or her own experiences with illness. From the examples presented in the chapter some nursing implications and general conclusions concerning the state of illness are derived. The reader is likewise encouraged to identify from his or her own experiences ways in which his or her nursing care might be improved. It is hoped that you will complete this chapter with a heightened appreciation of the feelings of ill persons and that you will have identified ways in which you can provide more thoughtful care.

This chapter concludes with a brief discussion of the stages of illness.

LEARNING ABOUT ILLNESS

Perhaps it seems strange to think of illness as a normal state of existence. However, a certain amount of illness is normal in that it is an unavoidable aspect of life. Everyone has had the flu, a cold or some other illness. As mentioned, it is possible for nurses to learn from their own experiences with illness and thereby improve nursing care. It is also helpful in this respect for nurses to read accounts of other persons' experiences with illness. Such accounts may be autobiographical, biographical or fictitious and may be found in professional literature as well as humanistic

literature. Ruffing writes of the value of illness-experience literature for nurses in her article "Literature by Consumers for Nursing." She observes:

Reading first-hand accounts of illness, disability, and other human crises prepares both the seasoned and the neophyte nurse for encounters with individuals coping with similar problems. The activity can provoke continuing insight, adding dimension and color to the special needs and concerns. Moreover, as an activity which accentuates the humanistic foundation of nursing practice, the reading is both engrossing and memorable.[3]

We strongly encourage readers of this text to broaden their knowledge of the experience

ing care to patients whose experiences appear to be similar to yours.

of illness by reading personal accounts of these experiences. To facilitate this activity we have incorporated selected appropriate entries into the bibliographies of following chapters.

At this point let us begin this chapter's consideration of the existence of the ill by reflectively thinking about our own experiences with illness. We should be able to identify some important "nursing insights" about how patients commonly experience illness, what they require and find helpful and possibly why some patients act as they do. For example, nausea is an uncomfortable sensation that occurs with many illnesses. By recalling her own experience with this distressing symptom, a nurse can give more sensitive, complete care to nauseated patients. Possibly the nurse would recall that sudden movements and the presence of strong odors worsened the nausea and that closing her eyes and taking slow, deep breaths helped her relax and relieved acute moments of nausea.

> While it is true that each of us responds individually to illness, it is also true that there are similar feelings experienced by many ill people. A nurse can give better patient care by recalling her own feelings and actions when ill.

Pause now and carefully try to recall your experiences with a recent illness—perhaps "the flu." Possibly you would find it helpful to conduct this exercise with classmates, talking together in small groups about your experiences with illness. Whether you follow this activity by yourself or with others, think specifically about the following three areas: (1) your mood and feelings during illness; (2) how medications affected you; and (3) your interests and sense of awareness when ill. Take a few minutes to think through and briefly write out your recollections in these three areas.

Now, let us continue by briefly considering some hypothetical situations depicting these topics and discuss some nursing insights derived from these examples. Compare your notes about your experiences with illness with the examples given and derive additional nursing insights from the uniqueness of your own recollections. Identify ways in which you can give more thoughtful, complete nurs-

MOOD AND FEELINGS DURING ILLNESS

Possibly your moods and feelings while ill were somewhat like those described below:

I felt that no one knew how uncomfortable I really was and that no one really cared. I was alone in my illness. No one was experiencing it except me. Although my moods fluctuated, generally I was somewhat depressed and quite irritable. Because of my illness I had plans that would not materialize and obligations that I could not fulfill. *Why me?* Why did *I* have to get sick, and why just *now*? Deep inside I recognized some angry feelings about being "struck down" with this illness and I was in part sorry for myself. Also, I felt powerless over the course of my life. How long would I have to feel like this? Would I feel even worse before I felt better again? What would the course of the illness be like?

It was an effort not to be short-tempered with others who were trying to help me. Somehow I felt as if my "caretakers" had let me down because they couldn't make me feel well. Everyone seemed to be full of energy and having a good time—except me. I was depressed and I resented others' trying to cheer me up. On the other hand, I resented it if they seemed "long-faced" and "crept" around me. In truth, I often didn't know what I wanted from one moment to the next. An extra blanket seemed necessary one moment, and too heavy and warm the next. Just when I thought I was feeling better, my stomach would cramp and I would get nauseated again and throw up. Oh . . . not again! My stomach ached like a boil. It hurt to move. My head ached so badly I thought it would split. Bright lights and noise made it worse. It was discouraging. I felt I just wanted to be left alone, and yet when I was alone I felt neglected and restless. If only I could sleep until I could be well again.

I found it difficult to be dependent and ask for things. I thought how nice it would be if someone could just "read my mind and know what I need when I need it." (A cool fresh cloth would feel comforting over my eyes. Won't someone shut off that television? I feel thirsty and dehydrated, yet am afraid to drink. I can't stand to throw up again.)

My body ached all over. My elbows soon were sore from rubbing on the sheets. I was discontent. Rapidly my body and spirit grew weary of being ill and being in bed. I didn't like myself mentally or physically. It seemed there was very little about me that was likable and I found I was poor company —even for myself.

What nursing insights into patient's moods and feelings can we derive from these recollections?

Nursing Insights. It is impossible to really know the experiences of another person, e.g., how a patient *really feels*. However, it is possible to try to *understand* and *appreciate* the feelings of others, by trying to mentally put oneself in the others' situations and by recalling one's own similar experiences.

> *Illness is often accompanied by mood and behavioral fluctuations.*

The insightful nurse *expects* that patients' moods and feelings (and hence their behaviors) will be affected by illness. Such a nurse realizes that sick people simply do not act as they would if they felt well. *Remember that illness causes both psychologic and physiologic changes*, i.e., changes in thoughts and feelings as well as physical changes. At times these changes are reflected as observable behavioral or mood fluctuations. For example, a patient's mood may fluctuate rapidly, perhaps from an attempt at gaiety one moment to tears the next. Illness is often an unsettling, "undoing" experience in which routine life patterns "fall apart." Frequently illness prevents people from doing what they want to do and often from being at home or where they want to be. Frustrated people who do not feel well are irritable, and irritable people often have rather rapid mood fluctuations. Since behaviors in part serve to express moods, rapid behavioral fluctuations may also occur among ill persons. Serious illnesses cause persons experiencing them to grieve. The grieving may be over various losses or potential losses, e.g., loss of health, loss of body parts, impending loss of life. (Grieving behaviors are discussed in Chapter 48.)

Illnesses often cause people to think more deeply than usual about life's inconsistencies and human fragility, e.g., the fact that human beings are mortals who often suffer without apparent reason and eventually will die. These thoughts may evoke deep anxieties. Learning that one has a deforming, life-threatening or chronic illness deals a severe blow. Later chapters will discuss reactions to confirmation of illness (Chap. 11), disturbances of body image (Chap. 15) and terminal illness (Chap. 49).

It is not uncommon for a sick person to have a low self-esteem and feel anxious, depressed, discouraged, restless, angry, powerless, dependent and frustrated. Such complex, varied feelings are often expressed directly or indirectly toward significant others in a patient's life (e.g., family, friends, nurses) or onto the environment. Feelings may also be internalized, i.e., directed inward onto the patient himself. The direction of feelings is discussed further below.

Often people feel *angry* because they are ill, and they may *project* this feeling (or other feelings) onto persons they care about (life partner) and/or persons caring for them (nurses, doctors). The "projection" of feelings means that unacceptable feelings such as anger are denied by the person as his own and are instead blamed or attributed (projected) to someone else. Projection is a mental mechanism (used to varying degrees by all of us) that is sometimes referred to as the "blaming" mechanism (see also Chap. 8).

It is helpful to both nurse and patient if a nurse *recognizes* and *anticipates* that an ill person often projects his feelings. The nurse is then not surprised when such projection occurs and does not tend to misinterpret it. It is important for a nurse to guard against being so hypersensitive that she takes patients' anger, tears, general irritability or other expressions of mood or emotion personally.

This does not mean, however, that the nurse simply overlooks or dismisses patients' projective behaviors. Instead, the caring nurse tries to evaluate objectively whether she actually did have a part in precipitating the reactions observed or whether they are attributable to other causes. At times it is helpful to the nurse if she can share her concerns with colleagues and ask for their impressions (feedback) of her behavior and that of the patient. There is a difference between this kind of professional review of nurse-patient experiences and gossip about patients' behaviors (see also Chapter 3).

If as a result of her evaluation a nurse finds she has been nontherapeutic with a patient, the nurse plans an appropriate approach to clarify the situation with the patient and to try to prevent its recurrence. For example, let us say that a patient became angry with a nurse. Upon evaluating the situation the nurse suspects she was preoccupied with another problem and was thoughtlessly abrupt with the patient, thereby making him angry. It would be appropriate for the nurse to return to the patient and clarify with him what she thinks happened between them. She might say something like: "I've been thinking about our last time together, and I realize now that I was abrupt with you. I *am* sorry that occurred. I had another concern in my thoughts at that moment and I wasn't listening carefully to what you were saying. I realize that my behavior might have made you angry." These kinds of self-disclosing statements by the nurse open the way for further discussion if the patient wishes.

The hypersensitive nurse who takes personally and is upset by patients' expressions of mood or emotion when she is not responsible for having caused them finds it difficult to be therapeutic. She often adds to the frustrations of persons in her care by making them feel bad for "upsetting the nurse." Or patients may be fearful that the "hurt nurse" will angrily, defensively retaliate and/or take advantage of their dependent positions. Often a hypersensitive nurse conveys to patients the unfortunate impressions that: (a) if they are "good" and don't upset her she will take care of them; but (b) if patients forget to say "thank you," cry, become angry or display other disturbing emotions, the nurse will have hurt feelings or will feel uncomfortable and will leave them alone or worsen their situations. These impressions place patients under severe emotional strains, causing them to feel that they cannot unburden themselves of their concerns or fears. Instead, patients in such situations feel they must act in appeasing ways and must internalize or not reveal their true emotions, i.e., that they must *suppress* their true feelings by voluntarily pushing them out of consciousness.

> *When people must suppress their true feelings, physiologic functions may be adversely affected.*

We know that physiologic functioning may be affected unfavorably when emotions such as anger and resentment are suppressed. Suppressed emotions may be expressed physiologically through such symptoms as increase in angina attacks (acute chest pains produced by interference with the heart's blood supply); elevations of blood pressure in persons who are hypertensive (whose blood pressures are abnormally high); precipitation of asthmatic attacks (attacks of varying severity characterized by a sense of chest constriction, wheezing and difficulty in breathing); or an increase in inflammation, irritation or ulceration in diseased stomachs or colons.

> *A nurse's moods and behaviors may actually increase the suffering of some patients physically as well as psychologically and may delay their recovery!*

What behavioral qualities might patients find helpful in a nurse? Frequently people who are ill want to be cared for by a person who is accepting, thoughtful, gentle, nurturing, kind, genuine, emotionally warm, caring and giving (see also Chap. 3). Often it helps the ill person to relax and feel better if his needs can be anticipated by others.

Nursing requires the abilities to listen carefully to patients and to accept them during both pleasant and unpleasant moments. The nurse who listens attentively allows the patient to put his feelings into words. The nurse also conveys to the patient the feeling that she will consider and respond to anything the patient has to say and that she will try to talk with the patient about anything he wishes to discuss. In other words, the helpful nurse's words and behaviors convey to the patient that his verbal and nonverbal expressions of his thoughts and feelings will not be devastating to her or provoke in her behaviors that are not in the patient's best interest. The nurse demonstrates to the patient that she is able (a) to hear what he has to say, (b) to consider and respond to the patient's words and (c) to notice and consider the patient's appearance and actions (physical condition and nonverbal behaviors) and respond in helpful ways.

At times, a nurse may feel a sense of discomfort in response to what a patient is saying or the *specific* manner in which he is acting; however, she still strives to convey a *general* acceptance of the patient as a person. That is to say, the attitude the nurse tries to convey to the patient is: "I care about you even though these particular words or this specific behavior of yours makes me feel uncomfortable." This acceptance of the patient as a person requires that the nurse demonstrate a genuine appreciation of the patient's situation rather than only looking at his behavior by itself and reacting to it without attempting to understand what prompts the behavior.

Assessing the Patient's Behaviors and Moods. We should add that while it is necessary to make allowances for a patient's behaviors and moods because he is ill, it is also necessary to evaluate or assess such behavior. Such assessment is done by keeping in mind the fact that *excessive and/or prolonged behaviors or mood swings may indicate severe emotional difficulties requiring psychiatric aid.* In addition, we do not mean to imply that the nurse should simply accept behaviors of an extreme nature. Obviously behaviors that are harmful to the nurse or patient cannot be tolerated. We are merely pointing out that genuine feelings of caring and acceptance are important in a helpful relationship, accompanied by a sincere desire to attempt to understand *why* the patient is acting as he is and then to be helpful.

In trying to assess a particular patient's moods and behaviors it is best if the nurse has some idea of what his *pre-illness personality* was like. If there is doubt about whether or not a patient's behavior is seriously "abnormal" (i.e., represents a gross deviation from his usual behavior), it is advisable to ask friends and family to describe the patient's pre-illness personality.

Realistically we expect mood fluctuations to occur even when we feel well; we feel more irritable one day than another. Sometimes we feel in harmony with everyone, and at other times everyone seems to misunderstand us. Patients cannot be unrealistically expected to behave "better" when they are sick than they would if they were well. A patient once said, "I am expected to be more pleasant than the staff and yet I'm the one who is sick!"

Because the hospitalized patient is under constant supervision 24 hours a day, his behavior may be subject to overevaluation. To appraise a patient's behavior realistically the nurse should remember that if her own behavior were under 24-hour surveillance, aspects of it might appear extreme. Whereas she can leave the presence of others if she feels upset, the patient has no place to go to be alone. Because of the lack of privacy, being hospitalized is like being in a fish bowl.

Finally, in assessing a patient's mood and behavioral fluctuations the nurse needs to be cognizant of the *mental stresses*, *physical fatigue* and *discomforts* he may be undergoing. Keep in mind how tired ill persons become from (1) worries and fears; (2) disrupted sleep; (3) noise and interruptions (from staff, other patients, visitors, telephones); (4) physical immobilization (from confinement to bed, traction, casts, dressings); (5) pain; (6) nausea and vomiting; and (7) numerous other discomforts, e.g., excessive gas formation in the stomach or intestine (flatulence), muscle cramping and sore skin. Of course, excessive stresses, fatigue and discomforts tend to make us all irritable.

> *The hallmark of a truly professional nurse is not merely her ability to take care of patients whom she personally likes and whose pleasant moods and behaviors make her feel good. The professional nurse has the ability to also care for, and about, those patients (often called "difficult") whom she may find personally upsetting.*

Such a nurse does not expect everyone to be of a similar disposition or even that a given individual will be consistently pleasant, nor does she expect other people to consistently attune their moods to hers. A sensitive nurse is adaptable to patients' moods. She learns to sense when levity might be enjoyed, for example, and when it is out of place; when patients need to be alone as well as when her presence can be helpful. The professional nurse views mood fluctuations as a normal occurrence in the existence of the ill. She attempts to evaluate and understand the moods and behaviors of patients in terms of her knowledge of the behavioral sciences and her own life experiences.

In summary, the knowledgeable nurse recognizes that *illness is physically and emotionally stressful to experience.* Moods and behaviors may be expected to vary in illness from what they are in health. With illness, many indications of frustration, anxiety and irritation may be noted. Such behavioral expressions need to be evaluated in light of both (a) the psychologic and physiologic stresses to which a given patient is subjected and (b) the patient's pre-illness personality.

Let us continue now to examine the existence of ill persons so that we might better understand this experience and provide more comprehensive, therapeutic nursing care.

EFFECTS OF MEDICATIONS DURING ILLNESS

Now, recall again your own experiences with "the flu." This time think about how medications affected you and made you feel. Does this sound familiar?

I didn't take many medications. Really the medicines were a problem in some ways. I had a headache, but anything I took for that upset my stomach. I vomited a lot and had diarrhea. I was given some liquid medication to stop the diarrhea, but it coated my mouth and the taste nauseated me. I had some pills which were to help to prevent nausea, but at first when I took them I vomited them back. Later, when they did stay down I felt so terribly drowsy from them that it was an effort to be awake and I felt unpleasantly groggy. The medicine certainly did affect how I felt; sometimes it made me feel better, but at times it also made me feel worse. On the whole, I felt weak, shaky and very tired. I had been awake a lot at night because I was sick. One night I took something to help me to sleep. It really hit me. When I got up to go to the bathroom I felt dizzy and unreal. I almost stumbled and fell.

Let us abstract some nursing implications from these experiences and see how we might better understand patients in terms of their experiences with medications.

Nursing Insights. A major component in understanding the experience of ill persons is understanding how specific patients are being affected by their medications. We are not referring to the precise physiologic actions of medications; these are discussed in texts focusing on pharmacology, medical-surgical nursing, etc. We refer here mainly to some psychologic effects of medications—e.g., alterations of alertness, mood, and behavior—and to some general ways that medications may make a person feel physically—e.g., dizzy, drowsy, nauseated. These effects are often minimized or overlooked and may be significant factors in accidents (e.g., patient falls) or misunderstandings (e.g., patient failing to follow instructions) that are disruptive to recovery.

For example, let us say that a drug causes a patient to feel mentally "groggy" and somewhat out of touch with his environment. If the nurse is unaware that the patient feels as he does, and moreover that medication is the cause of these feelings, she might make some of the following misinterpretations: (1) She might not realize that the patient requires safety precautions in his care and he might fall, choke, roll over on his IV, be burned, or otherwise be injured or interfere with his treatment. (2) She might interpret his vague disinterest in his surroundings, and in her, as rudeness or unfriendliness on his part; that is, she may incorrectly infer that he is alert but is deliberately choosing to be uncommunicative. (3) She may think this patient is depressed because he sleeps a great deal or is unusually quiet. (4) She may believe that his physical condition is becoming more serious and that he is becoming unresponsive. These are all serious misinterpretations.

Almost all medications have effects that may be unpleasant for the patient; therefore, he may become discouraged with his treatment and wonder if it's all worth it. Because the doctor has ordered the medication and because the nurse gives it to him, the patient may feel resentful toward those caring for him and may feel at times that they are adding to his misery rather than diminishing it. This is particularly true if the doctor and nurse appear disinterested in administering the medication or in how the medication is making the patient feel. The skillful administration of injectable medications reduces the amount of pain the patient must experience. This is very important, especially for persons who must have numerous injections or venipunctures. (Administration of injectable medications is discussed in Chap. 38.) Supportive concern and recognition of the patient's feelings also can do much to help him accept his prescribed medication.

Discussion with the patient can elicit information about the undesirable effects of his medications as well as benefits he is noticing. For example, while some analgesic medications may relieve pain, they may also cause constipation and feelings of unreality, which some persons find unpleasant. *There are times,* of course, *when the side effects or untoward actions of medications warrant discontinuation of the treatment.* In such situations, a nurse's observations (written and verbal) are often helpful in deciding whether or not this is advisable.

Medications may precipitate extreme behavioral changes in patients who are debilitated, very weak or aged. For example, it is not uncommon for a sedative to produce a gross confusion and disorientation in an aged patient. In such a situation the patient may not know where he is and may fall trying to leave his bed or the care facility. The patient may also panic and become combative, harming himself and/or others. (Care of confused or disoriented patients is discussed in Chap. 14.)

As the factors discussed in this section demonstrate, medications play a significant and varying role in the existence of the ill.

Remember: *Behavioral assessments and evaluations of how a patient feels generally must always be made carefully, giving full consideration to all medications the patient is receiving and their possible beneficial and harmful effects.*

INTERESTS AND AWARENESS DURING ILLNESS

As a final recollection on your part, try to remember what your interests and awareness were like during your own experience with illness. Again let us imagine that the following description is by a "typical" person with the "flu":

I noticed that it was difficult to be very interested in other people, or in what they were doing or talking about. I was mainly interested in *me* and how I felt from one moment to the next. I was constantly assessing my feelings, e.g., *"Do* I feel like turning over? Do I feel better or worse?" I was certainly more aware of my body than I usually am. Certain body functions and parts of my body seemed magnified in my mind, as if they were "blown up" out of all proportion, and occupied all my attention.

When I felt sick to my stomach I felt as if I were all one stomach and it was all I could think about; when my head ached I felt as if I were all head. I also noticed that I was acutely aware of sensations, e.g., odors, movements, lights, noises. At times I felt too nauseated to move. Sudden movements by others irritated me; noises and light seemed magnified in my senses and intensified my headache and irritability. Finally, I noticed that my awareness of time was altered. I experienced "time warps" . . . "time blurs." I dozed a lot, and since I was sick day and night for a couple of days, the light and darkness seemed all foggy and blended together. Somehow it was worse to be sick at night. I felt more alone. When I was sickest, and sleeping a lot, the time seemed to pass rather quickly and all run together. However, as I recovered and had a little energy, the time dragged and I felt discouraged that I didn't get well faster. Although I was feeling better, I wasn't able to pursue my normal activities. I was bored.

Once again, using this as an example of a "typical" experience while ill, let us see what can be drawn from this example and applied to understanding patients generally.

Nursing Insights. As our example indicates, *the ill person's interests are constricted and he is primarily interested in and concerned about himself;* i.e., he is egocentric. This is to be expected for several reasons, the first of which is the fact that *illness may threaten survival.* When survival is threatened, all a person's adaptive skills are mustered and self-interest becomes paramount; the animal-like reaction of "every beast for himself" comes forth.

A second reason for self-interest in the ill is simply the fact that *when we are in psychologic or physical pain it is most difficult to think of others.* Thus, at such times, one becomes "inner-directed" to the self rather than "outer-directed" to others. When we are suffering, our energies are directed toward obtaining relief.

Because the ill person is inner-directed, most conversations with him (and this is most certainly the case with the acutely or critically ill) center on the patient himself. This is as it should be. A patient should not feel pressured to talk about the state of the world, the nurse's life and interests or other topics. Likewise, he should not feel pressured to talk about himself but should be encouraged to do so if he wishes. In sum, the patient who talks about himself and his condition is not egocentric, rude or selfish; he is attempting to adapt to illness. The nurse will find that what a patient says helps her to understand him better; it also helps him to more effectively tolerate his situation.

A third reason for patients' self-interest is the fact that *areas of bodily concern tend to be magnified during illness and thus are difficult to put out of mind.* We all know that a tiny foreign particle in the eye seems much larger than it actually is, and removing that particle becomes our major concern. We are immobilized in terms of other tasks or interests until our discomfort is relieved. This mental magnification of physical problems is probably adaptive in nature, helping us survive; however, it is often helpful to the patient if the nurse helps to keep his problems in a somewhat "normal" perspective rather than adding to the magnification of them.

For example, if a patient has an abdominal incision he may frequently feel aware only of that incision (it is magnified in his mind and dominates his attention) and thus he may say, "I'm afraid to move because that operation might break open." Although the nurse gives recognition to how he feels and does not belittle him for feeling as he does, she helps the patient to put the incision in perspective with the rest of his body and his total wellbeing. "I think I know how you feel, but your operation area is secure. It is important that you move about so that you will recover more rapidly. It hurts at first, but the pain will lessen and your abdomen will actually become stronger than if you just lie still. I want you to try to think about your legs and your lungs as well as your abdomen. By moving your legs around in bed you help your blood circulation, and by coughing and deep breathing you help to keep your lungs free from infection." Having broadened the patient's perspective, from his incision to his total body, the nurse then proceeds to teach him exactly what he can do to help himself.

A fourth reason why self-interest is so predominant in the ill is that their *senses are often heightened,* again as a protective means of adaptation. As a nurse proceeds with her activities at the bedside she constantly strives to reduce unpleasant odors, disturbing noises, harsh lights and sudden, jerky movements on her part. All these factors can be irritating to patients who are experiencing heightened sensitivities. The nurse who smells of cigarette smoke, strong perfume or breath or body odors often cannot be tolerated by patients for these reasons. Such a nurse should have little cause to wonder why she evokes some of the responses she does from patients and co-workers.

> *Smooth, confident movements, accompanied by explanations of what is going on and what a patient can do to help, are learned skills of immeasurable value in nursing practice.*

Sudden, rough and jarring movements make a patient tense and frightened. Such movements cruelly insult a patient's integrity, causing him to feel unvalued. Of course, movements of this nature may also be physically painful.

Finally, in addition to being heightened, *senses may be distorted during illness*. This is true of the sense of time. With illness, time may take on new meanings. It may seem more precious than ever or it may be cursed; it may seem to fly by, with the patient virtually unconscious of its passage, or, for the patient locked in agonizing suffering, it may seem motionless. A distorted sense of time can contribute to confusion or disorientation.

In sum, we have noted the following major insights into patients' interests and awarenesses during illness:

▶ The ill person is primarily concerned about himself, because illness may threaten survival.

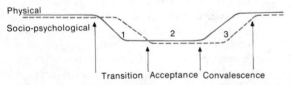

The solid line represents a normal level of physical well-being; the broken line represents a corresponding degree of socio-psychological integration. Lederer refers to the areas between the arrows, from left to right, as the period of transition from health to illness, the period of accepted illness, and the period of convalescence. During the first period, socio-psychological functioning may for a time persist at or near usual levels as the patient attempts to deny his illness and carry on as usual. Physical, social, and psychological aspects of his life come into close correspondence again during the period of accepted illness, though at a lower level of integration. During convalescence, physical improvement usually occurs first. For a time the patient may cling to the regression of illness, accounting for the lag in socio-psychological reintegration.

Figure 9–1. Stages of the experience of illness.

(From Martin, H. W., and Prange, A. J., Jr.: The stages of illness—psychosocial approach. Copyright © March 1962, The American Journal of Nursing Company, printed in *Nursing Outlook, 10*:168–171, March 1962.)

▶ When in pain or experiencing discomfort it is difficult to be "other-directed."

▶ Areas of bodily concern tend to be magnified during illness.

▶ Senses are often heightened during illness.

▶ Senses may be distorted during illness.

STAGES OF THE EXPERIENCE OF ILLNESS

Lederer and Martin and Prange discuss the general pattern of those illnesses which result in recovery as proceeding through three overlapping yet clearly demarcated stages: (1) stage of transition; (2) stage of acceptance; and (3) stage of convalescence (Fig. 9–1).

▶ *Stage of transition.* During this stage the individual passes from a state of health into illness. The illness may begin with vague, nonspecific symptoms that the individual may psychologically attempt to deny. The person experiences a "felt need" upon first noticing something is wrong or when he is first motivated somehow to seek treatment. With symptom progression, the person eventually acknowledges emotionally the fact that he is ill.

▶ *Stage of acceptance.* During this stage the individual has typically given up his attempts to deny illness. He is "defined" as sick and takes on the sick role. (The sick role is discussed in Chapter 13.) The patient has a prevailing self-concern, usually recognizes his dependent position and regresses into a state in which he has fewer and fewer psychologic responses available to him. The individual is now in a state of physiologic and psychologic dependence.

▶ *Stage of convalescence.* As the balance tips in favor of recovery the stage of reintegration proceeds. The individual passes through a transition from illness to health. In some instances it is difficult for the convalescent to leave the attentions and protections he has received while ill and reenter a situation in which he must once again tend to his own responsibilities and meet his needs. Usually the resolution of the physical illness proceeds somewhat ahead of the reintegration of the individual's psychologic and social functioning. It is important during this time that nursing staff recognize this lag and not push a patient into resuming self-care and self-responsibilities too early. Likewise, it is important not to prolong the state of regression, making it difficult for a patient to reintegrate and move ahead into the stage of convalescence and recovery.

BIBLIOGRAPHY

1. Lederer, H. D.: How the sick view their world. *Journal of Social Issues*, 8:4–15, 1952.
2. Martin, H. W., and Prange, A. J., Jr.: Stages of illness: a psychosocial approach. *Nursing Outlook, 10*:168–171, March 1962.
3. Ruffling, M. A.: Literature by consumers for nursing. *Nursing Forum, 14*(1):87–94, 1975.
4. Wu, R.: *Behavior and Illness.* Englewood Cliffs, NJ, Prentice-Hall, 1973.

CHAPTER 10

RECOGNIZING THE
NEED FOR HEALTH CARE

When an individual learns that he has manifestations of an illness, or when he begins to experience unusual sensations or impairment of customary function, his behavior will change correspondingly. He will begin to engage in activity either to deny the uncomfortable sensations or to define his state of health and to discover a suitable remedy.[35]

OVERVIEW AND STUDY GUIDE

This chapter focuses on some of the ways people respond to indications (i.e., "symptoms") of disorders in themselves, and it considers some reasons why persons with symptoms may delay seeking professional health care. Additionally, persons who seek health care more often than they actually appear to need it are discussed.

In studying this chapter you are encouraged to consider your own previous help-seeking behaviors in response to symptom development. If possible, also recall instances in which you developed symptoms and did *not* seek health care. In the latter instance can you identify the reasons why you did not seek aid?

Before reading the chapter, pause and identify your feelings about "hypochondriacs." What impression do you have about people described by this term? Can you identify how you developed your impressions about "hypochondriacs"? Imagine that you are assigned to care for a patient and before meeting him you are told, "He is really just a hypochondriac." How might this comment affect your prejudgment of this patient and your subsequent responses to his comments about his symptoms, e.g., pain?

After reading this chapter summarize in your own words some reasons why people might not seek health care as soon as they ideally should. If possible, recall examples of help-seeking or failure to seek health care from people you know, e.g., patients, family, friends. As appropriate, while caring for patients in the future, discuss with them the process they went through in seeking health care after they began to notice symptoms. Finally, after reading this chapter, briefly summarize what you have learned about persons who apparently seek health care more often than their condition requires. Also, reconsider your opinions about the usefulness of the term "hypochondriac."

INTRODUCTION

Health care personnel who routinely see patients (clients) may unfortunately tend to forget that often it is *not* "routine" for the patient to come for help. Indeed, for the patient the visit may be highly stressful and very important. The realization that one needs health care is generally a gradual process rather than a sudden revelation. Persons experiencing sudden, acute disorders or accidents may be brought by others to the health professional for care and treatment. These patients may welcome the assistance they are given. However, often it is extremely difficult for people to seek out health care on their own and submit to the necessary diagnostic and treatment activities.

By the time a patient reaches a doctor's office, clinic or hospital he may have experienced a great deal of anxiety and conflict about his condition. Weeks, months and even years may pass between the beginning of a mental or physical disorder and the time when some patients finally appear before health care personnel.

Sometimes they arrive in an ambulance and sometimes their arrival is too late for help to be given.

What has kept these persons from obtaining help? What behaviors have they been engaging in, in response to their disorders? Why have they now appeared for help? The experienced nurse does not belittle such patients or "scold" them for "not coming in sooner" once they do come to her attention. Instead, she tries to be of help to each patient and attempts to understand his behavior. Remember:

> *All behavior is purposeful and meaningful and can be understood.*

The knowledgeable nurse recognizes that an apparent symptom is not always the real reason a patient seeks help. Physical symptoms may be discussed in place of a patient's interpersonal or social problems. For example, it may seem easier and more acceptable to a patient to talk about his frequent headaches and backaches (and indeed he may have these symptoms) than it is for him to discuss his possible feelings of social isolation, impaired sexual functioning, rejection and anger. Yet the latter problems may well be the problems that are most disturbing to the patient and the real basis for his help-seeking behavior.

A nurse is frequently in the unique position of being able to serve in her community as a "bridge" between patients and health care specialists, e.g., doctors. Because of her place in the health professions, the nurse who recognizes how difficult it is for many people to seek appropriate aid can be of assistance to patients in this activity. Often people feel more comfortable in talking with a nurse than with a doctor. At home and in her community a nurse frequently may be approached by people asking her if *she* thinks they ought to go to a doctor, dentist or psychiatrist. In effect, they are asking her to make their decisions for them; also, however, they are asking for her support. Many people find it easier to go to a doctor or phone him, for example, if they can say, "A nurse I talked with thought I should come in." Often, after talking about his condition, his fears and other concerns with a nurse, a patient is relaxed enough and supported enough that he feels able to proceed with seeking help in more direct ways. A nurse can thus provide a valuable service by helping people obtain appropriate health care.

BEHAVIORAL RESPONSES TO CUES OF ILLNESS

Wu observes that, "In response to the cues of illness, the individual may engage in one or more of the following behaviors: (1) take action to relieve the symptoms; (2) take no action; (3) remain in a state of flux in which he vacillates between taking and not taking action; or (4) take counteraction in opposition to the cues."[35] Examples of these behaviors are provided in Table 10–1. Most of this table is self-explanatory. Let us clarify, however, two points Wu makes concerning seeking provisional validation and taking counteraction.

TABLE 10–1. BEHAVIORAL RESPONSES TO CUES OF ILLNESS

BEHAVIOR	EXAMPLES
1. Person takes action to relieve the symptoms.	1. Person takes actions that may be healthy, constructive, unhealthy or even harmful. Such actions may include seeking qualified practitioner; consulting a "quack"; self-diagnosis; self-treatment; home remedies; self-medication; seeking "provisional validation" from others about one's state of health (see text).
2. Person takes no action to relieve the symptoms.	2. Person delays action, adopts a "wait and see" attitude, procrastinates, rationalizes that his symptoms are not serious enough to require medical attention, delays seeking treatment.
3. Person remains in a state of flux, vacillating between taking and not taking action to relieve the symptoms.	3. Person considers taking action, experiences ambivalent feelings about seeking help ("*yes* I want to; *no* I don't want to") and conflicting desires (desire to avoid present discomfort and desire to avoid process of diagnosis, treatment, illness).
4. Person takes counteraction in opposition to the cues.	4. Person tries to prove that his symptoms are imaginary. He may increase his activities; deny and refuse to accept presence of illness; be confident everything is "OK"; "shop" for practitioners (qualified and/or quacks) to support his belief that he is not ill (see text).

Source: Based on information in Wu, R.: *Behavior and Illness.* Englewood Cliffs, NJ, Prentice-Hall, 1973, Chapter 8.

The person experiencing symptoms may talk with others about his symptoms, i.e., he attempts to obtain *"provisional validation"* of his state of health. "These discussions are not only to gain advice and information but also to obtain permission to suspend normal obligations and activities. Seeking care and assistance from others must be done in a way that is acceptable to the group."[35]

Persons appearing to be taking counteraction in the presence of cues of illness require careful assessment to separate *real ignorance* (failure to realize that the symptoms represent illness) from *psychological denial* (denying the presence of symptoms which are perceived as indications of illness).[35]

FACTORS AFFECTING WAYS INDIVIDUALS DEAL WITH SYMPTOMS

Numerous variables might influence ways in which people deal with symptoms (indications of organic or psychic malfunctioning) or seek help for health problems they cannot manage alone. Some of these variables are presented below. Many of them have been identified by Mechanic[24] and have been discussed by Wu[35] and others. Unfortunately, space does not permit detailed discussion of each variable.

Perceived seriousness of the abnormality or disorder.   Frightening, serious symptoms may prompt the person experiencing them to rapidly seek health care, while those symptoms perceived as neither incapacitating nor serious may be underemphasized and arouse less concern. Perceived seriousness of symptoms tends to vary with socioeconomic differences. Sometimes it is difficult to estimate the seriousness of the condition. It takes time to determine whether a disorder will require professional treatment, or whether it will "clear itself up." A period of time may thus pass while the person observes and evaluates his symptoms to decide whether he is getting better or worse.

Some people experience *doubt as to whether or not the symptoms are real* or only imagined. It is rather common today to hear people preface a discussion of their ailments with statements such as, "Maybe I'm neurotic, but . . ."; or "Maybe it's all in my head; however . . ."; or "I guess I'm just another hypochondriac; nevertheless . . ." Such statements reflect the fact that currently many people in our society

have a little bit of knowledge about anxiety, hypochondriasis, neuroticism, psychosomatics, and so forth and, on the basis of their incomplete knowledge, become fearful that their symptoms might be "imaginary." Such people may be reluctant to seek medical evaluation because of worry that the doctor may find nothing wrong with them and they will feel embarrassed for taking up his time. These patients are also concerned that they might be labeled as "neurotics," "hypochondriacs" or "malingerers." Unfortunately, fears of this nature are not uncommon and keep some people from seeking treatment for serious disorders (e.g., heart conditions, diabetes, malignancies) until their conditions pass beyond the treatable phase and death or permanent disability ensues. Other people may spend long periods of time suffering from disorders that could be alleviated rapidly with proper treatment.

Persons with some psychiatric disorders may be *out of contact with reality,* or their *abilities to accurately evaluate the seriousness of their disorders are impaired* in other ways. In situations such as these an affected individual may be unable to seek help on his own and may instead come to the attention of health professionals through the efforts of others, e.g., family, friends, police. Persons who are alcoholics or drug abusers may also appear for help through the efforts of others. The alcoholic or the drug abuser himself may have difficulty recognizing and accepting the serious nature of these conditions.

Children are unable to accurately assess the seriousness of disorders they have and are unable to seek out health care. Mature persons are responsible for performing these functions for children and for others (e.g., intellectually handicapped persons, confused and disoriented persons, and individuals with impaired states of consciousness) who are unable to assess their own disorders and seek help.

It is interesting that the "seriousness" of a disorder does not necessarily mean that a disorder is life-threatening. For example, in societies in which physical attractiveness is highly valued, persons whose physical characteristics deviate from the "attractive" standards may seek help for disorders that are otherwise rather minor.

In the early stages of chronic illnesses, symptoms may persist over a period of time without necessarily becoming worse or interfering with usual activities. Thus, persons in the early stages of chronic illness may not think of themselves as ill and may delay seeking early diagnosis and treatment. This is an unfortunate situation because chronic illnesses are increasing in frequency.

We have considered a variety of reasons why

it may be difficult to determine the seriousness of a disorder. Let us now proceed to review some other factors influencing an individual's judgment as to whether he views himself as ill and whether he will seek professional health care.

Pressure from family members. Help tends to be sought sooner when family members exert pressure in this direction. Additional significant others (peers, friends, teachers) also may exert pressure prompting the person experiencing the symptoms to seek aid.

Extent to which the disorder interferes with the individual's ability to engage in his usual social activities. Concern is heightened over those symptoms that are most likely to disrupt social functioning, e.g., family functioning. Disorders may be perceived as more serious if it appears they will have disruptive or serious consequences to the group.

The place "health" occupies in the individual's (or group's) value system. Symptoms may not be attended to until after some other need, which is valued more than health, is met. Some obese persons, for example, may value overeating more than they value weight loss.

Tendency of the individual to be concerned with abnormalities (disorders) and his tolerance of abnormalities (disorders). Some persons focus more than others on factors such as physical or mental symptoms or illnesses. Tolerance of these disorders in oneself and others also varies from person to person. Cultural factors may influence tolerance of symptoms, e.g., pain.

Information the individual has concerning the disorder. The type of information appears to be as important as the amount of information in determining the behavior of a person with a disorder. It seems important for persons to know when a given dysfunction is abnormal. Beyond this, increasing knowledge or providing added information to the person does not predictably influence resultant behavior.

Cultural background and value system of the individual who has a disorder. Cultural influences and the importance of values have been mentioned briefly before. Zola,[37, 38] among others, has noted that ethnic origin is important in determining when an individual will seek help for a perceived dysfunction. Zola's work compares the decisions of Irish, Italian and Anglo-Saxon Americans concerning when medical care should be sought.

Leininger writes of the relevance of the culture concept to nursing:

Individuals from different cultures perceive and classify their health problems in specific ways and have certain expectations about the way they should be helped. To ignore such cultural differences may seriously interfere with the nurse's ability to help a patient, and can limit the patient's progress toward *his* culturally defined health state. Moreover, what may seem to the nurse to be resistance or uncooperativeness of the patient to nursing or medical help could well be traced to the cultural background differences between the patient and nurse.[17]

Groups tend to ignore some symptoms and to agree on the need for help for others. Some group behaviors are governed in part by *ideologic beliefs*, e.g., persons of Christian Science belief may not seek aid from medical health care workers.

Social characteristics of the individual experiencing the disorder. Some men view illness as an indication of femininity and weakness and may thus be reluctant to seek help for disorders. Older persons, with symptoms viewed as not incapacitating and not serious, may tend to attribute their symptoms to the process of aging. Persons in lower social classes appear to be less likely to seek help than persons in higher social classes.

Visibility, recognizability or conspicuousness of the disorder. An individual may tend to experiment more with self-treatment in external, observable disorders (e.g., external bleeding) because the treatment alternatives are limited. On the other hand, alternative treatment forms are far more numerous in covert, ill-defined, ambiguous disorders (e.g., indigestion).[5] Help may be more readily sought for visible abnormalities against which there is *social prejudice* than for those not experienced in this manner.[19] Atypical behaviors are less readily defined in large, less intimate communities and may thus be more tolerated or ignored than in small, intimate communities.

Frequency, intensity, persistence and recurrence of the disorder. The more frequent, annoying, persistent or constant the disorder, in spite of attempts at self-treatment, the more likely the person will seek professional help. When a disorder markedly deviates from societal norms, increased social pressure is applied to get the affected individual to seek help.

Availability of treatment resources and health care personnel. We have previously indicated that some persons may need professional help but not realize that they have this need. Others may know they need help but are unable to make the effort or go the necessary distance to obtain help. The *physical proximity* of the treatment facility and *ability of the helpee to travel* are thus important. *Complex referral systems, specialization of services, malpractice* and *high mobility* are all factors that may cause problems in seeking help. Some people know they need help but do not know where to go to find it; others go to places where they may not be accepted for treatment.

A person needing help may be reluctant to get caught up in a time-consuming, expensive referral system and may not know which specialist to see first. "I don't know which doctor to start with. I'm sure that whichever one I see will just refer me to some others." Also, patients who are new to a community may not know which health professionals have a good, safe reputation; they may fear they will choose someone who is incompetent or unsafe. Some people may be unable to pay for the type of health care they would like to receive. Others may feel unable to "take the time to be sick." Many people feel they simply cannot afford to be sick and lose time from work or caring for a family, pay doctor and hospital bills, buy medications, etc. Thus, they postpone seeking help in the vain hope that their condition will improve.

We have mentioned that *time, effort, cost, inconvenience* and *lack of knowledge about health care facilities* and personnel are all factors that may influence a person's perception of the "availability" of these necessary resources. An additional factor is simply how comfortable the patient (client) feels with the health care personnel available to him—in other words, the *degree of interpersonal comfort* that exists between the patient and the doctor, nurse, dentist, etc. You will know from your own experiences that you tend to go more comfortably and more readily to a doctor or dentist you personally "like." This "personal availability" or "approachability" is an important quality in health care personnel if they truly want to be comfortably sought out by persons needing their help.

Let us next examine some attitudes toward a patient or his condition that might be detrimental to him once he has reached the doctor or nurse—attitudes that might make him feel uncomfortable about having come in. (1) *Scolding* the patient for not coming in sooner is obviously embarrassing to him and might make him reluctant to return the next time for fear of further reprimands. (2) Any sign of irritation *minimizing* the patient's concerns, so that he is made to seem "silly" for being worried and coming in for care, is rude and belittling. Im-

plying that he "pampers" himself and "gives in" to illness too readily or that he is overly concerned with his health will make it much more difficult for him to seek care again. Examples of statements that minimize the patient's concerns are: "You mean this is all that's bothering you?"; "Couldn't this have waited a day or so?"; or (in an irritated tone) "Everything has been checked out, nothing is wrong, you worry too much." (3) On the other hand, an attitude that *overalarms* the patient about his symptoms may frighten him away from further medical care by making him decide, "It's worse than I thought. There's no telling what will have to be done to me. Maybe it's too late anyway." (4) Finally, an attitude that is *too casual* and *joking* about a patient's condition may make him feel that his condition is not being taken seriously enough.

> The attitude a nurse takes toward a patient's symptoms can be important in determining the patient's future help-seeking behaviors. For example, a warm, concerned attitude may help a patient feel more comfortable in reporting future symptoms.

The help-seeker's various personal concerns, fears and previous experiences. The development of mental and/or physical symptoms creates a series of concerns and conflicts in an individual's life. Among these are: "Should I seek out a professional who will diagnose and treat my disorder? If I do seek out someone, should I accept their diagnosis and the treatment they suggest?" Private concerns, fears and previous experiences are all active as the affected person acts to resolve these conflicts.

Some persons avoid seeking medical care because of the *previous unfortunate experiences* they, or others whom they know, have had with doctors, medicine and surgery. Sometimes the criticisms leveled against the medical profession, nurses and hospitals are justified; at other times they appear not to be. The important point, in terms of this discussion, is the feeling that one cannot trust those persons needed to give care. And, on the basis of this, even when feeling ill, people may not seek necessary medical care. Persons who feel that doctors and nurses have been rude, callous, incompetent and indifferent to them will naturally be reluctant to seek out what they view as "more of the same." Winning back the confidence of such injured persons is a difficult task, but it is not an impossible one. Patients who feel they cannot trust us are frightened, and justly so, for they often place their lives in our hands.

In such a situation, it is most important to let the person talk about what happened in the past and to remain nonjudgmental yet supportive. The listener should not rush to the immediate defense of the doctor, nurse or hospital being criticized with statements such as: "I'm sure they were just doing what had to be done and what was right . . . after all, the doctor or nurse knows best," or "It was probably hospital policy to do it that way." Reacting in this manner will cause the patient to feel that it is useless to talk further because the listener appears to have already made up her mind that no matter what the situation may be, the staff is always right.

Instead of leaping to judgmental statements, such as those above, it is often most helpful to begin by attempting to find out all the information the person has about the situation, and thus to generally encourage discussion of the incident, rather than implying that you are certain that the "medical people" were right and you don't want to discuss it further. Often broad, supportive statements are helpful, such as, "So much about illness is frightening, isn't it?" or "It's upsetting to hear about an incident like your friend's experience." It is possible to encourage the person to think more critically about what he heard, saw, or experienced by saying something like, "It is difficult to understand such occurrences. What do you think was actually happening?"

After the person has been allowed to talk about the incident that frightened him, it is helpful to proceed to talk about his own current situation. For example, if he has just learned that he is going to need surgery, and he has told you about the frightening things that happened to his friend who had surgery, you can say something like, "I guess you must be wondering what will happen to you now after hearing about your friend's experience." Then it is possible to begin to talk about how his experience and condition may differ from his friend's, and to identify some of his specific fears and concerns. Often what one imagines and anticipates is more frightening than the actual experience.

> *A physical examination, diagnostic procedure or treatment that seems "routine" or "minor" to a health professional may seem very unusual, complex, frightening and serious to the patient and his family.*

The psychologic discomfort of having to submit to a *physical examination* and a discussion of one's *intimate life history* are also factors that keep some persons from seeking medical evaluation. For many the physical contact necessary during a physical examination is sexually threatening or otherwise disturbing and emotionally charged. People dislike being poked, probed, peered into and exposed and often have feelings of helplessness, fear and resentment toward the examiner. Submitting to diagnostic procedures also may be dreaded because of fear of pain, exposure and the unknown. The nurse can be of direct assistance to patients and help to relieve or minimize fears and anxiety in all these areas.

> *Too often physicals, histories, and diagnostic examinations are conducted in a manner embarrassing and dehumanizing for patients.*

As in assembly line fashion, patients may be unhappily processed through the "mill of medical science." They are asked to talk and then are thoughtlessly interrupted; they are excluded from conversation and "talked around and about" even though they are often lying in the middle of the group and the conversation is about them; they are vacantly stared at, or gazed through, as if they were lifeless; they are crudely and needlessly exposed; they are whisked out of their rooms without explanation; they are bluntly asked tactless questions and subjected to rude comment, often in front of a group, as their private life and distresses are made public. When people are expected to surrender all claims to human sensitivity, as in the above instances, it is no wonder that many delay seeking "medical assistance and care" as long as possible. Needless to say, none of these examples constitutes acceptable medical or nursing practice. If we really want to understand why patients are reluctant to seek medical aid and accept nursing care, we must look with honesty and sensitivity at existing practices.

There are still other reasons why people may not seek health care even though they believe that something is wrong with them. Some persons neglect finding out what their problems are because they *dread receiving a diagnosis that is unacceptable to them.* For some persons this may mean they do not want to hear the words, *"Everything seems to be all right; the diagnostic tests and examinations reveal no problem."* This paradoxical situation may occur for a variety of reasons. For example, a patient may not want to hear that he is capable of working when he does not want to work. Or a person who receives a great deal of attention because of his symptoms may not want to hear that there is no demonstrable basis for the symptoms. These problems are complex and, in some instances may indicate that the patient has psychosocial problems that merit investigation.

Mechanic[24] reported that interpersonal stress is an important determinant in seeking medical attention. Persons with high levels of stress (as indicated by frequency of nervousness and loneliness) were noted to visit physicians more often because of symptoms than those persons with lower stress levels. While stress may produce physical symptoms, it may be difficult to establish that symptoms are definitely stress-related. Stress may also accentuate a person's sensitivity to any pre-existing symptoms he may have.

Some individuals put off seeking health care because they *fear the worst.* They try to hope that by ignoring the trouble, it will resolve itself; they live with trying to ignore or wish away their difficulty. It is tragic that many people live in this state of fearful uncertainty. They dread the worst rather than seeking a professional opinion. Sometimes the illness does prove to be serious and the physician's diagnosis, when finally obtained, coincides with the patient's fears; i.e., he does need surgery or has cancer, syphilis or the heart problem he feared. Reluctance to learn of such problems is understandable. However, more often than not, the diagnosis will be of a less severe problem than that imagined or of an entirely different nature from what the patient imagined.

With any treatable condition, the sooner the treatment can begin, the better it is for the patient's well-being. It should also be recognized that medicine and nursing can provide helpful palliative and comfort measures for those with incurable illnesses.

Some persons delay seeking health care because they *fear admission to a hospital or long-term care facility.* These fears may cause some persons to not seek professional help even though they have urgent, serious symptoms. Some people fear that if they are admitted to a care facility, they will die there, or they may fear they will not survive surgery. Of course, in some instances these concerns are realistic.

Finally, some people delay seeking professional help, in spite of the presence of symptoms, because they are *reluctant to assume the "sick role"* (see Chap. 13).

Let us turn now from our consideration of some reasons that may cause delays in seeking professional health care and consider the other side of the coin as we briefly discuss further those persons who seek medical attention more often than their condition warrants.

PERSONS WHO SEEK MEDICAL ATTENTION MORE OFTEN THAN APPARENTLY NEEDED

For a variety of complex reasons, some people seek medical attention more frequently than their physical condition might "normally" warrant. Some individuals suffer from *self-induced disorders.* Others compulsively seek surgical procedures; these multi-operated persons have been said to suffer from *mania operativa* (surgical addiction).[9] More commonly, the professional health care worker might care for persons (often rather loosely referred to as *"hypochondriacs"*) who (a) give matters of health a high priority and a lot of attention, (b) show heightened sensitivity to changes in body functions and body structure and (c) have a tendency to more rapidly define themselves as "ill" than do others who lack these attributes.[35]

The term "hypochondriasis" is frequently heard in lay discussions. As far as professional usage goes, this term is generally considered to be of little value (except historically) and is actually a generic, descriptive one rather than a distinct nosologic entity. It is still found in some literature, however, and generally refers to persons who have a tendency to show somatic (bodily) "overconcern" and who have physical symptoms with no basis in demonstrable organic changes. Thus, the concept is somewhat synonymous with psychogenic functional disorders. The classification of "hypochondriasis" does not appear in the standard nomenclature of the American Psychiatric Association.

Let us strongly caution the reader that it can be damaging to a patient to apply any of the labels indicated above. Patients may accurately be said to suffer from self-induced disease or surgical addiction only after a thorough history and diagnostic work-up has been conducted by a qualified professional. It is then up to the discretion of that professional to determine the proper course of subsequent action for the treatment of these infrequent disorders. Likewise, describing a person as having hypochondriacal tendencies should be done only after a qualified professional has conducted a careful assessment of that individual. In all instances presented above, it would be improper for health care personnel to indiscreetly discuss these disorders or to discuss the diagnostician's impressions with the patient unless specific plans had been made to do so in conjunction with the attending physician and a treatment plan.

Instead of using "labels" such as the term "hypochondriasis," we prefer to describe the behaviors observed in given patients. Thus, we would say that some individuals show a very high level of concern and preoccupation with their body functions. Such persons may seek out medical attention far more often than their physical condition appears to warrant.

Persons of this type may be a source of frustration to professionals who desire to "cure" people. At times one notes these persons referred to as "perennial patients" or "professional patients."[31] Although patients of this kind are frustrating and irritating to some health care personnel, several factors must be kept in mind: (1) At least these patients do seek out health evaluations, and it is important that they do. They can develop serious physical ailments as readily as anyone else; therefore, they should not be discouraged from asking for care. (2) These persons *are* ill and *are* in need of care, for their bodily concerns signify high levels of anxiety, and in fact, they do not feel well. Persons who seek health care more often than physical symptoms indicate may be helpfully directed to psychiatric aid.

BIBLIOGRAPHY

1. Allodi, F. A., and Coates, D. B.: Social stress, psychiatric symptoms and help-seeking patterns. *Canadian Psychiatric Association Journal,* 18:153–158, April 1973.
1a. Altman, N.: Helping the hypochondriac. *American Family Physician,* 17:107–112, June 1978.
2. Antonovsky, A.: The image of four diseases held by the urban Jewish population of Israel. *Journal of Chronic Disease,* 25:375–384, 1972.
3. Apple, D. (ed.): *Sociological Studies of Health and Sickness.* New York, McGraw-Hill Book Co., 1960.
4. Baumann, B.: Diversities in conceptions of health and physical fitness. *Journal of Health and Human Behavior,* 2:39, Spring 1961.
5. Blackwell, B. L.: Anticipated pre-medical care activities of upper-middle class adults and their implications for health education practice. *Health Education Monograph,* No. 17, pp. 17–36, 1964.
6. Brodie, B.: Views of healthy children toward illness. *American Journal of Public Health,* 64:1156–1159, Dec. 1974.
7. Burgess, A. C., and Burns, J.: Why patients seek care. *American Journal of Nursing,* 73:314, Feb. 1973.
8. Campbell, J. D.: Illness is a point of view: the development of children's concepts of illness. *Nursing Digest,* 4:56–59, Summer 1976.
9. Chertok, L.: *Mania operativa:* surgical addiction. *Psychiatry in Medicine,* 3:105–118, April 1972.
10. Faces of Hypochondriasis (editorial). *Canadian Medical Association Journal,* 109:673, Oct. 20, 1973.
11. Fisher, J. V., Mason, R. L., and Fisher, J. C.: Emotional illness and the family physician. *Psychosomatics,* 16:171–177, Oct.-Dec. 1975.

12. Geertsen, H. R., Gray, R. M., and Ward, J. R.: Patient non-compliance within the context of seeking medical care for arthritis. *Journal of Chronic Diseases,* 26:689–698, Nov. 1973.
13. Hurtado, A. V., Greenlick, M. R., and Colombo, T. J.: Determinants of medical care utilization: failure to keep appointments. *Medical Care,* 11:189–198, May-June 1973.
13a. In sickness and in health. *Emergency Medicine,* 9:61, May 1977.
14. Kasl, S. V., and Cobb, S.: Health behavior, illness behavior, and sick role behavior. *Archives of Environmental Health,* 12:240–266, Feb. 1966.
15. Kirscht, J. P.: Social and psychological problems of surveys on health and illness. *Social Science and Medicine,* 5:519–526, Dec. 1971.
16. Koos, E. L.: Illness in regionville. *In* Apple, D. (ed.): *Sociological Studies in Health and Sickness.* New York, McGraw-Hill Book Co., 1960, Chap. 1, pp. 9–14.
17. Leininger, M.: The culture concept and its relevance to nursing. *Journal of Nursing Education,* 6:27–37, April 1967.
18. Lipsitt, D. R.: Psychodynamic considerations of hypochondriasis. *Psychotherapy and Psychosomatics,* 23:132–141, 1974.
19. MacGregor, F. C.: Some psychological hazards of plastic surgery of the face. *In* Apple, D. (ed.): *Sociological Studies of Health and Sickness.* New York, McGraw-Hill Book Co., 1960, Chap. 11, pp. 145–153.
20. Mark, H., et al.: Factors affecting patients' comprehension of illness and treatment at an urban medical center. *Journal Medical Society New Jersey,* 72:493–498, June 1975.
21. Martin, H. W., and Prange, A. J., Jr.: The stages of illness—psychosocial approach. *Nursing Outlook,* 10:168, March 1962.
22. McBroom, W. H.: Illness, illness behavior and socioeconomic status. *Journal of Health and Social Behavior,* 11:319–326, Dec. 1970.
23. McMichael, A. J., and Hetzel, B. S.: Patterns of help-seeking for mental illness among Australian university students: an epidemiological study. *Social Science in Medicine,* 8:197–206, April 1974.
24. Mechanic, D.: The concept of illness behavior. *Journal of Chronic Disease,* 15:189–194, Feb. 1962.
25. Mechanic, D.: The influence of mothers on their children's health attitudes and behaviors. *Pediatrics,* 33:444–453, March 1964.
26. Reader, G. G., and Schwartz, D.: Developing patients' knowledge of health. *Hospitals, J.A.H.A.,* 47:111–114, March 1, 1973.
26a. Rittelmeyer, J. F., Jr.: Caring for the hypochondriac. *American Family Physician,* 14:98–101, Sept. 1976.
27. Salerno, E. M.: A family in crisis. *American Journal of Nursing,* 73:100, Jan. 1973.
28. Suchman, E. A.: Stages of illness and medical care. *Journal of Health and Human Behavior,* 6:114–128, Fall 1965.
29. Sweetser, D. A.: How laymen define illness. *Journal of Health and Human Behavior,* 1:219, 1960.
30. Travis, T. A., Clancy, J., and Noyes, R., Jr.: The hysterical personality. *Postgraduate Medicine,* 54:221–225, Nov. 1973.
31. von Mering, O.: The diffuse health aberration syndrome: a bio-behavioral study of the perennial outpatient, *Psychosomatics,* 13:293–303, Sept.–Oct. 1972.
32. Wadsworth, M.: Health and sickness: the choice of treatment. *Journal of Psychosomatic Research,* 18(4):271–276, 1974.

33. Waitzkin, H., and Stoeckle, J. D.: The communication of information about illness. *Advances in Psychosomatic Medicine*, 8:180–215, 1972.

34. Wilson, J. T.: Compliance with instructions in the evaluation of therapeutic efficacy. A common but frequently unrecognized major variable. *Clinical Pediatrics*, 12:333–340, June 1973.

35. Wu, R.: *Behavior and Illness.* Englewood Cliffs, NJ, Prentice-Hall, 1973.

36. Zborowski, M.: Cultural components in response to pain. *In* Apple, D. (ed.): *Sociological Studies of Health and Sickness.* New York, McGraw-Hill Book Co., 1960, pp. 118–133.

37. Zola, I. K.: Pathways to the doctor—from person to patient. *Social Science and Medicine*, 7:677–689, 1973.

38. Zola, I. K.: Studying the decision to see a doctor. *Advances in Psychosomatic Medicine*, 8:216–236, 1972.

CHAPTER 11

PSYCHO-BEHAVIORAL REACTIONS TO THE CONFIRMATION OF ILLNESS

Illness lays bare the character of what may be called the patient's "security system." By this is meant the adequacy of the patient's behavior patterns in relationship to the demands of his environment. A weak security system is made even weaker by illness or disability, a strong security system is made even stronger. That is to say, illness is a crisis in the life of the individual, and any crisis serves to test and to display the strength of the person's resources for dealing with his world.

REINHARDT AND MEADOWS[61]

INTRODUCTION AND STUDY GUIDE

What are some typical reactions to diagnosis and illness? What are some of the general factors that contribute to how a patient thinks about his illness and reacts to it? These questions are the concern of this chapter.

The ways in which people react to the knowledge that they are ill are extremely variable and individualized. Suppose, for example, that you have just been told by your doctor that you have diabetes. You are to enter the hospital for a few days in order for your condition to be stabilized and for a treatment plan to begin. Pause, trying to *really* imagine that this is happening to you. What are your reactions to this news? What problems would this diagnosis pose for you? What plans do you need to make in order to go into the hospital tomorrow for several days? Identigy the "losses" you will experience as a result of the news the doctor has just given you.

Consider the various ways in which your friends and relatives have reacted to illness in the past. In giving patient care, attempt to identify how your patients each seem to be reacting *specifically* and *individually* to diagnosis and the state of illness. Look for evidence of the specific reactions discussed in this chapter.

GENERAL FACTORS INFLUENCING REACTIONS TO DIAGNOSIS AND ILLNESS

We could say, generally, that four factors combine to determine how a patient reacts to his diagnosis or illness: (1) the nature of the illness; (2) the nature of the patient; (3) the attitudes of others toward the illness; and (4) the patient's own attitudes toward the illness. Let us consider each of these factors in turn.

1. The Nature of the Illness. Illnesses have become departmentalized and differentiated within hospitals by the formation of special wards, and they have been segregated by professional persons into areas of specialization or interest, but illnesses cannot be categorized in terms of patient response to them. Each response is unique; the same illness holds different *"meanings"* for different individuals. The unique meaning of a given illness for a patient will, in part, determine his reaction to that illness. The disease or illness that one person dreads is not necessarily frightening to someone else; conditions that may seem minor in nature to a professional person may be of major concern to a patient—in fact, may panic him. The type of illness that an individual has is thus of great personal importance to him. The prognosis, severity, and expected length of illness are additional factors of great concern to an ill person.

2. The Nature of the Patient.   Individual responses to illness are largely determined by the characteristic responses to anxiety that every individual has developed during his life. Each person's pattern of using mental defense mechanisms (Chap. 8) actually becomes his characteristic *personality pattern.* An individual will therefore respond to the anxieties of illness as he has responded to other anxiety-provoking situations, in accordance with his basic personality traits. One individual may calmly accept his fate and treatment, whereas another with the same diagnosis may become disorganized in behavior, depressed, argumentative and resistive to medical care. We shall discuss some examples of specific defensive behavior later in this chapter.

In addition to his unique pattern of mental defense, an individual's *ideas about himself,* i.e., his self-concept, and his *personal philosophy of life* will also determine in part his reaction to his diagnosis and illness. A part of this general feeling about oneself and one's life is a feeling of motivation toward either health or sickness. These are subtle kinds of feelings that most of us are not even conscious of. Nonetheless, such feelings become apparent when life histories are subjected to careful evaluation. For example, we all know some people who tend to be ill more or less continually and others who are almost always well. For some people illness is more a life pattern than health is; it is actually a more manageable way of life for them than a healthy state. We do not mean to imply that all people who are ill at any given time are motivated to illness. We are referring instead to life-styles, or long-range patterns. This motivation toward health or illness is a crucial factor in an individual's reaction to illness, and in his recovery pattern.

Other factors that influence individual reactions to illness are age, social class, general state of personal happiness, financial position and number of past illnesses. Some brief examples of the influence of such factors follow: (a) *Age:* an older person may be able to accept an illness with a poor prognosis more calmly than a younger person. (b) *Social class:* certain diseases tend to be accepted more readily in one social class than in another. (c) *General state of personal happiness:* persons who are happy and feel loved may find illness and hospitalization difficult to bear because it means separation from home and loved ones; on the other hand, lonely, unhappy people may feel that they receive more attention, and are the object of more concern, when ill than when they are well. (d) *Financial position:* for persons of low to middle income, with no health insurance, an illness may rapidly plunge them into overwhelming debt, while well-to-do persons do not have this concern. (e) *Number of past illnesses:* One's first experience with major illness may seem almost unreal, because it brings the shocking realization of one's vulnerability to illness.

3. The Attitudes of Others Toward the Illness. The attitudes of others toward a patient's illness are readily communicated to him and will, in turn, influence his own reaction to his illness. For example, some illnesses are more socially *acceptable* than others, and these are less anxiety-provoking for the patient. If the patient's illness is of an *unacceptable* nature, he may feel rejected, "dirty" and victimized. Some illnesses are *threatening* to other people. Communicable diseases like tuberculosis and leprosy provoke fear in many people as a threat to their own health; they may, therefore, shun a patient with these illnesses. Conditions that are mutilating and disfiguring—e.g., burns, accidents, skin conditions, open ulcers, gangrene—may evoke strong reactions of *disgust, fear* and *revulsion* in others. (See Chap. 15 for a discussion of body image.) The same is true of conditions with offensive odors which may cause strong reactions in others. Obviously such reactions are apparent to the conscious patient and decidedly mar his self-image and influence his reaction to his illness.

4. The Patient's Own Attitudes Toward the Illness.   Illness is a major disruption to normal living for a patient and is disturbing to his self-image. His self-concept may undergo rapid and extreme alterations as a result of the physical and mental effects of the illness and its effects upon others in his life. If he is to live a life that is at all satisfactory during his illness and afterward, a patient must adapt psychologically; he must regain the psychologic equilibrium that his illness has disrupted.

A sick person is called upon to adjust his needs to the demands that his illness imposes. He will attain psychologic equilibrium during illness (if he can) in exactly the same ways he has at other times in his life: through the trial-and-error process of learning. Those caring for him must give him the time to learn and must be patient with him as he undergoes the trials and errors of adaptation.

It has been observed[53] that everywhere in life, whenever disruption of functions takes place, spontaneous synthesis and regeneration occur. This is true of both mind and body. Just as the body immediately begins to try to protect itself and heal when it suffers an insult, so the mind begins to strive for adaptation when illness strikes. For successful recovery to take place, *both* physical and mental adaptive mechanisms must function successfully and have sufficient time to do so. Some individuals recover physically from a critical illness or injury but are unable to regain a healthy level of psychologic adaptation; others adjust to the reality of their infirmity with amazing psychologic tenacity and grace, but die.

Some of the early attempts that a person makes at psychologic adaptation to his illness, or to the knowledge of his diagnosis, may be impulsive and irrational in nature. He may be attempting to solve this problem by defensive patterns that have worked for him in the past but are inappropriate in this new situation. Indeed, some of the early or most immediate behavioral responses to an illness may not seem to be at all in a person's best interest, since his behavior may actually alienate him from those upon whom he depends for cure and care. Also, under the stress of illness a patient may be unable to think rationally or to make sound decisions. However, whether these early attempts at adaptation appear "ideal" or not, the initial reactions to his illness are probably the most protective patterns of behavior upon which the patient can draw at the time.

SPECIFIC REACTIONS TO DIAGNOSIS AND THE STATE OF ILLNESS

In order for you to more readily comprehend the situations about to be discussed, pause to imagine that you have had back pain over a period of time and it has been growing steadily worse. You have had some diagnostic tests and are now hearing the results from your doctor. He tells you that there is no doubt about it, *you* appear to have cancer of the spine! Before reading further, stop to think about this situation. Similar situations happen to people daily. What influence would this have on your life, right now? How does it make you feel? What might your response or reply to the doctor be? What is *your* reaction to the diagnosis?

Anxiety. The predominant early responses to diagnosis and illness are physical and mental feelings of anxiety (see also Chap. 8). Why does this anxiety occur? Probably the fundamental basis for feeling anxious at such times is that "any disease is a failure, more or less complete, of the organism. Complete failure, of course, is death. From the start, therefore, illness is allied

with anxiety, and it tends to arouse all the anxiety-laden feelings of the patient."[61] Anxious feelings, then, are actually feelings of concern for one's life and well-being.

The specific causes of anxiety are variable from person to person and are probably associated with the fact that the situation in which the person finds himself provokes into action many unconscious thoughts and feelings that have been repressed and inhibited up to that time. Fantasies, fears, dreams and bits of repressed reality are all uncomfortably stirred up as awareness of an illness penetrates the mind.

> *High levels of anxiety are capable of increasing physiologic and psychologic pain. We also know that high levels of anxiety can affect the course of treatment adversely.*

It is becoming increasingly clear, for example, that patients who are extremely anxious prior to surgery are poorer surgical risks and tend to have a stormier postoperative course than patients who are relatively at ease preoperatively.

Shock. Many people experience a period of shock when they first learn of their diagnosis, particularly if it is serious in nature. They feel immobilized; things seem unreal and dreamlike. Even their own behavior may seem unreal to them, as if they were watching a motion picture of themselves and time has slowed down.

> *Often shock makes people incapable of thinking clearly or acting rationally. For a period of time their behavior may make no sense to themselves or to others; they may act automatically and like robots.*

For example, a patient when told that she has cancer may vacantly reply, "Yes—well, I'd better go and get the grocery shopping done." Indeed she may then walk out of the doctor's office, do the grocery shopping, and not even recall for a period of time what she has been told. She retreats for a time into the protective insulation of a dream-like state. When the period of shock begins to end, however, and an awareness of reality returns, she may collapse and sob or suddenly become extremely depressed, perhaps even suicidal. Individuals in a state of shock need protective care and understanding and must be supported especially as the shock lessens.

Denial.   The person in shock is denying his illness. Denial of illness, however, may continue after the initial shock has passed. "I'm really not sick." "How could *I* possibly have cancer? I don't believe it!" These are examples of verbal denial. The reasons why it is necessary for an individual to deny his illness are many. Whatever the reasons, the nurse should bear in mind that:

> *The denying patient is not being stubborn. What may appear to be obstinate behavior is generally a frightened attempt, on the patient's part, to fend off overwhelming threats.*

Denial is protective, and one must proceed with care in deciding how to approach this protective shield. Forcing a patient to lay down his armor too soon and "face facts" may mean making him vulnerable to a painful reality that he may be unable to endure.

The adaptive value of denial can be seen in the daily practice of nursing. For example, it is not uncommon to meet patients who deny a serious illness for a period of time and then, upon finally accepting it, rapidly die. The process of denial appears to have been life-sustaining for such persons. Instances have been cited in which patients have committed suicide when they have finally come to "accept" their diagnosis. Is it wrong for such people to *live* in the dream that they are healthy? Some patients die denying that they are ill, and this has possibly been therapeutically best for them. Their denial is left uninterrupted. Other patients are slowly helped to accept the reality of their illnesses and to adapt to them even though they may be fatal. The physician commonly determines how a patient's denial should be treated.

As we have seen, denial must be handled gently, for it is often a safety valve that prevents the emergence of sheer panic and terror. When you see a patient denying his condition you may think he is merely "pretending" that he doesn't believe what he knows is true. The denying patient is not trying to fool anyone. In true denial the patient honestly believes that he does not have the problem that he is denying. He feels convinced that others are wrong and will search desperately for evidence to support his belief. This quest for supportive evidence may lead such a patient to distort what he sees or hears, and therefore, he may misquote you or his doctor. If this occurs, try to understand that the patient's goal is not to make life difficult for anyone, but rather to make life bearable for himself.

Like any other behavior, denial occurs in various degrees. *Forgetting* is a mild form of denial; forgetting to take one's medication, forgetting to keep a doctor's appointment, or forgetting to stay on a prescribed diet are all mild forms of denial of illness. It is mentally convenient to "forget" what it is uncomfortable to remember.

In situations of more extreme denial we find that, in a pathetic struggle to prove that they are well, some people will push themselves into states of overexertion or make hopeless pilgrimages from one consultation room to another. They are trying to reassure themselves that they are not ill and do not have the disease that has been diagnosed. The danger of such actions is, of course, that they may prove fatal to the patient or may result in impairment that might have been prevented.

As we have said, at times a patient may be allowed to continue to deny his actual diagnosis; when little hope or treatment can be offered, nothing would be gained in bringing him to an acknowledgment of his fate. The nurse must respect such a decision and reinforce it. As for those patients who die because their denial causes them to overexert or avoid treatment, who can judge their actions? Certainly the nurse cannot. For some people serious illness may mean invalidism, weakness, dependency—all unacceptable ways of life for them. Each patient's life is his own and how he chooses to live or die is his choice. Although a nurse makes every attempt to help a patient accept treatment that will help him, she cannot force treatment or make decisions that are not hers to make.

Denial is very much a part of life. We all try to deny much of the unhappiness, suffering and apparent waste of life that we know exists throughout the world. You, as a nurse, will find much that you may want to deny. However, nursing actions must be based on reality. Giving up denial means facing truths that are often difficult to accept. In nursing it means facing life as it is and then trying to do what can be done to make some of life's harsh realities more bearable.

Suspicion.   Some people react to their diagnoses with suspicion. These feelings are closely related to those of denial, but the patient who is suspicious has not *completely* closed his mind to the possibility that his diagnosis may be true. He tries, however, to find many possible reasons for doubting the diagnosis. Suspicious statements will sound like these: "I'm fine—that doctor is just out to make some money." "The family just wants to put me in the hospital and be done with me." "The laboratory made a mistake; that report must be about someone else." "You are all lying to me, but I know what you're up to." You will find that some patients will be suspicious of their diagnosis if it *is* serious in nature, whereas others will be suspicious if their diagnosis does *not* prove to be serious. Therefore, one patient may say, "I don't believe you; it's not as serious as you make out," and another will say, "I don't believe you, this can't be all that's wrong with me. I know you're keeping something from me."

As we have said, adjustment and adaptation take time. If a person's life pattern has been one founded on suspicion, that is, "Everyone tries to take advantage of me," his initial reaction to the anxiety of illness and diagnosis will undoubtedly be one of suspicion. Some doubt is reasonable, but suspicion can grow out of proportion, so that the person becomes suspicious about everything. "My bill is going to be padded." "I don't believe that that medicine is for what you say it is." "Everyone is talking about me." "I know they're going to do more in surgery than they said they would." Extreme suspicion is a serious, reportable condition.

> *Patients who are suspicious are not just complaining; they are frightened and feel that they must be on their guard or they will be hurt and taken advantage of.*

The suspicious person lacks trust in others, and the person who lacks trust asks a lot of questions. This may prove to be irritating; however, patience is necessary, since trust is not easily or rapidly built.

Questioning. "Why me? Why did I have to get this? Why do I have to suffer?" People who are ill often scan their lives trying to find the answers to such questions and believing that there must be a reason for or a purpose to their illness. While some can find no answers to explain their misfortune of being ill, others find a variety of explanations such as illness is a punishment for sin; illness results from neglect of one's health; or illness is predestined and is in one's best interest. Still other patients may view their illness scientifically in biologic or psychologic terms. Another answer to the question "Why me?" is simply that illness is a part of life, something we are susceptible to and which occurs purely as a random phenomenon of nature.

Regardless of the answers, there are many questions about illness that evoke anxious feelings. For example, why does one person have a cancer confirmed at surgery while another's condition proves to be benign? Why does one person recover while another dies? Why does one person escape from a serious accident unscathed while another is mutilated?

Insignificance and Loneliness. Illness makes one feel insignificant, like a grain of sand on a beach. It also causes one to feel alone in facing his problems. Illness brings with it the realization that we all pass through life in separate orbits. We cannot move out of ours and into that of another person if we find our journey is frightening or is soon to end. Patients often feel trapped in their illness. "I can see what is happening to me. I know what will happen to me. But I can't alter it and neither can anyone else."

Regression and Dependency. Regression is a common reaction to illness; it is a natural reaction, when not extreme, since it facilitates recovery by allowing the patient to be more dependent than usual. By allowing himself to rest and be cared for, the patient can restore his strength and can progress to health.

It has been pointed out by Meerloo[53] that regression often serves as a defensive device against stress. Under stress all organisms tend to assume a less differentiated, more primitive way of life. On the microscopic level, multicellular organisms may become unicellular at times of stress or danger. In the body, "A temporary regression takes place when an injury occurs; more primitive cells, the fibroblasts, take over for regeneration and repair as if they temporarily returned to a state of omnipotent capacity."[53] Meerloo further points out that a different management of energy takes place with regression; the regressive principle leads the organism by means of the path of least resistance to a phase of greater inertia but regained stability. Regression thus helps in the process of attaining greater stability and better adaptation both physiologically and psychologically. It is a kind of "strategic retreat of the organism in order to mobilize new forces of resistance and regeneration."[53] Therefore:

> *In illness it should be expected that patients will regress to levels of behavior that are not as mature as those which they assume when well. They need to be allowed sufficient and appropriate regression and dependence upon others.*

Emotional regression (going back to earlier stages of psychologic development) may produce conflict for a patient if he realizes that although he is an adult, and thus "should" act as an adult, he wants or needs to act in rather child-like ways.

> *Ill persons have a strong need for security. Warm, friendly interactions and familiar settings promote feelings of security.*

In their search for security patients often hope to find in nurses the reassuring qualities of sympathy, tenderness, understanding and gentleness tempered with firmness. The careful reader will observe that these are qualities often attributed to the "ideal mother figure." Similarly, patients may expect physicians to possess "father-like" qualities, e.g., dominance, strength, protectiveness. The patient thus often looks to his doctors and nurses for protection from life's adversities. The regressed patient, seeking those qualities of ideal parents in staff members, is disappointed by the absence of such qualities. Likewise, patients long for familiar settings, objects and associations and may therefore critically compare their present situation with absent familiar situations.

The concerned nurse realizes that a patient's frequent "complaints" about relatively insignificant matters may indeed be superficial indications of his more serious, deeper concerns. Thoughtful health professionals strive to enhance patients' feelings of security and worth by helping to make the environment (shared by both staff and patients) as comfortable and emotionally warm as possible. For some patients, e.g., patients in long-term care facilities, staff members become "pseudo-family members." These patients (and others, of course) look to the staff for the protection, warmth, guidance, support, modeling, expectations and judgments they would hope to receive from their family. Security is enhanced for patients when staff members meet the patients' expectations of them. It is thus desirable for health professionals to assess a patient's expectations of them and to identify ways in which these expectations can be dealt with constructively.

Shame and Guilt. When patients believe that their illness is a punishment for sin or wrongdoing (either imagined or real), they may react with feelings of shame and guilt. Also, certain diseases may make an individual feel disgraced or ashamed, depending upon his family and cultural background. Some people feel that they shame their family by having certain "unacceptable" conditions (e.g., mental disorders, epilepsy, venereal disease, tuberculosis) and they may feel unrealistically responsible for having brought on the condition. Such feelings of shame and guilt related to illness are damaging to the self-concept. In some conditions, such as alcoholism, the patient may be viewed by others as weak-willed, or he may think of himself in those terms.

Rejection. Illness may precipitate feelings of being rejected. Although some of these feelings of rejection may be imagined, often they are partially based on reality, since illness does actually cause one to be removed from his usual life patterns and state of health. Those illnesses that are socially unacceptable or socially threatening, e.g., communicable disease, cause a patient to be rejected and isolated even more. Prolonged illnesses create many feelings of rejection in a patient's personal life, as friends and loved ones may begin to take the illness for granted and proceed with their own lives. Because illness does cause a patient to be shut out from many activities of life, it is especially important to him to have warm relationships with those caring for him.

At times patients may imagine that they are rejected because of illness when this is really not the case. In such situations the patient may be using his illness as an excuse for not receiving the attention of others instead of looking objectively at his behaviors.

Fear. The specific fears that accompany the realization that one has a dreaded illness are many and have been discussed in previous chapters. Here we present a brief list of some specific fears that often accompany illness:

▶ fear of a strange place, e.g., the hospital, nursing home, and so forth

▶ fear of equipment—"Will it hurt me? What if it doesn't run right?"

▶ fear of pain, loss of body parts, or mutilation

▶ fear of being "experimented" on

▶ fear of having to suffer as punishment for past misbehavior

▶ fear of treatments and diagnostic processes, e.g., surgery, cardiac catheterization

▶ fear of being abused or neglected; of having one's feelings hurt; or of being treated impersonally

▶ fear of being left alone or isolated from loved ones

▶ fear of loss of function or loss of self-control

▶ fear of death

▶ fear of burdening others

Many of these fears begin in childhood and accompany us, in various forms, throughout our lives. They are the subject of our fantasy and discussion, and as we observe manifestations of these fears in others, they gradually become part of our own feelings. Much of this mental activity is repressed until illness, with its accompanying anxiety, reaches the deeper levels of our minds and such fears resurface and magnify.

Often it is true that what is imagined and anticipated is more frightening than the actual experience; nevertheless, the dread is there.

> *The fearful person may be hostile to others; he is on the defensive and is trying to protect himself. He is ready to fight, but often he cannot identify what he should strike out at. Fear and hostility are often interrelated.*

Attempting to guess what a patient's fears may be is not good practice; through guessing you may suggest fears that he hadn't thought of but that will now disturb him. For example, suppose you are talking with a patient who is about to go to surgery. He appears fearful and so you guess at what his fears are and say, "Perhaps you're worried that you'll choke while you're unconscious because you can't swallow. Don't worry. Someone will suction you out until you are awake." If the patient didn't have that in mind before, he will now! Let the patient tell you what he is fearful of. You may make general comments, however, such as, "It isn't unusual to be frightened at a time like this. In fact it's perfectly normal. If you would like to talk about how you feel, I might be of some help to you."

Withdrawal and Depression

The actions of withdrawal by human beings are numberless: fantasy, autistic image-making, inferiority feelings, shyness, delusions, illusions, melancholia, anxieties, fears, self-incriminations, and so on. The individual thus turns to an internal drama, with isolating themes, wish-fulfilling thoughts and actions, and actors formed in the molds of unrestrained impulse.[61]

Withdrawal and depression commonly occur as reactions to diagnosis and illness. Like most of the other reactions discussed so far, we expect some of this behavior to accompany illness. Excessive or prolonged withdrawal or depression, however, is a cause for real concern, and observations of these conditions should be reported.

Let us briefly consider some common experiences and expressions during depression. The depressed person typically appears sad or shows little expression. The forehead is furrowed, the mouth turned down. Personal hygiene may be neglected; e.g., hair is uncombed, make-up is not applied, typical shaving patterns are neglected.

Physically, during depression the body as a whole appears to be "slowed down" or not working properly. This general slowing down process affects bowel function, the menstrual cycle and sexual interest. Food may seem tasteless, and the appetite is poor. The depressed person often loses weight and may suffer from a feeling of choking or tightness in the throat and a hollowness in the stomach. Sleep disturbances may occur, with insomnia and early morning wakening. When sleep does come, it is often broken or disturbed by bad dreams and nightmares, and the person awakens fatigued. Often such a patient awakens in the early morning hours filled with self-torturing thoughts or, in the presence of illness, to the reality of illness and suffering. In a desperate attempt to escape both his physical and mental anguish he may attempt to take his life.

With depression there are often evidences of sloth, weariness, exhaustion, persistent lassitude, inner tension, inertia and a general lack of energy. However, in states of *agitated depression,* the patient may be hyperactive: pacing, moving about, picking rapidly at the bed clothing and so on. Patients in states of agitated depression should be protected against suicidal attempts. Some additional typical signs of depression are sighing, wringing the hands, slow speech and frequent weeping.

The severely depressed person longs for an escape from his life situation, which he feels is intolerable. He may, therefore, be preoccupied with thoughts of death and/or suicide. Often it is difficult for a depressed individual to concentrate, and he may have difficulty remembering. His affect centers primarily around feelings of despair, hopelessness, isolation and desolation. The depressed person often withdraws from others. He may pull the shades, turn out the lights, pull the covers up around his head and shoulders, and not respond to the presence of others. He is suffering and in need of medical and/or psychiatric aid.

It is not uncommon for people under the stress of serious or terminal illnesses to express fears of "losing their mind" because they are unable to take their minds off themselves and their troubles. They may feel that they cannot endure their state. These troubled persons should not have their concerns minimized; they need opportunities to discuss how they feel and what they are worried about. Sometimes just talking about the pressures they are under is of help. Notation should be made of such a patient's distress, for he may benefit from skilled psychiatric evaluation and consultation. Some patients find relief in talking with their spiritual adviser or the hospital chaplain.

Paradoxical Reactions. At times patients respond to their diagnoses in ways that are paradoxical, that is, not at all what we might expect. For example, they may joke about their condition, even though it is extremely serious. Individuals with neurotic tendencies may appear relieved to learn that they are ill or that they require surgery. These are not expected reactions and may catch the nurse unaware of what is happening. Like all other reactions, these should be viewed as the individual's unique reaction to stress.

SUMMARY

In this chapter we have discussed some various ways in which people react to a diagnosis and the state of illness. We identified four general factors that influence these reactions: (1) the nature of the illness; (2) the nature of the patient; (3) the attitudes of others toward a patient's illness; and (4) the patient's own attitudes toward his illness. The specific reactions to diagnosis and the state of illness that were discussed include (1) anxiety, (2) shock, (3) denial, (4) suspicion, (5) questioning, (6) feelings of insignificance and loneliness, (7) regression and dependency, (8) shame and guilt, (9) rejection, (10) fear, (11) withdrawal and depression, and (12) paradoxical reactions.

BIBLIOGRAPHY

1. Barbour, T.: I traveled the mastectomy road. *Supervisor Nurse,* 6:40–43, March 1975.
2. Barckley, V.: The crises in cancer. *American Journal of Nursing,* 67:278–280, Feb. 1967.
3. Bayley, E. W., et al.: Burns: breaking the anger-despair cycle. *Nursing '75,* 5:42–49, May 1975.
4. Benfield, R. M., and Russell, F. F.: Hypervalinemia: a family's reaction, a nursing challenge. *Nursing Forum,* 14(2):130–144, 1975.
5. Bergeron, J. H.: A patient's plea: tell me, I need to know. *American Journal of Nursing,* 71:1572, Aug. 1971.
6. Bragg, T. L.: Psychological response to myocardial infarction. *Nursing Forum,* 14(4):383–395, 1975.
7. Brooks, B. R.: Aggression. *American Journal of Nursing,* 67:2519, Dec. 1967.
8. Bowden, M. L., and Feller, I.: Family reaction to a severe burn. *American Journal of Nursing,* 73:317, Feb. 1973.
9. Busch, K. D., and Gallo, B. M.: Emotional response to illness. *In* Hudak, C. M., Gallo, B. M., and Lohr, T.: *Critical Care Nursing.* Philadelphia, J. B. Lippincott Co., 1973.
10. Chaney, P. (ed.): Surviving. *Nursing '76,* 6:41–50, April 1976.
11. Coburn, D.: Anticipating breast surgery. *American Journal of Nursing,* 75:1483, Sept. 1975.
12. Crate, M. A.: Nursing functions in adaptation to chronic illness. *American Journal of Nursing,* 65:72–76, Oct. 1965.
13. Craven, P. K.: A facade for fear. *A.N.A. Clinical Sessions,* 1966, p. 28.
14. Croushore, T.: That abnormal finding was *mine. Nursing '77,* 7:96, March 1977.
15. Daly, K. M.: Don't wave good-bye. *American Journal of Nursing,* 74:1641, Sept. 1974.
16. De Young, M. A.: On the other end of the buzzer. *Nursing '77,* 7:96, Feb. 1977.
17. Dillon, A. M.: Nursing care of the patient with multiple sclerosis. *Nursing Clinics of North America,* 8:653–664, Dec. 1973.
18. Dixson, B. K.: Dealing with passive-aggressive behavior. *Nursing Forum,* 8(3):276–285, 1969.
19. Does anybody care? *American Journal of Nursing,* 73:1562, Sept. 1973.
20. Drake, R. E.: Guidelines for helping patients and families cope with traumatic illness. *In* Reinhardt, A. M., and Quinn, M. D. (eds.): *Family-Centered Community Nursing: A Sociocultural Framework.* St. Louis, The C. V. Mosby Co., 1973.
21. Educational Design Program: Understanding hostility—programmed instruction. *American Journal of Nursing,* 67:2131–2150, Oct. 1967.
22. Field, M.: *Patients are People,* 3rd ed. New York, Columbia University Press, 1967.
23. Foster, S., and Andreoli, K. G.: Behavior following acute myocardial infarction. *American Journal of Nursing,* 70:2344–2348, Nov. 1970.
24. Forster, B., and Forster, F.: Nursing students' reaction to the crying patient. *Nursing Research,* 20:265–268, May–June 1971.
25. George, M. M.: Long-term care of the patient with cancer. *Nursing Clinics of North America,* 8:623–631, Dec. 1973.
26. Hamburg, D. A.: Coping behavior in life-threatening circumstances. *Psychotherapy and Psychosomatics,* 23:13–25, 1974.
27. Harker, B. L.: Cancer and communication problems: a personal experience. *Psychiatry in Medicine,* 3:163–172, April 1972.
28. Harrell, H. C.: To lose a breast. *American Journal of Nursing,* 72:676, April 1972.

29. Hecht, A.: Questions relatives ask. *Geriatric Nursing,* 4:23, Feb. 1968.

30. Heller, S., et al.: Psychological outcome following open-heart surgery. *Archives of Internal Medicine,* 134:908–914, Nov. 1974.

31. Herth, K.: Beyond the curtain of silence. *American Journal of Nursing,* 74:1060, June 1974.

32. Hugos, R.: Living with leukemia. *American Journal of Nursing,* 72:2185, Dec. 1972.

33. Jackson, J. K.: The role of the patient's family in illness. *Nursing Forum,* 1:119, Summer 1962.

34. Johnson, D. E.: Powerlessness: a significant determinant in patient behavior? *Journal of Nursing Education,* 6:39, April 1967.

35. Jones, L. A.: Myasthenia and me. *RN,* 39:50–55, June 1976.

36. Jontz, D. L.: Prescription for living with M. S. *American Journal of Nursing,* 73:817, May 1973.

37. Kahana, R. J.: Personality and response to physical illness. *Advances in Psychosomatic Medicine,* 8:42–62, 1972.

38. Kee, J. L., and Hamilton, M. L.: Mr. Myers played the buzzer game. *Nursing '76,* 6:14–16, May 1976.

39. Kiely, W. F.: Coping with severe illness. *Advances in Psychosomatic Medicine,* 8:105–118, 1972.

40. Kiening, S. M. M.: Denial of illness. *In* Carlson, C. E. (ed.): *Behavioral Concepts and Nursing Intervention.* Philadelphia, J. B. Lippincott Co., 1970.

41. King, J. M.: Denial. *American Journal of Nursing,* 66:1010, May 1966.

42. Kornfeld, D. S.: The hospital environment: its impact on the patient. *Advances in Psychosomatic Medicine,* 8:252–270, 1972.

43. Larter, M. H.: "M.I. wives" need you. *RN,* 39:44–48, Aug. 1976.

44. Lederer, H. D.: How the sick view their world. *Journal of Social Issues,* 8(4):4–15, 1952.

45. Lee, J. M.: Emotional reactions to trauma. *Nursing Clinics of North America,* 5:577–587, Dec. 1970.

46. Leininger, M.: *Nursing and Anthropology: Two Worlds to Blend.* New York, John Wiley & Sons, 1970.

47. Levine, M. E.: The intransigent patient. *American Journal of Nursing,* 70:2106–2111, Oct. 1970.

48. Livsey, C. G.: Physical illness and family dynamics. *Advances in Psychosomatic Medicine,* 8:237–251, 1972.

49. Lord, E. A.: My crisis with cancer. *American Journal of Nursing,* 74:647, April 1974.

50. Luckmann, J., and Sorensen, K. C.: What patients' actions tell you about their feelings, fears and needs. *Nursing '75,* 5:54–61, Feb. 1975.

51. Mancino, D. J., and Harmon, V.: Visiting trends and gift giving. *Nursing Forum,* 11(3):264–272, 1972.

52. Martin, H. A., and Prange, A. J., Jr.: Human adaptation—a conceptual approach to understanding patients. *Canadian Nurse,* 58:234–243, March 1962.

53. Meerloo, J. A. M.: *Illness and Cure.* New York, Grune & Stratton, 1964.

54. Miller, M. B., Bernstein, H., and Sharkey, H.: Denial of parental illness and maintenance of familial homeostasis. *Journal American Geriatric Society,* 21:278–285, June 1973.

55. Neu, C.: Coping with newly diagnosed blindness. *American Journal of Nursing,* 76:2161, Dec. 1975.

56. Peterson, M. H.: Understanding defense mechanisms—a programmed instruction unit. *American Journal of Nursing,* 72:1651, Sept. 1972.

57. Petrillo, M., and Sanger, S.: 8 types of families . . . and how they affect your job. *Nursing '73,* 3:43–47, May 1973.

58. Prange, A. J., Jr., and Martin, H. W.: Aids to understanding patients. *American Journal of Nursing,* 62:98, July 1962.

59. Radulovic, P. O.: Under the cover of his charm. *American Journal of Nursing,* 73:1731, Oct. 1973.

60. Reeves, R. B., Jr.: What it is like to be a patient. *Delaware Medical Journal,* 45:12–15, Jan. 1973.

61. Reinhardt, J. M., and Meadows, P.: *Society and the Nursing Profession.* Philadelphia, W. B. Saunders Co., 1953.

62. Robinson, L.: *Liaison Nursing: Psychological Approach to Patient Care.* Philadelphia, F. A. Davis Co., 1974, Chap. 18.

63. Robinson, L.: The demanding patient. *Nursing '73,* 3:20–24, Jan. 1973.

64. Rosillo, R. H., Welty, M. J., and Graham, W. P., III: The patient with maxillofacial cancer. II. Psychologic aspects. *Nursing Clinics of North America,* 8:153–158, March 1973.

65. Rzepka, D.: We were no match for "Zorba the Greek"! *Nursing '75,* 5:26–29, Sept. 1975.

66. Savoie, S. M. R.: The person before the disease. *Journal of Nursing Education,* 6:11, Aug. 1967.

67. Saxton, D. F., and Haring, P. W.: *Care of Patients with Emotional Problems.* St. Louis, The C. V. Mosby Co., 1975.

68. Schnaper, N.: The psychological implications of severe trauma: emotional sequelae to unconsciousness: a preliminary study. *Journal of Trauma,* 15:94–98, Feb. 1975.

69. Schwartz, L. H., and Schwartz, J. L.: *The Psychodynamics of Patient Care.* Englewood Cliffs, NJ, Prentice-Hall, 1972.

70. Servatius, D.: Easing the shock of a radical vulvectomy. *Nursing '75,* 5:26–31, Aug. 1975.

71. Shontz, F. C.: The personal meanings of illness. *Advances in Psychosomatic Medicine,* 8:63–85, 1972.

72. Sproul, C. W.: Behavior responses in emergency situations. *In* Sproul, C. W., and Mullanney, P. J. (eds.): *Emergency Care: Assessment and Intervention.* St. Louis, C. V. Mosby Co., 1974.

73. Stryker, R. P.: *Rehabilitative Aspects of Acute and Chronic Nursing Care,* 2nd ed. Philadelphia, W. B. Saunders Co., 1977, Chap. 4, Psychological Reactions to Physical Disability.

74. Suggs, K. M.: Coping and adaptive behavior in the stroke syndrome. *Nursing Forum,* 10(1):100–111, 1971.

75. Thomas, B., and Carol, A.: Psychological aspects of physical trauma. *AORN Journal,* 15:45–50, Feb. 1972.

76. Thomas, M. D.: Anger in nurse-patient interactions. *Nursing Clinics of North America,* 2:737, Dec. 1967.

77. Tiedt, E.: The psychodynamic process of the oncological experience. *Nursing Forum,* 14(3):264–277, 1975.

78. Ujhely, G. B.: Two types of problem patients . . . and how to deal with them. *Nursing '76,* 6:64–67, May 1976.

79. Van Kaam, A. L.: The nurse in the patient's world. *American Journal of Nursing,* 59:1708–1710, Dec. 1959.

80. Verwoerdt, A.: Psychopathological responses to the stress of physical illness. *Advances in Psychosomatic Medicine,* 8:119–141, 1972.

81. Walker, J.: Dealing with . . . rage! *Nursing '75,* 5:24–29, Oct. 1975.

82. Warnes, H.: The traumatic syndrome. *Canadian Psychiatric Association Journal,* 17:391–394, Oct. 1972.

83. Wu, R.: *Behavior and Illness.* Englewood Cliffs, NJ, Prentice-Hall, 1973.

CHAPTER 12

WORRIES ILLNESS BRINGS

The startling strokes of fate bring mental conflict to man.

I CHING

INTRODUCTION AND STUDY GUIDE

Various sections of this text discuss some of the worries that accompany illness. This chapter focuses specifically on ways in which illness can interfere with usual patterns of need gratification. These disruptions cause worries. As you give nursing care, recall the major points made in this chapter and try to identify how a specific patient's illness has interfered with his usual patterns of meeting his needs. Then *plan* ways of appropriately helping to meet the patient's needs. Proceed to carry out this process for each patient in your care.

Earlier in this text (Chap. 1) we mentioned briefly some basic human needs, which were presented diagrammatically in the form of a hierarchy (Fig. 1–1). A simplified version of that hierarchy of needs is presented in Figure 12–1. In this chapter we discuss these common groups of human needs more carefully and identify typical examples of some concerns frequently expressed by patients as a result of the frustration of various need gratifications because of illness. As stated in Chapter 1, basic needs, i.e., survival needs, must be reasonably satisfied before it is possible to satisfy needs higher on the hierarchy. The degree to which needs are met varies; that is, needs may be totally unmet, partially met or totally met. Figure 12–2 illustrates a continuum ranging from "need satisfaction" to "need deprivation."

With illness, the relative importance of needs may fluctuate markedly from one hour to the next. For example, some needs, which were satisfied with ease and only passing attention in health, may increase in importance and demand considerable attention in illness. Much nursing expertise involves the skillful recognition of impaired need gratification, a recognition of the effect of this on the patient, and the identification and implementation of precise actions designed to remedy the thwarted satisfaction of needs. Realistically the nurse cannot meet *all* of a patient's needs, just as no one person can ever do this for another. However, it is important to realize that nursing is concerned with the total picture of a patient's needs and a consideration of all of them. Nursing care does not focus exclusively on physiologic survival needs.

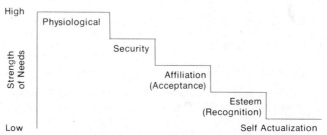

Figure 12–1. Maslow's hierarchy of needs. (Data [for diagram] based on Hierarchy of Needs in "A Theory of Human Motivation" from Motivation—Personality, 2nd Edition, by Abraham H. Maslow. Copyright © 1970 by Abraham H. Maslow. By permission of Harper & Row Publishers, Inc.)

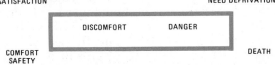

COMPLETE NEED
SATISFACTION

COMPLETE & PROLONGED
NEED DEPRIVATION

DISCOMFORT   DANGER

COMFORT
SAFETY

DEATH

Figure 12–2. Continuum from need satisfaction to need deprivation. (From Fischer, V. G., and Connolly, A. F.: *Promotion of Physical Comfort and Safety,* 2nd ed. Dubuque, Iowa, W. C. Brown Co., 1975, p. 34.)

SURVIVAL NEEDS IN ILLNESS

In health, survival needs may receive relatively little conscious attention and are usually not a source of concern. We eat, breathe, eliminate, get a drink of water and go to bed without realizing that we are actually doing these things to stay alive. In illness, however, we become acutely conscious of the life-sustaining necessity for survival needs to be met and regulated. A bout of diarrhea, for example, makes one keenly aware that elimination requires regulation, and at such a time, the need for balanced or controlled elimination occupies one's attention. We fear exhaustion and depletion.

Survival needs are essentially physiologic or bodily needs, for example, food, air, water, appropriate temperature, elimination, rest and pain avoidance. *The survival needs are thus the needs of major concern in critical illness.* In this respect sickness is comparable to the experiences of early childhood, which also focus on bodily processes. When ill, one's primary worries for a period of time may thus be bodily worries: for example, "Can I pass gas? Can I keep this food down? Will bowel movements hurt after surgery?" Much nursing time is occupied with attempts to help patients to meet their survival needs comfortably and safely and, therefore, to lessen their worries in this area.

Patients' bodily concerns may often center around worries about how much pain and suffering they will have to endure. Accompanying these worries are fears that they will not be able to bear their pain in a manner acceptable to themselves and others. Patients, especially men, often worry that they will cry or act "weak." These fears of loss of behavioral control are also part of the worries that many preoperative patients have: namely, that they will "talk" or "fight" as they come out of the anesthetic.

Impaired survival needs naturally bring worries about the future. Patients may be deeply concerned about the future well-being of their families and loved ones since the illness also affects them. Future debts resulting from the illness are often the source of patients' worries. Indeed, some patients are realistically concerned about whether or not they have a future, for when survival needs cannot be met, the patient knows he is in danger of dying. Worries about dying, or living in a crippled state, i.e., "just surviving . . . like a vegetable," are basic concerns that accompany serious illnesses.

Patients may respond to worries like those described above by displaying a concern for their bodily processes that is exaggerated or disproportionate to the seriousness of the illness. Thus, the nurse often cares for patients who have a heightened concern for their pulses, breathing, bowel movements and so on. Because these patients are unable to distinguish between what is important and what is not in regard to their body functions, they try, almost frantically at times, to observe and question anything they notice about their condition. Recognizing that these actions are an expression of the patient's fear and anxiety, the helpful nurse discusses the patient's concerns with him, provides appropriate reassurance, and helps rule out unnecessary concerns.

STIMULATION NEEDS IN ILLNESS

Although survival needs may come dramatically to the fore with illness, it should not be forgotten that other needs are also present. The needs for sexual activity, novelty, manipulation and exploration may be suppressed during critical illness, but these stimulation needs do not entirely disappear. Although illness and hospitalization may block the overt expression and satisfaction of some needs, for example, the need for sexual activity, evidence of the continued presence of such needs may appear in sublimated forms. Thus, a male patient may joke and otherwise sexually banter with a female nurse, expressing his sexual need in ways that he views as socially acceptable.

When stimulation needs are denied their normal expression because of illness, many worries related to the individual's life situation may develop. Patients whose marriages are based primarily on sexual experience may worry that their marriage partner will be sexually unsatisfied while they are ill and may even be unfaithful while they are hospitalized. Certainly operations that interfere with attractiveness or sexual function will cause concern for the patient. (See discussion of body image,

Chap. 15.) In addition, patients who are accustomed to an active sexual life may find prolonged illnesses that require rest, restriction of sexual activity and confinement difficult to bear; they naturally become restless and "on edge."

When needs for novelty, activity, manipulation and exploration are thwarted by illness, people may become bored, depressed and even disoriented. (See discussion of disorientation, Chap. 14.) Man is generally an active being. Inactivity spawns introspection, and for many, introspection is depressing. Patients worry about how long they will have to be inactive and whether or not they will be able to return to their pre-illness level of activity. Just as inactivity can cause the muscles to contract and atrophy, it also can cause mental activity to become restricted.

Frustration of stimulation needs becomes manifest in a convalescing patient's boredom and his attempts to introduce something new into his environment. Perhaps he plays a trick on the nurse or decorates "his space" in the ward by hanging up cards, ribbons, creepy-crawlies and so on. Orthopedic wards, occupied by many patients passing time while bones slowly heal and muscles strengthen, are often scenes of pranks as well as creative activities. In these situations the skillful nurse taxes her ingenuity to combat patients' boredom and to help patients take their minds off their aching, often confined, bodies. Occupational therapy is of great help in such situations. Some patients also enjoy visits with chaplains or volunteers.

SAFETY AND SECURITY NEEDS IN ILLNESS

In illness, typical day-to-day patterns that one has established for feeling safe and secure are interrupted. Accidents and illnesses, in themselves, bring the realization that one is not invulnerable to suffering and death; confidence is shaken at the daily assumption that one will always be alive and well is jolted. Such realizations make the ill person feel unsafe and insecure. He realizes that he truly lives his life alone. Even though he may have lived with loved ones, who protected him from many of life's unhappinesses, he now knows that these protectors cannot shield him from illness, accident or death and that they cannot experience for him the treatments he must undergo.

Nevertheless, the ill person continues to want protection, and he now looks to his doctors and nurses to protect him from life's adversities and uncertainties. The ill person may think of a nurse as his protector in much the same way that he thought of his mother in this role. Thus, he may try to ascribe superhuman powers to the nurse. For example, in his state of wishing for protection, he may expect that his nurse will be omniscient, or "all-knowing," so that she can see his future, protect him from harm or make the right decisions for him. Obviously a nurse does not have such superhuman powers. However, she can recognize when a patient is looking for strengths in those caring for him, and realizing this, she can be appropriately supportive and protective.

When illness threatens safety and security needs, a patient often becomes worried about being *left alone.* As we have said, he finds himself alone in his state of illness, often in the hospital, while those persons he is normally with are away from him. He goes to surgery alone—they wait; he feels pain alone—they look on; he gasps for breath—they breathe easily but cannot breathe for him. Nurses can help patients to feel less lonely in numerous ways. (See discussion of the nurse-patient relationship, Chap. 3.)

Illness also makes patients feel *helpless,* and they worry about what will happen to them in their helpless state. Will an accident occur during their treatment? In this era of mass communication almost everyone knows that medical and nursing accidents happen. Many people are coming to feel that hospitals are places of "hazards rather than havens." They are aware of infections and malpractice, and fear being the victims of carelessness. "Do these people taking care of me know what they're doing?"

Every attempt must be made to help the patient to feel and to be safe and secure.

Patients fear being *abandoned by loved ones* during their illness. As we mentioned earlier, the attitudes of others are readily communicated to patients. Some families feel relieved to have the ill person "taken off their hands," and once they have taken him to the hospital, they may feel relieved of their burden. Such people often do not visit or even telephone to inquire about the patient. Older patients particularly worry that they will be rejected by their families and "dumped into a nursing home where no one cares."

At the other extreme, some patients worry

that they will be sent home or taken home before they are ready to go. For example, patients may fear that they will be denied the care they need because of the cost involved. Indeed, this may happen, since at times, family members may pressure the doctor to send the patient home because of the cost. Cost cannot be minimized, but it is unfortunate when it interferes with the necessity for care. Another concern in this area is that of running out of money or insurance, having to go on welfare, and being sent to a "welfare ward." Often "welfare wards" are equated in patients' minds with neglectful care.

LOVE NEEDS IN ILLNESS

Separation from one's usual companions and way of life means that needs for love, belonging, and closeness are severely threatened in the existence of the ill. We are referring not only to romantic or physical love but also to those strong feelings of affection, concern, kindness, closeness and understanding that one shares with significant others close to him. These shared feelings are essential for a feeling of well-being; and therefore, their absence creates a most unhappy situation. When ill and away from those persons they care about, patients obviously worry: "Will loved ones change? Will they no longer want me? Am I an unattractive burden?"

Like the stimulation needs and the needs for safety and security, the needs for love and belonging are present in all patients. These important needs are not vaporized by illness. In fact, they may be intensified by the uncertainty of illness and by illness itself. As we mentioned, the persons who provide gratification of needs may shift somewhat with illness: when he was well, the patient's needs were gratified by individuals in his private life; with illness he now looks to those in the health care professions for need gratification.

We do not mean to imply that staff members can ever take the place of friends and relatives for the patient; nor do we mean to imply that loved ones cease to provide need gratification for the ill. However, staff members *are* needed to contribute to the ever-present needs for safety, security, love and belonging that continue into a patient's existence in a care facility. In these settings staff members may be with a patient more than loved ones are; also, they are often with him during "crisis moments" in his life and illness when loved ones may be excluded from his presence, e.g., surgery, intensive care, isolation and emergencies.

> *A patient is not truly "taken care of" unless the nurse helps him to feel safe, secure, loved and as one who "belongs" rather than as an outsider who is viewed as an intruder.*

Patients worry about being treated impersonally. A touch of the hand, a stroke on the brow, a look, a pat, the way a patient is handled, made comfortable, and helped can all contribute to making him feel valued and close to those caring for him. In all these "loving-caring gestures" the nurse remembers that her actions should not be seductive in nature but rather are a sincere expression of appropriate concern.

ESTEEM NEEDS IN ILLNESS

If a patient's needs for love, closeness and belonging are relatively satisfied through the concern and interest of health care personnel, then he has also been helped to meet another group of needs: the needs for esteem and self-esteem. Because he receives love, concern and respect from others, and because he feels he "belongs" and "is one" with others, the patient's feelings of self-esteem are enhanced. *He* is important enough that others care about *his* feelings. He is not overlooked or impersonally treated as if he is merely one person out of many whose weight will leave an indistinguishable imprint on the mattress he lies on; he does not feel forgotten before he has even left the care facility. The person who has an appropriate sense of esteem feels that he is regarded by others as an individual of worth and value, and he also has these feelings about himself.

Illness can markedly interfere with the gratification of esteem needs. The ill person often does not feel that he is of worth and value to others, or to himself, but instead he feels he is a "drag on life," a burden, and an unpleasant reminder of those aspects of life that people prefer not to think about. All these feelings create intense worries.

In our society our bodies are seldom viewed by strangers and we are not usually touched by them except perhaps in a handshake. With illness comes the realization that one's body will be viewed and handled by strangers, and feelings of esteem may be threatened by such experiences. Once again, realizing the prevalence of worries about being physically handled and visually inspected, we emphasize the following rule:

> *Minimize exposure of the patient by means of proper draping and make physical contact of a firm, but gentle, professional quality.*

Observance of this rule is a prime obligation of all medical personnel, since few experiences are more disheartening or humiliating to a patient than to be the subject of indifferent exposure and careless handling. We also emphasize this rule:

> *Always* introduce yourself by name to patients *when you first meet them.*

It is appalling to observe how frequently health personnel fail to perform even this common courtesy with patients and their significant others!

SELF-ACTUALIZATION NEEDS IN ILLNESS

Probably the most difficult group of needs for a patient to satisfy during illness are self-actualization needs. By these needs we refer to (1) expressing one's personality and (2) developing one's abilities. Illness makes it difficult for a person to be the kind of person he *really* is rather than the person he thinks others want him to be. Because he is dependent upon others for care and does not wish to arouse their displeasure, a patient often feels forced to succumb and act like the person others want him to be. He feels helpless to stand up and be himself because to oppose those caring for him means risking being cut off from their care and attention. Many of a patient's concerns thus center around trying to please all the staff members. Patients also find it difficult to meet self-actualization needs because of other patients who may exert pressure on them to act in one way or another.

Illness may also severely curtail a patient in making maximum use of his abilities by preventing him from using and developing his personal talents. In some accidents or illnesses a patient may be left in a state in which he can never again use abilities that he has developed; he may be blind, paralyzed, without a limb, without a voice, or permanently weakened. Meeting self-actualization needs may also be very difficult for persons confined to long-term care facilities. A large part of our unique identity and personality consists of how we use our individual abilities and talents; therefore, such losses are hard to bear and cause great concern.

SUMMARY

We have reviewed some typical worries and concerns of the ill that result because illness interferes with normal need gratification. In order to identify those worries that are fairly representative of ill persons, we have reviewed common groups of human needs. The *specific* worries and concerns of any given patient will depend largely upon the way in which his specific needs are blocked or frustrated by his specific illness. Nursing involves attempting to identify and understand such personal concerns and to provide supplementary need gratifications when the normal avenues of satisfaction are impaired.

BIBLIOGRAPHY

1. Adler, M. L.: Kidney transplantation and coping mechanisms. *Psychosomatics, 13*:337–341, Sept.–Oct. 1972.
2. Barnes, E.: *People in Hospital.* New York, St. Martin's Press, 1961.
3. Bettice, D., et al.: Cardiac patients' feelings about monitors. *American Journal of Nursing, 70*:1950–1952, Sept. 1970.
4. Blacher, R. S. (interview): Waking under the knife. *Emergency Medicine, 8*:132, Jan. 1976.
5. Black, K.: Social isolation and the nursing process. *Nursing Clinics of North America, 8*:575–586, Dec. 1973.
6. Blanchard, M. G.: Sex education for spinal cord injury patients and their nurses. *Supervisor Nurse, 7*:20–28, Feb. 1976.
7. Bronner-Huszar, J.: The psychological aspects of cancer in man. *Psychosomatics, 12*:133–138, March–April 1971.
8. Burnette, B. A. S.: Family adjustment to cystic fibrosis. *American Journal of Nursing, 75*:1986, Nov. 1975.
9. Burton, G.: Families in crisis: knowing when and how to help. *Nursing '75, 5*:36–43, Dec. 1975.
10. Chaney, P. (ed.): Ordeal. *Nursing '75, 5*:27–40, June 1975.
11. Cohen, R. G.: Providing emotional support for the seriously ill. *RN, 37*:62–70, Oct. 1974.
12. Craven, R. F., and Sharp, B. H.: The effects of illness on family functions. *Nursing Forum, 11*(2):186–193, 1972.
13. Dericks, V. C., and Donovan, C. T.: The ostomy patient really needs you. *Nursing '76, 6*:30–33, Sept. 1976.
14. Fives, B.: Support your patient's family—with a chaplain. *RN, 40*:58–59, March 1977.
15. Flynn, E. D.: What it means to battle cancer. *American Journal of Nursing, 77*:261, Feb. 1977.

16. Foster, S., and Andreoli, K. G.: Behavior following acute myocardial infarction. *American Journal of Nursing,* 70:2344–2348, Nov. 1970.

16a. Giacquinta, B.: Helping families face the crisis of cancer. *American Journal of Nursing,* 77:1585–1588, Oct. 1977.

17. Golub, S.: When your patient's problem involves sex. *RN,* 38:27–31, March 1975.

18. Greco, R. M.: Have you been a patient lately? *Supervisor Nurse,* 5:30–35, May 1974.

19. Hackett, T. P., Froese, A. P., and Vasquez, E.: Psychological management of the CCU patient. *Psychiatry in Medicine,* 4:89–105, Winter 1973.

20. Heller, S. S., Frank, K. A., Kornfeld, D. S., Malm, J. R., and Bowman, F. O., Jr.: Psychological outcome following open-heart surgery. *Archives of Internal Medicine,* 34:908–914, Nov. 1974.

21. Hickman, B. W.: All about sex . . . despite dialysis. *American Journal of Nursing,* 77:606, April 1977.

22. Higgins, S. H.: Your patient's illness is a family affair. *RN,* 39:48–49, Nov. 1976.

23. Houston, C. S., and Pasanen, W. E.: Patients' perceptions of hospital care. *Hospitals, J.A.H.A., 46*:70–74, April 16, 1972.

24. Jacobson, L.: Illness and human sexuality. *Nursing Outlook,* 22:50–53, Jan. 1974.

25. Kiely, W. F.: Coping with severe illness. *Advances in Psychosomatic Medicine,* 8:105–118, 1972.

26. Klein, R. F.: The patient's feelings. *American Family Physician,* 10:198–200, Nov. 1974.

27. Kornfeld, D. S.: The hospital environment: its impact on the patient. *Advances in Psychosomatic Medicine,* 8:252–270, 1972.

28. Kraegel, J. M., et al.: A system of patient care based on patient needs. *Nursing Outlook,* 20:257, April 1972.

29. Langlois, P., and Teramoto, V.: Helping patients cope with hospitalization. *Nursing Outlook,* 19:334–336, May 1971.

30. Larson, V.: What hospitalization means to patients. *American Journal of Nursing,* 61:44, May 1961.

31. Lawrence, J. C.: Homosexuals, hospitalization, and the nurse. *Nursing Forum,* 14(3):304–317, 1975.

32. Lee, R. E., and Ball, P. A.: Some thoughts on the psychology of the coronary care unit patient. *American Journal of Nursing,* 75:1498, Sept. 1975.

33. Lefebvre, P., Nobert, A., and Crombez, J. C.: Psychological and psychopathological reactions in relation to chronic hemodialysis. *Canadian Psychiatric Association Journal,* Special Supplement II, *17*:SS–9, 1972.

34. Levitas, I. M.: Treating hospital patients like people. *Medical Economics,* 43:85, Dec. 12, 1966.

35. Livingston, W. K.: What is pain? *Scientific American Reprint,* March 1953.

36. Livsey, C. G.: Physical illness and family dynamics. *Advances in Psychosomatic Medicine,* 8:237–251, 1972.

37. Long, E. S.: How to survive hospitalization. *American Journal of Nursing,* 74:486, March 1974.

38. Marram, G. D.: Patients' evaluation of their care. *Nursing Outlook,* 21:322–324, May 1973.

39. McPartland, T. S.: Patient care—psychological needs. *Hospital Progress,* 46:86–90, Dec. 1965.

40. Meerloo, J. A. M.: *Illness and Cure.* New York, Grune & Stratton, 1964.

40a. Miller, J.: Cognitive dissonance in modifying families' perceptions. *American Journal of Nursing,* 74:1468–1470, Aug. 1974.

41. Mitchell, M.: Rx for your patient's family. *Supervisor Nurse,* 7:42–43, Feb. 1976.

42. Muslin, H. L.: The emotional response to the kidney transplant: the process of internalization. *Canadian Psychiatric Association Journal,* Special Supplement II, *17*:SS–3, 1972.

43. Nicholson, E. M.: Personal notes of a laryngectomee. *American Journal of Nursing,* 75:2157, Dec. 1975.

44. O'Donovan, T. R.: Dealing with impact needs. *Supervisor Nurse,* 4:30–41, Feb. 1973.

45. Perrine, G.: Needs met and unmet. *American Journal of Nursing,* 71:2128, Nov. 1971.

46. Peterson, B. H.: Psychological reactions to acute physical illness in adults. *The Medical Journal of Australia,* 1:311–316, March 2, 1974.

47. Puksta, N. S.: All about sex . . . after a coronary. *American Journal of Nursing,* 77:602, April 1977.

48. Reinhardt, J. M., and Meadows, P.: *Society and the Nursing Profession.* Philadelphia, W. B. Saunders Co., 1953.

49. Ritvo, M. M.: Who are "good" and "bad" patients? *The Modern Hospital,* 100:79–81, June 1963.

50. Robinson, L.: *Psychological Aspects of the Care of Hospitalized Patients,* 2nd ed. Philadelphia, F. A. Davis Co., 1972.

50a. Rose, M. A.: Problems families face in home care. *American Journal of Nursing,* 76:416–418, March 1976.

51. Roy, S. C.: Adaptation: a basis for nursing practice. *Nursing Outlook,* 19:254, April 1971.

52. Santopietro, M. S.: Meeting the emotional needs of hemodialysis patients and their spouses. *American Journal of Nursing,* 75:629–632, April 1975.

53. Skipper, J. K., and Leonard, R. C. (eds.): *Social Interaction and Patient Care.* Philadelphia, J. B. Lippincott Co., 1965.

54. Smith, D. W.: Patienthood and its threat to privacy. *American Journal of Nursing,* 69:509–513, March 1969.

55. Smith, M. C.: Patient responses to being transferred during hospitalization. *Nursing Research,* 25:192–196, May–June 1976.

56. Smith, S.: The psychology of illness. *Nursing Forum,* 3(1):34–47, 1964.

57. Spiegel, A. D., and Demone, H. W., Jr.: Questions of hospital patients—unasked and unanswered. *Postgraduate Medicine,* 43:215, Feb. 1968.

58. Suggs, K. M.: Coping and adaptive behavior in the stroke syndrome. *Nursing Forum,* 10(1):100–111, 1971.

59. Susser, M., and Watson, W.: *Sociology in Medicine.* New York, Oxford University Press, 1963.

60. Tarnower, W.: The needs of the hospitalized patient. *Nursing Outlook,* 13:28, July 1965.

61. Van Bree, N. S.: Sexuality, nursing practice, and the person with cardiac disease. *Nursing Forum,* 14(4):396–411, 1975.

62. Van den Berg, J. H.: *The Psychology of the Sickbed.* Pittsburgh, Duquesne University Press, 1966.

63. Van Kaam, A.: The nurse in the patient's world. *American Journal of Nursing,* 59:1708, Dec. 1969.

64. Velazquez, J. M.: Alienation. *American Journal of Nursing,* 69:301, Feb. 1969.

65. Volicer, B. J.: Patients' perceptions of stressful events associated with hospitalization. *Nursing Research,* 23:235–238, May–June 1974.

66. Williams, F.: The crisis of hospitalization. *Nursing Clinics of North America,* 9:37–45, March 1974.

66a. Wiley, L. (ed.): Emphasizing the positive. *Nursing '77,* 7:30–34, Sept. 1977.

67. Zalar, M.: Human sexuality—a component of total patient care. *Nursing Digest,* 3:40–43, Nov.–Dec. 1975.

CHAPTER 13

THE SICK ROLE;
THE IMPAIRED ROLE

INTRODUCTION AND STUDY GUIDE

This chapter discusses the "sick role" (occupied by persons who accept the fact that they are ill and desire to recover) and the "impaired role" (occupied by disabled or chronically ill persons experiencing a state of wellness that is compatible with their handicapped status).[78] If one hopes to more completely understand the existence of the ill, it is necessary to examine the sick role in our society.

This chapter presents the four classic components of the sick role and reviews some typical sick role behaviors. It is equally important for a nurse to examine the roles occupied by chronically disabled persons who feel well (i.e., are not "ill") although they are handicapped. Some assumed characteristics of the impaired role are presented in the latter part of this chapter. It is important that health care workers maintain realistic expectations of persons occupying sick or impaired roles; unrealistic expectations can be a needless source of frustration to such individuals. Of course, all ill or disabled persons do not oc-

cupy *typical* sick roles or impaired roles. The knowledgeable nurse thus also needs to be aware of examples of deviant sick roles and deviant impaired roles. Such examples are provided in this chapter, along with a general introduction to role theory.

After reading this chapter the student is encouraged to:

1. State in your own words what is meant by a "role."

2. Identify four common expectations we tend to have of persons occupying the sick role.

3. Cite two examples of persons in deviant sick roles.

4. Write down and review the assumed characteristics of the impaired role presented in this chapter.

A suitable topic for group discussion would be identifying ways in which a nurse's role perceptions of patients might influence nursing care.

INTRODUCTION TO ROLE THEORY

Briefly stated, a social role is a pattern of *expected behavior;* therefore, the sick role is the pattern of behavior we expect from persons whom we view as "sick." We tend to mentally categorize people into various roles all the time, e.g., sexual roles, status roles, work roles, family roles. This process usually takes place more or less unconsciously.

The nurse, therefore, constantly is mentally assigning patients to various roles; often she is unaware of doing this. However, the superior nurse tries to become aware of this process, realizing that the roles she assigns to patients (e.g., the way she thinks of them) affect her expectations of them and her attitudes and actions toward them.

One problem we often experience in relation

to roles is that of deciding whether or not a given person should be placed in a particular role. Once we have mentally categorized an individual in terms of a given role, we react toward him and hold certain expectations of him in terms of this role. With a patient, our problem may not be one of knowing how to react to him when he is sick; rather, the problem may lie in deciding in the first place if he really should be considered sick. Problems in defining illness have been discussed in Chapter 10.

Roles are *learned.* Just as a nursing student learns the nursing role from the nurses with whom she associates, so have we all learned the sick role from our associates in life. We formed our expectations of sick people and learned sick role behaviors as we grew and observed how significant others in our lives reacted toward the ill or how they themselves behaved when ill. We have also learned ways of behaving when we were ill. Naturally, patients have all undergone experiences similar to these, and each has a concept of how he believes he is expected to behave and what he expects of those caring for him.

> *From the cultural norms surrounding us as we grew, we all learned what the rules of behavior, the rights, and the obligations of the ill are in our social group.*

We all tend to feel more comfortable when we know what behavior is expected of us in any given situation. If we feel we are not behaving as others expect us to, or if they are not behaving as we expect them to, uneasiness results and misunderstandings occur.

> *Patients feel uncomfortable when they are not sure what behavior is expected of them or if they do not feel like behaving as others expect them to. Also, patients feel uncomfortable when health care personnel do not perform according to the role expectations that patients hold for these care-givers.*

At times, conforming to one's expected role may be difficult, or the role itself may not be clear. For severe or critical illnesses, when the prognosis is clearly serious or is uncertain, the sick role definition is more likely to be clear cut. In this situation the sick role is quite evident.

People who do not act in accordance with the role in which we have placed them are disturbing to us. For example, a patient who is obviously ill but who refuses to cooperate in his treatment (so that he can recover) is disturbing to us if we expect that everyone who is ill will want to get better. Similarly, it is disturbing to patients when nurses fail to act in ways expected of them. (Chap. 4 discusses nurses' roles.) For example, a patient who expects a nurse to bathe him may be upset if the nurse says he can bathe himself.

THE SICK ROLE

Once an individual defines himself as ill, with or without validation from a doctor, family member, or friend, he will begin to engage in activities congruent with his perception of the sick role. He is said to be occupying a special position accorded by society to those defined as sick and thus is entitled to play the sick role.[78]

The Components of the Sick Role

For centuries people have had ideas about how the ill can be expected to behave, and, in turn, how to behave toward them. However, it was not until the early 1950's, with the classic published work of Talcott Parsons,[50] that the formalized concept of the sick role began to receive attention. Parsons made four major statements about the behavioral expectations that are relative to the sick role. These are summarized in Table 13–1. See if your ideas about sick people agree with his observations.

First, Parsons pointed out that *sick persons are exempt from normal social role responsibilities.* This exemption varies in degree, depending upon the nature and severity of the illness. For example, sick persons are not expected to do their usual work or to carry out their duties of father, mother, husband, or wife, as the case may be. The physician is often called upon to act as a legitimatizing agent for this suspension of obligations, e.g., to say about the patient, "He *is* sick and must have a rest and go to the hospital for treatment." Once the patient is told this by an authority, his claim to exemptions from his usual duties is typically viewed as legitimate by himself and by others. He has been told that he is sick and can act sick.

There are objective tests and criteria for the determination of whether or not one is ill, how sick one is, and what the nature of the illness is. Parents may serve as legitimatizing agents for children. A child may ask his mother to legitimatize his illness. Thus, he goes to her, says he is sick and doesn't feel like going to school, and then he waits to hear from her whether or not she says he is sick. She may say,

TABLE 13–1. MAJOR BEHAVIORAL
EXPECTATIONS RELATIVE TO THE "SICK ROLE"
(Identified by Talcott Parsons[50])

1. Sick persons are exempt from normal social role responsibilities.
2. Sick persons cannot be expected to "pull themselves together" and get well merely by acts of will or decisions on their part.
3. There is an obligation on the part of sick persons to "want to get well," for the state of being ill is defined as being an undesirable situation.
4. There is an obligation for sick persons to seek technically competent help, usually from a physician, and to cooperate with him in the process of trying to recover.

"I don't know whether you are sick or not. I'll take your temperature." Thus she looks for objective criteria to help her in her validation. If she says he is sick, he is exempted from his usual duty to go to school.

Although illness and the sick role may enable the ill person to be excused from his usual social role, it also can place an obligation on him, since others may tell him how he should act. For instance, when he is sick others can tell him that he *ought* to rest, stay in bed, not eat, take medicine, stay home, take care of himself, and so on, depending upon his illness. A patient may not want to give up his usual responsibilities and assume these new obligations that are part of the sick role. Also, these obligations may prove a source of difficulty in the transition period from illness to health, for as the patient recovers, he may no longer want to do what others believe he "ought" to do; e.g., he may want to be out of bed while others think he should still remain in bed.

Second, *it cannot be expected that the sick person could "pull himself together" and get well merely by an act of will or decision on his part.* Because he cannot "help" being ill, the sick person must be "taken care of." And because the illness itself is "not his fault," the sick role once again excuses the ill person from his usual responsibilities in life. Even though an ill person may have been partially responsible for the fact that he did become ill or injured, now that he *is* sick he is incapable of terminating his "condition"; the illness is beyond his control. The condition itself must either heal of its own accord or be acted upon. The patient is viewed as "entitled" to help, for he cannot, by his own will, make himself recover. Just as he cannot recover by using his own *will,* the sick person also cannot heal himself by his own *knowledge;* he is not competent to diagnose and treat himself. He does not know what needs to be done.

Third, *there is an obligation on the part of the sick person to "want to get well," for the state of being ill is defined as being an undesirable situation.* Illness is a strain that involves discomfort, disability, suffering, the possibility of death, and of course, its reality at times. In most instances it is to a patient's best self-interest to get well. There are problems, however, that can prevent a sick person from wanting to get well. Because the sick role is composed, in part, of privileges and exemptions from responsibilities for the ill person, these factors may become sources of "secondary

gain" toward which the patient often is unconsciously motivated. When this is the case, individuals may not be motivated to "get well" as strongly as they are to "stay ill or become ill." They wish to remain in the sick role and enjoy its privileges.

The fourth and final observation that Parsons made concerning the sick role was that *there is an obligation to seek technically competent help, usually from a physician, and to cooperate with him in the process of trying to recover.* This obligation varies in proportion to the severity of the condition. The patient is thus expected to act as he is directed to, even though the directions may require him to suffer or to risk death, disability or financial loss. He may be expected to cooperate even as life slowly leaves him and he eventually dies.

While the ill are expected to seek competent help, they are often in the difficult position of not really knowing who is a competent doctor (or nurse). Therefore, they often select such "helpers" in random ways, such as picking a name out of the phone book or going to their neighbor's doctor. Thus, without really *knowing* the competency of those caring for him and asking him to risk suffering or death, the patient is expected to cooperate fully in whatever he is asked to do. The patient is, therefore, often expected to assume "on faith" that those caring for him know what they are doing and that they have his best interests in mind at all times. This puts him in a most difficult position and creates problems of trust.

These are the major aspects of the sick role that Parsons identified. They are the patterns of behavior we commonly tend to expect from persons whom we view as sick. Let us now examine more closely some of the behaviors typical of persons in the sick role.

Sick Role Behaviors

Wu describes typical sick role behaviors, observing that such behaviors may fall into two major groups:[78] (1) actions prescribed to deal with the signs and symptoms of the illness and (2) behaviors that do not act directly upon the illness or its symptoms but rather provide those conditions believed to facilitate recovery.

Behaviors in the first group are directed toward health restoration and symptom relief. These include self-prescriptions and medical prescriptions directed toward cure, e.g., taking medicines, changing activities of daily living, increasing rest hours, decreasing work hours.

Examples of sick role behaviors directed at providing conditions that may facilitate recovery are[78] (a) total or partial *withdrawal* by the sick person from his usual role responsibilities; (b) focusing of the sick person's *attention on his body and its functions* when the signs and symptoms that are manifestations of illness are sufficiently disturbing or intense; (c) *regression* by the sick person as evidenced by an increase in his dependent behaviors; and (d) *compliance* by the sick person with prescribed medical regimens necessary for recovery.

Deviant Sick Roles

It has been observed that in order for an individual to properly qualify for the sick role he must (a) accept the fact that he is indeed ill and (b) have the desire to get well. Persons who do not meet these two conditions are not in the acceptable sick role but are instead in deviant sick roles. An example of a person in a deviant sick role is the individual who acknowledges that he is ill but who wishes to remain ill and does not try to comply with prescribed treatment. (*Noncompliance* is a serious problem in treatment and is receiving increasing attention in health care literature.) Other examples of deviant sick role behaviors are the following: (a) an individual using his illness for secondary gains other than for gains to recover (e.g., the patient who uses his sickness to gain power that he would not otherwise have); (b) an individual, reluctant to accept responsibilities, for whom the attention and protection afforded through illness serve as a refuge; and (c) an individual who no longer appears to care whether or not he will recover and becomes submissive, indifferent, withdrawn, uncommunicative and lacking in enthusiasm and initiative ("prisoner of war syndrome").[78]

THE IMPAIRED ROLE

The sick role pattern seems to apply most clearly when the prognosis is believed to be uncertain or serious. Other sets of behavioral expectations tend to occur in disorders in which the prognosis is believed to be known or is not serious. Authorities in role theory state that the prognosis of an illness is one deciding factor that helps us determine who is "sick" and who is merely "impaired." Thus, persons we think of in the sick role are viewed as having disorders that are more serious, more incapacitating and more life-threatening than those of persons in the impaired role. Of course, prognosis is not always a clear-cut factor, and so we may be uncertain at times whether a person is sick or impaired. Also, prognosis can change for the better or worse, and with such changes our view of the individual should change, e.g., from "sick" to "impaired" as he gets better. As we have indicated, along with such a change of view, our expectations of the individual also change.

In general, the role expectations for the impaired role tend to be more supportive of normal behavior than those of the sick role. We expect the impaired person to act more normally than the sick person. While in the sick role, the person is viewed and treated as dependent or sick; the impaired role reflects tendencies to (1) encourage independence in the person with respect to his personal care and social responsibility and (2) encourage *him* to seek appropriate medical care rather than assuming this responsibility for him.

The impaired role may be occupied by persons who perceive "no impairment of capacity to perform social roles and valued tasks"[78] and who feel fine, although they may be handicapped (e.g., blind), disabled or chronically ill. Such persons may experience a state of wellness that is congruent or compatible with their handicapped status in society.[78] While we give the person in the sick role a great deal of extra care, the individual in the impaired role is encouraged to do things for himself. Moreover, in the impaired role, the individual is encouraged to do some of his usual work. However, this does not mean that he is expected to fully assume the daily responsibilities associated with a normal healthy state. Medical personnel and family keep responsibilities and worries away from the person in the sick role. This is not always the situation with persons in the impaired role. Also, significant others (e.g., friends, family, doctors) usually do not need to be kept completely informed regarding the total condition of the person in the impaired role. Conversely, in the sick role there is a desire to have complete information regarding the sick person's condition.

Impaired persons are not typically insulated from the well population as are persons in the sick role. Also, impaired persons "cannot fulfill the obligation to 'want to get well' in terms of a cure as implied in the sick role norms."[78]

Wu defines impaired role behavior as:

"... any activity undertaken by a disabled person who no longer views himself as ill, but is restricted physically and/or psychosocially, for the purposes of maintaining control of his impaired condition, prevention of complications attending such conditions, and resuming role responsibilities commensurate with his controlled or convalescent state. It includes activities directed towards resumption of normal behaviors and the full realization of one's potentialities. It incorporates the concepts of rehabilitation and peak wellness for the disabled. In contrast, the individual who is unable to accept the disability and attending limitations will behave in a manner that interferes with the goals of maintenance and prevention and therefore is defined as deviant.[78]

In summation, the social pressures of the impaired role serve to maintain and aid normal behavior, while those pertinent to the sick role serve to discourage normal behavior, thus protecting and insulating the ill person. Also, the tendency to treat a person as dependent often appears directly related to the uncertainty and seriousness of the prognosis.

NURSING IMPLICATIONS

It is important for a nurse to pause and consider whether she is thinking of a given patient as "sick" or "impaired" and to determine her role expectations of him. A nurse's views of the sick role and impaired role will greatly influence her approach to individuals with whom she works as patient-clients. The superior nurse tries to realistically determine each patient's condition rather than haphazardly guessing about his assets or limitations, his need for dependence or independence, etc. At times a nurse may incorrectly think of a given patient as "impaired" rather than "sick," with the result that she expects too much of him; at other times she might mistakenly consider a patient as "sick" when he is, in fact, only "impaired," and thus she might be overly protective, to the patient's detriment.

Finally, if a nurse thinks of a particular patient as "impaired" (e.g., not seriously ill) but he acts as if he were "sick," she may feel upset and angry with him for wanting those privileges of the sick role to which the nurse feels he is not entitled.

Of course, the concepts of sick role and impaired role are important in a patient's interactions with his significant others. For example, a patient may want to move into an impaired role, but his family members may continue to treat him as sick. Or, conversely, an impaired individual may become sick, and his significant others may fail to acknowledge that he needs to be cared for and to be permitted to move into the sick role.

BIBLIOGRAPHY

1. Andersen, M. D. C., and Pleticha, J. M.: Emergency unit patients' perceptions of stressful life events. *Nursing Research, 23*:378–383, Sept.–Oct. 1974.
2. Bauman, B. O., and Kassenbaum, G. G.: Dimensions of the sick role in chronic illness. *Journal of Health and Human Behavior, 6*:16–27, Spring 1965.
3. Becker, M. H., and Maiman, L. A.: Sociobehavioral determinants of compliance with health and medical care recommendations. *Medical Care, 13*:10–24, Jan. 1975.
4. Becker, M. H., Drachman, R. H., and Kirscht, J. P.: A new approach to explaining sick-role behavior in low-income populations. *American Journal of Public Health, 64*:205–216, March 1974.
5. Berkman, P. L.: Survival and a modicum of indulgence in the sick role. *Medical Care, 13*:85–94, Jan. 1975.
5a. Brink, P. J.: Patientology: Just another ology? *Nursing Outlook, 26*:574, Sept. 1978.
5b. Cawley, M.: No cure, just care. *American Journal of Nursing, 74*:2010–2013, Nov. 1974.
6. Christman, L.: Assisting the patient to learn the patient role. *Journal of Nursing Education, 6*:17, April 1967.
6a. Cole, S. A.: Liminality and the sick role. *Man and Medicine, 2*:41–53, No. 1, 1976.
7. Copp, L. A.: Illness-sustaining role prescriptions. *Nursing Forum, 10*(1):36–48, 1971.
8. Craven, R. F., and Sharp, B. H.: The effects of illness on family functions. *Nursing Forum, 11*(2):186, 1972.
9. Croog, S. H., and Ver Steeg, D. F.: The hospital as a social system. *In* Freeman, H. E., Levine, S., and Reeder, L. G. (eds.): *Handbook of Medical Sociology*, 2nd ed. Englewood Cliffs, NJ, Prentice-Hall, 1972.
10. Derdiarian, A., and Clough, D.: Patients dependence and independence levels on the prehospitalization-postdischarge continuum. *Nursing Research, 25*:27–34, Jan.–Feb. 1976.
11. Duff, R., and Hollingshead, A. B.: *Sickness and Society*. New York, Harper & Row, 1968.
11a. Eggert, G. M., et al.: Caring for the patient with long-term disability. *Geriatrics, 32*:102–114, Oct. 1977.
12. Eisler, J., Wolfer, J. A., and Diers, D.: Relationship between need for social approval and postoperative recovery and welfare. *Nursing Research, 21*:520–525, Nov.–Dec. 1972.
13. Fabrega, H., Jr.: Toward a model of illness behavior. *Medical Care, 11*:470–484, Nov.–Dec. 1973.
14. Folta, J., and Deck, E. (eds.): *A Sociological Framework for Patient Care*. New York, John Wiley & Sons, 1966.
15. Franklin, B. J.: Birth order and tendency to "adopt the sick role." *Psychological Reports, 33*:437–438, 1973.
16. Freeman, H. E., Levine, S., and Reeder, L. G. (eds.): *Handbook of Medical Sociology*. Englewood Cliffs, NJ, Prentice-Hall, 1963.
17. Freeman, V. J.: Human aspects of health and illness: beyond the germ theory. *Journal of Health and Human Behavior, 1*:8, 1960.
18. Geertsen, H. R., Gray, R. M., and Ward, J. R.: Patient non-compliance within the context of seeking medical care for arthritis. *Journal of Chronic Diseases, 26*:689–698, 1973.
19. Gerson, L. W.: Expectations of "sick role" exemptions for dental problems. *Journal Canadian Dental Association, 38*(10):370–372, Oct. 1972.
20. Gerson, L. W., and Skipper, J. K., Jr.: A conceptual model for the study of the health action process. *Canadian Journal of Public Health, 63*:477–485, Nov.–Dec. 1972.
21. Gilson, B. S., et al.: The sickness impact profile: development of an outcome measure of health care.

22. Gold, N.: The doctor, his illness and the patient. *Australia New Zealand Journal of Psychiatry,* 6(4):209–213, Dec. 1972.

23. Gordon, G.: *Role Theory and Illness: A Sociological Perspective.* New Haven, CT, College and University Press, 1966.

24. Gould, D.: Power and sickness. *New Statesman,* 74:13, July 7, 1967.

25. Hallauer, D. S.: Illness behavior—an experimental investigation. *Journal of Chronic Diseases,* 25:599–610, 1972.

26. Hyman, M. D.: Social psychological factors affecting disability among ambulatory patients. *Journal of Chronic Diseases,* 28:199–216, 1975.

27. Imboden, J. B.: Psychosocial determinants of recovery. *Advances in Psychosomatic Medicine,* 8:142–155, 1972.

28. Johnson, D. E.: Powerlessness: a significant determinant in patient behavior? *Journal of Nursing Education,* 6:39–44, April 1967.

28a. Jones, B. E., and Miles, J. E.: The nurse and the hospitalized mentally ill physician. *American Journal of Nursing,* 76:1314–1317, Aug. 1976.

29. Jones, S. J.: Orthopedic injuries: illness as deviance. *American Journal of Nursing,* 75:2030, Nov. 1975.

30. Kahana, R. J.: Personality and response to physical illness. *Advances in Psychosomatic Medicine,* 8:42–62, 1972.

31. Kasl, S. V., and Cobb, S.: Health behavior, illness behavior and sick role behavior. *Archives of Environmental Health,* 12:531–541, April 1966.

32. Kasl, S. V., Cobb, S., and Gore, S.: Changes in reported illness and illness behavior related to termination of employment: a preliminary report. *International Journal of Epidemiology,* 1(2):111–118, Summer 1972.

33. Kennedy, D. A.: Perceptions of illness and healing. *Social Science and Medicine,* 7(10):787–805, Oct. 1973.

34. King, S. H.: Social-psychological factors in illness. *In* Freeman, H. E., Levine, S., and Reeder, L. G. (eds.): *Handbook of Medical Sociology,* 2nd ed. Englewood Cliffs, NJ, Prentice-Hall, 1972, pp. 129–147.

35. Knutson, A.: *The Individual, Society and Health Behavior.* New York, Russell Sage Foundation, 1965.

35a. Krupp, N. E.: Adaptation to chronic illness. *Postgraduate Medicine,* 60:122–125, Nov. 1976.

36. Kurtz, R. A., and Giacopassi, D. J.: Medical and social work students' perceptions of deviant conditions and sick role incumbency. *Social Science and Medicine,* 9:249–255, 1975.

37. Lesser, M. E.: Perceptions of illness at a therapeutic community for ex-drug addicts. *Social Science and Medicine,* 8:575–583, 1974.

38. Lewis, F. C.: Patients who want to be sick. *Today's Health,* 46:21, Jan. 1968.

38a. Levinson, R.: Sexism in medicine. *American Journal of Nursing,* 76:426–431, March 1976.

39. Livsey, C. G.: Physical illness and family dynamics. *Advances in Psychosomatic Medicine,* 8:237–251, 1972.

40. Martin, H. W., and Prange, A. J., Jr.: Human adaptation—a conceptual approach to understanding patients. *The Canadian Nurse,* 58:234–243, March 1962.

41. Martin, H. W., and Prange, A. J., Jr.: The stages of illness—psychosocial approach. *Nursing Outlook,* 10:33–44, March 1962.

42. Maxson, K. W.: Assuming the patient role. *Perspectives in Psychiatric Care,* 12:119–122, July–Sept. 1974.

43. McKinlay, J. B.: The concept "patient career" as a heuristic device for making medical sociology relevant to medical students. *Social Science and Medicine,* 5:441–460, Oct. 1971.

44. McKinlay, J. B.: The sick role—illness and pregnancy. *Social Science and Medicine,* 6:561–572, 1972.

45. Mechanic, D.: The concept of illness behavior. *Journal of Chronic Disease,* 15:189, Feb. 1962.

46. Mechanic, D., and Volkart, E. A.: Stress, illness behavior and the sick role. *American Sociological Review,* 26:51, Feb. 1961.

47. Merrington, H. N.: Personal disability and the family group: a two-way interaction. *Medical Journal of Australia,* 2(16):606–609, Oct. 19, 1974.

48. Nathanson, C. A.: Illness and the feminine role: a theoretical review. *Nursing Digest,* 4:74–77, Summer 1976.

49. Ossenberg, R. J.: The experience of deviance in the patient role—a study of class differences. *Journal of Health and Human Behavior,* 3:277–282, 1962.

49a. Owen, B. D.: Coping with chronic illness. *American Journal of Nursing,* 75:1016–1018, June 1975.

50. Parsons, T.: *The Social System.* Glencoe, IL, The Free Press, 1951.

50a. Perry, S. E.: How to make a sick nurse a happy patient. *RN,* 40:42–44, June 1977.

51. Petroni, F. A.: Preferred right to the sick role and illness behavior. *Social Science and Medicine,* 5:645–653, Dec. 1971.

52. Reeves, R. B., Jr.: What it is like to be a patient. *Delaware Medical Journal,* 45:12–15, Jan. 1973.

53. Richardson, S. A., et al.: Cultural uniformity in reaction to physical disabilities. *American Sociological Review,* 26:241–247, April 1961.

54. Richardson, S. A., et al.: Age, sex difference in values toward physical handicaps. *Journal of Health and Social Behavior,* 11:207–214, Sept. 1970.

55. Schmale, A. H.: Giving up as a final common pathway to changes in health. *Advances in Psychosomatic Medicine,* 8:20–40, 1972.

55a. Schmieding, N. J.: Relationship of nursing to the process of chronicity. *Nursing Outlook,* 18:58–62, Feb. 1970.

56. Schuettler, J. L.: Emily said one thing—but did another. *Nursing '77,* 7:42–43, April 1977.

57. Shuval, J. T., Antonovsky, A., and Davies, A. M.: Illness: a mechanism for coping with failure. *Social Science and Medicine,* 7:259–265, April 1973.

58. Shontz, F. C.: The personal meanings of illness. *Advances in Psychosomatic Medicine,* 8:63–85, 1972.

59. Siegler, M., and Osmond, H.: The "sick role" revisited. *Hastings Center Studies,* 1(3):41–58, 1973.

60. Sigerist, H. E.: The special position of the sick. *In* Roemer, M. (ed.): *Henry E. Sigerist on the Sociology of Medicine.* New York, M. D. Publications, 1960.

61. Smith, D. W.: Patienthood and its threat to privacy. *American Journal of Nursing,* 69:509, March 1969.

62. Smith, S.: The psychology of illness. *Nursing Forum,* 3(1):34–47, 1964.

62a. Taylor, C. M.: Caring for the chronically ill—one day at a time. *Nursing '78,* 8:59–60, Sept. 1978.

63. Taylor, C.: *In Horizontal Orbit.* New York, Holt, Rinehart and Winston, 1970.

64. Thomas, E. J.: Problems of disability from the perspective of role theory. *Journal of Health and Human Behavior,* 7:2–14, Spring 1966.

65. Tracy, G. D.: Prolonged disability after compensable injury. *Medical Journal of Australia,* 2(23):1305–1307, Dec. 2, 1972.

66. Turner, R. H.: Role taking: process versus conformity. *In* Rose, A. (ed.): *Human Behavior and Social Process.* Boston, Houghton Mifflin Co., 1962, pp. 20–38.

67. Twaddle, A. C.: Illness and deviance. *Social Science and Medicine,* 7:751–762, Oct. 1973.

68. Twaddle, A. C.: The concepts of the sick role and illness behavior. *Advances in Psychosomatic Medicine,* 8:162–179, 1972.

69. Verwoerdt, A.: Psychopathological responses to the stress of physical illness. *Advances in Psychosomatic Medicine,* 8:119–141, 1972.

70. Vincent, P.: The sick role in patient care. *American Journal of Nursing,* 75:1172–1173, July 1975.

71. von Mering, O.: The diffuse health aberration syndrome: a biobehavioral study of the perennial outpatient. *Psychosomatics,* 13:293–303, Sept.–Oct. 1972.

72. Waitzkin, H.: Latent functions of the sick role in various institutional settings. *Social Science & Medicine,* 5:45–75, Feb. 1971.

73. Weijel, J. A.: The influence of social security in an affluent society on illness behaviour. *Psychotherapy and Psychosomatics,* 23:272–282, 1974.

74. Williams, J. I.: Disease as deviance. *Social Science & Medicine,* 5:219–225, June 1971.

75. Wilson, J. T.: Compliance with instructions in the evaluation of therapeutic efficacy. A common but frequently unrecognized major variable. *Clinical Pediatrics,* 12:333–340, June 1973.

76. Wise, T. N.: When a patient drops out. *Emergency Medicine,* 7:48–56, March 1975.

77. Wright, B. A.: *Physical Disability, A Psychological Approach.* New York, Harper & Row, 1960.

78. Wu, R.: *Behavior and Illness.* Englewood Cliffs, NJ, Prentice-Hall, 1973.

79. Zola, I. K.: Pathways to the doctor—from person to patient. *Social Science in Medicine,* 7:677–689, Sept. 1973.

80. Zola, I. K.: Studying the decision to see a doctor. Review, critique, corrective. *Advances in Psychosomatic Medicine,* 8:216–236, 1972.

CHAPTER 14

DISORGANIZED BEHAVIOR AND THOUGHT PROCESSES ACCOMPANYING ILLNESS

INTRODUCTION AND STUDY GUIDE

Because of the physiologic and psychologic stresses and the social isolation that illness often imposes, various aberrations of behavior and disorganized thinking processes may accompany illness. When behavior becomes disorganized it is not directed toward achieving reality goals; the behavior does not correspond with what is culturally expected and what would be in accordance with reality. Disorganized thinking processes fail to keep the patient in contact with reality and fail to help him to function effectively. The nurse needs to be knowledgeable about various types of disorganized thoughts and behavior, the causes of such disorganization, and the appropriate methods of prevention and treatment.

This chapter focuses on problems such as confusion or disorientation, hallucinations, illusions and delusions. These are *common* problems in nursing care. Because space does not permit detailed discussion of these phenomena, an extensive bibliography is provided. The reader is encouraged to do additional reading from the sources listed.

As you read this chapter, clarify in your mind what is meant by confusion or disorientation. Can you give an example of a hallucination, an illusion, and delusional thinking? As you meet confused or disoriented patients try to identify what is causing their confusion or disorientation. Review the medical histories of these patients and their diagnoses; evaluate their environments and the interactions they have with others. Incorporate into your nursing care of these individuals appropriate suggestions from this chapter and nursing literature.

SOME GENERAL CAUSES OF DISORGANIZED THOUGHTS AND BEHAVIOR

Many different *psychologic stresses* may cause various forms of disorganized thought and behavior. Such stresses are not so clearly understood as are those stresses that are basically physiologic. It is increasingly recognized that *social and sensory deprivation* can precipitate disorganized behavior.

Some of the *physiologic* stresses that may cause disorganized behavior and thought processes during illness are temperature elevations; nutritional, fluid-electrolyte, and acid-base imbalances; impaired renal function; lack of sleep; and cerebral hypoxia interfering with the metabolic processes of the brain's cerebral neurons.[27] Older persons may be particularly susceptible to this last-mentioned type of confusion; indeed, older persons have been described as "living on the edge of cerebral hypoxia."[60] Noxious agents can also produce reversible or irreversible damage to cerebral neurons and thereby cause disorganized behavior. Numerous diseases that attack nervous tissue can cause behavioral changes. Although the precise etiologic mechanisms are poorly understood, a distended bladder or fecal impaction may have noxious effects upon brain cells, precipitating temporary confusion or delirium. Acidosis and increased levels of carbon dioxide are common causes of confusion. Also, hypertension contributes to brain ischemia.[27]

169

INDICATIONS OF DISORGANIZED BEHAVIOR

Some manifestations of disorganized behavior and thinking are confusion or disorientation, hallucinations, illusions and delusional thinking. Terms such as these often are not correctly applied or uniformly understood. For example, what one person means when she says a patient is "disoriented" may be very different from what another person thinks of as disoriented behavior. Thus, accurate terminology must be used appropriately in describing behavior and thought processes that are disorganized.

CONFUSION (DISORIENTATION)

The terms *"confusion"* and *"disorientation"* can be used interchangeably, and it is repetitious to use them both and say that a patient is "confused *and* disoriented." Confusion[35] generally refers to a state of disordered orientation; it represents a disturbance of consciousness in the sense that awareness of time, place or person is unclear. Confusion may be due to organic or psychic causes. Disorientation[35] likewise refers to impairment in the understanding of temporal, spatial or personal relationships. The confused or disoriented patient thus may not know who he is; what time of day or what day, month or year it is; or where he is.

Confusion, or disorientation, is not the same as delirium; a delirious patient may appear confused or disoriented, but not all confused or disoriented patients are delirious. Also, a comatose or semicomatose patient should not be called confused or disoriented. A person in a coma is unconscious and cannot be aroused even by powerful stimuli. A semicomatose person is in a mild coma. Before a patient can be described accurately as confused or disoriented he must be awake enough so that he can be expected to be properly oriented to his environment.[48]

Confusion or disorientation represents less severe alterations in brain function than does coma or delirium. With confusion or disorientation there is a loss of the higher nervous activity within the central nervous system. This high level nervous activity typically functions to enable one to maintain normal relationships within one's internal and external environments. Loeser observes that while the dysfunctions within the brain during confusion or disorientation are minor, the social dysfunction is devastating: "One doesn't need a very severe brain injury or a very severe alteration in the metabolism of the brain cells to result in what is functionally an essentially useless human being. If you don't know where you are or what to do, you are of little value to yourself or to the rest of the world, in spite of the fact that the amount of dysfunction within your central nervous system is minimal."[48]

With confusion or disorientation there is loss of ability to adapt and to respond to normal stimuli and to maintain the normal cyclic patterns of day and night. Thus, it is not uncommon to find that the confused patient may want to sleep during the daytime and then is hyperactive at night.

> *The confused patient is not comatose; he can perceive what is happening in his environment. He can hear and see, and can speak and respond in some way to what is happening around him. However, if we compare what is viewed as "normal" behavior with that of the confused patient, we find that what he says and does is not the appropriate or culturally expected behavior.*

Evaluating the Confused or Disoriented Patient. Confusion may be a transitory state that comes and goes and thus may be difficult to evaluate. The state may last minutes, hours, months or years. One cannot decide on the basis of one question or one observation whether a patient is confused; a *series* of questions and observations (of both verbal and nonverbal behavior) are needed. In the process of evaluation you might observe if the patient can find his way back to his room and his bed; if he appears to recognize his doctor and you; and if he seems to understand why he is in the hospital. Does he seem to know what time of day it is and where he is? How aware of current events is he? Does he know who the President is? If he has just listened to the news, does he seem to remember what he heard? Does he remember whether his doctor visited today, what he had for breakfast, or when he last saw visitors in the hospital? Much of this information can be obtained, without directly questioning the patient, by listening closely to what he says and by observing his behavior. At times, however, specific questions are necessary.

The following guidelines will help you in interviewing a patient to evaluate whether he is confused. In general, do not ask questions to which the patient can simply reply "Yes" or "No." His correct answer to such a question may only be a guess on his part or an attempt to cover up his confusion. For example, do not say, "Do you know where you are?" for the patient may say, "Yes," although he doesn't really know where he is. Instead say, "Tell me the name of this hospital and what city it is in."

Also, in attempting to determine whether or not the patient is oriented to time, person and place, evaluate your interviewing of the patient in light of the following.[48]

► Is the patient being asked realistic questions? What is his level of intelligence? What have his experiences been? How long has he been hospitalized?

► Is the patient fully awake when he is talked to or is he groggy and only half awake?

► Does he have the aids to orientation and expression that he requires? For example, is he exposed to radio, television, newspapers, calendars? Does he have a clock or watch? Does he have his glasses on? Are his dentures in so that he can speak clearly? Does he require a hearing aid? If so, is it turned on?

► Do you have the patient's attention when talking to him? (You may want to touch him before speaking to gain his attention.) Are you giving the patient your attention and really trying to communicate with him?

► Does he speak English or are you talking to him in a language he does not understand?

► Can he speak? Is he perhaps aphasic, i.e., capable of receiving stimuli for speech but unable to handle symbolic expression through language? (A patient may be aphasic and not be confused.) Has he had a laryngectomy? Is he deaf? Is he mute?

► Does the patient have memory difficulties? (The confused patient cannot function appropriately here and now. Someone with memory difficulties may not be confused; he may be able to function appropriately here and now but cannot remember.) It is important to know if the patient is aware of his intellectual deficit. A person with memory difficulties may say, "I don't know the date. I can't remember things." A confused patient may say, "It is 1926."

In describing the confused or disoriented patient, it is often best not to use the terms "confused" and "disoriented," since these terms may mean different things to different people. It is much clearer, and more accurate, if you state as simply as possible (1) how the patient appeared; (2) what you did to stimulate him; and (3) what his response was. For example:

"While Mr. Smith and I were walking down the hall, I asked him if he could tell me how he happened to come to the hospital. He replied: 'I don't know where I am. How long have I been here?' "

Some Causes of Confusion or Disorientation. Confusion is a common sign of both physical and mental illness. Causes of confusion include the following:

Congenital causes: relatively rare.

Degenerative causes (in any age group): relentlessly progressive diseases that may involve confusion, e.g., Huntington's chorea.

Infections (viral, bacterial, fungal): confusion may result from fever or infection.

Neoplasms (in brain or metastatic to brain): some tumors occur without neurologic findings but with confusion, e.g., frontal lobe, slow-growing tumors.

Vascular lesions: the most common cause in geriatric patients, e.g., repeated small strokes slowly destroying brain cells; ruptured aneurysms; arteriovenous malformations.

Trauma: mechanical deformation of the brain.

Metabolic factors: most commonly found causes in hospitalized patients, resulting from diabetes, electrolyte imbalance (prolonged vomiting), hormonal disturbances, hypothyroidism, drugs (side effect of steroids and some drugs used to treat Parkinson's disease; side effect of narcotics and sedatives and psychedelics). Alcohol is *the most common cause* of confusion found in the general hospital.

Seizures: confusion may occur during or following seizures.

Psychiatric causes: these may be numerous.

Sensory deprivation

Effects of Sensory Deprivation. Studies in sensory deprivation have established that when people are deprived of sensory stimulation they may develop confusion, inaccurate perception, faulty reasoning, impaired memory and even hallucinations. In spite of this fact, confused patients are frequently restrained and isolated from others by being placed in a room alone or by having curtains pulled around their cubicles. Confused patients' perceptual fields are actually further decreased by such "treatment," and they are placed in a situation that actually fosters the perpetuation of confusion. "When you take a confused patient, tie him down in bed, all fours splayed out, looking up at a white ceiling and leave him alone, you are just putting him through more sensory deprivation."[48]

Blindness and deafness are principal causes of sensory deprivation and, hence, confusion; the individual whose senses are impaired, e.g., because of cataracts and/or partial deafness, is more likely to become confused than a person with intact sensation.

It is not surprising to learn that darkness and loss of spatial image can precipitate or intensify a state of confusion. Studies in sensory deprivation (in which the subjects wore various kinds of goggles) demonstrated that fewer hallucinations occur with complete darkness (or with opaque head coverings) than if the visual field is generalized with translucent goggles that let in some light but that do not allow patterns to be seen. Also, when slight stimulation is allowed, e.g., a low sound or low ambient light, there is a greater amount of distortion and hallucinatory activity than in the total absence of stimulation. Presumably there must be some kind of stimulus before it can be distorted.[16]

Emphasis has also been placed on the importance of *meaningful* contact with the environment in minimizing sensory deprivation. Some investigators believe that it is the restriction of meaning that is mainly responsible for the effects of sensory deprivation, rather than the quantitative physical limitation of stimuli per se.[21] Thus:

> *Patients need to have* meaningful *contact with their environment and with persons in their environment.*

Nursing Care of Confused or Disoriented Patients

Confusion (or disorientation) is completely disabling to a patient; he is dependent on others for care and protection. Let us now examine some ways in which nurses may help these patients. There are three *major goals* to keep in mind in the care of confused patients: (1) prevent or modify disorganization; (2) support and protect the patient during aberrant behavior; and (3) reorient him to reality.[27] It is desirable to evaluate the patient's level of comprehension and his emotional state before attempting to orient him to reality, since a sedated, drugged, highly anxious patient will not be susceptible to reorientation efforts until his level of anxiety and his medications are reduced.[27]

Prevent or Modify Disorganization. It is helpful if a confused person can be assigned to the care of the same nurse for consecutive days. Everything is bewildering enough for such a patient without adding to it the presence of many different people. For the confused patient one assigned nurse fulfills the role of an "anchor person" by serving as a steady point of reference.[68] Authorities suggest that this "anchor nurse" should be generally good-natured and even-tempered, available and accessible, noncoercive, and patient. The nurse should consider her posture, voice and gestures when with the patient and make sure that these are friendly rather than threatening. Her movements should be slow and deliberate rather than sudden and sporadic. In her activities the nurse should strive to include rather than exclude the patient. That is, she should tell the patient what she will be doing and talk with him as she proceeds rather than remaining silent and simply doing things *to* him. This point will be discussed further later.

With professional skill a nurse can alter, manipulate, and plan the environment of patients in her care. The nurse governs "environmental input and output" and combats sensory saturation as well as sensory deprivation. She can alter the patient's physical environment to some extent and she can markedly alter his interpersonal environment. The professional nurse sets a "tone" of emotional care and respect for the disturbed patient. Others will be encouraged to follow her example, since the nurse serves as a model of behavior for other staff members and for a patient's friends and relatives. If a professional nurse treats a confused patient in a depersonalized, hopeless manner and makes fun of his behavior, then other people will follow the example that she has set. If the nurse shows respect for the patient, others will also.

Support and Protect the Patient. A confused patient may say or do things that are foreign to our experience; he makes us feel uncomfortable and may appear to be teasing or funny. He may remind us of people "acting silly" or of comedians. However, unlike the clown or comedian, the confused patient is *not* acting or performing for our benefit. He is with us to receive professional care, understanding and protection during his confusion. The comedian feels uncomfortable if we do *not* laugh at him; the disoriented patient feels uncomfortable if we *do* laugh at him, and he will become louder the more deeply confused he becomes. Unlike the comedian who can choose how he will communicate, the confused patient has no conscious choice regarding his communication. Laughing at or making fun of such a person is cruel. Also, joking about the confused patient within the hearing of other patients or their friends or relatives makes these other persons uncomfortable because they sense your lack of compassion and feel that you lack understanding of them.

How can a nurse helpfully regulate a disoriented patient's physical environment? Studies in sensory deprivation help a great deal and their findings can be implemented. A room should have adequate light, and the light should vary between night and day. Night lights should be left on in the patient's room. Shades should not remain down during the daytime. As mentioned earlier, the patient should have the normal aids to orientation available and in use: e.g., radio, television, newspapers, magazines, a calendar, an accurate clock or watch, glasses, dentures, and a hearing aid if required. To be used properly the radio must be clearly tuned in to programs in keeping with the patient's interests, if possible, and loud enough to be understood (too loud or too soft will be annoying); the television must be in focus as well as close enough to see and loud enough to hear; radio and television should not be left on hour after hour or the patient becomes fatigued and may attempt to mentally tune them out (perhaps lapsing more deeply into confusion); newspapers and magazines must be in good repair and current; a calendar must be where it can be viewed and large enough to be seen clearly, and turned to the correct day, week, or month; clocks and watches must be kept wound, accurately set and placed so the patient can easily see them; glasses must be clean and in use; hearing aids need to be properly placed, maintained with batteries, and turned on when in use.

Other manipulations of the physical environment that the nurse can carry out include rearranging furniture for the patient's benefit so he can see outside or into the halls; placing the call bell within reach; and arranging flowers, or some of the patient's familiar belongings. Familiar objects can help orient a confused patient, and colorful robes, curtains, bedspreads, pictures and wall paint are visually stimulating.

Further physical management includes moving the patient himself. Again, studies of sensory deprivation guide the nurse's action. People become confused when they do not move, do not touch themselves, and are not touched by others. (Consider here the detrimental effect of wrist restraints that restrict movement and do not allow the patient even to touch himself.) Enclosure in a confined space for a period of time can cause confusion. The nursing implications of these studies begin with the nurse's recognition that touching and movement are very important for orientation and include plans for the integration of these activities into nursing care.

Touch the patient when talking to him and when caring for him. Movement is helpful in maintaining orientation to body image: therefore, passive exercises, encouraging the patient to move, turning and positioning the patient, rolling the bed up or down for various periods, and getting the patient out of bed and out of his room as much as possible are essential nursing actions. It is important also to reduce noises, shadows and drafts that might disturb the patient or that he might misinterpret. Again, these are areas within the control of the nurse.

Because a confused person cannot respond appropriately to his needs, he must be periodically taken to the toilet, given fluids to drink, be supervised during meals, and helped to rest. Without such care the forgetful person can become impacted, incontinent, dehydrated, malnourished, and excessively fatigued. Intake and output records should be kept for all confused patients.

Incontinence contributes to confused patients' regression, feelings of helplessness, and lowered self-esteem. Every effort must be made to retrain the incontinent patient to normal bowel and bladder elimination or at least to prevent incontinence. The disoriented patient is not unconscious; he is not insensitive to the manner in which he is regarded or treated. If he is allowed to remain incontinent, the feeling communicated to him is one of hopelessness and degradation; his "animal nature" is allowed to take precedence over his "human na-

TABLE 14–1. SUGGESTIONS FOR NURSING INTERVENTION DURING SENSORY DEPRIVATION

PATIENT BEHAVIOR	NURSING INTERVENTION
Boredom, inactivity	Provide a variety of activities that allow patient to *explore* environment
Slowness of thought, daydreaming	Through goal-directed conversation with patient, focus his thinking on meaningful topics
Thought disorganization	Provide organization of patient's time through consistent interaction and orient him to time through use of clocks
Anxiety, panic	Provide a bench mark or reference point that patient can use to assess movement toward a goal that will increase security
Hallucinations	Provide reality validation so that patient does not have to read into the environment false stimuli that do not exist

ture." If he is roughly washed and diapered after incontinence he will not be encouraged to regain bowel and bladder control; he will instead actually be trained to be incontinent.

Contrast this type of "care" with an atmosphere of: (1) Staff *recognition* that confusion means a lack of appropriate response to time. (2) Staff *expectation* that the patient may be incontinent unless they assume for him a "time awareness" regarding his needs to void or defecate; the confused patient cannot plan ahead and therefore once he is aware of having to eliminate he may not have time to find the toilet or to get help. (3) Staff *awareness* that they must form a retraining plan and keep records on all shifts in an attempt to determine the patient's pattern of bowel and bladder function. (4) Staff *acceptance* of this area of need for care. (5) Staff *enthusiasm* that the confused incontinent patient *can* be trained or at least that they themselves can be trained to anticipate and respond to the patient's pattern of intake and output so that he will not be incontinent. What a difference in atmosphere for the patient; the difference between feeling that one is a chore and an animal, and the feeling that one is a person who is in need of help, can benefit from help, and is receiving it!

Reorientation.   All the nursing actions that have been mentioned thus far can be carried out without staff members ever talking to the patient. His furniture can be rearranged, his radio turned on, his elimination care given—all without ever talking to him, or at most giving only a few commands. However, if such is the situation, the patient's care is inadequate.

> *A major portion of the plan of care for confused patients must be directed toward thoughtful, preplanned, verbal communication—talking that is directed toward meeting the patient's need for reorientation.*

Confused patients are uncertain about what is real, and so nursing efforts are directed toward helping to re-establish with these patients the elements of reality that we share with one another. Reality comprises a mental experience or inner life that is private to each individual as well as aspects of life that are shared in common with others. For example, when a nurse sits at a desk, the nurse and the desk are obvious to all—they are a part of the "shared reality" that is available to everyone's experience; however, the nurse's thoughts as she sits at the desk are a part of her own inner reality. Her thoughts are not shared or obvious to the onlooker unless the nurse verbalizes what she is thinking. It is the shared facts of daily reality that the nurse may focus on initially in attempting to reorient the confused patient and to make him more comfortable.

Some important shared, basic factors in everyone's orientation are agreements about time, persons and places. As we have indicated, an individual is confused when he doesn't know what time it is; what day, month or year it is; who he is; who others are; where he is; and the geography and location of surrounding areas. In our waking lives we have mutual agreements in these areas; this constitutes an important part of reality, the awareness of which keeps us oriented.

If a nurse's goal is to focus on the shared elements of reality (e.g., concerning time, place and person), it is in these areas that she will plan her "verbal care" of the patient. How? Instead of talking about abstract things she will talk about the *real things* in the environment and the *facts* that she knows about the patient. For example, instead of feeding the patient in silence, the nurse who is trying to reorient the patient verbally will talk about what the foods are, what meal it is, the tray, the dishes, and so on. Instead of saying, "Have some of this," she will say, "Would you like some of these green beans?" In stressing shared time she will identify the meal being served. Instead of saying, "It's time to eat," she will say, "It is Tuesday morning. I have brought you some breakfast."

In a continuing attempt to reorient the confused patient the nurse directs her comments to reality. She will *repeatedly* identify herself to the patient (because he does not remember) and she will focus on what time it is, who the patient is, where he is, and why he is there. Speaking slowly, so that the patient will have time to think about what is being said and have time to ask questions, the nurse moves from topic to topic. If the patient misunderstands she will attempt to clarify briefly. The nurse should not contribute to a patient's disorientation by agreeing with his misinterpretations and she should not upset him by arguing but rather, work to understand what the patient may mean. The patient should be corrected gently and the comments refocused as appropriate. For example, if the patient says, "Aren't you Sister Mary?" She may respond, "No, I am Miss Thomas, your nurse at General Hospital. Who is Sister Mary?"

When you are going to speak to the confused patient, gain his attention, look into his eyes when you speak so he can watch your lips move, and speak clearly, slowly, and in an appropriate tone and volume of voice. Talk to the patient as an adult, not with "baby talk." You may find initially that it is difficult to talk to people if they make no reply to what you have said or if their replies don't make much sense. Lack of response may make you feel that you want to stop talking, or it may embarrass you. Confused people are sometimes a threat to our own reality and thus cause us to feel like retreating from them for fear that we also may become confused. Resist such feelings and try to understand them. Other feelings that you may have with a disoriented patient are: concerns that he may say something embarrassing to you; a belief that he may stay quiet and tranquil if you don't disturb him by talking; and worries about what other people will think about your attempts to communicate with the patient. Analyze such feelings, remembering that the confused patient needs your communication with him. It takes real effort to try to communicate with confused people, but it is of prime importance in their care.

Because confused people lose their awareness of the cyclic movement of time, they should be helped to dress in the daytime rather than remaining constantly in sleeping attire, which they may associate with night. Since medications such as sedatives may intensify confusion, first use other nursing measures to help restless, confused patients to sleep. For example, a brief talk, a back rub, a cup of warm milk, a trip to the bathroom, washing the hands and face can all help to relax a patient sufficiently so that sleep is possible without medication. Sedation may be contraindicated in patients who have impaired renal or cerebral functions.

Combat social isolation by stopping in the confused patient's room frequently; bringing the patient's chair (or bed) into the doorway of his room or out into the hall or by the nursing station (during the day, evening or at night); taking the patient for frequent walks or wheelchair rides; and encouraging visiting by friends, relatives, volunteers, staff or other patients.

The confused patient's coherence and thinking ability are dulled; he is bewildered and forgetful and perceives inadequately. Also, he may be inattentive, have sleep disorders, hallucinate, become agitated, talk incoherently, wander about or get lost.[60] Such a patient obviously needs protective care. The confused person is a frightened person. He often feels defenseless in his bewilderment and is afraid of being taken advantage of. He tries to protect himself when he feels threatened and at such times may refuse care and may try to keep people away from him. Forcing this patient or restraining him will add to his fear and aggres-siveness. Often the more fearful and upset the patient becomes, the more confused and defensive he becomes.

Restraint policy varies from one hospital and one physician to another; however, the trend is to forbid the use of restraint or to use it only according to definite procedures which ensure protection of the patient. If restraints are used they should be applied only after a decision is carefully made that the restraints are necessary for the *patient's well-being* and not for the convenience of the staff. Some general points to bear in mind concerning restraints are as follows: (1) Let the patient know that he is not being punished; inform him that he is being restrained for his own well-being so that he will not fall or injure himself. (2) Never place restraints around a patient's neck; he may suffocate. (3) Apply restraints snugly so the patient cannot get out of them or become entangled in them; however, do not impede the circulation. (4) Body restraints are preferable to wrist and ankle restraints because they allow greater freedom of movement. (5) Change the restrained patient's position often. (6) Remove the restraints frequently to give skin care and to allow the patient to move. (7) Put padding under the restraints to protect the skin. (8) *Carefully supervise the restrained patient.* Remember that the restrained person is totally dependent on others for his safety and care. This is a frightening condition for the patient and a situation of responsibility for the nurse.

Both physical restraint and the use of drugs to chemically restrain the patient can contribute to a patient's confusion by impairing reality testing and communication. Remove restraints as soon as possible.

HALLUCINATIONS, ILLUSIONS AND DELUSIONAL THINKING

Hallucinations, illusions and delusional thinking are other examples of disordered behavior and thought disturbances. Let us briefly consider these problems.

Hallucinations. Hallucinations[35] are sensory impressions occurring in the *absence of external stimuli*, whether or not accompanied by insight into their unreal nature on the part of the subject. Any of the senses may be affected, and so hallucinating patients may believe that they see, hear, smell, feel or taste objects or stimuli that are not actually present. The hallucinated stimuli (whether a vision, a sound, an odor or a taste) have no source in the environment; instead they are sensations arising within the patient himself.

The presence of visual hallucinations suggests that a patient's problem may be an organic disease of the brain rather than functional mental illness. Visual hallucinations most typically occur in the deliria of acute infectious diseases or toxic psychoses and most often occur with acute, reversible organic brain disorders. A variety of drugs may also cause visual hallucinations; such drugs include not only exotic drugs, e.g., mescaline, but also prescribed medications, e.g., amphetamines and antiparkinsonism medication. Also, the withdrawal of some drugs, e.g., alcohol and barbiturates, can produce visual hallucinations.[9]

Some additional causes of visual hallucinations with an organic basis are listed below:[9]

▶ Brain tumors and other space-occupying lesions

▶ The aura of an epileptic attack or migrainous headaches

▶ Metabolic disorders, e.g., adrenal insufficiency, dehydration, hypoparathyroidism, pernicious or addisonian anemia, hypoglycemia, anorexia, and uremia

▶ Trauma

▶ Collagen diseases

▶ Cerebrovascular accidents

▶ Degenerative diseases, e.g., Pick's and Alzheimer's diseases

Visual hallucinations are associated with mental illness as well as organic problems. Generally visual hallucinations are associated with the acute psychoses and auditory hallucinations with the chronic psychoses. Visual hallucinations may also occur as a result of sensory deprivation.[21]

Illusions. Illusions[35] differ from hallucinations in that with an illusion *a real stimulus is present* but the person *misinterprets* the actual stimuli from the environment. For example, a shadow may be present on the wall, but the patient misinterprets the shadow and believes that he sees a person standing by the wall. Whenever possible, try to identify the stimulus that the patient is misinterpreting; then control, reduce or remove this stimulus. Also, decrease other environmental stimuli in an attempt to control the patient's overresponsiveness.

Delusional Thinking. "Delusional thinking"[35] refers to thoughts or beliefs that are false; that is, they are contrary to demonstrable fact. For example, a person may believe that he is being persecuted by the police when this is not true.

BIBLIOGRAPHY

a. Angel, R. W.: Understanding and diagnosing senile dementia. *Geriatrics,* 32:47–49, Aug. 1977.
1. Arie, T.: Dementia in the elderly: diagnosis and assessment. *British Medical Journal,* 4:540–543, Dec. 1, 1973.
2. Blustein, J., and Seeman, M. V.: Brain tumors presenting as functional psychiatric disturbances. *Canadian Psychiatric Association Journal,* Special Supplement II, 17:SS-59, 1972.
3. Burnside, I. M.: Clocks and calendars. *American Journal of Nursing,* 70:117–119, Jan. 1970.
4. Bolin, R. H.: Sensory deprivation: an overview. *Nursing Forum,* 13(3):240–258, 1974.
5. Braun, A.: Some remarks on persecution pathology. *Psychotherapy and Psychosomatics,* 24:106–108, 1974.
6. Buchan, T.: Organic confusional states. *South African Medical Journal,* 46:1340–1343, Sept. 16, 1972.
7. Budd, S. P., and Brown, W.: Effect of a reorientation technique on postcardiotomy delirium. *Nursing Research,* 23:341–348, July–Aug. 1974.
8. Burnside, I. M.: Sensory stimulation: an adjunct to group work with the disabled aged. *Mental Hygiene,* 53:381, July 1969.
8a. Katzman, R.: Dementias. *Postgraduate Medicine,* 64:119–125, Aug. 1978.
9. Charlton, M. H.: Visual hallucinations. *Psychiatric Quarterly,* 37:489, 1963.
10. Chedru, F., and Geschwind, N.: Disorders of higher cortical functions in acute confusional states. *Cortex,* 8:395–411, Dec. 1972.
11. Chodil, J., and Williams, B.: The concept of sensory deprivation. *Nursing Clinics of North America,* 5:453, Sept. 1970.
12. Ciccone, J. R., and Racy, J.: Psychotic depression and hallucinations. *Comprehensive Psychiatry,* 16:233–236, May–June 1975.
13. Danto, B. L.: The violent patient: a medical emergency. *Clinical Medicine,* 82:18–22, Feb. 1975.
14. Dolan, M.: A return to laughter . . . and tears. *Nursing '76,* 6:43, Nov. 1976.
15. Downs, F. S.: Bed rest and sensory disturbances. *American Journal of Nursing,* 74:434, March 1974.
16. Dunham, J.: Perception and Sensory Deprivation. Presented at the Institute, "The Unconscious Patient and the Disoriented Patient," sponsored by the University of Washington School of Nursing, April 14, 1966.
17. Elia, J. C.: Cranial injuries and the post concussion syndrome. *In* F. Lane (ed.): *Medical Trial Technique Quarterly 1975 Annual.* Chicago, Callaghan & Co., 1975.
18. Ellis, R.: Unusual sensory and thought disturbances after cardiac surgery. *American Journal of Nursing,* 72:2021, Nov. 1972.
19. Field, W. E., and Ruelke, W.: Hallucinations and how to deal with them. *American Journal of Nursing,* 73:638, April 1973.
20. Fine, J., and Finestone, S. C.: Sensory disturbances following ketamine anesthesia: recurrent hallucinations. *Anesthesia and Analgesia* (Cleveland), 52:428–430, May–June 1973.

21. Flynn, W. R.: Visual hallucinations in sensory deprivation. *Psychiatric Quarterly, 36*:55, 1962.

22. Folsom, J. C., and Folsom, G. S.: The real world. *Mental Health, 58*:29–33, Summer 1974.

23. Fort, J.: Comparison chart of major substances used for mind alteration. *American Journal of Nursing, 71*:1740, Sept. 1971.

24. Fowler, R. S., Jr., and Fordyce, W. E.: Adapting care for the brain-damaged patient, Part I. *American Journal of Nursing, 72*:1832, Oct. 1972.

25. Fowler, R. S., Jr., and Fordyce, W. E.: Adapting care for the brain-damaged patient, Part II. *American Journal of Nursing, 72*:2056, Nov. 1972.

26. Garfield, J. M.: Psychologic problems in anesthesia. *American Family Physician, 10*:60–67, Aug. 1974.

27. Gerdes, L.: The confused or delirious patient. *American Journal of Nursing, 68*:1228, June 1968.

28. Glassman, A. H., Kantor, S. J., and Shostak, M.: Depression, delusions and drug response. *American Journal of Psychiatry, 132*:716–719, July 1975.

28a. Guze, S. B.: Acute brain syndrome. *Hospital Medicine, 13*:63–69, April 1977.

29. Haase, G. R.: Diseases presenting as dementia. *In* Charles E. Wells (ed.): *Dementia.* Contemporary Neurology Series (9). Philadelphia, F. A. Davis Co., 1971.

30. Hacker, C.: Do you have a bad trip if you go to hospital? *The Canadian Nurse, 67*:39–44, June 1971.

31. Hashizume, S.: She asked: "Am I going crazy?" *Nursing '75, 5*:12–15, Feb. 1975.

32. Havens, A.: Care of a depressed medical-surgical patient. *American Journal of Nursing, 70*:1070–1072, May 1970.

33. Hefferin, E. A., and Hunter, R. E.: How we turned the idea into a program: reality orientation. *Nursing '77, 7*:89–93, May 1977.

34. Henry, W. D., and Mann, A. M.: Diagnosis and treatment of delirium. *Canadian Medical Association Journal, 93*:1156, Nov. 27, 1965.

35. Hinsie, L., and Campbell, R. J.: *Psychiatric Dictionary,* 4th ed. New York, Oxford University Press, 1970.

36. Hirschfels, M.: The cognitively impaired older adult. *American Journal of Nursing, 76*:1981, Dec. 1976.

37. Holland, J., Fasanello, S., and Ohnuma, T.: Psychiatric symptoms associated with L-asparaginase administration. *Journal of Psychiatric Research, 10*:105–113, 1974.

38. Ianzito, B. M., Cadoret, R. J., and Pugh, D. D.: Thought disorder in depression. *American Journal of Psychiatry, 131*:703–707, June 1974.

39. Jana, D. K., and Romano-Jana, L.: Hypernatremic psychosis in the elderly. *Journal American Geriatric Society, 21*:473–477, Oct. 1973.

40. Jennett, B., and Plum, F.: Persistent vegetative state after brain damage. *RN, 35*:ICU-1, Oct. 1972.

41. Kerstein, M. D., and Isenberg, S.: Dealing with confused elderly patient. *Hospital and Community Psychiatry, 25*(3):160–161, 1974.

42. Kiersnowski, C., Martsolf, D., and O'Brien, P.: Miss Green thought we were "torturing" her. *Nursing '76, 6*:58–60, Sept. 1976.

43. Knicely, K. H.: The world of distorted perception. *American Journal of Nursing, 67*:998, May 1967.

44. Kornfeld, D. S.: The hospital environment: its impact on the patient. *Advances in Psychosomatic Medicine, 8*:252–270, 1972.

45. Kral, V. A.: Senile dementia and normal aging. *Canadian Psychiatric Association Journal, 17*:SS-25, 1972.

46. Levy, R.: Immobilized patient and his psychological well-being. *Postgraduate Medicine, 40*:74, July 1966.

47. Lipowski, Z. J., and Kiriakos, R. Z.: Borderlands between neurology and psychiatry: observations in a neurological hospital. *Psychiatry in Medicine, 3*:131–147, April 1972.

48. Loeser, J.: The Disoriented Patient: Causes and Effects. Presented at the Institute, "The Unconscious Patient and the Disoriented Patient," sponsored by the University of Washington School of Nursing, April 15, 1966.

49. Lyon, G. G.: Stimulation through remotivation. *American Journal of Nursing, 71*:982, May 1971.

50. MacDonald, D. J.: Psychotic reactions during organ transplantation. *Canadian Psychiatric Association Journal,* Special Supplement II, *17*:SS-15, 1972.

51. Matefy, R. E., and Krall, R. G.: An initial investigation of the psychedelic drug flashback phenomena. *Journal of Consulting and Clinical Psychology, 42*:854–860, Dec. 1974.

52. McCown, P. P., and Wurm, E.: Orienting the disoriented. *American Journal of Nursing, 65*:118, April 1965.

53. Meinhart, N. T., and Aspinall, M. J.: Nursing interventions in hypovigilance. *American Journal of Nursing, 69*:994, May 1969.

54. Morris, M., and Rhodes, M.: Guidelines for the care of confused patients. *American Journal of Nursing, 72*:1630, Sept. 1972.

55. Morse, R. M., and Litin, E. M.: The anatomy of a delirium. *American Journal of Psychiatry, 128*:143–147, July 1, 1971.

56. Moses, D. V.: Reality orientation in the aging person. *In* Carlson, C. E. (ed.): *Behavioral Concepts and Nursing Intervention.* Philadelphia, J. B. Lippincott Co., 1970.

57. Myers, R. S.: Whatever is bad by day is worse at night. *Modern Hospital, 110*:91, Jan. 1968.

58. Ohno, M. I.: The eye-patched patient. *American Journal of Nursing, 71*:271, Feb. 1971.

59. Olson, E. V.: Immobility: effects on psychosocial equilibrium. *American Journal of Nursing, 67*:794, April 1967.

60. Patrick, M. L.: Care of the confused elderly patient. *American Journal of Nursing, 67*:2536, Dec. 1967.

61. Patrick, M.: Little things mean a lot in geriatric rehabilitation. *Nursing '73, 3*:7–9, Aug. 1973.

62. Peterson, H. W., and Martin, M. J.: Organic disease presenting as a psychiatric syndrome. *Postgraduate Medicine, 54*:78–82, Aug. 1973.

63. Philip, S., et al.: *Sensory Deprivation.* Cambridge, MA, Harvard University Press, 1961.

64. Phillips, D. F.: Reality orientation. *Hospitals, J.A.H.A., 47*:47, July 1, 1973.

65. Post, F.: Paranoid disorders in the elderly. *Postgraduate Medicine, 53*:52–56, April 1973.

66. Post, R. M.: Cocaine psychoses: a continuum model. *American Journal of Psychiatry, 132*:225–230, March 1975.

67. Raft, D. D., Newmark, C., and Toomey, T.: The organic brain syndrome. *American Family Physician, 10*:119–123, Nov. 1974.

68. Reusch, J.: Psychotherapy for the well and psychotherapy for the ill. *Psychotherapy and Psychosomatics, 13*:68, 1965.

69. Robinson, L.: Coping with psychiatric emergencies. *Nursing '73, 3*:42–44, July 1973.

70. Robinson, L.: *Psychological Aspects of the Care of Hospitalized Patients,* 2nd ed. Philadelphia, F. A. Davis Co., 1972, Chap. 6, The Disoriented Patient.

71. Royalty, D. C.: "Try to keep her clothes on," that was the staff's only goal. *Nursing '76, 6*:38–40, April 1976.

72. Sanders, R. A.: Improvement in time orientation in hospitalized geriatric patients. *Journal of American Geriatric Society, 13*:1013, Dec. 1965.

73. Scarbrough, D. R.: Reality orientation: a new approach to an old problem. *Nursing '74, 4*:12–13, Nov. 1974.

74. Schnaper, N.: The psychological implications of severe trauma: emotional sequelae to unconsciousness. *Journal of Trauma, 15*:94–98, Feb. 1975.

75. Schultz, D. P.: *Sensory Restriction: Effects on Behavior.* New York, Academic Press, 1965.

76. Slaby, A. E., Lieb, J., and Tancredi, L. R.: *Handbook of Psychiatric Emergencies.* Flushing, NY, Medical Examination Publishing Co., 1975.

77. Spencer, D. J.: Cannabis-induced psychosis. *The International Journal of the Addictions, 6*:323–326, June 1971.

78. Stevens, C. B.: Ben was some "vegetable"! *Nursing '77, 7*:96, Jan. 1977.

79. Stevens, C. B.: Breaking through cobwebs of confusion in the elderly. *Nursing '74, 4*:41–48, Aug. 1974.

80. Taylor, D. A., et al.: Personality factors related to response to social isolation and confinement. *Journal of Consulting and Clinical Psychology (Washington), 33*:411, Aug. 1969.

81. Thomson, L. R.: Sensory deprivation: a personal experience. *American Journal of Nursing, 73*:266, Feb. 1973.

82. Ujhely, G. B.: Nursing intervention with the acutely ill psychiatric patient. *Nursing Forum, 8*(3):311–325, 1969.

83. Wang, H. S., and Busse, E. W.: Dementia in old age. *In* Wells, Charles E. (ed.): *Dementia.* Contemporary Neurology Series (9). Philadelphia, F. A. Davis Co., 1971.

84. Wells, C. E.: Clinical management of the patient with dementia. *In* Wells, Charles E. (ed.): *Dementia.* Contemporary Neurology Series (9). Philadelphia, F. A. Davis Co., 1971.

85. Wells, C. E.: The symptoms and behavorial manifestations of dementia. *In* Wells, Charles E. (ed.): *Dementia.* Contemporary Neurology Series (9). Philadelphia, F. A. Davis Co., 1971.

85a. Wells, D. A.: Dealing with delirium and dementia. *Consultant, 17*:207, Jan. 1977.

86. Weymouth, L. T.: The nursing care of the so-called confused patient. *Nursing Clinics of North America, 3*:709–715, Dec. 1968.

87. Wiley, L. (ed.): The perfect explanation may not be right at all. *Nursing '76, 6*:52–57, Sept. 1976.

88. Wolf, V. C.: Some implications of short-term, long-term memory theory. *Nursing Forum, 10*(2):150–165, 1971.

89. Zubek, J. P. (ed.): *Sensory Deprivation: Fifteen Years of Research.* New York, Appleton-Century-Crofts, 1969.

CHAPTER 15

DISTURBANCES OF BODY IMAGE

One of the fascinating paradoxes of the human condition is that the human body, which unites and identifies man as a biologic species, gives rise, in each of us, on a psychologic level, to a body image that is one of the subtly unique features of the individual personality.[47]

OVERVIEW AND STUDY GUIDE

Our approach to this chapter is to begin with a general introduction to the concept of body image and then to proceed to look more closely at (a) the development of body image, (b) disturbances of body image, (c) adaptation to body image changes, and (d) helping the patient to accept his changing body image.

As you read through this chapter, pause and reflect on any significant body image changes you have experienced. Consider also body image changes you have noticed in others. Can you identify your reactions to your own body image changes and to such changes you have observed in others? Recall one or two people in your past or present experience who have undergone the greatest body image changes. Think of ways in which these persons were helped by others and supported through their body image changes and ways in which these persons were frustrated or hurt emotionally by others during these changes.

As you continue to give nursing care, strive to be sensitive to body image alterations that patients in your care are experiencing. If your assessment of a given patient indicates he is undergoing body image alterations that are significant to him, identify appropriate nursing actions to help the patient with this change. We have concluded this chapter with a presentation of some ways a nurse can help a patient to accept his changing body image; can you identify ways not presented in our discussion? (This would be a suitable topic for group discussion.)

INTRODUCTION

Each of us carries in our minds an image of our own body; this organic picture is called *body image*. Body image forms an integral part of an individual's perception of himself, e.g., his conception of his personality, his worth, his ability to perform, his relations with other people. One's total body image defies description. Body image is so complex that it is impossible for an individual to describe his total body image. Body image is ultimately an intrapersonal experience of an individual's attitudes and feelings toward his body and the way one organizes these feelings.[46] Norris provides us with the following definition of body image:

Body image is the constantly changing total of conscious and unconscious information, feelings and perceptions about one's body in space as different and apart from all others. It is a social creation, developed through the reflected perceptions about the surfaces of one's body and responses to sensations originating from the inner regions of the body as the individual copes with a kaleidoscopic variety of living activities. The body image is basic to identity and has been referred to as the somatic ego.[46]

Have you ever tried to do a quick drawing of your total body? Pause for a moment and do so. As you made your drawing, were you aware of any particular parts of the drawing as being more meaningful to you than others?

A variety of "labels" and "meanings" are assigned by us to particular parts of our own

179

bodies. Likewise we tend to mentally categorize certain characteristic body images we observe in others. For example, one hears the character trait of "jolly" associated with "fat," or one hears "weak" associated with a "receding chin." Labeling of this nature is unfortunate, for it results in generalizations that may impede the process of knowing individuals as themselves . . . as they *really* are. Likewise, body language (gestures, facial expressions, postures) may be perceived as an indication of one's femininity or masculinity, one's aggressiveness or submissiveness, etc. Often such labeling of others takes place without our awareness of this process. Of course, the ways in which we mentally label or categorize others affect our interaction with them. As you give patient care, try to be aware of the various "labels" you assign to individual patients and how these labels might be affecting your nurse-patient communication. Pause for a moment and think of other examples of body image characteristics to which you assign various meanings. Consider factors such as size, movements, distortions, age and sex. You might find this an interesting topic for group discussion.

Paul Schilder[56] is an important contributor to our present knowledge of body image. According to him, body image is a *gestalt,* or a unified pattern for organizing sensory input. Although body image has a physiologic basis, it is composed of physical, psychologic and social experiences. Thus, body image not only includes an individual's personal and psychologic investment in his body and its parts but also has a sociologic meaning for both the individual and society. Body image is, to Schilder, a tridimensional unity involving interpersonal, environmental and temporal factors.

The concept of body image provides a way of thinking about one's body and how, through the body, one relates to the environment. This complicated internal mental representation of one's body slowly evolves during the normal processes of growth and development. Body image is a fluid, not a static, entity. "It is dynamic, i.e., everchanging, evolving, expanding or contracting, progressive or regressive, but goal-directed in terms of forming newer, more stable systems in the organism."[46]

Body image helps with the localization on the body surface of incoming sensory impulses and makes possible the performance of motor activities through the constant relationship of the body to other objects. The body image and the corresponding body boundaries thus function, in part, to help one maneuver in the external world. For example, knowledge of one's size or body boundaries is necessary in judging whether or not one can fit into a given space.

Objects that are attached to the body or participate in the body's movement (e.g., a cane, wheelchair or eyeglasses) are often viewed as part of the body image.

Body image is related to a variety of diverse phenomena, such as *sexual behavior, level of aspiration, ability to tolerate stress* and *style of life.* Body image is also related to choice of *"psychosomatic" symptoms.* For example, research with Rorschach responses demonstrates that persons whose symptoms involve the body's exterior (e.g., rheumatoid arthritics) tend to perceive their body boundaries as being firm and as a defense against the environment, while patients with symptoms involving the body's interior (e.g., patients with peptic ulcers) are likely to perceive their body boundaries as being infinite, vulnerable and easily penetrated.

Disturbances of body image are believed to underlie many clinical syndromes of bodily dysfunction. Illness, surgery, accidents and personality disorders can distort the body image, making necessary its reorganization. The nurse who is familiar with the concept of body image and who appreciates its importance can help patients with the distresses they may suffer from body image distortion. The knowledgeable nurse helps patients themselves but also with their significant others. It is important that nurses be aware of the potential and actual impact of nursing activities and diagnostic and treatment procedures that may threaten or alter patients' body images.

Knowledge of the body image concept has been used in psychiatry to gain an additional understanding of phenomena associated with acute and chronic brain disease and various degenerative, toxic and metabolic states. Body image theory is also useful in furthering understandings of preoccupations with the body which occur with disorders such as involutional psychoses, hypochondriasis, neurasthenias and the schizophrenias.[32]

DEVELOPMENT OF BODY IMAGE

Even during embryonic and infantile states multiple sensory impressions begin to lay the foundation for the formation of body image. As an infant grows into a child, and on through the life of that individual, his body image continues to be susceptible to new information. Gradually new, developing neural functions are laid over and inhibit earlier, more primitive structures within the nervous system. As a part of these developments the body image evolves, and one comes to have a composite of feelings and perceptions about one's body, its form and position. Typically this view is clearer for the external body than for internal body structures. Usually internal organs are only vaguely incorporated into the body image except when pain or discomfort is referred to the body's surface.

Infancy and *childhood* are periods of direct exploration of one's body surface and body orifices. An awareness of internal organs comes from sensations of discomfort. Early sensory experiences (e.g., pain, touch, temperature) are extremely important in the development of body image. Sensory messages from the body's inner surfaces are important in body image development as well as those from the body's outer surface contact with the environment. Movement, play, viewing oneself, experimentation, exploration, comparing and contrasting one's body with others—all these activities are important in the development of body image formation. The processes of interacting with others—socialization and culturalization—are also essential for the successful development of *body image integrity.*

As one grows over the years, the body image is continuously modified and the mental images of the body and body parts that are developed remain as memory traces within the nervous system. In addition to gaining knowledge about his own body, the growing child perceives the bodies of others and how others view their bodies. The child compares himself with these other persons and identifies with them. He learns to have certain attitudes toward his body and bodily functions, e.g., urination, defecation, salivation. Such attitudes and affects are generally related to the individual's sex and are acquired through the process of socialization. The attitudes of significant persons in a child's environment are very important during this socialization process.

Parental attitudes strongly influence what a child perceives as "good, clean, loved and pleasing" about his body and body parts and what he views as "bad, dirty, disliked or repulsive." During the developmental process a value comes to be attached to the body as a whole. However, "the psychic investment in some parts of the body appears to be greater than in others, and this differential evaluation appears to be related to the meaning which these particular parts have in the life of the individual."[15] As individuals we thus tend to place individualized *meanings* and *values* on certain parts of our bodies more than others:

e.g., one person highly values his penis, while another places high value on his strong legs; one person values her small waist, while another values her long straight nose.

> Body protuberances and body orifices are highly important in orienting one to his own body as well as to his environment and to the bodies of others.

At these points communication with the body, other persons and the environment is most direct and closest. Therefore, body protuberances and orifices have particular value and meaning in one's body image.

As the child grows, his body image continues to develop through activities in which he compares his body with others, observes the reactions of others toward his body, and gains control of his body through mastering new tasks and exploring his environment. The normally curious child enjoys looking at pictures of the human body and is fascinated with knowledge of body functions.

Body image is highly important to the *adolescent.* Numerous physical and psychologic changes occur during this period of rapid growth and development. The adolescent is highly concerned with developing in a normal, attractive manner. A great deal of attention is focused on one's growth changes and appearance. Comparisons with one's peers are commonly and frequently made. *Young adults* may also be quite concerned with their body images and may make frequent comparisons of these images against the cultural norms of attractiveness. Western cultures tend to place high values on maintaining a youthful image. This poses problems for some persons in their *middle* to *late adult* years as hormonal changes and other physical changes occur with normal aging.

Thus, throughout one's life, one's body image continues to evolve. New experiential data are constantly bombarding one's nervous system and are audited there. "In illness and health there is a wide variety of messages about the body being constantly fed into the system, either for interpretation-acceptance with integration into the self or for rejection and revision."[46] As the reader can see, from even this brief introduction, body image is a complex phenomenon.

SITUATIONS CAUSING BODY IMAGE DISTURBANCES

Table 15–1 provides examples of normal and pathologic changes that can affect body image. It will be noted that this table focuses more on body image disorders than on normal body image.

Body image disturbances may be classified as consequent to the following categories of illnesses: "(1) disorders following *neurologic diseases* and affecting any part of the sensory or motor system connected with movement and posture, whether involving the peripheral or the central nervous system; (2) disorders occurring with changes in the body structure as an expression of acquired or induced *toxic or metabolic disorder;* (3) disorders consequent to *progressive deformation*, occurring either late or early in life caused by other somatic diseases; (4) disorders after *acute dismemberment;* and (5) disorders of *personality development*, including the psychoses, psychoneuroses, and psychopathic states."[32]*

_____
*Italics added.

TABLE 15–1.   EXAMPLES OF SITUATIONS AFFECTING BODY IMAGE

NORMAL SITUATIONS
Normal growth and development of infant, child, adolescent
Normal changes with pregnancy and aging

ELECTIVE SURGICAL CHANGES
Plastic surgery procedures that alter appearance, e.g., facelift, rhinoplasty, scar revision
Transsexual surgical procedures
Abortion

DISEASE OR OTHER DISORDER
Loss of body function, e.g., cerebrovascualr accident ("stroke"), paraplegia, quadriplegia, laryngectomy, epileptic seizure, bowel/bladder incontinence
Impaired organ function, e.g., coronary ("heart attack"), asthma attack, pneumonia
Pathophysiologic changes in body size and proportion, e.g., obesity, gigantism, acromegaly, emaciation
Alterations in skin color, e.g., chronic dermatitis, Addison's disease
Alterations in skin texture, e.g., scar formation, thyroid conditions, chronic skin ulcers, exfoliative and excoriative dermatitis
Psychopathologic disorders, e.g., schizophrenia, anorexia nervosa, hysteria, hypochondriasis
Disease-produced alterations that are visible (e.g., leprosy, cancer of the face) or affect internal organs, e.g., tuberculosis (lungs), cancer (bone, brain, uterus, pancreas); some patients with cancer, gangrene, tuberculosis or decubitus ulcers say they feel as if they are "rotting away" or being "eaten up"
Birth defects or anomalies, e.g., large birthmarks, cleft lip, extra body parts, absence or malformation of body parts or organs
Painful body part, e.g., migraine headaches, chronic pain problems such as phantom limb pain
Alterations in joints and muscles with atrophic and hypertrophic arthritis
Development of characteristics common to other sex, e.g., hirsutism in females, enlarged breasts in males

SURGERY OR TRAUMA
Loss of obvious body part traumatically or surgically, e.g., major body part (limb); sexually characteristic body part (vulva, penis, female breast); other obvious body parts (eye, nose, hair, teeth)
Loss of internal body part surgically, e.g., gallbladder, stomach, lung, kidney
Surgical replacement of body organ, e.g., kidney
Surgical change in relationship of body parts, e.g., gastrostomy, colostomy, ileostomy, ureteroenterostomy
Traumatic disfigurement resulting in body distortion and/or scars, e.g., burns, cuts, crushing injuries
Loss or alteration of internal body parts that have sexual significance, e.g., tubal ligation, hysterectomy, vasectomy, laryngectomy
Violent physical assaults, e.g., rape, shooting, knifing

DRUGS
Side effects of drug therapy, e.g., striated skin, "moon face," loss of hair, hirsutism
Drug-induced states, e.g., LSD, delirium tremens

SOCIAL INFLUENCE
Sexual performance, e.g., feelings of loving one's sexual partner well and of being well loved by that partner, or feelings of rejection sexually or dissatisfaction in sexual performance, e.g., impotence, frigidity, premature ejaculation, painful coitus
Sociocultural concepts of physical attractiveness and normality

Source: Prepared in part from material presented in Norris, C. M.: The professional nurse and body image. *In* Carlson, C. E. (coordinator): *Behavioral Concepts and Nursing Intervention.* Philadelphia, J. B. Lippincott Co., 1970.

Body image disturbances can also be classified according to whether the body image is[14] (1) *exaggerated*, e.g., during pain or with hypochondriasis; (2) *diminished*, e.g., following cerebral vascular accidents; (3) *distorted*, e.g., with drug intoxication, migraine headaches, vertigo or syncope; or (4) *phantom*, e.g., phantom pain, phantom limb or following mastectomy.

Intrusive nursing activities (e.g., body temperature measurement, insertion of nasogastric tube, catheterization of urinary bladder, suctioning of tracheobronchial tree or mouth or nose, and administration of injections and intravenous fluids) and *intrusive diagnostic or monitoring activities* (e.g., bronchoscopy, cystoscopy, sigmoidoscopy, gastroscopy, cardiac catheterization, dilatation and curettage) may be threatening to body image. Similarly, *surgical procedures* and *dental procedures* may be perceived as threats to body image since they cause alterations in body image. Nonsurgical treatment procedures can also cause changes in body image. For example, *side effects of medications* can cause changes in secondary sex characteristics or the development of facial changes such as "moon face"; or changes may occur in skin color as a result of *radiation*.

REACTIONS TO ALTERATIONS IN BODY IMAGE

A variety of factors influence a patient's *adaptation to body image* changes. Among these factors are[46] (a) reactions of significant others to the alteration in body image; (b) the patient's own coping ability; (c) the nature and meaning of the threat; and (d) the rate at which the body image change occurs and the extent or degree of change.

The *reaction of significant others* is an important factor in the adaptation of patients to body image changes. For example, while some patients receive support and encouragement from significant others, other patients are deserted by significant others and left to face their alteration in body image alone. Other factors affecting a patient's adaptation to changes in body image are the *patient's own coping ability* and *the nature and meaning of the threat*. "The person who has limited coping abilities to deal with stress, and who is easily made to feel helpless and powerless, will experience greater threat with a change in his body image. To understand the nature of the threat, then, one needs to know the pattern of adaptation, the value of this pattern for the particular individual, and what coping abilities he has."[46] Numerous *small* changes in body image which

are spread out over a longer period of *time* tend to be less threatening than one sudden, *large* body image change.

> *Acute disturbances of body image may occur following surgical or traumatic dismemberment when the basic body image persists in spite of the visible or apparent loss of a body part.*

The individual whose body image is distorted feels like a stranger to himself and to others. "I look different. Will I be loved and accepted? Have I become repulsive and ugly? How changed am I?" Anxieties of this type are deep-seated and can be relieved only by loving and accepting responses from significant persons in the individual's life.[51]

> *A distortion of one's customary body image is experienced as a distortion of the self. A disfigured person may fear separation from and rejection by significant persons upon whom he is dependent.*

Adaptation to alterations in one's body image may lag far behind the physical changes that have occurred, particularly if the changes occur traumatically or if they are undesirable. As mentioned earlier, individual reactions to alterations in body image are variable, depending in part upon a given individual's coping abilities and patterns of adaptation. (Anxiety and use of mental defense mechanisms are discussed in Chap. 8; behavioral reactions to the confirmation of illness are discussed in detail in Chap. 11.)

Francis and Munjas[20] divide ego adaptations following body image alteration into "expected ... more useful reactions" and "less healthy ... reactions." Reactions that may be expected and are not indicative of emotional pathologic disturbances include (a) *mourning* (see Chap. 48), (b) *fear of rejection by others*, (c) *hostility* and (d) *"phantom"* sensations of missing body parts. While these reactions may be expected, they should be assessed in terms of their degree and persistence. Less healthy ego adaptations include (a) *denial*, (b) *severe depression* and (c) *failure to reintegrate*. Norris[46] notes that *shame* may be a response to those body image alterations that cause an individual to lose control of one's self or of one's immediate space, e.g., persons with impaired neuromuscular activity who have difficulty manipulating their bodies and performing the activities of daily living.

In our society, physical disfigurement is generally viewed with disapproval, repulsion and rejection. Deformity and disfigurement are therefore anxiety-provoking. "Despite evidence of social, vocational, and intellectual competency, the deformed are exposed to a kind of stereotyping which is socially disadvantageous. Pervasive as these attitudes are, there is a reality basis for the high concern manifested by patients with physical deformities."[32] In other words, many physically deformed persons *do* experience *rejection by others.* As a part of separation anxiety, deformed persons may feel *hostile* toward significant others. Also, they may feel hostile toward surgeons and other people (e.g., nurses) involved in their care.

Distortions of body image also modify a patient's unconscious mental life. Thus, he may *repeatedly dream* of the incident that caused his disfigurement and/or may have a wish-fulfilling dream life in which the lost part plays an active role. In some patients the threat or actuality of trauma associated with surgical procedures may reawaken *repressed fantasies of personal mutilation.* It is not unusual for patients who are to have limb amputations to be concerned about how the separated limb will be handled and disposed of. Sometimes actual *psychotic reactions,* related to distortions of body image, follow acute trauma or prolonged somatic disease.[32]

Because disturbances in body image are threatening and anxiety-provoking, *denial* is frequently used by these patients. For example, paraplegic patients may deny that their paralysis is permanent. *Depressive reactions* also occur frequently following disfigurement.

Alterations in body image have been demonstrated[3] to occur as a result of long-term confinement to a wheelchair. Because a wheelchair is present between the body and the external world, the body itself ceases to perform its normal function of contact with the environment; body image boundaries deteriorate because of disuse, and judgments about body boundaries become inaccurate. In this situation, body image boundaries no longer have the needed contact with the environment that provides the body with the feedback necessary for a continuing evaluation of its status and boundaries.

Following cerebrovascular accidents resulting in paralysis of limbs, the patient often feels as if the paralyzed limb were not a part of himself or as if it were gone, even though it is still a part of his body. Following amputation, the opposite occurs: the patient generally feels as if the missing body part were still present; he experiences a persisting *"phantom"* of the body part. Phantom sensations (occurring as if present in the missing part) may or may not be painful. While phantoms of amputated limbs are the most frequently encountered, phantoms may also occur following removal of other body protuberances (e.g., nose, eyes, teeth, nipples, breasts, penis) and other body parts of which one has conscious awareness.

The importance of body image and its distortion in illness can be illustrated by considering facial or mouth pain. Because of its importance in our communication with others, the face may frequently be involved in difficulties that we have with self-concept and in communicating our needs to others. The face becomes almost synonymous with the self.[51] When pain of the face or mouth occurs, therefore, the particular emotional significance of these body areas must be considered in understanding the total problem. Face pain after traumatic alteration of the facial configuration—i.e., through accident or surgery—may persist markedly past the time it might be expected to on the basis of the organic pathology. Such pain is understandable if we realize that the patient interprets the damaged face as damaged "self."

Body image and self-image are also of importance in understanding the problem of obesity. In some instances the obese individual's self-image may provide an important cornerstone for his emotional adjustment, so that weight loss, with its accompanying change in self-image, is anxiety-provoking and perhaps is emotionally detrimental. Mathis comments on this:

It is not enough to recognize that psychogenic factors exist. It is necessary to understand that although overeating has a significant meaning to the patient, the resulting obesity also may serve an important function. It is quite irrational to tamper with the overeating unless one is also prepared to deal with the function of the excessive weight. It is quite similar to the symptoms of a neurotic illness in that their removal without attention to the basic cause may produce more discomfort than the original symptoms. This means that the physician may at times decide that weight reduction is not in his patient's best interest, or that it should be combined with psychiatric assistance.[37]

Bellak[5] observes that when a person is ill with heart disease or disease of some other organ, the patient develops a special image of the involved organ which could be called an *"organ image."* When this occurs the organ looms predominantly in the patient's thoughts, and his attitude toward the sick organ may change in such a way that the organ itself becomes *anthropomorphized* in his thinking; i.e., he thinks of the organ as something independent, needing special care. The patient's attitude toward his sick organ (and thus, toward himself) may become overprotective and oversolicitous.

When an individual fails to reorganize his body image over a period of time following distortions or changes in his body, he has not made an appropriate psychologic adaptation. Such *maladaptive states* often occur in individuals for whom the integrity of the pre-illness or pre-accident body image was overvalued in maintaining self-esteem. For example, limb amputees generally adapt poorly to limb loss if the integrity of a limb symbolizes either masculinity or femininity to them. Thus, the *meaning* of the bodily defect to the individual is highly important. Kolb comments, "Depending upon the individual, the loss may have any meaning such as heroic sacrifice or a deserved punishment, a realization of helplessness and vulnerability, a conviction of loathsomeness, a despicable mutilation to be hidden or accepted, or a rejection of the part with defiance toward society and social customs."[32]

Because they emulate the generally rejecting attitudes of their families, peers and society as a whole, most patients with body defects manifest unhealthy attitudes and behavior in relation to their bodies. *Indications of rejection of one's body image include:*[32]

▶ Reluctance to meet others

▶ Reclusive tendencies

▶ Unwillingness to look into mirrors or to look directly at one's altered body part

▶ Unwillingness to discuss the deformity

▶ Unwillingness to accept corrective surgery, corrective aids, vocational rehabilitation, or other devices that aid rehabilitation

ASSISTING PATIENTS WITH BODY IMAGE CHANGES

When I got up at last . . . and had learned to walk again, one day I took a hand glass and went to a long mirror to look at myself and I went alone. I didn't want anyone . . . to know how I felt when I saw myself for the first time. There was no noise, no outcry; I didn't scream when I saw myself. I just felt numb. That person in the mirror *couldn't* be me. . . .

Over and over I forgot what I had seen in the mirror. It could not penetrate into the interior of my mind and become an integral part of me. I felt as if it had nothing to do with me; it was only a disguise . . . put on me without my consent . . . as I looked in the mirror . . . I saw in the place where I was standing a

stranger, a little pitiable, hideous figure. . . . It *was* only a disguise, but it was on me for life. It was there, it was real. Every one of those encounters, each time I looked in the mirror was like a blow on the head. They left me dazed and dumb and senseless every time, until slowly and stubbornly my robust persistent illusion of well-being and of personal beauty spread all through me again, and I forgot the irrelevant reality and was all unprepared and vulnerable again.[63]

Millions of persons must face the psychic trauma of unwanted changes in body image. Each of these individuals undergoes a personal crisis at such a time and is in need of the help and support of his significant others. Often it is nurses who are looked to first for assistance with the crisis that must be faced. Caring for patients undergoing body image changes requires all the skills, sensitivities and compassions health care professionals may have. It is in this area of care in which we try perhaps to heal the deepest wound of all—the wound to one's self-image. (See Chap. 3 for discussion of therapeutic nurse-patient relationship.)

The patient who has undergone traumatic body image assault may pass through the following four stages[47] as he moves toward acceptance of his body image changes: (1) impact, (2) retreat, (3) acknowledgment and (4) reconstruction.

Impact.　This stage is often experienced as a state of shock in which the person depersonalizes the experience. Significant others may also be in a state of shock. The nurse (a) establishes priorities of care (first priority is to sustain the patient's life), (b) examines her own feelings about the trauma and how it was caused, and (c) recognizes that she is involved in a high anxiety situation. In the last two instances the nurse is aware that patient, family and friends may quickly pick up on any expressions that are judgmental or indicate negative feelings such as repulsion. Also, the nurse works to reduce anxieties by not demanding decisions from patient or family and by providing appropriate brief yet truthful answers to questions.

Retreat.　Retreat is the second phase and is characterized by a period in which both patient and family have very high anxiety levels, which cause them to withdraw or flee. Reality is pushing forward on its own; the nurse should not force reality during this period but rather helps the patient and family accept it in small amounts. Denial may occur. It should be accepted but not reinforced. The period of retreat helps the patient and family reorganize their inner forces and prepare to move ahead.

Acknowledgment. During this stage the patient mourns the losses, which he now acknowledges. The patient may withdraw, isolate himself and refuse treatments, interactions, etc. (See discussion of grieving, Chap. 48.) He may be argumentative, sarcastic and possibly suicidal. At times he may lapse back into denial. Family members must change their concept of the patient. Some family members attach themselves to the staff; others withdraw. The helpful nurse remains available to the patient and family to provide appropriate support in movements toward acceptance of the patient's condition. This help includes exploration with the patient and family of the meaning(s) of the patient's change in body image. The nurse also assesses the patient's level of depression and is aware of the possibility of suicide attempts in the presence of moderate to severe depression. Whenever possible the patient is included in treatment plans and activities.

Reconstruction. Reconstruction is the final phase passed through by persons who have undergone traumatic body changes. This is a period of adjustment to technical devices or procedures, reorganization of social values and reintegration of the altered body image. The nurse's support and counsel continue to be invaluable to both patient and family. Future goals are established. Interpersonal relationships between the patient and his significant others are re-examined and reoriented; future goals and plans are made. Some regression may occur.

Crowley[14] comments: "In working with the patient who is suffering from a serious disturbance in body image, one's goals are to reduce anxiety to the point where [the] patient is able to view his situation comfortably and support him as he begins the task of reconstructing or changing his body image."

Nursing assessment of a patient with altered body image focuses heavily upon trying to identify the meaning(s) of the change to the individual patient. Assessment thus includes consideration of factors discussed earlier in this chapter, such as (a) the patient's developmental level (e.g., age); (b) the patient's self-concept in terms of such characteristics as attractiveness, strengths, individuality; (b) the patient's perception of the body image change; (c) perception of the patient's body image change by his significant others; (d) sociocultural views of the kind of body image alteration experienced by the patient; (e) the patient's occupation or other major life roles; and (f) the patient's preparation for the body image change.

Whenever possible patients should be psychologically prepared in advance of procedures that may change their body image severely, e.g., elective surgical procedures, radiation, chemotherapy for cancer. Examples of surgical procedures that change body image markedly include radical mastectomy, hysterectomy, colostomy, ileostomy, abdominal-perineal resection and radical excisions of the head, face and neck.

Summarized below are some additional nursing activities of importance in the care of persons experiencing body image changes:

▶ Recognize that persons subjected to sudden, unexpected, marked body image changes have not had any opportunity to prepare themselves mentally for these changes before they occur. The shock of the alteration may thus be experienced more intensely than occurs with persons who have undergone elective surgical procedures. Persons undergoing planned (elective) surgery usually have had the opportunity to consider possible body image alterations that will be present postoperatively.

▶ Consider the patient's typical patterns of adaptation and his coping capacities. Body image changes tend to pose a greater threat to persons with limited coping abilities for dealing with stress. The superior nurse is aware of the kinds of coping mechanisms that people tend to use following body image alterations. Thus, when possible, she plans care directed toward *preventing* less healthy ego adaptations by providing appropriate support and by recognizing and relieving anxieties experienced by patients and their significant others.

▶ Assist the patient to gradually look at visible changes to his body, e.g., following trauma or surgery. The sensitive nurse is aware of a patient's peeks at his incision during dressing changes or his glances at himself in the mirror. Be supportive of the patient during these activities and recognize that the patient is obtaining important visual feedback of his altered body.

▶ Assist the patient's significant others in their adjustments to the patient's altered body image by preparing them for the changes before they visit the patient. Provide opportunities for them to discuss their concern and express their feelings.

▶ Offer appropriate encouragement to the patient to express his feelings and concerns about his altered body image.

▶ Listen to the patient to identify areas of confusion and to become aware of how his behavior makes sense to him.

▶ Reduce the patient's anxiety by supporting areas of healthy coping and avoiding confrontation in troubled areas.

▶ Assist the grieving patient to adjust to his losses relating to body image alterations (see Chap. 48).

▶ Assist the patient to regain a balanced view of himself by not giving exaggerated attention to the altered body part.

▶ Respect the patient's need for privacy.

▶ Communicate, through your nursing care, your concern for and interest in the patient's body. Through your ability to care for and respect a patient's mutilated or otherwise changed body, he can learn to reassess his own possible feelings of dislike and revulsion concerning his body.

▶ Touching the patient's altered body part in appropriate ways can give the patient sensory input (perceptual feedback) that is helpful in his body reorientation.

▶ Encourage the patient to move. Movement helps to build body image by bringing the body into new relationships with itself, other people and the environment. Either passive or active movement of affected parts can provide this important kinesthetic feedback. When performing passive movements provide the patient with verbal feedback of movements being performed, e.g., "I'm lifting your arm off the pillow. Now I'm bending your elbow."

▶ Help the patient to become involved in caring for his body so that he can learn to love his body as it now exists. Through self-care, the patient directly increases those visual, tactile and proprioceptive* stimuli that help him learn to know his body once again.

▶ Show your respect for the patient's body by helping with matters of personal cleanliness and by performing activities that improve the patient's appearance; e.g., shampoo and set hair, supply clean gowns, offer cosmetics, apply deodorants. Of course, if the patient is capable of performing these ac-

Proprioceptive stimuli arise within bodily tissues (primarily the muscles, tendons and labyrinth) and provide information about the body's position and movement.

tivities, he should be encouraged to do so. (Chap. 27 discusses basic patient hygiene.)

▶ Provide clear explanations of body image changes that result in changes of body functioning.

Open discussions of body image changes that affect sexuality are helpful when the patient is ready. The nurse who lets her own modesty stand in the way of providing the patient with frank, clear discussions of his sexual functioning and other aspects of his sexuality is doing the patient a great disservice. The patient is in need of an informed professional person who can comfortably and clearly discuss all aspects of sexual expression. Appropriate areas of discussion might include (a) effect of the body image change on ability to reproduce; (b) modifications in intercourse following radiation, trauma or surgery; and (c) problems related to cosmetic appearance, e.g., scarring, alopecia (loss of hair), hirsutism (abnormal growth of hair), severe acne, need for prostheses (e.g., artificial breast or limb), altered innervation (paralysis), altered appearance due to dissipation or disability.

Discussions of possible problems that may occur during first attempts at intercourse following body image changes might include such topics as preliminary stimulation, lubrication and alternative positions. The interested, concerned nurse who is well informed can do a great deal to help persons with body image changes to regain pleasurable feelings of sexuality and to re-experience fulfilling sexual expression. Often it is desirable to have discussions relating to sexuality with both the patient and his sexual partner. In this way both the patient and the partner begin to realistically view the patient's body image alterations, and they begin to re-establish their lives in meaningful ways.

During all interactions with the patient, be certain you are using language the patient can understand. This requires careful assessment on your part. Helpful interaction requires more than simply making "telling" (informing) kinds of statements. However, when making statements that provide the patient with information, be sure to use language he is likely to understand. Also, don't assume that the patient "understands" what you have told him simply because you have "told" him.

Encourage the patient to interact with other

people. Experiencing the reaction of others to one's body and one's reaction to theirs is important in altering body image. The patient must learn to relate to others with his changed body. Initial interactions may be very difficult for a patient (and his significant others) when deforming body image changes have occurred. Once again, the nurse's support is essential in helping the patient with altered body image to continue to meet his needs for self-actualization, self-esteem, security, inclusion, affection and control.

The skillful nurse identifies a patient's feelings of isolation, rejection, shame, helplessness, discomfort and grief. Furthermore, she knows that *any one* of these feelings can be emotionally painful and that when they occur in combination (as they often do) they can be crushing.

Some body image disturbances can be prevented by measures such as providing appropriate counseling services to avoid genetic and constitutional defects and by providing safer work and social environments to minimize accidental trauma. Nurses may participate in all these activities.

BIBLIOGRAPHY

1. Ammon, L. L.: Surviving enucleation. *American Journal of Nursing*, 72:1817–1821, Oct. 1972.
2. Anderson, E. K.: Sensory impairments in hemiplegia. *Archives of Physical Medicine and Rehabilitation*, 52:293–297, July 1971.
3. Arnhoff, F. N., and Mehl, M. C.: Body image deterioration in paraplegia. *Journal of Nervous and Mental Diseases*, 137:88, July 1963.
4. Basch, S. H.: The intrapsychic integration of a new organ. A clinical study of kidney transplantation. *Psychoanalytic Quarterly*, 42:364–384, 1973.
5. Bellak, L. (ed.): *Psychology of Physical Illness.* New York, Grune & Stratton, 1952.
6. Blaesing, S., and Brockhaus, J.: The development of body image in the child. *Nursing Clinics of North America*, 7:597–607, Dec. 1972.
7. Brown, F. L.: Knowledge of body image and nursing care of the patient with limb amputation. *Journal of Psychiatric Nursing*, 2:397–406, July–Aug. 1964.
7a. Bucy, N., Unruh, I., and McFadden, G. A.: Lead your maimed patient back to independence. *RN*, 40:29–32, June 1977.
8. Cardone, S. E., et al.: Psychophysical studies and body-image. IV. Disturbances in a hemiplegic sample. *Archives of General Psychiatry*, 21:464, Oct. 1969.
9. Compton, C. Y.: War injury: identity crisis for young men. *Nursing Clinics of North America*, 8:53–66, March 1973.
10. Corbeil, M.: The nursing process for a patient with a body image disturbance. *Nursing Clinics of North America*, 6:155–163, March 1971.
11. Costello, A. M.: Supporting the patient with problems related to body image. *Proceedings of the National Conference on Cancer Nursing, Chicago, September, 1973.* American Cancer Society, 1974.
12. Craft, C. A.: Body image and obesity. *Nursing Clinics of North America*, 7:677, Dec. 1972.
13. Crate, M. A.: Nursing functions in adaptation to chronic illness. *American Journal of Nursing*, 65:72–76, Oct. 1965.
14. Crowley, D.: Body Image. Presented at the Institute, "The Unconscious Patient and the Disoriented Patient," sponsored by the University of Washington School of Nursing, April 14, 1966.
15. Crowley, D.: *Pain and Its Alleviation.* Los Angeles, University of California School of Nursing, 1962.
16. Dempsey, M. O.: The development of body image in the adolescent. *Nursing Clinics of North America*, 7:609–615, Dec. 1972.
17. Donovan, M. I., and Pierce, S. G.: *Cancer Care Nursing.* New York, Appleton-Century-Crofts, 1976, pp. 204–254.
18. Dorpat, T. L: Phantom sensations of internal organs. *Comprehensive Psychiatry*, 12:27–34, 1971.
19. Fisher, S., and Cleveland, S. E.: *Body Image and Personality.* Princeton, NJ, D. Van Nostrand Co., 1958.
20. Francis, G. M., and Munjas, B.: *Promoting Psychological Comfort.* Dubuque, Iowa, Wm. C. Brown Co., 1968.
21. Fujita, M. T.: The impact of illness or surgery on the body image of the child. *Nursing Clinics of North America*, 7:641, Dec. 1972.
22. Gallagher, A. M.: Body image changes in the patient with a colostomy. *Nursing Clinics of North America*, 7:669–676, Dec. 1972.
23. Gardner, W. H.: Adjustment problems of laryngectomized women. *Archives of Otolaryngology*, 83:31–42, 1966.
23a. Gold, D. D., Jr.: Psychologic factors associated with obesity. *American Family Physician*, 13:87–91, June 1976.
24. Gorman, W.: *Body Image and the Image of the Brain.* St. Louis, Warren Green, 1969.
24a. Hill, S.: The child with ambiguous genitalia. *American Journal of Nursing*, 77:810–814, May 1977.
25. Hirt, M., et al.: Attitudes to body products among normal subjects. *Journal of Abnormal Psychology*, 74:486, Aug. 1969.
26. Hogan, R. M.: Mr. O'Brien's beard. *American Journal of Nursing*, 77:61, Jan. 1977.
27. Iffrig, S. M. C.: Body image in pregnancy. *Nursing Clinics of North America*, 7:631, Dec. 1972.
28. Jordan, H. S., and Cypress, R. M.: All-around care for the leg amputee. *Nursing '74*, 4:51–55, April 1974.
29. Kaufman, R. V.: Body-image changes in physically ill teen-agers. *Journal American Academy of Child Psychiatry*, 11:157, Jan. 1972.
30. Kikuchi, J.: A preadolescent boy's adaptation to traumatic loss of both hands. *Maternal Child Nursing Journal*, 1:19–31, Spring 1972.
31. Kneisl, C. R.: Body image, its meaning to the self. *Journal of New York State Nurses Association*, 2:29, Spring 1971.
32. Kolb, L. C.: Disturbances of the body-image. *In* Arieti, S. (ed.): *American Handbook of Psychiatry*, 2nd ed., Vol. IV. New York, Basic Books, 1975.
32a. Lee, D. C., and Harlan, W. R., Jr.: Medical sculpture: A valuable aid to patient rehabilitation. *American Family Physician*, 15:110–114, Feb. 1977.
33. Lee, J. M.: Emotional reactions to trauma. *Nursing Clinics of North America*, 5:577–587, Dec. 1970.
34. Leonard, B. J.: Body image changes in chronic illness. *Nursing Clinics of North America*, 7:687–695, Dec. 1972.

35. Loxley, A. K.: The emotional toll of crippling deformity. *American Journal of Nursing*, 72:1839–1840, Oct. 1972.
36. Mamaril, A. P.: Preventing complications after radical mastectomy. *American Journal of Nursing*, 74:2000, Nov. 1974.
37. Mathis, J. L.: Obesity—sin or savior? *Psychosomatics*, 6:171, May–June 1965.
38. Mayer, D. D.: Skin grafts: the patient. *American Journal of Nursing*, 64:98–101, Nov. 1964.
39. McCloskey, J. C.: How to make the most of body image theory in nursing practice. *Nursing '76*, 6:68–72, May 1976.
40. Meyer, J. K., et al.: Is plastic surgery effective in the rehabilitation of deformed delinquent adolescents? *Plastic and Reconstructive Surgery*, 51:53–58, Jan. 1973.
41. Miles, M. S.: Body integrity fears in the toddler. *Nursing Clinics of North America*, 4:39–51, March 1969.
42. Mosey, A. C.: Treatment of pathological distortion of body-image. *American Journal of Occupational Therapy*, 23:413, Sept.–Oct. 1969.
43. Murray, R. L. E.: Foreword: Symposium on the concept of body image. *Nursing Clinics of North America*, 7:593, Dec. 1972.
44. Murray, R. L. E.: Body image development in adulthood. *Nursing Clinics of North America*, 7:617–630, Dec. 1972.
45. Murray, R. L. E.: Principles of nursing intervention for the adult patient with body image changes. *Nursing Clinics of North America*, 7:697–707, Dec. 1972.
46. Norris, C. M.: The professional nurse and body image. *In* Carlson, C. E. (ed.): *Behavioral Concepts and Nursing Intervention*. Philadelphia, J. B. Lippincott Co., 1970.
47. Olson, E. V.: Immobility: effects on psychosocial equilibrium. *American Journal of Nursing*, 67:794–796, April 1967.
48. Orbach, C. E., and Tallent, N.: Modification of perceived body and body concept. *Archives of General Psychiatry*, 12:126–135, 1965.
49. Parkinson, M. H.: Is it . . . or isn't it? *New Zealand Nursing Journal*, 65:10–11, Oct. 1972.
50. Peterson, B. H.: Psychological reactions to acute physical illness in adults. *Medical Journal of Australia*, 1:311–316, March 2, 1974.
51. Pilling, L. F.: Psychosomatic aspects of facial pain. *In* Alling, C., III, et al. (eds.): *Facial Pain*. Philadelphia, Lea & Febiger, 1968.
52. Plutchik, R., et al.: Studies of body image: 1. Body worries and discomforts. *Journal of Gerontology*, 26:344–350, July 1971.
53. Riddle, I.: Nursing intervention to promote body image integrity in children. *Nursing Clinics of North America*, 7:651–661, Dec. 1972.
54. Rubin, R.: Body image and self-esteem. *Nursing Outlook*, 16:20–23, June 1968.
56. Schilder, P.: *The Image and Appearance of the Human Body*. New York, International Universities Press, 1950.
57. Schwab, J. J.: Body image and medical illness. *Psychosomatic Medicine*, 30:51–61, 1968.
58. Slade, P. D., and Russell, G. F. M.: Awareness of body dimensions in anorexia nervosa: cross-sectional and longitudinal studies. *Psychological Medicine*, 3:188–199, May 1973.
59. Smith, C. A.: Body image changes after myocardial infarction. *Nursing Clinics of North America*, 7:663, Dec. 1972.
60. Smith, E. C., et al.: Reestablishing body image. *American Journal of Nursing*, 77:445, March 1977.

61. Spire, R. H.: Photographic self-image confrontation. *American Journal of Nursing*, 73:1207, July 1973.
62. Stutz, S. D.: The nursing challenges of OB: when the baby isn't normal. *RN*, 34:40–43, Nov. 1971.
63. Thomas, B., and Carol, A.: Psychological aspects of physical trauma. *AORN Journal*, 15:45–50, Feb. 1972.
64. Tiedt, E.: The psychodynamic process of the oncological experience. *Nursing Forum*, 14(3):264–277, 1975.
65. Tierney, E. A.: Accepting disfigurement when death is the alternative. *American Journal of Nursing*, 75:2149–2150, Dec. 1975.
66. Tomlinson, W. K.: Psychiatric complications following severe trauma. *Journal of Occupational Medicine*, 16:454–457, July 1974.
67. Trowbridge, J. E.: Caring for patients with facial or intra-oral reconstruction. *American Journal of Nursing*, 73:1930–1934, Nov. 1973.
68. Ullman, M.: Disorders of body image after stroke. *American Journal of Nursing*, 64:89, Oct. 1964.
69. Vernon, A.: Explaining hysterectomy. *Nursing '73*, 3:36–38, Sept. 1973.
70. Waechter, E. H.: Developmental consequences of congenital abnormalities. *Nursing Forum*, 14(2):108–129, 1975.
71. Wapner, S., and Werner, H.: *The Body Percept*. New York, Random House, 1965.
72. Welty, M. J., Graham, W. P., and Rosillo, R. H.: The patient with maxillofacial cancer. II. Psychologic aspects. *Nursing Clinics of North America*, 8:152–164, March 1973.
72a. Wiley, L. (ed.): Battered body: A teenage amputee taught us four tips for better long-term care. *Nursing '78*, 8:36–41, Jan. 1978.
73. Wiley, L. (ed.): Psoriasis: don't add to its heartbreak. *Nursing '76*, 6:35–39, Nov. 1976.
74. Wiley, L. (ed.): The defeated patient: her worries come first. *Nursing '77*, 7:28–33, April 1977.
75. Williams, B. P.: The problems and life-style of severely burned man. *In* Bergersen, B. S., et al. (eds.): *Current Concepts in Clinical Nursing*, Vol. II. St. Louis, The C. V. Mosby Co., 1969.
76. Williams, R. L., and Krasnoff, A. G.: Body image and physiological patterns in patients with peptic ulcer and rheumatoid arthritis. *Psychosomatic Medicine*, 26:701–709, Nov.–Dec. 1964.
76a. Winkler, W. A.: Confronting one's changed image: choosing the prosthesis and clothing. *American Journal of Nursing*, 77:1433–1436, Sept. 1977.
77. Wolf, E. S.: Nursing care of patients with breast cancer. *Nursing Clinics of North America*, 2:587–596, Dec. 1967.
78. Zalewski, N., Geronemus, D., and Siegel, H.: Hemipelvectomy—the triumph of Ms. A. *American Journal of Nursing*, 73:2073–2077, Dec. 1973.
79. Zavertnik, J.: Emotional support of patients with head and neck surgery. *Nursing Clinics of North America*, 2:503–510, Sept. 1967.
80. Zimny, G. H.: Body image and physiological responses. *Journal of Psychosomatic Research*, 9:185, Oct. 1965.

ESTABLISHING MEDICAL-NURSING DIAGNOSES; PLANNING AND PROVIDING CARE

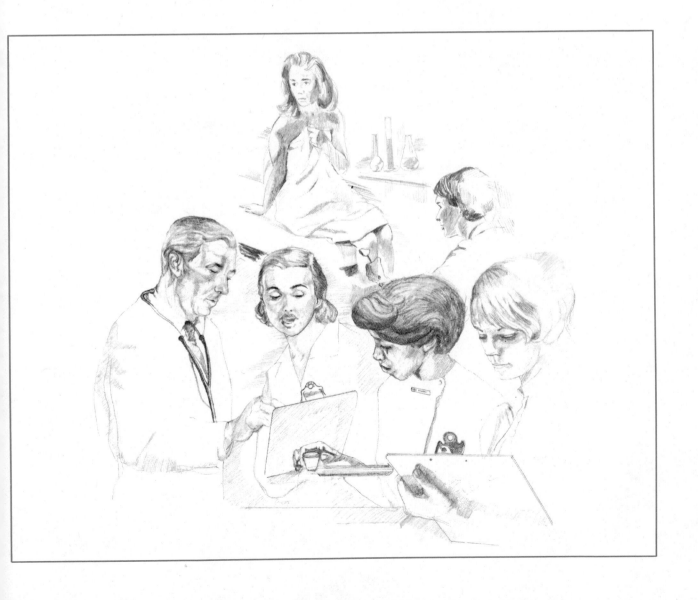

CHAPTER 16

DIAGNOSIS, TREATMENT AND REHABILITATION

INTRODUCTION AND STUDY GUIDE

Clearly, it is always more desirable to *prevent health problems* than to allow them to develop and then treat them. However, prevention is not always possible. Chapter 10 discussed recognizing the need for health care. This chapter considers the point at which the patient comes to a qualified health worker to have his symptoms diagnosed and treated.

This chapter focuses on some introductory concepts essential to the processes of diagnosis, treatment and rehabilitation. These often complex processes are best carried out by a multidisciplinary team of health professionals working in close cooperation with the client and his significant others. Clinical practices are increasingly becoming highly specialized. A variety of health workers may, therefore, participate in a client's plan of care. Specifically which person plans and administers the care varies, depending on factors such as the client's age, condition and location and on the availability and skills of the workers. As mentioned in Chapter 4, nurses may function in independent roles as private practitioners or therapists administering primary care. Most typically physicians prescribe diagnostic and therapeutic-rehabilitative procedures. They may carry out some of these activities themselves (often in consultation with physician specialists) or delegate them to other persons, e.g., the patient, family, nurses, or other professionals such as physical therapists.

As Chapter 4 has indicated, there are currently attempts under way to clarify nurses' roles in health assessment, illness prevention, diagnosis, treatment-rehabilitation, patient-family education and other areas of responsibilities and decision making. Areas being studied include: the review and updating of the laws under which nurses work (e.g., nurse practice acts); the establishment of nursing standards, nurse certification programs and intensive programs of professional nurse education; and the identification and implementation of patients' rights (Chap. 20).

> *Typically the basic health team consists of the patient, his significant others, the nurse and the doctor.*

The *patient* is the central figure in all of the health professionals' activities that affect him. *He* alone experiences the processes of health counseling, diagnosis, and treatment-rehabilitation. *He* interacts with the persons who are active in these processes; *his* life, mind and body are affected by the activities of health workers and the outcomes of these activities.

> Remember:
> *Ultimately it is always the right of the patient or his parents or guardian (as appropriate) to approve, accept or reject the plan of care proposed for him by health professionals. A patient's cooperation and understanding and the involvement of his significant others are essential for the effective planning, implementation and outcome of a program of care.*

Failure of a patient to adhere to prescribed treatments (patient noncompliance) is a problem that health professionals often encounter. Such situations must be carefully investigated with the patient to ensure development of a plan of care acceptable to him.

During the diagnosis and treatment-rehabilitation processes, assessment of the client's insight into his condition is an essential ongoing activity. Too often an unbalanced emphasis is placed on a patient's physical condition (when his most outstanding health problem is of a physical nature) and his psychosocial needs fail to be adequately recognized and met. The opposite may occur in patients whose health problems are most obviously of a psychosocial nature.

It should be noted that there are numerous diagnostic and therapeutic procedures in which it is necessary to have the patient's *informed consent* prior to carrying out the procedure. Examples of some of these procedures are endoscopy (visualization of the interior of the body), radiographic maneuvers involving the insertion of catheters, and all surgical procedures, including biopsies of tissues. Informed consent involves more than having the patient sign a form authorizing the performance of the recommended procedure. It also means that the patient must clearly understand the risks involved in the procedure. It is thus essential that the patient be given a clear explanation of the procedure to be performed, in language that he understands.[196] (See also Chaps. 19 and 20.)

This chapter is divided into three major sections: diagnosis, treatment, and rehabilitation. This division and sequence does not mean that we view rehabilitation as the third phase, or final stage, of a treatment program. On the contrary, our view is that rehabilitative activities should be appropriately integrated into all aspects of health care and should occur during all client-practitioner contacts. Such practices can prevent the development of many problems that might lengthen the period a client remains passively dependent and/or might result in permanent disabilities. Not only may the patient be subjected to unnecessary suffering, but also the financial costs of his health problem may be unnecessarily increased.

The rising costs of diagnostic and treatment-rehabilitative procedures pose serious problems and dilemmas. Health professionals are placed in the difficult position of trying to provide a client with the most thorough diagnostic work-up and best care possible, while also trying to keep the costs of such activities minimal or at best moderate. In some situations clients will neglect seeking necessary health care because of their concerns about cost. (Chap. 7 discusses changing concepts of health, disease and health care.)

STUDY GUIDE

This chapter contains a great deal of important information that you will need to study carefully, possibly repeatedly. The following study guide should prove helpful as you proceed:

Review carefully the comprehensive *bibliography* of this chapter and use it for reference as you seek additional information.

Because of the nature of this chapter, many *terms* and *phrases* are presented that may be new to you. We define in context as many of these as space permits; others you will need to look up. Perhaps you will want to prepare cards with definitions for study purposes. It is suggested that you learn the following:

informed consent	provisional diagnosis
history	definitive diagnosis
physical examination	lesion
diagnosis	sign
prognosis	symptom
clinical	objective
bacteriologic	subjective
physical diagnosis	localized
anatomic diagnosis	generalized
differential diagnosis	pathology

autopsy	supine position
holistic	prone position
ancillary examinations	dorsal recumbent position
adjuvant examinations	lateral
acute disorder	medial
chronic disorder	frontal plane
organic disorder	superior
functional disorder	inferior
prodromal symptoms	sagittal plane
cardinal symptoms	transverse plane
local symptoms	epigastric
constitutional symptoms	umbilical
syndrome	suprapubic (pelvic)
nursing history	hypochondriac
stethoscope	flank
otoscope	iliac
ophthalmoscope	inguinal
bronchoscope	roentgenography
cystoscope	radiopaque substances
laryngoscope	contrast studies
sigmoidoscope	fluoroscopy
speculum	CAT scan
fiberoptic scope	tomograms
sphygmomanometer	radioactive isotopes
thermometer	scan
tonometer	biopsy
inspection	clinical laboratory
palpation	pathology laboratory
percussion	physiatrist
auscultation	psychopharmacology
reflex hammer	iatrogenic disorder
density	preventive medicine
tuning fork	rehabilitation
Sims position	restorative phase
knee-chest position	social matrix
lithotomy position	

Suggestions for studying this chapter:

In your own words give some examples of different uses of the word *diagnosis*.

Differentiate between *signs* and *symptoms* and make a list of 10 possible signs and 10 possible symptoms.

As you study this chapter and Chapter 17, identify some differences between a *nursing prognosis* and a *medical prognosis* and between a *nursing history* and a *medical history*.

Familiarize yourself with the common abbreviations presented.

Identify the two major sets of activities in the diagnostic process and carefully review the steps under each of the major activities.

In your own words, discuss some factors that may make it difficult to establish a diagnosis.

Why is it important to establish an orderly sequence when conducting a history interview or performing a physical examination?

How might information about a patient's disorder be "indirectly" obtained?

Describe common activities in the diagnostic assessment of a patient with a psychiatric disorder.

In your own words, discuss five factors that may affect the way in which a patient gives his history and discusses his present symptoms. Provide at least one example of each of these factors. (This exercise would be suitable for group discussion.)

Familiarize yourself with major components of

medical and psychiatric histories. Carefully review the histories of patients in your care.

Numerous examples of disorders are provided in the sections of this chapter that discuss history taking and performance of physical examination. You may want to begin to look up information on those conditions that interest you. Again, preparing definition cards for review might be helpful.

Cite examples of how specific diagnostic tools can "extend the examiner's senses." Why is this important?

How are mirrors useful as diagnostic tools?

List four areas of the body that may be examined with a speculum.

What is the typical sequence in performing a physical examination and why is the sequence not used when examining the abdomen?

Why is it important to quantify observations whenever possible during physical examination? What are five measurements which might be made during physical examination?

Is it best to palpate tender areas first or last during physical examination?

List six characteristics that may be assessed by palpation. Which parts of the examiner's hand are best suited to assessing the six characteristics?

Familiarize yourself with common situations in which nurses employ inspection, palpation, percussion and auscultation.

In your laboratory and clinical experiences, practice inspection, palpation, percussion and auscultation. During percussion try to elicit and familiarize yourself with flat, dull, resonant, and hyperresonant sounds. (This will take time.) During auscultation, concentrate on frequency, intensity, quality and duration of sounds. Ask persons with skills in percussion and auscultation to help you learn.

Identify important factors in selecting and using a stethoscope.

Identify important nursing activities related to ancillary physical examinations.

What are some ways in which x-rays, radiopharmaceuticals, sound, temperature and electricity are used diagnostically?

What are "batteries" of laboratory tests?

Review carefully various uses of the word "treatment."

What considerations are important in deciding on optimum treatment?

Identify examples of patient compliance and noncompliance with treatment. Consider examples from your own experiences as a patient. Also, recall experiences of friends and relatives and patients you have cared for in your clinical experience. (This topic is appropriate for group discussion.)

What is meant by "therapeutic use of self"?

Familiarize yourself with various ways of classifying surgical procedures and various purposes of surgery.

What are four major treatment approaches used in psychiatric therapies? Provide at least two examples of each.

Familiarize yourself with areas of practice which are important in preventive medicine.

Provide some examples of irreversible, temporary and potential health problems.

What is a goal for rehabilitation in nursing?

Why is it important *not* to view rehabilitation as the final stage of treatment?

Distinguish between temporary, progressive and permanent health problems and the appropriate rehabilitation emphasis for each type of problem.

What are "self-help groups"? Find out what kinds of groups are available in your community, and if possible, arrange to attend some of their meetings.

Identify various local, state and national rehabilitation programs. You may wish to begin a card file of these programs for use in your practice. (This could be a group project.)

Consider what is meant by the nurse acting as "care coordinator" and "patient advocate" during rehabilitation activities.

In your clinical practice, assess each patient's needs for rehabilitation and implement appropriate plans. THINK REHABILITATION!

DIAGNOSIS

... it is easy for the most sensitive and compassionate of us to become too accustomed to patient examination, to treat it as an academic fact-finding tour and forget fears hidden behind those frequent patient smiles. It is similarly easy for us to take for granted the rare privilege extended to us by society and the individual patient when they permit us, even encourage us, to examine and question in a manner which if employed by another, unlicensed person would probably lead to arrest, jail, and conviction for assault and battery.[48]

Before therapeutic measure can be applied it is necessary to obtain a *history* (Hx) of the disorder and examine the patient. The examination process may combine a *physical examination* (PE) with various *special diagnostic techniques* and *laboratory studies*. As a result of this investigation the examiner hopes to learn about the source of the patient's disorder and the metabolic, chemical or pathologic structural changes caused by the disorder. *Care* and *treatment* (Rx) are then planned, based upon the *diagnosis* (Dx).

> *In the process of making a diagnosis, the patient's history, appearance, behavior and description of symptoms are assessed along with results of a physical examination and data from special diagnostic tests, e.g., laboratory, x-ray, pathology.*

Once the patient's problem is diagnosed, an

assessment is made of the *prognosis* (Px) of the condition, i.e., the probable outcome of the disorder. (Chap. 17 discusses prognosis further and compares the medical and nursing prognoses.) It is important to view diagnoses and prognoses as educated predictions rather than as absolute certainties.

Terminology

Diagnosis generally refers to the identification of a disease by the investigation of its manifestations, i.e., its signs and symptoms. However, the student of nursing soon observes that the term "diagnosis" is (a) often preceded by various qualifying adjectives and (b) used in ways that may or may not refer to a disease process. Such usage can be confusing, and an effort must be made to understanding the precise meaning of the phrase being used.

For example, a *medical diagnosis* typically refers to a disease and is usually expressed in terms based on anatomic concepts and words, e.g., duodenal ulcer. On the other hand, a *nursing diagnosis* describes the identification of "nursing problems," i.e., difficulties a patient and his significant others are experiencing in managing the satisfaction of one or more basic human needs. (See Chap. 17 for additional discussion.)

Psychiatric diagnoses are sometimes expressed in behavioral terms (e.g., reactive depression), or the primary difficulty the client is having may be stated more clearly in simple words (e.g., despondency following death of a loved one). The latter statement is more meaningful to the client should he read his chart or when his diagnosis and symptoms are discussed with him, e.g., during treatment.

You will encounter the term "diagnosis" used in still other ways, for example, in phrases referring to the diagnostic method: physical diagnosis, anatomic diagnosis, laboratory diagnosis, clinical diagnosis, bacteriologic diagnosis. In these examples the word "diagnosis" pertains to the result of observations made by particular methods; however, it does not necessarily identify a disease process. A *physical diagnosis*, for example, encompasses a group of procedures that focus on determining the normal or abnormal state of various organs. An *anatomic diagnosis* typically is a brief descriptive summary of the major anatomic lesions seen during an autopsy. A disease may or may

not be identified by the lesions listed in such a summary.

The term "diagnosis" may also be used in a variety of phrases indicating various levels in the steps of the diagnostic process or indicating the degree of certainty of the diagnosis. For example, one often sees on a patient's record the term *differential diagnosis*, followed by a list of several possible diagnoses. This list encompasses all of the diseases or conditions that are being currently considered and that are in the process of being systematically "ruled out" (R/O) or confirmed. Another common phrase is *provisional diagnosis*. A provisional diagnosis is a temporary, "working" diagnosis, based upon findings from the patient's history and physical examination. Such a diagnosis may later prove to be correct, or it may be replaced with a more accurate diagnosis, i.e., a *definitive diagnosis*, reached after reviewing findings from special diagnostic procedures. Figure 16–1 summarizes one view of the steps of diagnosis.

As mentioned previously, medical diagnoses are commonly expressed in terms based upon anatomic concepts. Many of these disorders are never directly observed in an ill person. For example, instead of actually seeing lobar pneumonia (inflammation and consolidation of one or more lobes of the lung) in a patient, the clinician observes the signs and hears about the symptoms produced by the pneumonia, e.g., fever, coughing, breathing difficulty, weakness, chill, pain in the side.

History-taking (i.e., talking in an organized way with a patient about the onset of his disorder) is used to obtain information about the patient's symptoms—how his disorder is causing him to feel. The signs of a disorder, on the other hand, are identified by the process of

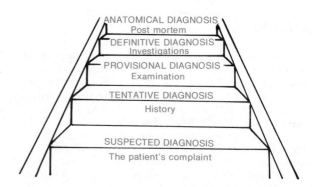

Figure 16–1. The steps of diagnosis. A suspected diagnosis, tentative diagnosis or provisional diagnosis may each be viewed as a "working" (temporary) diagnosis. (From Gelfand, M.: *Diagnostic Procedures in Medicine.* London, Butterworth & Co., Ltd., 1974, p. 35.)

physical examination, in which the examiner uses her own senses to study the "objective tracks"[48] of a disease.

Therefore, *signs* of illness technically are those observations of an ill person that the clinician makes during the physical examination of the patient. *Symptoms* are the patient's own recognitions that something is abnormal; his "complaints" or statements about what he is experiencing, e.g., pain, dizziness, nausea, fatigue, anxious feelings. Signs of illness are thus *objective* findings, while symptoms are *subjective* reportings. Subjective information refers to things that only the individual perceives, i.e., what he thinks, sees, feels, smells, hears, tastes.

It is important that subjective information be clearly identified as being reported by the patient and arising from within him. In communicating such information, the nurse can begin with statements such as, "The patient reports he is experiencing. . . ." or "Mr. Jones says he is noticing. . . ." (The terms subjective and objective are discussed further in Chap. 17.)

In practice one frequently finds that the terms "signs" and "symptoms" are not used precisely and often are not separated. Signs are frequently included in discussions of symptoms. Some use the phrase *subjective symptom* in place of symptom and *objective symptom* instead of sign.

Listed below are abbreviations for some terms commonly used with reference to history-taking, diagnosis and physical examination:

Abd.	abdomen
Ant.	anterior
AP	anteroposterior
CC	current complaint
CNS	central nervous system
Dx	diagnosis
HEENT	head, eyes, ears, nose, throat
Hx	history
L	left
Lab.	laboratory
Lat.	lateral
LLQ	left lower quadrant
LUQ	left upper quadrant
L&W	living and well
MSE	mental status examination
PE	physical examination
PI	present illness
Post.	posterior
PERRL	pupils equal, round, regular and react to light and accommodation
Px	prognosis
R	right
RLQ	right lower quadrant
R/O	rule out
RUQ	right upper quadrant
Rx	treatment
Sx	symptom
WN	well nourished
WNL	within normal limits
WNWD	well nourished, well developed

Development of the Science of Diagnosis

The ability to make an accurate diagnosis with reliable regularity is actually quite new. It is of interest to realize that physicians did not know the primary cause of a single important disease as recently as 100 years ago.

Disease was considered to be supernatural in origin throughout roughly the first half of written history. Development of the process of physical diagnosis began when the Greeks concluded that disease was not divine in origin but of natural origin. They reasoned that if disease was natural in origin, it could be studied and its course predicted. Thus, the first conceptual leap in the history of medicine was made.

Errors in theories of disease were slowly corrected. Eventually it was concluded that diseases might arise *locally,* with *generalized* manifestations. This idea was the opposite of that previously held, and the new concept encouraged development of the sciences of pathology, anatomy and physiology.

The 19th century was a period of intensive study at the autopsy table. These investigations were combined with more careful study at the bedside, i.e., clinical study. Correlations thus began to be discovered between pathologic anatomic changes and the clinical manifestations of disease. The normal functions of normal structures were investigated along with the impaired functions of abnormal structures, i.e., disease processes. The origin of disease slowly became pinpointed to increasingly finer sublevels, e.g., from organs, to tissues, to cells, to subcellular levels.

Major diagnostic developments have occurred in the present century in laboratory techniques and other special diagnostic aids, e.g., specialized x-ray techniques, electrocardiography and hematology. Such advances are indeed of substantial importance. An inherent danger exists, however. With the continual refinement of investigative procedures there is a temptation to lose sight of the whole person within his complete life situation and to focus instead upon the microcosm of the disease process. Health professionals would do well to combine the specific skills and knowledge of the present with the holistic wisdom of the past.

The Diagnostic Process

The diagnostic process can be viewed in terms of two major sets of activities: (1) collecting the facts and (2) analyzing the facts.[83]

Steps in Diagnosis*

1. *Collect the facts*
   A. Obtain clinical history.
   B. Perform physical examination.
   C. Carry out ancillary examinations, e.g., laboratory, x-ray.
   D. Observe the course of the disorder.

2. *Analyze the facts*
   A. Evaluate critically the collected data.
   B. List reliable findings in order of apparent importance.
   C. Select one or preferably two or three central features.
   D. List disorders in which these central features are encountered.
   E. Reach final diagnosis by selecting from the listed disorders either (1) the single disorder that best explains all the facts or, if this is not possible, (2) several disorders, each of which best explains some of the facts.
   F. Review all evidence (positive and negative) with the final diagnosis in mind.

---

*Adapted from p. 7 of Harvey and Bordley.[83]

Diagnostic errors may occur as a result of inaccuracies in any of the above steps. "Working diagnoses" direct the diagnostic activities and are revised as appropriate after each successive step in the diagnostic process.

The diagnostic process varies in complexity and duration. Some diagnoses are simple or immediately apparent; others are complex or elusive. For example, with acute disorders or following accidents the processes of history-taking and examination are quite brief, and a diagnosis may be made rapidly. In other situations, such as long-term (chronic) illnesses, the history and examination process may be quite lengthy. A thorough history is important in chronic diseases of organic origin and in psychiatric disorders.

In making diagnoses it must be remembered that some disorders imitate others and that a given disorder may present symptoms that vary from one individual to another. Of course, it is easier to diagnose conditions that occur commonly than to identify those which are rare and obscure. Also, it is not unusual for a given person to have several disorders present at the same time.

Signs and symptoms are usually closely correlated in the presence of *organic disorders*. The signs found by an examiner during a physical examination, therefore, commonly correspond with the symptoms mentioned by the patient during the history-taking process. Such

clear-cut patterns, however, are not always present. For example, a highly anxious patient may experience symptoms (e.g., upset stomach) for which no demonstrable signs are present. In other words, the patient may be experiencing the distress of indigestion even though the physical examination does not demonstrate physical (organic) findings which might explain the symptom of indigestion. In this instance the patient may eventually be diagnosed as having a *functional disorder*, i.e., a nonorganic difficulty. Let us emphasize that a functional diagnosis is not made without an extensive investigation of the patient's symptoms, i.e., it is not made merely on the basis of a physical examination. Laboratory and radiologic studies (x-rays), may also be done, for example.

An orderly, thorough approach to diagnostic activities is essential to ensure that nothing of significance is overlooked.

The expert clinician thus acquires the habit of doing a physical examination, mental status examination or history interview in exactly the same sequence. (These activities are all discussed in following pages.) The routines are modified only in special circumstances, e.g., emergencies when rapid assessment is essential, with unconscious patients. Clinicians typically develop their individualized sequence of examination and interview. It is not unusual for some history-taking to be combined with the physical examination. The skillful examiner improvises and builds on what her findings are as she proceeds with the examination. One finding alerts the examiner to other important observations.

Experts agree that *it is dangerous to jump to conclusions, establish mental blocks, or play hunches in formulating a diagnosis.* All of these activities can be misleading, drawing the clinician away from the correct diagnosis.

The diagnostic process is an ongoing, fluid process rather than a fixed, "one-time-only" activity. The pieces of the initial diagnostic puzzle gradually fall into place, often to be replaced later with additional diagnostic puzzles in the same patient. As the treatment plan proceeds, relationships change between the puzzle's pieces—symptom intensity varies, new symptoms may develop while others disappear, complications develop, cures occur. Periodic re-examinations are thus important.

Tentative diagnostic opinions usually are formed and then subjected to further testing until a refined, complete diagnosis is obtained. Such a diagnosis not only identifies (classifies) a patient's disorder but also may state the extent of involvement. Some diagnoses are ruled out (R/O), others are confirmed. Multiple diagnoses may be made in a given patient and combined treatment programs instituted.

> *Periodic reassessments of diagnosis and treatment are essential to monitor a patient's condition during the course of therapy.*

The process of making a diagnosis depends upon more than the diagnostician's technical knowledge. Keen clinical observations and thoughtful personal interaction cannot be replaced by sophisticated clinical laboratory techniques or other advanced diagnostic aids. The outstanding clinician relies heavily on her thoroughness, accurate observations, perceptiveness, interpretive skills, accumulation of knowledge and experience, interpersonal rapport and communication skills.

Computers are now being used in some settings to assist with various aspects of the diagnostic process. They are useful in some ways and inadequate in others. For example, a computer can correlate or screen extensive amounts of information and maintain an enormous memory bank. However, it cannot perform subtle activities that are important in the diagnostic process, such as picking up nonverbal communication cues. The sensitivities of human intelligence and person-to-person interaction cannot be replaced by computers. Also, the contact between the patient and examiner during the process of obtaining a history and performing a physical examination provides an important basis for establishing a meaningful "partnership."[48] This partnership is highly important in future health-maintenance or treatment activities between the clinician and client.

The process of establishing a diagnosis has been compared to the process of solving a crime. *Interrogation* and *examination* are essential skills in both of the problem-solving activities. In the process of making a medical or psychiatric diagnosis the clinician ("detective") may seek information about the patient's disorder (e.g., symptoms) *directly* from the patient, by taking a verbal or written history, or *indirectly,* by talking with the patient's significant others, other health care workers, etc. These activities are part of the "interrogation" process. (History interviews are discussed later in this chapter.)

Diagnostic *medical* examinations proceed along various lines, e.g., physical, chemical. For example, the patient's body may be examined by means of a physical examination. The examiner uses her own senses (e.g., vision, hearing, touching) as well as special diagnostic equipment, e.g., stethoscope. (Physical examination is detailed later in this chapter and an overview is given in Table 16–5.)

Findings from the history and physical examination direct the investigator toward other diagnostic methods (*ancillary examinations* or *adjuvant tests*) to be used. For example, if a patient gives a history of coughing and difficulty breathing, and the physical examination reveals that his lungs contain fluid, the examiner may decide to order x-ray studies of the lungs and a laboratory examination of sputum coughed up by the patient. Subsequent diagnostic procedures may include passing a scope (bronchoscope) into the lungs through the mouth to look at the inside of the tracheobronchial tree, removing a small portion of tissue (biopsy) with a needle or through the scope for laboratory study, or surgically opening the chest to directly explore the lung (exploratory thoracotomy).

Diagnostic activities can be time-consuming, inconvenient, expensive and uncomfortable for the client; therefore, patients should not be subjected to a particular diagnostic procedure unless it appears reasonably certain that clinically helpful information will be obtained. Special diagnostic tests should be chosen carefully on the basis of the relationship of their potential findings to the patient's suspected diagnosis. The test results are then used to assist in making a diagnosis or to confirm a suspected diagnosis.

The complete diagnostic assessment of a patient with a *psychiatric disorder* includes a history interview, mental status examination, assessment of pertinent social environmental factors and a complete physical examination. Other specialized diagnostic procedures such as those mentioned above (e.g., clinical laboratory tests) may be employed as appropriate. Psychologic testing, administered by a qualified psychologist, may be helpful in assessing some persons who present diagnostic problems. (Further discussions of a psychiatric history, mental status examination and psychologic testing are presented later in this chapter.) The physical examination includes related appropriate laboratory and other special studies, used to clarify and support initial diagnostic impressions. Consultation with a neurologist may be obtained, and a thorough neurologic examination may be performed.

Symptoms

Symptoms are common topics of both professional and nonprofessional communication. Nursing and medical literature contains countless books and articles focusing on symptoms. In this chapter we provide only the merest introduction to symptom assessment. Throughout your career you will continue to learn about symptoms on a professional level. On a personal level, quite possibly you will spend time listening to friends discussing their symptoms or time discussing your own symptoms. Even as you thumb through a magazine or watch television your attention is often directed to "symptoms" in commercials and advertisements.

How can you begin to make sense out of the information a patient presents as he tells you his symptoms during history taking? Possibly the following points will prove helpful.

▶ *Pinpoint as early as possible the body system or organ involved.*

▶ *Consider the relationship of the symptom to the structure and function of the organ involved.* Each of the body's various organ systems produces characteristic symptoms in the presence of disorders. For example, nausea, vomiting, constipation or diarrhea may occur in disorders in the stomach and intestinal tract. The presence of these symptoms thus directs the clinician's attention to assessment of the gastrointestinal system.

▶ *Identify what worsens (aggravates) or relieves (alleviates) the symptom.* For example, does the patient's chest pain become more severe when he is physically active? Is it relieved when he rests?

▶ *Consider the symptom in relationship to time.* For example, how long have symptoms been present? How have the symptoms changed with the passage of time? How often do the symptoms occur? Do the symptoms awaken the patient from sleep? These temporal relationships of symptoms, that is, the course of an illness, are important to assess. Such an assessment may involve making repeated clinical observations and diagnostic tests.

▶ *Assess associated events or symptoms.* Some disorders produce symptoms in a variety of body parts. For example, conges-tive heart failure may produce swelling of the ankles and abdomen and shortness of breath. Exploration of associated events may be highly revealing diagnostically. For example, it might be found that the acutely ill child has eaten a poisonous substance or the desperately ill adult might have been traveling recently and developed malaria or some other regional disorder. It might be learned that the patient with severe abdominal pain ate a very large meal, high in fat content, prior to developing his attack.

▶ *Realize that symptoms may signal the presence of a disorder that is more serious than the symptom itself,* e.g., constipation may indicate rectal cancer.

▶ *Recognize that patients may not mention their less dramatic symptoms because they do not view these symptoms as important,* e.g., constipation. Also, patients may be reluctant to mention symptoms that are *embarrassing* to them.

▶ *Use clear, correct terminology when referring to symptoms.* Psychologic and symptomatic terms used as symptoms must be clearly defined or understood. Examples of such terms are "depression" and "dyspnea." If such terms might be misunderstood, it is better to describe the symptom instead of—or in addition to—only using the term. This is a good practice! You will want to know the following general terms: (a) *prodromal symptoms,* those symptoms indicating the onset of an illness and noticed prior to the actual development of the illness, (b) *cardinal symptoms,* those symptoms of greatest significance in identifying the disorder, (c) *local symptoms,* those limited to particular body parts, and (d) *constitutional symptoms,* symptoms affecting the whole body, e.g., fever.

▶ *Recognize that characteristic symptom patterns are produced by some disorders and familiarize yourself with these patterns.* For example, local infection typically produces redness, swelling, temperature elevation and local pain.

Symptom patterns and symptom combinations often indicate specific diagnoses.

While one symptom may be predominant, symptoms usually do not occur alone, but rather are present in combination with other symptoms. The term *syndrome* refers to a group of symptoms that characterize a specific disorder. For example, a throat infection typically produces swollen neck glands, pain in the throat and fever. Thus, in assessing a disorder, it is helpful to look for familiar "clusters" of symptoms. Also, it is useful to identify *symptom patterns* and factors that change these patterns.

A final point concerning symptom evaluation is that it is helpful to remember a simple statement: *the most common disorders occur most commonly.* Headache, for example, is more likely to be caused by tension than by brain tumor, although it is symptomatic of both disorders. True, less common disorders must be kept in mind; however, the more common disorders are best considered first when assessing a patient's symptoms. Taylor[195] reminds us of an old proverb: *When you hear hoof-beats, don't look for zebras!* In other words, look first for what is most likely to be present.

A patient's symptoms are often of greater importance than physical examination or laboratory tests in the early stages of an illness. Indeed in some disorders, e.g., tension headache, the physical examination and laboratory tests may be normal. Diagnosis in these instances depends on a thorough evaluation of the patient's subjective complaints.

The following summary may be valuable as you practice symptom assessment:

ANALYSIS OF A SYMPTOM*

1. Total duration
2. Onset
   a. Date of onset (also determines total duration)
   b. Manner of onset (gradual or sudden)
   c. Precipitating and predisposing factors related to onset (emotional disturbance, physical exertion, fatigue, bodily function, pregnancy, environment, injury, infection, toxins and allergies, therapeutic agents)
3. Characteristics at onset (or any other time)
   a. Character (quality)
   b. Location and radiation (for pain)
   c. Intensity or severity
   d. Temporal character (continuous, intermittent, rhythmic; duration of each; temporal relationship to other events)
   e. Aggravating and relieving factors
   f. Associated symptoms
4. Course since onset
   a. Incidence
      (1) Single acute attack
      (2) Recurrent acute attacks
      (3) Daily occurrences
      (4) Periodic occurrences
      (5) Continuous chronic episode
   b. Progress (better, worse, unchanged)
   c. Effect of therapy

---

*From Hochstein, Elliot and Rubin, A. L. *Physical Diagnosis: A Textbook and Workbook in Methods of Clinical Examination.* New York, the Blakiston Division of the McGraw-Hill Book Company, 1964, p. 6. Used with permission of McGraw-Hill Book Company.

As a patient states his symptoms during the history interview, the interviewer must make important decisions about which of the symptoms presented she will select for further elaboration and possible investigation. Hodgkin[92] comments that if the symptoms chosen for elaboration are relatively insignificant, time will be wasted and possibly wrong conclusions will be reached. "It is possible for two doctors to interview a single patient and to obtain different histories because they have elaborated different symptoms." Hodgkin provides the following general rules about selection of the significant symptoms for elaboration:[92]

1. Elaborate those symptoms for which there is objective proof, i.e., if the patient says his skin itches and you can see signs of a rash.
2. Elaborate those symptoms that are localized to specific body parts or organs, e.g., diarrhea, cough, pain in knee.
3. Elaborate all symptoms that have obvious clinical relationships, e.g., cough and hemoptysis (coughing up and spitting blood from the respiratory tract).
4. Elaborate symptoms that are known to usually indicate serious disease, e.g., convulsions (involuntary muscle spasm or contraction, commonly called "seizures") or diplopia (double vision).
5. Put aside temporarily those symptoms known to occur in many disorders or those which are vaguely defined, e.g., listlessness, dizziness, headache, anorexia in children.
6. Put aside temporarily symptoms arising from causes that are unrelated to the main complaint and that can be managed separately, e.g., toothache in a patient with dyspnea (labored or difficult breathing). Remember that symptoms are only temporarily put aside and may later prove to be significant.

Medical and Psychiatric Histories

Typically when a patient first meets with a health clinician the clinician conducts an interview directed at identifying the patient's health history (clinical history) and present status, e.g., health disorders. This interview focuses on obtaining a *medical history* for patients with disorders essentially of a medical or surgical nature. Persons with primarily psychiatric disorders are interviewed to obtain a thorough *psychiatric history.*

While "medical model" history-taking is of vital importance in the diagnostic-treatment process, nurses need to remember that other information is necessary if comprehensive nursing care is to be offered. The additional information that a nurse needs includes such things as: (a) the habitual daily living patterns of an individual and his significant others and (b) the basic human needs that a patient is presently having difficulty satisfying. Such information can be obtained through a *nursing history*. A nursing history refers to the assessment and data-collection process a nurse uses when making a nursing diagnosis. Thus, a nursing history involves seeking information about more than a patient's symptoms. (See Chap. 17 for discussion of nursing history and nursing diagnosis.)

Concepts in History-Taking. History-taking obtains significant information about a patient in an organized manner. This information helps identify the patient's problems and provides data that serve as clues for proceeding with the physical examination and the selection of additional diagnostic activities.

A history that is well done provides an important data base for all members of the health team. Careful history-taking can, at relatively low cost, provide the greatest amount of information about a patient for the amount of time used. An axiom familiar to diagnosticians is: *Listen to your patient. He is telling you the diagnosis.*

The tone that an interviewer sets is highly important. The first 5 minutes of a history interview are very significant. Ideally a tone should be established that conveys to the client that the interviewer is concerned, attentive, trustworthy and skilled. The interviewer tries to let the patient know that his condition is being considered in a confidential, serious manner. A quiet, well-lit setting facilitates the interview. (Chap. 3 discusses the therapeutic relationship; Chap. 17 contains additional material about interviewing.)

The skillful interviewer is as concerned with what the patient may be trying to conceal as she is with what he is revealing. Remember, of course, that all of a client's omissions in history are not necessarily intentional. Some details may simply be forgotten (as you will discover if you try to reconstruct your own detailed medical history). The skilled interviewer (realizing that words are not all that is important in an interview) notices and evaluates obvious omissions, sudden shifts of subject matter, shying away from topics and nonverbal cues, e.g., facial expression, gestures, tone of voice.

A patient's account of his history and present symptoms is affected by such factors as his: (a) hopes and fears, (b) confidence in and reactions to the interviewer, (c) mental competence, (d) view of what actually is a reportable health disorder and (e) ability to observe and describe his life events.

Whenever possible a patient's physical discomforts, e.g., need to urinate, should be relieved before beginning the interview. If the patient is uncomfortable, he will have difficulty attending thoughtfully to the interview and his replies may be affected, e.g., he may give short, clipped, incomplete answers to questions.

During the history-taking interview the clinician not only begins to formulate ideas of possible diagnoses, but also assesses and records impressions of the patient's reliability. Patient reliability is important not only in regard to evaluating the information he is giving but also in considering how well the patient may cooperate with treatment plans.

Two objectives are important when taking a history: "(1) convince the patient of the importance and relevance of the questions being asked and (2) ascertain the complete sequence of events leading up to the present illness."[210] To meet the first objective, it is helpful to begin by focusing first on the patient's chief complaint, i.e., his present illness or reason for seeking health care. This demonstrates the clinician's interest in what is currently of greatest concern to the patient and elicits the patient's cooperation. After the patient is allowed time to briefly summarize, in his own words, without interruption, the reasons for his present contact with the health worker, the interviewer proceeds to take a more formal history.

While discussion of a patient's present disorder is of major interest in taking a history, it is also important to obtain information about the environment of the present illness. Thus, the clinician also discusses the patient's life-style, family history, and history of previous deviations from health. Finally, a thorough systems review is conducted to identify abnormalities in the various body systems. Questions asked in the systems review are important because they may detect disorders that the patient may not consider to be abnormal and has therefore not reported earlier in the history interview.

Medical History. A thorough, accurate history is highly important in establishing a diagnosis. In the practice of internal medicine, for example, it has been said that "a good history should be given the weight of 80 per cent of the weight in diagnosis, a good physical examination 15 per cent, and laboratory data, 5 per cent."[210] Knowledge of the natural history of disease is essential in taking a medical history. Gelfand comments: "I have usually found that the time taken for eliciting the patient's history should be three times as long as the physical examination, but this is not absolute. If the doctor can spend twenty minutes with his patient (and this may be the maximum time available in a busy practice) he should interrogate the patient for about fifteen minutes and spend five minutes on the physical examination. However, this is merely a guide. . . ."[73]

Summarized briefly below are *major components of a medical history:*

▶ *Chief complaint* (CC). Statement by the patient of his present major difficulty. Help the client be specific in describing his chief complaint. Chief complaints typically are observations made by the patient of a change from his usual condition, and/or the presence of dysfunction or pain. The chief complaint provides a broad, beginning data base concerning the patient's disorder. The data is then progressively refined and made more specific.

▶ *Present illness* (PI). Developed from the chief complaint. Provides information about reasons for the patient's current contact with the clinician. History of the present illness usually identifies the major disease mechanism or area of disorder (e.g., chest) and may even establish the diagnosis when symptoms are precise. Some general symptoms, such as weakness or fatigue, do not point to the basic disorder.

▶ *Personal history or patient profile.* Information about the patient as a person and about his life-style. Some of this information may be emotionally charged for the patient and difficult for him to relate. The interviewer's sensitivity and nonjudgmental approach are important here. Some information is obtained through relaxed conversation. Several interviews may be required before a complete profile is obtained.

▶ *Family history.* Past medical history of blood relatives, assessed with respect to patient's present illness and future health risks.

▶ *Past medical history.* Chronological review of previous disorders and contacts with health professionals.

▶ *Systems review.* Questions about the structure and function of the various systems. This review is undertaken to identify symptoms which the patient may or may not have previously reported, e.g., symptoms that were forgotten or considered unimportant, or symptoms that the patient simply does not view as symptoms.

A variety of printed *forms* are available for recording a patient's medical history. On some forms items are circled as part of the systems review, indicating they are a problem to the patient. Detailed notations and follow-up may then be made of circled items.

You may find it of interest to try taking your own medical history. Also, you may wish to practice your interviewing skills by doing a history on a friend.

The following outline presents information of importance to cover in taking a medical history. The patient's complete replies to queries provide the clinician with the beginnings of a comprehensive data base. (The reader is advised to look up new terms.)

Medical History (Sample Content)

A. *Date, hour, patient identification number*
B. *Patient personal identification.* Name, address, phone, sex, age, race, occupation, marital status, nearest kin or significant other, person to notify in case of emergency
C. *Chief complaint (CC).* Brief description in patient's own words of presenting disorder and duration
D. *Present illness history (PI)*
   1. Informant's name and reliability (informant may not be patient)
   2. Health status prior to onset of present disorder
   3. Immediate history of what brought patient to examiner
   4. Background history of present disorder, leading to immediate history
   5. Pertinent facts useful in making differential diagnosis, e.g., severity, duration, location, quality, radiation, continuity or intermittence of symptoms; chronologic history of disorder
E. *Personal history or patient profile*
   1. Residences over the years
   2. Education
   3. Employment (occupation)
   4. Diet
   5. Military service history
   6. Finances
   7. Marital history, e.g., information about spouse, children, previous marriages
   8. Home life, significant others
   9. Hobbies, interests
   10. Religious convictions
   11. Habits, e.g., energy, appetite, sexual activity, sleep, use of tobacco, alcohol, coffee, tea
   12. Weight, e.g., present, average, highest, lowest
   13. Drug use, e.g., medications, drug abuse
F. *Family history*
   1. Family tree
   2. Age and health status of mother, father and each sibling, or age at death and cause

3. History of disorders which may be influenced by heredity (familial disorders) or contact, allergies, deformities, serious illness

G. *Past medical history* (including psychiatric disorders)
   1. Previous hospitalizations: date, physician, disorder, hospital location
   2. Previous illness
   3. Previous operations
   4. Previous serious injuries
   5. Allergies, e.g., asthma, hay fever, food, skin, drugs (Make prominent note of drug allergies.)
   6. Disabilities
   7. Childhood diseases, immunizations

H. *Systems review*
   1. *Head:* Trauma, headaches, sinus pain, abnormal contour, hair
   2. *Eyes:* Visual changes, glasses, contact lenses, diplopia, photophobia, excessive lacrimation, eye pain or discharge, date of last eye examination
   3. *Ears:* Hearing changes, ear pain or discharge, tinnitus, vertigo, mastoiditis
   4. *Nose:* Smell, epistaxis, discharge, obstruction, pain, trauma, polyps, hay fever, sinusitis, head colds
   5. *Mouth and throat:* Taste, teeth or dentures, sore mouth, lips, gums (bleeding), tongue, voice change, sore throat, laryngitis, speech defect, dysphagia
   6. *Neck:* Neck swelling, goiter, pain, stiffness
   7. *Cardiopulmonary:* Chest pain, cough, expectoration, hemoptysis, dyspnea, orthopnea, night sweats, asthma, palpitation, murmur, peripheral edema, claudication, cramps, varicosities
   8. *Gastrointestinal:* Anorexia, food intolerance, nausea, vomiting, pain, flatulence, heartburn, use of antacids, hematemesis, melena, dysphagia, jaundice, color and form of stools, changed bowel habits, use of laxatives, diarrhea, constipation, hematochezia, rectal pain, hemorrhoids
   9. *Genitourinary:* Dysuria, polyuria, oliguria, frequency (volume), hematuria, nocturia (volume), pyuria, hesitancy, retention, urgency, incontinence, dribbling, stones, force and fullness of urine stream, venereal disease
      a. *Male reproductive:* Testes (mass, pain), potency, sexual habits
   10. *Breasts:* Breast mass, breast discharge, breast pain
   11. *Gynecologic (female reproductive)*
      a. *Menses:* Age at menarche, menstrual cycle, regularity, duration, amount, date of last menstrual period, irregular bleeding (spotting), dysmenorrhea, menorrhagia, discharge, itching, metrorrhagia, flushes, menopause (age), dyspareunia, pelvic pain
      b. *Sexual history:* Birth control (method), sexual habits, sexual dysfunction
      c. *Obstetrical history:* Number of pregnancies (gravida), children (para), abortions, complications during pregnancy and labor
   12. *Skin:* Pigmentary changes, pruritus, rash or other eruptions, ulcers, allergies, jaundice, hair or nail changes
   13. *Metabolic:* Changes in weight, appetite
   14. *Endocrine:* Changes in skin color or texture, hair distribution, sexual vigor, growth, voice, speech, goiter, excessive thirst
   15. *Hematologic (blood):* Bleeding tendency or blood disorder, anemia, bruising, sickle cell disease, lymphadenopathy
   16. *Musculoskeletal (locomotor):* Joint or muscle pain or stiffness, arthritis, joint deformity, coldness, muscle weakness, atrophy, dislocation, fracture
   17. *Neurologic-psychiatric:* Sensory and motor disturbances (e.g., increased, decreased or new sensations, paresthesia, paralysis, incoordination, abnormal gait, tremor, twitching), seizure (convulsions), headache, fainting, vertigo, extreme nervousness, sleeping irregularities, loss of consciousness, memory change, personality change, emotional instability, previous mental illness

Psychiatric History. In doing psychiatric interviews it is helpful to let the client initially talk about his problems in an unstructured manner without interruption from the interviewer. As necessary the interviewer may control a client's long, rambling comments by subtly interjecting questions and focusing on key words or phrases.

At times it is essential to obtain additional historical information from a patient's significant others. A family interview may be held for this purpose. During such an interview the clinician would observe the client's interactions with his significant others. These observations may provide helpful diagnostic information as well as indicating approaches that may be therapeutically useful.

Psychiatric History (Sample Content)

A. Disorder (complaint) as described by the patient
B. Present disorder, evolution of present disorder
C. Previous disorders, their natures and extent of treatment
D. Family history (important in assessing family influences and genetic disorders)
E. Personal history, including childhood development, adolescent adjustment and adult coping patterns
F. Current life functioning including social, educational, vocational and avocational areas

Common Diagnostic Tools

The progression of knowledge concerning disease processes occurred not only because of the increasing study of human anatomy through dissection after death, but also because tools were developed to explore the living body. Such tools were essential for the advancement of techniques of physical diagnosis because of the placement of vital organs within the body. Pause to realize that the vital organs (e.g., heart, brain, lungs, liver) are not accessible for examination by means of palpation (feeling) or inspection (looking). In fact, the vital organs are often encased within protective bony structures.

Diagnostic tools, such as the stethoscope, and diagnostic maneuvers, such as percussion (thumping), brought the inaccessible vital organs into contact with the senses of the examiner. Diagnostic tools can thus be viewed as extensions of the examiner's senses. Figure 16–2 depicts several of the diagnostic tools mentioned in this section.

A *stethoscope* is an instrument with two ear pieces connected by flexible tubing to a cone or bell and is used to listen to and amplify sounds produced by internal organs, e.g., lungs, heart, intestine. (The use of the stethoscope is described under *Auscultation*, later in this chapter.) The original stethoscope, invented by Laennec in 1816, was a wooden tube.

Various kinds of "scopes" have been developed for looking inside of structures. The *ophthalmoscope* was developed for examination of the interior of the eye. With it, information could be obtained not only about the eye, but also about the central nervous system and the blood vessels. (The latter information is obtained by inspecting the fundus of the eye.) An *otoscope* is used to examine the eardrum and exterior ear canal. Ophthalmoscopes and otoscopes are attached to a light source and are routinely used during physical examination.

Specialized scopes have been developed for the investigation of other body areas, e.g., *bronchoscope* (to observe the interior of the tracheobronchial tree), *cystoscope* (to inspect the interior of the urinary bladder via the urethra), *laryngoscope* (to visualize the larynx) and *sigmoidoscope* (for direct examination of the sigmoid colon via the rectum).

As can be seen, the complete name of a scope often identifies the body structure that the scope is used to visualize. Some scopes are designed for use with various special attachments that permit the examiner to grasp structures (grasping forceps), suction (suction tip), biopsy (biopsy forceps) or cauterize (cautery tip) once the scope is inserted.

Some scopes are rigid and others are flexible. The recent development of *flexible fiberoptic scopes* permits greater ease of insertion, greater maneuverability and a considerably increased range of visibility. Such scopes contain an ingenious optical system which enables visual images to be transmitted through a bundle of tiny glass fibers. One example of such a scope is the flexible fiberoptic bronchoscope.

Mirrors of various kinds, e.g., head mirror (worn by the examiner) and laryngeal mirror, are used during the examination to direct light into body areas such as the throat. Some instruments contain built-in mirrors and light

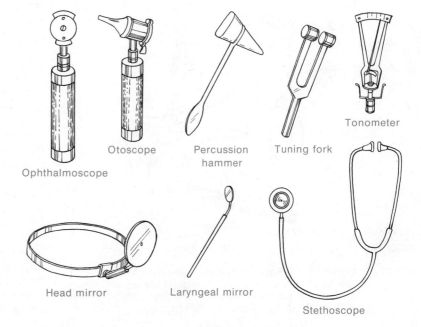

Figure 16–2. Common diagnostic tools.

Ophthalmoscope

Otoscope

Percussion hammer

Tuning fork

Tonometer

Head mirror

Laryngeal mirror

Stethoscope

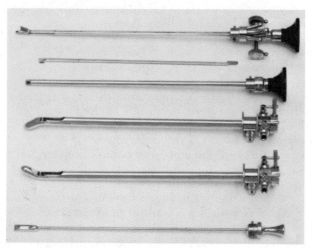

Figure 16–3. Cystoscope with lighting system. (Courtesy of American Cystoscope Makers, Inc.)

sources to facilitate inspection of internal body spaces. A cystoscope, for example, is a hollow metal tube with an electric bulb at its end. The bulb illuminates the inside (interior) of the urinary bladder. *Special lenses* (magnifying lenses) and mirrors within the cystoscope make possible detailed examination of the interior of the bladder (Fig. 16–3).

A *speculum* is an instrument used to distend or open a body orifice (passage, opening) or cavity, thus permitting visual inspection of the interior. A variety of these instruments have

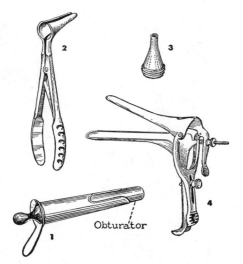

Figure 16–4. Specula: 1, rectal (David); 2, nasal (Vienna model); 3, ear (Boucheron); 4, vaginal (Pederson). (From *Dorland's Illustrated Medical Dictionary,* 25th ed. Philadelphia, W. B. Saunders Co., 1974, p. 1446.)

been developed for use in examining areas such as the rectum, inner nose, inner ear and vagina (Fig. 16–4).

Several *instruments of measurement* may be used during the process of physically examining the body. For example, a *scale* is used to weigh the patient and a *height measurement rod* (often attached to the scale) measures the patient's height. A blood pressure cuff attached to a *sphygmomanometer* (see Chap. 29) is used to measure the patient's blood pressure and a *thermometer* is used to measure body temperature (see Chap. 28). The patient's *pulse* and *respirations* are counted, using a watch with a second hand, and recorded (Chap. 29). A special instrument called a *tonometer* is used to measure pressure within the eyeball (intraocular pressure). Prior to placing this instrument on the eye's surface, a mild anesthetic solution is placed in the eye. A *tape measure* or *ruler* may be used to make linear measurements or measurements of circumference. Many other specialized diagnostic tools and tests are available for use in the diagnostic (and treatment) process.

Diagnostic Maneuvers

Inspection, palpation, percussion and auscultation are basic diagnostic maneuvers performed by an examiner during the physical examination process. These maneuvers are also used by nurses for physical assessment while giving patient care. The examiner may also use her sense of smell for diagnostic purposes.

As previously emphasized, a *systematic approach* to the process of physical examination is important to prevent omissions. Thus the examiner systematically applies her own special senses to each of the patient's areas or systems. *The usual sequence of activities is to* (1) *look* (inspect), (2) *feel* (palpate), (3) *tap or thump* (percuss) and (4) *listen* (auscultate). These diagnostic activities are discussed in detail below. Not all of the activities are used in examining each body part; suitable activities are selected according to the anatomy of the part.

The typical sequence of inspection, palpation, percussion and auscultation is not used during examination of the abdomen; instead the sequence used is to inspect, auscultate, percuss and, finally, palpate. Palpation is performed last in this instance because feeling a sensitive abdomen may produce additional symptoms, e.g., suppress early bowel sounds, trigger painful spasms.

Let us now examine more carefully the techniques of inspection, palpation, percussion and auscultation in physical examination.

Inspection (Discriminative Looking). As you inspect (look at) an area, try to develop in your mind a *visual description* of what you are seeing. Observe events (e.g., movements), colors, contours and symmetry or asymmetry. Some observations made during inspection can be quantitated by making *measurements*, e.g., with a soft tape measure or small ruler. Good lighting and adequate (but not excessive) exposure of the appropriate area facilitate proper inspection.

> Remember:
> *You must expose that which you wish to look at; you cannot inspect that which is not visible.*

Whenever possible, observations should be quantified by performing measurements. This permits the patient's findings to be evaluated by comparison with established "normals." Also, it provides a data base against which to compare future measurements. During physical examination, measurements are commonly made of the patient's height, weight, body temperature, and vital signs (i.e., pulse, respirations, blood pressure). Other measurements might include measuring the circumference of the head or a limb or the diameter of a lesion.

Palpation. Palpation refers to feeling with one's fingers and one or both hands. Skill and gentleness are important during palpation. The degree of pressure applied during palpation varies, depending upon factors such as the tenderness of the area being palpated and the depth of palpation required. In palpating the abdomen both *light* and *deep* palpation may be employed. Successful palpation may be difficult to perform on patients who are: (a) anxious or tense, (b) experiencing physical discomfort, (c) obese or (d) ticklish. It is helpful with ticklish or tense patients for the examiner to place the patient's hands beneath her own during initial palpations. Additionally, it is helpful to examine tender areas last and to observe the patient's face for nonverbal responses during the examination, e.g., grimacing, smiling.

During examination by palpation the patient may tell you of feelings of discomfort (e.g., pressure, fullness, tenderness) or pain that he experiences when you touch certain places on his body.

Palpation confirms data that have been gathered by means of inspection, helping to provide information about a part's structure or function. Numerous characteristics may be assessed by touching a patient's body with different parts of the examiner's hand and by exerting varying amounts of pressure. For example:

▶ *Temperature changes* can be detected by running the backs of the fingers or the dorsum of the hand over the skin. Cool areas may indicate reduced blood flow, and inflammation may increase skin warmth.

▶ *Moisture* may be felt while lightly stroking the patient's skin.

▶ *Events* (vibrations such as bruits and voice sounds, crepitus, pulsations, spasticity, rigidity, elasticity or other movements or qualities of movements occurring under the examiner's hand) can be detected by using the fingers and entire palm or hand. Vibrations are best felt with the lateral aspect of the hand or palm.

▶ *Textures* (e.g., unevenness) can be noted using the fingertips. The fingertips are very sensitive to touch because they have numerous nerve endings.

▶ *Locations and dimensions or contours* can be assessed by using several fingers, or one or both entire hands, depending upon the size of the body part being examined. For example, swelling may be felt and organ sizes and locations assessed. Firm, deep pressure is required to palpate deep organs such as the kidneys, spleen or liver. Light touch, on the other hand, is used to gently palpate the eye.

▶ *Consistencies* (hard, soft, rubbery, flaccid, tense) can be determined best by using the fingertips.

Sensitivity to touch perception in the examiner's fingers is reduced during the application of firm pressure, e.g., during palpation of deep organs. To counteract this problem it is helpful if the examiner uses both hands when it is necessary to apply firm pressure. The lower hand (touching the patient) is relaxed. Pressure is applied by placing the other hand on top of the resting hand. The upper hand also directs exploratory movements of the relaxed lower hand on the patient's body.[74]

Commonly nurses use palpation when taking a patient's pulse (to feel blood pulsating through blood vessels) and during breast examination. However, all accessible body parts may be examined by palpation—blood vessels, organs, skin, muscles, bones, glands. It is also possible to feel the vibrations of some body sounds, e.g., thrills, tactile fremitus.

Percussion. Percussion is a diagnostic maneuver which makes it possible for an examiner to obtain more information about internal organs or structures than can be obtained by merely feeling or looking at the outside of the body. Percussion is accomplished by the skillful "thumping" or "tapping" of a body surface with an instrument (rubber percussion hammer, also called reflex hammer) or the examiner's hand or fingers.

Percussion is performed to assess the density (relative solidness or hardness or fullness) of the cavity or organ underlying the surface being percussed. The location and size of underlying organs can also be determined. The sound produced by the thumping is carefully evaluated and deductions are made about the condition of the body part being assessed.

The experienced examiner knows that percussed sounds differ in various body areas, depending in part upon the density of underlying structures. The sounds produced when percussing over solid structures differ from those over hollow structures. Sounds in various body areas range from *flat* (nonresonant) through *dull, resonant, hyperresonant* and *tympanic*.[99] Tympanic sounds occur over hollow or gas-filled organs; solid tissue, e.g., muscle or solid organs, is flat. By percussion it is possible, for example, to differentiate between normal air-filled lung tissue and diseased, solidified lung tissue. Frequently nurses percuss a patient's abdomen for distention and his urinary bladder to assess the amount of urine within.

A quiet setting is necessary for the examiner during both percussion and auscultation, discussed in the next section. Both of these techniques require instruction and practice; both are valuable diagnostic maneuvers that can provide a great deal of information during the physical assessment of a patient.

To the novice, percussion seems a crude and awkward exercise, and he is likely to wonder if it can ever be more. At this point he is well advised to recall his

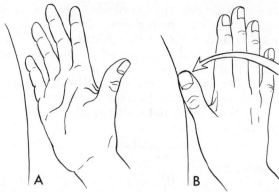

Figure 16–5. Direct percussion. *A,* The thumb is raised approximately 4 inches from the surface to be percussed. *B,* The thumb strikes the surface, and the resultant sound is assessed.

first kiss with malice aforethought, and how rapidly he improved with practice. The method can be remarkably productive in seasoned hands. Lacking the eye of the x-ray, some nineteenth century physicians became incredibly expert at the art of percussion. Necessity is the mother of perfection as well as invention.[48]

Percussion may be direct or indirect (Figs. 16–5 and 16–6). *Direct percussion* is accomplished by the examiner striking her fingers directly against the patient's skin. With *indirect percussion* the examiner places the first phalanx (i.e., terminal phalanx) of the middle finger of one hand (the nondominant hand) firmly against the patient's skin and then strikes that phalanx (just behind the fingernail bed) with the end of the middle finger of the dominant hand. Important points to remember in this activity are: (a) do not allow other fingers of the nondominant hand to touch the patient (if they do they will dampen or suppress the percussed sound), (b) hold the forearm of the dominant arm steady and use a quick, flicking wrist action from a flexed wrist for the striking force, (c) quickly withdraw the striking finger to avoid dampening the percussed sound, and (d) strive for a brief, intense tap. You will want to practice

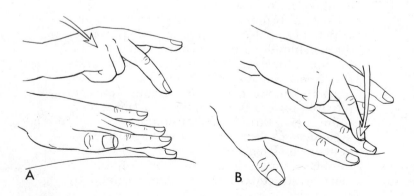

Figure 16–6. Indirect percussion. *A,* First phalanx of middle finger of nondominant hand is placed firmly on patient's skin. *B,* Phalanx on skin is struck with end of middle finger of dominant hand. (See text.)

percussion often. Why not try it today on a classmate or other friend?

Auscultation. When performing auscultation, the examiner carefully listens to and assesses the sounds produced by various body organs and tissues, e.g., heart, lung, bowel.

Auscultation is highly important in the diagnosis and treatment of a number of medical and surgical disorders. Auscultation of the lungs and heart is routinely performed not only as a preliminary scanning procedure but also during the ongoing assessment of a patient receiving treatment. Auscultation of the abdomen and peripheral blood vessels also is frequently important. Blood vessels in the neck and head are auscultated at times, e.g., if a brain aneurysm is suspected.

Auscultation can be performed by either direct or indirect methods. The less commonly used *direct method*, also called "immediate auscultation," involves the examiner simply placing her ear directly against the patient's body surface. The method has serious limitations because the sounds are too diffuse and too soft, especially if a patient is obese. The *indirect method* is the usual method of auscultation. It is performed with a stethoscope.

A quality *stethoscope*, having both a bell and a flat diaphragm, is recommended. When gently placed against the patient, the *bell* collects low pitched sounds, permitting the escape of high frequency sounds. It is thus best for perceiving low pitched sounds. The *flat diaphragm*, when firmly placed, excludes low frequency sounds and responds best to high pitched sounds.

Clinicians often purchase their own stethoscopes, thereby having readily available an instrument suited to their individual needs. Ear pieces should fit comfortably in the examiner's ears without totally occluding sound passage. The ear pieces should be kept clean, maintaining unobstructed openings. The tubing should be about one foot long and be free of leaks; a tight fit of the tubing onto the head (the portion applied to the patient) and the ear pieces is essential. During auscultation nothing should touch the tubing (otherwise, distracting noises are produced), and the patient should remain silent unless following the directions of the examiner to speak, cough, breathe deeply through open mouth, etc. For reasons of medical asepsis the patient should be asked to turn his head away from the examiner's face and cover his mouth when coughing and deep breathing. A tissue should be given the patient for mouth coverage.

Four sounds are typically listened for during auscultation. These are: (a) *frequency*, e.g., high pitch, low pitch, (2) *intensity*, e.g., loud sounds, soft sounds, (3) *quality*, e.g., the characteristic differences between two sounds of equal pitch and intensity which are coming from differing sources such as the lungs and bowels and (4) *duration* or length of the sound.

As with other techniques of physical examination, auscultation should be performed in a systematic manner. The ability to auscultate skillfully is invaluable during physical assessment, and nurses frequently auscultate while giving patient care. The reader is advised to devote time and concentration to the development of this skill.[114, 119]

Olfaction (Smelling). Tasting was at one time an important activity in the process of physical examination. For example, in ancient times a person called a "piss prophet" tasted urine in an attempt to identify disease. Esteemed in his day, such an individual would no doubt be viewed as offensive today. However, examiners still employ their sense of smell.[151] Olfaction, along with identification of other signs of a disorder, may help in the detection of many disorders, some of which are serious. Listed in Table 16–1 are some characteristic odors and their possible causes.

Physical Examination

Purposes. Physical examinations are given to identify deviations from "normal" findings. Skilled nurses increasingly are performing physical examinations. This professional activity requires knowledge of basic anatomy and physiology as well as possible pathology or abnormalities. As with other skills, the successful performance of a physical examination depends upon thoughtful practice and the accumulation of experience.

Physical examinations may be given in the presence of symptoms (to help identify the disorder so that appropriate treatment can be started) or in the absence of symptoms, e.g., as a routine health maintenance examination, preemployment examination. Whatever the reason for the examination, it provides an excellent opportunity for the health professional to establish important contact with the patient, build a successful patient-practitioner relationship, and provide appropriate patient education, e.g., teaching women breast self-examination.

Assisting with Physical Examination. If you are assisting a physician or another nurse to give a physical examination you may perform

TABLE 16–1.   CHARACTERISTIC ODORS DETECTABLE DURING PHYSICAL EXAMINATION
AND THEIR POSSIBLE CAUSES

CHARACTERISTIC ODOR	POSSIBLE CAUSE
Alcohol, liquefied Sterno, lighter fluid	Intake of these substances
Ammoniacal urine (ammonia-like odor)	Urinary tract infection with urea-splitting bacteria
Bitter almond odor	Cyanide poisoning
Body odor (general)	Poor hygiene; excessive perspiration (hyperhidrosis); foul-smelling perspiration (bromhidrosis)
Burnt rope odor	Marijuana
Camphor odor	Mothball ingestion
Fecal odor (in older patient)	Wound infection; abscess
Feculent odor	*Bacteroides* abscess
Fetid breath	Lung abscess
Foul-smelling stools (infant)	Malabsorption syndrome, e.g., cystic fibrosis
Garlic odor	Arsenic poisoning
Halitosis ("bad breath")	Poor dental and oral hygiene
"Horsey" or musty odor (infant)	Phenylketonuria (PKU)
Ketone, acetone, sickening sweet odor	Diabetic acidosis
Musty "new-mown clover" odor (fetor hepaticus)	Liver disease, hepatic coma
Nasal malodor (foul odor from nose)	Foreign body in nose; pharyngitis; chronic postnasal drip; nasal crusts; allergic, atrophic or chronic rhinitis
Paraldehyde odor	Acute poisoning
Stale urine odor	Uremic acidosis
Sweet, heavy, thick odor	*Pseudomonas* infection
Vaginal odor	Fungal infection; poor hygiene

the following activities as modified by agency policies:

► Assemble equipment and linens. Prepare examination room or patient's unit.

► Prepare patient physically and psychologically for examination.

► Perform some parts of the examination process, e.g., weigh and measure patient and obtain vital signs.

► Change draping as appropriate and assist patient into desired positions as necessary.

► Anticipate examiner's need for specific diagnostic tools and supplies. Keep these close at hand and pass them to examiner. Dispose of soiled items in appropriate manner.

► Caution and protect patient from falling. Examining tables may be relatively high and narrow compared with the patient's bed. Assist patient with use of sturdy stepstool if necessary for him to get on and off table.

► Assess need to remain with patient at all times, e.g., consider patient's age, orientation, level of consciousness, balance, cooperativeness. Commonly a female nurse is expected to be present during examination of a female by a male examiner (for reasons of legal protection and for the patient's psychological comfort).

► Label and handle specimens appropriately.

► Enter the examination procedure and specimen collections in patient's record.

► Perform aftercare for patient and equipment.

Ensuring Patient Comfort.   The sensitive examiner remembers that the patient is usually anxious about being examined. This anxiety is not only uncomfortable for the patient but may also distort the physical findings of the examination. It is therefore not only kind but also clinically important to minimize the patient's anxiety and help him relax. Factors which promote this include providing a comfortable, private setting for the examination and encouraging the patient to talk at times during the examination. Remember to close the door to the examining room or screen the patient.

A suitable *drape* is used to cover the patient during the physical examination, and the patient may wear a *gown* which opens in the back. *Exposure of the patient is kept minimal*, i.e., limited to the area being examined. However, one cannot properly examine a patient by reaching under his clothing, bedlinens or drapes. *Appropriate draping and appropriate exposure are both necessary!*

Drapes and gowns may be either of linen or of disposable paper. Linen (e.g., sheet, bath blanket, draw sheet) is more comfortable generally and less wasteful. A patient should not become chilled during examination. Keep a lightweight blanket available, and check with the patient if he is warm enough. Prevent drafts in the examining room. Elderly or ill patients may chill easily.

The examiner's hands should be warm, smooth and clean. Remember to make certain that your fingernails are clean, relatively short, and smooth when you perform physical examinations. The examiner's hands should be washed just prior to beginning and again immediately after completing the examination. For the patient's comfort, instruments used during the examination should be warmed as appropriate; e.g., the bell of a stethoscope can be warmed by rubbing it between your hands before placing it on the patient.

It is helpful to talk with the patient about examination activities as preparations are made to carry them out, e.g., "I'm going to listen to your chest now." Also, provide the patient with instructions about what he can do to assist with the examination, e.g., "Breathe in and out slowly and deeply through your open mouth." During the examination the clinician needs to be aware of her nonverbal communication (e.g., frowning, looks of concern) and its possible effects on the patient. A relaxed, friendly yet professional attitude on the examiner's part often helps put the client at ease.

Additional Pre-examination Preparation. Prior to beginning the examination encourage the patient to go to the toilet. This not only makes the patient more relaxed, but also facilitates examination of the abdomen, male genitals, vagina and rectum. *Urine* and *feces specimens* are collected at this time if required. Be certain to give the patient clear instructions about specimen collection, take the specimen from the patient as soon as it is ready, and promptly label it.

Before beginning the physical examination, the patient's *temperature* and *vital signs* may be taken and he may be weighed and his height measured. Place a clean paper towel on the scale for the patient to stand on with his bare feet. *Height* and *weight* measurements may be omitted if the patient is quite ill. (Chap. 28 discusses measurement of body temperature; Chap. 29 focuses on measurement of pulse, respiration and blood pressure.)

Instruments and equipment used during physical examination should be assembled close at hand and ready for use (i.e., in working order) to minimize disruption of the examination process.

Physical Examination Equipment. The equipment and instruments used for physical examination vary, depending upon the purpose and thoroughness of the examination and the patient's condition. Summarized below is a list of typical supplies:

Blood pressure cuff (sphygmomanometer)
Container for soiled instruments
Cotton applicators
Cotton balls in antiseptic solution or prepackaged antiseptic pledgets
Disposable pad (Chux)
Drapes (sheet, bath blanket)
Ear speculum
Eye chart, e.g., Snellen chart
Feces container and form
Flashlight and spotlight or gooseneck light
Forms, e.g., laboratory, x-ray, chart, physical exam, pathology
Gloves (sterile or clean)
Gown for patient
Guaiac test reagents
Head mirror
Laryngeal mirror
Lightweight blanket
Lubricant
Nasal speculum
Ophthalmoscope
Otoscope
Papanicolaou smear slides and request form
Paper towels
Percussion (reflex) hammer
Scale with height measure rod
Skin pencil
Stethoscope
Tape measure
Thermometer
Tissues and waste container
Tongue blades (depressors)
Tonometer and appropriate ophthalmic mild anesthetic solution
Tuning fork
Urine specimen bottle and form
Vaginal speculum

Additional items are required if a *neurologic examination* is to be given. These items might include: (a) audiometer, watch or some other item for assessing hearing, (b) containers of sugar and salt for testing taste, (c) dry cotton balls for testing corneal reflex and touch sensation, (d) safety pin for testing touch and pain sensations, (e) test tubes (two) filled with cold and hot water for testing temperature sensation, (f) vials (closed) containing fresh materials with easily recognizable odors, e.g., onion, orange extract, peanut butter, vanilla and (g)

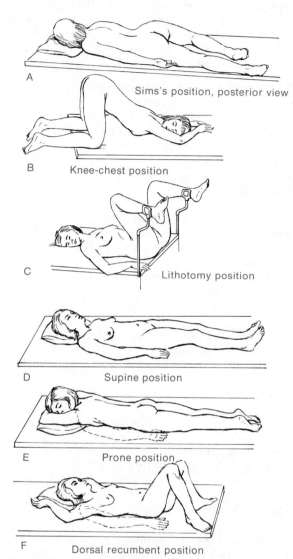

Figure 16–7. Various positions used for examination or treatment. Note alternate positions of patient's arms in prone and dorsal recumbent positions. (A, B and C from *Dorland's Illustrated Medical Dictionary,* 25th ed. Philadelphia, W. B. Saunders Co., 1974.)

A   Sims's position, posterior view

B   Knee-chest position

C   Lithotomy position

D   Supine position

E   Prone position

F   Dorsal recumbent position

various objects of differing easily recognizable textures and shapes, e.g., piece of silk cloth, block of wood, key, coin, bell, ball, bottle cap. The latter items are for testing texture discrimination and stereognosis (ability to recognize an object by feeling it) while the patient keeps his eyes closed.

Patient and Examiner Positions. Figure 16–7 illustrates various positions that the patient may be asked to assume during the course of a physical examination or during special examinations or treatments. Some of these positions, e.g., lithotomy and knee-chest, are embarrassing and uncomfortable for the patient. Thus, the patient should be kept in them no longer than necessary. Give the patient clear instructions about which position he is to assume and help him assume and maintain the position as necessary.

The examiner typically positions herself at the patient's right side when she is not standing in front of or behind the patient during the examination. Examination of the patient's right side first is easier for most right-handed clinicians. Also it is frequently more successful to feel for the position of the spleen or apex when the patient is examined from the clinician's right side.

Figures 16–8 and 16–9 and Tables 16–2 and 16–3 summarize positions of the ambulatory patient and the bed-bound patient and the examiner during the physical examination.

Approach to Physical Examination. When a serious disorder is present, a complete physical examination is indicated. For minor disorders, the examination is often limited to the body part affected.

Physical examination begins the moment the patient is first seen. Important "first impressions" include observations of the patient's general appearance, physique, gait, handshake, orientation and communication. These observations are sometimes referred to as a *noninvasive physical examination.* The *invasive* physical examination typically follows obtaining of the history. Burnside notes: "Invasive is a correct term, for psychologists tell us that the physical approach of one person to another to a distance of less than 2 feet is always interpreted by the subconscious as invasion. It may be seen as intimate invasion or threatening invasion but always it evokes a heightening of awareness."[25] Physical contact with the patient is best initiated in nonthreatening ways, e.g., by a careful inspection of the patient's hands. (Systemic diseases may cause changes in the hands.)

In performing physical examination the examiner makes frequent comparisons between the two sides of the body, e.g., noting symmetry or lack of symmetry. For descriptive purposes the body is divided into *planes* (Fig. 16–10); various body parts may be further subdivided. Fig. 16–11 illustrates *regions of the abdomen.* Table 16–4 provides an overview of the organs normally found in each abdominal quadrant. The content and order of the adult physical examination is summarized in Table 16–5.

Postexamination Activities. Immediately following completion of the examination the pa-

Text continued on page 224

Figure 16–8. Positions of examiner and ambulatory patient during the physical examination. (From Morgan, W. M., Jr., and Engel, G. L.: *The Clinical Approach to the Patient.* Philadelphia, W. B. Saunders Co., 1969, p. 91.)

General
inspection and vital
signs

Head
Neck

Back, posterior
thorax and lungs

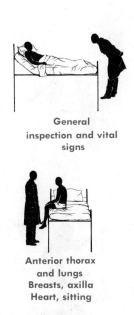

Anterior thorax
and lungs
Breasts, axilla
Heart, sitting

Breasts,
axilla
Heart,
recumbent

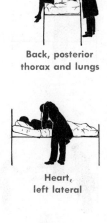

Heart,
left lateral

Abdomen

Extremities

Extremities

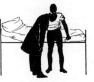

Extremities
Male
genitalia

Female
genital tract

Rectum

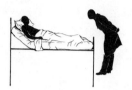

General
inspection and
vital signs

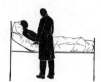

Head, right

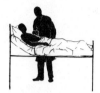

Head, left

Neck

Back,
posterior
thorax and lungs

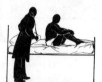

Back,
posterior
thorax and lungs

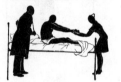

Back,
posterior
thorax and lungs

Anterior
thorax and lungs
Breasts, axilla
Heart, recumbent

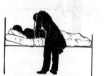

Heart, left
lateral

Figure 16–9. Positions of examiner
and bed-bound patient during physical
examination. (From Morgan and
Engel: *The Clinical Approach to the
Patient*, p. 93.)

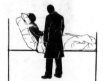

Heart, sitting

Abdomen

Extremities
Male
genitalia

Female
genital tract

Rectum

TABLE 16–2.   A SUMMARY OF THE EXAMINER'S AND PATIENT'S POSITIONS
DURING THE PHYSICAL EXAMINATION*

THE AMBULATORY PATIENT

Region	The Examiner's Position	The Patient's Position
1. General inspection and vital signs	Standing before the patient and moving as needed.	Sitting, or lying on the bed or examining table.
2. The head	Standing, facing the patient.	Sitting on the side of the bed or examining table.
3. The neck	Standing, facing the patient, then moving behind him.	Sitting on the side of the bed or examining table.
4. The back; posterior thorax and lungs	Standing behind the patient.	Sitting on the side of the bed or examining table.
5. The anterior thorax and lungs	Standing, facing the patient.	Sitting on the side of the bed or examining table.
6. The breasts and axillary regions	Initially facing the patient, then examining from the patient's right side.	Sitting, facing the examiner, then lying supine.
7. The heart	Standing at the patient's right.	In three positions: sitting, lying on his back, and on his left side.
8. The abdomen	Standing at the patient's right.	Lying on his back.
9. The extremities	Standing, facing the patient, and moving to the patient's right.	Lying flat, then sitting on the side of the bed, and finally standing.
10. The male external genitalia	Standing before the patient and slightly to his right.	Standing, facing the examiner.
11. The female genital tract	Sitting on a stool facing the perineum, and standing for part of the examination.	Lying on her back on an examining table with both knees flexed and her feet in stirrups.
12. The rectum	Standing, facing the buttocks.	Bending at the hips over the bed or examining table. The female retains the same position used in the examination of the genital tract.

*From Morgan, W. M., Jr., and Engel, G. L.: *The Clinical Approach to the Patient*. Philadelphia, W. B. Saunders, 1969, pp. 90–91.

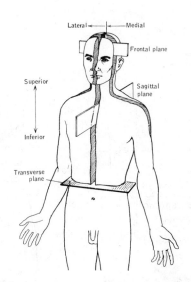

Figure 16–10.   Planes of the body (Davenport). Anterior view, in the anatomical position, with standard planes of reference shown by cleavages. (From *Dorland's Illustrated Medical Dictionary,* 25th ed. Philadelphia, W. B. Saunders Co., 1974).

TABLE 16–3. A SUMMARY OF THE EXAMINER'S AND PATIENT'S POSITIONS DURING THE PHYSICAL EXAMINATION*

THE BED-BOUND PATIENT

Region	The Examiner's Position	The Patient's Position
1. General inspection and vital signs	Standing at the foot of the bed.	Lying on his back with the head of the bed slightly elevated.
2. The head	Standing at the right side of the bed, then moving to the left side.	Lying on his back with the head of the bed slightly elevated.
3. The neck	Standing at the right side of the bed.	Lying on his back with the head of the bed slightly elevated.
4. The back; posterior thorax and lungs	Standing at the right side of the bed, examining across the bed, *or* from the right posterior oblique side of the chest.	Sitting on the left side of the bed with his back to the examiner *or* sitting up in bed with assistance.
5. The anterior thorax and lungs	Standing at the right side of the bed.	Lying on his back.
6. The breasts and axillary regions	Standing at the right side of the bed.	Lying on his back.
7. The heart	Standing at the right side of the bed.	In three positions: lying on his back, on his left side, and sitting.
8. The abdomen	Standing at the right side of the bed.	Lying on his back.
9. The extremities	Standing at the right side of the bed.	Lying flat on his back, then on his abdomen; if able, sitting on the side of the bed facing the examiner.
10. The male external genitalia	Standing at the right side of the bed.	Lying on his back.
11. The female genital tract	Sitting on a stool facing the perineum, and standing for part of the examination.	Lying on her back obliquely across the bed, with both legs flexed.
12. The rectum	Standing at the right side of the bed.	Lying on his left side with both legs flexed at the hip.

*From Morgan, W. M., Jr., and Engel, G. L.: *The Clinical Approach to the Patient*, Philadelphia, W. B. Saunders, 1969, pp. 92–93.

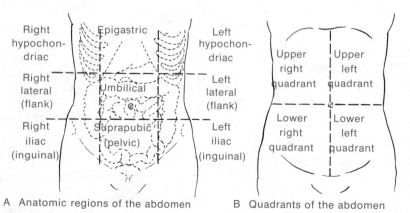

A Anatomic regions of the abdomen   B Quadrants of the abdomen

Figure 16–11. Terminology used with reference to abdominal anatomy.

TABLE 16–4. ORGANS FOUND IN EACH ABDOMINAL QUADRANT*

RIGHT UPPER QUADRANT (RUQ)	LEFT UPPER QUADRANT (LUQ)
Adrenal gland (right) Colon (hepatic flexure and portions of ascending and transverse) Duodenum Kidney (portion of right) Liver Gallbladder Pancreas (head) Pylorus	Adrenal gland (left) Colon (splenic flexure and portions of transverse and descending) Kidney (portion of left) Liver (left lobe) Pancreas (body) Spleen Stomach

Loops of small intestine in all quadrants

RIGHT LOWER QUADRANT (RLQ)	LEFT LOWER QUADRANT (LLQ)
Appendix Bladder (if distended) Cecum Colon (portion of ascending) Kidney (lower pole of right) Ovary (right) Salpinx (uterine tube; right) Spermatic cord (right) Uterus (if enlarged) Ureter (right)	Bladder (if distended) Colon (sigmoid and portion of descending) Kidney (lower pole of left) Ovary (left) Salpinx (uterine tube; left) Spermatic cord (left) Uterus (if enlarged) Ureter (left)

*Adapted from DeGowin, E. L., and DeGowin, R. L.: *Bedside Diagnostic Examination,* 2nd ed. New York: Macmillan Publishing Co., Inc., 1969.

TABLE 16–5. OVERVIEW OF ADULT GENERAL PHYSICAL EXAMINATION*

AREA	PATIENT POSITION	METHOD OF EXAMINATION	OBSERVATIONS/EXAMPLES
General Appearance Survey	Sitting if possible. Walking for gait observations	Inspection (begin assessment from moment first see patient) Palpation (shake hands)	Consciousness, state-of-awareness: comatose, stuporous, drowsy, inattentive, alert Mood, manner, relationship to surroundings: pleasant, angry, tearful, suspicious Dress, grooming, personal hygiene Facial expression: relaxed, anxious, depressed Posture, gait, other motor activity Age category, age communication Overall apparent state of health: acutely ill, chronically ill, frail, appears healthy Signs of distress: indications of pain or anxiety, cardiorespiratory distress Skin color: pale, flushed, cyanotic, jaundiced, irregular pigmentation Breath or body odor: alcohol, oral infection, acetone Speech: clarity, pitch, pace, content
		Observe and measure	Stature and habitus: height, body build, gross deformities Weight

*Space does not permit detailed discussion of the physical examination. The interested reader is referred to specialized physical examination texts (see bibliography) or a textbook of medical-surgical nursing, e.g., Luckmann, J., and Sorensen, K. C.: *Medical-Surgical Nursing: A Psychophysiologic Approach.*

Table continued on the following pages

TABLE 16–5. OVERVIEW OF ADULT GENERAL PHYSICAL EXAMINATION (*Continued*)

AREA	PATIENT POSITION	METHOD OF EXAMINATION	OBSERVATIONS/EXAMPLES
Extremities (musculoskeletal and peripheral vascular and neurologic) Integrate assessment of extremities with other assessments, e.g., general appearance survey, skin, musculoskeletal and neurological examinations.	Sitting to assess head, neck, hands, wrists, elbows, shoulders Supine to assess feet, ankles, knees, hips Standing	Compare *bilaterally* Inspection Palpation Percussion Reflex hammer may be used to test reflexes	General observations: symmetry; proportion of extremities to trunk; size and shape of arms, hands, legs, feet; range-of-motion; joint size, shape, tenderness, enlargement; deformity; scars, lesions, nodules, ulcers; temperature, swelling, tenderness, edema; pigmentation, color (e.g., redness); pulses; clubbing of fingers; involuntary movements; sensation; crepitation; muscle strength and size Legs: palpate for edema and signs of deep phlebitis; inspect for varicose veins; palpate dorsalis pedis and posterior tibial pulses; note alignment of legs and feet; test lower reflexes (knee jerk, ankle jerk, plantar reflex); inspect feet for calluses Arms: assess grip; test biceps, triceps and radial reflexes
Vital Signs (see Chaps. 28 and 29)	Sitting, supine, prone (as indicated)	Inspection Palpation Auscultation Measurement with thermometer, stethoscope, sphygmomanometer, clock	Respiratory rate, quality Pulse Blood pressure Body temperature
Skin and Nails	Sitting if possible (also, continue assessment as patient is supine)	Inspection Palpation (Continue skin assessment throughout examination. Begin with hands, forearms and face)	General appearance, color, icterus (jaundice), vascularity, moisture (sweating), temperature, hair distribution, edema, texture, tenderness, thickness, lesions, masses, eruptions, pigmentation, contusions, turgor and mobility, nail condition, fingernail color and contour
Lymph Nodes	Sitting if possible (also continue as patient is supine)	Inspection Palpation (Continue assessment throughout examination)	Occipital, cervical, supraclavicular, axillary, epitrochlear, inguinal Presence of enlargement
Head	Sitting if possible Supine, head of bed slightly elevated if possible.	Inspection Palpation Auscultation (stethoscope)	Position, movement, proportion to rest of body (size), hair distribution, scalp and skull condition, contour, presence of trauma Bruit
Face	Sitting if possible	Inspection Palpation	Size, symmetry, appearance, configuration, movement, facial expression, tenderness, swelling
Temporal Arteries	Sitting if possible	Palpation	Palpations

TABLE 16–5. OVERVIEW OF ADULT GENERAL PHYSICAL EXAMINATION (*Continued*)

AREA	PATIENT POSITION	METHOD OF EXAMINATION	OBSERVATIONS/EXAMPLES
Eyes	Sitting if possible (applies to all parts of eye examination, except where noted	Compare *bilaterally* as follows:	
1. Position		1. Inspection	1. Gross position and alignment of eyes
2. Eyelids		2. Inspection Gentle palpation	2. Position, ptosis, edema, lesions, infection, color, palpebral fissure
3. Lacrimal system		3. Inspection Gentle palpation	3. Discharge, tearing, inflammation
4. Visual acuity		4. Snellen test chart	4. Compares subject's ability to read lines of letters from a distance with previously determined normal
5. Visual fields		5. Examiner's finger is moved slowly into subject's field of vision laterally while subject maintains fixed focus	5. Identifies marked restriction of peripheral vision
6. Eyeballs	(Supine for tonometry)	6. Inspection Gentle palpation Tonometer	6. Appearance Tension (note positive family history of glaucoma; tonometry should be performed every 1–2 years on adults)
7. Ocular movements		7. Subject follows movements of examiner's finger	7. Paired movements of eyes, nystagmus, diplopia
8. Pupils		8. Inspection Flashlight	8. General inspection of size, shape, equality. Flashlight used to test reaction to light (light reflex). Accommodation tested by examiner bringing finger to bridge of subject's nose.
9. Conjunctiva		9. Inspection	9. Color, hemorrhage, injection, masses, foreign bodies.
10. Sclera		10. Inspection	10. Hemorrhage, jaundice, foreign bodies
11. Cornea		11. Inspection	11. Edema, lesions, clouding, macula, foreign bodies, ulceration
12. Iris		12. Inspection	12. Appearance, lesions, symmetry, foreign bodies
13. Anterior chamber		13. Inspection via ophthalmoscope	13. Pus, blood
14. Lens		14. Inspection via ophthalmoscope	14. Opacities
15. Fundus		15. Inspection via ophthalmoscope	15. Retina, optic disc, blood vessels, color, shape, size, exudate, hemorrhage
Ears		Compare *bilaterally* as follows:	
1. Auricle (pinnae)	Sitting if possible	1. Inspection Palpation	1. Masses, deformity, tenderness
2. Hearing acuity		2. Whispered word Ticking clock Tuning fork	2. Sound perception. In presence of reduced acuity, check lateralization and compare air and bone conduction. Rinne test; Weber test
3. Canal		3. Inspection via otoscope	3. Wax, discharge, color, mobility with swallowing, foreign bodies, masses, texture
4. Tympanic membrane (eardrum)		4. Inspection via otoscope	4. Color, bulging, perforation, discharge, fluid, scars, opacities

Table continued on the following pages

TABLE 16–5.   OVERVIEW OF ADULT GENERAL PHYSICAL EXAMINATION (*Continued*)

AREA	PATIENT POSITION	METHOD OF EXAMINATION	OBSERVATIONS/EXAMPLES
Nose and Sinuses	Sitting if possible	Inspection with flashlight and nasal speculum Substance to test smell	External nose: shape, size, deformity, asymmetry, masses Mucosa: discharge, bleeding, color, secretions Septum: straight, deviated, perforated Turbinates: thickness, size Nasal canal: patency, obstruction, polyps, drainage Frontal and maxillary sinuses: tenderness, thickening, secretions Sense of smell
Mouth	Sitting if possible	Inspection with flashlight and tongue depressor	Breath: aroma (odor) Lips: symmetry, color, moisture content, lesions, fissures, crusts, scars Teeth: alignment, caries, placque formation, missing teeth, deformities, dental restorations, dentures Gums or gingiva: appearance, color Mucosa: appearance, color, lesions, masses Palate: appearance, color, lesions, movement Tongue: appearance, color, lesions, masses, mobility, tremor, deviation, atrophy, enlargement, protrusion
		Substance to test taste	Sense of taste
Throat and Neck	Sitting if possible	Inspection with flashlight and tongue depressor Palpation Laryngoscope (if indicated)	Tonsils: appearance, color, enlargement, exudate Pharynx: appearance, color Larynx: appearance, color Musculoskeletal structure: nuchal rigidity (stiffness), range-of-motion, shape, symmetry, pain, swelling Lymph nodes and salivary glands: enlargement, distribution, tenderness, consistency, mobility Trachea: deviation from midline, tug Thyroid: enlargement, bruit, nodules Vessels: appearance, volume, symmetry, pulsation, bruit, murmur
Back and Spine; Posterior Thorax and Lungs	Standing if possible (spine) Sitting if possible with arms folded across chest (posterior thorax)	Inspection Palpation Percussion Auscultation (stethoscope)	Symmetry and strength of upper back muscles, posture, spinal profile (curvatures), spinal range-of-motion (mobility), skin condition, masses, muscle tone, pain, tenderness (e.g., costovertebral angle, spinous process, paravertebral muscles) See discussion of anterior thorax and lungs below

TABLE 16–5.   OVERVIEW OF ADULT GENERAL PHYSICAL EXAMINATION (*Continued*)

AREA	PATIENT POSITION	METHOD OF EXAMINATION	OBSERVATIONS/EXAMPLES
Breasts and Axillae	Sitting position first if possible, then supine (see far right column)	Compare *bilaterally* Inspection Palpation	*Female breasts:* inspect with subject sitting with arms relaxed at sides, then sitting with arms elevated over head, finally sitting with hands pressed against hips. Other positions may be: sitting hands clasped behind head; standing, leaning forward with arms outstretched, hands resting on chair back. Place small pillow under shoulder (with patient supine) of side being examined Breast observations: symmetry, contour, dimpling, size, level, tenderness, masses, nodules, skin color, vascular patterns, surface irregularity, rashes, skin retraction, ulceration, nipple inversion and/or discharge Axillary observations: (sitting position preferable) skin lesions, furuncles, rashes, enlarged axillary nodes
Anterior Thorax and Lungs	Sitting position at first (if wish) then supine	Compare *bilaterally* Inspection Palpation Percussion Auscultation (stethoscope) Measure chest diameter with tape measure if indicated	Thorax (chest): contour, size, shape, symmetry, deformity, slope of ribs, anteroposterior and lateral diameters, chest expansion (maximal circumference upon forced inspiration and expiration), boundaries of thoracic cavity, costal angle, rib or sternum tenderness, skin condition, masses, sinus tract, lesions, abnormal pulsations, mobility, respiratory motions (e.g., prolonged expiration, difficulty inspiring), abnormal chest movements (e.g., use of accessory muscles, intercostal muscle retraction or bulging, local lag or impairment in respiratory movement) Lungs: rate and quality of respiration, consolidation, cough, sputum, diaphragmatic level and movement (excursion), breath sounds and extra sounds, resonance, fremitus, rales, friction rubs
Heart	Supine (May wish to elevate upper body 35–40 degrees; may wish patient to sit up and lean forward or lie on left side)	Inspection Palpation Percussion Auscultation (stethoscope)	*Inspection:* pulsations (correlate findings with jugular venous pulse & carotid artery pulse), record jugular venous pulsations with patient sitting at 40° angle, measure height above sternoclavicular joint, point of maximum impulse (PMI), apical impulse *Palpation:* Locate PMI (localized or diffuse), apical impulse, thrill, palpable heart movements, intensity of left and right ventricular thrust, diastolic gallop, pericardial friction rub

Table continued on the following pages

TABLE 16–5.   OVERVIEW OF ADULT GENERAL PHYSICAL EXAMINATION (*Continued*)

AREA	PATIENT POSITION	METHOD OF EXAMINATION	OBSERVATIONS/EXAMPLES
Heart			*Percussion:* Estimate heart (cardiac) size *Auscultation:* heart sounds' rate, rhythm, intensity; first and second heart sounds; splitting of S_2; extra heart sounds (e.g., clicks, friction rub, opening snap, S_3 or S_4 gallop); murmurs (e.g., intensity, quality, location, radiation, timing)
Arteries		Compare *bilaterally:* Inspection Palpation Percussion Auscultation (stethoscope)	Presence, absence or diminution of expected arterial pulsations Arterial pulses (carotid, brachial, radial, femoral): rate, rhythm, volume, equality, pulse deficit Vessel walls, arteriosclerosis, bruit, capillary pulsation, blood pressure in popliteal arteries in presence of diastolic hypertension
Abdomen	Supine	Inspection Auscultation Percussion Palpation (light & deep)	Liver, spleen, kidneys, stomach, sigmoid colon, caecum, bladder, aorta, lymph nodes Appearance, contour, scars, lesions, subcutaneous fat, masses, organ enlargement, tenderness, pain, muscle tone, rigidity, tympany, dullness, distention, edema, abnormal pulsations, collateral circulation Hernias Intestinal activity: motility, pitch, frequency of bowel sounds
Genitals and Rectum Genital and rectal exams are often combined. Details of general rectal exam are in "C" below. Note presence or absence of secondary sex characteristics during examination.			
A. *Male genitalia*	Supine Standing or left lateral decubitus position (lying on left side) for rectal	Inspection Palpation	Penis, prepuce (retract and examine), testes (compare bilaterally) Masses, scars, lesions, discharge, tenderness, size, swelling, atrophy, enlargement, thickness, epididymitis, varicocele, hydrocele, spermatocele During rectal, examine prostate (size, shape, nodules, consistency, tenderness) and seminal vesicles

TABLE 16–5. OVERVIEW OF ADULT GENERAL PHYSICAL EXAMINATION (*Continued*)

AREA	PATIENT POSITION	METHOD OF EXAMINATION	OBSERVATIONS/EXAMPLES
B. Female genitalia	Supine Lithotomy	Inspection (vaginal speculum used for vaginal exam) Palpation (gloves) Materials for bacteriologic cultures and Papanicolaou smears	Vaginal speculum and bimanual examination, Papanicolaou smear, vaginoabdominal and rectovaginal examination *External genitalia* appearance, mons pubis, labia, clitoris, Skene's and Bartholin's glands, urethral orifice, vaginal opening (introitus): inflammation, ulceration, enlargement, swelling, nodules, discharge *Vagina* (discharge, hymen, color, ulcers, masses, inflammation, retrocele, cystocele); *cervix* (color, position, consistency, outlet, ulcerations, nodules, discharge, bleeding, tenderness, mobility, masses); *uterus* (contour, size, position, consistency, masses, tenderness, mobility); *adnexa* (tenderness, masses)
C. Rectum	*Male:* Various positions may be used, e.g., standing (bending at hips over bed or examining table), lateral *Female:* lithotomy or lateral	Inspection Palpation (gloves, lubrication) Proctoscope may be used to visualize rectum	Inspect perianal and sacrococcygeal areas at this time for rash, inflammation, lumps, cysts, sinus Anal sphincter tone, rectal prolapse, polyps, hemorrhoids (internal, external), bleeding, discharge, feces, mass, nodule, ulceration, tenderness, fistula, fissure
Nervous System and Musculoskeletal System	During a general physical examination the examiner does a screening of the nervous and musculoskeletal systems. These initial screening activities are followed by complete examinations of these systems if indicated. Activities which may be included in the *preliminary screening:* (a) assessment of patient's abilities to grip examiner's fingers, maintain arms held forward, do a knee bend, hop and walk on toes and heels and (b) evaluation of gait and Romberg's sign. A *complete neurologic examination* commonly tests the following six functions: (1) cerebral, (2) cranial nerve, (3) cerebellar, (4) motor, (5) sensory and (6) reflex. Neurologic examination might include various special diagnostic tests, e.g., brain scan, electroencephalography (EEG), computerized axial tomography (CAT scan, EMI), echoencephalography, pneumoencephalography, cerebral angiography, myelography.		

tient's drape is removed (without exposing the patient) and he is assisted with clothing and bedlinens as necessary. The rectal and perineal areas may need cleansing to remove lubricant or body secretions. Used linens, pads, and equipment are dealt with as appropriate, and the examining room or patient's unit is left in order. If the patient is in bed, leave him safe and comfortable.

Various *forms* are available for *recording findings* of the total physical examination, or the findings may be written out in an essentially narrative, outline format. If the nurse has not performed the physical but is recording in the patient record that a physical examination was performed, the following information might be noted: time of examination, name of examiner, pertinent observations made by the nurse that will assist in planning nursing care, specimens collected and disposition of specimens, e.g., sent to clinical laboratory.

In recording findings of a physical examination the examiner typically uses a comparison chart for recording various *reflexes*. The chart may be a simple figure drawing on which the right (R) and left (L) are indicated and the degree of reflex activity (on a scale of + to + + + +, i.e., 1 plus to 4 plus) is marked for the reflexes tested. An alternate method of recording reflexes is on a simple chart such as:

Reflexes	Right	Left
Biceps	+ + + +	+ + +
Triceps	+ + + +	+ +
etc.		

Ancillary (Adjuvant) Examinations*

Scopes, mirrors and specula are useful in visualizing many structures; however, some structures do not lend themselves to any of these approaches, e.g., kidneys, brain, heart, liver, bone, muscle. A mushrooming number of *specialized diagnostic tools and procedures* are useful in evaluating these and other structures

---

*Space does not permit detailed discussion of diagnostic techniques. The interested reader is referred to specialized texts and/or a textbook of medical-surgical nursing, e.g., Luckmann and Sorensen *Medical-Surgical Nursing: A Psychophysiologic Approach.* See also this chapter's bibliography.

and in studying those disorders which produce changes that cannot be seen, felt or heard, e.g., diabetes. Examples of such specialized devices and activities are: x-rays (roentgenography), nuclear medicine diagnostic activities, electrodiagnostic procedures, surgical biopsies, pathology techniques, cardiopulmonary laboratory tests and clinical laboratory tests. A mental status examination and various psychologic tests may be used to facilitate diagnosis in persons with primary psychiatric or neurologic disorders.

Collectively we refer to all of these as *ancillary examinations.* This phrase simply means examinations that supplement the findings in a patient's history and physical examination. For purposes of discussion, we have separated the specialized diagnostic examinations into "psychiatric-psychologic ancillary examinations" and "physical ancillary examinations."

Psychiatric-psychologic Ancillary Examinations. A *mental status examination* is highly important in establishing a psychiatric diagnosis. It consists of: (a) informal observation of the client and the content of his remarks during the interview and (b) direct questioning, focusing mainly on evaluating the patient's sensorium. Major areas covered in a mental status examination are listed below.[110] In recording findings, it is typical for the heading to be listed, followed by appropriate comments.

▶ *Appearance,* e.g., make up, mode of dress

▶ *Activity and behavior,* e.g., gestures, gait, coordination of bodily movements

▶ *Affect,* e.g., lack of emotional response or presence of outward manifestations of emotions such as fear, anger, depression, elation, resentment

▶ *Mood,* e.g., observable emotional manifestations, inward feelings, sum of statements

▶ *Speech,* e.g., spontaneity, coherence, articulation, duration of utterance, latency of response (pause before answering)

▶ *Thought content,* e.g., preoccupations, associations, delusions, depersonalization, obsessions, hallucinations, unusual experiences, anger, fear, paranoid ideation

▶ *Sensorium*

1. Orientation to person, place, time and circumstances
2. Recent and remote memory and recall
3. Calculations, digit retention (forward and backward), serial 7's and 3's
4. General fund of knowledge (well-

known leaders, places, events, distances)

5. Ability to do abstract thinking, e.g., to explain a common proverb.

▶ *Judgment*, e.g., concerning common problems such as what to do if you run out of medicine.

▶ *Insight*, e.g., into nature and extent of present disorder and its ramifications.

As previously mentioned, *psychologic tests* are valuable in assessing some persons with psychiatric or neurologic disorders. Such tests may: (a) differentiate between organic and psychic disorders, (b) measure intelligence, and (c) provide information about psychopathology, psychodynamics, personality and feelings. Psychologic tests may be classified as either "objective" or "projective."[110]

Objective tests are qualitative evaluations in which a client's responses are compared to standard, established norms. Examples of objective psychologic tests are:

▶ Vocational aptitude and interest tests

▶ Intelligence tests, e.g., Wechsler Adult Intelligence Scale (WAIS)

▶ Minnesota Multiphasic Personality Inventory (MMPI)

Projective psychologic tests reflect a client's fantasies and individual modes of adaptation and are of limited usefulness. Examples include sentence completion tests, Draw-a-Person tests, Rorschach Psychodiagnosis (interpretation of inkblots), and the Thematic Apperception Test (TAT), which calls for interpretation of people in various situations. Psychologic tests must be administered and interpreted by skilled psychologists.

In addition to being used to assess primary psychiatric disorders, some psychological testing may be given to clients having symptoms with a large psychic component, e.g., pain.

Physical Ancillary Examinations. In the course of establishing a diagnosis, ancillary physical examinations may be performed which will: (a) identify the source of the disorder, i.e., the "causative agent," (b) assess structural pathologic changes in the patient's body, (c) assess the patient's physiologic responses to the disorder and (d) assess the patient's functional impairments related to the disorder. (In the presence of neurologic problems, as pointed out above, the patient's psyche may also be investigated.) During the course of treatment some of these same examinations may be repeated to evaluate the patient's response to the treatment being given.

Ancillary physical examinations investigate not only the body's systems, organs and tissues, but also its fluids, excretions, cells and subcellular levels. Table 16–6 summarizes various physical ancillary examinations.

It is vitally important that all diagnostic test forms, specimens and test results be properly identified and handled. This ensures that the correct test is performed on the correct patient and that the findings of each patient's tests are accurately recorded. It also ensures that the laboratory receives fresh specimens.

Close cooperation is necessary between health team members during diagnostic testing to prevent serious mistakes. The attending physician, surgeon, radiologist, pathologist and clinical laboratory technician must closely coordinate their efforts. Often the accuracy of these diagnostic procedures depends upon proper scheduling of the tests and proper preparation of the patient (physically and psychologically) for the tests. Nurses play important roles in these activities. Commonly patients look to the nurse for instruction about: (a) what a specific test is, (b) what preparation is necessary (what do they need to do before the test, what will others do to them before the test), (c) what will happen to them during the test, what instruments will be used, and what sensations they might experience during the test (Will it hurt? Will I get a shock from it? Will I be put to sleep? Will I be stuck with any needles? Where will the catheter be put? What *is* a catheter?), (d) what will the test findings be likely to show and (e) what will happen after the test (Can I eat right away? Will I have to stay longer? Will they do anything else? How will I find out what they found and when will I hear?). The nurse's role in patient education is discussed in Chap. 17.

Patients are often highly anxious while diagnostic tests are being performed. Naturally they are worried about the possible findings and what those findings might mean—prognosis and treatment. Nurses can and should perform a valuable and expected service to patients by helpfully discussing the patients' concerns with them (refer to Chaps. 3, 10, 11, and 12).

In addition to the previously mentioned activities, nurses often are responsible for the aftercare of patients following diagnostic testing. This may include providing immediate aftercare (ensuring the patient's comfort, preventing complications, observing for untoward effects) and assisting with future referrals, tests or treatments.

The informed nurse is aware of potential hazards and complications associated with diagnostic physical examinations; for example, the cumulative effect of radiation must be considered, special waste precautions may be necessary following radioisotope studies, contrast dyes may cause untoward reactions.

All diagnostic tests should be entered into the patient's record: time and place of test, person performing test, special preparations and aftercare, findings.

Table 16–7 summarizes basic laboratory data and other tests commonly performed with physical examinations. As noted, not all of these tests are required for every patient.

EXAMINATIONS BY X-RAYS. *Roentgenography* refers to passing x-rays through the body for purposes of taking pictures (x-ray films or roentgenograms) of internal body structures (Fig. 16–12). The x-rays, after passing through the body, act on specially sensitized film.

X-rays (also called "roentgen rays") are electromagnetic radiation with extremely short wave lengths. The short wave lengths give x-rays special penetrating abilities. X-rays pen-

TABLE 16–6.   EXAMPLES OF DIAGNOSTIC PROCEDURES

Cardiovascular and Hematopoietic Systems

Ballistocardiography
Blood pressure measurement
Blood tests
Bone marrow aspiration
Cardiac blood pool scan
Cardiac catheterization { intracardiac pressure / intra-arterial pressure }
Circulation time
Dynamic blood flow studies (radionuclide angiography)
Echocardiography
Electrocardiogram (ECG or EKG)
Exercise tolerance
Ophthalmoscopic examination
Pericardium scan
Perthes' test
Phonocardiography
Plethysmography
Pulse assessment
Regitine test
Trendelenburg test
Tourniquet (capillary fragility) test
Ultrasound (heart; aorta)
Urinalysis
Venous pressure measurement
X-ray examinations: fluoroscopy (orthodiagraphy); intravenous angiocardiography; cardioangiography; aortography; arteriography; lymphangiography; venography (lower extremity phlebography); thoracic, abdominal and peripheral angiography

Digestive System

Feces examination (chemical, macroscopic, microscopic)
Gallbladder ultrasound
Gastric analysis (direct via nasogastric tube or indirect with dye)
Gastroenteroscopic examinations: colonoscopy with fiberoptic scope; esophagoscopy; gastroscopy with fiberoptic scope; peritoneoscopy; proctoscopy; upper GI endoscopy; sigmoidoscopy
Liver examinations: biopsy; excretory function tests; metabolic function tests, scan, serum protein tests, ultrasound
X-ray examinations: cholangiography, intravenous cholangiography (IVC), postoperative (T-tube) cholangiography, percutaneous transhepatic cholangiography; cholecystography, oral; colon series or barium enema; endoscopic pancreatocholangiography; esophagoscopy (barium swallow); hypotonic duodenography; upper GI series (UGIS) and small bowel examination

Kidney and Urinary Tract

Blood tests
Cystometry
Cystoscopy (cystourethroscopy)
Electronic evaluation of urinary flow rate
Kidney function tests (clearance, concentration, excretion)
Nephrotomography
Renal biopsy
Renal scan
Renogram
Urethral calibration
Urine examination
X-ray examinations: excretory urography (intravenous pyelography [IVP]); retrograde urography (pyelography); retrograde urethrography; voiding cystourethrography (VCU)

Musculoskeletal System

Aspiration of synovial fluid
Biopsy (muscle)
Blood tests
Bone scan
Cultures, e.g., skin lesions
Electromyography
Knee arthrography
Metabolic tests
Urine tests
X-ray examinations of bones and joints

TABLE 16–6.   EXAMPLES OF DIAGNOSTIC PROCEDURES (*Continued*)

Respiratory System

Bronchoscopy (fiberoptic or rigid scope)
Blood tests
Gastric contents analysis
Lung scan
Nasal and throat swabbings for smear and culture
Pulmonary function tests (PFT's)
Respiration assessment
Skin tests
Sputum examination (smear, culture)
Thoracentesis (obtain pleural fluid for examination)
X-ray examinations: AP chest film; bronchography; fluoroscopy, tomograms

Nervous System

Caloric test
Cerebrospinal fluid examination
Cisternal puncture
Echoencephalography
Electroencephalography (EEG)
Electromyography (EMG)
Intrathecal (subarachnoid) scan
Lumbar puncture (spinal tap)
Neurologic physical examination
Psychologic examinations
Sweat test
X-ray examinations: angiography of head and neck; cerebral angiography; computerized transaxial tomography (CAT scan); myelography; pneumoencephalography (PEG); ventriculography

Reproductive System

Female:
  Amniocentesis
  Hysterosalpingography
  Mammography
  Papanicolaou smear
  Placental scan
  Smear and culture
  Ultrasound
Male:
  Examination of spermatozoa
  Smear and culture

Endocrine System

Basal metabolic rate (BMR)
Glucose tolerance test (GTT)
Pancreas scan
Spleen scan
Thyroid hormone tests
Thyroid scan

---

etrate substances to varying depths, depending upon the densities of the various substances and the voltage used. The exposure of an x-ray film is determined by the differing amounts of radiation reaching the film.

Very dense structures (opaque structures) block the passage of the x-rays onto the film by absorbing more rays. Thus, the film underlying bones and other dense structures, such as foreign objects, is not heavily exposed and therefore remains lighter in color. The reverse is true with less dense (more translucent) structures such as soft tissue, internal organs, skin, muscles, body fat. Because the x-rays easily penetrate structures of this kind, they expose the underlying film, turning it darker.

Sometimes *radiopaque substances* are introduced into the patient before x-ray films are taken. Because radiopaque materials block x-rays, they can serve as "contrast media" in the patient, by clearly outlining the structures in which they are x-rayed. The contrast medium is particularly helpful because it creates a contrast on the x-ray film between two structures that would otherwise be difficult to tell apart because they are equally dense.

For example, in Figure 16–12 the patient was administered barium (a radiopaque substance) prior to a series of x-ray films. As the barium passes through the patient's digestive system, x-ray films are taken at one-hour intervals over a three-hour period. The barium clearly outlines the patient's intestines, which would otherwise not be visible on the x-ray films be-

TABLE 16–7.   BASIC LABORATORY DATA AND OTHER TESTS COMMONLY PERFORMED WITH PHYSICAL EXAMINATION*

AP chest x-ray
Electrocardiogram
Hematology, e.g., white blood count (WBC) and differential (diff), hematocrit (Hct), red blood cell morphology, platelet estimate
Indexes
Skin test with purified protein derivative (PPD)
Sputum smear
Stool guaiac
Urinalysis

*Not all of the above are required for every patient. (Adapted from Krupp, M. Q., et al.: *Physician's Handbook*, 18th ed. Los Altos, CA, Lange Medical Publications, 1976.)

cause they are soft tissue surrounded by other soft tissue.

A wide variety of *contrast studies* (such as the barium series just discussed) can be performed. Other examples are: cerebral angiogram (to visualize cerebral blood vessels), myelogram (to visualize the spinal subarachnoid space) and bronchogram (to visualize the tracheobronchial tree). The contrast media used are usually either a heavy metallic salt or a gas. These media are introduced in differing ways depending upon the test to be performed. For example, barium (for demonstrating the gastrointestinal tract) may be swallowed or given by enema; dyes may be introduced intravenously or swallowed in tablet

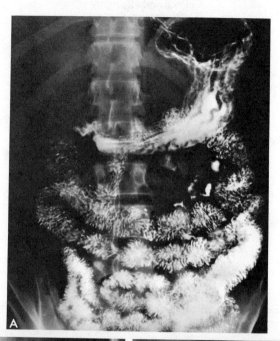

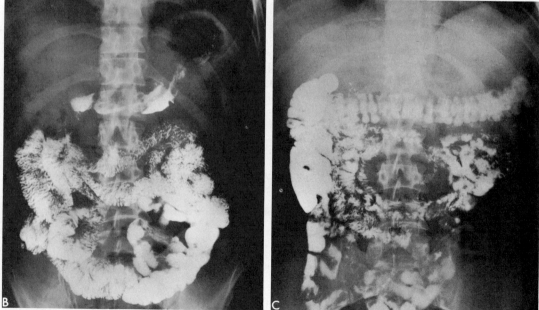

Figure 16–12. Frequent-interval film and fluoroscopy method for examination of the small intestine. *A,* At 1 hour after administration of the barium; *B,* at 2 hours; *C,* at 3 hours. (From Meschan, I.: *Radiographic Positioning and Related Anatomy,* 2nd ed. Philadelphia, W. B. Saunders Co., 1978.)

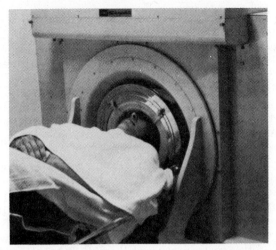

Figure 16–13. Computerized axial tomography (CAT). (From Reeves, K. R.: This CAT is a revolutionary scanner. *RN, 39*:41, Aug. 1976.)

form; air may be injected through a needle (pneumoencephalogram).

Fluoroscopy uses x-rays to observe the body's deep structures (e.g., joints, organs, systems) in motion. The patient is positioned between a fluorescent screen and the x-ray source (x-ray tube) and images of the moving internal structures are projected onto a screen. A darkened room facilitates observation of the screen. Often a radiopaque medium is given to the patient to help distinguish the structure

being assessed. Fluoroscopy reveals the size, shape and movements of organs such as the heart, lungs, stomach and intestines.

Computerized transaxial tomography (abbreviated various ways, e.g., CT, CAT, CAT Scan) is a relatively new, safe, diagnostic x-ray procedure. In essence the machine channels x-rays through the patient (at differing planes) and into a computer (Fig. 16–13). A 180-degree scan of the structure is made in three or four different planes. The computer records the "absorption potentials" of various tissues at various planes and supplies a printout which represents the structure studied (Fig. 16–14).

As mentioned earlier, body tissues vary in density. For CAT computer purposes, the various tissue densities are assigned numbers arbitrarily. These numbers (called "absorption coefficients") range from +500 (most dense) for bone, down to −500 (least dense) for air. Note the numbers in Figure 16–14 *A*.

In addition to providing computer printouts, photographs are taken of the image on the screen (Fig. 16–14 *B*). Color photographs are possible, but most are produced in varying shades of gray, e.g., bone appears black, soft tissues are differing gray tones, air is white.

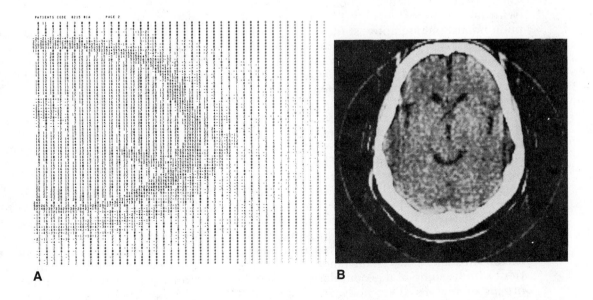

A   **B**

Figure 16–14. *A,* CAT computer printout. (From Skydell, B., and Crowder, A. S.: *Diagnostic Procedures: A Reference for Health Practitioners and a Guide for Patient Counseling.* Boston, Little, Brown & Co., 1975, pp. 44 and 45.) *B,* Polaroid photograph of EMI scan. (From Reeves, K. R.: This CAT is a revolutionary scanner.)

While conventional skull films are taken in lateral, anterior or posterior views, the CAT x-ray image gives a view as if one were looking down through the top of the head.

X-ray films taken at varying depths of the same structure produce pictures which visually "section" or "slice" the structure at different levels, e.g., the structure is divided by a series of x-rays into horizontal slices. Such x-ray films are called *tomograms* and may be produced not only by a CAT, but also by other x-ray machines. Tomograms give the radiologist the opportunity to visually slice apart a living, intact and functioning organ for study in a manner that formerly only the pathologist was able to do with a knife at autopsy.

Tomograms produced by a CAT are greatly superior to those taken by conventional x-ray machines. Because the CAT is 100 times more sensitive to differences in tissue densities, it makes it possible for the radiologist to visualize structures which cannot be seen on a standard x-ray film.[195] In some cases dye is injected to enhance visualization.

CAT's have most commonly been used to visualize the brain, although there are now whole-body CAT's that can produce tomograms from any level of the body. In some facilities CAT brain scans are replacing less safe procedures such as nuclear brain scans (with radioisotopes), cerebral angiograms and pneumoencephalography studies. Because a CAT scan uses x-rays and not radioactive tracer substances (used in nuclear brain scans), the patient is subjected to no more radiation than he would receive with conventional skull x-rays.

EXAMINATION BY RADIOACTIVE MATERIALS. *Radioisotope-tracer materials* may be used to test some organ functions and to identify the location of some malignancies. This is possible because radioactive isotopes (also called "radionuclides" or "radiopharmaceuticals") give off radioactivity as they transform, or decay, at constant, predictable rates. A wide variety of radioactive tracer substances are available for diagnostic uses. After one of these tracer substances has been placed in the patient's body, some of it accumulates in specific organs or regions. That body area's structure and function can then be assessed by (a) placing detectors over the area of radioactive tracer accumulation and measuring the area's radioactivity or (b) extracting samples (such as blood, urine, or stool) from the body and measuring the sample for radioactivity.

Two basic types of detectors commonly used are: (a) the reticular scanner (has a relatively small viewing field) and (b) the gamma camera or scintillation camera (combines a scanner with a camera and has a larger viewing field).[185] Both types detect emissions from a radioactive source and convert the emissions into signals which can be recorded and studied. In other words, the detectors are similar to sophisticated Geiger counters.

The gamma camera makes it possible to view on an oscilloscope screen the accumulation and distribution of the radioisotopes. Photographs (scintiphotographs) of the image are then periodically taken. The gamma camera actually produces an image without scanning. However, this instrument is still commonly referred to as a "scan" device.[222]

The reticular scanner must be moved back and forth (horizontally or vertically) across the organ being scanned. This movement is done at predetermined distances and rates. The scanning is then done line by line as the radiation emissions are converted into electrical impulses and counted.

Scanning is possible in structures and organs such as the brain, bone, lungs, liver, kidneys, spleen, pericardium and thyroid. As the tracer substance collects in the structure being assessed, it is possible to obtain a visual representation of the distribution of the tracer. In some areas of the body the radioisotopes will be more highly concentrated than in others. The skilled interpreter of nuclear scans can make assessments about an organ's size, shape, position and function from the pattern of distribution. It is also possible to identify the presence and size of abnormalities such as malignant tumors.

Examples of radiopharmaceuticals which may be used as tracers are: xenon 133 (^{133}Xe), iodine 131 (^{131}I), technetium 99m pertechnetate (^{99m}Tc pertechnetate), radioiodinated serum albumin (^{131}RISA), mercury 197 chlormerodrin (^{197}Hg chlormerodrin), radioiron (^{59}Fe), ^{131}I-rose bengal dye, ^{198}Au (gold) colloid, and ^{131}I with human serum albumin ([^{131}I]HSA).

OTHER ANCILLARY EXAMINATIONS

▶ *Ultrasonic waves* (sound waves too high in frequency for the human ear to detect) are used diagnostically to evaluate various body structures. The waves are directed at the organ or structure to be evaluated. As the waves vibrate back from their target they are transduced into oscilloscope tracings. Pathologic changes in muscles and joints may be studied by using sound. The brain (*echoencephalography*) and the heart (*echocardiography*) can also be studied.

Other examples of the diagnostic use of sound are: (a) *audiometry*, to assess hearing sensitivity and discrimination and (b) palencephalography (use of extremely sensitive microphones) to assess blood flow in the head.

▶ The temperature of various body areas can be assessed by the use of *thermography*. The resultant record of the test is called a "thermogram." Thermography may be employed to assess tumors, blood vessels and inflammatory processes.

▶ *Cardiopulmonary laboratories* are specialized to study the functions of the heart and lungs. For example, in studying the lungs, various pulmonary ventilatory capacity measurements may be made by using equipment such as spirometers.

▶ *Electrodiagnosis* means using electricity for diagnostic purposes. Examples of electrodiagnostic procedures are: *electrocardiography* (ECG or EKG, assesses heart function), *electroencephalography* (EEG, assesses brain function) and *electromyography* (EMG, assesses muscle function). Graphic recordings are produced with each of these diagnostic procedures. These records become part of the patient's record and are interpreted ("read") by specialists.

▶ A *biopsy* is the procedure of obtaining tissue from the living body for microscopic examination. Biopsies are commonly performed to look for evidence of malignancy or infection in the tissue specimen. The tissue sample may be obtained by: (a) puncture, needle or aspiration, (b) endoscopy or (c) surgical excision.

To perform a *needle biopsy* of an internal organ (e.g., liver) a special hollow needle is inserted through the body wall and into the organ being tested. Bone marrow may also be obtained by needle biopsy. *Endoscopy*, as mentioned, refers to the use of specially designed scopes for direct visual examination of the interior body structures. Special instruments may be inserted through these scopes to obtain a biopsy. *Excision biopsies* (e.g., muscle biopsy, breast biopsy) are performed by surgical cutting. With any biopsy, it is important that the specimen be obtained from the exact area in question and that the tissue specimen be properly handled once obtained, e.g., placed in special solution.

▶ *Tissue specimens* are sent to a *pathology laboratory* for detailed examination by a pathologist, who studies the specimen for structural alterations produced by disease.

LABORATORY TESTS. Specimens of *body fluids, exudates and excretions* may be obtained during the diagnostic (and treatment) process and sent to a *clinical laboratory* for study by laboratory technicians. In the laboratory, chemical, physical and microscopic methods are used to analyze the various specimens. Clinical laboratory tests evaluate abnormal body function in biochemical or physiologic terms.

Examples of substances that are studied in a clinical laboratory are: blood, sputum, urine, feces and cerebrospinal fluid (c.s.f.). Other body fluids may also be studied, e.g., pleural fluid, synovial fluid, amniotic fluid, peritoneal fluid, pericardial fluid, gastrointestinal secretions, perspiration. Contents of abscesses or cysts may be aspirated for study. Swabs may be used to obtain specimens of tissue exudate, nasopharyngeal discharge and vaginal and cervical discharge.

Any specimen must be carefully handled. This means proper specimen collection and labeling as well as delivery of the specimen to the laboratory while it is fresh. In some instances, a special preservative or some other agent is added to the specimen container. It is always important to know the temperature at which a specimen should be kept once it is collected: some are refrigerated, others are iced, still others are kept at room temperature. Failure to handle a specimen properly can distort the findings and make it necessary to obtain another specimen. For the patient this may mean repeating all the preparations, returning to the health care facility, and enduring the discomfort of another specimen being collected. Such errors are costly in terms of worry, inconvenience, time and money. Possibly even more serious is the error of putting one patient's name on another patient's specimen. Pause and consider some possible consequences from such an error!

Some basic laboratory tests are so important that they may be recommended in the initial work-up of all patients. Among these are: blood smear; total white cell count and differential; hematocrit; and urinalysis, including microscopic examination of a fresh specimen.[110]

Information technology using computers has entered the medical care field in several areas. One of these is in laboratory data systems. Currently, laboratory tests are more commonly produced as *batteries* instead of being ordered and reported singly. The *M-6* is one common blood test combination; it determines serum sodium, serum potassium, carbon-dioxide combining power, serum chloride, blood urea nitrogen, and glucose tolerance. More detailed

SMA-12 are that the test is: (a) convenient (one venipuncture produces 12 separate pieces of information and provides a complete biochemical profile), (b) fast (12 analyses are made in 60 seconds), (c) economical (the cost of the SMA-12 is less than if the 12 tests were done separately), (d) comprehensive (the results can reveal unsuspected malfunctions or abnormalities that may not be evident from the patient's history or physical examination and (e) easily interpreted (abnormal findings can be noted at a glance). It must be remembered, however, that different combinations of tests may be included among the 12 in different institutions. Also, additional follow-up tests may be necessary.

Batteries of tests, such as the SMA-12, are commonly used during hospital admission as a routine screening device. The practice of ordering batteries of tests is supported by some and cautioned against by others. However, whether batteries of tests are used or not, medical experts appear to agree that one "must not give undue weight to reports or opinions received from laboratory sources. Such reports are liable to a variety of errors of observation and interpretation. The results acquire true significance only when correlated with the clinical observations."[110]

Because the ranges of normal values can vary from one clinical laboratory to another (depending upon the laboratory methods), one should know the normal range of an individual laboratory before assessing the laboratory findings for a given patient.

Additionally, it is of importance to note that laboratory tests can be affected by drugs which the patient has taken in the 72 hours prior to the specimen collection. For example, low dosages of salicylates may elevate the blood uric acid level and corticosteroids may markedly elevate

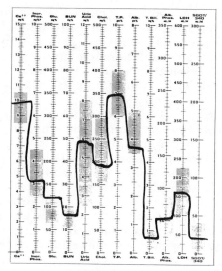

Figure 16–15. SMA 12/60 Serum Chemistry Graph. (From Elsberry, N. L.: Lab report. SMA-12: here's one way to interpret it. *Nursing '75*, 5:70, May 1975.)

combinations are also available. One is the *SMA-12* (sequential multiple analysis of 12 separate laboratory blood tests). The results of this test are printed on a sheet of paper in a series of bar graphs. Each bar has a shaded portion that indicates the normal level for that particular test (Fig. 16–15). Table 16–8 summarizes the measurements made in one SMA-12 and the major area which is assessed by each of the various tests.

Elsberry[57] notes that advantages of the

TABLE 16–8.   SMA–12 MEASUREMENTS*

Substance Measured	Major Area Assessed
Glucose (Glu.) Cholesterol (Chol.) Total Protein (T.P.) Albumin (Alb.)	Nutritional Status
Bilirubin (T. bill.)	Liver Function
Blood urea nitrogen (BUN) Uric acid	Kidney Function
SGOT L.D.H. Alkaline phosphatase (Alk. Phos.)	Tissue Injury
Calcium (Ca++) Phosphate (Inor. Phos.)	Parathyroid Function

*Based on Elsberry, N. L.: Lab report. SMA–12: here's one way to interpret it. *Nursing '75*, 5:70, May 1975.

the white cell count, lower the sedimentation rate and cause a diminution in the eosinophil count. A sampling of normal values for clinical laboratory tests is presented in Appendix I.

TREATMENT

> To cure sometimes,
> To relieve often,
> To comfort always.*

Treatment is based upon a patient's diagnosis or apparent needs. The first part of this chapter looked extensively at the diagnostic process. In this section we take a rather general look at the treatment process—some of the forms treatment may take and some problems actually caused by treatments. Preventive medicine is also briefly considered.

We view treatment as the "management and care of a patient or the combating of disease or disorder."[133] The word "care" is important in this definition. Throughout all types and phases of treatment, "caring for" and "caring about" the patient are central activities. As shown in the quotation above, "cure" is not always the goal of treatment. Some persons have disorders that cannot be cured. However, it *is* always possible to comfort and frequently it is possible to provide relief. In fact, it is in "caring" that the truly skilled nurse has most expertise (see Chap. 4).

You will spend a great deal of time studying treatments. Most of the remainder of this text discusses nursing activities related to treating patients. Indeed, most of your formal nursing education may focus primarily on learning how to care for patients undergoing a variety of treatments. In some instances you will be the person administering the specific treatment (e.g., medication, catheterization, wound care); at other times you will be caring for the patient before and after the primary treatment (e.g., surgery, radiation) has been performed by someone else.

Terminology

The word *treatment* (like the word "diagnosis") is used in a variety of ways. Some of the more general (broader) uses are with reference to: (a) the *goal, direction* or *basis* of treatment (see box below), (b) the *form, modality* or *route* of treatment, e.g., physical, intravenous, chemical, dietary, surgical, group, electroconvulsive, radiation (discussion of these begins on p.

---

*Quotation on statue in honor of the physician Edward Trudeau at Saranac Lake.

234), and (c) the *professional group* supervising or administering the treatment, e.g., nursing, medical, dental.

Terms used with Reference to the Goal, Direction or Basis of Treatment

Causal treatment: *directed at the cause of the disorder.*

Conservative treatment: *designed to conserve the body's vital powers until clear indications of the specific disorder develop, or directed at avoiding radical surgical or other radical therapeutic measures, e.g., in elderly or debilitated patients.*

Curative treatment: *directed at eradicating the patient's disorder by curing the existing disease, i.e., the opposite of palliative treatment.*

Empiric treatment: *employs methods that experience has shown to be helpful.*

Palliative treatment: *does not attempt a cure, but rather is directed at relieving pain and distress.*

Preventive treatment: *directed at preventing the occurrence of a particular disorder.*

Rational treatment: *employs therapies based upon knowledge of disease and knowledge of action of the particular remedies used.*

Specific treatment: *effective against the organism causing the disease, i.e., treatment especially adapted to the specific disease being treated.*

Symptomatic treatment: *(also called expectant treatment) directed at obtaining relief of symptom rather than at cure of a specific cause.*

Some more specific uses of the word treatment are in terms of: (a) the particular *type of disorder* being treated, e.g., reactive depression, cancer, spinal fracture, burn and (b) the *functional area* or *specific body function* being treated, e.g., occupational, speech, respiratory, dental, ocular. Some overlapping may occur. For example, dental treatment may refer to the professional group administering the treatment or to the functional area being treated. Likewise, medical treatment may refer to the professional group supervising the treatment or to the form of treatment. Commonly the word "therapy" is used interchangeably with "treatment."

Treatment Process

Professional practitioners involved in treating patients must be aware of the following as related to their own area of practice: (a) current acceptable therapies and trends toward new treatment modalities, (b) advantages and disadvantages (including possible complications and hazards) of the various treatments, (c) legal and professional aspects of therapy (Chap. 19), (d) how to select optimum treatment methods and supplementary treatment activities, (e) how to appropriately administer and assess treatment, (f) how to participate effectively in the total team approach to patient care, (g) how to utilize one's self therapeutically, (h) how to elicit effective patient cooperation and (i) patient rights concerning treatment. Let us briefly examine some of these factors more closely.

Decision making is an important part of the treatment process. (See discussions of decision making and problem solving in Chap. 17.) Individualized treatments must be decided upon for each specific patient. Because a patient's condition undergoes constant change, his treatment plan must be reassessed and restructured frequently. (Chap. 17 discusses assessment.) It is necessary for the health practitioner to be familiar with the new treatments constantly being introduced. Obviously, the treatment of a disorder is not static but rather varies from one time to another within a profession. Treatment also varies from patient to patient as well as for the same patient at different times.

In deciding on the optimum treatment for a given patient the health practitioner considers the cause of the disorder, the type of complications present, and the specificity and safety of available treatments. While some treatments are quite precise and specific in their actions, others have more general effects.

It is not uncommon for some form of treatment to be started before a definitive diagnosis is reached, e.g., lifesaving measures (Chap. 35) or comfort measures may be instituted before a patient's specific problem is identified. It is important, however, that medications not be given which may interfere with diagnosis.

Also, it is not uncommon for a given patient to be undergoing several treatments, for various disorders, at the same time. When this happens, the effect of the different treatments on each other requires careful forethought and ongoing evaluation. Many treatments have disadvantages or drawbacks. Iatrogenic disorders are discussed later in this chapter.

Just as a patient has the right to know his diagnosis and prognosis, it is also his right to be informed about treatments that he will undergo. *An informed patient is likely to be a more cooperative patient,* and patient participation is a vital part of successful treatment. (Patient rights are discussed in Chap. 20; patient-family education is discussed in Chap. 17.)

Preparation of a patient for treatment often involves both psychological and physical preparation. The patient should be informed of the reason for treatment, potential risks associated with treatment, the expected outcomes from treatment and his role in the treatment process. Nurses are commonly the health worker with whom patients feel most comfortable in discussing their treatment plans and their concerns about the entire illness-treatment experience (see also Chap. 3).

A patient who fails to comply with treatment instructions (e.g., a patient who takes more or less medication than the prescribed amount) may seriously jeopardize the treatment outcome. A patient's compliance with treatment is carefully assessed in deciding how much responsibility he can assume in his treatment plan. For example: Will the patient exercise as prescribed? Will he stay on the diet ordered for him? Will he stay on the proposed medication regimen? Will he return for follow-up care?

Every person involved in a treatment process needs to be aware of her own effectiveness as a therapeutic agent and needs to use the power of positive therapeutic suggestion with sensitivity and skill. It is well-recognized that the therapist who is enthusiastic about expected treatment results often obtains better results than one who is unenthusiastic, possibly even negative, about the possible benefits of a treatment.

Nurses who use themselves as therapeutic agents are commonly able to enhance the effectiveness of treatments they administer. This practice is called therapeutic use of self.

Types of Therapies

"In this century more new effective therapeutic agents have been developed than in all times past."[210] In addition to a myriad of advances in the more "routine" aspects of medication administration, surgery, psychotherapy, physical medicine and dietetics, the past few decades have seen dramatic therapeutic advances in areas such as: hemodialysis, organ transplantation, crisis intervention, operant conditioning, biofeedback, joint replacement, surgery on vital organs, self-help groups, blood administration, genetics, cardiopulmonary therapy, emergency care, fluid-electrolyte acid-base therapy, and nuclear medicine. Hypnosis has resurfaced as a therapeutic technique. Additionally, Western medicine has become interested in the therapeutic benefits of techniques long used in Eastern civilizations, such as yoga and acupuncture. Space does not permit exploration of all of these fascinating avenues of treatment. Instead, we present here a basic overview of therapeutic radiation, surgery, physical medicine and psychiatric therapies. Other types of treatments will be discussed in later chapters of this text.

Therapeutic Radiation. Therapeutic radiation or radiotherapy refers to the application of radiation for treatment purposes. The radiation may be in the form of radioactive substances or x-rays. Radiation occurs in nature or may be man-made. Artificial *radioactive substances* are created by producing nuclear reactions in stable elements.

Radiation is used therapeutically (in treating tumors and other medical disorders) because of its abilities to penetrate and be absorbed into matter and to change the basic structure of body cells. (The diagnostic use of radiation and x-rays was discussed earlier in this chapter.)

Various forms of cancer are the most common diseases treated by radiation. Radiation may be employed as the treatment of choice or in combination with chemotherapy or surgery.

Medication Administration. An important form of therapy, and one that has undergone dramatic changes in recent years, is the administration of medication. All aspects of health care have been touched by the tremendous increase in the number and kinds of drugs manufactured and prescribed. A wide range of medications are administered today for an incredible diversity of purposes: from the commonplace oral contraceptives and antibiotics to the most advanced immunosuppressive drugs used to retard homograft rejection in transplant surgery. Chapters 31, 32 and 38 discuss the principles of medication therapy and present in detail the nurse's role in safe and responsible administration.

Surgery. On the basis of a patient's history, physical and psychosocial assessment, and diagnostic test results a surgeon considers: (a) whether or not this patient may benefit from surgery, (b) which type of operation is most desirable and what are the goals of the surgery, (c) when surgery should be performed and (d) what potential risks are involved.

In assessing the *surgical risk* the surgeon looks for potential problems related to: (a) infection, (b) decreased blood volume, (c) coagulation defects, (d) dehydration and malnutrition, (e) fluid-electrolyte acid-base imbalances, (f) reduced cardiac or pulmonary reserves, (g) kidney or liver disorders, and (h) extremes of age. When risks are present, appropriate preoperative, operative and postoperative management must be directed at removing or modifying the risk.

Surgical procedures may be classified according to: (1) the *seriousness* of the procedure, e.g., major or minor surgery; (2) the *urgency* of the operation, e.g., urgent or elective surgery, and (3) the *reason* for the surgery or the *purpose* of the surgery. Another way surgeries are classified is according to whether they are "scheduled" (planned) or "unscheduled" (unplanned).

These classification systems often are used in combination and sometimes they overlap. For example, a patient may be said to have undergone "major emergency surgery." This tells us that the surgery was a serious procedure which was unscheduled and was performed immediately to save the patient's life. The opposite would be a "minor, scheduled elective" surgical procedure such as revision of a scar. *Elective* means the surgery was optional, not urgent, and thus was not necessary to prevent additional problems, e.g., tissue destruction, tissue death, impairment of function. Examples of emergency surgical situations include: traumatic wounds, perforation of abdominal organs, hemorrhage and some obstructions.

Surgical procedures may be performed for various diagnostic, palliative, prophylactic, cosmetic or curative purposes. Table 16–9 provides examples of some principal purposes of surgery and typical surgical procedures. Some overlap occurs in actual practice. For example, a patient may undergo a *diagnostic* breast biopsy followed immediately (while the patient is still anesthetized) by removal of the breast if the biopsy reveals cancerous tissue. The breast removal (an *extirpative* procedure) may be performed in such a manner as to also achieve the best possible *cosmetic* results.

A particular operation may be done for different reasons on different patients. For example, a colostomy may be performed as a curative procedure on one patient and as a palliative procedure on another.

Astonishing advances in surgical procedures

TABLE 16–9. PRINCIPAL PURPOSES OF SURGERY

PURPOSE OR REASON	EXAMPLES OF SURGICAL PROCEDURES
Relieve symptoms (palliative procedures)	Urinary diversion (to remove diseased bladder), colostomy (to relieve intestinal obstruction), neurosurgery to relieve pain.
Prevent disease (prophylactic procedures)	Removal of precancerous tissue, removal of ovaries to prevent breast cancer recurrence
Alter appearance (cosmetic and/or reconstructive procedures)	Face-lift, rhinoplasty, scar revision, transsexual surgery, skin grafts, breast reconstruction
Remove, repair or reconstruct traumatized or malfunctioning structures or tissues (extirpative, reparative or reconstructive procedures)	Amputation, hysterectomy (removal of uterus), wound debridement, internal fixation of fractures, appendectomy, repair of cardiac congenital defects, colostomy, splenectomy (removal of spleen), nephrectomy (removal of kidney), mastectomy (removal of breast)
Visualize internal structures for diagnostic reasons (exploratory or diagnostic procedures)	Exploratory laparotomy (incision of abdominal wall), exploratory thoracotomy (incision of chest wall), exploratory craniotomy (opening of the skull)
Obtain tissue specimen for diagnostic examination (diagnostic biopsy procedures)	Excisional biopsy, punch biopsy, frozen-section biopsy
Replacement of malfunctioning structures or organs (transplant or replacement procedures)	Kidney transplant, cornea transplant, total hip replacement, arthroplasty (plastic repair of joints)

have occurred since the middle of the 19th century when the significant discoveries of anesthesia and asepsis took place. Anesthesia made it possible to operate without causing immediate pain; asepsis gave the surgeon the ability to operate without simultaneously introducing hazardous (often fatal) infections. The protective mantles of anesthesia and asepsis gave peace and life to millions of patients, and endowed surgeons with seemingly unlimited opportunities to expand their creativity and skills.

More recent advances in preoperative, operative and postoperative care have continued to expand the range of surgical practice. Among these advances are: (a) discovery of roentgenography and other diagnostic techniques, (b) control of infection with specific antibacterial drugs, (c) ability to provide vital nutritional support through parenteral avenues (Chaps. 22, 23, and 38), (d) knowledge of fluid-electrolyte acid-base management (Chap. 24), (e) ability to maintain or restore an effective blood volume (Chap. 39), (f) ability to prevent complications of immobility (Chap. 33), (g) development of advanced techniques of anesthesia and pain control (Chap. 34) and (h) bioengineering developments that have produced sophisticated operating equipment, such as that used for microsurgery or to provide adequate cardiopulmonary support.

Advances such as these benefit general medical practice as well as surgical practice. In rela-

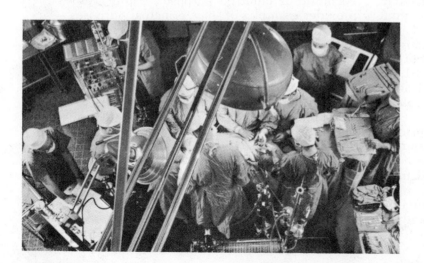

Figure 16–16. Open heart surgery in progress. (From *Nursing Care of the Patient in the O.R.,* p. 74. Copyright © Ethicon, Inc., 1973.)

tion to surgery they have reduced risks, increased the scope of new operative procedures, and simplified older, established surgical procedures.

Physical Medicine.   Physical medicine can be defined as "that branch of medicine using physical agents, such as light, heat, water and electricity, and mechanical agents in the management of disease."[109] As with other areas of medical practice, the field of physical medicine is rapidly enlarging. Examples of some techniques used in physical medicine include: diathermy, massage, therapeutic exercise, electrical stimulation and iontophoresis, ultraviolet therapy, hydrotherapy (Fig. 16–17), occupational therapy, training for functional independence, and homemaking activities. A physician who specializes in physical medicine and rehabilitation of the handicapped is called a *physiatrist.*

Psychiatric Therapies.   Four major therapeutic approaches used in varying combinations in psychiatric therapies are: (1) psychologic techniques, e.g., individual, group and family therapies, (2) medical approaches, e.g., psychopharmacologic therapy, convulsive therapy, (3) behavioral techniques, e.g., operant conditioning, desensitization, role playing and (4) social interventions, e.g., milieu (environmental) therapy, day care, halfway houses.

Psychologic techniques are numerous and varied in their philosophies and methods. Some focus on individual therapy, in which a therapist interacts with one client; others take a group approach in which a therapist works with two or more clients.

Examples of groups that may be formed for *group therapy* are: (a) *individual groups* composed of unrelated clients who observe and discuss each other's behaviors (i.e., provide "feedback") and practice new behaviors, (b) *couples groups,* made up of two or more couples, which function similarly to individual groups and (c) *family groups,* composed of an entire family, which look at interaction patterns, work to relieve symptoms and practice more effective ways of dealing with stresses. One or more therapists (i.e., co-therapists) meet with each type of group.

Family therapy is relatively new. This approach, now becoming more and more prominent, focuses essentially "on the threefold perspective of the patient's dynamics and role, the sociological approach, and the cultural dimension; this is clinically manifested through identification of areas of health and pathology, focus on communicating and sharing, and movement toward the ecological model of community psychiatry."[136]

Individual therapies (one-to-one) range from short-term *crisis intervention,* through intermediate-term *eclectic psychotherapy,* to long-term *psychoanalytic therapy.* (Crisis intervention is discussed in Chap. 5.) Verbal interaction is the primary technique used in all of these therapies, although the emphasis of the discussions varies. For example, crisis therapy primarily focuses on resolving a present crisis (i.e., a highly stressful situation which interferes with normal functioning activities) and

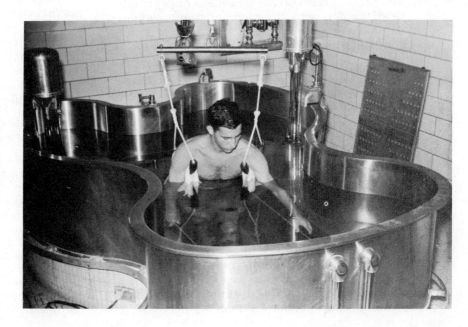

Figure 16–17. Hubbard tank therapy in the walk-in tank. Partial weight bearing is permitted by buoyancy effect of water and underarm support. (From Krusen, F. H., Kottke, F. J., and Ellwood, P. M., Jr.: *Handbook of Physical Medicine and Rehabilitation,* 2nd ed. Philadelphia, W. B. Saunders Co., 1971, p. 354.)

psychoanalysis mainly focuses on resolving conflicts in one's past. Crisis intervention may consist of only a few meetings over a period of weeks; psychoanalysis may involve daily sessions for years. Regardless of the approach, the goals of individual therapies are to help the client obtain relief from psychologic symptoms, learn patterns of behavior which are more adaptive and develop knowledge of himself which is meaningful to him emotionally.[21]

Both individual and group therapy may use several different techniques, e.g., relaxation, psychodrama, role reversal, hypnosis.

Traditional psychotherapies often assume that an individual's psychologic and behavioral difficulties arise from within him, and his symptoms are formulated by his particular basic adjustive techniques (defense mechanisms). More recent therapies show a change of emphasis, however. They state that causative factors in symptom formation are the relationships existing between the client and his cultural and environmental backgrounds.

Examples of some specific therapies frequently encountered are: transactional analysis (TA), gestalt therapy, encounter groups (T groups, human potential groups, sensitivity training groups), reality therapy and existential therapy.

Medical approaches used in psychiatric therapy may include the administration of medications or convulsive therapy. Psychopharmacologic therapy has had a highly beneficial impact on the treatment of psychiatric disorders, permitting many patients to lead useful lives who would have formerly been confined to institutions.

As with many physical diseases, the realistic objective of psychiatric treatment is often not a complete remission but rather the restoration of an adequate level of basic functions necessary for a satisfying and productive existence. When this therapeutic goal is attained, the medication must not be discontinued abruptly. The idea that the patient can become well, or stay well, "without a crutch" and "on his own" is erroneous. In psychiatric illness, as in many physical diseases, maintenance therapy may be both legitimate and necessary.[95]

Examples of psychopharmacologic drugs are: (a) antipsychotics ("major tranquilizers," neuroleptics), (b) lithium, (c) antidepressants (tricyclic compounds and monoamine oxidase inhibitors [MAOI]) and (d) sedative-hypnotics ("minor tranquilizers," antianxiety agents).

Convulsive therapies produce a grand mal seizure either electrically, through electroconvulsive therapy (ECT), or chemically, by administration of flurothyl or pentylenetetrazol. The reasons why convulsive therapy is effective are not known. However, it is helpful in treating selected patients.

Surgical treatment, i.e., *psychosurgery* performed with stereotactic techniques, is used occasionally in psychiatric treatment for some patients with severe disorders.

Behavioral therapies are currently being given considerable attention, although psychiatrists often view the therapeutic successes as transient and superficial.[136] Behavioral therapies are based upon conditioning (or conditional) learning theory and reinforcement theory. All behavior is assumed to be learned behavior and is believed to continue because of positive reinforcements.

Behavior therapists view themselves as teachers and believe there is far more to their role than merely "conditioning" their clients to bring about desired changes. Consistency is essential in responses to those behaviors upon which a client is working. This requires careful goal identification, planning and cooperation among all persons working with the client, e.g., staff members, patient's significant others.

In behavior therapy emphasis is placed on factors such as: the client-therapist relationship; bringing about direct changes that will broaden the client's adaptive behavioral skills; and identifying and unlearning unproductive or harmful behaviors (this is the major area of emphasis). Specific techniques used in behavior therapies include role playing, modeling, flooding, aversive conditioning, operant conditioning, extinction, desensitization and emotive imagery.

Social interventions may be used in psychiatric treatment in combination with medical, psychologic and behavioral techniques. Social interventions alter maladaptive factors in the client's environment in an attempt to modify the client's behaviors and attitudes. Examples of social interventions are:

▶ Establishing *minor changes in family or school activities*

▶ Use of *special services organizations*, e.g., family service groups, legal aid societies, consumer credit organizations, church-sponsored agencies, crisis centers, clinics, genetic counseling services, Planned Parenthood services, adult protective services, Travelers Aid, Homemaker Services, Visiting Nurse Services, Meals On Wheels

▶ Joining *nonresidential self-help organizations* composed of people who have certain problems in common and who want to help others cope with the shared problem, e.g., Schizophrenics Anonymous, burn recovery groups, friendship centers, Alcoholics Anonymous, the epilepsy society (Self-help groups are discussed later in this chapter, under *Rehabilitation*.)

▶ Living in *substitute "home-like" environments*, e.g., "crash pads" for young people, foster homes for children, family care homes for adults, board and care homes or mental care homes for the physically or mentally disabled

▶ Living in *residential self-help communities*, e.g., alcoholic residences, church-sponsored residences, Synanon for persons with narcotic problems

▶ Experiencing a *part-time hospital environment*, e.g., partial day care hospitalization, day hospitalization, night hospitalization

▶ Experiencing *full-time residence in a hospital*. The recent trend is toward keeping the client in the community as much as possible, rather than hospitalized for long periods of time. (In the past, persons with psychiatric disorders were often sent away from their community to live for long periods of time in isolated mental institutions). Today, when hospitalization is necessary, clients are often admitted for brief, intensive treatment to a psychiatric ward in a general hospital. As soon as possible, the client is discharged to the next appropriate treatment level. Most clients no longer require admission to inpatient psychiatric facilities.[95]

In commenting generally on psychiatric therapies, Brophy observes, "Regardless of the methods employed, treatment must be directed toward an objective, i.e., goal oriented. This usually involves (1) active patient cooperation; (2) establishing reasonable goals and modifying the goal downward if failure occurs; (3) emphasizing positive behavior (goals) instead of symptom behavior (problems); (4) delineating the method; and (5) setting a deadline (which can be modified later)."[21] Active participation of persons significant in the client's life is almost always an important ingredient in psychiatric therapies.

Iatrogenic Disorders

As previously mentioned, many treatments have disadvantages or drawbacks. As new treatments are put into use, the complications that occur with them are discovered. "Iatrogenic disorders" thus sometimes develop along with a patient's treatment. Iatrogenic disorders are produced inadvertently as a result of treatment being given for some other disorder—the treatment, in other words, actually creates new problems for the patient.

For example, because ionizing radiation is harmful to living tissue, the therapeutic application of radiation can create iatrogenic disorders resulting from tissue damage—radiation injury to the skin, radiation cataracts in the eyes, interruption of bone marrow function, production of congenital malformations in fetuses. In addition, the patient undergoing treatment may experience radiation syndrome ("radiation sickness") with symptoms such as malaise, nausea, vomiting, hemorrhage, inflammation of the throat and mouth, and diarrhea.

> *Possible iatrogenic disorders associated with therapies must be thoughtfully considered prior to initiating therapy and must be carefully watched for during and following therapy.*

The seriousness of possible iatrogenic problems must be carefully weighed against the possible benefits of the treatment and the patient's need for treatment. Alternate treatment approaches are also considered.

Havard comments on the incidence of iatrogenic disorders:

It is not surprising that the introduction of so many potent and toxic chemicals into clinical use has been accompanied by an alarming increase in drug-induced disease. Iatrogenic disease now accounts for 10 per cent of hospital admissions in the United Kingdom. A drug is to blame in 1 out of 10 patients admitted to hospital with jaundice, and 40 per cent of patients with severe hepatic necrosis have received drugs known to damage the liver. We live in an era of safe surgery and dangerous medicine.[84]

Other examples of drug-related iatrogenic problems are the development of vaginal fungal infections during treatment with antibiotics and the development of suprainfections related to antibiotic administration.

Serious adverse reactions can also occur from the interaction of drugs (see Table 16–10). Many examples of therapeutic, chemical and physical incompatibilities in medication could be cited. Examples of some medications which are contraindicated in certain physical conditions are: corticosteroids in peptic ulcer,

TABLE 16–10.   DRUGS IN COMBINATION*

DRUG	IN CONJUNCTION WITH	EFFECT
Alcohol	Antihistamine, barbiturates, hypnotics	Enhanced depressant effects on CNS
Amphetamines (including appetite suppressants and other cerebral stimulants	(a) Hypotensive agents (b) Monoamine oxidase inhibitors	(a) Antagonism of hypotensive effects (b) Risk of hypertensive crisis
Anticoagulants	Anabolic agents Clofibrate Phenylbutazone Salicylates	Enhanced anticoagulant effect
Oral hypoglycaemic agents	Monoamine oxidase inhibitors Propranolol Phenylbutazone Salicylates Sulphonamides	Enhanced hypoglycemic effect
Digitalis	Thiazides	Increased risk of toxicity due to hypokalemia
Imipramine and related antidepressants	(a) Monoamine oxidase inhibitors (b) Hypotensive agents	(a) Risk of hyperthermia, coma and convulsions (b) Antagonism of hypotensive effect
Monoamine oxidase inhibitors	(a) Amphetamines, sympathomimetic drugs, foods containing tyramine (b) Oral hypoglycemic agents (c) Imipramine and related antidepressants (d) Hypotensive drugs	(a) Risk of hypertensive crisis (b) Enhanced hypoglycemic effect (c) Risk of hyperthermia, coma and convulsions (d) Enhanced hypotensive effect
Phenothiazines	Alcohol, barbiturates, hypnotics, reserpine	Enhanced depressant effect on CNS
Probenecid	Salicylates	Antagonism of uricosuric action
Propranolol	(a) Oral hypoglycemic drugs (b) Quinidine (c) Ether	(a) Enhanced hypoglycemic effect (b) Depressant effect on myocardium (c) Increased risk of cardiac arrhythmia
Tetracycline	Oral iron	Reduced absorption and hence lower blood levels of antibiotic

*From C. W. H. Havard (ed.): *Current Medical Treatment*, 4th Ed. Bristol: John Wright & Sons Ltd., 1976, p. 37.

testosterone in prostatic carcinoma, oxytocin in severe toxemia, oxyphencyclimine in glaucoma, sulfonamides in the newborn, neostigmine in urinary tract infections and tridihexethyl chloride in pyloric obstruction.[153]

Health practitioners are advised to read carefully product information sheets, enclosed in drug packages, before administering medications to make certain that new contraindications have not been discovered or that recommended doses have not been changed. This is especially important when administering infrequently used or new medications.

> *Throughout your nursing career as you learn about treatments, always identify potential associated iatrogenic problems.*

Preventive Medicine

In closing this discussion of treatment, we want to mention once again that it is always better to prevent an illness than to cure one. *Preventive medicine* (or conservation of health) is all-important, and it is often complex and difficult to practice successfully. The prevention of health problems depends to a large extent on effective patient-family education and on dedication, by both the client and the health practitioner, to health maintenance. The client must want to remain well and must be informed about what actions he can take in an attempt to achieve this goal. The clinician must be dedicated to health maintenance activities, including patient-family education.

Some areas of importance in preventive medicine are:

▶ *Patient-family health education* (also discussed in Chap. 17)

▶ *Medical research* directed at illness prevention, e.g., medical genetics, continued attempts to identify the cause of common illnesses such as cancer, heart disease, Parkinson's disease.

▶ *Prophylaxis (prevention) of infectious diseases.* Smallpox, diphtheria, measles, whooping cough and poliomyelitis have almost been eliminated by immunization programs. Other disorders, e.g., food and water-borne infections, tuberculosis, influenza, typhoid, rubella, can be prevented through effective public health programs.

▶ *Presymptomatic diagnosis and screening programs.* (a) Primary screening in which health practitioners identify persons in high-risk groups, encourage them to take appropriate batteries of tests, and encourage those with positive test results to accept treatment. (b) Secondary screening in which health practitioners perform appropriate screening tests when a patient is being seen for other health reasons.

▶ *Early diagnosis and treatment* of health disorders when they do occur in order to prevent any further consequences of the disorder.

REHABILITATION*

As mentioned in Chapter 4, the specific task of a nurse is to help an individual attain satisfaction of basic human needs and to facilitate his doing this in as independent a fashion as possible. The concept of rehabilitation is inherent in this process. Rehabilitation, therefore, is central to the practice of nursing and is the vital issue in *all nursing practice*.

---

*This section was prepared by Margaret Helen Parkinson, R.N., R.M.N., Dip.N., B.Soc.Sc., M.N.

A nurse is concerned with facilitating optimal independence for a patient whether the patient is experiencing a long-term *irreversible* health problem, a short term *temporary* health difficulty, or even anticipating and trying to eliminate the effects of a *potential* health concern.

> *The primary function of a nurse is to support and build on a patient's strengths so that he can live his life in a satisfying style for as long as possible. In this sense, the primary function of a nurse is rehabilitation.*

The term "rehabilitation" has been defined in many ways. Some definitions focus on the restoration of independence after physical trauma (e.g., following limb amputation) or severe emotional illness (e.g., psychosis). Others stress the achievement of maximal physical potential for persons affected by long-term, chronic disabilities, e.g., multiple sclerosis, arthritis. The most complete definitions, however, include emotional, social and intellectual aspects of the patient as well as the physical. Krusen, Kottke and Ellwood provide this useful definition: "Rehabilitation involves treatment and training of the patient to the end that he may attain his maximal potential for normal living physically, psychologically, socially and vocationally."[109]

A nurse must always remember that what *she* views as "normal living" may not be the lifestyle the patient desires. Every person defines normal in a unique way. A *goal* for rehabilitation in nursing is to help a patient achieve a daily living pattern that facilitates a high level of self-esteem and creates individual satisfaction. To achieve this, the nurse and the patient must plan together.

The Rehabilitation Process

> *Rehabilitation begins when a patient first comes in contact with a health professional. It is not the final stage of treatment. On the contrary, rehabilitation is the underlying theme of all nursing and medical care.*

Rehabilitation involves *assessment* of the patient's physical and psychosocial needs and abilities. Both short-term and long-term assessment are necessary. For example, suppose

Ms. Smith, a nurse, is taking care of Mr. Anderson, a 20-year old man who has experienced a motor vehicle accident that has rendered him a paraplegic, i.e., he is permanently paralyzed from the waist down. In the first week of care, Ms. Smith is concerned with assessing Mr. Anderson's *current* physical and psychosocial needs. At this time she may well have to take responsibility for many of Mr. Anderson's basic physiologic needs, e.g., elimination and hygiene. She does this in a way that takes into consideration Mr. Anderson's desires and preferences. Ms. Smith also remains aware of the psychologic effects of the sudden and devastating trauma that Mr. Anderson has experienced. She attempts to assess and understand Mr. Anderson's emotional responses to his recent and present life events. Additionally, Ms. Smith also tries to identify the people who are most important in Mr. Anderson's life and to include them in the planning and giving of his care.

At the same time, Ms. Smith is thinking of the *long-term* consequences of Mr. Anderson's accident. She keeps informed of the patient's physical and emotional condition and developing prognosis. She gathers information about Mr. Anderson's habitual life-style, social circumstances, vocational ambitions, previous health history and patterns of handling prior life stresses. Such information forms the foundation (data base) for the long-term planning of Mr. Anderson's care. Making appropriate post-discharge referrals is one aspect of long-term planning. This activity establishes "bridges of care" between a patient's care in a health care facility and his home care.

Complementary short-term and long-term rehabilitation plans are developed *simultaneously*. Continuous assessment leads to the development and implementation of a comprehensive nursing care plan with short- and long-term goals. In the *acute stage* such plans focus on the satisfaction of the patient's needs while he recovers from his illness or injury. This is done in such a way that complications and secondary disabilities are avoided.

Residual disabilities can often be prevented or greatly reduced by thorough and skilled nursing care in the acute phase of illness.

The acute phase of illness is followed by a *restorative* and often a *retraining phase*. At this time the patient gradually takes more responsibility for his daily activities and for designing his ongoing life-style. The nurse now concentrates on developing the patient's knowledge, attitudes and skills to facilitate as complete a return to healthy living as possible. The skillful nurse involves the patient's significant others in this process.

Through support and teaching, the nurse ensures that the patient and his significant others have adequate *knowledge* about the patient's present and future physical and psychosocial potentials. By careful listening to the concerns of the patient and his significant others and by realistically focusing on positive aspects of the patient's situation, the nurse encourages the development of *attitudes* that facilitate healthy physical and psychosocial functions. The nurse also ensures that the patient and his significant others develop the *skills* or obtain help from others (professional or nonprofessional) that will enable them to live the kind of life they choose.

Every nurse must know the importance of evaluation in the nursing process (Chap. 17). The value of rehabilitation is greatly reduced if careful evaluation is not carried on throughout the nurse-patient relationship. A skillful nurse consistently evaluates the care she gives in relation to the previously identified, individualized patient needs and the goals. The nurse does this by reviewing objective data of the patient's progress or regression, by peer review with other professionals and by seeking the patient's evaluation of his situation and the care he is receiving. Further planning takes place on the basis of such evaluation.

Rehabilitation and Categories of Health Problems

Health problems have been traditionally categorized as *acute* or *chronic*. These labels are too broad to be particularly functional. We find the terms temporary, progressive and permanent more useful because they give a clearer concept of duration and prognosis.

A *temporary health problem* is one of relatively short duration from which the patient can typically expect complete return to his previous health status, e.g., appendicitis, reactive depression. A *progressive health problem* is one that may well continue throughout the patient's life. The patient can expect persistent alterations and possible deterioration in his physical and/or psychologic state, e.g., multiple sclerosis, Parkinson's disease, organic brain syndrome. A *permanent health problem* is one which cannot be reversed but does not necessarily worsen, e.g., blindness, amputation, paraplegia. The patient may not remain "ill;" however his activity status may be in some way impaired or altered. It will be seen that temporary, progressive and permanent health problems call for differing emphases in rehabilitation. (See also Chap. 13 for discussion of patient roles.)

▶ *Temporary health problems:* As stated, temporary health problems are of relatively short duration. They end either with the patient's death or with his return to his pre-illness life-style. When there is no fear of death occurring, the rehabilitation of patients experiencing temporary health problems is relatively easy provided the patient and his significant others are well informed of: the disease process, present and projected treatment, followup treatment and care, and preventative measures to avoid future recurrences of the problem.

▶ *Progressive health problems:* Progressive health problems are ones which, once they occur, exist in a dynamic form throughout the patient's life. The condition is not curable and the patient may well experience periods of exacerbation (increased severity of the disorder or symptoms) and remission (decreased or arrested symptoms) on a continuing basis. Effective rehabilitation is planned on a long-term basis and focuses on reducing the disabling effects of present symptoms and helping the patient live with persistent and possibly unpredictable changes in his physical and emotional status. The rehabilitative activities discussed below, concerning persons experiencing permanent health problems, also apply to persons experiencing progressive problems. However, the unpredictability of the disorder (e.g., changing symptom patterns) places an additional stress upon patients with progressive disorders. This stress makes their long-term adjustments to life change extremely difficult.

▶ *Permanent health problems:* Permanent health problems involve one or more irreversible disabilities. The primary task facing the patient is coping physically and psychologically with the permanency of the disorder. The effective nurse works with a person experiencing a permanent health disorder to assist him in adjusting his environment in such a way that his self-defined "normal" pattern of daily living is possible. This may involve such things as making alterations in the structure of the living environment, teaching the patient to use rehabilitative aids (e.g., specially designed equipment to assist the patient's physical

activities), and retraining the patient for remunerative occupation. Some rehabilitative aids are pictured in Figures 16–18 and 16–19.

Through a consistent therapeutic relationship, the nurse encourages persons disabled by progressive or permanent disorders to view their difficulties in terms of alterations in lifestyle rather than illnesses. These health problems are more usefully viewed as causing the affected persons to take on *"impaired social roles"* rather than *"patient/sick roles."* (Chapter 2 discusses the therapeutic relationship.)

Regardless of whether a patient is experiencing a temporary, progressive or permanent health problem effective two-way communication, including patient-family education, is of prime importance. The patient and his significant others should be well-informed of all aspects of the condition and treatment and they should be involved in all decisions affecting them.

> *An informed and involved patient is a person with a sense of personal control. A person who experiences control over his life and circumstances is more likely to make healthy adjustments to difficulties.*

Psychosocial Adjustment to Disability

A superficial view of the rehabilitation process focuses on adjustment and compensation for physical handicap only. While these aspects are of great importance, they are not enough for a disabled person to achieve a satisfying living pattern. In fact, achievements in physical rehabilitation may be rendered useless unless the patient is motivated toward success, has a hopeful mental attitude and has a supportive social environment.

Psychologic Factors. Health problems, especially those of a progressive or permanent kind, have significant psychologic effects on the patient. The emotional reaction which the patient may experience is very similar to a grief reaction. This phenomenon is easily understood when it is remembered that health problems usually involve a loss of some kind. This may be (a) a physical loss, e.g., loss of a limb, (b) loss or impairment of body function, e.g., paralysis, (c) loss or change of a psychological nature, e.g.,

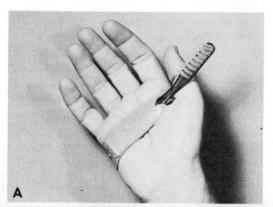

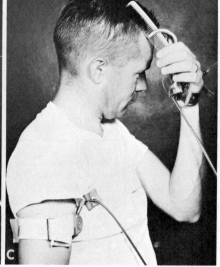

Figure 16–18.   *A.* Cuff with pocket to hold the handle of a toothbrush. *B.* Finger flexion splint activated by wrist extension to hold a razor or other equipment for daily self-care. *C.* Robin-Aid splint hook attached to the hand for prehensile activities. The hook is closed by elastic bands and opened by abduction of the opposite arm. (From Krusen, et al.: *Handbook of Physical Medicine and Rehabilitation,* 2nd ed., p. 478.)

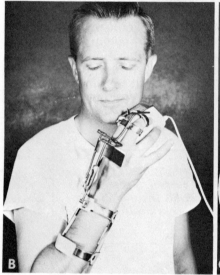

Figure 16–19.   Powered hand splint, activated by a McKibben carbon dioxide artificial muscle, to provide grasp for a flail hand. (From Krusen, et al.: *Handbook of Physical Medicine and Rehabilitation,* 2nd ed., p. 482.)

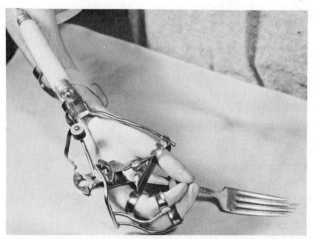

altered body image following severe burns, (d) social loss, e.g., loss of occupation, change of residence, change in interpersonal relationships or (e) varying combinations of the above. Whatever the nature of a loss, if it is significant it will be accompanied by a psychologic reaction. (See also Chapters 11, 15 and 48.)

If the patient is sensitively supported and understood and if he is allowed to express his feelings in a nonjudgmental environment, he is likely to reach a stage when he can *accept* his life changes and begin to make plans to create a satisfying life-style for himself. A genuine, empathic and warm nurse-patient relationship is of the utmost importance. Nurses often find these components of caring more difficult than the physical aspects of caring. It is unfortunate that patients are often denied the psychologic support they so vitally need and can rightfully expect to receive from nurses.

Social Factors. A nurse should always remember that a health problem very rarely affects just the patient alone. Every individual has a group of people with whom his life is interwined—his significant others. A *social matrix* is a group of people who are significant to each other. When something happens to one member of such a system, all other members are affected in some way. The effective nurse identifies early in her relationship with the patient the group of people who are significant for that patient. It is important to remember that such people may or may not be persons making up the traditional family. (*General systems theory* is useful material to review for a more complete understanding of a social matrix.)

> *Once a patient's social matrix is identified, the nurse offers these people therapeutic support and concern in much the same ways that she offers these to the patient.*

During the rehabilitation process the nurse remembers that a patient's significant others are probably experiencing the same stages of shock, disbelief and depression that the patient himself experiences before a healthy state of acceptance can be reached. The excellent nurse includes a patient's whole social system into the therapeutic arena. She does not concentrate on the patient in isolation from his significant others.

Successful rehabilitation depends upon both the *internal and external factors* impinging on the patient. Internal factors include the patient's physiologic status, emotional responses, cognitive abilities and his perception of reality. A patient's behavior reflects his subjective experiencing of internal factors. External factors include the physical nature of the patient's living conditions and community and the nature and strength of his support systems. The nurse offering a comprehensive rehabilitation plan must be aware of and coordinate the multifaceted nature of these factors.

The Team Approach to Rehabilitation

As with most health care, rehabilitation is best achieved by a *multidisciplinary approach.* A rehabilitation program should be developed for every patient entering the health care system. The nature and extent of the program depends on the type of health problem the patient is experiencing and the possible long-term effects it will have on his life-style. A rehabilitation program is best developed by the patient in cooperation with a team of professionals in a specialized rehabilitation center or within a general health care facility. Either way, the program should extend into the community in which the patient lives.

The team of professionals participating in rehabilitation most usefully includes nurses and physicians as well as various specialists such as clinical psychologists, psychotherapists, members of the clergy, social workers, nutritionists, physical therapists, occupational therapists, recreational therapists, stoma therapists and occupational (vocational guidance) counselors. Some therapists and teachers are highly specialized in working with persons with impaired speech, sight or hearing and with clients who have cerebral palsy or are mentally retarded. Technicians also bring to rehabilitation a wide variety of specialized skills, e.g., fitting artificial limbs (prostheses). Engineering specialists, who design equipment for use by physically impaired persons, are making significant, innovative contributions to rehabilitation. Social and behavioral scientists are also providing helpful knowledge. The specialists included in a specific client's treatment-rehabilitation team depend upon the needs of the individual.

Self-Help Groups

These nonprofessional, nonmedical groups spring from the need for help by persons having certain shared life experiences that are causing problems for them. All members of the group have a common basic problem; the nature of that problem varies from group to group. For example, one type of self-help group consists of women who have all had a breast removed surgically (mastectomy). Other postsurgical groups include persons (ostomates) who have had colostomies or ileostomies performed or persons who have had laryngectomies (removal of the larynx).

Other groups focus on behavioral difficulties such as drug abuse (including alcoholism), inability to control gambling or smoking, experiences with psychiatric hospitalizations, and experiences with grieving. Weight Watchers is a well known self-help group for persons experiencing difficulties with weight control. The names of other self-help groups with which you may be familiar are Alcoholics Anonymous, Gamblers Anonymous, Parents Without Partners, and Synanon. Some groups consist of the relatives or friends of the individual experiencing the basic problem.

Self-help groups may be highly effective in treatment-rehabilitation and in providing long-term support. These groups offer the vital, unique, realistic bonds which spring only from shared despairs and shared triumphs.

One of the most valuable services that a nurse can provide for certain patients is to refer them to appropriate self-help groups. Of course, this means the nurse must obtain information about the groups in her community. Many groups have national as well as local organizations. Community service organizations can often supply you with the names, locations and phone numbers of self-help groups.

The Nurse's Role in Rehabilitation

The nurse's role in a rehabilitation program reflects the intimate and personalized nature of the nurse-patient relationship. It is the nurse who has the skills and opportunities to appreciate the patient in a holistic way. The nurse, then, is the most appropriate professional to act as the *care coordinator* and the *patient advocate.*

Frequently a nurse spends more time with a patient than any other health professional. The nurse offers physical care of a personalized nature as well as ongoing emotional and social support. She has the generalized skills to help a patient with physical difficulties, social or psychiatric stresses, and combinations of these. The skillful nurse is thus probably the person best able to coordinate all aspects of the treatment-rehabilitation program and to discuss the plan of care with the patient and his significant others in a holistic and understandable fashion.

For the same reasons, the nurse is often the professional who can best be an advocate for the patient, by understanding his point of view and expressing it to other professionals when the patient cannot do this for himself; she also can interpret the services of other professionals to the patient and to his significant others in a way they can understand. As with all other areas in which nurses work, the nurse's place in a rehabilitation program is to support the patient, doing for him what he cannot do for himself, and facilitating his involvement and self-determination in his life events.

1. A day hospital for rehabilitation. *American Journal of Nursing,* 73:1900, Nov. 1973.
2. Abramson, A. S., and Kutner, B.: A bill of rights for the disabled. *Archives of Physical Medicine and Rehabilitation,* 53:99–100, March 1972.
3. Alexander, M. M., and Brown, M. S.: The why and how of physical examination. Parts 1 through 17. *Nursing '73,* July 1973 through *Nursing '76,* June 1976.
4. Anderson, N.: Rehabilitative nursing practice. *Nursing Clinics of North America,* 6:303, June 1971.
5. Armstrong, M. E.: Acupuncture. *American Journal of Nursing,* 72:1582, Sept. 1972.
6. Barrins, P. C.: What nurses need to know about hypnosis. *RN,* 38:37, Jan. 1975.
7. Bates, B.: *A Guide to Physical Examination.* Philadelphia, J. B. Lippincott Co., 1974.
8. Bayer, M.: Easing mental patients' return to their communities. *American Journal of Nursing,* 76:406, March 1976.
9. Beeson, P. B., and McDermott, W. (eds.): *Textbook of Medicine,* 14th ed. Philadelphia, W. B. Saunders Co., 1975.
10. Behrens, C. F., King, E. R., and Carpender, J. W.: *Atomic Medicine.* Baltimore, The Williams & Wilkins Co., 1969.
11. Beland, I. L., and Passos, J. Y.: *Clinical Nursing: Pathophysiological and Psychosocial Approaches,* 3rd ed. New York, Macmillan Company, 1975.
12. Belcher, E. H., and Vetter, R. (eds.): *Radioisotopes in Medical Diagnosis.* London, Thornton Butterworth, Ltd., 1971.
13. Benjamin, R. R., and Shapiro, S.: Counseling as preventive medicine. *Hospitals, J.A.H.A.,* 47:105–108, March 1, 1973.
14. Beyers, M., and Dudas, S.: *The Clinical Practice of Medical-Surgical Nursing.* Boston, Little, Brown & Co., 1977.
15. Bircher, A. U.: On the development and classification of diagnoses. *Nursing Forum,* 14(1):10–29, 1975.
16. Blahd, W. H.: *Nuclear Medicine.* New York, McGraw-Hill Book Co., 1971.
17. Blumhardt, R., and Nusynowitz, M. L.: A guide to bone scanning. *American Family Physician,* 9:153–157, Jan. 1974.
18. Brown, E. L.: *Newer Dimensions of Patient Care* (Parts 1 through 3). New York, Russell Sage Foundation, 1965.
19. Brown, M. S., and Alexander, M. M.: Physical examination. Parts 3 through 15. *Nursing '73,* Sept. 1973 through *Nursing '76,* March 1976.
20. Bumbalo, J. A., et al.: The self-help phenomenon. *American Journal of Nursing,* 73:1588–1591, Sept. 1973.
21. Brophy, J. J.: Psychiatric disorders. *In* Krupp, M. A., and Chatton, M. J.: *Current Medical Diagnosis & Treatment 1977.* Los Altos, CA, Lange Medical Publications, 1977.
22. Brunner, L. S., and Suddarth, D. S.: *Textbook of Medical-Surgical Nursing,* 3rd ed. Philadelphia, J. B. Lippincott Co., 1975.
23. Brunner, L. S., et al.: *The Lippincott Manual of Nursing Practice.* Philadelphia, J. B. Lippincott Co., 1974.
24. Burkhalter, P. K.: Cancer quackery. *American Journal of Nursing,* 77:451, March 1977.
25. Burnside, J. W.: *Adam's Physical Diagnosis,* 15th ed. Baltimore, The Williams & Wilkins Co., 1974.
26. Byrne, J.: Lab report. Hematologic studies. Parts 1 through 9. *Nursing '76,* Oct. 1976 through *Nursing '77,* June 1977.

27. Byrne, J.: Lab report. Liver function studies. Parts 1 through 5. *Nursing '77*, July 1977 through *Nursing '78*, Jan. 1978.

28. Carruth, B. F.: Modifying behavior through social learning. *American Journal of Nursing*, 76:1804, Nov. 1976.

29. Chapman, W. E., III (ed.): Physiologic monitoring. *Postgraduate Medicine*, 54:119–122 (Part 1) and 225–227 (Part 2), 1973.

30. Chatton, M. J.: *Handbook of Medical Treatment*, 14th ed. Los Altos, CA, Lange Medical Publications, 1975.

31. Christopherson, V. A., Coulter, P. P., and Wolanin, M. O.: *Rehabilitation Nursing: Perspectives and Applications.* New York, McGraw-Hill Book Co., 1974.

32. Churchill, E. D.: Surgery in the twentieth century. *In* Nardi, G. L., and Zuidema, G. D. (eds.): *Surgery: A Concise Guide to Clinical Practice*, 2nd ed. Boston, Little, Brown and Co., 1965, Chap. 1, pp. 1–8.

33. Cobb, A. B.: *Medical and Psychological Aspects of Disability.* Springfield, IL, Charles C Thomas, Publisher, 1973.

34. Condon, R. E., and Nyhus, L. M.: *Manual of Surgical Therapeutics.* Boston, Little, Brown & Co., 1972.

35. Conn, H. F. (ed.): *Current Therapy 1977.* Philadelphia, W. B. Saunders Co., 1977.

36. Conn, H. F., and Conn, R. B.: *Current Diagnosis 5.* Philadelphia, W. B. Saunders Co., 1979.

37. Cononi, G. A., and Siler, M.: Automated multiphasic health testing in the hospital setting. *Journal of Nursing Administration*, 2:70, Nov.–Dec., 1972.

38. Copp, L. A.: The waiting room—a health teaching site. *Nursing Outlook*, 19:481–483, July 1971.

39. Corrington, C.: Consultation. Facts about colonoscopy. *Nursing '76*, 6:53–55, Aug. 1976.

39a. Costrini, N. (ed.): *Manual of Medical Therapeutics*, 22nd ed. Boston, Little, Brown & Co., 1977.

40. Crane, J.: Physical Appraisal: An Aspect of the Nursing Assessment. *In* Sana, J., and Judge, R.: *Physical Appraisal Methods: Nurse Evaluation of Patients.* Boston, Little, Brown & Co., 1975.

41. Dalrymple, G. V., et. al. (eds.): *Medical Radiation Biology.* Philadelphia, W. B. Saunders Co., 1973.

42. Davidson, I., and Henry, J. H. (eds.): *Todd-Sanford Clinical Diagnosis by Laboratory Methods*, 15th ed. Philadelphia, W. B. Saunders Co., 1974.

43. Daylight on prescription prices. *Nursing Forum*, 11:346, No. 4, 1972.

44. Deaton, J. G.: Fingerprinting: New way to track down disease. *Consultant*, 14:87–89, Jan. 1974.

45. DeGowin, E. L., and DeGowin, R. L.: *Bedside Diagnostic Examination*, 3rd ed. New York, Macmillan Publishing Company, 1976.

46. De Hoff, J. L.: What you should know about interpreting cardiac enzyme studies. *Nursing '76*, 6:69–70, Sept. 1976.

47. Delaney, M. T.: Assessment: help yourself to help the patient by examining the chest. Parts I and II. *Nursing '75*, 5:12–14 and 41–46, 1975.

48. Delp, M. H., and Manning, R. T. (eds.): *Major's Physical Diagnosis*, 8th ed. Philadelphia, W. B. Saunders Co., 1975.

49. Donaldson, S. B.: Therapies for disease. *In* Moidel, H. C., Giblin, E. C., and Wagner, B. M.: *Nursing Care of the Patient with Medical–Surgical Disorders*, 2nd ed. New York, McGraw-Hill Book Company, 1976.

50. Downer, A. H.: *Physical Therapy Procedures.* Springfield, Charles C Thomas, Publisher, 1970.

51. Downey, J. A., and Darling, R. C.: *Physiological Basis of Rehabilitation Medicine.* Philadelphia, W. B. Saunders Co., 1971.

52. Dunphy, J. E., and Way, L. W.: *Current Surgical Diagnosis and Treatment*, 2nd ed. Los Altos, CA, Lange Medical Publications, 1975.

53. Eastham, R. D.: *A Laboratory Guide to Clinical Diagnosis.* Baltimore, Williams & Wilkins Co., 1973.

54. Eisenberg, L.: Psychiatric intervention. *Scientific American*, 229:116–127, Sept. 1973.

55. Elder, A. T., and Neill, D. W. (eds.): *Biomedical Technology in Hospital Diagnosis.* New York, Pergamon Press, 1972.

56. Elliott, C. S. J.: Radiation Therapy: How You Can Help. *Nursing '76*, 6:34, Sept. 1976.

57. Elsberry, N. L.: Lab report: SMA-12, Here's one way to interpret it. *Nursing '75*, 5:70–71, May 1975.

58. Engel, G. L., and Morgan, W. L., Jr.: *Interviewing the Patient.* Philadelphia, W. B. Saunders Co., 1973.

59. Eymontt, M. J., and Eymontt, D.: Preparing your patient for nuclear medicine. *Nursing '77*, 7:46, Dec. 1977.

60. Feinstein, A. R.: Clinical judgment in the era of automation. *Annals of Otology Rhinology Laryngology*, 79:728–738, Aug. 1970.

61. Finland, M.: Superinfections in the antibiotic era. *Postgraduate Medicine*, 54:175–183, Oct. 1973.

62. Fitzgibbons, D. J., and Hokanson, D. T.: The diagnostic decision-making process: factors influencing diagnosis and changes in diagnosis. *American Journal Psychiatry*, 130:972–975, Sept. 1973.

63. Folsom, J. C.: From custody to therapy. *Military Medicine*, 137:209–214, June 1972.

64. Fowles, W. C., Jr., and Hunn, V. K.: *Clinical Assessment for the Nurse Practitioner.* St. Louis, C. V. Mosby Co., 1973.

65. Frankel, S., et al. (eds.): *Gradwohl's Clinical Laboratory Methods and Diagnosis*, 7th ed. (Vols. 1 and 2) St. Louis, C. V. Mosby Co., 1970.

66. French, R. M.: *The Nurse's Guide to Diagnostic Procedures*, 4th ed. New York, McGraw-Hill Book Co., 1975.

67. Friedman, H. H. (ed.): *Problem-Oriented Medical Diagnosis.* Boston, Little, Brown & Co., 1975.

68. Friedmann, L. W.: Medicine, nursing and physical therapy. *Archives of Physical Medicine and Rehabilitation*, 52:404–406, Sept. 1971.

69. Froemming, P., et al.: Teaching health history and physical examination. *Nursing Research*, 22:432–434, Sept.–Oct., 1973.

70. Fry, J., and Majumdar, B.: Basic physical assessment. *Canadian Nurse*, 70:17–22, May 1974.

71. Gaul, A. L., Thompson, R. E., and Hart, G. B.: Hyperbaric oxygen therapy. *American Journal of Nursing*, 72:892, May 1972.

72. Geddes, D.: *Physical Activities for Individuals With Handicapping Conditions.* St. Louis, C. V. Mosby Co., 1974.

73. Gelfand, M.: *Diagnostic Procedures in Medicine.* London, Butterworth & Co. (Publishers) Ltd., 1974.

74. Gilles, D. A., and Alyn, I. B., *Patient Assessment and Management by the Nurse Practitioner.* Philadelphia, W. B. Saunders Co., 1976.

75. Goodman, L. S., et al. (eds.): *The Pharmacologic Basis of Therapeutics*, 5th ed. New York, Macmillan Publishing Co., 1975.

76. Gordon, E. E.: Rehabilitation: philosophy and practice. *Hospitals, J.A.H.A.*, 44:50–53, Oct. 1970.

77. Gorton, J. V.: *Behavioral Components of Patient Care.* New York, Macmillan Publishing Co., 1970 (Chap. 3, Crisis Intervention).

78. Gottlieb, M. E.: Mental status examination. *American Family Physician,* 9:109–113, Feb. 1974.

79. Griffin, W., Anderson, S. J., and Passos, J. Y.: Group exercises for patients with limited motion. *American Journal of Nursing,* 71:1742, Sept. 1971.

80. Guild, C. G., III: Surgical intervention. *Scientific American,* 229:91098, Sept. 1973.

81. Halpern, H. A.: Crisis theory: a definitional study. *Community Mental Health Journal,* 9(4):42–349, 1973.

82. Hartmenn, K., and Bush, M.: Action oriented family therapy. *American Journal of Nursing,* 75:1184, July 1975.

83. Harvey, A. M. G., and Bordley, J., III: *Differential Diagnosis: The Interpretation of Clinical Evidence.* 2nd ed. Philadelphia, W. B. Saunders Co., 1970.

84. Havard, C. W. H. (ed.): *Fundamentals of Current Medical Treatment,* 4th ed. Bristol, John Wright & Sons Ltd., 1976.

85. Hazzard, M. E., and Scheuerman, M.: Family system therapy. *Nursing '76,* 6:22, July 1976.

86. Heller, V.: Handicapped patients talk together. *American Journal of Nursing,* 70:332–335, Feb. 1970.

87. Henderson, V.: *The Nature of Nursing.* New York, Macmillan Publishing Co., 1966.

88. Henderson, V., and Nite, G.: *Principles and Practice of Nursing,* 6th ed. New York, Macmillan Publishing Co., 1978.

89. Henriques, C. C., et al.: Performance of adult health appraisal examinations utilizing nurse practitioners–physician teams and paramedical personnel. *American Journal of Public Health,* 64:47–53, Jan. 1974.

90. Hitchcock, J. M.: Crisis intervention: the pebble in the pool. *American Journal of Nursing,* 73:1388, Aug. 1973.

91. Hobson, L. B.: *Examination of the Patient; A Text for Nursing and Allied Health Personnel.* New York, McGraw-Hill Book Co., 1975.

92. Hodgkin, K.: *Towards Earlier Diagnosis,* 3rd ed. London, Churchill Livingstone, 1973.

93. Holley, L.: The physical therapist—who, what, and how. *American Journal of Nursing,* 70:1521, July 1970.

94. Holmes, J. E.: The physical therapist and team care. *Nursing Outlook,* 20:182, March 1972.

95. Holvey, D. N., and Talbott, J. H. (eds.): *The Merck Manual of Diagnosis and Therapy,* 12th ed. Rahway, NJ, Merck Sharp & Dohme Research Laboratories, 1972.

96. Hotchins, E. A.: Helping psychiatric outpatients accept drug therapy. *American Journal of Nursing,* 77:464, March 1977.

97. Hussar, D. A.: Drug interactions: good and bad. *Nursing '76,* 6:61–65, Sept. 1976.

98. Isler, C.: Transplant surgery and its special problems. *RN,* 35:OR-8, Nov. 1972.

99. Jarvis, C. M.: Perfecting physical assessment. Parts 1 through 3. *Nursing '77,* May through July, 1977.

100. Jarvis, C.M.: Vital signs: how to take them more accurately . . . and understand them more fully. *Nursing '76,* 6:31, April 1976.

101. Judge, R. D., and Zuidema, G. (eds.): *Methods of Clinical Examination: A Physiologic Approach,* 3rd ed. Boston, Little, Brown & Co., 1974.

102. Kalkman, M. E.: Recognizing emotional problems. *American Journal of Nursing,* 68:536–539, March 1968.

103. Kamenetz, H. L.: Selecting a wheelchair. *American Journal of Nursing,* 72:100, Jan. 1972.

104. Kampmeir, R. H., and Blake, T. M.: *Physical Examination in Health and Disease,* 4th ed. Philadelphia, F. A. Davis Co., 1970.

105. Kasanof, D. (ed.): Biofeedback: therapy with electronic teaching aids. *Patient Care,* 9:164, Aug. 1975.

106. Kelly, P., Sr.: Diagnostic tests: what shall we tell the patient? *Nursing '74,* 4:15–16, Dec. 1974.

107. Keys, J. W., et al.: *CRC Manual of Nuclear Medicine Procedures,* 2nd ed. Cleveland, CRC Press, 1973.

108. Kratzer, J. B.: What does your patient need to know? *Nursing '77,* 7:82, Dec. 1977.

109. Krusen, F. H., Kottke, F. J., and Ellwood, P.M., Jr.: *Handbook of Physical Medicine and Rehabilitation,* 2nd ed. Philadelphia, W. B. Saunders Co., 1971.

110. Krupp, M. A., and Chatton, M. J.: *Current Medical Diagnosis & Treatment 1977,* 16th Annual Revision. Los Altos, CA, Lange Medical Publications, 1977.

111. Krupp, M. A., et al.: *Physician's Handbook,* 18th ed. Los Altos, CA, Lange Medical Publications, 1976.

112. Kuenzi, S. H., and Fenton, M. V.: Crisis intervention in acute care areas. *American Journal of Nursing,* 75:830, May 1975.

113. Kyle, J. R., and Savino, A. B.: Teaching parents behavior modification. *Nursing Outlook,* 21:11, Nov. 1973.

114. Lehman, S. J.: Auscultation of heart sounds. *American Journal of Nursing,* 72:1242, July 1972.

115. Lemaitre, G. D., and Finnegan, J. A.: *The Patient in Surgery: A Guide for Nurses,* 3rd ed. Philadelphia, W. B. Saunders Co., 1975.

116. Lewis, B. M.: Two simple tables for interpreting blood gas measurements. *Postgraduate Medicine,* 53:195–199, April 1973.

117. Lewis, L. V. W.: *Fundamental Skills in Patient Care.* Philadelphia, J. B. Lippincott Co., 1976.

118. Lipkin, M.: *The Care of Patients: Concepts and Tactics.* New York, Oxford University Press, 1974.

119. Littmann, D.: Stethoscopes and auscultation. *American Journal of Nursing,* 72:1238, July 1972.

120. Loebl, S., George, S., and Wit, A.: *The Nurse's Drug Handbook.* New York: John Wiley & Sons, 1977.

121. Lowman, E. W., and Klinger, J.: *Aids to Independent Living: Self-Help for the Handicapped.* New York, McGraw-Hill Book Co., 1969.

122. Luckmann, J., and Sorensen, K. C.: *Medical-Surgical Nursing: A Psychophysiologic Approach.* Philadelphia, W. B. Saunders Co., 1974.

123. Lynaugh, J. E., and Bates, B.: Physical diagnosis: a skill for all nurses? *American Journal of Nursing,* 74:58–59, Jan. 1974.

124. MacBryde, C. M., and Blacklow, R. S.: *Signs and Symptoms.* Philadelphia, J. B. Lippincott Co., 1970.

125. Martin, E. W., et al. (eds.): *Techniques of Medication.* Philadelphia, J. B. Lippincott Co., 1969.

126. McAllister, B.: Liberation time for the handicapped! *RN,* 39:57–60, March 1976.

127. McGehee, H. A., et al. (eds.): *The Principles and Practice of Internal Medicine,* 18th ed. New York, Appleton-Century-Crofts, 1972.

128. McGuckin, M. A.: Lab report: microbiologic studies. Parts 1 through 5. *Nursing '75,* Dec. 1975 through *Nursing '76,* April 1976.

129. McLaughlin, L.: Nursing in telediagnosis. *American Journal of Nursing,* 69:1006–1007, May 1969.

130. McLean, E. R., Rockhart, J. F., and Chaney, J. H. G.: Questionnaire becomes preadmission tool. *Hospitals, J.A.H.A.,* 47:56–59, June 1973.

131. McVan, B. (ed.): What the nose knows: odors. *Nursing '77,* 7:46–49, April 1977.

132. Mellinkoff, S. M.: Chemical intervention. *Scientific American,* 229:103–111, Sept. 1973.

133. Miller, B. F., and Keane, C. B.: *Encyclopedia and*

Dictionary of Medicine and Nursing, 2nd ed. Philadelphia, W. B. Saunders Co., 1978.

134. Mitchell, P. H.: *Concepts Basic to Nursing*, 2nd ed. New York, McGraw-Hill Book Company, 1977.

135. Moidel, H. C., et al. (eds.): *Nursing Care of the Patient With Medical-Surgical Disorders*, 2nd ed. New York, McGraw-Hill Book Company, 1976.

136. Mora, G.: Recent psychiatric developments (since 1939). *In* Arieti, S. (ed.): *American Handbook of Psychiatry*, Vol. I, 2nd ed. New York, Basic Books, Inc., 1974.

137. Morgan, W. L., Jr., and Engel, G. L.: *The Clinical Approach to the Patient*. Philadelphia, W. B. Saunders Co., 1969.

138. Murray, J., and Smallwood, J.: CVP monitoring: side-stepping potential perils. *Nursing '77*, 7:42–47, Jan. 1977.

139. Murray, R., and Zentner, J.: *Nursing Assessment and Health Promotion Through the Life Span*. Englewood Cliffs, NJ, Prentice-Hall, Inc., 1975.

140. Murray, R,. and Zentner, J.: *Nursing Concepts for Health Promotion*. Englewood Cliffs, NJ, Prentice-Hall, Inc., 1975.

141. Neff, W. S.: *Rehabilitation Psychology*. Washington, D.C., American Psychological Association, Inc., 1971.

142. Nemiah, J. C.: Psychological aspects of surgical practice. *In* Nardi, G. L., and Zuidema, G. D. (eds.): *Surgery: A Concise Guide to Clinical Practice*, 2nd ed. Boston, Little, Brown & Co., 1965.

143. Olson, M. H.: Managing the complications of radiotherapy. *American Family Physician*, 9:137, April 1974.

144. Paltrow, K. G., and Brophy, J. J.: Review of areas/a key to diagnosis. *Postgraduate Medicine*, 42:A-137, December 1967.

145. Parker, W. A.: Medication histories. *American Journal of Nursing*, 76:1969, December 1976.

146. Patient assessment (programmed instruction series). *American Journal of Nursing*, 74:293 (Feb.), 1679 (Sept.), and 2039 (Nov.), 1974 and 75:105 (Jan.), 457 (March), and 839 (May), 1975.

147. Peck, R. E.: Automated psychiatric screening. *American Family Physician*, 9:134–138, No. 2, 1974.

148. Peterson, H. O. (ed.): Symposium: current concepts in radiology, Part I. *Geriatrics*, 29:47, March 1974.

149. Piazza, D., and Jackson, B. S.: Sara N.—an anxious patient undergoing cardiac catheterization. *RN*, 39:41–47, Nov. 1976.

150. Pinard, G., and Tetreault, L.: Concerning semantic problems in psychological evaluation. *Pharmacopsychiatry*, 7:8–22, 1974.

151. Plaisted, L. M.: The clinical specialist in rehabilitation nursing. *American Journal of Nursing*, 69:562–564, March 1969.

152. Potchen, E. J., et al.: *Principles of Diagnostic Radiology*. New York, McGraw-Hill Book Co., 1971.

153. Prior, J. A., and Silberstein, J. S.: *Physical Diagnosis: The History and Examination of the Patient*, 4th ed. St. Louis, C. V. Mosby Co., 1973.

154. Rae, J. W.: Rehabilitation: today's responsibilities and challenges. *Archives of Physical Medicine and Rehabilitation*, 54 (Suppl.):605–607, Dec. 1973.

155. Raeburn, J., and Soler, J.: Behavior therapy approach to psychiatric disorder. *The Canadian Nurse*, 67:36–38, October 1971.

156. Raft, D.: How to refer a reluctant patient to a psychiatrist. *American Family Physician*, 7:109–114, May 1973.

157. Raus, E., and Raus, M.: *Manual of History Taking, Physical Examination and Record Keeping*. Philadelphia, J. B. Lippincott Co., 1974.

158. Reader, G. G., and Schwartz, D.: Developing patients' knowledge of health. *Hospitals, J.A.H.A.*, 47:111–114, March 1973.

159. Reeves, K. R.: This CAT is a Revolutionary Scanner. *RN*, 39:40–43, Aug. 1976.

160. Rhoads, J. E., et al.: Surgical philosophy. *In* Moyer, C. A., et al.: *Surgery: Principles and Practice*, 3rd ed. Philadelphia, J. B. Lippincott Co., 1965.

161. Riffle, K. L.: Rehabilitation: the evolution of a social concept. *Nursing Clinics of North America*, 8:665, Dec. 1973.

162. Roach, L. B.: Assessment: assessing skin changes: the subtle and the obvious. *Nursing '74*, 4:64–67, March 1974.

163. Roach, L. B.: Assessment: color changes in dark skin. *Nursing '77*, 7:48–51, Jan. 1977.

164. Roberts, S. L.: Skin assessment for color and temperature. *American Journal of Nursing*, 75:610–613, April 1975.

165. Robinault, I. P.: *Functional Aids for the Multiple Handicapped*. New York, Harper and Row, 1973.

166. Robinson, L.: *Liaison Nursing: Psychological Approach to Patient Care*. Philadelphia, F. A. Davis Co., 1974 (Chap. 9, The patient with an undiagnosed illness).

167. Rodger, B. P.: Therapeutic conversation and post-hypnotic suggestion. *American Journal of Nursing*, 72:714, April 1972.

168. Rosenfeld, M. G., ed.: *Manual of Medical Therapeutics*. 20th ed. Boston, Little, Brown & Co., 1971.

169. Rusk, H. A.: *Rehabilitation Medicine*. St. Louis, C. V. Mosby, 1971.

170. Safilios-Rothschild, C.: *The Sociology and Social Psychology of Disability and Rehabilitation*. New York, Random House, 1970.

171. Samuels, M., and Bennett, H.: *The Well Body Book*. New York, Random House, 1973.

172. Sana, J. M., and Judge, R. D. (eds.): *Physical Appraisal Methods in Nursing Practice*. Boston, Little, Brown & Co., 1975.

173. Schanche, D. A.: What your hands tell a doctor about your health. *Today's Health*, 53:14–19, April 1975.

174. Schiller, R., Sr.: The dietitian's changing role. *Northwest Medical Journal*, 1:22–27, January 1974.

175. Schlesinger, A. D.: Health education. *Hospitals, J.A.H.A.*, 47:137–140, April 1973.

176. Schumann, D.: Doing it better—tips for improving urine testing techniques. *Nursing '76*, 6:23–27, February 1976.

177. Seedor, M. M.: *The Physical Assessment. A Programmed Unit of Study for Nurses*. New York, Teachers College Press, 1974.

178. Seward, C. M.: *Bedside Diagnosis*. Baltimore, Williams & Wilkins Co., 1971.

179. Shader, R. I. (ed.): *Manual of Psychiatric Therapeutics: Practical Psychopharmacology and Psychiatry*. Boston, Little, Brown & Co., 1975.

180. Shanks, S., and Kerley, P. (eds.): *A Textbook of X-Ray Diagnosis*, 4th ed. Philadelphia: W. B. Saunders Co., 1971.

182. Sheline, G. E., and Phillips, T. L.: Radiation therapy: *Journal of Nursing*, 77:246, Feb. 1977.

182. Sheline, G. E., and Phillips, T. L.: Radiation therapy: basic principles and clinical applications. *In* Dunphy, J. E., and Way, L. W.: *Current Surgical Diagnosis and Treatments*, 2nd ed. Los Altos, CA, Lange Medical Publications, 1975.

183. Sherburne, P.: Nursing in spite of technology. *Supervisor Nurse*, 4:26–29, Jan. 1973.

184. Sherman, J. L., and Fields, S. K.: *Guide to Patient Evaluation*. Flushing, NY, Medical Examination Publishing Co., 1974.

185. Skydell, B., and Crowder, A. S.: *A Manual of Diagnostic Procedures for Patient Teaching.* Boston, Little, Brown & Co., 1975.

186. Slessor, G.: Auscultation of the chest—a clinical nursing skill. *Canadian Nurse,* 21:40–43, April 1973.

187. Smith, D. W., and Germain, C. P. H.: *Care of the Adult Patient: Medical-Surgical Nursing,* 4th ed. Philadelphia, J. B. Lippincott Co., 1975.

188. Sommer, P. K.: Operative cholangiography: its pros and cons. *RN,* 39:38–39, Oct. 1976.

189. Sterman, L. T.: A review of clinical biofeedback. *American Journal of Nursing,* 75:2006, Nov. 1975.

190. Stevens, P., and Conkling, V.: We Teach Breast Self-Examination to Hospital Patients. *RN,* 40:25–31, Jan. 1977.

191. Stimson, G. V.: Obeying doctor's orders. *Nursing Digest,* 3:29–31, Nov.–Dec. 1975

192. Stohl, D. J.: Preserving home life for the disabled. *American Journal of Nursing,* 72:1645, Sept. 1972.

193. Stryker, R. P.: *Rehabilitative Aspects of Acute and Chronic Nursing Care.* Philadelphia, W. B. Saunders Co., 1972.

194. Tarver, J., and Turner, A. J.: Teaching behavior modification to patients' families. *American Journal of Nursing,* 74:282, Feb. 1974.

195. Taylor, R. B.: *A Primer of Clinical Symptoms.* New York, Harper & Row, 1973.

196. Thorn, G. W., et al. (eds.): *Harrison's Principles of Internal Medicine,* 8th ed. New York, McGraw-Hill Book Company, 1974.

197. Tracht, M. E.: Biopsy: how and where to proceed. *Consultant,* 14:49–52, April 1974.

198. Traver, G. A.: Assessment of thorax and lungs. *American Journal of Nursing,* 73:466–471, March 1973.

199. Troupin, R. H.: *Diagnostic Radiology in Clinical Medicine.* Chicago, Year Book Medical Publishers, Inc., 1973.

200. Uhley, H. N.: Automatic monitoring for all patients. *Hospitals, J.A.H.A.,* 47:101–102, Nov. 1973.

201. Valadez, A. M., and Anderson, E. T.: Rehabilitation workshops: change in attitudes of nurses. *Nursing Research,* 21:132–137, March–April 1972.

202. Wagner, H. N., Jr. (ed.): *Principles of Nuclear Medicine.* Philadelphia, W. B. Saunders Co., 1968.

203. Walker, H. K., Hall, W. D., and Hurst, J. W.: *Clinical Methods* (Vols. 1 and 2). Boston, Butterworths, 1976.

204. Wallach, J.: *Interpretation of Diagnostic Tests.* Boston, Little, Brown & Co., 1970.

205. Watson, E. M.: Clinical laboratory procedures. *Canadian Nurse,* 70:25, Feb. 1974.

206. Weinstock, F. J.: Tonometry screening. *American Journal of Nursing,* 73:656–657, April 1973.

207. Weiss, J. M.: Psychological factors in stress and disease. *Scientific American,* 226:104, June 1972.

208. West, W. L.: Occupational therapy—philosophy and perspective. *American Journal of Nursing,* 68:1708, Aug. 1968.

209. Widmann, F. K.: *Goodale's Clinical Interpretation of Laboratory Tests,* 7th ed. Philadelphia, F. A. Davis Co., 1973.

210. Wilkins, R. W.: Internal medicine. *In* Keefer, C. S., and Wilkins, R. W. (eds.): *Medicine: Essentials of Clinical Practice.* Boston, Little, Brown & Company, 1970. (Ch. 1, pp. 1–5)

211. Willard, H. W., and Spackman, C. S.: *Occupational Therapy.* Philadelphia, J. B. Lippincott, 1971.

212. Wilson, J. T.: Compliance with instructions in the evaluation of therapeutic efficacy. *Clinical Pediatrics,* 12:333–340, June 1973.

213. Wilson, P.: Evaluating chest films. *Nurse Practitioner,* 2:6, Jan.–Feb. 1977.

214. Wilson, R. L.: An introduction to yoga. *American Journal of Nursing,* 76:261, Feb. 1976.

215. Wintrobe, M. M., et al. (eds.): *Harrison's Principles of Internal Medicine,* 7th ed. New York, McGraw-Hill Book Co., 1974.

216. Wolf, W.: Radiopharmacy: a new profession. *Hospitals, J.A.H.A.,* 47:64–68, Sept. 1973.

217. Wu, R.: *Behavior and Illness.* Englewood Cliffs, NJ, Prentice-Hall, Inc., 1973.

218. Wyler, A. R., et al.: Magnitude of life events and seriousness of illness. *Psychosomatic Medicine,* 33:115, March–April 1971.

219. Young, C., Sr.: Exercise: how to use it to decrease complications in immobilized patients. *Nursing '75,* 5:81–82, March 1975.

220. Zaslow, S.: New touches in caring for preemies. *RN,* 39:31–36, Feb. 1976.

221. Zilva, J. F., and Pannall, P. R.: *Clinical Chemistry in Diagnosing and Treatment.* Chicago, Yearbook Medical Publishers, 1971.

222. Zimmerman, C. E.: *Techniques of Patient Care.* Boston, Little, Brown & Co., 1970.

CHAPTER 17

THE NURSING PROCESS: PROBLEM SOLVING IN ACTION

INTRODUCTION AND STUDY GUIDE

The nursing process is one of the most important nursing subjects you will ever study. The nursing process is so significant because it forms the basis both for nursing education and for nursing practice and consequently for your career in professional nursing. Throughout your life as a health professional, you will use the nursing process daily as you plan and care for patients and their families. What, then, is the nursing process and what makes it such a vital force in nursing?

Essentially, a process is a series of planned steps, methods or operations that produce a particular end result. We speak of the process of making something, carrying out activities, traveling, working and so forth. The nursing process is a series of planned steps and actions directed toward meeting the needs and solving the problems of patients and their families. More specifically, the nursing process is systematic problem solving; it is a scientific method adapted to the often unpredictable conditions of human life and applied to human beings who need nursing care.

We find it convenient to discuss the nursing process as a two-phase, five-step process. The two phases of the nursing process are (1) nursing assessment and

TABLE 17–1. NURSING PROCESS TERMS

TERM	DEFINITION
Nursing process	A series of planned steps and actions directed toward meeting the needs and solving the problems of patients and their families; systematic, scientific problem solving in action.
Assessment	A two-step process that enables the nurse to identify the patient's needs and problems. The first step is data gathering, and the second step is making a nursing diagnosis.
Data gathering	Gathering of information concerning the patient's physical health, mental outlook, social circumstances, family and community life, and other factors.
Nursing diagnosis	A statement of (a) the patient's current and potential problems and (b) the causative and contributing factors resulting in development of the problem.
Nursing management	A process involving direction and guiding of the nursing staff and the patient toward the resolution of the patient problems diagnosed during the assessment phase.
Nursing care plan	A detailed written guide for patient care which is directed toward (a) enabling the patient to reach his goals and objectives and (b) coordinating the nursing staff in their efforts to help the patient fulfill his health needs.
Implementation	Putting the nursing care plan into action; carrying out nursing actions (or interventions) which focus on assisting the patient to cope successfully with his problems and meet his goals and objectives.
Evaluation	Assessing the results of the care plan and the patient's progress toward his health goals; evaluation also indicates those areas in which the patient's care needs to be reappraised and modified.

(2) nursing management. The five steps are (1) data gathering, (2) stating the nursing diagnosis, (3) planning patient care or intervention, (4) implementing the care plan or intervention, and (5) evaluating and modifying the plan or intervention as necessary (Fig. 17–1 and Table 17–1).

As you study Figure 17–1, observe that the collection of data and statement of the diagnosis make up the assessment phase and that planning, implementing and evaluating make up the nursing management phase. Also note that the process (as shown by arrows) is continuous and cyclical and has no absolute beginning or end; evaluation (step 5) leads not only to further collection of data but also to a redefinition of the patient's problem and to the planning of new intervention or treatment. These ideas will all be covered in detail later in the chapter.

Upon completion of this chapter you should be able to define the following terms:

process
nursing process
problem solving
trial and error
hypothesis
input
output
feedback
assessment
data base
data gathering
subjective data
objective data
validation
primary sources
secondary sources
interview
assessment interview
problem-seeking interview

problem-solving interview
directive-interrogative interview
nondirective open-ended interview
open questions
closed questions
direct questions
indirect questions
primary questions
secondary questions
the patient history
the medical history
the nursing history
nursing diagnosis
medical diagnosis
problem
need
health standards
actual problem
potential problem
predictable problem
atypical problem
nursing management
medical prognosis
nursing prognosis
goal
objective
nursing care goals
nursing care objectives
expected patient outcomes
nursing orders
nursing care plan
target dates
outcome criteria for discharge
nursing intervention
dependent action
independent action
interdependent action
learning
patient learning goal
patient learning objectives
evaluation
accountability
nursing audit
modification

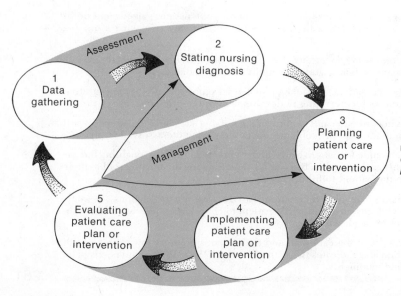

Figure 17–1. A two-phase, five-step model of the nursing process. (Adapted from Block, D.: Some crucial terms in nursing. What do they really mean? *Nursing Outlook, 22*:689, Nov. 1974, p. 693.)

You should be able to answer these questions and discuss these concepts:

1. What are the two major phases of the nursing process? What are the five steps of the nursing process?

2. List and discuss six methods of problem solving.

3. What are the seven steps constituting the scientific method of problem solving?

4. Give five reasons why it is necessary for health professionals to modify the classic scientific method of problem solving.

5. What are the three major elements in a cybernetic system?

6. List four barriers to problem solving.

7. Why do nurses gather data? Why must the data base be accurate, complete and up to date?

8. What are the four major purposes of data gathering?

9. What are the differences between subjective and objective data, and how does the nurse validate one type of data against the other?

10. List the sources of both primary data and secondary data.

11. List six methods of data gathering.

12. Give seven purposes of the interview.

13. Discuss the major types of interviews and their uses.

14. Discuss why it is difficult for many nurses to act in the official role of patient interviewer.

15. List the four phases of the interviewing process.

16. How does the nurse prepare herself, the patient, and the environment for the interview?

17. Describe several techniques for opening a patient interview.

18. Describe the three general categories of interview questions.

19. In what ways can the nurse use nonverbal responses to help the patient talk more openly during an interview?

20. Discuss methods for interviewing patients suffering from serious illness, hearing difficulty, dysphasia, language barriers, mental depression or conditions of the larynx.

21. What are the purposes of the nursing history?

22. Compare the areas covered in a nursing history with the areas covered in a medical history. How are they similar? How different?

23. Discuss three methods for systematic inspection and examination of the patient.

24. What observations should be made and recorded concerning the patient's psychologic and mental health status?

25. What resources for consultation are available to the nurse?

26. Why is it essential for the nurse to thoroughly review the literature? What is the best procedure for reviewing the literature?

27. Compare and contrast the medical diagnosis with the nursing diagnosis. How do these two types of diagnoses differ in focus, goals and objectives?

28. Discuss the two major components of the nursing diagnosis. Give examples of a problem statement and a statement of causality.

29. How does a problem differ from raw data? from a diagnostic statement?

30. Discuss the three major steps that the nurse must take to make a nursing diagnosis.

31. List the seven major steps that the nurse follows when planning patient management.

32. Describe three methods for setting priorities for patient care.

33. Discuss the five areas that the nurse must assess in order to analyze the patient's personal resources and deficiencies.

34. Discuss similarities and differences between the medical prognosis and the nursing prognosis.

35. How is a nursing prognosis established? In what ways can the nursing prognosis be used to improve patient care?

36. Describe the difference between a nursing care goal and a nursing care objective. What are the three major criteria for well-conceived nursing care goals and objectives?

37. Why is it important, when planning action, to generate as many alternative actions as possible?

38. Discuss methods for analyzing alternatives and choosing the best alternative.

39. What is a nursing care plan and what are its purposes?

40. What are some of the practical and philosophical problems which keep nurses from making full use of care plans?

41. Describe the five components of a complete, well-written nursing order. Discuss other attributes of the ideal nursing order.

42. What are the behaviors that the patient should ideally manifest when he is ready for discharge?

43. Differentiate between dependent, independent and interdependent nursing actions.

44. What are the characteristics of purposeful, efficient nursing actions?

45. Describe six specific methods that the nurse employs when implementing a plan of care.

46. Discuss eleven principles of learning. In what ways do each of these principles facilitate learning?

47. Describe five barriers to learning.

48. Describe each of the five major steps that are involved in developing a patient teaching plan.

49. Describe five different teaching activities and the purposes and advantages of each. List several useful teaching aids.

50. When is it necessary to modify a teaching plan?

51. What are the purposes of evaluation? Who is primarily responsible for evaluating patient care and the patient care plan? When must evaluation be performed?

52. Discuss the five steps of the evaluation process.

53. What is the nursing audit and what are its purposes?

54. List seven possible outcomes that can be generated by the evaluation process? If the patient has been unable to reach his health objectives, what are some reasons for this failure?

55. List guidelines for correcting and modifying a patient care plan.

You should be able to perform the following nursing activities:

1. Conduct a purposeful, helpful assessment interview.

2. Write a complete nursing history.

3. Assess the patient's physical, mental and psychologic status (at a basic level).

4. Write a nursing diagnosis.

5. Write a nursing care plan that is based upon the principles of good management and that is clear, precise and realistic.

6. Write and implement a patient teaching plan that is based upon a thorough assessment of the patient's learning needs and capabilities.

7. Evaluate the nursing care plan and the teaching plan objectively and accurately.

8. Modify the care plan and teaching plan as necessary.

BASIC CONCEPTS

Problem Solving: The Foundation of the Nursing Process

As emphasized earlier, the basis or foundation of the nursing process is problem solving. Before one can analyze the nursing process, one must first discuss what constitutes a problem, how problems arise from unmet needs, and what the process of problem solving involves.

In her article, "This Thing Called Problem Solving," Francis describes these concepts philosophically. She states:

> . . . life is a process of satisfying needs. A need is a condition requiring supply or relief. As we move along the continuum from recognizing a need to relieving, we encounter problems. Problems are unsettled questions. . . . The procedure for overcoming difficulties of all kinds is called problem solving.[36]

There are several methods of problem solving, the choice of which depends both on the seriousness of the problem and on the experience, skill, energy and intelligence of the problem solver. Common methods of problem solving (arranged from the least to the most sophisticated processes) are described below.

Unlearned Problem Solving. This form of problem solving merely involves mechanical reflexive reactions to problems. Unlearned problem solving is used by lower animals to solve problems of obtaining food or shelter and by humans in startling new situations.

Trial and Error Problem Solving. This method of problem solving involves trying out possible solutions without forethought and also without recording the outcome—which solutions fail and which succeed. In this form of problem solving, the solver basically does not know why certain of her actions work while others fail. This method means guessing, and guessing by nurses involved in patient care can be dangerous. If the trial solution works, the patient is lucky; if the solution fails, a patient could pay for the error with his life.

Intuitive Problem Solving. Intuition, or a strong hunch about a problem, arises when one has had some experience with similar problems in the past. Unfortunately, intuitive feelings are often based upon inconclusive or erroneous data and emotional responses to persons and situations. For example, have you ever had a teacher whom you "intuitively" disliked at the beginning of the semester but liked and admired by the end of the semester? What created the negative first impression and what factors changed it? Possibly your teacher resembled in looks or mannerisms some disliked individual from your past; a particular tone of voice, a hand gesture or a posture could have triggered unpleasant memories. Once you attended classes for a while, however, you discovered that the new instructor was actually very different from your first impression and from the person he seemed to resemble. Consequently, you were forced to reverse your original, intuitive opinion.

Traditionally, nurses have relied heavily upon intuition to evaluate patients and their problems. Nurses developed their intuitive powers by working with numerous patients in similar situations over the years. While experience with many patients obviously has merit, it is no substitute for systematic evaluation of *each* patient's unique situation and problems. Using intuition to evaluate a patient can be as faulty as using intuition to evaluate a new teacher or acquaintance. Hunches can be right and they can be wrong. For this reason, hunches must always be followed up with data; intuitive feelings must be substantiated with facts.

As you study the scientific method of problem solving, you will find that developing hunches is one of the first steps in scientific problem solving. For this reason, experience and intuition will always be valuable assets to a nurse. However, the professional person cannot stop at this level of problem solving. Instead, to help a patient solve problems satisfactorily, she must work through all the steps of the scientific process that follow the "hunch" stage.

Scientific Method of Problem Solving. The scientific method is a logical and systematic procedure for solving problems. Scientific problem solving is an outgrowth of Western civilization and is the foundation of much of our medicine and technology. The scientific method can be taught, and, indeed, it must be mastered by students of nursing.

Basically, the scientific method of problem solving can be broken down into the following seven distinct steps:

1. Recognition of the *general problem*, including defining the problem and developing hunches about its basis and solution.

2. Collection of *data* from all relevant sources.

3. Formulation of a *hypothesis*, or theory, which is defined in Webster's new *Dictionary of Synonyms* as "... an inference from data that is offered as a formula to explain the abstract and general principle that lies behind the data and determines their cause, their method of operation or their relationship to other phenomena."

4. Preparation of a *plan* for testing the hypothesis.

5. *Testing* the hypothesis.

6. *Interpretation* of test results and *evaluation* of the hypothesis.

7. *Termination* of the study or *modification* of the plan, based on further data collection.

To ensure accurate results, the problem solver must carefully *record* her data, hypotheses, plan, test results, evaluation and final plans for her study.

Modified Scientific Method of Problem Solving. Health professionals use a modified form of scientific problem solving in their work with patients. In Table 17–2 the classic and the modified formats for scientific problem solving are compared. Note that physicians use an examination–diagnosis–planning–medical treatment approach while nurses use a data gathering–nursing diagnosis–planning–nursing intervention or nursing care approach to problem solving.[36]

Nurses and physicians must modify the scientific method when working with patients for a number of reasons. First, scientists and health professionals typically work in different *environments* and have different *goals*. The scientist is often found in a laboratory, experimenting under controlled conditions with various chemicals, apparatus or laboratory animals. Typically, he is searching for new knowledge, which may be purely esoteric or theoretical. In contrast, doctors and nurses usually work in hospitals, clinics, offices, schools, and in patient's homes. Their goals are to help patients solve their immediate and long-range problems and to prevent further serious problems from arising.

Second, scientists and health professionals work within *different time frames*. Scientists sometimes take years to gather data, plan changes, and evaluate results. Doctors and nurses obviously have a limited time to work on a patient's problem, before the problem *must* be resolved. For example, if a patient is suffering from severe vomiting and diarrhea, he must be treated soon or he may develop dehydration and other problems. In this critical situation, the staff cannot spend days or even hours gathering data about the patient's symptoms; instead they must start corrective action immediately.

A third reason health professionals must modify the scientific method is that scientists have far greater *control* over their work than do nurses and doctors. For example, if a scientist places a laboratory rat on an experimental reducing diet, he can be sure that the rat will eat only the foods allowed on the diet. Because the scientist controls the feedings, he can expect to produce accurate results. If the rat fails to lose weight, the scientist knows that the diet is at fault and not the rat. On the other hand, when a nurse instructs a patient about a reducing diet, she can only hope that the patient will follow the diet. If the patient fails to lose weight, the nurse cannot know for certain if the problem lies with the diet or with the patient's failure to follow the diet. Furthermore, the nurse cannot control the patient's eating behavior; the patient has a right to control his own activities even though some of his activities may be unhealthy. For some health professionals, this lack of control in the clinical situation can be very frustrating.

Differences in the *complexity* of their tasks creates the fourth difference between the scientist's and the health professional's approach to problem solving. The scientist typically can choose to work on *one* problem at a time. When one problem is solved, he can work on the next. Because doctors and nurses work with human beings, they must apply problem-solving techniques to numerous interrelated problems at once. When a person is ill, he usually has both physical and psychological problems; he may also face economic and family troubles. Furthermore, often medical interventions themselves produce complications, e.g., many medications have side effects that are almost as severe as the condition they are prescribed to treat. Thus, for nurses and doctors, the question is not What problem shall I solve? but *Which* problem shall I work on first?

Finally, the problem-solving process proceeds in a *less orderly* fashion for the health professional than it does for the research scientist. It is usually possible for the laboratory scientist to follow the scientific method in a step-by-step fashion. Indeed, most scientists can at least hope that projects will proceed according to plan. Doctors and nurses can afford no such hopes. Within the hospital setting, emergencies frequently arise, patients suddenly "take a turn for the worse," and unexpected problems develop which need immediate solutions. For this reason, health professionals cannot always follow the steps of the scientific method in order. Instead, they must be able to adapt the method to any situation which arises and pursue those steps that will help solve the immediate problem.

TABLE 17–2.   COMPARISON OF THE CLASSIC SCIENTIFIC METHOD WITH THE MODIFIED SCIENTIFIC APPROACH USED BY DOCTORS AND NURSES

CLASSIC SCIENTIFIC METHOD	MEDICAL (CLINICAL) PROCESS	NURSING PROCESS
Recognizing a general problem area; broadly defining and describing the problem and developing "hunches"	a. Recognizing a patient's general health problems b. Reviewing why patient is being seen c. Developing "impressions" concerning patient's situation and symptoms	a. Recognizing a patient's need for help in certain general problem areas b. Reviewing background information about the patient c. Developing "impressions" concerning patient's problems
Collecting data from all relevant sources	Developing data base a. Medical history b. Physical examination c. Laboratory studies d. Other diagnostic studies, e.g., radiology, biopsy e. Consultation f. Review of the literature	Developing data base a. Nursing history b. Physical examination c. Review of laboratory test findings d. Review of diagnostic studies e. Consultation f. Review of the literature
Formulating a hypothesis	a. Analyzing and interpreting the medical data; making inferences b. Identifying the underlying disease processes causing symptoms (medical diagnosis) c. Developing the problem list and setting priorities	a. Analyzing and interpreting the nursing data; making inferences b. Defining the patient's problems and stating the impact of these problems upon the patient's life situation (nursing diagnosis) c. Developing the problem list and setting priorities
Preparing a plan for testing the hypothesis	a. Stating goals of medical care b. Developing a therapeutic plan of care, i.e., planning medical interventions	a. Stating patient's goals or behavioral objectives b. Developing total nursing care plan, i.e., planning nursing interventions
Testing the hypothesis	Implementing the medical care plan a. Writing physician's orders b. Performing procedures c. Educating the patient d. Referrals, etc.	Implementing the nursing care plan a. Writing nursing orders b. Administering or supervising nursing care c. Teaching the patient d. Referrals, etc.
Interpreting test results and evaluating the hypothesis	a. Establishing standards or criteria for evaluation of medical program and patient's progress, e.g., return to normal laboratory findings b. Recording patient's progress on chart c. Evaluating medical management and determining if goals are being achieved	a. Establishing standards or criteria for evaluation of nursing care plan and patient's progress, e.g., lessened pain upon movement b. Recording patient's progress on chart and care plan c. Evaluating nursing management and interventions and determining if goals are being achieved
Terminating the study or modifying the plan of action based upon further data collection	Terminating, modifying or continuing medical plan of care depending upon findings from evaluation process	Terminating, modifying, or continuing nursing care plan depending upon findings from evaluation process

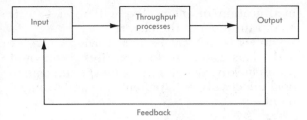

Figure 17–2. Major elements in a cybernetic model. (From Bailey, J. T., and Claus, K. E.: *Decision Making in Nursing: Tools for Change.* St. Louis, C. V. Mosby Company, 1975, p. 19.)

In sum, a health professional's work requires a problem-solving approach that is systematic and scientific and, at the same time, sufficiently flexible to deal with emergencies, unforeseen events, patient personalities, family misunderstandings, and multiple problems. As you will see, the nursing process appears to be such a problem-solving approach—a way of linking the scientific method with human realities.

The Systems Approach to Problem Solving.[8, 99] The systems method of problem solving uses concepts derived from both the scientific method and from systems theory. In this particular context of problem solving, a system can be defined as ". . . a way of thinking and acting which analyzes and integrates knowledge and information for the purpose of improving performance or producing order."[8]

You will recall from Chapters 1 and 6 that systems are composed of separate but interrelated subsystems or components that are linked together by a communications network. In addition, the activities of systems are directed toward certain goals.

A *cybernetic* system (which can help us in problem solving) depends on *feedback* to monitor and control its activities. In Chapter 6 we described feedback as involving reinserting (or feeding back) into an organism or a machine the results of its past performance in order to control its present and future performance.

Figure 17–2 shows the major elements in a cybernetic model: (1) *input:* information entering the system, (2) *throughput* processes: goal-directed activities going on within the model, (3) *output:* end-product of the system, and (4) *feedback:* information about the state of achievement of the system in relationship to the system's goal. Feedback is used to guide the system's future activities.

In their book, *Decision Making in Nursing: Tools for Change,* Bailey and Claus present a systems model for solving problems that is a cybernetic system with a feedback loop (Fig. 17–3). This model can be used for solving all

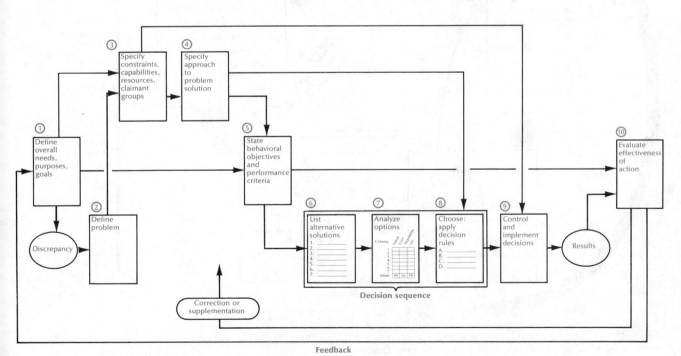

Figure 17–3. Claus-Bailey systems model for problem solving. (From Bailey and Claus: *Decision Making in Nursing: Tools for Change.*)

types of nursing problems, whether they are related to patient care or to ward and hospital management.

The steps of the Claus-Bailey systems model for problem solving are very similar to the steps of the scientific method and the modified medical and nursing processes shown in Table 17–2. However, this systems model of problem solving may be more helpful to some students than the outlines presented earlier for four reasons: (1) it gives the solver a complete, graphic, and map-like overview of the whole process of scientific problem solving; (2) the step-by-step format presented in linear fashion helps the solver to think clearly and systematically about problems; (3) its layout almost guarantees that steps will not be missed; and (4) it emphasizes the feedback process for evaluation and modification of plans. We will refer to this model throughout the chapter.[8]

Barriers to Efficient Problem Solving.[8] Bailey and Claus point out four barriers to efficient problem solving that nurses must overcome to deal effectively with patient care and management.

▶ Failing to specify purposes and goals

▶ Plunging into action before considering relevant alternatives

▶ Jumping to conclusions as to the cause of the problem and proceeding on a course of action (often costly) that may or may not solve the problem.

▶ Failing to look at probable consequences of actions

The use of a systematic scientific process of problem solving can help the nurse overcome these barriers and make logical decisions concerning patient care.

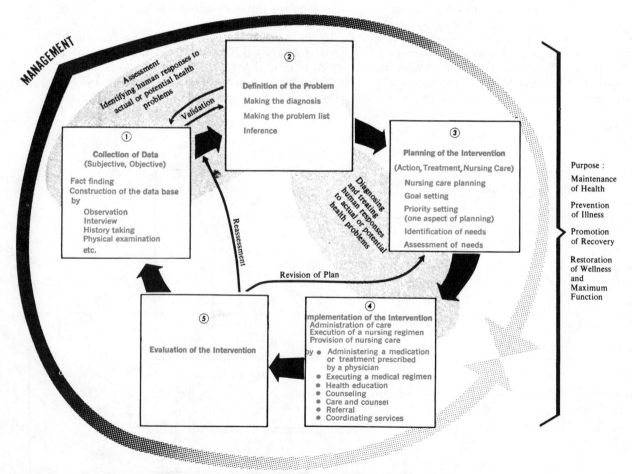

Figure 17–4.   Model of the nursing process: purpose and steps. (From Block, D.: Some crucial terms in nursing. What do they really mean? *Nursing Outlook, 22*:689.)

As shown earlier, the nursing process is a kind of problem-solving process. It is the approach expert nurses use to work with patients and their significant others, in finding new and more satisfactory ways to satisfy basic human needs.

The five basic steps of the nursing process we discussed earlier (Fig. 17–1) are, in turn, broken down into multiple smaller steps, as shown in Figure 17–4. As you study this model of the nursing process,[17] note the following attributes:

▶ The four *purposes* of the nursing process are maintenance of health, prevention of illness, promotion of recovery, and restoration of wellness and maximum function.

▶ The steps of the process are *interrelated*. Also, the arrows uniting the steps flow back and forth within the system, emphasizing that the system is *fluid* rather than static.

▶ The system is *open* and flexible, allowing for new input of ideas and information.

▶ *Assessment* is shown as a two-step process involving both (1) collecting data (subjective and objective) and (2) defining the problem and making the diagnosis.

▶ *Feedback* is emphasized, e.g., results of step 5 (evaluation of the intervention) are fed back into the system, leading to either a reassessment of the patient's problem or a revision of the care plan.

▶ The concept of *validation* is included. Thus, it is necessary to use data to confirm the definition of a problem; conversely, the definition of a problem must be verified by data.

▶ The system allows for *maximum creativity* on the part of the nurse as well as maximum use of her education and skills.

▶ The ultimate focus of the system is directed toward *better patient management*.

The entire system is constructed to help the patient solve his problems; consequently, the patient must be involved in each step of the process. Be sure to keep this in mind as you study the following sections of this chapter, which consider in detail each of the five steps of the nursing process.

STEP 1: NURSING ASSESSMENT—DATA GATHERING

Basic Concepts

Definitions and Purposes. Assessment is a two-step process that enables the nurse to iden-

tify the patient's needs and problems. The first step of the assessment process is *data gathering,* and the second step is *problem identification* or *diagnosis*. We define data gathering as the gathering of information about the patient's physical health, mental outlook, social circumstances, family and community life, and other factors.

> *The gathering of data is the most important aspect of the problem solving process. If the data gathered about a patient is sketchy or inaccurate, the diagnoses based on the data will be incorrect, the care plan will be faulty and interventions will be inadequate or harmful.*

Why do nurses gather data? One reason is to prepare the data base. A *data base*, which is part of the patient oriented record, is defined as information derived from the patient which serves as a starting point for planning nursing care and for identifying important patient problems.* A typical data base includes the following:

1. Patient's vital statistics, e.g., age, address, place of birth
2. Patient's present symptoms and complaints
3. Patient's reactions to his illness and expectations and goals regarding health care
4. Patient profile: includes a description of the patient and his average day
5. Social and cultural history: includes description of the patient's occupation, education, family members, significant others in the patient's life, church and social affiliations
6. Past medical history: includes discussion of previous hospitalizations, surgeries and illnesses, medications taken, chronic health problems, allergies
7. Family medical history: includes causes of death in close family members, chronic illnesses in family members
8. Interpersonal and communication patterns and skills
9. Activities of daily living and ability to function in each: eating habits, rest and sleep patterns, elimination patterns, hygiene and grooming, breathing, mobility, safety practices, sensory status (vision, hearing, speech, ability to speak, ability to feel pressure, heat and cold),

---

*The problem oriented record and data base are discussed in detail in Chapter 18. The medical data base is considered in Chapter 16.

sexual patterns, menstrual patterns (frequency and duration of menstruation and difficulty with menstrual periods)

10. Mental and emotional status: reactions to stress, general affect or mood, self-concept, body image, special fears, thought processes (disordered, ordered or rational), interests and motivations, willingness to take risks, nonverbal behavior (posture, hand motions), awareness of feelings of sadness, fear or happiness and manner of managing these feelings, mood-altering medications (e.g., tranquilizers)

11. Review of body systems and physical examination

12. Review of laboratory and diagnostic tests

The data for a *child* is similar to this, except that the parent-child relationship, the child's adjustment to school, relationships with peers, and developmental growth are included.

In addition to forming the data base, data gathering is used to (a) follow the progress of the patient in a treatment and care program, (b) evaluate effectiveness of nursing care that has been planned and is being implemented, and (c) redefine patient problems and status as they change over time. Types of data gathered for these purposes include the following: changes in elimination habits, vital sign patterns during hospitalization, increases or decreases in activity, lessening of symptoms, development of new symptoms, changes in emotional status (e.g., development of a depressed mood). Thus, data gathering never stops with the data base; it is an ongoing and continuous process.

> *Patient data requires constant updating if it is to be current and thereby useful in planning patient care.*

Remember that data gathering does *not* include interpretation or analysis of the information gathered. Interpretation of data and the deriving of conclusions constitutes the second step of the assessment phase—problem identification or diagnosis.

> *You must guard against jumping to conclusions (rushing into step 2—problem identification) before sufficient data has been gathered.*

The data gathered should include two kinds of statements: what the patient says about himself (subjective data) and what the health practitioner observes about the patient (objective data).

Subjective and Objective Data.   It is important to distinguish between objective and subjective data and to validate or check both types of data against each other before including them in the data base. *Subjective data* is basically what *patients tell you* they are experiencing, feeling, seeing, hearing or thinking; they are the personal expressions of patients about themselves and the environment. The following statements are examples of subjective data expressed by patients:

"I feel very depressed today."

"I don't feel like eating or doing anything."

"I feel very warm; in fact, I think I may have a fever."

"I haven't moved my bowels in days. I must be getting constipated."

Subjective data is usually obtained by the nurse when writing up the nursing history; it is also obtained during daily contacts with the patient. When recording subjective data, it is essential to write exactly what the patient says. For example, it is correct to chart "The patient states 'I feel very depressed today.' " It is incorrect to write "Patient appears depressed today." The latter is *your impression* of how the patient feels rather than a statement made by the patient concerning his or her own feelings.

Objective data, on the other hand, is information about the patient obtained by the *health practitioner* by observation via the senses (i.e., visual observations; listening to the patient's chest through a stethoscope; palpation of the body parts; feeling the patient's skin for warmth, dryness, or moistness; smelling the patient's breath for the odor of alcohol). These are examples of recorded objective data.

"Patient crying; refused breakfast tray; drank few sips of water."

"Patient's skin warm and dry to touch. Temperature 38°C. orally."

"No bowel movements recorded for 3 days. Hard mass of stool felt upon digital rectal examination."

Objective data is usually gathered during the physical examination or functional assessment. However, objective data gathering is also a continuous process, requiring daily and sometimes hourly or even minute-to-minute updating, depending on the condition of the patient.

When gathering objective and subjective data, it is essential to *validate the data* by (a) checking your observations with the patient and (b) checking what the patient says against your own observations. For example, consider how subjective data is checked with objective data. If a patient says, "I feel very warm, I think I may have a fever," the nurse must validate this subjective statement with objective data. She should feel the patient's skin and take his temperature to see if indeed the patient is feverish. If a patient says, "I feel constipated," the nurse should check the chart for the last recorded bowel movement and should perform a digital rectal examination for the presence of a fecal mass.

It is also necessary to validate objective data with subjective data. For instance, if a nurse observes that a patient has a forlorn expression, is tearful, and is anorexic (lacks appetite) she needs to *check her observation* that the patient seems depressed *with the patient*. The nurse might say to the patient "You seem depressed today. I notice you've been crying and you didn't touch your tray." The patient may confirm the nurse's observation or may deny it. In the latter case, the patient might say "I'm *not* depressed; I'm in pain! That's why I'm crying and why I can't eat." If the nurse had failed to validate her observations, she could have misinterpreted the patient's behavior and the patient would have continued to suffer pain needlessly.

Remember:
Validation of both subjective and objective data is the cornerstone of accurate diagnosis.

Sources of Data. There are two major sources of data: the primary source and the secondary source. The *primary source* is, of course, the patient. *Secondary sources* include the following:

▶ The patient's significant others, e.g., family, friends, business associates

▶ Hospital and clinic records—developmental records, charts from former hospitalizations, old care plans, current hospital records which contain medical and nursing histories and care plans, computer memories.

▶ Laboratory and diagnostic reports

▶ Other members of the health team—the doctor, the social worker, psychiatrist, dietician, physical therapist, other nurses

▶ Medical and nursing literature, notes from classes and lectures, educational films and tapes.

The subjective data that the patient (primary source) supplies is an invaluable part of the data base. For this reason, patients should be encouraged to participate in the data-gathering process whenever possible. However, there are a number of factors that influence the patient's ability to act as a willing and reliable source of data. Patient factors that must be evaluated include:

▶ Desire and need for medical and nursing care.

▶ Former experience as a patient.

▶ Language and communication skills. The patient who speaks only Spanish may have difficulty communicating with English-speaking personnel; the patient who has suffered a stroke may not be able to speak.

▶ Age. An infant or a senile person obviously cannot act as a data source.

▶ Physical condition. Very ill persons, highly sedated persons or patients in great pain are often unable to speak coherently.

▶ Mental condition. A patient who has a very low IQ or who is disoriented as to time, place or person cannot give reliable data.

▶ Emotional state. A depressed person may be unable or unwilling to speak; a patient in a manic (extremely hyperactive) state may be too agitated to give information.

▶ Fears concerning diagnosis. For example, many people have a great dread of cancer and will consciously or unconsciously withhold information that they fear might indicate the presence of cancer.

▶ Fears concerning legal implications or possible job loss. A pilot, for instance, may fear that he will lose his job if his symptoms indicate a severe heart condition.

▶ The patient's fear of supplying data that could lead to painful or embarrassing examinations or treatments. A woman may minimize her menstrual problems because she dreads undergoing a pelvic examination.

▶ Fear of criticism or loss of face with family or friends. A patient with venereal disease may be reluctant to discuss sexual contacts, because this information could adversely affect interaction with significant others.

It is, of course, valuable to use the patient as a data source, but secondary sources must be used whenever age or condition prevents the patient from giving data. Even when the patient is able to speak coherently, *secondary sources should always be used* because they supply a picture of the patient from other viewpoints (the family's, the doctor's). Since patients may be reluctant to supply certain types of information for the kinds of personal reasons we have discussed, a family member or friend may be a better source of pertinent data. In addition, secondary sources such as laboratory studies, diagnostic test results, conferences with expert consultants, and readings from the literature must always be used to verify the subjective data given by the patient.

Two points must be emphasized about sources. First, most people will give information about themselves, family members, and friends if they feel that the information will remain *confidential*. No matter what the potential benefit of data collecting, it is still an intrusion into the patient's personal life and feelings. In a hospital or clinic, a patient is asked to tell strangers about his life, problems, fears, and most intimate feelings. Before we ask patients to lower defenses and discuss themselves honestly, we must guarantee that (a) privacy will be respected and (b) statements will be read and discussed only by the professional persons concerned with their care.

Second, when gathering data from any source, you must always consider the factor of *human bias*. Human emotions color what we say about ourselves and how we perceive other people. For this reason it is difficult or impossible for most people to be totally objective when disclosing information of a personal nature. Fear and anxiety may distort a patient's perception of circumstances; guilt may cause significant others to hide their feelings about a patient. Health professionals, too, can be highly biased. For example, if a nurse's mother is an alcoholic, the nurse may carry a deep bias against all women patients who suffer from alcoholism. This bias may express itself in distorted observations of alcoholic patients and consequently may result in inaccurate patient profiles. If a nurse strongly dislikes a patient (or class of patients), she must, in the patient's best interest, be honest with herself and delegate the patient's care to a person who can be more objective.

Methods of Data Gathering

Methods of data collection include the following:

1. The interview
2. The nursing history
3. The physical examination
4. The psychologic and mental health examination
5. The consultation
6. Review of the literature

The methods of data gathering are listed in this order for purposes of discussion. In actual practice, the order depends on the patient's immediate situation. The nurse must have a thorough but flexible approach and be able to set priorities based on the patient's condition and the time available for data gathering. For example, if a patient is admitted to the hospital for elective surgery the next morning, the nurse has adequate time to follow the data collecting format in sequence. Of course, it is usually more productive for nurse and patient if the nurse begins data gathering by discussing the area of *greatest interest to the patient*— whatever that may be—and then proceeds to other assessment areas.

In contrast, for a patient in the emergency room after an automobile accident, time is of the essence and data gathering must focus on the immediate problem. The nurse and doctor must immediately conduct a physical examination to assess the patient's injuries and to evaluate blood loss, degree of shock, severity of pain, the possibility of concussions or fractures, and the adequacy of respiratory and cardiovascular functions. During the physical examination, the nurse should also interview the patient and significant others for the relevant information vital to prescribing emergency treatment: What were the circumstances of the accident? Does the patient have any allergies? Does he have a history of heart disease, diabetes, epilepsy, or other conditions which require ongoing care and medications? Later, after the patient's immediate injuries have been treated and pain and shock relieved, a more detailed history and physical and psychologic examination must be completed. In addition, consultants may be called upon for their opinion of certain patient problems, and the literature may be more extensively researched concerning the patient's diagnosis or problems.

It is vital that the nurse eventually gather data in every *assessment area, utilizing* all *the data gathering methods. If data is not collected in all areas, important patient problems will be missed.*

The failure to collect data in all assessment areas is particularly a problem for nurses who work in specialized fields of health care. For example, nurses who work on psychiatric or obstetric wards may tend to concentrate on collecting data pertaining to their specialty and fail to ask more general questions. A medical nurse specialist may focus on the patient's medical history, symptoms and problems and may slight the psychologic history and evaluation. This can be a dangerous practice, producing a lopsided patient profile. Health practitioners must guard against the tendency to dichotomize the patient into a "mind" versus a "body" and instead must use the techniques of data gathering to help evaluate and treat the *whole* individual.

The Interview

Purposes of the Interview. The nurse-patient interview constitutes the basis of the nursing process and the heart of the data-gathering procedure. Through the interview the sensitive nurse learns about the patient's social network and background, about feelings, fears, hopes, limitations, and potential strengths and assets. The interview supplies the raw data that the health practitioner will later compile into a composite diagnostic picture of the patient and his problems. Thus, the first step in becoming expert at the nursing process is to develop one's interviewing skills and techniques.

Exactly what is an interview and how does it differ from social conversation? An interview is a purposeful, highly specialized, goal-directed interaction between two persons—one who acts as interviewer and one who is the interviewee. Social conversation, on the other hand, tends to be random in subject matter, is typically without a specific purpose or goal, and takes place between friends, acquaintances or colleagues in an unstructured situation.

The interview, within the context of the nurse-patient relationship, includes the following seven purposes:

1. To establish and maintain a positive and open relationship between patient and nurse

2. To gather information from the patient

3. To provide information to the patient

4. To create an opportunity for the nurse to observe the patient's behavior and nonverbal communication

5. To counsel the patient concerning problems which have been identified

6. To teach the patient and significant others about his condition and its treatment

7. To enable the health practitioner and patient to develop a contractual agreement in which mutual expectations and purposes are clearly delineated

The *assessment interview*, which we discuss here, concentrates on (a) establishing a positive nurse-patient relationship, (b) gathering information for planning patient care, and (c) observing the patient's behavior. The principles and techniques of interviewing also apply to teaching and counseling, which we consider later in the chapter. In this chapter we outline some of the techniques involved in interviewing. These details should be considered along with the principles of a therapeutic nurse-patient relationship discussed in Chapter 3.

Types of Interviews. Interviews can be either problem seeking or problem solving. According to Yarnall and Atwood, the *problem-seeking* interview focuses on gathering data to uncover problems that the patient needs to resolve. The *problem-solving* interview, on the other hand, focuses on specific problems that have already been identified. In this case, the interviewer tries to learn more about the patient's problems and how they can be resolved, e.g., by gathering detailed information about the onset, characteristics, frequency and duration of the problem, factors that precipitate or aggravate it, and procedures and approaches that seem to alleviate the problem.[118]

Another way to classify interviews is as either directive-interrogative or nondirective–open ended. When using the *directive* approach, the interviewer typically asks a long series of prepared questions. The questions can often be answered by "yes" or "no" or with a few words. This interrogative method of interviewing is sometimes called the "Mr. District Attorney" approach. When this method is used, the patient plays a passive role while the interviewer has an active authoritarian role. The highly structured directive interview is useful in obtaining certain types of factual information, e.g., statistical data such as the patient's age, occupation, number of children. It is not effective in deriving information of an intimate, personal or emotionally charged nature.[16]

The *nondirective open-ended interview* is characterized by an open-ended *discussion* between the interviewer and the interviewee rather than by a staccato question and answer session. When this approach is used, the interviewee plays an active role in the interview while the interviewer's primary job is to offer leading statements and guide the conversation. This type of interview typically opens with a broad, open-ended statement or question, e.g., "I am here to discuss the problems which have brought you to the hospital" or "Tell me about your accident." Note that this type of statement is very different from directive statements, e.g., "When were you admitted to the hospital? What were your symptoms upon admission? Do you have any pain now? Where exactly is the pain?" In the nondirective interview, "Facts are not actively sought, they are permitted to emerge."[34]

During the nondirective interview, the nurse-interviewer (a) offers leads, (b) clarifies the patient's statements, (c) observes the patient's nonverbal behavior, and (d) helps the patient reach his own conclusions about his problems and find his own solutions. This type of interview is ideal for teaching and counseling purposes; it is also useful for gathering data about the patient's feelings, relationships and attitudes.

Both the directive and the nondirective interviews have their place in the data gathering process, and the two interviewing styles are usually used in combination. For instance, the interviewer may begin the interview with a general statement and then follow up the patient's answer with some specific questions. By using both types of questions in an appropriate way, the interviewer gains a fuller picture of the patient's life-style and problems.[16, 34]

The Nurse as Interviewer. Being cast in the role of interviewer is a new experience for nurses. Likewise, being interviewed by a nurse is a new experience for many patients. Until very recently, the typical graduate nurse was not trained in interviewing techniques. Even today, nurses are not generally portrayed as interviewers on television or in popular literature. The public image of the nurse (and consequently the patient's view) is out of step with many of the nurse's new professional responsibilities, e.g., interviewing and diagnosing. For this reason, it is essential for the nurse *to clarify her position as interviewer to the patient.* The nurse might say something like this: "I am your nurse, Miss Jones, and I will be talking with you today about any health problems that you might be having. Also, I will be asking you some questions about your daily habits like your mealtimes and your sleeping patterns. Our talk today will be the first of many talks we will have while you are in hospital so that you can be involved in planning the nursing care you will receive."

In addition to explaining her role as interviewer to the patient, the nurse must also *in-corporate this role into her own self-image.* It is difficult for many nurses to feel comfortable in the position of patient interviewer; new student nurses especially may feel awkward about questioning patients. This sense of discomfort has its roots in tradition. The nurse has been conditioned to view herself as a person who *assists* the physician while *he* takes the patient's history and conducts the physical examination. Thus, it may be difficult for nurses to see themselves as professional persons who, in conjunction with the physician, interview patients and perform physical assessments for *nursing* purposes.

Furthermore, some nurses have problems with the interview role because they initially relate to patients as friends rather than as strangers to whom they have a responsibility. Treating patients as friends endangers the professional purposes of the nurse-patient relationship and confuses the objectives of the interview. As Peplau emphasizes:

The nurse and patient are not friends; they are strangers to each other. If the nurse does not see the patient as a stranger, about whom she knows nothing but can learn much, then she is distorting the facts of the situation. She can distort in different ways. She might look upon the patient as a friend, seeking in him familiar elements that she has previously experienced with friends in other nonclinical situations. Or she can look upon the patient in light of her own need or wish to have friends, thus relating to him primarily to fulfill her own wishes. Such wishes for friends ought to be realized in the social life of the nurse outside the hospital.[88]

It is important to understand that Peplau's emphasis *does not* advise that a nurse is to remain distant in her interactions with patients. The statement that "the nurse and the patient are not friends" does not mean that the nurse should not be *friendly* to the patient. We are not giving the traditional advice that a good nurse must not become involved with the patient. This is false and dangerous teaching. On the contrary, a good nurse does become involved with patients. She does this best when she approaches each patient as a unique individual, living life within a unique and specific social matrix. The good nurse does not make unvalidated assumptions.

Finally, the student interviewer, in particular, may become uncomfortable during an interview because she senses that she is prying into the patient's personal life. Some students wonder if they have a right to ask the patient about his sexual activities, elimination patterns, past illnesses, and other such intimate concerns. To remedy this concern, it is helpful to keep the purpose of the assessment interview clearly in mind at all times.

Remember: *The purpose of the assessment interview is to gather information in all spheres of the patient's life in order to plan care that will enable him to regain his physical and emotional equilibrium. Indeed, if questions do not relate to this purpose, they should not be asked.*

If the interviewer words questions and statements in a clear, sensitive and compassionate manner, the patient will probably not feel that the nurse is prying; instead he will be assured of her desire to help him.

Phases of the Interview. The interviewing process can be divided into the following distinct phases:

1. Preparation and planning phases

2. Opening the interview

3. Conducting the interview: developing, exploring, directing

4. Closing the interview

Preparation and Planning for the Interview.[12, 13, 16] Interviews are purposeful, goal-directed conversations; consequently, the successful interviewer prepares for each interview with great care. The nurse interviewer prepares for the patient interview (a) before initially contacting the patient for interviewing purposes and (b) after greeting the patient, but before beginning the actual interview session.

Ideally, *before* meeting with the patient, the nurse should know who the patient is, precisely why she is meeting the patient and specifically what she wants to accomplish during the meeting. At the same time, the excellent nurse avoids developing preconceived ideas about the patient and resists developing rigid expectations regarding the process or outcomes of the interview. With these reservations in mind the nurse may make the following preparations:

▶ Review the patient's past history, chart, and care plan (if available) to learn about the patient's past illnesses and treatments

▶ Review the patient's present admission and hospitalization record

▶ Consult with the physician concerning the patient's condition, symptoms and problems

▶ Formulate (preferably in writing) specific objectives and goals for the interview; decide on exactly what is to be accomplished during the interview

▶ Formulate some initial leading questions and statements, worded to steer the interview in the right direction and to help pa-

tient and nurse focus on possible and potential problem areas

Once this initial preparation is completed, the nurse enters the second preparatory phase which involves *physically preparing the patient, the environment and herself* for the interview. At this time she will take measures to make certain that the meeting area (often the patient's room) has a quiet private atmosphere and that the patient is as comfortable and relaxed as possible.

▶ Reduce distractions in the environment. Turn off the radio and television; if possible, turn off the phone.

▶ Provide for "psychologic privacy." Request that other people leave the interview area if possible; the presence of others may inhibit the patient.

▶ Provide for geographic privacy. Close the patient's door; pull the curtains around his bed if he is on a ward.

▶ Prevent interruptions during the interview if possible. Avoid interviewing at times the patient will be involved in treatments or other types of patient care; avoid interviewing during visiting hours.

▶ Consider the patient's physical discomfort. If appropriate, ask him if he needs to use the bedpan or bathroom before starting. If he's thirsty, make certain that he has water or juices. Check whether he seems comfortable. If a patient is not comfortable, he will be thinking more about his discomfort than about what is being said.

Finally, the nurse must prepare herself physically and psychologically. It is important for the nurse also to be at ease during the meeting. She should have a comfortable chair near the patient and good lighting for taking notes. Also, she should make every effort to relax and to clear her mind of other concerns—plans for other patients, work left to be done. Concentrating on the task at hand will enable the nurse to conduct a successful interview and to truly "tune in" to what the patient is saying and feeling.

Opening the Interview. Remember that "you never get a second chance to make a good first impression." Clearly, the patient's first impression of the nurse interviewer significantly affects the outcome of the interview. If the nurse begins an interview in a rushed or brusque manner, the patient may respond by being uncommunicative throughout the session, thus dooming the interview to failure. Conversely, if the nurse *initially* creates an atmosphere of warmth and acceptance, the patient will usually be more open and communicative and the interview will proceed smoothly.

Fortunately, there are specific techniques that make opening an interview easier. We should all be warned, however, that specific techniques without genuine care, concern and warmth are useless. First, it is essential for the nurse to *address the patient by his name;* this small act conveys to the patient that the nurse sees him as a person and not as a hospital number or diagnosis. Next, as we pointed out earlier, the nurse should introduce herself and clarify her position as interviewer to the patient. She should explain (a) the purpose of the interview, (b) the ways in which data gathered during the interview will be used in planning care and (c) how the patient can be most helpful during the interview. It is essential to stress to the patient that he may ask questions and seek clarification about anything he doesn't understand. If the patient seems apprehensive, it sometimes helps to start the interview with some general remark such as "My, those are lovely flowers" as long as the interview does not drift off into general conversation. Once the patient seems relaxed and receptive, the interviewer can begin with a broad, open-ended statement such as, "I would like to hear about how you are finding things at present." Such a statement gives the floor to the patient and allows him to focus on those areas which are of interest and concern *to him.*

Conducting the Interview. Once the interview is in progress, the interviewer's task is to guide it toward her objective, e.g., to gather data about the patient's personal habits, to explore a problem identified by the patient. She must keep her ears, eyes and mind focused on the three elements that characterize interview interactions: (1) questions, (2) responses, and (3) nonverbal patterns of communication.

QUESTIONS.[12, 13] Questions can be rather difficult to use well. Few people really like to be questioned about all aspects of their life—their eating habits, their elimination patterns, their daily consumption of alcohol. Nonetheless, the nurse interviewer must sometimes ask questions if she is to learn about the patient. Because being questioned can make some

people feel anxious, hostile or inadequate, queries must be carefully thought out and skillfully worded. Therefore, the nurse interviewer must know (a) the purpose of the questions, (b) what types of questions should be asked and (c) techniques for wording and asking questions that will elicit complete and honest patient responses.

The *primary purpose* of asking questions during the assessment interview is to gather data about the patient in order to plan care. Other, more specific purposes include (1) to focus the interview upon a particular topic, (2) to seek clarification when the nurse has been unable to hear or understand the patient, (3) to determine whether the patient has understood the nurse's questions, (4) to help the patient further explore a certain point or problem and (5) to increase the nurse's own understanding of the patient's situation.

The *types of questions* to be asked fall into the following general categories: open questions vs. closed questions, direct questions vs. indirect questions, and primary questions vs. secondary questions. Characteristics and examples of each type are shown in Table 17–3. While each of these types of questions has a place in the interview, it is generally best to use open, indirect questions instead of closed, direct questions—particularly at the beginning of the interview. Open, indirect queries typically bring fuller, more honest responses from patients and are less threatening. Direct and/or closed questions can make the patient feel defensive. Sometimes, of course, the nurse must ask direct questions to obtain specific information from the patient.

A number of *techniques* to help word and ask questions effectively are summarized below:

1. *Word questions simply and concisely.* Wordy, complicated questions are confusing and are difficult to answer.

2. *Ask one question at a time and allow the patient sufficient time to answer each question before proceeding to the next.* Avoid double questions such as "Do you have pain before dinner or after dinner?" Also, never bombard a patient with questions. Some people feel under attack when forced to answer long strings of inquiries. In this situation, says Benjamin, the "interviewee is caught in a hailstorm of questions, and if he runs to the nearest shelter we can only admire his urge to survive."[13]

3. Use *broad, indirect and open questions* when beginning the interview. Then, if necessary obtain further data with direct closed questions.

4. *Word questions in terms that the patient understands.* Gear your vocabulary to the patient's age, education and general background.

TABLE 17–3.   TYPES OF INTERVIEW QUESTIONS: A COMPARISON

	OPEN QUESTIONS	**CLOSED QUESTIONS**
Characteristics:	Broad, unstructured questions that allow interviewee to state his opinions, views, and feelings	Narrow, restrictive questions that limit interviewee's responses to a few choices, e.g., *yes* or *no*
Examples:	How are you feeling today? What would you like for breakfast?	You are feeling better today, aren't you? Do you want cereal or toast for breakfast?
	How would you describe your pain? You have a lot of visitors. How does that feel to you?	Is your pain in your right wrist? Is your wife coming to visit today?
	DIRECT QUESTIONS	**INDIRECT QUESTIONS**
Characteristics:	Straightforward queries that go directly to the issue; may be either open or closed	Roundabout queries that are posed without appearing to be questions; an open-ended statement requiring an answer
Examples:	How well do your new dentures fit? Is it difficult to plan for the arrival of a new baby at this time?	Tell me about your new dentures. I wonder how it feels to be having another child right now.
	PRIMARY QUESTIONS	**SECONDARY QUESTIONS**
Characteristics:	Questions worded to initiate a new topic or subject	Questions worded to obtain more detailed information in respect to the primary question
Examples:	Why were you admitted to the hospital this time?	Patient: I was admitted because I have a lump in my other breast. Nurse: Oh! When did you first notice this lump?

Of course, you would avoid using medical terms with a patient who does not understand them; on the other hand, do not use lay terms when talking to a patient who does have some medical knowledge. In sum, neither talk down to patients nor use language which is unfamiliar to them.

5. Whenever possible, *use the patient's own terms when wording questions*. Also, *clarify what those terms mean to the patient*. Clarification is discussed in the next section, *Responses*.

6. Keep questions which can be answered with a simple "yes" or "no" to a minimum. "Check list" questions are better employed on written questionnaires than in the interview situation, where they tend to thwart communication. This type of questioning forces the patient to respond in a highly specific way and to "pigeonhole" responses. Persons who communicate well may overcome this problem and provide information about themselves spontaneously. However, more uncommunicative persons tend to remain silent between these types of questions.

7. Word questions carefully so that they *do not prejudice the patient's responses*. Questions that are the worst offenders for introducing bias are multiple-choice type questions and questions that call for a "yes" or "no". For example, a question such as "Do you experience stomach pain before, after, or during your meals?" forces the patient to respond in a way that corresponds with the interviewer's concept of the patient's problem rather than with the patient's viewpoint. In this situation, it would be better to ask "Have you been having any problems with your digestion?" This query allows the patient to speak freely about his symptoms. The multiple-choice question forces him to state that his symptoms are connected with his stomach and with mealtimes, neither of which may be true. An assertive patient might challenge a multiple-choice question and respond, "My pain isn't only in my stomach and it doesn't necessarily occur around mealtimes."

A shy patient, however, would be tempted to simply answer the nurse interviewer even though the question didn't allow him to explain the nature of his pain.

8. *Avoid, whenever possible, the use of "how" and "why" questions.* "How" questions demand that the patient supply specific information concerning a process that he may not know or may not be able to explain. "Why" questions tend to force the patient into giving explanations and reasons for his actions and life-style. Many people do not know why they do certain things and asking them a direct "why" simply frightens or antagonizes them; in essence, it puts the patient "on the spot." Furthermore, overuse of "why" may make the patient feel that the nurse disapproves of him and his actions; sensing this, the patient may either become hostile or withdraw from further questioning. "Why" may be used *occasionally* in interviews if it is employed to obtain factual information and if it is asked in a nonthreatening and friendly manner.

9. *Use secondary questions to clarify the patient's answers to initial questions.* As Becknell warns,

Do not be content with vague answers. When the patient uses terms such as sometimes, often, little, and much, clarify what is meant by them and record only this specific information. A response which is open to more than one interpretation does not supply the data necessary to plan effective nursing care.[12]

RESPONSES. The nurse interviewer's responses to the patient must be as carefully thought out and worded as her questions. Ten different types of responses* that are made during an interview are as follows:[12, 13, 16, 34, 72]

1. *Silence.* Silence is an important nonverbal response that can communicate warmth and understanding between patient and nurse but can also communicate misunderstanding, confusion or boredom. Properly employed, silence can be used during the assessment interview to (a) give the patient time to gather his thoughts and recall needed information, (b) give the patient the sense that he is being truly listened to, (c) give the nurse time to organize her thoughts

*Several of these responses have been discussed in terms of communication skills in Chapter 3. In this chapter we reconsider these topics from the standpoint of the assessment interview. We suggest that the student review Chapter 3 before reading this section.

in terms of further questions and to record data, and (d) give the nurse time to note how the patient communicates nonverbally. Finally, there is one situation during which it is *essential* for the nurse to remain silent. Silence is required whenever a patient stops speaking because he is overcome by emotion—usually weeping. If the nurse breaks this silence prematurely, the patient may feel thwarted in the expression of strong feelings and may hold any emotions inside rather than releasing them in a healthy way. The nurse can best help the patient express emotions by showing concern and support—not necessarily with words, but with a gesture, a nod, or a touch.[35]

As we stated in Chapter 3, many nurses do not feel comfortable with silences; many patients feel equally uncomfortable. In fact, in our culture, people grow restless if there are silences during ordinary conversation. Thus, it is wise, unless the nurse is quite experienced in employing silence, to avoid long silences. As Benjamin points out, ". . . a minute of meaningful silence is quite lengthy."[13]

Fortunately, there are a number of graceful ways to *break silences* during an interview. For example:

"Is there anything else you would like to say about this? (pause) If not, then I'd like to consider another point with you."

"You seem very quiet. Would you like to tell me what you're thinking about right now?"

"It seems to be difficult for you to talk about this problem. I wonder if we can try to explore the difficulty you're having."

"Can you try to tell me more about this problem which is bothering you?"

When a patient suddenly grows silent in the middle of a topic or in the middle of a sentence, the nurse can help him resume talking by saying "And?" or "Then?" or by simply restating words from the last sentence spoken by the patient (see *Restatement* below).

2. *Mm-hm.* While not a word, "mm-hm" is a highly significant human sound. Uttered during an interview, "mm-hm" generally implies that the nurse is listening to the patient in a permissive way and that she wants the patient to continue talking about the topic under consideration. "Mm-hm" also has other meanings, for example, "I approve of what you are saying." Conversely, "mm-hm" can express disapproval; the tone of "mm-hm" can say to the patient, "I don't like what you're saying!" Finally, "mm-hm" can express "suspended judgment" or indecision on the part of the interviewer; in essence, it can mean, "I'm not quite sure how I feel about what you're saying." All in all, the "mm-hm" is a highly expressive syllable. Used in a permissive, nonjudgmental way, "mm-hm" can be helpful, but

remember its precise meaning may be unclear to the patient.

3. *Restatement.* Restatement is a technique in which the interviewer restates or repeats the patient's words or phrases. By echoing the patient's words, the nurse attempts to help the patient examine and explore a certain topic more fully. When using the restatement technique, the nurse must remain a totally objective observer, i.e., she must not interpret his words or guess at underlying meanings; her task is to *repeat key words* from the patient's statements. According to Benjamin, there are four basic ways to use the restatement technique:[13]

A. Restating what the patient says *exactly.* This method is rarely used because it seems somewhat artificial and stilted.

Patient: I have a lot of pain.
Nurse: I have a lot of pain.

B. Restating what the patient says except for *changing the pronoun.*

Patient: I have a lot of pain.
Nurse: You have a lot of pain.

C. Restating what appears to be the *most important part* of what the patient says.

Patient: I was in the hospital for three months last year and I don't know how I'm going to stand to be admitted here again!
Nurse: You don't know how you're going to stand being admitted.

D. Restating in a *summary fashion* what the patient has said about a certain topic. Again, the nurse simply summarizes what the patient has said *without* interpreting his statements.

Patient: When I was in the hospital last year, I went through so much, nurse! After my operation, the pain was just terrible. And I could hardly move without feeling I was ripping apart. The thought of another operation just makes me sick. I almost told my doctor "Just forget it, Doctor! I'm not going to suffer like that again."
Nurse: When you were in the hospital last year, you underwent a lot of pain from your operation. Now you feel that you can hardly bear to undergo another surgery.

4. *Focusing.* Focusing is used during the assessment interview to keep the interview centered around the topics that need to be covered. Focusing statements are useful when talking with very anxious patients or confused patients who tend to "wander" when answering questions. This technique can also be employed when the patient suddenly changes the subject instead of answering the nurse's question. In this situation, the nurse must realize that she may be taking the patient's communication in a direction he doesn't really want to go (Chap. 3, p. 43).

5. *Clarification.* This technique enables the nurse to clarify vague, incomplete or ambiguous statements by the patient. There are certain *common words* which must always be clarified, e.g., small, large, a lot, some, somewhat, usually, often, many, few. Other terms which require clarification are those which have a *personal meaning* for the patient, e.g., "I'm sick to my stomach," "I feel funny," "I'm really on a bum trip today." Finally, medical or quasi-medical terms must be clarified, e.g., tumor, operation, nervous breakdown, spells, fits. The patient must always be asked to describe what is meant by the medical term he is using and the symptoms of the disease that he states he has had.[72] This is necessary because any terms can have different meanings for different people and patients are sometimes confused about their own medical history and previous diagnoses and, as a result, unknowingly give the nurse inaccurate data.

In the process of clarifying, then, the nurse needs to learn exactly what the patient means by the terms he uses. Thus, she might say:

"You say you drink a little every day. Could you be more explicit and tell me what type of liquor you drink? (pause for reply) How many glasses do you have a day?"

"Could you explain to me what you mean by 'a bum trip'?"

"Tell me more about the 'funny feeling' you are having."

"You say that you have had a nervous breakdown. Could you describe the symptoms which you had during that period? (pause for reply) Do you remember what medications you were taking at the time?"

6. *Summarizing.* The technique of summarizing the patient's ideas and statements may be done throughout the assessment interview as well as at the end of the session. Recall from Chapter 3 (p. 43) that summarization acts to pull together, into a brief coherent whole, the ideas and feelings the patient expressed and those feelings he portrayed nonverbally. When summarizing, the nurse may simply restate the most important aspects of the patient's conversation without any interpretation or she may stress certain aspects of the patient's discussion and behavior to the exclusion of others. Whenever she summarizes material, the nurse

must *verify* with the patient that her summarization correctly represents what he has been saying and feeling.

7. *Confrontation.* According to Enelow and Adler, "Confrontation directs the patient's attention to something that he may not be aware of—or, at best, dimly aware of . . . . In confrontation the interviewer describes to the patient something striking about his verbal or nonverbal behavior."[34] For example, "You sound very tired," "You look exhausted today" or "I notice that you've been biting your nails."

There are certain times during an interview when it is helpful to confront a patient. One such time is when the patient's *nonverbal behavior and body language do not coincide with his verbal communication.* What he says doesn't match his expression or his actions. Examples of confrontations in this situation are:

"You're telling me that you're happy about this pregnancy and yet you look very upset."

"You say that you feel calm and yet I notice that you're flushed and you're wringing your hands."

Second, it is valuable to confront a patient whose actions, voice and posture portray *anger, fear or anxiety.* Thus, the nurse might say, "You look very angry," "You sound frightened" or "You're pacing the floor like you really feel upset."

Like the technique of silence, the technique of confrontation is a difficult one for the beginning student to master. In our society, confronting other people with their behavior is considered an impolite if not hostile act. And yet, confrontation of a patient can be very helpful if it is done infrequently and in a kind and sympathetic manner. Like periods of silence, confrontation should not be overused. As you possibly know from your own experience, being constantly confronted with your actions can be very irritating. Therefore, for positive results, use confrontation only when necessary, and then, with tact and sensitivity.

8. *Supportive Responses.* A supportive response is one which indicates to the patient that the nurse is interested in him and understands how he feels, e.g., "I know how you feel" or "I understand." In regard to giving support, Enelow and Adler warn:

It must be clearly understood that supportive words without a supportive attitude on the part of the interviewer will sound hollow and will fail to accomplish their intended purpose. Without a genuine interest in the patient, a feeling of friendliness, and a desire to be helpful, supportive words are simply not supportive.[34]

9. *Reassurance.* The reassuring response can be either truthful and genuine or it can be false and phony. A patient who feels genuinely reassured by the nurse feels that his nurse respects him and his viewpoints. Ways to give a truly reassuring response include the following: (a) listening carefully to the patient and acknowledging that he has some distressing problems, (b) giving the patient correct information, (c) referring the patient to persons who are particularly equipped to help him with his problems and (d) being quietly supportive when the patient is frightened or in great pain.

In contrast to reassurance, false or inappropriate reassurance fails to make the patient feel better about himself and his problems. Failure results because this response "denies, in effect, that the patient has a problem and suggests that he need not feel as he does."[16] In essence, the use of false reassurance is a way of telling the patient to *not discuss* his concerns (because they are upsetting to the staff) and to either keep them to himself or forget about them. As Bernstein concludes "For this reason, it has been stated that a reassuring response serves to protect the feelings of the members of the health team and not those of the patient."[16] Examples of ways in which nurses use false reassurance are as follows (also see Chapter 3):

▶ Trying to cheer a patient up by making trite remarks.

▶ Inappropriately changing the topic of conversation, thereby lessening the nurse's anxiety rather than the patient's anxiety.

▶ Introducing irrelevant topics to distract the patient from the emotionally charged areas that he wants to discuss.

▶ Falsifying information to pacify the patient. For example, a nurse might falsely say to a dying patient "Of course you're not going to die. Don't even discuss such nonsense." This type of response stops a patient from talking about a real concern.

10. *Reflection of Feelings.* Restatement, discussed above, may be described as a mirroring of interview content. In contrast, reflection is a mirroring by the nurse of the *patient's feelings.* For example, a patient might say, "I simply can't stand to go down to physical therapy today. I get so exhausted there and besides it's not doing me a bit of good." The nurse, as she reflects the patient's feelings, might say, "You sound very tired and discouraged today."

Reflecting patient's feelings takes skill on the part of the nurse. Basically the technique involves (a) careful listening, (b) observing the patient's nonverbal behavior for signs of agitation, anger, depression, and other emotions and (c) choosing words or phrases which most succinctly capture the meaning and emotion *behind* the patient's words and actions. When wording a reflective response, it is essential to avoid the use of stereotyped phrases and cliches. Some suggested introductory phrases for reflective statements are:

"You think that. . . ."
"You seem to feel. . . ."
"You apparently believe. . . ."
"In other words. . . ."
"What I hear you saying is. . . ."
"I understand you to say. . . ."

Repeated use of the phrase "You feel . . ." should be avoided because it tends to irritate some patients, thereby nullifying the beneficial effect of the technique.[12]

> *It is important when using the technique of reflection to reflect both the patient's positive and his negative feelings. Reflection of negative feelings should be done in a noncritical, nonjudgmental manner.*

Finally, reflection is most effective when accompanied by nonverbal gestures on the part of the nurse that signal acceptance of the patient's feelings. Methods for using nonverbal techniques during the interview are briefly considered below.

Nonverbal Communication. The attentive nurse-interviewer is aware not only of the patient's words but also of his expressions and body language. Specifically, the nurse should look for (a) frequently repeated nonverbal signals, e.g., crying each time a particular topic is mentioned, (b) physical gestures that portray confidence, anxiety, anger, defensiveness, fear, sorrow and (c) gestures and facial expressions that are inconsistent with the patient's words (as discussed under the confronting response). These observations can help bring to light problems that the patient finds difficult or frightening to discuss.

In addition, the nurse must be attuned to her own nonverbal communication. She can convey the gamut of human feelings (both negative and positive) by the way she sits, holds her head and uses eye contact. Indeed, warmth, understanding, fatigue, boredom, irritation and anger can be portrayed more dramatically in a facial expression, a glance, a touch or a shrug of the shoulders than they ever can in words. For this reason, the nurse needs to know how to use nonverbal communication to facilitate verbal communication during an interview rather than to halt it. Positive ways to use nonverbal responses during the interview are as follows:

▶ Nodding coupled with a sympathetic facial expression may enable the patient to talk more freely about himself.

▶ Sitting close to the patient or touching him may help him talk about difficult or painful subjects.

▶ Sitting quietly reduces distractions which may disturb the patient.

▶ Maintaining eye contact with the patient usually helps him feel that the nurse is attentive to what he is saying.

Closing the Interview. The closing of the interview sets the stage for future interviews and discussions. Thus, it is essential that the interview end in a manner that clearly indicates to the patient that the interview is closing on a warm and friendly note.

It is just as important to *plan* the closing of an interview as it is to plan interview content. Some suggestions for a successful closing follow:

▶ Prepare the patient (and yourself) in advance for closing by informing him *at the beginning* of the interview how long the interview will last. For instance, "Mr. Jones, we'll be talking together for around a half hour today. We should finish about 3 o'clock."

▶ Always clearly indicate to the patient that the session is now coming to an end, e.g., "We'll be finished in just a few minutes."

▶ Do not introduce any new material at closing time. If the patient brings up new points he wishes to discuss, schedule a second interview. It is important to stop at the planned time because if you continue to talk with the patient when you need to do other work you may appear rushed, inattentive or irritated.

▶ It is sometimes helpful to state that you now have enough information to plan the patient's nursing care. You might say, "Mr. Jones, thanks for being so helpful. You've told me a lot about yourself and your illnesses. I appreciate that. You and I should be able to plan some good nursing care for you."

▶ Summarize the content of the interview at closing time. Also, try to reflect the patient's general feelings during the session. Finally, remember to verify with the patient that your summarization is accurate.

▶ Refer to your future plans with the patient

and for the patient. For example: "Mrs. Clare, I'll be seeing you tomorrow morning at 9 o'clock to discuss your surgery in more detail. In the meantime I will do as we have decided and call the social worker and make an appointment with her to see you. I'll arrange for the Lutheran chaplain to visit you soon."

▶ Give the patient a task to do between interview sessions. Using this technique, the nurse might say, "You seem to have a lot of concern about going into labor. I plan to visit you tomorrow morning. I'll leave you a sheet of paper and a pencil. Between now and tomorrow, I want you to jot down all your questions about labor and delivery. When I see you in the morning, we'll discuss what you've written down."

Interviewing Patients Who Have Special Problems.[72] Thus far, we have discussed interviewing patients under relatively good conditions. However, within the clinical situation, conditions are often far from good for interviewing. Quite often you will encounter patients who are difficult to interview because of serious illness, hearing problems, speech impairment due to stroke, a language barrier, mental depression, or disorders of the larynx.

Serious illness can make the interview difficult because the patient may be suffering from weakness, fever and exhaustion, severe pain, diarrhea, vomiting, nausea, or difficulty in breathing. Try to make the patient comfortable; check his position and whether he needs any medication. Obtain information relevant to the immediate illness first, asking short, specific questions that the patient can answer easily. Obtain only as much information at one time as the patient's condition permits; schedule several short (10 to 15 minutes) interviews to complete the data base.

Deafness or hearing impairment can mean that the patient has difficulty responding to the nurse's questions. Find out if the patient has a hearing aid (check if it is turned on) or whether one can be brought to the hospital for him. Face the patient so that he can watch your lips and expression; use gestures. Use short sentences and phrases rather than single words or long sentences; short phrases give more clues about what is being asked than single words do.

Dysphasia (impairment of speech) due to cerebral injury can result in lack of coordination in speech, failure to arrange words in proper order, inability to find the words to express needs, and in some cases, total unresponsiveness. Ask short questions that can be answered with "yes" or "no" or with a nod. Give the patient enough time to answer and be understanding and empathic; the patient may be extremely frustrated by his difficulty answering your questions. Never make injudicious remarks about the patient in his presence. Remember that a dysphasic patient can hear even if he cannot speak!

A language barrier—the patient cannot speak the language of the nurse and is unable to understand what is being said around him. The nurse can use gestures and observe the patient's gestures and nonverbal behavior. Do not shout or use "pigeon English," but speak to the patient in a normal tone of voice. Find an interpreter in the hospital or find out if any member of the family can interpret for the patient.

A depressed patient may show slowed speech, brief responses, and little or no verbal spontaneity. It may be difficult to interview him because of his poor concentration, feelings of worthlessness, preoccupation with pessimistic or suicidal thoughts, or exhaustion from inability to sleep or eat well. Use a kindly but firm attitude. Give support and genuine reassurance; help the patient feel that he is not worthless and that you want to spend time with him. Ask short questions that can be answered "yes" or "no." Accept silences when they occur, but do not permit lengthy silences. Persist with the interview even though the patient seems distracted and preoccupied.

Conditions of the larynx may mean that the patient is unable to speak or that he is very hoarse when he speaks. Give the patient a "magic slate" to write out his answers; encourage him to use sign language to answer you.

Recording the Interview. The ability to take accurate notes during an interview, without interfering with the flow, is an important skill to develop. Points about recording the interview that need stressing are as follows:

▶ Tell the patient that you plan to write down information, and explain that the information you are recording will be used to plan his care.

▶ Record data the patient gives you *during the session*. Recall of information following an interview is usually poor. There is, however, one exception to this rule: If you plan to record something about the patient that you are not prepared for him to see, wait until *after* the interview to write those notes.

▶ Listen attentively to the patient. Try not to appear more interested in note taking than in listening.

▶ Summarize the data before writing your

notes. Do not try to write down verbatim what the patient says; this is neither possible nor helpful. Also, do not attempt to write finished polished sentences.

▶ Make every effort to ensure that notes concerning the patient remain confidential. Do not leave your notes where anyone can read them.

▶ Be honest with the patient about your notes. If you are using them in a research project or for a classroom assignment, tell him so. Also, if you cannot guarantee that the notes will remain confidential, it is best to tell the patient the truth.

There are a number of printed forms available for recording assessment data, e.g., assessment forms, history forms, review of systems forms. In the sections to come we will present examples of standard forms.

The Nursing History

Definition and Purposes.   The major purpose of the assessment interview (which we have just discussed in detail) is to obtain and write up the patient's nursing history. The *patient history* (whether medical or nursing) is basically "a description of the patient's chief complaint, patient profile, history of the present problem or problems, past health history, family and a review of systems."[87] A *nursing* history, in contrast to the medical history, centers on descriptions of the patient's physical, mental and emotional reactions to illness and hospitalization and the resultant changes in his lifestyle. It focuses on collecting information about the ways a patient normally gets his basic human needs met and on identifying obstacles (problems) to that normal process in the present. The *medical* history (discussed in Chap. 16) concentrates on the patient's symptoms and the progress of his disease. Thus, while medical and nursing histories are based upon similar content, they focus upon different aspects of the patient's life.

The nursing history, taken by a skilled interviewer, is a valuable assessment tool. Essentially, the nursing history:

▶ Constitutes the first stage of problem solving and planning for immediate and long-term patient care

▶ Establishes an information base upon which the nursing diagnosis and the plans for treatment can be built

▶ Helps the nurse initiate a positive, helpful and communicative relationship with the patient

▶ Allows the nurse to observe the patient's verbal and nonverbal communication and his general behavior

▶ Gives the patient an opportunity to discuss *his* feelings about himself and his current problems as well as his expectations about himself and about the health professionals caring for him

▶ Reveals the patient's past, present and potential problems concerning the meeting of basic human needs

▶ Helps the patient remember events and symptoms which he may have forgotten or repressed

▶ Provides a written format in which to record information about the patient's physical, functional, mental and emotional status

▶ Creates a reference point from which the nurse can measure the patient's progress throughout his hospitalization

Nursing History Formats.   There are many different types of nursing history formats, structured to meet the particular needs of the nurses who work with them. In this chapter we describe three basic types of nursing formats along with some hints for using them. They are (1) the structured check list format for the general hospital patient, (2) the specialized history format (in this example, a pediatric history) and (3) an unstructured open-ended format.

THE STRUCTURED NURSING HISTORY.   An excellent example of a structured nursing history format is shown in Figure 17–5. This format, developed by Eggland, is structured for completeness and ease of use by the nurse. Even though this history form is essentially a check list, Eggland warns that it is important to avoid sounding as though a check list is being used. In other words, don't ask the patient questions in an insensitive, rote fashion; take the time to use the interviewing skills that we emphasized earlier. For example, instead of opening the interview with the section on vital statistics, begin with broad questions such as "How are you feeling?" or "What brings you to the hospital?" In this way, you begin the patient's history with the area of greatest concern to him, and you learn about his *chief complaint.*[32]

As you study Figure 17–5 note that the major areas covered in a nursing history form are essentially the same as the areas covered in the medical history except that the nursing history

Patient: _Merion Miller_

Address: _2654 N. 76th St._

Vital statistics:

Age: _35_   B.P. _126/78_

Ht: _64"_   P _78_

Wt: _130 lbs._   R _18_

Diagnoses: _Rheumatoid Arthritis_

known by: _Entire family_

Chief complaint: _1. Dizziness_
2. Joint pain
3. Fatigue

History of present illness:
lightheaded, loses balance 4-5 times per day for last 2 years. Diagnosed 2/15/76. NOT related to any special activity, but is hungry after "attack". Takes candy which relieves symptoms.

Past history:

Allergies: Food _No_
Drug _No_
Other _None_

Major illnesses, operations and hospitalizations (include dates):
1972 Delivered male child
1975 Delivered female child

Hospital of choice: _Mercy_

REVIEW OF SYSTEMS:

VISION:
No diff. ✓ glasses____ last checked____ blurring____ diplopia____ pain____ inflammation____ cataracts____ glaucoma____
Comments: _____

HEARING:
No diff. ✓ limited____ aid____ pain____ tinnitus____ discharge____
Comments: _____

SPEECH:
No diff. ✓ language____ aphasic____ can understand____ can express____
Comments: _____

RESPIRATORY:
No diff. ✓ pain____ dyspnea____ cough____ sputum____ sinusitis____ epistaxis____ colds freq.____
last chest X-ray____ results____
Comments: _____

CIRCULATORY:
No diff. ✓ edema____ numbness____ syncope____ dizziness____ cyanosis____ anemia____ bruising____
chest pain____ palpitations____ cong. defect____
Comments: _____

GASTROINTESTINAL:
Nutrition:
No diff. ✓ appetite _good_ adeq. food ✓ adeq. fluid _6-7 glasses_ difficulty chewing _no_ dental status _good_
diet _Reg. and increased CHO_ due to:____ meal/snack pattern _3 meals + 4/5 snacks_ dysphagia _no_
nausea _no_ vomiting _no_
Comments: _____
Elimination:
No diff. ✓ stool _q 2-3 days_ constipation____ diarrhea____ incontinence____ ileostomy____ colostomy____
who cares for:____
Comments: _____

Treatment of current illness:

Medication: _Aspirin 600 mg with meals and @ bedtime._

Treatments: _Occasional use of dry heat to painful knees._

Physician(s): _Dr. John James_

Last appt. _6 months_   Next appt. _Will Call_

Care being given by: _Self_

Capability of caregiver: _Satisfactory_

Adequacy of care: _Satisfactory_

Other services involved: _No_

Equipment and prosthesis: _None_

Condition and care: _____

Family history

Hereditary illnesses: _None_

Family members in home:

Name	Age	Health	Occupation
Husband	36	good	sales
daughter	2y	good	—
son	5y	good	—

Changes: in family routine, employment, relationships, or prior goals/values:
None

Figure 17–5. Example of a structured nursing history format. (From Eggland, E. T.: How to take a meaningful nursing history. _Nursing '77,_ 7:23, July 1977.)

Figure continued on the opposite page

URINARY:

No diff. ✓ urine *Clear, Amber* incontinence_____ nocturia_____ hematuria_____ UTI_____ stones_____

dribbling_____ catheter type_____ size_____ reason_____ date inserted_____ removed_____

Comments: _____

NEUROLOGICAL:

No diff. ✓ incoordination_____ convulsions_____ paralysis_____ parasthesia_____ weakness_____

Comments: _____

MUSCULOSKELETAL:

No diff._____ deformities_____ pain ✓ stiffness ✓ *on arising* contractures *none* arthritis ✓ exercises *3 x day*

done by *self*

Comments: _____

REPRODUCTIVE:

No diff. ✓ menses problem_____ last Pap test *1/15* results *Neg* menopause_____ self-breast check ✓ infection_____

prostate problems_____

Comments: _____

SKIN:

description (dryness, color, turgor) *oily, good color, firm*

rashes *none*   location_____

lesions *none*   location_____

lotions or aids *Hand lotion*

Comments: _____

Activities of Daily Living:

Needs assistance in:

mobility ✓ transfers_____ hygiene_____ dressing ✓ feeding_____ meal prep_____ shopping_____ housework ✓

laundry ✓ banking_____

Comments: _____

Sleep:

hours *7-8* naps *sometimes* aids *No* insomnia *No* due to:_____

Comments: _____

Activities:

reading ✓ TV ✓ games_____ cards ✓ handwork ✓

limitations imposed by illness *handwork, housework, child care*

visitors _____

Comments: _____

Habits:

alcohol *NO* tobacco *NO* drugs *NO*

Comments: _____

Psychosocial history:

Present mental status:

alert ✓ confused_____ memory_____ orientation *good*

Comments: _____

Present behavior:

cooperative ✓ anxious_____ depressed ✓ demanding_____ distrustful_____ lethargic_____ talkative ✓

withdrawn_____

Comments: *worries about possibility of further disability.*

Mental status and behavior prior to illness: *good*

Reaction to illness and care: *Well-adjusted to illness*

Expectations for self: *Maintain self sufficiency*

Expectations of doctors and nurses: *Teach and guide in nutrition. Support*

Environment:

adequate space ✓ cleanliness *yes* safety hazards *no*

Comments: _____

Financial status:

a family concern *no* job *not employed* education *College (2 years)*

Employment:

interruption for patient due to illness_____ interruption for family to give care_____ emotional reaction_____

Comments: _____

Figure 17–5 Continued

contains a section entitled "Activities of Daily Living." Moreover, as emphasized earlier, the nursing history focuses on the patient's reactions to his problems and symptoms rather than on the disease underlying the symptoms. Because medical and nursing histories are similar, emphasize to the patient that you do not plan to simply repeat the doctor's questions. Explain that you are seeking information that will help you plan his *nursing care* rather than his medical care. During your conversation show him how you intend doing this.

Learning how the patient feels about himself, his family and his symptoms is not always easy. Fortunately there are helpful techniques for approaching the different areas listed on the history. Below we have presented some leading questions and statements which you may use to open the various areas of discussion.

▶ *History of present illness.* "Tell me as much as you can about your symptoms." "What were the circumstances when you first experienced symptoms?" "Are you under stress when you develop symptoms?" "If so, what kind of stress?" "In what ways do your symptoms affect your activities?" "How are you presently coping with your symptoms?" "What is your doctor doing about your symptoms?" "Has your doctor told you about your diagnosis?"

▶ *Past history.* "How has your health been in the past?" "Tell me about any major illnesses or operations which you have had?" "Do you have any history of allergy?"

▶ *Family history.* "How has this illness changed your life and your family's life?" If a family problem is mentioned, Eggland suggests asking, "How are you coping with this problem?"[32]

▶ *Review of systems.*[32] Begin with broad categories and then ask about specific symptoms. For example: "How is your vision?" "Do you have any trouble with your eyes?" "Any blurring of vision or eye pain?" "How about your hearing?" "Any discharge from your ears?" "Do you ever experience problems breathing?" If the patient *does* have a symptom, Eggland suggests asking what he is doing about the symptom, e.g., "Have you told your doctor about your shortness of breath?" "What did the doctor say?" "Did he prescribe any medications?" If the patient has *not* seen a doctor, you might inquire, "Is there some reason you have not seen your doctor about this problem?"

▶ *Activities of daily living.* "In what ways are your symptoms affecting your activities and daily routine?" "What are your typical sleeping habits?" "Have you noticed any change in your sleeping patterns since you developed your symptoms?"

▶ *Psychosocial history.* "What were you like before your illness and what's the difference now?"[28] This question enables the patient to discuss his self-image and ways in which it has changed since the development of illness; it also helps to clarify the patient's reactions to illness. To learn about the patient's *goals and expectations* for himself, you might ask: "Ideally, how do you see yourself feeling and functioning by the end of your hospitalization? By the end of the year?" "If everything doesn't proceed ideally, what level of activity would you be willing to accept?"[60] It is also important to ask the patient what he *expects of the health professionals* who are caring for him. Thus you might inquire: "In what ways can we (doctors and nurses) help you the most?" "How do you feel about the care that you are receiving?" "Do you feel that everything possible is being done to help you?" "Do you have any criticism of your care thus far?"

▶ *Financial status.* "Has money become a concern since your illness developed?" If so, ask: "Are you using community resources to help you through this period?"

As you discuss each area of the history with the patient, it is important to make liberal use of the comment sections. Use comments to describe and elaborate on particular symptoms and concerns. It is especially important to describe *pain* in complete detail, e.g., location, duration, type of pain, and what relieves the pain.[7] The comment section is most useful if you *directly quote* the patient rather than writing down your interpretation of what the patient says.

> *Remember that the nursing history is strictly a device for gathering data; it must not be used for interpretation of data.*

Thus the comment section should be primarily employed to describe how the patient views himself and his situation rather than how you view the patient.

THE SPECIALIZED NURSING HISTORY. Specialized services (e.g., pediatrics, obstetrics, psychiatry and communicable diseases) usually have specialized history formats. Figure 17–6 exemplifies the type of historical data needed to complete a child's nursing history. Note that the history forms for both child and adult are similar in basic content, e.g., chief complaint, present illness, family history, review of systems. The pediatric history, however, is addressed principally to the child's parents and focuses primarily on the birth, growth, and development (physical, mental and social) of the child. The even more specialized history format for obstetrics is structured around such topics as the woman's menstrual periods, previous miscarriages, consumption of medication which might affect her pregnancy, and genetic background. On a psychiatric service, emphasis is placed on the patient's history of childhood development, adolescent

adjustment, and coping mechanisms (see Chap. 16).

To obtain a good history on a specialized service, it is essential to learn about the patient's *general* medical background as well as his special needs and problems. Failure to obtain a *full* picture of the patient's overall health and illness patterns may result in incorrect or missed diagnoses—sometimes with dangerous consequences.

THE UNSTRUCTURED HISTORY. The almost totally nonstructured assessment form developed by Little and Carnevali constitutes a

---

PATIENT: Susan R. Born 10/15/68.
PROBLEM #1: Well-baby care. First visit 7/17/73.

PAST HISTORY

Prenatal – Mother's second pregnancy. She was in good health throughout. From 3rd to 9th month she was followed at DGH (Denver Gen'l Hosp.). She reported no infections, illnesses, hospitalizations, X-rays or accidents during the pregnancy. Her doctor placed her on vitamins and iron tablets for the entire pregnancy. Both she and the baby's father have RH positive blood types. She followed her normal diet except for slight sodium restrictions during the final trimester. She has had no abortions or miscarriages. She has two other children.

Natal – Labor lasted 5 hours. Her husband was able to be with her most of the time. She received a caudal anesthetic and the baby was delivered by vertex. Baby born DGH. Birth weight 7 lbs. 4 oz. She cried spontaneously and did not need oxygen.

Postnatal – Nursery stay uneventful with mother and infant going home after 3 days. Infant exhibited slight jaundice on 3rd or 4th day, but no cyanosis or rashes. She lost 3 oz. during first week. Breastfeeding was initiated in hospital and went well-- she was hungry and sucked well and the breasts withstood the firm pressure.

Allergies – No allergic reactions to medications, insects, animal or seasons. Breaks out in fine, macular, itchy rash 12 hours after eating tomatoes.

Accidents – None.

Illnesses – Chickenpox at 2½ years. Rubella at 3 years.

Operations – Tonsils removed at 3½ years. Stayed in hospital one night. No adverse reactions.

Immunizations – DPT #1 1/1969
              DPT #2 2/1969   Given by private pediatrician,
              DPT #3 3/1969   Kansas City.
              DPT booster 3/1970 CGH Clinic
              Trivalent polio 1/1969
              Trivalent polio 2/1969 Given by private pediatrician, Kansas City
              Trivalent polio 4/1969
              Trivalent polio booster 5/1970
              Tine test 7/1969 (negative) CGH Clinic
              Measles-rubella-mumps vaccine 6/1972

Family History – Mother – 30 yrs., good health
                Father – 35 yrs., back treated at work clinic
                Siblings: Jane – 3 yrs., good health
                         John – 6 yrs., partially deaf, attends special school

Family Diseases – No nose bleeds, sinus problems, glaucoma or cataracts. No tuberculosis, hypertension, heart murmurs, strokes, anemia, rheumatic fever, asthma, leukemia or pneumonia. Mother has hayfever in springtime. No ulcers or colitis. Mother had kidney infections with each pregnancy and is still seen in UTI clinic for recurring problem. No arthritis, club feet or congenitally dislocated hips. No convulsions, mental retardation, mental problems, coma or epilepsy. No diabetes, cancer or tumors. Older sibling partially deaf, maternal aunt totally deaf from birth.

Social – Family of 5 live in small, 2-bedroom house with no basement and tiny yard. Father works nights as trainman and sleeps during day. Mother home with children. Family struggles to keep within a budget and recreational activities limited. Father becoming more interested in helping with children as they get older.

REVIEW OF SYSTEMS

EENT – No persistent nosebleeds, frequent colds or earaches. Had 5 strep throat infections year of tonsillectomy.

Cardio-Resp – No trouble breathing, turning blue or choking. Keeps up with other children, runs stairs.

GI – No problems with diarrhea, constipation, bleeding, bloody stools, pain, vomiting, encopresis.

GU – No problems with frequency, pain, bleeding, enuresis.

Neuro – No convulsions, fits, seizures, blackouts, dizzy spells, epilepsy.

Skeletal – Broke right middle finger in fall from tricycle in 1970. No complaints of joint pain or swelling.

Senses – Mother feels she hears and sees; no vision or hearing testing ever done.

HABITS

Eating – Good appetite. Eats most foods. Eats cereal, milk, fruit, vegetables, and meat daily. Eggs 4-5 times per week. Likes snacks of fruits, cookies, juices, candy.

Bowels – Mother unsure of pattern since child goes by herself and rarely complains of problems. No recent diarrhea or constipation. Toilet trained since early 3's.

Sleep – Generally in bed by 8 or 9 and up by 6:30 or 7. Will sometimes take short nap in afternoon. Sleeps in top bunk bed in children's bedroom. No problems with nightmares or night terrors.

Development – Friendly, outgoing little girl who gets along well with most people. Has several girl friends on block. Knows her name, can dress herself, can count to 5 and is looking forward to school next year.

OBJECTIVE – Wt. 36 lbs. Ht. 41"
Physical Examination – (Total explanation of physical findings would be written into this area.)

PLAN

Impression – Healthy 4 yr. old.

Therapeutic – DT booster and polio booster given. DDST done. Hct. done. Urinalysis done. Vision tested, normal. Hearing tested, normal.

Education – 1) Discussed eating and snacking. Limiting candy intake and watching tooth brushing. 2) Discussed getting ready to go to school – learning to cross streets, tie own shoes, knowing home address and phone number, etc. 3) Return to clinic in 1 year for health check -- all screening, check on school readiness.

Figure 17–6. Pediatric history format. (From Alexander, M. M., and Brown, M. S.: Physical examination. *Nursing '73, 3*:35, Aug. 1973.)

listed down one side (i.e., breathing/circulation, elimination). These broad categories serve to remind the nurse interviewer of major potential problem areas for patients. Observe that the nurse who wrote up the assessment for A. Longbranch discusses only some of the suggested categories recorded; also the categories which are discussed are not recorded in any definite order.

According to Little and Carnevali, the major

rather radical departure from the structured check list history format that we have discussed thus far.[60] As you can see in Figure 17–7, this assessment form is really an almost blank piece of paper with some assessment categories

---

SAMPLE NURSING ASSESSMENT FORM

Name _Arthur Longbranch_   Age _47_   Date _6/22/75_

Prefers to be called _"Art"_   Assessment made by _Jill Sutter_ RN

Areas	Subjective/Objective Data
Client perceptions of: Current health status Goals Needed/usable services **Functional Abilities:** Breathing/Circulation Elimination Emotional/cognitive Mobility/safety Nutrition Hygiene/grooming Sensory input Sexuality Sleep/rest **Resources & Support Systems:** Environmental Personal/social Other	_Perceived health status_: Rt inguinal hernia repair in A.M. Hosp (Subj) stay expected: 3–4 days. Older brother had same surg. 6 mo. ago — no prblms. no prev. hosp admissions. Expects spinal anesthesia — some concern re aftereffects. MD told him he was in good cond. No other med. prblms. Objective: uses medical terminology _Goals_: To be out of hosp in 3–5 days, up day of surgery, To (Subj) ret to job as accountant in 2 wks & to his golf game in 6 wks. _Expected care_: Dr will order Rx to control pain & sleep prn. (Subj) Brother said backrubs @ HS → relaxation. ō limitations on visitors _Hygiene/grooming_ (Subj) Usually showers ā bkfst/q̄ d. shaves 2x daily ā bkfst & p̄ supper. (objective:) Trimmed moustache — long side burns Toupee _Sensory Input_: (Subj) glasses for close work — none for distance, checked 6 mo ago. No difficulty hearing. _Sleep/Rest_: Usual sleep pattern 10³⁰p to 6³⁰a s̄ waking. (Subj) Usual Rx for Sleeplessness: reading & hot cocoa sleep not often a problem unless worrying. _Nutrition_: 3 meals 7³⁰a, 12 noon 6p no snacks except (Subj) coffee. Drinks 10–12 cups/day Dislikes: strong vegetables, mayonnaise, casserole dishes. No food allergies. (objective:) Ht 6' Wt 180#. Looks well nourished _Elimination_: BM p̄ bkfst. q̄ d. Rx for constipation: 1c prune (Subj) juice in a.m. No nocturia, frequency or burning. _Social/Rec_: (subj) Plays bridge 1x wk c̄ fellows in office. Plays golf 2x wk. Enjoys lake fishing, boating, reading (mysteries) Gardening — roses, orchids (Objective) Has Sports Illustrated, US News and World report, Newsweek at bedside

Figure 17–7. Completed sample nursing assessment form. (From Little, D. E., and Carnevali, L. D.: _Nursing Care Planning,_ 2nd ed. Philadelphia, J. B. Lippincott Co., 1976, p. 145.)

Figure continued on the opposite page

advantage of this type of format is that it grants more freedom of expression to nurse and patient than does a check list. Also, this form removes any temptation on the nurse's part to simply ask questions about items on a list regardless of whether or not those items have significance for the patient. In essence, without the crutch of a check list of "prefabricated questions" the nurse is forced to be more selective, sensitive and creative in her interviewing style.[60]

Recording the Nursing History. Becknell and Smith list a number of suggestions for complete, clear, objective and accurate recording of the nursing history.[12] They are as follows:

▶ Write as concisely as possible. Sentences do not have to be complete as long as they are accurate and clear (see Figs. 17–5 and 17–7).

▶ Write legibly; spell accurately; use acceptable grammar; employ only standard medical abbreviations.

▶ Avoid long, technical phrases or words unless absolutely necessary for preciseness. Never use a word unless you understand its meaning.

▶ Be factual in your descriptions. Avoid the use of words which need interpretation, e.g., good, bad, thin, fat.

▶ Describe the patient's behavior rather than attempting to interpret his behavior. Avoid labeling the patient, e.g., "belligerent," or "depressed."

▶ Whenever possible, support your observations of patient behavior and communication patterns with examples of what the patient actually does and says.

The Physical Examination*

Preparation for the Physical Examination. Nurses, like physicians, must be able to accurately assess the patient's physical condition. Upon admission to a hospital, the patient is always physically examined by the physician and often by the nurse as well. Today, public health nurses and family nurse practitioners routinely conduct physical examinations in the hospital, in clinics, in schools and in the patient's home. Following an initial physical examination, the hospital patient's physical condition is assessed on a daily or even more frequent basis depending upon his condition.

Prior to examining the patient, lay out the equipment that you will use during your examination, e.g., a stethoscope, sphygmomanometer, thermometer, flashlight, tongue blade and gloves. Next, explain to the patient what you plan to do during the examination and why. Help the patient relax as much as possible. Insure his comfort. Ask him to urinate prior to the examination. Make certain that the examination room is quiet, warm and well lighted. Before beginning the examination, wash your hands in the patient's presence even if your hands are clean. This simple act increases the

---

*The physical examination is described in Chapter 16. Detailed discussions of the nursing physical examination are presented in bibliographic entries 1, 2, 10, 46, 47, 78. We recommend that you read further on this vital subject.

Support Systems: (subj) Wife, employed school teacher. Married 20 years 2 daughters 16 y.o. @ home 18 y.o. away @ Univ. Family will visit evenings. Hospital Ins. & Sick leave. (Objective) Picture of wife & daughters outside their home on bedside stand.

Breathing: (Subj) Does not smoke. No hist. of chronic resp. disease. (Objective) R 14 No Sx of resp. infection.

Figure 17–7 Continued

patient's confidence in you as a conscientious professional person.[46]

Physical Examination Skills. To conduct a nursing physical examination, the nurse must become proficient in the following six basic skills: (1) measurement, (2) inspection, (3) palpation, (4) percussion, (5) auscultation and (6) detection of odors. These skills require the trained use of one's eyes, ears, hands and nose. Now, let's consider each of these skills briefly.

Measurement involves determining the magnitude of a certain structure or function and then recording the findings numerically. Measurement is one of the most basic of scientific skills. To be useful, measurements must be accurate and precise. Data obtainable during the physical examination by measurement include the patient's blood pressure, temperature, pulse rate, respiratory rate, height, weight and the circumference of body parts (e.g., the abdomen or leg), as well as the length or diameter of certain bony structures (measuring the pelvic outlet is part of the prenatal examination). Measurements taken during the patient's initial physical examination form a valuable baseline of information to which the nurse can refer throughout his hospitalization.

Inspection or *observation* involves "visually assessing the patient."[46] More specifically, inspection is a highly critical and detailed visual examination of the patient's general physical appearance and specific body parts—noting such characteristics as size, color, position, symmetry and degree of movement. Inspection can be performed while looking at and talking to the patient; it can also be done while performing the other physical examination skills.

Palpation (feeling), *percussion* (tapping with the fingers) and *auscultation* are discussed in Chapter 16.

The *detection of abnormal odors* is a final and extremely important diagnostic skill. Indeed, McVan points out in her article devoted to patient odors that "odors . . . can be just as important as vital signs." Odors can help the nurse identify many different types of disorders. Characteristic odors detectable during physical examination and their possible causes are described in Table 16–2, Chapter 16.

The Systematic Examination. To perform a careful and complete physical examination, one must use a systematic approach. With this end in mind, educators and clinicians have attempted to devise methods for systematically inspecting and examining the patient.

The use of a *body systems approach* is one suggested method. Using this method, the nurse observes and records data about each of the body systems, e.g., the respiratory system, neurologic system, cardiovascular system. The *Review of Systems* that we considered in our discussion of the nursing history is based on this concept.

A second method involves *inspecting the patient from head to foot.* Wolff and Erickson have developed a special pictorial device for helping the nurse make a head-to-toe assessment called the "Assessment Man" (Fig. 17–8A). To use this tool, one begins with the patient's head (noting mental and emotional status, vision, hearing, the mouth) and proceeds down the body to his extremities (noting movement and sensation). As the nurse gathers her data she can enter her observations into the series of boxes depicted in Figure 17–8B. Each box represents a category (mental status, emotional status) into which raw data can be sorted and classified.[116]

A third systematic method has been developed by McCain and her colleagues—a detailed tool for assessing the *functional abilities* of the patient. This form is completely oriented to nursing and in no way duplicates the medical history and medical physical examination. To date, these nurse researchers have identified 13 functional areas which are considered as separate items for purposes of assessment: social, mental, emotional, body temperature, respiratory, circulatory, nutritional, elimination status, reproductive status, state of rest and comfort, state of skin and appendages, sensory perception and motor ability. Table 17–4 gives a sampling from their extensive list of functional factors. McCain points out that all the factors listed may not be applicable to every patient and that the nurse must judge which items are appropriate to the situation.[74]

The Psychologic and Mental Health Examination

Learning about the patient's mental and psychologic status is just as important as learning about his physical condition. It takes as much skill and sensitivity to note a patient's mood, manner and speech as it does to observe skin color, vital signs, breast lumps and tissue changes. Bates instructs:

Conduct your assessment of mental status with the same acceptance and respect for the patient that you show in other portions of the examination. At the same time, do not avoid possibly significant areas because of your own anxieties or fears of upsetting the patient.[10]

Ideally, the nurse should assess the patient's psychologic and mental health status through-

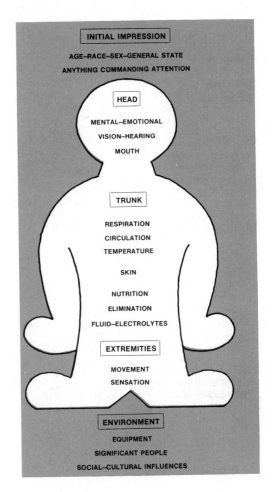

Figure 17–8A. "The Assessment Man"—a head-to-toe assessment tool. (From Wolff, H. and Erickson, R.: The assessment man. *Nursing Outlook, 25*:103, February 1977, p. 105.)

MENTAL STATUS	RESPIRATION	NUTRITION	SENSATION
EMOTIONAL STATUS	CIRCULATION	ELIMINATION	EQUIPMENT
VISION and HEARING	TEMPERATURE	FLUID and ELECTROLYTES	PEOPLE—SOCIAL—CULTURE
MOUTH	SKIN	MOVEMENT	LEARNING

Figure 17–8B. The method for recording data from the "Assessment Man."

Mental Status

State of consciousness
    Alert and quick to respond to surroundings
    Drowsy and slow to respond
    Semiconscious and difficult to arouse
    Comatose and unable to arouse
    State of automatism
Orientation
    To time
    To place
    To person
Intellectual capacity
    Level of education
    Ability to recall events: recent; past
Attention span
Vocabulary level
    Use of simple, nontechnical words
    Use of complex, technical words
Ability to understand ideas
    Slow to learn meaning and make relationships
    Quick to gain meaning and make relationships
    Insight into health problems

Emotional Status

Emotional reactions
    Mood
    Presence or absence of anxiety
    Defenses against anxiety: such as aggression;
        depression; fantasies; identification;
        rationalization; regression; repression;
        sublimation
Body image
    Effect of illness on self-concept
    Adaptation of self-concept to reality demands
Ability to relate to others
    To family
    To other patients
    To health team members

Sensory Perception

Hearing
    Sensitivity to sound
        Voice tone that distinguishes sounds: low;
            moderate; loud
        Distance that sounds distinguished
        Need to see speaker to distinguish
            sounds
    Presence of impairment
        Partial or complete
        Unilateral or bilateral
        Ability to lip read
        Use and effectiveness of supportive aid
Vision
    Acuity
    Presence of impairment
        Partial or complete
        Unilateral or bilateral
        Type: hyperopia; myopia; astigmatism;
            color-blindness; diplopia; photophobia;
            nyctalopia; other
        Use and effectiveness of supportive aid
    Enucleation
        Unilateral or bilateral
        Use of prosthesis

Speech
    Has auditory expression
    Aphasia
        Verbal defect
        Syntactical defect
        Nominal defect
        Semantic defect
    Anarthria
    Mute
    Laryngectomy
        Use and effectiveness of esophageal speech
    Unusual speech patterns: such as lisping;
        repetitive; staccato; stammer; stutter
Touch
    Hyperesthesia
    Anesthesia
    Paresthesia
    Paralgesia
Smell
    Anosmia
    Hyperosmia
    Kakosmia
    Parosmia
Taste
    Distinguishes: sweet; salt; sour; bitter
    Aftertaste present

Motor Ability

Mobility
    Complete bed rest
    Bed rest with bathroom privileges
    Sit in chair
    Ambulatory
        Without assistance
        With supportive aids: person;
            crutches; walker
        Use of wheel chair
        Use of stretcher
    Posture
        In bed
        Upright
Range of motion
    Passive
    Active
Gait
Equilibrium
Abnormal movement
    Clonic
    Tonic
    Spastic
    Flaccid
    Tic
    Ataxia
Muscle tone
    Spasm
    Contractures
    Weakness
Paralysis
    Hemiplegia
    Paraplegia
    Quadriplegia
Loss of extremity
    Location
    Extent
    Use and effectiveness of prosthesis

*From McCain, R. F.: Nursing by assessment—not intuition. *In* Marriner, A.: The Nursing Process: A Scientific Approach to Nursing Care. St. Louis, C. V. Mosby Co., 1975, p. 34.

out the assessment interview and physical examination. Specifically, the following observations should be made and recorded:[7, 10]

▶ *General appearance and posture:* Note patient's personal hygiene, appropriateness of dress, manner of standing, sitting and walking.

▶ *Motor activity:* Observe for signs of agitation or hyperactivity. Note inability to relax or undue tenseness and restlessness.

▶ *Facial expression:* Watch for inappropriate expressions or changes in expression when new topics are introduced.

▶ *Speech patterns:* Listen to the patient's voice for loudness, clearness, inflection, pace of speech and organization and coherence of sentences.

▶ *General mood and manner:* Observe particularly for signs of depression, anger, fatigue, disinterest. Note if the patient seems open and easy to talk to or guarded and withdrawn.

▶ *Memory:* Test for memory of past events (anniversaries, past history) and recent events (events of the day). Elderly patients and those with organic brain disease usually have a poor memory for recent events.

▶ *Orientation:* Determine if the patient is oriented to *time* (the date, the year, time of day, day of the week), *place* (address of home, name of hospital) and *person* (patient's name and names of family and friends).

▶ *Thought content:* Attempt (tactfully) to determine (a) the types of things which the patient thinks about or worries about and (b) if he has any repetitive or highly disturbing thoughts which are linked to his illness or hospitalization.

▶ *Thought processes:* Observe the patient's thought patterns as he discusses himself and family. Note if he seems to be thinking in a logical and coherent manner.

Consultation

Consulting with other sources of information is an important way to test the validity and enlarge the scope of what you have learned about your patient thus far. What resources for consultation are available to the nurse?

Experts, of course, can provide a great deal of information about certain *specific aspects* of the patient's condition. For example, you may want to discuss the patient's diagnosis and symptoms with his doctor; results of his tissue biopsy with a pathologist; the patient's dietary indiscretions with a dietician and his financial woes with a social worker. You may also want to consult other nurses who have contacted the patient to see if your impression of the patient is similar to their impressions.

Another source to consult is *patient records,* e.g., his old chart, current health records, and care plans from earlier hospitalizations. When reviewing health records, carefully study the medical and nursing histories, laboratory studies, progress and nursing notes as well as any statements from consultants (neurologists, psychiatrists, physical therapists).

Recall that talking with the patient's *significant others* also may reveal important data that the patient either forgot to tell you or perhaps deliberately withheld. Indeed, consulting with the patient's significant others is essential for understanding the patient's home, life-style and "world."

Review of the Literature

Review of the literature is a task which can be undertaken not only while assessing the patient but through each and every step of the nursing process. A thorough search of the literature for information about the patient's diagnosis, symptoms, medications, functional disabilities and rehabilitation needs serves several purposes.

First of all, the literature presents a "textbook" picture of the patient's general condition against which you can compare the patient's actual experience. Also, selected readings help you to *expand your knowledge* of the patient's medical diagnosis and medications. In addition, reviewing nursing literature can provide you with insights for making *your own diagnosis* of the patient's problems and their causation. Finally, a careful survey of current readings creates a solid theoretical basis for planning and evaluating nursing interventions.

When reviewing the literature, it is easiest to start with a general textbook that gives basic information about the patient's condition. Next, consult journal articles and specialized textbooks for more specific information and studies relevant to your patient's problems. Finally, you may want to listen to some taped lectures by physicians and nurses who are well known in their fields. Most health science libraries have tape libraries which cover a myriad of subjects and often present information which cannot be found in books or articles.

After the review of literature and completion of the data gathering process, you are ready to proceed to the second stage of assessment and to the second step of the nursing process—establishing a nursing diagnosis.

STEP 2: NURSING ASSESSMENT—THE NURSING DIAGNOSIS

Introductory Concepts[28, 58, 73, 119]

While nurses have always *acted* as diagnosticians, the term "nursing diagnosis" is almost newborn. As Yura states, "For a number of years, *diagnosis* was a charged and forbidden word in nursing."[119] Until recently, nurses carefully chose their words (both written and spoken) to avoid being accused of the "crime" of diagnosing patient symptoms. For example, a few years ago, if a nurse observed that a patient was literally gasping for breath, she was forbidden to chart "patient dyspneic." Instead she had to chart "patient *appears* to be dyspneic." In conversing with physicians about patients, the nurse was forced to watch her words so that in no way could she be accused of treading on what doctors considered their exclusive territory—namely patient diagnosis.

Today, the situation is changing. Now it is recognized that diagnosis is *not* the exclusive domain of physicians or even of health professionals. If a diagnosis is "essentially an inference about a state that is undesirable" then lawyers, social workers, telephone repairmen, police detectives and auto mechanics all make diagnoses.[73] Clearly, nurses share with these experts from other fields the common diagnostic activities associated with uncovering problems and discovering their causation—gathering facts, organizing data, seeking patterns and drawing and stating conclusions. Of course, nursing diagnoses deal with *patient* problems rather than with legal, telephone or mechanical problems.

Nursing diagnoses can also be compared and contrasted with medical diagnoses. Medical and nursing diagnoses are *similar* in that the same basic procedures underlie both processes: taking a history, performing the physical examination, analyzing and synthesizing the data obtained. Both doctors and nurses need identical types of skills to make diagnoses, e.g., interviewing skills, physical assessment skills, observational skills. Moreover, the purpose of diagnosis is the same for both professions—developing a plan of patient care that is based on the scientific method of problem solving.

Nursing diagnoses differ from medical diagnoses in their *focus* and consequently in their *goals and objectives. Physicians* are primarily interested in diagnosing the patient's *disease* and the *underlying pathologic processes.* Recall from Chapter 16 that the physician "examiner hopes to learn about the source of the patient's disorder and the metabolic, chemical or pathologic structural changes caused by the disorder." For example, a medical diagnosis might read: "Profound normocytic anemia due to acute hemorrhage." *Nurses* on the other hand, focus their diagnostic skills on defining the patient's *presenting problems* (i.e., difficulties in getting basic human needs met), along with their causation and their effect on the patient's life-style. In essence, the nursing diagnosis focuses upon the *patient's response* (both physical and emotional) to his disease and to its underlying pathology. A nursing diagnosis might state: "Severe weakness and fatigue resulting in inability to perform routine housekeeping tasks due to heavy blood losses during menstrual periods."

It is essential to remember that both forms of diagnosis are necessary for a total plan of patient care. To successfully develop a patient's total diagnostic picture, nurses and physicians must work together as well as separately; above all else they must communicate their findings to one another.

Definition and Clarification of the Nursing Diagnosis

Nursing diagnosis is a complex concept to define. Mundinger and Jauron define it as follows:

Nursing diagnosis is the statement of a patient's response which is actually or potentially unhealthful and which nursing intervention can help to change in the direction of health. It should also identify essential factors related to the unhealthful response.[73]

A well-developed diagnostic statement is composed of the following components: (1) a statement of the problem and (2) a statement of causality.

A Statement of the Problem. This is a description of current and potential patient problems (i.e., unhealthy or maladaptive patient responses or functional disabilities) that can be alleviated by nursing interventions. The accompanying tentative list of patient problem statements was developed by participants in the First National Conference on the Classification of Nursing Diagnoses in St. Louis. It represents a first step in the development of a nursing nomenclature for classifying unhealthy patient responses. Note that items described in the list below as "nursing diagnoses" are described in this text as "patient problem statements." In this chapter, nursing diagnoses are defined as containing *both* a statement of the patient's problem and a statement of causality.

Tentative List of Nursing Diagnoses[39]

Alterations in faith
Altered relationships with self and others
Altered self-concept
Anxiety
Body fluids, depletion of
Bowel function, irregular
Cognitive functioning, alteration in the level of
Comfort level, alterations in
Confusion (disorientation)
Deprivation
Digestion, impairment of
Family's adjustment to illness, impairment of
Family process, inadequate
Fear
Grieving
Lack of understanding
Level of consciousness, alterations in
Malnutrition
Manipulation
Mobility, impaired
Motor incoordination
Non-compliance
Pain
Regulatory function of the skin, impairment of
Respiration, impairment of
Respiratory distress
Self-care activities, altered ability to perform
Sensory disturbances
Skin integrity, impairment of
Sleep/rest pattern, ineffective
Susceptibility to hazards
Thought process, impaired
Urinary elimination, impairment of
Verbal communication, impairment of

A Statement of Causality. This is a description of the causative or contributing factors resulting in the development of the problem. This statement is linked to the problem statement with a "due to" or "related to" clause. The statement of causality is very important because it usually contains clues to the types of nursing interventions needed.[20] For example, consider this nursing diagnosis: "Reluctance to cough and deep breathe following surgery due to pain in incision." If the patient doesn't want to cough "due to pain in incision," it is evident that nursing measures must be

taken to relieve the incisional pain, e.g., administration of a pain medication 15 minutes prior to the coughing session, splinting the wound.

Before discussing the process of diagnosing, we must distinguish among some terms that are *not interchangeable* even though they are often used interchangeably. Below we briefly consider the terms *problem, need, diagnosis* and *data* in relationship to each other.

▶ *Problem* vs. *need.* A *problem* is defined as "a discrepancy which exists between what actually is and what should be or could be."[8] *Needs* are those physiologic, environmental, and sociopsychologic components required by the human organism for survival and for physical and mental health. Important patient needs are diagrammed in Figure 17–9 (see also pp. 9–10). A problem

PATIENT NEEDS

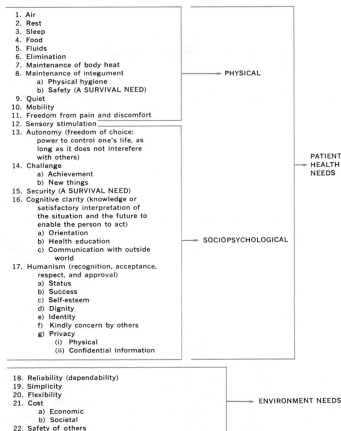

Figure 17–9. Patient needs. (From Kraegel, J. M., et al.: A system of patient care based on patient needs. *Nursing Outlook, 20:*257, April 1972, p. 259.)

arises when a need fails to be met or is blocked in any way, i.e., a discrepancy arises between what the patient should have or would like to have and what he actually has.

▶ *Problem* vs. *diagnosis*. A *problem* statement is only the first part of the diagnostic statement. A *diagnosis* contains both a statement of the patient's problems and a clause concerning causation.

▶ *Data* vs. *problem* vs. *diagnosis*. *Data* are facts recorded without any attempt to relate them to a cause, e.g., "patient's mucous membranes dry; lips crusted; skin dry and scaly, weight 110 pounds—3 pounds less than yesterday's recorded weight; almost continuous elimination of diarrhea stool." A *problem*, on the other hand, is an interpretation of the data. Interpreting the data above, the nurse could state that the patient's problem is dehydration. To expand this problem statement into a *diagnosis*, the nurse would write: "Dehydration due to severe diarrhea."

Making the Nursing Diagnosis

The process of making a nursing diagnosis is similar to the process of making a medical diagnosis (see Chap. 16) except that the nurse concentrates on the patient's problems whereas the physician focuses on the patient's pathology.

Major steps in making the nursing diagnosis are:

1. Analyzing the data

2. Stating the problem

3. Stating the cause of the problem or contributing factors

Below we outline in detail the major components of each step.

1. *Analyze the data* from the interview, history, physical examination, consulting with experts, and review of the literature.
   A. *Classify* the data. Sort the data into boxes or functional areas (see Fig. 17–8B).
   B. *Note gaps* in the data. Ask yourself: Am I missing or slighting any assessment areas? For example, fluid and electrolyte balance? cardiovascular function? patient's health goal? Note if any information recorded is irrelevant.
   C. *Fill in any gaps* in the data by repeating or expanding on the data gathering activities as needed.

D. *Apply standards* to the data. *Health standards* are criteria against which a patient's functional abilities, behavioral responses and mental acuity can be measured to determine whether a patient's responses are adequate in terms of established norms for a given population. (Recall from Chapter 7 that standards of health and disease vary from population to population, from social class to social class and from person to person.)
   (1) Compare the patient's data to *health standards formulated by health professionals*. To estimate the degree of sickness, one must know standards of "wellness." Textbooks, periodicals and government publications contain standards for average weight, height, blood pressure and laboratory findings for different ages and populations. Standards are also available for measurements such as cardiac function, motor function and exercise tolerance. Olebaum has formulated a set of criteria for determining *levels of wellness* in adults, based on three premises: (a) a healthy adult is able to meet his own needs without encroaching on the rights of other people; thus he displays independence and competence in his daily activities; (b) all the functions listed in Figure 17–10 are influenced by the individual's emotions, social learning, external influences, and physiology; and (c) "these functions and behaviors are not the fruits of wellness; rather they are the maintenance of work, the dues of wellness."[83]
   (2) Compare the patient's data *to his own standards for optimum physical, mental and emotional functioning*. It is important to know how the patient feels about himself; how he saw himself before his illness, how he sees himself now and the kind of person he would ideally like to be. Remember that a patient's standards for himself may vary greatly from textbook standards for the population and from *your* standards for him.
   (3) Determine the patient's areas of *ability* and *disability* by noting differences between standards for "normal" responses and performance and the patient's responses and performance.
E. *Synthesize the data*. "Sift" the data for patterns and look for connections between the development of the patient's symptoms and certain *events* in the patient's life. For example, does the patient always develop indigestion, stomach cramps and belching after eating certain foods? Note similarities and differences between the patient's presenting symptoms and *textbook descriptions* of those symptoms. At this point, you can begin to make generalizations about the patient's symptoms and abnormal responses, draw conclusions, make inferences (educated guesses), and in essence, state your own *interpretation* of the data.
F. *Validate your conclusions* about the data. Check your conclusions about the patient's symptoms with various reliable sources. Does

AN ADULT IN OPTIMAL HEALTH

A. performs Activities of daily living

B. has a stable Body image perceived as being socially acceptable

C. provides for his own Comfort and relaxation (psychological and physical)

D. efficiently Disposes of metabolic wastes

E. obtains and maintains an Environment conductive to well-being

F. has an appropriate intake and healthy distribution or excretion of Fluids and electrolytes

G. Guards himself against overwhelming changes. Regulatory and defense systems intact and helpful

H. maintains good Hygiene

I. Builds and maintains meaningful Interpersonal relationships. Is comfortable with interdependence

J. Juxtaposes the tasks of his various life roles with minimal conflict while keeping in touch with his own needs

K. accumulates Knowledge and skills that bring him success in his chosen life roles and self-esteem

L. holds expectations and makes decisions reflecting understanding of his own Limitations and situational realities

M. maintains optimal Motor function (strength, range of motion, locomotion, gross and fine coordination)

N. obtains, digests, and metabolizes appropriate amounts of foods that promote good Nutrition

O. efficiently utilizes Oxygen

P. demonstrates Personality growth and creative expression appropriate to his developmental level and prized by his culture

Q. demonstrates high Quality cerebral functioning (to remember, think abstractly, transfer knowledge, concentrate, and solve problems)

R. mobilizes Resources to meet his needs (internal, significant others, community). Begins by expressing his needs freely to an appropriate person

S. receives and recognizes Sensory input (the five senses, balance, proprioception, and body scheme)

T. is a Team member of his own prevention/rehabilitation team. Has sufficient understanding, initiative, self-control, and financial resources to maintain health

U. recognizes and cherishes the Uniqueness of his own identity and the Uniqueness of each other person

V. demonstrates functional Verbal and nonverbal communication

W. attains healthful balance of productive Work and rest

X. humanistically eXpresses his love and respect for all life and the quality of that life

Y. may have symptoms, but they are Yielding to prescribed therapy. Uses therapies to help him carry out his wellness work

Z. demonstrates a Zeal for living

Figure 17–10. Criteria for determining levels of wellness in adults. (From Oelbaum, C. H.: Hallmarks of adult wellness. *American Journal of Nursing, 74*:1623, Sep. 1974, p. 1623.)

the doctor hold a similar view? Does the patient agree with you? Does the literature confirm your findings? Other sources may validate your conclusions. However, remember, just because other people do not agree with your hypotheses does not necessarily mean you are wrong. Disagreement with other sources indicates that you need to recheck your interpretation of the patient's data to see if you still arrive at the same conclusion.

2. *State the problem.* Cady *et al.* define a patient problem as a "difficulty or concern experienced by the patient at a given point in time."[20] Earlier we described a patient problem as an unhealthy or maladaptive response. In order to state the problem, the nurse must first make the following determinations based on her analysis of the data:

A. Determine whether or not a problem exists.

B. If a problem *does exist*, decide if the problem is actual or potential. *Actual* problems are those "which are currently being experienced by the patient, e.g., 'pain', 'impaired mobility,' 'fatigue'". *Potential* problems are those "which the patient is at high risk for developing unless preventative measures are identified and implemented, e.g., potential skin breakdown due to poor protein intake."[20]

C. Decide if the problem is predictable or atypical. A *predictable* problem is one that you expect most patients to develop given the same circumstances. For example, a certain amount

of pain is predictable for most patients during their postoperative period. *Atypical problems* are difficulties and concerns which *do not* normally develop among all patients given the same circumstances. For instance, infection is *not* a typical development following surgery, although it is always a possibility.[20]

D. Determine, if possible, *the impact of the problem upon the patient's life-style and activities of daily living.* For example, is depression upsetting the patient's relationships with his family? Is fatigue affecting the patient's ability to work regularly? In these cases, the problem statement might read: "Depression due to death of best friend resulting in reduced communications with family members." "Fatigue due to chronic loss of sleep resulting in patient losing at least 15 hours weekly from 40 hour per week job."[60]

3. *State the cause of the problem (if possible) or contributing factors.* As we have said earlier, it is important to learn the cause of a problem because it is then easier to propose interventions. The causes of some simple problems are readily apparent. However, in more complex problems (especially of a psychologic nature), the causes can be highly obscure. These situations call for systematic detective work; Bailey and Claus[8] suggest the disciplined approach shown in Figure 17–11.

A. The first step is to *narrow down the facts* about

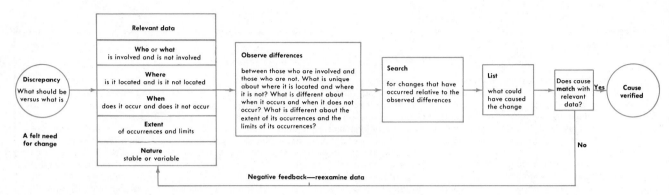

Figure 17–11. A systems model of the problem identification process. (From Bailey and Claus: *Decision Making in Nursing: Tools for Change.*)

the problem by answering the questions shown in the "relevant data" box in Figure 17–11. Answers to these questions help the nurse separate data that *is* related to the problem (and is thus involved in its causation) from data that is *not* related to the problem. In performing this step, it is ideal to draw up two lists: one of problem-related data and one of non–problem-related data. Then carefully compare the lists and note differences between them.

B. Next, note any *changes* in the patient's lifestyle, environment, significant others, physiologic processes, body structure, finances and other concerns that occurred prior to or at the time the problem developed. This step is essential because the causes of most problems are rooted in some kind of change—usually changes which lead away from the norm. Observe *magnitude* of the change and *how* the change occurred.

C. Make a list of all the *possible causes* of the changes.

D. *Match* each possible cause on the list with the list of problem-related data you compiled in Step A. As an aid, Bailey and Claus suggest asking yourself this question: "Could this cause have yielded all these results?" If the answer is "yes," you have verified the cause. If the answer is "no" to all your hypothesized causes, you must reexamine the data and develop new hypotheses. As an exercise, select an unsolved and complex problem in your own life and try to isolate its cause using this model.

E. Once you have determined the cause of the problem, add the cause—in the form of a "due to" or "related to" clause—to the problem statement. This completes the process of stating the nursing diagnosis.

We have recorded a procedure for making *one* nursing diagnosis. In actual practice, a patient may have from five to ten nursing diagnoses. Furthermore, because the patient's situation is in a constant state of flux, *nursing diagnoses change from day to day.* In Durand's words,

A nursing diagnosis tends to reflect the progress of the patient. Whereas a medical diagnosis may remain the same until the patient has recovered or died, a nursing diagnosis indicates the significant responses the patient makes at the stages of his illness and therefore may change with daily changes in the patient.[28]

In sum, the process of making a nursing diagnosis is a highly complex one, requiring the nurse to delineate multiple problems, continuously collect new data, modify old diagnosis and develop new diagnoses as the patient's condition changes.

Evaluating Diagnostic Statements[20, 60, 99, 103]

Once you have written the nursing diagnoses for a patient, it is important to evaluate your diagnostic statements by asking yourself the following questions:

▶ Are diagnostic statements written in *clear,* simple language?

▶ Are diagnoses *precise?* Does each diagnostic statement present the patient's unique situation at this point in time? Is each diagnosis developed separately?

▶ Are statements *concise?* Are symbols and abbreviations used appropriately? A set of symbols and abbreviations helpful in writing concise diagnostic statements are illustrated in Table 17–5.

▶ Are diagnoses worded in *neutral* terms? Have you avoided labeling the patient with such negative terms as manipulative, hypochondriac, difficult or chronic complainer?

▶ Are problem statements always followed with a *causality* phrase, i.e., "due to" phrase? If you do not know the cause yet, follow the problem statement with a question mark, i.e., "due to?"

▶ Have you stated whenever possible the *impact* of the patient's problem upon his *lifestyle and activities of daily living?*

▶ Have you tried to be *objective* and *factual* in stating your diagnoses? Have you tried to state what you know to be true about the patient rather than what you think *might* be true?

▶ Are nursing diagnoses composed in terms of *abnormal patient responses* and not patient needs? For example, "Need for more frequent postoperative turning and deep breathing" is not as well stated as "Inadequate postoperative turning and deep breathing due to pain in area of incision." This last statement, by clarifying the cause of the problem, enables the nurse to immediately plan appropriate interventions.

▶ Have you avoided diagnosing as problems those patient responses which *may be of value* to the patient at certain points in his illness? For example, in some situations it is appropriate—even healthy—for a patient to be angry or to grieve over losses or to temporarily withdraw from other people.

▶ Are diagnoses stated as *patient problems* and not as medical diagnoses or nursing problems? For example, "Patient has difficulty turning" is a patient problem; "Pa-

tient is difficult to turn" is a nursing problem.

▶ Can the patient problems that you have diagnosed be *resolved by nursing interventions alone?* Diagnosis of a patient problem that requires medical intervention to be resolved is *not* a nursing diagnosis.

▶ Are the diagnoses also addressed to the needs and problems of the *patient's family?*

▶ Does the list of nursing diagnoses contain *potential patient problems* as well as actual problems?

▶ Does the list of nursing diagnoses encompass the patient's psychologic, physical, social and financial difficulties?

▶ Have you arranged the patient's nursing diagnoses in *order of immediacy?* Some patient problems are life-threatening; others are less urgent. All of the patient's nursing problems should be considered, but in order of priority.

Uncertainty and the Diagnostic Process

Every diagnostician, no matter how knowledgeable and skilled she is, faces the possibility that her carefully formulated diagnosis may be in error. As Delp explains,

The possible error inherent in every diagnosis arises from the fact that all knowledge of human origin is uncertain. The distinguishing characteristic of scientific knowledge is not that it is more certain than nonscientific knowledge but that the degree of uncertainty can be rather well determined.[26]

Because nurses and doctors are human beings caring for other human beings with complex

TABLE 17–5. ABBREVIATIONS AND SYMBOLS USED IN WORDING DIAGNOSTIC STATEMENTS

leads to	→	with	$\overline{c}$
resulting from		without	$\overline{s}$
or secondary to	← or 2°	equal	=
increased	↑	unequal	≠
increasing	↗	degree of	o
decreased	↓	complains of	c/o
decreasing	↘	shortness of breath	SOB
greater than	>	complaints	Cx
less than	<	diagnosis	Dx
before	$\overline{a}$	prescriptions	Rx
after	$\overline{p}$	activities of daily living	ADL

problems, the risk of making a mistake in diagnosis is always present. Nonetheless, if nurses are to develop as independent diagnosticians, they must be willing to take risks and to live with the uncertainty and doubt that are part of all endeavors to interpret patient data.

STEP 3: NURSING MANAGEMENT— PLANNING NURSING CARE

The term "management" invokes the connotations of directing, steering, guiding and controlling. *Nursing management* involves directing, steering and guiding the nursing staff and the patient toward the resolution of problems diagnosed during the assessment phase. The nurse manager also controls the program of patient care by (a) planning patient goals and specifying time limits for their accomplishment, (b) planning, administering and supervising therapeutic activities and (c) developing criteria for evaluation and possible modification of care. Thus nursing management encompasses the last three steps of the nursing process— namely, planning, implementing and evaluating. In this section, we consider the mechanics of management underlying *planning*. When planning, the nurse analyzes the patient's problems, develops goals and objectives for the patient, sets deadlines for resolution of his problems, and prescribes actions for meeting the objectives and the deadlines.

In the past, patient care planning was frequently haphazard. Plans for patient care were not carefully thought out nor were they based upon problem-solving techniques. Nurses often failed to work as a team in planning patient care and seldom consulted with other health professionals. As a consequence, nursing actions were at times ineffectual or even harmful.

However, with the development of team nursing, primary nursing and the health care team, new ideas about patient care planning began to evolve. Today, disciplined managerial planning is replacing the routine planning that centered around carrying out doctor's orders. Currently, nurses who plan patient care draw from the principles and techniques used in modern business and personnel management—principles which advocate using problem-solving methods and tailoring actions to meet objectives.

Because the activities involved in current patient care planning are built upon management

theory, the following discussion of planning is broken into two sections: the *theory* of planning nursing management and the *practice* of planning nursing management.

Under *theory*, we consider the major steps that are involved in planning solutions to problems. This section presents a disciplined way to *think* about problems and their resolution. Under *practice* of planning, we describe how to write a nursing care plan which utilizes the principles discussed under management theory.

The Theory of Planning Nursing Management

Ideally, planning solutions to patient problems involves the following seven steps:

1. Set priorities
2. Research the problem
3. Analyze the patient and total situation
4. Establish the nursing prognosis
5. Develop goals and objectives
6. Set deadlines
7. Formulate a plan of action

Set Priorities

The first step in planning patient care is to decide which problems need attention immediately and which problems can wait for attention without harm to the patient. In other words, the nurse needs to rank the patient's problems in order of priority.

One convenient method for ranking problems is to *assign a rating* to each problem listed, i.e., high priority, medium priority and low priority.[119] *High priority* patient problems are those which are *life-threatening* and as such require *immediate* professional attention. Examples of high priority problems include respiratory obstruction, severe hemorrhage, threatened or attempted suicide, and cardiac arrest. In emergency and critical care situations, a patient can develop several high priority problems at the same time and the nurse must quickly summon help so that all the patient's life-threatening problems can be dealt with at once. *Medium priority* problems do not directly threaten the patient's life although they may result in unhealthy or destructive physical or emotional changes. For example, immobility can lead to many serious complications, none of which are immediately life-threatening, e.g., decubitus ulcers (bedsores), renal stones, contractures (shortening of a muscle), mental depression. *Low priority* problems include problems that develop when the patient must cope with changes arising from normal growth and development. Low priority must also be given to those problems which the patient can handle by himself with minimal assistance from the nurse.

When setting priorities, it is also helpful to consider *Maslow's hierarchy of human needs* (see Chap. 1). Note that in patient care the lower level needs must be met before the higher level needs can really be considered. Problems involving man's "higher needs" for esteem and self-actualization may have low priority if a patient is critically ill. (The excellent nurse, however, will always attend a patient in such a way that his dignity and individuality is preserved.)

Establishing the patient's *nursing prognoses* for his various problems is also helpful in establishing priorities. The nursing prognosis, which is essentially a prediction as to the possible outcome of a problem, is considered on p. 292.

Priorities change daily as the patient's condition worsens or improves. For the patient who is critically ill, survival is of the highest priority. When the patient's condition improves, higher needs become more important and low priority problems gain a higher priority. Thus in her planning of care, the nurse must assess the patient daily and assign nursing care priorities in accordance with his condition.

Research the Problem

In nonemergency situations it is essential to carefully research each patient problem before planning action. To this end the nurse must pursue a *second review of the literature*. In her review the nurse should concentrate on (a) the nature of the problem (Is it a response to normal life events, illness, or disability?), (b) causative and contributory factors, (c) problem-related theories, hypotheses and studies, (d) methods for treating the problem and (e) recommendations for nursing care, rehabilitative activities and patient education.

In addition, the nurse needs to obtain *opinions of experts* concerning the patient's problems and their solutions. Doctors, medical specialists, dieticians, and physical therapists can all offer useful and timely information about specific patient problems.

Analyze the Patient and the Total Situation

The next step in planning nursing management is to study the patient and the health care system upon which his welfare ultimately depends. First, consider the patient's strengths and weaknesses in terms of the extent to which he can help resolve his own problems. Assess the patient's resources and deficiencies in the following five areas:

1. *Physical Structure and Function.* Note the patient's general state of health, the intactness of his limbs, and the functional levels of his physiologic systems, e.g., respiratory and cardiovascular systems. Patients who suffer paralysis, traumatic loss of limbs, recent blindness or deafness, severe cardiac symptoms, great difficulty breathing upon exercise, and muscle weakness and atrophy will undoubtedly find it difficult or impossible to participate in the resolution of certain problems. On the other hand, patients who have some degree of mobility, adequate use of their senses, and who are free of severe cardiovascular or respiratory symptoms may be able to participate actively in their treatment program.

2. *Emotional Status.* Analyze how the patient feels about his particular problem. Does it make him angry? Depressed? Apathetic? Or does he feel optimistic about his ability to solve the problem? Does he seem motivated toward positive change? Also evaluate the patient's need to be dependent versus his desire for independence. A person who longs to be cared for and "pampered" by others may resist any activities that encourage him to become more self-reliant. Conversely, a patient who is strongly independent may resist plans of care which force him to curtail his activities and rely upon the services of others. The patient's general state of emotional health or illness must also be taken into consideration. A patient with a mental illness such as schizophrenia or deep depression may be unable to consider options or cooperate with prescribed therapies. At the same time most patients can participate in the planning of their own care to some extent and should be encouraged to do so.

3. *Intellectual Status.* Observe whether the patient is oriented to time, place, and person. Note whether he is able to (a) remember your discussions concerning his problems, (b) ask intelligent questions about his situation and (c) think through solutions to basic problems. The oriented patient with a good memory and adequate problem-solving skills should be able to decide (with you) on realistic goals for himself, accurately follow his treatment regimen, question recommendations that he doesn't understand, and care for himself when he goes home. In contrast, patients who are mentally

confused or mentally retarded may require almost continuous nursing direction and supervision, lest they become hazards to themselves and others.

4. *Financial Resources.* Tactfully inquire into the patient's economic situation. For instance, gather information (from patient, chart, family or social worker) concerning the patient's health insurance coverage, his financial responsibilities and the stability of his employment. The amount of money and the type of insurance plan a health consumer has decrees the type of health care he can afford to purchase. Unfortunately, even the person with some funds can suffer financial hardships if he requires long-term care, extensive surgeries, or lengthy rehabilitation services. Furthermore, some patients face the additional trauma of job loss due to severe illness. Other patients are disqualified from their occupation because of disabilities, e.g., a truck driver who loses his legs will be forced to train for a new occupation—a lengthy and costly endeavor. Thus, learning about a patient's present and future financial situation places you in a better position to plan his care realistically, in keeping with his economic resources.

5. *Human Resources.* As you care for the patient, observe whether he has visitors, the visitors' relationship to the patient and their attitude toward him. Note if the patient is receiving any phone calls, cards or flowers. Some patients have numerous visits and calls; others have virtually no one who visits or even inquires about them. All patients need the love and care of other people as they encounter the crisis of illness. Indeed, as we pointed out in Chapter 5, a person's chances for successfully coping with crisis increase if he has the support and concern of his significant others.

Having considered the patient and his situation, next analyze the resources of the *health care facility* that is responsible for his care. Consider exactly what this health care agency can and cannot offer the patient in terms of treatment and nursing care. To formulate a realistic care plan, it is essential to consider and weigh the following factors:

▶ Size of nursing staff

▶ Availability of specialized consultants

▶ Equipment and facilities (modern? antiquated? deficient?)

▶ Floor or ward count of patients (patient load)

▶ Ratio of nurses to patients

▶ Institutional funds and grants available for special patient services and equipment

▶ General philosophy of care of the institution

▶ Category of institution (acute, chronic, rehabilitative)

Establish the Nursing Prognosis

The term "prognosis" comes from a Greek word meaning "foreknowledge." Dorland's Medical Dictionary defines *medical prognosis* as "a forecast as to the probable outcome of an attack of disease; the prospect as to recovery from a disease as indicated by the nature and symptoms of the case." In other words, a medical prognosis attempts to predict the probable outcome for a particular disease or pathologic entity that the doctor has diagnosed.

Like the medical prognosis, the *nursing prognosis* is a predictive statement. Unlike medical prognoses, nursing prognoses forecast the outcome of particular patient *problems* rather than diseases. Also, nursing prognoses help to *establish the rationale* for assigning patient care priorities and directing nursing therapy.

Nursing prognoses are distinct from nursing diagnoses. As Ware writes, "...while the nursing diagnosis identifies 'what is wrong' the nursing prognosis aids with answering the question, 'What is the likelihood of somehow altering the outcome?'"[114] The outcome could be either the outcome of the disease or the outcome of a particular problem.

How is a nursing prognosis established? Nursing prognoses are based on the following: (a) the nurse's total patient assessment, (b) the patient's overall health status, (c) the patient's resources, abilities and strengths, (d) the nurse's knowledge of and experience with similar problems, (e) clinical and laboratory information, (f) current knowledge concerning the typical course of the illness or problem and (g) nursing resources available within the health care facility.

Table 17–6 presents an example of ways in which the nursing prognosis can be used to improve patient care. The patient, in this case, has a medical diagnosis of carcinoma of the head of the pancreas. His medical prognosis is grave, i.e., probably death. Observe that the prognoses for the patient's four nursing diagnoses tend to be "good" given certain conditions, i.e., relief of current pain, support of chemicals. In the third column of Table 17–6, note how these nursing prognoses have been used to substantiate both the ranking of nursing priorities and the prescribed program of nursing therapy.

Nursing prognoses need to be shared with the patient, his family and members of the health care team. Shared knowledge concerning prognoses ensures greater continuity of patient care. Sharing also helps all persons involved in the patient's care program (including the patient) to appreciate the rationale underlying the program.

Develop Goals and Objectives

The next step in the management process is developing goals and objectives with and for the patient. The terms "goal" and "objective" are frequently used interchangeably, but strictly speaking they express *different concepts*. In Storlie's words: ". . .goals refer to an end state, a point we want to reach. Objectives ask how. . . ."[108] For example, if you are a student, your overall long-term goal is to graduate from a school of nursing. Your objectives are to satisfy all science requirements, complete your nursing courses with passing grades, and complete laboratory and clinical work satisfactorily.

Within the nursing process, *nursing care goals* are the ultimate aims towards which the patient's entire nursing care plan is directed.

These goals focus primarily upon "the solutions of patient problems involving effective coping with impaired health, the daily demands of living, and the stresses of illness and treatment."[60] *Nursing care objectives* are the day to day levels of performance which the patient must reach in order to eventually attain his long-range goals.

To be useful, nursing objectives cannot be written in a loose, nonspecific fashion. Loosely worded objectives leave both nurse and patient without any sense of direction. Helpful nursing objectives are clearly stated in terms of *expected patient outcomes*. Expected patient outcomes spell out, in observable, measurable terms, the expected patient behaviors or clinical manifestations which should develop as a result of planned therapy.

This is an example of a poorly worded objective: "Control of diarrhea." Correctly written,

TABLE 17–6. RELATIONSHIP OF NURSING DIAGNOSIS AND PROGNOSIS TO PRIORITIES FOR DIRECTING NURSING THERAPY*

MEDICAL DIAGNOSIS	MEDICAL PROGNOSIS		
Carcinoma of head of pancreas	Probable death		
NURSING DIAGNOSIS	NURSING PROGNOSIS		PRIORITY AND RATIONALE FOR DIRECTING NURSING THERAPY
1. Questionable acceptance of death	1. Good	4th	Overwhelming, but his ability to wrestle with this issue is dependent on his being reassured about his financial security and the control of his pain prior to learning acceptance of his death.
2. Increasing concern over financial situation	2. Depends on rate disease progresses	2nd	Readily taken care of when energies are not overtaxed; therefore, number of stresses could be reduced by attending to this secondly.
3. Increasing pain	3. With support of chemicals, good	1st	Even though not primary nor necessarily most important, it is the most recurrent in demand of energy reserves, therefore relief is essential for physical comfort and utilization of energies for other major concerns.
4. Fear of future pain	4. With relief of current pain, good	3rd	Will dissipate with continued adequate control of present pain and with patient learning methods of pain control.

*From Ware, A. M.: Nursing prognosis: a necessary chain to nursing therapy. To be published by the *American Journal of Nursing*.

the nursing objective states: "Decrease in number of stools to one daily. Stools of normal consistency." Note that the latter statement is worded in such a manner that the nurse and patient can *observe and measure* whether or not diarrhea is controlled. Expected patient outcomes are discussed again when we consider how to write a nursing care plan.

Nursing care goals and objectives must be (a) realistic, (b) acceptable to the patient and his family and (c) coordinated with the goals of the entire health team. First, *realistic* nursing care goals and objectives are based upon a review of everything known about the patient and his problems. As you consider possible goals, you must carefully evaluate the patient's resources, his disabilities, the types of problems he faces, and his medical and nursing prognoses. For example, one overall goal for a middle-aged sedentary patient with heart disease would be to increase his tolerance to physical exercise. Next you must think about how to realistically program objectives so that the patient can safely meet his overall goals. It would be not only unrealistic but dangerous to expect this patient to jog for a mile on the first morning of an exercise program. The patient may *eventually* be able to jog a mile without cardiovascular symptoms but to try to do so too soon could prove fatal. A realistic objective might be to expect the patient to walk one full block every morning for the first week, two blocks the second week and so forth until he finally gains the stamina to jog.

Second, if goals are to be workable, they must be planned not only for the patient but *with the patient*. The nurse's goals for the patient must be acceptable *to him* because it is the patient and not the nurse who must live with the goals—often for a long time. If the nurse and patient do not agree on goals, the ensuing conflict of ideas may result in the patient's refusal to cooperate with the nurse's program of care. According to Little and Carnevali, the patient often signals his disenchantment with the nurse's goals in the following ways:[60]

▶ A lack of enthusiasm for ideas or activities

▶ An absence of questions

▶ Nodding compliance

▶ Failure to take any initiative

▶ Failure to contribute any ideas about how to fit actions or desires into the proposed plan

▶ Expressions of guilt at failure to comply

The nurse may also express her irritation with the patient's goals and with his failure to comply with her aims for him. She may become angry with the patient or withdraw from him or attempt to make him feel guilty. Obviously, this type of patient-nurse conflict is destructive for both parties. To resolve their differences, nurse and patient must talk frankly, negotiate and compromise.

In addition, it helps to involve the patient's *family* in setting therapeutic goals and objectives. Significant others are often responsible for carrying out the nursing program once the patient is discharged. They may be more willing to continue the patient's regimen at home if they agree with the nurse about the goals of the program and if they understand the objectives.

Finally, during goal setting, the nurse may consult with the *physician and other members of the health care team* about their goals for the patient. Whenever possible, team members (nurse, doctor, physical therapist) need to coordinate their aims and plans for the patient.

Set Deadlines

After developing objectives for the patient's therapeutic program, the nurse plans deadlines for meeting the objectives. Deadlines serve several purposes:

1. Deadlines act to "pace" the patient's nursing care program; pacing helps keep the patient's progress on target.

2. Deadlines serve to motivate people to strive toward their goals and objectives; they endow patient care activities with a greater sense of purpose and urgency.

3. Deadlines, when met satisfactorily, provide the staff and patient with a sense of accomplishment.

4. Deadlines, when *not met* on time, act as a "red flag" to the staff, indicating that either the deadlines are unrealistic or the objectives of the program are not workable and need to be modified.

Clearly, it is essential to develop realistic deadlines or deadlines may be missed. If deadlines are missed often, the patient and staff may become discouraged with themselves and with the therapeutic program. Realistic deadlines are based upon the following: (a) the typical course of the patient's problem and the speed with which problem-related symptoms are usually controlled, (b) the resources, capabilities and energy levels of the patient and staff and (c) the patient's own inner time clock and rhythms. (Chapter 6 discusses the variety in patients' patterns of healing, rest and activity, and sleep and elimination.)

The nurse has finally learned enough about the patient and his problems to formulate a plan of action. This step in the management process involves selecting actions that will enable the patient to achieve the objectives of the nursing program. These selected actions, when written on a nursing care plan, are usually called *nursing orders*.

The development of a plan of action is basically a two-step process. The first step is to develop alternatives, and the second step is to select the best alternative.

DEVELOP ALTERNATIVES. Develop as many alternative plans for solving the patient's problems as possible. Generating many different options is advantageous in at least three ways. First, if one option fails to solve the problem, alternatives can be tried and one of them may succeed. In addition, by having a "pool" of alternatives readily available, the patient is protected from dangerous lapses in his nursing care. Finally, researching various alternatives stimulates the nurse to develop a creative approach to patient care rather than relying on a few basic routines and procedures.

How are alternatives developed? According to Bailey and Claus, "Alternatives are generated through applying skills of information processing and creativity. Experiences, knowledge, and relevant information and facts need to be synthesized."[8] Specific ways to develop alternatives for solving problems include the following:

1. Recall ways in which you handled a similar patient problem in the past
2. Consider the problem from various angles and in different ways
3. Fantasize how you would ideally like to see the patient's problem resolved
4. Talk with a colleague or meet with a group of colleagues and "brainstorm" possible solutions to the problem
5. Obtain expert advice and recommendations

Ideally, the consideration of numerous alternatives results in a creative solution to the patient's problem. To arrive at a creative solution, one must feel free to think in new ways and express different ideas—even if those ideas seem unrealistic and farfetched. Only by considering the *entire range* of possible solutions to a problem can one hope to select the one solution most likely to solve the problem.

SELECT THE BEST ALTERNATIVE. The next step is to analyze the various alternatives and choose the one that seems best. In most patient care situations, the best alternative is the action plan which promises the greatest benefit and the least risk. To select such an alternative, you must systematically examine all of the available options. Ask yourself the following questions and try to answer them objectively:

▶ Has this type of plan been used before in a similar situation? If so, what were the results?

▶ Does this particular alternative enable the patient to meet his objectives and goals within the proposed time limits?

▶ Does this proposed plan take into consideration the patient's age, sex, life-style, attitudes, religious and cultural traditions, social resources and ability to cope?

▶ Is the proposed plan realistic in terms of health facility resources? Is equipment, staff time, staff size, and funding adequate?

▶ What might be some undesirable consequences if this alternative is selected? Would this particular solution to the problem bring more problems in its wake?

Remember that all decisions concerning human problems are made at risk and that some uncertainty underlies all aspects of patient care planning. If your chosen plan fails, review the alternatives you considered earlier, develop some new alternatives and select another "best" alternative for testing and evaluation. If this solution also fails, proceed through the planning process again! Eventually, with sufficient patience and determination, you will discover an action plan that works.

The Practice of Planning Patient Care

Thus far, we have primarily concentrated on the theory of patient management planning and—more specifically—on management by objectives. In this section, we discuss how to

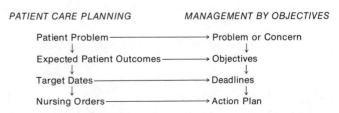

Figure 17–12. Correlation between patient care planning and management by objectives. (From Cady, J. W., Freshman, D. J., and Norby, R. B.: *Taking the Pain Out of Care Planning.* Chicago, Medicus/Nursing Care Systems, 1975, p. 63.)

apply these management principles to the actual practice of patient care planning, i.e., writing a nursing care plan. Note in Figure 17–12 the correlation between patient care planning and management by objectives. As you see, the steps are basically the same. Patient care planning is the practice of organizing and crystallizing plans for the patient and writing them down in a format all members of the nursing staff can understand and follow.

Introduction to the Nursing Care Plan

What is a nursing care plan? Ryan defines the nursing care plan as follows:

A *nursing care plan* is an information receiving, processing, sending, and evaluating center initiated by the professional nurse through the use of specialized assessment, diagnostic, communication, and judgmental skills and compiled as a guide for directing nursing activities toward the fulfillment of health needs of the patient and the achievement of related nursing goals.[99]

Ideally, the specific *purposes* of the nursing care plan (also referred to as the patient care plan) are to:

▶ Provide a detailed guide for patient care

▶ Put patient goals, objectives, priorities, deadlines and nursing actions in writing

▶ Individualize patient care

▶ Coordinate the efforts of all nursing team members

▶ Provide a source of information and a line of communication for nursing team members

▶ Guarantee continuity of patient care

▶ Develop patient care activities which are based upon scientific principles and upon the process of systematic problem solving

▶ Assist the staff in meeting the patient's psychosocial needs

▶ Encourage patient and family participation in the nursing program

▶ Construct a program for patient family health education

▶ Ensure adequate discharge planning

The concept of the written nursing care plan dates back to the late 1940's. Before that time, nurses' plans for patients were communicated verbally. However, modern nursing practice, with its emphasis on comprehensive patient care, requires the disciplined, coordinated approach to patient care that can only be provided by *written* plans.

Since the 1940's, nursing care plans have gradually evolved from a list of routine orders to increasingly sophisticated and detailed management guides. Once primarily a planning tool for academic nursing students and clinical nursing specialists, the care plan is now widely recognized by general practitioners as an indispensable basis for nursing care. Today, the Joint Commission on Accreditation of Hospitals upholds the nursing care plan and states that it has a definite place in the complete patient care record.

Despite its wider acceptance, the nursing care plan is still in a state of evolution. The comprehensive nursing care plan which fulfills all of the purposes listed above is an ideal rather than a reality. For instance, one author who studied nursing care plans (Ciuca) found that the nursing care plans in his sample of 235 nursing care plans "with minor exceptions did not reflect the comprehensive approach to patient care that is so evident in the literature."[22] Instead, the plans he studied served "mainly as a quick reference for the functional, mechanical tasks of administration of medications and treatments, monitoring the vital signs, intake and output, and diagnostic studies."[22]

Several factors have kept the nursing care plan from reaching its full potential as a force in nursing. Time and work pressures, lack of administrative support for care plans, and the inability of some nurses to view themselves as competent managers have all contributed to the reluctance of many nurses to accept care plans. In addition, as emphasized earlier, the process of planning care—like the process of diagnosis—is laced with uncertainty and risk. Clearly, it is not possible to predict exactly how a particular patient is going to react to a particular nursing care plan. Because of the unpredictability of patient outcomes, many nurses resist putting their plans for patients in writing.

Stevens emphasizes that physicians can plan patient care with a greater sense of certainty than can nurses.[106] For example, doctors write many of their medication and treatment orders on the basis of specific and often indisputable laboratory and diagnostic test results. On the other hand, nurses must base the majority of nursing orders upon their sometimes fallible assessment of the patient's physical, mental and emotional status. Unfortunately, there are no laboratory findings that can guide the nurse in helping a patient accept his amputated legs or live with a painful chronic illness.

In sum, in writing care plans, as in all other nursing activities, the nurse must learn to cope with the problem of insecurity and the fear of failure. Thus Stevens advises: "The solution to this problem obviously requires an altered concept of nursing intervention."[106] Nurses must come to truly accept that: (a) there is no *one* right plan; (b) patient behaviors and outcomes are ultimately unpredictable; (c) even a "good" plan of care can fail to help the patient under certain circumstances; and (d) plans can always be revised and changed when the need for revision arises. Keep these concepts in mind as we discuss nursing care plans.

Types of Care Plans

As you care for patients in various hospitals and health care facilities, you will discover a variety of nursing care plans, in many different formats. Two basic types of care plans are (1) institutional (staff) care plans and (2) student care plans.

Institutional (Staff) Care Plans. The most commonly used type of staff care plan is the *Nursing Care Card* or *Kardex*. Figure 17–13 illustrates the format for nursing care cards on the PM&R (Physical Medicine and Rehabilitation) ward at University Hospital, Seattle. Note that this particular care card is broken down into five major sections: (1) basic information about the patient (name, age, diagnosis), (2) sustanal care (supportive care), (3) remedial care (care which treats or cures disease), (4) restorative care (care which helps the patient return to a normal life style) and (5) preventative care. Moreover, this care card contains space for patient problems and approaches, activities, teaching, patient goals and special interests and discharge plans. In addition to a nursing care card, the typical Kardex also lists the patient's medications and treatments on a separate card. Advantages of a Kardex format are: (a) it gives written information concerning the patient's problems and his medical and nursing orders; (b) it is clear and concise and provides for a quick review of the patient's status and (c) its use ensures continuity of patient care from shift to shift. The Kardex care plan should be initiated upon the patient's admission to the health care facility. Upon discharge of the patient, the plan should be filed as part of the patient's permanent hospital record. Some institutions use a computerized type of nursing care plan, and others have devised a variety of individualized forms.

Student Care Plans. Each school of nursing typically has a care plan format developed by the faculty for student use. Because student plans are used as learning tools, they are usually more elaborate than the concise practical plans used by hospital staffs. As you study the following section on writing nursing care plans, it might help you to look at the care plan used in your school or facility.

Writing a Nursing Care Plan

In essence, a well-written nursing care plan condenses the data concerning a patient (his problems, resources, prognoses, goals, objectives and therapeutic activities) into concise statements that clearly communicate the patient's current status and needs to all nurses responsible for the patient. Table 17–7 illustrates a care plan written for a patient who is in a nursing home and who is recovering from a cerebral vascular accident (stroke) with resultant mild left hemiparesis (paralysis affecting the left side of the body). Using this sample, we will discuss guidelines for skillfully developing and writing each section of the care plan. We will also consider how to establish expected patient behaviors for discharge.

Writing Nursing Diagnoses. You will recall that a nursing diagnosis is composed of (1) a statement of the problem (unhealthy or maladaptive patient responses or functional disabilities) that can be alleviated by nursing interventions and (2) a statement of causality (i.e., a description of the causative or contributing factors resulting in the problem). Note that the nursing diagnoses listed in Table 17–7 have the attributes of well-written diagnostic statements. In other words, they (a) are patient centered, (b) are clear and concise, (c) contain "due to" clauses and (d) are specific and descriptive, e.g., "Difficulty ambulating due to decreased muscle strength on Ⓛ side following CVA." Observe also that each problem is dated according to when it was first diagnosed.

Patient Strengths and Weaknesses. This section of the care plan summarizes the patient's (1) strengths, abilities and resources that can be used to deal with a particular problem and (2) weaknesses and disabilities that might thwart plans for solving the problem. Recall that the third step of planning nursing management was to analyze the patient's personal resources and deficiencies in terms of his physical structure and function, emotional status, intellectual status, financial resources and human resources. Patient strengths and weaknesses must be worded in clear, concise and objective

NURSING CARE CARD   PM&R

CAUTION:

Name:

Age: Diagnosis:

Room:

Classification:

Phones: OR Procedures: Nsg. Hx:

Religion: Care Review:

Occupation: PHR:

SUSTANAL CARE

Diet: Positioning:

  Feeding: Special Equipment:

  Adaptive Equipment: Sitting Tolerance:

Fluids: Frequency_____ _____hrs.

  I&O   Skin Tolerance

Oral Hygiene: Back_____   R. Side_____

Bathing: Abdomen_____   L. Side_____

                                                        Turn Schedule:

Dressing:

PROBLEM: APPROACH: Ambulation-Transfers:

                                                    Bed_____   W/C_____

                                                    Commode_____   Tub_____

                                                    Shower_____   Toilet_____

                                            Bowel Program:

                                                    Frequency_____   Time_____

                                                    Procedure:

                                            Bladder Program:

                                                    Catheter Change_____   Size_____

                                                    Procedure:

REMEDIAL CARE: GRAPHICS:

  P.T.:

  O.T.:   Vital Signs:

  Speech: TPR

                                                        B/P

DAILY PROCEDURES:

RESTORATIVE CARE: Wt.

  Activity: PREVENTATIVE CARE:

  R.T.:   Pt. Goals:

  Grounds Pass:

Teaching: Special Interests:

                                                        Discharge Plans:

Figure 17–13.   Nursing Care Card—Kardex. (Courtesy of University Hospital, Seattle.)

terminology. Written correctly, this description of the patient should guide the nursing staff in their endeavors to help the patient overcome his problems and reach his objectives.

Writing Expected Patient Outcomes.[20]   Earlier, when we discussed the development of patient goals and objectives, we emphasized that objectives must be stated as expected patient outcomes to be useful. Expected patient outcomes express, in measurable terms, exactly what a patient should feel like, look like, act like and say once his problem is resolved or is progressing toward resolution. Study the examples of expected patient outcomes in Table 17–7. Note that the expected outcomes are:

▶ Phrased *clearly* and *concisely*

▶ Written in terms depicting *patient action*, e.g., "washes hands and face after meals"

▶ *Realistic* and *obtainable*, e.g., "↑ in endurance to 7 to 8 min. of walking s̄ resting"

▶ *Specific* and *concrete*, e.g., "Attendance at exercise session at 9:30 AM qd"

▶ Directly *observable* by use of the five senses, e.g., "changes underclothes when soiled," "↓ in # of complaints of fatigue," "absence of halitosis"

▶ *Patient centered* rather than nurse centered; e.g., "Obtains urinal or requests help to bathroom upon need to void" is *patient* centered while "Offers urinal or assists to bathroom upon patient's need to void" is *nurse* centered.

▶ *Problem oriented*, e.g., "Increase in range of motion (ROM); improved muscle strength and tone on (L) side, less reliance on wheelchair and rails in hall" clearly indicates at least partial resolution of the specific problem of "Difficulty ambulating due to decreased muscle strength on (L) side following CVA."

One final characteristic of well-developed expected patient outcomes is that they are *acceptable to the patient and his family.* As we indicated earlier, for a care plan to be successful, the patient and nurse must agree upon the goals and objectives of the plan.

Writing Projected Dates and Scheduled Times. Note in Table 17–7 that the projected dates/times are written to establish the following two separate time requirements:

1. The *projected date or deadline* by which an expected patient outcome is to be achieved; e.g., the expected patient outcome of "Attendance at exercise session at 9:30 AM qd" (2c), written 4/16, should be resolved by 4/17.

2. *Scheduled hours and lengths of time* for

observing the patient, making progress notes on his chart, giving nursing care, and assisting the patient in the performance of tasks developed to help him progress toward obtainment of his health goals and objectives. For instance, Mr. Williamson's expected outcome is "increase in ambulation time to 2 hours per day." Note that ambulation times are scheduled for every 2 hours starting at 7 AM and continuing to 7 PM. Also notice that nursing order 2a and b further crystallizes these time requirements by specifying a graduated time schedule for ambulation activities. We discuss timing and nursing orders in more detail below.

Writing Nursing Orders.   Nursing orders are defined as nursing actions or interventions designed to help the patient achieve specific patient outcomes (or objectives) by specified deadlines or projected dates. You will recall that the nurse develops nursing orders or actions by (1) generating alternatives and (2) selecting the best alternative.

It is important to realize that the term "nursing order," like the term "nursing diagnosis," is quite new. Before the term "nursing order" came into being, nurses used vague terms such as "nursing approaches," "suggested approaches" or "nursing activities" to label their actions. Thus Little and Carnevali write:

Nursing orders are only recently coming into their own as a legitimate part of the health care record system. Many nurses have not believed in them; and this lack of conviction did not generate much interest in them or sense of importance for them in other parts of the health care system. Even the labels— "Suggested Approaches" or "Actions"—had a slippery, elastic quality that negated accountability for either the prescriber or the implementer.[60]

At this time, however, nursing orders are a bona fide part of most nursing care plans. Nurses are expected to write clear, intelligent orders that they and other nurses can carry out independently of the physician. Today, the nurse who writes and signs an order is *morally and legally responsible* for that order.

Basically, a complete well-written nursing order is composed of the following five components:[60]

1. Date

2. Specific action verb (instruct, place, supervise, compliment, observe) and occasionally a modifier (actively, softly, gently)

TABLE 17–7. NURSING CARE PLAN

Last Name: Williamson   **First Name:** John   **Room Number:** 401E   **Age:** 72

Sex: M ✓   F   **Doctor:** Rubens   **Date of Admission:** April 15, 1978

Diagnoses: Cerebral vascular accident, mild left hemiparesis, arteriosclerosis (hardening of arteries)

DATE	NO.	NURSING DIAGNOSES	STRENGTHS? WEAKNESSES?	EXPECTED PATIENT OUTCOMES	PROJECTED DATES/ SCHEDULED TIMES	NURSING ORDERS
4/16	1	Poor personal hygiene due to lack of interest in self-care and forgetfulness	**Strengths:** 1. Cooperates when asked to change clothes and wash. 2. Is able to carry out self-care with minimum of assistance **Weaknesses:** 1. Moves very slowly, especially left arm and leg 2. Tires easily 3. Does not verbalize needs but responds to questions 4. Occasionally incontinent of urine	1a. Washes hands and face after meals b. Changes underclothes when soiled c. Shaves self daily Brushes hair daily d. Brushes dentures after each meal; absence of halitosis e. Obtains urinal or requests help to bathroom upon need to void	4/30 tid qd qd tid	1a. Give verbal reminders after meals to wash hands and face; have soap and washcloth handy b. Give verbal reminders to change underclothes; offer assistance if necessary but encourage maximum independent action c. Keep shaver and mirror within easy reach d. Instruct on importance of oral hygiene; show proper way to clean denture and gums; offer supervision as necessary e. Place urinal near bedside at night with tissue handy Ask if need to go to BR before meals and after meals Instruct on importance of keeping skin in perineal area clean and dry *J. Jones R.N.*

TABLE 17–7. NURSING CARE PLAN (*Continued*)

| 4/16 | 2 | Difficulty ambulating due to decreased muscle strength on (L) side following CVA | **Strengths:**

1. Dislikes being dependent

2. Fairly alert, intelligent

3. Right side unaffected by CVA

4. Aware of physical limitations and need to compensate for them

Weaknesses:

1. Lack of confidence in ability to balance self

2. Lack of interest in walking and increasing level of ambulation.

3. Weight gain of 10 pounds probably due to inactivity

4. Under effect of tranquilizer (Valium)

5. Poor physical endurance

6. Little emotional support from family members who do not realize extent of impairment following CVA | 2a. ↑ in ambulation time to 2 hours per day

b. ↑ in endurance to 7 to 8 min. of walking s̄ resting

c. Attendance at exercise session at 9:30 AM qd

d. ↑ in number of activities which involve walking and exercise

e. ↑ in range of motion (ROM); improved muscle tone and strength on (L) side; less reliance on wheelchair and rails in hall

f. Loss of 10 lbs. gained during period of inactivity

g. ↓ in # of complaints of fatigue when ambulating to no more than 2 by end of ambulating session | 5/1
q2h 7AM
–7 PM

5/1

4/17
qd

4/17

5/1

5/30

5/1 | 2ab. Supervise periods of ambulation q2h throughout day
   Start c̄ 5 min. periods and gradually ↑ to 15 min. periods; ↑ walking time by 1–2 min. per day depending upon pt's tolerance to activity

   c. Encourage to attend group exercise session under Ms. Jones at 9:30 AM qd

   de. Encourage activities which involve physical action; e.g., exercises in pool, gardening. Refer to physical therapist & occupational therapist. Perform ROM's daily to improve muscle tone.

   f. Instruct patient concerning special 900 calorie reducing diet ordered by Dr. Encourage intake of high protein foods, fruits and vegetables. Explain relationship between lack of exercise & weight gain.

   g. Compliment pt each time he completes activity program with no more than two complaints of fatigue.

J. Jones R.N. |

3. Prescribed activity, e.g., "Keep shaver and mirror within easy reach"

4. Time units, e.g., "Supervise periods of ambulation q 2 h throughout day"

5. Signature of nurse writing order

As you study the nursing orders in Table 17–7, observe that each order contains all five of the required components. Also, note that these orders are:

▶ *Independent or interdependent nursing activities* which can be performed either without a doctor's orders or in conjunction with a physician's orders. The majority of the orders written for Mr. Williamson are prescriptions for independent nursing activities. Order 2f is written in conjunction with a physician's order for a special reducing diet, i.e. "Instruct patient concerning special 900 calorie reducing diet ordered by doctor. . . ."

▶ *Itemized* and *numbered* for greater clarity and precision.

▶ *Specific* and *precise,* e.g., "Supervise periods of ambulation q 2 h throughout day. Start c̄ 5 min. periods and gradually ↑ to 15 min. periods; ↑ walking time by 1 to 2 min. per day depending upon pt's tolerance to activity." This order is sufficiently clear and precise that all persons reading the order should interpret it the same way. On the other hand, the following order would be subject to serious misinterpretations: "Supervise periods of ambulation throughout the day; increase walking time according to patient's tolerance."

▶ *Realistic* and *achievable.* All of the orders written for this sample nursing care plan are achievable; none appear to place unrealistic demands upon either the patient or nursing staff.

Finally, a well-conceived nursing order takes into account, whenever possible, the *patient's personal desires and preferences.* Also nursing orders include plans for *patient education.*

Writing Expected Patient Behaviors for Discharge.   Discharge planning is a vital component of comprehensive patient care. Planning for a patient's discharge (or transfer to a less acute ward, rest home or other extended-care facility) involves, first of all, establishing expected patient behaviors for discharge. Expected patient behaviors for discharge "outline what the patient's status should be at discharge,"[20] and thus these patient outcomes are really long-term patient health goals. Discharge behaviors, within the care plan, state long-term *nursing* goals, not medical goals—although medical and nursing goals for patients ideally complement each other.

In the majority of cases, expected patient behaviors for discharge revolve around the following behaviors:

1. The patient shows no evidence of acute symptoms or complications (severe pain, dehydration).

2. The patient is able to discuss: (a) his illness and its ramifications upon his life-style, (b) signs and symptoms (signaling complications) that should be reported to his doctor, (c) his home care regimen including diet, activities and rest, (d) his schedule of follow-up appointments with doctors, public health nurses and clinics and (e) his plans for future rehabilitative and preventative care.

3. The patient and his family are able to demonstrate skills in performing procedures that are part of the home-care regimen, e.g., changing dressings, taking blood pressure readings, transferring from bed to wheelchair.

Like expected patient outcomes, expected patient behaviors upon discharge must be written in clear, precise, measurable and observable terms; discharge criteria must also be realistic. For example, consider the writing of outcome criteria for discharge for a woman who has had a mastectomy (removal of the breast). Here is a poorly worded and probably unrealistic discharge goal for such a patient: "Demonstrates acceptance of mastectomy."

Compare this vague statement with these more precise outcome criteria for discharge:

1. Views mastectomy site without expression of disbelief or distaste

2. Discusses plans for obtaining information about various types of breast prostheses, new bras and clothing

3. Recalls information about complications following mastectomy and how to prevent them

4. States willingness to follow the recommended medical and nursing regimens upon discharge

5. Talks openly about the loss of her breast and states confidence in her ability to cope with the loss; names persons she can talk with concerning emotional problems should they arise.

These patient behaviors can be directly observed (i.e., seen or heard) by the nurse; also, all are obtainable goals for most patients following mastectomy.

Once outcome criteria are developed, the next step is to assess whether these criteria are being met. Assessment is based upon observation of the patient and careful review of progress notes in the patient's chart. If discharge criteria have not been met, the patient may have to be discharged later. In other cases, the nurse may refer the patient to an outpatient care facility or to a health practitioner (e.g., visiting nurse) who can assist him in achieving his long-term goals following discharge.

STEP 4: NURSING MANAGEMENT— IMPLEMENTING THE CARE PLAN

Once the patient's care plan has been formulated and written, the next step is to activate and implement the plan. To implement the plan, the nurse (a) carries out nursing orders (performs nursing interventions or actions) and (b) carries out physician's orders, thereby helping activate the medical care plan.

The process of implementation clearly requires that the nurse exercise all of her management skills. The major managerial duties involved in implementing decisions concerning patient care include:

1. *Planning* the exact strategy for carrying out therapeutic orders with other members of the nursing team.

2. *Organizing* the planned activities, e.g., identifying activities that can be performed close together in time or location.

3. *Assigning* and *delegating* activities, as appropriate, to other nurses and to the patient, his family, and friends.

4. *Leading* and *directing* the *counseling* of the patient, family, and other team members; this activity requires not only managerial skills but communication and teaching skills as well.

5. *Scheduling* activities for maximum nurse efficiency and maximum patient benefits.

6. *Controlling* the implementation process by developing and using evaluation procedures.

Throughout the implementation process, the nurse continues to assess the patient, evaluate the results of both medical therapy and nursing therapy and modify the nursing care plan as necessary. Although the nurse cannot change the medical care plan directly, she definitely can and should consult with the physician about the patient's progress and suggest changes in the medical regimen when necessary.

Types of Nursing Interventions

Basically, nursing interventions are nursing actions which focus on assisting the patient to cope successfully with his problems and meet his goals and objectives. Nursing interventions or actions are often classified as dependent, independent and interdependent. Let us briefly define these terms.

Dependent action involves carrying out the physician's orders, e.g., giving prescribed medications; performing prescribed treatments and procedures. However, as you perform these dependent activities, do remember this warning:

> *Dependent functioning does not imply following orders blindly and without question. Critical thinking and sound judgment must be exercised to make decisions about what, when, how much, and in what manner.*[119]

For example, nurses must be alert to possible errors in doctors' prescriptions for medications. In addition, nurses must exercise their own judgment concerning the administration of medications and treatments. For instance, before a nurse gives a pain medication to a new postoperative patient, she needs to carefully assess the patient's level of consciousness, the patient's blood pressure (pain medications can drastically lower blood pressure following surgery), and the location and severity of the pain. If the nurse decides to give the pain medication, she must next decide whether to give the whole dose or only a partial dose. Once the medication is given, the nurse must carefully assess the patient's response to the medication and talk with the surgeon if she feels that the medication order needs to be modified.

Independent actions involve carrying out the nursing orders written on the nursing care plan. As implied earlier, these activities do not require a physician's order and may be performed completely independently of the doctor. Recall that during the planning stage, in Table 17–7, the nurse ordered many different nursing actions for Mr. Williamson. Now, during the implementation stage, it is the nurse's responsibility to do one of the following: (a) carry out the orders herself, (b) perform the nursing actions in collaboration with the patient and possibly his family or (c) delegate the various nursing activities to appropriate nursing personnel.

Interdependent actions are activities which are performed by the nurse in collaboration with other members of the health care team. For example, the nurse may work with a physician in setting up a teaching program for a group of patients. While establishing the program, the nurse may delegate various tasks to other health professionals. For example, she may ask a dietician to teach a certain aspect of a course or a technician to demonstrate laboratory procedures for the patients.

Guidelines for Nursing Actions

To really help the patient attain his objectives, nursing actions must have certain characteristics. Ideally, nursing actions are:

▶ Consistent with the nursing care plan and with the medical care plan

▶ Planned on the basis of problem-solving techniques and scientific principles

▶ Therapeutically safe and effective

► Individualized to treat each patient problem

► Geared to use all appropriate health facility resources, e.g., staff, specialists, equipment

► Developed to maximize patient resources and capabilities

► Scheduled to coincide with the patient's needs for rest, activity, food, sleep, recreation, and other activities

► Organized to allow the patient and his family to participate in the therapeutic program

► Used whenever possible to teach the patient how to care for himself and how to avoid complications and setbacks

► Continuously updated in accordance with changes in the patient's condition and situation.

Specific Methods of Implementation

As the nurse's professional role enlarges and her responsibilities grow, nursing interventions likewise tend to increase in number and complexity. Below we list and briefly discuss some of the major nursing interventions that nurses use daily. These nursing interventions include the following:

1. Carrying out independent, dependent and interdependent nursing actions.

2. *Counseling* of the patient and his significant others concerning his illness and the resultant problems. Counseling in *acute* situations may require using crisis intervention techniques (see Chap. 5). Counseling is also employed to help patients with *long-term chronic illness* and disabilities come to terms with their condition. In this case, the nurse counselor allows the patient to talk out his concerns in a warm nonthreatening atmosphere. Another form of counseling focuses on assisting the patient to *participate more fully* in his therapeutic program. To insure patient participation, the nurse counselor may draw up a *contract* between herself and the patient. Written contracts (or formalized agreements) clarify the objectives of the therapeutic program as well as the exact roles and duties of the nurse and patient within the program. To be workable, contracts must be clearly stated, explicit, and realistic. Counseling also involves helping patients *cope successfully* as they pass through the *various developmental stages* of a normal

life, e.g., childhood, adolescence, pregnancy, childbearing, retirement. In this case, the counselor not only discusses the patient's personal problems at different developmental stages, but she also talks about the many normal changes which occur as a person performs each of life's developmental tasks.

3. *Supervision* of the patient and his family and other nursing team members in the performance of patient care activities.

4. *Coordination* of the patient's total health care program throughout his hospital stay. Specific activities for which the nurse coordinator is responsible include: (a) meeting with other health team members concerning the patient's program, (b) scheduling all of the patient's activities (e.g., his visit with the dietician, daily hour in the physical therapy department for rehabilitative exercises, meetings with the occupational therapist, (c) discussing the patient's care program with his family and (d) planning for the patient's discharge and postdischarge activities, e.g., arranging for clinic appointments, visiting nurse.

5. *Teaching* the patient and his family about health care. Because of its tremendous importance, patient-family education is discussed in detail in the next section.

6. *Referring* patients who require continuing care to other health professionals or health care facilities. Referrals may be written on special forms, given on the phone or requested in person. Most health care institutions have a definite referral system that simplifies the transfer of information about the patient from one health care facility or department to another. Patients are typically referred to dieticians, social workers, psychiatrists, clergymen, physical therapists, occupational therapists and various organizations such as Alcoholics Anonymous, clinics, nursing homes, rehabilitation centers or public health nursing departments. Referrals must always be made thoughtfully and carefully or they may become more of a problem to the patient than a help. Thus Marriner cautions:

Sometimes referrals are made rashly without consideration of the consequences to the patient. They are not practical if the patient cannot get to the clinic to which he has been referred because he has no transportation. Occasionally they are made in a routine manner without consideration of the patient as a unique individual.[65]

In essence, before making a patient referral, assess the patient carefully in terms of his unique personality, needs, resources and disabilities. Next, assess the facility or group to whom you are referring the patient in terms of its resources and objectives. Then ask yourself: Can the needs of my patient really be met by this institution or group or person? Talk with the patient and his family about the possible referral. If the patient feels that he is willing to work further on his problem in the way you suggest, then make the referral. However, remember to tell the patient if there are other options available if this particular referral does not work out satisfactorily.

7. *Recording and reporting* the nursing actions performed and the patient's response to each aspect of his therapeutic program. Also, the nurse maintains a complete record of the patient's daily progress toward his goals. Recording and reporting are discussed in detail in Chapter 18.

Patient-Family Education

Among members of the health care team, nurses carry the primary responsibility for patient-family education. While health education is a vital aspect of total patient care, it has unfortunately been somewhat neglected until very recently. Storlie explains the problem this way:

Teaching, learning, and listening are important parts of nursing care. Because they are difficult to document and even harder to measure, they are not always emphasized to the extent that clinical procedures are. Nor is patient teaching practiced consistently by all members of the profession. However, the nurse who recognizes the patient's dignity, rationality, and individuality will include teaching in her daily care of patients as regularly as she does charting.[108]

In this text, we cannot give as much space to exploring the subject of patient teaching as we would like. Here, we consider the highlights of the subject; there are many excellent books and articles on patient teaching and on general learning theory and teaching methods.* A more thorough study of this important topic will be of definite value to you.

Principles of Learning

Learning is an experience that encompasses a person's total being. In essence, learning involves not only acquiring new knowledge, information and skills but also *changing one's behavior.* When a person truly learns, he may change his attitudes, life-style and method of solving problems as a result. Because the act of learning takes great energy and concentration, helping patients who are experiencing illness, anxiety and pain to learn is a true nursing chal-

---

*Note bibliographic references 41, 52, 56, 57, 62, 63, 81, 95, 101, 102, 105, 107, 108, 111, 113.

lenge. To meet this challenge, it is essential to understand what factors facilitate patient learning and which factors hinder learning.

Factors that Facilitate Patient Learning

1. The patient must be *ready to learn, both physically and emotionally.* A patient who is in severe pain or frightened, restless, or anxious is obviously not going to profit from a teaching session no matter how well it is presented. In addition, the patient must be able to comprehend the information and ideas being discussed. Thus if a patient is suffering from an oxygen lack to the brain with a resultant poor concentration and memory loss, it is best to postpone teaching sessions until the patient is better able to comprehend.

2. The patient will learn more if he feels *a genuine desire to learn.* People differ greatly in the amount of information about their illness or behavior that they can tolerate. Some patients become anxious if they feel "in the dark" about their illness; they want to know as much as possible about its cause, prevention and possible cure. Other patients become extremely anxious if the nurse tries to talk with them concerning their disorder. When an anxious patient resists instruction, it is best not to push him into listening to ideas that he is not ready for. Instead, wait until the patient approaches *you* with questions about his condition. By this point, his anxiety may well have lessened and he will be ready to take in new information.

3. Patients learn best in a *warm, accepting atmosphere.* The patient needs to feel that the nurse is genuinely interested in helping him learn and that he can take his time assimilating new facts and performing new tasks. Patients should not be criticized if they cannot recall everything they have been taught. Remember how anxious you were during your first few days in the school of nursing and how overwhelmed you felt (and may still feel) by the enormous volume of new words and concepts that must be learned. In this respect, patients are no different from yourself. They need time to assimilate ideas and develop new skills. Patients should have the right to make mistakes and even to fail at a task without losing face. The nurse's role is to act as an instructor and not as a judge.

4. Learning is facilitated in a *pleasant quiet environment, free from distractions.* The teaching area or classroom should be well lit, moderately cool, and if possible, away from the area of heavy ward activity.

5. Material is learned more easily when it is presented in a form that has meaning for the patient. You might ask the patient what he understands about his health problem already and what in particular he would like to discuss and learn about at this time. Throughout a teaching session you need to check that the patient is understanding and whether you are still discussing material that is relevant for him.

6. The patient will be more successful in *remembering and assimilating well-organized materials which proceed from the simple to the complex*. In a well-developed teaching plan, each concept presented is based upon a broader and more fundamental concept. Clearly one cannot understand abnormalities of function without first understanding normal function. One cannot comprehend the treatment and prevention of a disease without first learning about the cause of the disease. Thus, to teach a patient about his illness and its care, it is best to begin with a broad discussion of the normal anatomy and physiology of the diseased organ or system, proceed to a description of those factors which cause the disease, and finally end the discussion with a presentation of how the patient can assist in his treatment and rehabilitation program.

6. Learning is *strengthened and reinforced when positive patient behaviors are rewarded*. We are all more motivated to study and learn when we know that our efforts will be rewarded. For students, the reward typically is a high grade. For patients, incentives and rewards center around (a) control of their pain and other symptoms, (b) returning to a normal or near-normal life-style, (c) avoiding complications and (d) pleasing the nurse instructor or the doctor. In addition, remember that *immediate* rewards reinforce positive behaviors far more than do delayed rewards. Therefore, it is important to compliment a patient immediately after he asks a thoughtful question or demonstrates that he has read about his illness or performs a procedure satisfactorily.

7. Patients learn more when they are encouraged to *actively participate in their health education program*. Active participation generates interest in learning whereas absence of participation results in boredom. Who hasn't read an article and forgotten most of the subject matter because the passive act of reading was not supplemented with the active act of discussion? Who hasn't almost fallen asleep during a long tedious lecture? Who hasn't doodled and daydreamed during classes conducted by teachers who never ask questions or call for a discussion? As Marriner emphasizes, "The more the teacher teaches the less the student may learn."[65]

There are a number of ways to encourage patient participation. For instance, as you present new material, check with the patient to make certain that he understands the subject matter. Discuss all written materials and brochures with the patient; do not assume that if you hand a patient a list of instructions he will necessarily follow them. Patients usually require discussion as to *why* those particular instructions are so vital. If you demonstrate a procedure to a patient, have the patient give a return demonstration as soon as possible. Better yet, if extra equipment is available, allow the patient to work through each step of the procedure *with you* rather than waiting to redemonstrate the entire procedure later.

8. *Repetition of key facts and concepts* reinforces the learning of facts and principles. *Frequent practice* reinforces the learning of skills and facilitates the performance of procedures. Reviewing materials presented earlier prepares the patient for learning new materials.

9. Patients retain information and skills longer when they are allowed to *immediately* put new information skills into practice. When patients are not allowed to use their knowledge, they tend to quickly forget what they have learned. For example, in many obstetric wards, it is now common practice for new mothers to begin almost immediately to care for their babies. While on the ward, mothers learn, under supervision, to bathe, feed and diaper their offspring. In the past these procedures were usually demonstrated by the nurse, but the mothers had to wait until they went home to perform the procedures themselves. By the time of discharge, many of the young women with first-born babies had already forgotten important points about caring for their infants. Currently, patients are being allowed to return demonstrations almost immediately—under supervision—instead of being sent home to flounder alone.

10. Patients may occasionally reach *learning plateaus*. At this time, the patient may appear to have lost interest in learning or he may seem quite discouraged. Learning plateaus, as you know from your own educational experiences, are normal. To help the patient surmount the plateau, you might use visual aids, movies, or other stimulating methods of presentation. Also you might give the patient a brief break from lessons and not present any new materials until he recaptures his interest in learning.

1. *Physiologic barriers.* Patients experiencing critical illness, severe pain, restlessness, oxygen deprivation, fatigue, weakness, deafness, or visual problems will have difficulty learning. These physiologic states act as barriers to learning because they reduce the patient's ability to concentrate and deplete his energy.

2. *Emotional barriers.* Psychologic stresses also interfere with the patient's powers of concentration. Patients who feel anxious, fearful of the unknown, and angry because they are ill may be too psychologically stressed to learn.

3. *Cultural barriers.* Learning and teaching problems arise when patients speak a different language from the nurse, have a different educational background, are of a different race or ethnic group, or have a different value system from the nursing staff. Unfortunately, nurses have been known to reject and consequently avoid teaching patients who are part of the counterculture, for example, ex-convicts or individuals who are part of the drug culture. Nurses must avoid such differential treatment.

4. *Environmental barriers.* Lack of privacy, a noisy environment, and numerous interruptions tend to seriously disrupt patient teaching sessions.

5. *Inadequate or poor teaching.* The nurse herself may be a barrier to patient learning. Teaching problems that hinder a patient from learning include lack of knowledge and preparation on the instructor's part, lack of planning, overuse of technical words, the delivery of poorly prepared or fragmented lectures, unwillingness to draw the patient into discussion, hurried or poorly planned demonstrations, and a condescending attitude on the part of the nurse toward the patient.

Principles of Teaching

In order to teach, one must first make three important decisions: (a) what to teach, (b) when to teach, and (c) how to teach.

What to Teach. The patient may be interested to learn about the following:

1. The basic normal anatomy and physiology of his body

2. The underlying pathology which is causing his symptoms

3. The rationale for his treatment program

4. Complications, limitations, and changes in his life-style which may develop due to his illness

5. His probable prognosis

6. The purpose of his medications, their safe administration, and any possible side effects

7. The cost of his care

8. The expected duration of his care—short-term or long-term care

9. Nature of the diagnostic tests and studies that he will be undergoing—the preparation for those tests and the meaning of test results

10. Preventative and rehabilitative measures which will help prevent and overcome complications

11. The hospital environment in which he resides, e.g., the bedside equipment and how it works; the location of bathrooms, the cafeteria, and the chapel; hospital policies and routines

12. The hospital staff who will be assisting him to recovery, e.g., the names of the nursing supervisor, the head nurse, dietician, and team leader and the name and telephone number of the chaplain and others whose services the patient may desire.

In addition, the patient may have other topics in mind that he may wish to pursue. Ask the patient what he wants to learn more about. Listen for clues that will help you recognize the patient's areas of greatest interest and concern.

When to Teach. It may help to have patient teaching deliberately scheduled, or during the course of a nurse's hectic day, it may be given a low priority or even forgotten. Instruction may be given at specific times that are formally designated by the nurse or presented throughout the day, when a patient asks questions or when new experiences occur for the patient that require explanation.

How to Teach. The teaching method selected depends both upon the subject matter and upon the patient's background, personality and needs. Teaching may be done by means of formal lectures and procedural demonstrations. Informal discussions with patients either individually or in a group may be more appropriate however. Audio-visual aids and printed information may be useful for many patients.

In whatever way teaching is done, however, it must (a) center on patients' learning needs, (b) communicate accurate, current and relevant information and (c) be conducted by a warm and enthusiastic person.

Developing a Teaching Plan

A nurse should never attempt to teach a patient without first assessing the patient's learning needs and devising a teaching plan to fit his needs. Like the patient care plan, the patient teaching plan is based upon the problem-solving method. One type of printed form for preparing a formal teaching plan is shown in Figure 17–14. The systematic approach to patient teaching includes the following major steps:

1. Assess the patient's learning needs and capabilities

2. Develop teaching goals and objectives

3. Decide on subject content, teaching activities and learning resources

4. Evaluate the patient's progress and the overall teaching plan

5. Modify the teaching plan as necessary

Assess the Patient's Learning Needs and Capabilities

To assess a patient's learning needs and capabilities, the nurse must carefully gather data about the patient's physical and mental status, his background and his unique situation and life-style. The patient's concerns, of course, establish the content of his lesson. The presentation of the content, in turn, is determined by the following:

▶ *The patient's level of education.* The vocabulary used to instruct the patient with a college background may be different from that used to teach a person with a fifth-grade education. Furthermore, less educated patients may need concrete and practical answers and examples, while more educated people can sometimes learn better from more abstract statements and examples. Reading ability is often correlated with educational background. A poor reader will benefit little from being handed sophisticated reading materials about his illness; however, he might learn well from audiovisual presentations and from demonstrations.

▶ *Pre-existing knowledge.* It is important to determine what the patient already knows

---

Name: _____

Room: _____

Overall goal (nursing staff): _____

_____

_____

Diagnosis: _____

Overall objective (patient or other significant person):
Upon discharge from the hospital,
the patient (or other responsible person) will be able to:

_____

_____

Intermediate Objectives	Related Content	Teaching Activity	Resources	Patient Evaluation (return Demonstration)	Date	Nurse

Figure 17–14.   Patient Teaching Plan. (From Gulko, C. S., and Butherus, C.: Toward better patient teaching. *Nurses' Drug Alert I*:49, March 1977, p. 56.)

about his condition. The best way to find this out is to ask!

▶ *The patient's age.* Children and the elderly require somewhat specialized teaching approaches. Children are usually receptive to instruction which involves playing games and role-playing. The child who is going to surgery can be taught with colored pictures or with dolls upon which an incision has been hand drawn. A child with heart or kidney disease might enjoy working with plastic models of the heart and kidney. When instructing elderly patients, always evaluate their hearing and visual acuity. Also, remember that some elderly people have a shorter attention span than do young and middle-aged adults.

▶ *Motivation to learn.* Recall the principle of learning that a patient who is in great pain or who is critically ill or disoriented is not capable of learning until his condition improves. In general, the best candidates for in depth patient teaching include patients who are preoperative, convalescing, participating in rehabilitation programs or awaiting discharge. However, patients at all stages of illness need and have a right to explanations and information about themselves and what is happening to them.

▶ *Psychologic status.* Before beginning a teaching program, evaluate the patient's attitude toward his illness. Attitudes change during the course of a serious illness. Typically, patients first experience a sense of disbelief—often accompanied by anger and denial. Next, they may progress to a beginning awareness of the disorder and its ramifications. Later they come to accept the illness, and finally they learn to adapt to it. It is impossible to teach a patient about his disorder when he is in the stage of denying that he has a disorder. However, once the patient becomes aware that he really is ill, he may be willing to accept some instruction.

▶ *Expected prognosis.* Teaching content is greatly influenced by the patient's medical and nursing prognoses. For example, a patient who is terminally ill has different learning needs and capabilities than the patient who is not facing death. Unfortunately, because the learning needs of the dying patient *are* different, they are often ignored altogether. Dying persons and their families do have many questions and concerns and they have a right to learn the answers.

The approach to teaching is influenced first by the teacher's ability to use or alter that approach to meet her own needs and those of the patient. Some nurses find it difficult to formally

lecture; others are uncomfortable demonstrating a procedure in front of a group but can work comfortably with an individual patient. Second, the teaching approach is influenced by interference factors. For instance, a classroom may not be available and may not be appropriate for formal teaching; equipment for demonstrations may not be accessible; the nurse's time may be limited.

Develop Learning Goals and Objectives

What we said earlier about nursing care goals and objectives generally applies to patient learning goals and objectives. A *patient learning goal* is a broadly stated directive that sums up the overall aim of the patient's educational program. *Learning objectives* spell out in clear specific terms what the patient should know and be able to do at various stages of his educational program. Learning objectives must be realistic and in keeping with the patient's age, intelligence and educational level. In addition, learning objectives should be stated in *behavioral terms* so that the patient's progress toward his objectives can be measured and evaluated. For example, consider these two learning objectives—one vague and one which states clearly and exactly what the patient is to learn.

Vague objective: Patient should understand special diet prior to discharge.

Specific objective: The patient is able to (a) list foods allowed on special diet as well as foods that are forbidden and (b) discuss the health benefits that he will receive if he remains on his diet and complications which will develop if he does not abide by the diet.

Sometimes it is helpful when writing learning objectives to assign a deadline for the attainment of each objective. For example, "By the end of the first lesson, the patient will be able to list the foods allowed on his special diet."

Decide on Subject Content, Teaching Activities and Learning Resources

After deciding on goals and objectives, the next step is to develop the body of the teaching plan. As we stated earlier, the *content* taught and the level of its presentation will depend upon the patient's disorder as well as his condition, age, and prognosis. In addition, content is also based on the patient's goals and objectives.

Teaching activities vary with the content to be taught and with the patient's learning needs and capabilities. Types of teaching activities include the following:

▶ *One-to-one instruction.* This method may be formal or informal and allows the nurse to pace the learning content and activities to the individual patient's learning rate. Also, the nurse can modify her program in keeping with the patient's learning progress.

▶ *Group instruction.* This method requires that the nurse arrange for a meeting place, prepare handout materials in advance of the meeting, prepare a meeting agenda and a lesson plan, arrange seating to facilitate group interaction (e.g., putting the chairs into a circle), lecture on major topics, lead a discussion, review major points covered in the discussion and arrange for the next meeting. The major advantages of group instruction are that (a) it is economical in terms of the teacher's time and (b) patients with similar problems can share experiences, viewpoints and opinions with each other. Disadvantages include: (a) the nurse must pace her instruction to the level of the group rather than to the individual patient and (b) some patients are intimidated by a group and find it difficult to ask questions or enter into a discussion.

▶ *Lectures.* Lectures are usually delivered in a group setting. This method is useful for quickly delivering large amounts of factual information to a group.

▶ *Discussion.* We stated earlier that discussion is an important teaching activity because it encourages the patient to actively participate in his health education program. You can draw patients into a discussion by asking them for their responses to the content, asking for examples of ways in which the content is applicable to their lives, and by calling for personal experiences and opinions. For instance, in a class for cancer patients, a patient might discuss how he dealt with the problem of baldness following radiation therapy. In a postnatal class, an experienced mother might describe (for the benefit of new mothers) the "three-day blues" that most mothers feel following the birth of a child and the ways she coped with them.

▶ *Demonstration.* Demonstrations are typically used to teach *motor skills*, e.g., how to give a self-injection of medication, transfer safely from bed to wheelchair. To prepare for a demonstration (a) organize your notes and thoughts so that you can accompany the demonstration with a discussion of the procedure; (b) assemble the equipment and make certain that it works properly; (c) if possible, prepare a handout that outlines the procedures for the patient so that he can follow the demonstration more easily and (d) practice the demonstration until you feel comfortable doing it. When giving the demonstration, make certain that the patient is able to see you perform each step. Proceed slowly and allow time during the demonstration for questions. Following the demonstration, have the patient *return* the demonstration as soon as possible so that he does not forget what he has seen and learned.

Teaching activities can be enlivened by the proper use of *teaching aids.* Useful teaching tools include pamphlets, hand drawings, models of organs, charts, graphs, audiotapes, bulletin boards, a blackboard, posters, pictures, the overhead transparency projector, slide shows, films, film strips, closed circuit television, flash cards, programmed instructions and games.

The use of *resource persons* is an extremely helpful adjunct to regular teaching activities. For example, when teaching patients about a special diet, ask the dietician to attend the session and share her knowledge with the patients. Physicians, physical therapists and occupational therapists can all make significant contributions to a patient lecture or discussion.

Evaluate the Patient's Progress and the Overall Teaching Plan

The patient and the nurse must evaluate the teaching program and the patient's progress *together.* Thus they must ask themselves: Has the *patient* met his learning goals and objectives? Is he more knowledgeable about his concerns? Is he able to demonstrate the skills necessary for him to care for himself? Have his attitudes changed toward his illness? Is he more positive, confident and self-assured? Can he cope with the limitations that his illness may have brought into his life? Do the patient's significant others understand his problems and do they know what to do to help him best?

Was the *content* of the lessons in sufficient depth? Was the content clear? Was the information presented at the patient's level of education and understanding? Was the information taught in an interesting way? Were teaching aids and resources used as appropriate?

Did the *nurse* meet her objectives for teaching the patient? Did the patient perceive her as interested in the material and in him? Did she encourage questions and discussion? Did she allow the patient to give a return demonstration as soon as possible following her demonstration of a procedure? Was she supportive, warm, accepting and encouraging toward the patient? Did she involve the patient's significant others in the lessons as often as possible? Did she give the patient frequent feedback as to his progress? Did she arrange to teach in a quiet area free from distractions? Was instruction individualized and modified to match the patient's learning rate and learning interests?

If the nurse develops the patient's learning objectives properly (i.e., in behavioral terms) the actual process of writing the evaluation section of the teaching plan should not be difficult. For instance, to evaluate the learning objective "The patient is able to list foods allowed on special diet as well as foods that are forbidden," the nurse simply asks the patient to list the foods. If the patient can perform this verbal task, the nurse knows that this aspect of her teaching is successful. If the patient can list only a few foods or none at all, the nurse must find another way to present the information to the patient—perhaps with flashcards or posters.

Modify the Teaching Plan as Necessary

The teaching plan will need to be modified if (a) the patient has not reached all of his learning goals and objectives or (b) the patient's learning goals have changed due to the resolution of some problems or the development of new problems. To modify the teaching plan, the nurse will need to reassess the patient's learning needs, draw up new goals and objectives, devise new teaching activities and re-evaluate the patient and the plan. This process continues until the patient finally achieves his learning goals.

STEP 5: NURSING MANAGEMENT— EVALUATION AND MODIFICATION OF THE PATIENT CARE PLAN

Evaluation: Basic Facts and Concepts

After the patient's needs have been assessed, his problems diagnosed, his care planned and his plan of care put into action, it is time to ask these questions:

▶ Is the care plan really working?

▶ Is the patient progressing steadily toward his long-term health goals?

▶ Is the patient accomplishing his short-term behavioral objectives? Is he meeting the deadlines for these objectives?

▶ Have the patient's problems been totally or partially resolved?

▶ Were any problems incorrectly diagnosed?

▶ Have new problems arisen since implementation of the plan? Were any of these problems a direct result of the care plan?

To answer these critical questions accurately and truthfully, one must employ the evaluation process. To begin to understand the evaluation step, it is necessary to first pursue a few more important questions.

What Exactly Is Evaluation?   One dictionary defines evaluation as "the accurate appraisal of value." Phaneuf writes more specifically: "Evaluation requires appraisal of the extent or degree to which stated objectives are attained."[90] Bailey and Claus describe evaluation in managerial terms. They state: "Evaluation involves comparing results to standards, reviewing all deviations including those within the tolerances, and applying judgment with respect to the seriousness of the discrepancies and needs for correction."[8] Ryan discusses evaluation from the standpoint of systems theory:

Evaluation, within the context of systems theory is characterized as the feedback capability of the system. It identifies deviations or deficiencies within the system and moves the system toward fixing responsibility and controls. As a feedback and control process, it involves measurement and the comparison of resulting measures against standards. Standards may be desired outcomes, expected outcomes, predicted outcomes, norms and other forms of criteria.[99]

Finally, Marriner defines evaluation as a form of nursing assessment or reassessment. She writes:

Evaluation is the process of assessing (1) the patient's progress toward health goals, (2) the quality of patient care in an institution by means of the nursing audit, (3) the quality of individual nursing care through self-evaluation as well as (4) overall personnel performance.[65]

Why Evaluate?   As you can see from Marriner's nursing oriented definition, evaluation of patient care can be pursued on both an individual and an institutional level. On the *individual* level, the major purposes of evaluation are to determine: (a) the extent to which the nursing care plan is really working, (b) the progress which the patient is making toward the behavioral goals and objectives of the plan, (c) the quality of patient care which the patient is receiving and (d) the status of the patient's problems (any problems resolved? any new problems?). The evaluation process also helps to pinpoint errors in patient assessment and diagnosis which can result in faulty patient management.

On the *institutional level,* evaluation proceedings are used to determine if patient care (as depicted in patient records) meets legal and professional standards. This formalized evaluation procedure is called *nursing audit.* (See Figure 17–16 and the accompanying discussion later in this chapter.) In addition, evaluation techniques are used in health care facilities to rate the performance of health professionals and other personnel.

Who Evaluates?   On the *individual* patient level, the professional nurse who assesses the patient and plans his care is primarily responsible for evaluating the extent to which her plan for the patient is working. Those nurses who assist in the implementation phase of the nursing process should also participate in the evaluation procedure. In addition, physicians can contribute to the evaluation process by stating their opinions concerning the patient's progress under the current nursing care plan. And, last but not least, the patient and his family must be allowed a voice in the evaluation process—since in all truth the patient has the most to gain from competent well-planned nursing care and the most to lose if care planning has been inadequate or faulty.

On the *institutional level,* the nursing audit is usually performed by an audit committee composed of a group of professional nurses. Nursing supervisors and head nurses evaluate patient care on their ward or floor as well as the performance of the nurses under their supervision.

Evaluate How Often?   Ideally, evaluation is an ongoing process that takes place on a *continuing basis* throughout the patient's hospitalization or home-care program. However, some patients need more frequent and careful evaluation than do others. For example, the critically ill patient or the new postoperative patient needs almost constant reassessment of his condition and his response to planned nursing care. On the other hand, the patient who is on a rehabilitation service or who is on a minimum care ward requires less frequent reassessment. However, *all* patients, regardless of their status or condition require a periodic thoughtful reappraisal of their needs, problems, care plan and progress.

Guidelines for Effective Evaluation

According to Bailey and Claus, the evaluation process should be conducted in accordance with certain guidelines. Thus, evaluation should be (a) planned in advance, (b) conducted in terms of objectives and purposes, (c) objective, (d) verifiable, (e) a cooperative effort, (f) specific (pinpointing strengths and weaknesses, achievements and deficiencies), (g) quantitative, (h) feasible and (i) productive of useful information.[8]

Steps in the Evaluation Process

There are five major steps in the evaluation process, as follows:

1. Establish standards or criteria for evaluation

2. Assess existing conditions and compare findings with standards

3. Summarize outcomes of the evaluation.

4. Identify reasons for patient's failure to achieve expected patient outcomes stated in care plan

5. Take corrective action and modify the care plan

STEP 1: ESTABLISH STANDARDS OR CRITERIA FOR EVALUATION

Dorland's Medical Dictionary defines a standard as "something established as a measure or model to which other similar things should conform." Another dictionary states: "*Standard* applies to an authoritative rule, principle, or measure used to determine the quantity, weight or extent or especially the value, quality, level or degree of a thing." In nursing, patient care standards are basically rules or measures which have been developed for the purpose of judging the quality of patient care.

To be of value, standards must be realistic, attainable and reasonable, as well as understandable and acceptable to those persons using the standards. Ideally, standards should not be narrow or rigid. Instead, they should be broad enough to encompass a myriad of individual problems and flexible enough to be adapted to changing and fluctuating situations.

The ANA has developed a set of broad standards which can be used to evaluate the extent to which the nursing process is being used in the planning of patient care.

ANA's
Eight Standards of
Nursing Practice*

1. The collection of data about the health status of the client/patient is systematic and continuous. The data are accessible, communicated and recorded.

2. Nursing diagnoses are derived from health status data.

3. The plan of nursing care includes goals derived from the nursing diagnoses.

4. The plan of nursing care includes priorities and the prescribed nursing approaches or measures to achieve the goals derived from the nursing diagnoses.

5. Nursing actions provide for client/patient participation in health promotion, maintenance and restoration.

6. Nursing actions assist the client/patient to maximize his health capabilities.

7. The client's/patient's progress or lack of progress toward goal achievement is determined by the client/patient and the nurse.

8. The client's/patient's progress or lack of progress toward goal achievement directs reassessment, reordering of priorities, new goal setting, and revision of the plan of nursing care.

Note the following correlations between these standards and the steps of the nursing process.

▶ Standard 1 correlates with step 1, data gathering.

▶ Standard 2 correlates with step 2, making the nursing diagnosis.

▶ Standards 3 and 4 correlate with step 3, planning nursing care.

▶ Standards 5 and 6 correlate with step 4, implementing the care plan and performing nursing interventions.

▶ Standards 7 and 8 correlate with step 5, evaluation of the patient's progress and modification of the patient's care plan and implementations as necessary.

Because the ANA's Standards of Nursing Practice are broad, they can be applied to all

*American Nurses' Association Congress for Nursing Practice, copyright © American Nurses' Association, 1973.

groups of patients. However, in addition, more specialized standards are needed to evaluate the status and progress of *special groups* of patients, e.g., neurologic patients, postoperative patients, patients who have suffered a myocardial infarction ("heart attack"). For instance, one standard of care for a patient following a myocardial infarction might be: "Collection of data about the status of the patient includes assessment of presence and degree of cardiac pain, stability of pulse and blood pressure, presence of arrhythmias, feelings of fear and anxiety." This type of data, then, must be collected on all patients following a myocardial infarction for their nursing care to be "up to standard."

STEP 2: ASSESS EXISTING CONDITIONS AND COMPARE FINDINGS WITH STANDARDS

This step of the evaluation process involves measuring the results of the patient care plan, the nursing interventions and the patient's activities by (a) gathering data and (b) comparing the observable patient behaviors and condition and/or the nurse's performance against established standards and criteria. As implied earlier, the evaluation process can be conducted at the level of the individual patient or on an institutional level for groups of patients. Below, we briefly consider each of these evaluation levels.

Evaluation of the Individual Patient's Progress. To evaluate a patient's progress within a nursing care program, the nurse must determine the extent to which the goals and objectives of the care plan are being met by the patient. To perform this step, the nurse must evaluate (1) the patient's physiologic and behavioral responses and the degree to which they conform to the expected patient outcomes outlined in the patient care plan and (2) the care plan itself.

EVALUATE THE PATIENT'S RESPONSES. To evaluate the patient's responses, the nurse can do the following:

1. Review, in the patient's care plan, the *expected patient outcomes* and their *projected dates* for accomplishment. As we stated earlier, expected patient outcomes must express in clear, measurable terms exactly what a patient should feel like, look like, act like and say once his problem is resolved or is progressing toward resolution. In addition, well-stated expected outcomes indicate those clinical manifestations that should be present as a result of therapy.

2. *Observe* the patient's *physiologic and behavioral responses.* Physiologic responses include clinical measurements such as vital signs, skin condition, and body weight loss or gain. Behavioral responses include both verbal statements and nonverbal activities.

> Remember *that the patient's responses to his plan of care must be evaluated at least* each day *and* not *just on the projected date by which the expected outcome is to be achieved.*

3. *Compare* the patient's responses with the expected patient outcomes and *look for discrepancies.*

As an example of this process, turn back to Mr. Williamson's care plan (Table 17–7). Recall that one of Mr. Williamson's nursing diagnoses was "Poor personal hygiene due to lack of interest in self-care and forgetfulness." The expected patient outcomes for this problem (written 4/16) state that by 4/30 Mr. Williamson will wash his hands and face after meals, change his underclothes when soiled, shave himself daily, etc. If by 4/30, the nurse finds that Mr. Williamson is indeed washing his hands and face after meals, changing his underclothes when soiled, and shaving himself daily, she knows that the expected patient outcomes and projected dates were realistic and that the nursing orders accomplished their intent. On the other hand, if the nurse assesses Mr. Williamson's progress at designated times between 4/16 and 4/30, and if she finds that his personal hygiene is *not* improving and is even growing worse, then the nurse has evidence that the patient is not meeting the objectives of the care plan. She also knows that the care plan (in particular the patient outcomes, projected dates and nursing orders) will need to be reviewed, revised and re-implemented.

EVALUATE THE PATIENT CARE PLAN. The patient care plan needs frequent and careful re-evaluation. Questions the nurse must ask herself are: Is the care plan complete? Does it clearly communicate the patient's needs, goals and activities? Is it realistic? Is it helping the patient reach his objectives? Is it completely up to date? Is it being revised as necessary in keeping with changes in the patient's needs, problems, objectives and behaviors? A strategy for planning and evaluating nursing care plans is presented in Table 17–8. Note particularly the standards and criteria for care plan evaluation.

Evaluation of Institutional Patient Care by Nursing Audit. As implied earlier, the nursing audit is a systematic procedure for (a) evaluating patient care within an institution and (b) judging whether or not the patient care given meets established standards. The nursing audit, like other forms of audit (e.g., tax audit, bookkeeping audit) involves the inspection and review of records. In essence, then, the nursing audit "is a method for evaluating quality of care through appraisal of the nursing process as it is reflected in the patient care records for discharged patients."[90] The audit is conducted by an audit committee composed of professional nurses. Records reviewed include the patient's legal record (chart), his nursing care plan and his Kardex. Audits are conducted in hospitals, nursing homes, public health nursing agencies, and other organizations.

The major goals of the nursing audit are to:

▶ Improve the quality of health care throughout the nation

▶ Improve the quality of nursing care throughout all health care facilities

▶ Promote improved communication among nurses as well as all members of the health care team

▶ Detect and analyze problems and errors within the health care system and develop measures for preventing future errors

▶ Insure that nurses are accountable or answerable for the care that they give their patients. *Accountability* is "the state of being accountable, responsible, liable."[75] Phaneuf explains professional accountability and its relationship to the nursing audit and the nursing process in this way:

Evaluation is a part of professional accountability. Nurses are answerable to themselves as practitioners; to patients and families; to physicians and others who participate in the care of patients; to the institutions and agencies in which they practice; to the community; and to the nursing profession which is in turn accountable to society. The audit is one way through which nurses can help to satisfy the accountability that is inherent in professional practice. It entails rigorous assessment of the nursing process actually used in patient care.[90]

There are a number of nursing audit formats in use. Figure 17–15 illustrates the audit form or instrument developed by Phaneuf. Part I of the audit instrument is directed toward an assessment of whether or not institutional procedures and policies governing patient care are being followed. This section can be filled out by a trained clerk.

Part II of the form is called the *Nursing Audit Chart Review Schedule.* This section of the

TABLE 17–8. STRATEGY FOR PLANNING AND EVALUATING NURSING CARE PLANS*

UNITS IN SEQUENCE	ELEMENTS	ACTIVITIES	STANDARDS (EXPECTED OUTCOMES)	CRITERIA
Total nursing care plan	Nursing assessment Nursing diagnosis Nursing objectives Nursing orders	Analyze Synthesize Decide Direct Coordinate Instruct	Communicates information about individual patient and his environment which guides nursing team in care of that patient	Initiated on admission of patient Initiated, compiled and written in pencil by professional nurse Contains these components: Nursing assessment, diagnosis, objectives, orders Readily available to nursing staff Used in nursing rounds and team conferences Updated periodically
Nursing assessment	Personal identifying factors about patient Orientation to environment Perceptions Expectations Preferences Habits of daily living	Interview Observe Describe Sort Classify Report Record	Records identifying information permitting immediate development of a plan for nursing care including patient's perceptions, preferences and expectations	Permits immediate development of beginning individualized care plan Contains personalized identifying information Describes patient's perceptions of his own needs and problems Includes patient's preferences Includes patient's expectations about his illness and therapy Is not duplicated in medical records
Nursing diagnosis	Statements describing patient's current and potential problems, strengths, and deficits	Analyze data Predict outcomes Make inferences Hypothesize Determine needs Identify problems Establish priorities Record	In terse statements describes patient's current and potential problems	Contains short statement of patient's current and potential problems Statements are arranged in order of immediacy Identifies strengths and deficits of coping responses Considers lack of health information a problematic area Shows discrepancies between current behavior and expected outcomes
Nursing objective	Statements identifying desirable behavioral changes, treatment goals, or intended results of intervention	Translate needs/problems into target behaviors Formulate goals Determine conditions which must exist to precipitate change	Concise statements describing target behavior, treatment goals, or intended results of nursing intervention	Identifies target behaviors Desirable outcomes are derived from identified needs/problems Statements are phrased succinctly in action terms
Nursing orders	Directions Schedules Procedures Principles	Specify nursing actions Determine when, who, and where Translate principles into concrete directions	Prescribes nursing intervention in action terms formulated to carefully direct the nursing team toward progressive, continuous and personalized nursing care	Describes nursing intervention techniques behaviorally Considers patient preferences Plans for teaching health care Schedules treatment events Revised as behavioral change indicates Includes patient, family, community participation in current and after-care plans Initiated by author

*From Ryan, B. L.: Nursing care plans: a systems approach to developing criteria for planning evaluation. *Journal of Nursing Administration*, May–June, 1973, p. 57.

audit is designed to evaluate not only patients' charts but also the patient care plan and Kardex. The Chart Review Schedule is based upon what Phaneuf views to be the seven functions of nursing—functions which "are considered to be the components of the nursing process, and as such, they are subject to measurement."[90] Note that the seven functions of nursing listed in Figure 17–15 are:

1. Application and execution of physician's legal orders

2. Observation of symptoms and reactions

3. Supervision of the patient

4. Supervision of those participating in care (except the physician)

5. Reporting and recording

6. Application and execution of nursing procedures and techniques

7. Promotion of physical and emotional health by direction and teaching

Observe that the five steps of the nursing process as presented in this chapter are integrated throughout this list of professional nursing functions.

Finally, Part III of the audit instrument states the final patient care score for the chart reviewed: excellent, good, incomplete, poor, unsafe. This section of the audit tool is also used

PART I. HOSPITAL OR NURSING HOME AUDIT

Data must be held in STRICT confidence and MUST NOT BE FILED with patient's record.

All Entries To Be Completed By Trained Clerk

1. Name of patient: 2. Sex 3. Age 4. Date admitted 5. Discharge date

(LAST)   (FIRST)

6. Name of institution: 7. Floor 8. Medical supervision Private ☐ Ward ☐ OPD/Clinic ☐

9. Complete diagnosis(es):

10. Admitted by referral from: Physician on staff ☐ M.D. not hospital affiliated ☐ Clinic/OPD ☐ 11. Via emergency ☐

12. Patient discharged to: Self-care ☐ Family care ☐ PHN Agency ☐ Other specify: ☐ Died ☐ Unknown ☐

13. If patient died: M.D. present ☐ M.D. promptly notified ☐ Family present ☐ Family promptly notified 14. If patient Catholic: Last rites given: YES ☐ NO ☐

15. All nursing entries signed by name and dated: YES ☐ NO ☐ 16. Nursing entries show whether made by professional, practical, student nurse, or other: YES ☐ NO ☐

17. Patients' clothing, valuables, and other personal items were accounted for in accordance with policy: YES ☐ NO ☐

	YES	NO
18. Operative and other patient or family consent forms completed as required by policy	—	—
19. A. Were there any accidents or other special incidents?	—	—
B. If yes, chart indicates report was submitted to administration	—	—
C. Or, report is part of chart	—	—
20. A. Kardex in use	—	—
B. If yes, Kardex becomes part of permanent chart	—	—
21. Nursing care plan is recorded in the chart	—	—
22. A. Nursing admission entry shows assessment of patient's condition: physical	—	—
emotional	—	—
B. Nursing discharge entry shows assessment of patient's condition: physical	—	—
emotional	—	—

Figure 17–15. The nursing audit instrument. (From Phaneuf, M. C.: *The Nursing Audit: Profile for Excellence.* New York, Appleton-Century-Crofts, 1972, p. 21.)

Figure continued on the opposite page

PART II. NURSING AUDIT CHART REVIEW SCHEDULE

All Entries To Be Completed By A Member Of the Nursing Audit Committee

(Please check in box of choice; DO NOT obscure number in box.)

Name of patient: _____
                        (LAST)   (FIRST)

		YES	NO	UNCERTAIN	TOTALS
I.	APPLICATION AND EXECUTION OF PHYSICIAN'S LEGAL ORDERS				
1.	Medical diagnosis complete	7	0	3	
2.	Orders complete	7	0	3	
3.	Orders current	7	0	3	
4.	Orders promptly executed	7	0	3	
5.	Evidence that nurse understood cause and effect	7	0	3	
6.	Evidence that nurse took health history into account	7	0	3	
	(42) TOTALS		0		

		YES	NO	UNCERTAIN	TOTALS
II.	OBSERVATION OF SYMPTOMS AND REACTIONS				
7.	Related to course of above disease(s) in general	7	0	3	
8.	Related to course of above disease(s) in patient	7	0	3	
9.	Related to complications due to therapy (each medication and each procedure)	7	0	3	
10.	Vital signs	7	0	3	
11.	Patient to his condition	7	0	3	
12.	Patient to his course of disease(s)	5	0	2	
	(40) TOTALS		0		

		YES	NO	UNCERTAIN	TOTALS
III.	SUPERVISION OF THE PATIENT				
13.	Evidence that initial nursing diagnosis was made	4	0	1	
14.	Safety of patient	4	0	1	
15.	Security of patient	4	0	1	
16.	Adaptation (support of patient in reaction to condition and care)	4	0	1	
17.	Continuing assessment of patient's condition and capacity	4	0	1	
18.	Nursing plans changed in accordance with assessment	4	0	1	
19.	Interaction with family and with others considered	4	0	1	
	(28) TOTALS		0		

		YES	NO	UNCERTAIN	TOTALS
IV.	SUPERVISION OF THOSE PARTICIPATING IN CARE (EXCEPT THE PHYSICIAN)				
20.	Care taught to patient, family, or others, nursing personnel	5	0	2	
21.	Physical, emotional, mental capacity to learn considered	5	0	2	
22.	Continuity of supervision to those taught	5	0	2	
23.	Support of those giving care	5	0	2	
	(20) TOTALS		0		

		YES	NO	UNCERTAIN	TOTALS
V.	REPORTING AND RECORDING				
24.	Facts on which further care depended were recorded	4	0	1	
25.	Essential facts reported to physician	4	0	1	
26.	Reporting of facts included evaluation thereof	4	0	1	
27.	Patient or family alerted as to what to report to physician	4	0	1	
28.	Record permitted continuity of intramural and extramural care	4	0	1	
	(20) TOTALS		0		

Figure 17–15 *Continued*

Figure continued on the following page

PART II.   NURSING AUDIT CHART REVIEW SCHEDULE (*Continued*)

VI. APPLICATION AND EXECUTION OF NURSING PROCEDURES AND TECHNIQUES	YES	NO	UNCERTAIN	TOTALS	DOES NOT APPLY
29. Administration and/or supervision of medications	2	0	0.5		2
30. Personal care (bathing, oral hygiene, skin, nail care, shampoo)	2	0	0.5		2
31. Nutrition (including special diets)	2	0	0.5		2
32. Fluid balance plus electrolytes	2	0	0.5		2
33. Elimination	2	0	0.5		2
34. Rest and sleep	2	0	0.5		2
35. Physical activity	2	0	0.5		2
36. Irrigations (including enemas)	2	0	0.5		2
37. Dressings and bandages	2	0	0.5		2
38. Formal exercise program	2	0	0.5		2
39. Rehabilitation (other than formal exercise)	2	0	0.5		2
40. Prevention of complications and infections	2	0	0.5		2
41. Recreation, diversion	2	0	0.5		2
42. Clinical procedures - urinalysis, B/P	2	0	0.5		2
43. Special treatments (e.g., care of tracheotomy, use of oxygen, colostomy or catheter care, etc.)	2	0	0.5		2
44. Procedures and techniques taught to patient	2	0	0.5		2
(32) TOTALS		0			

VII. PROMOTION OF PHYSICAL AND EMOTIONAL HEALTH BY DIRECTION AND TEACHING	YES	NO	UNCERTAIN	TOTALS	DOES NOT APPLY
45. Plans for medical emergency evident	3	0	1		3
46. Emotional support to patient	3	0	1		3
47. Emotional support to family	3	0	1		3
48. Teaching promotion and maintenance of health	3	0	1		3
49. Evaluation of need for additional resources (e.g., spiritual, social service, homemaker service, physical or occupational therapy)	3	0	1		3
50. Action taken in regard to needs identified	3	0	1		3
(18) TOTALS		0			

TOTAL SCORE

FINAL SCORE

Figure 17–15 *Continued*

PART III.   AUDIT RESULTS

All Entries To Be Completed By A Nursing Audit Committee Member

Record reflects service as:

EXCELLENT (161-200)   GOOD (121-160)   INCOMPLETE (81-120)   POOR (41-80)   UNSAFE (0-40)
☐   (   )   ☐   (   )   ☐   (   )   ☐   (   )   ☐   (   )

Record did not permit appraisal   ☐   Why?

Remarks (including criticisms/questions pertinent to policy procedures, practices as shown in Parts I and II):

_____   _____
Signature of Nursing Audit Committee   Date:
member who reviewed the record.

for the auditors' remarks concerning the patient's care as documented on the chart and the general policies and procedures of the institution. For instance, the auditor might comment on unusually good nursing practice, errors which need correction, or instances in which patient rights were ignored. Ultimately, the nursing audit, by pointing out the strengths and weaknesses of nursing care within health care facilities and by recommending needed changes, raises the standards and practice of the nursing profession and of the individual nurse.

STEP 3: SUMMARIZE OUTCOMES OF THE EVALUATION

Once the patient's progress has been assessed, the next step is to summarize the findings from the evaluation process. Possible outcomes of the evaluation procedures are as follows:[119]

1. The patient's problems are *resolved:* he has achieved the expected patient outcomes by the projected date and he is reaching his long-range goals.

2. *Some* of the patient's problems are resolved and he has achieved some of the expected patient outcomes. However, other problems still remain unresolved.

3. The patient's problems have *not* been resolved, and he has not achieved the expected patient behaviors.

4. *New* problems are evident. These new problems may have arisen from:
   (a) Untoward changes in the patient's condition
   (b) More astute observations of the patient and further research on the part of the nursing staff
   (c) The therapy program (i.e., iatrogenic problems)

5. The *nursing diagnosis is in error.* Some patient problems are wrongly labeled or the "due to" clauses (pointing to causation) are incorrect.

If the patient's problems have all been resolved and he is meeting his health goals, the next two steps of the nursing process are unnecessary. In this case, the nurse can proceed with the current plan—remaining alert, however, to the possibility that parts of the care plan may and probably will need revision in the future. On the other hand, if evaluation reveals that problems remain unresolved and new problems are developing, then it is essential to proceed to step 4 of the evaluation process discussed below.

STEP 4: IDENTIFY REASONS FOR PATIENT'S FAILURE TO ACHIEVE EXPECTED PATIENT OUTCOMES STATED IN CARE PLAN

There are numerous reasons why patients fail to achieve the objectives formulated in their care plans. Some basic reasons for failure include the following: (a) an erroneous, incomplete or unrealistic care plan, (b) an outdated care plan, (c) uncooperative attitudes on the part of the patient or nursing staff, (d) conflicts between the patient and the nursing staff, (e) conflicts between the nursing staff and the medical staff concerning the patient's care, (f) conflicts between the patient and his family, (g) failure by the patient or the staff to closely follow the care plan and (h) faulty or inadequate implementation of the care plan.

As you research the reasons why *your* patient has not reached his behavioral objectives, attempt to be as objective as possible about the patient, the nursing staff, the care plan and yourself. Also try to accept the fact that no care plan is perfect and no nursing action is infallible. Most care plans and patient care situations require careful reassessment, problem and error identification, and modification before all or even a majority of a patient's problems can be resolved. The process of care plan modification is briefly considered below.

STEP 5: TAKE CORRECTIVE ACTION AND MODIFY THE CARE PLAN

The nursing care plan and nursing interventions must be corrected and modified if (a) the care plan is failing to help the patient achieve his objectives, (b) the patient's condition has changed or (c) the nursing staff has gained new insights into the patient's background and behavior.

To modify the patient's care plan, the nurse may need to reassess the patient's current status, assets and deficiencies; develop new nursing diagnoses; draw up fresh goals and objectives; update and implement the nursing orders; and evaluate, once again, the patient's progress under the new revised care plan. This cycle of activity then continues until the patient at last achieves the realistic goals which he and the nurse have set together.

BIBLIOGRAPHY

1. Alexander, M. M., and Brown, M. S.: Physical examination: the why and how of examination. *Nursing '73*, 3:25, July 1973.
2. Alexander, M. M., and Brown, M. S.: Physical examination. Part 2: history taking. *Nursing '73*, 3:35, Aug. 1973.
3. Altman, G. B.: Implementation of nursing audit. *Nurse Practitioner*, Jan.–Feb. 1976.
4. Archer, C. O., and Swearingen, D.: Application of Benjamin Franklin's decision-making model to the clinical setting. *Nursing Forum*, 26:319, 1977.
5. Aspinall, M. J.: Nursing diagnosis—the weak link. *Nursing Outlook*, 24:433, July 1976.
6. Assessing vital functions accurately. *In Nursing Skillbook, Nursing '77 Books.* Horsham, Pa., Intermed Communications, 1977.
7. Baer, E. D., et al.: How to take a health history. *American Journal of Nursing*, 77:1190, July 1977.
8. Bailey, J. T., and Claus, K. E.: *Decision Making in Nursing: Tools for Change.* St. Louis, C. V. Mosby Co., 1975.
9. Barba, M., et al.: The evaluation of patient care through use of ANA's standards of nursing practice. *Supervisor Nurse*, 9:42, Jan. 1978.
10. Bates, B.: *A Guide to Physical Examination.* Philadelphia, J. B. Lippincott Co., 1974.
11. Beaumont, E., and Claypool, S.: Have you tried health hazard appraisal? *Nursing '75*, 5:75, May 1975.
12. Becknell, E. P., and Smith, D. M.: *System of Nursing Practice: A Clinical Nursing Assessment Tool.* Philadelphia, F. A. Davis Co., 1975.
13. Benjamin, A.: *The Helping Interview*, 2nd ed. Boston, Houghton Mifflin Co., 1974.
14. Berg, H. V.: Nursing audit and outcome criteria. *Nursing Clinics of North America*, 9:331, June 1974.
15. Berni, R., and Fordyce, W. E.: *Behavior Modification and the Nursing Process*, 2nd ed. St. Louis, C. V. Mosby Co., 1977.
16. Bernstein, L., Bernstein, R. S., and Dana, R. H.: *Interviewing, A Guide for Health Professionals*, 2nd ed. New York, Appleton-Century-Crofts, 1974.
17. Block, D.: Some crucial terms in nursing. What do they really mean? *Nursing Outlook*, 22:689, Nov. 1974.
18. Brown, M. M.: The epidemiologic approach to the study of clinical nursing diagnoses. *Nursing Forum*, 13:346, 1974.
19. Buffaloe, N. D., and Thorneberry, J. B.: *Concepts of Biology: A Cultural Perspective.* Englewood Cliffs, NJ, Prentice-Hall, 1973.
20. Cady, J. W., Freshman, D. J., and Norby, R. B.: *Taking the Pain Out of Care Planning.* Chicago, Medicus/Nursing Care Systems, 1975.
21. Carrieri, V. K., and Sitzman, J.: Components of the nursing process. *In* Marriner, A.: *The Nursing Process: A Scientific Approach to Nursing Care.* St. Louis, C. V. Mosby Co., 1975, p. 8.
22. Ciuca, R. L.: Over the years with the nursing care plan. *Nursing Outlook*, 20:706, Nov. 1972.
23. Copp, L. A.: Improved patient care through evaluation. Part 3: your plan of nursing care. *Bedside Nurse*, 5:25, 1972.
24. Cornell, S. Z., and Brush, F.: Systems approach to nursing care plans. *American Journal of Nursing*, 71:1377, June 1971.
25. Daubenmire, M. J., and King, I. M.: Nursing process models: a systems approach. *Nursing Outlook*, 21:512, Aug. 1973.
26. Delp, M. H., and Manning, R. T.: *Major's Physical Diagnosis*, 8th ed. Philadelphia, W. B. Saunders Co., 1975.
27. Donaldson, S. K., and Crowley, D. M.: The discipline of nursing. *Nursing Outlook*, 26:113, Feb. 1978.
28. Durand, M.: Nursing diagnosis: process and decision. *In* Marriner, A.: *The Nursing Process: A Scientific Approach to Nursing Care.* St. Louis, C. V. Mosby Co., 1975, p. 60.
29. Dutton, C. B., and Steinhart, M. J.: Symptoms—physical or functional? Part 2: psychologic symptoms of organic disease. *Consultant*, April 1977.
30. Easton, R. E.: *Problem-oriented Medical Record Concepts.* New York, Appleton-Century-Crofts, 1974.
31. Eddy, L., and Westbrook, L.: Multidisciplinary retrospective patient care audit. *American Journal of Nursing*, 75:961, June 1975.
32. Eggland, E. T.: How to take a meaningful nursing history. *Nursing '77*, 7:23, July 1977.
33. Ellis, J. R., and Nowlis, E. A.: *Nursing: A Human Needs Approach.* Boston, Houghton Mifflin Company, 1977.
34. Enelow, A. J., and Adler, L. M.: Basic Interviewing. *In* Enelow, A. J., and Swisher, S. N.: *Interviewing and Patient Care.* New York, Oxford University Press, 1972, p. 29.
35. Enelow, A. J., and Swisher, S. N.: *Interviewing and Patient Care.* New York, Oxford University Press, 1972.
36. Francis, G. M.: This thing called problem solving. *In* Marriner, A.: *The Nursing Process: A Scientific Approach to Nursing Care.* St. Louis, C. V. Mosby Co., 1975, p. 5.
37. Fredette, S.: The art of applying theory to practice. *American Journal of Nursing*, 74:856, May 1974.
38. Fuller, D., and Rosenaur, J. A.: A patient assessment guide. *Nursing Outlook*, 22:460, July 1974.
39. Gebbie, K., and Lavin, M. A.: Classifying nursing diagnoses. *American Journal of Nursing*, 74:250, Feb. 1974.
40. Gillies, D. A., and Alyn, I. B.: *Patient Assessment and Management by the Nurse Practitioner.* Philadelphia, W. B. Saunders Co., 1976.
41. Gulko, C. S., and Butherus, C.: Toward better patient teaching. *Nurses' Drug Alert*, 1:49, March 1977.
42. Hardiman, M. A.: Interviewing? Or social chit-chat? *American Journal of Nursing*, 71:1379, July 1971.
43. Helfer, R. E., Weil, W. B., et al.: Interviewing children. *In* Enelow, A. J., and Swisher, S. N.: *Interviewing and Patient Care.* New York, Oxford University Press, 1972, p. 125.
44. Henderson, V.: *ICN Basic Principles of Nursing Care.* London, International Council of Nurses House, 1960.
45. Hoyman, H. S.: Models of human nature and their impact on health education. *Nursing Digest*, Sept.–Oct. 1975.
46. Jarvis, C. M.: Perfecting physical assessment: part 1. *Nursing '77*, 7:28, May 1977.
47. Jarvis, C. M.: Perfecting physical assessment: part 2. *Nursing '77*, 7:38, June 1977.
48. Johnson, D. E.: Development of theory: a requisite for nursing as a primary health profession. *Nursing Research*, 23:372, Sept.–Oct. 1974.
49. Kelly, N. C.: Nursing care plans. *In* Marriner, A.: *The Nursing Process: A Scientific Approach to Nursing Care.* St. Louis, C. V. Mosby Co., 1975, p. 83.

50. Kesler, A. R.: Pitfalls to avoid in interviewing outpatients. *Nursing '77*, 7:70, Sept. 1977.
51. Kraegel, J. M., et al.: A system of patient care based on patient needs. *Nursing Outlook, 20*:257, April 1972.
52. Kratzer, J. B.: What does your patient need to know? *Nursing '77*, 7:82, Dec. 1977.
53. Lambertsen, E. C.: Evaluating the quality of nursing care. *Hospitals, JAHA*, 39:61, Nov. 1965.
54. Langford, T.: The evaluation of nursing: necessary and possible. Supervisor Nurse, 2:65, Nov. 1971.
55. Lee, W.: *Decision Theory and Human Behavior*. New York, John Wiley & Sons, Inc., 1973.
56. Levin, L. S.: Patient education and self-care: How do they differ? *Nursing Outlook*, 26:170, March 1978.
57. Lewis, K. M.: Teaching teamwork: a key to better pre-op teaching. *RN*, 37:61, May 1974.
58. Little, D. E.: Physicians and nurses: a communication gap. *Northwest Medical Journal*, March 1974, p. 3.
59. Little, D., and Carnevali, D.: Nursing care plans: let's be practical about them. *In* Marriner, A.: *The Nursing Process: A Scientific Approach to Nursing Care*. St. Louis, C. V. Mosby Co., 1975, p. 90.
60. Little, D. E., and Carnevali, D. L.: *Nursing Care Planning*. 2nd ed. Philadelphia, J. B. Lippincott Co., 1976.
61. Luciano, K. B.: Components of planned family-centered care. *In* Marriner, A.: *The Nursing Process: A Scientific Approach to Nursing Care*. St. Louis, C. V. Mosby Co., 1975, p. 141.
62. Mager, R. F.: *Goal Analysis*. Belmont, CA, Fearon Publishers, 1972.
63. Mager, R. F.: *Preparing Instructional Objectives*, Palo Alto, CA, Fearon Publishers, 1962.
64. Marram, G. D.: Patients' evaluation of their care: importance to the nurse. *Nursing Outlook, 21*:322, May 1973.
65. Marriner, A.: *The Nursing Process: A Scientific Approach to Nursing Care*. St. Louis, C. V. Mosby Co., 1975.
66. Marshall, J. C., and Feeney, S.: Structured versus intuitive intake interview. *Nursing Research, 21*:269, May–June 1972.
67. Mayers, M. G.: A search for assessment criteria. *Nursing Outlook*, 20:323, May 1972.
68. Mayers, M. G.: *A Systematic Approach to the Nursing Care Plan*. New York, Appleton-Century-Crofts, 1972.
69. Mayers, M., and El Camino Hospital: *Standard Nursing Care Plans*. Stockton, CA, KP Medical Systems, 1974.
70. Mayers, M., and El Camino Hospital: *Standard Nursing Care Plans, Volume II: ICU, CCU, Emergency, Psychiatric, Hemodialysis*. Stockton, CA, KP Medical Systems, 1974.
71. Moidel, H. C., Giblen, E. C., and Wagner, B. M.: *Nursing Care of the Patient with Medical-Surgical Disorders*, 2nd ed. New York, McGraw-Hill Book Co., 1976.
72. Morgan, W. J., and Engel, G. L.: *The Clinical Approach to the Patient*. Philadelphia, W. B. Saunders Co., 1969.
73. Mundinger, M. O., and Jauron, G. D.: Developing a nursing diagnosis. *Nursing Outlook*, 23:94, February 1975.
74. McCain, R. F.: Nursing by assessment–not intuition. *In* Marriner, A.: *The Nursing Process: A Scientific Approach to Nursing Care*. St. Louis, C. V. Mosby Co., 1975, p. 34.
75. McClure, M. L.: The Long Road to Accountability. *Nursing Outlook*, 26:47, Jan. 1978.
76. McFarlane, J.: Pediatric Assessment and Intervention. *Nursing '74*, 4:66, Dec. 1974.
77. McGuire, R. L.: Bedside Nursing Audit. *American Journal of Nursing*, 68:2146, Oct. 1968.
78. McVan, B.: Odors. *Nursing '77*, 7:46, April 1977.
79. Neelon, F. A., and Ellis, G. J.: *A Syllabus of Problem-oriented Patient Care*. Boston, Little, Brown and Company, 1974.
80. Nicholls, M. E.: Quality control in patient care. *American Journal of Nursing*, 74:456, March 1974.
81. Nursing Care Systems: *A Realistic Approach to the Teaching and Implementation of Care Planning*, Chicago, Medicus Systems Corporation, 1975.
82. Nursing Care Systems: *Patient Care Planning Syllabus*. Chicago, Medicus Systems Corporation, 1974.
83. Oelbaum, C. H.: Hallmarks of adult wellness. *American Journal of Nursing*, 74:1623, Sept. 1974.
84. Orovan, S. K.: Patients help plan nursing care. *The Canadian Nurse*, 68:46, Sept. 1972.
85. Palisin, H. E.: Nursing care plans are a snare and a delusion. *American Journal of Nursing, 71*:63, Jan. 1971.
86. Passos, J. Y.: Accountability: myth or mandate? *Journal of Nursing Administration*, May–June 1973.
87. Patient assessment: taking a patient's history: programmed instruction. *American Journal of Nursing*, 74:293; Feb. 1974.
88. Peplau, H. E.: Talking with Patients. *In* Marriner, A.: *The Nursing Process: A Scientific Approach to Nursing Care*. St. Louis, C. V. Mosby Co., 1975, p. 61.
89. Phaneuf, M. C.: The nursing audit for evaluation of patient care. *Nursing Outlook, 14*:51, June 1966.
90. Phaneuf, M. C.: *The Nursing Audit: Profile for Excellence*. New York, Appleton-Century-Crofts, 1972.
91. Plummer, E. M.: The clinical conference discussion leader. *Nursing Forum*, 13:94, 1974.
92. Pope, S. S.: The "problem" of nursing care plans. *Supervisor Nurse*, 8:25, Jan. 1977.
93. Ramey, I. G.: Setting nursing standards and evaluating care. *Journal of Nursing Administration*, May–June 1973.
94. Randolph, B. M., and Bernau, K.: Dealing with resistance in the nursing care conference. *American Journal of Nursing*, 77:1955, Dec. 1977.
95. Richards, N. D.: Methods and effectiveness of health education: the past, present and future of social scientific involvement. *Social Science and Medicine*, 9:141, 1975.
96. Rinaldi, L. A., and Rubin, C. F.: Adding retrospective audit. *American Journal of Nursing*, 75:256, Feb. 1975.
97. Roy, Sister C.: The impact of nursing diagnosis. *Nursing Digest*, Summer 1976.
98. Rubel, Sister M.: Coming to grips with the nursing process. *Supervisor Nurse*, 8:30, Feb. 1976.
98a. Russo, N. G.: Protocol: women's health assessment. *Nurse Practitioner*, 3:23, Aug. 1978.
99. Ryan, B. J.: Nursing care plans: a systems approach to developing criteria for planning and evaluation. *Journal of Nursing Administration*, May–June 1973.
99a. Ryden, M. B.: Energy: a crucial consideration in the nursing process. *Nursing Forum*, 26:71, 1977.
100. Schick, D.: Steps for evaluating patient care. *AORN Journal, 20*:237, Aug. 1974.
101. Sharp, A. E.: Four steps to better patient-teaching. *RN*, 37:62, May 1974.
101a. Shipley, R. H.: Applying learning theory to nursing practice. *Nursing Forum*, 26:83, 1977.

102. Smith, D. M.: Writing objectives as a nursing practice skill. *American Journal of Nursing, 71*:319, Feb. 1971.

103. Smith, D. W., and Germain, C. P. H.: *Care of the Adult Patient: Medical–Surgical Nursing*, 4th ed. Philadelphia, J. B. Lippincott Co., 1972.

104. Snyder, J. C., and Wilson, M. F.: Elements of a psychological assessment. *American Journal of Nursing, 77*:235, Feb. 1977.

105. Staton, T. F.: *How to Instruct Successfully*. New York, McGraw-Hill Book Co., 1960.

106. Stevens, B. J.: Why won't nurses write nursing care plans? *In* Marriner, A.: *The Nursing Process: A Scientific Approach to Nursing Care*. St. Louis, C. V. Mosby Co., 1975, p. 97.

107. Storlie, F.: A philosophy of patient teaching. *Nursing Outlook, 19*:387, June 1971.

108. Storlie, F.: *Patient Teaching in Critical Care*. New York, Appleton-Century-Crofts, 1975.

109. Tabiason, S. J.: The indexes to nursing literature. *Supervisor Nurse, 9*:23, Jan. 1978.

110. Taylor, J. W.: Measuring the outcomes of nursing care. *Nursing Clinics of North America, 9*:337, June 1974.

111. Ulrich, M. R., and Kelley, K. M.: Patient care includes teaching. *Hospitals, JAHA, 46*:59, April 1972.

112. Vitale, B. A., Schultz, N. V., et al.: *A Problem Solving Approach to Nursing Care Plans: A Program*. St. Louis, C. V. Mosby Co., 1974.

113. Waitzkin, H., and Stoeckle, J. D.: The communication of information about illness. *Advances in Psychosomatic Medicine, 8*:180, 1972.

114. Ware, A. M.: Nursing prognosis: a necessary chain to nursing therapy. Accepted for publication in 1978 by *The American Journal of Nursing*.

114a. Wiley, L.: Coping with a seductive patient. *Nursing '78, 8*:41, July 1978.

114b. Wiley, L.: 10 commonsense tips for a better unit. *Nursing '78, 8*:89, March 1978.

115. Will, M. B.: Referral: a process, not a form. *Nursing '77, 7*:44, Dec. 1977.

116. Wolff, H., and Erickson, R.: The assessment man. *Nursing Outlook, 25*:103, Feb. 1977.

117. Wooley, F. R., Warnick, M. W., et al.: *Problem-Oriented Nursing*. New York, Springer Publishing Co., 1974.

118. Yarnall, S., and Atwood, J.: Problem-oriented practice for nurses and physicians. *Nursing Clinics of North America, 9*:215, June 1974.

119. Yura, H., and Walsh, M. B.: *The Nursing Process— Assessing, Planning, Implementing, Evaluating*, 2nd ed. New York, Appleton-Century-Crofts, 1973.

120. Zimmer, M. J.: Guidelines for development of outcome criteria. *Nursing Clinics of North America, 9*:317, June 1974.

121. Zimmerman, D. S., and Gohrke, C.: The goal-directed nursing approach: it does work. *In* Marriner, A.: *The Nursing Process: A Scientific Approach to Nursing Care*. St. Louis, C. V. Mosby Co., 1975.

CHAPTER 18

REPORTING AND CHARTING

By Rosemarian Berni, R.N., M.N.

INTRODUCTION AND STUDY GUIDE

This chapter looks at the value of sharing information for the purposes of implementing high quality patient care and providing legal protection to patients, health care workers and health care institutions. The chapter describes two forms of communication—oral reporting and written documentation. The differences between the source-oriented health care record and the problem-oriented health care record are also considered. The legal aspects of the record are discussed.

The major goals of this chapter are (1) to facilitate the process of communication and (2) to facilitate the process of understanding during health care. "Communication" implies the giving or the exchanging of information, and "understanding" implies that the receiver of the information has comprehended the sender's meaning. Both processes are important for the welfare of the patient (consumer) and the welfare of the health care practitioner (provider). Patients need to receive excellent, safe care, and practitioners need to maintain high quality, safe practices in order to survive in the modern health care system. Students require a clear perspective of both needs. Clear communication is essential in these activities.

The achievement of satisfactory communication and understanding in health care requires certain behaviors of the nurse: (1) to write and speak honestly; (2) to write and speak clearly; (3) to write and speak concisely but thoroughly; (4) to write and speak relevantly; (5) to write and speak systematically; (6) to write and speak from the level of one's competence; and (7) to begin to utilize a systematic recording system for the advocacy of the patient and his nurse.

The following *study guide* is presented to help you meet the objectives of this chapter.

Before you begin reading, ask yourself the following questions:

1. Do I have something important to say when I care for patients?
2. How can I help people *understand* me as well as *hear* me?
3. What happens to the patient if I communicate clearly?
4. What happens to the health care team if I communicate clearly?
5. What happens to me if I communicate clearly?
6. What happens to the progress of health care if I communicate clearly?

As you read the chapter, familiarize yourself with the following terms:

communication
understanding
documentation
accountability
liability
chart
legal record
source record
problem-oriented record
data base
problem list
initial plan
progress notes
flow sheets
audit
computerized charting
reinforcement

Carefully consider the following statements in relation to reporting and charting: (1) personalized, oral communication is useful; (2) organization promotes learning; (3) direct accountability to the patient/consumer is the professional nurse's right and responsibility; and (4) systematic positive reinforcement promotes learning and productivity.

Following your reading of the chapter, attempt to answer the following questions:

1. What is the difference between "reporting" and "recording" in many nursing environments today?
2. What are the benefits and risks of personalized, oral communication?
3. What are the benefits and risks of written communication?
4. What are the benefits and deficiencies of the source record?
5. What are the benefits and risks of the problem-oriented record?

6. What are the four parts of the problem-oriented record?

7. What are the five parts of an initial plan?

8. What are the four parts of the problem-oriented progress note?

9. What is a flow sheet?

10. How can the use of the computer help nurses and patients in the process of record keeping?

11. How can patient and family teaching be evaluated from the record?

12. How can one test the integrity of the written records?

13. How can a systematic record help the patient and the health care team learn?

14. What is the difference between communication and understanding?

15. How do you follow a patient's problem from (a) identification to (b) treatment to (c) response to treatment to (d) modification of treatment?

16. What precautions do you take when writing on a legal document?

COMMUNICATION*

> *Generally the word "reporting" is used for oral communication and the word "documentation" is used for written communication.*

Traditionally, nurses have been assigned tasks orally by the head nurse at change-of-shift time. Much of early nursing's communication patterns consisted of oral, face-to-face instruction and exchange of information. At present, however, a *"change-of-shift report"* may be given during *"walking rounds"* (when staff members walk through a care facility together to visit patients and plan care) or via *audio tape recordings, telephone calls* or *written communication.* It is not uncommon for a mixture of these methods to be used.

A change-of-shift report is the exchange of information by nurses (or other staff members) between shifts or tours of duty, e.g., between nurses who have been on duty during the day and those who are coming on duty to continue the nursing care during the afternoon and night shifts. The major purpose of a change-of-shift report is to provide continuity of nursing care by sharing important patient care information. Information that may be given in a change-of-shift report includes a review of each patient's general condition, problems and special care needs, such as special emotional needs, dietary restrictions, intravenous therapy, significant medication changes, activity and teaching plans, surgical procedures, and prognosis.

> *Discussions about patients should always be conducted in a dignified manner. Conduct this personalized oral communication carefully and quietly in order to protect the patient's privacy.*

---
*Communication is also discussed in Chapter 3; interviewing is discussed in Chapter 17.

It is highly distressing for patients and visitors to overhear staff members "gossiping" or "joking" about their work, e.g., about patient behavior. Such unethical conduct is totally unnecessary and out of place. Nurses serve as role models for nonprofessional members of the health care team. The tone of the nurses' communication is thus important.

Personalized, *oral communication* has many benefits, such as providing the opportunity for immediate response or feedback. Nonverbal communication is also possible with face-to-face reporting. Additionally, people have an opportunity to learn to know each other when they exchange information face to face.

Oral communication is not without problems, however. Careless, lengthy discourse can interfere with quality of care. Even careful, concise oral communication can be forgotten. Since both speaker and listener may have difficulty remembering what was said, responsibility and accountability for actions may be difficult.

Written communication, on the other hand, has the value of permanence, particularly if entries are written in black ink in the permanent chart (patient health care record) on official, permanent record pages. Black ink photographs best and should be used when the chart information will be stored on film for the purpose of conserving space. Written information is accessible to many health care team members and is becoming increasingly available to the patient. *Confidentiality is an absolute requirement.* Nurses are often the only persons who can protect patients' records from unauthorized readers. Another asset of written permanent information is that such information can be *"audited"*; i.e., the record can be analyzed and used as a tool for evaluation of care. (Auditing was discussed in Chap. 17.)

Written information about the health care process is necessary in order for a patient to receive optimum health care. The patient benefits from *coordinated, accurate, complete, cost-effective, competent* and *cohesive* health care over the years. Written records are often the "watch dogs" for such good health care in the same way that written financial ledgers are the "watch dogs" for good business practice. However, this is true only if the written records are of high quality. Fortunately, increasingly better record systems are being developed to improve record keeping as well as to facilitate record auditing.

The patient and his next of kin, or legal advocate, have the right to determine the following information from the patient's record:

▶ Was the care coordinated so that the right people did the right things at the right time?

▶ Was the care accurate? Were the plans of care carried out correctly?

▶ Was the care complete? Was the total plan of care finished?

▶ Was the care cost-effective? Was the care efficient and not wasteful?

▶ Was the care competent? Were personnel properly trained for the care they were providing?

▶ Was there continuity of care? Were the proper referrals made?

The health care provider has the right to determine the same information from the record. Complete records that reflect high quality care can protect a nurse from litigation, i.e., law suits. More important, accurate, complete records help improve quality care by enabling team members to share their expertise and by facilitating the process of clinical research.

> *Nursing recording should be legible, concise, complete, organized, objective, nonjudgmental and competent.*

Figure 18–1 presents two examples of nursing recording. You will observe that Sample A is much less helpful and less precise than Sample B.

Written communication is not without problems, e.g., lengthy run-on sentences, poor penmanship, usage of vague terminology, irrelevant or inaccurate information, or informa-

---

Sample A. General recording and no documentation of a plan.

	Progress Notes
8 PM 11/22/77	Pt. had a better night. She was more cooperative about getting ready for bed. Incontinent of urine just p̄ being assisted to bed p̄ going to toilet. Speaks a little better. J. Jones RN

In Sample A, no flow sheet (tabulated record) was utilized by the nurse.

Sample B. Specific recording and documentation of a plan.

	Progress Notes
8 PM 11/22/77	#4 Urinary incontinence Wet bed approx. 200 cc., 15 min. p̄ toileting c̄ 75 cc. void. Started double-void technique q̄ void trial. See flow sheet (tabulated record) at bedside. J. Jones RN

Sample B flowsheet at the bedside (tabulated record) was utilized by the nurse.

Flowsheet (Patient Problems and Nursing Plans)

Date	#4 Urinary Incont.	#4 →	#5 ↓ ADL	#6 Communication	Comments
	Toilet q̄ 2 h. while awake & record q̄ double-void amount. // Praise each void trial.	Record q̄ incont. amount // Neutral response if pt. is incont.	Teach and record undressing skill h.s.	Review speech bk. c̄ pt. h.s. List new words spoken approp.	
11/22/77		8 PM Approx. 200 cc.	8 PM O.K. except tight slacks	8 PM "toilet"	
11/22/77	10 PM 50 cc. 10:15 PM 150 cc.	0̄			↓J. Jones RN

Figure 18–1. Comparison of nursing records.

tion that might adversely implicate the institution or staff without just cause.

ABBREVIATIONS USED IN CHARTING

Abbreviations are useful in efficient charting, saving time and space and providing a common language. Each facility should display an approved list. The nurse is responsible for seeking out and learning acceptable abbreviations. A partial list of some common abbreviations follows:

LATIN AND GREEK TERMS

Abbreviation	Derivation	Translation
a.	ante	before
a.c.	ante cibum	before meals
ad lib.	ad libitum	at pleasure, as much as one pleases
aq.	aqua	water
b.i.d.	bis in die	twice a day
c, c̄	cum	with
caps.	capsula(e)	capsule(s)
elix.	elixir	elixir
et	et	and
gel.	gelatum	a gel, jelly
gtt.	gutta(e)	drop(s)
h., hr.	hora	hour
h.s.	hora somni	at bedtime
no.	numero	number
noct.	nocte	at night
o.d.	oculus dexter	the right eye
o.l.	oculus laevus	the left eye
o.u.	oculi uterque	each eye
p., p̄	post	after
p.c.	post cibum	after meals
per rect.	per rectum	rectally
p.o.	per os	by mouth
p.r.n.	pro re nata	as needed, as occasion rises
q.	quaque	each, every
q.h.	quaque hora	every hour
q.i.d.	quater in die	four times a day
q.s.	quantum sufficit	as much as is sufficient
Rx	recipe	take thou
s., s̄	sine	without
sig.	signa, signetur	write, let it be written
sol.	solutio	solution
s.o.s.	si opus sit	if necessary
ss, s̄s̄	semis	one-half
stat.	statim	immediately
suppos.	suppositorium	suppository
syr.	syrupus	a syrup
tab.	tabella(e)	tablet(s)
t.i.d.	ter in die	three times a day
tinct., tr.	tinctura	a tincture
ung.	unguentum	an ointment

GENERAL MEDICAL NOTATION

BMR	basal metabolic rate
B/P	blood pressure
c/o	complaint of
CSF	cerebrospinal fluid
CVA	costovertebral angle (or cerebrovascular accident)
D & C	dilatation and curettage
DOE	dyspnea on exertion
GI	gastrointestinal
IM	intramuscular
IV	intravenous
PMD	past (previous) medical doctor
PTA	prior to admission
Px	prognosis
SC	subcutaneous
SOB	shortness of breath
Sx	symptom
TPR	temperature, pulse, respiration
vs	vital signs (B/P and TPR)

TERMS USED IN SPECIALIZED AREAS

Hematology

CBC	complete blood count (includes Hct and WBC count)
ESR	erythrocyte sedimentation rate (reflects inflammation)
Hct	hematocrit (percentage of total blood volume composed of blood cells)
Hgb, Hb	hemoglobin (oxygen-carrying component of RBC's)
RBC	red blood cell
WBC	white blood cell

Chemistry

Cl^-	chloride (an electrolyte)
BUN	blood urea nitrogen (reflects kidney function)
FBS	fasting blood sugar
GTT	glucose tolerance test
2h. p.c. BS	blood sugar level 2 hours after a meal (screening test for diabetes)
HCO_3^-	bicarbonate ion
K^+	potassium (an electrolyte)
Na^+	sodium (an electrolyte)
NPN	nonprotein nitrogen (test of kidney function)
pH	hydrogen ion concentration (reflects acidity and alkalinity of blood)
PT	prothrombin time (test of blood clotting; reflects liver function)
Cl, HCO₃, K, Na or Lites	serum electrolytes (includes chloride, bicarbonate, potassium, and sodium)
UA	urine analysis (shows pH, presence of red or white blood cells or sugar)

Functional Tests

C_{cr}	creatinine clearance (test of renal function)
circ. time	circulation time (test for congestive heart failure)
PBI	protein bound iodine (test of thyroid function)
RAI uptake	radioiodine uptake test (thyroid function test)

Special Tests

CMG	cystometrogram (urinary bladder muscle activity)
ECG, EKG	electrocardiogram (electrical activity of heart)
EEG	electroencephalogram (electrical activity of brain)

EMG	electromyogram (electrical activity of muscle)
LP	lumbar puncture (spinal tap) (for obtaining sample of CSF)
NCV	nerve conduction velocity

X-rays

BaE	barium enema (for lower GI tract)
CUG	cystourethrogram (lower urinary tract)
IVP	intravenous pyelogram (kidney structure and function)
UGI	upper GI series

RECORD-KEEPING SYSTEMS

Two systems of written record keeping used in health care facilities are (1) *the source record* and (2) *the problem-oriented record*. These systems are discussed in the following sections of this chapter. An introductory comparison of the major components of these record-keeping systems is provided in Table 18–1.

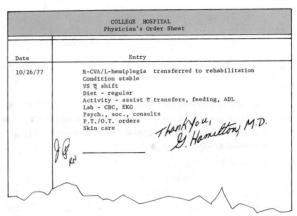

Figure 18–2. Sample physician's order sheet.

The Source Record ("Traditional Chart")

The source record is the traditional chart and is still used by many institutions. Each discipline or department records information on a separate sheet, e.g., physician's order sheet, physician's progress notes, nurse's notes, physical therapy record, x-ray findings, laboratory data. The *advantage* of this organization is that each discipline can easily find the proper place to write its entries. However, *disadvantages* are that the record is fragmented and the entries of various disciplines of the health care team are isolated from each other. In the traditional chart it is difficult to identify (a) the patient's problems and how these problems are being managed in an interdisciplinary manner and (b) the patient's responses to the health care team's problem-solving interventions. Also, information on patient and family teaching and the response to this teaching is often obscured or absent. Finally, a continuous log that has been simultaneously recorded in separate areas of the chart is difficult to audit when the effectiveness of patient care is being evaluated by

TABLE 18–1.   TABULATED COMPARISON OF THE MAJOR COMPONENTS OF THE TRADITIONAL RECORD AND THE PROBLEM-ORIENTED RECORD

TRADITIONAL (SOURCE) RECORD	PROBLEM-ORIENTED RECORD
1. Data base: history, physical examination, etc.	1. Data base: history, physical examination, etc.
2. No formal problem list	2. Formal, numbered problem list
3. No formal initial plans	3. Problem-oriented initial plans and multidisciplinary orders
4. Source-oriented sheets Physician's order sheet Physician's progress notes Nursing notes Physical therapy record Occupational therapy record Respiratory therapy record Enterostomal therapy record Nutritional therapy record	4. Multidisciplinary progress notes
5. Flow sheets	5. Problem-oriented flow sheets
6. Laboratory summaries	6. Laboratory summaries
7. Correspondence	7. Correspondence
8. Discharge and referral summaries	8. Problem-oriented discharge and referral summaries

peers or by auditing officials. A sample physician's order sheet is shown in Figure 18–2.

The Problem-Oriented Record

The problem-oriented record, introduced and developed by Dr. Lawrence Weed, is rapidly replacing the source record as the charting method of choice. The *benefits* of the problem-oriented record arise from the fact that this record is oriented to the patient's needs or problems rather than to the convenience of the health care team's members. The problem-oriented record is an integrated system. When executed properly, this record fosters efficiency, thoroughness, reliability and analysis during patient care.

The four major parts of the problem-oriented chart are (1) data base, (2) problem list, (3) initial plans and (4) progress notes and flow sheets.

Data Base.   The data base is information that is compiled from the nursing and medical histories, the physical examination and all other assessment tools, e.g., laboratory records. (See Chapters 16 and 17 for discussions of these areas.) From this information a patient's specific problems and needs are identified. The data base should list a patient's abilities as well as his disabilities.

Problem List.   The problem list serves as the "table of contents" of the patient's record. As such, it labels problems that interfere with the patient's well-being and quality of life (see Fig. 18–3). These problems may involve signs and symptoms as well as the need for more effective health care team effort. Deficiencies in the

health care system often become problems for the patient.

Each problem on a problem list has a number assigned to it. The numbers indicate the chronological order in which the problems were identified, not the priority or severity of the problem. The problem list is the index or table of contents to a systematic record. If a problem is solved or resolved, a line is drawn through the problem listed and the date of problem resolution is noted (Fig. 18–3). The number attached to a resolved problem is not used for any other problem. For example, in the problem list in Figure 18–3, the patient has the following unresolved problems: #3, right cerebral vascular accident with left hemiplegia; #4, decreased mobility; #5, decreased activities of daily living; #6, ischemic ulcer of the right anterior superior iliac spine; and #7, disposition after discharge from hospital. Problems 1, fractured right humerus, and 2, bowel incontinence, have lines drawn through them because they have been resolved and information about them has become part of the data base, perhaps during a previous admission.

Initial Plans.   The initial plans are the "beginning plans" for problem solution. When a member of the health team enters a problem on the problem list, that person is obligated to write an initial plan, at the writer's level of competency, for the problem's solution or management.

A complete initial plan has five elements: (1) diagnosis, (2) treatment, (3) patient/family/staff education, (4) evaluation of the plan, and (5) the goal, or predicted outcome. We will consider these elements in the following example of a patient with a decubitus ulcer: (1) *diagnosis* includes whatever additional information is currently needed for the diagnosis, such as testing a new patient's ability to use a hand mirror to check the condition of the skin on his buttocks and other bony prominences; (2) *treatment* would involve a skin check $\bar{q}$ h.s.,

COLLEGE HOSPITAL Problem List			
Date of Onset	Number	Problem	Date Resolved
1970	~~1~~	~~Fractured R-humerus~~	1970
1970	~~2~~	~~Bowel incontinence~~	1970
10/13/77	3	R-CVA, L-hemiplegia	
10/26/77	4	↓ Mobility	
10/26/77	5	↓ ADL	
10/12/77	6	Ischemic ulcer, R-ant. sup. iliac spine	
10/26/77	7	Disposition $\bar{p}$ discharge from hosp.?	

Figure 18–3.

washing c̄ soap and water b.i.d., no dressing, etc.; (3) *patient/family/staff education* might include a behavior modification program to reinforce the patient's learning to check his skin for redness regularly with a hand mirror; (4) *evaluation* of the plan requires measuring and recording the circumference and depth of the decubitus ulcer upon admission and thereafter at regular intervals; and (5) the *goal* or *predicted outcome* might state that barring unusual circumstances, this particular decubitus ulcer should heal in 2 weeks.

The goal or predicted outcome is developed from an acceptable standard of treatment; it is not based on the available level of care. Deficient or incomplete treatments due to lack of staff, incompetence, insufficient equipment, insufficient supplies, patient noncompliance, or other problems or complications are noted as barriers to adequate care if they occur as the record unfolds. The goals or predicted outcomes written in a particular problem-solving initial plan are based upon adequate care, not upon substandard care. It is important to write a competent initial plan because this helps the patient and the health care team to guide their efforts in an efficient and logical manner. When the physician starts to write the initial medical plan, a list of medical orders is included (see Fig. 18–2). Orders written by nurses are usually found in their written plans and flow sheets.

Progress Notes. The fourth part of the problem-oriented record is the progress notes (also called "narrative notes"). This section includes information presented in a narrative format and multi-itemed information charted on flow sheets. Progess notes are written for the purpose of modifying the initial and subsequent problem-solving plans or for summary purposes as required by some regulatory bodies. There are four labeled parts to the problem-oriented progress note. These parts are represented by the acronym "SOAP," in which the letters stand for subjective data, objective data, assessment, and plan. *Subjective data* is information from the patient that cannot be measured, e.g., a statement by the patient such as "I'm mad that I have a bed sore!" Objective data is information that can be measured, e.g., "The decubitus ulcer is superficial, round, and 2.5 cm. in diameter. Patient eats protein only for breakfast." *Assessment*, or *analysis*, is the opinion of the health care team member after analyzing the data, e.g., "The slow healing of the decubitus ulcer as measured and recorded on the flow sheet is most likely due to insufficient protein intake." The *plan* has the same elements to be considered as in the initial plan; e.g., is *more information* needed? In the example in Figure 18–4, the nurse does not feel this is necessary and thus has not included that element. Is there need for a *treatment* change? The nurse thinks so and has ordered large portions of protein for the patient at breakfast. Is there need for a change in the *evaluation, education* or *goal* setting elements of the plan? The nurse has written that she has reviewed the need for adequate protein intake with the patient and his friend and has added protein intake monitoring to the flow sheet. She has revised the goal for healing to an additional one week.

Note: The nurse thinks "SOAP" but writes only what is pertinent. If there is no subjective data, none is recorded. Usually a progress note is written only when the plan needs to be modified. Flow sheets usually meet the requirement for ongoing summaries.

Figure 18–5 is an example of a *problem-oriented flow sheet* in which problems are labeled as in the problem-oriented nursing care plan. Examples of other types of flow sheets are temperature, pulse and respiration graphs; diabetic management graphs; and hourly logs of leisure time activities for patients needing to improve their quality of life.

Each time a problem is written about in the progress notes, its number and title are included first. This allows the health care team to easily identify a problem and follow the problem-solving process efficiently instead of searching through pages of unidentified and unorganized narrative script. The team members have the opportunity to learn from each other because their planning and evaluation of implementation of care are included in one organized location, the *patient's* problem-oriented progress notes. The flow sheets help the patient, family and team learn about the progress or lack of progress in the problem-solving process. Flow sheets are often kept on clipboards at the bedside, and patients are able to have active involvement in their own problem-solving process.

The *computer terminal* is becoming a common sight in some health care settings. Patient care information is rapidly stored in computers and is available for instant retrieval. Concise, organized record-keeping methods help nurses utilize computers more easily. On national levels computerized information may become increasingly helpful in health care management because the total population may eventually be utilized as a massive sample for health care research.

		COLLEGE HOSPITAL Progress Notes*
Date/Time	Problem	Notes
10/26/77 2 PM	3	*R-CVA, L-hemi.* Pt. transferred from acute care to rehabilitation. Monitor B/P and TPR q̄ shift.
	4	↓ *Mobility* Review goal of self-transfer training c̄ patient ante each physical therapy session. Help practice *minimal* assisted transfers q̄ transfer c̄ safety belt. Also use safety belt in W.C. for now.
	5	↓ *Activities of daily living* Review goals of self-feeding and self-dressing ante each occupational therapy session. Help practice *minimal* assisted feeding, dressing and undressing when on ward.
	6	*Ischemic ulcer, R-ant. sup. iliac spine* Test ability to use a hand mirror for skin checks. Skin check q̄ h.s. (assist for now). Wash ulcer c̄ soap and water b.i.d., no dressing—monitor size of ulcer. Use special praise h.s. skin checks and keep log for friend and pt. to see. Superficial ulcer should heal in 2 weeks.
	7	*Disposition p̄ discharge from hosp.?* Neighbor reports pt. will be admitted to the Danish Home if he can transfer, feed and dress himself. Goal = success in 3 weeks. R. Brown, R.N.
10/27/77 2 PM	5	↓ *ADL* Holding note. Evaluation and program will follow. Plate guard left in bedside stand. B. Black, OTR
10/31/77 10 AM	6	*Ischemic ulcer, R-ant. s. i. spine* Pt. said, "I'm mad I have a bed sore!" The ulcer is superficial, round, diameter = 2.5 cm and has not ↓ since baseline 10/26/77. Eats protein only at breakfast. Slow healing due to ↓ protein intake. Large portions of protein ordered for breakfast. Reviewed need for protein c̄ patient and friend. Protein intake monitored. Goal = healed by 11/16. M. Smith, R.N.

*Brief description of patient: 87-y-o widowed male found on the floor by neighbor and brought to the hospital 10/13/77 in acute distress. Lives alone, no living relatives.

Figure 18–4.

Problem	#3 R-CVA, L-hemi	#3	#3	#4 ↓ Mobility	#5 ↓ ADL	#6 Ulcer R-AS	#6 Log Protein	Comments
Date	V.S. q shift AM	→ PM	→ noct.	P.T. 11a & 4p Assist self-trans c̄ belt in W.C.	O.T. 9a & 2p Assist self-feed & dress on ward	I Spine Measure qd. Wash bid —air ↑ skin qhs c̄ mirror log at bedside	q̄ d 10/31/77 RB	
10/26/77	37-80-22 120/70 RB	37-82-20 118/70 SS	36-80-18 116/70 BK	RB SS	RB SS	RB 2.5 cm. SS		
10/27	37-84-22 124/72 RB	37-80-20 120/72 SS	37-82-20 114/68 BK	RB SS	RB SS	RB 2.5 cm. SS		
10/28	37-80-20 122/70 RB	37-82-22 122/74 SS	37-80-18 114/68 BK	RB SS	RB SS	RB 2.5 cm. SS		Uses hand mirror well for skin SS
10/29	37-80-22 124/74 JS	37-84-22 124/74 PP	37-80-16 114/70 OO	JS PP	JS PP	JS 2.5 cm. PP		Uses plate guard well JS
10/30	37-82-20 120/70 JS	37-80-20 118/70 PP	37-78-16 116/70 OO	JS PP	JS PP	JS 2.5 cm. PP		
10/31	37-80-20 124/74 RB	37-80-16 116/68 SS	37-80-16 116/70 BK	RB SS	RB SS	RB 2.5 cm. SS	AM—All RB P—0 SS N—0 BK	See progress note RB

Flow Sheet/Progress Notes
Key: RB = R. Brown RN   OO = Olive Olson LPN
SS = Sue Smith RN   JS = Jane Somer
BK = Betty Knight RN   PP = Pat Parker

Name
John Doe

Number
22-33-45

Figure 18–5.

ACCOUNTABILITY*

Nursing has evolved from doing tasks for the physician (a master-servant accountability relationship) to a professional relationship of direct accountability to the consumer of health care, the patient. (Chap. 4 discusses nursing roles.) The nurse's behaviors and records are sometimes reviewed in courts of law. Therefore, the nurse's records must be accurate, clear, complete, concise and permanent, and they must reflect the entire nursing process from assessment to re-evaluations of patient responses. Problem-oriented records, with flow sheets written in ink, provide a system through which nurses are able to systematically describe the nursing process and consumers' responses to that process. Patients' charts are legal records. That is one reason why it is important that the nurse's written actions and written observations of the patient's responses to these actions should not be discarded or altered. Permanent problem-oriented flow sheets help organize large amounts of data in relatively small amounts of space and should be retained in the legal record. Nurses' records reveal the professional nursing process and should be retained for the protection of the patient, the health care system and the nurse.

The question often arises as to whether a nurse should carry out a physician's orders that are merely given verbally instead of being properly written out and signed by the physician. The nurse is responsible for her own actions. If she carries out orders that are not put in writing, there is no evidence that the order was actually ever given by a physician. Legally, the nurse thus becomes *solely* responsible for this action.

Realistically, certain situations (e.g., emergencies) do not permit time for the physician to write out his orders. Verbal orders given by a physician during an emergency should be repeated clearly out loud by the nurse before she takes action. If at all possible, the nurse should jot down in brief script the verbal orders as she carries them out, particularly medication orders. Then, as soon as possible, the verbal orders should be transcribed to the permanent record and signed by the physician. Some nurses request a third person who has heard the physician's verbal orders to cosign the order as a witness. Some hospitals have emergency flow sheets, which are checked off and signed by

*See also Unit V.

emergency team members, thus facilitating the procedure of recording orders and actions.

The nurse is advised to always familiarize herself with the verbal order policies of the setting in which she works and to *always* remember that she is ultimately legally responsible for her own actions.

Intermittent review of record keeping at the time it is being accomplished is useful in demonstrating the integrity of the record and provides an opportunity for immediate recognition of work well done.[11] This is one form of audit.

If initials of nurses are utilized in a patient's record, a key with the complete signatures must be on each page. The record must be concurrent. No blank lines are permitted; thus, any blank space inadvertently present should be crossed off. The chart must be the original record; errors are never blocked out; instead, they are crossed through and signed and dated by the person making the correction.

If the record is *complete* and *organized*, the responses to patient and family teaching will be retrievable because the teaching goals will be documented and the outcomes to the teaching will be found readily under the problems involved.

The legal requirements affecting medical records vary from state to state. Some general practices are enumerated in the following:

1. The record is truthful.
2. The record is complete.
3. The record is legible.
4. The record is confidential.
5. The record is retrievable.
6. The record is comprehensible.
7. The record is a formal document.
8. The record is written in chronological order as to date and time.
9. The record is continuous with no blank spaces.
10. If blank spaces occur in the record, they are crossed out, dated and signed.
11. If errors occur in the record, they are crossed out, dated and signed.
12. Brief corrections of the record are written and signed and dated within the text of that entry.
13. Lengthy corrections of the record are written as amendments.
14. No erasures or blocking-out mechanisms may be applied to the record.
15. The record is written in black ink or typed for better legibility if microfilming is utilized.
16. Only appropriate abbreviations are used in the record.
17. All entries into the record with the exception of data summaries are dated and signed by the author.
18. The person who signs any entry into the record is accountable for the entry.

SUMMARY

Communication implies the giving or the exchanging of information, and understanding implies that the receiver of the information has comprehended the meaning of the sender. Oral communication can be useful for immediate feedback and interchange. Written communication helps prevent misunderstanding or omission and provides a permanent record. A systematic, logical, concise, complete and organized permanent record is useful to all members of the health care team as well as the patient.

BIBLIOGRAPHY

1. Abdellah, F. G., and Chow, R. K.: The long-term care facility improvement campaign: The PACE project. *Association of Rehabilitation Nurses Journal*, Nov.–Dec. 1976.
2. Atwood, J., Mitchell, P. H., and Yarnall, S.: The POR: a system for communication. *Nursing Clinics of North America*, 9:229–234, June 1974.
2a. Baumann, B. A.: The integrated progress record. *Supervisor Nurse*, 8:29, Aug. 1977.
3. Berni, R., and Readey, H.: *Problem Oriented Medical Record Implementation: Allied Health Peer Review*. St. Louis, The C. V. Mosby Co., 1974.
4. Berni, R., and Nicholson, C.: The problem-oriented record: a tool in rehabilitation and patient-teaching. *Nursing Clinics of North America*, 9:265–270, June 1974.
5. Berni, R.: The problem-oriented record. *In* Marriner, A. (ed.): *The Nursing Process; A Scientific Approach to Patient Care*. St. Louis, The C. V. Mosby Co., 1975.
6. Berni, R.: The problem-oriented record and nursing audit. Part I. *The Nurse Practitioner*, 1(1):29–38, Sept.–Oct. 1975.
7. Berni, R.: The problem-oriented record and nursing audit. Part II. *The Nurse Practitioner*, 1(2):79–85, Nov.–Dec. 1975.
8. Berni, R., and Fordyce, W. E.: *Behavior Modification and the Nursing Process*, 2nd ed. St. Louis, The C. V. Mosby Co., 1977.
9. Bloom, J. T., et al.: Problem-oriented charting. *American Journal of Nursing*, 71:2144, Nov. 1971.
10. Bonkowsky, M. L.: Adapting the POMR to community child health care. *Nursing Outlook*, 20(8):515–518, Aug. 1972.
11. Corbus, H. F., et al.: The problem-oriented medical record in long-term facilities: a teaching method. *Journal of Gerontological Nursing*, 3(4):24–31, July–Aug. 1977.
11a. Creighton, H.: The diminishing right of privacy: computerized medical records. *Supervisor Nurse*, 9:58, Feb. 1978.
12. Dinsdale, S. M., et al.: The problem-oriented medical record in rehabilitation. *Archives of Physical Medicine and Rehabilitation*, 51:488, Aug. 1970.
13. Esley, C. E.: Medical records. *Hospitals, J.A.H.A.*, 46:135–140, April 1972.
14. Howard, F., and Jessop, P.: Problem-oriented charting—a nursing viewpoint. *The Canadian Nurse*, 69:34–37, Aug. 1973.
15. Hurst, J. W.: Ten reasons why Lawrence Weed is right. *New England Journal of Medicine*, 284:51, Jan. 7, 1971.
16. Hurst, J. W., and Walker, H. K. (eds.): *The Problem-Oriented System*. New York, MEDCOM Press, 1972.
17. Hurst, J. W., et al.: More reasons why Weed is right. *New England Journal of Medicine*, 288:629, March 22, 1973.
18. Kerr, A. H.: Nurses notes: that's where the goodies are! *Nursing '75*, Feb. 1975.
19. LaVoie, D. J., and Foley, A.: How to make change-of-shift reports more meaningful. *Nursing '73*, 3:55–56, April 1973.
20. Mitchell, P. H.: A systematic nursing progress record: The problem-oriented approach. *Nursing Forum*, 12:187, 1973.
21. Monson, R. A.: The POMR and the physician. *Hospitals, J.A.H.A.*, 49:51–53, April 16, 1975.
22. Niland, M. B., and Bentz, P. M.: A problem-oriented approach to planning nursing care. *Nursing Clinics of North America*, 9(2):235–245, June 1971.
22a. Pepper, G. A.: Bedside report: would it work for you? *Nursing '78*, 8:73, June 1978.
23. Phaneuf, M. C.: *The Nursing Audit: Profile for Excellence*. New York, Appleton-Century-Crofts, 1972.
24. Phillips, D. F.: Medical records: the problem-oriented system. *Hospitals, J.A.H.A.*, 46:84–88, July 16, 1972.
25. Phillips, D. F.: Some POMR criticism clearly misdirected. *Hospitals, J.A.H.A.*, 49:58–61, April 16, 1975.
26. Schell, P. L., and Campbell, A. T.: POMR—not just another way to chart. *Nursing Outlook*, 20(8):510–514, Aug. 1972.
27. Springer, E. W. (ed.): *Automated Mecical Records and the Law*. Pittsburgh, Aspen Systems Corporation, 1971.
28. Thomas, D., and Pittman, K.: Evaluation of problem-oriented nursing notes. *Journal of Nursing Administration*, 72:50, May–June, 1972.
29. Vaughan-Wrobel, B. C., and Henderson, B.: *The Problem-Oriented System in Nursing: A Workbook*. St. Louis, The C. V. Mosby Co., 1976.
30. Wakefield, J. S., and Yarnall, S. R. (eds.): *Implementing the Problem-Oriented Medical Record*. Seattle, MCSA Publications, 1973.
31. Weed, L. L.: Medical records that guide and teach. *New England Journal of Medicine*, 278:593 (March 14) and 278:652 (March 21), 1968.
32. Weed, L. L.: *Medical Records, Medical Education, and Patient Care*. Chicago, Year Book Medical Publishers, 1971.
33. Weed, L. L.: Quality control and the medical record. *Medical Record News*, Oct. 1971.
34. Yarnall, S. R., and Atwood, J.: Problem-oriented practice for nurses and physicians—general concepts. *Nursing Clinics of North America*, 9(2):215–227, June 1974.

INTRODUCTION TO LEGAL CONCEPTS

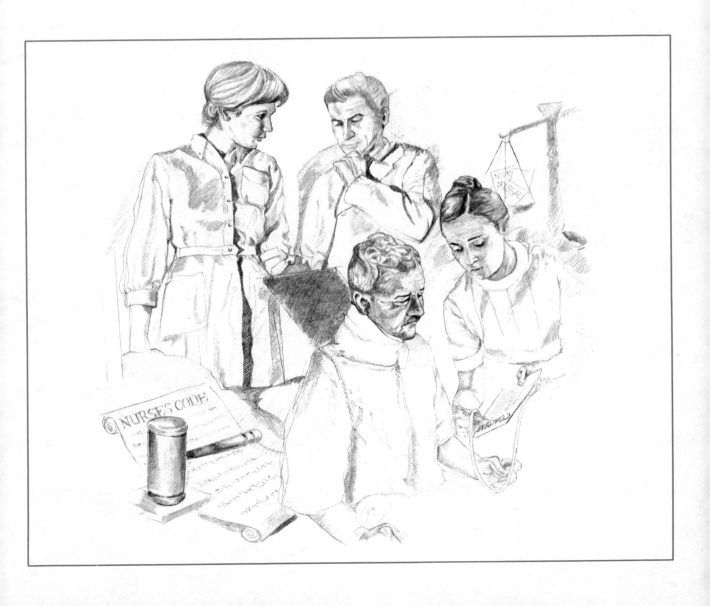

CHAPTER 19

LEGAL AND ETHICAL ASPECTS OF NURSING

By George R. Nock, B.A., J.D.

INTRODUCTION AND STUDY GUIDE

It is not unreasonable for the nurse to think of the law as an enormous pain in the neck. Because the law is a response to human imperfections, it offers constant, unpleasant reminders of our individual imperfections. It also imposes obligations that the nurse might consider distractions from her efforts to give the best possible health care. The other side of the coin is that the law is designed both to prevent human error and, when it occurs, to ameliorate its effects. Properly understood, it can be used as an effective tool to enhance health care. But no matter what you think of it, it is there, and the nurse can no more safely ignore it than a drowning person can ignore water.

One purpose of this chapter is to give the nurse the barest nodding acquaintance with some of the legal principles she is most likely to encounter in the practice of her profession. This chapter fails dismally if it induces any reader to believe that it gives her adequate knowledge of this enormously complex subject. It fulfills its purpose if it enables her to recognize a legal problem and identify the steps she must take—often including consultation with an expert—to solve it.

Ethics are also treated in this chapter, because of their inseparability from law. We will be discussing two kinds of ethics. Professional ethics are those applicable to all nurses, whether they are set out in formal codes or merely part of a common professional understanding. Personal ethics are those of individual nurses, derived from religious beliefs or other professionally unrelated sources, and may not be shared by the profession as a whole. We will explore some areas of potential tension between legal duties and personal ethics.

While reading this chapter, you should try to answer the following questions:

1. How can I protect myself against charges of negligence or malpractice?

2. Why is it legally important for me to keep detailed records and make certain reports?

3. What are the potential legal consequences of failing to obtain the patient's consent to treatment?

4. Why is it important for me to be very careful in discussing a patient's affairs with others?

5. What must I take into consideration in deciding whether to apply restraints to a patient?

6. What kinds of professional conduct may I legally engage in as a student nurse? As a graduate nurse?

7. What should I do if asked to witness a will?

8. What should I do if directed to remove life-support systems from a terminally ill patient?

9. May I legally refuse to participate in an abortion and still keep my job?

SOURCES OF THE LAW

Statutes. When most people speak of "laws," they have in mind those laws enacted by legislative bodies. Such laws are called *statutes* when enacted by Congress or state legislatures, and *ordinances* when enacted by local governing bodies, such as city councils. Statutory law makes up a great deal of the law, and because it is enacted by bodies elected by the people, it is the most democratic part of the law. But statutes are by no means the only important source of the law.

Administrative Regulations. When a legislative body does not have enough information to make necessary detailed regulations of certain kinds of conduct, it often sets up a board or administrative agency, one of whose functions

337

is to devise and issue such regulations. These regulations have the force of law as long as they are not in conflict with other kinds of law. For example, a state legislature may, by statute, create a nurse licensure board. The board will promulgate (officially announce) detailed regulations for the licensure and professional conduct of nurses. These regulations are valid as long as they are within the scope of the board's statutory powers and do not conflict with any statute the legislature might itself enact with respect to nursing practice.

Common Law. Law began in the English-speaking world before there were any statutes. Courts had to decide cases brought before them as best they could. When courts decided individual cases, they often wrote opinions explaining the bases for their decisions, including such legal principles as they were able to devise or discover. Each such opinion in turn became precedent for the decisions of future cases. Over the centuries, a huge body of legal principles was built up. They are collectively known as the "common law," an institution unique to the English-speaking world. The common law is valid to the extent that it is not in conflict with statutory or constitutional law. Most of the legal concepts and principles covered in this chapter were developed through the common law.

Constitutional Law. The United States Constitution states that it is the supreme law of the land. This means that the courts can declare any federal or state statute or other law, or even a state constitution, to be "unconstitutional." This gives the courts, particularly the United States Supreme Court, great power to restrict the rights of Congress and of the states to make laws. The theory is that if the court finds a conflict between a law and the Constitution, the supreme nature of the Constitution requires the courts to refuse to enforce the conflicting law.

AREAS OF POTENTIAL LEGAL LIABILITY FOR THE NURSE

Torts and Crimes. A *crime* is an offense against society. A *tort* is an offense against one or more individuals. Crime is punished by prosecution brought by the state. A tort is redressed by civil action brought by the person injured. This is true even though the same act may be both a crime and a tort. The key to understanding the difference between crimes and torts is to remember the difference between their purposes. The purpose of the criminal law is to protect society; its focus is thus on prevention. The purpose of tort law is to determine whether the victim of an injury should have to suffer its consequences, or whether the person or persons who caused the injury should be required to bear some of the burden of it by paying damages to the victim. The differences of purpose explain many of the differences of approach between criminal and tort law, and should be carefully borne in mind throughout this chapter.

Negligence, Including Malpractice. Negligence is neither a tort nor a crime, but a type of conduct that may form the basis for tort or, less frequently, criminal liability. Negligence is failure to discharge a duty to use reasonable care. There must first be a duty to the victim (or "plaintiff," as he is called if he is the party bringing a lawsuit). A nurse has no legal duty to the public at large to use reasonable care in the practice of her profession. But she does have a duty to her patients and perhaps to others as well. If a person having such a duty fails to discharge it by using reasonable care, he is negligent.

"Reasonable care" is that which would be used by a mythical creature of the law known as the "reasonable man of ordinary prudence." In the nursing context, this refers to that care which would be exercised by a reasonably competent nurse. If the negligence of a person (the defendant) is found to be the legal cause of actual damage to the plaintiff, all the elements are present to make the defendant liable to the plaintiff in tort.

It is important to remember that there is no tort liability for negligence unless the plaintiff is actually damaged. Nurses on countless occasions fail in their duty to use reasonable care toward their patients but escape legal liability because no damage results. A nurse who ignores a patient's signal light for several hours is certainly acting negligently. But if he pressed the button merely because he was bored and wanted to chat with the nurse, he has suffered no legal damage from her negligence. Similarly, even if her negligent behavior contributes to actual damage on his part, if her contribution is too indirect and remote, she will not be liable.

There are countless obvious ways in which a nurse can incur liability for negligence. She may fail to make a timely check of a patient's vital signs, or fail to note or report to a physician certain signs or symptoms that a reasonably competent nurse would know demand attention. She may inject the wrong medication, or the wrong dosage of the right medication, because of a misinterpretation of a physician's order or a misreading of a medication label. Or she may simply be careless in the handling of a patient's property, with the result that the property is lost.

A nurse can also be negligent in some ways that are not so obvious. She is negligent if she assigns a patient-care task to any person who she knows or ought to know is incompetent or not legally qualified to perform that task. For example, if a registered nurse tells a licensed practical nurse to start an intravenous injection in the absence of an RN, she acts negligently. If the LPN misses the vein and damages the patient, the RN is liable to the patient for negligence—in this case, her negligence in assigning the procedure to an unqualified person. Of course, the LPN may also be liable for negligence for accepting the assignment, knowing of her lack of qualifications to perform it.

A nurse may even be negligent in carrying out a clear, direct order of a physician, if a reasonably competent nurse would be expected to question the order. For example, a reasonably competent nurse would not administer what she knows or should know is a lethal dose of a narcotic, no matter what she is told by a physician. Nurses trained in the old school of unquestioning obedience to the physician[2] should be aware that there may be an overriding legal duty to question, or even to refuse to execute, a physician's order. The fact that a physician may be negligent in giving an order does not relieve the nurse of legal liability for carrying it out. Also, the nurse who fails to perform an act she should perform is not relieved of liability simply because a physician negligently failed to leave an order for its performance.

It should be obvious from the foregoing that the nurse may not avoid responsibility by pointing out that someone else's negligence was partly responsible for damage to the patient. Each person whose negligence contributes substantially to damage to the patient is liable for that damage.

The standard of care which a nurse must use in order to avoid being negligent is basically that which a reasonably competent nurse is trained to use. Of course, she has an obligation to keep up with advances in nursing practice, because a reasonably competent nurse does so, and she will be held to the standard of care current in the nursing profession. If she consistently carries out her duties as she has been taught to do, she has little fear of legal liability.

The term "malpractice" should be mentioned. Although it is used by courts, it has no precise legal meaning. Courts and health care professionals alike use it in a variety of senses.

Its two most prominent meanings are (1) negligence in the practice of one's profession and (2) any kind of professional misconduct giving rise to legal liability. The latter is somewhat broader than the former because it includes certain torts, such as assault, battery and false imprisonment, which are at least technically distinct from negligence (see discussion of these torts below). The term "malpractice" is legally superfluous. The legal liability of health practitioners and other professionals is determined by traditional principles of negligence and the various intentional torts; there is no separate theory of malpractice liability.

Gross Negligence. Our discussion of negligence has heretofore centered on "ordinary" negligence, i.e., failure to use reasonable care. There is also a concept known as *gross negligence,* defined, with splendid imprecision, as a gross deviation from the standard of conduct expected of a reasonably prudent person. Conceivably, a nurse's failure, over a period of several hours, to notice a compound fracture in a patient's exposed forearm might constitute gross negligence. Gross negligence has several implications for civil liability, some of which will be discussed below, but it also raises the specter of criminal liability. Ordinary negligence is, for all practical purposes, never the basis for ciminal liability. Gross negligence can be the basis for criminal liability, but only if it results in death or, in some states, a battery (see below). Gross negligence resulting in death is normally manslaughter, a serious crime. Although criminal prosecutions of health practitioners for manslaughter on a theory of gross negligence are rare, they do occur. The nurse should be aware of this possible consequence of a grave breach of her duty to use reasonable care.

Professional Liability Insurance. The best way for the nurse to protect her patients from harm and herself from legal liability is simply to do her job properly. However, if a nurse cannot be certain that she will unfailingly meet the standard of reasonable care, she can protect both herself and her patients from financial loss by carrying malpractice insurance, or as it is more precisely called, professional liability insurance. In exchange for a regular premium, the insurance carrier will provide legal representation to the nurse in the case of a lawsuit and will pay any judgment against her, up to the limits of the policy.

In deciding whether to carry professional liability insurance, the nurse ought to understand another legal concept, called *respondeat superior*. Under this concept, an employer is liable in damages for the conduct of his employee in the scope of the employment, regardless of whether or not the employer personally is negligent or otherwise culpable (at fault). The law regards employees as extensions of the employer, for purposes of liability. Since the employees are advancing the employer's interest, he is responsible for compensating anyone to whom they incur legal liability.

In practice, the doctrine of *respondeat superior* means that if a nurse is a hospital employee and incurs liability for negligence while engaged in hospital business, the hospital will be liable for the damages. *But the nurse is also personally liable* for the full amount of the damages attributable to her. The plaintiff will sue the hospital, the nurse, and everyone else connected with the case. Let us assume that he recovers a judgment against the nurse and the hospital. If the hospital pays the judgment, the nurse's liability is extinguished.

Since hospitals nearly always carry professional liability insurance, the practical effect of *respondeat superior* is that the hospital nurse usually does not have to pay damages for her own negligence. She thus may get away without carrying insurance. Furthermore, some hospitals have insurance policies that specifically cover nurses and other employees as well as the hospital. Such a policy guarantees both to provide legal representation to the nurse and to pay a judgment rendered against her. Even if she works for a hospital providing such insurance coverage, however, the nurse may want to take out her own policy. For the hospital's policy will cover her for negligence only while she is on duty; if she engages in any private practice, including giving medical advice to a friend, that policy will not cover her for liability incurred in the course of such private practice.

It goes without saying that a nurse who has no employer must provide her own insurance coverage if she is to have any insurance protection.

Some nurses feel that they can avoid carrying professional liability insurance because they are "judgment-proof." This means that they do not have enough money or other assets to be able to respond in damages for any civil liability they may incur. Bankruptcy is available for the discharge of most debts, including civil judgments for damages. The bankrupt person gives up all his nonexempt assets, if any, which are divided among his creditors, and is discharged from all his debts. One may obtain a discharge in bankruptcy as often as once every 6 years. In a state having liberal exemption statutes, a person in modest circumstances (most nurses can be so characterized) can often keep all or nearly all his assets and discharge his debts in bankruptcy. Plaintiffs will often not bother to sue nurses who do not have insurance, on the sensible ground that one cannot draw blood from a turnip.

But refusal to carry insurance on the cynical ground that one is too poor to pay damages for one's mistakes raises serious ethical questions. Although no formal ethical principle governs, there is widespread agreement within the profession that a nurse's moral duty to her patients includes a duty to protect them against the financial consequences of her errors. Professional liability insurance provides such protection. The nurse who sees no need for it might question whether she has enough compassion for her patients to be an effective health care worker.

In determining whether to carry professional liability insurance, the nurse should first determine what protection, if any, is provided by her employer. She should then weigh her and her patients' need for coverage against the cost involved. The cost is presently nominal, but could skyrocket, like physicians' insurance premiums, if successful claims against nurses multiply. She should bear in mind that, without insurance coverage, she is responsible, if sued, for her own legal fees. These are always very high, from the nurse's point of view. If she elects to obtain coverage, she should try to get a policy that provides coverage as broad as possible; i.e., "coverage for damages arising out of 'the performance of professional services' by the insured nurse in the practice of her profession."[9] She should make sure that she is not protected merely against "negligence," since a nurse may readily incur liability for conduct that is considered an "intentional tort," and thus outside the realm of negligence.

Professional liability insurance is available at low cost through most associations of nurses or student nurses. Coverage is also available through insurance brokers and agents.

Good Samaritan Laws. Under Anglo-American law, one has no general duty to go to the aid of another in distress. This means that if the nurse (or physician) is driving to work and sees an accident victim at the side of the road, blood welling from his leg, she has every legal right to drive by and let him exsanguinate—

even if she could quite easily stop the bleeding. Indeed, under common law, driving by was the "smart" thing to do; for under common law principles, if the nurse stopped to render aid, she assumed a duty to the victim to use reasonable care and incurred legal liability if her failure to use such care caused damage to the victim.

There are few, if any, cases in which an accident victim sued a physician or nurse who rendered emergency aid without an obligation to do so, but health practitioners were nonetheless fearful of such suits. Perceiving themselves as having nothing to gain and everything to lose from rendering emergency care at the scene of an accident, they often "drove by." To try to change this attitude, most states have passed "Good Samaritan laws," which modify the common law principle by giving immunity from damages for the rendition of emergency aid, except for gross negligence or more serious misconduct. All such laws cover physicians, but only about half cover nurses. Some cover "any person." It should be noted that these laws still create no duty to stop and render aid. Furthermore, they leave open the possibility of liability for serious misconduct. Thus, the only way to be completely safe is still to "drive by."

But once again, ethical considerations intrude. The personal ethics of most nurses, and to a lesser extent, the informal ethical standards of the profession, impel a nurse to use her professional skills in aid of the injured wayfarer, in the manner of the original Good Samaritan (Luke 10:30–37). These laws give her every encouragement to do so. In a state where she is covered by a Good Samaritan law, the nurse has no moral excuse for failing to honor her ethical impulse to render aid.

Reporting Requirements. The law imposes several reporting requirements on the nurse or other health practitioner. The first is the reporting, to appropriate personnel, of accidents in the hospital or other place of employment. The importance of making a prompt report of an accident, from the health care perspective of attempting to lessen the consequences of the accident, is obvious. Even if there is no specific legal duty to make such a report, failure to make it may amount to negligence. The nurse should be aware of other legal aspects of reporting accidents. The report alerts appropriate authorities and thus facilitates the gathering of evidence while it is still fresh. The outcome of a lawsuit may hang on the presence or absence of such freshly gathered evidence. And the report itself, if reduced to writing, may become important evidence in the lawsuit.

The law also imposes specific duties to report certain things to the authorities. Most states now have laws requiring nurses and physicians to report to the local police any suspected cases of child abuse they might observe. Various states have other reporting laws, requiring reports to health authorities of such conditions in newborns or infants as ophthalmia neonatorum or phenylketonuria. Cases of communicable diseases, particularly venereal diseases, may have to be reported. Births out of wedlock or gunshot wounds may be subject to reporting requirements.[4] The nurse should ascertain what reporting requirements exist in her state, county and city and should learn how to fulfill them. If there is no specific reporting requirement, she is under no legal duty (but may be under a moral one) to report anything to the authorities. Statutes that impose reporting duties usually provide some immunity from damages for defamation or invasion of privacy (see below) for those under a duty to make the reports.

Records. Nurses must keep extensive records, particularly patients' charts. Since these records are often the primary means of communication between nurse and physician, their importance in the patient's treatment is obvious. But their legal importance, if less obvious, is no less great. For one thing, failure to keep proper records is plainly negligent and may easily be the basis for tort liability. Failure to note and chart symptoms and signs, or to do so accurately, can obviously impair proper diagnosis and treatment and result in legally cognizable damage to the patient or even to others, such as potential victims of a communicable disease, the symptoms of which a nurse fails to chart.

Records have legal importance in other ways. Witnesses who testify in lawsuits will rely on a nurse's records to refresh their recollection of the events on which the suit is based—events often occurring years before trial. The accuracy of their testimony may depend on the accuracy of their records. Often the witness will be the person who made the records. You may wish to spare yourself the irony of being sued for negligence and losing because you did not make prompt and complete records and therefore could not testify with certainty as to the crucial events.

Finally, the record itself may become evidence in a court of law, as a result of what is known technically as the business records exception to the hearsay rule. In order to qualify for admission in evidence under this rule, the record must have been made in the ordinary course of business, soon after the occurrence of the events recorded. If the court concludes that the record was made at a later time, and particularly if it was made long after the fact and in anticipation of the coming lawsuit, it will be inadmissible. The medical record might be the key evidence supporting the position of the hospital, physician or nurse. Thus, the nurse who fails to keep prompt and accurate records might lose thousands or millions of dollars in a lawsuit for herself, her employers or her associates. Charting may not be the most exciting part of a nurse's job, but she should be properly terrified of the potential consequences of neglecting it.

Assault and Battery. *Battery* is the unconsented touching of another person. It is both a crime and a tort. Assault is also both a crime and a tort, but criminal assault and tort assault use different definitions. A *criminal assault* is an attempt to commit a battery. A criminal battery thus always involves an assault—though an assault does not always involve a battery, since the attempted battery might not be successful. A *tort assault* is intentionally placing one in apprehension of receiving an immediate battery—i.e., making one think he is about to be struck or otherwise receive a battery. A mere threat is not enough.

These terms may not seem to mean very much, but their legal importance for the nurse is enormous. First of all, assault and battery are intentional torts, which means that the person who commits them is legally liable even if the victim is not damaged. Second, virtually any kind of touching of a patient by a nurse or physician is a battery unless the patient consents to it—and the acts leading up to the battery may constitute an assault if the patient realizes what is happening. Thus, the administration of an injection without consent is a battery. The nurse who approaches the unconsenting patient, hypodermic syringe at the ready, commits an assault. Although criminal prosecutions of health practitioners for assault and battery committed during the course of diagnosis or treatment are extremely rare, civil suits for assault or battery under such circumstances are not.

Since virtually all diagnosis and treatment requires some physical contact with the patient, it is obvious that the practitioner's protection against liability for assault or battery depends on the patient's consent to the touching.

Consent is presumed if the patient is an adult (or a child being examined or treated in the presence of a parent or adult guardian), is informed and aware of what the physician or nurse is going to do, and makes no objection. If the patient is unconscious or otherwise unable to communicate, his consent to lifesaving treatment will be presumed in the absence of any indication of lack of consent. Otherwise, the consent must be expressed, and is much more easily proved if given in writing.

Consequently, all hospitals and many clinics and physicians ask patients to sign broadly worded consent forms, which are valid until revoked in some manner. A patient has a perfect legal right to refuse, and a parent or guardian of a minor patient has a perfect legal right to refuse, consent even to routine lifesaving measures, such as blood transfusions.

Occasionally, particularly in the case of a minor, a court will issue an order allowing treatment without consent. Without such an order, actual consent or some special circumstance such as the patient's danger to others, touching the patient is legally actionable. Although a patient whose life was saved by treatment administered over his objection may not recover substantial damages, his ability to win a lawsuit and recover nominal damages may bring endless grief to those responsible for providing such treatment.

False Imprisonment. False imprisonment consists of unjustifiably restraining another person by force or threats of force. It may be a problem for the nurse in two situations. The first arises when a patient wants to leave the hospital and the hospital does not want him to leave, either because his physician advises that he should remain hospitalized or because he has not paid his bill. In *neither case* may he legally be detained by force or threats of force. In the former case, he is customarily asked to sign a statement that he is leaving against medical advice and absolving the hospital of liability for damages caused by his early departure. But he cannot be detained even if he refuses to sign such a statement. And in the latter case, the hospital does not have even an arguable claim to detain him. Telling him that he cannot leave the hospital might, under the circumstances, be construed as a threat of force, and is hence risky.

The other situation concerns the application of restraints. If use of restraints is reasonably necessary to protect the patient or others, it is justifiable, and hence not false imprisonment. At the same time, failure to use restraints when they are required is negligence. But any unnecessary use of restraints constitutes false imprisonment. Application of restraints directly to the patient's body will also amount to a battery, unless there is justification. It is obvious that the nurse must exercise a careful professional judgment concerning the need for restraints. False imprisonment is another intentional tort for which the plaintiff can recover without proof of damage.

Defamation. Defamation is the generic term which includes libel and slander. Both consist of making remarks about another person, to a third person, which tend to degrade or damage the reputation of the object of the remarks. If the remarks are made orally, they are called *slander;* if they are stated in writing, or perhaps on radio or television, they are considered *libel.* Libel, and some cases of slander, give rise to liability even if the plaintiff (the object of the defamation) was not actually damaged. There are two defenses to an action for defamation: truth and privilege. If the defendant can prove that what he said was true, he wins the lawsuit. Even if what he said was not true, he may win if he can show that he was privileged to say it. There are two kinds of privilege: absolute and qualified. A nurse would probably never enjoy an absolute privilege to defame unless she was a witness in a legal proceeding; a witness's statements on the stand are absolutely privileged. But there are circumstances in which she would have a qualified privilege.

A qualified privilege exists when there is a limited communication for a legitimate reason. For example, a nurse might conclude that a patient was suffering from a venereal disease. Disclosure of that to another person would be libel or an actionable slander, for which the patient could recover without showing damage. Quite apart from the defense of truth, however, the nurse who made the disclosure could claim a qualified privilege if she, in good faith, made the disclosure to a physician or supervisor for the purpose of aiding in the treatment of the patient or limiting his social contacts, to the health authorities in accordance with a statutory reporting requirement, or perhaps even to another patient whom she reasonably believed the infected patient was trying to seduce. She would not be privileged if she made the disclosure, over coffee, to a nurse from a different service for the purpose of having a good laugh.

Physicians and nurses have extraordinary opportunities to learn unflattering facts about their fellow human beings. Persons in the health care professions are subject to a clear ethical duty to keep their mouths shut about what they learn, in the absence of a very good reason for disclosing it. The law of defamation, in certain circumstances, makes this duty a legal one as well. Failure to observe it may be very costly to the nurse. The fact that hospitals and physicians' offices are notorious gossip mills does not alter the fact that much of that gossip is both illegal and unethical. As a matter of common decency, ethical obligation and legal prudence, it is well to remember the observation of the person who said, "I've never been hurt by what I didn't say."

Invasion of Privacy. This tort consists of unjustifiably publicizing private or derogatory information about another person, even if the information is true. The defenses are somewhat broader than those applicable to defamation, but obviously truth is not one of them. Generally, there is no invasion of privacy if the material has been recently and widely publicized, if it is legitimately newsworthy, or if the plaintiff is a public figure and has a limited right to privacy.

Nurses are apt to commit this tort in one of two general ways. The first consists of releasing medical information about a patient without his consent. In the case of press releases issued by the hospital giving periodic reports of the condition of a prominent patient, the patient has usually consented and his status as a public figure usually means that there is a legitimate public interest in his condition. But there are limits. Even a President of the United States might justifiably complain about the issuance of a medical bulletin announcing to the world that the President is under observation for tabes dorsalis.

The second consists of simply discussing the patient's medical condition with persons who have no business hearing it. As with defamation, when there is no legitimate reason to disclose certain information about a patient, there is no privilege to do so. Under the tort of invasion of privacy (for which the plaintiff can also recover without proving that he has been damaged), the fact that the information is entirely accurate provides no protection against a successful lawsuit.

Narcotics and Other Controlled Drugs. Here we usually deal not with torts, but with crimes, some very serious. Nurses have special opportunities to commit these sorts of crimes, and a correlative obligation to take special care not to commit them.

There are certain drugs that no one may legally possess, except under certain extremely rare circumstances. They include marijuana and heroin. The nurse has no special opportunities to possess these drugs, since they are not ordinarily to be found in a hospital drug locker. But she should be aware that possession of heroin is normally a felony (a crime carrying a possible prison sentence) and that possession of marijuana is typically a misdemeanor. A conviction for possession of either can do serious damage to a nurse's career.

There are also a number of narcotic drugs that may be legally prescribed by a physician. Possession of such drugs without a prescription is a crime. The nurse's proper role in the administration of such drugs is quite limited: she may administer them solely on the order of a physician. Under most narcotic statutes, she may not possess these drugs for any purpose other than such administration, and may not even "dispense" them. Dispensing is a function reserved to the pharmacist.

With respect to non-narcotic prescription drugs, the nurse's proper legal function is similarly limited to that of administration. It is unfortunately common for hospital nurses to go into the pharmacy and take such drugs when they are needed. This is a risky practice. Though not a serious crime, it would amount to unlawful practice of pharmacy. Even if we assume that a prosecutor would not bring criminal charges under those circumstances, there might be other legal consequences. If the nurse made an error in dispensing the drug, causing harm to a patient, the fact that she was acting in excess of her proper function would be strong evidence of negligence.

THE LEGAL LIMITS OF A NURSE'S FUNCTION

Areas of Nursing Function. Every nurse wants to know the precise legal limits of her proper function. Unfortunately, an exact legal definition of the practice of nursing is not to be had. Most states have statutes (nurse practice acts) that try to define the practice of nursing. But these are deliberately vague because new developments in medicine and nursing change the profession's perceptions of what a nurse can properly do. If a statute were drawn in such a way as specifically to define all areas of nursing practice, the statute would have to be changed frequently—a difficult process—or areas of nursing function would be frozen. The disadvantage of vague statutes is that they offer very little help in resolving many specific questions about what a nurse can and cannot legally do.

Most statutes are based loosely upon the American Nurses' Association model definitions of professional and practical nursing. These generally permit the professional nurse to perform any acts in the observation, care and counsel of patients; health maintenance; supervision of others; or administration of medications and treatments prescribed by physicians or dentists. The professional nurse's functions require substantial specialized judgment and skill, and the knowledge of biologic, physical and social science. Practical nursing permits the performance of "selected acts" of health care and does not require the skill and knowledge required for professional nursing. Neither type of nurse is permitted to make medical diagnoses or to prescribe treatment, although some state statutes permit a professional nurse to make a "nursing diagnosis."[1, 4]

The statutory definition of nursing practice may be supplemented by administrative regulations promulgated by the state board of nursing licensure or registration. When a serious legal question arises as to whether a given act is within the scope of the nurse's function, the state attorney general may render a formal opinion on the question. Such an opinion, while technically not having the force of law, is usually treated by the profession as stating the law.

Finally, the definition of legally permissible nursing practice may be shaped by court decisions. For example, if a patient sued a hospital for damages caused by improper insertion of an intravenous needle by a registered nurse, the question of negligence of the nurse or her supervisor might depend on whether a registered nurse is legally qualified to start intravenous injections. The court's decision on that question would determine the law for that state on whether registered nurses may legally perform that particular function. Similarly, a decision that a physician is necessarily negligent in allowing a licensed practical nurse to administer inoculations constitutes a legal determination that inoculations are outside the scope of a licensed practical nurse's function. Thus, "the operational definition of professional nursing in a particular state is the synthesis of legislation, administrative determinations and judicial decisions."[8] The inevitable consequence of such a system is to leave unanswered, at any given time, questions about the legality of certain acts on the fringes of the nursing function.

Legal Status of the Student Nurse. There is normally no attempt whatever to define by statute the permissible limits of a student nurse's function. She is not a licensed professional nurse, and if she performs a function legally reserved to such a nurse, she is technically guilty of practicing nursing without a license. However, there appears to be no case of prosecution of a student nurse for this offense, and she thus need have no realistic fear of criminal punishment. As long as she discharges her duties under the supervision and direction of a physician or licensed professional nurse, and follows the instructions she is given, she should be quite safe from any charges of unauthorized practice.

But the courts are in agreement that, for purposes of tort liability, if the student nurse is performing the functions of the licensed professional or practical nurse, she is held to the same standard of conduct as such a licensed nurse. This would be a harsh rule if it operated for the purpose of punishing a student nurse who exceeds her proper function. However, although a student who is found liable for damages because she performed the duties of a registered nurse without using the care expected of such a nurse may feel punished, in law she has not been. Remember, the purpose of tort law is not to punish but to determine whether a person who has sustained a loss should be compensated for it. The patient has the right to expect that anyone performing functions legally reserved for a professional nurse will do so as well as a professional nurse should. If his expectations are not fulfilled, and he suffers damage, it makes excellent sense that those responsible for the damage should lift its financial burden from his shoulders.

Nurse Practice Acts. There have historically been two kinds of nurse practice acts. *Permissive* acts provide for registration or licensure of nurses, but allow anyone to practice nursing as long as a title such as "registered nurse" is not used by an unregistered or unlicensed person. *Mandatory* acts require licensure of nurses and forbid the practice of nursing by unlicensed persons. The original nurse practice acts were permissive. But when it became clear that permissive acts, since they did not prevent unqualified persons from practicing nursing, offered no protection to the public, states began to enact mandatory acts. Most, if not all,[3, 4] states now have mandatory acts.

A mandatory act necessarily requires a statutory definition of professional nursing. Such definitions have already been discussed. It should be noted that a definition which is broad enough to provide the necessary flexibility to permit proper development of the concept of the nursing function may be so vague as to give the public no notice of what a nurse legally can and cannot do. If so, the statute becomes unenforceable, as violative of the Due Process Clause of the United States Constitution. For this reason, nursing groups drafting proposed nurse practice statutes or statutory amendments should consult with expert legal counsel, who will advise them of potential constitutional problems.

Licensure. Nurses are licensed by state boards, composed wholly or largely of nurses, whose principal function is determining which persons are legally qualified to practice as licensed nurses. The requirements for licensure as a registered nurse normally include graduation from an approved school of nursing (most schools approved by one state are approved by all states), proof of moral character and attaining a minimum score (the minimum score needed varies from state to state) on a nationally administered examination.

The license must be renewed, for a small fee, at regular intervals. Nurses who fail to renew their licenses on time risk the board's refusal to permit their renewal, or a requirement of retaking the examination. There is a recent trend among the states to require nurses to submit proof of continuing professional education before their licenses will be renewed.

A license may be revoked or suspended by the board for acts of misconduct or even incompetence. The nurse who suffers such revocation or suspension may seek review in the courts to determine the legality of the disciplinary action.

A licensed nurse who moves to a new state is usually licensed to practice in her new state of residence by "endorsement." She need only present her license from her former state of residence, her test score on the national examination and possibly proof of moral character. Some states, however, will not license by endorsement.

The student nurse should decide in which state she wishes to be initially licensed and should make sure that she is preparing to satisfy the licensure requirements of that state. Her school of nursing may offer assistance in ascertaining these requirements, but she has the ultimate responsibility for both ascertaining and meeting them.

SOME SPECIAL LEGAL ASPECTS OF THE NURSE-PATIENT RELATIONSHIP

Wills. Because nurses are intelligent, sober, readily locatable throughout their professional lives, and available when patients begin to realize their mortality, they are often asked to witness wills. Witnessing is a simple procedure. There should be two, or preferably three, witnesses present at the same time. They should all watch the person making the will (the *testator*) sign the will, declare that it is his, and ask the witnesses to witness it. That done, they should sign their names as witnesses in the designated place. It is not necessary for the witnesses to read the will or know its contents. A witness may later be required to testify that the testator signed the will. If the will is contested, the witnesses may be called on to testify as to the testator's apparent mental or physical condition. The testimony of the nurse or other health practitioner will be particularly valuable. Consequently, she should note on the patient's medical record any observable facts bearing on his mental competency to make the will.

A beneficiary of a will must not witness it. If a person named in the will witnesses it, the gift to him is void. This means that you should not witness a will if you know or suspect that you are a beneficiary. In addition, if you are named in a patient's will and are neither a relative nor a long-time friend of the patient, legal and ethical problems will result. If an old man leaves his fortune to his nurse, rather than to his children, the latter will surely contest the will on the theory that the nurse took advantage of the testator's weakened condition and improperly persuaded him to make the legacy. If the nurse has in fact done so, she has obviously committed a grave breach of ethics by abusing her position of trust and confidence. On the other hand, a dying person might readily disdain a group of grasping relatives in favor of a dedicated nurse who may have been the only person in years to show a genuine interest in him. There is no impropriety in her accepting a legacy under such circumstances. The best the nurse can do is to make sure that she gives no one grounds to claim overreaching on her part.

Privileged Communications. The nurse has a clear ethical duty to keep confidential any communication from a patient—particularly if its disclosure would in any way embarrass the patient. Because it is important to the patient's welfare that he frankly communicate any relevant facts about his condition, he should be encouraged to do so by being given assurance that what he says will be treated in confidence. Accordingly, the law in most states recognizes a privilege on the part of the physician to refuse

to testify as to what the patient has told him in confidence. Clergymen, lawyers and others enjoy a similar privilege. Unfortunately, in most states, nurses do not.[5] In a state where she does not have such a privilege, a nurse called upon to testify as to what a patient told her may face an ethical problem. It is not a problem likely to arise often, because in most cases the patient, by putting his medical condition in issue in court, is deemed to have "waived the privilege." But where there has been no waiver, a nurse may find a conflict between what she considers an ethical duty of confidentiality and a legal duty of disclosure. In such a case, she may wish to seek advice of counsel.

If a nurse discloses a confidential communication in response to a direct order of a judge, she will presumably be protected against any charge of breach of professional ethics. But she may feel that her personal ethics require her to keep the communication confidential. If so, she confronts a severe dilemma, because refusal to testify in the face of a direct order to do so is contempt of court, which is punishable by fine or imprisonment. Investigative reporters often face a similar dilemma and thus must decide whether to refuse an order to testify in order to protect the confidentiality of a news source. In such a case, a nurse's lawyer can tell her of her legal rights and obligations, but only her conscience can resolve the dilemma of a conflict between her legal duty and her personal ethics.

EUTHANASIA AND THE "RIGHT TO DIE"

One of the great public and legal controversies of the day concerns euthanasia, in its "active" and "passive" forms. *Active euthanasia* is a euphemism for "mercy killing," i.e., taking positive steps to kill a person in order to end his suffering or for other assertedly noble motives. The legal status of active euthanasia is clear: it is murder. Indeed, it normally fulfills the definition of first-degree murder in that it is a willful, deliberate and premeditated murder. The killer's "noble motives" are legally irrelevant and provide neither justification, excuse, nor mitigation in the eyes of the law. Juries may be reluctant to convict a sincere mercy killer, but his legal status is still that of a murderer. No sensible nurse should have any part in active euthanasia, for she is guilty of murder if she knowingly participates in mercy killing, even under the direct order of a physician.

Passive euthanasia is more complex. This is typically exemplified by the removal of life-support systems in order to allow the patient to die naturally. Its legal status is unsettled. One who removes life-support systems or otherwise discontinues treatment designed to prolong life, with the result that the patient dies, has clearly killed the patient. Whether this killing is criminal depends on whether the killer is under a legal duty to continue the treatment. The legal controversy concerns whether this duty exists. A physician, for example, clearly has no legal duty to treat a person who is not his patient and can thus, with impunity, allow that person to die. But it has been strongly argued that once the physician-patient relationship has begun, the physician (and also the nurse, if there is a nurse-patient relationship) is under a duty to use reasonable means to prolong life. Because a person may not legally consent to his own death, under traditional principles, the physician may not discontinue life-prolonging treatment even if the patient begs him to do so.

The much-publicized recent case of Karen Ann Quinlan[12] attempts to resolve that issue. Quinlan had been comatose for months. In the opinion of her physicians, she would never regain consciousness and would die without the use of life-support systems. Her father asked the physicians to withdraw these systems and allow her to "die with dignity." When they refused, he brought a lawsuit, asking to be named his daughter's guardian (she was not a minor) for the purpose of giving consent to the withdrawal of these systems. Since she was not dead by any medical definition, the question of what legally constitutes "death" for the purpose of allowing discontinuation of treatment was not presented. The state attorney general intervened in the lawsuit, contending that it would be murder to discontinue treatment and announcing his intention of prosecuting the physicians if they did so. The trial court ruled against the father. The Supreme Court of New Jersey reversed the decision. It held that under certain circumstances, a terminally ill person has a constitutional right of privacy broad enough to allow him to withdraw consent to life-prolonging treatment, absolving his physicians of any legal duty to continue such treatment. If the patient is unconscious, a guardian may make the decision to discontinue treatment. The trial court was ordered to appoint the father as guardian and require the physicians to respect and carry out his decision regarding discontinuance of treatment, guaranteeing them immunity from civil or criminal liability for doing so.

This case should be viewed with caution. Although it represents an interpretation of the United States Constitution, it is binding only in the state of New Jersey; the United States Supreme Court has the last word on constitutional interpretation, and it has not acted in this area. This decision also represents a significant departure from traditional legal principles. Any

nurse who is directed to participate in the discontinuance of treatment of a terminally ill person should be aware that she faces some risk of legal liability for doing so unless she acts in response to a valid court order.

A number of persons have signed what are known as "living wills," in which they stipulate that if they become terminally ill, no extraordinary measures should be used to prolong their lives. Unless a state has expressly recognized the validity of such "living wills," their legal status remains uncertain, and nurses should be wary of carrying them out.

ETHICS

Every nurse is guided by two sets of ethics: her own personal morality, as applied to the decisions she makes in the practice of her profession; and the ethics, formal and informal, common to the profession as a whole. Informal ethical standards are not readily capable of being reduced to writing; the nurse absorbs them during her training and practice in the same way she learned as a child to distinguish between right and wrong in her daily life. Formal ethics are represented by written ethical codes. There is no complete agreement on their contents, but the several codes reflect general agreement on basic principles. None of these codes has the force of law, and a violation of a purely ethical standard is not grounds for criminal prosecution. But such a violation may be considered in determining whether to revoke or suspend a nurse's license to practice, and may bear on the question of whether a nurse's conduct amounts to negligence or whether she has forfeited a legal privilege, as in the case of defamation or invasion of privacy. Violation of an ethical code may also subject her to censure, a formal condemnation by her professional association.

There are several formal ethical codes. The best known is the *Code for Nurses* adopted by the American Nurses' Association. Its 1976 version, together with interpretive statements, is provided at the end of this chapter and should be carefully studied. The underlying theme of the *Code* is that the nurse makes her ethical decisions in the interests of her patients and with full accountability to them. One of its primary purposes is to provide a framework for the nurse to make these ethical decisions.

The International Council of Nurses (ICN) first developed and adopted an ethical code for nurses in 1953. The code was revised in 1965 and again at the ICN Congress in 1973. The 1973 revision of the ICN Code is included here:

CODE FOR NURSES—ETHICAL CONCEPTS APPLIED TO NURSING*

The fundamental responsibility of the nurse is fourfold: to promote health, to prevent illness, to restore health and to alleviate suffering.

The need for nursing is universal. Inherent in nursing is respect for life, dignity and rights of man. It is unrestricted by considerations of nationality, race, creed, colour, age, sex, politics or social status.

Nurses render health services to the individual, the family and the community and coordinate their services with those of related groups.

Nurses and People
The nurse's primary responsibility is to those people who require nursing care.

The nurse, in providing care, promotes an environment in which the values, customs and spiritual beliefs of the individual are respected.

The nurse holds in confidence personal information and uses judgement in sharing this information.

Nurses and Practice
The nurse carries personal responsibility for nursing practice and for maintaining competence by continual learning.

The nurse maintains the highest standards of nursing care possible within the reality of a specific situation.

The nurse uses judgement in relation to individual competence when accepting and delegating responsibilities.

The nurse when acting in a professional capacity should at all times maintain standards of personal conduct which reflect credit upon the profession.

Nurses and Society
The nurse shares with other citizens the responsibility for initiating and supporting action to meet the health and social needs of the public.

Nurses and Co-Workers
The nurse sustains a cooperative relationship with co-workers in nursing and other fields.

The nurse takes appropriate action to safeguard the individual when his care is endangered by a co-worker or any other person.

Nurses and the Profession
The nurse plays the major role in determining and implementing desirable standards of nursing practice and nursing education.

The nurse is active in developing a core of professional knowledge.

The nurse, acting through the professional organization, participates in establishing and maintaining equitable social and economic working conditions in nursing.

The nurse must make ethical decisions daily. For some of them, formal codes will provide no definite answer. Each nurse should try to develop a rational basis for making ethical decisions that will further the ends of the profession and enable her to live with her own conscience. Murphy and Murphy have suggested an excellent basis for such decision making: their article is highly recommended to the reader.[7]

Abortion: An Ethical Problem.   There will seldom, if ever, be a conflict between a nurse's professional ethical obligations and her legal duties. The profession would undoubtedly resolve any such conflict in favor of obeying the law. But there might arise conflicts between the law and a nurse's personal ethics. One such conflict, in the area of privileged communications, has already been considered. Another potential conflict lies in the area of abortion. It is useful to consider this question not only because it presents some problems for the individual nurse but also because it provides an illustration of another phase of the legal process.

In 1973, the Supreme Court of the United States held that the constitutional right of privacy gives a woman in the early stages of pregnancy a constitutional right to control her own body to the extent of aborting her embryo or fetus, and that the state has no compelling interest in preventing the abortion which outweighs this right. As a result, any laws prohibiting or regulating abortion, except to the extent that they require the abortion to be performed by a licensed physician, during the first trimester of pregnancy, are unconstitutional and thus may not be enforced. The state has a more substantial interest in controlling abortion during the later stages of pregnancy. Consequently, during the second trimester, the state may regulate abortion in ways reasonably related to the mother's health, and during the third trimester, may prohibit abortion altogether.[10, 13]

Although the Supreme Court has held that a public hospital need not perform abortions on indigent women, thus depriving many such women of any method of actually obtaining an abortion,[11] it is also clear that the state may not interfere in the decision of a woman and her physician that her pregnancy be terminated in its early stages. This raises a question as to the legal rights of the substantial number of health practitioners who have strong personal ethical objections to abortion. The crucial question concerns whether a nurse or physician may constitutionally be fired for refusing to participate in an abortion. The answer is not yet clear, although one court has stated that such a nurse or physician has a constitutional right to refuse to participate.[14]

If the health practitioner's ethical objection to abortion springs from religious belief, he will claim the protection of the right to free exercise of religion guaranteed him by the First Amendment to the United States Constitution. This must be balanced against a pregnant woman's constitutional right, if such there be, to an abortion. Her constitutional right would be meaningless if she could find no one to perform the abortion. A large public hospital with a substantial nursing staff could probably find a number of nurses who would participate in abortions without ethical qualms. In such a case, the hospital would have a very weak justification for firing a nurse who refused to participate. On the other hand, if a gynecologist in private practice, who readily performed abortions in his office, were forced to hire or retain a nurse who refused, on religious grounds, to participate in such procedures, the rights of the physician and his patients would be adversely affected—the physician would have to either hire another nurse for the sole purpose of assisting him in abortions or give up performing them altogether. The courts would be reluctant to state that she had a constitutional right to compel him to do either.

But the courts have not ruled on this problem, and the answer is far from clear. It is mentioned only to illustrate one aspect of the legal process and the importance of the nurse's seeking expert legal advice when confronted with an ethical dilemma of this sort.

CODE FOR NURSES WITH INTERPRETIVE STATEMENTS*

Introduction

The development of a code of ethics is an essential characteristic of a profession and provides one means for the exercise of professional self-regulation. A code indicates a profession's acceptance of the responsibility and trust with which it has been invested by society. Upon entering the profession of nursing, each person inherits a measure of the responsibility and trust that has accrued to nursing over the years and the corresponding obligation to adhere to the profession's code of conduct and relationships for ethical practice.

The *Code for Nurses*, adopted by the American Nurses' Association in 1950 and periodically re-

*Copyright © American Nurses' Association, 1976. ANA Publication Code No. G-56R 25M 4/77.

vised, serves to inform both the nurse and society of the profession's expectations and requirements in ethical matters. The *Code* and the Interpretive Statements together provide a framework for the nurse to make ethical decisions and discharge responsibilities to the public, to other members of the health team, and to the profession. While it is impossible to anticipate in a code every type of situation that may be encountered in professional practice, the direction and suggestions provided here are widely applicable.

The *Code for Nurses* and the Interpretive Statements are both directed toward present-day practice. Previous *Codes* have been more prescriptive, identifying codes of both personal and professional behavior, describing appropriate relationships with physicians and other health professionals, and identifying certain responsibilities of the nurse as a citizen, an employee, and a person. The present *Code*, while remaining prescriptive, depends more on the nurse's accountability to the client, and, in that sense, represents a change to an ethical code.

The requirements of the *Code* may often exceed, but are never less than those of the law. While violations of the law may subject the nurse to civil or criminal liability, the constituent associations may reprimand, censure, suspend, or expel ANA members from the Association for violations of the *Code*. The possible loss of the respect and confidence of society and one's colleagues are serious sanctions which may result from violation of the *Code*. Each nurse has a personal obligation to uphold and adhere to the *Code* and to insure that nursing colleagues do likewise. Guidance and assistance in implementing the *Code* in local situations may be obtained from the American Nurses' Association or its state constituents.

The *Code for Nurses* is based on belief about the nature of individuals, nursing, health, and society. Recipients and providers of nursing services are viewed as individuals and groups who possess basic rights and responsibilities, and whose values and circumstances command respect at all times. Nursing encompasses the promotion and restoration of health, the prevention of illness, and the alleviation of suffering. The statements of the *Code* and their interpretation provide guidance for conduct and relationships in carrying out nursing responsibilities consistent with the ethical obligations of the profession and quality in nursing care.

Code for Nurses with Interpretive Statements

1. **The nurse provides services with respect for human dignity and the uniqueness of the client unrestricted by considerations of social or economic status, personal attributes, or the nature of health problems.**

1.1 SELF-DETERMINATION OF CLIENTS

Whenever possible, clients should be fully involved in the planning and implementation of their own health care. Each client has the moral right to determine what will be done with his/her person; to be given the information necessary for making informed judgments; to be told the possible effects of care; and to accept, refuse, or terminate treatment. These same rights apply to minors and others not legally qualified and must be respected to the fullest degree permissible under the law. The law in these areas may differ from state to state; each nurse has an obligation to be knowledgeable about and to protect and support the moral and legal rights of all clients under state laws and applicable federal laws, such as the 1974 Privacy Act.

The nurse must also recognize those situations in which individual rights to self-determination in health care may temporarily be altered for the common good. The many variables involved make it imperative that each case be considered with full awareness of the need to provide for informed judgments while preserving the rights of clients.

1.2 SOCIAL AND ECONOMIC STATUS OF CLIENTS

The need for nursing care is universal, cutting across all national, ethnic, religious, cultural, political, and economic differences, as does nursing's responses to this fundamental need. Nursing care should be determined solely by human need, irrespective of background, circumstances, or other indices of individual social and economic status.

1.3 PERSONAL ATTRIBUTES OF CLIENTS

Age, sex, race, color, personality, or other personal attributes, as well as individual differences in background, customs, attitudes, and beliefs, influence nursing practice only insofar as they represent factors the nurse must understand, consider, and respect in tailoring care to personal needs and in maintaining the individual's self-respect and dignity. Consideration of individual value systems and lifestyles should be included in the planning of health care for each client.

1.4 THE NATURE OF HEALTH PROBLEMS

The nurse's respect for the worth and dignity of the individual human being applies irrespective of the nature of the health problem. It is reflected in the care given the person who is disabled as well as the normal; the patient with the long-term illness as well as the one with the acute illness, or the recovering patient as well as the one who is terminally ill or dying. It extends to all who require the services of the nurse for the promotion of health, the prevention of illness, the restoration of health, and the alleviation of suffering.

The nurse's concern for human dignity and the provision of quality nursing care is not limited by personal attitudes or beliefs. If personally opposed to the delivery of care in a particular case because of the nature of the health problem or the procedures to be used, the nurse is justified in refusing to participate. Such refusal should be made known in advance and in time for other appropriate arrangements to be made for the client's nursing care. If the nurse must knowingly enter such a case under emergency circumstances or enters unknowingly, the obligation to provide the best possible care is observed. The nurse withdraws from this type of situation only when assured that alternative sources of nursing care are available to the client. If a client requests information or counsel in an area that is legally sanctioned but contrary to the nurse's personal beliefs, the nurse may refuse to provide these services but must advise the client of sources where such service is available.

1.5 THE SETTING FOR HEALTH CARE

The nurse adheres to the principle of non-discriminatory, non-prejudicial care in every employment setting or situation and endeavors to promote its acceptance by others. The nurse's readiness to accord respect to clients and to render or obtain needed services should not be limited by the setting, whether nursing care is given in an acute care hospital, nursing home, drug or alcoholic treatment center, prison, patient's home, or other setting.

1.6 THE DYING PERSON

As the concept of death and ways of dealing with it changes, the basic human values remain. The ethical problems posed, however, and the decision-making responsibilities of the patient, family, and professional are increased.

The nurse seeks ways to protect these values while working with the client and others to arrive at the best decisions dictated by the circumstances, the client's rights and wishes, and the highest standards of care. The measures used to provide assistance should enable the client to live with as much comfort, dignity, and freedom from anxiety and pain as possible. The client's nursing care will determine to a great degree how this final human experience is lived and the peace and dignity with which death is approached.

2. The nurse safeguards the client's right to privacy by judiciously protecting information of a confidential nature.

2.1 DISCLOSURE TO THE HEALTH TEAM

It is an accepted standard of nursing practice that data about the health status of clients be accessible, communicated, and recorded. Provision of quality health services requires that such data be available to all members of the health team. When knowledge gained in confidence is relevant or essential to others involved in planning or implementing the client's care, professional judgment is used in sharing it. Only information pertinent to a client's treatment and welfare is disclosed and only to those directly concerned with the client's care. The rights, well-being, and safety of the individual client should be the determining factors in arriving at this decision.

2.2 DISCLOSURE FOR QUALITY ASSURANCE PURPOSES

Patient information required to document the appropriateness, necessity, and quality of care that is required for peer review, third party payment, and other quality assurance mechanisms must be disclosed only under rigidly defined policies, mandates, or protocols. These written guidelines must assure that the confidentiality of client information is maintained.

2.3 DISCLOSURE TO OTHERS NOT INVOLVED IN THE CLIENT'S CARE

The right of privacy is an inalienable right of all persons, and the nurse has a clear obligation to safeguard any confidential information about the client acquired from any source. The nurse-client relationship is built on trust. This relationship could be destroyed and the clients' welfare and reputation jeopardized by injudicious disclosure of information provided in confidence. Since the concept of confidentiality has legal as well as ethical implications, an inappropriate breach of confidentiality may also expose the nurse to liability.

2.4 DISCLOSURE IN A COURT OF LAW

Occasionally, the nurse may be obligated to give testimony in a court of law in relation to confidential information about a client. This should be done only under proper authorization or legal compulsion. Privilege in relation to the disclosure of such information is a legal right that only the patient or his representative may claim or waive. The statutes governing privilege and the exceptions to them vary from state to state, and the nurse may wish to consult legal counsel before testifying in court to be fully informed about professional rights and responsibilities.

2.5 ACCESS TO RECORDS

If, in the course of providing care, there is need for access to the records of persons not under the nurse's care, as may be the case in relation to the records of the mother of a newborn, the person should be notified and permission first obtained whenever possible. Although records belong to the agency where collected, the individual maintains the right of control over the information provided by him, his family, and his environment. Similarly, professionals may exercise the right of control over information generated by them in the course of health care.

If the nurse wishes to use a client's treatment record for research or nonclinical purposes in which confidential information may be identified, the client's consent must first be obtained. Ethically, this

insures the client's right to privacy; legally, it serves to protect the client against unlawful invasion of privacy and the nurse against liability for such action.

3. The nurse acts to safeguard the client and the public when health care and safety are affected by incompetent, unethical, or illegal practice of any person.

3.1 ROLE OF ADVOCATE

The nurse's primary commitment is to the client's care and safety. Hence, in the role of client advocate, the nurse must be alert to and take appropriate action regarding any instances of incompetent, unethical, or illegal practice(s) by any member of the health care team or the health care system itself, or any action on the part of others that is prejudicial to the client's best interests. To function effectively in the role, the nurse should be fully aware of the state laws governing practice in the health care field and the employing institution's policies and procedures in relation to incompetent, unethical, or illegal practice.

3.2 INITIAL ACTION

When the nurse is aware of inappropriate or questionable conduct in the provision of health care, concern should be expressed to the person carrying out the questionable practice and attention called to the possible detrimental effect upon the client's welfare. When factors in the health care delivery system threaten the welfare of the client, similar action should be directed to the responsible administrative person. If indicated, the practice should then be reported to the appropriate authority within the institution, agency, or larger system. There should be an established mechanism for the reporting and handling of incompetent, unethical, or illegal practice within the employment setting so that such reporting can go through official channels and be done without fear of reprisal. The nurse should be knowledgeable about the mechanism and be prepared to utilize it if necessary. When questions are raised about the appropriateness of behaviors of individual practitioners or practices of health care systems, documentation of the observed behavior or practice must be provided in writing to the appropriate authorities. Local units of the professional association should be prepared to provide assistance and support in reporting procedures.

3.3 FOLLOW-UP ACTION

When incompetent, unethical, or illegal practice on the part of anyone concerned with the client's care is not corrected within the employment setting and continues to jeopardize the client's care and safety, additional steps need to be taken. The problem should be reported to other appropriate authorities such as the practice committees of the appropriate professional organizations or the legally constituted bodies concerned with licensing of specific categories of health workers or professional practitioners. Some situations may warrant the concern and involvement of all these groups. Reporting should be both factual and objective.

3.4 PEER REVIEW

In addition to the role of advocate, the nurse should participate in the planning, establishment, and implementation of other activities or procedures which serve to safeguard clients. Duly constituted peer review activities in employment agencies directed toward the improvement of practice are one example. This ongoing method of review is based on objective criteria, it includes a mechanism for making recommendations to administrators for correction of deficiencies, it facilitates the improvement of delivery services, and it promotes the health, welfare, and safety of clients.

4. The nurse assumes responsibility and accountability for individual nursing judgments and actions.

4.1 ACCEPTANCE OF RESPONSIBILITY AND ACCOUNTABILITY

The recipients of professional nursing services are entitled to high quality nursing care. Individual professional licensure is the protective mechanism legislated by the public to ensure basic and minimum competencies of the professional nurse. Beyond that, society has accorded to the nursing profession the right to regulate its own practice. The regulation and control of nursing practice by nurses' demands that individual professional practitioners of nursing bear primary responsibility for the nursing care clients receive and be individually accountable for their practice.

4.2 RESPONSIBILITY

Responsibility refers to the scope of functions and duties associated with a particular role assumed by the nurse. As nursing assumes functions, these functions become part of the responsibilities or expectations of performance of nurses. Areas of responsibilities expected of nurses include: data collection and assessment of the health status of the client; determination of the nursing care plan directed toward designated goals; evaluation of the effectiveness of nursing care in achieving the goals of care; and subsequent reassessment and revision of the nursing care plan as defined in the ANA Standards of Nursing Practice. By assuming these responsibilities, the nurse is held accountable for them.

4.3 ACCOUNTABILITY

Accountability refers to being answerable to someone for something one has done. It means providing an explanation to self, to the client, to the employing agency, and to the nursing profession. Over and above the obligations such accountability imposes on the individual nurse, there is also a liability dimension to accountability. The nurse may be called to account to be held legally responsible for judgments exercised and actions taken in the course of nursing practice. Neither physician's prescriptions nor the employing agency's policies relieve the nurse of ethical or legal accountability for actions taken and judgments made. Accountability, therefore, requires evaluation of the effectiveness of one's performance of nursing responsibilities.

4.4 EVALUATION OF PERFORMANCE

Self-evaluation. The nurse engages in ongoing evaluation of individual clinical competence, decision-making abilities, and professional judgments. The nurse also engages in activities that will improve current practice. Self-evaluation carries with it the responsibility for the continuous improvement of one's nursing practice.

Evaluation by peers. Evaluation of one's performance by peers is a hallmark of professionalism, and it is primarily through this mechanism that the profession is held accountable to society. The nurse must be willing to have practice reviewed and evaluated by peers. Guidelines for evaluating the appropriateness, effectiveness, and efficiency of nursing practice are emerging in the form of revised and updated nurse practice acts, ANA's Standards of Nursing Practice, and other quality assurance mechanisms. Participation in the development of objective criteria for evaluation that provide valid and reliable data is the responsibility of each nurse.

5. The nurse maintains competence in nursing.

5.1 PERSONAL RESPONSIBILITY FOR COMPETENCE

Nursing is concerned with the welfare of human beings, and the nature of nursing is such that inadequate or incompetent practice may jeopardize the client. Therefore, it is the personal responsibility and must be the personal commitment of each individual nurse to maintain competence in practice throughout a professional career. This represents one way in which the nurse fulfills accountability to clients.

5.2 MEASUREMENT OF COMPETENCE IN NURSING PRACTICE

Competence is a relative term, and an individual's competence in any field may be diminished or otherwise affected by the passage of time and the emergence of new knowledge. This means that for the client's optimum well-being and for the nurse's own professional development, nursing care should reflect and incorporate new techniques and knowledge in health care as these develop and especially as they relate to the nurse's particular field of practice.

Measures of competence are developing; they include peer review criteria, outcome criteria, and ANA's program for certification.

5.3 CONTINUING EDUCATION FOR CONTINUING COMPETENCE

Nursing knowledge, like that in the other health disciplines, is rendered rapidly obsolete by mounting technological advances and scientific discoveries, changing concepts and patterns in the provision of health services, and the increasing complexity of nursing responsibilities. The nurse, therefore, should be aware of the need for continuous updating and expansion of the body of knowledge and skills current. The nurse should assess personal learning needs, should be active in finding appropriate resources, and should be skilled in self-directed learning. Such continuing education is the key to maintenance of individual competence.

5.4 INTRAPROFESSIONAL RESPONSIBILITY FOR COMPETENCE IN NURSING CARE

All nurses, be they practitioners, educators, administrators, or researchers, share responsibility for quality nursing care. Therefore all nurses need thorough knowledge of the current scope of professional nursing practice. Advances in theory and practice made by one professional must be disseminated to colleagues. Since individual competencies vary in relation to educational preparation, experience, client population and setting, when necessary, nurses should refer clients to and/or consult with other nurses with expertise and recognized competencies, e.g. certified nurses and clinical specialists.

6. The nurse exercises informed judgment and uses individual competence and qualifications as criteria in seeking consultation, accepting responsibilites, and delegating nursing activities to others.

6.1 CHANGING FUNCTIONS

Because of the increased complexity of health care, changing patterns in the delivery of health services, continuing shortages in skilled health manpower, and the development acceptance of evolving nursing roles, nurses are being requested or expected to carry out functions that have formerly been performed by physicians. In turn, nurses are assigning some nursing functions to variously prepared ancillary personnel. In this gradual shift of functions, as the scope of practice of each profession changes, the nurse must exercise judgment in seeking consultation, accepting responsibilities, and assigning responsibilities to others to ensure that clients receive quality care at all times.

6.2 JOINT POLICY STATEMENTS

Nurse practice acts are usually expressed in broad and general language in order to provide the necessary freedom for interpretation of the law so that future developments, new knowledge, and changing roles will not necessitate constant revision of the law. The nurse must not engage in practice prohibited by law or delegate to others activities prohibited by practice acts of other health care personnel or by other laws. Recognition by nurses of the need for a more definitive delineation of roles and responsibilities, however, has resulted in collaborative efforts to develop joint policy statements. These statements may involve other health care providers or associations and usually specify the functions that are agreed upon as appropriate and proper for the nurse to perform. Such statements represent a body of expert judgment that can be used as authority where responsibilities are not definitively outlined by legal statute.

6.3 SEEKING CONSULTATION

The provision of health and illness care to clients is a complex process that requires a wide range of knowledge and skills. Interdisciplinary team effort with shared responsibility is the most effective approach to provision of total health services. Nurses, whether practicing in clearly defined or new and emerging roles, must be aware of their own individual competencies. When the needs of the client are beyond the qualifications and competencies of the nurse, consultation must be sought from qualified nurses or other appropriate sources.

Discretion must be exercised by the nurse before intervening in diagnostic or therapeutic matters that are not recognized by the nursing profession as established nursing practice. Such discretion should be based on education, experience, legal parameters, and professional guidelines and policies.

6.4 ACCEPTING RESPONSIBILITES OR DELEGATING ACTIVITIES

The nurse should look to mutually agreed upon policy statements for guidance and direction; but even where such statements exist, personal competence should be carefully assessed before accepting responsibility or delegating activities. Decisions in this area call for knowledge of and adherence to joint policy statements and the laws regulating medical and nursing practice as well as for the exercise of informed nursing judgments.

6.5 ACCEPTING RESPONSIBILITY

If the nurse does not feel personally competent or adequately prepared to carry out a specific function, the nurse has the right and responsibility to refuse. In so doing, both the client and the nurse are protected. The reverse is also true. The nurse should not accept delegated responsibilities that do not utilize nursing skill or competencies or that prevent the provision of needed nursing care to clients. Inasmuch as the nurse is responsible for the client's total nursing care, the nurse must also assess individual competence in assigning selected components of that care to other nursing service personnel. The nurse should not delegate to any member of the nursing team a function for which that person is not prepared or qualified to preform.

7. The nurse participates in activities that contribute to the ongoing development of the profession's body of knowledge.

7.1 THE NURSE AND RESEARCH

Every profession must engage in systematic inquiry to identify, verify, and continually enlarge the body of knowledge which forms the foundations for its practice. A unique body of verified knowledge provides both framework and direction for the profession in all of its activities and for the practitioner in the provision of nursing care. The accrual of knowledge promotes the advancement of practice and with it the well-being of the profession's clients. Ongoing research is thus indispensable to the full discharge of a profession's obligations to society. Each nurse has a role in this area of professional activity, whether involved as an investigator in the furthering of knowledge, as a participant in research, or as a user of research results.

7.2 GENERAL GUIDELINES FOR PARTICIPATING IN RESEARCH

Before participating in research the nurse has an obligation:
1. To ascertain that the study design has been approved by an appropriate body.
2. To obtain information about the intent and the nature of the research.
3. To determine whether the research is consistent with professional goals.

Research involving human subjects should be conducted only by scientifically qualified persons or under such supervision. The nurse who participates in research in any capacity should be fully informed about both nurse and client rights and responsibilities as set forth in the publication *Human Rights Guidelines for Nurses in Clinical and Other Research* prepared by the ANA Commission on Nursing Research.

7.3 THE PROTECTION OF HUMAN RIGHTS IN RESEARCH

The individual rights valued by society and by the nursing profession have been fully outlined and discussed in *Human Rights Guidelines for Nurses in Clinical and Other Research;* namely, the right to freedom from intrinsic risks of injury and the rights of privacy and dignity. Inherent in these rights is respect for each individual to exercise self-determination, to choose to participate, to have full information, to terminate participation without penalty.

It is the duty of both the investigator and the nurse participating in research to maintain vigilance in protecting the life, health, and privacy of human subjects from unanticipated as well as anticipated risks. The subjects' integrity, privacy, and rights must be especially safeguarded if they are unable to protect themselves because of incapacity or because they are in a dependent relationship to the investigator. The investigation should be discontinued if its continuance might be harmful to the subject.

7.4 THE PRACTITIONER'S RIGHTS AND RESPONSIBILITIES IN RESEARCH

Practitioners of nursing providing care to clients who serve as human subjects for research have a special need to clearly understand in advance how the research can be expected to affect treatment and their own moral and legal responsibilities to clients. Here, as in other problematic situations, the practitioner has the right not to participate or to withdraw under the circumstances described in paragraph 1.4 of this document. More detailed guidance about the rights and responsibilities of nurses in relation to research activities may be found in *Human Rights Guidelines for Nurses in Clinical and Other Research.*

8. The nurse participates in the profession's efforts to implement and improve standards of nursing.

8.1 RESPONSIBILITY TO THE PUBLIC

Nursing has the responsibility to admit to the profession only those who have demonstrated a capacity for those competencies believed essential to the practice of nursing. Areas of concern for nursing competence should include adequate performance of nursing skills, academic achievement, humanitarian concern for others, acceptance of responsibility for individual actions, and the desire to improve nursing practice. Nurses involved in the evaluation of student attainment carry a primary responsibility for ensuring that the profession's obligation[s] to the public relative to entry qualifications for practice are met.

The nursing profession exists to give assistance to those persons needing nursing care. Standards of nursing practice provide guidance for the delivery of quality nursing care and are a means for evaluating that care received by clients. The nurse has a responsibility to the public for personally implementing and maintaining optimal standards.

8.2 RESPONSIBILITY TO THE DISCIPLINE

The professional practice of nursing is founded on an understanding and application of a body of knowledge reflected in its standards. As the profession's organization for nurses, ANA has adopted standards for nursing practice, nursing service, and nursing education. The nurse has the responsibility to monitor these standards in everyday practice and through voluntary participation in the profession's ongoing efforts to implement and improve standards at the national, state, and local levels.

8.3 RESPONSIBILITY TO NURSING STUDENTS

The future of nursing rests with new recruits to the profession. Nursing has a responsibility to maintain optimal standards of nursing practice and education in schools of nursing and/or wherever students engage in learning activity. This places a particular responsibility on all nurses whose services are concerned with the educational process.

9. The nurse participates in the profession's efforts to establish and maintain conditions of employment conducive to high quality nursing care.

9.1 RESPONSIBILITY FOR CONDITIONS OF EMPLOYMENT

The nurse must be concerned with conditions of economic and general welfare within the profession. These are important determinants in the recruitment and retention of well-qualified personnel and in assuring that each practitioner has the opportunity to function optimally.

The provision of high quality nursing care is the responsibility of both the individual nurse and the nursing profession. Professional autonomy and self-regulation in the control of conditions of practice are necessary to implement standards of practice as established by organized nursing.

9.2 COLLECTIVE ACTION

Defining and controlling the quality of nursing care provided to the client is most effectively accomplished through collective action. Collective action may include assistance and representation from the professional association in negotiations with employers to achieve employment conditions in which the professional standards of practice can be implemented and which are commensurate with the qualifications, functions, and responsibilities of the nurse. The Economic and General Welfare program of the professional association is the appropriate channel through which the nurse can work constructively, ethically, and with professional dignity. This program, encompassing commitment to the principle of collective bargaining, promotes the right and responsibility of the individual nurse to participate in determining the terms and conditions of employment conducive to high quality nursing practice.

9.3 INDIVIDUAL ACTION

A nurse may enter into an agreement with individuals or organizations to provide health care, provided that the agreement is in accordance with the Standards of Nursing Practice of the American Nurses' Association and the nurse practice law of the state and provided that the agreement does not permit or compel practices which are in violation of this Code.

10. The nurse participates in the profession's effort to protect the public from misinformation and misrepresentation and to maintain the integrity of nursing.

10.1 ADVERTISING SERVICES

A nurse may make factual statements that indicate availability of services through means that are in dignified form, such as:

A professional card identifying the nurse by name and title, giving address, telephone number, and other pertinent data.

Listing name, title, and brief biography in reputable directories and reputable professional publications. Such published data may include the following: Name, address, phone, field of practice or concentrates; date and place of birth; schools attended, with dates of graduation, degrees, and other scholastic distinctions; offices held; public or professional honors; teaching positions; publications; memberships and activities in professional societies; licenses; names and addresses of references.

A nurse shall not use any form of public or professional communication to make self-laudatory statements or claims that are false, fraudulent, misleading, deceptive, or unfair.

10.2 USE OF TITLES AND SYMBOLS

The right to use the title "Registered Nurse" is granted by state governments through licensure by examination for the protection of the public. Use of that title carries with it the responsibility to act in the public interest. The nurse may use the title "R.N." and symbols of academic degrees or other earned or honorary professional symbols of recognition in all ways that are legal and appropriate. The title and other symbols of the profession should not be used, however, for personal benefit by the nurse or by those who may seek to exploit them for other purposes.

10.3 ENDORSEMENT OF COMMERCIAL PRODUCTS OR SERVICES

The nurse does not give or imply endorsement to advertising, promotion, or sale of commercial products or services because this may be interpreted as reflecting the opinion or judgment of the profession as a whole. Since it is a nursing responsibility to engage in health teaching and to advise clients on matters relating to their health, it is not unethical for the nurse to utilize knowledge of specific services and/or products in advising individual clients. In the course of providing information or education to clients or other practitioners about commercial products or services, however, a variety of similar products or services should be offered or described so that the client or practitioner can make an informed choice.

actively seek to promote collaboration needed fo[r] ensuring the quality of health services to all persons.

10.4 PROTECTING THE CLIENT FROM HARMFUL PRODUCTS

It is the responsibility of the nurse to advise clients against the use of dangerous products. This is seen as discharge of nursing functions when undertaken in the best interest of the client.

10.5 REPORTING INFRACTIONS

Not only should the nurse personally adhere to the above principles, but alertness to any instances of their violation by others should be maintained. The nurse should report promptly, through appropriate channels, any advertisement or commercial which involves a nurse, implies involvement, or in any way suggests nursing endorsement of a commercial product, service, or enterprise. The nurse who knowingly becomes involved in such unethical activities negates professional responsibility for personal gain, and jeopardizes the public confidence and trust in the nursing profession that have been created by generations of nurses working together in the public interest.

11. The nurse collaborates with members of the health professions and other citizens in promoting community and national efforts to meet the health needs of the public.

11.1 QUALITY HEALTH CARE AS A RIGHT

Quality health care is mandated as a right to all citizens. Availability and accessibility to quality health services for all citizens require collaborative planning by health providers and consumers at both the local and national level. Nursing care is an integral part of quality health care, and nurses have a responsibility to help ensure that citizens' rights to health care are met.

11.2 RESPONSIBILITY TO THE CONSUMER OF HEALTH CARE

The nurse is a member of the largest group of health providers, and therefore the philosophies and goals of the nursing profession should have a significant impact on the consumer of health care. An effective way of ensuring that nurses' views regarding health care and nursing service are properly represented is by involvement of nurses in political decision making.

11.3 RELATIONSHIPS WITH OTHER DISCIPLINES

The complexity of the delivery of health care service demands an interdisciplinary approach to delivery of health services as well as strong support from allied health occupations. The nurse should

11.4 RELATIONSHIP WITH MEDICINE

The interdependent relationship of the nursing an[d] medical professions requires collaboration around the need of the client. The evolving role of the nurs[e] in the health delivery system requires joint practic[e] as colleagues, deliberations in determining func[-] tional relationships, and differentiating areas of prac[-] tice between the two professions.

11.5 CONFLICT OF INTEREST

Nurses who provide public service and who hav[e] financial or other interests in health care facilities o[r] services should avoid a conflict of interest by refrain[-] ing from casting a vote on any deliberation affectin[g] the public's health care needs in those areas.

CONGRESS FOR NURSING PRACTICE

Ingeborg G. Mauksch, Ph.D., R.N., F.A.A.N., Chairperson
Morris Miller, B.S., R.N., Vice Chairperson
Lucy Brand, M.S., R.N.
Raymond G. Cink, M.P.H., R.N.
Betty Evans, Ph.D., R.N.
Jeanne Margaret McNally, Ph.D., R.N.
Wanda C. Nations, L.L.B., R.N.
Sister Marilyn R. Schwab, M.S.N., R.N.
M. Elaine Wittmann, Ed.D., R.N.

AD HOC COMMITTEE TO REVISE THE CODE

Kathleen Sward, Ed.D., R.N.
Rose C. Dilday, M.S., R.N.
Barbara Durand, M.S., R.N.
Shaké Ketefian, Ed.D., R.N.
Lois R. Jorgenson, B.S.N., R.N.

BIBLIOGRAPHY

a. Beletz, E. E.: Some pointers for grievance handlers[.] *Supervisor Nurse*, 8:12, Aug. 1977.
b. Creighton, H.: Allowing relatives to help patients[.] *Supervisor Nurse*, 9:104, May 1978.
c. Creighton, H.: Countersuits. *Supervisor Nurse*, 9:64[,] Jan. 1978.
1. Creighton, H.: *Law Every Nurse Should Know*[.] Philadelphia, W. B. Saunders Co., 1975.
1a. Creighton, H.: Slander. *Supervisor Nurse*, 9:64, Apri[l] 1978.
1b. Creighton, H.: The right of privacy: cases and research problem. *Supervisor Nurse*, 8:62, Nov. 1977.
2. Crowder, E.: Manners, morals, and nurses; an historica[l] overview of nursing ethics. *Texas Reports on Biolog[y] and Medicine*, 32:173, 1974.
3. De Young, L.: *The Foundations of Nursing*, 3rd ed. St[.] Louis, The C. V. Mosby Co., 1976.
4. Health Law Center: *Nursing and the Law*, 2nd ed[.] Rockville, MD, Aspen Systems Corporation, 1975.
5. Hershey, N.: When is a communication privileged[?] *American Journal of Nursing*, 70:112, Jan. 1970.

5a. Horsley, J. E.: How to keep consent forms from be-
    coming hot potatoes. *RN, 41*:33, May 1978.
6. Kelly, C.: *Dimensions of Professional Nursing;* 2nd ed.
    New York, The Macmillan Co., 1968.
6a. Langford, T.: Establishing a nursing contract. *Nursing
    Outlook, 26*:386, June 1978.
6b. Mancini, M.: Laws, regulations, and policies. *Ameri-
    can Journal of Nursing, 78*:681, April 1978.
6c. McCartney, M. L.: In the witness box: how to give
    nursing testimony, *Nursing '77, 7*:89, April 1977.
7. Murphy, M., and Murphy, J.: Making ethical de-
    cisions—systematically. *Nursing '76, 6*:CG13, May
    1976.
7a. Rozovsky, L. E.: Answers to the 15 legal questions
    nurses usually ask. *Nursing '78, 8*:73, July 1978.
8. Spaulding, E.: *Professional Nursing: Foundations,
    Perspectives and Relationships,* 8th ed. Philadelphia,
    J. B. Lippincott Co., 1970.
9. Williams, B.: How good is your insurance protection?
    Nursing '76, 6:81, Jan. 1976.

Legal Cases

Note: Legal cases are cited according to a special
methodology. First, the name of the case (usually the names
of the plaintiff and defendant) is given. The name is followed by a number representing the volume of the designated reports in which the case will be found. Next is an
abbreviation representing the name of the series of reports.
The number after this abbreviation represents the page on
which the case begins. There may follow, in parentheses, the
date of the case and possibly the designation of the particular court that decided it. The parenthetical information is not
required in finding the case. Sometimes, as in the *Quinlan*
case below, the same case will be found in two series of
reports; either may be used. The meanings of the abbreviations used below are as follows: U.S., United States Reports; N.J., New Jersey Reports; A.2d, Atlantic Reports,
Second Series; F.2d, Federal Reporter, Second Series;
L.W., United States Law Week; S. Ct., Supreme Court
Reporter. Any law librarian will be able to show you how to
find any case you might want to read.

10. Doe v. Bolton, 410 U.S. 179 (1973).
11. Poelker v. Doe, 97 S.Ct. 2391 (1977).
12. *In re* Quinlan, 70 N.J. 10, 355 A.2d 647 (1976).
13. Roe v. Wade, 410 U.S. 113 (1973).
14. Wolfe v. Schoering, 45 L.W. 2149 (6th Cir. 1976).

CHAPTER 20

PATIENTS' RIGHTS

By James C. Hanken, J.D.

INTRODUCTION AND STUDY GUIDE

One purpose of this chapter is to inform the student about the nature of patient rights and to present the theories and analyses that underlie those rights.

Another purpose is to establish that these rights exist apart from a statement published by any organization or professional society. The rights actually spring from the legal relationships or contracts that exist in the situation. The *statement* of patient rights is a method by which those rights can be demonstrated to the patient in order to educate him and to establish for his peace of mind the basis by which he will deal with health care professionals.

The third purpose of this chapter is to present the need for a continued study of the subject of patient rights, recognizing that there is a concern when those rights are stated exclusively by either a provider or user of health care. The object is to help you understand that these rights are arising from a developing area of the law wherein the relationships are constantly being restudied and re-evaluated.

Before you begin your reading ask yourself the following questions:

1. What do the words "patients' rights" mean to me?

2. What have I already read and heard about patients' rights?

3. What rights would I anticipate having should I be admitted to the hospital?

4. How much can I ask of the hospital or the doctor as to the course and conduct of my treatment?

5. Can I be an object of experimentation?

6. May the information accumulated about my care be utilized to develop new and different treatment methods?

You should become familiar with the following terms, which are utilized throughout this chapter:

    informed consent
    malpractice
    privacy
    confidentiality
    patient-physician relationship
    self-determination
    liability
    standard of care

Following your reading, attempt to answer the following questions:

1. Does the potential patient have a right to know in advance what rights are afforded him as a patient at a medical facility?

2. Does the patient have a right to prompt attention in an emergency situation?

3. Does the patient have a right to know the identity and level of professional training of all those providing treatment?

4. Does the patient have a right to have every form that he must sign carefully explained and to have the significance of each consent clarified?

5. Does the patient have a right to a review of his preliminary diagnosis to protect himself against premature labeling of his condition?

6. Does the patient have a right to a clear, complete, and accurate evaluation of his condition?

7. Does the family of the patient have a right to a clear, complete, and accurate evaluation of his condition?

8. Does the patient have a right to a copy of all the information contained in his medical record?

9. Does the patient have a right to a detailed explanation, in layman's terms, of every diagnostic test, treatment, procedure, or operation, including alternative procedures, costs, risks, and the identity and qualifications of the person actually performing the procedure?

10. Does the patient have a right to know whether a particular test or procedure is for his benefit or for educational purposes?

11. Does the patient have a right to refuse any particular drug, test, or treatment?

12. Does the patient have a right to both personal and informational privacy with respect to the hospital staff, other doctors, residents, interns, medical students, any type of researcher, nurses, and other patients?

13. Does the patient have a right to continuity of care by means of access to the doctors who provided treatment while he was in the health care facility?

The most significant movement in the law during the 20th century has been the recognition of individual rights. The first significant situation was the civil rights movement, which had its initial success in Brown v. The Board of Education, 347 U.S. 483 (1953). With this success and under the auspices of the Warren Supreme Court, the rights movement was under way. Although the early successes were in civil rights, it was not long before the movement expanded into other areas. "Women's rights" and "consumer rights" are other expressions that indicate that the law gives recognition to rights of individuals in certain situations identifiable in our society.

A parallel development in recent years has been the beginning of a more general and widespread understanding and concern about the true cost of our health care delivery system. Inasmuch as a patient is a *consumer* of health services, it has followed that the patient has been recognized as a particular type of consumer—with specific rights in this role.

Only recently have these rights been given detailed description. The American Hospital Association (AHA) adopted a "Patient's Bill of Rights" (PBR), which has received widespread approval. Hospitals across the country began to individually formulate particular statements of rights that they present to patients as part of the admission procedure. The report of the Commission on Medical Malpractice[10] recommended that "hospitals and other health care facilities adopt and distribute a statement of patient's rights in a manner which most effectively communicates these rights to all incoming patients." This Commission went on to cite with approval the statement distributed by Boston's Beth Israel Hospital and by Cleveland's Hugh-Norwood Family Health Center. The Joint Commission on Accreditation of Hospitals includes in its current accreditation manual a statement of patient rights that are to be observed by accredited hospitals.[22] Both Minnesota and California have adopted specific statutes recognizing rights for patients.

All these efforts are restatements of rights generally already judicially recognized. What are these rights? Where do we find them?

GENERAL PATIENT RIGHTS

The fact that a "patient's bill of rights" has been proposed or adopted by various government agencies and professional associations does not change the fact that the law already has accorded rights to patients. The law provides that a patient is entitled to proper medical care

from a physician. When proper care has not been delivered, this is described as *malpractice* (Chap. 19). The law provides a patient the right to be informed of the nature of the treatment he is to receive, possible alternatives and the risks to be accepted. This is called *informed consent.*

The analysis behind these legal doctrines is basically simple. Malpractice law requires that a patient is entitled to receive that level of care from the health care practitioner that is ordinarily employed under similar conditions and circumstances by a reasonable man. The doctrine of informed consent stresses that the patient is entitled to full disclosure in terms he can understand about the treatment, risks and alternatives available to him.[24]

However, partially as an outgrowth of the consumer protection movement, a need was felt for a precise statement of rights between the patient and the health care providers. The AHA Patient's Bill of Rights was thus drafted. Where did these rights originate?

Patient rights were originally analyzed from the contractual standpoint. This approach arose from the traditional consensual relationship between physician and patient. Thus the statement of rights covered those rights that a patient could claim based upon the nature of the contractual relationship. The contract was generally an implied one and required the practitioner to provide care consistent with good medical practice. This analytic approach gave rise to the ability to establish contractual limitations upon what can be expected, through an implied limitation of agreements. However, the weakness of this analysis concerns the patient who has not consented to treatment. One such situation is an emergency in which the patient is unconscious and receives medical care. There has been no consensual approach giving rise to an implied agreement. The courts, rather than creating a contract in this situation, have sought to establish a different analysis of the relationship.

Our legal system provides certain basic rights to its participants. These include the rights that flow from the United States Constitution. There are rights that arise from recognized relationships such as husband and wife or landlord and tenant. These relationships create rights and responsibilities. In patient-physician relationships, the situation between the person who is ill and the health care provider is that of dependency and commitment from the patient toward the physician.

Under the patient-physician relationship, a health care practitioner who undertakes to render care to a person thereby creates a professional relationship with a corresponding duty of care to the recipient. This responsibility arises from the dependency of the patient upon the skills and involvement of the health care provider. The law has found that the patient must necessarily place his trust and confidence in the practitioner because of his own lack of knowledge and skill in the field. The courts then place the health care provider in a fiduciary role, requiring him to act with the utmost good faith with the patient in providing the appropriate standard of care.

It is obvious that these legal analyses offer little specific detail that is readily understandable to the layman. The patient wants to know what he can expect from his doctors, hospital, and nurses. This Patient's Bill of Rights is an attempt to list what the patient has a right to expect.

A Patient's Bill of Rights

Approved by the House of Delegates of the American Hospital Association, February 6, 1973

The American Hospital Association presents a Patient's Bill of Rights with the expectation that observance of these rights will contribute to more effective patient care and greater satisfaction for the patient, his physician, and the hospital organization. Further, the Association presents these rights in the expectation that they will be supported by the hospital on behalf of its patients, as an integral part of the healing process. It is recognized that a personal relationship between the physician and the patient is essential for the provision of proper medical care. The traditional physician-patient relationship takes on a new dimension when care is rendered within an organizational structure. Legal precedent has established that the institution itself also has a responsibility to the patient. It is in recognition of these factors that these rights are affirmed.

1. The patient has the right to considerate and respectful care.

2. The patient has the right to obtain from his physician complete current information concerning his diagnosis, treatment, and prognosis in terms the patient can be reasonably expected to understand. When it is not medically advisable to give such information to the patient, the information should be made available to an appropriate person in his behalf. He has the right to know, by name, the physician responsible for coordinating his care.

3. The patient has the right to receive from his physician information necessary to give informed consent prior to the start of any procedure and/or treatment. Except in emergencies, such information for informed consent should include but not necessarily be limited to the specific procedure and/or treatment, the medically significant risks involved, and the probable duration of incapacitation. Where medically significant alternatives for care or treatment exist, or when the patient requests information concerning medical alternatives, the patient has the right to such information. The patient also has the right to know the name of the person responsible for the procedures and/or treatment.

4. The patient has the right to refuse treatment to the extent permitted by law, and to be informed of the medical consequences of his action.

5. The patient has the right to every consideration of his privacy concerning his own medical care program. Case discussion, consultation, examination, and treatment are confidential and should be conducted discreetly. Those not directly involved in his care must have the permission of the patient to be present.

6. The patient has the right to expect that all communications and records pertaining to his care should be treated as confidential.

7. The patient has the right to expect that within its capacity a hospital must make reasonable response to the request of a patient for services. The hospital must provide evaluation, service, and/or referral as indicated by the urgency of the case. When medically permissible a patient may be transferred to another facility only after he has received complete information and explanation concerning the needs for and alternatives to such a transfer. The institution to which the patient is to be transferred must first have accepted the patient for transfer.

8. The patient has the right to obtain information as to any relationship of his hospital to other health care and educational institutions insofar as his care is concerned. The patient has the right to obtain information as to the existence of any professional relationships among individuals, by name, who are treating him.

9. The patient has the right to be advised if the hospital proposes to engage in or perform human experimentation affecting his care or treatment. The patient has the right to refuse to participate in such research projects.

10. The patient has the right to expect reasonable continuity of care. He has the right to know in advance what appointment times and physicians are available and where. The patient has the right to expect that the hospital will provide a mechanism whereby he is informed by his physician or a delegate of the physician of the patient's continuing health care requirements following discharge.

11. The patient has the right to examine and receive an explanation of his bill regardless of source of payment.

12. The patient has the right to know what hospital rules and regulations apply to his conduct as a patient.

No catalogue of rights can guarantee for the patient

the kind of treatment he has a right to expect. A hospital has many functions to perform, including the prevention and treatment of disease, the education of both health professionals and patients, and the conduct of clinical research. All these activities must be conducted with an overriding concern for the patient, and, above all, the recognition of his dignity as a human being. Success in achieving this recognition assures success in the defense of the rights of the patient.

The AHA version of the Patient's Bill of Rights reflects in its twelve separate provisions four general topics:
1. Right to adequate health care
2. Right to information
3. Right to privacy
4. Right to self-determination

The first means that the patient is entitled to that medical attention that is necessary and that the health care provider is capable of rendering. The second is to give recognition that the patient is entitled to receive health care with understanding and knowledge so that he may properly participate. The third provides the patient with the fundamental right of human dignity while going through the indignity of illness. The final aim is to recognize that health care is a *service* the patient desires and requests and not something inflicted on him.

THE RIGHT TO ADEQUATE MEDICAL CARE

The principal legal right any patient has upon entry into a hospital or on becoming the patient of any health care practitioner is the right to receive adequate medical attention. We may ask, however, what is adequate? Does it depend upon the circumstances of each individual case? The fact that the ultimate result is an unfavorable one does not indicate the inadequacy of the treatment.

This right is dealt with rather vaguely in the AHA Patient's Bill of Rights. The very first enunciated right reads that "The patient has the right to . . . care." A later paragraph states that "the hospital must make reasonable response to the request of that patient for services. The hospital must provide evaluation, service, and/or referral as indicated by the urgency of the case" (AHA PBR No. 7). There is also the recognition that "The patient has the right to expect reasonable continuity of care" (AHA PBR No. 10). These statements somewhat tentatively convey the basic recognition that care is the ultimate purpose behind the relationship.

George J. Annas, the Director for the Center

for Law and Health Services of the Boston University School of Law, has stated it much more affirmatively in his proposed bill of rights for patients.[4, 5] The Annas proposal states that a patient has the right to "access to the highest degree of medical care without regard to source of payment for that treatment and care." He adds that the patient has the right "to prompt attention, especially in an emergency situation." This, of course, adds a qualitative factor to the patient's right to care and will be affected by the development and formulation of the PSRO and peer review of health care.

PSRO (Professional Standards Review Organization) and peer review have been imposed by federal legislation as a means of qualitative evaluation of health care. PSRO and in-house peer review mechanisms attempt to monitor and improve the quality of care by (a) studying services as they are provided to the patient and (b) retrospectively analyzing care based on documentation in the patient's medical record.

Fundamentally, all of this is based on the existing law of malpractice, which clearly requires adequate health care. But the law of malpractice is the product of the common law, which means it develops from a case-by-case analysis by the courts. This allows the law to develop a pattern of requirements that will be imposed upon the health professions from each new factual situation brought to court. It would seem to be in the best interests of the health professions to formulate a clear, accurate, precise and enforceable statement of the patient's right to adequate medical treatment. This would establish a standard that would not be changed with each new case. If the health professions provided a clear and intelligible statement of the patient's right to adequate care, the courts would be more ready to use such a statement than the rather vague statements that exist in the AHA version.

THE RIGHT TO INFORMATION

One of the most frequently cited causes for malpractice litigation has been the ignorance of the patient as to what he has undergone and his inability to obtain information about it. A confused and uninformed patient who has a bad result is likely to be a patient who will commence litigation. He may attack by a malpractice action or by a claim that he never gave informed consent. Informed consent, discussed above, has been identified in the AHA Patient's Bill of Rights as a fundamental right of the patient.

However, one criticism of the AHA version of the Patient's Bill of Rights has been that in it the responsibility to supply information to the patient lies with the physician without any recognition of the hospital's responsibility in this respect. The statement of patients' rights formulated by George J. Annas, mentioned earlier, provides stronger emphasis on the responsibility of the hospital.[4, 5] In addition Annas would establish a patients' rights advocate as a part of hospital procedure. The purpose of this advocate is to represent the interest of the patient to the institution in an ombudsman fashion. Annas proposes that the hospital has a responsibility to provide a mechanism for the implementation of patients' right under any rights proposal.

One of the most controversial rights often discussed was not provided for in the AHA version. This is the right of the patient to receive a copy of his medical record at the conclusion of his treatment, for his own use or information. Several states require that this be provided. Annas has clearly stated that the patient has this right. This is one of the areas in which substantial development is still under way. It certainly appears that the trend is toward providing a patient with access to his own individual records, although this is not a uniformly recognized right.

The HEW report on medical malpractice has explicitly stated in its recommendation the following:

> The commission finds that patients have a right to the information contained in their medical records and recommends that such information be made more easily accessible to the patients and the commission further recommends that states enact legislation enabling patients to obtain access to the information contained in their medical records through their legal representatives, public or private, without having to file a suit.[10]

The AHA Patient's Bill of Rights explicitly confirms that the patient is entitled to know the basis on which charges are made for his treatment, whether or not he is responsible for those charges (AHA PBR No. 11). Furthermore, the patient is entitled to know the individual relationships between those professionals who are working in conjunction to provide his treat-ment (AHA PBR No. 8). Thus the statement provides an explicit expression and recognition of patients' rights in this regard.

THE RIGHT TO PRIVACY

A patient coming to a hospital is generally ill and is thus in an emotionally and psychologically vulnerable position. His very role as a patient makes him subject to emotional and psychologic damage. The patient needs to be protected in this situation through the recognition of his basic human dignity and by according him privacy and courtesy.

The various patients' bills of rights have all given some recognition to this essential ingredient. The AHA version commences with the recognition that the patient is entitled to "considerate and respectful care" (AHA PBR No. 1). It goes on to provide that the patient is to receive "every consideration of his privacy concerning his own medical care program" (AHA PBR No. 5). It also requires those not directly involved with his care have to have the express consent of the patient to be present (AHA PBR No. 5). Furthermore, it requires that all communications and records be kept confidential (AHA PBR No. 6).

These statements underline the application of the right of privacy in the hospital setting. The concept of the right of privacy is a very recent development in law. It fundamentally springs from the recognition that the individual's dignity is legally protected. The development of this concept has been widespread in recent years. It has been given constitutional underpinnings in the abortion[33] and birth control[19] cases.

In 1973 in Roe v. Wade, 410 U.S. 113 (1973), the United States Supreme Court, basing its decision on a fundamental constitutional right of privacy, authorized abortions despite criminal laws to the contrary. This statement of individual dignity and right of self-determination must be recognized as having even broader application than as applied in that case.

Based on these concepts, the statement of these rights in the AHA Patient's Bill of Rights provides a sound expression of what should be available to the patient. There are two fundamental protections. First, the health care provider must maintain the confidentiality of information concerning the individual. Second, the basic human dignity of a person is not to be lowered or diminished by making him a subject of experimentation, a teaching tool for medical students, or a "thing" to be treated without his permission and approval. While the busy modern health practitioner may be applauded for his efficiency in clinical practice, the loss of human involvement and personal relationships has created an element of distance and lack of warmth that gives rise to potential litigation.

THE RIGHT OF SELF-DETERMINATION

An individual who comes to the health care professional for treatment is by that decision placing himself in the hands of professionals for consideration and judgment as to what treatment should be carried out. However, this does not imply a surrender of the power to make decisions or a surrender of the right of determination. Thus, all decisions that affect bodily or emotional health of the patient must be the choice of the patient. In other words, the patient must consent to his treatment and has the right to refuse treatment. He especially is entitled to refuse to become an object of experimentation and education of learning professionals. This right is thus closely allied with the right of information.

The AHA Patient's Bill of Rights gives specific recognition to these principles (AHA PBR Nos. 3, 4, 9). The purpose behind the recognition of the patient's right to self-determination is to acknowledge that the patient is the proper decision maker. The fact that the doctor possesses superior knowledge does not transfer the decision-making process to him. It is the duty of the doctor to adequately inform the patient of what is involved and to permit the patient to make the decisions. It is the patient's right to refuse treatment and to terminate his stay in a hospital. There is no public duty imposed on a patient to become a basis for experimentation or a visual aid for education. It is true that experimentation and education have a significant role in health care delivery, but the patient's right to willingly and knowingly participate must be respected.

These rights have unfortunately been sometimes ignored in the past. Revelations of government-sponsored medical experiments performed without consent and frequently without even informing the patient are shocking and are contrary to these rights.

CONCLUSION

The relationship between the patient and the health care professionals is a consensual relationship. Through that relationship the patient seeks the aid and assistance of the health care delivery system to better his physical or psychological well-being. In seeking this assistance, he does not surrender his basic rights. In fact he has the right to anticipate adequate health care, the right to full disclosure of all information that affects his well-being, the right to determine the course of action that will affect his well-being and the right to maintain his integrity as a person in our society. These basic rights cannot be withdrawn or withheld. Any system for the delivery of health care must recognize and encourage these rights.

BIBLIOGRAPHY

1. Abdellah, F. G.: Approaches to protecting the rights of human subjects. *Nursing Research*, 16:316, 1967.
2. American Hospital Association: *A Patient's Bill of Rights*, 1972.
3. American Nurses' Association: *The Nurse in Research: ANA Guidelines on Ethical Values*, 1968.
4. Annas, G. J.: The patient rights advocate; can nurses effectively fill the role? *Supervisor Nurse*, 5:20, 1974.
5. Annas, G. J., and Healy, F. X.: The Patient Rights Advocate: Redefining the Doctor-Patient Relationship in the Hospital Context. *Vanderbilt Law Review*, 27:243, 1974.
6. Baldwin: Confidentiality between physician and patient. Maryland Law Review, 22:181, 1962.
7. Bastiansen, S.: Psychotherapy and the autonomy of the individual. *Psychotherapy and Psychosomatics*, 24:399, 1974.
8. Battistella, R. M.: The right to adequate health care. *Nursing Digest*, 4:13, 1976.
9. Bernstein, A. H.: Law in brief: access to physician's hospital records. *Hospitals, J.A.H.A.*, 45:148, 1971.
10. Department of Health, Education and Welfare, Pub. No. OS73–88, *Report of the Secretary's Commission on Medical Malpractice*, 1973.
11. Dornette, W. H.: Medical records. *Clinical Anesthesia*, 8:285, 1972.
12. Ederma, A. B.: Confidentiality of medical records and invasion of privacy. *Journal of Occupational Medicine*, 11:200, 1969.
13. Epstein, R. L., and Benson, D. J.: Drug abuse treatment and parental consent. *Hospitals, J.A.H.A.*, 47:63, 1973.
14. Epstein, R. L., and Benson, D. J.: The patient's right to know. *Hospitals, J.A.H.A.*, 47:47, 1973.
15. Epstein, R. L., and Benson, D. J.: The patient's right to refuse. *Hospitals, J.A.H.A.*, 47:39, 1973.
16. Fleisher, L.: Ownership of hospital records and roentgenograms. *Ill. Continuing Legal Ed.*, 4:73, 1966.
17. Freeman, F.: Significant changes in two decades of hospital-doctor-patient relation. 617 *Trial Lawyer Quarterly* 617:34, 1969–70.
18. Gavin, M. P.: Consumer services: inhospital reachout. *Hospitals, J.A.H.A.*, 49:65, 1975.
19. *Griswold v. Connecticut*, 381 U.S. 485 (1963).
20. Holle, M. L.: Public relations in nursing service. *Supervisor Nurse*, 6:33, 1975.

21. Jacobson, S. F.: Ethical issues in experimentation with human subjects. *Nursing Forum, 12*:58, 1973.
22. Joint Commission on Accreditation of Hospitals, *Accreditation Manual for Hospitals Preamble* 1–2, 1970, updated 1973.
23. Kelly, L. Y.: The patient's right to know. *Nursing Outlook, 24*:26, 1976.
24. King, J. H.: *The Law of Medical Malpractice in a Nutshell*. St. Paul, MN, West Publishing Co., 1977.
25. Kramer, M.: The consumer's influence on health care. *Nursing Outlook, 20*:574, 1972.
26. Lee, A. L., and Jacobs, G.: Workshop airs patients' rights. *Hospitals, J.A.H.A., 47*:39, 1973.
27. Lewis, E. P.: The health care consumer: compliant captive? *Nursing Outlook, 23*:21, 1975.
28. Marram, G. D.: Patient's evaluation of their care: importance to the nurse. *Nursing Outlook, 21*:322, 1973.
29. Nations, W. C.: What constitutes abuse of patients? *Hospitals, J.A.H.A., 47*:51, 1973.
30. Porte, F. X.: The multifaceted PR role. *Hospitals, J.A.H.A., 47*:115, 1973.
31. Quinn, N., and Somers, A. R.: The patient's bill of rights. A significant aspect of the consumer revolution. *Nursing Outlook, 22*:240, 1974.
32. Rogatz, P.: Patient care evaluation. In the light of public scrutiny. *Hospitals, J.A.H.A. 47*:42, 1973.
33. *Roe* v. *Wade*, 410 U.S. 113, (1973) *Doe* v. *Bolton*, 410 U.S. 179 (1973).
34. Ryan, J. L.: The single room: a right for every patient's privacy. *Nursing Digest, 3*:46, 1975.
35. Storlie, F.: Bridging the information gap. *Supervisor Nurse, 3*:59, 1972.
36. Warren, S. D., and Brandeis, L. D.: The right to privacy. *Harvard Law Review, 4*:193, 1890.
37. Wren, G. R.: Protecting the patient's right to privacy. *Hospital Topics, 47*:49, 1969.

APPLICATION OF BIOMECHANICS TO NURSING

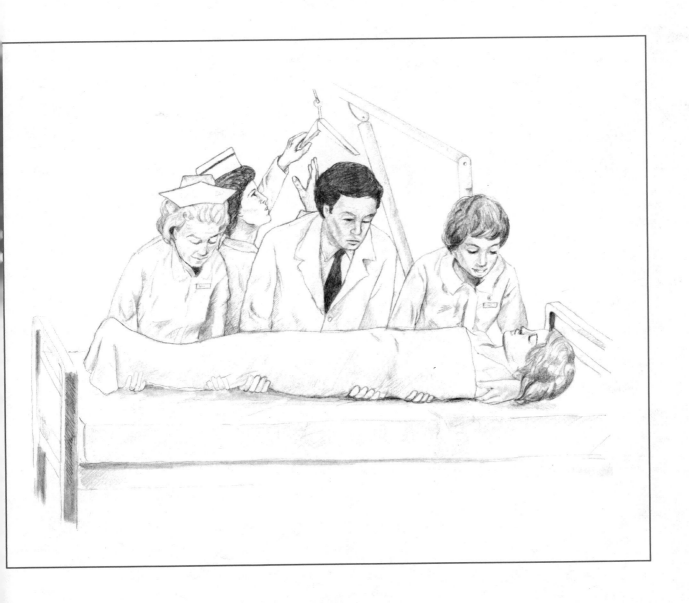

CHAPTER 21

BASIC BIOMECHANICS FOR NURSES

By Doris I. Miller, Ph.D.

OVERVIEW, STUDY GUIDE AND GENERAL CONCEPTS

Biomechanics represents that branch of science in which the principles of mechanics are applied to the study of living organisms. As the term implies, biomechanics is interdisciplinary in nature; it combines the fundamentals of anatomy and physiology with those of statics and dynamics. Working from this common, although rather widespread, knowledge base and utilizing similar instrumentation, biomechanics researchers investigate a variety of problems involving both human beings and animals. Their findings are applied to numerous fields including biotechnology, sports, space exploration, dentistry and medicine. Within the health sciences, biomechanics plays an important role in orthopedics, rehabilitation, prosthetics, orthotics, physiotherapy and nursing.

RATIONALE

This chapter is intended to familiarize the student with the basic principles of biomechanics and their application in various nursing situations. The forces most commonly encountered by the nurse are described, and examples of their influence are cited. Concepts of forces producing changes in linear and angular motion are explained. Detailed discussions of stability, friction, pressure, lifting and specific procedures dealing with the moving of patients are provided. This approach, which focuses upon force, is not the traditional one encountered in most nursing texts, but it is not new. It follows the model provided in mechanics in which emphasis is placed upon general principles and mechanisms underlying motion.

If the student has a solid understanding of the mechanical principles influencing the motion of persons and inanimate objects, she will be able to apply them to numerous situations. This approach

has a distinct advantage over attempting to memorize rules that fit specific cases, since the nurse rarely encounters identical circumstances in positioning, moving, lifting or transferring patients. As a professional, the nurse must appreciate the reasons for using given procedures. Only then can she make modifications to suit individual needs and be effective in the teaching of aides, patients and family.

MEASUREMENT SYSTEM

Although the majority of the material in this chapter is qualitative in nature, a limited amount of quantitative data is provided to help clarify mechanical concepts. In keeping with the current conversion to the metric system, the measurements are given in SI (le Système International) units. In this absolute measurement system, force is expressed in newtons (N.), mass in kilograms (kg.), length in meters (m.) and pressure in pascals (Pa.). One newton is the force required to accelerate a mass of one kilogram one meter per second squared (kg. $\times$ m./s.^{2}). By way of conversion among force units:

$$1 \text{ N.} = 0.102 \text{ kg. force} = 0.224 \text{ lb. force}$$

$$1 \text{ kg. force} = 9.8 \text{ N.} = 2.2 \text{ lb. force}$$

$$1 \text{ lb. force} = 4.45 \text{ N.} = 0.45 \text{ kg. force}$$

One pascal is defined as the pressure exerted by a force of one newton acting on an area of one square meter. Since this is an extremely small amount of pressure, it is more convenient to speak in terms of kilopascals (kPa.), or thousands of pascals.

Commonly used pressure units are related as follows:

$$1000 \text{ Pa.} = 1 \text{ kPa.} = 10.19 \text{ Gm./cm.}^2$$
$$= 0.145 \text{ lb./in.}^2 = 7.48 \text{ mm. Hg}$$

Admittedly, these measurement units may be new to the majority of students. Most medical journals and scientific periodicals, however, now require data to be reported in SI units. Therefore, they will be encountered with increasing frequency by those in the nursing profession, and it is to the student's advantage to have a working knowledge of this measurement system. To ease the transition somewhat, values in the more familiar metric units and in English units are provided in parentheses following their SI equivalents.

GLOSSARY

Since some of the terms encountered in this chapter may also be unfamiliar, the following glossary is provided. The student may wish to glance through it before proceeding, in order to gain an introduction to the terminology. In most instances, these words or phrases are explained when they are first used in the text. Subsequently, if their meaning is not clear, reference can be made to the glossary. After completing the chapter, the student should (a) have a working knowledge of each of the following terms and (b) where appropriate, be able to provide examples of their application to nursing practice. In this way, the glossary can also serve as a review of the material related to biomechanics.

angle of pull—the angle between the line of action of a force and the object to which it is being applied.

axis of rotation—a stationary reference line or point around which a body (or body segment) or object rotates. For the purpose of simplification, a joint axis is assumed to be fixed.

base of support—the area defined by the contact(s) of an object or person with the supporting surface.

biomechanics—the science that investigates the effect of internal and external forces on living bodies in motion and at rest.

body segment—a functional part of the human body, such as the head, trunk, forearm, upper arm, hand, thigh, lower leg or foot.

center of gravity (or **center of mass**)—the point where the mass of a body would be located if all of the mass were concentrated in an infinitely small volume (a point).

component—a force component represents a part of the force. It is common to divide a force into two components directed at right angles to one another. These components are usually either vertical and horizontal or at right angles to (normal) and along (tangential) the surface.

equilibrium—a balanced condition in which the sum of the forces acting upon an object in any direction equals zero and the sum of the moments of force about any axis or point equals zero.

force—energy (e.g., a push or pull) expended to change the state of rest or motion of a body. A *compression* force pushes against an object, while a *tension* force exerts a pulling effect. A *shear*, or tangential, component of force acts along the surface.

friction—the tangential component of the reaction force. It opposes motion or impending motion. Friction is proportional to the force pressing the surfaces together (normal reaction) and the physical nature (e.g., roughness) of the contacting surfaces (coefficient of friction).

HAT—head, arms and trunk; approximately 68 per cent of body weight.

leverage—see *moment of force*.

moment of force—the tendency of a force to produce *rotation*. It is equal to the magnitude of the force multiplied by the perpendicular distance from the axis of rotation to the line of action of the force. This term is used interchangeably with *torque* and *leverage*. The moment arm, or *lever arm*, is the perpendicular distance from the axis of rotation to the line of action of the force. A disrupting moment is a moment of force that is great enough to cause a body to assume a new position. In contrast, a restoring moment causes a body to return to its original position.

momentum—the "quantity of motion." *Linear momentum* is equal to the mass of a body multiplied by its velocity. *Angular momentum* is dependent upon the mass of the body, mass distribution with respect to the axis of rotation, and the angular velocity of the body.

muscle torque (or the **moment of muscle force**)—the tendency of a muscle to produce rotation of a limb about a joint axis. If a muscle produces a torque that exceeds the torque produced by a resistance or load, the muscle contracts concentrically, or shortens. If, on the other hand, the torque generated by the muscle is less than the torque of the resistance or load, the muscle contracts eccentrically, or lengthens.

Newton's laws of motion

I   Every body remains at rest or in uniform motion in a straight line unless it is compelled by some external force to change that state (law of inertia).

II The acceleration is proportional to the applied force and takes place in the direction in which the force acts (law of acceleration).

III For every action (force) there is always an equal but opposite reaction (force) (law of action and reaction).

normal—at right angles (perpendicular) to a surface.

pressure—total force divided by the area over which the force is applied.

reaction force—an external force acting upon a body by virtue of the body's contact with an external structure or surface. It is often divided into normal and tangential (friction) components.

resultant—the sum of two or more vector components.

rotation—includes flexion-extension, abduction-adduction, medial-lateral rotation when used in the context of body segment motion.

summation of forces—determination of the resultant force by considering the magnitude and direction of the components of forces.

tangential—along the surface.

torque—see *moment of force*.

vector—a quantity that has magnitude, direction and dimension, e.g., force, velocity, acceleration.

weight—the gravitational force acting upon a body.

The weight vector always acts vertically downward from the center of mass toward the center of the earth. Its line of action is referred to as the *line of gravity*.

GENERAL FORCE CONCEPTS

The term "force," which has an intuitive meaning to most people, may be operationally defined as *a push or pull that produces or tends to produce a change in the state of rest or motion of a body or object*. In other words, force is necessary to initiate, stop or alter movement. To understand how the motion of a nurse, patient or object such as a bed or instrument tray is influenced in a given situation, we must identify the major forces acting upon these systems. These forces include weight and reaction (or contact) forces, which are external, and in the case of living organisms, muscle forces, which are internal (within the body).

All forces are vector quantities; that is, they have (a) magnitude, (b) direction and (c) point of application. A fourth characteristic, (d) the line of action, can be determined if both the direction and point of application are known. If we wish to influence straight line motion in a given direction, we must exert force in that direction. For example, to lift a tray, the nurse must provide an upward force that is greater than the weight of the tray. To produce a change in rotational motion, a force must act at some distance from the axis about which rotation occurs. Thus, to propel his wheelchair, a patient must push along the rim of the wheel rather than downward in the direction of the axle. To move a bed so that the side rather than the head is against the wall, the nurse would unlock both wheels at the foot of the bed and the one wheel at the head on the side that is to be away from the wall. She would then push against the foot of the bed in the direction shown in Figure 21–1.

When a force acts upon a body for a period of time, it imparts momentum to that body. Momentum can be thought of as the *quantity of motion*. Linear momentum is a function of both the mass and the velocity of the body. A heavy patient in a wheelchair rolling out of control down a steep ramp would have considerable linear momentum! Angular momentum, or the *quantity of angular motion*, is generated by a force acting at a distance from the axis of rota-

tion. Thus, if a nurse pushed against a heavy swinging door, the door would acquire angular momentum with respect to the vertical axis through its hinges. Muscles continuously produce angular momentum of the limbs.

In the following sections of this chapter, both external and internal forces are examined in detail, and these general force concepts are explained more fully as they relate to practical situations in nursing.

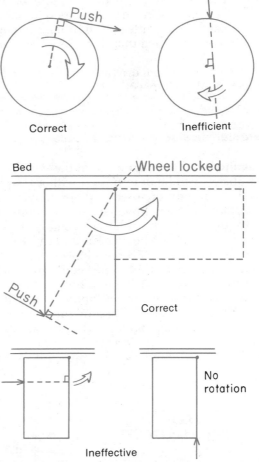

Figure 21–1. Force producing rotation about an axis. (*Note:* to produce effective rotation, the line of action of the force is as far away from the axis of rotation as possible.)

WEIGHT

Although each body or object exerts a force of attraction upon every other body, such a force is significant only if the mass of one of the bodies is extremely large. For example, we cannot ignore the force with which the earth attracts the objects on its surface. This force of attraction, known as the weight, acts upon all the particles composing a body or object. Weight is therefore termed a *distributed force*. To simplify consideration of this force, it is customary to represent weight by its resultant, that is, one single force that has the same effect as all the individual particle weights combined (Fig. 21–2). The point at which the resultant weight acts is designated the *center of gravity*, or *center of mass* (these terms are used interchangeably). Since every object, body, or body segment has weight, this force must be taken into account in any analysis of human movement. Nurses should also be aware that the moment of the total body weight is intimately related to stability and that the moments of individual segment weights have implications for proper patient positioning if myostatic contractures are to be prevented. These concerns are discussed in detail in the following sections.

Characteristics of the Weight Force

Magnitude.   The magnitude of the weight of most objects can be determined with a simple household or bathroom scale. When moving or supporting a patient, however, it is also important to appreciate the relative weights of the body segments.[5] The head, neck and trunk represent approximately 58 per cent of the body weight; each upper limb 5 per cent; and each lower limb 16 per cent. Thus, a nurse performing range of motion exercises for the lower limb of a 775 N. (79 kg., 174 lb.) patient must support about 124 N. (13 kg., 28 lb.). Also, the lumbosacral junction in the vertebral column must continually withstand over 60 per cent of the body weight. Little wonder this region of the body is often the site of pain.

Direction.   The weight force always acts vertically downward. Thus, if unopposed, a body will seek its lowest possible position of stability. A weak or helpless patient left near the edge of the bed should be protected by raising the side rails. Otherwise, a loss of balance could result in the patient's falling to the floor and sustaining injury. When a patient is in a sitting position, the weight of the upper limbs pulling downward may cause excessive stress on the superior joint structures of the shoulder. It is therefore important to provide adequate support under the forearms.

Point of Application.   As indicated previously, the center of gravity of a body or object is the point at which the resultant weight force acts. This point of application can be thought of as a balance point. If the object is of uniform composition, the center of gravity will be located at its geometric center. The center of gravity of a person in anatomic position (erect with forearms supinated) is commonly cited as being at about 55 per cent of the standing height in women and slightly higher in men (56 to 57 per cent).[19] It is important to realize that this location refers to one specific (and not very common) body orientation. When the relative position of the body segments changes, the location of the center of gravity reflects these changes. For example, if the arms are raised above the head, the center of gravity will be elevated slightly. While not a fixed anatomic point, for practical purposes, the center of gravity can be assumed to lie within the hip region.

It should also be indicated that each body segment has its own center of gravity. Cadaver studies have shown that for the upper arm, forearm, thigh and lower leg, it is approximately 43 per cent of the length of the particular segment from the proximal end.[5] For example, the center of gravity of a 0.5 m. (20 in.) long thigh is about 0.2 m. (8.6 in.) down the thigh from the hip joint.

Line of Action.   The line of action of the weight (also known as the line of gravity) is vertically downward from the center of gravity. Lifting a person or object opposes the direction of the weight and requires the application of an upward force greater than the weight. Whenever possible, nurses should avoid or at

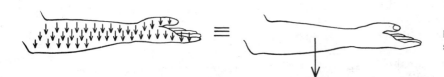

Figure 21–2. Distributed weight force represented by its resultant.

least minimize lifting, since this action works against gravity. Therefore, transfer and working surfaces should be at the same height so that such objects as instrument trays need not be habitually lifted when moving them from one area to another. Similarly, when assisting a patient into bed, the bed should be lowered as much as possible. This reduces the distance the patient's center of gravity has to be raised and thereby requires less effort on the part of the patient and the assistant.

The line of gravity of the body is also of considerable importance in standing and sitting postures. If it is too far forward as a result of slouching or the head being forward, there is a greater tendency for the body to fall forward. As a consequence, increased levels of back extensor muscle activity are required to maintain equilibrium, and undesirable compression of the anterior portions of the intervertebral discs may result.

Moments Produced by Weight

In the absence of external supporting forces, the stability of a person or object depends upon the relationship between the line of gravity and the base of support (the area of contact of the object or person with the supporting surface). If the line of gravity falls within the base of support in the original position, the weight will have a restoring moment of force with respect to the axis of rotation, and the body will return to its original position. If the line of action of the weight, however, falls outside the base of support, the weight will have a disrupting moment, and the body will tend to assume a new position (Fig. 21–3).

> The concept of moment of force (also referred to as torque or leverage) deals with the potential of a force to produce rotation about an axis. The magnitude of the moment of force with respect to a particular axis is equal to the magnitude of the force multiplied by the perpendicular distance from the axis of rotation to the line of action of the force. Thus, the greater the force or the longer the perpendicular distance (called the moment arm or lever arm), the greater the tendency to initiate, stop or alter rotary motion (see Fig. 21–1).

Stability. The four principles of stability relate directly to the concept of disrupting and restoring weight moments. They are the (a) weight of a person or object, (b) size of the base of support, (c) height of the center of gravity and (d) distance between the line of gravity and the edge of the base.

Stability is directly proportional to the weight of an object. Many people have observed that it requires less force to knock over a light chair than a heavy one. In other words, more force is required to tip the heavy chair to a position in which its weight provides a disrupting moment. With this in mind, nurses should avoid transferring patients to chairs of light weight unless these chairs are braced firmly against a wall or some other reliable supporting structure.

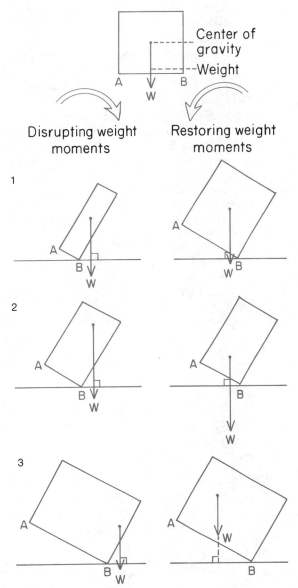

Figure 21–3. Disrupting and restoring moments of the weight force with respect to an axis through *B*.

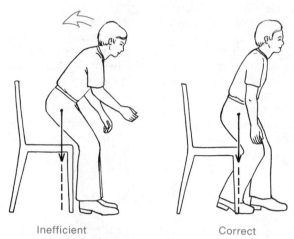

Figure 21–4. Moment of the weight when rising from a chair.

Inefficient   Correct

Other things being equal, stability is directly proportional to the size of the base of support. As is evident from Figure 21–3 *(1)*, the object with the larger base is experiencing a restoring moment, while the weight of the one with the smaller base is producing a disrupting moment. Thus, a supine or prone position is more stable than a side-lying position unless the upper arm and leg are supported by pillows or other suitable padding. Similarly, the base of support, and therefore the stability, of a weak or elderly patient can be increased with a cane or walker. Further, when rising from a chair, it is important that the individual first shift the body weight forward toward the edge of the chair and

place one foot back and the other slightly forward so that the line of gravity falls within the area outlined by the feet. Unless these preliminary adjustments are made, the weak person is likely to experience a restoring weight moment that will return him to the original sitting position (Fig. 21–4).

In most instances, a nurse or reasonably active patient is able to change the size of the base of support by moving the feet or grasping an external object to maintain a stable position. The individual may also alter the relative orientation of the body segments so that the line of gravity remains within the base. The latter situation is particularly evident when carrying a heavy load. If the load is held directly in front of the body, it is necessary to increase the lumbar curve so that the shoulders can be thrown back and thus permit the combined line of gravity of the weights of the body and load to fall within the area outlined by the feet. Carrying the load slightly to the side reduces this hyperextension of the spine but requires equivalent lateral compensation. If possible, the load should be divided into two parts of equal weight with one being carried by each hand. Failing this, if the load can be adequately supported in one arm, the other arm can be extended to the side for balance rather than bending the trunk laterally. A nurse should avoid carrying objects habitually on the same side of the body, but rather should make a conscious effort to alternate between the left and right sides so that the same tissues are not subjected to continual stress.

As illustrated in Figure 21–3(2), stability is inversely proportional to the height of the center of gravity above the base of support. Thus, patients with upper body casts lose their balance more readily than those with casts of equivalent weight on the lower body. In situations in which the maintenance of a stable posi-

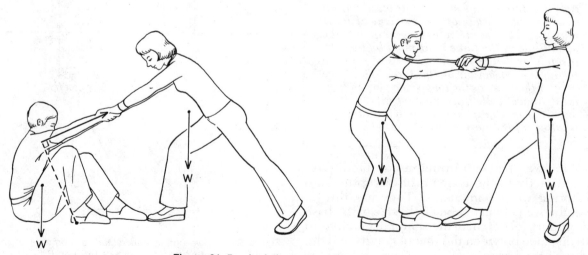

Figure 21–5. Assisting patient from the floor.

tion is important, the center of gravity should be lowered by flexing at the hips and/or knees as well as increasing the base of support. Consider, for instance, the nurse's position when assisting a patient to transfer from bed to chair. The knees are flexed and the base enlarged in the direction of the transfer.

Stability in a given direction is proportional to the distance of the line of gravity from the edge of the base of support in the direction in which stability is desired (Figure 21–3, 3). When assisting the patient from the floor, the nurse (standing in front of the patient) assumes a position that enlarges her base of support in a forward-backward direction with the center of gravity initially close to the forward edge of the base. In contrast, the patient is encouraged to maintain a sitting position, with the buttocks as close to the heels as possible. When the nurse pulls on the patient's arms to assist him from the floor, her center of gravity can be shifted backward while she remains in balance. Meanwhile the patient's line of gravity soon falls in front of his rear heel and within his new base of support outlined by his feet. Had the patient been in a sitting position with his knees almost completely extended, it would be much more difficult to assist him to his feet (Fig. 21–5).

Another example of the application of this principle is the pull maneuver, discussed on page 374.

> *Stability is intimately related to weight and particularly to the relationship between the position of the center of gravity and the base of support. The principles outlined, however, seldom act independently. Thus, to achieve increased balance in a given direction, the base of support is increased in that direction, the center of gravity is lowered and moved as far away from the edge of the base of support in the direction in which stability is desired. If a position is to be changed most easily, the opposite adjustments should be made.*

Positioning. The nurse must understand that individual body segment weights can produce moments of force about their respective joints. This has particular relevance for positioning the patient. When a person is lying on the back, the weight of the feet tends to produce rotation about the ankle joint, resulting in plantar flexion. The amount of plantar flexion is limited by the joint structure of the ankle, namely, the shape of the bony articular surfaces and their associated joint capsule, tendons and ligaments. The calf muscles (soleus and gastrocnemius), however, are in a shortened position, and a foot-drop muscle contracture may result.

A properly placed *footboard* can prevent this from occurring. Similarly, the weight of the lower limb creates a moment of force with respect to the long axis of the limb and tends to cause the thigh to rotate laterally (external rotation) when a patient is in a supine position. A *trochanter roll* at the hip therefore may be required to maintain normal alignment. The student should be able to identify other examples in which the weight of a body segment tends to produce undesirable moments of force about a joint axis and should be able to explain what measures must be taken to reduce stress on the joint and to prevent muscle contractures.

CONTACT OR REACTION FORCES

In accordance with Newton's third law of motion, when a person (or object) "acts" or exerts force upon the surroundings, the surroundings "react" at the points of contact with forces of equal magnitude but opposite direction. Thus, the nurse carrying an instrument tray experiences reaction forces from the floor and from the tray. A patient being assisted to a standing position from a chair initially is in contact with the chair, the floor and the nurse or aide. Reaction forces from all these sources influence his motion. The nurse in Figure 21–6 is affected not only by the weight of her body but also by reaction forces from the

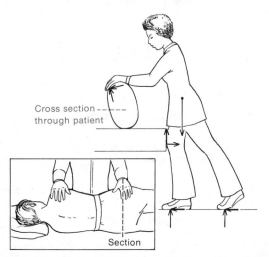

Cross section through patient

Section

Figure 21–6. Contact or reaction forces acting upon the nurse.

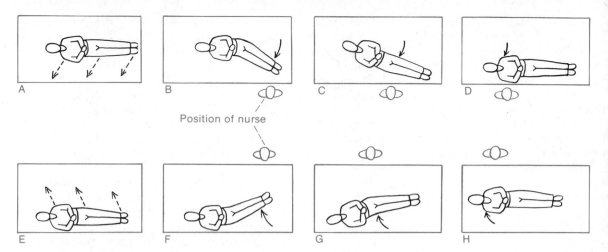

Figure 21–7. One helper pull maneuver. In *A*, patient is at foot of bed. The nurse pulls patient toward her in three segments (*B, C, D*). She then moves to the other side of the bed and repeats the pulling motions (*F, G, H*) until in *H* the patient is at the head of the bed. Procedure 1, p. 385 explains this zigzag pattern and other pull maneuvers in detail. Below is explained how the nurse uses her body effectively in performing pull maneuvers.

PULL MANEUVER

The execution of a pull maneuver illustrates the principle that *stability in a given direction is proportional to the distance of the line of gravity from the edge of the base of support in the direction in which stability is desired.* At the beginning of the maneuver, the nurse's center of gravity is close to the forward edge of the base of support. The result is good stability for movement in the backward direction (the direction in which the nurse moves in a pull maneuver) but great instability in the forward direction. This means that the nurse's center of gravity can shift backward a substantial distance before the moment of the weight becomes a disrupting moment with respect to the rear edge of the base. In contrast, only a small forward displacement of the center of gravity will result in a disrupting moment of the weight with reference to the forward edge of the base.

A pull maneuver is used for moving patients in bed or along other flat surfaces. A force that is safe for the nurse and effective in moving the patient is produced. Pulling includes an upward force component, which reduces friction between the patient and the bed or supporting surface.

SUGGESTED STEPS	RATIONALE/ASSESSMENT
1. Assume a wide-based forward-backward stance in the direction of movement.	1. The force can be applied over a greater distance when the base of support is enlarged in the direction of the movement.
2. Flex knees and hips in order to extend arms on the bed.	2. This permits a more horizontal and less upward direction of force application. Thus, the force of the patient's weight is not opposed significantly.
3. Place arms under body part to be moved with fingers flexed on the far side,	3. The force is transmitted to the patient by means of the hands. Sliding (kinetic) friction occurs between the nurse's arms and the sheet rather than between the patient's skin and the sheet. Thus, potential damage to the patient's skin is lessened.
or grasp rolled turning sheet with pronated hands at bed level.	A turning sheet likewise protects the patient from friction.
4. Contract the muscles of arms, shoulders and fingers statically (isometrically).	4. Arms serve as rigid connections between the nurse's body and the part of the patient to be moved.
5. Contract the abdominal and gluteal muscles statically.	5. Contraction of the abdominal muscles raises the pressure within the abdominal cavity and reduces compression on the lumbar intervertebral discs.
6. Push down and forward against the floor with the forward foot by contracting the strong knee and hip extensor muscles so that the center of gravity shifts backward and the task is accomplished by pulling rather than lifting.	6. The patient is pulled in the same direction in which the nurse is moving. The horizontal component of the ground reaction force acting toward the nurse provides the linear momentum necessary to move the patient.

floor on both her feet, from the bed on her right thigh, and from the patient on her hands.

To facilitate our understanding of such reaction or contact forces, it is helpful to divide them into normal and tangential components. By definition, a normal component of force acts at right angles to the surface, while a tangential component acts along the surface. Since these two components are perpendicular to one another, they act independently.

> *It is important to realize that the tangential component of the reaction force is also referred to as the* friction or shearing *force, while the normal component is responsible for creating pressure against the surface.*

In the example of the nurse in Figure 21–6, friction or tangential components act along (a) the surface of the floor, (b) the nurse's thigh and (c) her hands. The normal components, acting at right angles to the surfaces indicated, are directed (a) vertically upward through the feet, (b) back into the thigh from the bed and (c) into the palms of the hands. In the following sections, the significance of these reaction force components is examined.

Tangential Component—Friction

Friction always acts along the surface in a direction that opposes motion or impending motion between the contact surfaces. For example, during the push-off phase of walking, the ball of the foot thrusts downward and backward and the surface reacts upward and forward with a force of equal magnitude. The tangential or friction component acts forward against the foot. In this case, although there is no movement of the contact surfaces, there is a tendency for the foot to slip back (impending motion). The friction or tangential component opposes this tendency.

Although other kinds of friction exist, we are concerned here with only three types of dry friction—static, kinetic and rolling.

> Static friction *implies a nonslip condition, while* kinetic friction *is characterized by a sliding of the contact surfaces.* Rolling friction *refers to the resistance encountered by a circular object to its rolling motion.*

In general, the amount of friction experienced is related to both the component of the reaction force normal to the surface (which re-flects the force pressing the two surfaces together) and the coefficient of friction (which depends upon the nature of the contacting surfaces). The symbol for normal force is N (not to be confused with the abbreviation for newton) and the coefficient of friction is represented by the Greek letter μ (*mu*). Dry and rough surfaces have higher coefficients of friction than smooth and lubricated surfaces.

Static Friction. When a force such as a push or pull is applied to move an object or person, some resistance to this effort is experienced. For example, a patient will not begin to move up in bed the instant that the nurse pulls in that direction. In fact, until movement occurs, the resistance encountered will be directly related to the force applied (Fig. 21–8). In other words, the static friction or tangential force opposing the impending motion equals the component of the applied force acting along the surface. If the nurse pulls toward the head of the bed with 98 N. (10 kg., 22 lb.) of force (which is not sufficient to move the patient) and is resisted by 98 N. of force, the patient will not move.

The maximum static friction force (which occurs just in an instant before the surfaces begin to slip) is expressed as the coefficient of static friction (μ_s multiplied by the normal component of the reaction force (N):

$$\text{Maximum static friction force} = \mu_s \times N$$

For a given pair of surfaces, the coefficient of static friction is slightly larger than the coefficient of kinetic (sliding) friction. Thus, it requires a greater force to initiate motion than to continue it. Once an object has begun to slide on a surface, it takes less effort to get it to its destination if it is kept in motion rather than if a series of starts and stops are employed.

In nursing, there are numerous instances when it is desirable to have as large a maximum static friction force as possible to prevent slipping. The tips of canes and crutches are constructed to increase the coefficient of static friction. A patient, however, should not position them too far in front or to the side, since the magnitude of the normal reaction will then be reduced, and slipping will be more likely. As another example, a heavy chair elicits a higher reaction force component normal (at right angles) to the floor than does a light one. Therefore, a large force is required to move heavy furniture.

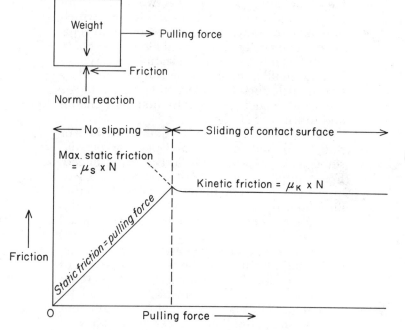

Figure 21-8.   Friction relationships.

When a patient moves up in bed, instruct him to push his feet down into the mattress as well as toward the end of the bed (Fig. 21–9). The downward component of the push causes an equal and opposite upward force from the mattress. The maximum static friction force is directly related to the magnitude of this normal reaction. The harder he pushes down, the less chance his feet will slip. If the component of

force the patient exerts along the mattress is less than the maximum static friction force, the static friction holds his feet in position and assists him in moving up in bed. If, however, the tangential force component he exerts is greater than the maximum static friction force, his feet slip. Thus, the downward push with its associated upward normal reaction is essential to prevent slipping, and the part of the push toward the foot of the bed elicits a reaction that assists the patient in moving up in bed.

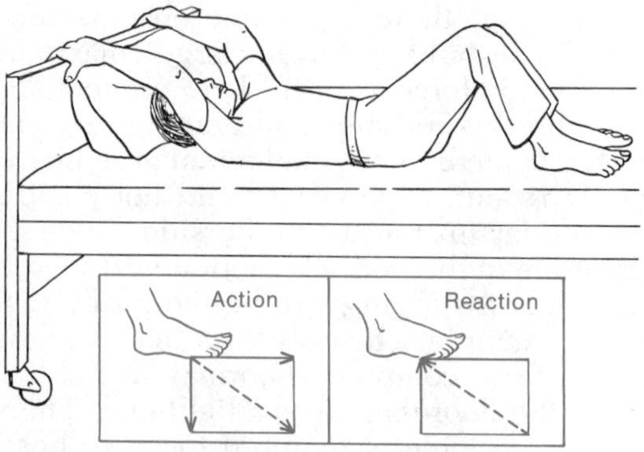

In some cases, it is desirable to reduce the maximum static friction so that an object can be started moving easily along a surface. In these instances, the contact surfaces should be smooth and/or lubricated and the pressure between the surfaces reduced. Consider, for example, the use of plastic beneath a slip sheet under a heavy patient.

Kinetic Friction.   The kinetic friction force, which is present when slipping occurs, is always equal to the product of the coefficient of kinetic friction and the normal reaction:

$$\text{Kinetic friction force} = \mu_k \times N$$

Thus, kinetic friction acts in a direction that retards sliding between surfaces.

Figure 21-9.   Components of reaction force.

To facilitate slipping, the kinetic friction that impedes the motion should be lessened. This can be accomplished by reducing the coefficient of kinetic friction and/or decreasing the normal reaction. For instance, smooth articular cartilage and lubricating synovial fluid within a synovial joint very effectively minimize kinetic friction. Plastic under a slip sheet can serve a similar function.

Utilizing a pull rather than a push when moving a patient generally decreases the normal reaction of the supporting surfaces on the patient. A pull tends to have a slight upward component and therefore reduces the pressure between the patient and the bed or chair. As a result, kinetic friction is reduced. In contrast, a push exerted on a patient is usually accompanied by a downward component, which increases the pressure between the patient and his supporting surface and therefore increases the kinetic friction. Since a patient is not a rigid body, pushing also tends to produce undesirable compression of the tissues and joints. When attempting to move an inanimate object such as a bed, chair or nightstand, however, it is generally more efficient to push against it, taking care not to exert any force downward and to push as near to the level of the center of gravity of the object as possible. In this case, the individual is able to utilize the strong hip and knee extensor muscles more effectively, and since the object is rigid, compression is not a consideration.

An excessive shear force can damage a patient's skin and predispose the affected areas to tissue breakdown and pressure sores. This shear may be static or kinetic friction. The nurse must bear this in mind when moving and positioning a patient and should pay particular attention to the heels and sacral area, which are prone to damage from shear.

In other instances, the objective is to maximize kinetic friction. An example of this is applying the brakes to a moving wheelchair. The brake-wheel interface has a high coefficient of kinetic friction. Applying the brake increases the normal reaction on the wheel by the brake. The greater the kinetic friction, the more quickly the wheelchair will come to a stop.

Rolling Friction. Rolling friction is the resistance to the rolling of a circular object. No slipping, however, occurs between the wheel and the floor or supporting surface. Although many variables such as the size of the wheel, its rate of rotation and the properties of the contacting surfaces influence the rolling friction force in a rather complex manner, it is known that the coefficient of rolling friction is substantially less than the coefficients of static and kinetic friction, and other things being equal, rolling frictional resistance is smaller than resistance to static and kinetic forces. Therefore, it requires much less force to push a bed with casters or wheels than to push one that is not so equipped. Similarly, experience tells us that it is easier to push a wheelchair along a smooth floor than along a rug because of the nature of the contacting surfaces. The roughness of the carpet increases the friction coefficient, and as a consequence, the friction resistance increases.

Friction is the component of the reaction force that acts along the surface, opposing the tendency of one object to slide on another. The movement of a wheel that rolls without slipping is resisted by rolling friction; and the slipping of an object on a surface is slowed by kinetic friction. If motion is impending but no sliding takes place, the friction is termed static. All three of these friction forces can be increased by making the contact surfaces rougher (increasing the coefficient of friction) and by increasing the force pressing them together (normal reaction). All things being equal, maximum static friction is greater than kinetic friction, which in turn exceeds rolling friction. In nursing, all three types of resistance will be encountered. Whether or not the friction should be increased or decreased will depend upon the requirements of the situation.

Normal Component—Pressure

By definition, the normal component of any reaction force acts at right angles to the contact surface. In virtually all cases, this force component is directed inward against the skin of an individual and therefore tends to compress the underlying tissue. Whether or not the tissue is damaged and pressure sores (decubitus ulcers) develop depends upon pressure exerted and the length of time it is applied. Pressure is defined as force divided by the area over which it is exerted.

To illustrate the concept of pressure, consider a 535 N. (54.5 kg., 120 lb.) individual standing in a stationary position. This person experiences a normal reaction force of 535 N. acting upward on the soles of the feet, which have a total area of approximately 0.027 m.² (42.in.²). The pressure is therefore:

$$\frac{535 \text{ N.}}{0.027 \text{ m.}^2} = 19{,}814.8 \text{ Pa.} = 19.8 \text{ kPa.} = 148 \text{ mm. Hg}$$

or

$$\frac{54.5 \text{ kg.}}{0.027 \text{ m.}^2} = 2018.5 \text{ kg./m.}^2 = 201.85 \text{ Gm./cm.}^2$$

or

$$\frac{120 \text{ lb.}}{42 \text{ in.}^2} = 2.86 \text{ lb./in.}^2$$

If the individual balanced on only one foot, the pressure would increase to 39.6 kPa. No wonder a small pebble in the shoe causes so much discomfort! Pressure on the foot during walking has been estimated by Brand[2] to be between 100 and 500 kPa. (approximately 1000 and 5000 Gm./cm.^{2}). These high values are the result of normal ground reaction force components slightly in excess of body weight acting over relatively small areas of the foot. It must be kept in mind that the soles of the feet are specially adapted to withstand relatively high pressures and that, in most cases, they are subjected to intermittent rather than continuous pressure.

It has been estimated that a prolonged pressure of 10.7 kPa. (109 Gm./cm.^{2}, 80 mm. Hg) will cause tissue necrosis.[21] Such a pressure is more than three times the mean capillary pressure of 25 mm. Hg and as a result occludes the circulation, depriving the underlying surface tissue of the blood supply required for its survival. When an 800 N. (81.5 kg., 179 lb.) patient lies in bed or sits in a chair, he experiences an 800 N. normal reaction upward against his body. At the extreme, imagine that this patient were supported in only one small area 1 cm. × 1 cm. (0.0001 m.^{2}). In this region, he would be subjected to 8000 kPa. (~80,000 Gm./cm.^{2}) pressure. If the individual were lying supported evenly at 10 such points, the pressure would reduce to 800 kPa. and would further decrease to 80 kPa. if 100 similar contact areas were provided. Maximum pressures of 13.34 kPa. (100 mm. Hg) have been measured in the ischial tuberosity region of individuals lying in a supine position on a compliant surface and 12.67 kPa. (95 mm. Hg) in the trochanteric region when lying on the side. In seated individuals, these values were 20 kPa. (150 mm. Hg) and 66.7 kPa. (500 mm. Hg) on compliant and hard surfaces respectively.[10] These values all exceed the 10 kPa. level, which if maintained even a few hours, will cause tissue breakdown and pressure sores. (Refer to Chapter 33 for further discussion of decubitus ulcers.)

The importance of providing a large area over which the normal reaction force can be distributed should be appreciated by the nurse. When positioning a patient, it is essential to protect bony prominences and support body hollows. If this is done correctly, the normal force of the bed or chair upon the patient will be distributed over a large area and the pressure on the skin reduced.

> Remember: *Even relatively small pressures, if acting over a long period of time, will restrict blood flow and lead to tissue damage. The position of a patient must therefore be changed frequently to avoid this damage.*

MUSCLE FORCE

Coordinated and purposeful movement of the human body is produced by the action of muscles exerting tension (pulling) forces upon bones causing movement of these bones about joint centers. In this section, the characteristics of muscle force and muscle torque are considered with respect to their relevance to specific nursing tasks.

Characteristics of Muscle Force

Point of Application. Most muscles attach to bones by means of tendons. Their points of application on the bone are referred to as proximal and distal attachments, or origins and insertions. The proximal attachment (origin) is the one closer to the midline of the body.

Direction. The direction of a muscle force is taken to be along a straight line joining its origin and insertion. When a muscle contracts, it pulls toward its center, exerting tension (i.e., pulling force) on its connections with the bone. A muscle cannot generate a compression or pushing force against the points to which it attaches. The old adage that you can't push on a string applies in this case.

The motion produced at the joint by the contraction of the muscles crossing it depends upon the action of external forces as well as stabilization of the attachments. The latter can be illustrated by the hip flexor muscle action in three different cases. Imagine a person lying on the floor about to perform a sit-up exercise. If the feet are held against the ground and the hip flexors contract, the upper body is lifted from the ground. If the shoulders are held down, however, the lower limbs are raised. Therefore, when a muscle shortens, the unstabilized attachment approaches the one that is stabilized. If neither the upper body nor lower limbs are secured, the individual tends to move into a V-sit or pike position in which both muscle attachments move closer to one another. It is thus evident that either muscle attachment does not necessarily remain fixed.

In addition to the role of muscles in active contraction, the nurse must also be aware of the passive function of muscles in limiting motion. For example, before using the head gatch to raise the upper body of the patient into a sitting or Fowler's position, the patient's knees should be flexed slightly to relieve the strain on the hamstring muscles. The hamstrings, which cross both the hip and knee joints at the back of the leg, are stretched if the knees are extended at the same time the hips are flexed. Thus if, while sitting, a patient's legs are supported on a footstool (knee extension), less padding is required in the lumbar (low back) area, since the passive pull of the hamstrings tends to rotate the pelvis upward and reduce the lumbar curve more than if the patient's feet were on the floor.

Magnitude. The generation of muscle tension is a mechanical event produced by neuromuscular electrochemical interactions. Since the maximum force a muscle can produce at its optimal length is proportional to the number of contractile (actin and myosin) filaments within it, the potential of a muscle to develop isometric or static tension can be estimated from its physiologic cross section (i.e., the cross-sectional area of its fibers). On the basis of experimental studies, Elftman[7] stated this value to be approximately 34.6 N./cm.² (3.5 kg./cm.², 50 lb./in.²). Thus, the quadriceps femoris (the hip flexor–knee extensor muscle group on the front of the thigh) is capable of exerting greater force than its counterpart in the upper limb (i.e., triceps brachii).

To stress the comparatively high forces muscles can generate, Elftman pointed out that if all the muscles of the body were to contract simultaneously while at their optimal length, the 3.3 m.² (6 ft.²) total physiologic cross section would develop a force of about 22 tons! This situation, of course, would never occur, and the fact that the lines of action of the various muscles are not the same would reduce the resultant force produced in any given direction. The illustration does serve to emphasize the fact that muscle forces are considerably higher than is commonly thought. The amount of tension (i.e., pulling force) actually exerted depends upon the (a) number of motor units (motor neurons and the muscle fibers they supply) recruited; (b) temporal sequence of motor unit activation; (c) frequency with which these units are activated or fired; (d) physiologic state of the muscle at the time of activation; and (e) muscle length (the degree of overlap of the contractile elements within a muscle cell). The last point (e) deserves further discussion.

When a muscle is at its "resting length" the muscle will be capable of producing greater tension than if it were in a more shortened or elongated condition. The resting length is related to an optimum overlap of the contractile filaments within the muscle cell or sarcomere and is the physical length a muscle would adopt if freed from its attachments. The successive linking and breaking of the actin-myosin cross-bridges to produce shortening (i.e., force) can be likened to pulling down a retractable ladder. Resting length (optimal overlap) would be obtained by having your hands grasp the bottom rungs of the ladder and, by a hand-over-hand action, pulling the end of the ladder down to the ground. The ladder represents the actin; the legs and trunk are the backbone of the myosin; the arms stand for the cross-bridges; and the hands are analogous to the binding sites. Extreme muscle stretch (beyond filament overlap) is similar to having the ladder suspended slightly above your reach so that you are unable to grasp the end and as a result cannot pull it down (insufficient overlap decreasing the number of actin-myosin binding sites). A muscle in an excessively shortened condition can be compared to a ladder that has been fully extended to the ground so that you would not be able to pull it down any further (too much overlap again decreasing the number of binding sites). For example, it is more difficult to use the hamstrings (knee flexor–hip extensor group behind the thigh) to extend the hip when the knees are flexed than when they

When a muscle contracts, it exerts a force upon the bones to which it is attached. Because the line of action of the muscle force is at some distance from the joint axis, the muscle produces a moment of force or torque with respect to the joint. The associated bones, therefore, have a tendency to rotate (i.e., flexion-extension, abduction-adduction, medial-lateral rotation) about the joint axis. As a consequence of the shallow angle of muscle pull, the moment arm of the muscle force with respect to the joint is extremely short. For example, the moment arm of the erector spinae is approximately 5 cm. (2 in.).[15]

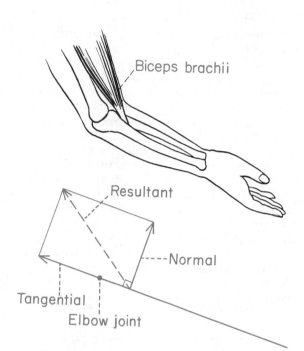

Figure 21–10.   Components of muscle force.

> *Since torque depends upon the magnitude of the force and the length of the moment or lever arm, the muscle force must be comparatively large to compensate for the small moment arm if adequate levels of muscle torque are to be produced to permit coordinated movements of the body.*

are extended because in the former case the hamstrings are shorter than their resting length. Therefore, if a nurse must kneel on the bed to assist in moving a patient (refer to Procedure 3, B) most of the force to extend the nurse's trunk and hips will have to come from the back extensor muscles with little assistance from hamstrings.

Line of Action.   In most instances, a muscle pulls at a very shallow angle with respect to the bone to which it attaches. Although this angle of pull alters slightly as the joint moves through its range of motion, the line of action of the muscle force is always very close to the joint.

If a muscle force were divided into two independent components acting at right angles to each other, one tangential (along) and the other normal (at right angles) to the bone, the tangential component would almost invariably be the larger of the two and would be directed toward the joint to stabilize it (Fig. 21–10). Thus, the tangential portion of muscle force is often termed the *stabilizing component.* Since it acts through the joint, the tangential component is incapable of producing rotation of the limb with reference to the joint. The normal part is referred to as the *rotary component,* since it acts at right angles to the bone in a direction that produces muscle torque.

Concentric.   In slow (quasi-static) movement, if the moment or torque produced by the muscle force with respect to the joint axis exceeds the moment of the resistance, then the muscle will shorten (Fig. 21–11). In this type of contraction, which is termed concentric, the cross-bridges between the actin and myosin filaments within the sarcomere move closer together. When lifting, the quadriceps femoris (knee extensor muscle group on the front of the thigh) contract concentrically, extending the knee joint. Concentric torque is also referred to as *positive work.*

Static.   If the moments of the muscle force and external resistance with respect to the joint are equal, there will not be any perceptible movement of the limb, and to the naked eye, the muscle length will remain unchanged. In this instance, the contraction is said to be static or isometric (i.e., same length). As Andersson et al.[1] have pointed out, to prevent fatigue, static muscular activity of the postural muscles should be minimized in everyday tasks. To accomplish this, the moments of the body segment weights and other resistance forces about the respective joints must be reduced by keeping the limbs and external objects that are being supported as close to the midline of the body as possible. On the other hand, in some nursing tasks such as the pull maneuver, certain muscle groups should be contracted statically (referred to in some sources as "setting" the muscles). For example, static contraction of the muscles of the nurse's upper limbs permits the backward movement of the nurse generated by the strong knee extensor muscles to be transferred directly to the patient. Muscles tend to produce maximum static torques somewhere near the middle of the joint's range of motion. For example, knee extensors generate maximum static torque when the angle between the thigh and the lower leg is about 120 degrees.[11, 13, 23] Thus, it is difficult to lift a heavy burden from the floor when the knees are fully flexed.

Eccentric. Finally, if the muscle torque is less than the torque of the resistance with respect to the joint, the muscle lengthens and is unable to perform its agonistic (prime mover) function. Although it continues to apply tension (i.e., pull on the bone), its rotational tendency is overcome by the resistance and it contracts eccentrically. The cross-bridges within the muscle cell break and reattach, but in this case the ends of the sarcomere move further apart. This could be likened to the movement of the hands in climbing down a ladder. Eccentric torque is also referred to as *negative work.*

Comparative Values. At any given muscle length, torque is greatest when the muscle is contracting eccentrically (i.e., lengthening) and is least when the muscle is contracting concentrically (i.e., applying tension while shortening). If the isometric or static torque is considered the reference standard and is designated 100 per cent, then corresponding eccentric and concentric values would be approximately 120 and 75 per cent, respectively.[18] The practical implications for the nurse are wide-ranging. A patient who is capable of lowering himself into a chair (an action that involves eccentric contraction of the knee and hip extensors as well as the elbow extensors if the arms of the chair are utilized for support) may be unable to get up without assistance, since the concentric torques generated by these muscles may not be sufficiently large. Similarly, a nurse who is able to safely lower a fainting patient to the floor, or even support the patient statically until help arrives, may require assistance in getting the patient up from the floor. Patients who are too weak to sit up without help should still be encouraged to actively participate in lowering themselves back to supine position, an action requiring eccentric contraction of the abdominal and hip flexor muscle groups.

LIFTING

This section discusses the relevance of muscle force, weight, and reaction force to the nursing activity of lifting. It incorporates biomechanical concepts already presented in the chapter.

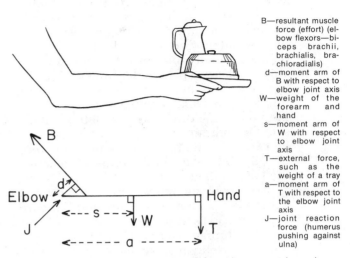

B—resultant muscle force (effort) (elbow flexors—biceps brachii, brachialis, brachioradialis)
d—moment arm of B with respect to elbow joint axis
W—weight of the forearm and hand
s—moment arm of W with respect to elbow joint axis
T—external force, such as the weight of a tray
a—moment arm of T with respect to the elbow joint axis
J—joint reaction force (humerus pushing against ulna)

Figure 21–11. Conditions for concentric, eccentric and static muscle contraction. Assume:

d = 3 cm. (1.2 in.)
s = 15 cm. (5.9 in.)
a = 30 cm. (11.8 in.)
W = 20 N. (2 kg.; 4.5 lb.)
T = 50 N. (5 kg.; 11.2 lb.)

(Both W and T provide resistance to elbow flexion.)

Concentric muscle contraction: moment of muscle force with respect to the joint axis must be greater than the moments of the resistance forces.

$$B \times d > (W \times s) + (T \times a)$$
$$B > \frac{(W \times s) + (T \times a)}{d}$$
$$B > \frac{(20 \times 15) + (50 \times 30)}{3}$$
$$B > \frac{300 + 1500}{3}$$
$$B > 600 \text{ N. (61 kg.; 135 lb.)}$$

The elbow flexors must provide a force greater than 600 N. if the elbow joint is to flex.

Static muscle contraction: moment of muscle force with respect to the joint axis must equal the moments of the resistance forces. Therefore, B must equal 600 N. to keep the forearm in a horizontal position.

Eccentric muscle contraction: if B is less than 600 N., the forearm will be lowered. Note that even though the muscle force can be considerably higher than the resistance forces (e.g., 500 > 70), the muscle still lengthens because its moment of force with respect to the joint is less than the resistance moments.

Background

Statistics reveal that low back pain and injury continue to be major causes of work days lost in industry as well as the source of considerable personal discomfort. These problems affect young individuals between 20 and 35 years of age as well as older persons. In fact, some researchers estimate that between 70 and 80 per cent of all workers will suffer low back symptoms at some time during their careers.[4] In a number of individuals this disability is thought to be linked to lifting or associated activities and may be the result of chronic injury (i.e., continued minor insults that individually would not cause pain or disability). Since nursing personnel are commonly involved in lifting, it is particularly important to understand the problem and to consider methods that are safe for both nurse and patient. As one of the first steps in attempting to achieve this objective, a brief review of the relevant anatomy of the back is in order.[22]

The spinal column, which is called upon to withstand compression, tension, shearing, bending, and twisting forces, consists of 24 presacral vertebrae (7 cervical, 12 thoracic and 5 lumbar vertebrae) separated by intervertebral discs. At the base of the column are the sacrum and coccyx, made up of 5 and 4 fused vertebrae, respectively. The bodies of the vertebrae become progressively more massive from the first cervical (C1) vertebra down through the last lumbar (L5) vertebra, since each in succession must bear a greater proportion of the upper body weight when an individual is in an erect or sitting position.

> Because the lumbosacral (L5–S1 junction) has to accommodate more weight than all those above it, this joint and the others associated with the low back region seem particularly susceptible to injury and are commonly the sites of pain.

Injury to the Low Back

Considerable indirect evidence implicates the lower lumbar intervertebral discs as the site of low back pain.[17] The discs, which account for approximately 25 to 30 per cent of the length of the vertebral column, play a major role in shock absorption and force transmission. Each disc consists of three parts. Tightly bound to the adjacent vertebral bodies by ligaments is an outer ring of fibrocartilage and collagenous tissue known as the anulus fibrosus. Within this ring but not completely separate from it is an oval semigelatinous mass known as the nucleus pulposus, which contains 75 to 90 per cent water by weight. Cartilaginous end plates are found on the superior and inferior surfaces of the disc separating it from the adjoining vertebral bodies.[14]

There is considerable individual variability in the exact compressive force at which the lumbar discs are damaged. Older persons and those with previous history of back injury or pain cannot sustain as much force as younger individuals with intact vertebrae and discs. In general, however, the spine is well adapted to safely bear large compressive forces but is much more susceptible to damage from shearing (along the surface of the disc) and torsional (twisting) forces.[20]

The vertebral column is able to withstand high forces for extremely short periods of time without injury, while lesser forces acting over a longer period of time are injurious. We are therefore able to land safely from a jump but may suffer structural damage to the cartilaginous structures from continual poor posture or repeated lifting of comparatively light objects in an incorrect manner.

Forces in Lifting

Even a rather superficial analysis of lifting requires a consideration of (a) muscle forces; (b) intra-abdominal and intrathoracic pressures; and (c) weights of the load and body segments. Let us briefly examine their influences and interactions in the recommended "crouch" or "leg" lift (knees flexed, trunk almost erect) (Fig. 21–12) and the "stoop" or "back" lift (knees straight, hips flexed) considered dangerous by most authorities.

If the trunk is nearly erect, most of the weight of the upper body and load being lifted is directed down through the vertebral column, stabilizing it and causing some compression of the discs. By contrast, with the trunk horizontal,

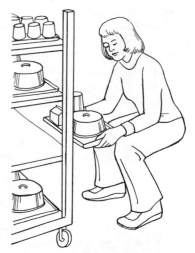

Figure 21–12. An efficient and safe lifting position. (*Note:* when removed from cart, tray will be moved close to the trunk.)

these weights produce a shearing force rather than compression on the disc. Recall that discs are more susceptible to damage from shear.

The moments of the weights of the upper body and load with respect to the lumbosacral junction also influence the magnitude of the compressive force on the discs. If these moments or torques are large, they will have to be overcome by a large moment of force by the back and hip extensor muscles. Since muscle moment arms are characteristically short, this means extremely high muscle forces. In the case of the erector spinae, over 95 per cent of the muscle force is directed along the spine, resulting in compression of the disc. Nachemson[16] indicated that when a 687 N. (70 kg., 154 lb.) person lifts a 196 N. (20 kg., 44 lb.) weight with the back straight and knees bent (crouch lift), the approximate load on the third lumbar disc exerted 2060 N. (210 kg., 462 lb.) of force. When the back was bent and the knees straight during the lift (stoop technique), the force on the disc increased to 3335 N. (340 kg., 748 lb.).

While it is sometimes assumed that these weight moments are large in the stoop method of lifting and small when using the crouch technique, the latter cannot be taken for granted.[3] For the moment of the load with respect to the lumbosacral joint to be small (and it should be), the load must be lifted from a position close to the body; for example, between the knees rather than in front of them. Competitive weightlifters are acutely aware of this and start their lift with their feet actually beneath the bar.

At the beginning of a lift, there is a characteristic elevation of intra-abdominal and intrathoracic pressures (known as the "snatch" pressure). The heavier the weight lifted and the more flexed the trunk, the higher the intra-abdominal pressure (IAP). This elevation in pressure is accomplished largely as a result of contraction of the oblique abdominal and the intercostal muscles at the end of inspiration. The glottis is closed to help contain the pressure. (More information on this Valsalva maneuver is provided in Chapter 33.) In a longitudinal direction, the elevated pressure relieves some of the compression on the discs created by the erector spinae muscles, since it tends to force the vertebrae apart. Eie[6] suggested that there may be up to a 40 per cent reduction in compressive force as a result of this "extensor" mechanism. In an anteroposterior plane the IAP also serves to reduce the shearing force when the trunk is flexed since it pushes back against the lumbar discs.

Research therefore supports the superiority of the crouch method of lifting from the standpoint of safety. Dangerous shear forces are less, and provided that the load is kept close to the body, compressive forces on the discs are also less than when using a stoop technique. Most of the vertical movement in the crouch lift is achieved through contraction of the quadriceps femoris muscles (strong knee extensor group) with less reliance on the hamstrings (hip extensors) and erector spinae (back extensors). To maximize the potential of the quadriceps, however, the nurse should begin the lift with an angle of approximately 120 degrees between the thigh and lower leg. This is usually not feasible if an object is lifted from floor level. It is therefore important to store heavy items on elevated shelves if they have to be lifted to be moved.

Practical Lifting Advice

When moving and lifting persons and objects, the following points should be kept in mind:

1. A mechanical hoist should be employed to lift a large patient or heavy object.
2. A heavy load should be divided into several smaller parts which can be moved separately.
3. Heavy objects should be moved by sliding them along the floor or tipping them from corner to corner rather than lifting them. If these objects require frequent moving, they should be equipped with casters.
4. Assistance should be requested when lifting or moving a heavy patient or object.

If an individual must perform a lift, the following guidelines should be followed:

1. Plan the move ahead of time and be sure the path is clear.
2. Face the direction in which the move will be made to avoid twisting the vertebral column when carrying the load.
3. Place the feet comfortably apart to provide a stable base of support.
4. Flex the knees and keep the trunk as vertical as possible.
5. Keep the load close to the body.
6. Lift by extending the knees and keeping the back almost vertical.
7. Avoid jerking and twisting during the lift.

The need to develop and practice these correct lifting techniques even with relatively light loads cannot be overstressed. In addition, nurses should exercise regularly to strengthen and stretch the muscles involved in lifting, specifically the back, hip and knee extensors as well as the oblique abdominals, which are used to increase the intra-abdominal pressure and relieve some of the pressure on the discs.

APPLICATION OF BIOMECHANICAL PRINCIPLES TO SPECIFIC NURSING PROCEDURES

Having read the preceding overview of biomechanics, you should now appreciate the relevance of biomechanics to nursing practice. You should also be able to recognize the forces influencing the movement of both patient and nurse. Before proceeding further, read Procedures 1 through 5 carefully and attempt to identify how the anatomic and mechanical principles previously discussed apply in the practical situations of moving and lifting patients. Once this has been done, compare your responses with those provided in the comments for each procedure. Keep in mind that many of the stated principles apply to more than one procedure.

Efficient performance of the procedures that follow require considerable skill. In order to develop such skill you will need to practice each procedure many times. It would be helpful for you to take the role of both the patient and the helper(s). This way you will learn what it feels like to have the procedure done to you as well as to do it to someone else. Ask for feedback from a colleague or teacher as you practice. Most important, ask for feedback from the person who is taking the role of the patient during your practice performances. Be patient with yourself. It takes time to develop the psychomotor skills needed in these procedures. It will probably be most helpful for you to try to remember the *principles* involved rather than trying to memorize the steps. Eventually your movements will become smooth and you will be gentle and supportive with the patient.

1.   MOVING HELPLESS PATIENT IN BED

By Jean Saxon, R.N., M.N.

Definition and Purposes.   *These methods will enable one or more workers to move a dependent patient's body either in segments or as a whole.* They are used to correct patient's body alignment, prepare for position change, remove hazards or prevent complications, e.g., inadequate chest expansion, pressure from side rails or foot of bed. Nurse modifies procedure to utilize patient's capabilities and according to sizes of patient and nurse.

Contraindications and Cautions.   Patients with recent spinal injuries or spinal surgery need to be moved by two or more people to maintain alignment. Nurse should obtain help to move heavy patients. The pull sheets beneath the patient easily become wrinkled and can traumatize tissue. Also, prolonged skin contact with plastic can cause skin burns because dissipation of body heat is prevented. Thus, these items should not be left under the patient for too long.

Patient-Family Teaching Points.   Provide the patient and family with the following information: (a) encourage patients to move themselves if they are able, thereby maintaining present muscle strength or increasing strength of their muscles; (b) even if the patient appears to be unconscious, explain how the move is to be accomplished and what signal will be given to initiate the move; (c) emphasize that correct body mechanics will prevent injury to the worker; (d) emphasize that it is more effective to pull the patient into position than it is to push him.

PRE-PROCEDURE ACTIVITIES

PRELIMINARY PATIENT ASSESSMENT

Includes determination of:
- diagnosis and activity orders
- level of consciousness
- abilities and limitations concerning movement
- presence of skin, muscle or bone lesions

PRELIMINARY PLANNING

Includes:
- type and method of move to be accomplished and ways personnel can participate
- bed linens and gown if needed
- comfort and safety of patient
- number of personnel required to safely move patient

EQUIPMENT

- firm bed (bed board if needed), tight bottom linen
- 6 mm. thickness vinyl plastic, 4 ft. × 4 ft.
- folded draw sheet or pull sheet
- side rails, footboard

PREPARATION OF PATIENT

- Discuss with patient and other personnel how move is to be accomplished
- Avoid drafts, provide privacy
- Adjust bed to working height, lower side rails, lock bed wheels
- Fan-fold top linen to foot of bed or loosen top linen and expose extremities
- Change wet or soiled linen
- Place pull sheet with plastic sheet under it beneath patient if needed
- Remove head pillow and place against head of bed
- Remove all pillows, bolsters or other positioning aids
- Place patient's arms on chest
- Unless contraindicated, bed should be level or at 20-degree angle (Trendelenburg position). (When gravity is used to assist movement, less force is needed to move patient.)

PROCEDURE

SUGGESTED STEPS

RATIONALE/DISCUSSION

Moving Patient Up in Bed

A. Moving patient *up* in bed by *one worker* who moves patient's body diagonally in sections. To move patient up in bed, move his legs first. (To move patient down in bed, move head and shoulders first.) (Fig. 21–7, p. 374.)

A. Used when helpless patient can be moved with ease by one worker.

1. Slide patient's legs diagonally toward head of bed, using pull maneuver (see p. 374).

1. Worker faces foot of bed at 40-degree angle. Diagonal pull allows for pull in direction of force.

2. Slide patient's hips toward head of bed; using diagonal pull maneuver.

2. Movement brings patient's hips in line with feet near edge of bed. Pull sheets are advantageous for heavy patients or patients with skin lesions on back.

Procedure continued on the following page

SUGGESTED STEPS	RATIONALE/DISCUSSION

Moving Patient Up in Bed (Continued)

3. Slide patient's head, shoulders and chest toward head of bed, using diagonal pull maneuver. Support patient's head on worker's arm nearest the head of bed; worker's hand reaches under and around patient's far shoulder.	3. Support of patient's head prevents hyperextension and lateral flexion of neck during pull maneuver. Worker's hand around patient's shoulder provides surface upon which pull force is exerted. Patient's body is now on side of bed near worker and has been moved upward in bed.
4. Raise side rail next to patient and go to other side of bed.	4. Protects patient from falling.
5. Repeat diagonal pull of body sections as described above.	5. Move patient diagonally upward and to other side of bed.
6. Pull patient to edge of bed on alternate sides of bed until desired height in bed is reached.	6. Patient is gradually moved up in bed by being moved from one side of the bed to the other in a "zigzag" pattern.
7. Slide patient to center of bed, using a right angle (90-degree) pull of body sections.	7. Protects patient from falling. Worker faces longitudinal center of bed. Pull is in direction of force.
8. Align patient's body.	8. Assess patient for straight spine and alignment of legs and arms.

B. Moving patient *up* in bed by *two workers* working from the same side of the bed.	B. Used when patient is too heavy for one worker.
1. Slide patient's legs first, then move remainder of body in unison upon count of "3." Use diagonal pull maneuver toward head of bed.	1. Does *not* maintain spinal alignment because leg movement causes torsion of spine. (Pull sheets may be used as in "C" below.)
2. Repeat on alternate sides of bed until patient is at desired height in bed.	
3. Slide patient to center of bed using right angle (90-degree) pull maneuver.	3. Assess patient for correct body alignment.

Position of helpers

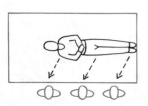 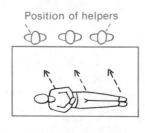 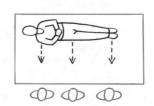

Figure 21–13. Three helper pull maneuver used to move patient up in bed.

SUGGESTED STEPS	RATIONALE/DISCUSSION

Moving Patient Up in Bed *(Continued)*

C. Moving patient *up* in bed by *three workers* working from the same side of the bed. (Fig. 21–13.)

C. Used when patient's body must be maintained in alignment during move (e.g., spinal disorders, fractures) or when patient is too heavy for one worker.

1. Each worker assumes responsibility for supporting one of patient's body sections. Areas to be supported are
▶ head, shoulders and chest
▶ hips
▶ thighs and ankles
Pull sheets may be used. When used, one worker supports patient's head and shoulders and grasps sheet and plastic at midchest level, another at iliac crest and thigh, while the third supports knees and ankles.

1. All body sections are supported by three workers simultaneously.

2. Signal by count of 1, 2, 3; at count of "3," pull in unison to slide patient's body by using diagonal pull maneuver.

2. Pulling in unison maintains patient's spine in correct alignment.

3. Repeat maneuver on alternate sides of bed until patient is at desired height in bed.

4. Slide patient to center of bed using right angle (90-degree) pull maneuver.

4. Protects patient from falling. Assess patient for correct body alignment.

Moving Patient to Side of Bed

D. Moving patient to *side* of bed by *one or more* workers.

D. Used to move helpless patient to side of bed.

1. *One worker* moves patient to *side* of bed by moving body sections (as described in A), using a right angle (90-degree) pull maneuver.

1. Worker faces longitudinal center of bed. Pulls are in direction of force.

2. *Two workers* move patient to side of bed by sliding his legs first and then his head and trunk in unison (as described in B) using a right angle (90-degree) pull maneuver.

2. Used when patient is too heavy for one worker. Does *not* maintain spinal alignment.

3. *Three workers* move patient to *side* of bed by moving patient's body sections in unison (as described in C), using a right angle (90-degree) pull maneuver.

3. Used when patient's spine must be maintained in alignment.

Procedure continued on the following page

POST-PROCEDURE ACTIVITIES

Check patient for correct body alignment; replace head pillow and other bolsters as needed; cover patient; raise rails; lower bed.

Aftercare of Equipment.   Store unneeded bolsters and plastic squares (if removed); discard laundry.

Final Patient Assessment.   Assess patient for pain or discomfort caused or relieved by move; assess skin condition after moving. *Chart/Report:* Final assessment data and patient-family teaching.

COMMENT ON PROCEDURE 1: MOVING HELPLESS PATIENT: UP IN BED; TO SIDE OF BED*

Among the biomechanical principles applied in this procedure are the following:

1. The bed is raised to a height that permits the nurse to keep her back as erect as possible when moving the patient. This reduces the moment of both the nurse's upper body weight and the external reaction force of the patient with respect to the nurse's lumbosacral joint. As a result, there is less compression and less shear on the intervertebral discs, particularly in the lumbar region.

2. The nurse "faces" in the direction of the intended movement so that twisting of the vertebral column is avoided while she is moving the patient. Intervertebral discs are more likely to sustain damage during a combination of torsion (twisting) and compression than when they are subjected to compressive forces alone.

3. Force is exerted in the direction of the desired movement as in the diagonal pull maneuver.

4. The patient is pulled rather than pushed so that the slight upward force reduces the normal component of the reaction of the bed on the patient. This in turn decreases both the maximum static friction between the patient and the bed (which must be overcome to initiate the movement) and the kinetic friction force (which must be exceeded to continue the movement). The decrease in the friction or shear force on the patient's skin lessens the chance of damaging these tissues. In addition, the pulling action avoids compression of the patient's joints and tissues.

5. The smooth plastic under the tight pull sheet reduces the maximum static friction and the kinetic friction between these two surfaces. Therefore, less effort is required on the part of the nurse to move the patient.

6. The patient is aligned in a way that prevents undue stress upon the joint structures.

Figure 21–14 shows two methods by which the nurse can help a patient who is not totally helpless to move himself up in bed.

Figure 21–15 shows a method by which two persons can move a patient to the edge of the bed using the pull maneuver.

---

*Comments on procedures are by Doris I. Miller

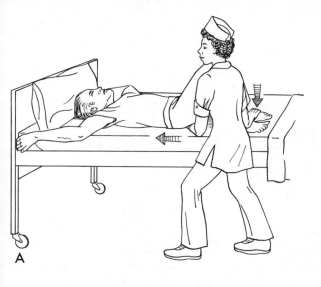

A

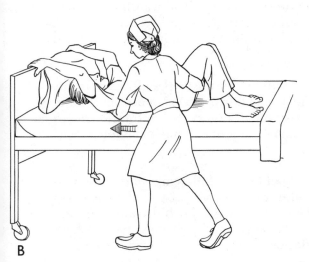

B

Figure 21–14.   Assisting patient to move himself up in bed (two methods). *A,* Moving patient up in bed with patient assisting with strong arms. Nurse stabilizes patient's feet and provides assistance at patient's sacrum (buttocks). *B,* This method is inefficient because the nurse's left arm is not needed under patient's shoulders. Weight of buttocks on bed will impede movements.

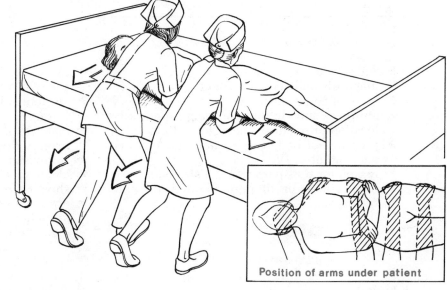

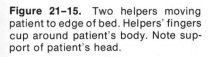

Figure 21–15.   Two helpers moving patient to edge of bed. Helpers' fingers cup around patient's body. Note support of patient's head.

Position of arms under patient

2.   TRANSFER OF HELPLESS PATIENT FROM BED TO STRETCHER

By Jean Saxon, R.N., M.N.

Definition and Purposes.   *Three-person carry of patient to stretcher is accomplished by three (or more) helpers lifting the patient from one side of the bed and then carrying him to the stretcher. A helpless patient can also be transferred to a stretcher by three or four helpers lifting and sliding him from bed to stretcher on a draw sheet or by using a draw sheet with a short roller bar.* This transfer is used to move a patient who is helpless, sedated, and/or unresponsive because of injury, illness, medication or anesthesia. The nurse determines the method of transfer and number of helpers.

Contraindications and Cautions.   If patient has unstabilized injury to his spinal cord, maintain alignment of his spine during transfer. Do not use short roller bar for patients with spinal injuries or chest or spinal surgery. Never transfer such a patient without physician's written permission except in extreme emergency, e.g., fire.

Patient-Family Teaching Points.   Provide the following information as appropriate: (a) explain reason for transfer to stretcher; (b) explain transfer procedure, mentioning that signals will be given to accomplish the move; (c) use mechanical lifts when patient is too heavy for workers to lift safely; and (d) have patient assist in transfer if he can safely do so.

PRE-PROCEDURE ACTIVITIES

PRELIMINARY PATIENT ASSESSMENT

Includes determination of:
▶ diagnosis and activity orders
▶ level of consciousness
▶ abilities and limitations, e.g., paralysis, location of fractures, need for splints
▶ presence of body lesions and attachments, e.g., catheter, IV
▶ reason for transportation via stretcher
▶ medications or therapy needed prior to transfer

EQUIPMENT

▶ draw sheet or plastic sheet under draw sheet
▶ stretcher (IV pole, holder for drainage bag, linen)
▶ clamps for disconnecting tubing or closing urinary drainage tubing
▶ pillows and other position aids
▶ clean sheet or bath blanket
▶ short roller bar
▶ equipment to accompany patient on stretcher after transfer is accomplished, e.g., chart, medications

PRELIMINARY PLANNING

Includes:
▶ Deciding on method of transfer

PREPARATION OF PATIENT

▶ Provide privacy
▶ Explain destination and method

PRELIMINARY PLANNING

▶ selection of number of helpers needed (three or more if patient is heavy or has IV or other attachments)
▶ organization of unit
▶ determination of equipment to be disconnected or to hold IV or drainage apparatus
▶ designation of team leader and signals she will use during move (best to have helper who supports greatest amount of patient's weight be leader)

PREPARATION OF PATIENT

▶ Clamp catheter (do not disconnect) to prevent backflow of urine during transfer
▶ Hang IV and drainage bag on side of bed from which patient will be lifted
▶ Fan-fold linen and cover patient with bath blanket or sheet
▶ Clamp and disconnect nasogastric tube and other tubes if permitted
▶ Place patient's arms on his chest (secure with draw sheet if necessary)
▶ Lock stretcher *and* bed
▶ Raise bed to stretcher level (slightly higher for draw sheet transfer)
▶ Level mattress if tolerated by patient

PROCEDURE

SUGGESTED STEPS	RATIONALE/DISCUSSION

Three-Person Carry

A. *Three-person carry* of helpless patient from bed to stretcher is accomplished by three helpers (working on the same side of the bed) lifting and carrying patient to stretcher.

A. Enhances good body mechanics for helpers; is safe and comfortable for patient. (If patient is excessively heavy, use four helpers or mechanical lift.)

1. Position stretcher at right angle to head or foot of bed (Fig. 21–16).

1. Gives room for helpers to move; shortens distance to carry patient.

2. Move patient to edge of bed from which he is to be lifted. (See Procedure 1.)

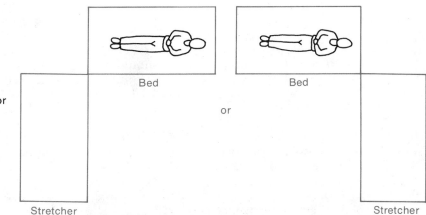

Figure 21–16. Positioning of stretcher for three-person carry.

Procedure continued on the following page

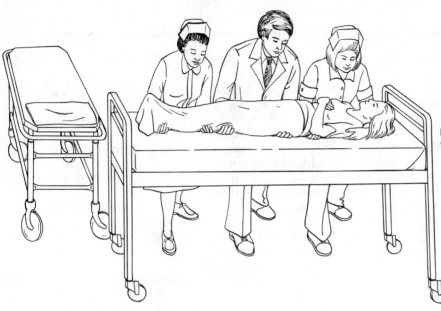

Figure 21–17. Position of helpers for three-person carry.

SUGGESTED STEPS	RATIONALE/DISCUSSION

Three-Person Carry (Continued)

3. Three helpers position themselves at bedside along same side of bed. (See Fig. 21–17.) Each helper assumes responsibility for supporting one of the following body sections of the patient: (a) head, shoulders and chest; (b) hips; and (c) thighs and ankles. Strongest helper stands beside male patient's head and shoulders or beside female patient's hips.

3. Each section of the helpless patient's body will be adequately supported during transfer. Strongest helper can more safely lift heaviest section of the patient's body.

4. Helpers assume wide-based, forward-backward stances with knees flexed.

4. Provides a stable base in the direction of intended backward motion. Flexed knees bring helpers' arms to bed level and place helpers in position to lift with strong leg muscles.

5. Helpers place their arms on bed, sliding them under patient's head, shoulders and chest; hips; and legs. Next helpers flex their fingers securely around far side of patient's body.

5. Flexing of helpers' fingers places patient's weight within a forearm lever, thereby enabling efficient use of force during lifting. Helpers' elbows serve as fulcrum.

6. At the leader's count of "1" helpers simultaneously roll patient to their chests, keeping their elbows on bed.

6. Brings patient's weight within helpers' base of support.

7. On count of "2" helpers stand, holding patient securely against their chests.

7. Use of helpers' strong hip and leg muscles provides safest and most efficient lifting force.

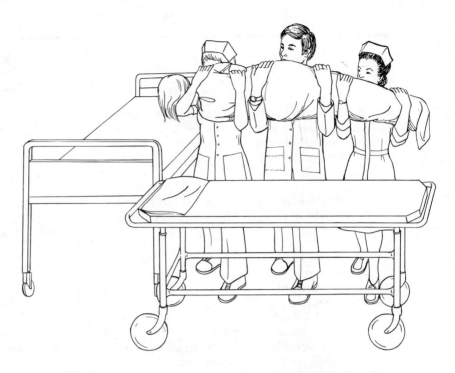

Figure 21–18. Proper support of patient during three-person carry.

SUGGESTED STEPS	RATIONALE/DISCUSSION

Three-Person Carry (Continued)

8. On count of "3" helpers step backward, then pivot toward stretcher and walk to side of stretcher. (See Fig. 21–18.)

8. Helpers must move in unison to maintain patient's alignment and to prevent injury or discomfort to patient or themselves.

9. On count of "4" helpers flex hips and knees (while in a wide-based, forward-backward stance) in order to lower their elbows to stretcher edge.

9. Patient's weight is maintained within helpers' base of support. Helpers' strong leg muscles support patient's weight.

10. On count of "5" helpers lower patient to back-lying position by slowly straightening their knees and lowering their forearms onto the stretcher.

10. Provides controlled movement of patient's weight as he rolls away from helper's chests and onto his back.

Draw Sheet Transfer

B. *Draw sheet transfer* of helpless patient to stretcher requires three or four helpers. Even more helpers may be needed to safely transfer a heavy patient or a patient encumbered with excessive tubing and/or equipment.

> Caution: *Without adequate help*, draw sheet transfers *can produce back injuries to helpers because helpers must reach beyond their base of support.*

1. Loosen draw sheet on both sides of bed and roll draw sheet close to patient on both sides. Place turning sheet if draw sheet not present.

1. Draw sheet or turning sheet (with plastic if needed) is used throughout transfer.

Procedure continued on the following page

SUGGESTED STEPS   RATIONALE/DISCUSSION

Draw Sheet Transfer (Continued)

2. Three helpers stand at side of bed from which patient is to be moved. Using 90-degree pull maneuver, helpers pull patient to edge of bed. (See Procedure 1 and p. 374.)

2. Pull maneuver is safest method for helpers and is comfortable for patient.

3. First helper goes to far side of bed and holds patient in position along edge of bed.

3. Protects patient from slipping off bed. Important to support patient's arm and leg nearest edge of bed.

4. Second and third helpers position stretcher parallel to bed, against side of bed nearest patient. (Lock wheels of bed and stretcher.)

Caution: *To prevent patient injury always lock wheels of bed and stretcher prior to transferring patient.*

5. Raise head of stretcher (or place pillows on stretcher equal to head elevation of bed) if patient requires head and chest elevation.

5. Elevation of patient's head and chest is necessary to facilitate breathing for some patients with lung and/or heart disorders.

6. Pad space between stretcher and bed to bridge the two surfaces.

6. Deep depression or hump between stretcher and bed will impede slide of patient.

7. Place clean sheet over empty half of bed.

7. Protects helper's clothing from contamination by patient's bottom sheet.

8. First helper kneels on sheet-covered bed at level of patient's waist and grasps rolled draw sheet with one hand at patient's mid-chest and other hand at patient's hips. Helper's hips are flexed in preparation for the lift, which will be accomplished by straightening hips.

8. If patient is heavy, an extra helper kneels on sheet-covered bed. One helper grasps rolled draw sheet at patient's shoulder and waist; the other helper grasps rolled draw sheet at patient's iliac crest and mid-thigh.

9. Second helper stands at corner of stretcher at an angle to the patient's head. She reaches across the head of the stretcher, supports patient's head with one hand and with other hand grasps rolled draw sheet at patient's shoulder. Prepares to use 90-degree pull maneuver. A fourth helper may support the head of a very helpless or heavy patient.

9. If patient is able to support his own head, or if a fourth helper supports head from top of stretcher, second helper shifts her position. Second helper then stands at side of stretcher, reaches across stretcher and grasps draw sheet at patient's shoulder and waist.

10, Third helper, standing at foot of stretcher, moves patient's legs to edge of stretcher near bed. Helper then moves to side of stretcher, reaches across stretcher and grasps rolled draw sheet at patient's iliac crest and at top of patient's thigh. Prepares for 90-degree pull maneuver.

10. Prior movement of patient's legs reduces drag of lower extremities. Draw sheet is grasped as close to patient's body as possible.

SUGGESTED STEPS   RATIONALE/DISCUSSION

Draw Sheet Transfer (Continued)

11. First helper (leader) counts "1, 2, 3"; at count of "3" first helper lifts by straightening hips; second and third helpers pull. Helpers move in unison.

11. The first helper's lift action reduces friction and permits an efficient pulling force by the second and third helpers.

12. Place patient's legs in line with his body at center of stretcher.

Caution: *Do not pull patient beyond center of stretcher.*

Roller Bar Transfer

C. *Roller bar transfer* uses a draw sheet between patient and roller bar. A roller bar (manufactured under several trade names) is a metal frame containing metal rollers covered with plastic fabric. Fabric rolls around the frame when weight (patient) is placed on it, and the weight is pulled. Roller bars vary in length (30 to 60 inches); the shorter model is used more frequently and is discussed below.

C. *Roller bar with a draw sheet transfer is preferred over draw sheet transfer alone* because patient's weight is supported on roller bar. Pulling requires less force than lifting, and lifting is not required when using roller bar. Nonetheless, it is desirable to use three helpers for this transfer.

Caution: *Do not use roller bar of any kind for patients with spinal injuries. The short roller bar produces hyperextension of the thorax and is contraindicated in patients with chest surgery.*

1. First helper works on far side of bed; second and third helpers work on side from which patient will be moved.

1. First helper remains on far side of bed throughout transfer.

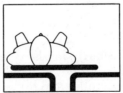
Davis Patient Roller is placed beneath patient. Draw sheet technique is recommended.

Patient is gently rolled across D.P.R. from bed or O.R. Table to stretcher and vice versa.

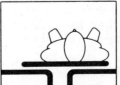
After transfer is complete, draw sheet technique is again employed and Roller removed.

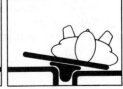
Gaps and varied height levels are bridged by using a pillow beneath the Roller.

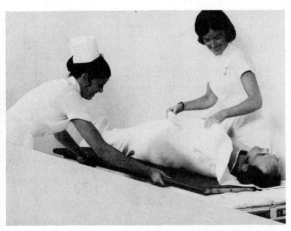

Figure 21–19. The Long Davis Patient Roller. (From Chick Orthopedic, Oakland, CA.)

Figure 21–20. The Chick Davis Patient Roller. (From Chick Orthopedic, Oakland, CA.)

Procedure continued on the following page

SUGGESTED STEPS	RATIONALE/DISCUSSION

Roller Bar Transfer (Continued)

2. Loosen draw sheet on both sides of bed or place turning sheet under patient if draw sheet not present.	2. Draw sheet or turning sheet is used throughout transfer to protect patient's skin from roller bar.
3. First helper reaches across patient, grasps draw sheet and rolls patient toward her. Helper next smoothes draw sheet over patient's back and supports patient on side.	3. Permits placement of roller bar under patient. Smooth draw sheet protects skin on patient's back. Helper's body protects patient from falling.
4. Second helper places short roller bar on bed, behind patient at level of his hips, while patient is on his side. Second helper is the leader.	4. Roller bar supports majority of patient's weight. Leader controls movement.
5. Helpers lower patient backward, onto roller, by guiding him with taut draw sheet (or turning sheet). Second helper holds roller bar in place with one hand.	5. Provides for controlled movement of patient from side-lying to supine position on roller bar.
6. Roll draw sheet toward patient on both sides so that it does not hang over the sides of bed and the roll is within easy reach of helpers.	6. Prevents catching draw sheet between bed and stretcher. Draw sheet is not rolled to the patient (as in B, 1) because helpers must reach across the stretcher (see step 9 below) and across bed (see step 12 below) during the transfer.
7. Second and third helpers position stretcher parallel to and in contact with bed. Lock wheels of bed and stretcher; pad space between stretcher and bed.	7. Helpers work quickly because roller bar is uncomfortable. Locked wheels prevent movement of bed or stretcher during transfer. Padding bridges surfaces.
8. First helper maintains taut draw sheet throughout move.	8. Provides smooth draw sheet to protect patient's skin; maintains weight on roller bar.
9. Second helper (leader) stands at side of stretcher, grasps draw sheet at levels of top and bottom edges of roller and prepares for 90-degree pull maneuver.	9. Roller bar supports most of patient's weight.
10. Third helper stands at head of stretcher. Reaching under draw sheet, worker uses one arm to support patient's head and far shoulder and her other hand to support patient's near shoulder.	10. Supporting patient's shoulders under draw sheet helps maintain smooth draw sheet. Helper stands at head of stretcher to reduce reaching distance.
11. Leader gives signal by counting "1, 2, 3."	11. Provides for simultaneous action by helpers.
12. On count of "3" second helper pulls draw sheet and third helper guides head and shoulders as first helper maintains taut draw sheet.	12. Roller bar remains under patient, supporting his weight as he rolls from bed onto stretcher.

SUGGESTED STEPS	RATIONALE/DISCUSSION

Roller Bar Transfer (Continued)

13. Helpers maintain grasp on draw sheet until patient is in center of stretcher.	13. Prevents patient from falling off stretcher.
14. Unlock stretcher and move it away from bed. Relock stretcher. Protect patient from falling while moving stretcher.	14. Work quickly because roller bar produces pressure on body tissues once tension is released on draw sheet.
15. With a helper on each side of stretcher, turn patient on his side with the draw sheet and remove roller bar. Remove draw sheet if not needed.	15. Roller bar is uncomfortable, therefore is removed quickly.

> Caution: *Stretcher is narrow. Support patient on stretcher during turn to his side.*

16. Align patient's head, body and legs on center of stretcher.

POST-PROCEDURE ACTIVITIES

Remove draw sheet (and plastic sheet) if appropriate; smooth surface beneath patient; establish correct body alignment for patient, e.g., place head pillow and other bolsters as needed; cover patient for privacy and warmth; raise side rails or fasten stretcher straps; check IV for correct flow rate; attach urinary drainage bag below bladder level *and unclamp tubing;* reattach other equipment which must accompany patient; obtain equipment and supplies to be sent with patient, e.g., chart, linen.

Aftercare of Equipment. Place bed and unit in order for patient's return. Return roller bar to storage area.

Final Patient Assessment. Determine patient's comfort and safety. *Chart/report:* Time patient sent by stretcher, where he went and who accompanied him, according to agency policy.

COMMENT ON PROCEDURE 2: TRANSFER OF HELPLESS PATIENT FROM BED TO STRETCHER

In addition to many of the biomechanical principles pointed out in the previous procedure, the following are used in the transfer of a helpless patient.

Three-Person Carry

1. The patient is moved to the edge of the bed before the lift is initiated so that the nurses can keep their trunks more erect than would be possible if they attempted to lift the patient from the middle or from the far side of the bed. As already indicated, the nearly vertical trunk orientation reduces the moments of the weights of the patient and the nurse's upper body with respect to the lumbosacral joint. In addition, since most of the upward movement is achieved by utilizing the knee and

Text continued on the following page

COMMENT ON PROCEDURE 2: TRANSFER OF HELPLESS PATIENT FROM BED TO STRETCHER

Three-Person Carry (Continued)

hip extensor muscles, less back extensor muscle force is required. As a result of both these factors, compression of the nurse's lumbar intervertebral discs is reduced and injury to this area of the back is less likely.

2. The strongest individuals are positioned to support the patient's trunk. This is done because the trunk of the human body represents approximately 58 per cent of the total weight.

3. The base of support is enlarged in the direction of intended motion as indicated by the forward-backward stride position assumed by the nurses.

4. The patient is rolled toward the nurses before the lift is executed so that the moment of the patient's weight with respect to the nurses is reduced as much as possible.

5. Each nurse involved in the transfer turns his or her body as a single unit rather than twisting the trunk as the pivot is made to take the patient to the stretcher.

6. Lowering the patient to the stretcher involves eccentric contraction of the nurses' knee and hip extensor muscles.

Draw Sheet Transfer

1. The wheels of bed and stretcher are locked. Since the maximum static friction far exceeds the rolling friction, the nurses are able to exert force against the bed and stretcher without moving them.

2. Using the 90-degree pull maneuver, the nurses apply force in the direction they wish to move the patient.

3. The space between bed and stretcher is padded to provide a smoother surface over which to move the patient.

4. Extreme caution is advised when the helper on the bed pulls up on the draw sheet. Since the helper's knees are flexed, the hamstrings are in a somewhat shortened position, and they cannot generate maximum hip extensor torque. Although the gluteal muscles may aid in extending the hips, it is likely that most of the upward motion will be the result of back extension. In addition, the helper is unstable because her line of gravity will be close to the forward edge of the base of support (i.e., the knees). Therefore, the helper can easily lose balance in the forward direction and may not be able to recover by increasing the base in that direction. Because of these problems, this procedure should be avoided if at all possible.

5. The helper stands at the end of the bed and stretcher while moving the patient's feet. An individual who must reach across the stretcher to move the patient's legs is in an unstable position and risks low back injury as a result of compressive and shearing forces on the lumbar discs.

Roller Bar Transfer

1. The roller bar takes advantage of the fact that the coefficient of rolling friction is considerably less than the coefficient of kinetic (i.e., sliding) friction.

2. The nurses do not have to "work against gravity" when using this device.

3. The first helper, in reaching across the patient to grasp the draw sheet, exerts a moment of force with respect to the axis around which the patient will turn (i.e., the side of the patient). During the initial part of this pull, the "disrupting moment" provided by the nurse is opposed by a "restoring moment" of the pa-

Roller Bar Transfer (Continued)

tient's weight. The latter torque becomes progressively smaller as the patient is rolled onto his side because the moment arm of the patient's weight with respect to the turning axis becomes less. As a result, correspondingly less torque needs to be applied by the nurse as the patient approaches a side-lying position.

4. When the patient is on his side, while the roller bar is being placed or removed, he must be supported by a nurse. Recall that the base of support in such a side-lying position is comparatively small. In the absence of a stabilizing external force, if the patient's line of gravity should fall outside either edge of this base, he would roll to a supine or a prone position depending on the direction of the weight moment with respect to the axis of rotation.

5. The patient should be removed from the roller bar as quickly as possible to prevent the restriction of blood flow to the skin at the points of contact. Because the roller bar surface is solid, it exerts considerable pressure on the bony prominences and thus could cause tissue damage.

3.   ASSISTING PATIENT TO SIT ON SIDE OF BED: TO "DANGLE"

By Jean Saxon, R.N., M.N.

Definition and Purposes.   *One method of assisting a patient to move from supine to sitting position on the edge of the bed with feet supported on floor or footstool.* Used by one worker to assist a weak, paralyzed or postoperative patient to sit on edge of bed in order to cough; deep breathe; increase muscle activity; assist in overcoming orthostatic hypotension; prepare for chest examination, transfer or ambulation activities; and relearn independent movement. This method reduces stress on abdominal surgical incisions. The nurse modifies the procedure to utilize the patient's capabilities.

Contraindications and Cautions.   Patients with impaired balance may be injured unless supported while in the sitting position. Patients with severe orthostatic hypotension require special preconditioning and supportive devices, e.g., elastic stockings, prior to "dangling." (See Chap. 33.) Do not maintain fainting patient in sitting position.

Patient-Family Teaching Points.   Provide the patient and family with the following information as appropriate: (a) encourage patients to use their own muscle power to maintain and strengthen muscles; (b) explain that self-movement is less uncomfortable than being moved by others; (c) explain that muscular inactivity (e.g., due to fear of pain or falling) may contribute to forgetting how to perform various movements; (d) explain that giving verbal instructions and touching the patient on the body part to be moved will help the patient to learn and perform each step of the procedure; (e) emphasize that family, patient and staff should

Procedure continued on the following page

use the same procedure; (f) explain that having the patient roll to his side prior to sitting minimizes tissue trauma and stress (e.g., minimizes trauma to scrotum and ischial tuberosities and reduces stress on abdominal and perineal wounds); and (g) explain that prior to discharge the patient needs to practice the method he will use to sit up in his bed at home.

PRE-PROCEDURE ACTIVITIES

PRELIMINARY ASSESSMENT

Includes determination of:
▶ diagnosis and activities orders
▶ ability to follow directions
▶ abilities and limitations concerning movement, e.g., orthostatic hypotension, paralysis, weakness
▶ presence of skin, muscle, bone lesions
▶ "dangling" procedure taught to patient by physical therapist
▶ adaptability of "dangling" procedure to patient's home environment (if applicable)

PRELIMINARY PLANNING

Includes:
▶ side of bed to be used (right or left)
▶ comfort and safety of patient, e.g., pre-medication for pain, side rails, slippers, robe
▶ arrange unit to provide space for worker to assist and protect patient

EQUIPMENT

▶ firm bed (hi-low bed if possible)
▶ footstool if bed is high or patient is short
▶ slippers
▶ paper or sheet to protect bottom sheet from soil of slippers
▶ robe or bath blanket if needed for warmth
▶ pillow and/or arm sling as needed

PREPARATION OF PATIENT

▶ Discuss with patient how move to "dangle" position will be accomplished
▶ Fan-fold top linen to foot of bed
▶ Place paper under patient's feet (to protect sheet from contamination by patient's slippers)
▶ Put on patient's slippers
▶ Lift half side rail (if present and needed) on the side on which patient will sit
▶ Level and lower bed; *lock bed wheels*
▶ Position footstool (if needed)

PROCEDURE

SUGGESTED STEPS	RATIONALE/DISCUSSION
Dangle Positions	
A. "Dangle" position for *weak* or *postsurgical patient.*	A. For patient who has use of extremities.
1. Tell patient to move toward the edge of bed in a supine position. (Procedure 1, instruct to move body sections.)	1. Patient in supine position moves close enough to bed edge to allow his knees to bend over mattress edge when sitting.
2. Worker stands at side of bed at level of patient's waist.	2. Protects patient from rolling out of bed; positions worker to assist patient.
3. Tell patient how to roll to his side. During instruction, touch each body part he will move.	3. Touching body parts to be moved reinforces verbal instruction. Patient's use of his own muscles increases his strength.

SUGGESTED STEPS	RATIONALE/DISCUSSION

Dangle Positions (Continued)

a. Tell patient to bend his knees as your hand is placed under them; on command have patient lift his far leg over his near leg.	a. Assist in movement only if necessary. Patient's far leg serves as a long lever force.
b. Tell patient to move his near arm away from his side and to grasp side of mattress. On command have patient reach for side rail (or mattress edge) with his far arm.	b. Prevents rolling on near arm, causing possible injury. Touching patient's hands reinforces instructions. Far arm serves as a long lever force.
c. Tell patient to pull on side rail (or mattress edge) with far hand and simultaneously lift far leg over near leg (Fig. 21–21A).	c. Simultaneous movement of patient's far arm and far leg produces most effective pulling force. Maintains spinal alignment, minimizes stress on abdominal muscles. Worker assists by pulling patient's far arm and leg if needed.
4. Tell patient how to assume sitting position on side of bed.	4. Method minimizes stress and trauma on abdominal muscles, scrotum, ischial tuberosities and perineal wounds.
a. Tell patient to slide his heels off edge of mattress on command.	a. Weight of legs acts as a counterweight and pulls trunk upright. Worker places hands around patient's knees to reinforce directions and assist if needed.
b. Tell patient to push fist of upper arm into mattress; pull with lower arm by grasping mattress edge, then roll upward on elbow on command.	b. Produces force for lateral movement of trunk to upright position. Worker assists by pulling under lower shoulder if needed.

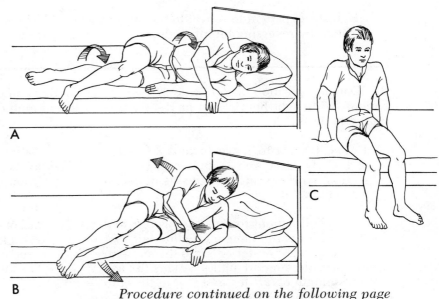

Figure 21–21. Weak or postsurgical patient helping himself to a sitting position on edge of bed, i.e., to "dangle." Patient first moves himself to edge of bed. *A,* Patient rolls onto his side by using his far arm and leg as levers to turn his body. *B,* Patient assumes sitting position by pushing fist of far arm into mattress while grasping mattress edge with near hand and sliding his heels off mattress edge. *C,* Patient maintains upright position by pushing fists into mattress (arms behind and to sides of buttocks) and keeping feet flat on floor.

Procedure continued on the following page

SUGGESTED STEPS	RATIONALE/DISCUSSION

Dangle Positions (Continued)

c. Tell patient to push, pull and roll upward with arms as heels and legs go over the edge of mattress (see Fig. 21–21*B*).	c. Simultaneous movement of arms and legs maintains spinal alignment and utilizes gravity from weight of patient's legs.
5. When upright position is attained, tell patient to push his fists into mattress to assist in maintaining sitting position. (Patient may grasp side rail with near hand for support.)	5. Strengthens arm muscles. Use of fists increases length of arms and provides stability for sitting balance (see Fig. 21–21*C*).
6. Tell patient to place both feet flat on floor (or footstool).	6. Assess for absence of pressure behind knees (at popliteal area). (Pressure may injure nerves and blood vessels.) Stabilizes sitting position.
7. Ask patient how he feels. Observe for symptoms (e.g., pallor) of orthostatic hypotension.	7. Assess patient for lightheadedness, fainting, dizziness, sweating (diaphoresis).
8. Tell patient to alternately flex each foot up and down (i.e., dorsiflex and plantarflex feet) if there are symptoms of orthostatic hypotension.	8. Provides pumping action of leg muscles to support venous return.
9. Place patient in supine position if orthostatic hypotension persists and apply elastic stockings or Ace bandages to lower legs and abdominal belt or binder.	9. Prevents pooling of venous blood in legs and abdomen.
10. Help patient to put on robe and/or cover with bath blanket.	10. Maintains body warmth.
11. Instruct patient to return to the supine position by reversing the procedure.	11. Provides controlled movement by the patient, avoids jarring by sudden loss of balance.
B. "Dangle" position *on left side of bed* for patients with right hemiplegia or right leg or right arm disability.	B. Recommended in the literature as preferred method for right hemiplegia.
1. Tell patient to move toward *left* edge of bed. Instruct him to move each body section. Worker stands at left side of bed at patient's waist.	1. Patient is in the supine position. Worker protects patient from rolling off bed; positions worker to assist the patient.
a. Tell patient to (1) slide his *left* foot under his right knee; (2) slide *left* foot down right posterior leg to the ankle to provide support under ankle; (3) use strength of *left* leg and foot to lift both legs toward edge of bed (Fig. 21–22).	a. Worker touches patient's *left* foot and guides his movements to reinforce verbal instructions. Strong leg is used to lift impaired leg.

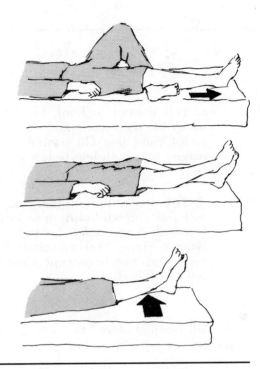

Figure 21–22. Patient moving impaired right leg to side of bed. Strong left leg is slid under knee and down to ankle of weak right leg. Then strong left leg lifts and moves weak right leg. (Adapted from *Strike Back at Stroke,* distributed by the American Heart Association.)

SUGGESTED STEPS	RATIONALE/DISCUSSION

Dangle Positions (Continued)

b. Tell patient to move his buttocks toward edge of bed by pushing into mattress with foot of flexed *left* leg and his *left* shoulder. If assistance is needed, worker lifts "dead weight" of patient's right buttock from right side of bed (using her elbows as a fulcrum).

b. Allows elevation of left buttock to decrease friction and therefore requires less of the patient's energy to move. Assistance of worker reduces friction caused by weight of right buttock.

c. Tell patient to pull his head and shoulders into line with rest of body by grasping mattress edge or half side rail with *left* hand.

c. Touching patient's hand reinforces verbal instruction.

2. Tell patient how to roll to *left* side, touching each part to be moved. Worker stands on *left* side of bed at patient's waist.

2. Worker stands in a protective position, within easy reach to reinforce movement by touching patient.

a. Tell patient to grasp right arm at wrist with *left* hand and to pull right arm over chest as far as possible.

a. Brings weight of arm toward center of gravity; therefore, weight of arm will not impede turn.

b. Tell patient to grasp *left* side rail at mattress level with his *left* hand (or to grasp the mattress edge) and push *left* shoulder under body on command. (If assistance is needed, worker places hand on patient's right shoulder blade and rolls patient on his left side.)

b. Patient's movement assists in turning trunk; assistance of worker turns upper trunk.

Procedure continued on the following page

SUGGESTED STEPS	RATIONALE/DISCUSSION

Dangle Positions (Continued)

c. Tell patient to hook his *left* foot under his right ankle and use left foot to lift right leg. On command, have patient turn both legs to left side.

c. Provides long lever force to turn trunk. Patient's *left* foot and leg provide the power for the turn. Patient's legs are flexed at knees.

d. Tell patient to simultaneously push with *left* arm while lifting and turning legs with power of *left* leg to *left* side-lying position. Worker stands in protective position to prevent patient from rolling off bed.

> Caution: *Patients with right-sided extremity disorders are in danger of falling out of bed when turning to the left side. For example, "dead weight" of paralyzed limbs or weight of plaster casts on limbs makes it difficult for the patient to control his turn because his "good" side is not in a position to control the movement.*

3. Tell patient how to assume sitting position on *left* side of bed (Fig. 21–23).

a. Tell patient to (1) grasp edge of mattress or mattress level of side rail with *left* hand; (2) roll up on *left* elbow; then (3) push with *left* hand until trunk is upright on command.

a. Worker assists by pulling with her hand under patient's *left* shoulder. It is difficult for patients to learn this movement because arm strength must be developed.

b. Tell patient to hook his right foot with his *left* foot and then slide heels of both feet off edge of mattress on command.

b. Weight of legs assists in pulling trunk upright. Worker guides patient's legs off bed by supporting under patient's knees.

c. Tell patient that as his legs go over edge of mattress he should simultaneously roll up on his *left* arm and push his trunk upright. Worker stands in front of patient with feet in forward-backward wide-based stance, facing head of bed with outside foot forward.

c. Worker assumes position to assist patient. (Patients often need help in starting momentum.) Patient's impaired right arm should be across his chest and worker's hands should be placed to support patient's left shoulder and knees (Fig. 21–24).

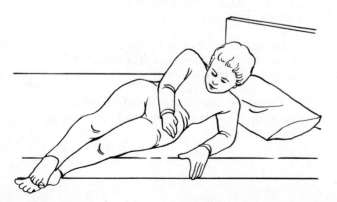

Figure 21–23. Person with right-sided disability (right hemiplegia or right leg or right arm disability) assisting self to sitting position. Patient rolls up on strong arm as weight of legs pulls her upright. Strong left leg controls right leg. Patient's body should be close to edge of bed when beginning this activity.

SUGGESTED STEPS	RATIONALE/DISCUSSION

Dangle Positions (Continued)

4. Instruct patient to support his trunk by grasping side rail or pushing *left* fist into mattress.

5. Instruct patient to guide his right foot with *left* foot to a position flat on floor; then he should unhook *left* foot and place it flat on floor to provide balance.

6. Worker helps patient to dress in robe and/or covers him with bath blanket.

7. Instruct patient to position right arm on pillow or in lap. If patient's sitting balance is poor, worker supports patient's right arm and hand with pillow and/or sling.

4. Use of *left* arm to support balance increases arm strength. Strong arm will be needed for transfer and walking activities.

5. Sitting balance is enhanced by placing feet apart and flat on floor. If patient's right arm is disabled, it should be supported while patient is in "dangle" position; patient should grasp side rail with strong left hand to maintain balance.

6. Robe and covers maintain body warmth. After patient has developed sitting balance, he is taught to dress himself.

> Caution: *To prevent injury, position paralyzed arm correctly. Also, do not place covers over paralyzed arm because this impairs observation of arm by worker and patient.*

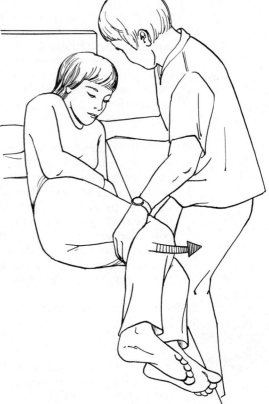

Figure 21–24. Worker assisting patient who has right-sided impairment to sitting position. Patient is being helped to a sitting position on the edge of the bed, i.e., "to dangle." Patient's impaired right arm is across her chest and worker's hands are placed in a position of support under patient's left shoulder and knees.

Procedure continued on the following page

SUGGESTED STEPS	RATIONALE/DISCUSSION

Dangle Positions (Continued)

8. Worker remains with patient throughout "dangle" period, standing or sitting in front of patient. Check patient's pulse and blood pressure if indicated.	8. Protects patient from falling out of bed. Assess patient for orthostatic hypotension and excessive weakness.
9. Instruct patient to return to the supine position by reversing the procedure.	9. Patient may need assistance to lift his legs to bed level.
C. "Dangle" position on *right side of bed* for patients with right hemiplegia or right leg or right arm disability.	C. Provides greater control of movement for right hemiplegia. Recommended by author.
1. Tell patient to move toward the right edge of bed. Teach him how to move each body part. Worker stands at right side of bed at patient's waist.	1. Patient is in the supine position. Worker protects patient from rolling out of bed; positions worker to assist the patient.
a. Tell patient to (1) slide his *left* foot under his right knee; (2) slide his *left* foot down the posterior right leg to the ankle; and (3) use strength of *left* leg to lift both legs toward the edge of bed.	a. Worker guides movement of *left* leg to reinforce verbal instructions.
b. Tell patient to assist in moving his buttocks toward the edge of bed by pushing foot of flexed *left* leg and *left* shoulder into mattress to lift *left* buttock. Worker places hands under buttocks and utilizes 90-degree pull maneuver (see p. 374) to move buttocks to edge of bed.	b. It is more difficult for patient with right hemiplegia to move to the right because of the dead weight of the buttock on the paralyzed side. As the patient gains strength in the left side, he will be able to lift himself high enough to clear the right buttock.
c. Tell patient to grasp his right arm at wrist with his *left* hand and pull right arm across chest. Then tell patient to push his head and shoulders to the right by pushing against the *left* side rail or mattress with his *left* hand and arm. Worker assists by placing hands under patient's shoulders and waist, then using pull maneuver to move patient's upper trunk to right side of bed.	c. Patient's actions remove weight of impaired right arm and shoulder, which would impede move. Prevents injury to impaired arm. As patient gains strength in *left* arm, he will be able to slide to the right on his *left* shoulder.
2. Tell patient how to roll to *right* side, touching each part to be moved.	2. A patient with right hemiplegia can roll to the right side easier and with more control than he can to the left.
a. Tell patient to grasp right arm at the wrist with his *left* hand and to move his right arm to the right side of the bed, extending it away from his body.	a. Prevents rolling onto impaired arm, causing possible injury to the arm or hand.

SUGGESTED STEPS	RATIONALE/DISCUSSION

Dangle Positions (Continued)

b. Tell patient to lift his *left* leg over his right leg on command.	b. Provides a long lever force.
c. Tell patient to reach with his *left* arm over to right mattress edge or right side rail at mattress level on command.	c. Provides a long lever force.
d. Tell patient to simultaneously lift his *left* leg and *left* arm, controlling the speed of the turn by the rapidity of movement of leg and arm.	d. Force obtained from long levers provides efficient movement. Assistance by worker is not required.
3. Tell patient how to assume sitting position on *right* edge of bed.	
a. Tell patient to place fist of *left* hand on mattress at chest level and push.	a. Provides momentum for elevation of trunk. Worker assists by pulling with hand under right shoulder.
b. Tell patient to hook right foot with *left* foot and move feet off mattress edge.	b. Weight of legs assists in pulling trunk upright. Worker assists by guiding legs off bed by holding under patient's knees.
c. Tell patient to push down on mattress with his *left* fist and simultaneously move his legs off edge of bed.	
4. Instruct patient to support trunk by pushing *left* fist into mattress.	4. Use of fist elongates arm and provides better support.
5. Instruct patient to guide right foot with *left* foot to a position flat on the floor; then unhook *left* foot and place it flat on floor.	5. Sitting balance is enhanced by placing feet apart and flat on floor.
6 to 9. Same as in B.	

D. "Dangle" position on *left side of bed* for patients with left hemiplegia or left leg or left arm disability. Follow instructions in C above, substituting "right" for "left" and "left" for "right" arms and legs.	D. Disabled side is under patient when he is turned to his left side.

E. "Dangle" position on *right side of bed* for patients with left hemiplegia or left leg or left arm disability. Follow instructions in B above, substituting "right" for "left" and "left" for "right" arms and legs.	E. Disabled side is up when patient is turned to his right side.

Procedure continued on the following page

POST-PROCEDURE ACTIVITIES

Worker stays with patient during entire time he is in "dangle" position. Check patient's pulse and observe reaction to activity. Return patient to supine position if there is any untoward reaction. Observe time in dangle position. Assist patient as necessary to return to supine position. Remove abdominal and leg supports if used. Ensure patient's good body alignment, comfort and safety. Cover patient.

Aftercare of Equipment.   Place unit in order; store pillow, sling and abdominal and leg supports.

Final Patient Assessment.   Determine patient's tolerance to activity and his comfort and safety. *Chart/report:* Length of time patient "dangled," amount of assistance and instruction needed, pulse rate, B/P (if taken), reaction to activity and recommendations for progressive activity and independence. Also chart/report evidence of orthostatic hypotension, corrective measures used to raise blood pressure (e.g., exercises, supports) and effectiveness of these measures.

COMMENT ON PROCEDURE 3: ASSISTING THE SEMI-HELPLESS PATIENT TO SIT ON SIDE OF BED: TO "DANGLE"

When assisting a semi-helpless patient to sit on the side of the bed, the nurse should recognize these principles of biomechanics:

1. The patient is encouraged to use his capabilities to come to a sitting position on the side of the bed. Although this activity (or ADL) alone will not put the joints through a complete range of motion or require sufficient muscle involvement to take care of all the individual's exercise needs, it does make a contribution toward these ends.

2. In rolling to the side before sitting, there is less possibility of injuring the tissues in the buttocks area than in sitting and then pivoting around. While the body cannot exactly be considered a circular object, the friction encountered by rolling onto the side before sitting up will be considerably less than the kinetic friction between the patient's skin and the bedclothes, which would have to be overcome to pivot while in a sitting position. Also, if the patient encountered static friction between his skin and the bed at the beginning of the pivot (i.e., no slipping of these surfaces), considerable stretching of the skin would result.

3. The patient should wear slippers or shoes that provide a high static coefficient of friction with the floor. This type of slipper furnishes a high maximum static friction force and thus helps to prevent slipping.

4. The patient should pull on the side rail with his far hand. This action provides a moment of force with respect to the turning axis along the side of the patient's body. Using the far hand rather than the one closest to the edge of the bed provides a larger moment arm with reference to the turning axis.

5. Once the patient's heels are off the bed, the weight of his legs provides a moment of force with respect to the axis of rotation through his hips and at right angles to the edge of the bed. This, in addition to the moment of force provided by pushing the upper arm down into the bed, causing rotation in the same direction, assists the patient to sit up. The patient should either use the lower arm for stabilization or push down into the mattress with it to provide an additional, although rather small, moment of force to assist in sitting up.

6. The patient grasps the side rail or places fists on the bed to increase his base of support in the sitting position.

7. The hemiplegic patient uses his strong foot to push downward into the mattress and slightly away from the edge to which he is moving. This provides a sideward reaction force component to move him toward the edge of the bed and an upward force component to lift his hips.

4. MECHANICAL PATIENT LIFTS

By Jean Saxon, R.N., M.N.

Definitions and Purposes.   *A mechanical patient lift consists of a portable or stationary jack on a fixed base or a wheeled base with special attachments for lifting helpless persons. A wind-up, electric or hydraulic jack may be used to which is attached canvas, mesh or a nylon sling or frame to support the patient.* These devices are used to lift dependent patients from bed to chair, stretcher, toilet, bathtub, car or swimming pool; off the floor; or back to bed or to obtain the patient's weight safely and with a minimum of physical effort. The nurse determines which type of sling or frame to use for safety and comfort.

Contraindications and Cautions.   Follow manufacturer's directions for operation of lift. Do not lift patients who exceed the weight limit specified. Determine if severely spastic or handicapped patients can be lifted safely. Test operating functions of lift by raising and lowering patient over bed before moving patient away from safety of bed. Sitting slings should not be used for patients with unstable spinal injuries. Keep base of lift widened for stability.

Patient-Family Teaching Points.   Provide the patient and family with the following information as appropriate: (a) teach and supervise patient and family about operation of the mechanical lift prior to independent use; (b) explain value of the mechanical lift for patient's comfort and safety; (c) explain that the mechanical lift protects helpers from back injuries and requires a minimum of physical effort; (d) explain that one person can lift and move a patient safely with the correct sling design for the patient's handicap, a flat surface for the base and knowledge of the patient's behavior in the lift.

PRE-PROCEDURE ACTIVITIES

PRELIMINARY PATIENT ASSESSMENT

Includes determination of:
▶ diagnosis and activity orders
▶ level of consciousness
▶ movement capabilities and limitations, e.g., blood pressure changes with position change, occurrence of muscle spasms, ability to support head
▶ presence of body lesions (e.g., decubiti) and attachments (e.g., catheter)

EQUIPMENT

▶ mechanical lift (with scale for weight)
▶ appropriate straps, chains or frame
▶ appropriate sling, e.g., nylon or net sling for bathing or swimming; canvas or nylon comfort seat with opening for buttocks for toilet, commode or bedpan use; wire loop frame sling for head support; stretcher sling (Fig. 21–25).

Procedure continued on the following page

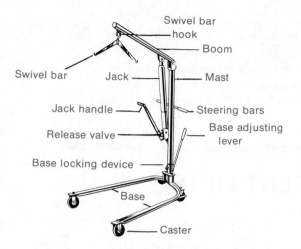

Figure 21–25. Parts of Hoyer Patient Lifter. (From *Instruction Manual for Hoyer Patient Lifter,* Form 10M 1-76, p. 2.)

PRELIMINARY ASSESSMENT

▶ read Kardex for type of sling, attachments, and length of chains or straps used previously
▶ reason for transfer

PRELIMINARY PLANNING

Includes:
▶ obtain mechanical lift, sling and attachments
▶ obtain equipment to which patient is to be transferred, e.g., stretcher, wheelchair
▶ obtain supplies as indicated, e.g., linen, pillows
▶ organize unit to accommodate lift
▶ select assistant for transfer (worker steadies sling and keeps patient's body centered over base while assistant operates lift); one individual can operate a mechanical lift when worker is familiar with the patient and equipment

EQUIPMENT

▶ commode, toilet, bathtub, wheelchair, chair, etc., according to reason for transfer
▶ linen supplies as needed, e.g., gown, towels, bath blanket, positioning devices
▶ clamps and plugs for closing or disconnecting tubes
▶ portable IV infusion stand
▶ restraints as appropriate

PREPARATION OF PATIENT

▶ Provide privacy
▶ Explain transfer to patient even if he is unresponsive
▶ Place drainage bags, IV, etc. on side of bed from which patient will be transferred
▶ Disconnect or clamp tubes as appropriate
▶ Fan-fold top linen and cover patient
▶ Raise bed to working height

PROCEDURE

SUGGESTED STEPS	RATIONALE/ASSESSMENT
Mechanical Patient Lifts	
1. Center sling under patient (with smooth side up) by rolling him from side to side.	1. Assess placement of sling under patient for (a) equal distance from side to side and (b) support of patient's weight. Hems of sling are rough and cause skin abrasions.

SUGGESTED STEPS	RATIONALE/ASSESSMENT

Mechanical Patient Lifts (Continued)

2. Widen the base with the base adjusting lever and lock the lever.

     2. The base of the lift must be as wide as possible to maintain stability. The base is narrowed only temporarily to go through narrow doorways or around nonmovable equipment.

3. Position base of lift under bed with boom centered over sling.

     3. Patient's weight will be balanced over the lift's base.

4. Lower boom far enough to attach sling by opening release valve and depressing boom manually. Do not allow boom or swivel bar to injure patient.

     4. Allows for effortless and safe attachment of boom to sling.

5. Attach ring of webbing straps (or chains) to swivel bar with S hooks facing away from patient. Shorter straps (or chains) will attach to the portion of the sling which supports the patient's back.

     5. S hooks should face away from patient to avoid injury. Sling support will form a "bucket" seat.

6. Attach webbing straps (or chains) to sling with S hooks all the way through the holes in the sling; shorter portions of straps (or chains) go into holes of the back support and longer portions go into the holes of the seat support.

     6. Assess for security of attachments and equal distance between chains or webbing straps on right and left sides of patient. Patient may be tipped out of side of sling if support is not even.

7. Place patient's arms on his chest or allow him to grasp the straps or chains.

     7. Patient's arms may be injured going through narrow spaces. Provides the patient with a sense of security.

8. Close or tighten release valve and then pump or wind the jack high enough to allow the sling to clear the bed.

     8. Assess for balance of patient's weight in sling. If not balanced, slowly lower patient to bed and readjust sling or attachment.

> Caution: *Each time the worker uses a particular lift for the first time or whenever a patient is apprehensive,* slowly *lower the patient to the bed to demonstrate safe operation of the lift.*

Valves vary in their tightness, even among similar types of lifts. Sudden release of a valve could frighten, drop or injure the patient.

9. Hang urinary drainage bag on steering bar and place IV on portable IV stand.

Procedure continued on the following page

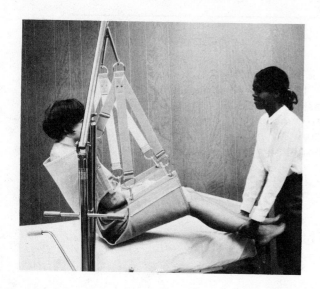

Figure 21–26. Assistant lifting patient's legs off bed while using Hoyer lift. (From *Instruction Manual for Hoyer Patient Lifter*, Form 10M 12-77, p. 7.)

SUGGESTED STEPS	RATIONALE/ASSESSMENT

Mechanical Patient Lifts (Continued)

10. Worker wheels the lift by holding the steering bars while assistant guides the patient's legs off the bed and turns the patient to face the jack and mast (Fig. 21–26).

11. Worker wheels the lift to the destination as assistant steadies patient.

12. Worker slowly lowers the patient by opening release valve (or unwinding the jack) and adjusts the position of the lift's base to destination (e.g., chair, stretcher) to compensate for the changing position of the boom. Simultaneously, the assistant guides the patient to protect his feet and legs and then guides the patient into position on the chair, stretcher, etc.

13. Hang urinary drainage bag below bladder level and position other attachments appropriately.

14. Detach sling from straps or chains and remove lift unless continued support is necessary.

10. Assess for maintenance of patient's weight over base of lift. In sitting slings the patient's heels will rub on the bed if not supported. Protect patient's feet and legs from injury. Use of two helpers ensures patient's safety.

11. Movement of the sling can be frightening to the patient, and sudden movements can unbalance lift.

> Always *use assistant to steady patient if the lift is being used to transport the patient more than 10 ft.*

12. The patient's distance from the jack and mast changes as he is raised and lowered. In the high boom position the patient is close to or touching the jack and/or mast.

14. Support may be needed to maintain patient's head above water in a bathtub.

SUGGESTED STEPS	RATIONALE/ASSESSMENT

Mechanical Patient Lifts (Continued)

15. Remove sling under these circumstances: when patient is moved to a flat surface (e.g., bed, stretcher, treatment table); when patient has enough strength to lift himself for replacement of the sling while in a chair, wheelchair or commode.

15. Patient should not be left on the sling because wrinkles or seams of sling will cause localized pressure on the skin.

16. Leave the sling in place under the patient when patient cannot be repositioned easily on the center of the sling in a sitting position (e.g., very weak, paralyzed or obese patient). Smoothe wrinkles in sling to provide an even surface under the patient.

16. It is difficult to center the sling under a patient who is in a chair or wheelchair; there is danger of unbalancing the patient if the sling becomes displaced. It is important that the sling is smooth when left under the patient to decrease localized skin pressure.

17. Position patient correctly and ensure his safety, e.g., apply restraints as needed.

17. Assess patient for comfort, safety and good body alignment.

18. Repeat steps to return patient to bed.

19. Record on Kardex (if not previously recorded) the lengths of chains or straps at which sling was positioned for transfer. Count loops of chain, measure straps and record which holes are used on sling.

19. Length of chains or straps and holes of sling are adjusted for the individual patient. Provides for efficient, safe use of mechanical lift.

Modifications of Mechanical Lift Procedure

1. Transferring from *bed* to *commode* or *toilet* using portable lift.

   a. Use comfort sling for elimination.

   a. Hole in sling for buttocks allows for elimination.

   b. Adjust the patient's clothing prior to placing the sling under the patient.

   c. Place commode to allow sufficient room for lift base, for privacy with curtains or closed door, and near signal device.

   c. Signal device allows communication without disturbing privacy.

   d. Wheel base of lift around sides of toilet or commode.

   e. Assistant guides patient's buttocks far back onto seat of commode or toilet by grasping sling at patient's hips and guiding the sling or by pushing patient's knees.

   e. Patient's posture is corrected from a semisitting position (which occurs when sitting in sling) to the desired upright sitting position on the commode or toilet.

Procedure continued on the following page

SUGGESTED STEPS	RATIONALE/ASSESSMENT

Modifications of Mechanical Lift Procedure (Continued)

f. Detach S hooks from sling and remove lift.

g. Assure patient's safety. Give signal device.

2. Transferring to *open platform tub* using a portable lift.

> Note: *Portable lifts* cannot *be used for transfers to pools or two-H or three-sided closed tubs. Use a fixed lift in these situations.*

a. Use nylon or net comfort slings.

a. Water drains away from such slings when patient is removed from water.

b. Transport patient to tub via portable lift from bed or stretcher.

b. Two workers are required to transport the patient in a portable lift.

c. Lift patient in sling high enough to move his buttocks over tub side.

d. Turn patient in the sling to face foot of tub. Since patient's body is near mast and jack, guide the turn carefully.

d. Avoid injury to patient's head, arms and feet during turning in sling.

e. Lower the patient into the water by *slowly* opening release valve and then guide patient into correct position by moving sling if using fixed base lift or guiding base if using portable lift. Do not detach sling if patient cannot support his head to keep it out of the water.

e. Patient's head and chest are supported when necessary by keeping sling attached to lift.

f. Upon completing bath, lift patient from water and dry him. Wrap a bath blanket around the patient and the sling. Return the patient to bed or stretcher.

f. Patient quickly loses body heat when wet skin is exposed to air.

g. Remove wet sling and bath blanket quickly by rolling sling in bath blanket as patient is turned from side to side. Complete drying patient.

g. Bath blanket absorbs moisture from sling. Bed will stay dry if bath blanket and sling are removed quickly. Follow agency policy on care of wet sling.

3. Transfer into *island tub*

a. Worker and assistant transport patient to tub via portable lift and elevate him high enough to move his buttocks over tub side.

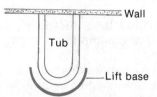

Figure 21–27. An island tub (at 90-degree angle to wall) provides working space on both sides and end. Tub may be elevated on solid base of flush with floor. Portable lift base fits around free end of tub.

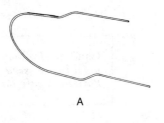
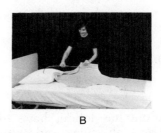
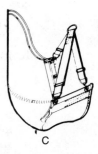

Figure 21–28. Wire loop head support for Hoyer Patient Lifter sling. *A,* Wire head support loop. *B,* Maneuver in which loop is inserted in sling pocket in back of sling. *C,* Sling with wire head support loop inserted. (*A* and *C* from *Hoyer Parts Catalogue,* Form 10M 11-77, p. 5. *B* from *Instruction Manual for Hoyer Patient Lifter,* Form 12–77, p. 8.)

SUGGESTED STEPS	RATIONALE/ASSESSMENT

Modifications of Mechanical Lift Procedure (Continued)

b. Assistant turns patient in the sling 180 degrees so that patient's back is to the jack and mast. (Patient faces the faucet/drain end of the tub.)	b. Allows orientation of the patient's position, allowing him to be placed in the tub with feet toward faucet/drain. Avoid injury to the patient's head while turning him in sling, since boom is in high position.
c. Worker steers base of lift around open end of tub as assistant lifts patient's legs over edge of the tub.	c. Suspends patient over tub. Patient's legs must be lifted to level of his buttocks to clear rim of tub.
d. Worker lowers patient into water by *slowly* releasing valve and simultaneously backing base of lift away from the end of the tub. Assistant guides sling.	d. Base of lift must be backed away from end of tub because boom places patient toward foot of tub as boom is lowered. Prevents injury to patient's feet from pressure on front of tub.
4. Use of *head support sling* (Fig. 21–28)	4. This special attachment provides security and comfort for patients who cannot support head against gravity.
a. Select sling that will accommodate wire loop head support.	
b. Place sling under patient.	
c. Insert wire loop ends into pockets at upper sides of sling and snap canvas around loop, thus forming the head support.	c. Wire loop is inserted into pockets on underside of sling after patient is centered on sling.
d. Attach straps or chains and proceed as previously described.	

Procedure continued on the following page

SUGGESTED STEPS	RATIONALE/ASSESSMENT

Modifications of Mechanical Lift Procedure (Continued)

5. *Lifting patient from floor*

> Caution: *Following a fall, possible injury must be assessed prior to moving the patient. Patient is safe on the floor.*

a. If patient has fallen, have him examined by a physician and obtain permission for lifting him.

b. Place sling under patient and slide patient away from walls or fixed equipment.

    b. Provides room for base of lift to fit around patient without injury to patient.

c. Wheel base around head or feet of the patient.

d. Assistant guides patient past base of lift as patient is raised from floor. Assistant then turns patient to face mast and jack.

    d. Prevents patient from bumping against any part of lift.

e. Raise patient above bed level, move lift base under bed and lower patient to bed.

6. *Weighing the patient*

a. Obtain lift with beam scale. Attach sling and straps or chains to swivel bar. Balance scale on zero.

    a. This action subtracts weight of equipment by balancing scale *after* equipment is attached but *prior* to lifting patient.

b. Place sling under patient and attach chains or straps to sling and swivel bar.

c. Raise patient over bed and measure his weight.

d. Lower patient to bed; remove sling.

e. Subtract weight of linen prior to recording patient's weight.

POST-PROCEDURE ACTIVITIES

Remove sling and place in patient's unit if it is to be used again. Discard sling in laundry if soiled or will not be used regularly for this patient. Position patient in correct body alignment. Inspect patient's skin for evidence of excoriation or pressure from sling. Rehang bladder drainage bag below bladder level. Check IV for rate of flow and inspect IV site for abnormalities. Reattach other tubing and remove clamps. Cover patient, raise side rails and lower bed.

Aftercare of Equipment.   Return mechanical lift with straps, chains and frames to storage area.

Final Patient Assessment.   Determine patient's comfort and safety. *Chart/ report:* Type of sling or frame used; length of chain or straps and their points of attachment to sling; precautions needed for patient; patient's tolerance for activity.

COMMENT ON PROCEDURE 4: USE OF MECHANICAL PATIENT LIFTS

The use of a mechanical lift to move a patient should bring to mind these concerns:

1. The possibility of injury to the nurse is minimized by having the mechanical device provide the force for the lift.

2. The patient must be properly balanced in the sling and, in many cases, further stabilized by means of contact forces supplied by an assistant.

3. The patient's line of gravity must fall within the base of support of the lift.

4. A mechanical device accomplishes a patient lift primarily by applying a force that is normal (at right angles) to the patient's skin. The tangential or shear force on the patient's skin which is present in manual lifts is largely avoided and the skin is thereby protected.

5. The head of a weak patient must be supported. Otherwise, its weight will cause it to drop until restrained by joint structures, causing undue stress and perhaps injury to these tissues.

6. Wheels on the mechanical lift minimize the friction opposing its motion (i.e., rolling friction) and facilitate its movement. It would take a great deal more effort to slide rather than roll such a device along the floor.

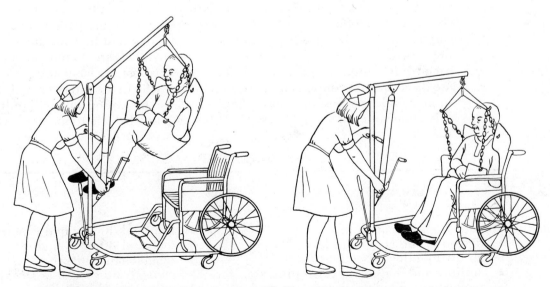

Figure 21–29. Use of mechanical patient lift. The patient's distance from jack and mast changes as patient is lowered to the wheelchair.

5.   TRANSFER OF SEMI-HELPLESS PATIENT FROM BED TO CHAIR OR WHEELCHAIR

By Jean Saxon, R.N., M.N.

Definition and Purposes.   *These methods are used to assist a semi-helpless patient in transferring from bed to a chair or wheelchair.* They can be used by one helper to assist a patient who has generalized weakness due to prolonged bed rest or surgery; hemiplegia (weakness or disability of one side of the body); or one leg that is non–weight bearing because of hip, leg, knee or ankle fractures or surgery (including amputation). The procedure is used for patients who are learning to accomplish independent transfers; the patient does not pull or hang on to helper. The nurse modifies the procedure to utilize the patient's capabilities.

Contraindications and Cautions.   One helper should not attempt to transfer a patient who cannot follow directions. Use standby assistance of another worker until patient is strong enough to be transferred safely by one helper. The method of transfer discussed here cannot be used with a patient who lacks sitting balance. A patient with severe orthostatic hypotension requires special preconditioning prior to this method of transfer. Do not use ambulation belts over surgical wounds or skin lesions. Secure bed and chair by locks, blocks or other firm supports, e.g., wall or furniture.

Patient-Family Teaching Points.   Provide the patient and family with the following information as appropriate: (a) encourage patient to use his own muscle power to maintain and strengthen muscles; (b) explain that muscular inactivity may contribute to forgetting how to perform various movements; (c) explain that giving verbal instructions and touching the patient to reinforce the desired movement helps the patient to learn and perform each step of the procedure; (d) emphasize that correct body mechanics will prevent injury to the patient and helper; (e) emphasize that the patient will progress to independent transfer quickly by using this procedure; (f) explain that street shoe(s) provides a firm foundation for standing balance; (g) emphasize that the physical therapist, family, staff and patient should use the same procedure; and (h) explain that moving in the direction of the patient's stronger side is safest and most efficient because his strong side will pull his weak side along and the weak side will not become an obstacle to movement.

PRE-PROCEDURE ACTIVITIES

PRELIMINARY ASSESSMENT

Includes determination of:
► diagnosis and activity orders
► ability to follow directions
► abilities and limitations concerning transfer movements (Kardex for previous method)
► presence of skin, muscle, bone lesions

EQUIPMENT

► firm bed (hi-low bed if possible)
► footstool if bed is high or patient is short
► wheelchair with wheel locks or *arm*chair
► shoe(s) and sock(s) or stocking(s)
► colored sock, felt boot or slipper for non–weight-bearing foot

PRELIMINARY ASSESSMENT

▶ presence of IV, urinary drainage, nasogastric tube, etc.
▶ transfer method taught to patient by physical therapist

PRELIMINARY PLANNING

Includes:
▶ method of transfer to be accomplished, e.g., non–weight-bearing, hemiplegic
▶ need for one additional helper to safely move patient, e.g., if patient confused or extremely weak or if equipment is attached
▶ comfort and safety of patient, e.g., side rails, chair or wheelchair to fit patient, street shoes, robe, belt, sling, brace, restraints, pillows or wedges for positioning
▶ arrange unit to provide space for helper to assist and for correct placement of wheelchair or chair
▶ determination of equipment to be disconnected or to hold IV or drainage equipment

EQUIPMENT

▶ ambulation belt, e.g., Posey Walking Belt or Special Gait Belt (see Figs. 21–30 and 21–31)
▶ half side rail (if needed)
▶ bath robe, bath blanket
▶ paper or sheet to protect bottom sheet from shoes
▶ IV pole (if needed)

PREPARATION OF PATIENT

▶ Discuss transfer procedure with patient
▶ Place wheelchair (with wheels locked) or chair (with legs blocked or placed against solid object) parallel to head or foot of bed (next to patient's strong side)
▶ Lower bed; *lock bed wheels*
▶ Position footstool (if needed)
▶ Remove or fan-fold top linen to foot of bed
▶ Place paper under patient's feet to protect sheet from contamination by patient's shoe(s)
▶ Put colored sock, felt boot or slipper on patient's non–weight-bearing foot
▶ Put different sock(s) or stocking(s) and street shoe(s) on weight-bearing foot
▶ Disconnect nasogastric tube and other tubes if allowed

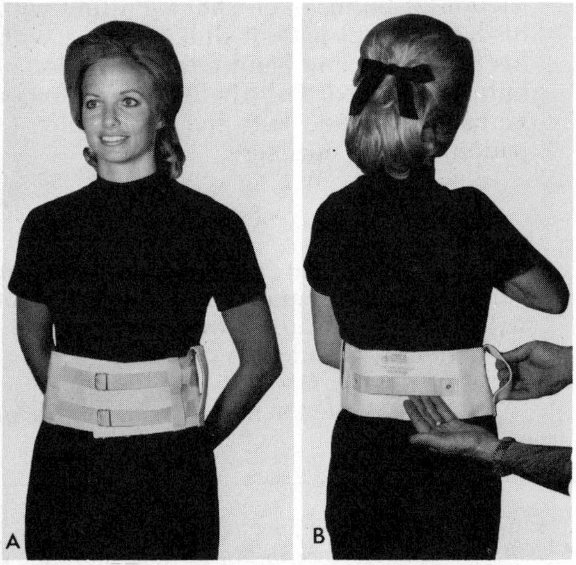

Figure 21–30. A walking belt may be worn by a patient who is crutch walking for the first time. There are side and back handles that may be held by the nurse to prevent the patient from falling. (From *J. T. Posey Catalog.* J. T. Posey Co., Pasadena, CA, 1974.)

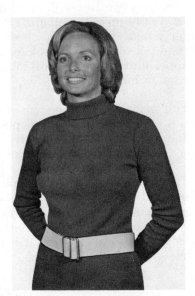

Figure 21–31. The Posey Special Gait Belt. (From J. T. Posey Co., Pasadena, CA.)

Procedure continued on the following page

PREPARATION OF PATIENT

▶ Hang urinary drainage bag on wheelchair or chair
▶ Attach IV pole to wheelchair or place bed IV pole so that tubing will not be displaced during transfer
▶ Lift half side rail (if present and needed) on side from which patient will transfer
▶ Apply ambulation waist belt if possible

PROCEDURE

SUGGESTED STEPS	RATIONALE/DISCUSSION

Transfer from Bed to Chair

A. Transfer of *weak* or *postsurgical* patient to chair or wheelchair.

    1. Tell patient to "dangle" on side of bed from which he will transfer (see Procedure 3, A).

    2. Helper assumes forward-backward stance, in front of and facing the patient.

    3. Tell patient to slide his buttocks close to edge of bed by shifting his weight alternately from right to left buttock as he (a) pulls his body forward with hands over mattress edge; (b) pushes with both fists on mattress; or (c) pushes with one fist on mattress and pulls on side rail with other hand. Helper assists by pulling alternately on right and left side of waist belt (or right and left upper buttock) using pull maneuver in direction of movement.

    4. Tell patient to place his feet in a forward-backward wide-based position on the floor (or footstool if necessary) with his strongest foot back slightly under bed.

    5. Tell patient to lean his trunk forward. Helper pulls patient's trunk forward (a) by grasping center of belt; or (b) with helper's arms under the patient's arms and palms of helper's hands over patient's shoulder blades.

    6. Tell patient to push his fists into edge of mattress (or grasp top of side rail with near hand) on command.

A. For patient who has use of his extremities.

    1. Determine which side of bed is best for transfer by assessing placement of IV, urinary drainage, unit arrangement, etc.

    2. Position protects patient from falling and ensures helper's correct body mechanics.

    3. Positions patient's trunk at edge of bed. Rocking motion lifts weight on alternate buttocks, enhancing sliding by reducing friction of buttocks on sheet. Pulling with his hands helps patient slide; pushing with his fists or fist and hand reduces friction of buttocks on bed. Pull by helper reinforces verbal instruction and gives assistance to patient's weak muscles.

    4. Provides wide base of support for patient's weight upon standing. Back foot will provide upward-forward force needed for patient to stand up.

    5. Brings patient's trunk within base of support.

> Caution: *Do not support patient under his armpits (axillae), since injury to major nerves and blood vessels can occur.*

    6. Provides leverage for upward movement.

SUGGESTED STEPS

RATIONALE/DISCUSSION

Transfer from Bed to Chair (Continued)

7. Tell patient to stand, on command, by simultaneously leaning forward, pushing with his fists and pushing with his back foot as he straightens his legs.

7. Patient's simultaneous movements provide the forward-upward force needed to stand.

8. Helper commands "stand" and shifts her weight from her forward to backward foot as she pulls patient forward and upward with belt (or with her hands over patient's shoulder blades).

8. Helper's action provides reinforcement to patient to lean forward. This is the most difficult action for patients to remember.

9. Tell patient to stand up straight and balance himself in standing position with hands on armchair, side rail or mattress. Helper continues to face patient and assists by placing one knee against patient's forward knee and guides patient's trunk by holding belt (or with hands over shoulder blades).

9. Helper's action stabilizes patient's upright position by bracing one of his legs and pulling his trunk forward. Weak patients tend to buckle at the knees, and fearful patients tend to fall backward.

10. Ask patient how he feels. Observe for symptoms of orthostatic hypotension. (Orthostatic hypotension is discussed in Chapter 33.)

10. Assess patient for lightheadedness, fainting, dizziness, sweating (diaphoresis).

11. Tell patient to sit on bed (or helper pushes patient back onto bed) if symptoms of orthostatic hypotension develop. Then helper uses remedial measures as described in Chapter 33.

> Caution: *Do not risk danger of patient fainting and falling to floor.*

12. If footstool is used, tell patient to place his dominant foot in center of footstool, step to floor with his other foot and then lower strong foot to floor. Helper uses belt to assist.

12. Patient's dominant leg is used to lower body during step, since muscle power is needed to bend leg as the body is lowered.

13. Tell patient to place his near hand on far arm of chair or wheelchair as he pivots on the balls of his feet. Helper continues to hold belt (or keeps her palms over patient's shoulder blades) and guides patient's hand to arm of chair. Helper pivots with the patient.

13. Patient's action provides support needed to maintain his balance and to position his body in preparation for sitting. Helper assists in maintaining patient's balance as necessary, reinforces instruction and remains in position in front of patient.

14. Tell patient to step back to chair until he is close enough to touch seat with his leg and grasp the other arm of the chair or wheelchair with other hand. Helper places her knee against patient's forward knee and continues to hold belt (or keeps palms over shoulder blades).

14. Patient's action places feet in forward-backward stance. Helper braces patient's knee and uses belt to assist patient to maintain balance.

Procedure continued on the following page

SUGGESTED STEPS	RATIONALE/DISCUSSION

Transfer from Bed to Chair (Continued)

15. Tell patient to lean forward and lower his buttocks slowly to the seat by bending knees and elbows. Helper pulls patient's trunk forward and gradually releases pressure against patient's knee.	15. These actions maintain patient's center of gravity over his feet and control movement to prevent patient from falling back into seat.
16. Tell patient to push his buttocks to the back of the seat by leaning trunk forward, pushing on chair arms and pushing with his feet. If necessary, helper pulls patient's trunk forward by pulling on patient's shoulder blades or on belt. Simultaneously, helper pushes on patient's knees with her knees or hand.	16. Patient's action of leaning forward brings weight over his ischial tuberosities; pushing on chair arms reduces the amount of weight to be moved; and pushing with his feet provides the force for sliding. Patients tend to incorrectly lean *back*, thereby pushing their buttocks forward instead of backward.
17. Ask patient if he is comfortable. Observe for correct sitting posture.	17. Assess patient's body alignment, comfort and safety.
18. Reverse procedure to return patient to bed.	
19. If footstool is used to return to bed, tell patient to step up with dominant leg.	19. Muscle power is needed to lift body.

B. Transfer of patient with *right hemiplegia or right-sided disability* from the *left side of bed* to chair or wheelchair (Fig. 21–32).	B. Wheelchair or chair is placed with back toward head of bed. Placement of colored sock or slipper on patient's right foot reminds him not to bear weight on his right leg if it is non–weight bearing.
1. Tell patient to "dangle" on *left* side of bed (see Procedure 3, B).	1. Positions patient with his *strong left side* next to wheelchair or chair.

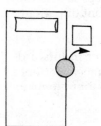

Figure 21–32. Patient moving from left side of bed to chair on left, his strong side.

SUGGESTED STEPS	RATIONALE/DISCUSSION

Transfer from Bed to Chair (Continued)

2. Helper assumes a forward-backward stance in front of the patient's *weak right side.*	2. Places helper in a position to assist patient and promotes correct body mechanics.
3. Tell patient to slide his buttocks closer to edge of bed by tipping his trunk from side to side while pushing down on side rail or pushing on mattress edge with his *left* hand. Helper assists by pulling on *left* side of waist belt; she also utilizes belt to maintain patient's trunk balance. In addition, helper assists by pulling at patient's *right* upper buttock with her left palm.	3. Encourages patient to use muscles of *strong left side* to maintain and increase muscle strength. Helper's assistance is needed to compensate for right-sided weakness while patient is learning. As patient develops added strength in his strong *left* side, he will be able to transfer independently.
4. Tell patient to place his feet (foot) on the floor. Helper guides patient's right foot to a wide base with her right foot.	4. Patient will bear his weight on his strong *left* leg.
5. If footstool was used for "dangle" position, helper pushes stool aside. Tell patient to slide off edge of bed until his feet (foot) touch floor.	5. Stepping off a footstool is too difficult for patient until he has skill on stairs with use of a four-legged cane, crutches or prosthesis.
6. Tell patient to lean trunk forward. Helper pulls on center of waist belt.	6. Brings patient's trunk over base of support.
7. Tell patient on command to push on top of side rail or on near arm of wheelchair or chair. Helper pulls upward on waist belt.	7. Provides leverage for upward movement and balance.
8. Tell patient to "stand." Helper blocks patient's right foot with her right foot and pushes on patient's right knee with the side of her right knee.	8. Helper stabilizes patient's right foot and leg to help him maintain his balance. If patient is an amputee or is non–weight bearing, only the belt is used to help maintain balance.
9. Tell patient to reach for far arm of chair or wheelchair with his *left* arm.	9. Provides a point of balance for patient.
10. Tell patient to pivot on ball of *left* foot until his back faces chair or wheelchair. Helper pivots with patient.	10. Patient's action drags right leg into position. Helper maintains forward-backward stance in front of patient's right side in order to assist patient while using good body mechanics.

Procedure continued on the following page

SUGGESTED STEPS	RATIONALE/ASSESSMENT

Transfer from Bed to Chair (Continued)

11. Tell patient to lean forward and slowly lower his buttocks to chair seat by bending his *left* knee and elbow. Helper stabilizes the patient's right foot and knee with her right foot and knee and/or guides patient with the belt.

11. Provides for slow controlled movement.

> Caution: *Patient may be injured by falling backward into wheelchair or chair.*

12. Tell patient to lean forward and push with his *left* foot and arm to place buttocks at the back of the seat. Helper assists by pushing on patient's right knee with her knee.

12. Provides good sitting balance.

> Caution: *Helper does not push on patient's knee if patient has hip, thigh or knee disability.*

Helper then assists by pulling up and back on belt behind patient.

13. Ask patient if he is comfortable. Observe for correct sitting posture. Check for correct alignment of right extremities, e.g., position of sling, placement of pillows, adequate circulation, feet on foot rests of wheelchair, need for restraints.

13. Assess body alignment, comfort and safety.

> Caution: *Patients who cannot remember they are disabled require restraints to remind them to request help in getting out of chair or wheelchair.*

14. When returning patient to bed, the wheelchair or chair must be moved to the *left side of the foot end of the bed* or the *right side of the head end of the bed.*

14. Positions patient with his *strong left* side next to bed.

15. Using the techniques discussed above, return patient to edge of bed. (If entering bed on right side see C, 2 below.)

16. If bed is too high, patient must be lifted onto side of bed by two helpers or a mechanical lift.

16. Footstool cannot be used until patient can bear weight on right side or can use crutches or four-legged cane.

17. To return to supine position, use Procedure 3, B and C.

17. Assess for comfort and safety.

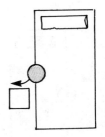

Figure 21–33. Patient moving from right side of bed to chair on the left, his strong side.

SUGGESTED STEPS	RATIONALE/ASSESSMENT

Transfer from Bed to Chair (Continued)

C. Transfer of patient with *right hemiplegia or right-sided disability* from *right side* of bed to chair or wheelchair (Fig. 21–33).

1. Tell patient to "dangle" on *right* side of bed. (See Procedure 3, C.)

2. Repeat steps 2 to 13 as in B, above, except instead of placing hand on side rail, patient places his hand on arm of chair or presses his fist into mattress.

3. When returning patient to bed, the wheelchair or chair *must be moved to the right side of the head of the bed* or *the left side of the foot of the bed.*

4. Using previously discussed techniques, return patient to bed.

C. Wheelchair or chair is placed with back toward foot of bed.

1. Positions patient with his strong left side next to wheelchair or chair.

2. In "dangle" position on right side of bed, side rail is on patient's disabled side and cannot be used by him. Fist elongates arm for leverage.

3. Positions patient with his *strong left* side next to bed.

D. Transfer of patient with *left hemiplegia* or *left-sided disability* from *left side of bed* to chair or wheelchair. Use procedure C above, substituting "right" for "left" and "left" for "right" arms and legs (Fig. 21–34).

D. Wheelchair or chair is placed with back toward foot of bed.

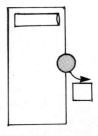

Figure 21–34. Patient moving from left side of bed to chair on right, his strong side.

Procedure continued on the following page

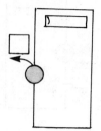

Figure 21–35. Patient moving from right side of bed to chair on the right, his strong side.

SUGGESTED STEPS	RATIONALE/ASSESSMENT

Transfer from Bed to Chair (Continued)

E. Transfer of patient with *left hemiplegia* or *left-sided disability* from *right side of bed* to chair or wheelchair. Use procedure B above, substituting "right" for "left" and "left" for "right" arms and legs.	E. Wheelchair or chair is placed with back toward head of bed.

POST-PROCEDURE ACTIVITIES

Check patient's pulse and observe reaction to activity. Observe length of time in wheelchair or chair. Ensure patient's comfort and safety: check IV for correct flow rate; attach urinary drainage bag below bladder level; reattach other equipment; position patient in correct body alignment; remove belt, shoes, socks, robe and sling; place call bell for patient's use; and raise side rails.

Aftercare of Equipment. Place unit in order; store belt, wheelchair (chair), sling, etc.

Final Patient Assessment. Determine patient's tolerance to activity, comfort and safety. *Chart/Report:* Length of time patient was up in wheelchair or chair; amount of assistance and instruction needed; and pulse rate. Record evidence of orthostatic hypotension, corrective measures used to raise blood pressure and effectiveness of these measures. Record patient's reaction to activity and recommendations for progressive activity and independence.

COMMENT ON PROCEDURE 5: TRANSFER OF SEMI-HELPLESS PATIENT FROM BED TO CHAIR OR WHEELCHAIR

In transferring a semi-helpless patient from the bed to a chair, the following biomechanical principles are evident:

1. The patient is encouraged to assist as much as possible. Patient activity helps to maintain and perhaps increase existing levels of muscular strength.

COMMENT ON PROCEDURE 5: TRANSFER OF SEMI-HELPLESS PATIENT FROM BED TO CHAIR OR WHEELCHAIR

2. The wheels on the wheelchair are locked before transferring the patient. This increases the maximum static friction between the wheels and the floor. Under normal circumstances, the pushing force of the patient or nurse against the chair will be less than the maximum static friction force, and the chair will not slip.

3. The patient's street shoes are worn because they have a higher coefficient of friction with the floor than do stockings or bare feet. As a result, the danger of the patient slipping on the floor is lessened.

4. A forward-back stance is used to increase stability in that direction, which coincides with the direction of the motion.

5. When the patient alternately shifts his weight from side to side in moving toward the edge of the bed, he should pull against the mattress with his right hand and/or the nurse should pull forward on the patient's right side when the patient's right buttock is lifted off the mattress. This takes advantage of the reduced friction on the right side. The same procedure, of course, applies to the left side.

6. Before attempting to stand, the patient leans forward to bring his line of gravity over the base of support provided by the feet.

7. The patient pushes down and back into the mattress with his fists and into the floor with his strong leg. In reaction, the upward and forward force on his body helps him to assume a standing position.

8. The patient must possess sufficient strength in his knee extensor muscles (quadriceps femoris) to permit a controlled lowering of the body since stepping downward onto a stool or the floor requires eccentric, or lengthening, contraction of this muscle group. Because the maximum force generated by a muscle eccentrically exceeds that produced concentrically, the patient may be able to step down onto the stool but may not have enough strength to step back up because the latter action requires a concentric contraction of the quadriceps.

9. The patient increases his base of support by holding onto the edge of the bed or the arm of the chair.

10. The chair must be of sufficient weight so that it does not tip when the patient pushes down on its arm. In other words, the moment of force of the weight of the chair must be greater than the moment of force applied by the patient with respect to the edge of the base (or axis) about which the tipping would take place.

11. To sit back in the chair, the patient must push forward and downward against the arms of the chair with his hands and against the floor with his feet. In reaction, the upward force lifts the hips and thereby reduces the friction between the patient's trunk and the chair, and the backward force moves the body in the desired direction.

BIBLIOGRAPHY

1. Andersson, B. J. G., Ortengren, R., Nachemson, A. L., Elfstom, G., and Broman, H.: The sitting posture: an electromyographic and discometric study. *Orthopedic Clinics of North America*, 6:105–109, 1975.
2. Brand, P. W.: Pressure sores—the problem. *In* Kenedi, R. M., Cowden, J. M., and Scales, J. T. (eds.): *Bedsore Biomechanics*. Baltimore, University Park Press, 1976.
3. Chaffin, D. B.: On the validity of biomechanical models of the low-back for weight lifting analysis. American Society of Mechanical Engineers Paper 75-WA/Bio-1, 1975.
4. Chaffin, D. B., and Park, K. S.: A longitudinal study of low-back pain as associated with occupational weight lifting factors. *American Industrial Hygiene Association Journal*, 34:513–522, 1973.
4a. Ciuca, R., and Bradish, J.: Passive range-of-motion exercises: a handbook. *Nursing '78*, 8:59, July 1978.
4b. Ciuca, R., Bradish, J., and Trombly, S. M.: Active range-of-motion exercises: a handbook. *Nursing '78*, 8:45–49, Aug. 1978.
5. Dempster, W. T.: Space Requirements of the Seated Operator. Wright Air Development Center Technical Report 55–159, 1955.

6. Eie, N.: Load capacity of the low back. *Journal of the Oslo City Hospitals, 16*:73–98, 1966.

7. Elftman, H.: Biomechanics of muscle. *Journal of Bone and Joint Surgery, 48A*:363–377, 1966.

8. Ford, J. R., and Duckworth, B.: Moving a dependent patient safely, comfortably: Part 1—positioning. *Nursing '76, 6*:27–36, Jan. 1976.

9. Ford, J. R., and Duckworth, B.: Moving a dependent patient safely, comfortably: Part 2—transferring. *Nursing '76, 6*:58–65, Feb. 1976.

10. Fergusson-Pell, M. W., Bell, F., and Evans, J. H.: Interface pressure sensors: existing devices, their suitability and limitations. *In* Kenedi, R. M., Cowden, J. M., and Scales, J. T. (eds.): *Bedsore Biomechanics.* Baltimore, University Park Press, 1976.

11. Haffajee, D., Moritz, U., and Svantesson, G.: Isometric knee extension strength as a function of joint angle, muscle length and motor unit activity. *Acta Orthopaedica Scandinavica, 43*:138–147, 1972.

11a. Hefferin, E. A., and Hill, B. J.: Analyzing nursing's work-related injuries. *American Journal of Nursing, 76*:924–927, June 1976.

12. Hutton, R. S., and Miller, D. I.: Length-torque measurement: an integration of neuromuscular physiology and biomechanics. *Journal of Physical Education and Recreation, 46*(2):81–87, 1975.

12a. Klabak, L.: Getting a grip on the transfer belt technique. *Nursing '78, 8*:10, Feb. 1978.

13. Lindahl, O., Movin, A., and Ringquist, I.: Knee extension. *Acta Orthopaedica Scandinavica, 40*:79–85, 1969.

13a. Long, B. C., and Buergin, P. S.: The pivot transfer. *American Journal of Nursing, 77*:980–982, June 1977.

14. Markolf, K. L., and Morris, J. M.: The structural components of the intervertebral disc. *Journal of Bone and Joint Surgery, 56A*:675–687, 1974.

15. Morris, J. M., Lucas, D. B., and Bresler, B.: Role of the trunk in stability of the spine. *Journal of Bone and Joint Surgery, 43A*:327–351, 1961.

16. Nachemson, A.: Towards a better understanding of low-back pain: a review of the mechanics of the lumbar disc. *Rheumatology and Rehabilitation, 14*:129–143, 1975.

17. Nachemson, A.L.: The lumbar spine—an orthopaedic challenge. *Spine, 1*:59–71, 1976.

18. Rasch, P. J.: The present status of negative (eccentric) exercise: a review. *American Corrective Therapy Journal, 28*:77–78, 90–94, 1974.

19. Rasch, P. J., and Burke, R. K.: *Kinesiology and Applied Anatomy*, 5th ed. Philadelphia, Lea & Febiger, 1974.

20. Roaf, R.: A study of the mechanics of spinal injuries. *Journal of Bone and Joint Surgery, 42B*:810–823, 1960.

21. Scales, J. T.: Pressure on the patient. *In* Kenedi, R. M., Cowden, J. M., and Scales, J. T. (eds): *Bedsore Biomechanics.* Baltimore, University Park Press, 1976.

22. Schultz, A. B.: Mechanics of the human spine. *Applied Mechanics Reviews, 27*:1487–1497, 1974.

23. Williams, M., and Stutzman, L.: Strength variation through the range of joint motion. *Physical Therapy Review, 39*:145–152, 1959.

24. Works, R. F.: Hints on lifting and pulling. *American Journal of Nursing, 72*:260–261, 1972.

UNIT

VII

PROVIDING FOOD AND FLUIDS

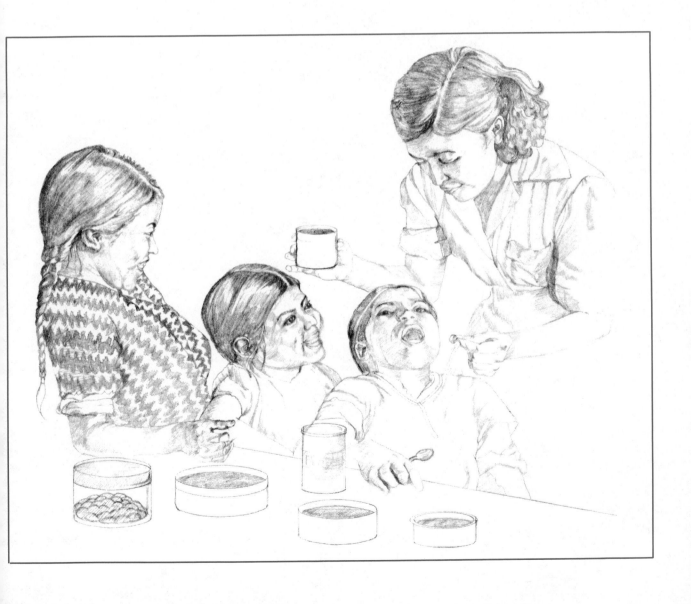

CHAPTER 22

BASIC DIET MANAGEMENT

By Bonnie Worthington, Ph.D.

OVERVIEW AND STUDY GUIDE FOR CHAPTERS 22 AND 23

The focus of Chapters 22 and 23 is to convey basic information about the role of nutrition in maintenance of health and prevention of disease. Discussion of elementary principles of nutrition is followed by a synopsis of current nutritional controversies, food habits and methods of assessing nutritional status. Chapter 23 covers special dietary needs during each stage of the life cycle and in various disease states and the nurse's role in optimizing nutritional care. After completing these chapters the student should be able to accomplish the following:

1. Define in simple terms the basic functions of the major nutrients, vitamins, minerals and fluid
2. Evaluate the dietary intake of a patient and judge its adequacy
3. Critique the hypotheses that

all food additives are very dangerous

organic foods are nutritionally superior to "regular" foods

food supplements are necessary for optimal health

all people need to take vitamins daily

4. Define the various factors that influence food choices and affect nutritional status
5. Recommend a plan for evaluation of nutritional status
6. Describe special nutritional needs during each stage of the life cycle
7. Define basic dietary approaches to specific diseases such as

diabetes mellitus

ulcer

diverticulosis

celiac disease

regional enteritis

ulcerative colitis

hepatitis

cirrhosis

cholelithiasis (gallstones)

atherosclerosis

congestive heart failure

hypertension

glomerulonephritis

nephrotic syndrome

kidney failure

gout

hypoglycemia

phenylketonuria

allergy

8. Define the options in feeding when standard oral meals cannot be tolerated
9. Describe the role of the nurse in assuring that nutritional needs of the patient are met
10. Formulate a list of recommendations that might be provided to a patient regarding community sources of help with diet

To assist in your study of these chapters, consider and answer the following questions:

1. What are the Recommended Dietary Allowances and how should they be used?
2. What are the major functions of each of the nutrients?
3. What are food additives and for what purposes are they used?
4. What is meant by the term "organic food"?
5. For whom might you recommend vitamin or mineral supplements?
6. Who needs protein supplements?
7. What factors affect food choice for an individual?
8. What circumstances adversely affect nutritional status?
9. How might a patient's diet be evaluated?
10. What other factors need consideration in evaluating nutritional status?
11. What milks are appropriate for feeding infants?
12. What are expected food-related behaviors of preschool children?
13. What nutritional problems may develop during school age and adolescence?
14. What is the "prudent diet"?
15. What are the recommended added calorie and protein needs for pregnant and lactating women?
16. What are the basic hospital diets and for what purposes are they used?
17. What are basic strategies in management of obesity?

18. What types of tube feedings are available?

19. For what purposes might intravenous hyperalimentation be used?

20. How might you improve a patient's appetite?

21. How may nausea and vomiting be minimized?

22. How is choking or dysphagia managed?

BASIC CONCEPTS OF GOOD NUTRITION

Introduction

Good nursing care demands careful attention to the patient's nutritional requirements. With the support of the dietitian and other members of the health care team, the nurse must see that adequate and appropriate foods, fluids, and/or nutritional supplements are provided to the patient on a regular basis. This is obviously true in the hospital setting in which medical problems of major significance are routinely encountered. Beyond this basic area of disease management and cure, however, it is essential that health care in general focus on the goal of prevention of disease whenever possible. Consequently, nutritional care in the form of ongoing consultation should be an integral part of total medical service based upon the needs of the individual patient or family. *Health*, by definition, encompasses good nutritional status; the nurse must therefore aggressively support all clinical and community activities that are aimed at accomplishing this end.

Nutrition has been defined as the sum of processes by which a living organism ingests, digests, absorbs, transports, uses and excretes nutrients. With the proper nutritional support in the form of raw materials, the organism can grow, function and reproduce. Body defense mechanisms, wound healing phenomena and a variety of other vital processes require an optimum nutritional environment. For many years, nutritionists have studied the nutritional needs of man and other animals and have attempted to learn about the multiple effects of environment, metabolism, disease and activity on these needs. As a result, we now know that man requires over 35 nutrients for growth and function; we also know that his needs may change with disease, activity or environmental stress. Logically, then, it is easy to understand that suboptimal provision of the essential nutrients leads to deterioration in body function and in overall health and vitality.

In accepting the responsibility of providing care for the patient as an individual, the nurse accepts the responsibility for applying the principles of nutrition. In addition, the nurse serves as a liaison between the patient and other professional people in interpreting the patient's nutritional and dietary problems. The perceptive nurse identifies problems, seeks solutions and incorporates the findings into the nursing care plan. In order to carry out this function, the nurse must acquire knowledge of the principles of nutrition; she must also develop appreciation of food composition and an understanding of the roles food plays in the lives of individuals and groups. Beyond these basic issues of importance, the nurse must maintain an appreciation of specific modifications of diet and food behavior as they relate to the total therapeutic regimen that is planned for the individual patient and his family.

Recommended Dietary Allowances

In 1941, the Food and Nutrition Board of the National Academy of Sciences developed its first listing of dietary recommendations for daily intake of specific nutrients. Since that time, these recommendations, called the Recommended Dietary Allowances (RDA), have been revised every 4 years in accord with new research data on human needs during the life cycle. As they now stand, in the judgment of the Food and Nutrition Board, the *Recommended Dietary Allowances are the levels of intake of essential nutrients considered, on the basis of available knowledge, to be adequate to meet the known nutritional needs of almost every healthy person.*[26] Therefore, except for calories, the RDA do not represent minimal or average nutritional requirements of individuals; they designate instead the minimal need plus a margin of safety sufficient to accommodate the normal variations observed in a healthy population.

Considerable use is made of the RDA in assessing dietary adequacy of populations and of individuals. This listing provides a rough standard against which one can compare dietary intake data of clients or groups. In using this standard, however, one must keep in mind that malnutrition may not necessarily exist whenever the recommendations are not completely met. On the other hand, the recommendations may not be high enough for individuals depleted by disease, traumatic stresses, specific drug therapy or chronic dietary inadequacies. Use of the RDA therefore demands that common sense be applied in the overall dietary evaluation. In general, if the patient under consideration is distinctly different anatomically or physiologically from the average, healthy person described by the Food and Nutrition Board, the RDA as a standard of reference may prove to be of limited value.

Calories and Their Relationship to Body Weight

All foods supply a source of energy to the body in the form of calories. A *calorie* is the amount of heat needed to raise the temperature of 1 Gm. of water 1 degree Celsius. Calorie needs vary with age, sex, rate of growth, body size, activity level and other factors. Energy is needed constantly by the body to maintain the circulation, respiration, muscle tone, body temperature and other vital processes. The basal energy requirement is related to the amount of muscle tissue present in the body, and this can be predicted from body weight data. Calorie needs generally are expressed as the number of kilocalories (kcal.) needed per day. Adult basal needs may be estimated quickly by multiplying the ideal body weight (in pounds) by 10 kcal. for women and by 11 kcal. for men. Ideal, or normal, weight, which is calculated according to height, is always used, since excess body weight is generally composed of adipose tissue, which requires very little energy for maintenance. For example, suppose a man's ideal body weight is 180 lb. His basal energy needs would then be estimated as follows:

$$180 \text{ lb.} \times 11 \text{ kcal./lb.} = 1980 \text{ kcal.}$$

People of similar size have similar *basal* energy needs, but *total* energy requirement is dependent on physical activity. Total energy requirement may vary widely among individuals and for the same individual day by day because the total energy requirement is dependent on the vigor with which muscles are used and total body mass is moved. Since the average adult in most developed societies spends a great deal of time sitting, lying or standing, the recommended calorie allowances are based on this sedentary life pattern.

The daily energy requirements of man are met by regular consumption of foods and fluids in sufficient quantities. The basic energy-yielding nutrients are protein, carbohydrates and fat. These nutrients supply calories in the following amounts:

Fat	9 kcal./Gm.
Carbohydrate	4 kcal./Gm.
Protein	4 kcal./Gm.

In many developed countries, approximately 10 per cent of dietary calories are supplied by protein, with 40 and 50 per cent being derived from fat and carbohydrate, respectively. Alcohol, which furnishes 7 kcal./Gm., may also provide a significant source of calories in the diets of some people; if used in excessive amounts, however, nutrition and health status may be seriously impaired.

Fuel supplied to the body in the form of calories is utilized as required to support physiologic functions. Excess calories are converted into body fat and stored in the various fat depots (fat pads). Storage of a limited supply of body fat is desirable for maintenance of health; fat generally provides padding for vital organs and nerves and insulates the body against rapid temperature changes or excessive heat loss. Under typical circumstances, approximately 25 to 30 per cent of the female body is fat, while only about 14 per cent of the male body is fat.

Ideally, daily energy intake is just sufficient to meet the body's requirements. When intake of calories exceeds energy needs, gain in weight gradually takes place as a result of deposition of adipose (fat) tissue. Overweight or obesity may eventually develop if action is not taken to reverse this trend. On the other hand, a diet deficient in calories leads to loss of body weight over time. Eventually this phenomenon may result in the development of serious malnutrition, emaciation and increased susceptibility to disease. Both underweight and overweight endanger life and health. Even moderate obesity may tax the cardiovascular system over a long term. It complicates gallbladder disease, diabetes and a multitude of other conditions. Extreme obesity may even disturb brain function by compromising adequate oxygen supply to the lungs and hence the brain. Extreme underweight strains the body's ability to rebuild and maintain itself. It can affect all systems and may even cause death when effort to reverse the progressive debilitation is late in coming or insufficient in magnitude.

Obesity. The term "obesity" is used to indicate the presence of excess body weight of 15 per cent or more above the ideal. Determining and "ideal," however, is a difficult problem, and generally it is defined in reference to average weight according to height and frame. Unfortunately, persons vary widely in these anthropometric parameters. Thus, assessment of body composition is of critical importance in judging the existence and/or significance of obesity in a patient. It should be remembered that a large person is not necessarily obese because his weight is high in proportion to his height and frame; such an individual may support a substantial muscle mass instead of fat pad and thus would not be a candidate for aggressive weight control therapy. Similarly, the patient who "looks fat" even though his weight is not high in proportion to height and frame may, in fact, have much fat and little muscle on his frame. Under such circumstances, weight control therapy may be advisable even though it is not dictated precisely by body weight/height/frame evaluations.

Much remains to be learned about the causes and management of obesity. There clearly are many forms of obesity and many reasons why it develops in some individuals and not in others. Accumulation of excessive body fat may begin as a result of simple overfeeding in childhood, or it may develop as a result of intense and frequently repeated episodes of emotional stress later in life. It may be complicated by low levels of physical activity and high levels of social and cultural pressure in a food-oriented environment. Once established, obesity may lead to progressive deterioration of self-image and continual utilization of food as a means of providing satisfaction in a world that otherwise is disappointing and devoid of pleasure.[5]

Obese patients must be managed on an individual basis, at least in the beginning. Treatment under any circumstance is always difficult, but treatment without thorough understanding of the significant causative factors involved is certain to fail. Before any therapy program is instituted, great effort should be made to develop a clear understanding of the duration of the problem and the relevant factors involved. Specific problems related to food and food consumption should be defined so that a therapy program can be structured to overcome the major food-related encounters during the day. Ideally, an interdisciplinary health care team can participate in assessment and management of the patient. A physician, nurse, nutritionist and psychologist may all serve important roles in determining the best overall approach to treatment.

In most cases of obesity, some form of dietary regulation is required in order that reasonable weight loss can occur over time. The basic principles are limited in number and straightforward in application. The diet that is selected should meet all the nutritional needs of the patient if at all possible. A vitamin and/or mineral supplement may be required in some cases. Specific food items which are allowed should be planned in accord with the patient's culture or life-style; strong emphasis should be placed on nutritious foods that are reasonably low in calories but enjoyable and satisfying. Efforts to increase exercise levels and modify inappropriate food-related behaviors should be made in most circumstances. With some individuals, behavior modification programs may be very effective. A slow loss of body fat over a long period of time is encouraged and therefore should be anticipated by both client and therapist. Ideally this is accompanied by improvement in self-image and development of a sound and sensible eating pattern that is conducive to maintenance of normal body weight in the future.[4]

Underweight. Loss of body weight as a result of insufficient calorie intake frequently accompanies many chronic disease processes. The basis for the weight loss is simple: an inadequate amount of food is consumed to provide for daily energy needs of the body, and thus the body begins drawing on its own reserves, specifically adipose tissue and lean body mass. Mild weight loss in most healthy individuals can be tolerated reasonably well without impairment of body defense mechanisms and overall physiologic operation. With substantial weight loss, however, the following problems develop:

decreased resistance to disease
impaired wound healing
retarded physical growth
reduced physical activity
increased vulnerability to environmental insults

These effects are especially significant in the person who enters the period of chronic undernutrition with little caloric reserve. With such an individual, death is a certain consequence unless aggressive effort is made to reverse the weight loss through appropriate nutritional support via oral or intravenous routes.

Carbohydrates

Carbohydrates are one of the major energy sources in the diets of all people around the world. Carbohydrate-containing foods are widely available, since carbohydrate is the predominant compound in grains, vegetables, fruits, and other plants. Generally, such foods are low in cost and often can be easily stored for relatively long periods. In some countries, carbohydrate foods make up almost the entire diet. In developed countries, about 50 per cent of the total calories are derived from this source, with the remainder coming from fats and proteins.

The three major groups of carbohydrate foods are monosaccharides, disaccharides and polysaccharides.

> Monosaccharides *are the simple sugars, glucose, fructose and galactose. By combining two monosaccharides, a* disaccharide *is formed. The major disaccharides include sucrose (glucose plus fructose), lactose (glucose plus galactose) and maltose (glucose plus glucose).* Polysaccharides *are complex carbohydrates made up of many units of one monosaccharide, usually glucose. Significant dietary polysaccharides include starch, dextrins, cellulose, pectins and glycogen.*

Most dietary carbohydrate is found in the form of polysaccharides and disaccharides, but a limited number of foods contain free monosaccharides.

The energy-producing systems of body cells are designed to utilize glucose. This compound is made available to body cells by several mechanisms: (1) it is consumed as such in food; (2) it is released in the intestines by digestive processes that break down polysaccharides and disaccharides and (3) galactose and fructose are converted into glucose in the liver. Provision of sufficient glucose to the body therefore necessitates that digestion and absorption in the small intestine are proceeding normally. Since only monosaccharides can be absorbed from the intestine, absence of digestive enzymes such as amylase, lactase, sucrase and maltase prevents normal polysaccharide and/or disaccharide breakdown and thus prohibits normal uptake into the body.

As mentioned previously, the *primary function of carbohydrates in human nutrition is to provide a major source of energy.* Although fat is also a fuel, it is primarily a storage form, and the body may function adequately without a daily supply of fat in the diet. The body tissues, however, require a constant dietary supply of carbohydrates to survive, since the amount of carbohydrate held in the body at any time is relatively small. A total of about 350 Gm. is stored in the liver and the muscle tissues as glycogen and another 10 Gm. are present as circulating blood sugar. This available carbohydrate provides only about 1400 kcal. This amount is sufficient to maintain the normal human organism for only 12 to 15 hours.

Carbohydrates are also important for their *protein-sparing action* and their valuable *antiketogenic effect.* That is, a sufficient intake of carbohydrate for energy prevents significant utilization of protein for this purpose. This protein-sparing action of carbohydrate allows the major portion of protein entering the body to be used for its basic purposes of building lean body tissue and synthesizing numerous enzymes, hormones and other regulatory compounds. The amount of carbohydrate available also determines how much fat will be broken down in the body. Thus, it affects the formation and disposal of ketones. Ketones, which are the immediate products of fat metabolism, normally are broken down or excreted. In extreme conditions, however, such as starvation or uncontrolled diabetes in which carbohydrate supply is inadequate or unavailable, these ketones accumulate and produce a condition called *ketosis.* Thus, the antiketogenic effect of carbohydrates prevents a damaging excess of ketone formation and accumulation in the body.

The continual presence of glucose in the body is essential for *functioning of several vital organs.* The glycogen stored in the cardiac muscle is an important emergency source of energy. In a damaged heart, poor glycogen stores related to a low carbohydrate intake may cause cardiac dysfunction or angina. A constant supply of glucose is also necessary for proper functioning of the central nervous system. The brain contains no storage supply of glucose and thus is dependent on a minute-to-minute basis for a supply of glucose from the bloodstream. Sustained and profound hypoglycemic shock (sudden development of low blood glucose level) may cause irreversible brain damage, since glucose is indispensable for functional integrity.

Once in the cell, glucose must undergo a series of chemical reactions to produce energy for the body's various demands. This energy is produced through three basic processes, which occur in the following order:[28]

Process 1: production of a common compound. Through the action of a series of enzymes in the cellular cytoplasm, the glucose molecule is gradually broken down into a smaller fragment called *acetyl coenzyme A (acetyl CoA).*

Process 2: the energy cycle. Acetyl CoA moves into the energy-producing organelle, the mitochondrion, where it is converted into energy compounds. This series of reactions is commonly called the *Krebs cycle,* or the *tricarboxylic acid (TCA) cycle.*

Process 3: production of compound with stored energy. Another series of enzymes in the mitochondria traps the energy that is produced and stores it in a compound that can be readily broken down when energy is needed. This energy-binding compound is called *adenosine triphosphate* (ATP).

Fats

Fat is another energy source available to the body, and among its assets is its concentrated form. While carbohydrate provides 4 kcal./Gm. of material, fat provides 9 kcal./Gm. An additional advantage of fat is its almost unlimited storage capacity in the body as adipose tissue.

Fats (or lipids) are found in several forms in the diet, i.e., solids, oils, waxes and related compounds. They are all greasy to the touch and insoluble in water. Some foods consist almost entirely of fat. These include butter, margarine, oil, salad dressings, bacon and cream. Other foods contain substantial fat but in a form that is less obvious. Foods in this category include egg yolk, meat fats, olives, avocados and nuts.

The significance of fat as an energy source in the diet varies according to country. People living in the most developed countries consume a relatively large amount of fat, so that 35 to 40 per cent of the daily calories may be derived from this source. In many developing areas, fat and fatty foods are relatively expensive, and thus they provide a limited calorie contribution to the diets of most individuals in these regions.

Fat in the diet comes in several chemical forms, the most common of which are tri-

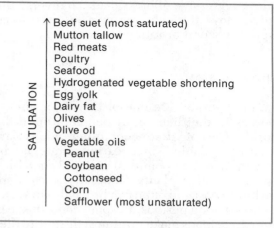

Figure 22–1. Distribution of food fats according to their degree of saturation. Animal fats are saturated; most fats derived from plants are unsaturated.

glyceride and cholesterol. *Triglyceride* consists of glycerol and three fatty acids. Fatty acids are composed of long chains of carbon atoms with attached hydrogen atoms. If all the carbon atoms are connected by single bonds, the fatty acid contains much hydrogen and is said to be *saturated.* If there are double bonds in the carbon chain, less hydrogen is present, and the fatty acid is said to be *unsaturated.* Triglycerides with unsaturated fatty acids tend to be soft or fluid substances. Triglycerides with saturated fatty acids tend to be hard and solid. In general, animal fats are saturated and vegetable fats (oils) are unsaturated, but individual fats vary in the degree to which they manifest these characteristics (see Fig. 22–1). It is also possible to convert unsaturated fat into saturated fat by the introduction (under pressure) of hydrogen into the available double bonds. This process, known as *hydrogenation,* is utilized to convert vegetable oil into solid hydrogenated vegetable shortening.

Utilization of dietary triglyceride necessitates (1) its digestion in the small intestine, (2) the absorption of its breakdown products by the small intestine absorptive cells, (3) its resynthesis within the absorptive cells into triglyceride compounds and (4) its final release into the circulation (via the lymphatics) in the form of protein-fat complexes called *lipoproteins.* These lipoproteins leaving the small intestinal cells are frequently referred to as *chylomicrons.* Chylomicrons are one of several types of lipoproteins that circulate in the bloodstream. The other lipoprotein forms originate in the liver.

In the cells, fatty acids are used as concentrated fuel to produce energy. The production of energy from fat follows the same general pattern as that of carbohydrate. Fatty acids are first broken down into the common fragment acetyl CoA, which then enters the mitochondria and is burned (metabolized) to produce energy through the Krebs cycle. The energy is stored for future use in the form of ATP. When there is sufficient glucose available to keep the Krebs cycle running properly, the fatty acid fragments are oxidized normally and the intermediate products, the ketone bodies, do not accumulate. In the presence of insufficient glucose, however, routine acetyl CoA processing is impaired, and ketone bodies form and accumulate. The fatty acids that are not used for energy in body cells are then used in the synthesis of various structural compounds or are stored in adipose tissue where they are converted into triglycerides for future use.

Cholesterol is the other major form of dietary fat. It is a steroid compound and is largely present in egg yolk, liver and other organ meats, and fatty dairy products such as butter. Cholesterol is absorbed intact without prior digestion. The level in the diet appears to affect the level in the bloodstream, but since the liver also synthesizes cholesterol and releases it into the circulation, the relative role of dietary sources in modifying blood cholesterol level is the subject of much debate. Cholesterol is utilized in the body for the synthesis of various membranous components of body cells.

Proteins

While the major role of fats and carbohydrates is the provision of energy, the *major role of proteins is the supply of building blocks for body tissues and regulatory compounds.* Proteins make up the basic structure of all living cells and are the essential life-forming and life-sustaining ingredients in the diets of all animals. The amount of dietary protein varies in different cultures, but in countries where adequate nutritional provisions are available, it contributes about 10 to 15 per cent of the total calories.

Proteins are found in most animal and plant foods. They consist of chains of amino acids, which are released during digestion in the small intestine. A given protein contains a specific number of individual amino acids linked in a specific sequence. Amino acids, the structural units of proteins, have been termed essential or nonessential on the basis of whether or not the body can manufacture them. Eight amino acids cannot be synthesized by man and thus must be obtained from the diet. The 11 remaining amino acids can be synthesized by man and thus are nonessential in the

TABLE 22–1. ESSENTIAL AND NONESSENTIAL AMINO ACIDS

ESSENTIAL	NONESSENTIAL
Threonine	Glycine
Leucine	Alanine
Isoleucine	Aspartic acid
Valine	Glutamic acid
Lysine	Proline
Methionine	Hydroxyproline
Phenylalanine	Cystine
Tryptophan	Tyrosine
	Serine
	Arginine
	Histidine

diet; these amino acids, however, are important and necessary for synthesis of body proteins (see Table 22–1).

According to the amount of essential amino acids they contain, protein foods are broadly classified as complete or incomplete. *Complete protein foods* are those that contain all the essential amino acids in sufficient quantity and ratio to supply the body's needs. These proteins are of animal origin and include meat, milk, cheese and eggs. *Incomplete protein foods* are deficient in one or more of the essential amino acids. These foods are of plant origin and include grains, legumes, seeds and nuts. In a mixed diet, animal and vegetable proteins complement each other. Even in a totally vegetarian diet, plant proteins can be appropriately mixed to provide a balanced ratio of essential amino acids.

It is therefore important to consider the quality and sources of dietary protein in arriving at a recommendation for adequate daily protein intake. All the essential amino acids must be provided in sufficient amounts. The better the quality of the protein or protein mixtures, the less the amount needed to meet body needs.

> *Securing sufficient protein in the daily diet is one of the most significant world health problems existing today.*

Protein is vital to life and health, but it is scarce and expensive. Protein deficiency affects millions of children in developing nations around the globe; protein deficiency (along with calorie deficiency) is the major cause of growth retardation, poor resistance to disease and death among children in these populations.

The primary function of dietary protein is to provide necessary amino acids for growth and maintenance of proteins in body tissues. Amino acids also contribute to the body's overall energy metabolism. After removal of the nitrogenous portion (the amino group) of the amino acid, the remaining part may be converted to fat or carbohydrate. If there is not sufficient carbohydrate or fat in the diet for energy, then as much as 58 per cent of the total dietary protein becomes available for oxidation and energy production. Therefore, sufficient nonprotein calories are needed in the diet to ensure that protein is used for its primary building purpose and is not broken down to yield energy. Using protein is an expensive way to run the energy-requiring machinery of the body.

Since protein is such an important nutrient for tissue building and rebuilding, much study has been given to how much protein the body actually requires. General recommendations for dietary protein intake have been developed on the basis of research pertaining to all age groups.[26] Survey of this information reveals an increased need for protein per pound of body weight during childhood. During adulthood, the recommended amount levels off for maintenance and repair of body tissues.

To maintain life and health over time, multiple body processes involving energy production and tissue building must proceed in an organized fashion. Such order requires the participation of a variety of control agents. Vitamins and minerals are two types of control agents that operate in important roles as coenzymes or cofactors. A *coenzyme* is an organic molecule, usually containing phosphorus or a vitamin, that is required for activation of a basic enzyme or enzymes. A *cofactor* is a mineral that is needed for the action of an enzyme.

A vitamin is a vital organic compound required in small amounts for coenzyme functions in biochemical pathways. Vitamins must be ingested, since the human body is not able to manufacture them.

Vitamins are usually classified according to their solubility in either fat or water. The *fat-soluble vitamins* include vitamins A, D, E and K. *Water-soluble vitamins* include vitamin C and the B-complex group. Usually, with limited planning, sufficient amounts of all the vitamins can be obtained in the daily diet. However, under unusual conditions (i.e., stresses such as illnesses, debilitation, alcoholism, drug therapy, severe calorie restriction), dietary vitamin sources may be insufficient and supplementation of the diet with appropriate vitamin preparations may be in order. Pertinent points about each vitamin are provided in Tables 22–2, 22–3, and 22–4.

TABLE 22–2.   BASIC INFORMATION ABOUT FAT-SOLUBLE VITAMINS

VITAMIN	FUNCTION	RESULTS OF DEFICIENCY	SOURCES
Vitamin A (retinol), provitamin A (carotene)	Vision cycle—adaptation to light and dark Tissue growth, especially skin and mucous membranes Toxic in large amounts	Night blindness Xerophthalmia Susceptibility to epithelial infection; changes in skin and membranes and in tooth formation	Retinol (animal food): liver, egg yolk, cream, butter or fortified margarine, whole milk Carotene (plant foods): green and yellow vegetables and fruits
Vitamin D (calciferol)	Absorption of calcium and phosphorus Calcification of bones Toxic in large amounts	Rickets Faulty bone growth; poor tooth development	Fortified or irradiated milk, sunshine, fish oils
Vitamin E (tocopherol)	Antioxidant—protection of materials that oxidize easily Normal growth Reproduction (in animals)	Protection of vitamin A and unsaturated fatty acids Breakdown of red blood cells, anemia Sterility (in rats)	Vegetable oils, vegetable greens
Vitamin K (menadione)	Normal blood clotting Toxic in large amounts	Bleeding tendencies, hemorrhagic disease	Green leafy vegetables, cheese, egg yolk, liver, synthesized by intestinal bacteria (main source)

Modified from Williams, S. R.: *Essentials of Nutrition and Diet Therapy.* St. Louis, The C. V. Mosby Co., 1974.

TABLE 22–3.   BASIC INFORMATION ABOUT SELECTED B-COMPLEX VITAMINS

VITAMIN	FUNCTION	RESULTS OF DEFICIENCY*	FOOD SOURCES
Thiamine (vitamin B_1)	Normal growth Coenzyme in carbohydrate metabolism Normal function of heart, nerves and muscle	Beriberi GI: loss of appetite, gastric distress, indigestion, deficient hydrochloric acid CNS: fatigue, neuritis, paralysis CV: heart failure, edema of legs especially	Pork, beef, liver, whole or enriched grains, legumes
Riboflavin (vitamin B_2)	Normal growth and vigor Coenzyme in protein and energy metabolism	Ariboflavinosis Wound aggravation, cracks at corners of mouth, glossitis (smoothness of tongue), eye irritation and sensitivity to light, skin eruptions	Milk, liver, enriched cereals
Niacin (nicotinic acid)—precursor: tryptophan	Coenzyme in energy production Normal growth, health of skin, normal activity of stomach, intestines, and nervous system	Pellagra Weakness, lack of energy and loss of appetite Skin: scaly dermatitis CNS: neuritis, confusion	Meats, peanuts, enriched grains
Pyridoxine (vitamin B_6)	Coenzyme in amino acid metabolism: protein synthesis, heme formation, brain activity Carrier for amino acid absorption	Anemia CNS: hyperirritability, convulsions, neuritis Pregnancy: anemia	Wheat, corn, meat, liver
Pantothenic acid	Coenzyme in formation of active acetate: fat, cholesterol, and heme formation and amino acid activation	Unlikely due to widespread occurrence and intestinal bacteria synthesis	Liver, eggs, milk, beef, cheese, legumes, broccoli, kale, sweet potatoes, yellow corn, synthesized by intestinal bacteria
Folic acid	Growth and development of red blood cells	Certain types of anemia, e.g., megaloblastic (large immature red blood cells) anemia	Liver, green leafy vegetables, asparagus, eggs
Cobalamin (vitamin B_{12})	Normal red blood cell formation, nerve function, and growth	Pernicious anemia	Liver, meats, milk, eggs, cheese

*Key: GI, gastrointestinal; CNS, central nervous system; CV, cardiovascular.
Source: modified from Williams, S. R.: Essentials in Nutrition and Diet Therapy. St. Louis, The C. V. Mosby Co., 1974.

TABLE 22–4.   BASIC INFORMATION ABOUT VITAMIN C (ASCORBIC ACID)

FUNCTIONS	CLINICAL APPLICATIONS	FOOD SOURCES
Intercellular cement substance; firm capillary walls and collagen formation Helps prepare iron for absorption and release to tissues for red blood cell formation	Scurvy (deficiency disease) Sore gums Hemorrhages, especially around bones Tendency to bruise easily Stress reactions Growth periods Fevers and infections Wound healing; tissue formation Anemia	Citrus fruits, tomatoes, cabbage, potatoes, strawberries, melons, chili peppers, broccoli, chard, turnip greens, green peppers, asparagus

Source: modified from Williams, S. R.: Essentials in Nutrition and Diet Therapy. St. Louis, The C. V. Mosby Co., 1974.

sometimes defined to include those minerals about which little is known in terms of human physiology. These three groups of minerals are listed below with their chemical symbols:

Minerals

The remaining nutrients essential to man are minerals. *Minerals are inorganic elements acting in the body as control agents in a variety of processes involving energy production as well as body building and maintenance.* While only small amounts of all vitamins and most minerals are necessary in the body, some minerals are required in large amounts. Calcium, for example, accounts for 2 per cent of body weight, largely because of its predominance in skeletal tissue. An adult weighing about 150 lb. has about 3 lb. of calcium in his body. On the other hand, iodine is present in very small amounts in the body. This same 150 lb. adult contains only a small fraction of an ounce of this mineral.

It is consequently understandable that the body minerals are generally classified in two main categories—the major minerals and the trace elements. In addition, a third group is

Group I: *Major minerals*
    Calcium (Ca)
    Magnesium (Mg)
    Sodium (Na)
    Potassium (K)
    Phosphorus (P)
    Sulfur (S)
    Chlorine (Cl)
    Fluorine (F)
Group 2: *Trace minerals*
    Iron (Fe)
    Copper (Cu)
    Iodine (I)
    Manganese (Mn)
    Cobalt (Co)
    Zinc (Zn)
    Molybdenum (Mo)
    Chromium (Cr)
Group 3: *Minerals whose functions are poorly understood*
    Aluminum (Al)
    Boron (B)

TABLE 22–5.   BASIC INFORMATION ABOUT SELECTED ESSENTIAL MINERALS

MINERAL	FUNCTION	RESULTS OF DEFICIENCY	SOURCES
Calcium (Ca)	Bone formation Tooth formation Blood clotting Muscle contraction and relaxation Heart action Nerve transmission	Rickets Porous bones Poor tooth formation Delayed blood clotting Tetany, decrease in free serum calcium	Milk and milk products, cheese, green leafy vegetables, whole grains, egg yolk, legumes, nuts
Phosphorus (P)	Bone formation Metabolism of carbohydrates and fat	Rickets Poor growth	Milk, cheese, meat, egg yolk, whole grains, legumes, nuts
Sodium (Na)	Water balance, osmotic pressure Acid-base balance	Imbalances in water shifts and control Imbalances in buffer system	Table salt (NaCl), milk, meat, eggs, baking soda, baking powder, carrots, beets, spinach, celery
Potassium (K)	Water balance in cells Acid-base balance Muscle and nerve action Protein synthesis	Water imbalance Heart action (irregular beat, cardiac arrest) Tissue breakdown	Whole grains, meat, legumes, fruits, vegetables
Iron (Fe)	Hemoglobin formation, carrying oxygen to cells for oxidation of nutrients to produce energy	Anemia Poor growth Inability to meet demands of pregnancy	Liver, meats, egg yolk, whole grains, enriched bread and cereal, dark green vegetables, legumes, nuts
Iodine (I)	Synthesis of thyroid hormone, which regulates basal metabolic rate, cell oxidation	Goiter Impaired metabolic rate	Iodized salt, seafood
Fluorine (F)	Dental health, prevention of dental caries by application to formed teeth	Excess causes dental fluorosis (mottled teeth)	Fluoridated water (1 ppm)

Source: modified from Williams, S. R.: *Essentials in Nutrition and Diet Therapy.* St. Louis, The C. V. Mosby Co., 1974.

Selenium (Se)
Cadmium (Cd)
Vanadium (V)

Table 22–5 summarizes significant data about each of the minerals for which accepted information has been accumulated.

Fluids*

Maintenance of life and health demands that water balance be kept within closely defined limits at all times. *Water is an essential nutrient that is basic to life, and its overall balance within the compartments of the body is regulated by various physiologic processes.*

Water *enters* the body (1) as preformed water in liquids that are drunk, (2) as preformed water in foods that are eaten and (3) as a product of cell oxidation. Water *leaves* the body through the kidneys, the skin and the lungs and in the feces. These routes of water intake and output must be in constant balance to avoid dehydration or its opposite, water intoxication. Since most of the major minerals required by the body are dissolved in the body fluids as electrolytes, fluid imbalance involves imbalances in these elements as well.

Fluid and electrolyte imbalances are likely to occur in many types of illnesses. Imbalances may also result from the indiscriminate use of diuretics, vitamin D, salt, sodium bicarbonate, and plain water enemas. Most illnesses pose some threat to fluid and electrolyte balance.

Appropriate management of some patients entails ongoing monitoring of fluid intake (I) and output (O). Preciseness of monitoring depends upon the seriousness of the patient's condition. At times, rough estimates are adequate; at other times (e.g., a severely burned patient), precise measurement of fluid balance is essential. Assessment of fluid output involves collection and measurement of urine and feces and estimation of losses via the skin (perspiration) (about 450 to 600 ml./day) and lungs (about 350 to 400 ml./day). Assessment of fluid input requires measurement of all liquids the patient takes, including water and other fluid nourishment (milk, soup, coffee, tea, eggnog, soft drinks), soft solids (ice cream, gelatin, sherbet, thin cereals, thin puddings) and intravenous solutions. To assist in estimation of fluid input, health institutions generally provide the nursing staff with lists that define the amount of fluid that common serving dishes, glasses and cups contain. The unit of measure generally is a cubic centimeter (cc.) or milliliter (ml.). Additionally, if water containers are left at the patient's bedside, the nurse must learn to assess the amount of water taken by the patient.

In general, the nurse evaluates fluid consumption at intervals recommended by the agency in which she is employed. At certain times during the day, fluid intake is charted on input and output forms.[24] On the basis of this information, significant decisions are made about appropriate future care of the patient. If insufficient fluids are being taken, for example, the physician may order the administration of a defined amount of intravenous solution to supply needed fluid or electrolytes.

Under certain circumstances, the patient's fluid intake should be more or less than he typically consumes in a 24-hour period. It may be necessary, therefore, to *force fluids* or *restrict fluids* according to a given specification. Routinely, the amount of fluid which a patient should take is defined for the nursing staff. The fluid order might read that the patient is to have 3000 ml. of fluid each day, or if fluids are to be restricted, the amount might be 800 to 1000 ml. Fulfilling the directive may require considerable ingenuity on the part of the nursing personnel; provision of understanding, encouragement and support is a vital part of establishing optimal patterns.

Common sense dictates approaches to take in forcing or restricting fluids. Under either circumstance, careful records should be maintained of the actual fluid intake over time. *When fluid intake is to be high,* fluids are placed within easy reach at the bedside in containers that can be easily managed by the patient without assistance. A variety of fluids or soft foods should be provided at proper temperature, and goals are established for intake at regular intervals during the day. *When fluids are restricted,* they should be kept out of sight as much as possible, and when offered, they should be presented in small containers at pre-established intervals. Foods that are dry, salty or very sweet stimulate thirst and must be avoided during fluid restriction. Oral hygiene must be maintained as necessary, and lips may be kept lubricated with suitable cream. Regular rinsing of the mouth with water or chipped ice may also provide satisfaction to the patient.

---

*Fluid balance and imbalance is discussed in detail in Chapter 24.

POPULAR CONCERNS ABOUT DIET AND HEALTH

The regular consumption of foods containing appropriate amounts of vital nutrients is clearly essential to maintenance of health and recovery from illness. Unfortunately, however, the curative or therapeutic roles of food have been grossly exaggerated in recent years, and as a result it is estimated that 75 per cent of the population of the United States believes that extra vitamins provide more pep and energy. Additionally, 20 per cent of the population is estimated to believe that arthritis and cancer are due to vitamin or mineral deficiencies, at least in part. About 65 per cent of the population believes that a daily bowel movement is essential to health, and about 2.5 million adults use supplemental means to achieve this. Millions of individuals treat themselves without consulting physicians, and approximately 3 million adult Americans have worn brass or copper jewelry as treatment for arthritis and rheumatism. Finally, it is a widespread belief that a faulty diet is the cause of most health problems. It is justifiable to claim that "Americans love hogwash"[31] and consequently will pay almost anything to obtain a "magic potion" for their health problems.

The most widespread and expensive type of quackery in the United States today is the promotion of vitamin products, special dietary foods and food supplements. Millions of consumers are being misled concerning their need for such products. The food quackery situation today is much like the patent medicine craze, which reached its height in the last century. Not only is such food faddism misleading and costly for the average consumer, but in many instances it may be dangerous, especially if a "magic potion" is substituted for appropriate and effective health care procedures that are known to assist in the prevention or relief of specific disease entities.

Recent research into *food faddism* in developed societies has revealed five major origins of the problem.[31]

▶ philosophical-religious elements (such as those at the root of the Zen macrobiotic movement)

▶ hucksterism

▶ abandonment of medical aid in favor of unorthodox treatment (as represented by the widespread belief that vitamin E will cure heart disease in those who are seriously ill)

▶ the influence of the respected but somewhat adventurous or biased scientist

▶ distrust of the commercial food industry (as seen in many adherents of the organic food movement)

The nurse is in a good position to understand the causes of food faddism and to recognize their dangers. Her understanding of people should help her appreciate the peculiar appeal of such misinformation. Her scientific background should enable her to assess the potent effects of food faddism on the long-term health and well-being of people she contacts.

If headway is to be made, however, in the reversal of this trend toward widespread acceptance of food fads, the nursing and medical professions must become active in movements to protect the public from the effects of such propaganda. A four-point program seems in order to initiate this effort:[31]

▶ Health professionals must be aware that some of their own colleagues have disseminated useless substances or misinformation.

▶ Health nutritional professionals should be more willing to attack food faddism.

▶ Health professionals should not be careless in their own nutritional habits. They should instead present obvious examples of good health through good nutrition.

▶ Health professionals must educate themselves in the area of nutrition so that they are able to distinguish fact from fallacy.

In these four ways, health professionals can provide their patients with a clear understanding of correct nutrition along with suitable recommendations as to how optimal nutritional status can be maintained through sensible daily eating practices.

Food Additives

Food additives are substances added to foods to improve color, flavor, consistency or stability. Use of such additives is an old practice that was begun to help preserve foods for long periods of time. Many additives are still used for food preservation. Beyond their basic use as preservatives, however, many food additives now are used for aesthetic purposes much to the disapproval of a portion of the consumer market.[32]

Some food additives have come under criticism in recent years because of experiments on laboratory animals in which large amounts produced tumors. In humans, the long-term effects of *small* amounts of these same additives are unknown, but it has been suggested that gradual accumulation of such materials in body tissues might eventually be lethal. No proof of this suggestion has yet been presented, but even so, the food additive scare has been widespread. In looking rationally at the issue and attempting to take a stand, it seems reasonable that effort should be made to avoid use of unnecessary additive chemicals in the food supply whenever possible. Legitimately, however, if human beings are to survive, long-term preservation of our precious food commodities is essential to provide for the daily needs of people during seasons of plenty and famine. Use of preservatives is therefore essential.

Natural and Organic Foods

As the additive scare gained momentum during the past several years, distrust of the food industry increased, and efforts to avoid "processed" foods developed. Widespread enthusiasm for "*natural foods*" has been obvious and supermarkets as well as other specialty stores now maintain a substantial number of whole grain or minimally processed food products. By and large, these products are wholesome and certainly palatable; their nutritional composition, however, may not be much different from that of products which are not advertised as "natural." Table 22–6 provides a comparison of the nutritive composition of two representative cereal products on the market. It is clear that in terms of the nutrients indicated on the chart, the "processed" product is, in fact, superior in many ways.[10]

"*Organic foods*" have also risen to a position of substantial popularity in recent years. This movement, again, is the direct result of the popular dislike for widespread use of chemicals in food production and processing. *Organic foods,* by definition, are foods grown in the absence of "chemical" pesticides and fertilizers or animals raised without use of any "chemicals in their foods" or "injections" to promote or modify growth. Organic farming entails the use of organic fertilizers, like manure and compost, and no sprays or other such pest control agents are employed. Fresh organic foods are often very tasty and in many cases are quite superior to "standard" fresh foods in overall aesthetic quality. These foods, however, are not always superior nutritionally to comparable counterparts, and in some parts of the country their high cost and substantial deterioration and spoilage losses make it difficult

TABLE 22–6.   NUTRIENT VALUES OF A TYPICAL "NATURAL" CEREAL COMPARED WITH A POPULAR CONVENTIONAL CEREAL

	QUAKER 100% NATURAL	CHEERIOS
Serving size	1 oz. (¼ cup)	1 oz. (1¼ cups)
Calories	120	110
Nutrient composition (percentage of Recommended Dietary Allowances)		
Protein	2	6
Vitamin A	*	25
Vitamin C	*	25
Thiamin (vitamin B_1)	2	25
Riboflavin (vitamin B_2)	*	25
Niacin	2	25
Calcium	2	4
Iron	2	25
Vitamin D	*	10
Vitamin B_6	†	25

*Contains less than 2 per cent of RDA.
†Value not given.

to justify purchase of these foods in this age of rising food prices and worldwide food shortages.

There is no reliable evidence that organic fertilizers are better than inorganic fertilizers in providing essential elements for plants and in turn for people. The principal advantage of organic fertilizers is that they improve the physical properties of the soil. Most commercial farms use large quantities of inorganic fertilizers and in their soil management return organic residues such as cornstalks, straw, or livestock manure to the fields in quantities that often exceed the harvested portion of the crop. These residues are worked into the soil where they decay by microbial action. Thus major quantities of organic matter become part of the soil and any comparison of commercial fertilizer use with so-called "organic farming" is frequently a comparison of two systems of farming that both utilize large amounts of organic matter in crop production.

Food Supplements

A variety of food supplements now on the market are proclaimed as vital additions to the poor nutritional staples consumed by the average person in today's world of processed foods and high stresses. Many of these products are high-protein materials with or without the added bonus of several vitamins and minerals. The advertising releases related to these products attempt to convince the consumer that his normal diet is poor and that "optimum health and performance" can be achieved only with sufficient dietary supplementation. These products are frequently expensive, and individuals with limited financial resources must sacrifice other necessities in order to purchase them. However, of people who decide that these products are essential for their health, 99 per cent really do not need dietary supplementation at all. This is especially true in the case of protein; it is the rare individual in developed societies who actually obtains insufficient protein in the daily diet to meet physiologic needs. If protein supplements are taken under circumstances of a protein-sufficient diet, the extra protein (amino acids) will be deaminated and the residual compounds burned for energy or stored as fat. The occasional malnourished individual who needs to consume an increased amount of protein daily is best advised to select an acceptable food source of protein and consume it on a regular basis; in most cases the cost would be less, and the pleasure obtained through daily food-related experiences might very well be therapeutic itself.

Vitamin and Mineral Supplements

Use of vitamin and mineral supplements is now widespread and most likely will continue in the future. While a large number of people who take vitamins really do not need them, a certain portion of the population probably benefits from this regular practice. In general, a well-planned, balanced diet composed of typical foods available in local markets meets the daily vitamin and mineral needs of most people. Those people, however, who exist on chronic weight reduction diets may not be consuming enough food to obtain these needed nutrients. The same may be said for alcoholics and persons with chronic disease and anorexia or chronic malabsorption and intestinal upsets. In these circumstances, vitamin and mineral supplementation may be beneficial, especially if dietary improvement cannot be accomplished.

Unfortunately, millions of people take vitamins each day "just to be sure their needs are met." When winter rolls around, some stock up on vitamin C. Others consume large amounts of

vitamin E in hopes of improving sexual performance or vitality. Persons with rashes, diarrhea, constipation or headaches may also be unwary victims of propaganda emphasizing that vitamins are good for them; they may assume that the more they take, the better off they will be. The Food and Drug Administration has developed regulations designed to (1) prohibit false and misleading promotional and labeling claims about vitamins and minerals and (2) distinguish between vitamins and minerals that are dietary supplements and those which should be sold as drugs. However, substantial educational effort is required on the part of the public if citizens are to learn what vitamins can and cannot accomplish.

Many sources and combinations of vitamin supplements are available on the market. Some people decide it is necessary to "go back to nature" and use "natural" vitamins, but this often proves to be expensive. Some individuals pay close to $5 for 100 tablets of vitamin C from pure rose hips, from acerola berries, or from a host of combinations with natural ingredients, such as honey. In fact, the same amount of pure ascorbic acid can be bought for under $1.

Two major fallacies lie behind the rush for so-called "natural" vitamins. The first fallacy is the belief that natural vitamins are superior to those synthesized by man. Actually, each vitamin has a specific molecular structure that remains the same, regardless of how the vitamin is produced. The body cannot distinguish in any way between vitamin A present in liver and vitamin A produced in a laboratory; only the wallet "knows for sure."

A second misconception about natural vitamins is the belief that "natural" vitamin products do not contain synthetic ingredients. In fact, some of the synthetic ingredients many persons are trying to avoid are present in the "natural" products. In processing tablets and capsules, for example, vitamin manufacturers must use excipients and binders, such as ethyl cellulose, polysorbate 80 (a synthetic emulsifier), and gum acacia.

> *Most "natural" products are therefore not natural at all but instead contain a number of necessary "chemical" constituents.*

One last issue related to vitamins is worthy of emphasis at this point. Vitamins are by no means so benign that large amounts can be taken without fear of toxic effects. It is a known fact that large amounts of several vitamins can cause serious anatomic and physiologic damage. This is especially true for vitamins A and D and possibly for vitamin C. Limited knowledge is available about the potential undesirable side effects of large intakes of niacin, vitamin B₆ and vitamin E (Table 22–7).

Supplementation of the diet with *iron* is a practice with considerable merit in many circumstances. This is especially true for adult premenopausal women whose regular diets may be relatively low in calories. Even with careful planning of daily menus and reasonable daily consumption of calories, obtaining 18 mg. of iron from the diet is difficult. The daily iron need of the individual woman relates directly to the volume of her monthly menstrual blood (iron) loss. Those women with regular blood loss of more than 30 to 40 ml. per month are good candidates for iron supplements. Women on chronic low-calorie (low-iron) diets might also profit from iron supplements. This is especially true in women with a history of iron deficiency anemia. If iron supplementation is recommended, an appropriate (absorbable) form of iron should be selected. The ferrous salts are more readily absorbed than the ferric compounds and should be recommended in all cases at a level approximating the RDA for adult women (18 mg./day).

Use of *calcium* supplements for prevention or amelioration of osteoporosis is subject to much debate. Some physicians and nutritionists believe that regular calcium supplementation through adulthood in women may assist in the construction of a sturdy skeleton that is somewhat more resistant to the bone-resorptive tendencies that develop in middle age. While this idea seems attractive and is supported by clinical reports, much controversy still exists about the long-term effectiveness of this practice.

Special Foods

The idea has prevailed for years that some foods possess certain "magic" characteristics that make them especially desirable in the daily diet for preventive or therapeutic purposes. Included in this category are honey,

TABLE 22–7. KNOWN INFORMATION ON VITAMIN TOXICITY

VITAMIN	RANGE OF TOXICITY	REPORTED SYMPTOMS
Vitamin A	Greater than 30,000 I.U. daily for at least 3 months	Fatigue, lethargy, insomnia, anorexia, abdominal discomfort, weight loss, bone and joint pain, loss of body hair, headaches, liver dysfunction
Vitamin D	Greater than 2000 I.U. daily	Anorexia, nausea, vomiting, drowsiness, headache, pallor, diarrhea, polydipsia, polyuria, fever, hypertension, renal damage, calcium deposition in soft tissues with hypercalcemia and hypercalciuria
Vitamin E	Greater than 800 I.U. daily	Weakness, fatigue, nausea, intestinal distress, headaches, giddiness, blurred vision, inflammation of mouth, chapping of the lips, muscle weakness, low blood sugar, increased bleeding tendency, reduced human gonadal function
Vitamin C	Greater than 1000 mg. daily	Rebound scurvy, inaccurate urinary glucose assay, menstrual bleeding in pregnant women, hemolytic reaction in people with G-6-P-dehydrogenase deficit, oxalate kidney stones, false negative tests for stool blood, destruction of vitamin B₁₂ in food
Niacin	Greater than 1 Gm. daily	Flushing, itching, dermatoses, hyperbilirubinemia, liver damage, elevated blood sugar, elevated blood uric acid with gouty arthritis, peptic ulceration, cardiac arrhythmias, gastrointestinal problems

data related to their derivation, nutritional composition, and role in the diet.

wheat germ, brewer's yeast, seaweed, lecithin, blackstrap molasses and fertilized eggs. All these foods are nutritious and contribute significant amounts of certain nutrients to the daily diet. None, however, possesses special curative properties and none is superior to many other foods in the ease of digestion, absorption and/or metabolism. Table 22–8 provides a listing of some of these foods along with

Separating Fact from Fallacy

Among the many services a skilled nurse must provide is assistance in evaluating the proliferation of claims and fads related to diet and health. In order to accomplish this task, the nurse must remain knowledgeable about the current findings and controversies. This can be done by participating in available continuing education programs, reading available review articles and establishing a list of resource per-

TABLE 22–8.   THE FACTS ABOUT SOME "SPECIAL" FOODS

Food	Source	Nutritional Composition	Pertinent Information
Brown sugar	A refined sugar product with small amounts of mineral residue from the original molasses preparation	410 kcal./½ cup 2.6 mg. iron/½ cup	Almost identical to white sugar in nutrient content (negligible) and calories (high)
Honey	A sweet material produced by bees from the nectar of flowers	65 kcal./T. 0.5 mg. iron/5 T.	Supplies carbohydrate largely in the form of glucose and fructose; not significantly easier to tolerate or digest than refined sugar; no special curative properties for fatigue, colic, sleeplessness, coughs, or a variety of other problems
Sea kelp/seaweed	Marine plants that grow in the sea	100 Gm. contains 312 kcal. 756 mg. calcium 7.8 mg. iron Good source of iodine Fair source of some trace elements	Nutritious but has no special curative properties; for those who meet their iodine needs by use of iodized salt, expenditure for these products to obtain iodine seems wasteful
Desiccated liver	Dried and powdered form of beef liver	Excellent source of vitamin B_{12} and some other nutrients	Does not necessarily prevent or cure pernicious anemia; taken in large amounts, it might mask the hematologic signs of pernicious anemia and allow the degenerative neurologic changes to progress unnoticed
Wheat germ	The central germ portion of wheat kernels	Good source of B vitamins, vitamin E and protein	Nutritious but unable to increase strength and endurance, prevent aging, cure muscular dystrophy or heart disease
Lecithin	A natural emulsifier found in egg yolks and soybeans	Phospholipid	Role in dissolving calcium and cholesterol plaques in blood vessels not clearly proved; in health, lecithin is produced in the body

sons in the community who can assist in answering difficult questions.

FACTORS THAT INFLUENCE FOOD INTAKE, DIETARY PATTERNS, AND NUTRITIONAL STATUS

A variety of factors determine the amounts and types of foods an individual will consume. The following factors are considered:

▶ appetite

▶ financial status

▶ geographic location; cultural background

▶ religion; social circumstances

▶ age

▶ individual differences and preferences

▶ physiologic and sensual reactions

▶ special physiologic conditions, i.e., pregnancy, lactation

▶ the media and the medicine man

▶ use of alcohol and drugs

▶ illness and injury

TABLE 22–8.   THE FACTS ABOUT SOME "SPECIAL" FOODS (*Continued*)

FOOD	SOURCE	NUTRITIONAL COMPOSITION	PERTINENT INFORMATION
Raw milk	Unpasteurized cow milk	Basically the same as pasteurized milk with no vitamin D; slightly higher vitamin C content	No special health benefits; may easily become contaminated if not kept in sterile containers at proper temperature
Yogurt	A fermented, cultured form of milk	Similar in composition to milk; may have considerable amount of added sugar	No special health benefits; no easier to digest; may alter gut flora favorably by supplying bacteria that produce B vitamins and vitamin K
Blackstrap molasses	Molasses syrup formed in the process of refining sugar	1 T. contains 45 kcal. 137 mg. calcium 3.2 mg. iron	Potent-flavored concentrated calorie source with no special curative properties; good source of iron
Brewer's yeast	By-product of the beer brewing industry	Good source of some B vitamins, amino acids, and some minerals 1 T. contains 1.4 mg. iron 1.25 mg. vitamin B_1 0.34 mg. vitamin B_2 3.0 mg. vitamin B_3	A nutritious food supplement but has no special curative properties
Gelatin	A glutinous material (colloidal protein) obtained from animal tissues	Incomplete protein	*Alone*, it is useless in building body protein; not necessary for strong nails, since nail formation is also influenced by general body nutrition, health, environment, local nail care and many other factors *In conjunction with other dietary amino acid sources*, it may provide useful sources of amino acids for body proteins
Fertilized eggs	Eggs produced by hens kept with roosters	Similar nutritionally to unfertilized eggs	No special health benefits; do not contain "special hormones" that commercial eggs lack; more expensive than unfertilized eggs

Appetite

While a wide variety of factors determines an individual's choice of foods, the basic sensation of "hunger" is certainly influential. The mechanisms that regulate hunger and satiety in the human body are poorly understood, but certain factors are now known to play a significant part. It is theorized that there are centers in the brain's hypothalamus that regulate food intake. Experiments have shown that injury of the ventromedial part of the hypothalamus results in overeating, while injury to the lateral regions promotes undereating. Clearly, however, other factors are involved: these include blood sugar level, gastric secretions, gastric motility, hormonal factors, and responses of the autonomic nervous system. For most people, the body adjusts ingestion of food to meet the requirements of health, proper functioning and growth. Occasionally this homeostatic mechanism does not operate properly, and excessive or insufficient hunger develops, with obesity or emaciation as long-term results.

Financial Status

It goes without saying that the amount of money you have to spend will influence what and how much you purchase. This is certainly the case for food. Families with middle or high incomes are generally able to purchase whatever they desire in the way of food items. In poor families, however, the limited amount of money available for food must buy a sufficient quantity to prevent hunger. Of necessity, foods of moderate to low price predominate in the diet, although there may be periodic "splurges," which can provide some variety and may even be a reasonably low-cost form of entertainment.

Geography

The specific location in which an individual resides will have a distinct effect on the types of foods he consumes. This is less true in developed societies where food preservation, packaging and transportation are sophisticated. Even under these circumstances, however, geographic location definitely affects the availability of many fresh food items, meats and other more labile materials. It is a sound prac-

tice for health professionals to keep abreast of the changing food supply in local markets during the year. If this is done, reasonable suggestions can be made to patients about food items available for use in special dietary regimens which are prescribed.

Culture

Eating habits are generally learned in early life and reflect very definitely the cultural influences that predominated in the home at that time. Eating habits as well as child-rearing practices vary from culture to culture; eating utensils, meal times, and food service patterns differ; many other features about food and eating are unique to specific cultural groups. One of the best publications summarizing significant issues in this area is the pamphlet, "Cultural Food Patterns in the U.S.A."; it is available through the American Dietetic Association in Chicago, Illinois.

Religion

Religious practices often dictate what a person will and will not eat, how he will prepare his food and when he will eat it. The Jewish and Islamic religions are particularly rich in food-related traditions. Those who carefully follow the teachings of the Old Testament will not eat meat and dairy products together. Those who follow Islam celebrate religious holidays with long periods of fasting followed by enormous feasts.

The Seventh Day Adventists and the Church of Jesus Christ of the Latter Day Saints support the philosophy that dietary practices are an integral part of religious beliefs. According to their doctrines, the best diet is the original vegetarian diet prescribed by God for good health. The diets of these peoples, therefore, are typically based on grains, fruits, vegetables and nuts, but dairy products and eggs may also be consumed. Tea, coffee, alcoholic beverages and strong spices and condiments may be eliminated in the interest of maintaining optimum health and preventing disease.

Social Circumstances

In most societies, social gatherings revolve around food and drink. The items served on these special occasions often are determined by tradition or custom dictated by the cultural group involved. Eating and drinking offer a significant means of socialization with friends and family. When opportunities for this source of enjoyment are eliminated (as may be the case for most hospitalized or many elderly citizens), the pleasure of eating may be much reduced. Appetite may become poor (or nonexistent) and serious malnutrition may develop. Great effort must be made by friends and caretakers to provide lonely persons with appropriate social contacts on a regular basis, especially during meals. This one effort may have a sizable impact on the eventual status of health and well-being of the individual involved.

Age

The age of an individual influences not only the types of foods he prefers but also the amount of food and specific nutrients required on a daily basis. Clearly those persons who are growing most rapidly (i.e., infants and adolescents) have the highest nutritional demands per kilogram of body weight; persons growing slowly (preschoolers and school age children) require less nutritional support per unit of body weight. Adults who are simply maintaining a stable body structure require the least nutritional support per unit of body weight until some special condition develops. Pregnancy and lactation both increase nutritional requirements substantially. Trauma, surgery, serious illness and other disease circumstances may also augment daily nutritional needs. As the adult becomes older, his calorie needs per day decrease but his requirement for all other nutrients stays approximately the same. It may require special ingenuity to plan acceptable daily menus that provide appropriate nutritional support within a limited calorie allotment. (See also Chap. 23.)

Individual Differences and Preferences

Within the framework of one's culture and life-style, eating patterns and nutritional requirements vary further in relation to individual preferences and physiologic differences. Choice of specific foods in the final analysis is an individual matter and relates to taste, texture and flavor preferences, which are based on experience with foods in the home and elsewhere. Likewise, each human being is unique in his specific nutritional requirements for optimum function. Recognition and appreciation of these highly important individual characteristics are vital if the nurse is to provide sound dietary advice and overall high quality health care.

Physiologic and Sensual Reactions

Some persons respond unfavorably to consumption of specific foods or beverages. The unpleasant sensations take the form of nausea, vomiting, diarrhea, headache or a variety of symptoms which fall within the category of "allergic responses." It stands to reason that foods which provoke these undesirable reactions are generally excluded from an individual's diet as a means of preventing this obvious distress. Again, appreciation for these problems when they occur must be developed by the sensitive nurse, and effort must be made to assist the patient in obtaining foods that will not cause undue distress.

Pregnancy and Lactation

Pregnancy and lactation are associated with increased nutritional needs and frequently are accompanied by altered eating patterns.[35] These patterns of eating may be related to specific appetite changes and food-related cultural practices believed to be conducive to the health of the infant and mother. Many traditions, superstitions and prejudices determine what foods are "acceptable" for the pregnant or lactating woman in most cultures. In parts of the South Pacific, for example, pregnant women are advised not to consume shellfish so that the baby will not develop scales on the head. In Ethiopia, it is traditionally believed in some areas that eating roasted meat during pregnancy will cause spontaneous abortion. In many cultures, women may consume a variety of nonfood items (clay, dirt, starch, ashes) for the purpose of easing the delivery, preventing birthmarks on the infant, or otherwise improving the circumstance of mother and infant before or after birth. Understanding the solid cultural basis for many of these practices is essential in formulating an approach to the situation. If the unusual practice does not appear to compromise the health of the woman involved, it may be unwise to recommend discontinuance of the practice, strange as it may seem.

The Media and the Medicine Man

The media and the traveling "medicine man" have dramatic influences on the eating patterns and supplementation regimens of people in most societies of the world. Radio, television, newspapers, magazines and similar media for information distribution reach many people and are very influential. New food products, food supplements, food service outlets and other innovations are appealingly introduced to the public on a regular basis. So ingenious are most of the advertisements that a listener who has no apparent interest in the product may be stimulated to purchase the item at the earliest opportunity.

Similar appeal is also conveyed by the traveling huckster who is out to sell a new food or supplement with or without an accompanying book on the virtues of the product in optimizing health. Since good health and prevention or cure of disease are desired by almost everyone, it is easy to understand how a smooth-talking, suave salesman can convince a gullible public to buy his line. All too often, this phenomenon takes place among people who think they know

better than to become entrapped. The influence of this form of persuasion is highly significant in affecting food practices of individuals in most societies.

Use of Alcohol and Drugs

Regular use of both alcohol and drugs can significantly modify appetite and food intake over time. *Moderate* drinking (and use of some drugs) may be accompanied by increased appetite along with an undesirable gain in body weight. On the other hand, *heavy* use of alcohol and some drugs may depress appetite to such an extent that malnutrition eventually develops if management of the drinking or drug ingestion is not accomplished. Many drugs, including alcohol, damage the mucosal linings of the stomach and bowel and thus prevent efficient use of the limited nutrients that are consumed; in such cases, malnutrition is especially likely.

Additionally, some drugs when present within the body are antagonistic to the functioning of specific vitamins or interfere with the normal metabolic processes in which the vitamins participate.[30] Consequently, use of such drugs may promote clinical signs of vitamin

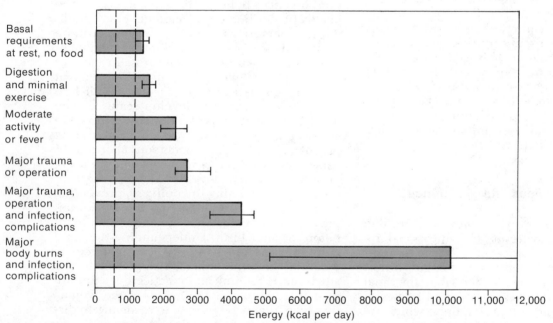

Figure 22–2. Metabolic energy requirements for the average adult under various conditions of stress are shown by the bars in this graph. The black lines indicate the range of variation for different individuals. The basal requirement of an adult at rest and not eating is about 1400 kcal per day. Standard intravenous feeding with 5 per cent dextrose can supply about 600 kcal per day. When the solution concentration is doubled to 10 per cent, feeding through a peripheral vein can provide only about 1200 kcal per day. With total intravenous feeding the patient can normally obtain 3000 kcal per day and in some cases up to 4000 kcal per day. Intake of 10,000 kcal per day has been possible only with a combination of oral food intake and total intravenous feeding. (Data from Lieber, C. S.: The metabolism of alcohol. *Scientific American, 234*(3):25, March 1976.)

deficiency even though the dietary quality appears satisfactory. By way of example, Aminopterin is an antagonist of folic acid; patients using Aminopterin may demonstrate folic acid deficiency.

Illness and Injury

Disease and trauma can markedly affect both appetite and nutritional requirements.[3] Nutritional status will gradually degenerate if appropriate nutritional care is not provided to patients under these conditions. Most people who are sick or injured have a poor appetite. At the same time, nutritional needs are frequently higher than usual because of the increased metabolic work required during fever, wound healing, and combating infection (see Fig. 22–2). Nutritional needs may be further elevated by sizable daily nutritional losses in the urine or from a bleeding or weeping wound. It is the responsibility of the health care team to evaluate the ongoing condition of each patient and estimate daily nutritional needs on the basis of clinical, anthropometric and laboratory data. Nutritional support through intravenous or tube feeding may be required instead of or in addition to the standard oral diet.

ASSESSMENT OF NUTRITIONAL STATUS

Evaluation of nutritional status is an important part of total patient evaluation and provides essential information for differential diagnosis. Recognition of nutritional deficits, excesses or imbalances can be of particular importance in determining the management and therapy of a patient and in returning him to health as quickly as possible. The *major features of nutritional evaluation* are not unlike those of general evaluation: (1) observing the patient's general appearance, (2) obtaining careful medical and dietary histories, (3) performing a thorough physical examination and (4) assessing selected laboratory measurements.[7] The kind of information that might be collected during a nutritional evaluation is provided in the following simple outline:

I. Dietary data
  A. Usual food patterns
    1. Duration of meal
    2. Kinds of foods eaten
    3. Amounts of foods eaten
    4. Items used regularly in large amounts
    5. Times during day when eating occurs
    6. Other pertinent features
  B. Use of dietary supplements (type, dose, time taken, specific preparation)
  C. Previous experience with modified diets
  D. Specific food likes, dislikes, intolerances
  E. General state of appetite
  F. Money available for food
  G. Transportation and facilities available for food purchasing, preparation and storage

II. Health history (as a partial indicator of past nutritional status)
  A. History of current illness
  B. History of past illness and recovery from surgery
  C. History of past pregnancy and outcome
  D. History of bleeding problems
  E. Drug use (what, when taken, why taken)

III. Physical condition and anthropometric data
  A. Height, weight, skinfold thickness
  B. Muscular development
  C. Neurologic condition
  D. Status of eyes, skin, tongue, mouth
  E. Dental status

IV. General biochemical measurements
  A. Urinalysis
  B. Stool assay (blood, fat, etc.)
  C. CBC, blood indices
  D. Serum proteins and lipids
  E. Serum electrolytes, blood pH
  F. Liver function studies
  G. Blood sugar, BUN, creatinine
  H. Nutrient absorption studies

V. Special biochemical measurements
  A. Nutrient and/or metabolic excretion after fasting or provision of test dose
  B. Concentration of nutrient in blood, plasma, RBC, WBC or other tissue
  C. Activity of specific enzymes (which suggest availability of certain nutrients, especially vitamins)
  D. Excretion of abnormal metabolites

Dietary Evaluation

Dietary studies are used to determine the sources and amounts of nutrients consumed on a daily basis by the individual or group under consideration. These studies can by no means be taken as absolute indications of adequate nutrition, but they are widely used to obtain presumptive evidence of dietary inadequacies or excesses. Information related to diet is useful in assessing need for nutritional intervention programs or for special feeding programs within homes or entire communities. Additionally, however, knowledge of existent dietary practices is an absolute necessity if recommendations for dietary modifications are to fit appropriately into the existent conditions and life-style of the patient.

Methods of Dietary Evaluation. Several methods of assessing dietary patterns are currently available, and each has its assets and problems in routine clinical use. The *three major means of diet evaluation* are the dietary history, the food record and the 24-hour recall. The first two methods take considerable time to accomplish. Therefore, if a limited amount of time is available for dietary assessment, these methods may be undesirable. The 24-hour recall (or a modification of it) can be completed easily and rapidly and may thus, at times, be the method of choice.

In taking the *dietary history* the interviewer discusses in depth the use of food in typical daily routines and in past circumstances. Great effort is made to fully understand the present and past bases for current eating patterns. Questions are asked in an informal, relaxed conversation in the clinic office or in the home. This information is generally used along with food record data to assess the dietary patterns of the patient and to make appropriate recommendations for modifications, if necessary.

The *food record* is a more quantitative evaluation of food consumption than the dietary history. That is, it provides more precise information on the amounts of specific nutrients consumed daily. The food record requires cooperation of the person in the household or institution responsible for food preparation. The client is instructed to keep a careful record of the amounts of each type of food consumed within a period of 3 or 7 days. This record is then given to a health care team member, e.g., dietitian, who determines the average daily intake of specific nutrients as reported in the food record. The average daily intake of specific nutrients is then compared with the Recommended Dietary Allowances for an individual of the same age and sex. Significant deviations from the RDA may suggest inadequate nutrition. This information is integrated with all of the client's other data instead of being used in isolation.

The *24-hour recall* is a relatively rapid assessment procedure which entails acquiring information from the client about his specific food intake during the previous 24 hours. These data are obtained during a short interview with the client. In some cases the client's memory permits him to accurately recall a representative day's food consumption. Not infrequently, however, the client may have considerable difficulty remembering what was consumed during the time period, especially if he was unaware that this information would be requested. The 24-hour recall, therefore, is believed to be most useful when large numbers of people are to be questioned within a short period in an effort to develop a feeling about trends in food consumption patterns within a specific *group* under consideration.

Occasionally, modifications or combinations of the above methods are utilized when they seem to meet the needs of particular circumstances best. Most commonly, a diet history is completed with a food record to allow for both quantitative and qualitative assessment of the dietary adequacy. In some settings, use of a *food frequency score sheet* has proved to be the most useful and rapid method available. This tool assesses the weekly frequency of consumption of each food on a carefully selected list designed to contain all major food sources of key nutrients. Data obtained can be tabulated by a computer to provide a rough estimate of average daily consumption of major nutrients, vitamins and minerals.

Use of Food Composition Tables. Evaluation of recorded data from food records necessitates determination of the nutritional composition of selected foods. This can be accomplished by the use of available food composition tables.[8] Additionally, there is a variety of smaller, more limited booklets and tables which provide selected information about specific aspects of food composition (e.g., calories, sodium content, carbohydrate). While much printed data is available, most tables need constant updating.

Changing Food Patterns. Not infrequently, dietary assessment of an individual suggests that the average daily intake of specific nutrients is not adequate to meet daily needs. The diets of some people, for example, completely exclude some types of foods or entire food groups, or the total food consumption may be inappropriately high or low. In such circumstances, the health professional suggests reasonable modifications in daily eating patterns to improve dietary quality or quantity. This practice is admirable and indeed necessary in some cases. It should be recognized from the beginning, however, that individual eating habits are very personal and in most cases are so ingrained within a person that efforts to alter them substantially may be fruitless. If dietary change is to be accomplished, it must be approached slowly, with recommendations for change presented only when firm justification is available. In addition, modifications that meet the cultural, personal and economic restrictions of the individual are much more likely to succeed. Change in food habits is not easy for anyone; when change is deemed necessary, it should be approached gradually with the full intention of adapting the proposed modifications easily into the client's life-style.

Clinical and Anthropometric Assessment

Clinical Patterns of Malnutrition. Physical signs and symptoms of malnutrition can be valuable aids in detecting nutritional deficiencies.[7] These may include delayed growth and development of children as determined by comparing growth data of an individual or a group with standard height/weight trends on growth charts. Other physical characteristics of malnutrition are pallor of the skin, atrophy of mucous membranes of the mouth and eyes, and degeneration of nail beds and palm surfaces. In the more serious cases of advanced protein-calorie malnutrition, hair discoloration and hair loss may accompany edema and delayed wound healing. Obviously, the sooner the diagnosis of poor nutritional status is made in individuals and in populations, the sooner clinical public health intervention programs can be formulated.

It must be emphasized that (1) signs of malnutrition may not be specific—that is, they may be related to non-nutritional factors such as poor hygiene or excessive exposure to the sun—and (2) they may not correlate with dietary intake data or the biochemical values in the individual or the population. This should not discourage the health worker from participating in the clinical evaluation of children and adults.

The World Health Organization Expert Committee has conveniently classified the *physical signs most often associated with malnutrition* into the following three groups:

Group 1—Signs that are considered to be of value in nutritional assessment. These are often *associated* with nutritional deficiency status. Signs of malnutrition may often be mixed and may be due to deficiencies in two or more micronutrients.

Group 2—Signs that need further investigation. They *may* be related to malnutrition, perhaps of a chronic type, but are often found in populations of developing countries where other health and environmental problems, such as poverty and illiteracy, coexist.

Group 3—Signs that have *no* relation to malnutrition, although they may be similar to physical signs found in persons with malnutrition and must be carefully delineated from them. This usually takes the particular expertise of a physician or other health worker expertly trained in nutritional diagnosis.

Although it is important to recognize that various signs have different degrees of reliability, signs of malnutrition falling in Groups 1 and 2 have been combined in Table 22–9 and are described in less technical terminology so that health workers of all categories may better understand their clinical significance. The WHO classification is particularly helpful in limited surveys that are aimed at rapid clinical screening of the community. The more reliable the signs and the more experienced the observer, the more definitive the nutritional diagnosis is likely to be.

Any physical finding that suggests a nutritional abnormality should be considered a "clue" rather than a "diagnosis," and as such, should be pursued further. Pallor, for example, should not be considered diagnostic of anemia but is a clue that could lead to laboratory confirmation of anemia. Similarly, epiphyseal enlargement or costochondral beading should not be interpreted as evidence of vitamin D deficiency without appropriate laboratory confirmation.

Finally, it should be recognized that the use of clinical methods in detecting nutritional deficiencies has definite disadvantages if used alone. When used in a cautious manner in connection with dietary and biochemical methods, clinical methods may greatly assist in providing a picture of the nutritional status of individuals or of a community. It is anticipated that as biochemical procedures become more refined and nutrition surveys are accomplished with more standardized formats, our increased knowledge will enable us to make more precise nutritional diagnoses.

Anthropometric Methodology. Anthropometric measurements include the determining of certain physical data showing the size and proportions of parts of the body. These measurements can be obtained with efficiency, speed, and accuracy by trained nonprofessional personnel. Measuring length and weight for gestational age and skinfold thickness in neonates, for example, is helpful in distinguishing infants with intrauterine growth retardation from small-for-gestational age, dysmature or postmature babies. The gathering of these anthropometric measurements on newborn infants is also helpful in identifying target populations and groups in need of nutritional assistance. In adults, discrepancy in height/ weight relationship suggests malnutrition or excessive fat stores. Skinfold thickness information may be very helpful in defining early onset of *excessive* adipose tissue deposition. Counseling, in such a case, is provided about modification of life-style and eating patterns to reverse the trend toward obesity.

In gathering anthropometric measurements as part of a data collection system, standardized equipment and procedures should be used. Appropriate reference standards for height, weight, head circumference, chest circumfer-

ence and skinfold measurements should be selected based on the following:

▶ Characteristics of the population being examined

▶ Availability of data on that segment of the population presumed to have achieved "optimal" growth

▶ Recommendations of various nutrition agencies which have endeavored to standardize anthropometric data collection from different parts of the world

Biochemical Assessment

Evaluating nutritional status by laboratory methods is a more objective and precise approach than the methods previously mentioned. It utilizes biochemical tests performed in a clinical laboratory to measure levels of nu-

TABLE 22–9. PHYSICAL SIGNS INDICATIVE OR SUGGESTIVE OF MALNUTRITION

BODY AREA	NORMAL APPEARANCE	SIGNS ASSOCIATED WITH MALNUTRITION
Hair	Shiny, firm; not easily plucked	Lack of natural shine; dull and dry; thin and sparse; fine, silky and straight; color changes (flag sign); can be easily plucked
Face	Skin color uniform; smooth, pink, healthy appearance; not swollen	Skin color loss (depigmentation); skin dark over cheeks and under eyes (malar and supraorbital pigmentation); lumpiness or flakiness of skin of nose and mouth; swollen face; enlarged parotid glands; scaling of skin around nostrils (nasolabial seborrhea)
Eyes	Bright, clear, shiny; no sores at corners of eyelids; membranes a healthy pink and moist; no prominent blood vessels or mound of tissue on sclera	Eye membranes (conjunctivae) are pale; redness of membranes (conjunctival injection); Bitot's spots; redness and fissuring of eyelid corners (angular palpebritis); dryness of eye membranes (conjuctival xerosis); cornea has dull appearance (corneal xerosis); cornea is soft (keratomalacia); scar on cornea; ring of fine blood vessels around corner of eye (circumcorneal injection)
Lips	Smooth, not chapped or swollen	Redness and swelling of mouth or lips (cheilosis), especially at corners of mouth (angular fissures and scars)
Tongue	Deep red in appearance; not swollen or smooth	Swelling; scarlet and raw tongue; magenta (purplish color) tongue; smooth tongue; swollen sores, hyperemic and hypertrophic papillae; atrophic papillae
Teeth	No cavities; no pain; bright	May be missing or erupting abnormally; gray, brown or black spots (fluorosis); cavities (caries)
Gums	Healthy; red; do not bleed; not swollen	"Spongy", bleed easily; recession of gums
Glands	Face and neck not swollen	Thyroid enlargement (front of neck); parotid enlargement (cheeks become swollen)

trients in biologic fluids (blood or urine) or to evaluate certain biochemical functions that are dependent on an adequate supply of essential nutrients. The interpretation of laboratory data, however, is often difficult and does not necessarily always correlate with either clinical or dietary findings.

Not all nutrients can or should be assessed by laboratory methods. In general, *laboratory methods are used to determine deficiencies* in the following:

▶ Serum protein, particularly albumin

▶ The blood-forming nutrients; iron, folate, vitamin B$_6$ and vitamin B$_{12}$

▶ Water-soluble vitamins: thiamine, riboflavin, niacin, vitamin C

▶ Fat-soluble vitamins A, D, E, K

▶ Minerals: iron, iodine, and other trace elements

▶ Levels of blood lipids such as cholesterol and triglycerides

▶ Glucose and various enzymes that are implicated in heart disease, diabetes and other chronic diseases

The use of laboratory tests has two primary functions. The first is to detect marginal nutritional deficiencies in individuals, particularly when dietary histories are questionable or unavailable. Their use is especially helpful before

TABLE 22–9.   PHYSICAL SIGNS INDICATIVE OR SUGGESTIVE OF MALNUTRITION (*Continued*)

BODY AREA	NORMAL APPEARANCE	SIGNS ASSOCIATED WITH MALNUTRITION
Skin	No signs of rashes, swellings, dark or light spots	Dryness (xerosis); sandpaper feel (follicular hyperkeratosis); flakiness; swollen and dark; red swollen pigmentation of exposed areas (pellagrous dermatosis); excessive lightness or darkness (dyspigmentation); black and blue marks due to bleeding (petechiae); lack of fat under skin
Nails	Firm, pink	Spoon-shaped (koilonychia); brittle, ridged
Muscular and skeletal systems	Good muscle tone; some fat under skin; can walk or run without pain	Muscles have "wasted" appearance; baby's skull bones are thin and soft (craniotabes); round swelling of front and side of head (frontal and parietal bossing); swelling of ends of bones (epiphyseal enlargement); small bumps on both sides of chest wall (on ribs), beading of ribs; baby's soft spot on head does not harden at proper time (persistently open anterior fontanel); knock-knees or bowlegs; bleeding into muscle (musculoskeletal hemorrhages); person cannot get up or walk properly
Internal systems Cardiovascular	Normal heart rate and rhythm; no murmurs or abnormal rhythms; normal blood pressure for age	Rapid heart rate above 100 beats/min. (tachycardia); enlarged heart; abnormal rhythm; high blood pressure
Gastrointestinal	No palpable organs or masses (in children, however, liver edge may be palpable)	Liver enlargement; enlargement of spleen (usually indicates other associated diseases)
Nervous	Psychologic stability; normal reflexes	Mental irritability and confusion; burning and tingling of hands and feet (paresthesia); loss of position and vibratory sense; weakness and tenderness of muscles (may result in inability to walk); decrease or loss of ankle and knee reflexes

Source: Christakis, G. (ed.): Nutritional assessment in health programs. *American Journal of Public Health*, Nov. 1973.

overt clinical signs of disease appear, thus permitting the initiation of appropriate remedial steps. The second function of the laboratory test is to supplement or enhance other studies, such as dietary or community assessment among specific population groups, in order to pinpoint specific nutritional problems. Laboratory investigation is of little use if it merely confirms a known clinical diagnosis.

Often, laboratory values suggest marginal or acute deficiencies when the patient appears clinically normal. This is because clinical signs usually occur only after prolonged inadequate intake or absorption of nutrients. The probability, then, is that the subject may be in a preliminary stage of depletion and if this state continues will become ill. Most important, a deficiency in one nutrient can be considered an almost certain indicator of other nutritional inadequacies; these too should be rigorously investigated.

BIBLIOGRAPHY

The references for this chapter will be found at the end of Chapter 23, page 475.

SPECIAL NUTRITIONAL CONSIDERATIONS

By Bonnie Worthington, Ph.D.

SPECIAL NUTRITION CONSIDERATIONS DURING THE LIFE CYCLE

Each stage of the life cycle brings with it a unique set of circumstances that dictate individual nutritional needs. Throughout infancy and childhood, significant nutritional support is necessary for normal growth and development. When growth ceases at the end of adolescence, nutritional needs decrease to a level sufficient to maintain optimal body status. With pregnancy come increased nutritional requirements to provide for maternal physiologic adjustments and fetal growth. During lactation, nutritional requirements increase significantly, largely because of the volume of milk produced each day. As age increases, especially beyond 50 years, overall nutritional needs remain approximately the same but calorie requirements usually decrease. Recognizing the basis for nutritional requirements during the various stages of the life cycle enables the nurse to provide appropriate guidance to clients of all ages.

Infancy

During the first year of life, the infant grows rapidly, with the rate tapering off somewhat in the later half of the year. By 6 months of age, birth weight generally has doubled, and by 1 year it probably has tripled. To support this rapid rate of tissue synthesis, sufficient calorie and protein intake is critical; the other nutrients also play an important supportive role in the growth process.

A variety of milks and solid foods are available for feeding infants in most countries.[12, 29]

The "ideal" food for young infants is breast milk, which potentially is available to 99 per cent of all babies. This milk contains everything the infant needs until about 4 to 6 months of age (Table 23–1). In addition to a satisfactory calorie content (20 kcal./oz.) and easily digestible forms of protein, carbohydrate and fat, breast milk has a low electrolyte load, a high vitamin content (if the mother's diet is adequate), an acceptable iron content (in absorbable form) and an abundance of "protective factors" such as immunoglobulins, macrophages and antiviral agents. *No artificial formula precisely duplicates human milk!*[18]

While human milk is clearly the most satisfactory food for human infants, breast feeding may not necessarily be the most acceptable method of infant feeding for a given mother. Ideally, all pregnant women are provided with sufficient information about all options in infant feeding. Under such circumstances, an intelligent choice can be made on the basis of individual conditions and life-styles. In the past, at least 50 per cent of young mothers selected bottle feeding simply because they were not given enough information about breast feeding to consider it a viable option. It is hoped that this situation will disappear as health professionals become more aware of the importance of allowing all women to choose their mode of infant feeding based on a thorough understanding of all possibilities.

A variety of commercial formulas on the market are designed to resemble human milk as closely as possible. Most of them contain about 20 kcal./oz. and provide the nutrients babies need (with the exception of iron in some cases) (Table 23–2). Adequate infant formulas can also be made in the home from evaporated milk, corn syrup and water. These preparations are

TABLE 23–1. COMPOSITION OF MATURE HUMAN MILK AND COW MILK

COMPOSITION	HUMAN MILK	COW MILK
Water (ml./100 ml.)	87.1	87.2
Energy (kcal./100 ml.)	75	66
Total solids (Gm./100 ml.)	12.9	12.8
Protein (Gm./100 ml.)	1.1	3.5
Fat (Gm./100 ml.)	4.5	3.7
Lactose (Gm./100 ml.)	6.8	4.9
Ash (Gm./100 ml.)	0.2	0.7
Proteins (% of total protein)		
Casein	40	82
Whey proteins	60	18
Nonprotein nitrogen (mg./100 ml.)	32	32
(% of total nitrogen)	15	6
Amino acids (mg./100 ml.)		
Essential		
Histidine	22	95
Isoleucine	68	228
Leucine	100	350
Lysine	73	277
Methionine	25	88
Phenylalanine	48	172
Threonine	50	164
Tryptophan	18	49
Valine	70	245
Nonessential		
Arginine	45	129
Alanine	35	75
Aspartic acid	116	166
Cystine	22	32
Glutamic acid	230	680
Glycine	0	11
Proline	80	250
Serine	69	160
Tyrosine	61	179
Major minerals per liter		
Calcium (mg.)	340	1170
Phosphorus (mg.)	140	920
Sodium (mEq.)	7	22
Potassium (mEq.)	13	35
Chloride (mEq.)	11	29
Magnesium (mg.)	40	120
Sulfur (mg.)	140	300
Trace minerals per liter		
Chromium (μg.)	—	8–13
Manganese (μg.)	7–15	20–40
Copper (μg.)	400	300
Zinc (mg.)	3–5	3–5
Iodine (μg.)	30	47*
Selenium (μg.)	13–50	5–50
Iron (mg.)	0.5	0.5
Vitamins per liter		
Vitamin A (I.U.)	1898	1025†
Thiamin (μg.)	160	440
Riboflavin (μg.)	360	1750
Niacin (μg.)	1470	940
Pyridoxine (μg.)	100	640
Pantothenate (mg.)	1.84	3.46
Folacin (μg.)	52	55
Vitamin B_{12} (μg.)	0.3	4
Vitamin C (mg.)	43	11**
Vitamin D (I.U.)	22	14‡
Vitamin E (mg.)	1.8	0.4
Vitamin K (μg.)	15	60

*Range 10 to 200 μg./liter.
†Average value for winter milk; value for summer milk, 1690 I.U./liter.
**As marketed; value for fresh cow milk, 21 mg./liter.
‡Average value for winter milk; value for summer milk, 33 I.U.
Source: Fomon, S.: Infant Nutrition, 2nd ed. Philadelphia, W. B. Saunders Co., 1974, pp. 362–363.

TABLE 23–2. CALORIE VALUE OF SELECTED MILK FORMULAS

MILK	KCAL./OZ.
Human	21–23
Cow's	20
Evaporated (diluted for formula)	21
Low fat, 2% (+ milk solids)	17
Skim (+ milk solids)	10
Enfamil	20
Similac	20
Lofenalac	20
SMA	20

nutritionally satisfactory except for their deficits of iron and vitamin C. Fresh homogenized milk is not appropriate for infants during the first 6 to 12 months of life; fresh cow's milk contains protein that causes a small amount of bleeding of the intestinal mucosa in the infant and thus may promote iron deficiency anemia. Skim milk should not be fed to infants under 1 year old. Not only is skim milk derived from "fresh" cow's milk but it contains only 10 kcal./oz. and thus cannot support optimum growth of young infants.

Textured foods should be added to the diet of the infant by about 4 to 6 months of age. *Most babies do not need solids before this time.* Early introduction of solid foods has been said to be the major reason for the development of obesity in infancy. Parents need to be advised to introduce solid foods when the baby needs additional calories in the diet. Iron-fortified rice cereal is a reasonable "first choice," with strained fruits and vegetables providing a further contribution. Babies do not need the numerous commercial baby foods; parents can easily prepare suitable foods for their infants from fruits, vegetables and other table foods. Strained foods should gradually be replaced by foods of lumpy texture and finally by fully textured foods that require considerable oral motor manipulation. In all cases, special attention should be given to provision of sufficient calories, iron, vitamin D and vitamin C. Some reasons inappropriate calorie support is provided include the following:

- High or low formula concentration

- Misinterpretation of "fussiness" to mean hunger

- Excessive "mothering" with food

- Excessive use of solids in the diet

- Multiple "feeders" in the family leading to overfeeding

- Stressful environment promoting poor appetite

▶ Chronic anorexia related to disease or drug therapy

▶ Excessive loss of calories by vomiting and/or diarrhea

Preschool Age

As the infant grows, he gradually becomes more independent and more capable of feeding himself. He develops his self-feeding skills by "regular practice" and thus needs to be provided with an opportunity to finger feed and manipulate feeding utensils. In the process of learning these necessary self-feeding skills, spills and messes should be expected. A parent who expects the young preschooler to avoid mishaps in the feeding process will be very frustrated. Parents should be encouraged to relax and let junior "do his own thing" because gradually he will become more coordinated and will be less likely to leave the feeding scene in a shambles. Some characteristics that affect the nutritional practices of the preschool child are given here:

▶ He is an individual.

▶ He develops at his own speed.

▶ He asserts his independence.

▶ He rejects new foods.

▶ He eats less some days than others.

▶ He rebels when forced to eat.

▶ He learns by experience with fingers before forks.

▶ He eats best when he is
　relaxed
　comfortable in a chair that fits
　provided small servings
　free to choose some foods for himself
　allowed to eat in a pleasant environment
　　with minimal distractions

With his increased interest in the world around him, the preschool child may not demonstrate as much interest in food as he did in infancy. Refusal of food is common, and the desire to consume the same food repeatedly during the day or week is also seen. Parents should be encouraged to offer a variety of food to their children at this age but should not be upset if it is not consumed but merely explored or nibbled at. Repeated exposure to certain foods generally brings about repeated trials so that gradually a new food may become totally acceptable. Preschool children learn very quickly that parents can be manipulated easily by rejection of foods. Parents should be warned to avoid becoming the victims of their clever children who take advantage of parents' desires to "make them happy" or "stop their begging or whining."

The young child should set his own goals concerning the quantity of food he consumes. The portions offered to him should be small. Often if the preschooler can pour his own milk from a small pitcher into a little glass, he consumes a greater amount. It is normal, however, for the quantity of milk consumed during this period to decline. It is also normal for the preschooler to imitate other significant persons in his environment. While mother often plays a major role in the "care and upkeep" of the young child, the father and siblings play an important part in influencing the feeding behavior of preschool children in the home.

School Age

The slower rate of growth demonstrated by the school age child results in a general decline in the food requirement per unit of body weight. This lower requirement continues until the onset of the adolescent growth spurt. Food likes and dislikes during this stage are the products of earlier years, but the eating behavior of peers and the constant media advertisements for specific foods have a strong influence. School age children become increasingly involved in school-related, sports-related and other social activities that compete effectively with the dinner hour. Meals may be hurried or skipped, and the older child may often be left alone to prepare food for himself. Consequently, snacks play a significant part in the total food intake. Parents should be encouraged to prepare nutritious snack foods that can be eaten at home or easily carried out and will contribute effectively to the child's total daily nutritional intake.

Adolescence

To support the rapid physical growth during this period, calorie needs increase to meet the metabolic demands, although individual needs vary and girls require fewer calories than boys. Calorie and protein needs are easily met unless poverty or purposeful dieting exists. Minerals particularly needed are calcium for support of long bone calcification and iron for maintenance of the increased red blood cell mass. Menstrual blood losses in the adolescent girl predispose her to iron deficiency anemia. Boys may suffer from the same condition if growth rate is high and limited income prevents purchase of iron-rich foods. Intakes of needed vitamin C and vitamin A may be low because of erratic food intake. Peer group pressure may lead to increased snacking and dependence on a limited number of foods.

Most surveys in developed societies show that the adolescent girl is the most vulnerable person nutritionally of all members of the population because of (1) her physiologic sex differences associated with fat deposits during this period and her possible comparative lack of physical activity (thus she gains weight easily) and (2) social pressures and personal tensions concerning figure control (leading to unwise, self-imposed crash diets for weight loss). As a result, she may become malnourished at this important time in her life when she is building nutritional reserves that may be used to support reproductive requirements later. Adolescent girls are thus in need of appropriate and responsible dietary counseling. Rigorous efforts to maintain an unreasonably low body weight should be discouraged. Recommendations for development of regular physical activity patterns should be provided as an optimal means of balancing calorie intake and output over time.

Adulthood

Normal adults require sufficient nutritional support to maintain themselves in good health. The number of calories required daily depends directly on the level of physical activity in the daily routine. The moderately or highly active adult has little difficulty meeting both calorie and nutrient needs unless poverty is existent. The adult who is very inactive and consumes a limited number of calories may not select foods of sufficiently high nutritional value to support nutrient needs. Such individuals, especially those who chronically undertake weight reduction regimens, may find themselves seriously malnourished unless organized effort is made to fulfill daily nutrient needs either by appropriate food intake or by use of nutritional supplements.

On the basis of available research and clini-

cal data, the "best" diet for the average adult would appear to be one containing all needed nutrients and providing approximately 30 per cent of the calories from fat, 55 per cent of the calories from carbohydrate and 15 per cent of the calories from protein. Ideally, the fat in the diet should be relatively low in saturated fatty acids, and the carbohydrate should be predominantly complex (such as starch) rather than refined sugar. Additionally, enough nondigestible material (fiber) should be included in the daily regimen to allow for maintenance of normal gut motility. In all cases, the calorie intake should not exceed the calorie needs to support normal basal metabolism and voluntary activities. Maintenance of appropriate body weight throughout adulthood should be a primary concern of every adult desirous of maintaining optimum health.

Pregnancy

Support of a normal, healthy pregnancy logically requires extra nutritional provisions to the adult woman during this time.[35] An increase of

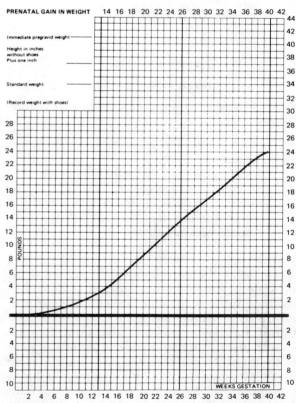

Figure 23–1. Pattern of normal prenatal weight gain. (From Committee on Maternal Nutrition, Food and Nutrition Board, National Research Council, National Academy of Sciences: *Maternal Nutrition and the Course of Pregnancy.* Washington, D.C., 1970.)

approximately 300 kcal. are needed each day, along with 30 Gm. of extra protein; an average weight gain of 25 lb. is recommended (Fig. 23–1). Small increases in amounts of the other vital nutrients are also necessary to meet the added demands of the fetus. In most cases, simple and sensible increases in daily food intake can accommodate the added nutritional needs of the pregnant woman. In some cases, however, iron, folic acid, or general vitamin supplements may be justified for individuals at high risk for malnutrition. High-risk women include adolescents, women with previous pregnancy difficulties, women pregnant after a very short interconceptional period, women from low socioeconomic levels, and women with heart disease, diabetes or other diseases associated with increased pregnancy risk. Prenatal nutritional counseling is a routine part of well-organized care for pregnant women in both private and clinic settings. Effort is made to provide reasonable guidelines for meeting nutritional needs within the framework of individual cultures and life-styles (Table 23–3).

Lactation

Daily production of 500 to 1000 ml. of milk for a growing infant clearly demands considerable input from the lactating mother. During lactation, nutritional needs relate directly to the amount of milk produced each day. The average lactating mother who is producing about 800 ml. of milk daily should consume an additional 500 kcal. and 20 Gm. of protein per day; moderately increased amounts of other essential nutrients should also be ingested (Table 23–3). The breast milk content of most vitamins reflects the level of maternal intake. The calcium content of breast milk is relatively stable, since maternal dietary calcium deficiency is rectified by withdrawal of calcium from skeletal stores. Malnourished women may continue to breast-feed, even under very adverse conditions. Under such circumstances, the overall milk supply is generally reduced and the mother suffers progressive debilitation from constant drain on limited nutritional reserves.[35]

Old Age

Nutritional needs of the average adult do not change much with increasing age. By and large, the metabolic machinery requires about the same level of nutritional input at age 70 as it does at age 40. However, daily calorie needs decrease with age in relation to a reduction in physical activity and reduced basal metabolic

TABLE 23–3.   RECOMMENDED DAILY DIETARY ALLOWANCE FOR FEMALES 19 TO 22 YEARS OF AGE

	NONPREGNANT	PREGNANT	LACTATING
Energy (kcal.)	2100	2400	2600
Protein (Gm.)	46	76	66
Vitamin A (I.U.)	4000	5000	6000
Vitamin D (I.U.)	400	400	400
Vitamin E (I.U.)	12	15	15
Vitamin C (mg.)	45	60	80
Folacin (μg.)	400	800	600
Niacin (mg.)	14	16	18
Riboflavin (mg.)	1.4	1.7	1.9
Thiamin (mg.)	1.1	1.4	1.4
Vitamin B_6 (mg.)	2.0	2.5	2.5
Vitamin B_{12} (μg.)	3.0	4.0	4.0
Calcium (mg.)	800	1200	1200
Phosphorus (mg.)	800	1200	1200
Iodine (μg.)	100	125	150
Iron (mg.)	18	18+	18
Magnesium (mg.)	300	450	450
Zinc (mg.)	15	20	25

rate associated with decreased amounts of metabolically active lean body mass. Daily calorie requirements decrease by about 7 per cent with each decade after age 25. It must be remembered, however, that considerable individual variation exists. Some active and healthy senior citizens continue to lead vigorous lives and maintain metabolically active lean body masses. Such persons clearly require more caloric support than the immobilized aged individual whose daily calorie needs are relatively low. A major difficulty encountered by the inactive older adult concerns obtaining the necessary *nutrients* from a diet sufficiently low in *calories*. Such a goal can be achieved if one attends closely to diet planning and omits the sources of "empty calories." For some people, however, this task is impossible, and in such circumstances, low-dose vitamin or mineral supplements may be justified.

SPECIAL DIETS

Basic Principles of Diet Therapy

Provision of appropriate nutritional support is basic to assuring overall optimal patient care. The primary objective of "diet therapy," therefore, is to meet the patient's nutritional needs within the framework of his individual preferences, problems, food tolerances, and overall program of management. Many types of dietary patterns may be "therapeutic" in their effects on groups of patients. The circumstance of each individual must be carefully judged by the health care team in order to define an appropriate diet prescription. Modification of the original diet order usually develops over time. As the patient improves, for example, his food tol-

erances may change rather rapidly. Effort should be made to provide the best possible oral feeding regimen.[9] Sometimes, however, this goal cannot be achieved, and tube or intravenous feeding programs may become necessary.

Standard Dietary Regimens in the Hospital Setting

In many cases, nutritional needs of the ill or hospitalized individual do not differ from those

TABLE 23–4. TYPES OF HOSPITAL DIETS

	CLEAR LIQUID DIET	FULL LIQUID DIET	SOFT DIET	REGULAR—HOUSE GENERAL—FULL
Characteristics	Temporary diet of clear liquids without residue; nonstimulating, nongasforming, nonirritating	Foods liquid at room temperature or liquefying at body temperature	Normal diet modified in consistency to have no roughage. Liquids and semisolid food; easily digested	Practically all foods; simple, easy-to-digest foods, simply prepared, palatably seasoned
Adequacy	Inadequate: deficient in protein, minerals, vitamins and calories	Can be adequate with careful planning: adequacy depends on liquids used	Entirely adequate liberal diet	Adequate and well balanced
Use	Acute illness and infections. Postoperatively. Temporary food intolerance. To relieve thirst. Reduce colonic fecal matter. 1 to 2 hour feeding intervals	Transition between clear liquid and soft diets. Postoperatively. Acute gastritis and infections. Febrile conditions. Intolerance for solid food. 2 to 4 hour feeding intervals	Between full liquid and light or regular diet. Between acute illness and convalescence. Acute infections. Chewing difficulties. Gastrointestinal disorders. 3 meals with or without between-meal feedings	For uniformity and convenience in serving hospital patients. Ambulatory patients. Bed patients not requiring therapeutic diets
Foods	Water, tea, coffee, coffee substitutes. Fat-free broth. Carbonated beverages. Synthetic fruit juices. Ginger ale. Plain gelatin. Sugar	All liquids on clear liquid diet plus: All forms milk. Soups, strained. Fruit and vegetable juices. Eggnogs. Plain ice cream and sherbets. Junket and plain gelatin dishes. Soft custard. Cereal gruels	All liquids. Fine and strained cereals. Cooked tender or puréed vegetables. Cooked fruits without skins and seeds. Ripe bananas. Ground or minced meat, fish, poultry. Eggs and mild cheeses. Plain cake and puddings. Moderately seasoned foods	All basic foods
Modification	Liberal clear liquid diet includes fruit juices, egg white, whole egg, thin gruels	Consistency for tube feedings: foods that will pass through tube easily	Low residue—no fiber. Bland—no chemical, thermal, physical stimulants. Cold soft—tonsillectomy. Mechanical soft—requiring no mastication. Light diet—intermediate between soft and regular. *Note:* Because of trend toward more liberal interpretation of diets and foods, soft diet may be combined with light diet in some hospitals	For a light or convalescent diet, fried foods, rich pastries, fat-rich foods, coarse vegetables, raw fruits may be omitted

Source: Miller, G. F., and Keane, C. B.: *Encyclopedia and Dictionary of Medicine, Nursing, and Allied Health,* 2nd ed. Philadelphia, W. B. Saunders Co., 1978, p. 293.

of everyone else. The routine hospital diet therefore is designed to be nutritionally adequate and palatable to the tastes and cultural backgrounds of the resident population. Most patients in the hospital receive the *general (house) diet.* This diet can be modified, however, to meet the needs of those individuals who cannot tolerate its texture, composition or other characteristics (Table 23–4).

Routine modifications of the house diet include the *light, soft, general (full) liquid* and *clear liquid diets.* The light diet excludes fresh fruits and vegetables with considerable fiber *and/or* seeds as well as whole grain breads and cereals. The patient with inadequate digestive or masticatory (chewing) skills to handle such foods might well prefer the light regimen. The soft diet is commonly required by the patient with problems in chewing or digesting the more "complex" and sometimes "rich" foods in the house diet; persons without teeth and those recovering from surgery are representative of the types of patients for whom a soft diet is recommended. Liquid diets may be used before and after surgery as well as in circumstances in which substantial oral or esophageal lesions compromise manipulation of solid foods. In the general (full) liquid diet any liquid material is allowed; a clear liquid diet provides only tea, broth, gelatin dessert, and other "clear" liquid items.

Diet Before and After Surgery

Degree of tolerance to the stress of surgery and rate of recovery are directly related to the initial nutritional condition of the patient. When time permits, therefore, nutritional preparation of the surgical candidate should correct any existing nutrient deficits. The diet should also provide for the establishment of optimum *reserves* to be used during surgery and the immediate postoperative period. Such stores can be developed for protein, calories, vitamins and minerals, all of which are required in increased amounts during and after any significant trauma. The time needed to prepare a given patient for surgery with minimal risk is related to his degree of debilitation. In some cases, several days may be satisfactory, while in others, many weeks may be necessary to rectify serious depletion.

Prior to the time of surgery, nothing is given by mouth for at least 8 hours. This ensures that the stomach has no retained food at the time of the operation, since food in the stomach may be vomited *and/or* aspirated during anesthesia or recovery from it. Additionally, any food present may increase the possibility of postoperative gastric retention or expansion or may interfere with the surgical procedure itself.

Optimum nutritional support in the *postoperative period* is vital for rapid healing. The patient should progress from clear to general liquids and then to a soft or regular diet as soon as possible. Nutrient stores deposited before surgery are rapidly depleted, especially if blood and fluid losses are substantial. Adequate protein intake in the postoperative period is of primary importance in order to replace losses and supply increased demands. A negative nitrogen balance of as much as 20 mg./day may occur during the peak time of stress; this nitrogen loss represents an actual loss in tissue protein of over 1 lb./day. In addition to the protein losses from tissue breakdown, plasma proteins are lost through hemorrhage, wound healing and exudates. Increased metabolic losses of protein also result from extensive tissue destruction, inflammation, infection and trauma. If there was any prior malnutrition or chronic infection, the patient's protein deficit may actually become severe and cause serious complications. Adequate protein along with sufficient calories (from carbohydrate or fat) is therefore critical to ultimate survival, but maintenance of satisfactory vitamin and mineral status is an additional goal of nutritional therapy.

Diet in the Management of Obesity

Appropriate management of the obese patient ideally involves planning by an interdisciplinary team.[4, 16] In most cases, a variety of problems can be identified in medical, social and psychologic evaluations. Optimal therapy requires that attention be given to all significant concerns, not only to excessive body fat. Diet may, however, be one important aspect of the total care plan.

Specific dietary guidelines must be developed for each individual on the basis of his existent eating patterns and identified food-related problems. *No one diet is appropriate for everyone!* Success in weight reduction can be achieved only if the "diet" is appropriate to the client's culture and life-style. Many patterns of eating can promote fat loss if the intake of calories is less than the caloric expenditure.

Some points to keep in mind about diets for weight reduction include the following:

▶ A diet must produce a negative caloric balance if any weight loss is to occur.

▶ No weight will be lost through any conceivable change in proportion, combination or omission of certain nutrients unless the calorie intake falls below the calorie requirement.

▶ An estimated average daily allowance of calories derived from a diet of mixed nutrients is the fundamental basis for lifetime control of obesity.

▶ Obesity of the common type should be considered controllable but not curable.

▶ Any individual who has ever developed a serious degree of obesity must watch his diet for the rest of his life.

▶ The loss of fat weight must be accomplished by a method in which the major factor is a diet that, once weight reduction has been achieved, can be easily adapted for permanent control and is not detrimental to health.

▶ Diets very low in carbohydrate or protein may seem more efficient in that they increase the weight loss for a given calorie deficit, but this is a transient illusion attributable to water loss or changes in water balance. Actually, no added loss of fat is produced.

▶ A diet based on such an unbalanced "magic formula" is plainly injurious to health if the patient adheres to it for any length of time because he is then, in reality, "dieting with malnutrition."

Relevant specifics to attend to in dietary planning for the overweight client include the following:

▶ Assure nutritional adequacy

▶ Balance calorie intake throughout the day

▶ Plan for snacks in the daily routine

▶ Choose low-calorie foods with high nutritional composition

▶ Deal with the environment (especially inappropriate food stimuli)

▶ Provide education on energy balance as needed

▶ Identify problem periods during the day

▶ Include exercise when possible

▶ Encourage family support

▶ Help patient build good self-image

▶ Recommend that the patient control food portion size and the number of portions, avoid hidden calories, eat more slowly, plan meals ahead and shop for food when he is not hungry

All these issues should be considered if optimal management is to be provided.

Diet in the Management of Diabetes Mellitus

Diabetes mellitus is an inherited disease in which lack of sufficient "functional" insulin is a primary defect. As a result of the existent "insulin deficiency," regulation of circulating blood glucose is impaired. Glucose has difficulty moving from the blood into body cells and consequently remains in the bloodstream in relatively high concentrations where it draws water from the cells. Eventually the glucose is removed by the kidneys and carries with it a substantial amount of water. As a result of poor glucose utilization and excessive fluid losses in the urine, the diabetic patient develops increased hunger and thirst. The body begins to burn large amounts of fatty acids for energy, and severe ketosis and even diabetic coma may eventually occur. Regulation of blood glucose level is thus a primary focus of patient care. In addition, avoidance of the long-term vascular complications of diabetes is highly desirable, but this is believed to be difficult (if not impossible). Optimum control of the diabetic symptoms is often associated with the best prognosis.

Methods of dietary management of diabetes differ from clinic to clinic and relate directly to the philosophy of the physician in charge. A trend toward more liberal dietary management has been seen over the past decade. Restriction in intake of refined sugar is a primary goal in all management programs. Some degree of regulation in intake of other carbohydrates and fats is observed, and considerable use is made of the Exchange System developed jointly by the American Diabetic Association and the American Dietetic Association. The Exchange System divides foods into six groups, or exchanges (Table 23–5). Foods in any one group can be substituted or exchanged for other foods in the same group. The exchanges within each group are approximately equal in amounts of calories, carbohydrate, protein and fat. In addition, each exchange contains similar amounts of minerals and vitamins. Precise guidelines as to how the Exchange System is used to assist diabetics in planning diets are provided in the new publica-

which is easily obtained by writing to the American Dietetic Association, 430 North Michigan Avenue, Chicago, IL.[1]

Diet in the Management of Gastrointestinal Disease

Since the function of the gastrointestinal system is to accept and process food for ultimate body use, it stands to reason that diseases, injuries or surgical procedures that compromise gut integrity may necessitate a temporary "special" diet. Overall, recent trends in dietary management of GI disease have been toward liberalization of old traditions. It is now the widespread belief that patient tolerance should dictate the degree of dietary restriction. A patient with a peptic ulcer, for example, may tolerate spicy food without difficulty. If this is the case, there seems little justification for routinely prescribing a bland diet.

The specific dietary modification chosen for a patient with GI disease is directly related to the type of lesion, its severity, its probable duration and a host of other individual variables. A wound, lesion or inflammatory process in the upper regions of the GI tract may require a bland diet, which will not irritate the lesion by excessive spices, temperature or texture. Constipation or diverticular disease may warrant a high fiber regimen. Partial gut obstruction, hemorrhoids or mucosal inflammation in the lower bowel may necessitate restriction of dietary fiber. Generally these modifications are implemented on a short-term basis, but in some cases, long-term dietary control is recommended. Table 23–6 summarizes some common GI diseases along with their "standard" dietary regulation.

TABLE 23–5.   THE SIX MAJOR EXCHANGE LISTS

List 1: Milk Exchanges	Nonfat, low-fat and whole milk
List 2: Vegetable Exchanges	All nonstarchy vegetables
List 3: Fruit Exchanges	All fruits and fruit juices
List 4: Bread Exchanges	Bread, cereal, pasta, starchy vegetables and prepared foods
List 5: Meat Exchanges	Lean meat, medium-fat meat, high-fat meat and other protein-rich foods
List 6: Fat Exchanges	Polyunsaturated, saturated and monounsaturated fats

TABLE 23–6.   DIETARY MANAGEMENT OF SELECTED GASTROINTESTINAL DISEASES

Disease	Description	Clinical Symptoms	Diet Therapy
Peptic ulcer	Excessive acid erosion of gastric or duodenal mucosa	Increased gastric contractions with pain	Individualized; often bland; avoid potential stimulants of acid production (alcohol, caffeine, meat extracts)
Diverticulosis, diverticulitis	Small protrusions from the intestinal lumen with or without inflammation	With inflammation: pain, tenderness, nausea, vomiting, distention, intestinal spasms, fever	Acute phase: liquid or low residue Chronic phase: high residue to reduce intraluminal pressure
Celiac sprue	Inherited intestinal sensitivity to the protein gluten	Diarrhea with multiple bulky, foamy, greasy stools; distended abdomen; malnutrition	Gluten-free diet (omission of wheat, oats, rye, and usually barley)
Regional enteritis	Regional inflammation and thickening of the wall with decrease in luminal diameter	Abdominal pain and diarrhea	Individualized; low residue if partial intestinal obstruction is suspected, otherwise, as tolerated
Ulcerative colitis	Mucosal inflammation in the lower bowel	Pain and mucosal bleeding with frequent loose stools	Individualized; reduced residue as required to minimize irritation of mucosa, especially before and after surgical repair
Hemorrhoids	Blockage of venous blood flow from the lower abdomen causes high portal and/or systemic venous pressure with dilatation of venous channels leading from the anus	Pain and bleeding related to defecation	Individualized; reduced residue when appropriate, especially before and after surgical repair

Diet in the Management of Liver and Gallbladder Disease

Hepatitis. The viral agents that induce hepatitis produce diffuse injury to liver cells. In milder cases, the tissue injury is largely reversible, but with increasing severity more extensive damage occurs. Consequently, clinical symptoms vary, depending on the degree of liver involvement. Jaundice (yellow pigmentation of the skin) is a common symptom, but general malaise, loss of appetite, diarrhea, headache, fever, and enlarged and tender liver and spleen may also occur. Treatment involves bed rest, avoidance of dehydration and provision of optimum nutrition to allow for recovery of the damaged liver tissue. Routine diet specifications call for frequent meals with high protein (75 to 100 Gm./day), high carbohydrate (300 to 400 Gm./day) and moderate fat (100 to 150 Gm./day). Nutritional therapy is the key to recovery. When a patient cannot eat voluntarily, it may be necessary to utilize tube or intravenous feeding.

Cirrhosis. Liver damage from a variety of sources may advance to the point where functional liver cells are replaced by inert scar tissue. Fatty liver frequently precedes cirrhosis and usually is accompanied by malnutrition. In developed societies, alcoholism is often the root of the difficulty, and fatty liver and early cirrhosis may appear within 5 years of the onset of obvious drinking problems. With continuous drinking, food intake often is neglected, resulting in multiple nutritional deficiencies that augment the rate of existent liver cell destruction. Early symptoms of liver damage include nausea, vomiting, loss of appetite, distention and epigastric pain; jaundice may eventually appear with weakness, edema, ascites and anemia from GI bleeding, iron and/or folic acid deficiency and hemorrhage.

Treatment is difficult when alcoholism is the underlying problem. Each patient requires individual supportive care, but usually therapy is aimed at correction of fluid and electrolyte imbalances and provision of nutritional support to encourage healing of the liver tissue as soon and insofar as possible. While a basic high-protein diet may be desirable in many cases, special clinical problems may necessitate specific modifications for individual patients:

▶ Sodium is usually restricted to 500 to 1000 mg. daily to reduce fluid retention when edema or ascites is present.

▶ If esophageal varices (enlarged veins) develop, it may be necessary to give soft foods that are smooth in texture to prevent rupture of these blood vessels.

▶ If liver function becomes seriously compromised (so that conversion of ammonia to urea becomes markedly reduced), dietary protein intake must be reduced substantially to avoid GI production of ammonia during protein digestion or consequent to bacterial action.

The amount of protein restriction will vary with the circumstances of the individual patient. An unconscious patient may receive no protein, but the usual amounts range from 15 to 50 Gm. daily, depending on whether the symptoms are severe or mild. Return to a normal diet is generally possible when liver function gradually improves. In some cases, however, the liver damage is so serious and irreversible that chronic protein restriction may be required to avoid hepatic coma.

Cholelithiasis (Gallstones). The gallbladder functions to concentrate and store bile from the liver and release it into the small intestine when stimulated to do so. Bile is rich in cholesterol, which normally is kept in solution by other bile components. When the surface of the gallbladder is inflamed or infected, however, the absorptive characteristics of the mucosa may be altered, and the solubility of the bile ingredients may change. Excess water or bile acids may be absorbed, and cholesterol may eventually precipitate and form stones. A high dietary fat intake over a long period of time predisposes to gallstone formation because of the constant stimulus to produce more cholesterol as a necessary bile ingredient to emulsify fat. When stones are present in the gallbladder, contraction from the cholecystokinin mechanism causes pain, which often is severe. The patient may report a sense of fullness and distention after eating, especially after eating fatty foods. Treatment may eventually involve surgical removal of the gallbladder, but this may be postponed until weight loss is achieved. Fat in the diet is generally reduced to minimize stimulation of the gallbladder. If weight loss is indicated, calories will be reduced according to need and the patient's life-style and culture.

Diet in the Management of Kidney Diseases

Various inflammatory and degenerative diseases may affect the kidney diffusely, involving entire nephrons and nephron segments. In such conditions, the normal functions of the nephron are disrupted, and nutritional disturbances in the metabolism of protein, electrolytes and water follow. Filtration and reabsorption frequently are disrupted. Symptoms result from either excessive "backup" of wastes in the circulation or excessive loss of vital blood components (i.e., protein) in the urine. Diet therapy therefore depends upon the specific nature of the lesion. With excessive urinary losses, dietary replacement is required. With impaired elimination of wastes, diet must be controlled to minimize the buildup of these compounds in the circulation. Acute glomerulonephritis, the nephrotic syndrome and chronic renal failure are three examples of kidney disorders; their features and dietary indications are summarized in Table 23–7.

Diet in the Management of Cardiovascular Disease

A number of conditions involve organs of the cardiovascular system—the heart, the blood vessels and the blood itself. Three basic problems are considered here: atherosclerosis, congestive heart failure and hypertension. Diet modification plays a role in the basic therapy indicated for each one.[21]

Atherosclerosis. Atherosclerosis is a complex disease involving the accumulation of lipid and other material in arterial walls. The cause of the disease has not yet been identified, but multiple risk factors have emerged as contributory components in the disease process. The nature of the underlying disease process has focused attention on fat metabolism. High intake of cholesterol has been associated with higher blood cholesterol levels. Large-scale studies have also demonstrated a definite association between other types of dietary fat and elevated blood lipid levels (*hyperlipidemia*). Hyperlipidemia seems to be linked to high fat intake that includes a large percentage of animal or saturated fat. Dietary substitution of foods high in polyunsaturated fatty acids for those high in saturated fatty acids has been effective in lowering these blood lipids, especially blood cholesterol. However, the importance of the lowered blood lipid levels in terms of the disease process is unknown at this point. Management of patients with atherosclerosis generally involves the following recommendations:

▶ Restrict fat intake to less than 35 per cent of total calories in the diet.

▶ Reduce the amount of saturated fat intake in relation to intake of polyunsaturated fat so that about half the calories supplied by fat come from each source.

▶ Restrict intake of cholesterol to less than 300 mg./day.

In the acute phases of cardiovascular disease, additional dietary modification may be indicated. The basic therapeutic objective is cardiac rest. Hence the purpose of all care is to fulfill this requirement for restoring the damaged heart to adequate functioning; the diet is therefore modified in energy value and texture. During the early recovery phases calories may be limited to 800 to 1200 kcal. daily to continue cardiac rest from metabolic loads. If the patient is overweight (as is frequently the case), this

TABLE 23–7.   DIET THERAPY IN DISEASES OF THE KIDNEY

DISEASE	BASIC DEFECT	CLINICAL SYMPTOMS	DIET THERAPY
Acute glomerulonephritis	Infection involving glomeruli; loss of glomerular function (especially filtration)	Blood and protein in urine, edema, hypertension, renal insufficiency	Adequate protein (unless renal failure develops), adequate sodium (unless edema or hypertension becomes serious), general nutritional support, water input adjusted to output
Nephrotic syndrome	Degeneration of capillary basement membrane with creation of "pores" that allow escape of protein	Massive albuminuria, low serum protein levels	High-protein, high-calorie diet; moderate to low sodium intake
Chronic renal failure	Degeneration of renal tissue with depression of all renal functions	Anemia; weakness; weight loss; hypertension; skin, oral and GI bleeding; muscle twitching; uremic convulsions	Protein restriction (unless dialysis is frequent), controlled intake of major electrolytes (K^+, Na^+) and water

calorie reduction may be continued for a longer period to bring about desired weight losses. Early feedings may consist of soft or easily digested foods to avoid effort in eating and chewing. Smaller meals served more frequently may provide needed nutrition without causing undue strain or pressure.

Congestive Heart Failure. When the heart's ability to maintain normal pumping activities is compromised, blood accumulates in the vascular system on the right side of the heart, causing right-sided heart failure. As a result, venous pressure rises, overcoming the balance of filtration pressure necessary to maintain the normal capillary fluid shift mechanism. In congestive heart failure, as a result of the failure of this mechanism, fluid that normally would flow between the tissue spaces and the blood vessels is held in the tissue spaces rather than being returned to the circulation. This accumulation of fluid in the tissues is called *edema*.

Because sodium ions in tissue fluids increase retention of fluid in this region, the diet for edema of cardiac failure restricts sodium intake. The main source of dietary sodium is sodium chloride (common table salt). Other high-sodium compounds, such as baking powder and baking soda, contribute small amounts. Sodium also occurs naturally in certain foods. Sodium-regulated diets may involve mild, moderate or severe sodium restriction. With moderate to severe restrictions, careful dietary planning is required; use of a variety of "salt substitutes" may assist in maintaining a palatable menu.[19]

Hypertension. Hypertension may be defined as persistent elevated levels of blood pressure above 150 systolic and 90 diastolic (see Chap. 31). In most cases the cause is unknown, but about 20 per cent of the population is affected. Since the disease is clearly familial, some persons are much more likely to demonstrate hypertension than others. The major objective of treatment is to lower the blood pressure to normal levels with the hope of relieving the symptoms and preventing vascular damage. The main treatment involves drug therapy, which may cause excessive potassium loss from the body. Thus, potassium replacement in food and medication is usually a part of treatment. Since the results of numerous studies have linked hypertension to a sensitivity to high salt use, reduction in salt intake is a major goal of dietary therapy. Severe sodium restriction is generally unnecessary, but most patients can benefit considerably from moderate limitation in daily sodium intake. General guidelines may call for a 2000 mg. sodium diet; recommendations for following such a regimen are provided in Table 23–8.

Diet in the Management of Selected Metabolic Disorders

Gout. The basic metabolic defect in gout has not yet been fully elucidated, but abnormal purine metabolism is clearly involved. Breakdown of the purines adenine and guanine typically leads to the production of uric acid. This compound is ordinarily excreted in the urine and is not accumulated in the bloodstream. The patient with gout, however, demonstrates a marked elevation in blood uric acid level, ultimately leading to the deposition of urate in joints and soft tissues. Management of the disease requires reduction in blood uric acid by use of appropriate drugs and dietary purine restriction. Purines are found in highest amounts in organ meats, but significant amounts are found in other meats as well.

Hypoglycemia. Various forms of hypoglycemia (low blood sugar) have been defined, but all are rare. Many types of hypoglycemia cannot be treated by dietary manipulation. Functional hypoglycemia, however, may occur in individuals who are poorly equipped to regulate blood sugar adequately after ingesting refined carbohydrate. Under such circumstances, the refined carbohydrate is quickly digested and absorbed, leading to a quick rise in

---

TABLE 23–8.   RESTRICTIONS FOR A MILD LOW-SODIUM DIET (2 TO 3 GM.)

Do not use:
1. Salt at the table (use salt lightly in cooking)
2. Salt-preserved foods such as salted or smoked meat (bacon and bacon fat, bologna, dried or chipped beef, corned beef, frankfurters, ham, kosher meats, luncheon meats, salt pork, sausage, smoked tongue), salted or smoked fish (anchovies, caviar, salted and dried cod, herring, sardines), sauerkraut, olives
3. Highly salted foods, such as crackers, pretzels, potato chips, corn chips, salted nuts, salted popcorn
4. Spices and condiments, such as bouillon cubes,* catsup, chili sauce,* celery salt, garlic salt, onion salt, monosodium glutamate, meat sauces, meat tenderizers,* pickles, prepared mustard, relishes, Worcestershire sauce, soy sauce
5. Cheese,* peanut butter*

*Dietetic low-sodium products may be used.

blood sugar level and a rapid insulin response. The insulin then promotes a rapid drop in blood sugar, which falls below the normal basal blood sugar level and remains low because of poor compensation by normal physiologic patterns. A patient with this functional hypoglycemia is advised to consume frequent *small* meals and avoid concentrated carbohydrates such as sugar, candy and jelly. If this is done, rapid rises in blood sugar level, along with the subsequent adverse reactions, will be avoided.

Diet in the Management of Special Diseases of Infancy and Childhood

Certain problems of infancy and childhood require special attention to dietary intake. Several of these problems are discussed here as examples of the circumstances that require attention during this phase of the life cycle.

Phenylketonuria (PKU). PKU is the best-known inborn error of amino acid metabolism. The child with PKU is born with little or no *phenylalanine hydroxylase,* an enzyme needed to convert phenylalanine to tyrosine in the body (see Fig. 23–2). Without this enzyme, the conversion cannot take place and high levels of phenylalanine remain in the circulation along with low levels of tyrosine. As a result, phenylalanine damages the brain and promotes severe mental retardation. Since tyrosine deficit compromises the production of melanin (a brown pigment), these children are often fair-skinned, blue-eyed and blond.

The response of this disorder to dietary management has been evaluated extensively. Prevention of brain damage can be achieved by regulation of phenylalanine intake in the diet. A special low phenylalanine diet is provided throughout infancy and childhood, and blood phenylalanine levels are monitored at regular intervals. Good dietary management has clearly been shown to allow normal mental and physical development of children with PKU. It is currently recommended that the special diet be maintained through at least age 6 years, and many professionals advocate its continuance (at least in part) for the years that follow.

Food Allergy. Allergy is an altered or abnormal tissue sensitivity to foreign substances. Any food substance is a potential allergen, but milk, egg, corn and wheat are the most frequently incriminated foods in infant allergies. Reactions to allergens may be manifest in a variety of symptoms such as vomiting, colic, diarrhea, irritability, fatigue, edema, urticaria (hives), allergic rhinitis or atopic eczema. Certain physiologic and psychologic states may produce food *intolerances* that are often misinterpreted as allergic reactions. Infant food intolerances may also result from overfeeding, underfeeding or feeding too rapidly. Management of food allergy or intolerance involves elimination of the problem foods or undesirable feeding practices. *Total* elimination of specific foods may be needed for a period of time, but gradually, as the child becomes older, reintroduction of these foods into the diet may be possible.

Psychologic and Sociologic Effects of Instituting Special Diets

Since food habits are an ingrained part of every individual's total character, modification in diet has a substantial influence on routine, food-related experiences. For some persons, a

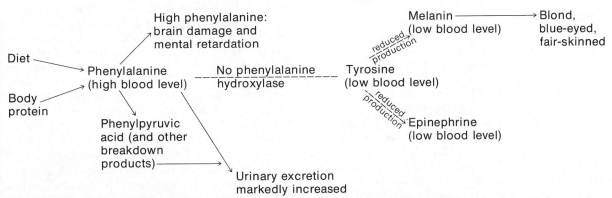

Metabolic Defect in Phenylketonuria

Figure 23–2. Absence of the enzyme *phenylalanine hydroxylase* prevents conversion of phenylalanine to tyrosine. Blood samples reveal high phenylalanine and low tyrosine. Urine samples show excessive phenylalanine and its breakdown products. Production of melanin and epinephrine is decreased. Mental retardation develops owing to the toxic character of high levels of phenylalanine in the brain.

special diet may seem impossible, especially when it excludes foods that have marked cultural significance. At best, special diets demand some readjustment in normal eating activities. Great effort may be required to substitute "restricted" foods with acceptable alternatives. Use of spices and condiments may "dress up" a meal that otherwise might seem uninteresting. Substitutes for rich "party" foods and alcoholic beverages may also be required. In any case, the psychologic and sociologic impact of modified dietary regimens should be recognized by all health professionals; great effort must be made in assisting the patient in restructuring his "food environment" to satisfy his needs for medical management and for cultural survival.

SPECIALIZED METHODS OF FEEDING

Ideally, the nutritional needs of a patient can be met through routine dietary means. In some circumstances, however, tolerance of food in its standard form is impaired. Under such circumstances, nutritional requirements still exist, and effort must be made to define a suitable mode of providing this nutritional support until "hospital meals" can again be used. Both tube feeding and intravenous hyperalimentation are employed when solid or liquid meals are not taken or are taken in inadequate quantities. Preparation of nutritionally complete tube and intravenous feeding mixtures has received considerable research attention over the past decade. A variety of commercial products that are now on the market fulfill these purposes, but some institutions still prefer to prepare their own products "in house."

Tube Feeding

The patient's nutritional needs may be met by either commercially prepared or blended (hospital-prepared) tube feedings. When commercially prepared tube feedings of any nature are used in hospital dietary departments, a decision must be made concerning purchase of appropriate products. Review of available product specifications is mandatory, and both nursing and medical staff should assist the dietitian in making appropriate decisions. The various categories of prepackaged defined formulas (e.g., milk-based, blended whole meals; elemental predigested diets; high-nitrogen elemental diets; semisynthetic diets) should be

examined in order to ascertain which are most appropriate for individual patients. A useful approach to comparative review of products is to analyze merits of individual diets of a certain type. Cost, packaging, shelf life, total nutrient content, nutritional precautions with use, nutrient omissions and osmolality all should be evaluated for each diet under consideration. Palatability is also of importance, since some formulas will be used occasionally for between-meal feeding. The unpleasant aftertaste that may occur with some tube or supplementary feedings is an undesirable characteristic that should be weighed as part of product evaluation.

On occasion, a feeding tube is placed directly into the pharynx (pharyngostomy), esophagus (esophagostomy), stomach (gastrostomy) or jejunum (jejunostomy). Lesions in the GI tract preceding the point of tube insertion are common causes for these special feeding procedures, although other factors may also dictate the decision. In most cases, tube feedings previously described are employed. Aspiration must be avoided with gastrostomy and esophagostomy, and hyperosmolar dehydration should be avoided with jejunostomy. In all cases, precise care of the insertion site is vital to avoid infection.

Intravenous Hyperalimentation

Early work on the development of suitable and complete intravenous solutions for use in humans began in the early 1960's at the University of Pennsylvania School of Medicine.[11] Since that time, considerable effort has been made to improve upon the original formulations so that optimum nutritional support can be provided to patients over long periods of time. Solutions currently available provide most of the calories in the form of carbohydrate; protein hydrolysates or free amino acid solutions supply the amino acid and nitrogen needs. A variety of salts, vitamins and trace elements are also included, and in some circumstances, intravenous lipid may be introduced to provide additional calories and essential fatty acids via a separate IV line. In any case, the solutions employed are designed to be "nutritionally complete." While appropriate levels of all nutrients have not yet been confirmed by repeated investigations, it is clear that long-term survival is possible with total maintenance on the intravenous formula. Careful patient monitoring is mandatory, of course, since variation in blood composition may occur dramatically within a short period of time when intravenous input is continuous. Care of the catheter site is also critical to avoid intro-

THE NURSE'S ROLE IN NUTRITIONAL MANAGEMENT OF THE HOSPITALIZED PATIENT

Food and the Hospitalized Patient

Optimum care of the hospitalized patient requires that attention be given to *all* his needs, including nutrition. Sufficient amounts of appropriate foods can best provide this nutritional support, but definition of the specific nutritional care plan requires input from all members of the health care team. The nurse, in consultation with the physician and the nutrition specialist, identifies the needs of the patient and a plan of care is outlined. Useful and necessary background knowledge may come from several sources including the patient, his chart, the family or other relatives, oral or written communication with other hospital personnel and related research. Past, present and future nutrition needs should be considered in arriving at a final plan for nutritional care.

While the nutritional needs of the patient may be clearly defined and a plan specified, a hospitalized person frequently suffers from some degree of gastrointestinal dysfunction or stress, and a desire for food and eating may be minimal. Meals may be refused or vomited, or diarrhea may further complicate the problem of improving nutritional status. Under such circumstances, members of the health care team need to utilize various tactics to improve the patient's appetite; if these efforts fail, alternative means of meeting nutritional requirements may be considered.

Maintaining or Improving the Patient's Appetite

A number of reasonable efforts can be made to optimize the condition of the patient and his feeding environment. The appetite of the patient may be significantly stimulated if his environment is clean and attractive, and if he is made comfortable before a meal is served to him.

Serving Food

Nursing responsibilities in relation to food service vary from institution to institution. Most hospitals employ a dietitian to organize a centralized food service; in large settings, a number of dietitians may be required to fulfill all the administrative and therapeutic responsibilities. In general, nurses are responsible for ordering and canceling diets for patients, for assisting with the serving of meals, for helping patients eat, and for recording information concerning how well the patient is eating.

In most circumstances, patients are served food at their bedsides. Some hospitals, however, have cafeterias for patients who are up and about, and some have areas where patients may eat together. Obviously, the more seriously ill the patient is, the more assistance he will require in the feeding process. The following ideas should be kept in mind in serving food to hospitalized patients:

▶ Check carefully to be sure that the name on the tray corresponds with the name on the patient's identification bracelet.

▶ Place the tray within easy reach of the patient.

▶ Remove covers from foods when required. Open milk cartons and cereal boxes, butter toast, cut meat, and otherwise assist *as indicated*. If the patient does not wish assistance, however, do not get in the way.

▶ Serve trays last to those patients who need the most assistance with eating.

▶ Record foods that are commonly left uneaten and attempt to define the reason for their rejection (e.g., uncomfortable dentures may prevent adequate chewing of meat).

▶ Judge the quantitative adequacy of the meal by determining whether the patient is satisfied afterward. If the patient is still hungry (and weight control is not a concern), arrange for a snack prior to the next meal. Also note if the servings appear to be too large and see that they are appropriately reduced or that more frequent smaller meals are provided.

▶ Encourage the involvement of the family in the meal situation if this arrangement is beneficial to the patient. Judge the suitability of foods brought to the patient from guests and record food intake from this source. If foods from friends do not support good nutritional status of the patient, they should be advised against.

▶ Remove trays as soon after eating as possible. Clean up any spills and change soiled linen if necessary. Leave the patient clean and comfortable.

▶ Offer the patient an opportunity to brush his teeth after eating and provide him assistance if needed.

Feeding Patients

Some patients need assistance with the process of feeding and frequently this task requires involvement of the nurse. A few recommendations for assisting with feeding are provided below:

▶ Help the patient position himself comfortably. Raise the head of the bed if required to establish a semisitting position, which aids in swallowing.

▶ Drape an unfolded napkin appropriately to protect bed linen and sleeping garments.

▶ Ready the food for eating and encourage as much independent feeding as possible.

▶ Provide a drinking tube for patients unable to use a cup.

▶ Provide relaxed and pleasant support of the patient during feeding and take the opportunity to improve nurse-patient relationships at this time. *Do not rush.*

▶ Make each bite a manageable mouthful to avoid discomfort and choking.

▶ Serve the food according to the order of preference of the patient. Offer liquids and solids alternately and allow sufficient time between bites for proper chewing.

▶ Try to stay with the patient throughout the feeding period.

▶ Initiate supportive and pleasant conversation.

▶ If the patient is blind, tell him what is being offered to him. Work out a system with the patient to dictate appropriate rate of feeding.

▶ Try at all times to make the mealtime as pleasant as possible.

Management of Patients with Special Problems

Nausea and Vomiting. For patients with a tendency toward nausea and vomiting special attention should be given to the issues mentioned in the foregoing discussions about feeding patients. Additionally, the following considerations are appropriate:

▶ Avoid abrupt movement and undue motion, which might provoke nausea.

▶ Encourage the patient to take deep breaths when nausea sets in.

▶ Limit food and fluid intake when discomfort is serious; then offer small amounts of fluid (or food) as tolerated.

▶ Offer foods with a bland character as opposed to those which are spicy or fatty; liberalize the diet as the patient tolerates.

▶ If the patient vomits, minimize the chances of vomitus entering to lungs. Turn the patient's head to one side while he is vomiting and is in the lying position. Elevate his head on a pillow or raise the head of the bed slightly. This position may help vomitus leave the mouth. In some cases when the patient is very weak or unconscious, it may be necessary to use a suction machine to remove vomitus from the mouth and throat to prevent choking.

▶ The patient with an abdominal wound or surgical repair site should be provided abdominal support while vomiting. A firm pillow or the nurse's hand may provide the needed relief under these circumstances.

▶ After vomiting, a patient should be assisted in oral hygiene immediately and effort should be made to replace soiled garments and linen.

▶ Help reduce sources of tension for the patient with a tendency toward vomiting.

▶ Record on the patient's chart the approximate amount, appearance and odor of the vomitus and send a specimen to the laboratory for evaluation when the circumstance dictates.

Choking. When a piece of solid food lodges in the patient's throat, immediate action must be taken to prevent loss of consciousness and eventually death. The nurse who is faced with such an emergency can take the following steps, proceeding from the first to the last only if necessary:

1. Position the victim over a chair or the side of the bed so that his head hangs face down and dependent. Deliver three sharp blows to his upper back. While this procedure is not often effective, occasionally it serves to dislodge a piece of meat from the throat.

2. Support the back of the patient's head, reach inside the mouth with one hand and try to

grasp the meat between the tips of the index finger and middle finger. Because the anoxic, unconscious patient is completely relaxed, this maneuver is often successful.

Instead of fingers, a pair of 9-inch plastic tweezers called "choke savers" may be employed. This instrument is made so that it should slip easily into the pharyngeal region to grasp the lodged food with its curved tips. It is a wise practice for restaurant supervisors to keep such devices on hand within easy reach; all employees should be carefully instructed in procedures for dislodging food in emergency circumstances.

3. As an alternative to the above approaches, a procedure called the Heimlich maneuver may be attempted. As the patient stands or sits with food obstructing the airway, the nurse approaches from behind and grasps him in a bear hug above the umbilicus and below the xiphoid process. After firmly adhering her right hand to her left wrist, a sudden strong upward pressure is exerted against the abdomen. This should cause compression of the lungs and subsequent dislodging of the food upward, restoring an open airway. If the patient is lying down, the nurse may kneel astride him; after placing her hands one on top of the other above the umbilicus, a quick upward thrust may be exerted against the abdomen.

4. When the circumstance dictates, insert a small needle percutaneously through the trachea in the midline, just above the suprasternal notch. Angle the needle caudally about 45° and push in until a distinct popping sensation tells you that you have passed through the anterior tracheal wall. Blow through the opening at a rate of about 20 times per minute until assistance arrives.

Dysphagia. Difficulty or discomfort in swallowing (dysphagia) poses a serious threat to maintenance of nutritional status. A variety of initiating factors have been identified, but regardless of the cause, normal feeding processes may be severely compromised. Tube or intravenous nutritional support may be utilized for a period of time but eventual use of routine oral feeding is essential to rehabilitation. Support of the dysphagic patient requires considerable skill on the part of the nurse who must learn to assist the patient in successful eating and eventually instruct him to proceed on his own.

The specific details associated with feeding the dysphagic patient cannot be covered in depth in the present synopsis. Suffice it to say, the patient must be placed in a comfortable upright position in a pleasant environment. He must be instructed about simple oral movements related to tongue and jaw manipulation. If the sucking mechanism is intact, fluids can be presented through a straw. Salivation may be stimulated by use of tart solutions. Swallowing may be initiated by assuring lip closure. In planning the modified diet, the normal diet should be used as the reference point. Adjustments in its consistency should be made in accord with the patient's individual level of tolerance. Gradual upgrading of dietary texture should be instituted as feeding skills improve.[2]

Cooperating with the Dietitian

Successful nutritional management of any patient relates directly to the quality of the interactions among physician, nurse and dietitian. Each of these team members is responsible for one or more aspects of nutritional care. In most settings, no one individual can handle the entire problem. The role of the dietitian is to maintain ongoing knowledge of nutritional condition of all patients for whom she is responsible. From the recommendations of the physician and the reported observations of the nurse, the dietitian plans an appropriate meal composition and feeding routine for each patient. Great effort is made to design the nutritional care plan so that it works well into the tolerance of the patient and the work routine of the nursing staff. Additionally, it must satisfy the specifications in the physician's prescription or in general meet the dietary guidelines for patients with given disease entities. Overall, the success in instituting an effective plan for nutritional care is based on the cooperation and profitable interchange between the health professionals involved. Without such communication and focus on the individual patient's needs, success in providing appropriate nutritional support may be minimal.

PATIENT AND FAMILY PREPARATION FOR DISCHARGE

Dietary Counseling

Helping the patient learn more about his diet and nutritional needs is an important part of his total care. If he is made aware of the role food plays in his health and in helping him to regain his strength or in minimizing the discomforts of his disease, he is more likely to accept his prescribed diet. If this basic understanding of appropriate diet is developed within the hospital, sensible eating habits may continue at home.

Nutrition education can be provided through a variety of mechanisms. Planned conversations with the patient can be arranged during which discussion of dietary issues in relation to the individual and his family can take place. The specific needs of the patient can be explored and questions related to the workability of a special diet can be dealt with. When choices are made from the hospital selective menu, there is an opportunity for providing sound guidance in appropriate meal planning. The health worker can make suggestions for food items that the patient may need more than others and can discuss the comparative food values.

Mealtime itself presents opportunities for teaching. When serving the patient his meal tray or assisting him with eating, the nurse or other team members can point out certain food items as examples of foods that supply specific nutrients to the body. For example, if the patient has been injured and requires protein to promote wound healing, the nurse can point out the protein-containing foods on the tray and suggest that he eat these important foods first while his appetite is best. Similar information can be provided about the other foods served. The health care worker should learn to take advantage of all opportunities to assist the patient in acquiring sensible food selection patterns.

Tips on Planning Special Meals in the Home Setting

Not infrequently, a patient is discharged from the hospital with a diet prescription that is reasonably different from his usual food patterns. If this new eating behavior is to be successfully initiated in the home, careful attention must be given to instructing the patient (or his caretaker) in meal preparation and planning along suitable lines. Often it is necessary to start from scratch and provide the patient or caretaker with basic instructions about food preparation using modified methods or ingredients. If a low-fat diet has been recommended, for example, means of preparing foods with low-fat composition must be designed. Use of fats and oils in cooking may need to be replaced by methods employing broiling, baking in lemon juice and/or thorough draining of fat before serving. If a major change in food preparation is required, much effort needs to be made

by the dietitian and other health professionals to arrive at acceptable cooking strategies.

The hospital dietitian is generally the best source of initial information about planning the special diet. Eventually, however, use should be made of printed materials designed to assist in instituting special cooking modifications within a given culture and life-style. There is a variety of brochures and books that relate to planning and preparing foods for special dietary regimens. Information about such publications is generally available through the dietitian or the local branch of the American Dietetic Association. Many distributors of special food products for restricted diets also publish helpful tips about cooking under various dietary prescriptions. Information about products and product distribution can also be obtained through these same professional and commercial sources.

In the end, one frequently finds that the ability of the patient to obtain satisfactory help and long-term support with nutritional therapy or rehabilitation relates directly to the assurance by the nursing staff that he can succeed. The friendly support and encouragement of the nurse therefore provide an integral part of optimal provision of total patient care.

Community Resources for Assistance with Dietary Problems

A patient who is discharged from the hospital on a special diet should recognize that a number of community resources provide special dietary assistance. Originally, all basic directions and justification for them should be provided by the attending physician or the dietitian from the hospital staff. Ideally the patient should leave the hospital with a clear understanding and appreciation of his nutritional care plan. Should questions arise in the home setting, the assistance of the original dietitian in the hospital should be sought. Considerable difficulty with dietary management may necessitate a visit to the hospital dietitian for additional one-to-one instruction.

When the dietary program requires ongoing supervision or frequent modification, the advice of a *consulting dietitian* in the community should be obtained. Recommendations of appropriate individuals within the local area can generally be obtained from the private physician, clinic physician or local dietetic association. Consulting dietitians are able to provide ongoing individual nutritional care for a variety of problems. With a clear understanding of the patient's medical problem(s) and a regular report of progress from the attending physician, the consulting dietitian is able to assist the patient over a long (or short) period of time such that appropriate diet therapy is achieved and maintained.

In addition to the consulting dietitian, other sources of help are available in some communities. A Dial-a-Dietitian telephone service has been established in many large cities. An interested party simply calls the appropriate number from the telephone directory to contact a dietitian who will answer his questions. In addition to this service, the state and local health departments also support dietary specialists. These persons are available to a limited extent to answer questions about special diets or food-assistance programs in the local area. The nutritionists in the local branches of the American Heart Association and the National Dairy Council provide useful assistance with some problems; other nonprofit organizations may also contribute help in some parts of the world. Finally, each community has its own unique services, which often include health care assistance services for various populations. Information about local nutrition services should be obtained through established dietetic associations or health care units.

BIBLIOGRAPHY: CHAPTERS 22 AND 23

a. Albanese, A. A.: Nutrition of the elderly. *Postgraduate Medicine*, 63:117, March 1978.
1. American Diabetes Association and American Dietetic Association: *Exchange Lists for Meal Planning*. Chicago, The American Dietetic Association, 1976.
2. Baltes, M. M., and Zerbe, M. B.: Reestablishing self-feeding in a nursing home resident. *Nursing Research*, 25:24, 1976.
3. Blackburn, G. L., et al.: Nutritional care of the injured and/or septic patient. *Surgical Clinics of North America*, 56:1195, 1976.
4. Bray, G. A., and Bethune, J. E.: *Treatment and Management of Obesity*. Hagerstown, MD, Harper & Row, Publishers, 1974.
5. Bruch, H.: *Eating Disorders*. New York, Basic Books, 1973.
6. Buckley, J. E., et al.: Feeding patients with dysphagia. *Nursing Forum*, 15:69, 1976.
6a. Busse, E. W.: How mind, body, and environment influence nutrition in the elderly. *Postgraduate Medicine*, 63:118, March 1978.
7. Butterworth, C. E., and Blackburn, G. L.: Hospital malnutrition and how to assess the nutritional status of a patient. *Nursing Digest*, Winter 1976.
7a. Caly, J. C.: Helping people eat for health: assessing adults' nutrition. *American Journal of Nursing*, 77:1605, Oct. 1977.
8. Church, C. F., and Church, H. N.: *Food Values in Portions Commonly Used*. Philadelphia, J. B. Lippincott Co., 1975.

9. Davies, G. J., et al.: Special diets in hospitals: discrepancy between what is prescribed and what is eaten. *British Medical Journal*, 1:200, 1975.
10. Deutsch, R. M.: *Realities of Nutrition*. Palo Alto, CA, Bull Publishing Co., 1976.
10a. Donovan, L.: Is the doctor starving your patient? *RN*, 41:36, July 1978.
11. Dudrick, S. J., and Rhoads, J. E.: Total intravenous feeding. *Scientific American*, 226:73, 1972.
12. Fomon, S. J.: *Infant Nutrition*, 2nd ed. Philadelphia, W. B. Saunders Co., 1974.
13. Fuerst, E. V., et al.: *Fundamentals of Nursing*, 5th ed. Philadelphia, J. B. Lippincott Co., 1974.
14. Garn, S.: Nutrition, growth, development and maturation: findings from the ten-state nutrition survey of 1968–1970. *Pediatrics*, 56:306, 1975.
15. Grant, J. A. N.: Patient care in parenteral hyperalimentation. *Nursing Clinics of North America*, 8:165, 1973.
16. Howard, L.: Obesity: a feasible approach to a formidable problem. *Nursing Digest*, Winter 1976.
17. Jeejeebhoy, K. N., et al.: Total parenteral nutrition: nutrient needs and technical tips. *Modern Medicine of Canada*, 29:832. Sept. 1974.
18. Jelliffe, D. B.: World trends in infant feeding. *American Journal of Clinical Nutrition*, 29:1227, 1976.
19. Johnston, B., and Koh, M.: *Halt! No Salt*. Bellevue, WA, Dietary Research, 1972.
20. Krause, M. V., and Mahan, L. K.: *Food, Nutrition and Diet Therapy*, 6th ed. Philadelphia, W. B. Saunders Co., 1978.
21. Kritchevsky, D.: Diet and atherosclerosis. *American Journal of Pathology*, 84:615, 1976.
22. Labuza, T. P.: *The Nutrition Crisis*. St. Paul, West Publishing Co., 1975.
23. Lappé, F. M.: *Diet for a Small Planet*. New York, Ballantine Books, 1975.
24. Lewis, L. V. W.: *Fundamental Skills in Patient Care*. Philadelphia, J. B. Lippincott Co., 1976.
25. Lieber, C. S.: *Metabolic Aspects of Alcoholism*. Baltimore, University Park Press, 1977.
26. National Academy of Sciences: *Recommended Dietary Allowances*. Washington, D.C., National Academy of Sciences, 1974.
28. Orten, J. M., and Neuhaus, O. W.: *Human Biochemistry* 9th ed. St. Louis, The C. V. Mosby Co., 1975.
29. Pipes, P.: *Nutrition in Infancy and Childhood*. St. Louis, The C. V. Mosby Co., 1977.
30. Roe, D.: *Drug-induced Nutritional Deficiencies*. Westport, CT, The Avi Publishing Co., 1976.
31. Rynearson, E. H.: Americans love hogwash. *Nutrition Review*, 32:1, 1974.
32. Whelan, E. M., and Stare, F. J.: *Panic in the Pantry*. New York, Atheneum Press, 1976.
33. Williams, S. R.: *Essentials of Nutrition and Diet Therapy*. St. Louis, The C. V. Mosby Co., 1974.
34. Williams, S. R.: *Nutrition and Diet Therapy*. St. Louis, The C. V. Mosby Co., 1977.
35. Worthington, B., et al.: *Nutrition in Pregnancy and Lactation*. St. Louis, The C. V. Mosby Co., 1977.

CHAPTER 24

FLUID AND ELECTROLYTE BALANCE AND IMBALANCE

There are many ways of looking at man. Poets, psychologists, and politicians have their ways. Physicians, at times, must consider him a complex biochemical system, reacting to a myriad of influences and, in turn, trying to maintain a state of balance known by the happy term "homeostasis." Nowhere is this better seen than in that field of science known as fluid and electrolyte metabolism.[27]

INTRODUCTION AND STUDY GUIDE

Fluid and electrolyte balance, like man himself, can be considered from many different aspects. From the viewpoint of a chemist, the term connotes a highly complex and technical field of study, often seemingly remote from man. To the physician, fluid and electrolyte metabolism is the study of chemical reactions in man; to him, the term symbolizes an ever-broadening field of research with vast therapeutic applications. To the nurse, the subject implies an exacting, sometimes burdensome, always vital part of the care of the whole patient. For her, the science of fluids and electrolytes involves the careful measurement of the patient's intake and output of fluid as well as the intelligent observation of a myriad of symptoms; it means alertness to the many subtle yet significant changes in the patient's psychologic affect and physiologic functioning. Finally, to the patient, fluid and electrolyte balance may mean a relative state of well-being, while severe imbalance may spell discomfort, mounting distress, coma and even death.

The study of fluid and electrolyte balance and imbalance, then, has numerous practical and vital implications for nurses and their patients. Nurses are continually involved with problems of balance and imbalance as they perform procedures such as the following:

▶ Measuring a patient's food and fluid intake and measuring output from urine, stool and vomitus as well as gastric, intestinal and bile drainage

▶ Weighing patients daily

▶ Starting intravenous infusions and adding electrolyte solutions and medications in intravenous infusions

▶ Checking the flow rate of intravenously administered fluids

▶ Irrigating nasal gastric suction tubes

▶ Recording fluid balance at the end of each 8-hour shift and each 24-hour period

▶ Reporting to the physician any deviation from normal fluid intake and output and any symptoms that might indicate a fluid or electrolyte imbalance

▶ Monitoring laboratory values and reporting to the physician any deviation from normal

These cardinal responsibilities, many of which may sound uninteresting, if not actually unpleasant, constitute some of the most significant services that patients require from their nurses. Although few patients actually die of fluid and electrolyte imbalance, such imbalances can influence the possible outcome of a disease process. That is why fluid and electrolyte therapy is always a part of the total therapeutic plan for patients. Because doctors base many therapeutic decisions upon nurses' records of a patient's fluid intake and output and weight, it is imperative that nurses understand the importance of these measurements.

To provide the basic principles of fluid and electrolyte physiology and pathology, this chapter will discuss the following major concepts:

°Dolly Ito, R.N., D.N.Sc., and Wanda Roberts, R.N., B.S.N., M.N., assisted with the revision of materials pertaining to normal fluid and electrolyte balance and critically reviewed content pertaining to fluid and electrolyte imbalances.

▶ Body water—its composition, volume, distribution, functions and homeostatic regulation

▶ Electrolytes and plasma proteins—their distribution, functions and measurement

▶ Water and electrolyte exchange between fluid compartments

▶ Homeostatic mechanisms that regulate water and electrolyte balance

▶ General concepts of fluid and electrolyte imbalance

▶ Specific fluid and electrolyte imbalances

▶ General principles of diagnosis, management and treatment of various imbalances

▶ The care of patients particularly susceptible to imbalances

Because the topics just listed are complex and require a precise grasp of technical material on the reader's part, we offer the following guides to help you gain the most from your reading:

Before you begin to study the material in this chapter, *review* the following chemical terms and concepts:

atom
element
molecule
compound
electrical charge
electrolytes
ions
ionization
cations
anions
the law of electrical neutrality
solutions
pH

As you study the chapter, familiarize yourself with the following terms:

semipermeable membrane
plasma proteins
osmolality
nephron
Bowman's capsule
ADH
aldosterone
volume deficit
volume excess
dehydration
water intoxication
circulatory overload
ascites
hypernatremia

hyponatremia
buffer
H^+ regulator
PO_2
PCO_2
acidosis
alkalosis
hyperkalemia
hypokalemia
tetany
hypoproteinemia
anasarca
edema
tissue turgor
Kussmaul respirations
parenteral hyperalimentation
osmotic diuresis

Upon completion of this chapter, you should be able to generally discuss the following concepts:

1. The percentage of water in the adult human body

2. Water distribution throughout the body's fluid compartments

3. The composition of the body fluids in each of these fluid compartments

4. Semipermeable membranes and control of body water distribution

5. The role of proteins in plasma and in cell protoplasm

6. The role of the kidney nephron in maintaining fluid and electrolyte balance

7. The important hormones involved in the maintenance of fluid and electrolyte balance

Upon completion of this chapter, you should be able to apply this knowledge to patients in your care. Thus, in the clinical situation:

1. Identify those patients assigned to you who are likely candidates for developing an imbalance.

2. *Prevent* imbalances from developing in your patients.

3. Look for the early signs of imbalance and report them accurately.

4. Assess patient's needs in terms of fluids and diet.

5. Begin to participate knowledgeably in the treatment of fluid and electrolyte upsets, being fully aware of the medical problems that medical treatment can create.

BODY WATER

Like a fish torn from the sea, a human being deprived of water cannot live for long. Without fluid, a person's skin dries and cracks, his temperature soars to burning heights, his mind deteriorates, his cells shrivel and, finally, he lies as withered and dead as an ancient Egyptian mummy. What, then, is this all-important substance so absolutely vital to life? What is its chemical makeup, and what are its functions? Where is water distributed in the body? How can water be lost from the body and, more vitally important, how can it be replaced? These are some of the important questions upon which our discussion will center.

Body Fluid and Body Water

Our cells depend upon an aqueous medium much as the bodies of our marine ancestors depended upon the sea for sustenance and for continued life. Like sea water, body fluid is not "pure," but contains both water and various "salts," which technically are termed *electrolytes*. Electrolytes are substances that dissociate into ions or electrically charged particles when placed in water. In this chapter, then, the term *body fluid* refers to *both* water and electrolytes, while the term *body water* refers to water alone.

Body fluid is in a state of balance when its water and electrolyte components are present in the proper proportions, when losses of body water and electrolytes are replaced, and when excesses are eliminated.

Total Body Water (TBW)

Water is the major constituent of the body; 60 to 70 per cent of the body of an adult male weighing approximately 75 kg. is composed of water (45 L.). The rest is composed of solids.[35] It is important to realize that these figures apply to the "average man" and that there are tremendous variations between individual men, between men and women, and between adults and children.

First, adults vary significantly in the amount of water their bodies contain. This variance is due mainly to the amount of body fat present, since fat is essentially water-free. Consequently, a thin individual will have more fluid per pound of weight than a fat individual.

Second, a woman's body contains a smaller percentage of fluid in relation to her total weight than does a man's. This is because a woman's body is composed of a larger amount of fat. It is estimated that the average female body contains 50 to 54 per cent water.

Finally, the percentage of fluid present in the bodies of infants and children varies significantly from that of adults. The figures in Table 24–1 compare the proportion of body water per pound of body weight at different ages. Note that the percentage of water *decreases* with age. Also, note that there are no differences in the percentage of body water between the male and female until late adolescence or early adulthood, when the female body increases in the proportion of fat.

Important implications for patient care rest upon these facts. First, fluid balance is of greater importance in the *infant* than in the adult because so much of a baby's body is composed of water. Small imbalances in children immediately become evident. *The younger the child, the more serious is any decrease in the vital body fluids.*

Second, the aged have slowly diminishing body fluids which frequently makes their skin dry and scaly; therefore, they do not need to be bathed as often as a younger person. The use of soothing skin lotions is far more satisfactory than the use of drying alcohol. It is important to realize that in addition to the normal percentage of body water depletion, the aged also may have an altered thirst mechanism that prevents adequate fluid intake. Thus, the geriatric patient may easily become dehydrated.[32] Indeed, a certain degree of dehydration appears to be always present in the very old, as typically evidenced by their lack of muscle tone, dry hair and wrinkles.

Water Distribution

Water and electrolytes (i.e., body fluid) are distributed between two fluid compartments: the *intracellular fluid* (ICF) *compartment* and the *extracellular fluid* (ECF) *compartment*. Seventy per cent of total body water is normally within the cells (in the ICF compartment), while 30 per cent of total body water is located outside the cells in the ECF compartment. Twenty-four per cent of the water in the ECF compartment occupies the tissue spaces (*interstitial* water), while 6 per cent appears in the

TABLE 24–1.   BODY WATER AS PERCENTAGE OF BODY WEIGHT AT VARIOUS AGES

	NEWBORN	6 MO.	2 YR.	16 YR.	20–39 YR.		40–59 YR.	
					M	F	M	F
Total body water (% of body weight)	77	72	60	60	60	50	55	47

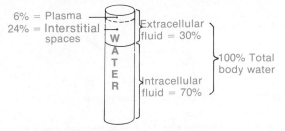

6% = Plasma
24% = Interstitial spaces
Extracellular fluid = 30%
Intracellular fluid = 70%
100% Total body water

Figure 24–1. Total body water distribution in the adult.

vascular space as plasma (Fig. 24–1). The body fluids are not static but *move freely* between all compartments and spaces. This appearance of uncensored movement is somewhat misleading, for water must obey laws. Its movement between the vascular and interstitial spaces is subject to Starling's forces, and its distribution between intracellular and extracellular spaces is governed by the law of osmosis.[13]

Despite the interchange between compartments, each type of fluid has its own particular functions.

▶ The *intracellular fluid* provides the cell with the internal aqueous medium necessary for its chemical functions.

▶ The *extracellular fluid* serves as the body's transportation system, carrying water, electrolytes, nutrients and oxygen to the cells and removing the waste products of cellular metabolism.

Extracellular fluid is composed of interstitial fluid and plasma.

▶ *Interstitial fluid* lies outside both the vascular space and the cells; it provides the cells with the external medium necessary for cellular metabolism.

▶ *Plasma,* which contains colloids or plasma proteins, is the liquid part of the blood; along with red blood cells, it maintains vascular volume.*

The Functions of Water

The most abundant component of all living matter is water. The functions of water are as follows:

▶ Provides an aqueous medium for cellular metabolism

▶ Transports materials to and from cells

▶ Acts as a solvent in which are dissolved the many solutes available for cell function

▶ Regulates body temperature

▶ Maintains the physical and chemical constancy of the intracellular and extracellular fluids

▶ Maintains the vascular (blood) volume

▶ Aids in the digestion of food through hydrolysis, which is the breakdown of molecules through the addition of water

▶ Provides a medium for the excretion of waste from the body

Water Balance*

Body water *balance* is dependent upon a balance between water intake and output, i.e., gains in body water must equal losses in body water. Thus, water *imbalance* exists when water intake and output are unequal and gains in body water exceed losses, or losses exceed gains. In water imbalance individuals can become subject either to water overload or to dehydration. If overload becomes too great, a person's lungs can fill with water and he may actually drown in his own fluids. If intake is not great enough or is entirely lacking, a person becomes dehydrated.

In Table 24–2 a typical 24-hour water balance record provides an example of *normal* intake and output, which would keep the body of an adult in normal water balance.

Note that our greatest single source of water *intake* is from water or liquids ingested as beverages, while our second greatest source is the "hidden" water in foods. Indeed, it may surprise you that lean meats contain 75 per cent water, while fruits and vegetables contain an even greater percentage. However, if the intake of "hidden" water in foods and the water of

---

*In discussing fluid and electrolyte metabolism, we are concerned only with the *plasma* component of the vascular compartment, since red blood cells do *not* move out of the vascular compartment and do not flow from one compartment to another.

*In discussing water balance, the authors have drawn extensively from personal communication with Joleen K. Heath as well as from her article, "A Conceptual Basis for Assessing Body Water Status."[18]

TABLE 24–2.   BODY WATER BALANCE IN THE ADULT OVER A 24-HOUR PERIOD

INTAKE		OUTPUT		
Oral fluids	1200 ml.	Urine	1500 ml.	
"Hidden" water from foods	1100 ml.	Water vapor from lungs	400 ml.	insensible water loss
Metabolic sources (water of oxidation):	300 ml.	Sweat	600 ml.	
Protein = 40 ml./100 Gm.				
Fat = 100 ml./100 Gm.		Feces	100 ml.	
Carbohydrate = 100 ml./100 Gm.				
Total	2600 ml.	Total	2600 ml.	

oxidation are combined, these two sources of water *exceed* the "beverage" intake.

> *Thus, to assess water balance, it is important to keep an accurate record of the intake of both solid foods and liquids.*

Turning next to *output*, note that the largest proportion of water is eliminated from the kidneys, moderate amounts of water are eliminated from the skin and lungs (insensible or evaporated water loss), and only small amounts of water are normally eliminated from the gastrointestinal tract. The elimination and conservation of water are homeostatically controlled by the kidneys, the gastrointestinal tract, various hormonal substances and nervous system. Because of the importance of the renal system in regulating output, it is possible to estimate the state of water balance by comparing the 24-hour intake volume with the 24-hour urine output volume, realizing that urinary output represents slightly over half the total water output in a normal adult.

Insensible water loss from the lungs and skin is not the same as visible sweating, or diaphoresis, which is an observable water loss. Insensible loss includes the 750 to 1000 ml. of water eliminated in the vapor of our breath and in the moisture that constantly forms on our skin, even though we may not be aware of it. These insensible losses are increased when body metabolism is accelerated as in fevers, when respirations are significantly increased as in pneumonia (especially in children), and in individuals living in hot climates before becoming acclimatized. Consequently, these insensible losses must be carefully estimated by

the doctor when attempting to correct water imbalances. Nurses should assess insensible losses by carefully noting and recording the patient's rate and depth of respiration and the presence of diaphoresis.

In summary, when a state of water balance exists, water intake—in the form of ingested food and fluid and oxidation—equals the water output through the kidneys, bowel, skin and lungs. Accurate assessment of intake and output must take into consideration *all* sources of water gains and losses.

Minimum Water Requirements for Survival

In reviewing the chart of typical water balance for 24 hours you will see that an "average" person should take in approximately *2600 ml. of fluid per day* to meet the body's water requirements. If this is the case, how much water does an individual need for *survival?*

Over the years scientists have tried to establish the minimum food and water requirements for human beings. It is recognized that men and women can survive for remarkably long periods (up to 45 days) without food. This survival is possible because the body is able to convert its stored protein and fat supplies into needed energy when food is not available. However, it is impossible to survive without water for even half this period. The maximum amount of water produced by oxidation of fat stores would barely equal the amount of water lost by insensible sweating. Consequently, man *must* obtain his water supply through sources outside his own body.

While a minimum of 2000 ml. of fluid intake per day is required for *normal* balance, 1500 ml. per day is the basal* requirement. This basal water requirement applies *only* if the individual is healthy, relatively inactive and living in a temperate climate. Under these conditions an individual could live for a period of time, but he would not be in optimal balance. Persons who live in a hot climate, who have high fevers with continued excessive perspiration, or who have a rapid respiratory rate may require up to *5000 ml. of water per day.* When these basal requirements are not met, *dehydration* is the inevitable result.

How long can a person live without *any* water? Adults can live up to 10 days and children up to 5 days, provided weather conditions are favorable. In the hot, drying desert, however, death may come within a few hours. With the loss of 1 per cent of body water a person feels thirsty. When he loses 5 to 8 per cent of his body water he becomes ill; he feels weary, his pulse rate rises, his temperature soars (because he can no longer sweat) and his mental processes deteriorate. With the loss of 11 to 15 per cent of water, he develops delirium, deafness and kidney failure. In the final stages of dehydration (more than 20 per cent), "his skin cracks, a blood-sweat oozes from his body, his eyes weep tears of blood, he becomes a 'senseless automaton,' digging desperately in the sand, and he passes beyond any possible revival by water."[45]

Death from dehydration can occur anywhere, especially among children and among the aged whose water intake is neglected. Children, because of their precise kidney function and greater metabolic rate, are particularly vulnerable. It is common to see young children develop severe dehydration rapidly (e.g., with minor gastrointestinal upsets).

> *Therapeutic intervention must be initiated* rapidly *to save a severely dehydrated child from certain death.*

ELECTROLYTES AND PLASMA PROTEINS

Equilibrium or homeostasis, in addition to water balance, depends on the proper balance of electrolytes and plasma proteins or colloids. Thus, it is important to consider the role of these substances in the body's physiology: namely, their chemical nature, functions, measurement, balance and concentration within the body's fluid compartments.

The Chemical Nature of Electrolytes*

An electrolyte is defined as a substance or compound composed of atoms, which, when placed in a solvent such as water, break up into separately charged particles called *ions*. Positively charged ions are called *cations*, and ions that are negatively charged are *anions*. Important cations in terms of body fluid metabolism are sodium (Na^+), potassium (K^+), calcium (Ca^{++}) and magnesium (Mg^{++}), while important anions are chloride (Cl^-), bicarbonate (HCO_3^-), phosphate ($HPO_4^=$), and sulfate ($SO_4^=$).

As a simple example of how ionization works, let us consider sodium chloride (NaCl). If we place NaCl into solution, it will dissociate or ionize into the positive cation Na^+ and the negative anion Cl^- ($NaCl \rightarrow Na^+ + Cl^-$). We can prove that sodium carries a positive charge and chloride a negative charge by placing sodium chloride in a wet electric cell and then passing an electric current through the solution; we then find that Na^+ (a cation) travels to the *negative* pole, or *cathode*, and Cl^- (an anion) travels to the *positive* pole, or *anode*.

Both anions and cations are contained in body water. Each cation is *always balanced chemically* by an anion. This relationship is expressed by Faraday's *law of electrical neutrality*, which states:

> *The sum of the number of negative electric charges must equal the sum of the number of positive electric charges in a solution.*

Thus, if the cations in our body fluids increase, the anions must increase; and if the cations decrease, the anions must also decrease. In this way the electrolyte balance is maintained.

Not all substances dissociate in solution. Substances that *do not ionize* and consequently do not carry an electric charge are called

---

*Basal requirements are those absolute minimums that will sustain cellular activity if the individual is totally at rest.

*We assume that the reader has taken at least one course in basic chemistry and consequently is familiar with the terminology used in describing chemical elements and processes as well as with some of the important chemical reactions that occur in the human body.

nonelectrolytes. An example of a nonelectrolyte is glucose, which remains a nondissociated, electrically neutral molecule in body fluid. Most organic compounds are nonelectrolytes.

The Chemical Nature of Plasma Proteins

Protein plays a significant role in fluid and electrolyte metabolism. It is found both in cells and in plasma. Protein within the protoplasm of the cells is called *proteinate* (an anion), while protein in plasma is in colloid form. Colloids are macromolecules that are usually unable to pass through an animal membrane because of their size, and consequently these plasma proteins tend to remain within the blood vessels rather than diffusing out into the tissues. Some authorities believe that plasma proteins tend to behave like anions, having a negative charge and being balanced electrically by cations. The most important plasma proteins are *albumin*, *globulin* and *fibrinogen*. These colloidal substances are synthesized in the liver.

The Physiologic Functions of Electrolytes and Plasma Proteins

Electrolytes and plasma proteins perform important physiologic functions within the body. The major functions of electrolytes are (1) the promotion of neuromuscular irritability, (2) the maintenance of body fluid osmolality, (3) the regulation of H^+ balance and (4) the distribution of body fluids between the fluid compartments.

Plasma proteins, like electrolytes, play an important role in body water distribution. Basically, plasma proteins hold water within the blood vessels, thereby preventing the leakage of excess water into the tissues and the subsequent development of edema. The basic functions of sodium, potassium, calcium, magnesium and protein, in conjunction with the major homeostatic regulators controlling these substances, are outlined in Table 24–3.

Measuring Fluids and Electrolytes

In nursing care of patients with fluid and electrolyte imbalances, the correct measurement of the fluids and electrolytes used in parenteral therapy is of great importance. Even small errors in measurement while preparing intravenous infusions can result in serious fluid and electrolyte imbalances.

The most important measurements used in working with fluids and electrolytes are the following:

1. The *liter* (L.) and the *milliliter* (ml.) (or cubic *centimeter*, cc.) are measures of *volume*. IV solutions are always measured in liters and milliliters. For example, the doctor may order 1 L. (1000 ml.) of normal saline for a patient with a fluid imbalance. (For all practical purposes the milliliter and cubic centimeter are equivalent, and fluid measurements are often expressed in cubic centimeters.)

2. The *gram* (Gm.) and the *milligram* (mg.) are units of *weight;* 1 Gm. equals 1000 mg. We can express serum electrolytes and plasma proteins in terms of percentages. This measurement tells us the number of grams or milligrams of an electrolyte or colloid in 100 ml. of fluid. For example, the normal plasma protein content of blood is 6 Gm./100 ml., or 6 Gm. per cent. In other words, there are 6 Gm. (6000 mg.) of protein in every 100 ml. of plasma.

3. The *milliequivalent* (mEq.) is the *measure of the chemical activity or chemical combining power of an ion.* In other words, the milliequivalent is a measure of the power of a cation to combine with an anion, thus forming a molecule. The milliequivalent system makes it possible to compare one compound with another. The electrolyte content within a water compartment can be most accurately expressed in terms of *milliequivalents per liter* (mEq./L.).

Although two different chemicals may have equal weights, one may have a greater chemical combining power or greater number of charges than does the other chemical. The opposite is also true. For example, 23 mg. of sodium, 39 mg. of potassium, 20 mg. of calcium and 4140 mg. of proteinate differ significantly by weight, yet each exerts only 1 mEq. of chemical activity. This is why ions are measured in terms of *milliequivalents* rather than milligrams (i.e., in terms of *chemical combining power* rather than weight).

Metheny and Snively have suggested the following analogy to clarify the concept of the milliequivalent:[28] In our civilization we use the word *horsepower* to designate physical power. For example, an old jalopy may have "30 horsepower," meaning it has the same amount of driving force as if 30 horses were pulling it. A powerful racing car, on the other hand, may have over 600 horsepower. The *weight* of the jalopy and the *weight* of the modern sports car have *nothing* to do with the *power* of these respective cars. Indeed, the slow jalopy will

TABLE 24-3. ELECTROLYTES: BASIC FUNCTIONS AND MAJOR HOMEOSTATIC REGULATORS

BASIC FUNCTIONS	MAJOR HOMEOSTATIC REGULATORS
Sodium (Na^+)	
1. Regulates fluid volume within ECF compartment 2. Increases cell membrane permeability 3. Maintains blood volume and controls size of vascular space 4. Controls body water distribution between ECF and ICF compartments 5. Acts as a buffer base (sodium bicarbonate), thereby helping to regulate H^+ concentration 6. Stimulates conduction of nerve impulses 7. Helps maintain neuromuscular irritability 8. Assists in controlling contractility of muscles—in particular, heart muscle	Aldosterone, a mineralocorticoid, controls Na^+ excretion and retention
Potassium (K^+)	
1. Regulates water and electrolyte content of cellular fluid 2. Helps promote transmission of nerve impulses, especially within the heart 3. Helps promote skeletal muscle function 4. Assists in transforming carbohydrates into energy and restructuring amino acids into proteins 5. Assists in regulation of acid-base balance by cellular exchange with H^+	1. The sodium pump conserves cellular K^+ by actively excluding Na^+ (see p. 486) 2. The kidneys (which excrete 80 to 90 per cent of K^+) conserve K^+ when cellular K^+ becomes depleted
Calcium (Ca^{++})	

1. Required for building strong and durable bones and teeth
2. Essential for blood coagulation
3. Decreases neuromuscular irritability
4. Promotes normal transmission of nerve impulses
5. Establishes thickness and strength of cell membranes
6. Assists in absorption and utilization of vitamin B_{12}
7. Activates enzymes that in turn activate chemical reactions within the body
	1. Regulated by parathyroid glands and by parathyroid hormone (parathormone)
	2. Level of serum calcium affected by level of serum phosphate
	  a. Increase in serum phosphate associated with decrease in serum calcium
	  b. Decrease in serum phosphate associated with increase in serum calcium
	3. Regulated by thyrocalcitonin hormone from the thyroid gland
	4. Vitamin D is necessary for absorption and utilization of calcium

Magnesium (Mg^{++})	
1. Activates many enzymes—in particular, those associated with vitamin B metabolism and the utilization of potassium, calcium and protein 2. Promotes regulation of serum calcium, phosphorus and potassium levels 3. Essential for integrity of neuromuscular system and function of heart	Regulated by parathyroid glands
Hydrogen Ion (H^+)	
1. Necessary for healthy cellular function 2. Promotes efficient functioning of enzyme systems 3. Necessary for the binding of oxygen by hemoglobin 4. Concentration of H^+ determines relative acidity or alkalinity of body fluids	1. *Buffering*, principally by the H_2CO_3:$NaHCO_3$ buffer system (the normal ratio of carbonic acid to sodium bicarbonate is 1:20) 2. The *lungs* regulate the carbonic acid side of the ratio 3. The *kidneys* regulate the sodium bicarbonate side of the ratio
Protein	
1. The most basic and vital constituent of living cells 2. Required for growth and development and for maintenance and repair of tissue 3. Forms the bulk of muscle, visceral and epithelial tissue and is a constituent of plasma and hemoglobin 4. Required for the manufacture of enzymes, hormones, many antibodies and some vitamins 5. Holds water within blood vessels and "sucks" back water that leaks from blood vessels (see discussion of plasma proteins and colloid osmotic pressure)	

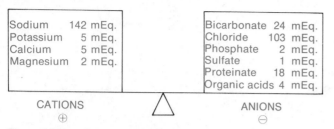

Sodium	142 mEq.
Potassium	5 mEq.
Calcium	5 mEq.
Magnesium	2 mEq.

Bicarbonate	24 mEq.
Chloride	103 mEq.
Phosphate	2 mEq.
Sulfate	1 mEq.
Proteinate	18 mEq.
Organic acids	4 mEq.

CATIONS ⊕   ANIONS ⊖

Figure 24–2. When their weights are written in milliequivalents, the cations and anions of extracellular fluid approximately balance each other. (Modified from Metheny and Snively.)

lyte, even though the *weights* of the two electrolytes may differ significantly. Moreover, the number of milliequivalents of cations in the body fluids must always balance the number of milliequivalents of anions for chemical neutrality to exist (Fig. 24–2). Chemical neutrality of the body fluids is essential for the maintenance of normal neuromuscular excitability.

Normal Electrolyte and Plasma Protein Balance

We normally obtain essential electrolytes and plasma proteins by ingesting a diet that is adequate in nutrients. A minimum daily intake of 2400 to 2600 ml. of water, 4.5 Gm. of sodium, 3 Gm. of potassium and 0.05 Gm. of protein per kg. of body weight is required for healthy balance.

It is important to remember that electrolytes are dissolved in the water that we lose through urination, defecation or sweating. Thus, whenever water is replaced, electrolytes must also be replaced, and vice versa, to maintain water and electrolyte balance.

undoubtedly be far heavier than the speedy convertible. Thus, the difference in physical activity and performance between these two automobiles is best measured in terms of *mechanical* power rather than weight!

In sum, 1 mEq. of *any* electrolyte is chemically equivalent to 1 mEq. of any other electro-

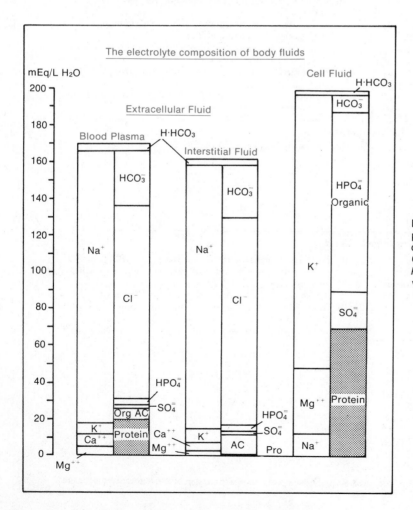

Figure 24–3. A comparison of the electrolyte composition of the extracellular and intracellular fluid compartments. (Modified, by permission, from Gamble, J. L.: *Chemical Anatomy, Physiology and Pathology of Extracellular Fluid.* Cambridge, Harvard University Press, 1947.)

Water and electrolytes are distributed throughout the body's fluid compartments. Extracellular fluids and intracellular fluids contain the *same* electrolytes but in different amounts. The electrolytes contained in the *intracellular* fluid include potassium, magnesium, phosphate, proteinate and traces of sodium and chloride. *Potassium* is the major cation of the ICF and *phosphate* is the major anion. The electrolytes contained in the *extracellular* fluid include sodium, chloride, bicarbonate and traces of potassium, magnesium, protein and phosphate. *Sodium* is the major cation of the ECF and *chloride* is the major anion. In Figure 24–3 the relative proportions of electrolytes are shown for both the intracellular and extracellular compartments.

Samples of *plasma* are used by laboratories to measure electrolytes in the *extracellular* fluid compartment. This is because the plasma component of the ECF compartment has almost the *same electrolyte composition* as does the interstitial component, except that plasma contains the plasma proteins (colloids). Normal approximate laboratory findings for electrolytes and plasma proteins within the plasma are as follows:

Sodium	140 mEq./L.
Potassium	5 mEq./L.
Chloride	103 mEq./L.
Bicarbonate	24 mEq./L.
Colloids	6 Gm/100 ml. (6 Gm. per cent)

While electrolyte concentration of the ECF is measurable, scientists are not as yet able to analyze the concentration of electrolytes in the intracellular fluid.

The *transcellular* fluids (e.g., urine, bile, saliva) each have their distinct electrolyte composition which tends, in health, to remain fairly stable. When illness strikes, the transcellular fluids may become depleted through vomiting, diarrhea, excessive perspiration, and so forth. When such depletion occurs, electrolytes are lost along with water. Both water and electrolytes, then, must be replaced for balance to be restored.

FLUID AND ELECTROLYTE MOVEMENT

A knowledge of fluid and electrolyte transport throughout the body and its regulation is basic to an understanding of such pathophysiologic concepts as edema, dehydration, circulatory overload and water intoxication as well as numerous other fluid and electrolyte imbalances. To understand fluid and electrolyte movement within the fluid compartments of the body, one must carefully consider the following two processes: (1) the transport of fluid and electrolytes between the intracellular fluid and extracellular fluid compartments and (2) the transport of fluids between the interstitial fluid compartment and the vascular compartment.

Fluid and Electrolyte Transport Between the Intracellular and Extracellular Fluid Compartments

The flow of fluids and electrolytes between the ICF and ECF compartments depends upon the *osmolality* of the fluid compartments and the phenomenon of *active transport*.

Osmolality. Osmolality is defined as the total number of dissolved particles (solute) per liter of solvent. When two solutions of different osmolalities (different concentrations of dissolved particles per liter) are separated by a membrane permeable to water, the *distribution* of water *shifts* so that the osmolalities of the two solutions equalize. Because water goes where the greatest number of electrolyte particles are, the solution with the greatest osmolality (greatest concentration of dissolved particles per liter) *gains* water while the solution with the lowest osmolality (lowest concentration of dissolved particles per liter) *loses* water. In the body, osmolality controls water distribution between the ICF and ECF compartments. Water is normally distributed between the compartments so that the osmolalities remain essentially the same in all the fluid compartments.

The dissolved particles within the body fluids are primarily electrolytes and colloids. Should the ICF develop a greater osmolality (more electrolytes per liter) than the ECF, water will shift from the ECF into the ICF and the cells will consequently *swell*. Conversely, should the ECF develop a greater osmolality than the ICF, water will shift from the cells into the ECF compartment, and the cells will *shrivel*. Thus, osmolar changes affect cell volume.

While osmolality controls water distribution, osmolality itself is principally regulated by water *intake* and *output*. Water intake is controlled by thirst, while water loss is controlled by the antidiuretic hormone (ADH), the kidney nephron and the gastrointestinal tract.

How is osmolality measured? Laboratories use the *serum sodium level* as a direct measure of plasma osmolality and as an indirect measure of ICF osmolality since both the ICF and ECF compartments have the *same* osmolality. The normal serum sodium level is 140 mEq./L. When sodium (the principal cation of the ECF) is elevated above normal limits, the osmolality of the plasma, and consequently of the body, is increased. When the serum sodium level is depressed below normal limits, osmolality is decreased.

The patient with an elevated serum Na+ level due to water depletion is suffering from a hyperosmolar imbalance; i.e., he has a decrease in water *relative* to particle concentration (hyperosmolality). Thus, his electrolytes are said to be concentrated. Conversely, when the patient has a lowered serum Na+ and /or an increase in body water due to water retention or overload, the patient has a *hypo-osmolar* imbalance; i.e., he has an *increase* in water *relative* to particle concentration (hypo-osmolality), and his electrolytes are diluted. The concepts of hyperosmolality and hypoosmolality are diagrammatically represented in Figure 24–4.

Active Transport. While osmolality controls *water* movement and distribution, active transport applies to the work (energy) required to *transport ions* across a cellular membrane against concentration or chemical or electrical gradients.

One special type of active transport dealing with sodium and potassium is the *sodium pump.* Recall that large amounts of sodium exist extracellularly and large quantities of potassium exist intracellularly. Since sodium and potassium both can diffuse through the cell wall, an active mechanism must operate to keep these ions in their respective compartments where they are critically needed. The sodium pump is this mechanism and is particularly important in preventing continual swelling of cells.

The cells contain many nondiffusible substances that tend to cause osmosis of water to their interior. The sodium pump opposes this tendency and prevents cellular distention.[3]

Fluid Transport Between the Vascular Compartment and Interstitial Fluid Compartment

To grasp how fluid exchange occurs between the vascular (blood) and the interstitial (tissue) fluid compartments, it is necessary to consider briefly the following factors: plasma proteins, capillary permeability, plasma osmolality, blood hydrostatic pressure, filtration pressure, colloid osmotic pressure and the role of the lymphatic system.

The *plasma proteins,* as we stated earlier, are negatively charged particles found mainly in the blood or intravascular compartment. The normal level of plasma proteins in the blood is 6 to 8 Gm./100 ml. *Albumin* makes up the largest fraction of plasma proteins.

Because they are large particles, the plasma proteins are generally unable to pass through the walls of the capillaries, although a small amount of protein does escape. While the capillary walls are *freely permeable* to water and to certain electrolytes, they are *not freely permeable* to protein, and the plasma protein concentration remains high. Thus, plasma normally has a 0.5 per cent *greater* osmolality than interstitial fluid; i.e., it has a 0.5 per cent greater capacity to attract and to hold water than interstitial fluid. Any reduction in plasma osmolality results in swollen tissues (edema) and loss of blood volume.

The three major factors involved in the maintenance of blood volume, and the prevention of edema, are blood hydrostatic pressure, colloid osmotic pressure and filtration pressure (also called Starling's capillary forces).

Blood hydrostatic pressure (BHP) is the pressure of the blood cells and plasma within the capillaries. Blood hydrostatic pressure is dependent upon the level of the arterial blood pressure, the rate of blood flow through the capillaries and the venous pressure. As you will recall from physiology, each of these factors is, in turn, influenced by other factors. Some of the major influences are diagrammed in Figure 24–5. The normal blood hydrostatic pressure within the arterioles is 32 mm. Hg, and within the venules it is 12 mm. Hg.

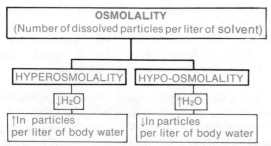

Figure 24–4. The concept of osmolality as applied to water depletion and water excess in human beings.

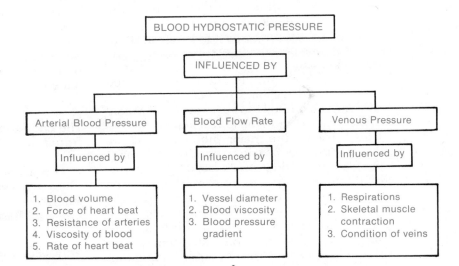

Figure 24–5. The major factors influencing blood hydrostatic pressure.

The next major factor in the transport of fluids between the vascular and interstitial compartment is the *colloid osmotic pressure* (also called "oncotic pressure," OP), or that pressure exerted by the plasma proteins. The plasma proteins work somewhat like a sponge, holding water within the vessels and sucking back that water which escapes from the vessels. Normally the colloid osmotic pressure within the capillary is around 22 mm. Hg.

Finally, the *filtration pressure* (FP) is the pressure of the blood in the blood vessels minus the colloid osmotic pressure (FP = BHP − OP). The filtration pressure in the arteriole is +10 mm. Hg (32 mm. Hg BHP − 22 mm. Hg OP = +10 mm. Hg FP). In the venule, the filtration pressure is −10 mm. Hg (12 mm. Hg BHP − 22 mm. Hg OP = −10 mm. Hg

FP). These figures demonstrate that at the arteriolar end of the capillary, the blood hydrostatic pressure, or pressure of blood within the capillaries, is *greater* than the colloid osmotic pressure. Fluid is thus *forced out of the capillaries* into the tissues. At the venular end of the capillary, the blood hydrostatic pressure is *less* than the colloid osmotic pressure, and the water is *sucked back* into the vessels. Thus, the filtration occurs at the arteriolar end of the vessel and reabsorption at the venular end of the capillary (Fig. 24–6). When blood hydrostatic pressure, and thus filtration pressure, exceeds the opposing, or reabsorptive forces of colloid osmotic pressure, fluid escapes into the tissues, and edema results. When blood hydrostatic pressure drops back toward normal values, the plasma protein sponge can soak up

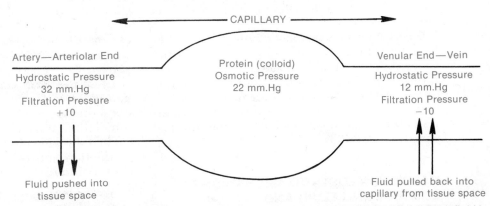

Figure 24–6. Pressure differences within the capillary function to push and pull fluid; fluid is pushed out of the capillary into the tissue spaces at the arteriolar end and is pulled back into the capillary from the tissue spaces at the venular end. (Modified from Dutcher and Fielo.)

the lost fluid, bringing it back into the bloodstream, and edema subsides.

A final factor influencing fluid transport between the plasma and interstitial fluid is the *lymphatic system*. This system functions to return excess fluid, protein and debris, filtered out of the capillary, back into circulation.

Having considered the major factors that control the *return* of fluid to the vascular system, let us next discuss the major problems that can influence the *loss of water* from the plasma.

Rise in Blood Hydrostatic Pressure. This raises the filtration pressure, causing fluid to be squeezed out into the tissues more readily. The result is edema or swelling of tissues. For example, a rise in the blood hydrostatic pressure occurs in hypertensive individuals and in those who receive an overload of intravenous fluids.

Drop in Colloid Osmotic Pressure. This reduces the rate of reabsorption of fluid that was filtered out at the arteriolar end of the capillary. Fluid will accumulate in the tissues, with resulting edema.

A decrease in the colloid osmotic pressure is usually the result of protein depletion. *Hypoproteinemia* (low plasma proteins) usually occurs in malnutrition, infection, hemorrhage, profuse serous drainage and severe burns; in instances of renal, cardiac or hepatic damage; and after lengthy operations. Patients afflicted with these conditions are usually edematous and perhaps *dehydrated* as well. Although patients with edema appear to have "too much water," they often actually suffer from the problem of water depletion. This is due to the shift of water from the intracellular compartments and the vascular spaces to the interstitial spaces. Thus, water is not circulated appropriately and is not available for the body to meet its various needs.

Obstruction in the Lymphatic System. This can lead to fluid retention within the interstitial spaces because fluid is blocked in its attempt to return to the venous circulation. For example, *lymphedema* can occur after a radical mastectomy, which involves removal of the lymphatics of the axilla. It can also result from tropical parasitic infections.

MAJOR HOMEOSTATIC MECHANISMS CONTROLLING FLUID AND ELECTROLYTE BALANCE

Water and electrolyte balance and their distribution throughout the body are homeostati-

cally regulated by the endocrine system, the gastrointestinal system, the renal and cardiovascular systems, the nervous system and the respiratory system. These systems exercise control over water and electrolyte intake and excretion. Moreover, these systems are the *only* controls over body water and electrolyte exchange. For this reason, even minor breakdowns in the function of any one of these systems can lead to water and electrolyte imbalances.

The Endocrine System as a Homeostatic Regulator

The major hormones maintaining fluid and electrolyte balance are the antidiuretic hormone (ADH), aldosterone, thyroid hormones, and parathyroid hormone (PTH).

ANTIDIURETIC HORMONE (ADH) OR VASOPRESSIN

As the name implies, ADH prevents the body, under certain conditions, from losing fluid. It is opposed to ("anti") fluid loss (diuresis). Some major facts concerning ADH are as follows:

> ### ADH
> Function: *maintains osmotic pressure within normal limits*
> Action: *controls water reabsorption*
> Site of action: *distal renal tubules and collecting ducts in nephrons*
> Formed: *by neurosecretory cells of hypothalamus*
> Stimulus: *increased osmolality of ECF*
> Released: *from posterior lobes of the pituitary gland (neurohypophysis)*

Hyperosmolality of ECF stimulates hypothalamic osmoreceptors, which in turn stimulate release of ADH from storage in the posterior pituitary. In sum, an *increase* in the osmolality of the ECF results in an *increased secretion* of ADH and a *decreased* urinary output. Conversely, a *decrease* in the osmolality of the ECF leads to a *decreased secretion* of ADH and an *increased* urinary output. For a diagrammatic illustration of the effect of osmolality on ADH release, see Figure 24–7.

The following circumstances stimulate ADH production and release (with resultant water conservation):

▶ Water loss that causes an increase in ECF osmolality

▶ Reduced circulating blood volume

▶ Presence of pain

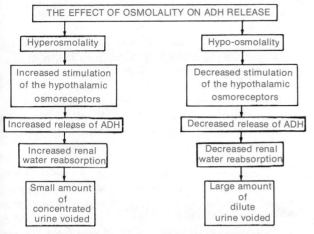

Figure 24–7. The effect of osmolality on ADH release and inhibition.

▶ Secondary to administration of drugs (e.g., morphine sulfate, barbiturates, anesthetic agents)

▶ Stress: emotional and physiologic (e.g., surgical trauma, accidental trauma, unusual and prolonged physical exertion)

It is particularly important to realize that the physiologic reaction to the stress of surgical or accidental trauma is to increase production and release of ADH. It appears that excessive stress, such as a surgical procedure, activates the patient's hypothalamic centers. Consequently, both ADH and ACTH are released in large amounts following injury. ACTH is one of the hormones involved in stress reactions. This

means that following surgery or accident, *urine volume is reduced regardless of intake!* Remember, then, the following important rule:

> *Administer fluids* cautiously *during early postoperative and post-trauma periods while ADH is being released.* "Forcing" *fluids can result in overhydration and drowning.*

Factors suppressing ADH formation are: (1) hypo-osmolality of the ECF or an increased water load, (2) increased blood volume, (3) exposure to cold, (4) acute alcohol ingestion, (5) CO_2 inhalation and (6) administration of diuretics. These conditions, then, cause an *increased urinary output.*

Diabetes insipidus is a disease caused by an inadequate quantity or quality of ADH production or secretion. This condition is characterized by extreme thirst, high fluid intake and the resultant daily voiding of large amounts of very dilute urine. For a diagrammatic summary of factors affecting ADH release, see Figure 24–8.

ALDOSTERONE

Aldosterone is the second hormone that helps maintain fluid and sodium balance. Whereas ADH maintains balance by regulating

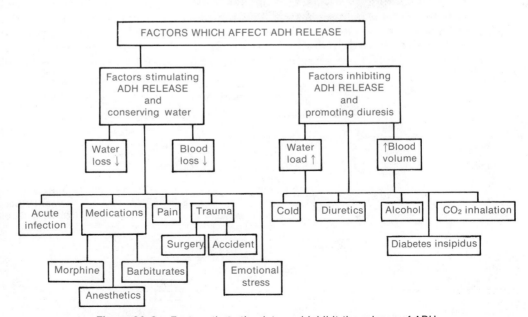

Figure 24–8. Factors that stimulate and inhibit the release of ADH.

water reabsorption or excretion, aldosterone maintains balance by regulating sodium ion concentration. Because sodium holds fluid in the body (more specifically, ECF), aldosterone maintains water balance by maintaining sodium balance.

Aldosterone

Major function: *regulates sodium ion concentration which in turn regulates ECF volume*
Formed and released: *zona glomerulosa of adrenal cortex; not dependent on pituitary function*
Stimulus: *decreased sodium ion concentration in ECF and renal hypoxia*
Site of action: *renal tubules*

There are at least six major factors that control the secretion of aldosterone.

Sodium Depletion. Sodium depletion appears to be the *greatest single stimulus* to aldosterone secretion. Sodium depletion occurs among people who are deprived of a sufficient NaCl intake, who sweat excessively, or who live in hot climates. These individuals suffer from a decrease in interstitial fluid and plasma volume, with a resultant reduced blood flow to vital organs such as the kidney.

Changes in the ECF Volume. Increased ECF volume, such as an increase in interstitial fluid volume (as with pitting edema), causes a decrease in aldosterone secretion, which results in an increase in renal sodium (and water) excretion. Conversely, a decrease in ECF volume (as with dehydration) causes an increase in aldosterone secretion, which results in a decrease in renal sodium (and water) excretion.

Changes in Intravascular Fluid Volume. These changes are of great importance in influencing aldosterone secretion and release. An acute *loss* of blood due to *hemorrhage* is a major stimulus for aldosterone release, resulting in renal tubular reabsorption of sodium, and water retention, which acts to keep the Na^+ in an isotonic solution.

Changes in the Electrolyte Composition of the Intravascular Fluid Compartment (Plasma). Increased aldosterone secretion results from decreased sodium ion concentration (secondary to increased sodium ion excretion) or increased potassium ion concentration (secondary to decreased potassium excretion and/or increased potassium intake).

Constriction of Two Major Arteries. Constriction of the carotid and the renal arteries stimulates an increased secretion of aldosterone.

Large Doses of ACTH. These also cause an increase in aldosterone secretion. This effect, however, is short-lived in human beings.

Other Factors Affecting Serum Levels of Aldosterone. Stress is a powerful stimulant to aldosterone secretion. Some examples of stress are nervous tension and anxiety, pregnancy, major surgery and trauma. Hepatic disease or failure influences serum aldosterone concentrations because degradation of the hormone occurs primarily in the liver. Thus, individuals with liver disease tend to suffer from edema because of excessive sodium and water retention.

As mentioned, the two major homeostatic hormones for maintaining water and sodium balance are the antidiuretic hormone (ADH, or vasopressin) and aldosterone. Two others, the thyroid hormone and the parathyroid hormone, will also be considered. The diuretic hormone (DH), or diuretic principle, has received some interest, but thus far, little is known. The role of these hormones is noted in Figure 24–9.

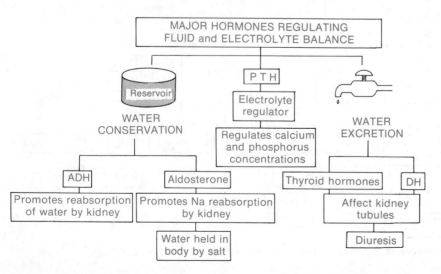

Figure 24–9. A summary of the major hormones that play a role in fluid and electrolyte metabolism.

The *thyroid* hormone is important for normal diuresis and calcium regulation and for release of the hormones tetraiodothyronine (T_4) and triiodothyronine (T_3).[17] These two hormones increase cardiac output sufficiently for adequate perfusion of the nephron as well as increasing the volume of glomerular filtrate, hence urinary output. The hormone *thyrocalcitonin* helps maintain calcium balance.[17]

The parathyroid gland secretes *parathormone*, which controls calcium and phosphate metabolism; that is, it regulates calcium and phosphate ion concentration by increasing or decreasing the ionization of calcium from bones to maintain normal serum calcium levels. An inverse relationship between serum calcium and phosphate is maintained to foster normal excitability of nerves and muscles.

SUMMARY

In summary, ADH and aldosterone prevent an excessive loss of water from the body. ADH regulates renal tubular reabsorption of water in relation to ECF volume, thereby controlling water metabolism. Aldosterone regulates renal tubular reabsorption of sodium ions in relation to sodium ion concentration of ECF, thereby controlling sodium metabolism and secondarily controlling water balance. Recall that water is reabsorbed along with sodium ions to maintain normal osmolality.

The Gastrointestinal Tract as a Homeostatic Regulator

The gastrointestinal tract plays a very important part in maintaining fluid and electrolyte balance because under normal conditions the gastrointestinal system is the sole route of intake for fluids and electrolytes. Thus, the major role of the gastrointestinal tract is the replenishment, by absorption, of the fluids and electrolytes lost from the body through the skin, respiratory tract and kidney. The intestinal tract absorbs the fluids from dietary intake, as well as approximately 7 to 9 L. of glandular and gastrointestinal tract secretions. However, out of this enormous amount of fluid, only 100 ml. of water are lost from the bowel daily; the rest is reabsorbed.

Moreover, fluids and electrolytes within the intestinal tract are subject to rapid transport across the intestinal mucosa in both directions. Approximately every 90 minutes a volume of fluid equal to the volume of the body's blood plasma (i.e., 3000 ml. in a 70-kg. man) passes through the intestinal mucosa. With such a rapid turnover of fluid, it is no wonder that the smallest upset in gastrointestinal tract function precipitates fluid and electrolyte imbalance.

> *The fluid imbalances most commonly encountered in clinical practice are gastrointestinal and cardiovascular in origin.*

The Renal System as a Homeostatic Regulator

The kidney, one of the most active and complex organs of the body, maintains a homeostatic internal environment by regulating water, sodium and hydrogen ions. To understand the work of the kidneys in maintaining fluid and electrolyte metabolism, we must review the anatomic structure of the kidney and those physiologic functions of the kidneys specifically concerned with water and electrolytes.

ANATOMIC STRUCTURE OF THE KIDNEY*

The *nephron* is the kidney's functional unit, serving to clear the blood of waste materials, form urine, and regulate both the fluid and electrolyte balance as well as maintain acid-base (H^+) balance of the body. Within each human kidney there are approximately 1,000,000 nephrons. Each nephron is composed of a glomerulus (with an afferent and efferent vessel), Bowman's capsule, proximal convoluted tubule, the loop of Henle, the distal convoluted tubule and the collecting tubule (see Fig. 24–10).

The work of the nephron in the formation of urine is as follows: blood flows into the kidney from the renal artery—an artery that is derived directly from the abdominal aorta. Upon reaching the kidney, the blood is channeled into a cluster of tiny capillaries called a *glomerulus*, a Latin word meaning "little ball." Each glomerulus, in turn, is partly encapsulated within a double endothelial capsule called *Bowman's capsule*. Filtration occurs because of the balance between the hydrostatic pressure (produced by the systolic thrust of the heart) of the blood within the capillaries and the oncotic

---

*The anatomy of the kidney will be discussed in greater detail in Chapter 30. In this chapter, we are mainly concerned with the kidney nephron, which is the structure most closely connected with fluid and electrolyte balance.

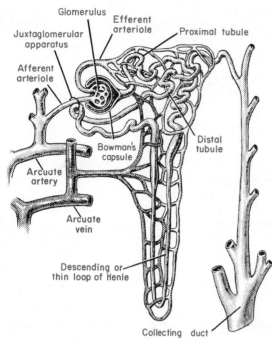

Figure 24-10. The nephron. (From Smith: *The Kidney: Structure and Functions in Health and Disease.* Oxford University Press, 1951.)

pressure of plasma proteins (review Starling's force of the capillaries). The ultrafiltrate is dilute, protein-free and similar to plasma; it contains waste products and is known as glomerular filtrate. Glomerular tufts produce approximately 120 ml. of glomerular filtrate each minute[5] which passes through the semipermeable membranes of Bowman's capsule.

Within the proximal convoluted tubules, active and passive reabsorption takes place; 80 per cent of sodium ions and almost all of the other substances are reabsorbed, including glucose, amino acids, some vitamins and chloride ions. Along with sodium ion reabsorption, there is an obligatory reabsorption of water *without regard* for the body's need for fluids and electrolytes. Within the *loop of Henle* further reabsorption of water occurs. The amount of reabsorption of fluids that takes place in the distal convoluted tubules and collecting tubules depends on the amount of ADH and aldosterone, which in turn depends on the body's requirement for fluids.

By the time the filtrate is ready to enter the *collecting tube,* where the process of urine formation will finally be completed, 98 per cent of the glomerular filtrate will have been reab-

sorbed! This means that out of every 100 ml. of fluid that pass through the glomerulus every minute, approximately 98 ml. will have been reabsorbed through the tubules, leaving only 2 ml. of filtrate to be carried to the renal pelvis and finally excreted as urine. Because of their abilities, the kidneys are called the master chemists of the body. Any upset or disease that destroys renal function wreaks havoc on the body's fluid and electrolyte balance.

PHYSIOLOGIC FUNCTIONS OF THE KIDNEY IN HEALTH AND DISEASE

The major functions of the kidney are briefly listed in the following box:

The Kidney
1. *Selects and rejects materials according to the body's needs*
2. *Removes wastes from the body*
3. *Controls H^+ balance*
4. *Regulates the composition of the blood and ECF*
5. *Maintains volume and concentration of urine*
6. *Regulates ECF sodium concentration*

Kidney Selectivity.   As you recall from our discussion of the structure of the nephron, most of the water, electrolytes and other substances that pass through the glomerulus are normally returned to the bloodstream. Concentrating ability is markedly altered in the very young and the very old. As previously noted, ADH and aldosterone are excreted under the stimulus of any kind of stress, be it burns, shock, or cardiovascular renal disease. Under these circumstances, both sodium ions and water tend to be retained at the expense of the body's osmolality. Thus, a state of overhydration or hypo-osmolality may occur.

Removal of Wastes.   The kidneys remove the waste products of metabolism, nitrogenous products, drugs, toxins and other foreign substances that have been absorbed by the digestive tract. This function will be considered in detail in Chapter 30.

H^+ Balance.   One vital role of the kidney is to maintain the blood at the slightly alkaline pH of 7.35 to 7.45. The kidney is able to control the alkalinity of the blood by controlling the *rate* at which H^+ is excreted from the body. (H^+ balance will be discussed later in this chapter.)

Blood Composition.   The kidney nephron, by means of its selective filtration process and its reabsorptive abilities, directly affects the composition of the blood and the ECF. By altering the osmolality (number of particles per liter) of he ECF, the kidney indirectly affects the osmolality of the ICF. For example, if the kidney becomes seriously damaged, blood composition may be radically changed because wastes and toxins, as well as excess acids, are not being excreted. This alteration in blood composition will eventually affect the water and electrolyte composition of the entire body—within the vascular system, within the tissues and within the cells.

Maintenance of Volume and Concentration of Urine.   Both the urine volume and the concentration of electrolytes within the urine vary widely from person to person as well as from day to day in the same person. For example, under extreme circumstances, urine volume output could vary from 200 ml. per day to 14 L. per day.

Electrolyte concentrations in the urine are equally variable. Sodium, chloride, potassium, calcium and phosphorus may appear in small or large amounts, depending upon the body's needs at the time. Thus, there are no set norms for the concentration of electrolytes within the urine—there are just minimum, optimum and maximum values.

This variability in urine volume and concentration is, with health, in keeping with the body's requirements at the time. If we ingest more fluids and electrolytes than our bodies need, *excretion* results; if we ingest fewer fluids and electrolytes than we need, *conservation* results. This means that if a healthy person ingests a large amount of fluid, he will excrete a large volume of dilute urine. Conversely, if he ingests a small amount of fluid, he will excrete a small volume of concentrated urine. If he has a decreased intake of *both* water and sodium chloride or an increased loss of these substances, only the minimum volume of urine necessary for eliminating the nitrogenous wastes accumulated from the day's metabolic activities will be excreted. This volume is approximately 500 ml. As you can readily see, the capacity of the kidney to alter the concentration and volume of urine to be excreted is highly adaptive for humans; without such a capacity we could not survive.

The ability of the kidney to concentrate urine is a good test of both kidney function and the state of the body's fluid balance. The normal kidney is able to concentrate urine up to a specific gravity of 1.030.* When a person has

*Specific gravity is the ratio of the weight of a substance to the weight of an equal volume of water. As a basis of comparison, laboratories use water as a constant against which to measure solutions such as urine. Distilled water has a specific gravity of 1.000 Gm./ml.; i.e., 1 ml. of water weighs 1 Gm. The normal range for the specific gravity of urine is from 1.012 to 1.022, although the healthy kidney has a range of 1.010 to 1.030. In the case of urine and certain other solutions, the term "specific gravity" is also used to indicate the concentration of that solution.

healthy kidneys, the degree of dehydration or overhydration can be determined by the specific gravity of excreted urine. That is, a dehydrated person will have low volume output with high specific gravity, and an overhydrated person will have high volume output with low specific gravity.

The test for the specific gravity of urine has important implications for the surgical patient. It is necessary to know the concentrating powers of a patient's kidneys *before* surgery in order to maintain his fluid balance *following* surgery. The preoperative patient with *normal* kidneys will be able to concentrate urine to a specific gravity of 1.030. This means that he will be able to excrete in a 24-hour period 35 Gm. of solutes in a liquid medium of 500 ml. This amount of solute waste is normal for a 24-hour period. If the preoperative patient has *impaired* kidneys, he may be able to concentrate urine to only 1.010; thus, he will require 1450 ml. of water to excrete the same 35 Gm. of solutes in 24 hours. Following surgery, the patient with damaged kidneys will have an even larger load of solute wastes owing to the trauma he has undergone. As a result, it may take an even greater amount of urine to excrete his solutes!

You will recall that ADH normally conserves water in the body following trauma or surgery. In the patient with renal disease this mechanism will not be operative, and consequently he may lose much more fluid than he should at this critical time.

In addition to renal disease, any serious illness tends to impair the functioning of the nephron. Thus, in diseases unrelated to the kidney, the patient may also be subject to dehydration because of the kidney's inability to concentrate the urine.

To summarize, the kidneys alter the volume and concentration of urine in keeping with the body's requirements. When the ability to concentrate urine is lost, as a result of kidney or other disease, there is danger of developing dehydration.

Sodium Regulation.   You will recall that sodium determines both the volume and the osmolality of the ECF; the kidney, which controls the delicate balance of sodium within the body, is precise in its capacity to conserve sodium. Over a 3- to 4-day period, *intake of sodium almost exactly equals output.* Moreover, out of the 24,000 mEq. of Na^+ filtered by the glomeruli daily, 99.5 per cent is reabsorbed in order to keep the body in a steady state.

What controls the kidney in its regulation of

sodium? Two factors seem important: first of all, aldosterone fosters sodium reabsorption; second, changes in body posture seem to be associated with changes in urine flow and sodium excretion. For example, when an individual first stands up after lying down, urine flow and sodium excretion are decreased. Conversely, if he has been standing up and then goes to bed, both urine flow and sodium excretion increase. These changes in posture have definite implications for patients on bed rest.* Individuals lying down may initially have a better urinary output than those standing for prolonged periods. Diuresis is thus temporarily facilitated by bed rest.

For purposes of simplification, we have discussed the kidney in isolation from the other organs of the body. Actually, the kidney is vitally linked with every other organ, particularly the hormonal and nervous systems. Moreover, the kidney forms a vital link between the cardiovascular and renal systems. Consequently, hormonal diseases (especially those involving ADH and aldosterone), nervous system disorders and cardiovascular disorders all affect kidney function and consequently fluid and electrolyte balance. Congestive heart failure, hypertension, diabetes insipidus and disorders of the adrenal cortex are a few of the numerous diseases that can impair the work of the kidney nephron.

---

*For a further discussion of bed rest, see Chapter 33.

While the kidney is characterized as the "master chemist" of the body, the brain and nervous system can be characterized as the "master switchboard," regulating the kidney as well as the rest of the body. The overall function of the brain as a homeostatic regulator is to centrally control water and sodium intake and excretion. The nervous system accomplishes its role by manufacturing and releasing ADH, which regulates changes in volume and osmolality of ECF.

Hormonal Production. The antidiuretic hormone (ADH) is secreted by the cells of the hypothalamus, a portion of the brain. ADH is stored in the posterior pituitary.

Regulation of Body Water Volume. The midbrain contains a *volumetric monitoring system* that responds to variations in extracellular fluid volume. This system evidently receives information about fluid volume from various receptors located in the walls of the great veins, the arteries and the atria. From the volumetric monitoring system, information concerning blood volume is relayed to those control systems that govern ADH release, thirst and the release of aldosterone.

How are these mechanisms stimulated and inhibited? You will recall that receptors in the hypothalamus are responsible for stimulating the release of ADH from storage in the posterior pituitary gland. The *thirst center* is also located in the hypothalamus and may be turned off and on by changes in body fluid osmolality. In addition, messages are somehow carried from the volumetric regulating center to the adrenal cortex for either the release or inhibition of

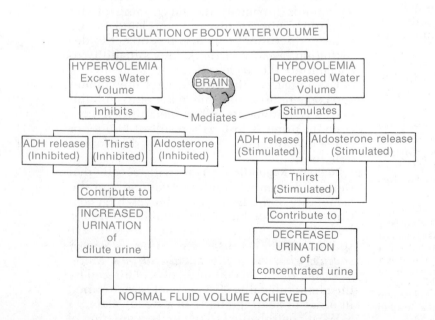

Figure 24–11. The regulation of body water volume depends upon ADH, thirst, and aldosterone. The release or inhibition of these mechanisms is mediated by the brain.

aldosterone—the body's conserver of sodium and, consequently, of water.

To illustrate how body water volume is regulated, consider the following examples of volume increase and decrease. When body water volume increases *(hypervolemia)*, ADH release is inhibited and aldosterone is not secreted. As a result, the individual urinates a large amount of fluid. Because he is not thirsty, he does not drink to replace the water he is excreting, and his body fluid regains its normal volume. Conversely, when body water volume decreases significantly *(hypovolemia)*, ADH is released. The thirst center is stimulated and the individual drinks; also, his urine decreases in amount and is more concentrated. Moreover, because of aldosterone release, sodium is conserved and water is held in the body; thus, water balance is again achieved (Fig. 24–11).

Regulation of Body Water Osmolality. While the *midbrain* apparently contains the volume receptors, the *hypothalamus* is believed to be the locus of activity for the regulation of body osmolality. First, the hypothalamus manufactures ADH and contains osmoreceptors that signal the posterior pituitary gland to release or to retain ADH as needed. Osmoreceptors in the hypothalamus are believed to shrink when the osmolality of the ECF increases and to swell when the osmolality of the ECF decreases. Consequently, an increased osmolality of the ECF (which causes the osmoreceptors to shrink) allows ADH to be released. Conversely, in patients in whom osmolality of the ECF is decreased, the osmoreceptors swell and ADH is not secreted.

Second, the *thirst center* is very sensitive to the osmolality of the body fluids. Basically, thirst results from (1) low water intake, (2) excessive water loss, (3) excessive Na^+ intake and (4) excessive intravenous infusion of hypertonic solutions.* These circumstances result in cellular dehydration, reduced blood volume (hypovolemia), and hyperosmolality of the ECF. These changes in osmolality stimulate the thirst center, and nerve impulses are conveyed to the higher brain centers which then create "the drive to drink"—a drive that is controlled, to some degree, by cultural norms.

On the other hand, thirst is *inhibited* by (1) a large water intake, (2) water retention within the body, (3) a low Na^+ intake and (4) excessive infusions of isotonic or hypotonic solutions.*

---

*An *isotonic solution* is one that has the *same* osmolality as another solution, i.e., normal saline, which contains 0.9 per cent NaCl, is isotonic with plasma. A *hypotonic solution* is one that has a *lower* osmolality than another solution to which it is compared. For example, distilled water is hypotonic to plasma. A *hypertonic solution* is one that has a *greater* osmolality than another solution to which it is compared. For example, a solution of 5 per cent NaCl would be hypertonic to plasma.

These circumstances result in hypotonic expansion of all compartments which in turn diminishes the desire to drink.

A patient's complaint of thirst is of practical importance because thirst is the major symptom that people are *consciously* aware of in fluid imbalance and dehydration. However, the presence or absence of thirst, in clinical situations, is *not always* a true indicator of the state of fluid balance for the following reasons:

1. *Edematous* individuals may be thirsty, although they appear to be overloaded with fluid. The thirst develops because the blood volume may actually be quite low as a result of the seepage of a large amount of plasma into interstitial spaces, thereby causing a type of dehydration. Sufficient fluid is not available in the bloodstream to effectively circulate to tissues and cells.

2. A *dehydrated* person may not be thirsty. For example, comatose or confused elderly patients may be severely dehydrated and yet have no drive to drink.

3. A person with *hypo-osmolality* of the ECF will not experience thirst even though the water volume of his body is lowered. In conditions in which the individual has lost more electrolytes than water, the drive to drink will be inhibited even though a state of dehydration exists.

4. An individual may be *either* dehydrated or in a state of fluid overload because his responses to the thirst drive are influenced more by his culture than by his actual fluid requirements. For example, in American culture it is customary to drink socially and at meals; we consider it impolite not to offer a guest a beverage. Consequently, at times, our drinking habits may be more influenced by social custom than by the physiologic need for fluid.

At this point, let us briefly review the mechanisms discussed. The overall functions of the brain in the control of homeostatic mechanisms are to ensure the proper intake and excretion of sodium and water. As we have pointed out, the brain performs these functions by means of hormonal production and secretion, and by the regulation of both body fluid volume and osmolality.

Two illustrations of how the brain normally responds to changes in fluid volume and osmolality follow: first, consider what happens to a man who is vigorously exercising and consequently is losing a great deal of water and some Na^+ in his sweat. This man loses a certain amount of his blood volume, which can be demonstrated by a definite loss in weight. The receptors in his vascular system consequently respond to the loss of blood volume and relay the message to the midbrain.

From the volumetric center in the midbrain, messages are conveyed to the hypothalamus, which then stimulates the release of ADH from the posterior pituitary gland, or neurohypophysis. Because the plasma is more concentrated than normal, fluid is pulled from the interstitial and intracellular compartments into the vascular system to equilibrate among compartments. Also, the hyperosmolality of the ECF stimulates osmoreceptors in the hypothalamus, which further contribute to ADH release. With the secretion of ADH, the desire to urinate is diminished, and the urine produced appears somewhat concentrated. Thirst and "salt hunger" increase. Thirst is in response to changes in body fluid volume and osmolality, which are conveyed to the thirst center, while "salt hunger" is apparently linked to stimulation of the volume receptors in the midbrain. As a result of the release of aldosterone any Na^+ that this individual ingests will be retained, and Na^+ retention, in turn, holds fluid within his body. Thus, at the end of his tasks, this man, weary from exercise and possibly pleased with his weight loss, will probably be found resting, having a large cold drink, eating potato chips and rapidly regaining both his fluid and weight losses!

Conversely, what happens to the individual who has a fluid overload, perhaps resulting from an evening out with friends and too much to drink? The changes that occur in the overhydrated man are the opposite of those present in the individual described above; in situations of fluid overload there are increased blood and interstitial fluid volumes. Volume receptors respond accordingly, and ADH and aldosterone

are not secreted. However, thirst and "salt hunger" are inhibited, and diuresis results. The overhydrated man, then, who has healthy nervous, renal and hormonal systems will urinate a large amount of dilute urine. As a result, his blood and interstitial fluid volumes are restored to normal.

HYDROGEN ION (ACID-BASE) BALANCE[25, 30, 36–38, 40, 41]

H+, Acids and Bases

The cation H^+ is the active component of all acids. The *greater* the amount of H^+ present in a solution, the *more acid* the solution. Conversely, the *less* H^+ present in a solution, the *less acid*—or *more alkaline*—the solution.

An *acid*, by definition, is a hydrogen ion (proton) *donor*; i.e., an acid loses hydrogen ions to a base, thereby neutralizing or lessening the strength of the base. On the other hand, a *base* is a hydrogen ion (proton) *acceptor*; i.e., a base accepts hydrogen ions from an acid, thereby causing the acid to become weaker (see Fig. 24–12).

For example, if a strong acid such as hydrochloric acid is added to a strong buffer* base such as sodium bicarbonate, the result is a weaker acid (carbonic acid) and a neutral salt (sodium chloride):

$$HCl \quad + \quad NaHCO_3 \quad \rightleftarrows$$

hydrochloric acid	sodium bicarbonate
(strong acid)	(strong buffer base)

$$H_2CO_3 \quad + \quad NaCl$$

carbonic acid	sodium chloride
(weak acid)	(neutral salt)

---

*Buffers are discussed later in this section.

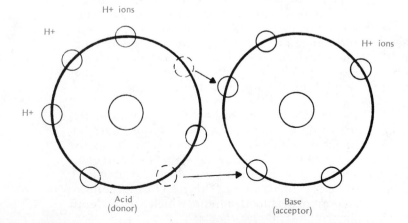

Figure 24–12. Schematic hydrogen ion donor-acceptor concept. (From Stroot, V., et al.: *Fluid and Electrolytes: A Practical Approach.* Philadelphia, F. A. Davis Co., 1974, p. 77.)

Hydrogen ions are normally present in the body fluids in a concentration of 0.00004 mEq./L. (between 0.0000001 and 0.00000001 Gm./L. of extracellular fluid). This vital ion is found in both cellular and extracellular fluids. Hydrogen ions play a vital role in the regulation of numerous biochemical and metabolic activities. (See Table 24–3.)

Because H⁺ circulates in the body fluids in such minute amounts, the hydrogen ion concentration of the body fluids (and of any solution) is measured in pH values rather than in Gm./L. or mEq./L.

> pH, then, measures the acidity and alkalinity of a solution.

Technically, pH is chemical shorthand for the *negative logarithm* of the hydrogen ion concentration. Neutral pH is a H⁺ concentration of 0.0000001 Gm./L., which is 10^{-7} Gm./L., or a pH of 7. The pH scale extends from 0 to 14, with 7 being neutral. For each pH interval there is a *tenfold difference* in the concentration of H⁺ in a solution. The *higher* the pH, the *lower* the H⁺ concentration of a solution and vice versa. A solution with a pH that is *less* than 7 is *acid;* when the pH is *greater* than 7 the solution is *alkaline.*

Different body fluids have different pH values. The pH of the blood is 7.40. Intracellular fluid pH ranges between 6.9 and 7.2. Urine pH is 6.0; cerebrospinal fluid pH is from 7.36 to 7.44; gastric juice pH is from 1.0 to 2.0; the pH of bile from the gallbladder is between 5.0 and 6.0.

The pH (H⁺ concentration) of the blood indicates whether the body is in a state of acid-base balance or imbalance.

> 1. *The range of blood pH compatible with life is from 6.8 to 7.8 (a tenfold difference in the number of H⁺ ions in the blood).*
> 2. Acidosis *exists when the blood pH drops below 7.40.*
> 3. Alkalosis *exists when the blood pH rises above 7.40.*

As you consider the pH of body fluids, realize that these fluids lie in both the acid and alkaline ranges. Snively and Roberts discuss this point:

Obviously, the normal pH of human body fluid is considerably to the alkaline side of what is usually regarded as neutrality—namely, pH 7.0. The metabolic waste products of the human, on the other hand, have an acid pH as reflected by the fact that normal urine lies on the acid side of neutrality. So

man, with his alkaline body fluid pH, produces more acid than alkali.[38]

Because the body fluids must remain on the alkaline side of neutral and because our bodies produce sizable quantities of acid, the body must be able to control H⁺ concentration and maintain the pH within the narrow range that is compatible with life.

Regulation of Hydrogen Ion Balance

The four regulatory systems (listed in order of activation) that control pH balance are (1) the buffers, (2) the lungs, (3) the cells and (4) the kidneys. Buffers are usually referred to as *chemical* regulators; the cells are called *biologic* regulators; the lungs and kidneys are classified as *physiologic* regulators.[25] Each of these vital homeostatic regulatory systems has a specific role.

The Buffers. "Buffers are chemicals that act as sponges which can give off or take on hydrogen ions as needed to maintain arterial blood pH at 7.35 to 7.45."[36] This sponge-like buffer action protects the body against dangerous fluctuations of H⁺ concentration when excess acids or alkali are added to the body fluids.

Within the body, the major buffer system is the *base bicarbonate* (HCO_3)/*carbonic acid* (H_2CO_3) *system.* This system acts to regulate H⁺ concentration of body fluids by maintaining a *ratio* of 20 parts (normally 20 mEq.) base bicarbonate to 1 part (normally 1 mEq.) carbonic acid (Fig. 24–13). If this ratio changes, acidosis or alkalosis results.

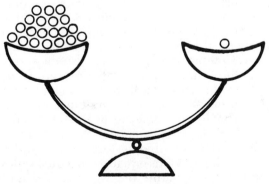

20 bicarbonates : 1 carbonic acid

Figure 24–13. Acid-base balance. Blood pH is 7.4. (From Stroot, V., et al.: *Fluid and Electrolytes: A Practical Approach.* Philadelphia, F. A. Davis Co., 1973, p. 79.)

This chemical buffer system has the advantage of being able to react *immediately* to acid or alkali excesses. It has a disadvantage in that it cannot sustain regulation. For more powerful and longer-lasting regulatory action, the body must rely upon the lungs and kidneys in its struggle to maintain H^+ balance. As you will see, the lungs and kidneys act to regulate the hydrogen ions that dissociate from the body's chemical buffer systems. This is illustrated in the following equation:[25]

$$CO_2 \quad + \quad H_2O \leftrightarrows H_2CO_3 \leftrightarrows \quad H^+ \quad + \quad HCO_3^-$$

| carbon di-oxide (volatile —regulated by lungs) | water | carbonic acid | hydrogen ion | bicarbonate ion (nonvolatile—regulated by kidneys) |

Note that the *lungs* regulate *volatile H^+* in the form of CO_2 while the *kidneys* regulate *nonvolatile H^+* in the form of bicarbonate (HCO_3^-).

The Lungs.   The lungs constitute the second line of defense against H^+ imbalances. The respiratory system (including its neurologic centers in the medulla) controls the H_2CO_3 component of the H_2CO_3:$NaHCO_3$ buffer system. The lungs regulate the carbonic acid level by *altering the rate and depth of respiration*. If the body is suffering an *acid* overload, the rate and depth of respiration *increases*, enabling the patient to "blow off" excess CO_2. The CO_2 combines with the breath vapor, forming H_2CO_3: $CO_2 + H_2O \rightarrow H_2CO_3$. Conversely, in the presence of a *base* overload, the rate of respiration *decreases*, and CO_2 is retained and combines with body fluid, which then increases the H_2CO_3 part of the ratio. Healthy lungs are *rapid* regulators, partially correcting H^+ irregularities within 1 to 3 minutes following their development.

The Cells.   The cells are capable of admitting or releasing excess hydrogen ions. Whenever excess hydrogen ions cross the cell membrane, they must be either (a) exchanged for ions of the same charge (usually Na^+ and K^+); or (b) accompanied by ions of the opposite charge. In this way, the cells maintain electrical neutrality. Compared to the buffer systems and the lungs, the cells are *slow* regulators, requiring 2 to 4 hours to control shifts in H^+ concentration.

The Kidneys.   The renal system constitutes the fourth line of defense against H^+ imbalance. The kidneys regulate $NaHCO_3$ in the H_2CO_3:$NaHCO_3$ buffer system. You should recall from the previous equation that the kidneys eliminate nonvolatile H^+, whereas the lungs eliminate volatile H^+. To compensate for H^+ imbalances, the kidneys alter the *rate of excretion* of H^+ in the urine. In *alkalosis*, the kidneys *retain* hydrogen ions and excrete bicarbonate ions. In *acidosis*, the kidneys retain bicarbonate ions and *excrete* hydrogen ions. The renal system is the *slowest* of all the regulating systems, taking from a few hours to several days to compensate for H^+ imbalances.

Failure of Hydrogen Ion Regulation

The maintenance of H^+ balance depends upon the healthy function of the kidneys, lungs and brain. These remarkable organs can normally adjust swiftly and efficiently to fluctuations of H^+ concentration. However, when subjected to *unusually heavy loads of acid or alkali*, or in the *presence of renal, respiratory or brain disease*, the body's ability to cope with H^+ regulation fails, and imbalances result. The two *major types* of imbalances are acidosis and alkalosis.

Acidosis *is a condition in which the H^+ concentration is elevated above normal or the alkali reserve of the body is reduced below normal.* Alkalosis *is a condition in which the H^+ concentration of the body fluid is decreased below normal or the body base concentration is increased above normal.*

Acidosis and alkalosis are further classified as metabolic or respiratory. *Metabolic* imbalances are caused by failure of the *renal* system to regulate H^+ balance. *Respiratory* imbalances are caused by failure of the *pulmonary* system to regulate H_2CO_3. All four of these imbalances are considered in Table 24–4.

FLUID AND ELECTROLYTE IMBALANCE*

Major Categories of Imbalances

Fluid and electrolyte imbalances can be organized into three major categories:

I. Imbalances caused by a *deficit or excess of water and/or electrolytes*
   A. Water-saline† imbalances
      1. Water deficit (dehydration, hypernatremia, hypertonic dehydration)
      2. Water excess (water intoxication, hyponatremia, hypotonic water excess)
      3. Saline deficit (extracellular volume deficit, hypovolemia, salt deficit)
      4. Saline excess (extracellular volume excess, hypervolemia, salt excess)
   B. Potassium imbalances
      1. Potassium deficit (hypokalemia)
      2. Potassium excess (hyperkalemia)
   C. Calcium imbalances
      1. Calcium deficit (hypocalcemia)
      2. Calcium excess (hypercalcemia)
   D. Magnesium imbalances
      1. Magnesium deficit (hypomagnesemia)
      2. Magnesium excess (hypermagnesemia)
   E. Hydrogen ion imbalances (acid-base imbalances)
      1. Metabolic acidosis (primary base bicarbonate deficit of extracellular fluid)
      2. Metabolic alkalosis (primary base bicarbonate excess of extracellular fluid)
      3. Respiratory acidosis (primary carbonic acid excess)
      4. Respiratory alkalosis (primary carbonic acid deficit)
II. Imbalances caused by *nutritional deficiencies*
   A. Protein deficiency (hypoproteinemia)
   B. Calorie deficiency‡
III. Imbalances caused by *shifts in the position of the extracellular fluid (ECF)*‡
   A. Plasma shifts to the interstitial spaces
   B. Interstitial fluid shifts into the plasma

---

*The subject of fluid and electrolyte imbalance is extremely complex. In this text, we present only the highlights concerning the causes, symptoms and treatment of various imbalances. For a comprehensive coverage of this topic, consult a medical-surgical nursing text or a text specifically devoted to fluids and electrolytes.

†Saline refers to a solution containing sodium, chloride and water.

‡Calorie deficiencies are described in Chapter 22. For a discussion of fluid shifts, consult a more advanced text.

Each of the imbalances (with the exception of calorie deficiency and fluid shifts) are briefly described in Table 24–4.

As you study Table 24–4, notice that fluid and electrolyte imbalances are basically triggered by the following causative factors:

I. *Deficiencies* of fluid and electrolytes due to:
   A. Inadequate dietary intake
   B. Excessive losses (diarrhea, vomiting, gastric suction)
   C. Accumulation of fluids and electrolytes within the body (Fluid can collect within the abdomen and within the tissue spaces. In both cases, fluids are lost from the general circulation.)
II. *Increased use* of fluids and electrolytes
   A. The healing process following injury
   B. Development of infection and high fever
III. *Excess fluid and electrolytes* in relation to the needs of the body
   A. Excessive intake (orally or parenterally) of fluids and electrolytes
   B. Inadequate excretion of fluid and electrolytes due to disease and breakdown of one or more of the body's homeostatic regulators (e.g., kidneys, lungs, brain, gastrointestinal tract, endocrine glands)

It should be emphasized that in the clinical situation patients are rarely admitted with one specific imbalance. Most patients have a mixture of imbalances. Furthermore, few patients display all the classic symptoms for each imbalance as described in Table 24–4. This table is intended to be a greatly oversimplified outline in which the various imbalances have been isolated and compartmentalized for easier learning.

Conditions Increasing Susceptibility to Fluid and Electrolyte Imbalances

Any person who is ill enough to be hospitalized is a candidate for the development of fluid and electrolyte imbalances. However, some patients are far more susceptible to various imbalances than others. Briefly, those persons who are most prone to fluid and electrolyte disturbances are as follows:

Patients with Diarrhea. Diarrhea is a common problem which varies greatly in severity from a mild condition to one that is life-threatening. Diarrhea is defined as

Text continued on page 504

TABLE 24–4. BASIC FEATURES OF FLUID AND ELECTROLYTE IMBALANCES[6, 7, 11, 28, 41]

ETIOLOGY	SIGNS AND SYMPTOMS	BASIC CLINICAL CARE
Water Deficit		
Water *decreases* in relation to sodium *Specific causes:* 1. Increased water output due to diarrhea; fever with profuse diaphoresis 2. Decreased water intake due to coma, unavailability of water, difficulty in swallowing 3. Impaired renal concentrating ability, such as occurs with chronic renal insufficiency 4. Iatrogenic solute loading such as excessive infusions of hypertonic solutions, excessive tube feedings of protein substances 5. Overeating highly salted foods	Thirst, dry mouth, dry sticky mucous membranes, tachycardia, oliguria, fever, apathy, stupor *Lab findings:* increased serum sodium concentration; increased urine specific gravity; increased hemoglobin concentration	1. Fluid replacement with sodium-free water 2. Observation for and treatment of shock and renal failure should they develop 3. Educating patients concerning problems connected with excessive use of salt in food (e.g., an increased incidence of hypertension occurs among heavy salt ingesters)
Water Excess (Water Intoxication)		
Water *increases* in relation to sodium *Specific causes:* 1. Excessive intake of water by mentally ill persons 2. Iatrogenic causation due to administering electrolyte-free water to sodium-depleted patients or patients with increased ADH secretion 3. Decreased water excretion due to renal disease 4. Increased water intake after loss of sodium-containing fluids, such as occurs after abdominal G.I. tract losses (e.g., diarrhea, vomiting, suction) or with diuretics, low-salt diet for cardiovascular or renal disease, frequent use of tap water enemas	*Moderate* water excess may be asymptomatic *Severe* water excess results in increased urine output, weakness, nausea, vomiting, disorientation and finally convulsions and coma due to swelling of brain cells with water *Lab findings:* decreased serum sodium concentration; decreased urine specific gravity; decreased hemoglobin concentration	1. Restriction of plain water intake; e.g., ice chips, IV solutions of 5% dextrose in water 2. Convulsions may require treatment with IV hypertonic salt solution 3. Administer sodium-containing fluids when appropriate
Saline Deficit		
Water and sodium *decrease together* *Specific causes:* 1. Large losses of body secretions and excretions due to vomiting, diarrhea, fistulous drainage, diaphoresis 2. Low salt intake while on diuretics 3. Large collections of fluid within the body, e.g., ascites (fluid collecting within the abdomen), edema (fluid collecting within tissue spaces)	Postural drop in blood pressure, loss of body weight, decrease in fullness of neck and hand veins, tachycardia, rapid respirations, fatigue, weakness, oliguria or anuria, shock (severe cases) *Lab findings:* hemoconcentration in severe deficit; low or normal plasma proteins	1. Replace fluids with IV infusions of isotonic solutions 2. Encourage sodium-containing oral fluids 3. Observe for shock or renal failure
Saline Excess		
Water and sodium *increase together* *Specific causes:* 1. Administration of excessive amounts of IV saline solutions 2. Diseases causing failure of homeostatic fluid regulation, e.g., heart disease, renal failure, liver disease 3. Administration of cortisone injections resulting in side effects of sodium and water retention	Peripheral edema (may be pitting), weight gain, puffy eyelids, pulmonary edema (excessive fluid in the alveolar spaces), ascites, distended neck veins, pleural effusion, distended hand veins *Lab findings:* decreased hematocrit; decreased plasma proteins	1. Restriction of fluids 2. Restriction of sodium 3. Administration of diuretics

TABLE 24–4.   BASIC FEATURES OF FLUID AND ELECTROLYTE IMBALANCES *(Continued)*

ETIOLOGY	SIGNS AND SYMPTOMS	BASIC CLINICAL CARE
Potassium Deficit		
1. Inadequate potassium intake due to poor diet or appetite 2. Excessive potassium loss due to diarrhea, vomiting, drainage from fistulas of small or large intestine 3. Iatrogenic causes, e.g., diuretic administration, prolonged administration of potassium-free IV solutions, excessive use of enemas and laxatives, which cause loss of potassium-containing mucus of colon	Malaise, weakness, lethargy; flabby, weak muscles of heart, intestines and respiratory system; arrhythmias; decreased intestinal motility culminating in abdominal distention and paralytic ileus; shallow respirations, which may result in apnea and respiratory arrest due to weakness of respiratory muscles; tingling and numbness of fingers and extremities *Lab findings:* decreased serum potassium below 4 mEq./L.	1. IV administration of potassium salts 2. Administration of oral potassium preparations 3. High-potassium diet, e.g., increased amounts of bananas, orange juice, coffee, tea, cola drinks, meat, chocolate
Potassium Excess		
1. Poor potassium output due to (a) renal failure or (b) oliguria following surgery 2. Excessive administration of IV solutions containing potassium 3. Excessive release of potassium from cells following severe burns, crushing injuries	Diarrhea, intestinal colic, oliguria progressing to anuria, bradycardia progressing to cardiac arrest *Lab findings:* elevated serum potassium above 5.6 mEq./L.	1. Restriction of oral and parenteral foods and fluids containing potassium 2. Hemodialysis or peritoneal dialysis may be necessary in severe cases involving renal failure
Calcium Deficit		
1. Poor dietary intake of calcium-rich foods, especially during pregnancy and lactation when calcium requirements are high 2. High losses of calcium in diarrheal stool or wound drainage 3. Disorders such as hypoparathyroidism, massive burns, pancreatitis, acute metabolic alkalosis 4. Accidental surgical removal of the parathyroid glands during thyroidectomy 5. Poor vitamin D intake and absorption	Tingling and numbness of fingers, muscle cramps, tetany, convulsions *Lab findings:* decreased serum calcium below 4.5 mEq./L.; elevated serum phosphorus	1. IV administration of a 10% solution of calcium gluconate 2. High-calcium diet 3. Oral administration of calcium lactate 4. Administration of vitamin D supplements 5. Administration of parathormone may be helpful
Calcium Excess		
1. Overactivity of parathyroid glands 2. Overconsumption of milk or mineral waters 3. Excessive movement of calcium out of bones (occurs in patients with multiple fractures and bone tumors)	Bone pain, osteoporosis, osteomalacia (softening of bone), pathologic fractures, relaxed muscles, renal stones, kidney infection, cardiac arrest *Lab findings:* elevated serum calcium concentration above 5.8 mEq./L.; decreased serum phosphate	1. Restriction of calcium intake 2. Treatment of parathyroid disorders 3. Administration of steroids, thereby lessening stress due to inflammation and resultant calcium mobilization out of bones 4. Administration of sodium sulfate and saline solutions to increase diuresis and consequent output of calcium
Magnesium Deficit		
1. Inadequate dietary intake of magnesium for a month or longer 2. Excessive losses of magnesium due to prolonged gastric suction 3. Chronic alcoholism 4. Severe renal disease 5. Prolonged administration of IV solutions without magnesium additives	Hypertension, tachycardia, tremor, twitching, pronounced neuromuscular irritability, tetany, disorientation, convulsions *Lab findings:* plasma magnesium concentration below 1.4 mEq./L.	1. Administer magnesium either in IV solutions or by IM injection 2. Increase intake of magnesium-containing foods, e.g., soybeans, cocoa, nuts, seafood, whole grains, peas, dried beans
Magnesium Excess		
1. Overdoses of magnesium in the treatment of magnesium deficit 2. Renal insufficiency resulting in magnesium retention	Decreased pulse rate, sedation deepening to coma, respiratory embarrassment, cardiac arrhythmias progressing to cardiac arrest	1. Treat underlying cause, e.g., renal failure 2. Stop all injections and infusions of magnesium

Table continued on the following page

TABLE 24–4.   BASIC FEATURES OF FLUID AND ELECTROLYTE IMBALANCES *(Continued)*

ETIOLOGY	SIGNS AND SYMPTOMS	BASIC CLINICAL CARE
Protein Deficit		
1. Inadequate intake of protein in diet 2. Abnormal losses of protein due to hemorrhage, burns, draining ulcers or wounds, ascites 3. Increased utilization of protein for rebuilding of tissues following trauma or burns 4. Increased protein catabolism as a result of elevated basal metabolism, infection, malignancy	Weight loss, loss of muscle mass and tone, fatigue, mental depression, lowered resistance to infection, anemia *Lab findings:* depressed hemoglobin, depressed hematocrit, lowered RBC count, decrease in serum albumin below 4 Gm./100 ml. (severe cases)	1. A high-protein diet that is adequate in calories and high in vitamins and minerals 2. Protein hydrolysates administered via tube feeding or parenterally
Metabolic Acidosis *(Primary Base Bicarbonate* *Deficit of ECF)*		
Basic causes: 1. Abnormal loss of $NaHCO_3$ which decreases pH of body fluids 2. An overproduction or overingestion of nonvolatile acids, overloading kidneys and resulting in failure of the renal tubules to secrete the excess H^+ *Specific causes:* 1. Abnormal losses of $NaHCO_3$ resulting from severe diarrhea; losses of pancreatic, biliary and lower bowel secretions; vomiting of *deep* GI contents 2. Overproduction of metabolically produced acids (occurs in diabetic acidosis, starvation, prolonged fasting) 3. Excessive ingestion of metabolic acids, e.g., (a) when patients are on high-fat, low-carbohydrate diets, (b) following ingestion of heavy doses of salicylic acid (salicylate intoxication), and (c) following overingestion of medications that cause H^+ overload, e.g., ferrous sulfate or paraldehyde (used to treat alcoholism) 4. Renal insufficiency (kidneys are unable to excrete overloads of acid; occurs in shock, toxic conditions, nephritis)	Deep rapid breathing (Kussmaul respirations), shortness of breath upon exertion, weakness, disorientation, sweet and fruity acetone odor to breath, coma *Lab findings:* urine pH usually below 6; plasma pH below 7.35; plasma bicarbonate below 25 mEq./L. in adults and below 20 mEq./L. in children; serum CO_2 level decreased below 22 mEq./L.	1. Treatment of underlying cause, e.g., discontinuation of high-fat diet or any drugs that are causing condition; treatment of kidney disease, diarrhea, etc. 2. Oral and parenteral fluids to correct dehydration resulting from diarrhea, vomiting, etc. 3. Fluid intake and output and daily weight records 4. Parenteral administration of a bicarbonate solution to neutralize the acid and correct the HCO_3^- deficit 5. Low-protein, high-calorie, high-carbohydrate diet

TABLE 24–4. BASIC FEATURES OF FLUID AND ELECTROLYTE IMBALANCES *(Continued)*

ETIOLOGY	SIGNS AND SYMPTOMS	BASIC CLINICAL CARE
Metabolic Alkalosis (Primary Base Bicarbonate Excess of ECF)		
Basic causes: 1. Abnormal rise in the base bicarbonate of plasma 2. Decrease in H^+ concentration of plasma, resulting in rise in blood pH *Specific causes:* 1. Ingestion of large amounts of alkali, e.g., baking soda for "acid stomach" 2. Excessive loss of H^+ from stomach due to severe vomiting or gastric suction 3. Diuretic therapy, which can cause loss of K^+ and Cl^- in urine with a compensatory increase in serum HCO_3^-	Nausea, vomiting, diarrhea, shallow slow respirations progressing to periods of apnea, cyanosis, muscle twitching, hypertonicity of muscles, tingling and numbness of fingers, tetany,* irritability, disorientation, rapid irregular pulse, convulsions *Lab findings:* pH level of serum above 7.45; urine pH often above 7; plasma bicarbonate above 29 mEq./L. in adults and above 25 mEq./L. in children; serum CO_2 increases above 32 mEq./L.; serum potassium below 4 mEq./L.	1. Correction of underlying cause, e.g., caution patient against self-treatment with alkali substances; treatment of vomiting; decrease diuretic dosage 2. Administration of appropriate replacement fluids to patient who is vomiting or receiving gastric suction 3. Administration of acidifying solutions either orally or parenterally, e.g., arginine chloride, ammonium chloride 4. Correction of potassium deficit 5. Correction of tetany (if it arises) with calcium gluconate IV
Respiratory Acidosis (Primary Carbonic Acid Excess)		
Basic cause: Respiratory abnormalities that result in failure to excrete CO_2 adequately; the retained CO_2 combines with water to form carbonic acid, causing an increase in H^+ content of blood *Specific causes:* 1. Voluntary breath holding, which can occur in children and disturbed adults 2. Chronic respiratory conditions, e.g., emphysema, asthma, bronchitis, bronchiectasis 3. Acute respiratory conditions, e.g., pneumonia, damage to brain's respiratory center 4. Overdosage with narcotics or sedatives, causing depression of medulla (respiratory center)	Difficulty in breathing, wheezing, tachycardia, cyanosis, restlessness, diaphoresis, disorientation *Lab findings:* urine pH below 6; plasma pH below 7.35; plasma bicarbonate above 29 mEq./L. in adults or 25 mEq./L. in children; blood gas carbon dioxide (Pco_2) above 38 mm. Hg	1. Correction (or at least control) of underlying respiratory condition 2. Improvement of ventilation and aeration by means of intermittent positive pressure breathing (IPPB), postural drainage, tracheostomy, use of respirator in critical cases (see Chap. 36) 3. Antibiotics to correct respiratory infections leading to occlusion of air passages
Respiratory Alkalosis (Primary Carbonic Acid Deficit)		
Basic cause: hyperventilation resulting in the excessive secretion of CO_2 leading to rise in blood pH *Specific causes of hyperventilation:* 1. Hysteria and anxiety reactions 2. Severe prolonged exercise 3. Anoxia at high altitudes, causing person to gasp for air 4. Salicylate intoxication (aspirin poisoning), which leads to overstimulation of respiratory center 5. Oxygen lack, fever, CNS diseases such as meningitis and encephalitis can all cause overstimulation of the respiratory center	Abnormally rapid respirations, lightheadedness, muscle twitch, tetany, generalized convulsions, unconsciousness *Lab findings:* urine pH above 7; plasma pH above 7.45; plasma bicarbonate depressed below 25 mEq./L. in adults and 20 mEq./L. in children; blood gas carbon dioxide (Pco_2) drops below 35 mm. Hg	1. Psychotherapy and sedation for hysterical patients 2. CO_2 treatments, e.g., ask patient to rebreathe own CO_2 from a paper bag; administer whiffs of 5% CO_2

*Tetany accompanied by muscle twitching, tingling and numbness of fingers may occur in severe metabolic alkalosis. Tetany develops because there is a marked decrease in the ionization of calcium when body fluids become alkaline. Calcium must be ionized in order to perform its functions within the ECF (e.g., reduction of neuromuscular irritability). For more details, consult a more advanced text.

the passage of liquid or unformed stool. Causes of diarrhea include emotional stress, intestinal infections, irritating foods (e.g., fried, greasy or spicy), some drugs, fecal impactions, ulcerative colitis, carcinoma and certain neurologic diseases. The three major fluid and electrolyte imbalances caused by diarrhea are (1) volume deficit; (2) potassium deficit; and (3) metabolic acidosis (see Chap. 30).

Patients Who Are Vomiting.   Like diarrhea, vomiting is an extremely common problem that accompanies numerous disorders. Causes of vomiting include emotional stress, drugs (e.g., morphine sulfate, codeine sulfate), febrile conditions, excessive alcohol intake, pain, surgery, motion sickness, pregnancy and mechanical obstruction of the gastrointestinal tract. Vomiting, if severe or prolonged, produces (1) fluid volume deficit; (2) potassium deficit; (3) magnesium deficit; (4) metabolic alkalosis; and (5) ketosis of starvation (see Chap. 23).

Patients Receiving Gastric Suction.   The purpose of gastric suction is to remove gaseous and liquid substances from the gastrointestinal tract. Postoperative patients often are placed on gastric suction; also, patients with any type of gastrointestinal obstruction may receive gastric suction. Gastric suction can potentially cause all the imbalances created by vomiting. These imbalances can be, at least in part, prevented by (a) irrigating the gastric tube with *isotonic* solutions and (b) giving the patient *isotonic* ice chips rather than ice chips made from tap water. Balanced intravenous solutions are essential for fluid and electrolyte replacement (see Chap. 41).

Patients Receiving Intestinal Suction.   Intestinal suction removes gas and liquid materials that accumulate in the intestinal tract in the presence of intestinal obstruction and/or absence of peristalsis. Intestinal suctioning can lead to metabolic acidosis and fluid volume deficit (see Chap. 41).

Patients Who Are Hemorrhaging.   Hemorrhage may follow severe burns, serious accidents, surgery and childbirth. In addition, patients who suffer from peptic ulcers, cancer, tuberculosis, esophageal varices (a complication of cirrhosis of the liver) and clotting disorders may periodically hemorrhage. Hemorrhage results in depletion of both extracellular and intracellular fluids as well as a percentage of all the electrolytes. Blood must be replaced quickly or shock will ensue.

Patients with a High Fever.   An elevated body temperature accompanies most infectious and toxic disorders. High fever may also complicate blood diseases (e.g., acute anemia and leukemia), some central nervous system disorders (e.g., head injury, upper spinal cord injuries), cancerous tumors, heat stroke, serum sickness and allergy. Furthermore, fever may be a side effect of some drugs (e.g., barbiturates, morphine, Dilantin). Prolonged fever can result in a fluid volume deficit and respiratory alkalosis due to overstimulation of the respiratory center in the medulla and the consequent increased loss of CO_2 from the lungs (see Chap. 28).

Patients with Large Draining Wounds.   Any patient with a large open wound is losing considerable amounts of fluid, protein and electrolytes. Continued heavy wound drainage eventually results in (1) protein deficit and (2) fluid volume deficit (see Chap. 42).

Patients with Edema.   Edema is the abnormal retention of fluid within the body's tissues. It is a symptom of many common diseases—e.g., congestive heart failure, hypertension, toxemia of pregnancy, burns, trauma, allergic reactions, malnutrition, kidney disease and liver disorders. Basically, edema results from (1) damage to the capillary walls, allowing fluid to drain from the vascular system; (2) interference with venous return to the heart; (3) decrease in the plasma proteins with consequent decrease in plasma oncotic pressure; (4) rise in blood hydrostatic pressure, which causes fluid to seep into the tissues; and (5) obstruction of the lymphatics. Edema can result in extracellular fluid volume deficit. As noted below, the treatment of edema can lead to further serious fluid and electrolyte problems of iatrogenic origin.

Patients Receiving Diuretic Therapy.[28]   Diuretics are prescribed to patients with edema to increase sodium and water excretion. Diuretic drugs are categorized into the following groups: (1) thiazides, (2) mercurials, (3) carbonic anhydrase inhibitors, (4) potassium-conserving diuretics and (5) other diuretics (e.g., Edecrin, Lasix). One unfortunate side effect of many diuretics is *hypokalemia* (potassium deficit). Diuretics that promote heavy potassium excretion are the thiazides, the mercurials, furosemide (Lasix), ethacrynic acid (Edecrin) and Diamox, which is a carbonic anhydrase inhibitor. Patients who are taking these diuretics must be encouraged to eat potassium-rich foods; in some cases, a potassium supplement is necessary.

Patients on Special Diets.   Special diets, because they lessen intake of certain types of foods and seasonings, predispose patients to imbalances. The *low-sodium diet* is often prescribed for patients with cardiovascular disease and kidney disease in order to control edema. Severe sodium restriction can result in saline deficit, especially if the patient is receiving diuretics at the same time he is on the diet. *Low-carbohydrate/high-protein diets,* popular in the treatment of obesity, can result in metabolic acidosis due to the accumulation of ketones in the blood and urine (see Chap. 23).

The Patient with Ascites. The abnormal accumulation of fluid and electrolytes within the abdominal cavity is called ascites. Ascites is commonly a complication of cirrhosis of the liver and congestive heart failure. Ascites varies in severity; however, as much as 20 L. of fluid can accumulate in the patient's abdominal cavity in a week, causing the patient to look "9 months pregnant." Ascitic fluid resembles plasma in its composition. Imbalances associated with ascites include (1) protein deficit, (2) water deficit, (3) fluid volume deficit and (4) shift of fluid from plasma to interstitial spaces.

Assessing and Diagnosing Patients with Suspected Imbalances

"The diagnosis of imbalances is the heart of any scheme of fluid and electrolyte balance."[6] Accurate diagnosis (both medical and nursing) depends upon a careful assessment of the patient's fluid and electrolyte status. The assessment process involves three crucial steps:

> 1. *Review of the patient's history*
> 2. *Analysis of signs and symptoms*
> 3. *Analysis of laboratory findings*

Each of these steps will be briefly considered.

The Patient's History. When reviewing the patient's history for evidence of possible imbalances, make special note of the following clues:

▶ Sudden weight gain or loss

▶ Gastrointestinal disturbances (e.g., prolonged vomiting, diarrhea, anorexia, ulcers)

▶ Disease conditions that could upset homeostatic balance (e.g., renal disease, endocrine disorders, neural malfunction, pulmonary disease)

▶ Fluid balance records that show a pronounced discrepancy between fluid intake and output

▶ Therapeutic programs that can produce imbalances (e.g., special diets, diuretic therapy, administration of drugs with emetic

action such as morphine, prolonged intravenous fluid administration, gastric suction, intestinal suction)

▶ Fever and diaphoresis

▶ Draining wounds, burns, trauma

Analysis of Signs and Symptoms. When assessing for fluid and electrolyte imbalances, the next step is to gather data concerning the patient's *signs and symptoms.* This information is based upon (a) conversations with the patient and family, (b) planned observations of the patient, and (c) the physical examination.

Turn again to Table 24–4 and note that each fluid and electrolyte imbalance is characterized by several signs and symptoms that affect *every* system of the body—cardiovascular, renal, integumentary, pulmonary, gastrointestinal, neurologic, endocrine and musculoskeletal. To further complicate the issue, several imbalances may have similar symptoms, and one imbalance can trigger the onset of another. Because the manifestations of fluid and electrolyte disturbances are so numerous, widespread, interrelated and (frankly) confusing, one must gather information about the patient with a suspected imbalance in a planned and systematic way. Therefore, as you gather data, there are a number of factors (all of which show characteristic changes in the various fluid and electrolyte upsets) to assess and evaluate. These factors are listed in Table 24–5 along with (a) significant deviations (signs and symptoms) that may signal a fluid and electrolyte disturbance and (b) examples of the fluid and electrolyte imbalances indicated by each symptom.

The majority of these factors are considered in various chapters throughout this text.* However, we will describe methods for assessing skin turgor and peripheral vein filling and emptying here.

Skin turgor describes the elasticity and shape of the skin. To assess skin turgor, pinch the patient's skin either over the clavicle (as shown in Fig. 24–14) or on the forearm. Next, observe how long it takes for the pinched skin to fall back to its original shape. Normally, the skin

---

*Vital signs are discussed in Chapters 28 and 29. Appetite is considered in Chapter 22, while thirst is discussed earlier in this chapter. Chapter 30 covers urinary and bowel elimination. Information concerning behavioral disturbances can be found in Chapter 14.

TABLE 24–5.   SYMPTOMS OF FLUID AND ELECTROLYTE IMBALANCES[6, 8, 9, 28]

SYMPTOM	RELATED FLUID AND ELECTROLYTE IMBALANCE
1. TEMPERATURE	
a. Elevated temperature	a. Water deficit
b. Subnormal temperature	b. Water excess
2. PULSE	
a. Increased bounding pulse (not easily obliterated)	a. Fluid volume excess
b. Increased thready, weak pulse	b. Fluid volume deficit
c. Weak, irregular pulse	c. Potassium deficit or excess
d. Tachycardia	d. Water deficit, magnesium deficit, fluid volume deficit
e. Bradycardia	e. Magnesium excess
3. RESPIRATIONS	
a. Deep rapid breathing (Kussmaul)	a. Metabolic acidosis, respiratory alkalosis
b. Shallow slow respirations progressing to intervals of apnea	b. Metabolic alkalosis, respiratory acidosis
c. Shallow slow respirations due to respiratory muscle weakness	c. Potassium deficit (severe) or potassium excess (severe)
d. Moist rales	d. Fluid volume excess, pulmonary edema
4. BLOOD PRESSURE	
a. Hypotension	a. Fluid volume deficit
b. Hypertension	b. Fluid volume excess, magnesium deficit
5. WEIGHT	
a. Rapid weight gain	a. Fluid volume excess
b. Rapid weight loss	b. Fluid volume deficit
c. Chronic weight loss	c. Protein deficit
6. THIRST	
a. Increased thirst	a. Decreased blood volume due to hemorrhage; water deficit resulting in hypertonic extracellular fluid
b. Absence of thirst	b. Water excess resulting in hypotonic extracellular fluid
7. APPETITE	
a. Loss of appetite (anorexia)	a. Potassium deficit; protein deficit
8. URINARY OUTPUT	
a. Decreased urinary output	a. Decreased blood volume resulting in increased secretion of ADH and aldosterone, water deficit, fluid volume deficit
b. Increased urinary output	b. Increased blood volume resulting in decreased secretion of ADH and aldosterone; water excess, fluid volume excess
9. STOOLS	
a. Hard, dry stools	a. Fluid volume deficit
b. Abdominal distention with few or no stools	b. Potassium deficit
c. Abdominal cramps accompanied by diarrhea	c. Potassium excess
10. ENERGY AND STAMINA LEVELS	
a. Easy fatigability and loss of stamina	a. Potassium deficit, water excess, protein deficit, fluid volume deficit

immediately returns to its original shape. However, skin with poor turgor (due to fluid volume deficit) tends to remain elevated in a slightly pinched position for several seconds.

Assessment of the *peripheral veins* and the speed with which they fill and empty upon changes in position also aids in evaluating a patient's state of hydration. To check peripheral vein emptying and filling, follow this simple procedure: (1) Have the patient raise his hand and hold it in an elevated position; (2) note how many seconds it takes for blood to empty from the hand veins (see Fig. 24–15); (3) have the patient lower his hand and keep it in a dependent position; and (4) note how many seconds it takes for blood to fill the veins. Normally, upon elevation of the hands, the peripheral veins empty in 3 to 5 seconds. Upon lowering the hands into a dependent position, the veins fill in 3 to 5 seconds. Veins take longer to

TABLE 24–5.   SYMPTOMS OF FLUID AND ELECTROLYTE IMBALANCES (Continued)

SYMPTOM	RELATED FLUID AND ELECTROLYTE IMBALANCE
11. FACIAL APPEARANCE a. Drawn facial appearance with sunken eyeballs b. Full, swollen appearing face with puffy eyelids	a. Severe fluid volume deficit b. Fluid volume excess
12. LEVEL OF CONSCIOUSNESS (CNS CHANGES) a. Apathy, lethargy, lassitude b. Disorientation and confusion c. Hallucinations d. Stupor terminating in unconsciousness	a. Fluid volume deficit, water excess, potassium deficit b. Water excess (water intoxication); severe potassium deficit, magnesium deficit, metabolic or respiratory acidosis c. Magnesium deficit, water excess d. Profound alkalosis, profound acidosis, shock
13. MUSCLE TONE a. Flabby muscles b. Flaccid paralysis c. Tetany d. Convulsions	a. Potassium deficit, protein deficit b. Severe potassium deficit or severe potassium excess c. Calcium deficit, metabolic alkalosis d. Magnesium deficit, calcium deficit, water excess (water intoxication), metabolic alkalosis
14. SENSATION a. Tingling and numbness of fingers b. Severe muscle cramps c. Sensation of numbness and deadness in extremities (prelude to flaccid paralysis) d. Numb extremities e. Deep bony pain and flank pain	a. Calcium deficit, metabolic alkalosis, potassium deficit b. Calcium deficit, potassium deficit c. Potassium deficit or potassium excess d. Calcium deficit, potassium deficit e. Calcium excess
15. TISSUE TURGOR a. Decreased skin turgor b. Edema of dependent parts of body c. Pitting edema d. "Finger imprinting" on sternum e. Mucous membranes dry and sticky f. Dry but otherwise normal axillae or groin (normally, apocrine sweat glands in axillae and groin are constantly producing moisture)	a. Fluid volume deficit b. Shift of fluid from vascular compartment into interstitial spaces c. Fluid volume excess d. Severe water excess e. Water deficit f. Severe water deficit
16. NECK VEINS a. Flat (collapsed) neck veins b. Distended neck veins	a. Fluid volume deficit b. Fluid volume excess
17. PERIPHERAL VEINS a. Increased vein filling time (veins not apparent) b. Increased vein emptying time (peripheral veins appear engorged)	a. Fluid volume deficit b. Fluid volume excess, shift of fluid from interstitial spaces into vascular compartment

fill when fluid volume is decreased and empty more slowly when fluid volume is excessive.

Analysis of Laboratory Findings.   Several types of laboratory tests are used to confirm or establish a diagnosis of fluid and electrolyte imbalance. *Standard diagnostic tests* include (a) a complete blood count, (b) hemoglobin estimates and (c) a complete urinalysis including a description of the odor of the urine, amount of sedimentation, urinary pH, specific gravity and tests for protein and glucose.* In addition,

there are many special diagnostic tests available for evaluating fluid and electrolyte balance.

First of all, measurements of *serum electrolyte concentrations* are essential for accurate diagnosis of electrolyte imbalances. The average values in health for the chemical constituents of plasma are listed in Table 24–6. Dangerously high and low levels of plasma sodium, potassium, calcium, magnesium, hydrogen ion (as pH) and protein are tabulated in Table 24–7.

Second, there are several laboratory tests available for measuring *hydration status* (i.e., *water-saline balance*). Note in Table 24–8 that

---

*Routine blood tests are listed in the appendix. The characteristics of urine are described in Chapter 30.

TABLE 24–6.   PLASMA CHEMICAL CONSTITUENTS: AVERAGE VALUES IN HEALTH

CONSTITUENT	NORMAL RANGE
Na^+	137–147 mEq./L.
K^+	4.0–5.6 mEq./L.
Ca^{++}	4.5–5.8 mEq./L.
Mg^{++}	1.4–2.3 mEq./L.
Cl^-	98–106 mEq./L.
HCO_3^-	Adults: 25–29 mEq./L.
	Children: 20–25 mEq./L.
Cl^- plus HCO_3^-	123–135 mEq./L.
$HPO_4^=$	1.7–2.6 mEq./L.
Protein	6–8 Gm./100 ml.
pH	7.35–7.45

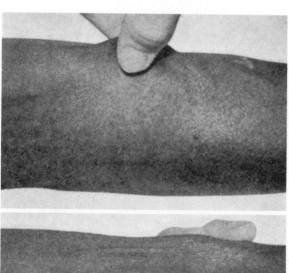

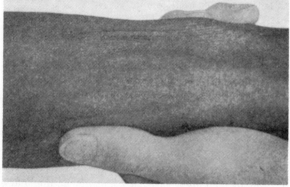

Figure 24–14.   Poor skin turgor. (Moyer, C. A.: *Fluid Balance, A Clinical Manual.* Chicago, Year Book Publishers, 1952, p. 71.)

these tests include serum osmolality, serum sodium, blood urea nitrogen, hematocrit and urine osmolality. In addition, specific gravity of urine measurements are performed to assess the patient's state of hydration. The specific gravity test indicates the degree of concentration of the urine, i.e., the amount of dissolved solids in the urine. Normally the specific gravity of urine ranges from 1.003 to 1.030. A low specific gravity develops in water excess, whereas a high specific gravity occurs in saline and water deficits. According to Grant and Kubo, "urine osmolality tests provide a more accurate measure of urine contents than do specific gravity measurements. Specific gravity is determined by the solute weight; urine osmolality describes the number of solute particles present."[14]

A third group of special laboratory tests involves determination of *blood gas values.*

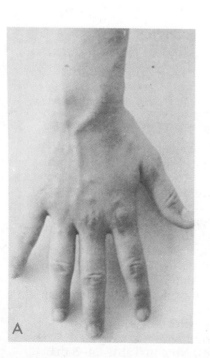

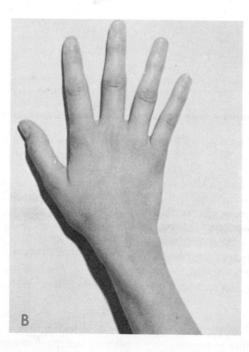

Figure 24–15. Appearance of hand veins when the hand is held in a dependent position (*A*) and in an elevated position (*B*). (From Metheny, N. M., and Snively, W. D.: *Nurses' Handbook of Fluid Balance,* 2nd ed. Philadelphia, J. B. Lippincott Co., 1974, p. 64.)

TABLE 24–7.   DANGEROUS HIGH AND LOW LEVELS OF SOLUTES IN PLASMA

	TOO HIGH		TOO LOW	
	Mild to Moderate Symptoms	*Severe Symptoms*	*Mild to Moderate Symptoms*	*Severe Symptoms*
Sodium (mEq./L.)	155–170	>170	120–130	<120
Potassium (mEq./L.)	7–9	>9	2.2–3.0	<2.2
Calcium (mEq./L.)	6–7	>7	3–4	<3
Magnesium (mEq./L.)	>5	>10(?)	1 and below (?)	<1(?)
Hydrogen ion, as pH	7.5–7.6	>7.6	7.0–7.5	<7.0
Glucose (mg./100 ml.)	1000 or above (?)	—	40–60	<40
Protein (Gm./100 ml.)	—	—	3.4–5	<3

Source: Keitel, H. G.: A primer for understanding and recognizing fluid and electrolyte imbalances. *Consultant,* 3:42–47, Feb. 1963.

These tests are used to diagnose hydrogen ion (acid-base) imbalances. As shown in Table 24–9, blood gas analysis measures blood pH, PCO_2 and PO_2.

Blood pH indicates the hydrogen ion concentration of the blood and is the most accurate measure of acid-base status. Note in Table 24–10 that the pH of the blood must be maintained within a very narrow range or severe imbalances (acidosis or alkalosis) followed by death may result.

PCO_2 is a measure of carbon dioxide tension (also called partial pressure of the blood gas carbon dioxide). Observe in Table 24–9 that the carbon dioxide tension of venous blood is higher than that of arterial blood. This test is

TABLE 24–8.   LABORATORY TESTS TO MEASURE HYDRATION STATUS

TEST	NORMAL VALUES	SIGNIFICANCE
Serum Osmolality		
Measure all particles exerting osmotic pull per unit of water; reflects total body hydration	270–300 mOsm./kg. water	Increases with dehydration; decreases with water excess
Serum Sodium		
Indirectly measures hydration because sodium is intricately related to water and fluid balance	135–147 mEq./L.	Hypernatremia indicates that water loss exceeds sodium loss Hyponatremia: false—sodium stores intact but water intake is excessive, renal blood flow is decreased true—excess loss of sodium without adequate replacement
Blood Urea Nitrogen		
Reflects difference between rate of urea synthesis and its excretion by kidney	6–22 mg./100 ml. serum	Increases with decreased renal blood flow or urine production, and in dehydration
Hematocrit		
Measures portion of blood volume occupied by RBC's	37–47 ml./100 ml. (females) 40–54 ml./100 ml. (males)	Decreases with decrease in RBC's or with normal hemoglobin and saline overload Increases with hemoconcentration, as in saline deficit
Urine Osmolality		
Measures number of particles per unit of water in urine	38–1400 mOsm./kg. water (varies greatly with diet; normal ratio of urine osmolality to serum osmolality is 4:1)	Reflects changes in urine contents more accurately than does specific gravity

Adapted from Grant, M. M., and Kubo, W. M.: Assessing a patient's hydration status. *American Journal of Nursing,* 75:1306, Aug. 1975.

TABLE 24–9.   NORMAL BLOOD GAS VALUES*

	pH	P_{CO_2}	P_{O_2}
Arterial blood	7.40	40 mm. Hg	100 mm. Hg
Mixed venous blood	7.36	46 mm. Hg	40 mm. Hg

*Average values for a 25-year-old person at rest.
Data taken from Murray, J. F.: The Normal Lung. Philadelphia, W. B. Saunders Co., 1976, p. 161.

used to help diagnose problems resulting in acidosis or alkalosis of either metabolic or respiratory origin. The P_{CO_2} is *elevated* when the H_2CO_3:$NaHCO_3$ ratio is increased and *acidosis* is present. The P_{CO_2} is *lowered* when the H_2CO_3:$NaHCO_3$ ratio is decreased and *alkalosis* is present.

P_{O_2} is the oxygen tension or the partial pressure of oxygen. In Table 24–9, observe that the P_{O_2} of arterial blood is much higher than the P_{O_2} of venous blood. A low P_{O_2} is found in patients who are hypoventilating or anoxic as a result of heart disease or respiratory disease.

Clinical Care of Patients with Fluid and Electrolyte Imbalances

Depending upon the severity of the imbalance, patients with fluid and electrolyte disturbances may have only a few mild symptoms or they may be desperately ill. Consequently, the various medical and nursing interventions used to correct fluid and electrolyte problems range from the simple to the complex.

In essence, the treatment of patients with fluid and electrolyte disturbances revolves around two concepts: (1) the *replacement* of fluids, electrolytes and nutrients and (2) the

TABLE 24–10.   pH LEVELS OF ACID-BASE BALANCE*

← 6.8	6.8–7.34	7.34–7.45	7.46–7.8	7.8 →
Death	Acidosis	Normal	Alkalosis	Death

*The narrow range of pH that supports life is between 6.8 and 7.8, but the even narrower range of normal pH is between 7.35 and 7.45.

Source: Sharer, J. E.: Reviewing acid-base balance. *American Journal of Nursing,* 75:980, June 1975; adapted from *Fluid and Electrolytes.* North Chicago, Abbott Laboratories, 1970, p. 23.

limitation of fluids and the correction of electrolyte excesses.

> Major goals of fluid replacement:
> 1. Correct pre-existing deficits *of water and electrolytes and restore, as quickly as possible, the* vascular fluid volume, *thus reducing shock and dehydration.*
> 2. *Meet the patient's* maintenance (*or life-sustaining*) *needs for fluids, electrolytes and calories.*
> 3. Replace dynamic or concurrent losses *of fluid and electrolytes from suctioning, vomiting, diarrhea and so forth.*

When fluids are ordered, the physician considers the following:

▶ The *patient:* appearance, complaints, daily weight, vital signs

▶ The *laboratory reports:* urine and blood studies

▶ The *diagnosis:* type of imbalance(s) present

▶ The daily *intake and output record*

▶ The *route* of fluid administration: by mouth, feeding tube, IV infusion, hyperalimentation, blood transfusion, bone marrow infusion

▶ The *type* of solution required: hypertonic, isotonic, hypotonic, nutrient

▶ The *rate* of fluid administration: rapid, slow, continuous

Conversely, the goal of *fluid limitation* is to reduce the fluid volume of the body in order to prevent such urgent problems as severe edema, pulmonary edema and circulatory overload. Fluids are limited in such conditions as fluid volume excess and in certain cardiac and renal disorders.

More specifically, treatment of patients with fluid and electrolyte imbalances is based upon the following measures: (a) recording intake and output and daily weights; (b) regulation of diet; (c) regulation of oral fluid intake; (d) administration of medications; (e) tube feeding; (f) intravenous infusions; (g) blood transfusions; (h) parenteral hyperalimentation; and (i) bone marrow transfusions.

Recording Intake and Output and Daily Weight.   The fluid balance record and the record of the patient's daily weight are valuable aids in diagnosing fluid and electrolyte imbalances and in calculating fluid replacement needs easily.

> *To obtain accurate* daily weight *measures, it is essential to weigh the patient at the same time every day (preferably before breakfast), on the same scale, in the same clothing and after the patient has voided.*

Patients who are rapidly losing weight are losing body fluid; patients who are rapidly gaining weight are retaining body fluid.

Although weight can easily be measured accurately, *fluid balance records* are notorious for being inaccurate and imprecise. Causes for error in recording intake and output include (a) failure on the part of the staff to comprehend the value of these records; (b) poor communication among staff members concerning which patients are on fluid balance; (c) guessing at measurements rather than actually measuring fluids, urine and liquid stools; (d) failure to estimate losses from perspiration, incontinence and wound exudate; (e) failure to measure fluids used to irrigate the patient's bladder, wound or gastric tube; and (f) failure to explain the fluid balance record and its importance to the patient and his family. The fluid balance record (intake and output record) is discussed further in Chapter 22.

Regulation of Diet. Planned changes in diet can correct some fluid and electrolyte imbalances. For example, patients with potassium deficit, calcium deficit or magnesium deficit may benefit greatly from *adding foods* containing the deficient electrolyte to their daily diet, provided that urine output is adequate; e.g., orange juice and bananas are high in potassium; milk, cheese and green leafy vegetables are high in calcium; soybeans, cocoa and nuts are high in magnesium. Likewise, patients suffering from a protein deficiency need to increase their consumption of meat, fowl, fish, eggs and other high-protein foods.

On the other hand, treatment of other imbalances depends upon the *restriction* of foods containing certain electrolytes. For instance, patients who suffer from salt excess or fluid volume excess will need to restrict salt. In some cases it may be enough to simply avoid adding salt to food during cooking or at the table. In other cases, complicated by heart or renal disease, it may be necessary to restrict foods containing large amounts of sodium, e.g., buttermilk, ice cream, bread. The low-sodium diet is discussed in Chapter 23.

Regulation of Oral Fluid Intake. Depending upon the imbalance, the intake of fluids by mouth may need to be either increased or restricted.

Oral fluids are *increased* ("forced") when (a) body fluids must be replenished or replaced, e.g., in water deficit, fluid volume deficit, hemorrhage; and (b) the patient is not vomiting, does not have dysphagia (difficulty in swallowing) and the situation is not an emergency. Medical and nursing orders for oral fluid replacement must be precise; i.e., they should state the *amount* of oral fluid the patient should receive each day as well as the *type* of fluid (water, juice, soup). In addition, intake and output records must be accurate to be useful in evaluating the patient's response to his fluid order.

Fluids are *restricted* in water excess, fluid volume excess and circulatory overload. Fluids must be carefully measured and spaced throughout the day so that the patient does not suffer unduly from thirst. Methods for forcing fluids and restricting fluids are discussed in Chapter 22.

Administration of Medications. A number of medications are available for correcting fluid and electrolyte imbalances. For example, diuretics are typically ordered to promote water excretion in fluid volume excess. Oral and IV potassium preparations help alleviate potassium deficit. Intravenous solutions of calcium gluconate and oral dosages of calcium lactate and vitamin D are administered in calcium deficit. Magnesium preparations given either IV or IM are prescribed for patients with magnesium deficit. Alkalizing preparations (e.g., sodium bicarbonate, 1 to 3 ampules) are given IV for persons with metabolic acidosis. Acidifying preparations (e.g., ammonium chloride or arginine chloride) are administered either orally or IV to patients suffering from metabolic alkalosis.

Tube Feeding. Tube feeding (or gastric lavage) is the administration of feedings into the stomach by means of a tube. Tube feedings are used to nourish those patients who are capable of digesting and absorbing nutrients but, because of their condition, are unable to eat normally. The specific conditions that indicate the need for tube feedings are as follows: (a) unconsciousness or semiconsciousness; (b) dysphagia (swallowing difficulties); (c) extreme anorexia; (d) extreme weakness and debility; (e) disorientation; (f) major psychoses; and (g) oral surgery.

For tube feedings to nourish a patient adequately, the feeding formula must contain sufficient calories, minerals, vitamins and water to accomplish the following:

▶ Meet the patient's *basal requirements* for calories, water, minerals and vitamins

▶ *Replace abnormal losses* due to vomiting, diarrhea, drainage, etc.

▶ Supply sufficient *protein* for tissue synthesis and repair

▶ Supply *electrolytes* and *vitamins* that are particularly necessary for cell growth and tissue healing (e.g., potassium, magnesium, vitamin C)

▶ Prevent solute overload

Tube feeding *formulas* fall into three basic categories:[19]

1. Tube feeding mixtures that are *commercially prepared* and sold (e.g., Sustagen, Meritine, Ensure). The protein in these mixtures is derived from milk. These nutrient solutions are either premixed or sold in powdered form, which is reconstituted with measured amounts of water. Diarrhea and expense are the two major disadvantages of commercially prepared tube feedings.

2. Tube feedings *prepared in a blender*, in which solid and semisolid foods are liquefied (Table 24–11). "Blenderized" feedings are preferable to commercially prepared feedings because they are less expensive, are often better balanced nutritionally and are better tolerated by most patients.

3. *Low-residue* (low-bulk) tube feedings that are *commercially prepared* (e.g., Vivonex, W-T, Flexical, Precision LR). Low-residue feedings supply protein in one of these forms: (a) crystalline amino acids, (b) casein hydrolysate and (c) egg albumin. These diets offer three advantages: (1) they are easily absorbed, (2) minimal digestion is necessary and (3) stool bulk is decreased (essential in some conditions of the colon).

Information concerning routes for tube feedings, types of feedings, methods of feeding, tube feeding complications and general nursing care can be found in Chapter 41, which discusses the clinical care of patients with gastric and intestinal tubes.

Intravenous Infusions. Because of the dangers inherent in parenteral (by injection) administration, fluids and electrolytes should be administered whenever possible by the *oral route* (either by mouth or by tube) rather than by the intravenous route.* However, when a patient *must* receive fluids, electrolytes or medications swiftly or (in some cases) over a long period of time, the method of choice is intravenous administration. More specifically, intravenous infusions are ordered for patients under these circumstances:

▶ Patients in *life-threatening situations* (e.g., hemorrhage, shock, severe burns). Under these drastic conditions, IV fluids (which directly enter the vascular system, thereby

---

*The venipuncture procedure and the complications of venipuncture are discussed in Chapter 38.

TABLE 24–11.   TUBE FEEDING PREPARED FROM FOOD

	DIET SUPPLYING 1 KCAL./ML.	DIET SUPPLYING 1.5 KCAL./ML.
Baby meat	210 ml.	210 ml.
Egg	50 ml. (frozen)	60 ml. (dried)
Applesauce	120 ml.	—
Orange juice	240 ml. (reconstituted)	100 ml. (concentrated)
Whipped potatoes	200 ml.	—
Refined cereal	100 ml.	—
Oil	45 ml.	45 ml.
Milk	960 ml.	480 ml.
Strained carrots	100 ml.	60 ml.
Dextrose	60 Gm.	12 Gm.
Skim milk powder	—	60 Gm.
Total amount	2000 ml.	1000 ml.
Percentage of total calories		
Protein	16%	23%
Fat	40%	46%
Carbohydrate	44%	31%
Osmolality	567 mOsm./L.	1000 mOsm./L.

Adapted from Hoffman, J. S.: Tube feeding. *In* Condon, R. E., and Nyhus, L. M. (eds.): *Manual of Surgical Therapeutics,* 3rd ed. Philadelphia, F. A. Davis Co., 1974, p. 215.

immediately increasing plasma volume) are absolutely necessary.

▶ Patients who may have *nothing by mouth* or who are *unable to ingest oral liquids* owing to prolonged nausea, vomiting, diarrhea, peritonitis, paralytic ileus or fistula.

▶ Patients who require *medications* that, if given orally, will be destroyed by the gastric juices or will not be absorbed by the gastrointestinal tract.

▶ Patients who, because of their condition, are *unable to digest or absorb a diet* administered by mouth or tube; e.g., individuals who do not have an anatomically and functionally intact intestinal tract because of burns, sepsis or neurologic disorders. Such patients may require the administration of IV fluids over a long period of time.

When selecting a *site* for administration of IV fluids, it is essential to consider (a) the condition of the vein (if collapsed or too small, it cannot be used), (b) the characteristics of the tissue over the vein (edematous, injured), (c) the purpose and duration of the infusion, (d) the type and amount of IV fluid ordered and (e) the diagnosis and condition of the patient. Stroot classifies the available sites for venipuncture this way:[41]

The available sites are the superficial veins of the extremities. The most commonly used veins in the order of the frequency of their use are as follows:
1. Veins of the forearm (basilic, cephalic)
2. Veins around the *cubital fossa* (antecubital, cephalic, basilic)
3. Veins in the radial area
4. Veins in the hand
5. Veins in the thigh (femoral, saphenous)
6. Veins in the foot
7. Veins in the scalp (infant and elderly)

Once a venipuncture site is selected, the *method* of venipuncture is decided upon. The chosen vein may be entered via (1) a small steel needle (butterfly, standard); (2) a plastic catheter or tubing threaded through a metal needle (Intracath); or (3) a catheter that is placed into the vein by means of a minor surgical procedure called a cutdown. These methods and the equipment used are discussed in Chapter 38.

The *type of intravenous solution* ordered will depend upon the patient's condition and the fluid and electrolyte imbalance. There are many substances that can be infused intravenously; e.g., carbohydrates, protein hydrolysates, electrolytes, alcohol, vitamins, water and some medications. In addition, parenteral fluids vary in their *tonicity;* thus IV fluids may be either hypotonic, isotonic or hypertonic. A summary of these three types of solutions is presented in Table 24–12. A list of some commonly used IV solutions, along with their purposes and tonicity, is presented in Table 24–13.

Because of the grave dangers inherent in parenteral therapy, the *physician's orders* for IV fluids and electrolytes must be as precise, clear and exact as are prescriptions for dangerous or potentially lethal medications.

Unfortunately, physicians, like nurses and other professional people, are sometimes careless or hurried and, as a result, neglect to write clear and complete orders. A *safe order* for parenteral infusions should include the following items:

1. The *specific solution* or solutions the patient is to receive; if more than one bottle of solution is to be given, the bottles should be numbered consecutively.

2. The *additive solutions*, if any, should be written out, as well as the number of milliliters or milliequivalents to be given. The doctor

TABLE 24–12. KEY FACTS ABOUT PARENTERAL FLUIDS

TYPE OF SOLUTION	EXAMPLE	DESCRIPTION AND USES	RATE OF INFUSION
Hypotonic	NaCl 0.45%	Will cause water to flow into cells by osmosis; can cause water intoxication	2 ml./min.
Isotonic	Dextrose 5% in water, normal saline—0.9%, lactated Ringer's,* dextrose 2.5% in 0.45% NaCl	Has the same osmotic pressure as plasma and body fluids	1–3 ml./min.
Hypertonic	Dextrose 10% in water, dextrose 5% in 0.45% NaCl or in normal saline, dextrose 5% or 10% in lactated Ringer's*	Will draw water out of cells, shrinking them; can cause dehydration	1–2 ml./min.

*Lactated Ringer's per 100 ml.: NaCl 0.6 Gm., KCl 0.03 Gm., CaCl 0.02 Gm., Na lactate 0.31 Gm.
Source: modified from Kee, J. L.: Fluid imbalance in elderly patients. *Nursing '73*, 3:42. 1973.

TABLE 24–13.   COMMONLY USED IV SOLUTIONS:
PURPOSES AND TONICITY

IV SOLUTIONS	PURPOSE	TONICITY
5% dextrose/0.45% saline	Hydrating	Hypertonic
5% dextrose/0.9% saline	Replacement	Hypertonic
5% dextrose/water	Fluid and calories	Isotonic
2.5% dextrose/0.45% saline	Hydrating	Isotonic
5% dextrose/0.25% saline	Hydrating	Hypertonic
10% dextrose/water	Fluid and calories	Hypertonic
lactated Ringer's	Replacement	Isotonic
1/6 molar sodium lactate	Replacement	Isotonic
0.45% saline	Hydrating	Hypotonic
0.9% saline	Replacement	Isotonic

(From Livingston.[26])

should specify whether the solution is to be added to the bottle or placed into the tubing.

3. A rough *time schedule* should be included if more than one IV is ordered.

4. If a single IV is ordered, either the time for its *completion* or the *drip rate per minute* must be specified.

5. A *maximum drip rate* should be ordered in case the IV (or IV's) get behind schedule.

The following is an example of an *acceptable order* for parenteral fluids:

8/17/78   #6 IV 1000 ml. 5% dextrose/water. Add to bottle KCl 20 mEq.
Start at 8 AM and run to 4 PM.
#7 IV 1000 ml. 5% dextrose/saline.
Start at 4 PM and run to midnight; then discontinue both IV's.
Run IV's #6 and #7 no faster than 150 gtt./minute even if behind schedule.

An example of a *questionable* order that you should *not* accept without further clarification from the doctor is:

8/17/78   #6 IV 1000 ml. 5% dextrose/water, add KCl 20 mEq.
#7 IV 1000 ml. 5% dextrose/saline.
Discontinue IV's following this infusion.

This order leaves far too much to the discretion of the nurse. A schedule, maximum drip rate, and instructions concerning additive medicines are all missing. With this order, it would be possible to either overload the patient with fluid or fail to hydrate him rapidly enough. Such serious errors can be avoided by clarifying with the physician any sketchy instruction concerning parenteral fluid infusions.

Keeping the IV *on schedule* (thereby avoiding overhydration or underhydration of the patient) is a major nursing responsibility. The most accurate way to regulate the flow of IV infusions, is to *mathematically calculate the rate of flow*. Formulas that can be used to calculate the rate of flow for IV fluids are as follows:[26]

$$\text{ml./hr.} = \frac{\text{total amt. fluid to be given (in ml.)}}{\text{total time for infusion (in hr.)}}$$

$$\text{gtt./min.} = \frac{\text{total vol. (ml.)} \times \text{drop factor (gtt./ml.)}}{\text{total time of infusion (in min.)}}$$

$$\text{gtt./min.} = \frac{\text{ml./hr.}}{60 \text{ min./hr.}} \times \frac{\text{gtt.}}{\text{ml.}}$$

Note that the IV flow rate in two of the formulas above have been computed on the basis of drops (guttae, abbreviated gtt.) of solution to be infused per minute. To compute the number of drops to be administered per minute, you must first check the *drop factor* for the particular type of IV set being used. The drop factor is usually given on the outside of the package containing the IV equipment. The drop factor is defined as *the number of drops necessary to deliver 1 ml. of fluid to the patient*. As implied above, the drop factor varies according to the pharmaceutical company that has produced the IV apparatus. Common drop factors are 15 drops/ml., 20 drops/ml. and 60 drops/ml. Sets that deliver *large* drops (15 and 20 drops/ml.) are called *macro-drip* sets, and are used for adults. Sets that deliver *small* drops (60 drops/ml.) are called *micro-drip* sets and are used for children.

Once the drop factor has been determined, it is fairly simple (with the use of a formula) to obtain the desired IV flow rate in drops per minute. Consider the two examples below.

Example 1
Amount and type of solution: 1000 ml. 5% dextrose/water
Time limit: to be infused in 8 hours
Drop factor: using macro-drip set, which requires 15 drops to deliver 1 ml. of fluid
Flow rate (gtt./min.)

$$\frac{1000 \text{ ml.} \times 15 \text{ gtt./ml.}}{60 \text{ min./hr.} \times 8 \text{ hr.}} =$$

$$\frac{15,000 \text{ gtt.}}{480 \text{ min.}} = 31 \text{ gtt./min.}$$

Example 2
Amount and type of solution: 500 ml. of 0.45% saline
Time limit: to be infused in 12 hours
Drop factor: using micro-drip set, which requires 60 drops to deliver 1 ml. of fluid
Flow rate (gtt./min.)

$$\frac{500 \text{ ml.} \times 60 \text{ gtt.}}{(60 \text{ min.} \times 12 \text{ hr.})} = \frac{30,000 \text{ gtt.}}{720 \text{ min.}}$$

$$= 42 \text{ gtt./min.}$$

A second (highly accurate) way to calculate IV flow rates is by means of *slide rule IV drop calculators,* which are available through some of the commercial drug houses, e.g., Abbott Laboratories, Cutter Laboratories, and Baxter Laboratories.

A third way to keep an IV on schedule is to place a *long strip of adhesive tape on the side of the IV bottle next to the milliliter calibrations.* The tape is then marked to show the amount of solution the patient should receive every hour in order to complete the IV on time. For example, if the patient is to receive 1000 ml. in 8 hours, you know that he will have to receive 125 ml. every hour. If the IV starts at 8 AM, the tape is then marked to show that by 9 AM 125 ml. should have been infused, and 875 ml. should be left in the bottle; by 10 AM 250 ml. should have been infused, with 750 ml. left, and so forth. This simple and practical method of IV scheduling is illustrated in Figure 24–16.

Finally, IV infusion pumps are used to deliver IV fluids precisely, at a preset drip rate.

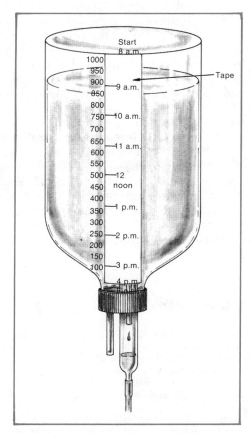

Figure 24–16. Tape attached to IV bottle to assist with keeping intravenous infusions on schedule.

Once the IV is started and throughout the period during which it is running, it is essential to make the following vital assessments:

1. The patient: *assess for signs of circulatory overload (headache, dizziness, difficult breathing) and reactions to medications within the infusion (e.g., K^+ excess, Ca^{++} excess).*

2. Urinary output: *assess for adequacy of renal function; poor urinary output could cause circulatory overload.*

3. The infusion site: *assess for (a) signs of infiltration of IV fluids into the tissues (swelling, hardness, pain at needle site, feeling of coldness around injection site, evidence of tissue necrosis) and (b) signs of thrombophlebitis (redness, warmth and tenderness at puncture site and along vein).*

4. The needle site: *observe if needle is in place and attached to IV tubing. Check if tape is adequately anchoring needle to skin.*

5. The flow rate: *make certain (a) that the flow rate has been properly calculated and (b) that the IV is dripping according to scheduled number of drops per minute. To check the flow rate, count the number of drops that fall into the "drip chamber" for 1 minute (or count drops for 15 seconds and multiply by 4).*

6. The IV bottle: *at beginning of your shift note the level of fluid in the bottle; also note which medications have been added to the bottle. Check fluid level frequently. If more than one IV is ordered, bring next bottle to bedside once fluid (currently running) has reached the neck of the bottle. Observe the height of the bottle; it should be about 3 ft. above the needle site.*

7. The IV tubing: *tubing should not be kinked because kinking reduces fluid flow.*

8. The armboard: *when an armboard is used, make certain that it is positioned comfortably and that it does not occlude circulation.*

Blood Transfusions. Blood transfusions are administered to restore blood volume following hemorrhage or severe trauma. Types of transfusions, blood group systems, typing and cross matching, safe blood administration, and transfusion reactions are discussed in detail in Chapter 39.

Parenteral Hyperalimentation.* Metheny and

---

*Parenteral hyperalimentation is also discussed in Chapter 23.

Snively define parenteral hyperalimentation as "a method of feeding a patient who cannot tolerate an oral feeding or in whom it is necessary to bypass the gastrointestinal tract.[28] When parenteral hyperalimentation is ordered, the patient is infused with large amounts of essential nutrients required by the body for tissue synthesis and growth and for anabolism.

Because they must meet the patient's total nutritional needs, *solutions* used for parenteral hyperalimentation contain far more nutrients and calories than do ordinary IV solutions. These solutions also contain vitamins and minerals; in addition, electrolytes can be added as necessary. Two examples of parenteral infusion solutions are (a) protein hydrolysate basic fluid and (b) crystalline amino acid solution.

A hyperalimentation IV is usually *administered* into the *subclavian vein*. According to Schulte, the central parenteral nutrition catheter is the patient's "lifeline." Consequently, this catheter must be inserted and cared for under strict aseptic technique; also, it must not be dislodged.[34]

Major *complications* of parenteral hyperalimentation include the following:

Sepsis: The *catheter* may become contaminated during insertion, or infection may develop around the catheter site when it is left in place for a long period of time. A further danger is that the *IV solution* may become contaminated due to breaks in sterile technique by ward personnel. It is essential that these solutions hang for no longer than 8 hours and that the tubing and filter are changed daily using meticulous sterile technique.

Catheter dislocation: If the catheter was improperly inserted, the patient may suffer pneumothorax, hydrothorax or air embolism, among other complications.

Osmotic diuresis: If the parenteral feeding is given too rapidly, the patient will develop a *glucose overload* and will consequently undergo excessive diuresis; if diuresis remains unchecked, extreme *dehydration* followed by shock and death will ensue. Signs precipitated by too rapid administration of hyperalimentation fluids include headache, nausea, and lassitude culminating in convulsions. In addition, urinary sugar content is greatly elevated.

When caring for patients receiving parenteral hyperalimentation, it is essential to make the following observations:

1. The patient: *check vital signs, urinary output (excessive?) and body weight. Carefully assess for signs of dehydration.*

2. Urine sugar and acetone: *a high urine sugar could signal osmotic diuresis.*

3. The infusion site: *check for signs of infection or inflammation.*

4. The IV solution: *make certain the infusion isn't flowing too rapidly. Also check that the bottle doesn't hang at the bedside for more than 8 hours.*

In addition, because parenteral hyperalimentation is a hazardous procedure, the observant nurse checks for signs that this therapy can be discontinued and the patient returned to oral or tube feedings. With this goal in mind, the nurse should note (a) the cessation of nausea and vomiting and (b) a willingness on the patient's part to drink and eat small amounts of nutrients.

Bone Marrow Transfusions. Bone marrow transfusions are currently being used in emergency situations in which the patient needs fluid *immediately* and it is not possible (owing to collapsed veins or limited time) to cannulate a vein. In a report by Valdez, a long, sharp 14-gauge needle was inserted into the bone marrow of a tibial malleolus (ankle) at an angle of 20 degrees. Apparently, the patient reported little pain during the procedure. During a 30-day period the patient's bone marrow was infused with approximately 42 L. of fluid. During this period not a single infection developed, nor were there any signs of embolism.[29, 43]

Nevertheless, when the bone marrow route is used for infusions, it is essential to observe for signs of infection and tissue slough around the site of injection as well as for embolism. Meticulous aseptic technique is mandatory both when inserting the needle into the bone marrow and while caring for the injection site. To keep the infusion open, the needle must be flushed daily with normal saline.

BIBLIOGRAPHY

1. Abbott Laboratories: *Fluid and Electrolytes.* Chicago, Abbott Laboratories, 1971.
2. Beland, I., et al.: *Clinical Nursing,* 3rd ed. New York, The Macmillan Co., 1975.
3. Beyers, M., and Dudas, S.: *The Clinical Practice of Medical Surgical Nursing.* Boston, Little, Brown and Co., 1977.
3a. Borgen, L.: Total parenteral nutrition in adults. *American Journal of Nursing,* 78:224, Feb. 1978.

3b. Brin, M., and Bauernfeind, J. C.: Vitamin needs of the elderly. *Postgraduate Medicine, 63*:155, March 1978.

4. Burke, S.: *The Composition and Function of Body Fluids,* 2nd ed. St. Louis, The C.V. Mosby Co., 1976.

5. Cameron, S., et al.: *Nephrology for Nurses.* Flushing, NY, Medical Examination Publishing Co., 1976.

5a. Cohen, S.: Metabolic acid-base disorders: part 3: Clinical and laboratory findings. *American Journal of Nursing,* 78:P.I. 1, March 1978.

6. Condon, R. E.: Fluid and Electrolyte Therapy. *In* Condon, R. E., and Nyhus, L. M. (eds.): *Manual of Surgical Therapeutics,* 3rd ed. Philadelphia, F. A. Davis Co., 1974.

7. Contiguglia, S. R., et al.: Electrolyte Disorders. *In* Friedman, H. H., and Papper, S. (eds.): *Problem-Oriented Medical Diagnosis.* Boston, Little, Brown and Co., 1975.

8. del Bueno, D. J.: Electrolyte imbalance: how to recognize and respond to it. Part I. *RN, 38*:52, Feb. 1975.

9. del Bueno, D. J.: Electrolyte imbalance: how to recognize and respond to it. Part 2. *RN, 38*:54, March 1975.

9a. del Bueno, D. J.: A quick review on using blood-gas determinations. *RN, 41*:68, March 1978.

10. Dickens, M. L.: *Fluid and Electrolyte Balance: A Programmed Text,* 3rd ed. Philadelphia, F. A. Davis Co., 1974.

10a. Dudrick, S. J.: A patient on I.V. therapy need not starve! *Consultant, 18*:142, Feb. 1978.

11. Friedman, H. H., and Papper, S.: *Problem-Oriented Medical Diagnosis.* Boston, Little, Brown and Co., 1975.

12. Ganong, W. F.: *Review of Medical Physiology,* 6th ed. Los Altos, CA, Lange Medical Publications, 1973.

13. Goldberg, M.: Water control and the dysnatremias. *In* Bricker, N. S. (ed.): *The Sea Within Us.* New York, Searle and Co., Science and Medicine Publishing Co., 1975.

14. Grant, M. M., and Kubo, W. M.: Assessing a patient's hydration status. *The American Journal of Nursing,* 75:1306, Aug. 1975.

15. Guyton, A. C.: *Textbook of Medical Physiology,* 5th ed. Philadelphia, W. B. Saunders Co., 1976.

16. Guyton, A. C., Taylor, A. E., and Granger, H. J.: *Circulatory Physiology II: Dynamics and Control of the Body Fluids.* Philadelphia, W. B. Saunders Co., 1975.

17. Hallal, J. C.: Thyroid disorders. *The American Journal of Nursing,* 77(3):417, March 1977.

18. Heath, J. K.: A conceptual basis for assessing body water status. *Nursing Clinics of North America,* 6:189, March 1971.

19. Hoffman, J.: Tube feeding. *In* Condon, R. E., and Nyhus, L. M. (eds.): *Manual of Surgical Therapeutics,* 3rd ed. Philadelphia, F. A. Davis Co., 1974.

20. Kee, J. L.: Fluid imbalances in elderly patients. *Nursing '73,* 3:49, 1973.

20a. Kemp, G., and Kemp D.: Diuretics. *American Journal of Nursing,* 78:1007, June 1978.

21. Klein, W.: Critical electrolyte problems. *Emergency Medicine,* July 1973, p. 79.

21a. Keitel, H. G.: A primer for understanding and recognizing fluid and electrolyte imbalances. *Consultant,* 3:42–47, Feb. 1963.

22. Krueger, J. A., and Ray, J. C.: *Endocrine Problems in Nursing.* St. Louis, The C. V. Mosby Co., 1976.

23. Leaf, A., and Cotran, R.: *Renal Pathophysiology.* New York, Oxford University Press, 1976.

24. Lee, C. A., et al.: Extracellular Volume Imbalance. *American Journal of Nursing,* 74:888, May 1974.

25. Lee, C. A., et al.: What to do when acid-base problems hang in the balance. *Nursing '75,* Aug. 1975.

26. Livingston, C.: Assisting with Intravenous Therapy. *Nursing Process II Syllabus.* Seattle, University of Washington School of Nursing, Summer 1975.

27. Medical Staff, Lilly Research Laboratories: Clinical application of fluid and electrolyte balance. *Physicians' Bulletin, 26*:2, Feb. 1961.

28. Metheny, N. M., and Snively, W. D.: *Nurses' Handbook of Fluid Balance,* 2nd ed. Philadelphia, J. B. Lippincott Co., 1974.

28a. Metheny, N. A., and Snively, W. D.: Perioperative fluids and electrolytes. *American Journal of Nursing,* 78:840, May 1978.

29. Michaels, R. M. (ed.): Bone marrow as an emergency route for fluids. *Nurses' Drug Alert, 1*:156, Nov. 1977.

29a. Murray, J. F.: *The Normal Lung.* Philadelphia, W. B. Saunders Co., 1976, p. 161.

30. Oakes, A., and Morrow, H.: Understanding blood gases. *Nursing '73,* 3:15, Sept. 1973.

31. Pitts, R. F.: *Physiology of the Kidney and Body Fluids.* Chicago, Year Book Medical Publishers, 1963.

32. Plumer, A. L.: *Principles and Practice of Intravenous Therapy,* 2nd ed. Boston, Little, Brown and Co., 1975.

33. Reed, G. M., and Sheppard, V. F.: *Regulation of Fluid and Electrolyte Balance: A Programmed Instruction in Physiology for Nurses.* Philadelphia, W. B. Saunders Co., 1971.

34. Schulte, W. J.: Parenteral nutrition (hyperalimentation). *In* Condon, R. E., and Nyhus, L. M. (eds.): *Manual of Surgical Therapeutics,* 3rd ed. Philadelphia, F. A. Davis Co., 1974.

35. Scribner, B. H. (ed.): *University of Washington Teaching Syllabus for the Course on Fluid and Electrolyte Balance,* 7th ed. Seattle, University of Washington School of Medicine, 1969.

35a. Shafer, N.: The puzzle of postural hypotension. *Consultant, 18*:66, May 1978.

36. Sharer, J. E.: Reviewing acid-base balance. *American Journal of Nursing,* 75:980, June 1975.

37. Slonim, N. B.: Blood-gas and pH abnormalities. *In* Friedman, H. H., and Papper, S. (eds.): *Problem-Oriented Medical Diagnosis.* Boston, Little, Brown and Co., 1975.

38. Snively, W. D., and Roberts, K. T.: The clinical picture as an aid to understanding body fluid disturbances. *Nursing Forum, 12*:133, 1973.

39. Spencer, R. T.: *Patient Care in Endocrine Problems.* Philadelphia, W. B. Saunders Co., 1973.

40. Stolar, V. (Consultant): *Human Acid-Base Chemistry: Programmed Instruction.* New York, The American Journal of Nursing Co., 1973.

41. Stroot, V., et al.: *Fluid and Electrolytes: A Practical Approach.* Philadelphia, F. A. Davis Co., 1974.

42. Tepperman, J.: *Metabolic and Endocrine Physiology,* 3rd ed. Chicago, Year Book Medical Publishers, 1973.

42a. Twombly, M.: The shift into third space. *Nursing '78,* 8:38, June 1978.

43. Valdez, M.: Intraosseous fluid administration in emergencies. *Lancet, 1*:1235, June 11, 1977.

44. Vander, A. J., et al.: *Human Physiology: The Mechanisms of Body Function,* 2nd ed. New York, McGraw-Hill Book Co., 1975.

45. Wolf, A. V.: Thirst. *Scientific American, 194*:70, 1956.

UNIT
VIII
BASIC CLINICAL CONSIDERATIONS

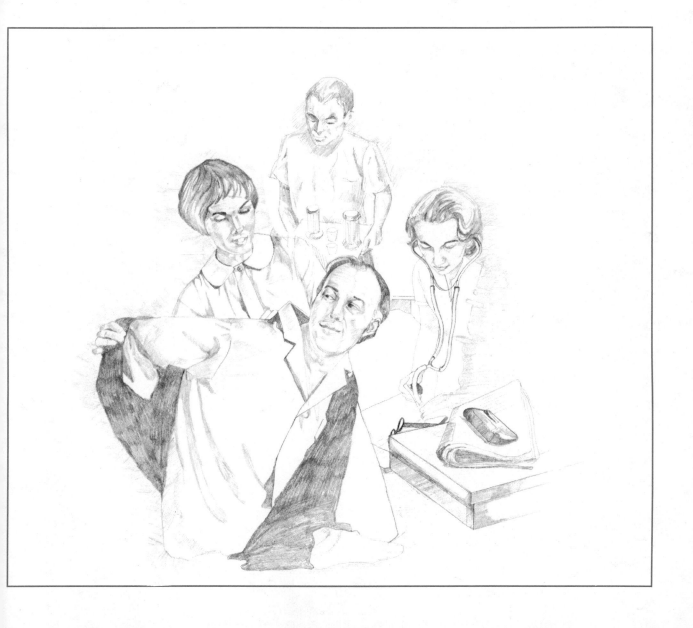

CHAPTER 25

PROVIDING A SAFE AND THERAPEUTIC ENVIRONMENT

By Mary A. Chelgren, R.N., Ph.D.

OVERVIEW AND STUDY GUIDE

Ill persons enter health care institutions for care, comfort and cure. The environment supporting the individual should be therapeutic. Key terms associated with this environment include the following:

antibiotics	isolation
antiseptic	reverse isolation
bacteria	laminar flow room
resident	microbes
transient	nosocomial
bactericidal	pathogens
contamination	sensitivity
disinfectant	sensory stimulation
epidemiology	deprivation
fomite	overload
germicide	sepsis, asepsis
humidity	sterile
immunization	virulent
infection	virus
infection chain	

Upon mastery of this chapter, you should be able to:

1. Describe factors composing a desirable therapeutic environment for ill persons.
2. Differentiate between environmental factors that can be easily manipulated (controlled) and those which cannot be manipulated.
3. Identify environmental factors that may have either positive or negative influence on the course of an individual's illness.
4. List links (elements) in the infection chain and at least two means by which each link may be broken.
5. Recognize and list comfort and safety hazards in an individual's therapeutic environment along with methods to alleviate the hazards.
6. Describe modifications that can be made to maintain a desirable therapeutic environment based on a person's age, culture, religion, treatment and illness status.
7. Identify special needs of individuals being cared for in unusual types of environments, e.g., ICU, CCU, isolation, reverse isolation.

INTRODUCTION

Entering a health care facility poses a crisis for the patient as well as for those persons physically and emotionally close to him. Since the health care facility is designed to support the patient during his crisis, certain conditions in both the personnel and the physical surroundings are desirable. The hospital milieu carries certain potential threats or hazards for the patient. Thus, it is important to consider *environmental factors* such as temperature, humidity, light, noise and dust; factors of *physical safety* such as fire, mechanical injury, chemical injury, electrical injury and radiation injury; *psychologic factors* such as the need for communication, concern about personal effects, fear, loneliness and anxiety; and factors of *bacteriologic safety*, including nosocomial and community-acquired infections. Health personnel can consciously minimize these threats and thus create a safe, helpful therapeutic environment.

Whenever a patient enters a health care facility, the surroundings as well as his *personal characteristics* must be considered. For exam-

521

ple, the needs and characteristics of an elderly person are different from those of a child. Likewise, persons with sensory deficits have needs different from those of persons without such deficits. In addition, religious preference, cultural background, type of illness and treatment protocol all influence the patient's stay in a given environment. The nurse again seeks to be aware of these factors in order to take advantage of and compensate for them as needed in relating to the patient and assisting in his care and adaptation.

HOSPITALIZATION

Regardless of the reason, hospitalization is always a personal crisis.[16] The level of crisis may be affected by (1) the type of hospital (admission to a general hospital carries different overtones than admission to a psychiatric hospital); (2) the circumstances of admission (emergency, major surgery or minor procedures); (3) previous hospitalizations (first vs. sequential); (4) the size of the health care facility (50 vs. 1000 bed institution); and (5) the location of the facility (near home or some distance away). For persons who usually adapt slowly to change the shock or crisis of admission may be more severe. Thus, the very young and the very old especially may have strong biologic (physiologic) as well as emotional reactions to admission to the hospital.

The speed with which hospitalization occurs influences the patient's response. For example, a person admitted to a hospital because of trauma (automobile accident, severe burns) or a psychiatric emergency may react with shock, anger or disbelief. When admission has been planned, the reaction may be less severe, depending on the nature of the illness. When the reason for hospitalization is sudden and life-threatening (stroke, heart attack, severe burns, severing of spinal cord) the patient may or may not be alert enough to respond, but those persons surrounding him perceive the stress, excitement and drama of the situation.

Initial impressions of the facility and personnel also affect the individual's response. The process of admission, types of questions asked, and responses to the patient's answers all give an impression to the patient. Rigid, forced conformity of behavior (e.g., all persons put to bed in a hospital gown immediately on admission) threatens the patient's sense of individuality and independence and may precipitate a sense of depersonalization. Once these feelings are established, it may take much longer to reverse them than it took to create them. Thus, the manner in which persons are treated initially is very important. Allowing a patient to make decisions regarding his care, treatment or environment supports his self-concept, sense of personal worth and sense of independence. Incidentally, the manner in which a person leaves the hospital (discharge procedure) also influences his overall response to the total hospital experience.

Health care personnel significantly affect the patient's response to hospitalization. Initially on admission and later as needed, personnel should be certain that each patient understands specifically who is caring for him and what he can expect from various members of the health team. The health team may include physicians (the patient's physician, consulting physician, resident, intern, medical student), registered nurses (head nurse, team leader, staff nurses), licensed practical (vocational) nurse, nurse's aides, orderlies, cleaning and maintenance personnel, dietary personnel, laboratory staff, pharmacy staff and others. Because the exact manner in which each of these people will interact with the patient differs, he needs to understand what each does and what expectations he can form for each.

> Remember: *Highly stressed persons recall only a fraction of what they are told when under stress. Therefore, the need for repeated explanations for such persons should be understood and accepted without accusing the patient of inattention.*

The room to which the patient is assigned is usually equipped with a bed, bedside stand, overbed table, occasional chair, lights, communication system and call bell. Special care units may have additional equipment such as sphygmomanometer, oxygen source, suction equipment and various types of monitors. All equipment should be explained and demonstrated, especially the means whereby the patient can call for assistance. It is important to explain the use of the call bell at the bedside as well as in the bathroom. (A further description of the typical patient unit is found in Chap. 27.)

Once he is assigned to a room, the patient immediately begins to establish *territorial rights* on *his* area of the room, *his* supplies, *his* bed.[10] Thus, imaginary boundaries are established, and infringement beyond these limits without permission is frequently perceived as an invasion of privacy. Considering this response, it is advisable for health personnel to knock before entering a patient's room, to ask permission to use his equipment or furniture and in other ways to let the patient truly assume responsibility for the territory that at least temporarily belongs to him.

The area in which a patient is placed is determined by the rules and regulations of that facility. Frequently this assignment is based on the primary reason for admission (e.g., medical or surgical care), and the severity of the patient's illness (e.g., intensive care or rehabilitation). In addition, it is common practice to separate children from adults. Regardless of his location, however, the patient needs the assurance that whoever can aid in his care *is* available to him. This includes laboratory personnel, medical specialists and administrative personnel. In other words, *the health care facility exists to serve the patient.*

THREATS TO COMFORT AND SAFETY OF THE HOSPITALIZED INDIVIDUAL

Influences of the External Environment

The inside of buildings can be manipulated in a variety of ways. Thus, the temperature, humidity, light and air most comfortable or desirable for the individual can be controlled.

The *room temperature* that is perceived as comfortable varies among individuals and according to one's culture. Older and inactive persons tend to prefer a higher room temperature. Generally, 20 to 22°C. (68 to 72°F.) is considered comfortable. It is desirable to maintain the temperature within this range because when temperature extremes occur, the body uses cardiovascular and pulmonary systems to maintain a comfortable internal temperature. If the patient suffers from dysfunction in any of these systems, the added burden of adapting to the external temperature may further threaten or delay recovery.

External (room) temperature is only one factor in the patient's sense of comfort. *Humidity,* or the amount of moisture in the air, affects the evaporation of moisture from the skin. Since this evaporation of skin moisture is an important means of heat regulation by the body, high humidity combined with high environmental temperature may cause physical discomfort. Conversely, when the temperature is low but the humidity is high, some people experience discomfort, especially in joints. If air-conditioning units manipulate temperature and *movement of air* but not humidity, excessive drying of the skin and mucous membranes may cause discomfort and irritation of the nose,

throat and bronchi. Therefore, air conditioners should have humidity controls to provide comfort.

The amount of *available light* is an important factor in comfort. When close work is attempted in dull light, eyestrain, headache or irritability may result. On the other hand, it is more difficult for a patient to rest when there is excessive light. Therefore, ideally, the health care facility should have a means of regulating the intensity of available light. In artificially lit rooms, when possible, it is desirable to duplicate day and night cycles by varying the intensity of the light. These contrasting periods of lighting assist the patient's orientation. Orientation is further encouraged when the patient's room has an outside window.

Noise (sudden, loud or distracting sounds) is irritating to well persons; even lower levels of noise may produce discomfort in persons who are ill, exhausted or in pain. However, absolute silence may also be undesirable. ("The quiet is so loud I can't sleep.") Hence, to ensure comfort for particular individuals, undesirable sounds or noise must be controlled.

Specific sounds may be more irritating to some people than to others. A sudden, loud noise universally produces a reaction of fright or disturbance. Measures must be taken to decrease the level of noise by reducing squeaks in equipment by lubricating friction points; avoiding dropping of objects; allowing the patient to personally control the volume of his radio or television; muffling telephone or communication equipment, especially at night; reducing talking or laughing within the hearing of ill persons; and constructing facilities with materials that limit sound conduction. Persons with impaired hearing or mechanical hearing aids may be especially sensitive to noise and may become confused by it, since their ability to differentiate sounds is reduced.

Dust is another important element in a patient's external environment. It poses significant hazards to persons with known allergies or with reduced pulmonary function. In addition, dust in hospitals may be laden with microorganisms, all of which carry the potential for producing infection, adding to irritation, or precipitating allergic reactions. Hence, it is important to avoid activities that stir up dust and to construct facilities so that air moves from areas of highest dust collection to the outside. (Research has demonstrated that a poorly planned ventilating system may actually spread infectious organisms throughout an institution.[11])

Additional activities to control dust include wet (not dry) dusting and cleaning; folding bed linens rather than shaking them; keeping doors closed between patient rooms and sterile areas (e.g., operating rooms); venting laundry centers to the outside (due to the high level of contamination from soiled linen); and separating soiled linen areas from places where clean linens are kept. Finally, air conditioners with special filters may be needed for persons suffering from severe allergies or pulmonary dysfunction.

Much has been written about the hazards of *cigarette smoking* to the smoker, but the effects of smoke on the nonsmoker must also be considered. Persons in a smoke-filled room may experience a headache; nose, throat and lung irritation; and/or an allergic response. Ill persons may also experience nausea. When a number of people smoke in a confined area, the carbon monoxide level may exceed the standard for safety established by the federal government. In addition, when a person is attempting to "kick" the smoking habit, being in the vicinity of smokers can be especially traumatic. Finally, the extreme fire hazard associated with cigarette smoking is another reason for limiting smoking in hospitals. (This is discussed further below.)

To further discourage smoking, many hospitals no longer sell cigarettes on the premises or permit smoking in public areas. Where more than one person occupies a room, assignment may be made according to whether or not the occupants smoke.

To summarize, temperature, humidity, light, noise, dust and smoke all affect the comfort and safety of the patient. The nurse can influence each of these factors by specific actions and thus enhance the comfort for both herself and the patient.

Threats to Physical Safety

The danger of fire is ever present. All institutions must have a well-understood, well-rehearsed plan for action in case of fire. This plan should include moving patients to safety, calling for aid and using fire extinguishers. Hospitals contain many combustible materials, including gases, oils, paper, bedclothes, lint and grease (from cooking). In addition, although oxygen itself is not combustible, it supports combustion. Operating rooms, intensive care units, gas storage areas, laundries and kitchens carry a heavy risk of fire.

> *Acquaint yourself with the location of fire call boxes, fire-fighting equipment and the fire safety plan of any facility in which you work.*

Cigarette smoking is extremely hazardous in hospitals. The ashes might ignite pajamas, bed linens or paper in waste baskets. Sudden eruption of flame will occur if a lighted match or cigarette is placed near oxygen. *If* smoking is permitted, ash trays must be readily accessible. In addition, if the level of orientation or strength of a smoker is in question, he should not be permitted to smoke, or a responsible person should hold his cigarette.

Two major problems associated with fire are heat and smoke. Smoke reduces oxygen and causes carbon dioxide to accumulate; heat causes tissue damage. In removing patients from the area of a fire, it is imperative to avoid both smoke inhalation and tissue damage. Careful study of the particular institution's plan in case of fire is important. Prevention is the first line of defense. Prompt, efficient, safe action by each person in case of fire must be the second line of defense. The nurse can use various methods for moving patients to safety; e.g., seriously ill persons may be dragged away from the fire on a blanket.

The nurse must be aware of other causes of *thermal injury*, such as scalding with hot liquid, overexposure to infrared lamps and application of overheated hot water bottles or heating pads. Careful placement of equipment along with frequent checking to note temperature and tissue response to heat will help prevent these types of injury.

Falls are probably the most common threat to physical safety in hospitals. Persons who are weakened by illness, taking new medications, experiencing new treatments, walking in unfamiliar areas and sleeping in unfamiliar beds are more susceptible to falls than well persons who are in a familiar environment. The careful nurse, aware of the dangers of falling, incorporates safety measures into plans for care.[9] Specific safety measures and the rationale for each are summarized below.

▶ *Raise side rails on bed and stretcher as appropriate.* Hospital beds are twin size and stretchers are very narrow. Rails also assist patient in turning.

▶ *Keep bed in low position except when giving patient care.* In case unattended patient attempts to get out of bed, the distance to the floor is reduced.

▶ *Keep floor uncluttered (no paper, water, electric cords, small objects in walkway).* Reduces chance of stumbling, tripping or slipping on objects.

▶ *Use a dim night light.* Facilitates safe patient and staff movement.

▶ *Suggest that patient wear slippers with nonskid soles.* The patient is less likely to slip when getting out of bed or walking.

▶ *Apply only nonskid wax to uncarpeted floors.* Reduces the risk of slipping.

▶ *Use nonskid tips on canes, crutches and walkers.* Supportive devices are less likely to skid.

▶ *Use braking devices on wheelchairs, stretchers and commodes.* Brakes aid in stabilizing rolling objects when patient gets on or off.

▶ *Provide personnel to support the patient who is in danger of falling.* A patient may be unaware of his own instability in the following situations:
   after being in bed a period of time
   after undergoing application of a cast or amputation
   after taking medication that may cause vertigo, hypotension or confusion
   after blood loss or severe pain
   after a stroke, with residual weakness of one side of the body
   after surgery

▶ *Open and pass through doors or around corners cautiously.* Reduces chance of injury due to fall or collision with another person.

▶ *Use special safety measures for the very young and for potentially suicidal patients. (Know the official policy of the institution.)* Prevents patients from injuring self.

▶ *Use properly applied restraint devices when indicated* (see Chap. 43). Restraints are used only as a last resort to keep patient from injuring himself.

In addition to falls, safety is threatened by *improperly functioning, broken* or *inadequately repaired equipment.* Broken glass or broken plastic with sharp edges should be removed immediately from the patient's environment. Young children, disoriented persons and very depressed persons must be protected from self-injury.

Chemical injury may be caused by all medications that are improperly used as well as by gases, oils, paints and cleaning compounds. Medications should be stored carefully and should not be within reach of ambulatory patients, especially those who are disoriented, confused and very young. When medications are given, it is imperative that the right person receive the right drug in the right dosage at the right time. Prompt reporting of misuse of drugs may avert extensive injury or prolonged discomfort.

An unexpected potential source of chemical injury is deteriorated or outdated medicine. Any drug that has changed in appearance, smell or consistency; has been kept past its expiration date; or has been stored in other than the specified manner should be discarded or checked by a qualified pharmacist before use, since its potency as well as chemical structure may have been altered. (See also Chaps. 31, 32, and 38.)

Noxious and *poisonous substances* also should be stored appropriately, i.e., in properly labeled, safe containers (preferably the original ones), away from drugs and food, and in places not accessible to young children or disoriented persons. Antiseptics and disinfectants to be used externally or, in diluted strength, internally merit safe care to avoid improper use.

Frayed cords, exposed wiring and improperly functioning *electrical equipment* should be repaired to avoid possible electrical shock or burn. Effects of electrical shock range from local discomfort to massive destruction of tissue. All electrical equipment should be properly grounded. (Most hospital outlets carry the three-prong opening.) It is advisable to have the ground wire source evaluated periodically to ensure that it is intact.[18]

Artificial *pacemakers,* which mechanically stimulate heart rate, are being used increasingly in selected persons. Thus, nurses often care for patients with recent implantation as well as patients with pacemakers who are receiving treatment for other disorders. Many pacemaker units function "on demand," namely, in the absence of a sensed electrical impulse from the heart. Consequently, if electrical impulses of similar wavelength are in the environment (from leaks in electrical equipment, e.g., microwave oven), the pacemaker will not activate a ventricular contraction. Hence, it is important to know where electrical leaks may occur and to warn pacemaker patients to stay away from these danger areas.

The use of *x-rays* or *radioactive substances* (isotopes) necessitates actions to protect the patient as well as personnel and visitors. Federal regulations guide the installation of x-ray equipment. The radiation on personnel working in the area is controlled by wearing shields (lead aprons, gloves, drapes) and reducing the time spent in close contact with radiation. These protective devices must be used consistently by personnel in the area, since the effect of radiation is cumulative; i.e., brief exposures over a long period of time may be as significant as a single long exposure.

When caring for patients receiving radiotherapy, the nurse needs to be aware of the source of radiation, its location and the method of administration (implantation and anchoring). Care should be well planned in order to reduce the length of time one is close to the patient. (Usually these patients are in private rooms.) Pregnant persons should avoid close contact if at all possible.

Shielding used during direct patient care is limited, but use of gloves and special tools is highly important in case a radioactive implant becomes dislodged or there is sudden direct exposure to radioactive substances through loss of body excreta (vomitus, wound drainage, urine, feces). Immediate assistance from the radiology department must be sought for guidance in limiting contamination while disposing of body excreta or dislodged implants.

Threats to Psychologic Safety

A patient removed from his usual setting is removed from his usual support systems. When admitted to a hospital, he is experiencing illness while adapting to the environment and culture of the hospital. The abrupt change from a familiar to an unfamiliar residence, along with the stress associated with illness and loss of support system, may precipitate a type of *cultural shock*. The farther the hospital from the patient's home, the greater the loss of support and, potentially, the greater the stress.

In the hospital "culture" are many factors that threaten the self-concept of the patient.[2] For example, medical terminology poses communication problems for the uninitiated. Terms such as *void, EEG, CCU* and *prep* are examples of commonly used words requiring translation. The patient faces many mechanical problems: He is confronted with buttons to call the nurse, to operate the bed, and to turn on the television. He must learn to manipulate a bedpan and to manage an IV bottle and tubing.

Removal of personal effects such as clothes, jewelry and money as well as medication from home disturbs the patient's sense of equilibrium. Being told when to get dressed and undressed, bathe, go to bed, take medicine and eat meals creates a sense of loss of independence and control. Is it any wonder that a degree of cultural shock is experienced by the person entering a hospital or other health care facility? The full impact of this shock may be partially reduced by the careful nurse who removes as many of the contributing factors as possible; e.g., she lets the patient wear his own clothes, determine the time for bathing and choose his menu and explains the meaning of medical and technical terms.

A crisis of any type may precipitate questioning of self-worth and the meaning of life. For some persons, illness leads to a search for meaning through religious expression. The observant, open nurse will be alert to the patient's request for religious support and will take appropriate actions to bring in a religious counselor as indicated. The hospitalized patient whose source of religious support is disrupted may ask directly to see his religious advisor, may want to discuss his religious feelings and needs with the nurse, or may simply "act out" his sense of loss and frustration and depend on the nurse to discern the need for religious guidance. In any instance, the nurse should respect the religious preference of the patient, readily consult the clergy as resource persons to assist in the care of the patient, and contact the religious advisor as appropriate, e.g., at the request of the patient, his significant others, or when circumstances clearly warrant it.

The adult who is suddenly forced to be served and directed, may experience a loss of *self-esteem.* He seeks to respond in a way that leads to his being labeled as cooperative, nice, pleasant, helpful and uncomplaining rather than uncooperative, grumpy, unpleasant, complaining or angry. Illness and treatment often precipitate a feeling of anger—and in some cases recovery would be enhanced if expression of the anger were allowed. Fear, loneliness and anxiety, all common reactions to loss of health, need expression in order for healing to occur on the emotional level along with the physical level. Finding an acceptable time, place and manner for expression of feelings is the challenge.[16] (See Chapter 3 for further discussion of the nurse-patient relationship.)

Psychologic safety is also threatened by exposure to unpleasant sights, smells and sensations. These situations occur sometimes as a result of thoughtlessness of personnel or accidents, or they may be side effects of the health care itself. If this type of discomfort can be avoided, every measure should be taken to control it. Generous use of screens, closed doors, and thoughtful manners can frequently keep unpleasant sights from the patient. If an accident or surgery has produced body disfigurement, time must be taken to prepare the patient for his first observation of the change in his body image. (Body image changes are discussed in Chap. 15.)

When undesirable smells cannot be removed, use of room ventilation and room deodorizers may be warranted. Room deodorizers are effective only insofar as their scent overrides the undesirable odor. Some deodorizers are of limited use, since the patient's response to that odor may be as negative as the response to the original one.

Unpleasant sensations on the body surface are usually related to bed linens and other materials in contact with the skin. Smooth and soft materials are more comfortable than harsh, hard textures, and they reduce the tendency to local skin irritation and breakdown. In cases in which skin irritation threatens to cause skin breakdown, a piece of synthetic sheepskin may be placed between the patient's skin and the bed linens.

Finally, psychologic comfort may be disturbed by factors influencing stimulation of the patient's senses.[5] In health, sensory stimulation (hearing, sight, smell) is voluntarily controlled; the individual may move toward or away from such stimulation as he deems necessary for comfort. In illness, particularly when the patient is hospitalized, this control is altered, especially in specialized care centers such as coronary care units, intensive care units, recovery rooms and isolation units. For example, care may necessitate monotonous lights, sound and smell 24 hours a day, without normal day and night variations. If such areas are designed so that patients cannot see natural diurnal changes, this adds to the monotony. In these situations, there may be *sensory deprivation* (less than optimum quantity or quality of stimulation) in some respects and *sensory overload* (excessive stimulation of the senses) in other respects. Either one may lead to confusion; loss of orientation, especially to time and place; alteration of sleep patterns; and dampened affect. The nurse is alert to situations with a potential for either deprivation or overload and will vary the environment wherever possible. When the environment cannot be adequately varied, use of clocks with day and night hours in different colors, large calendars on which each day can be marked, room decorations, visits from significant persons, diversional activities, and exercises may all help combat the problem. In addition, thoughtful actions such as touching the patient, identifying the time and place, describing outside environmental conditions, explaining care and treatment and listening to the patient may enhance the quality of care the patient perceives.

In summary, the nurse who is alert to the patient's need for psychologic comfort will use a variety of creative ways to incorporate such measures into her *caring* ministry.

Threats to Bacteriologic Safety

Wherever persons are grouped together (e.g., in hospitals, nursing homes, retirement homes, sports arenas, churches, schools), they are at risk to acquire others' illnesses or potential pathogens. This is especially true of ill persons, since illness increases the likelihood of acquiring a secondary infection. In addition, where ill persons are found in close proximity, the number of pathogenic organisms in the environment is multiplied, especially since the same nursing staff and medical staff care for persons with different types of illness and various degrees of resistance to illness. Finally, any highly stressful experience reduces the body's ability to resist infection. Thus, since illness is a stressful experience, organisms that normally do not cause illness may do so.

An illness produced by microorganisms or viruses is called an *infection*. For infections (systemic or local) to develop, there must be a series of orderly conditions or events: (1) an *infectious agent*, (2) a *reservoir* of organisms, (3) a *portal* (means) *of exit* from the reservoir, (4) a *means for* the organism to be *transmitted* (transferred), (5) a *portal* (means) *of entry* into another person (host), and (6) a person *susceptible* to the organism in the strength and amount contacting him. *If any of these six factors is absent, an infection cannot occur.* These factors might be considered as links in the infection chain (see Figs. 25–1 and 25–2 and Table 25–1).

Some persons enter the hospital specifically for treatment of a known infection. Other persons enter for some other type of treatment but may acquire an infection while in the hospital. An infection acquired in a hospital is called a *nosocomial infection,* as contrasted to the *community-acquired infection,* which is acquired away from the hospital.

The high incidence of nosocomial infections prior to Lister and the discovery of antisepsis kept many persons away from hospitals. Historically, with the introduction of antisepsis the incidence of infection fell, further decreasing significantly again when antibiotics were dis-

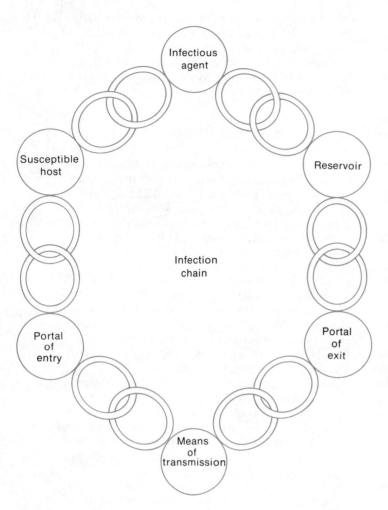

Figure 25–1. Links in the infection chain.

TABLE 25–1.   CHARACTERISTICS OF AND WAYS OF WEAKENING LINKS IN THE INFECTION CHAIN

LINK	CHARACTERISTICS OF LINK	WAYS TO WEAKEN LINK
Infectious agent (pathogen, etiologic agent): includes bacteria, viruses and fungi that normally inhabit or have recently been introduced into the body and on the skin	Has form capable of reproducing Requires food and proper temperature to grow; some (aerobic) require oxygen, others (anaerobic) require absence of oxygen Able to resist chemical and physical agents (e.g., heat, drying, chemicals) that threaten its life May or may not produce toxins (See a microbiology text for more detail.)	Use antiseptics to inhibit growth of organisms Use disinfectants to destroy microorganisms Use anti-infective agents of sufficient strength and for sufficiently long time to kill, mutate or weaken organisms
Reservoir: natural habitat of organisms (where they grow and reproduce)	May be on human beings, animals, soil, food, water or body excreta Human beings and animals can be reservoirs yet demonstrate no evidence of the disease (carrier)	One relates in self-protective ways to each type of potential reservoir Limit contact with exposed people (especially those exposed to viral infections, which may be highly contagious before the disease is recognized), particularly if own resistance is low

TABLE 25–1. CHARACTERISTICS OF AND WAYS OF WEAKENING LINKS IN THE INFECTION CHAIN (*Continued*)

LINK	CHARACTERISTICS OF LINK	WAYS TO WEAKEN LINK
Portal (means) *of exit:* the primary route of escape for the organism	Frequently related to site of growth and reproduction (reservoir) Examples: respiratory tract, GI tract (especially mouth, anus), body excreta (urine, feces, wound drainage) Spreading ultimately depends on ability of infectious agent to live outside the reservoir	Cover nose and mouth when sneezing or coughing Do not talk directly into face of another person Do not talk or breathe directly over open wound Careful handling of body exudate that may carry organism Proper disposal of dressings and wound coverings Careful handwashing after handling body excreta or drainage Isolation of persons with known infection
Means of transmission: method by which organisms are spread	Direct contact (kissing, intercourse) Via moist surfaces (water, water glasses, food, food utensils), hands, clothes, vectors (ticks, bats, mosquitoes), air movement, contaminated prepackaged supplies (IV solution or other supplies)	Avoid direct contact if infection is known Use disposable glassware and properly sterilized equipment Careful, proper handwashing Personal items should be used by only one person Control air movement by folding, not shaking, bed linens Quality check on sterility of prepackaged, presterilized materials Consider anything in contact with floor or infected person as carrying pathogens
Portal (means) *of entry:* frequently the same as the portal of exit	Any of the following may indicate entrance of pathogens into the body: unexpected temperature elevation, local tenderness, dysuria, diarrhea, skin lesions, purulent drainage, unexplained cough	Avoid break in skin whenever possible Carefully discard disposable syringes and needles to avoid accidental skin puncture Discard facial tissues, wound dressings and other body excreta without touching directly (use paper bags, gloves)
Susceptible host	As immunologic defenses are weakened, susceptibility to infection increases; high-risk persons include: Very young children in whom passive immunity from mother is lost but own immunologic defense is underdeveloped Very old persons in whom immunologic defenses are diminished Undernourished or malnourished persons Persons with chronic diseases such as uremia, diabetes, leukemia, other forms of cancer Persons receiving certain types of medical therapy, e.g., steroids, cortisone, antibiotics, irradiation Persons in shock	Maintain up-to-date immunologic program for all persons Separate high-risk persons from persons with known or potential infections Carefully screen visitors for high-risk persons Provide nutritional supplements for malnourished or undernourished persons

covered. Unfortunately, after the advent of antibiotics, the incidence of nosocomial infections again increased. Reasons suggested for this increase include laxity in handwashing, overuse of antibiotics, and the development of antibiotic-resistant strains of microorganisms. Certainly, the increase in the number and extensiveness of surgical procedures carried with it the increased risk of infection. In addition, because people live longer today, more older, debilitated persons with a high risk of infection are admitted to the hospital.

Whatever the reason for the discouraging statistics on infection control in hospitals, specific means must be used to keep the rate of infection as low as possible. These maneuvers include:

1. Use of enforced separation such as *isolation techniques* to keep one infected person away from others; *reverse isolation* to keep an especially susceptible person away from exposure to harmful as well as potentially harmful pathogens (see Chap. 45 for discussion of isolation procedure); *laminar flow rooms* that control movement of air out of the room in order to reduce airborne contaminants; and *life island techniques* to maintain a person in a sterile environment (see Chap. 45).

2. Careful and judicious handwashing technique, paying special attention to areas commonly missed. (See Procedure 6.)

3. Geographical grouping of patients to separate persons likely to have or to develop infections (burn patients, children) from high-risk persons (surgical patients, newborns).

4. Restriction of visitors with known or suspected infection from all patients, especially those in the high-risk group.

5. Careful attention to means of transmitting organisms from one person to another; e.g., sitting on the bed of one patient and later sitting on the bed of another; setting things on the floor and later placing them on the bed or furniture;

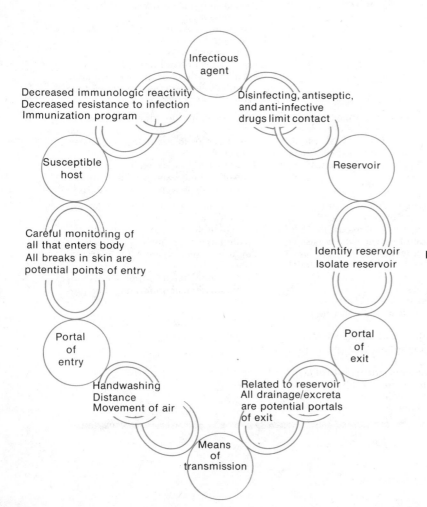

Figure 25–2. Disruption of the infection chain.

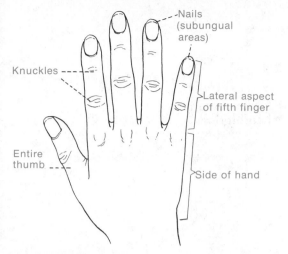

Nails
(subungual
areas)

Knuckles

Lateral aspect
of fifth finger

Entire
thumb

Side of hand

Figure 25–3. Areas commonly missed in handwashing. Special attention must be given to these areas in order to have effective handwashing technique.

giving care to patients with infections and then walking outside the hospital without either covering the uniform or changing into street clothes; placing duty shoes where they can contaminate new areas, e.g., on the bed or table;

permitting visitors or others to use the patient's personal items; and moving unused items from one patient's room to another.

6. In the original architectural design of the hospital, attention must be paid to movement of air and people. For example, air from the laundry, where soiled linen is collected and sorted, should be vented outside the institution and not through patient care areas. Also, one should traffic movement from outside directly to patient care areas and not through food areas, surgical areas, or other places where high-risk patients receive care.

Of all the means used to control infections, the most important one continues to be careful handwashing. In order to protect herself as well as her patients, the nurse should learn effective handwashing technique. This includes careful attention to those areas commonly missed in the handwashing procedure, namely, the thumb, knuckles, subungual areas, lateral aspect of fifth finger and side of hand (see Fig. 25–3).

6. HANDWASHING

By Jean Saxon, R.N., M.N.

Definition and Purposes. *Handwashing involves the removal of soil, debris and transient pathogens by means of friction, soap or detergent, and running water.* Careful handwashing reduces spreading of pathogens to other individuals, objects and self. Nurse adapts procedure according to degree of contamination and the subsequent activity to be performed.

Patient-Family Teaching Points. Explain and demonstrate correct method of handwashing and provide the patient and family with the following information as appropriate: (a) importance of handwashing to prevent "spreading germs" and to protect self and others; (b) importance of cleansing fingernails and of using friction over all surfaces of hands and wrists during handwashing; (c) times when hands should be washed, e.g., after elimination; (d) desirable water temperature (warm); and (e) importance of drying hands thoroughly after washing to prevent chapping.

PRE-PROCEDURE ACTIVITIES

PRELIMINARY ASSESSMENT/PLANNING	EQUIPMENT
Work area: ▶ check for location of sinks and presence of soap, paper towels and waste containers	▶ soap (or detergent) ▶ paper towels in dispenser ▶ sink with mixed hot and cold faucets *Procedure continued on the following page*

Procedure continued on the following page

PRELIMINARY ASSESSMENT/PLANNING

Nurse should
- pin rings with uneven surfaces inside pocket
- wear wrist watch 4 to 5 inches above hand or pin to blouse, shirt front or pocket
- inspect hands for dryness, cracking of skin, hangnails, cuts or abrasions (Intact skin is the body's first line of defense.)
- inspect fingernails to make certain they are short, smooth and free of chipped nail polish

EQUIPMENT

- waste containers
- hand lotion

PROCEDURE

SUGGESTED STEPS

A. Washing at beginning of day's activities and after gross soiling.

1. Assume a forward-backward wide-based stance at sink. Flex knees and bend at hips if sink is low.

2. Prevent clothing from becoming damp or touching sink; avoid splashing onto self and surrounding area, e.g., floor.

3. Water should be comfortably warm [about 40.5°C. (105°F.)]; wet hands and wrists.

4. Hold hands and wrists parallel to floor or lower than elbows throughout procedure.

5. Avoid touching sink with hands.

6. Add soap or detergent to hands. (Rinse bar soap before and after using and drop into soap dish.)

7. Rub palmar surfaces together to work up lather.

8. Using one lathered hand to wash the other, grasp one wrist and cleanse it by using friction to apply lather around it. Next, apply lather with friction over dorsum of the hand. Proceed to clean the dorsum of the fingers with fingers flexed to expose creases at knuckles.

9. Using friction, clean lateral aspects of fingers and hands by interdigitation; rub

RATIONALE/DISCUSSION

A. Washing hands reduces numbers of transient pathogens.

1. Good body alignment saves energy and reduces stress on bones, muscles and ligaments.

2. Pathogens can be transmitted via fluid; wet floors are dangerous.

3. Warm water has a lower surface tension than cold water, thereby increasing cleansing action.

4. Avoid dripping of suds or water containing microorganisms over clean skin or onto floor.

5. Sink and faucets are considered to be soiled. If you contaminate hands during procedure (e.g., touch sink or faucets), rewash hands.

6. Soap and detergents emulsify oil and lower surface tension of water.

7. Lather lifts soil and pathogens.

8. Wash one handbreadth above contamination to avoid recontamination of hands during rinsing or drying. Skinfolds harbor great numbers of transient pathogens that quickly become resident if not removed.

9. Concentrate on friction while reaching from wrist to thumb tip and from wrist to

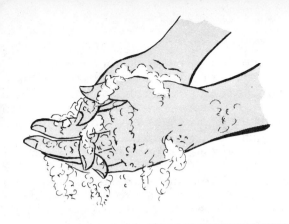

Figure 25-4. Handwashing, using friction and interdigitation. (From Leake, M. J.: *A Manual of Simple Nursing Procedures,* 5th ed. Philadelphia, W. B. Saunders Co., 1971, p. 11.)

SUGGESTED STEPS	RATIONALE/DISCUSSION
right thumb over left, then left thumb over right (see Fig. 25–4).	fifth digit tip on each hand. Lateral aspects of hands are most frequently missed areas in washing hands.
10. If wedding band is worn, move ring up finger and wash under ring.	10. Pathogens are harbored and grow in dark, moist area under ring.
11. Cleanse under nails (subungual areas) with a fingernail of the other hand.	11. Brushes, toothpicks, nail files and orange wood sticks may injure the skin and may be a source of contamination.
12. Rinse under nails, then over wrists and hands, using friction to remove suds.	12. Friction is the most important part of handwashing. Running water flushes off suds, soil and transient pathogens.
13. Repeat steps 1 through 10 and 12.	13. Additional pathogens are removed by repeated washings. (Repetition is needed when hands are grossly contaminated and prior to procedures requiring strict asepsis.)
14. Pat hands and wrists with towel to absorb water. Use second towel to complete drying.	14. Dry paper toweling rubbed on skin can cause abrasions. Skin left moist can become chapped.
15. Use dry side of second towel or a third towel to turn off faucets.	15. Faucets are considered to be contaminated. A dry barrier is needed to prevent transmission of pathogens.
16. Dispose of used towels in waste basket.	
17. Apply hand lotion.	17. Washing hands removes skin oil. Lotion replaces skin lubricant and prevents excessive dryness.
B. Washing before and after caring for patient, before handling clean supplies and charts, and at other times of minimal contamination.	B. Washing hands appropriately is the most important barrier to cross-contamination.
1. Follow all steps except 11 and 13 above.	1. Rapid friction movements with suds and running water can effectively cleanse hands of small to moderate amounts of transient bacteria and soil.

POST-PROCEDURE ACTIVITIES

If necessary, see that soap (detergent) and towels are replenished and waste container is emptied by reporting to appropriate individual. Note condition of floor around sink area. If floor is wet, see that floor is cleaned to prevent falls.

In summary, protecting the patient from bacteriologic threats to safety entails use of surgical and medical asepsis in order to control microorganisms. Surgical asepsis seeks to control and prevent-movement of all microorganisms, not only pathogenic ones. Various sterilization methods are utilized to achieve the goal of freedom from all microorganisms. (See Chap. 37 for a discussion of surgical asepsis and sterilization.)

Medical asepsis refers to measures taken to control and reduce the number of pathogenic organisms. It is sometimes referred to as *clean technique*. In medical asepsis, cleaning agents are used along with antiseptics, disinfectants and germicidal (germ-killing) agents to control pathogenic organisms. The perfect disinfectant—namely, one which is inexpensive, noncorrosive to metal (or other material), nonirritating to skin and mucous membranes, and effective in a strength that acts quickly to kill all pathogens—has yet to be found. The available disinfectants have limitations, and no single one is effective for all purposes.

In selecting a disinfectant for a particular situation, consideration must be given to the *strength* of the solution as related to its planned use, the period of *time* the item to be disinfected can be exposed to the chemical without ill effects, the *temperature* at which the solution is used and the *character of the material* to be disinfected. Items to be disinfected should first be cleansed of all body exudate or organic material (with soap or detergent if possible), since such exudate may render the disinfectant inert. Knowing the limitations of the chemical being used will help in achieving the goal of removing pathogens. (See Table 25–2 for evaluation of various types of disinfecting solutions.)

TABLE 25–2.   EVALUATION OF LIQUID GERMICIDES (BACTERIA ONLY)

COMPOUND	GENERAL USEFULNESS AS		EFFECTIVENESS AGAINST		OTHER PROPERTIES
	Disinfectants	*Antiseptics*	*Tubercle Bacillus*	*Spores*	
Mercurial compounds	None	Poor	None	None	Inactivated by organic matter; bland
Phenolic compounds	Good	Poor	Good	Poor	Bad odor; irritating; not inactivated by organic matter or soap; stable
Quaternary ammonium compounds	Good	Good	None	None	Neutralized by soap; relatively nontoxic; odorless; absorbed by gauze and fabrics
Chlorine compounds	Good*	Fair	Fair*	Fair*	Inactivated by organic matter; corrosive
Iodine and iodophors	Good	Good	Good	Poor	Staining temporary; relatively nontoxic; corrosive
Alcohols	Good†	Very good†	Very good†	None	Volatile; strong concentration required; rapidly cidal; inactivated by organic matter
Formaldehyde	Fair	None	Good**	Fair**	Toxic; irritating fumes
Glutaraldehyde	Good	None	Good	Good	Low protein coagulability; aqueous solution useful for lens instruments and rubber articles; limited stability; corrodes carbon steel objects after 24 hours exposure
Combinations					
Iodine-alcohol	Fair	Very good	Very good	None	Stains fabrics
Formaldehyde-alcohol	Good**	None	Very good**	Good**	Toxic; irritating fumes; volatile

*4 to 5% concentration.
†70 to 90% concentration.
**5 to 8% formaldehyde (12 to 20% formalin).

Source: Evans, M. J.: Some contributions to prevention of infections. *Nursing Clinics of North America*, 3:641, 1968; modified from Spaulding, E. H.: *Journal of Hospital Research*, 3:15, 1965.

PATIENT CHARACTERISTICS REQUIRING ADJUSTMENT OF ENVIRONMENT

The individual characteristics of a person determine the type of environment in which that person is safest and most comfortable. Specific characteristics directly affecting the environment vary with age, orientation and sensory acuity.

Age

Older persons constantly face the threat of falling. A fall may occur because the person's *posture* has been altered in such a way as to precipitate a loss of balance. Other causative factors include *orthostatic hypotension* following extended periods of time in a reclining or sitting position; *pathophysiologic changes* in the cardiovascular system, such as anemia or atherosclerotic changes; and *medical therapy* for hypertension or side effects of drugs used for other problems. When any of these conditions is present, assisted ambulation is warranted, especially if fainting is likely.

Disorientation to time, place and person may also characterize the older person. Causes of this include *cerebral hypoxia* from vascular changes; being placed in *unfamiliar places,* surrounded by unfamiliar persons; *medical therapy* such as sedatives, hypnotics, analgesics

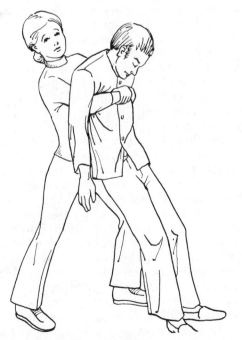

Figure 25–5. Supporting the fainting patient as he is lowered to the floor, sliding on nurse's leg.

and tranquilizers; and *impairment* of *vision* and *hearing.* Sudden change in the level of cerebral function (i.e., restlessness, confused ideas, garbled speech) warrants careful assessment of recent change in oxygen intake and carbon dioxide output. Either one of these may alter cerebration by reducing available oxygen to brain cells as well as altering the pH of body fluids. Environmental manipulation including careful lighting of walkways (especially to the bathroom at night time), placement of familiar objects within reach or sight and judicious monitoring of individual response to drugs may aid in providing safety and comfort for the individual.

Since many elderly persons adapt poorly to sudden and drastic external and internal temperature change, caution must be taken to avoid such extremes. A generous, readily available supply of blankets in order to avoid chilling is important. Use of air conditioners, fans and other means to reduce high room temperature is also warranted. This intolerance of external temperature extremes is directly related to the reduced cardiovascular and respiratory reserve, which makes internal adaptation slow, difficult or even impossible. Sudden onset of high or low body temperature in the older person may result in mental confusion, loss of balance and alteration of consciousness if the internal adaptive mechanisms are inadequate for coping with such rapid change. (See Chap. 47 for additional discussion of care of the elderly.)

Special consideration must also be given to the environment of the very *young.* In this age group, too, *falls* are common and must be prevented. Preventive actions include careful selection of the crib or bed, making certain it is the proper size for the size of the child; use of crib sides and even crib nets if the child tends to climb; and having a responsible attendant with the child when he is not safely in his crib or bed.

Mechanical injury must also be guarded against for the young, since they lack insight into potential hazards. *Dangerous equipment,* such as controls for a steam inhalator, must be kept out of children's reach. Electrical outlets should be plugged to avoid insertion of small objects into openings, and electrical cords (especially extension cords) should be stored where child cannot play with them. *Chemicals* must be kept in a locked or safe place, with child-proof caps on the tops of containers whenever possible.

Toys must be evaluated in light of the developmental age of the child. Items with loose or small parts are not safe for young children, who are prone to place such objects into the mouth or some other body orifice. Items with sharp edges or points might cut a child who is unable to use them appropriately, and materials that cannot be cleaned must be evaluated for possible transmission of infectious organisms.

In addition, it may be necessary for health personnel to have assistance when administering certain treatments to a child, since anxiety and fear may be expressed by vigorous voluntary and involuntary movement. A second adult may be needed to assist with parenteral injections to ensure safe and effective treatment. (See Chap. 46 for additional discussion of care of the young.)

Orientation

A patient's level of orientation (awareness) toward himself and his surroundings may also necessitate changes in the environment to keep it safe and helpful. Unconscious (comatose) persons need continuous surveillance, since they cannot meet their own basic needs. They must be turned frequently and regularly in order to maintain a patent airway, prevent pressure sores and reduce lung congestion. Since the swallowing reflex may be absent, careful assessment for choking and fluid collection in the throat must be made.

The recently paralyzed person may be so disoriented as to not realize that he has loss of muscle function and reduced sensation. These persons need protection from falls, burns and pressure sores. (See Chap. 33 for discussion of the complications of immobility.)

Very restless, mentally confused persons have special needs also. They may injure themselves by falling from mechanical devices or equipment. Restlessness and confusion may cause them to interfere with treatment through dislodging intravenous needles, nasogastric tubes, urinary catheters, wound dressings and drains. Purposeless movement may also lead to débridement of body surface through friction caused by rubbing on bed linens or other objects. If the cause of the restlessness can be determined (e.g., hypoxia, distended urinary

bladder, pain, drug reaction), it should be relieved, and precautionary measures should be taken. At times, providing additional light in the room and having a familiar person stay with the patient may help reduce restlessness and confusion. As a last resort, to avoid self-injury or injury to others, some means of body or extremity restraint may be used. (Chap. 14 discusses confusion; Chap. 43 discusses restraints).

Sensory Acuity

Alteration in the sensory acuity of an individual may also necessitate changes in the environment. Persons with impaired *hearing* may be able to understand verbal statements only with a mechanical hearing aid. If these individuals are unable to keep the earplugs free of wax and the batteries changed, health personnel must assist in order to maintain a functioning hearing aid. Other measures which may help in communicating with these persons include making eye contact or physical contact (touch) before beginning to speak; keeping light on the face of the speaker so lips can be seen; enunciating words clearly and slowly; using simple sentence construction; and using written means of communicating when spoken message is not understood. Shouting at persons with impaired hearing tends to exaggerate vowel sounds and has limited value in enhancing comprehension.

For persons with impaired *sight*, making verbal contact prior to touching the person might reduce fright. Persons with diminished sight need to be familiar with room arrangement and placement of personal effects to carry out their self-care and maintenance. If these cannot be maintained as arranged, informing the patient of change is very important to his safety and comfort. If impaired sight is due to cataracts, providing brighter light when the person is attempting to do close work may help.

As mentioned earlier, when persons have a reduced sense of *touch* or *position*, it is very important to take precautions to avoid falls, burns or other tissue damage. Tissue damage may be caused by too much cold applied to an area for too long as well as by too much heat. Hence, heating pads, hot water bottles, ice packs and ice caps should be used judiciously, if at all. (See Chap. 44 on use of heat and cold.)

These reduced sensations also predispose the individual to tissue breakdown from pressure on points of the body to the extent that blood supply (hence, oxygen) is reduced and pressure sores (decubiti) develop. Using alternating pressure mattresses and sheepskin pads, frequently changing position, and padding bony prominences may all help reduce the incidence of pressure sores. (See Chap. 33 for further discussion of pressure sores.) Maintaining adequate hydration and nutrition along with careful physical cleanliness may also be useful.

Residents of health care facilities may lose their sense of *taste* and *smell*. They may be most acutely aware of this at mealtime. Providing colorful, attractive meals may aid in overcoming the anorexia due to loss of taste and smell. With the loss of smell, these persons also have increased risk of personal injury through fire or burns, since smoke cannot be smelled and a fire might go unnoticed until flames or crackling bring it to attention. Careful placement of working smoke detectors is very important for the safety of these persons. Finally, if these persons have draining wounds or other conditions causing an odor, measures to control odors are warranted.

SUMMARY

When a patient enters a health care facility for care, comfort and/or cure, his environment and all its complexities must be considered. In this chapter we identified factors that affect the patient's well-being, noting ways a careful nurse might seek to establish and maintain a therapeutic as well as safe and helpful environment.

BIBLIOGRAPHY

a. Althouse, H. L.: How OSHA affects hospitals and nursing homes. *American Journal of Nursing*, 75:450–453, March 1975.
b. Beverley, E. V.: Reducing fire and burn hazards among the elderly. *Geriatrics*, 31:106–110, May 1976.
1. Bolin, R. H.: Sensory deprivation: an overview. *Nursing Forum*, 13(3):240–258, 1974.
2. Brink, P. J., and Saunders, J. M.: Cultural shock: theoretical and applied. *In* Brink, P. J. (ed.): *Transcultural Nursing: A Book of Readings*. Englewood Cliffs, NJ, Prentice-Hall, 1976, pp. 126–138.
2a. Breitung, J.: Are you fudging on hand-washing routines? *RN*, 40:71, June 1977.
3. Castle, M.: Isolation—precise procedures for better protection. *Nursing '75*, 5:51–57, May 1975.
3a. Feldtman, R. W., et al.: Hospital electrical safety. *American Family Physician*, 13:127–137, March 1976.
4. Fox, M. K., Langner, S. B., and Wells, R. W.: How good are handwashing practices? *American Journal of Nursing*, 74:1676–1678, Sept. 1974.

5. Harmer, B., and Henderson, V.: *Textbook of Principles and Practice of Nursing*, 5th ed. New York, Macmillan Co., 1955, pp. 193–200.
5a. Hirschfeld, M. J.: Care of the aging holocaust survivor. *American Journal of Nursing*, 77:1187–1189, July 1977.
6. Innes, B: Environmental status. *In* Mitchell, P. H.: *Concepts Basic to Nursing*. New York, McGraw-Hill Book Co., 1973, pp. 184–186.
6a. Jones, M.: Nurses can change the social systems of hospitals. *American Journal of Nursing*, 78:1012–1014, June 1978.
7. Kernaghan, S. G.: Health care supply—the industry that grew and grew. *Hospitals, JAHA*, 49:53–58, Aug. 1, 1975.
8. Kornfeld, D. S.: The hospital environment: its impact on the patient. *Advances in Psychosomatic Medicine*, 8:252–270, 1972.
9. Kukuk, H. M.: Safety precautions: protecting your patients and yourself. Part I. *Nursing '76*, 6:45–51, May 1976.
9a. Leadership at work: A patient's wealth can threaten his nursing care. *RN*, 41:145–146, Sep. 1978.
10. Levine, M. E.: The dimensions of the holistic response. *In* Levine, M. E.: *Introduction to Clinical Nursing*, 2nd ed. Philadelphia, F. A. Davis Co., 1973, pp. 443–486.
11. Litsky, B. Y.: Infection control and hospital design. *Supervisor Nurse*, 3:21–31, Feb. 1972.
11a. Myers, S. T.: You *have* to find time to nurse the mind too. *RN*, 41:63–64, Jan. 1978.
12. Niland, M., et al.: *Nursing Process I, N281 Syllabus*. University of Washington School of Nursing, Seattle, WA. Winter 1976, pp. 2–1 to 2–5.
13. Piepgras, R.: The other dimension. *American Journal of Nursing*, 68:2610–2613, Dec. 1968.
14. Porte, B.: The multifaceted PR role. *JAHA*, 47:115–116, Aug. 1, 1973.
15. Price, A. L.: *The Art, Science and Spirit of Nursing*, 2nd ed. Philadelphia, W. B. Saunders Co., 1959, pp. 184–186.
15a. Primeaux, M.: Caring for the American Indian patient. *American Journal of Nursing*, 77:91–94, Jan. 1977.
15b. Reuben, S., and Byrnes, G. K.: Helping elderly patients in the transition to a nursing home. *Geriatrics*, 32:107–122, Nov. 1977.
16. Schmieding, N. J.: The relationship of nursing to the process of chronicity. *Nursing Outlook*, 18:58–62, Feb. 1970.
17. Walker, P. H.: Detecting electrical hazards in the hospital. *Nursing Care*, 6:11–14, March 1973.
18. Wood, L. A. (ed.): *Nursing Skills for Allied Health Services*, Vol. I. Philadelphia, W. B. Saunders Co., 1972, pp. 123–137.
19. Wood, L. A. (ed.): *Nursing Skills for Allied Health Services*, Vol. III. Philadelphia, W. B. Saunders Co., 1975, pp. 1–19.
20. Woodward, J. A.: An ICU is a place to live—not just survive. *RN*, 41:62, Jan. 1978.

CHAPTER 26

PROMOTING REST AND SLEEP

By Sarah Sanford, R.N., M.A.

INTRODUCTION AND STUDY GUIDE

Rest and sleep are basic concepts in nursing. While they are interrelated, they are neither interchangeable nor identical. A certain amount of sleep is necessary in order to feel rested, but sleep is only one way of obtaining rest.

The primary purpose of this chapter is to examine each of the concepts of rest and sleep and to supply fundamental knowledge to be used as a basis for planning nursing care. Contextual definitions of these concepts are provided, along with a discussion of their roles in maintaining and promoting optimum mental and physical functioning.

A second purpose is to examine the process of sleep. In this discussion we identify the specific stages of sleep, the physiologic manifestations of these stages, the cyclic nature of the process as a whole and the many factors that influence sleep behavior. Since sleep is a universal occurrence, general theories of its function are also presented.

A third purpose is to examine disordered sleep. Sleep deprivation, primary alterations in sleep patterns and alterations in sleep due to other mental and physical conditions are discussed. In addition, methods of treatment for the various types of disordered sleep are included.

Finally, in this chapter we will explore the nursing role in promoting effective sleep and rest. The emphasis is placed on meeting individual needs for rest and sleep by taking a sleep and rest history and utilizing that information as the basis for formulating care plans. General categories of nursing actions provide the conceptual framework for planning specific patient interventions. Teaching implications for not only the patient and his family but also other health team members are presented.

Upon completion of this chapter, the student should be able to meet the following objectives.

1. Define the similarities and differences between rest and sleep.

2. List and explain the three prerequisite conditions necessary for obtaining the feeling of being rested.

3. Differentiate the contemporary view of sleep from the historical view of a uniformly quiescent state.

4. Name the two distinct types of sleep activity and compare the physiologic manifestations of each.

5. Identify the specific sleep stages and the order in which they normally occur.

6. Differentiate between the first and second portions of the sleeping period in terms of relative content of the two types of sleep activity.

7. Define the concept of synchronization in terms of circadian rhythm.

8. Discuss the effects of age and personality type on individual sleep patterns.

9. Describe the effects of L-tryptophan, exercise, prior sleep-wakefulness pattern and the environment on the sleep pattern.

10. Define the physical and mental changes associated with sleep deprivation.

11. Explain the rebound phenomena that occur with REM and stage 4 NREM deprivation.

12. Differentiate between primary and secondary insomnias.

13. Explain the syndrome of drug dependence insomnia.

14. Describe the effect of sleep activity on coronary artery disease, peptic ulcer disease and nocturnal dyspnea.

15. Identify the components of a sleep and rest history.

16. Identify and give examples of the three categories of nursing actions designed to meet the sleep and rest needs of patients.

17. Discuss teaching implications in the areas of sleep and rest for patients and other health team members.

18. Understand and be able to use correctly the following terms:

REST

The term "rest" connotes feelings of peace, relief and relaxation. Subjectively restful circumstances may also include physical situations such as inactivity after exercise, mental relaxation techniques such as meditation, reading, watching television and a break in the day's activities. Indeed, rest implies relief from anything that tires, disturbs or worries. No single definition could include all the individual modes and connotations inherent to rest. However, for the purposes of this chapter, rest is contextually defined as a state of relatively decreased bodily work, either physical, mental, or both, which leaves the individual feeling refreshed and revived. Rest, then, is obtained through a variety of methods, all of which are designed to have a recuperative effect.

During illness, bed rest is frequently prescribed as a part of the treatment plan. However, simply limiting physical activity by keeping patients in bed does not guarantee the state of rest. Although the medical goal of restrictions on activity is to decrease the physical and mental demands upon the body, such limitations may, in fact, trouble or worry patients to such a degree that emotional stress prevents effective rest and thus also prevents its recuperative effects.[15]

Role of Rest in Mental and Physical Functioning

Even in the absence of illness, adequate rest is necessary for general well-being. Lack of rest produces the physical symptoms of tiredness and fatigue: exhaustion after minimum muscle expenditure, difficulty in performing routine physical tasks and overall weakness. As weariness occurs, mental activities, too, become more difficult because of lapses of attention and a decreased ability to concentrate. Nervousness and irritability are not uncommon. Although not serious in themselves, these manifestations prevent high-level wellness and functioning at optimum levels.

During illness, adequate rest is crucial. Illness in itself is a stress and requires the body to mobilize all its physiologic and psychologic reserves to maintain its integrity. Without the recuperative effects and the feeling of well-being that rest provides, depression or disinterest can develop. These attitudes greatly hamper even the most aggressive attempts to re-establish health and functioning.

If illness requires hospitalization, the patient is particularly vulnerable to rest disorders. Already anxious because of the illness, he is also subjected to a new environment, new faces, loss of privacy and control, strange noises, plus frequent new procedures, many of which are painful. Perhaps the greatest challenge for nursing is to establish conditions conducive to rest in such a situation.

Prerequisites for Feeling Rested

Although each person's needs for rest are individual, there are several conditions that must be met before relaxation and, subsequently, a rested sensation can be obtained. These conditions can be categorized into three general areas and apply to almost all patient situations.

Adequate Sleep. The most basic prerequisite to feeling rested is adequate sleep. While the precise number of hours of sleep needed varies greatly, there is a minimum daily requirement necessary for any given individual to feel rested. When an individual fails to receive this minimum amount of sleep, feelings of irritability and tension accompany generalized fatigue; relaxation in this circumstance is difficult. Sleep loss, then, not only results in fatigue and irritability but also can accentuate them by making rest more difficult. Inability to sleep is a frequent complaint of patients in the hospital. The nurse's role in promoting sleep and rest is discussed in detail later in this chapter.

Decreased Tension, Worry, and Anxiety. After a rest period, an individual is more likely to have a sensation of being rested if he feels that things are under control, both in his personal life and in the health care setting. This includes believing that those caring for him are competent, available and willing to help him when he needs it. It also includes believing that he as an individual is important and that those involved in his care are concerned with and interested in helping him deal with personal problems that might interfere with his ability to relax. In addition, a person must understand what is happening to him; he therefore needs frequent explanations of procedures and information as to what is, and will be, happening to him. Finally, to avoid boredom and feelings of inadequacy, he must be able to engage in activities that he perceives as being purposeful.[31, 32]

Physical Comfort. Physical discomfort must be minimized before relaxation can occur. Obvious sources of pain must be removed or controlled. (See Chap. 34 for a more complete discussion of pain.) In addition to control of pain, general comfort measures include assisting with hygiene, positioning, and ensuring adequate warmth and privacy. The role of physical comfort in promoting relaxation and rest cannot be overemphasized.

SLEEP

Sleep has already been mentioned as a necessity for the subjective feeling of being rested. Sleep is also universal; it is something we all do and apparently need, since no individual has been documented as being able to function without it. Indeed, we each spend one third of our lives sleeping.

What Is Sleep?

An unequivocal definition of sleep does not exist despite voluminous reports in the literature of sleep research.[16] Historically, sleep has been viewed as a "uniformly quiescent state," a state of profound muscle relaxation and loss of ability to respond to the surrounding environment. Many early researchers likened sleep to coma or an anesthetic state.

Anthropologists have viewed sleep as early man's answer to his inability to cope with dangers imposed by darkness; i.e., a behavior practiced by man in a place where his predators could not reach him during those hours when his vision was impaired by darkness. Although this is a possible explanation for sleeping, it is not probable because as technology has advanced, making artificial illumination possible, the need for sleep has not disappeared.

The contemporary view of sleep has modified the historical definition. Research has now shown that sleep is a characteristic state of consciousness, not a type of unconsciousness, as previously believed.[16] Although perception of, and thus the ability to react to, the environment is decreased, it is not completely absent. Certain types of stimuli will arouse a sleeper, while others will not. A baby's cry will arouse its mother, but the telephone may not; a dog's barking may arouse its owner, but the alarm clock may not. It may be that selected stimuli are perceived more readily than others. While this awareness is related to the loudness or intensity of the stimuli, it is not solely dependent upon it.[10]

Research has also shown that sleep is a cyclic phenomenon. The period of sleep recurs cyclically, usually once a day. In addition, sleep is composed of distinct stages that follow a specific and repeating pattern throughout the sleep period (see Physiology of Sleep, below.)

With these contemporary views in mind, we can expand upon our contextual definition of sleep: it is a specific state of consciousness that occurs cyclically, is composed of distinct stages and can be characterized as a relative unresponsiveness to the surrounding environment.

Physiology of Sleep

Great advances have been made in the study of sleep during the last 15 years through the use of electroencephalograms (EEG), which record the electrical activity of the cerebral cortex; electro-oculograms (EOG), which record eye movements; and electromyograms (EMG), which record the tone of muscles. These recordings allowed researchers, for the first time, to obtain both qualitative and quantitative data about sleep.

Identification of Sleep Stages. Perhaps the biggest single advance in sleep research was the discovery that sleep is not a uniformly quiescent state. Specific stages of sleep are now known to exist and are classified as one of two types of sleep activity. The two major types of activity are known as REM and NREM sleep, the latter being further divided into four specific stages (see Table 26–1).

REM SLEEP. REM (rapid eye movement) sleep is often referred to as active or paradoxic sleep. It is characterized by extremely rapid eye movements (for which it was named) and a very active EEG much like that seen in waking. Small convulsive twitches of the muscles of the face may occur. However, the EMG reflects extremely low muscle tone—the lowest of all the sleep stages—which is associated with immobility much like paralysis in the large muscles that maintain posture.[10, 16] This immobility occurs as a result of hyperpolarization (overexcitation with subsequent failure to transmit impulses) of specific neurons in the brainstem.[10]

Physiologically, REM sleep is truly paradoxical. The body is essentially paralyzed, but body temperature, blood flow and oxygen consumption by the brain are all increased.[2, 10] The heart rate, blood pressure and cardiac output are also increased, often approaching levels seen during waking. Respiratory rate during REM alternates between very fast and very slow, and self-limiting apneic (nonbreathing) periods have been reported.[2, 10] Some researchers believe that the large-muscle immobility during REM is physiologically necessary to minimize use of body energy stores during this time when the brain's energy consumption and metabolism are elevated.

NREM SLEEP. NREM (non-REM) sleep is also referred to as slow-wave or quiet sleep. As an individual progresses through the four stages of NREM, he becomes increasingly more difficult to arouse. Stage 1 NREM is subjectively the lightest of all sleep stages and is frequently considered a transition state between waking and sleeping, for the EEG during this stage shows some characteristics also seen in waking. Stage 2 NREM is often referred to as the *door stage* because it occurs both before and after REM sleep. It is characterized by distinctive wave forms called "sleep spindles" and K complexes in the EEG. In stages 3 and 4 NREM, the EEG shows large, low-frequency, slow waves, called deltas. These final stages are thus frequently called "slow-wave sleep" and they differ from each other only on the basis of the number of delta wave forms on the EEG. This type of sleep is associated with slow, rolling eye movements, if they are present at all. There also is muscle relaxation but not immobility; this is reflected by an EMG higher than that during REM but lower than that of waking.

Physiologically, NREM sleep conforms to the classic view of sleep as a quiescent state. During this type of sleep, cardiac and respiratory rates decrease to basal levels.[16] There are also decreases in blood pressure, metabolic activity and body temperature.[16]

PERCENTAGES OF SLEEP TIME FOR EACH STAGE. In the young adult, REM sleep involves about 20 to 25 per cent of the total time spent asleep, stage 1 NREM involves roughly 5 per cent, stage 2 NREM composes 50 to 55 per cent, and stages 3 and 4 NREM each compose roughly 10 per cent of the total sleep time.[22] Changes in these percentages occur with age. (See Determinants of Individual Sleep Needs.)

REBOUND PHENOMENA. Both REM and NREM sleep are necessary for optimal mental and physical functioning. Two stages, however—stage 4 NREM and REM—are believed to be of particular importance. Selective

TABLE 26–1. NREM VS. REM ACTIVITY SUMMARY

FEATURES	NREM (NON-REM)	REM (RAPID EYE MOVEMENT)
Synonyms	Slow wave, quiet sleep (3 and 4)	Active, paradoxical sleep
Characteristics	Muscular relaxation Slow, rolling eye movements or no eye movement	Large muscle immobility Small convulsive twitches of face Rapid darting eye movements
Physiologic manifestations	Cardiac rate decreased Respiratory rate decreased	Cardiac rate, blood pressure and cardiac output increased Respiratory rate irregular Apneic periods
Percentages of sleeping time for young adults	Stage 1: 5 Stage 2: 50–55 Stage 3: 10 Stage 4: 10	20–25
Rebound	Stages 1, 2 and 3: None Stage 4: Yes	Yes
Dreams	Stages 1, 2 and 3: Probably not Stage 4: Realistic, like thought process	Vivid, full color with auditory component Emotionally charged

loss of either of these stages results in their occupying consistently greater (compensatory) percentages of total sleep time on subsequent (recovery) nights.[16] These compensatory increases, called *rebounds*, are thought to occur because the individual has developed a "debt" for them. Consequently, the individual repays the debt during the first subsequent night that sleep is undisturbed.

Cyclic Nature of Sleep

Circadian Rhythm. The term circadian rhythm is derived from the Latin roots *circa* meaning "about" and *dia* meaning "day." It refers to innate oscillations in physiological parameters which occur approximately every 24 hours and result in variations of both physical and mental function. Each day our body's functioning has high and low periods of mental and physical performance dictated by our inherent biologic clock, or circadian rhythm. It is no accident that circadian oscillations occur once a day: This is roughly the same time period of our daily light-dark pattern determined by the earth's rotation.[29] The human organism's need to function at optimum levels during the daylight hours and sleep during darkness may have been the reason that man's biologic clock originally synchronized itself with the physical environment.[7]

Researchers have found that individuals placed in an environment lacking any external information as to time of day (light or dark) continue to show the circadian oscillations. However, the length of a complete circadian cycle increases slightly to 25 hours, which conforms closely to the lunar calendar day of 24 hours and 50 minutes.[7] (For further information on circadian rhythm, the reader is referred to Chapter 6.)

For sleep to be of maximum benefit, it must occur during the low period of the circadian oscillation. Studies have shown that sleep is qualitatively rated poorest when the circadian rhythm, as measured by body temperature oscillation, is not synchronous with an imposed sleep-wakefulness schedule.[25] If an individual sleeps at an inappropriate time in his circadian rhythm, e.g., a period other than the low period, he is desynchronized. One of the most frequent causes of desynchronization is the "jet lag" syndrome.

Our society favors sleeping at night. Therefore, the majority of the population has synchronized its sleep-wakefulness schedule to being active during the day. Resynchronization must occur when an individual changes his sleep-wakefulness schedule; this process requires 3 to 5 days.[26] If the customary sleep-wakefulness schedule is oriented to working at night, resynchronization occurs. Unfortunately, in many instances the individual spends 5 days resynchronizing to a night activity schedule, only to spend his 2 days off sleeping at night. After the days off, he goes back to work and activity at night, therefore beginning the process of resynchronization all over again. The process of continual resynchronization can lead to chronic feelings of fatigue and may be involved in the general tendency of many to avoid night work.

Sleep Stage Cycling. In addition to occurring cyclically, sleep itself is composed of cycles (Fig. 26–1). Each cycle consists of ordered sleep-stage progressions that vary in length from 60 to 120 minutes but average 90 minutes.[25] The average adult exhibits four to six sleep-stage cycles per night. These cycles are the sleep correlates of basic rest activity cycles (BRAC's), which occur during both sleep and wakefulness. Like the circadian rhythms, BRAC's are endogenous and self-sustained oscillations that are reflected in alterations in the efficiency of physical and mental function. BRAC's may be the reason for alternating periods of alertness and drowsiness during the day.[26]

For the first 20 to 30 minutes following the onset of sleep, there is a general progression from stage 1 NREM into stages 2 and 3 NREM. An approximately 30-minute period of stage 4 NREM follows, after which the pattern reverses itself and the sleeper moves back

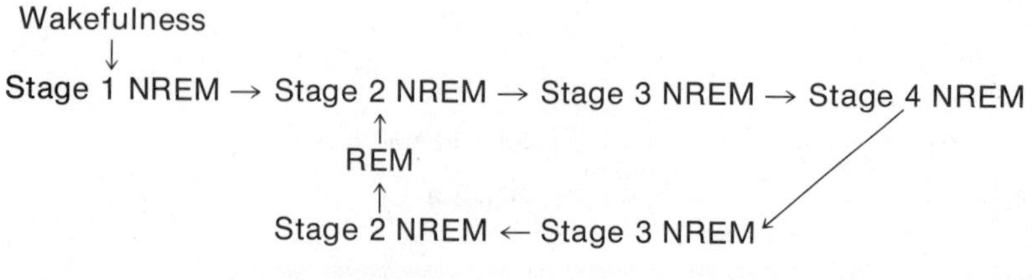

Wakefulness
↓
Stage 1 NREM → Stage 2 NREM → Stage 3 NREM → Stage 4 NREM
                        ↑
                      REM
                        ↑
      Stage 2 NREM ← Stage 3 NREM

Figure 26–1.   Sleep stage cycle.

through stage 3 and into stage 2. From stage 2, the sleeper then enters the first REM period, which lasts about 10 minutes and is followed again by stage 2 NREM. This pattern of both entering REM from stage 2 and returning to stage 2 at the completion of REM is the basis for calling this the "door stage." Once the sleeper returns to stage 2, he repeats the initial descending progression, and the cycle repeats itself. If the sleeper is aroused at any point during the progression of sleep-stage cycles, he does not return to the stage from which he was aroused but instead starts the initial descending pattern from the beginning.

As the night progresses, the amount of time spent in each stage changes. During the early part of the night, the 90-minute cycles are dominated by stages 3 and 4 NREM, with the REM periods lasting no more than 30 minutes. As the night progresses, however, REM periods increase in length and can last as long as 60 minutes; during this portion of the night, stages 3 and 4 NREM are shortened proportionately.[42] Thus, the majority of NREM sleep takes place in the first half of the night, while the majority of REM occurs during the last half.

Sleep-stage cycling also occurs during daytime naps, but the relative quantities of NREM and REM sleep depend upon the time of day in which the naps are taken. Morning naps, as if a continuation of the latter half of the night, are associated with large proportions of REM sleep and decreased amounts of NREM 3 and 4. Afternoon naps, on the other hand, are composed of proportionately more NREM sleep.[40] Because of their proportionately high content of NREM 3 and 4 sleep, afternoon naps can result in decreased amounts of these two stages in the early part of the subsequent night's sleep.[40]

The Mysterious Need for Sleep: Theories of Function

Despite aggressive study regarding the function(s) of sleep, research has yet to answer the question, "Why do we sleep?" Sleep experts generally agree that the process of sleep is restorative. However, the view that the primary function of sleep is to balance the effects of motor movement associated with the waking state has been altered. People confined to bed or immobilized due to spinal injuries have little motor movement; yet they still sleep and apparently need to do so. Even though illness and confinement to bed with little muscle movement can cause deterioration of muscle tissues, sleep time in healthy individuals is essentially unaltered by decreased muscle activity during waking hours. This was shown in studies done by the National Aeronautics and Space Administration. In these studies, astronauts placed in antigravity chambers had only minimal motor movement, and their need for sleep remained. In fact, minimizing motor movement in these healthy individuals did not remarkably change their sleep time.[11]

A Biochemical Theory of Sleep Function. Biochemical theories of sleep function have received much emphasis in sleep research. One of these theories has been called the "bottle theory," since it compares the brain and central nervous system to a bottle.[10] According to this theory, the waking state causes depletion of some unknown cerebral substance; i.e., the bottle is emptied. Sleep is initiated when this mysterious substance reaches a certain, presumably low, level; the process of sleep serves to replenish the supply. While admittedly vague, this theory is consistent with several observations: (1) When an individual sleeps longer than necessary, the excess sleep is generally nontherapeutic, often leaving the individual feeling tired, i.e., as if the bottle had overflowed.[17] (2) Levels of adenosine triphosphate (ATP) and other high-energy phosphate compounds are higher in animals allowed to sleep than in sleep-deprived animals. The incorporation of phosphorus into the intermediate substances (phosphoproteins and phosphopeptides) of these high-energy compounds is also increased during sleep. (3) Experimental seizures in animals produce marked depletion in high-energy phosphate levels; the postictal drowsiness and tendency to sleep may represent the need to refill the bottle.[10] The search for this substance has led researchers to the study of neurotransmitters (chemical substances that enable electrical impulses in the brain to be passed from neuron to neuron), but as yet no single substance has been identified. In the process of this research, sleep investigators have discovered that neurotransmitters are apparently involved in sleep staging. At the present time, it appears that REM sleep may be associated with the cerebral availability and mobilization of the catecholamines (epinephrine and norepinephrine), while serotonin may be involved with NREM sleep stages.[10, 43] For further information on the role of neurotransmitters in sleep activity the student is referred to the literature.[43]

Psychologic Theory of Sleep Function. The

belief that adequate sleep is necessary for general feelings of well-being and maintenance of mental and emotional equilibrium is supported by most sleep researchers.

SORTING AND STORING INFORMATION. Sleep is thought to be the time for processing information and reviewing the day's events. Contextual and conceptual input from the day's events is sorted and selectively stored in memory during sleep. In this way, each day's perceptions are "filed away" to make room for new ones. Evidence for this theory is based largely on the finding that disorientation and inability to appropriately categorize perceptions are common occurrences in sleep deprivation.

DREAMING. Dreaming is thought to be the actual activity during sleep in which this processing and rehearsing of perceptions takes place. The nature of dream activity is dependent upon the sleep stage in which it occurs. The relative importance of REM vs. NREM dreams is a source of controversy among sleep researchers.[8] Most researchers believe that REM sleep and its dreams are the key mechanisms necessary for maintenance of mental and emotional equilibrium.[3] This is because REM dreams are described as vivid, full-color experiences that frequently include auditory components and are highly emotionally charged. The hypothesis is that these dramatic dreams provide the psyche with the opportunity to deal with profound concerns and psychological perceptions, thus clearing these phenomena from the consciousness. NREM dreams, on the other hand, tend to be less dramatic, more realistic and more similar to normal thought processes.[41]

The exact role of each of these dreams in psychologic maintenance is not known. REM dreams are recalled more frequently than NREM dreams, but this could be a function of the vivid and dramatic nature of these dreams and not necessarily a function of greater relative importance. Although it is generally believed that everyone dreams and that variation occurs only in an individual's ability to recall them, sleep researchers cannot report this with certainty simply because dreams cannot be recorded or studied directly. However, self-classified nondreamers have been taught recall techniques and have consequently discovered that they do, in fact, dream. Dreams are probably the most mysterious aspect of sleep and continue to be studied extensively.

Sleep researchers have found that individuals develop characteristic patterns for the number of hours they sleep from night to night.[1, 24, 42] Although the mean number of hours per night for a healthy adult is 7½, the variation in sleep patterns is great. It has been documented that some people sleep as few as 3 hours and still report feeling rested.[35] Others sleep as many as 10 hours a night and complain of daytime fatigue. Precise reasons for the individual differences in day-to-day quantitative needs for sleep have not been clearly defined, but two factors—age and personality type—seem to be involved.

Age. The quantity of sleep varies with age. Infants sleep more than children, children more than young adults and young adults more than the elderly.[13] Total sleep time, which is high in childhood, shows a decline during adolescence, after which it plateaus and remains fairly constant until old age. The number of arousals in a given night also changes with age. Arousals increase even during those years when total sleep time is constant.[13] These findings have been interpreted as indications that the intensity of sleep activity diminishes steadily as age increases.

The percentages of time for the various stages also change with age. Neonates have been found to have unusually high levels of REM sleep; in premature infants REM levels are even higher. As the neonate reaches late infancy, REM percentages are only slightly greater than those in the adult.[13] Thus, the percentage of the total sleep time that consists of REM tends to decline from infancy to childhood. After a plateau during young adulthood, REM percentages show a further decline in the elderly.[13] These declines are due to decreases in the tendency to have REM periods of increasing length as the night progresses.

On the basis of these observations, sleep researchers have suggested that the main biologic function of REM sleep occurs in early development—during intrauterine development and shortly after birth.[36] Some researchers believe that REM provides stimulation required for cerebral neuron maturation.[36] Other researchers suggest that the inordinately high percentages of REM in the young merely reflect the immaturity (e.g., inefficiency) of the central nervous system rather than a specific biologic need for this stage of sleep.[36] Nonetheless, neither of these theories is consistent with the REM rebound phenomenon that is seen in all ages when REM sleep is lost. These consistent compensations for lost REM sleep imply that its functions in the mature individual are not trivial.[13]

Stage 4 NREM also declines dramatically with age. In contrast to the plateau maintained during young adulthood for total sleep time and REM sleep, stage 4 shows marked change throughout this period.[13] Concomitantly, both stages 1 and 2 NREM increase with age.

Overall changes in sleep patterns associated with age, then, can be described as (1) a decrease in total sleep time, manifested primarily by decreases in stage 4 NREM and, to a lesser extent, REM; (2) increases in the number of arousals during the sleep period; and (3) increases in stages 1 and 2 NREM.

Personality. Chronic nervousness, depression and introversion are believed to be involved in establishing characteristic sleep patterns. Total sleep time tends to be elevated in individuals exhibiting these tendencies, yet these people rarely report feeling refreshed. Researchers have documented that the increased sleep time in this type of individual is a function of increased REM sleep, the quantity of NREM sleep being essentially normal.[18]

Some researchers believe that increased REM sleep reflects an increased need for psychologic coping because mental and emotional concerns are not dealt with effectively during the waking hours.[18] This belief is certainly consistent with the psychologic functions thought to be performed by sleep and dreams.

General Influences on Sleep

Many influences other than age and personality can either enhance or impair the general sleep pattern. The presence of one or more of these factors in association with efforts to rest and sleep can affect the effectiveness of the sleep obtained.

One of the most frequent influences on sleep patterns is the amount of sleep received in the immediate past, e.g., the *prior sleep-wakefulness pattern*.[9] Sleep pattern alteration can therefore occur after parties, studying for an important exam, getting up early to go skiing or hiking, or other situation that infringes on the time normally spent asleep. The subjective feeling of tiredness after one or two nights of decreased sleep is related to the reason for the sleep pattern change.[9] *Stress* or anxiety associated with pressures of work, school or emotionally painful events further disturbs sleep that is already quantitatively altered, primarily affecting REM. This invariably leaves the individual feeling more nervous and irritable than if his decreased sleep were associated with recreational activities.[34]

Changes in the *sleep environment* can also alter sleep patterns, e.g., a different bed or pillow, sleeping alone instead of with a spouse, a different room or different degrees of ventilation, light or noise. Researchers have found changes in the NREM and REM proportions of sleep in the new environment. The characteristic changes consist of decreased REM, prolonged time needed to fall asleep, more awakenings, and decreased total sleep time.[6, 34]

Illness, which acts as a physiologic stressor, also changes sleep patterns. Individuals who are ill characteristically report trying to increase sleep time in an effort to obtain the feeling of being rested. If illness requires hospitalization, individuals are in double jeopardy—the need for sleep is increased and at the same time an altered environment impairs the ability to obtain it. Fortunately, altered sleep patterns due to changes in the sleep environment disappear after 1 or 2 days of adaptation to the new environment. As previously noted, naps taken during the afternoon can decrease the amounts of stages 3 and 4 NREM sleep during the night that follows.

Intake of selected substances can alter sleep behavior. L-*Tryptophan* is an essential amino acid present in a variety of foods such as meats, dairy products and legumes. This substance has been shown to enhance the ability to fall asleep, e.g., shorten sleep latency, and has for that reason been considered a natural hypnotic.[4, 21] The old custom of drinking warm milk before bed thus has basis in scientific fact. It may be that L-tryptophan is a contributing factor in the drowsiness frequently experienced following a large meal.

Two frequently consumed beverages also alter sleep. *Alcohol*, in small quantities, can promote relaxation and, thus, sleep; however, large quantities are associated with suppression of REM sleep.[11, 16] *Coffee*, because of its caffeine content, has been found to decrease sleep time, primarily during the latter half of the night.[5] If an individual is having difficulty obtaining effective sleep, it is suggested that intake of these substances be limited generally and avoided altogether within 4 or 5 hours of retiring.

Physical exercise also affects sleep. Some researchers have reported that exercise during the day increases the amount of stages 3 and 4 NREM sleep, but it also has been reported to decrease REM sleep.[37] However, a usual pattern of physical exercise several hours before the sleep period time tends to promote muscle relaxation and thus aid sleep.[37, 45] Sleep may be disturbed by excessive exercise in the unconditioned individual, since the resultant fatigue results in physiologic activation of the body and makes relaxation more difficult.[37]

Hormonal changes are also associated with alteration in sleep behavior. With menses there is a general tendency for women to complain of fatigue; they thus desire increased sleep in an attempt to compensate. Sleep disruptions are frequent complaints of menopausal women, and hormonal replacement therapy has been successful in alleviating some of these complaints. However, since menopause is frequently an emotionally charged time for many women, emotional stress is probably a component of the disturbed sleep patterns.

Finally, *medications* affect sleep, either immediately or on a long-term basis.[34] Changes can also occur when chronically used medications are withdrawn.[14] Barbiturates, morphine, imipramine (Tofranil) and its derivatives, monoamine oxidase (MAO) inhibitors, meprobamate (Equanil) and amphetamines all suppress REM sleep.[34]

A common tranquilizer, chlordiazepoxide (Librium), has been found to enhance falling asleep and increase total sleep time for the first few days of administration. After 3½ weeks of administration, however, this effect disappears and is replaced by a decrease in NREM, slow-wave, sleep.[20] Another commonly prescribed tranquilizer, diazepam (Valium), is also known to suppress selected stages of sleep. EEG studies on individuals receiving this drug have shown that the immediate effect is to suppress REM sleep; with chronic administration, REM returns to normal, but at the expense of stage 4 NREM sleep.[34] Thus, while both these medications may result in drowsiness and sleep, the sleep that is obtained can be qualitatively altered, both immediately and on a long-term basis.

Two medications, chloral hydrate (Noctec) and flurazepam (Dalmane), are thought to promote sleep without altering its patterns. When administered for periods as long as a month, chloral hydrate was an effective hypnotic and was not associated with disrupted sleep patterns.[20] The same is believed true of flurazepam if it is not administered in doses exceeding 60 mg./day; however, conflicting reports exist.[16, 20] Many believe it leads to qualitative sleep disruption.[16, 20, 23] A good general guideline is to use hypnotic medications only when all other methods of promoting sleep fail, and then for the shortest possible period of time.

Sleep is clearly a complex process. For it to supply the subjective feeling of being rested and consequently optimize physical and mental functioning, it must not only involve adequate hours but, in addition, be synchronized with the body's inherent circadian rhythm. Also, sleep staging activity must occur in a precise progression, such that each sleep stage occupies a fairly constant portion of the total sleep time.

Sleep Deprivation

Loss of Both Types of Sleep. Sleep deprivation clearly is a disorder of inadequate time; indeed, the only totally accepted function of sleep is to prevent the signs and symptoms of sleep deprivation. It has been documented that after 60 hours without sleep, decreased strength of neck flexion, hand tremors, awkwardness, nystagmus, ptosis (drooping eyelids), difficulty with speech articulation, difficulty concentrating, decreased facial movements and an overall appearance of apathy develop.[16, 27, 28] Beginning with the third day, changes in bodily sensations and visual illusions are exhibited. Behaviorally, as the time without sleep increases, declines in perceptual, cognitive and psychomotor functions occur.[27] Frightening visual hallucinations have been documented but are not a common finding. They seem to be more common in individuals who historically have manifested other types of psychic disruptions.[22, 28]

Recovery from sleep deprivation is associated with increased total sleep time, primarily due to a marked increase in the percentages of NREM 3 and 4 sleep. Total REM time is also increased on the recovery night, but because of the increased total sleep time, the percentage of REM is either unchanged or only slightly elevated.[16, 22] Sleep quantity and stage patterning return to pre-deprivation values after one recovery night.

Selective Sleep-Stage Deprivation. By awakening sleeping individuals as they enter a specific stage, researchers have been able to study the effects of deprivation of selected sleep stages. With selective loss of sleep, both the progression of stages and the percentages of total sleep time occupied by them are altered.

REM SLEEP DEPRIVATION. If individuals are continually awakened as they enter REM sleep, they progressively try to enter REM more often and require more intense stimulation in order to be aroused.[16] When allowed to sleep, individuals deprived of REM sleep exhibit consistent rebound phenomena. Formal psychiatric testing shows no consistent abnormalities, but subjectively, these individuals report increased appetites, increased suspiciousness and tendencies for withdrawal and introversion.[16, 39]

Clinically, selective REM loss can occur with the use of many hypnotic medications. As was previously noted, compensatory increases occur when such medications are withdrawn. Since REM sleep is associated with rather profound physiologic demands in terms of cardiac workload, these rebound situations can be significant and dangerous in cardiac patients. If subjected to these rebounds in REM sleep, cardiac patients can experience nocturnal angina (chest pain), myocardial infarctions (heart attack), and/or extensions of pre-existing infarctions.

STAGE 4 NREM SLEEP DEPRIVATION. As is true for REM sleep, stage 4 NREM sleep deprivation is associated with more frequent attempts by the sleeper to enter this stage.[30] A consistent rebound of this stage has been documented on the recovery night.[30] However, if both stage 4 NREM and REM loss occur after a period of total sleep deprivation, a consistent rebound of stage 4 NREM occurs.[30] Thus, in the situation of total sleep deprivation, compensation during recovery nights preferentially favors stage 4 NREM sleep.

Primary Sleep Disorders

Primary sleep disorders are conditions with no known physical or mental cause.[44]

Primary Insomnia. Primary insomnia is a syndrome involving difficulty falling asleep, many awakenings during the night, and/or early morning awakenings.[45] It is a chronic syndrome and is not to be confused with transient periods of sleep difficulty that accompany some physical or mental illnesses. EEG sleep records of primary insomniacs have shown that NREM 3 and 4 sleep, which usually dominate sleep during the early part of the night, are decreased.[45] Thus, the insomniac may experience not only quantitative sleep loss but qualitative abnormalities as well. Since this syndrome has no proven cause, treatment is only symptomatic and often includes exercise several hours before bedtime, establishing a relaxing bedtime routine that may or may not include ingesting some source of L-tryptophan, and search and treatment for undue psychologic stressors in the daily life style. Biofeedback and meditation techniques have been used with some success, but their role in long-term treatment of insomniacs has yet to be proved. As a last resort, hypnotic medications that do not in themselves alter sleep patterns have been used. Because of the chronicity of this disorder, insomniacs frequently are accustomed to taking many medications to help them sleep, but this practice frequently results in further alteration of sleep patterns and perpetuation of the problem.

Drug-dependence Insomnia. Although not technically a primary sleep disorder, drug-dependence insomnia is discussed at this point because of its frequent association with abuse of medications in primary insomnia. Excessive use of hypnotic medications not only fails to improve sleep but also results in alteration of sleep activity. EEG's of drug-dependent individuals show marked reductions in both REM and stages 3 and 4 NREM sleep.[23]

One of the first steps in the treatment of primary insomnia with drug dependency is the withdrawal of all drugs. However, if this is not done gradually, the withdrawal process results in central nervous system overexcitability and prolonged inability to sleep.[14] Withdrawal of drugs, even if gradual, is associated with an immediate and marked increase in REM sleep, with subsequent increased frequency and intensity of dream activity; stages 3 and 4 NREM sleep slowly return to normal levels without any rebound.[23] Treatment, then, even under the best conditions, is associated with disrupted sleep. Subjectively, when medications were gradually withdrawn, insomniacs reported no increase in their difficulty in sleeping, and some reported improvement.[23]

Narcolepsy. Narcolepsy is a specific disorder characterized by frequent, irresistible attacks of sleep of relatively short duration.[23] In approximately 70 per cent of the individuals with sleep attacks, there also occurs a phenomenon known as *cataplexy*. This manifests itself as partial or complete loss of muscle tone and can result in serious falls or injuries.[23] Vivid full-color and auditory hallucinations accompany the onset of sleep in about 25 per cent of those affected. After the sleep attacks, narcoleptics usually report feeling refreshed.

Sleep attacks are more frequent after meals, in boredom-producing situations, and toward the end of the day. The attacks accompanied by cataplexy are frequently preceded by emotionally charged events, either very happy or very upsetting. Needless to say, this disorder can be incapacitating. Unless diagnosed and treated properly, it can stigmatize the narcoleptic as being lazy, irresponsible or emotionally unstable.[23]

EEG studies on narcoleptics have shown that daytime sleep attacks, as well as the initial stage in nocturnal sleep, consist of REM sleep.[23] Narcolepsy therefore is believed to be a REM sleep disorder. It seems to be a phenomenon of inappropriate REM breakthroughs during the waking state with varying degrees of muscle immobility and hallucinatory episodes similar to REM dreams. Treatment is based on REM suppression through the use of medications such as amphetamines and methylphenidate (Ritalin).[23]

Hypersomnias. Hypersomnia is similar to narcolepsy in that excessive sleep is a symptom, but the desire to sleep is not irresistible. However, sleep is usually much longer, lasting several hours to several days, and is accompanied by extreme difficulty in awakening and by confusion.[23] Two periodic hypersomnias are the Kleine-Levin syndrome, which is also associated with morbid hunger, and Pickwickian syndrome, which is associated with morbid obesity and consequent respiratory insufficiency. The hunger and obesity aspects of these hypersomnias have prompted researchers to suspect a central nervous system disorder, involving either an anatomic or physiologic abnormality in the hunger-satiety center in the hypothalamus.[44] Hypersomnias have occurred with head injuries, cerebrovascular disorders and brain tumors. They have also been seen in psychologic disorders such as depression, in which sleep provides an escape from the stresses of daily life. Indeed, it has been found that many individuals who demonstrate characteristically prolonged sleep patterns have tendencies toward depression, introversion and withdrawal.[19] However, hypersomnias do occur in the absence of hunger, obesity and psychiatric conditions; the exact mechanism and cause remain a mystery.

EEG studies of hypersomniacs show that both the cyclic sleep-stage progression and the percentage of time for each of the sleep stages are within normal limits in spite of excessively prolonged periods of total sleep time.[23] Thus, the sleep in hypersomnia is essentially normal except in terms of duration. Treatment is therefore based on limiting the period of sleep and involves use of stimulant drugs.[23]

Sleep Apnea. Self-limiting apneic periods can occur during sleep activity.[2, 16] They are a usual occurrence in normal infants up to 3 months of age[23] and have been documented in individuals of all ages in conjunction with REM sleep. Percentage of the total sleep time spent in REM is high during infancy, which may account for the usual occurrence of these periods in this age group.

Apneic periods of excessive length or increased frequency have been implicated in the sudden infant death syndrome.[23] One study concerned the sleep of five infants who had demonstrated both frequent and prolonged apneic periods. REM sleep was indeed the stage during which these apneic periods most frequently occurred, and two of the five infants subsequently expired from what appeared to be the sudden infant death syndrome.[38] There is, unfortunately, no effective treatment of sleep apnea in infants; it characteristically either goes unnoticed or has fatal results.

Apneic periods have been documented in pickwickian hypersomnia, narcolepsy and, to a lesser extent, primary insomnia.[23] In these sleep disorders the apneic periods occur during both REM and NREM sleep.[23] If these periods are not corrected by attempts to normalize sleep patterns, treatment may require tracheostomy and artificial ventilation during sleep.

Parasomnias. In parasomnias, events occur during sleep that usually are seen only during waking.[44] Two types of parasomnias are somnambulism (sleepwalking) and enuresis (bed-wetting).

SOMNAMBULISM. Sleepwalking is a disorder seen primarily in children, and originally it was thought to be a process of acting out dreams. However, EEG studies have shown that sleepwalking occurs exclusively during NREM sleep, primarily stages 3 and 4, when mental recall of dreaming behavior is very low.[22] During the somnambulism incident, the sleepwalker functions at a very low level of awareness. He has total amnesia regarding the event when he is aroused, either during the incident or the next morning.[22] Treatment consists of protective measures such as removing dangerous objects from the sleeping environment and locking doors. If somnambulism is frequent or lasts several years, drugs capable of suppressing stage 4 NREM sleep, such as diazepam (Valium), may be used.[22]

ENURESIS. Bed-wetting is the most common and easily the most distressing childhood sleep disorder. Controversy reigns as to basis for this disorder, although repressed hostile or dependent feelings for parents may play a role in some cases.[22] The initial belief that enuretic episodes occur during dreams has been largely contradicted by sleep studies that show the majority of episodes to occur during nondreaming sleep, that is, during NREM stages 2 and

1.[23] Children generally outgrow this disorder; 90 per cent are dry by the age of 7, and 97 per cent by age 12.[23] Because parents are understandably concerned about enuresis, treatment usually involves educating parents to be patient and to avoid overreaction, which can produce anxiety and guilt in the enuretic child. Imipramine (Tofranil) has been used with some effectiveness, but there is a tendency for relapse when the drug is withdrawn.[23] The reader is referred to Chapter 30 for further information.

Secondary Sleep Disorders

Secondary sleep disorders are specific or nonspecific disturbances that accompany chronic clinical problems.[44]

Secondary Insomnia

TEMPORARY DISTURBANCES. Most individuals experience secondary insomnia at some time during their life, either in conjunction with travel, poor sleeping conditions or psychologic stress. Any condition involving pain or physical discomfort can also cause difficulty in sleeping. This type of insomnia is usually as transient as the condition that produces it, and treatment is based solely upon the cause.

PSYCHOTIC DISTURBANCES. Secondary insomnia accompanies some mental disorders. Psychotic depression has been found to be associated with difficulty in falling asleep, more time awake, decreases in stages 3 and 4 NREM, and decreases in total sleep time.[44] Schizophrenia has been found to be associated with decreased REM prior to and during acute episodes; it is postulated that schizophrenics develop a REM debit and that acute hallucinatory episodes are related to partial REM breakthroughs during wakefulness.[44] Treatment for secondary insomnia in these cases involves counseling and use of specific antipsychotic drugs. Evidence that the sleep pattern of individuals with these disorders is normalizing is frequently a gauge of the effectiveness of the treatment program.

CHRONIC RENAL INSUFFICIENCY. Secondary insomnia can result from chronic renal insufficiency. Such patients experience difficulty in falling and staying asleep at a frequency three times that seen in the general population.[44] The disturbed sleep patterns may be associated with above normal levels of creatinine and other end products of metabolic processes, but dialysis (a process that clears excess electrolytes and metabolites) fails to correct the difficulty. Treatment is difficult in these patients for several reasons: general disability often precludes exercise; intake of foods and fluids is often markedly restricted; these individuals are faced with many daily psychologic stresses associated with chronic illness; and finally, many hypnotic medications are usually excreted from the body by the kidney. Thus, use of these medications is difficult without exposing the patient to the danger of drug toxicity.

Alcoholism. Excessive intake of alcohol supresses REM sleep and is associated with a fragmented sleep pattern that lacks the usual specific progression.[11, 34] Subjectively, sleep is less refreshing, and the alcoholic frequently reports nervous irritability and fatigue. Acute withdrawal from alcohol is associated with a marked increase in REM, often to the extent that REM approaches 100 per cent of the sleep time.[11] The alcoholic must desire to quit drinking to be treated. Although withdrawal of alcohol is complete, the patient is treated with carefully administered hypnotic medications to decrease the physiologic disruption of the withdrawal process. Sleep normalizes in these individuals once the acute phase of alcohol withdrawal is over and the hypnotic medications have been gradually withdrawn.

Hypothyroidism. Insufficient thyroid hormone is associated with complaints of chronic fatigue and somnolence. It often presents with symptoms common to hypersomnia. EEG patterns of individuals with hypothyroidism show decreased stages 3 and 4 NREM sleep in spite of excessive total sleep time.[44] Unlike many sleep disorders, the sleep disturbances of hypothyroidism totally disappear with thyroid hormone replacement therapy.[44]

SLEEP EXACERBATED CONDITIONS

Not infrequently, individuals with medical illness experience some manifestations of that illness during sleep; in some cases, catastrophic illness appears in sleep.

Coronary Artery Disease

Myocardial infarctions frequently occur at night; because of this, researchers have studied sleep EEG's concomitantly with parameters of myocardial function, namely, the electrocardiogram (ECG).[22, 24, 33] One study showed that 82 per cent of the episodes of nocturnal angina occurred during REM sleep.[33] Also, the ECG during these episodes showed electrical changes associated with cardiac muscle strain.[33] Physiologically, this is consistent with increased cardiac demands that occur normally during REM.

Various hypnotic medications are administered to cardiac patients to decrease pain and anxiety and consequently promote rest and sleep. Not infrequently these medications include morphine and diazepam (Valium), both known suppressors of REM sleep. The value of suppressing REM, and thus decreasing its physiologic manifestations upon the myocardium, is not known. However, the benefit of REM suppression must be weighed against the potentially greater degree of physiologic strain that could occur in a REM rebound when these drugs are withdrawn.

Peptic/Duodenal Ulcer

Patients with peptic/duodenal ulcer have been found to secrete 3 to 20 times more gastric acid at night than normal individuals.[12] Simultaneous studies of sleep EEG's and gastric secretion rates in these individuals correlated the increases in gastric secretion to REM sleep.[24] This finding of increased gastric secretion is consistent with the clinical finding of nocturnal pain frequently reported by ulcer patients.

Nocturnal Dyspnea

Patients with chronic respiratory conditions such as emphysema or cor pulmonale frequently experience increased dyspnea (difficult breathing) at night.[44] This respiratory insufficiency has not been found to correlate with any specific sleep stage. It is believed to be the result of an increased blood return to the heart, which consequently causes pulmonary edema and congestion when the individual assumes a reclining position.[44] Dyspnea in these individuals can sometimes be minimized by having them sleep with the head elevated.

NURSING ROLE IN PROMOTING SLEEP AND REST

One of the most important responsibilities in nursing is to assist patients in all phases of ill-

ness to receive the beneficial and recuperative effects of rest and sleep. In order to meet this responsibility the nurse must use knowledge of the individual nature of obtaining rest and the patterns of sleep as the basis for informed nursing care and planning.

Sleep/Rest History

A nursing history is performed in nearly every health care setting. Information on individual patterns of rest and sleep is not always included but should be a high priority. Not only methods of resting such as reading, hobbies or specific relaxation techniques but also specific patterns regarding sleep behavior should be ascertained. Important data on the sleep pattern include the number of hours slept each day; usual times for going to bed and arising; usual number of awakenings during the night and the reasons; daily exercise pattern; number and length of daytime naps; and usual sleep environment, including type of bed, whether the individual sleeps alone or with someone, number of pillows and blankets and amount of ventilation, light and noise that is usually present. The nurse should also discern customary use of any aids for sleep, specifically defining any bedtime or pre-sleep routines, ingestion of snacks or beverages, taking a bath or shower, or the use of medications. Finally, the nurse must determine the individual's beliefs about the quantity of rest and sleep he needs to function at optimum levels. A summary of data to be gathered in the sleep and rest history is pre-

---

TABLE 26–2.   SLEEP AND REST HISTORY

A. Rest
  1. Methods (reading, specific meditation techniques)
  2. Time of day performed
B. Sleep patterns
  1. Number of hours per night
  2. Usual time of going to bed
  3. Usual time of arising
  4. Number of awakenings during night and reasons for them
  5. Daily exercise pattern
  6. Number and length of naps
  7. Sleep environment
     a. Type of bed
     b. Sleeping companion, if any
     c. Number of pillows and blankets used
     d. Ventilation
     e. Light
     f. Noise
  8. Usual bedtime routine
     a. Snacks
     b. Bath/shower
     c. Reading, watching television
  9. Medications for sedation/sleep
  10. Personal belief about sleep needs

sented in Table 26–2. Once the sleep and rest history is completed, a nursing care plan can be formulated that is capable of assisting the patient to meet his individual needs.

Nursing Actions in Meeting Rest and Sleep Needs

Specific actions taken to meet the sleep and rest needs of patients will vary and are based on the patient's situation and his degree of incapacitation due to illness. However, nursing actions in promoting rest and sleep can be divided into general categories to provide the student with a framework for formulating individualized plans.

Planning Activities around Customary Rest and Sleep Periods. The sleep and rest history will supply the nurse with information regarding the times of the day the patient is most active and the times he usually rests and sleeps. This information is the basis for care planning and should be analyzed and discussed with each patient so that necessary alterations in usual routines can be explained and minimized. The patient's understanding of imposed alterations and the demonstration by nursing personnel that they are willing to recognize his individuality in terms of rest and sleep needs and patterns will greatly decrease anxiety associated with those alterations.

Regardless of the patient situation, continual review of nursing procedures as well as the schedule of these activities is critical and should emphasize minimal disruption of periods of rest and sleep. Vital sign determination, intake and output recording, hygiene measures and linen changes are procedures that are often scheduled and performed without appropriate consideration of the patient situation. Does the patient need to have his vital signs taken every 2 hours, or could he be on a more infrequent schedule? Must he have his bath or shower at 7 AM or could it wait until 9 or 10? All too often the patient is awakened or interrupted for procedures that are not critical at that particular time. In scheduling patient activities, the nurse should remember that the average length of a sleep-stage cycle is 90 minutes, and therefore, rest and sleep periods should be at least that long.

Diagnostic procedures such as x-rays and laboratory tests are generally performed at times convenient for those departments; however, it is frequently possible to determine a time that is acceptable to both the department and the patient. When these procedures must be performed at an inappropriate time, forewarning the patient can greatly decrease the disruptive effects upon his routine.

Scheduling, planning and keeping the patient informed about not only the therapeutic plan but also its rationale will allow maximum use of periods of rest and sleep. In this way, the nurse potentiates specific measures being performed to regain and optimize health.

Regardless of whether daytime naps had been included in the patient's customary daily routine, during illness there is a general tendency for at least one nap. The nurse should remember that the time of day naps are taken determines the type of sleep obtained. Early morning naps are proportionately high in REM sleep, while afternoon naps are proportionately high in NREM. If the patient reports difficulty in sleeping at night, the nurse should review the time of any napping. Afternoon naps can result in decreased NREM sleep during the early part of the night (when NREM occurs in large quantities), thus altering appropriate sleep-stage progression and percentages. It may be necessary to discourage naps in the afternoon in favor of some other form of restful activity acceptable to the patient. It is important that the rationale for avoiding afternoon naps be explained and that the replacement activity is purposeful to the patient. If he fails to understand the reason for restricting such naps or is bored by the activity that is substituted, anger or inability to stay awake may result.

Promoting Relaxation. Regardless of individual methods of obtaining rest and patterns of sleep, neither rest nor sleep is likely to occur unless the patient first is able to relax. Efforts to promote both mental and physical relaxation are necessary if rest and sleep periods are to be used with maximum efficiency and supply maximum recuperative benefit.

MENTAL RELAXATION. The effects of tension, worry and anxiety on the individual's ability to rest were covered in the first section of this chapter. They are related to the patient's critical beliefs about his safety and his control of the situation.

Illness itself invariably implies alterations in life-style, not only in the immediate sense but also in terms of the future. A very real patient concern during illness is related to outcome. Often the patient must deal with fears of future disability or even death. Therefore, the nurse must learn the physiologic manifestations of the patient's illness so that appropriate explanations of therapeutic procedures and their rationale can be given. It is advisable to make maximum use of resources such as other nursing personnel, textbooks and the patient's doctor to ensure understanding of the seriousness and potential outcomes of each patient's condition. The nurse can also assist the patient in formulating and presenting questions he would like to ask his doctor. These measures assist the patient in development of a realistic understanding of his illness and its effects. The nurse is cautioned against making either intentional or inadvertent blanket reassurances to the patient that all will be well; indeed, this is not always the case, and the possibility of disability or death may have a basis in fact. In such cases social service or religious counseling referrals may be appropriate in order to assist the patient in coping.

Reassuring the patient that the nursing staff is available to him and that they are willing to help him deal with his concerns can greatly decrease the anxiety associated with illness. It is important to ensure that the call mechanism is not only working but within easy reach. Also, answering it without undue delay greatly aids the patient's ability to relax. Thus, the nurse must first recognize that fears and anxiety may be present and then demonstrate availability and willingness to assist the patient in coping.

PHYSICAL RELAXATION. Maximum use of periods for rest and sleep requires physical relaxation, which occurs more readily if physical discomfort is minimized. Measures to prevent and manage pain are a major component of minimizing physical discomfort and involve not only simply administering analgesic medication but careful planning so that it can exert maximum benefit, e.g., 30 minutes before painful procedures are expected. The reader is referred to Chapter 34 for other measures to prevent and manage this complex sensation.

Measures to minimize tissue irritation also favor physical relaxation and are especially important prior to patient attempts to rest or sleep. The skin should be clean and dry, and drainage tubes should be placed and anchored so that they function properly and do not pull, pinch or abrade tissue. The patient needs to be assisted in turning and supporting himself so that anatomic alignment is maintained and pressure points are protected. This is especially true for patients in casts and/or traction and should occur in conjunction with skin care and padding of these types of therapeutic equipment. Soiled dressings should be changed and binders rewrapped. Linen should be checked to make sure it is clean, dry and smooth. There should also be adequate covering to ensure warmth without causing the patient to feel too hot.

Nursing actions such as back rubs and massages are effective aids to decreasing muscle cramping and stiffness and thus favor relaxation. These actions are particularly effective if performed immediately prior to a rest or sleep period. The nurse may find that suggesting to the patient that he close his eyes, take several deep breaths, and make a conscious effort to loosen muscles during and after massages is helpful in promoting physical relaxation.

Establishing the Sleep Environment. Changing one's sleep and rest environment has been shown to decrease ability to rest and sleep. The nurse should explain this to the patient, informing him that it may take him longer to fall asleep and that he may have more awakenings and decreased total sleep time.[6] It is important to stress that these are normal adaptation effects and that such problems usually disappear after 1 or 2 days.

Environmental concerns involve not only the physical setting but also the ability to perform usual pre-sleep routines that have been successful in the past. Effective patterns of preparing for sleep and rest will be shown in the sleep and rest history and, in many cases, can be duplicated if such information is included in the nursing care plan. As the patient's condition permits, he should be allowed to have a bedtime snack, read or watch television, and take a warm bath or shower if he customarily does so. Even if the patient is not in the habit of customarily performing such activities, establishing a relaxing routine may assist him to rest and sleep in the health care setting. A knowledge of the various aids to sleep, such as L-tryptophan, and a relaxation-promoting bedtime routine, can potentiate all other measures the nurse performs to help her patients rest and sleep effectively.

Every effort should be made to duplicate the usual sleep setting. The sleep and rest history will provide much information that will enable the nurse to do so. The number of pillows and blankets, room temperature, ventilation, and amount of light should be adjusted whenever possible to conform to patient preferences.

Noise should be kept to a minimum. This involves noise from equipment, from other patients and their visitors and from hospital staff. A certain amount of noise is unavoidable. Common sources of noise include suction and monitoring equipment, housekeeping personnel performing their various duties, and the care of patients in the same room. Noise due to use of equipment should be explained and kept to a minimum. Housekeepers should be informed of rest and sleep periods so that their duties can be performed at a suitable time; this is easily accomplished by simply posting a sign on the door to the patient's room. Prior to sleep periods, care of patients in the same room should be planned so that, at its completion, both patients can be free from further interruption. If one of the patients must be interrupted for treatment procedures, these activities should be grouped so that they are performed no more frequently than every 90 minutes and as quietly and efficiently as possible. Noise from nursing staff is rarely intentional, but it disturbs patients, nonetheless. Staff should be frequently reminded that conversation, laughter and patient interruptions must be kept at minimum levels, in terms of both frequency and volume.

Noise and interruptions pose special problems in critical care settings such as intensive and coronary care units. Cardiac monitors, respirators and suction equipment are frequently necessities but are a source of noise and distraction. This type of equipment does, however, allow selected physiologic functions to be monitored without disturbing patients, a fact that can be considered in deciding whether the patient needs to be awakened for treatment procedures. Even though patients in critical care settings are seriously ill, the same measures regarding planning activity and rest periods and promoting relaxation apply. These types of nursing measures frequently require more organization and effort in the critical care setting, but the need for effective rest and sleep are also more important if maximum benefit is to be received.

Medications for promoting relaxation, rest and sleep may be necessary when nursing measures fail. The nurse should remember that many hypnotic medications interfere with appropriate sleep behavior and must make every effort to minimize the need for them. Medications should never be considered replacements for nursing measures. However, short-term administration of such medications can be of value when necessary.

Teaching Implications Regarding Rest and Sleep

It should now be clear that both rest and sleep are highly individual matters. Nurses should use this fundamental knowledge regarding normal rest and sleep and the factors that influence them as a basis for helping the individual in the health care setting to obtain maximum effectiveness from these processes.

Teaching implications for the patient and his family include reviewing the effects of age and personality on sleep patterns and the fallacy of the belief that every individual needs 8 hours of sleep each night. Knowing the effect of factors such as L-tryptophan and establishing a bedtime routine that promotes relaxation before sleep will allow the nurse to teach patients ways to maximize the benefits of the rest and sleep. In addition, the nurse's awareness of the effects of hypnotics and sedatives can serve as the basis for instructing patients in the most appropriate use of such medications. The nurse should emphasize the fact that while these medications may be effective on a short-term basis, they qualitatively disrupt sleep patterns. Patients need to be taught that routine use of medications is associated with loss of effectiveness and that such drugs should be used only when other methods of promoting sleep and rest have failed.

Teaching implications for other health team members include, in addition to the actions of hypnotic medications, the importance of allowing uninterrupted periods for rest and sleep. It must be remembered that the average sleep cycle lasts approximately 90 minutes. This information and the seriousness of the illness must form the basis for planning treatment and diagnostic procedures.

BIBLIOGRAPHY

1. Agnew, H. W., Wilse, M. A., Webb, W. W., and Williams, R. L.: Sleep patterns in late middle age males: an EEG study. *Electroencephalography and Clinical Neurophysiology*, 23:168, Jan. 1967.
2. Aserinsky, E.: Periodic respiratory pattern occurring in conjunction with eye movement during sleep. *Science*, 150:763, Nov. 5, 1965.
3. Berger, R. J.: The sleep and dream cycle. *In* Kales, A. (ed.): *Sleep Physiology and Pathology.* Philadelphia, J. B. Lippincott Co., 1969.
4. Brezinova, V., and Oswald, I.: Sleep after a bedtime beverage. *British Medical Journal*, 2:431, May 20, 1972.
5. Brezinova, V.: Effect of caffeine on sleep: an EEG study in late middle-age people. *British Journal of Clinical Pharmacology*, 1:203, March 1974.
5a. Brown, J., and Hepler, R.: Stimulation—a corollary to physical care. *American Journal of Nursing*, 76:578–581, April 1976.
6. Coble, P., McPartland, R. J., Silva, W. J., and Kupfer, D. J.: Is there a first night effect? (A revisit.) *Biological Psychiatry*, 9(2):215, Oct. 1974.
7. Conroy, R. T., Miles, W. L., and Miles, J. N.: *Human Circadian Rhythm.* London, J. & C. Churchill, 1970.
8. Cunningham, S. G.: Comfort and sleep status. *In* Mitchell, P. H. (ed.): *Concepts Basic to Nursing*, 2nd ed. New York, McGraw-Hill Book Co., 1977.
9. Dement, W. C., Mitler, M. M., and Zarcone, V. P.: Some fundamental considerations in the study of sleep. *Psychosomatics*, 14:89, March–April 1973.

10. Dement, W. C., and Mitler, M. M.: New developments in the basic mechanisms of sleep. *In* Usdin, G. (ed.): *Sleep Research and Clinical Practice.* New York, Brunner/Mazel Co., 1973.

10a. Dement, W. C., et al.: Narcolepsy: A major cause of excessive sleepiness. *Consultant, 17*:25–28, Dec. 1977.

10b. Garner, H. G.: You may have to leave the hospital to get well. *Supervisor Nurse, 9*:76–79, Sep. 1978.

11. Dement, W. C.: *Some Must Watch While Some Must Sleep.* San Francisco, W. H. Freeman and Company, Inc., 1974.

12. Dragstedt, L. R.: Causes of peptic ulcer. *Journal of the American Medical Association, 169*:203, Jan. 1959.

13. Feinberg, I.: Effects of age on human sleep patern. *In* Kales, A. (ed.): *Sleep Physiology and Pathology.* Philadelphia, J. B. Lippincott Co., 1969.

14. Fink, R. D., Knott, D. H., and Beard, J. D.: Sedative-hypnotic dependence. *American Family Physician, 10*(3):116, Sep. 1974.

15. Ford, A. B.: The meaning of rest. *Cardiovascular Nursing, 1*:11, Jan. 1965.

16. Freemon, F. R.: *Sleep Research: A Critical Review,* 2nd ed. Springfield, Charles C Thomas Co., 1974.

17. Globus, G. G.: A syndrome associated with sleeping late. *Psychosomatic Medicine, 31*:528, Nov.–Dec. 1969.

18. Hartmann, E., Blakeland, F., Zwilling, G., and Hoy, P.: Sleep need: how much sleep and what kind? *American Journal of Psychiatry, 127*:1001, Feb. 1971.

19. Hartmann, E.: Sleep requirements: long sleepers, short sleepers, variable sleepers and insomniacs. *Psychosomatics, 14*:95, March–April 1973.

20. Hartmann, E., and Cravens, J.: The effects of long term administration of psychotropic drugs on human sleep: I–IV. *Psychopharmacologica, 33*:153, April 1973.

21. Hartmann, E., Cravens, J., and List, S.: Hypnotic effects of L-tryptophan. *Archives of General Psychiatry, 31*:394, Sep. 1974.

22. Kales, A., and Kales, J.: Evaluation, diagnosis, and treatment of clinical conditions related to sleep. *Journal of the American Medical Association, 213*:2229, Sep. 1970.

23. Kales, A., and Kales, J.: Sleep disorders. *New England Journal of Medicine, 290*(9):487, Feb. 28, 1974.

24. Karacan, I., Eliot, R. S., Williams, R. L., Thornby, J. I., and Solis, P. J.: Sleep in post-myocardial infarction patients. *In* Eliot, R. S. (ed.): *Stress and the Heart,* Vol. 1. Mount Kisco, CA, Futura Publishing Co., 1974.

25. Kleitman, N.: *Sleep and Wakefulness.* Chicago, The University of Chicago Press, 1963.

26. Kleitman, N.: Basic rest-activity cycle in relation to sleep and wakefulness. *In* Kales, A. (ed.): *Sleep Physiology and Pathology.* Philadelphia, J. B. Lippincott Co., 1969.

27. Kollar, E. J., Namerow, N., Pasnau, R. O., and Naitoh, P.: Neurological findings during prolonged sleep deprivation. *Neurology, 18*:836, Sept. 1968.

28. Kollar, E. J., Pasnau, R. O., Rubin, R. T., Naitoh, P., Slater, G. G., and Kales, A.: Psychologic, psychophysiologic, and biochemical correlates of prolonged sleep deprivation. *American Journal of Psychiatry, 126*(4):488, Oct. 1969.

28a. Langrehr, A. A.: Social stimulation. *American Journal of Nursing, 74*:1300–1301, July 1974.

29. Levine, M. A.: *Introduction To Clinical Nursing,* 2nd ed. Philadelphia, F. A. Davis Co., 1973.

30. Moses, J. M., Johnson, L. C., Naitoh, P., and Lubin, A.: Sleep stage deprivation and total sleep loss: effects on sleep behavior. *Psychophysiology, 12*(2):141, March 1975.

31. Murray, M.: *Fundamentals of Nursing.* Englewood Cliffs, NJ, Prentice-Hall Co., 1976.

32. Narrow, B. W.: Rest is . . . *American Journal of Nursing, 67*:1646, Aug. 1967.

33. Nowlin, J. B., Troyer, W. G., and Collins, W. S.: The association of nocturnal angina pectoris with dreaming. *Annals of Internal Medicine, 63*:1040, Dec. 1965.

34. Oswald, I.: Drug research and human sleep. *Annual Review of Pharmacology, 13*:213, 1973.

35. Rechtschaffen, A. and Monroe, L. J.: Laboratory studies of insomnia. *In* Kales, A. (ed.): *Sleep Physiology and Pathology.* Philadelphia, J. B. Lippincott Co., 1969.

36. Roffwarg, H. P., Muzio, J. N., and Dement, W. C.: Ontogenetic development of the human sleep-dream cycle. *Science, 152*:604, April 29, 1966.

37. Shapiro, C. M., Griesel, R. D., Bartel, P. R., and Jooste, P. L.: Sleep patterns after graded exercise. *Journal of Applied Physiology, 39*:187, Aug. 1975.

38. Steinschneider, A.: Prolonged apnea and the sudden-infant-death syndrome: clinical and laboratory observations. *Pediatrics, 50*:646, Oct. 1972.

39. Vogel, G. W.: REM deprivation III: dreaming and psychosis. *Archives of General Psychiatry, 18*:312, March 1968.

40. Webb, W., Agnew, H. W., and Sternthal, H.: Sleep during the early morning. *Psychonomic Science, 6*(6):277, Oct. 25, 1966.

41. Webb, W.: *Sleep: An Experimental Approach.* New York, The Macmillan Co., 1968.

42. Williams, R. L., Agnew, H. W., and Webb, W. G.: Sleep patterns in young adults: an EEG study. *Electroencephalography and Clinical Neurophysiology, 20*:376, Feb. 1964.

43. Williams, H. L., and Coulter, J. D.: Monoamines and the EEG stages of sleep. *Activitas Nervosa Superior, 11*:188, Nov. 1969.

44. Williams, R. L., and Karacan, I.: Clinical disorders of sleep. *In* Usdin, G. (ed.): *Sleep Research and Clinical Practice.* New York, Brunner/Mazel Co., 1973.

45. Wyatt, R. J.: Treatment of insomnia. *Connecticut Medicine, 37*(10):493, Oct. 1973.

CHAPTER 27

PROVIDING BASIC PATIENT HYGIENE

By Maureen Niland, R.N., M.S.

OVERVIEW AND STUDY GUIDE

When a person becomes ill the need for hygiene may increase, yet the person's ability to take care of his own personal hygiene may decrease. A patient requires hygiene care for both physical and psychologic reasons. While assisting the patient with hygiene care, the nurse has an opportunity to (a) establish rapport and assess the patient's overall condition; (b) prevent infection; (c) provide cleanliness and comfort; and (d) teach hygiene principles.

Hygiene care and skills included in this chapter are as follows: assisting the patient with a bedpan, urinal or bedside commode and with handwashing; oral care; care of eyes, ears and nose; general skin care; bathing; perineal care; nail, foot and hair care; back massage; general grooming; and providing comfort and cleanliness for the patient in bed.

Before beginning this chapter, pause and think about your personal beliefs regarding hygiene. Your personal hygiene practices are derived from your cultural background and family teachings. Cultural practices tend to affect general hygiene habits more than scientific knowledge. *Your* feelings about cleanliness and privacy can influence those for whom you care. By keeping an open mind to hygiene practices that are different from your own and learning factual information as well as skillful methods, you can provide effective hygiene care.

STUDY GUIDE

Some basic knowledge of anatomy, physiology, microbiology and the social sciences is important for understanding the rationale for hygiene skills and assessing the need for hygiene. The following suggestions for review include examples of how the information is applied to hygiene care. Review the following:

1. Names and locations of *bones*. This information serves as a basis for relating the patient's condition to contraindications for movement during such activities as bathing and bedmaking.

2. Names and locations of *muscles* and *joints*. This knowledge assists you in performing good body mechanics, giving appropriate support of joints during bathing, and providing effective back massage.

3. Layers of the *skin;* normal appearance of skin; the mechanisms of secretion, excretion and heat regulation; and protective functions of the skin and its appendages. This background aids in assessing a patient's skin condition, judging when massage is needed and determining which hygiene agents to use in skin care.

4. Process of *circulation* and *respiratory* system. This is helpful for understanding specific points such as why gums are massaged during oral care, why some patients have difficulty lying flat during bedmaking and why assessment of nail beds is important.

5. *Gastrointestinal* and *genitourinary* systems. This helps in understanding the methods used in perineal care; why a male prefers to stand for voiding (passing urine); and why the sitting position is best for defecation (expelling feces, bowel movement).

6. Parts of the *infection chain* (host, agent, environment) and how *pathogens* are transmitted. This knowledge can be used to determine how to attack the weakest link in the infection chain. How can the worker alter the environment of the mouth when giving oral care? How are oral infections spread per facial sinuses to other areas of the body? Why is handwashing essential in all care?

7. Location of various parts of the eye: canthus, conjunctiva, lacrimal sac and sclera. This knowledge helps in preventing infections. Why wash the eyes from the canthus outward?

8. Inflammatory process. This helps in recognizing stages of the healing process. Is a lesion (damaged or altered tissue) becoming worse or improving? Lesions are frequently discovered during oral care, bathing or bedmaking.

9. General *psychosocial* principles and *communication* techniques. This background helps the nurse in responding appropriately to privacy needs,

understanding how general grooming affects self-image and facilitating therapeutic communication while giving physical care.

Be familiar with the following *terms* (directions/positions) before reading this chapter:

anterior   posterior
dorsal   prone
dorsal recumbent   superior
inferior   supine
lateral

Review the scientific facts and principles of the following concepts:

asepsis   privacy
body mechanics   safety
individuality   work organization

While reading this chapter, consider how each of the above concepts relates to hygiene care in general and specific hygiene skills, e.g., bedmaking. After completing this chapter, reflect upon how the excellent nurse applies scientific facts and principles during hygiene care.

INTRODUCTION

Each member of society views the need for privacy and hygiene differently. Although hygiene habits are highly individualized, hygiene practices are similar within societal groups. Hygiene preferences stem from cultural background, family practices, individual life-style, physical problems, emotional state, advertising, and cost.

Illness influences personal hygiene habits in various ways. For example, a man who usually bathes daily at home may change his personal hygiene habits in the hospital. When in the patient role, he may refuse to be bathed in bed because he feels dependent and embarrassed. Illness can affect a patient's physical condition, thereby altering one's hygiene requirements. For example, vomiting, diarrhea, excessive perspiration and prolonged immobility in bed can increase need for hygiene. Emotional problems also can change hygiene practices. A patient who is depressed may show little interest in personal hygiene.

During hygiene care (e.g., perineal care) organisms can be transmitted in exudate (fluid) draining from orifices (entrances or outlets). A nurse must be careful to avoid the spread of pathogenic organisms while giving hygiene care.

History

Throughout history emphasis on personal hygiene has varied. Factors that have historically influenced hygiene practices include social norms, religious rituals, the environment (e.g., availability of water for bathing), and the evolution of hygiene aids such as the bathtub, soap and electronic devices, e.g., hair dryers.

In the hospital setting, hygiene practices originated with the need to establish sanitary conditions that would promote healing and prevent spread of disease. Unfortunately, some hospital hygiene practices have become ritualistic tasks. An example of ritualistic practice is requiring a patient to bathe daily regardless of his need for bathing. Perpetuating these traditions does not always provide optimum care for patients.

Determining Need for Hygiene Care

Hygiene policies and practices vary from institution to institution. However, the excellent nurse provides care based not only upon institutional policies and practices but also upon (a) assessment of individual patient needs; (b) current scientific rationale; and (c) the purposes of hygiene care. Some of the purposes for providing hygiene care are:

▶ Comfort and relaxation, e.g., feeling refreshed and relaxing tense muscles

▶ Stimulating circulation, e.g., massage and friction

▶ Cleanliness, e.g., removing necrotic tissue, transient microorganisms, secretions and other debris

▶ Improving self-image, e.g., smell and appearance

▶ Conditioning the skin, e.g., cleansing, stimulating circulation and prevention of excessive dryness

Communication and Assessment

In addition to accomplishing the above purposes, other benefits can be gained during hygiene care. The skillful nurse also uses this time to communicate with the patient and make observations about his condition. The novice nurse may have difficulty in simultaneously performing new procedures, conversing with the patient and making appropriate observations. Initiating conversation with the patient before starting hygiene care can be relaxing for both nurse and patient. As the nurse gains skills, she will be able to focus more on the patient as a person and will become more sensitive to the patient's needs for privacy and learning.

Priorities of Care

Whether you are providing care for one or several patients, establishing priorities and work organization are essential for effective care. Several factors determine priorities of nursing care: (a) the patient's general physical condition; (b) individual hygiene requirements; (c) preferences and requests from the patient; and (d) the number of patients for whom you are caring. Depending upon the situation, hygiene care may take precedence over other needs or vice versa.

Assume that you are caring for the following patients. Think before acting: what care does each need, when and why? A short time spent planning can prevent many interruptions and frustrations for you and the patient. One patient is critically ill, and maintenance of physical integrity is paramount. A second patient is dying. Both physical and emotional care are important; for this patient, hygiene care that focuses on preventing additional discomfort is the first priority. For example, it may cause pain when you do perineal care, but care is necessary to prevent further excoriation and increased pain. Another patient is having several tests. Only short periods of time are available for hygiene between scheduled appointments. All of the patients require medications, other treatments and monitoring of their vital signs. How will you best assist these patients with their needs?

Some nurses allow themselves to be guided solely by patient preferences. Before fulfilling a patient's request, first consider whether it is therapeutic for him, know the daily activities, and discuss his request with the nurse in charge. For example, a patient may avoid oral care because of oral discomfort; he may not realize that oral care could decrease discomfort of a sore mouth. Providing for patient preferences is important; if you cannot fulfill a request, it is helpful to explain your reasons to the patient.

Types of Hygiene Care

Knowledge of usual hygiene activities performed in institutions plus assessing patient needs will help in establishing priorities for hygiene, organization and providing effective overall care. The following terms are commonly used in relation to hygiene care.

Complete morning care usually entails complete bathing and perineal care; back massage; oral, hair and nail care; and a complete change of bed linens.

Partial morning care usually involves washing the patient's face and hands and providing oral and hair care. Areas of the body that have the most secretions (e.g., axillae and perineum) are also usually bathed. Soiled linen and pillow case are changed.

Early morning care is often provided by the night staff to prepare patients for breakfast or early morning diagnostic tests. This usually consists of refreshing comfort measures such as washing face and hands, oral care and offering the bedpan or urinal.

H.S. care (hour of sleep care) is given in the evening or at bedtime (just before the patient retires for the night). This usually involves oral care; washing face, hands and back; back massage for relaxation; and changing soiled linen and gown.

Preoperative hygiene care. Some institutions have the patient bathe the night before surgery. The operative site is scrubbed with an antiseptic solution in the early morning before surgery. Dentures, contact lenses, wigs, hair pins, and make-up are removed for safety. The patient is offered an opportunity to void because bladder distention can be a problem during or following surgery. This is done just before the patient leaves his hospital room for surgery.

With each type of hygiene care the patient's bedside unit is straightened and cleaned, and necessary items are left within reach of the patient. The nurse who focuses on patient needs also will adapt these "routines" to the patient's habits as much as is feasible. For example, if a patient desires complete hygiene care at night rather than in the morning, the nurse will try to fulfill this request.

Patient Teaching of Hygiene Principles

Correcting misconceptions regarding hygiene and teaching new personal hygiene habits are difficult. Recall that hygiene practices are usually based on culture and customs, not scientific knowledge. Habits and attitudes become well established and change slowly.

For example, a person who has very dry skin and has used a particular soap will resist changing his soap even if told it is harmful to the skin. The following points are important in patient teaching: (a) know the scientific facts; (b) know teaching-learning theory, e.g., readiness for learning; (c) never tell a patient something is absolutely wrong, for this only reinforces the previous habit; (d) provide new information, e.g., explain the advantages of scientific methods; (e) incorporate teaching while providing hygiene care; and above all, (f) be pragmatic about what is realistic for this patient.

BASIC PATIENT UNIT

Most equipment and supplies needed for patient hygiene care are kept in the patient's unit. A *patient unit* consists of furnishings and items in the patient's immediate environment (see Fig. 27–1). Furniture in a basic patient unit typically includes the (a) hospital bed; (b) overbed table; (c) bedside stand; (d) lamp; and (e) chair. In addition to the furniture, a basic patient unit contains a call signal and various personal care items. The call signal should *always* be in working condition and within easy reach of the patient. Some personal care items are supplied by the institution, and others are brought from the patient's home. Personal care

items usually supplied by the institution include the (a) wash basin; (b) emesis basin; (c) soap and soap dish; and (d) bedpan or urinal. Some institutions also provide such items as toothbrush, toothpaste, mouthwash, skin lotion, tissues, deodorant and comb. However, such oral and hair care supplies are usually brought by the patient. A waste disposal bag is typically attached to the side of the bed.

Hospital Bed

Standard hospital beds are available in three types: manual, hydraulic, and electric. Each has a device for adjusting the position of the head, knees and height of the bed. *Manually* operated beds have hand cranks located at the foot of the bed. These cranks are turned clockwise to obtain various positions of the bed. The usual configuration for the hand cranks is right side (head crank), left side (knee crank) and center (adjusts height of the bed). *Hydraulic* beds are driven by air pressure. The plug attached to the bed can be placed into a wall outlet for compressed air. A push button is used by the worker to adjust positions of the bed. Some hydraulic beds have a foot pedal that can be used when no wall outlet is available for compressed air. Pumping the foot pedal creates a source of air pressure for changing positions of the bed. *Electric* beds operate by a motor that is electrically driven to adjust the bed to various positions. The electrical cord and plug are located at the head of the bed. Switches (levers or but-

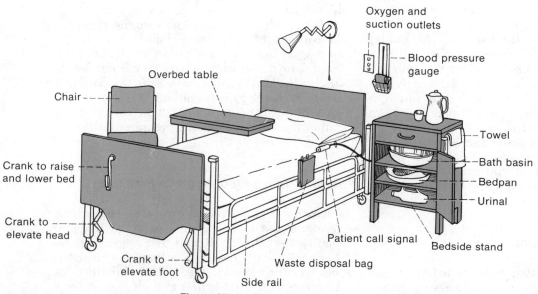

Figure 27–1. Basic patient unit.

tons) for changing bed positions may be located in various places on the bed (e.g., foot of bed, sides of bed). In addition, some electric beds have a control panel on the side of the bed or one that can be attached to bed linen. If the control panel is within easy reach for the patient, he can operate the bed himself to change bed positions.

Overbed Table

An overbed table is a small table supported by a bar attached to a wide-based bottom (see Fig. 27-1). The table is designed so the base can slide under the bed, thus positioning the table over the bed. The table also can be adjusted to various heights. The patient can use the overbed table for eating, reading and writing. The worker can use the table as a movable, hard, flat surface for placement of items while giving care. When the worker is assisting with hygiene care, the table usually is placed lengthwise beside the bed. Some overbed tables have a movable top that lifts or slides. Under the top may be a mirror and/or a storage area. The mirror enables the patient to perform self-care (e.g., oral and hair care) more easily. The storage area is most often used for make-up, hair care items and shaving equipment.

Bedside Stand

The bedside stand is also used to store the patient's personal items. To guide the worker in assessing the patient unit for hygiene supplies, one type of bedside stand and an arrangement of personal care items is included as a sample.

A bedside stand usually has one drawer and a cupboard with shelves (see Fig. 27-1). Typically, on top of the bedside stand is a water carafe, water glass, and possibly additional items such as a small radio. The top drawer usually contains tissues, personal possessions such as small amounts of money, and oral or hair care equipment. For aseptic reasons it is best to separate oral and hair care equipment. The first shelf in the bottom section contains a wash basin with soap and soap dish; emesis basin, which is placed inside the wash basin; oral care equipment, which is inside the emesis basin; skin lotion; other hygiene agents (e.g., deodorant); and a bath blanket. On the bottom shelf is elimination equipment, such as a bedpan, bedpan cover, urinal and toilet paper. Also, a robe and slippers may be found on the bottom shelf. Most bedside stands have a metal bar on the side or back of the stand for hanging a washcloth and towels.

Lamp

Some type of movable lamp usually is attached to the wall, head of the bed or bedside stand. The lamp must be safely positioned so that neither the patient nor the worker will bump against it, burning or bruising themselves. The lamp should allow the patient to come to a sitting position without hitting his head and should not cause glare. When correctly positioned, a good lamp can be useful in performing bedside procedures such as removing sutures.

Chair

Most patient units have at least one straight-back chair with or without arms. In addition to using the bedside chair for patient and visitors, it is used by staff. The chair seat is used for placement of clean linen while bathing the patient and changing bed linen. At such times, the chair seat is wiped off with a disinfectant before placing clean linen on it. This prevents contamination of clean linen by microorganisms. The chair back can be used for hanging a linen bag for soiled linen. Workers and visitors should sit on the chair, *not* on the bed. This decreases spread of organisms.

A patient's unit is most comfortable for him if he has within easy reach those items he most frequently uses and if he can easily reach storage areas in his bedside stand and overbed table. Some patients like to have one or two personal items (e.g., cards, photographs) placed for their viewing. The patient's environment can become cluttered unless all workers strive to neatly put away infrequently used items. Additionally, assessment of a patient's unit before collecting supplies eliminates accumulation of duplicate supplies in the unit.

ELIMINATION

Before starting hygiene care, offer the patient an opportunity to defecate (have a bowel movement) or void (urinate). Offering the patient time to use the toilet, commode, bedpan or urinal before other hygiene care helps the patient to feel more relaxed and comfortable and decreases the possibility of interruptions caused by the patient's need to eliminate during hygiene care.

The patient may have *elimination needs* at

any time, but the most frequent times are upon awakening, before and after meals, and before sleep. Many patients are reluctant to express the need for elimination because of embarrassment and lack of complete privacy. You can best assist a patient by (a) offering to provide for elimination *before* he has to ask; (b) having a casual yet professional approach concerning the need for elimination; (c) providing maximum privacy and comfort for the patient; and (d) knowing how to position a patient for the most effective evacuation if he must use a bedpan or urinal.

It is important to assess a patient's ability to meet his own elimination needs safely and in privacy. When a patient requires assistance in using the bedpan, commode or toilet, the worker considers the following factors in *providing patient comfort, safety and privacy and reducing possible embarrassment:*

▶ Provide adequate assistance to the patient as he (a) moves to and from a commode or toilet or (b) gets on or off a bedpan, commode or toilet.

▶ Secure commode wheels as the patient gets on and off the commode.

▶ Pad bedpan or commode for patients who are very thin or emaciated to prevent discomfort and skin breakdown.

▶ Stay with patients who are weak or in danger of falling off the toilet or commode. Secure safety belts as appropriate. Remember to frequently observe any restrained patient. Raise side rails as necessary for patients using a bedpan.

▶ Place call signal and toilet paper within easy reach of patients using elimination equipment.

▶ Close bathroom or patient room doors, pull curtains and close window drapes as appropriate to provide privacy.

▶ Ensure patient warmth, e.g., use patient's robe or place bath blanket around patient's shoulders. At times it is helpful to cover the patient's legs with a towel or bath blanket while on the commode or toilet.

▶ Be sure that patients getting up to use the commode or toilet wear shoes or slippers to prevent slipping and to provide warmth.

▶ Observe patient for hypotensive epsiodes (sudden drop in blood pressure). The pa-

tient may complain of dizziness, appear pale, feel clammy or have a thready pulse. This usually can be prevented by having the patient first sit on the side of the bed with pressure on his feet to aid in venous return and to allow the body time to adjust to position change.

▶ Observe patients frequently when elimination could cause excessive *tiredness* (e.g., weak patients); *pain* (e.g., patients with kidney stones or rectal surgery); or *severe complications from the strain of defecation* (e.g., some patients with heart or eye problems).

Weak or helpless patients should not be allowed to sit on commodes or bedpans for long periods of time. Being left in this state for longer than a reasonable amount of time not only is demeaning and uncomfortable for the patient but may promote skin breakdown due to shearing force on the patient's buttocks (see Chap. 33).

▶ When elimination creates unpleasant odors, promptly air the room withut chilling the patient and use room deodorizers appropriately. Conduct these activities in ways that do not embarrass the patient.

Bedpans and Urinals

A male patient confined to bed uses a bedpan for defecation and a urinal for voiding (see Fig. 27–2). A female patient typically uses the bedpan for both defecating and voiding. Female urinals are available but are not commonly used.

Bedpans. *Standard bedpans* are available in adult and pediatric (children's) sizes and are commonly made of plastic. Metal bedpans are used in some facilities, but they tend to be quite cold unless warmed prior to use. A pediatric bedpan is sometimes used for an adult with small hips or for a very thin adult. The smaller size conforms more comfortably to the buttocks of these patients; thus, it provides comfort and helps decrease potential skin breakdown that could be caused by a larger pan.

A *fracture bedpan* has a thinner rim than the standard bedpan. Although a fracture bedpan is more easily placed under the patient's buttocks, it is also easier to spill the contents of the fracture pan. Fracture pans are useful for a variety of conditions, including patients (a) who are paralyzed or who cannot be safely turned (e.g., spinal injuries); (b) with a body or long leg cast; (c) who are immobilized by some types of trac-

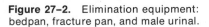

Figure 27-2. Elimination equipment: bedpan, fracture pan, and male urinal.

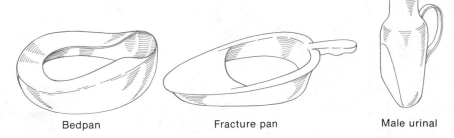

Bedpan   Fracture pan   Male urinal

tion; or (d) who are very thin or emaciated. If the patient is weak or helpless, two helpers should give and remove the bedpan. The use of two people saves the worker's back from strain, allows more accurate placement and is less traumatic for the patient. As emphasized earlier, do *not* leave a patient on a bedpan for extended periods of time, as this can cause tissue damage. If a patient desires to remain on a bedpan for a long time, insist on periodically removing the bedpan.

GIVING THE BEDPAN. Explain to the patient how to assist, elevate the bed to a comfortable working height, and assemble bedpan, bedpan cover and toilet paper. Fold top bed linen out of the way for visualization and moving the patient without unnecessary exposure. Raise the distal side rail for safety and as an aid for lifting or turning the patient.

Two methods can be used for giving a bedpan. For either method or any type of bedpan, the flattest and widest part goes toward the patient's head. The first method is used with the patient on his back (see Fig. 27-3A). Ask the patient to flex his knees, push down on the mattress with his feet, and raise his buttocks. The worker uses one hand to assist in elevating the buttocks and the other hand to slide the bedpan under the patient. The second method is used when the patient is turned to his side (see Fig. 27-3B). Ask the patient to turn toward the far side of the bed. Place the bedpan firmly against his buttocks. Next, place your palm firmly against the topside of the bedpan; push downward and toward the patient. Then have the patient roll back onto the bedpan, while holding the bedpan securely (see Fig. 27-3A and B).

After using either method to give the patient the bedpan, elevate the head of the bed to a near-sitting position. This provides the best position for gravity to aid in evacuation. To promote comfort and prevent the bed from becoming wet, check that the patient is correctly centered on the bedpan. Before leaving the patient, (a) place the call bell and toilet paper near the patient's hand for easy reach and (b) raise the side rails.

REMOVING THE BEDPAN. First lower the head of the bed. Ask the patient to push his feet against the mattress to lift his buttocks and slide the bedpan out. Another method is to have the patient roll toward the far side of the bed. Hold bedpan securely to prevent spillage while patient rolls to the side.

You may need to cleanse the patient's genital area, as reaching this area is difficult for a person who is in bed. In addition to toilet paper, it may be necessary to use soap and water for cleansing the genital area. If the patient is excoriated, warm water without soap is best for cleansing. To decrease the patient's feeling of dependency, explain that you are assisting with this care because self-help is difficult in bed. (See discussion of perineal care later in this chapter for correct method of cleaning the genital area.) Reposition the patient for comfort, lower the bed and provide handwashing for the patient.

Cover the bedpan and take it to the hopper, toilet, dirty utility room or other appropriate place for *disposal of excreta.* Be sure to measure and record liquid waste, if the patient's output is being measured. Perform necessary tests on urine and feces, and chart findings (see Chaps. 24, 30 and 40). Clean the bedpan with a disinfectant and return it to the bedside stand with a clean cover. Be sure to wash your hands after completing care.

Urinal. The standard urinal usually is made of plastic and is used by the male patient who is confined to bed or can only stand to void at the bedside. If the urinal is used in bed, remind the patient to tilt the closed end downward to avoid

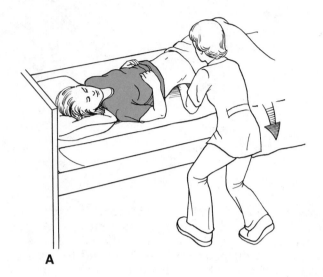

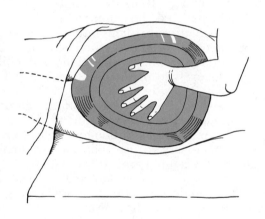

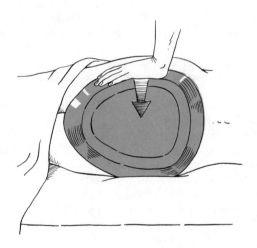

Figure 27–3. Two methods of giving bedpan to patient who can assist with lifting self. *A,* With patient on back. *B,* With patient on side.

spilling. When assisting the patient with standing to void at the bedside, use caution. The patient may be unsteady on his feet or may have a hypotensive episode. If the patient is unable to hold the urinal, the worker places the urinal between the patient's legs and positions the penis in the urinal. Provide privacy by covering the patient while the urinal is held in place for voiding.

A *female urinal* is shaped differently than a male urinal. The opening is larger, and the urinal has a wide, flat bottom. When a female urinal is used, it is held close to the perineum to prevent spillage. This type of urinal can be used in place of the bedpan for a female who has severe mobility restriction and cannot lift her buttocks.

Although some urinals have caps, they frequently do not close tightly. Do *not* leave partially filled urinals at the bedside for the following reasons: (a) asepsis; (b) aesthetic appearance; (c) unpleasant odor; and (d) potential spilling. Dispose of urine as discussed in the preceding section on the bedpan. Offer the patient handwashing, and wash your own hands after completing care.

Bedside Commode

The bedside commode is a chair or wheelchair that has an opening in the center of the seat (see Fig. 27–4). The underside of the seat has grooves for insertion of a bedpan. The bedside commode or toilet is always preferable to a bedpan because bedpans are uncomfortable,

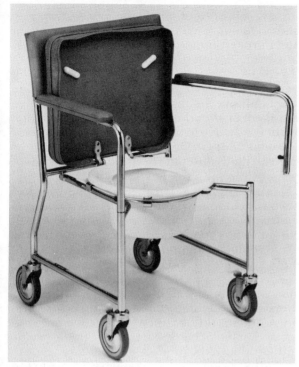

Figure 27–4. Bedside commode. (From Everest & Jennings, Inc., Los Angeles, CA.)

and it may be difficult for a patient to sit in a position that facilitates defecation or urination. Also, using a bedpan is embarrassing for many people. Bedpans should never be used simply for the convenience of nursing personnel. Patients should be encouraged to use a bedside commode or toilet unless such activity is contraindicated. When assisting a patient with a bedside commode:

▶ Apply the principles used for bed-to-chair transfer (see Chap. 21)

▶ Ensure patient privacy and safety

▶ Provide a lap cover, e.g., sheet or other linen over patient's lap

▶Observe and dispose of excreta as with the use of the bedpan

▶ Clean the bedside commode and return it to the appropriate place

▶ Offer the patient handwashing facilities and wash your own hands

Assisting the Patient in Handwashing

As discussed in Chapter 25, the use of effective handwashing technique is the best defense against transmission of organisms. Patients should be encouraged to wash their hands (a) prior to their oral care and meals and (b) after elimination.

> *Offering bedridden patients the opportunity to wash their hands is frequently neglected. Not only is this activity essential for cleanliness, but it also is refreshing and enhances the patient's self-esteem.*

When a patient cannot use a sink, provide a washcloth and towel for handwashing. Some institutions use disposable washcloths. If assisting a patient with handwashing, be sure to cleanse all surfaces of his hands and between every finger.

▶ Use wet washcloth with soap.

▶ Use friction by rubbing the washcloth against the skin surfaces.

▶ Rinse hands and rinse washcloth.

▶ Pat dry with towel.

ORAL CARE

Oral health is extremely important to physical and psychologic welfare. Oral problems can cause localized pain and systemic disease. Loss of teeth can affect self-image, and halitosis ("bad breath") can influence social interaction. Nutrition affects the condition of the oral cavity and general physical health; in turn, the condition of the oral cavity influences nutritional intake. Briefly, the persistence of dental problems stems from:

▶ Lack of knowledge regarding effective oral hygiene techniques

▶ Lack of knowledge as to how to prevent problems

▶ Poorly established patterns during childhood

▶ Poor nutrition and frequent snacking on "junk" foods

▶ Imbalances in the oral flora, allowing growth of harmful bacteria that cause caries

In spite of the importance of oral health, oral care is frequently neglected in everyday life. Many people neglect oral care because they are resigned to the outmoded belief that all teeth eventually must be removed. Through preventive care, teeth can be preserved throughout one's lifetime. Health care workers can encourage and provide effective oral care, but oral hygiene often is a neglected area of patient care. Some possible reasons for neglect of patients' need for oral care and health teaching are as follows:

▶ The assumption that the patient knows how to perform effective oral hygiene

▶ Lack of direct patient observation because most patients do self-care

▶ Lack of assessment of the oral cavity

▶ When the condition of the oral cavity has deteriorated or severe halitosis exists, this aspect of care is viewed as offensive

▶ Patient with a sore mouth may refuse care because they fear discomfort

▶ Lack of appreciation of the significance of oral care to overall well-being

Background knowledge of anatomy and the normal appearance of the oral cavity is necessary for assessment of the condition of the oral cavity. Both assessment and oral care require an understanding of medical asepsis. Thorough handwashing must be done to prevent transmission of organisms from the worker to the patient.

Oral Problems

> Dental caries *(cavities) and* periodontal disease *(affecting gums and tooth-supporting structures) are the two major types of oral problems.*

Dental caries is responsible for most of the tooth loss *before* age 35. *Periodontal disease* is the principal cause of tooth loss *after* age 35.[11] Dental caries and periodontal disease have existed throughout history and continue to be prevalent despite preventive efforts. While scientific knowledge has increased the means for prevention of dental caries, eating patterns have become more deleterious, and poor hygiene habits persist.

Both dental caries and periodontal disease involve a *host* (tooth and supporting structure) and an *agent* (dental plaque). The host, agent and the *oral environment* (e.g., amount and pH of saliva, presence of food) affect the progress of the disease processes. To break the chain of events involved in these disease processes, one must improve the resistance of the host, remove the agent or alter the oral environment so that it is not conducive to the development of disease.

Dental Caries. Dental caries is a disease of the calcified structure of the tooth. The agent responsible for dental caries is *dental plaque.* "Dental plaque is a dense, noncalcified mass of bacteria colonies in a gel-like intermicrobial matrix.[16] Freshly deposited plaque is transparent unless stained brown, e.g., by tobacco or tea. When old dental plaque is present, the teeth appear dull and dingy. *Cavitation* occurs as the result of a combination of bacterial enzymes within the dental plaque, fermenting dietary carbohydrates, and organic acids. The organic acids diffuse out of the plaque onto the tooth enamel (hard covering). These acids initiate decalcification of enamel and dentin. Once the cariogenic bacteria have access to the dentin matrix (tissue substance of tooth), the tooth starts to break down, resulting in cavitation.

Many theories exist as to the specific etiology of dental caries. Some researchers believe sucrose is the cause, while other investigators contend that multiple factors are involved in causing dental caries. Bibby, a proponent of the multiple factor theory, states, "Caries occurred before there were any refined carbohydrates." [2] Thus, Bibby questions whether sugars are the sole cause of dental caries. However, most health professionals agree that sugars play some role in the incidence of dental caries. While there remains some question concerning dietary sugars, all authorities agree that nutrition plays a significant role in whether or not dental caries develop. For example, the maturation of the tooth and tooth-supporting structures are influenced by nutrients such as calcium, phosphorus, fluoride, vitamins and proteins.

Adequate nutrition provides the susceptible host of the tooth with greater resistance to decay. A diet consisting of foods from the basic four groups is generally nutritious. However, dietary needs vary with such factors as age and general physical condition. For example, more protein may be needed when a person has a systemic infection, when a mother is nursing her baby, or during the growth years. "Considerations of the effects of nutrients on the decay process can become very complex when it is realized that in addition to a primary effect a given nutrient may have, it may also exert one or more indirect or secondary effects on the process of decay."[8] Modulation of the diet is probably a key factor, as both deficiencies and excess can decrease resistance to decay. The use of fluoridated water and inclusion of whole-grain foods, which contain phosphorus, can have a caries-inhibiting effect. Fats in the diet can be a barrier to acid penetration by forming an oily film on the surface of the tooth.

On the other hand, a low-protein, high-carbohydrate diet promotes proliferation of cariogenic bacteria in the flora of the oral cavity. Between-meal snacking is one of the major factors contributing to dental caries. Most between-meal snacks contain carbohydrates, which provide a medium for bacterial growth. The combination of nutrients influences the amount of plaque on the teeth and creates an oral environment, which can enhance or inhibit formation of dental caries.

If dental plaque and food remain in the mouth, this also provides an oral environment that is conducive to formation of dental caries. For this reason, a person's oral hygiene is a vital factor in the development of dental caries. Food debris that remains in the mouth after eating is removed by the self-cleansing action of the tongue and saliva. Additional food debris and materia alba can be removed only with vigorous rinsing. *Materia alba* is the loosely adherent white or grayish mass of oral debris and bacteria that lies over dental plaque. Dental plaque cannot be removed by rinsing, but can be removed by brushing and flossing. If the dental plaque is allowed to remain on the teeth it becomes calcified. This calcified, hard, tenacious material is called *calculus (tartar)*. Calculus cannot be removed by toothbrushing. Dental instruments are required to scrape off the hardened mass of calculus.

In summary, to decrease the incidence of dental caries, one must disrupt the chain of events in the disease process. The condition of the host (tooth) can be made more resistive to dental caries by (a) adequate nutrition; (b) the application of fluoride directly to the surface of the teeth by a dentist or hygienist; (c) the use of dentifrices containing fluoride; and (d) the ingestion of fluorine in water or juice. The agent (dental plaque) and the oral environment are dependent upon nutritional intake patterns and effective removal of debris and plaque before calculus forms. Corrective measures to remove existing dental caries and calculus usually improve the health of the host and the condition of the oral environment.

Periodontal Disease. The word "periodontal" (*peri*, "around" and *odous*, "tooth") means "situated or occurring around a tooth; pertaining to the periodontium."[5] The *periodontium* is the tissue that supports and surrounds each tooth. This tissue consists of *gingiva* (gums),

which firmly attaches around the neck of the tooth; *gingival papilla*, the projection of gingiva between the teeth; *periodontal membrane*, a fibrous network that attaches the tooth to the gingiva and supporting alveolar bone. Periodontal disease is a long-term process that involves destruction of the tooth-supporting structures (the periodontium). Detachment of the teeth occurs secondary to the atrophy of the supporting structures.

Periodontal disease is common among young adults. Often this is precipitated by emotional stress, which aggravates an inflammatory process. In the elderly population, the progression of periodontal disease leads to tooth loss. Periodontal disease usually progresses in four stages: (1) gingivitis; (2) periodontitis; (3) acute necrotizing ulcerative gingivitis; and (4) destruction of the tooth-supporting structure.[9] *Gingivitis* is a mild inflammatory process that is usually characterized by bleeding gums and halitosis. With *periodontitis* and *acute necrotizing ulcerative gingivitis* there is mobility of the teeth, purulent drainage at the margin of the gingiva, and severe tissue recession. A person with periodontitis may have little discomfort and may not notice the deteriorating condition of his mouth. On the other hand, the person with acute necrotizing ulcerative gingivitis may experience severe pain. In the fourth stage of periodontal disease, the periodontium atrophies to the point that the gum appears to have completely receded away from the tooth. Without adequate supporting structure the tooth becomes very loosely attached or falls out.

The exact etiology of periodontal disease is as yet unknown. However, "the most prevalent theory is that periodontal disease is initiated by the bacterial component of the dental plaque; however, no definitive microorganism has been identified."[12] The accumulation of dental plaque in the gingival sulcus (crevice) causes inflammation and bleeding. If the dental plaque remains on the tooth until calculus is formed, this causes abrasion and ulceration of the gingival sulcus. Food debris lodged between the teeth also can cause an inflammatory process. The exact part nutrition plays in the cause or prevention of periodontal disease is controversial. However, good nutrition definitely plays an important role in maintaining the tooth-supporting structures. In addition to the nutrients mentioned in the discussion of dental caries, the consistency of the diet can affect the host (tooth-supporting structure) and the oral environment. Firm-textured foods provide stimulation of the gingiva and are less likely to remain in the mouth. A fibrous diet also can help prevent atrophy of salivary glands and increase the protein content of saliva, which creates a "healthy" oral environment. A diet consisting of only soft-textured foods can increase plaque formation and lead to atrophy of the bone structure surrounding the tooth.

As with dental caries, oral hygiene is an important factor in the development or prevention of periodontal disease. Toothbrushing and flossing can remove the agent (dental plaque) and change the oral environment. Both toothbrushing and flossing can alter the condition of the host (tooth-supporting structures). Flossing is particularly helpful in providing gingival stimulation for the person with natural teeth. Patients with dentures and patients without teeth (edentulous) can stimulate their gingiva with gum massage. Some gingival tissue is very fragile. Therefore, the friction created by toothbrushing, flossing and gum massage should stimulate gingival circulation without causing irritation or abrasion of the gingival tissue.

Other Oral Problems.   Other conditions that commonly occur as the result of poor nutrition or irritation are as follows:

Cheilosis (cracking or ulceration of the lips and angles of the mouth) can be caused by riboflavin deficiency, excessive salivation or mouth breathing.

Erosion of the enamel and dentin can result from chemical irritants or mechanical factors such as a hard toothbrush or abrasive dentifrices. Severe erosion can expose retained roots and bone spurs.

Stomatitis is an inflammatory process of the oral mucosa and can result from irritants such as tobacco or drugs.

Systemic diseases and the *systemic side effects of drugs* also can cause oral manifestations (e.g., gingival hemorrhage, atrophic changes, excessive dental caries, stomatitis).

Finally, *oral malignancies* may appear as lumps or ulcerative areas in the mouth.

Assessment of the Oral Cavity

Preparation for Assessment.   An initial oral assessment is indicated whether the patient has natural teeth, dentures or no teeth at all. The first oral assessment provides (a) information on the condition of the oral cavity, (b) data on the effectiveness of past oral hygiene practices and (c) clues to systemic problems. This information combined with a history of the patient's oral hygiene habits provides the basis for health teaching and planning oral care. After the initial assessment, the nurse determines how often subsequent oral examinations should be performed (e.g., once daily, twice daily). The frequency of oral examinations depends upon the following:

▶ Findings on the initial assessment

▶ Need to monitor progress of oral problems

▶ Need to reinforce teaching

▶ Suspected new problems or patient complaints

To perform a good oral examination, the nurse (a) must be able to distinguish between normal and abnormal findings of the mouth and (b) must perform the examination systematically. By using a *systematic* approach, the nurse performs in a more efficient way; also, she is less likely to overlook an area of the mouth during the examination.

Only two basic pieces of equipment are needed for an oral examination:

Light source (overbed light, penlight, or flashlight). The light source must be bright enough to allow good visualization of the oral cavity.

Tongue blade. The tongue blade facilitates movement of the tongue and cheeks for maximum visualization of all areas of the oral cavity.

The condition of the host (tooth and supporting structures), the presence of the agent (excessive dental plaque) and the general oral environment all influence a person's appetite, sense of well-being and appearance. Therefore, a thorough assessment of the oral cavity and effective oral care are a must!

First explain to the patient what you will be doing and how he can assist. Position the patient for comfort and ease of visualization. Usually a Fowler's position (nearly sitting) in bed is best. One suggested sequence for the oral examination is as follows:

▶ Throat

▶ Tongue

▶ Cheeks, gums, condition of teeth

▶ Floor of the mouth

▶ Roof of the mouth

▶ Inner and outer aspects of the lips

If the patient has dentures, they must be removed *before* the oral examination. Dentures prevent the worker from examining the palates and gums of the patient. Before the dentures are removed, observe how well they fit (e.g., whether they adhere tightly or constantly move about as the patient talks). Some difficulty may be encountered in removing the upper dentures. A good way to break the denture seal is for the patient to close his mouth and puff out his cheeks. If the patient is unable to break the seal, the worker or the patient can place a finger above the edge of the denture and exert pressure to pull it away from the gum. If the patient still has difficulty, place one or more fingers of both hands inside the patient's lip and over the borders of the dentures on both sides. A *rocking motion* breaks the seal better than pulling on both sides at the same time. Lower dentures usually come out easily. If assistance is needed with lower dentures, place your fingers inside the patient's bottom lip and grasp the teeth of the denture.

After removing the dentures observe the appearance of the denture linings; look for calculus, dental plaque or food debris on the dentures; and check for broken or cracked areas. Then place the dentures in a denture cup or on a paper towel.

Observations and Method of Oral Examination. Ask the patient to slightly tilt his head backward and open his mouth. With the tongue blade in one hand and the light source in position for good visualization you are ready to begin the oral assessment. *Assess the condition of the oral mucosa* throughout the oral examination by observing for moistness, color and any inflammation, abrasions, lesions or ulcerative areas of the mucous membranes. The steps of the oral examination are as follows:

1. Use the tongue blade to depress the tongue while the patient says "Ah." This gives a clear view of the *throat.* Observe condition of the mucosa of the throat.

2. Ask the patient to protrude his tongue for observing the *top portion of the tongue.* Observe for moisture, color, eruptions and adhered debris.

3. With the tongue in a relaxed position, use the tongue blade to push the tongue to one side and then the other. Look at the *sides and the underside of the tongue.* Note abrasions, growths and enlarged or ruptured blood vessels. The sides of the tongue are common places for cancers to begin.

4. While holding the tongue to one side, observe the appearance of the *inner aspects of gums and teeth.* Palpation of the gums also may be necessary. Are the gums inflamed, bleeding or receding? Note any hyperplasia (increased size) of the gums, color and any drainage between the teeth. Observe the teeth for caries, calculus, debris and erosion. If the patient is edentulous, note any atrophy of the periodontium.

5. To look at the *external portion of the teeth and gums,* use the tongue blade to hold the cheek outward.

6. Observe the *mucosa of the cheeks.*

7. To observe the *floor of the mouth (palate),* ask the patient to touch the roof of his mouth with his tongue. Note growths and condition of mucosa.

8. To examine the roof of the mouth (palate), have the patient tilt his head in hyperextended position with his mouth opened widely. Note growths and condition of mucosa.

9. Observe *inner and outer aspects of the lips.* Note any dryness, lesions or cheilosis.

Assessing the Need for Oral Hygiene. The frequency, type of oral care, and assistance needed with oral hygiene are determined by (1) findings from assessment of the oral cavity; (2) ability for self-care; (3) assessment of health teaching needs; (4) knowledge of preventive measures, e.g., that removal of dental plaque retards caries and periodontal disease; (5) patient's general condition; (6) use of treatments or drugs (e.g., oxygen, atropine) that have a drying effect on oral mucosa.

Assessing Self-Care Abilities. Assessment of a patient's self-care abilities goes beyond just evaluating his physical ability to brush his teeth. For example, a patient's *ambulatory skills* must be assessed. Some patients will be able to get up to a sink for oral care. Bedridden patients who can do self-care will need all equipment placed within easy reach. Other bedridden patients will need total assistance with oral care. Assessment of *mental/emotional status* is also important. The patient who has memory deficits may need structured verbal guidance to perform self-care. Instruction will take more time on the part of the worker than actually giving total care. Nevertheless, as with every activity of daily living (ADL), the patient should be encouraged to perform as much as possible by himself.

Assessing the Need for Patient Teaching. The findings from the oral examination coupled with the patient's history regarding oral habits is used to assess the patient's need for health teaching. The worker can incorporate some patient teaching into discussion while giving oral care, e.g., encouraging more fluids because of noted dryness of the oral mucosa. The worker also can offer information, e.g., explaining that a particular drug the patient is receiving usually has a drying effect on the mucous membranes.

In addition, demonstration is a good method for teaching changes in oral hygiene practices. The worker might demonstrate toothbrushing or flossing technique to increase removal of dental plaque. A teaching aid, such as disclo-

sure tablets, can be used to supplement the demonstration. *Disclosure tablets* stain dental plaque red so that it can be easily seen. The patient is given one of the disclosure tablets to chew for about a minute. Then he rinses once with water. *Before* he starts to brush his teeth he is asked to look in a mirror to see the amount and location of the red-stained dental plaque. *After* he completes toothbrushing, he looks in a mirror to see if his technique has been effective in removing all the dental plaque. Caution the patient that it is not harmful if some redness remains on his tongue. Use of the disclosure tablet provides a means of reinforcing teaching and evaluating the patient's skill and learning.

TABLE 27–1.   ORAL CARE ASSESSMENT GUIDE

NUMERICAL AND DESCRIPTIVE RATINGS*

RATING PARAMETER	1	2	3
Mucous membranes	Moist; membranes intact	Dry; membranes intact	Dry with abrasive or ulcerative areas
Gums	No bleeding or noticeable recession	Slight recession or tendency to bleed	Noticeable recession or gums bleed easily or are swollen
Saliva	Moderate, clear	Scanty or excessive amount	Viscid or ropy
Palates	Moist; no debris or small amount	Dry; small or moderate debris	Dry or moist with large amount of debris
Tongue	Moist; small amount of coating	Dry or moderate amount of coating	Dry or moist with large amount coating or hairy tongue (yellow-black coating)
Odor	Absent or pleasant	Moderate, unpleasant	Pungent
Teeth/dentures	No materia alba; no dental caries or dentures fit well on gum borders	Small or moderate amount materia alba; no dental caries or drainage between teeth; or poorly fitting dentures	Large amount of materia alba; many cavities or purulent (pus) drainage between teeth or cracked/poorly fitting dentures
Plaque/calculus	No plaque and/or small amount calculus	Small or moderate amount plaque or moderate calculus	Large amount of plaque or calculus
Lips	Smooth, soft, no cracking	Rough, dry, small amount of crusting or cracking; tendency to bleed	Dry, cracked, and large amount of crusted secretion or easily bleed
Lesions (growths, sores)	None	Lesion on lips	Lesion in oral cavity
Self-care ability	Total self-care	Needs partial help or direction to complete care	Needs total assistance
Patient teaching	Most knowledge stems from fact; brushes effectively; flosses teeth	Some misconceptions; brushes effectively; never flosses	Many misconceptions; rarely cleanses mouth or brushes ineffectively; never flosses

= Total

*1 is the *best* rating and 3 the *worst* rating for each parameter. All items should be rated; the total number of points ranges from 12 to 36. The total score is viewed as a continuum, with patients scoring high requiring the most oral care.
Source: Adapted from Passos, J., and Brand, L.: Effects of agents used for oral hygiene. *Nursing Research,* 15:199, 1966.

Sometimes it is best to assess the patient's ability for self-care before determining needs for health teaching. For a variety of reasons the patient may not be capable of doing effective oral care.

ASSESSING THE PATIENT'S GENERAL CONDITION. As discussed under "Other Oral Problems," systemic diseases and drugs can produce oral symptoms; e.g., blood disorders can manifest as petechiae (tiny hemorrhagic spots) within the oral cavity, or stomatitis can stem from the side effects of drugs. Conversely, oral problems can cause abnormalities in various areas of the body, e.g., head and neck pain, enlargement of maxillary and other lymph nodes. These observations can be mistaken as originating in an area of the body other than the oral cavity. Dry oral mucosa can be related to mouth breathing, poor function of salivary glands, drugs or insufficient fluid intake.

Evaluation of Findings

Abnormal findings are recorded on the patient's progress notes. Ill-fitting or broken dentures and caries need referral for dental services. Other observations such as a frayed toothbrush or the need for using dental floss should be discussed with the patient. The patient's mental/emotional status (e.g., short attention span) will influence the method of teaching oral hygiene principles as well as the amount of assistance needed for oral care. Assessment will influence both the frequency and type of oral care. The guide in Table 27–1 can be used as an evaluation tool both prior to and after oral care.

Providing Oral Care

Patients with Natural Teeth. Regardless of the frequency or method used in providing oral care, the major concerns are thoroughness of cleansing and maintaining and improving the condition of the oral mucosa. *Equipment* needed for providing oral care in bed includes toothbrush, dentifrice, dental floss, tissues or face towel, a cup of water, and emesis basin. *Brushing* is usually done upon arising and at bedtime. By habit, some patients will be accustomed to brushing their teeth after each meal. Daily brushing of the tongue and flossing are usually recommended.

TYPES OF BRUSHES. Discourage patients from using frayed and uneven hard-bristle toothbrushes, as these are ineffective in cleansing, cause abrasion of teeth and traumatize the gingiva. Recommended features in toothbrush design are (1) straight handle; (2) size small

enough to reach all areas of the mouth easily; (3) even and rounded brushing surface; and (4) soft, multitufted nylon bristles. Rounded soft bristles provide gingival stimulation without causing abrasion. The even, multitufted design allows contact with all surfaces and is more durable. When an electric toothbrush is used, examine it for electrical hazards and caution the patient *not* to turn it on until it is in place in the patient's mouth. Some institutions have *toothettes* available. Toothettes are pieces of foam attached to sticks. They are used for patients who have very sensitive gingivae, after oral surgery, or for the patient who does not have a toothbrush.

DENTIFRICES. Most patients select a dentifrice based on convenience, habit, advertising claims and taste. A dentifrice that contains fluoride is helpful in prevention of dental caries. Although enamel is resistive to abrasion, long-term use of an abrasive toothpaste can cause damage to teeth. Toothpaste should be applied in a thin layer and worked into the bristles of the toothbrush.

BRUSHING TECHNIQUE

> *The most often recommended brushing method combines vibratory motion with massage of the gingiva.*

This technique allows removal of dental plaque on the teeth and beneath the gingival margin. When this method is used, a soft brush is needed. For cleansing the *outside surfaces of all teeth* and *inside surfaces of back teeth*, the bristles of the brush are at a 45-degree angle to the teeth. Place the brush with the tips directed slightly onto the gingival sulcus. Vibrate the brush back and forth with short strokes without disengaging the tips. The toothbrush will reach only two or three teeth at a time (see Fig. 27–5). After brushing one area, overlap placement with an adjacent position. For *inside surfaces of front teeth,* use the bristles on the end of the brush in a vibratory motion (see Fig. 27–5). To clean the *chewing surfaces*, brush back and forth.

After brushing the teeth, brush the *tongue*. This decreases the number of microorganisms and removes debris to retard dental plaque formation. Ask the patient to protrude his tongue. Holding the brush at a right angle to the length of the tongue, direct the tips of the bris-

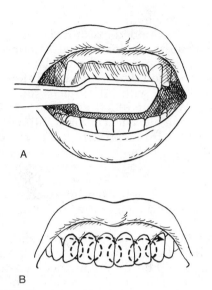

Figure 27–5. Tooth brushing for outer surface of upper teeth.

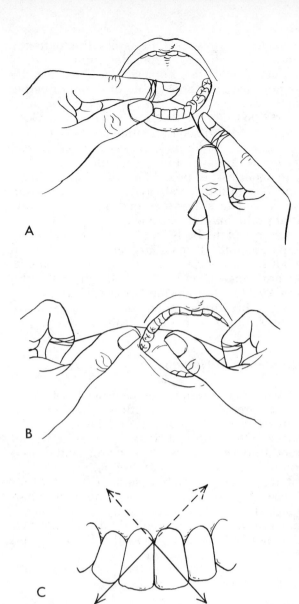

Figure 27–6. Flossing technique. *A,* Flossing bottom teeth. *B,* Flossing top teeth. *C,* Directions of flossing.

tles of the toothbrush toward the throat. With light pressure, bring the brush forward and over the tip of the tongue. Then brush the sides of the tongue. Now have the patient rinse his mouth thoroughly. Repeat brushing and rinsing as needed.

FLOSSING. Toothbrushing alone cannot remove all the dental plaque and debris in the gingival sulcus. When flossing is used correctly in addition to brushing, dental plaque between the teeth can be removed. Flossing not only helps prevent periodontal disease but also aids in removing materia alba and food debris, which can be a source of halitosis. If flossing is done *prior* to brushing but *after* applying dentifrice, the fluoride in the dentifrice can come in direct contact with the tooth surface. This aids in prevention of cavities. Unwaxed dental floss usually is recommended because it is thinner, slides easily between teeth and is more absorbent.

Learning to floss correctly requires instruction and practice. Loosely wrap floss about 12 to 18 inches long around index or middle finger of each hand. To clean the *lower* teeth, hold the floss so that the forefingers of both hands are on top of the strand. Loop the floss around a tooth and pull the ends forward to curve it into a C shape against the sides of the tooth; then slide the floss to the gum line. Move the floss back and forth to clean *both* sides of the tooth. Carefully work the floss under the gum until it meets

resistance. Then bring the floss toward the biting surface. To clean the *upper* teeth, hold the floss so that it is over the thumb of one hand and the forefinger of the other hand. The thumb is to the outside of the teeth to hold back the cheek. Work the floss between the teeth as done with the lower teeth. When the floss becomes soiled or frayed, move to a new section of the strand by slipping a turn of floss from the middle finger of one hand and adding a turn to the finger of the other. After flossing, rinse vigorously to remove loose debris. While firm pressure is needed against the sides of the teeth, caution the patient not to traumatize the gums.

Patients with Dentures. Debris, dental plaque and calculus collect on dentures as with natural teeth. The same type of brush that is used for natural teeth also can be used for dentures. Discourage the use of denture brushes with hard bristles because they wear grooves in dentures. Encourage patient to wear dentures during the day. This improves eating technique, speech, appearance and contour of the mouth. Some health professionals recommend removal of dentures at night for maintenance of the gums. When dentures are removed from the patient's mouth, they should be stored in a *labeled* denture cup to prevent loss and breakage. Ideally, dentures are cleaned after each meal. Cleanse the tongue and oral mucosa and provide massage for the edentulous patient at least daily.

CLEANSING AGENTS. Many denture cleaners are available. Meresene is most helpful in preventing fungal infections. Kleenite is *not* recommended for dentures with soft liners because it causes the liner to become brittle. Water used with soap or a mild cleansing agent cleans dentures without causing abrasion. One solution that can be prepared at home consists of 1 tsp. Clorox, 2 tsp. Calgon and ½ glass (4 oz.) warm water. Clorox can cause corrosion; therefore, Calgon is used as an anticorrosive agent.

BRUSHING DENTURES. Dentures should be brushed at the sink because of the advantage of having running water. Place a paper towel and a small amount of water in the sink. This serves as a cushion should you accidentally drop the dentures. While cleaning the denture, grasp it in the palm of one hand and brush with the other hand. Be sure all surfaces are brushed thoroughly. If the patient must remain in bed and is capable of self-care, place an emesis basin and container of water on the overbed table within easy reach of the patient. For ease of reinsertion, the dentures are rinsed with cold water before they are replaced in the patient's clean mouth.

CLEANSING THE MOUTH. Each time the dentures are removed, the patient's mouth should be rinsed with warm water. If a brush is used for cleansing the oral mucosa, it should be multitufted, soft nylon. Use long straight strokes from the posterior to anterior surfaces of the mouth. Toothettes or gauze also can be used. Remember to also cleanse the patient's tongue.

MASSAGE. Massage stimulates circulation and toughens the oral mucosa, thereby increasing resistance to trauma. If a toothbrush is used, apply the sides of the bristles in a vibratory motion. For digital massage, place thumb and index finger over the ridge of the gum. Use a press and release motion to massage. Rub the patient's palate with the end of the thumb. Keep thumbnail away from the palate to prevent mucosal trauma.

Patients with Excessive Dryness or Irritation of Oral Mucosa. Patients who have a dry oral cavity or dry lips may require oral hygiene every 2 to 8 hours to improve the condition of the oral mucosa. Rinsing the patient's mouth with water, mouthwash or saline usually refreshes the patient.

There are many varieties of *mouthwash*. Some mouthwashes are bactericidal. Unfortunately, these mouthwashes can destroy the normal bacterial flora of the mouth, resulting in overgrowth of fungus. On the other hand, the astringent effect of some mouthwashes can be beneficial. *Saline* (water and salt solution) is easy to make and soothing for many patients with mucosal irritation. For the patient who experiences pain with severe stomatitis, *anesthetic solutions* are available. Be sure to check for allergies before using drugs such as lidocaine (Xylocaine).

A dilute solution of *hydrogen peroxide* is effective in removing debris from the coated, dry tongue, and for patients with acute necrotizing ulcerative gingivitis. The effervescent action of this oxygenating agent is effective in débridement and decreasing anaerobic microorganisms. Because hydrogen peroxide removes necrotic tissue and organisms, it eliminates a source of halitosis. Continued use of hydrogen peroxide can lead to sponginess of the gingiva and decalcification of tooth surfaces. Thus, the mouth should be rinsed after using hydrogen peroxide.

The Comatose Patient. The external surfaces of the teeth of comatose patients can be brushed in the usual manner. To clean internal and chewing surfaces, some means must be used to keep the patient's mouth open. A mouth gag can be made by putting tongue blades together and covering them with gauze that is taped in place.

Never put your fingers in the patient's mouth. Human bites can be very painful and dangerous. The worker can become infected if there is a break in the skin and subsequent entry of organisms or can lose nerve sensation of the injured finger.

To cleanse the internal and chewing surfaces of the teeth, first put the mouth gag in place between the upper and lower teeth at the posterior, lateral section of the jaw. Use a toothbrush, cotton-tipped applicator (see Fig. 27–7),

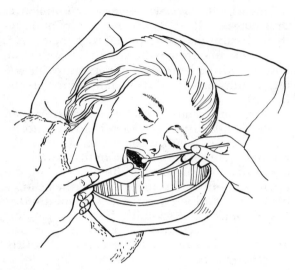

Figure 27–7. Mouth care being given to comatose or helpless patient.

or tongue blades covered with 4 × 4 gauze for cleaning. To cleanse the tongue, use the gauze-covered tongue blades with cleaning solution such as saline or hydrogen peroxide. Use only a small amount of solution on the gauze, as the patient can aspirate the solution because of a poor gag reflex. Use a moisturizing agent on the lips (e.g., white petroleum jelly) after completing oral hygiene.

SPECIALIZED SENSE ORGANS: EYES, EARS AND NOSE

The specialized senses of sight, hearing and smell help us to interact with the environment. Deficits in the function of these sense organs can contribute to disorientation and impede communication. Hygiene care of the eyes, ears and nose prevents infection and helps maintain function. Hygiene care of these sense organs is always done as part of the general bathing procedure whenever secretions or dryness are problems.

Eyes

When a patient has severe visual impairment or is blind, he requires thorough explanation of his surroundings in order to perform self-care and to avoid injuries from unfamiliar obstacles in the environment. Although all patients should receive an explanation from nursing personnel regarding the health care facility environment, this is essential for a visually impaired or blind person if he is to function at his maximum capacity. Inform the blind or visually impaired patient about the location of his room in relation to the nurses' station, toilet facilities and other significant areas in the hospital; describe and locate items in his immediate environment, e.g., describe the bedside stand while using the patient's hands to feel the outline of the item and its location; locate and discuss the use of the call signal; and discuss the usual activities of the facility (e.g., times of meals). When placing hygiene care items tell the patient what equipment is available, identify its location (e.g., beside your right hand), and explain what you expect him to do. If the patient is left alone for self-care, explain how to call for assistance and tell him when you will return.

Most blind patients can function as independently as patients with vision once they are provided with information about the environment. Many visually impaired or blind patients have imposed limitations of independent function because nursing personnel fail to provide a thorough explanation of the environment or assume a blind person is not capable of self-care.

When a patient has impaired visual function, he may display behavior of "confusion" or "disorientation," or appear clumsy, which may lead nursing personnel to believe the patient is mentally impaired. "Confusion" or "disorientation" most often are the result of misperception of the environment viewed through the blurring effect of poor vision or because the patient lacks the knowledge about his surrounding environment. Loss of peripheral vision contributes to "clumsiness" and can be a safety problem for the patient.

Hygiene care of the eyes aids in maintaining the function of the eyes and preventing eye infections and injuries as well as improving the patient's appearance. For example, heavy, crusted eye secretions impair the patient's ability to fully open his eyes, are a source of eye irritation and potential infection, and are aesthetically unappealing.

Assessment. When assessing the eyes, include the entire eye orbit, eyelashes and eyebrows in your examination. Note the following: (a) scaliness of skin underlying the *eyebrows;* (b) *eyelids*—edema, lesions, crusted secretion, inflammation; (c) *eyelashes* that might irritate eye surface, styes; (d) *lacrimal sac*—swelling, excessive tearing or absence of tears, crusting at inner canthus; (e) *sclera* or *conjunctiva*—color, inflammation; (f) *pupil*—size, shape, light response; (g) other problems

—eye movement, cataracts, drainage, complaints of burning, pain.

Hygiene Care of Eyes.   Eyes are cleansed from the *inner* to the outer canthus. This is the natural tract for removal of debris from the eye. Each eye is cleansed with a separate portion of the washcloth. This prevents potential spread of infection from one eye to the other. Soap causes eye irritation.

Never use soap for cleansing eyes.

For patients who have crusted secretions, place a *wet*, warm washcloth or cotton ball over the closed eye. Leave this in place until secretions become softened. Water or saline can be used. Repeat application of warm compresses until secretions are moist enough for easy removal without traumatizing the mucosa. Warm compresses also can be used for styes. This helps relieve pain and facilitates suppuration. When there is drainage from a stye or other infection, be very cautious not to spread the infection.

Eye Care for the Comatose Patient.   The comatose patient may require frequent eye care, as often as every 4 hours. The frequency of care depends on the general condition of the eye and the amount of moisture in the environment. Besides cleansing the eye, it is important to keep the eye moist and protected from the debris in the air. If the blink reflex is lost or decreased, the open eye can become dry from the air. This can lead to *corneal ulceration*. In some situations, liquid tear solution is instilled into the conjunctival sac or the eyes may be irrigated with a normal saline solution. If the corneal reflex is absent and the eyes remain open or appear irritated, close the eyes and cover them with a protective shield.

Eyeglasses.   Eyeglasses should be examined for cleanliness at least daily. Most patients do not ask to have their eyeglasses cleaned and will wear dirty glasses that impair vision. Cautiously handle eyeglasses to prevent them from breaking. When cleansing eyeglasses, avoid scratching the lens. Use warm water, mild soap and nonabrasive drying material. Label eyeglasses with the patient's name, and when not in use, store them in the top drawer of the bedside stand.

Contact Lenses or Artificial Eyes.   Contact lenses or artificial eyes are removed prior to surgery. An artificial eye can be cleansed with warm water and soap. Do not allow patients to wear contact lenses for long periods of time. Contact lenses need moisture to prevent friction.

Lack of moisture or wearing contact lenses for a lengthy period can cause corneal abrasions, which can be very painful.

When contact lenses are removed, place them in separate containers labeled "right" and "left" eye.

Ears

Hearing can be even more important than vision as a means of orientation to the external environment. Hearing loss restricts communication, creates safety hazards, and in part can account for some patients having paranoid ideas. Not hearing or knowing what is said makes the patient doubtful about people in his environment. If auditory stimuli are misinterpreted, the environment becomes distorted. Many older patients particularly have difficulty with background noise, which contributes to a muffling effect of normal conversation. The task of listening becomes more difficult if persons do not face the patient directly while speaking. The patient with hearing loss may tire easily because he has to listen carefully. This may decrease attempts at conversation, especially in the new, unfamiliar hospital environment. Many people feel embarrassed to point out that they have a hearing loss. The patient may not use his energy to listen carefully and may miss much of the usual conversation; this distorts his world. Thus, a patient with hearing loss may display behavior that appears related to mental or emotional problems (e.g., paranoia, confusion).

Accumulated wax in the ears and injuries can impair hearing. Many people remove wax from their ears by using sharp objects, which can traumatize the ear. The patient can also incur injuries to other parts of his body secondary to hearing loss. For example, the patient may not hear another person warn him to step out of the way of a moving wheelchair and may accidentally back into the wheelchair, falling or injuring his legs. Poor hygiene also can endanger the welfare of the patient. When there is poor hygiene of the ears, debris may accumulate behind the ear and in the anterior aspect of the external ear. This can lead to ulcerative areas and infection.

Assessment.   To assess the condition and

function of the ear, first examine the anterior and posterior aspects of the external ear for dryness, crusting, debris and drainage. Look for wax or drainage at the entrance to the ear canal. Gently palpate the tragus (anterior external cartilage area), which is a very sensitive area and can give clues to ear problems. Palpate lymph nodes for enlargement and pain. Note tophi (hard nodules) in helix (superior-posterior external cartilage area). Tophi are deposits of uric acid crystals characteristic of gout. Sebaceous cysts behind the ear are common. To test gross hearing, have the patient listen to a ticking watch or whisper in his ear. Test one ear at a time, while occluding the other ear.

Hygiene Care of the Ears.   The ear usually can be cleansed with a couple of movements of the washcloth-covered hand. To remove wax at the entry point of the ear canal, the worker's finger can be slightly depressed into the entrance of the ear canal.

> *Instruct patients never to use articles such as bobby pins to remove earwax. Insertion of such articles into the ear can cause trauma to the canal and middle ear.*

Hearing Aids.   If a patient uses a hearing aid, some special care is needed. Check that the appliance is functioning properly. Cleanse the external ear piece. Frequently the opening in the ear piece becomes blocked with wax and debris. Blockage of the opening impairs the functioning of the hearing aid.

Nose

Not only does the nose subserve the sense of smell, but it also serves a protective function. The mucoid secretions, cilia and specialized tissue in the nose aid in controlling temperature, humidity and entry of foreign particles into the respiratory system. Excessive accumulation of secretions can impair the sense of smell and breathing. If the patient is unable to sniff or blow his nose, secretions can become crusted and may obstruct the airways or irritate nasal mucosa. If the patient's sense of smell is impaired, he may be unable to detect various aromas of foods, thereby having a decreased appetite.

Assessment.   When inspecting the nose, examine for inflammation and moistness of the nasal mucosa; color, consistency and amount of nasal discharge; and position of nasal septum. Also note any bleeding or difficulty in breathing.

Hygiene Care of Nose.   Hygiene care can improve the functioning ability of the nose. A patient usually can remove nasal secretions by blowing his nose. This may be all that is needed for effective hygiene, other than cleansing the external opening and tip of the nose during bathing. Some patients must be cautioned against harsh nose blowing. To prevent increased pressure, gentle nose blowing is advised for patients who have had eye surgery and those for whom bleeding may be a problem, e.g., patients with bleeding disorders or patients taking drugs, such as aspirin, heparin or Coumadin, that increase bleeding tendency.

For patients who cannot remove nasal secretions, assistance may be needed to clear congestion and protect nasal mucosa. External crusted secretions can be removed with a wet washcloth or a cotton-tipped applicator moistened with water or normal saline. Use a moisturizing agent to keep the end of the nose from becoming dry and to prevent the skin from cracking. In some situations, suctioning is necessary to remove congestion for adequate breathing. *Never* suction a patient who has had brain surgery or a patient with a head injury.

SKIN CARE

The *skin* with its *appendages* (hair and nails) is commonly referred to as the *integumentary system.* As the external surface of the body, the skin is a protective barrier between the internal and external environments. Besides its protective function, the skin also serves as an organ for secretion, excretion, sense of touch and body temperature regulation.

Hygiene care provides cleansing and conditioning of the skin so it can effectively maintain the integrity of the body. *Bathing* may be the first type of skin care that comes to mind. However, several other aspects of hygiene care play a major role in maintaining the condition of the skin. *Hair* care serves to stimulate surrounding skin and remove sources of infections. *Massage* of skin on the back and around bony prominences stimulates circulation for improving nutrition to the skin and underlying tissue. Some hygiene care is directed toward conditioning the mucous membranes and skin of body orifices, such as the *mouth, eyes* and *nose.* Hygiene care of *nails, feet* and *perineal* area requires special emphasis because these areas are prone to skin breakdown and infection. Bed linen also can cause skin breakdown;

e.g., soiled, wrinkled sheets are a source of skin irritation. Heavy bed linen over sensitive, fragile skin can cause pressure that impedes circulation. In addition, various agents used in skin care can be protective or damaging to skin; e.g., some agents cause excessive dryness, leading to breaks in the skin.

Anatomy and Physiology of Skin

Anatomy of the Skin.   The skin is the largest organ of the body. It consists of three layers that are continuous with each other: epidermis, dermis, and subcutaneous tissue. The *epidermis* is the most superficial layer and in itself comprises several layers called *strata*. The outermost stratum of the epidermis contains dead cells that are continuously removed by friction or bathing and replaced by cells moving toward the surface from deeper layers. Melanin and keratin are formed in the inner cellular stratum of epidermis. *Melanin* (pigment) gives skin color and protection from ultraviolet rays of the sun. *Keratin* plays a role in the acidity of the skin surface.

The thin epidermis, which has no blood vessels, receives its nutrition from the underlying *dermis.* In addition to a good supply of blood vessels, the dermis consists of dense connective tissue, nerve fibers, sebaceous (oil) glands and some hair follicles. Sebaceous glands are present on all skin surfaces except the palms and the soles.[1]

Beneath the dermis is *subcutaneous tissue,* which provides support and a blood supply to the dermis. The subcutaneous tissue consists of loose connective tissue, blood and lymph vessels, fat, sweat glands and some hair follicles. *Eccrine sweat glands* are most numerous on the forehead, palms and soles. *Apocrine sweat glands* are found mainly in the axillae and genital areas.[1]

Functions of Skin.   The integumentary system serves several physiologic functions.

PROTECTIVE COVERING.   The skin normally has some bacteria (resident bacteria) on its surface. As long as the skin remains intact to prevent invasion of pathogens, these resident bacteria can prevent excess growth of fungi. The sebaceous glands secrete *sebum* (an oily substance), which has antibacterial and antifungal properties. Also, the normal acidity of the skin surface inhibits growth of pathogenic organisms. Besides resisting invasion from pathogens, intact skin protects underlying tissue from trauma.

BODY TEMPERATURE REGULATION AND SECRETION/EXCRETION.   Many factors contribute to body temperature regulation. The integumentary system has at least two ways of regulating body temperature: sebaceous and sweat glands. The sebaceous glands, by their secretion of sebum, provide a protective coating to prevent rapid water evaporation and skin dryness. Sweat glands, by the excretion of sweat, serve to regulate body temperature through water evaporation from skin surface. Heat dissipates from the skin when cutaneous blood vessels dilate so that more blood reaches the surface. This factor plus increased sweat gland secretion aids in lowering body temperature. To elevate body temperature, the cutaneous blood vessels constrict and sweat gland production decreases. The excretion of sweat also aids in removing waste products from the body.

SENSE ORGAN.   Because the skin has nerve receptors it serves as a sense organ for touch. This allows us to sense pain, pressure, heat and cold. The skin provides a tactile means of communicating with the external environment for protection and orientation to surroundings.

General Skin Care

The condition of the skin gives clues regarding a person's general health and need for hygiene. Although skin can be easily observed during hygiene care, assessment of abnormalities is difficult because many signs are subtle. The novice nurse, through practice in observation of skin and deliberateness in relating what is observed to anatomy and physiology, can become skilled at assessment of the skin. Principles related to skin care include the following:

▶ Intact skin is the first line of defense.

▶ Excessive dryness contributes to skin breakdown.

▶ Poor circulation impedes nutrition to the skin.

▶ Some bacteria are necessary for maintaining homeostatic environment on the skin surface.

▶ The greater the number of organisms, the greater the possibility of infection.

▶ Pathogens grow well in a warm, moist environment.

Assessment.   To effectively assess the skin, one needs a good light source for visualization.

Roach suggests that in addition to a light source (nonglare daylight or 60-watt bulb), position, environmental conditions such as temperature, amount of perspiration and sebum, edema (swelling), and pigmentation patterns all affect accuracy of assessment of skin.[15] The following discussion is by no means comprehensive, but it can serve as a basic reference for assessment of the skin.

COLOR.   The amount of melanin varies not only among races but within races. Blacks, Caucasians and persons with yellow, brown or red skin each have varying shades, tones and pigmentation patterns. Usually the most difficult patients to assess are those with very light or very dark skin. At first glance, the light-skinned person may appear ashen or cyanotic. The very dark-skinned person may have some conditions that go unnoticed. As Roach states, "The normal distribution patterns of pigment in dark-skinned persons may obscure certain color changes and lead to misinterpretation. . . ."[15] She also points out that with good technique, awareness of differences among people, and associating the patient's overall condition with skin color, the nurse can assess the dark-skinned person.[15] The descriptive terms for skin color are somewhat vague: pallor (pale); cyanotic (bluish); rubra or erythema (reddish); jaundice (yellowish); and ashen (grayish). Regardless of the amount of melanin, assess the patient for presence or absence of underlying red tones on skin surface and for the color of the sclerae, conjunctivae and mucous membranes in the oral cavity. Various types of *discoloration* also may be noted: ecchymosis (reddish purple blotch); petechiae (pinpoint reddish spots); purpura (reddish purple areas).

SKIN TEMPERATURE.   The temperature of the skin primarily gives clues to possible inflammatory processes and circulation problems. To evaluate skin temperature, place the back of your fingers against the patient's skin. Also note the patient's skin color and the room temperature. Skin temperature can be related to room temperature and correlated with skin color: cyanosis suggests a cold environment or circulatory problems, and erythema suggests a hot environment or inflammation.

SUPPLENESS.   Suppleness (pliability, ease of movement) of the skin is related to the amount of moisture and oil; general texture (smooth, rough); turgor (fullness of tissue); elasticity of fibers in the dermis layer; and edema. Lift a section of skin and observe for ease of movement and speed of return to original position. *Edema* (fluid in tissue) causes a change in color and a shiny appearance as the skin becomes taut.

INTACTNESS AND LESIONS.   Observe for breaks in the skin. Inspect and palpate for lesions and rashes, such as *macules* (flat spots), *papules* (raised lesions; pimples), *vesicles* (fluid-filled lesions) and *nodules* (solid, raised lesions). Note if lesions are localized or generalized over the body. An example of a condition related to hygiene care is a macular or papular rash on arms and legs caused by rubbing the skin against bed linens that have been cleaned with harsh detergents and disinfectants.

SENSATION.   Usually sensation can be evaluated while palpating the skin for lesions. When using light and firm pressure during palpation, ask the patient what he feels. In addition, the patient may comment that the worker's hands feel cold or hot. Decreased responses to temperature, pressure and touch can be manifestations of generalized or localized problems, e.g., a circulatory problem or callused skin. Knowledge of a patient's altered sensations is important when determining the temperature of water to be used for bathing as well as for protecting the patient during movement, e.g., bathing, bedmaking and treatments such as warm soaks. Complaints of itching may suggest lack of moisture or allergies. This is important for determining the agent for cleansing the skin and the frequency of bathing.

CLEANLINESS.   The patient's overall cleanliness is based upon the amount of moisture, dirt and oil on the skin and the presence of body odor.

Nursing Judgment.   Skin care most often is an independent nursing judgment. All the assessment factors have implications for type and frequency of hygiene care and should be noted before planning hygiene care or during care. Skin care is based on fulfillment of physiologic needs, assessment of the condition of the skin, hygiene practices and psychologic benefits to the patient.

Agents Used for Skin Care

The selection of an agent for cleansing and protecting the skin is based upon the condition of the skin (e.g., oily, dry, intactness), purpose of the skin agent, patient's preferences and availability of an agent.

Soaps.   Soap lowers the surface tension to aid cleansing. Some soaps cause excessive dryness by removing too much sebum on the skin surface. Caution is advised when using antibacterial soaps, which destroy most bacteria on the skin; although these soaps decrease odor caused by the bacteria, they alter the natural flora of the skin and can allow increased fungal growth. Some patients may require hypoallergenic soaps. For excessively dry or excoriated (loss of superficial layers) skin, *plain warm water* is an effective cleansing agent. Products containing a demulcent or emollient also can be used as protective skin agents.

Demulcents. Demulcents tend to coat skin and mucous membranes. When used over abrasive areas, this type of agent provides a mechanical means of protecting underlying cells from the drying effect of air and guards against irritants in the external environment. *Glycerin* is a frequently used demulcent. Although this can be effective as a protective agent, in high concentrations it can have an adverse effect by absorbing too much water. This can lead to dehydration and irritation of exposed tissue.

Emollients. Emollients are used to soften skin and mucous membranes by forming an oily film that prevents evaporation of water from underlying layers of skin. Two commonly used emollients are lanolin and white petroleum jelly.

Powders. Powders can be used to prevent friction and/or absorb moisture. Water-absorbent powders, when used sparingly, can decrease friction and retard bacterial growth. However, they should not be used on open, draining areas, since the powder can cake or crust, causing further skin irritation. Starches have a beneficial drying effect but can become doughy from absorbing moisture.

Nursing Judgment. The excellent nurse bases her selection of skin agents on assessment data and a knowledge of the purposes of various skin agents. Most health care facilities have one or two types of soaps plus some type of protective skin agent available for patient hygiene care. Although patient preferences are important, discourage use of agents that are contraindicated. For example, a patient may prefer a harsh detergent soap but may have very dry skin. In this situation, a mild soap, plain water or a product containing a demulcent or emollient should be encouraged.

BATHING

Bathing serves many purposes: it (a) cleanses the skin; (b) stimulates circulation to the skin; (c) provides exercise; (d) relaxes tense muscles; (e) improves sense of well-being; (f) provides physical and psychologic comfort; and (g) gives the nurse an opportunity to observe and converse with the patient. As with other hygiene

care, observation and communication may be difficult when first learning skills.

Principles applicable for all bathing are as follows:

▶ Promote safety and prevent falls.

▶ Assess psychologic and physical needs.

▶ Determine self-care abilities, know activity limitations, and encourage self-help unless contraindicated.

▶ Explain to the patient his role, what will be done and when.

▶ Patient teaching is individualized according to the patient's needs.

▶ Determine the purpose of bathing.

▶ Cleansing bath is for removal of dirt, excessive oil, perspiration, transient bacteria and dead epithelial cells.

▶ Frequency of bathing is based on the condition of the skin.

▶ *Not all* patients need daily bathing.

▶ If the patient has oily skin, is diaphoretic, or is incontinent of urine or feces, frequent bathing is necessary.

▶ Body excretions of urine and feces require immediate cleansing to prevent skin irritation.

▶ Do not apply soap to excoriated skin.

▶ Bathe from *clean to dirty* areas of the body.

▶ Use friction to stimulate circulation and remove debris, unless contraindicated.

▶ Provide warmth and privacy by covering and draping the patient.

▶ Use good body mechanics when assisting patients with bathing: keep back straight, use legs and abdominal muscles, and maintain a wide base of support.

▶ Collect all necessary items before starting care.

Reasons for Bathing

Bathing and application of skin preparations are tied to cultural influences more than any other hygiene practices. Many Americans adhere to the practice of daily bathing and apply oils or other skin preparations. Some people feel compelled to bathe daily regardless of need. As pointed out earlier in this chapter, in the hospital daily bathing has been a tradition. With increased emphasis on conservation of environmental resources and bathing based upon need, hygiene practices may change in the future.

Some people bathe for reasons other than cleansing the skin. A warm tub bath can be used as a comfort measure for sore, tense muscles. For some people, bathing is a time for being alone to screen out external stimuli or relieve generalized tension. For others, bathing is a stimulant to "get started in the morning." In the hospital setting, a patient's usual bathing practices frequently are altered because of the patient's physical condition or because the hospital routines interfere with his usual bathing habits. The patient's physical need for bathing is the primary consideration; whenever feasible, the adaptive nurse facilitates continuation of the patient's usual bathing practices.

Skin Protection

The amount of sebum on the skin surface varies among people. For people with very oily skin, sebum can accumulate to the point of causing skin irritation, clogged pores or blemishes. Frequent bathing with a detergent-type soap that causes dryness will best condition oily skin. If the patient is diaphoretic (perspiring excessively), frequent bathing is required to prevent skin breakdown from the moisture.

On the other hand, some people normally have dry skin. Skin may become dry from systemic changes, environmental conditions or drug therapy. Elderly people tend to have dry skin because of decreased secretions. Several options are available to the nurse who cares for the patient with dry skin. In addition to decreasing the frequency of bathing, plain water with friction can remove dead epithelial cells without causing excessive drying. Products such as Alpha Keri or Septi Soft, which contain demulcents and emollients, can be added to bath water or applied directly to the skin as a cleansing and protective agent. When these types of products are used, rinsing is eliminated. This allows an oily film to remain on the skin. Applications of lotion between bathings may be necessary. Soaps containing lanolin

also may be helpful. When using soap on any patient, it is important to rinse thoroughly since remaining residue can be a source of skin irritation.

Thorough drying of the skin is always important. Special attention is given to drying creased areas of the body (e.g., buttocks, under the breasts, between fingers and toes). It may seem unnecessary to mention this because you automatically dry after bathing, but many patients ignore drying because of physical difficulties. Also, some patients (e.g., patients with diabetes mellitus or other metabolic problems and immobilized patients) are particularly prone to skin breakdown and infections. They may not give attention to thorough drying because they lack an appreciation of how moisture can be a conducive environment for pathogenic growth. Thus, patient teaching may be indicated for this aspect of hygiene care.

Patient Teaching

Patients may not recognize their need to alter bath practices. Remember, people cling to usual bathing habits as with other hygiene practices. The excellent nurse relates patient teaching to observations about the patient. For example, if the nurse notices that a patient has very oily skin, she may state, "Your skin appears oily. Is this a problem for you?" The patient may respond with a comment such as, "It's not a problem when I'm able to shower every day" or "It's only a problem on my face." Recalling that both sebaceous and sweat glands are located in the area of the face, one expects increased secretions in that area. The nurse might suggest that the patient use soap when washing his face instead of cleansing only with water. In another situation, the nurse may notice a patient scratching and may observe flaky, dry patches of skin. The nurse can offer suggestions such as those discussed earlier for people with dry skin.

Some patients have misconceptions about bathing; e.g., they may believe that bathing is harmful during illness or that chilling during bathing causes a cold. Before responding to patients' misconceptions or providing care, find out why the patient has certain beliefs, the importance of various hygiene practices to the patient, the patient's usual bathing habits and contraindications based on the patient's condition.

Methods of Bathing

In addition to the usual methods of bathing at home in a shower or bathtub, a patient may be

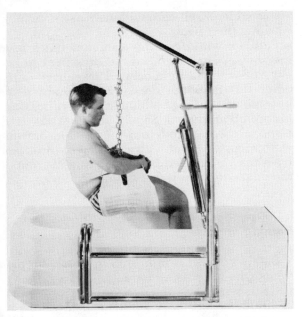

Figure 27–8. Mechanical device for lifting patient into bathtub. (From Invacare Corporation, Long Beach, CA.)

bathed in bed. Some patients may require a therapeutic bath for healing purposes. Regardless of the method of bathing (shower, tub, bed), the amount of self-care and assistance needed from the worker will vary. For example, the patient who showers may need assistance in washing his back, or the patient in bed may be able to bathe completely except for his feet or back.

In years past, most patients bathed in bed. As emphasis increased on preventing complications of immobility, more patients were encouraged to bathe at a sink or in the shower or bathtub. Today, certain patients still require bathing in bed, e.g., patients with casts, those in traction, and those on strict bed rest for energy conservation. Some weak or paralyzed patients can now shower because of new devices, e.g., chairs for showering or mechanical lifts that transfer a patient into a bathtub (see Fig. 27–8).

Providing for shower or tub bathing sometimes demands considerable time and energy from the worker, e.g., arranging to get help for transferring a patient into the bathtub. The physical and psychologic benefits to the patient should have priority over convenience for the worker. This demonstrates concern for the patient's needs. The method of bathing and the amount of assistance needed are nursing judgments based upon assessment of benefit to the patient, safety factors, patient preferences and contraindications.

Bathing in the Shower or Bathtub

Patients usually prefer to shower or use a bathtub rather than bathe in bed. Whether the patient uses bathtub, shower chair or standing shower, the most important principle for general patient welfare is *safety!* The following guidelines can assist the worker in organization and provide for maximum patient safety and comfort during bathing.

Schedule use of shower or bathtub. This prevents unnecessary frustration of waiting.

Explain to the patient how to use the call signal for assistance. Bathrooms are equipped with some type of signaling device. Most facilities have a pull cord or push button that shows as a red light in the hall or at the nurses' station and/or has a loud buzzer.

> *Patients need to be cautioned to call for help when feeling weak or faint.*

A patient may experience faintness or weakness because of vasodilatation from hot water (blood normally flowing to the brain shifts from the central nervous system to the periphery as environmental temperature increases). Problems also can occur because of prior periods of inactivity. The patient's body may be unable to compensate for the added physical stress, especially when showering.

Collect needed items: towel, washcloth, soap, clean gown or pajamas, personal toilet articles (e.g., deodorant, powder). Place these within easy reach to prevent possible falls from reaching for supplies.

Prepare shower/tub by checking if cleansing is needed; placing rubber mat on bottom of shower/tub; and placing paper bath mat or towel on floor beside shower/tub to prevent slipping and provide warmth.

Adjust room temperature, if feasible.

Place an occupied sign on door of bathroom for privacy. *Always knock* before entering an occupied bathroom.

Assist patient to bathroom as indicated to prevent falls.

Have patient wear robe and slippers on route to bathroom.

Adjust water temperature and pressure. Wait long enough for water temperature to stabilize at 41 to 46°C. Caution the patient not to readjust the water temperature. Burns can occur when the patient is unfamiliar with the faucets or illness has altered his sense of touch.

To *avoid falls,* instruct patient to use safety grab bars when getting in and out of the shower or tub.

After the patient is finished bathing, have bathroom cleaned and remove soiled linen and occupied sign on door.

Showering. A standing shower is usually unassisted, but the patient may require help in washing his back. The *shower chair* can be used for patients who are unable to tolerate standing and for patients who would otherwise require bathing in bed (e.g., confused or weak patients). Usually the shower chair or bathtub is the best choice for a patient who can sit and has no dressing or cast, which would be a contraindication. Most shower chairs have wheels and are made of plastic. A movable shower head or hand-held shower nozzle can be used to direct the water at an appropriate level.

The patient may be transported to the shower area in a wheelchair or the shower chair. Be sure the patient is kept covered with a robe or bath blanket for privacy and warmth. Use slippers for warmth and to prevent scraping the patient's feet on the floor.

> *If the patient is confused, paralyzed or weak, a restraining device is required to prevent him from falling or slipping out of the chair.*

Do not be misled into thinking that a restraining device is unnecessary because you are with the patient. Remember that you will be bathing the patient and may not be in a position to prevent him from falling out of the chair. Once the shower chair is in the desired position, set the brakes to keep it from rolling. Place a towel across the patient's lap for modesty.

Tub Bathing. In addition to other preparations for shower or tub bathing, half-fill the tub with water. Some patients use tub bathing for both cleansing and therapeutic effects. Caution the patient not to soak in the tub for longer than 20 minutes, since maximum vascular benefits are accomplished in 15 to 20 minutes, the patient may tire easily, and the bathroom usually is needed for other patients. If you are assisting the patient in and out of bathtub, provide support under axillae and have a chair close by for the patient to sit while drying. If assisting the patient with bathing, place a towel across the patient's lap for modesty. Many patients who

are capable of self-care will need assistance in washing their backs.

Patients with *dressings* can sometimes use the shower chair or tub if the dressing can be covered with plastic and taped to keep it dry. In other situations the dressing is permitted to become wet during bathing and a dry dressing is applied afterward. Some patients with *casts* also can be assisted into the tub or shower chair; e.g., a patient with a cast on his arm can have plastic secured over the cast and around the edges to keep it dry during bathing.

Bathing in Bed

Bathing in bed is indicated primarily for patients who have restricted mobility (e.g., *some* patients with casts, traction, or back problems) or limited exertion (e.g., some heart and respiratory conditions) and often for first-day postoperative patients who may experience hypotension or are very weak.

Assessment. While bathing a patient in bed the nurse has an excellent opportunity to assess various systems of the body and to communicate with the patient. The following assessment can be done while bathing the patient:

Respiratory—observe breathing with movement and the rate, quality and pattern of breathing at rest.

Cardiovascular—observe temperature, color of skin, circulation to extremities and nail beds; note complaints of coldness and changes in heart rate.

Musculoskeletal—evaluate joint mobility and muscle strength during range-of-motion exercises; note coordination.

Mental/emotional/social—note orientation, emotional state, ability to follow directions, personal concerns, complaints of discomfort, attitudes toward hygiene, cultural practices, feelings related to modesty, and reactions to illness and hospitalization.

Gastrointestinal—note any abdominal distention, fecal incontinence and bleeding from rectum; ask about bowel patterns.

Genitourinary—note bladder distention, urinary incontinence and complaints of difficulty in voiding.

Integumentary—note intactness of skin, general condition of skin and other skin factors listed earlier in this chapter; ask the patient about sense of touch, e.g., temperature of water, pressure with rubbing.

By being sensitive to the patient's statements and observant while bathing each part of the body, the nurse can assess general physical and psychologic needs plus needs for skin care and patient teaching. Through the use of touch dur-

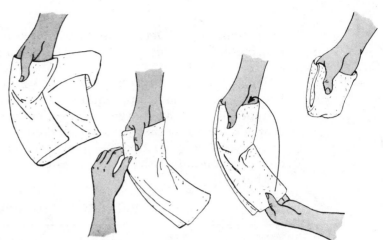

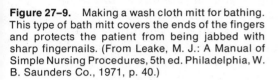

Figure 27–9. Making a wash cloth mitt for bathing. This type of bath mitt covers the ends of the fingers and protects the patient from being jabbed with sharp fingernails. (From Leake, M. J.: A Manual of Simple Nursing Procedures, 5th ed. Philadelphia, W. B. Saunders Co., 1971, p. 40.)

ing bathing, the nurse can convey an attitude of concern and can establish an effective nurse-patient relationship.

Types of Bed Baths. Several options are available for bathing a patient in bed. The choice of bed bath is a nursing judgment based on the patient's general condition, self-care abilities and comfort needs. For the *traditional complete bed bath*, the worker uses a washcloth, face towel, bath towel and wash basin to totally assist the patient in bathing. Another option in some facilities is the *towel bath*, in which a special towel is used and two workers bathe the patient. A *partial bed bath*, which may be done by the patient or the worker, involves cleansing areas where the most secretions accumulate, e.g., face, hands, axillae and perineal area. Sometimes the term *self-help bed bath* is used in situations in which the patient is confined to bed for bathing but is able to bathe himself completely except for his back and legs.

TRADITIONAL BED BATH.   The traditional method of bathing in bed currently is used more frequently than the towel bath. This procedure usually is completed in about 15 to 30 minutes. The traditional bed bath is presented in Procedure 7. Throughout most of the traditional bed bath procedure the *washcloth* is folded into a *mitt* (see Fig. 27–9). This prevents the ends of the washcloth from dragging over the patient's body, since they can feel cold to the patient. The mitt also facilitates more effective friction in washing.

> *To make a mitt (Fig. 27–9):*
> 1. *Grasp washcloth at edge and fold one-third over palm of your hand*
> 2. *Bring remaining opposite edge across palm and hold with your thumb*
> 3. *Bring extended end of washcloth up to palm and tuck edge under*

Practice making a mitt until you are able to fold the washcloth using one smooth motion.

7.   TRADITIONAL BED BATH

Definition and Purpose.   *Bathing a patient in bed with a washcloth and towel.* The purpose is to cleanse the skin of the patient who is confined to bed and who does not have the physical and/or mental capability of self-bathing.

Contraindications and Cautions.   Keep side rail up on the side away from worker during bath to (a) aid patient in turning and (b) prevent patient from falling off bed. Keep both side rails up when worker is away from bed. Use *no* soap when washing patient's eyes. Determine if patient has any allergies to soaps. If patient has a cast, protect cast from becoming moist, e.g., place plastic covering over edges of cast.

Patient-Family Teaching Points. Provide patient and family with the following information as appropriate: (a) amount of participation by patient that is therapeutic; (b) how energy conservation is related to patient's condition, if he is confined to bed for that purpose; (c) daily bathing may cause very dry skin and is discouraged unless patient perspires excessively or is incontinent; and (d) how to obtain community services if patient requires complete bathing at home upon discharge.

PRE-PROCEDURE ACTIVITIES

PRELIMINARY ASSESSMENT/PLANNING

▶ Check activity orders and specific precautions for patient movement and positioning
▶ Assess patient need for bathing
▶ Assess patient's physical capability to assist worker; plan to assist patient as appropriate

> *Incorporate passive range-of-motion exercises into bed bath procedure as appropriate for helpless patient.*

▶ Assess patient's ability to comprehend directions
▶ Check patient's preference regarding soap and other hygiene aids
▶ Check bedside stand for hygiene aids (if not available have family bring in)
▶ Check linen and equipment available in patient unit
▶ Check room temperature and ventilation (adjust as feasible); close windows and door to prevent drafts
▶ Wash hands prior to obtaining linen

PREPARATION OF PATIENT AND UNIT

▶ Explain how patient can assist
▶ Explain sequence of procedure
▶ Move unnecessary items out of work area
▶ Pull curtain and/or screen for privacy
▶ Place needed items on overbed table or bedside stand; adjust to comfortable work height
▶ Adjust bed to comfortable work height with side rails up as needed
▶ Place light away from patient
▶ Offer bedpan/urinal (wash hands after use)
▶ Position patient supine, if patient's condition permits

EQUIPMENT

▶ Wash basin
▶ Soap dish
▶ Linen hamper
▶ Laundry bag
▶ Bath blanket
▶ 2 washcloths
▶ 2 towels (bath)
▶ 2 towels (face)
▶ Gown
▶ Hygiene aids, e.g., soap, powder, deodorant, skin lotion

PROCEDURE

SUGGESTED STEPS	RATIONALE/DISCUSSION
A. Remove top linen and cover patient with bed blanket.	A. Top sheet can be used as cover when bath blanket unavailable.
1. Loosen top linen at foot of bed.	
2. Remove spread and blanket. If to be re-used, fold while removing (see Procedure 9).	2. To keep linen dry for replacement.
3. Place one end of bath blanket at patient's shoulders. Ask him to hold top edge of bath blanket in place if he can.	3. Bath blanket provides extra warmth during procedure. If patient unable to hold bath blanket in place, tuck top corners of bath blanket under patient's shoulders.
4. Moving from patient's shoulders to his feet, reach under bath blanket, grasp top edge of sheet and bring to foot of bed.	4. Keep patient covered with bath blanket while removing sheet. Maintain privacy and warmth.
5. Once at foot of bed, fold top sheet into bundle; place in laundry bag or fold for replacement.	5. If top sheet is clean, it can be replaced as the bottom sheet when bed is remade.
B. Position patient close to edge of bed nearest worker.	B. Prevents unnecessary reaching.
C. Remove patient's gown; keep him covered with bath blanket as you do so.	*If patient has IV, remove gown from arm with-out IV first, then lower IV container, slide gown up IV tubing and over IV container. Re-hang IV container and check rate of flow.*
D. Move overbed table or bedside stand within easy reach.	D. Avoids worker twisting and reaching unnecessarily.
E. Remove pillow if condition permits.	E. Pillow removal simplifies washing patient's neck and ears. Some patients (e.g., those with difficulty in breathing) require pillow at all times.
F. Place bath towel under head.	F. Protects bed from becoming wet.
G. Pull side rails up as needed for safety and obtain bath water.	G. Fill wash basin one-third to one-half full, with water temperature approximately 43 to 46°C. (109.4 to 114.8°F). Too little water in basin is inadequate for bathing and cools rapidly. Too much water may spill. Water that is too hot can cause discomfort or even burn patient. Cool water can chill patient. Determine water temperature by using wood-encased bath thermometer or placing worker's wrist in water.

Procedure continued on the following page

SUGGESTED STEPS	RATIONALE/DISCUSSION

H. Wash, rinse and dry patient's face and neck.

1. Wash around eyes *without* soap. With worker's hand in mitt, place index finger at inner canthus; then move toward outer canthus. Dry eyes thoroughly.

H. Encourage self-help if patient is capable.

1. Examine eyes. Using a separate section of mitt to wash each eye avoids spread of organisms. If patient washes own eyes, check that eyes are free of secretions or provide mirror for patient to check self. For removal of crusted secretions, see discussion of care for eyes.

> *Ask patient if soap is desired.*

2. Wash, rinse, dry forehead.

2. Observe for skin eruptions.

3. Wash, rinse, dry cheeks and nose.

3. If drainage from nares, note color.

4. Wash, rinse, dry around mouth.

4. Observe for parched lips. If lips have crusted secretions, soak lips with wet cloth before attempting to remove secretions. This decreases trauma to tissues.

5. Wash, rinse and dry ear with cloth over hand. Place two fingers in anterior external ear and thumb behind ear.

5. One smooth motion cleans anterior and posterior aspects of ear. Observe ears for secretions and condition of the skin.

6. Wash front and back of neck. Lift patient toward you, if necessary, to reach back of neck. Rinse and dry.

6. Observe for skin eruptions, scaling at hair line, and enlarged lymph nodes.

I. Remove bath towel under patient's head.

J. Wash, rinse and dry *arms.*

1. Move patient toward center of bed to clean arm nearest worker. To clean far arm, move patient to edge of bed nearest worker.

1. This allows ease of cleansing arms and good body mechanics.

2. Place bath towel lengthwise under arm. Position towel well up under axillae.

2. Protects bed from becoming wet and can be used to wrap arm for warmth between wash, rinse and dry.

3. Grasp wrist and elevate arm (see Fig. 27–10).

3. Provides maximum visualization and range of motion.

4. Use mitt to wash and rinse arms. Use long, firm strokes in direction toward shoulder and light strokes in direction toward hand. Be sure to cleanse axillae thoroughly.

4. Smooth, continuous motion; firmness creates friction for easy removal of debris and stimulates circulation to heart.

> *If IV present, be careful (a) not to place pressure over vein or over insertion site; (b) not to dislodge needle; and (c) to check IV flow after moving arm.*

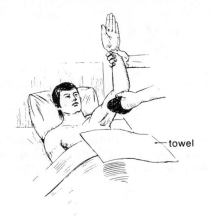
←towel

Figure 27–10.   Bathing arms of patient. (From Wood, L. A., and Rambo, B. J. (eds.): *Nursing Skills for Allied Health Services,* 2nd ed. Vol. 1. Philadelphia, W. B. Saunders Co., 1977, p. 248.)

SUGGESTED STEPS	RATIONALE/DISCUSSION
	Palpate for enlarged nodes in axillae. Note skin eruptions and dryness. Apply lotion as indicated.
K. Cleanse *hands*.	K. For cleansing nails, hands can be soaked now or at end of bath.
1. Wash without mitt.	
2. Support at wrist joint.	
3. Put hands in water with bath towel under basin. Wash with cloth, using firm strokes from fingertips toward hand. Wash all sides of each finger and move each finger at each joint.	3. Check circulation by observing temperature of hands and color of hands and nail beds. Necrotic tissue collects between fingers and may be difficult to remove. Firm strokes provide friction for debris removal and stimulate circulation. Moving joints provides range of motion.
L. Wash, rinse and dry *chest*.	
1. Place bath towel over chest and fold bath blanket down to patient's umbilicus.	1. Provides privacy and warmth while keeping bath blanket dry for later replacement over patient.
2. Hold one corner of towel away from chest. With other hand mitted, cleanse chest using firm, long strokes. Replace towel over chest between wash, rinse, and dry periods.	2. Allows visualization of area being washed while keeping rest of chest covered. Maintains privacy and warmth. Firm strokes stimulate circulation and decrease tickling sensation. Remember to wash under breasts. Assess condition of breast tissue, skin under breast and nipples; note depth and rate of breathing.
M. Wash, rinse and dry *abdomen*.	
1. Fold bath blanket down to pubic region; tuck sides around hips.	1. Assess for abdominal distention.
2. Place bath towel lengthwise or crosswise over abdomen.	2. For female, face towel can be placed across chest and bath towel across abdomen.

Procedure continued on the following page

SUGGESTED STEPS

RATIONALE/DISCUSSION

3. Lift bath towel up with one hand; use mitted hand to cleanse abdomen. Work from side to side, using long, firm strokes.

3. Give special attention to cleansing umbilicus and creased folds of abdomen. Firm strokes decrease tickling sensation.

4. Lower bath towel to abdomen between washing and rinsing.

5. Dry abdomen with bath towel.

6. Remove towel(s); reposition bath blanket at shoulder height.

N. Wash, rinse and dry *legs.*

Expose one leg at a time.

Prevent unnecessary exposure and provide warmth.

1. Move patient close to side of bed near worker; begin with farthest leg.

1. Decreases unnecessary reaching and motion.

2. Drape leg. Slide bath blanket toward hips, keeping blanket close to leg. Bring corner of bath blanket around thigh and hip; tuck corner under lateral thigh (see Fig. 27–11).

2. Draping prevents unnecessary exposure and drafts.

3. Securely position bath basin near foot to to be bathed.

3. Support basin with free hand while lifting foot. Prevents spilling.

4. Position your near arm under patient's leg; grasp heel; bend leg at knee. Slightly elevate leg off mattress; slide bath towel lengthwise under leg (see Fig. 27–11).

4. Lifting patient's leg in this manner supports joints. Placing towel on bed protects bed from spilled water.

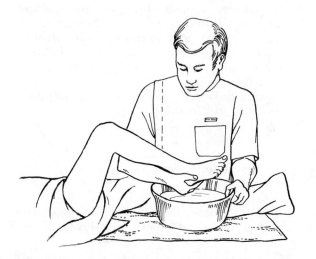

Figure 27–11.   Positioning leg and foot for bathing.

SUGGESTED STEPS	RATIONALE/DISCUSSION
5. Continue supporting leg and foot. With your free hand slide bath basin under lifted foot (see Fig. 27–11). Place patient's foot firmly on basin bottom.	5. Controls leg movement; prevents spilled water. Position foot to avoid pressure from edge of basin on calf of leg. Leave foot to soak, while bathing leg.
6. With mitted hand, use firm, long strokes to cleanse and dry leg.	6. Aids venous return.
7. Open washcloth and cleanse foot.	7. Use firm touch to decrease tickling sensation. *Cleanse and dry thoroughly between each toe* to prevent skin breakdown. Inspect skin. Clean and clip nails as needed.
8. Cleanse near leg and foot in the same manner as in steps 2 through 7.	8. For both legs and feet assess sensation, circulation, muscle strength and joint mobility. Provide range of motion for lower extremity joints unless contraindicated.
O. *Change water.*	O. For safety, raise side rails while away from bed; check temperature of water.
P. Wash, rinse and dry *back*.	
1. Turn patient to prone or side-lying position while keeping him covered with bath blanket.	1. When possible, the prone position is most relaxing.
2. Drape patient by sliding bath *blanket* from shoulder to thighs. Tuck blanket edges securely around thighs.	2. Decreases sense of exposure. Assess skin and circulation; note muscle tension; be alert for respiratory difficulty.
3. Place bath *towel* lengthwise over back.	3. Promotes warmth and privacy.
4. Use unmitted hand to hold towel away from back; use mitted hand to cleanse back with continuous, long, firm strokes. Work down from back of neck to buttock.	4. Bathe posterior thighs, if not cleansed during bathing of legs.
Q. Give *back massage* now or after completing bath.	Q. Sequence depends on purpose of back massage.
R. Obtain *clean* water for *perineal care.*	R. Assist patient with perineal care as needed.

POST-PROCEDURE ACTIVITIES

Offer patient opportunity to use personal care items, e.g., deodorant, powder, lotion. Assist with putting on clean gown. Provide hair care. For safety, replace call signal, lower bed, and replace bed cranks. Hang *clean* face towel, bath towel, and washcloth on bar of bedside stand. Changing bed linen may be necessary if damp or soiled.

Procedure continued on the following page

Aftercare of Equipment.   Disinfect bath basin. Replace basin, soap, soap dish and personal care items in bedside stand. Clean top of bedside stand and overbed table, and position within patient's reach. Take soiled linen to appropriate place.

Final Assessment of Patient and Unit.   Position patient for comfort and proper alignment. Remove unnecessary items and leave needed items (e.g., tissues, paper bag for trash, water) within *easy* reach of patient. *Charting:* Type of bath usually recorded on flow sheet. Chart abnormal findings on progress notes, e.g., skin breakdown, loss of motor strength, abnormal sensation, cool extremities, respiratory distress with change of position. Pertinent conversation, ability for self-care and patient preferences may be noted in nursing care plan.

TOWEL BATH.   The main advantages of the towel bath are (1) increased efficiency, (2) greater comfort for the patient, and (3) the use of a skin agent that conditions dry skin. Towel bathing in bed can be accomplished in about 2 to 10 minutes.

Preparation for the towel bath is similar to that for the traditional bed bath. Both procedures permit the worker to employ the principle of bathing from *clean* to *dirty* areas. In the traditional bed bath method, the worker moves from head (cleanest area) to foot (dirtiest area); however, for the towel bath, the patient is bathed from foot to head. In the towel bath method a clean section of the towel is used for each portion of the body.

Supplies: cleansing agent and 0.5 L. of water in pitcher, large plastic bag, large terry cloth towel, linen hamper and laundry bag, 2 washcloths and a bath towel, patient gown, and linen for bed change (see Procedure 9).

To prepare the patient, remove spread and blanket and patient gown, as in Procedure 9. Cover surgical dressings, casts and open skin areas with plastic. Place patient in supine position with legs apart and arms loosely at sides.

Prepare the towel as follows: fold towel in half, top to bottom; fold again in half, top to bottom. Fold in half again, side to side, and then roll towel, beginning with folded edges. Place rolled towel in plastic bag. Fill pitcher with 0.5 L. of water at 46 to 47°C. (114.8 to 116.6°F.; check temperature with bath thermometer); add cleansing agent. Pour solution over towel in plastic bag. Knead solution quickly into towel;

hold open edge of bag over sink and squeeze out excess solution. Take closed bag containing towel to patient's bedside.

Cleansing the Patient.   One worker pulls sheet to patient's waist as the other worker places the towel on one side of patient's chest with edges up and outward. Then open towel to other side of patient's chest (see Fig. 27–12A). Leave 20 to 25 cm. overlap at shoulder height to allow for washing face, neck and ears.

One worker unrolls the towel and opens it over patient's entire body, while the other worker simultaneously removes the top sheet. Keep the sheet close to towel to prevent unnecessary exposure. Tuck towel around the body (see Fig. 27–12B). Fan-fold the top sheet against foot of bed or remove it if soiled or excessively wrinkled.

With one worker on each side at the foot of the bed, begin bathing the patient by *moving together* toward the patient's head. As the patient is bathed *foot to chest,* use a *gentle massaging motion.* Use a *clean* section of the towel for *each* part of the body. As bathing continues, fold used sections of the towel upward and away from the feet.

As the towel is moved toward the patient's head, the fan-folded sheet or clean sheet is placed over the patient. Leave about 8 cm. between the towel and sheet to allow skin to air dry, provide privacy, and keep sheet from becoming wet. The exposed skin will air dry in seconds.

Wash patient's face, neck and ears with the overlapped sections of towel under the chin.

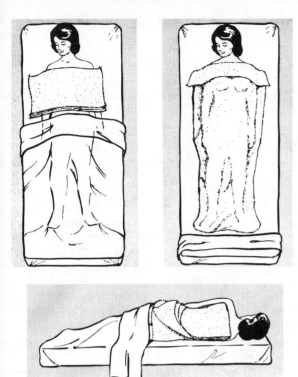

Figure 27–12. Placement of towel for bath procedure. *A,* Start by placing towel over chest. *B,* Towel tucked around patient's body for bathing and massage motion. *C,* Placement of towel for bathing back. (From Vestal Laboratories, Division of Chemed Corporation, St. Louis, MO.)

Wash the ears with corner sections of the towel, as in the traditional bathing procedure.

One worker grasps the towel in the middle, removing it from the patient. The towel is folded into quarters with the *soiled side turned in.* The other worker turns the patient toward his side.

Place the folded towel on the patient's back with selvage (hem) edge at the patient's sides and corners of open area covering buttocks. Bathe patient by moving from *shoulders* to buttocks (see Fig. 27–12*B*).

To clean patient's buttocks, turn first three layers of towel up and over patient's hips and use the remaining section for cleaning (see Fig. 27–12*C*). Use a *clean* section of the towel for *each* wipe. As a section of the towel becomes soiled, tuck it underneath and pull a clean area over buttocks.

Remove towel and place in laundry bag. Change bottom bed linen as done in Procedure 9. Offer the patient an opportunity to use deodorant, and assist with putting on clean gown or pajamas. Provide for other hygiene needs as appropriate, e.g., hair and nail care. Replace top linen as in Procedure 9.

Final assessment of patient and unit is the same as for the traditional bed bath.

Cleansing Agent Used for the Towel Bath. The liquid solution used for cleansing provides an oily film, moisturizes and leaves no alkali residue. To be effective for conditioning dry skin, the solution is allowed to dry on the skin *without rinsing.* Septi Soft concentrate is most commonly used, but other products such as Alpha Keri can be used as a skin protective and cleansing agent. Follow the manufacturer's directions for the amount of cleansing agent that is added to the water.

Use of the Towel Bath. Although two workers are needed for this method of bathing, the increased efficiency is more cost-effective. Not only does the procedure take less time but one worker can prepare the patient and unit while the other prepares the equipment. The terry cloth towel used in the towel bath procedure is 228 cm. × 91 cm. and weighs 0.2 kg. The towel is quite moist after completing the bathing process. If the facility sends linen to an outside laundry service which charges for laundering by weight, this does create an added expense.

The towel bath method is an alternative to but not necessarily a substitute for the traditional method of bathing in bed. The towel bath is used for patients who need the psychologic benefit of increased relaxation; in situations in which pain could be reduced by the decreased movement involved in this method; and/or for conditioning dry skin. The towel bath is particularly effective for patients with excessively dry skin or sore joints, such as in arthritis, or patients who need a cleansing bath but suffer increased pain from touch or movement. In one research study, patients reported no embarrassment, increased warmth, and less exhaustion with the towel bath versus the traditional method.[7]

Some workers consider the decreased time spent with the patient as a disadvantage of towel bathing, but the worker is free to spend more time with patients at other times without being involved with the physical task of bathing. Patients report feeling less rushed when the towel bath is used.[7] However, assessment of the patient is more difficult until the worker becomes skilled at observing quickly.

(Write-up on the towel bath is adapted from "Septi-Soft Towel Bath Procedures," Vestal Laboratories, Division of Chemed Corporation, St. Louis, Mo.)

Special Types of Baths

Medicated Baths. Medicated baths are given to cleanse the skin of previously applied ointments or creams; heal irritated skin; soften crusted debris for easy removal; relax the patient, and relieve itching and for their sedative or stimulant effect. *Agents used for a soothing effect* are oatmeal, cornstarch and sodium bicarbonate (baking soda). Examples of *agents used for a stimulating effect* are sodium chloride (saline) and dry mustard. Potassium permanganate is a caustic agent that is sometimes used to promote healing. It has an astringent, antibacterial and antifungal effect. Medicated baths are seldom ordered but are used for a variety of skin problems. The towel bath, in a sense, can be considered a medicated (use of skin protective agent) or therapeutic bath.

Therapeutic Baths. Therapeutic baths are provided for physical needs other than cleansing:

Relaxing tub bath—soaking in warm water (43°C. or 109.4°F.) to relieve tension.

Hot water tub bath—soaking in hot water (45 to 46°C. or 113 to 114.8°F.) to relieve muscle soreness.

Cooling bath—to relieve tension or to lower body temperature. The temperature of the water varies, depending upon the therapeutic effect desired and the method used. *Never* start with cold water. The body's homeostatic mechanisms require time to adjust to the change in temperature. Start with warm plain water and gradually cool the water. The cool water on the surface of the body and evaporation allow heat to dissipate. The cooling bath can be done by

sponging with a towel in bed or by putting the patient in a bathtub.

> *Check the patient's temperature* before *starting the bath and 30 minutes after* completing *the bath.*

This type of bath is particularly effective in lowering the body temperature in small children.

Soaks are used for removing necrotic (dead) tissue or softening crusted secretions. Soaks promote suppuration (pus formation) of wounds. *Asepsis* is very important because open or abraded areas of skin can be portals of entry for pathogens. It may be necessary to use sterile supplies, depending on the patient's condition and reason for the soak. Soaks also may be used on the skin over inflamed areas of the body, e.g., at an intravenous infusion site that has become irritated.

The sitz or hip bath provides moist heat to the perineal and anal area to cleanse, promote healing and drainage, or reduce soreness in these areas. The moist heat helps relieve vascular congestion and reduces inflammation. This type of bath is used mainly for patients who have had rectal surgery; female patients who have undergone pelvic surgery or delivery of a baby; and patients with hemorrhoids. Water temperature depends upon the purpose of the sitz bath and the condition of the patient's skin; usually the temperature is 43 to 45°C. (109.4 to 113°F.).

> *Although the patient may tell you the water temperature is too cool, warmer water is not used because sensitive skin and mucous membranes are easily burned.*

Most facilities have plastic disposable sitz baths that can be sent home with the patient upon discharge (see Fig. 27–13). This sitz bath device is placed over the toilet bowl and is partially filled with warm water. To maintain water temperature, a bag with tubing can be hung by the toilet with the tubing placed in the basin. Water is dripped into the basin as the temperature cools. Some facilities use a portable *metal* sitz bath device (see Fig. 27–13B), which is available with an electric motor to maintain water temperature. However, many of these have been found to be an *electrical hazard*. The treatment is given for about 15 minutes. Longer treatments will have a negative circulatory effect (see Chap. 44). Regardless of the sitz bath device used, position the

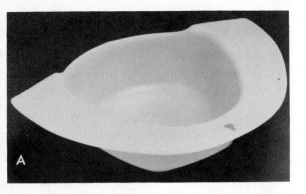

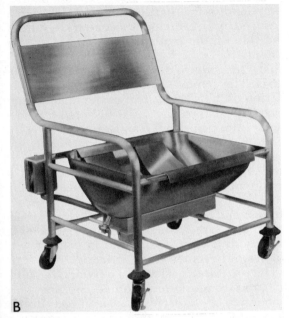

Figure 27–13. Sitz bath devices. *A,* Plastic disposable sitz bath. *B,* Metal sitz bath. (From Everest & Jennings, Inc., Los Angeles, CA.)

patient's buttocks into the hollowed area without causing pressure on the area being treated or on his back or legs; place a bath blanket around the patient to provide warmth and privacy; and after completing the treatment, clean the device with a disinfectant and rinse thoroughly.

PERINEAL CARE

Perineal hygiene involves cleansing the external genitalia and surrounding area. This may be done in conjunction with general bathing (see Procedure 7 for sequencing). Other indications for perineal care are as follows: genitourinary infection; incontinence (of urine or feces); excessive secretions or concentrated urine, causing skin irritation or excoriation; insertion of a Foley catheter; postpartum care

after vaginal delivery; after some types of surgery in the area.

Purposes of Perineal Care

The purposes of perineal care are to (a) prevent or eliminate infection and odor; (b) promote healing; and (c) promote comfort. Because this area of the body has several orifices it is a common portal of entry for pathogens. The perineal area is conducive to growth of pathogenic organisms because it is warm and moist and is not well ventilated. Thorough hygiene is essential in order to maintain the condition of the skin and protect the integrity of the body.

Anatomy of the Perineal Area

The perineal area is located between the thighs and extends from the top of the pelvic bones (anterior) to the anus (posterior). The perineum contains sensitive anatomic structures related to the functions of sexuality, elimination and reproduction. A brief discussion of female and male perineal anatomy follows.

Female Anatomy (Fig. 27–14).   Within the female perineal area is the *vulva* (external geni-

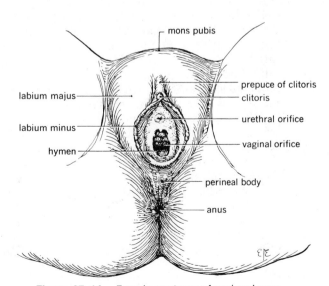

Figure 27–14. Female anatomy of perineal area.

talia), which consists of the mons pubis, prepuce, clitoris, urethral and vaginal orifices, labia majora and minora, sebaceous and Bartholin's glands, ducts, and vestibule. Several muscle groups and fasciae provide support for the pelvic floor and help maintain the contour of external genitalia. Fat and connective tissue serve to protect this area from trauma.

The most anterior area of the vulva is the *mons pubis,* which is a hair-covered pad of fatty tissue lying over the symphysis pubis. The *prepuce* is a fold of dense connective tissue that covers the clitoris. The *clitoris* consists of erectile tissue containing vascular spaces surrounded by muscles. The many nerve fibers in the clitoris make it very sensitive to stimuli. The *urethral orifice* (external urinary meatus) opens into an area between the clitoris and vagina. The bladder and urethra lie anterior to the vagina.

The *vagina* extends upward and backward between the urethra and rectum. The cervix of the uterus protrudes into the vaginal cavity. The skin surface of the vaginal orifice is normally somewhat moist. The vagina is kept moist by mucus-producing glands (Bartholin's glands) that are located laterally to the vagina. Endocervical glands secrete an exudate that collects various cells as it moves through the vagina. The secretion has a slight odor, which is due to the cells and normal vaginal flora. The amount of cloudy vaginal discharge (leukorrhea) varies with hormonal changes; e.g., it increases during ovulation and with sexual stimulation. Vaginal secretion is slightly acid, which inhibits bacterial growth.

The labia majora and minora together enfold the vulva. The *labia majora* consist of fatty tissue extending from the mons pubis laterally into the perineum (perineal body), which separates the vulva and anal area. Anteriorly, the labia majora unite to enfold the clitoris and prepuce. The skin of the labia majora is similar to other skin surfaces and is fairly resistive to trauma. The labia majora has hair follicles and sebaceous and apocrine (sweat) glands. Posterior to the clitoris the skin fold divides to form the *labia minora,* which extends downward and inward to enfold the vaginal orifice. Its modified skin surface is sensitive to external trauma and has only sebaceous glands. The *vestibule* is the area containing the urethral and vaginal orifices and is surrounded by the labia minora.

A small, moist surface area of perineum (*perineal body*) separates the vulva from the anal orifice.

Male Anatomy (Fig. 27–15). The *penis* is a structure which contains urethral pathways for urination and ejaculation through the *urethral meatus.* At the end of the penis is the *glans* covered by a skin flap called the *prepuce* (foreskin). The urethral orifice (meatus) is located in the center portion of the penis and opens at the tip of the penis. The shaft of the penis consists of columns of erectile tissue bound by the dense fibrous tissue of the prepuce. The skin on the penis is non–hair bearing and thin; thus, it is easily traumatized. Erection is caused by engorgement secondary to stimuli. The skin on the penis is loose and allows for distention.

The *scrotum* is located at the root of the penis. The scrotal sac contains testicles and a portion of the duct system of the male genital tract. The skin on the sac is bisected from the shaft of the penis to the anus. Each half of the scrotum contains a *testis* with *epididymis* and *spermatic cord.* The *vas deferens,* which is a cord-like structure, extends from the epididymis to the external inguinal ring. This area consists of blood and lymph vessels, nerves, and muscle. The scrotal skin surface contains a large number of apocrine glands. Because this skin is thin and in contact with clothes, it becomes easily irritated.

The *prostate* consists of a network of glands that produce prostatic secretion. The glands are embedded in muscles that contract during ejaculation to move the prostatic secretion through the ejaculatory ducts, which separate into posterior and median sections of the prostate, and into the prostate urethra. The posterior prostate surface is in close contact with the rectal wall.

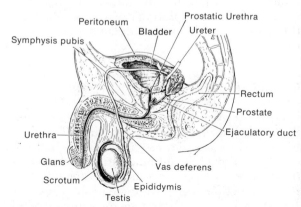

Figure 27–15. Male anatomy of perineal area.

The most pertinent principles for perineal hygiene are as follows: (a) bathe from clean to dirty areas; (b) body orifices are portals of entry for pathogens; and (c) warm, moist skin is conducive to pathogenic growth.

> *The* urethral *orifice is considered the* cleanest *area, and the* anal *orifice is considered the* dirtiest *area.*

Because the orifices in the perineal area are in close proximity, cross contamination is a potential problem. The normal flora of the urinary system is different from that in the gastrointestinal system. Entry of organisms from the anal orifice into the urethral orifice can cause urinary tract infections because these organisms are foreign to the urinary tract.

During perineal care, *completely cleanse* the skin around the urethral orifice first, and do not return to cleanse this area after cleansing the anal orifice. A separate portion of the washcloth is used for each wipe. Because the perineal area is a warm, moist environment it requires frequent cleansing with thorough rinsing and drying. An ill person is less resistant to infection, usually spends more time in bed, and receives less ventilation of the perineal area. The condition of the skin is more prone to breakdown, and the integrity of the body is jeopardized. The perineal area also has hair over portions of the skin surface. These hair follicles tend to harbor organisms, such as lice.

Need for Perineal Care

Assessment. Deterioration of the condition of skin may go unnoticed when the patient is doing his own perineal care. Listen for complaints of itching, burning with urination, and soreness. If the patient uses a bedpan or urinal, observe the perineal area while assisting with this care. When the patient has an unpleasant odor or concentrated urine is noted, examine the perineal area for retained secretions and skin irritation. Other findings can be noted by inspection and palpation. Assess for lesions; ulcers; scars; amount, color, odor and source of drainage; tenderness; inflammation; excoriation; edema; and enlarged lymph nodes.

Frequency and Type of Care. Assessment of the need for perineal care is based on the (a) patient's susceptibility to infection; (b) assessment of skin problems; and (c) need to remove sources of odors. Patients who are prone to skin breakdown include those with concentrated urine; fecal or urinary incontinence; Foley catheters; recent genitourinary or rectal surgery; diaphoresis; and metabolic disorders such as diabetes mellitus. Unpleasant odors may indicate infection or poor hygiene. Thorough perineal care and teaching the patient scientific principles of perineal hygiene can be primary means of preventing problems.

Approach to Care. Often the nurse or patient ignores perineal hygiene because of embarrassment. Assessment also may be neglected for the same reason. A professional attitude on the part of the nurse can reduce embarrassment for both patient and nurse. Whether the nurse is assessing the patient, having the patient do self-care in bed, or providing assistance with perineal care, she should use terminology the patient can understand.

Basic Perineal Care

Some workers prefer to wear gloves during perineal care for aesthetic reasons. Research indicates that many organisms are transmitted by the hands of workers (see Chap. 40). Thus, *clean disposable gloves* should be worn while assisting with perineal area. Use a mild soap with warm water (43°C. or 109.4°F.) for cleansing. If skin is excoriated, use only plain warm water. When soap is used be sure to rinse off residue for prevention of skin irritation. Since the perineal area is easily traumatized by friction and retains moisture, thoroughly pat dry all skin surfaces.

Positioning and Draping. Both female and male patients are placed in the dorsal recumbent position for the initial part of perineal care and in the side-lying position during the last part. To provide a sense of privacy and decrease exposure, drape the patient for assessment and perineal care. Before draping the patient to cleanse the genitalia, position the patient dorsal recumbent (female frequently is placed on the bedpan for perineal care).

One method of draping is to fan-fold a bath blanket or sheet to the patient's mid-thighs. Then place a towel on the abdomen slightly above the genitalia. Have the patient slightly flex the legs so that all areas can be effectively reached for cleaning.

A second method of draping, which provides a greater sense of security, involves wrapping the legs with a bath blanket. Place the bath blanket on an angle with one corner between the patient's legs and a corner to each side of the bed. Bring one side corner around the leg and tuck under the hip (see Fig. 27–11). Repeat this for the other leg. Then fold the corner from between the legs back onto the abdomen. Have the patient slightly flex the legs so that all areas can be cleaned.

When cleansing the anal area, drape the buttocks. The patient should be in a side-lying position with the buttocks toward the worker. Place a bath blanket or sheet over the thighs and tuck under the leg that is resting on the mattress.

Male Perineal Care.   If the patient has not had a circumcision, the prepuce (foreskin) must be retracted before starting perineal care. *Smegma* (a cheese-like substance), which is secreted by sebaceous glands, collects under the prepuce. Grasp the shaft of the penis in one hand, holding the washcloth in the other hand (see Fig. 27–16). Start bathing at the tip of the penis (cleanest area). Use a circular motion, cleaning from the center to the periphery, and use a separate section of the washcloth for each wipe. Thoroughly rinse this area. Then proceed washing down the shaft toward the body. Next wash the scrotum and perineum. Hold the scrotum so the perineum and all surfaces of the scrotal sac can be cleansed. Pat dry the penis and scrotum.

For ease in cleansing the rectal area, have the patient turn to his side unless this is contraindicated. Separate the buttocks with one hand and use the washcloth in the other hand to cleanse.

Female Perineal Care.   In some situations, more effective cleansing can be accomplished

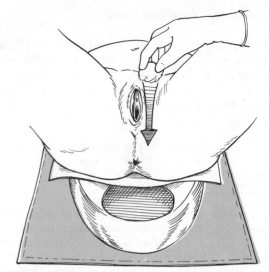

Figure 27–17.   Cleansing of the female perineum.

when the patient is placed on a bedpan for cleansing and rinsing the vulva and perineum. *Smegma* tends to collect on the inner surface of the labia. Use one hand to retract the labia. With the other hand wash from front to back (clean to dirty). Use a separate section of the washcloth for each wipe in a downward motion (see Fig. 27–17). Wash from the urethral to the vaginal orifice; then wash the labia. After bathing the vestibule, cleanse the perineum. The perineum may be easier to reach while the patient is lying on the side for cleansing the rectal area (dirtiest). Rinse and pat dry skin surfaces of vestibule, perineum and rectal area.

Special Perineal Care

If the patient has had genital or rectal surgery, sterile supplies may be required for cleaning the operative site. For example, sterile cotton balls can be used to gently cleanse the sensitive area (see Fig. 27–17). The operative site and perineal area sometimes are washed with plain water or a disinfectant such as Betadine. If Betadine is used, be sure to ask the patient if he is allergic to iodine. Sitz baths may be used for comfort and healing.

If the patient has a Foley catheter, basic hygiene care is provided, but additional precaution is needed to prevent infection. Crusted secretions can build up around the catheter at the urinary meatus. Use Betadine to cleanse the urinary meatus and around the portion of the catheter near the urethral orifice. Recommendations for the frequency of catheter care vary from every 8 hours to daily.

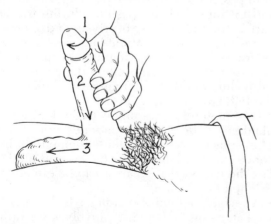

Figure 27–16.   Steps in cleansing male perineum.

Many people ignore nail and skin care of hands and feet until discomfort occurs. Problems commonly stem from neglect and abuse: biting nails and cuticles, improper trimming of nails, exposure to chemicals (e.g., household cleansers), frequent periods of immersion in water, trauma, ill-fitting shoes and inadequate hygiene. Some general constitutional factors and diseases (e.g., poor nutrition, arthritis and diabetes mellitus) make a person more prone to nail and foot problems. Poor circulation and altered metabolic function can lead to skin breakdown and infection. Nail and foot care is important to a patient's general health and comfort.

Etiology of Nail Problems

Nails serve as a hard protective covering (nail plate) over distal portions of extremities. As an extension (appendage) of skin on the dorsal surface of hands and feet, nails protect the underlying soft nail beds from trauma. The nail root grows distal to the matrix, which is nourished by blood vessels. Growth occurs at approximately 1 mm. per week. Poor circulation and/or poor general nutrition can impede nail growth and alter the texture of nails, e.g., making them brittle. Nails easily grow into soft tissue at the sides (ingrown nails), causing trauma to the tissue. Nail and cuticle biting as well as excessively long nails, which easily break and tear away from the skin, can lead to infections of nails and surrounding tissue. Fungal infections are common and may require extended periods of treatment. As an infectious process progresses, the nail sometimes loosens at the root. Infections can also cause the skin at the nail root to become swollen, tender and more susceptible to trauma from activities of daily living.

Etiology of Foot Problems

Carbary states: "Each week more than half a million people seek help for foot problems."[3] She goes on to comment that Americans spend over 1 million dollars on foot care products each year. Feet are more susceptible to trauma and prone to infection than other areas of the body. Stress on the many bones of the feet from being overweight or wearing ill-fitting shoes causes pressure and irritation that contribute to many foot problems. Dirty socks or stockings and poorly ventilated shoes create an environment that encourages bacterial and fungal growth.

Purposes of Nail and Foot Care

The primary purposes of nail and foot care involve prevention of the following: (1) infection and inflammation; (2) trauma from ingrown nails and long or jagged nails catching on linen, etc., and pressure on nails from long toenails rubbing against the end of shoes; (3) trauma secondary to nail care, e.g., improper trimming; and (4) accumulated debris in order to decrease odor and eliminate potential sources of infection. The excellent nurse appreciates the need for special attention to nail and foot care, provides thorough hygiene, and teaches patients the etiology and complications of problems as well as hygiene principles to prevent problems.

Assessment and Need for Care

Assessment of nails and surrounding tissue and determining need for care can be accomplished during general bathing, while talking with the patient or while providing other care. Assessment of circulation to hands and feet and observing for signs of inflammation and infection are paramount. Inspect fingernails and toenails for color, shape (contour), length and texture (pliability, brittleness, thickness). Depress the nail plate onto the nail bed to note blanching and speed of color return. This provides information regarding circulation. Also note the condition of the skin surrounding nails: swollen, inflamed, callused, abraded, dry patches, lesions, temperature and hair growth. Temperature and hair growth provide clues to nutrition and circulation to the distal portion of the extremities. Some people have scanty general body hair; this is taken into account when evaluating the amount of hair growth on fingers and toes. Especially, observe the condition of the skin between the fingers and toes, as these are particularly prone to retain moisture and undergo skin breakdown.

Most patients will not require extensive, repeated care. For example, long or jagged nails and removal of excessive debris usually are needed only once during a short hospitalization. Remember, nails grow slowly and patients usually are not involved in activities that produce excessive buildup of debris. Cleansing of nails and skin of hands and feet should be based on the assessed condition of nails and feet.

Care of Nails and Feet

Basic hygiene care of nails and feet includes trimming nails, cleansing under nails, and thoroughly rinsing and patting dry the skin on the hands and feet. Use extra caution to prevent trauma when caring for patients with diabetes mellitus. These patients are very susceptible to infections and other nail and foot problems as a result of circulatory and neurologic complications of their disease process. Nursing personnel frequently say, "I don't have time to give the patient nail and foot care." Neglect of this aspect of hygiene care is unwarranted! Hygiene care is the primary means of prevention and with good organization the worker can provide nail and foot care with very little effort. Some measures on the part of the worker can decrease foot odors, provide more effective aseptic conditions and safety for the worker and patient, enhance comfort for the patient, and increase the worker's efficiency.

Two measures that aid the worker when doing nail and foot care are wearing gloves and soaking the patient's hands and feet. For some workers, *wearing gloves* decreases the offensiveness of performing foot care. Gloves should always be worn by the worker when the patient has open skin lesions or an infection. This decreases the chance of cross contamination between patient and worker. *Soaking* hands and feet softens skin and nails and loosens debris. Soaking not only aids cleaning and trimming but is comforting and refreshing for the patient.

Organization of Care. Soaking hands and feet and trimming nails can be done at times other than during general bathing. To best organize care for several patients, intersperse soaking with other care and encourage patient participation in care. When a patient is given a *towel bath,* the skin agent helps to soften nails and skin. If the patient bathes in the *tub,* additional time for soaking can be allotted. Many patients can be provided with nail care equipment for cleaning their fingernails while you care for another patient, and you can later return to assist with nail trimming and foot care. If the patient is capable of *sitting* for a short period of time, position him comfortably in the bedside chair without pressure on the popliteal area. Place his feet in a wash basin of warm water (44°C. or 111.2°F.). Soap or emollient-demulcent products can be added to the water for softening skin and nails, removing debris and decreasing odor. Position the overbed table low and over the patient's lap. Use another wash basin or emesis basin, positioned on the overbed table, for soaking his hands. Place the basin so that the patient's arms rest comfortably on the overbed table without impeding circulation. If the call signal is left within reach of the patient and the patient is physically and mentally able to sit for a period of about 30 minutes, this leaves the worker free for other care. In most situations, the worker should return in about 15 minutes to rewarm the water. Soaking and other nail and foot care can be organized around the patient's and worker's other activities.

Cleansing and Trimming Nails. Nails do not always require soaking before trimming, but soaking makes brittle nails more pliable and therefore easier to trim. Nails are cut or clipped straight across to prevent ingrown nails. Avoid using scissors, and do not clip nails too close to the skin. While doing nail care, protect your eyes from flying nails. The safest nail care is provided by using a nail clipper for cutting, an orange stick for cleansing under nails and an emery board for shaping nails. If feasible, clip the cuticles around the side of the nails and push the cuticle back toward the nail root. A washcloth can be used to retract the cuticle.

Skin Care of Feet. Removing debris and some callused buildup on feet is best accomplished by vigorous scrubbing with a washcloth. Avoid friction over open areas of skin to prevent further trauma. *Never cut* callused areas, as this tends to leave scar tissue due to damage of the dermis layer of skin. Repeated soaking for several days is helpful in removing callused areas. Apply a lanolin-based lotion or petroleum jelly after each soaking to further soften callused areas and to moisturize dry skin. If the patient has a problem with excessive moisture, use a *small* amount of water-absorbent powder between toes. This not only decreases odor but aids in preventing skin breakdown.

Care As a Teaching Tool. Patients are appreciative of nail and foot care. Providing this aspect of care fosters the patient's sensitivity to the need for proper hygiene, and the worker's methods serve as a model for care. Whenever feasible, have the patient do at least a portion of the care so that his understanding and capabilities can be evaluated. For example, the worker may manicure one hand as a model and have the patient do his own care for the other hand. As you provide care, explain the reasons for your methods.

Summary

While nail and foot hygiene is comforting to patients and helps to prevent problems in these areas, it is essential to the well-being of the patient with decreased circulation. An infected toe of a patient with diabetes mellitus or peripheral vascular disease can lead to a gangrenous area and amputation of toe, foot or leg. The most important points to emphasize to the patient are to keep feet clean; keep areas between fingers and toes dry; properly trim nails; avoid injury to the skin surrounding nails; wear clean socks or stockings; and wear properly fitting shoes. *Nail and foot care is an essential part of hygiene, not a luxury.* Proper hygiene not only promotes comfort and prevents foot and nail problems but also decreases expenses for the patient. As pointed out earlier, Americans spend a lot of money on foot problems. Most of this expense is unnecessary when thorough hygiene is done regularly.

BACK MASSAGE

Massage of various areas of the body can be *stimulating* and *relaxing*, e.g., massaging the scalp or sore, aching feet will stimulate circulation as well as relax and comfort the patient. To some extent massage is accomplished by the rubbing action of washing the body during bathing. *Caution* is indicated when considering massage of limbs. *Never* massage a limb without a specific order, for this can have a detrimental effect. The lower extremities may have a thrombus (blood clot), which upon massage can become dislodged (embolus) and may travel to another area of the body. In most situations massage is an independent nursing judgment based on the patient's need for skin conditioning, relaxation, etc. The primary focus of this section is *back massage,* which includes the area from the neck and shoulders to the lower buttocks.

To effectively provide back massage, the nurse must know the location and directions of the major muscle groups involved: trapezius, deltoid, latissimus dorsi, external oblique and gluteal muscle groups. She must also keep in mind the location of bony prominences to avoid direct pressure over such areas, since it can result in damage to the underlying tissue.

Principles and Purposes of Back Massage

The principles and purposes of back massage are the same as for massage of any area of the body. The primary *principles* include the use of the following:

▶ *Aseptic* measures such as handwashing before and after massage and using a separate container of lotion for each patient

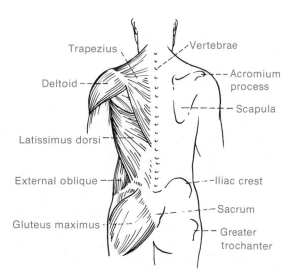

Figure 27–18. Muscles and bony prominences of the back.

▶ Proper *positioning* of the patient for good body alignment

▶ Appropriate *body mechanics* by the worker, e.g., use of strong leg muscles rather than weak back muscles and body weight as a force in the direction of movement

The major *purposes* of massage are to:

▶ Provide *physical contact* for both physical and psychologic benefits

▶ *Stimulate* and *relax* muscles

▶ *Increase circulation* for improving nutrition to cells

▶ *Reduce tension* associated with anxiety and stress

▶ *Condition the skin* for prevention of skin breakdown

Several methods can be used to achieve the purposes of back massage. One suggested method is discussed in Procedure 8.

Providing Back Massage

Back massage frequently is done in conjunction with morning care. When stimulation is desired, massage may be given after a bed bath and before changing bed linen. If massage is for relaxation, it is provided after completing other

H.S. (hour of sleep) care. The primary purpose of massage (stimulation or relaxation) determines not only when the massage is done but the types of strokes used (see Procedure 8).

Imagine yourself lying in bed all day. A nurse comes to your bedside and tells you she is going to give you a back massage. She squirts some lotion on your back and smoothes the lotion into your skin. Now imagine another nurse offering you a back massage the next day. This second nurse warms some lotion in her hands and then proceeds to massage all of your aching back muscles. Consider the difference between the first and the second nurse. The "laying on of hands" during back massage affords the patient and the nurse tactile contact. The second nurse most likely conveys a more "caring attitude" through this contact. Also, the second nurse provides more comfort by the smooth, rhythmic motion of massaging the back muscles.

Some nurses believe that only bedridden patients need back massage. Although the bedridden patient requires massage to prevent skin breakdown from pressure to the back from lying on the mattress, the ambulatory patient also needs back massage. The ambulatory patient may have been sitting for long periods or may be anxious about tests. For these types of patients, back massage can have an overall therapeutic effect by reducing stress and providing tactile contact.

Skin Agents for Back Massage

The most frequently used skin agent is a lanolin-based lotion. If the patient has excessively oily skin, powder may be the skin agent of choice. Some type of skin agent is needed to decrease friction between the worker's hands and the patient's back.

Assessment

Before and *after* back massage the nurse should assess the condition of the skin, especially noting erythema. Since massage normally produces cutaneous vasodilatation, one expects erythema following massage. Use the patient's verbal comments, nonverbal facial expressions, and change in tenseness of muscles as guides to the effectiveness of massage.

8.   BACK MASSAGE

By Jean Saxon, R.N., M.N.

Definition and Purposes.   *Back massage consists of the rhythmic rubbing, squeezing and stroking of the tissues of the back, buttocks, neck and upper arms.* It is used to provide physical and psychologic comfort and relaxation, increase local circulation (prevention and therapy for skin lesions or decubitus ulcers), stimulate general circulation and stimulate physical activity. Nurse adapts procedure to patient's individual needs.

Contraindications and Cautions.   Back massage may be contraindicated in the following situations: suspected or confirmed diagnosis of myocardial infarction (heart attack); trauma (accidental, surgical or pressure-induced) to superficial and deep tissues, e.g., fractures of ribs, back surgery, incisions, ulcers and skin lesions.

Patient-Family Teaching Points.   Present the following information as appropriate: (a) explain indications and contraindications for massage; (b) never massage limbs without a physician's or registered nurse's direction, and never massage limbs if sore spots develop after surgery or when a patient is on prolonged bed rest (danger of emboli); (c) do not use electric vibrators over bones, metal prostheses or bone fixation devices; (d) use other nursing measures as indicated to relieve pressure and muscle tension, e.g., frequent position changes, padding of bony prominences, maintenance of proper body alignment.

PRE-PROCEDURE ACTIVITIES

PRELIMINARY ASSESSMENT/PLANNING

Includes determination of
- ▶ diagnosis, activity orders, and psychosocial needs
- ▶ limitations of position and optimum position possible
- ▶ contraindications to massage or to particular massage techniques, e.g., stroking
- ▶ purpose of massage, e.g., to prevent skin lesions or prepare for sleep
- ▶ patient's post-procedure activities, e.g., rest, ambulation
- ▶ lubricant indicated by skin texture

PREPARATION OF PATIENT

- ▶ complete preliminary care; adjust bed to working height
- ▶ position patient with back, shoulders, upper arms and buttocks exposed
- ▶ position prone if possible, otherwise side-lying or supine; when possible move patient to edge of bed for best use of body mechanics by nurse (see Fig. 27–19)
- ▶ drape genitalia, legs, arms and front torso for warmth and modesty (bath blanket conforms and feels comfortable)
- ▶ avoid drafts and provide privacy

EQUIPMENT

- ▶ bath blanket
- ▶ bath towel
- ▶ pillows
- ▶ lubricant (lotion, alcohol, powder, vegetable oil, shortening or cream)

Note: Personal items carry patient's organisms, which can be transmitted to others; therefore, patient should have individual container of lubricant.

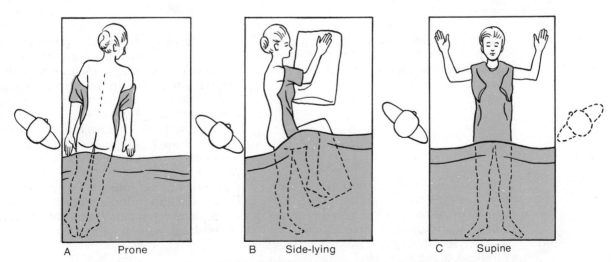

Figure 27–19.   Patient positions for back massage.

A   Prone   B   Side-lying   C   Supine

PROCEDURE

SUGGESTED STEPS	RATIONALE/DISCUSSION

A. *Prone position*

1. Warm hands; warm lubricant (under warm water or in hands) and rub lubricant between hands.

    1. Cold causes vasoconstriction and muscle tension.

2. Prepare patient for texture and temperature of lubricant; e.g., state lubricant may feel cool, wet or greasy.

    2. Knowledge reduces apprehension or startle response.

3. Apply lubricant to sacral area.

4. Stroking

    a. Stroke from base of buttocks up to shoulders, over upper arms and back to base of buttocks, keeping hands parallel to vertebrae.

    a. Long, continuous and rhythmic rubbing is soothing; pressure over bones (vertebrae) produces tissue injury; rubbing skin increases circulation to superficial tissues and produces blanching, followed by redness of tissue (alternate emptying and filling of arterioles, capillaries and venules). O_2 and nutrients are essential to tissue cell life and reach cells via the circulation.

    b. Use palmar surface of hand for stroking.

    b. Large surface contact reduces stimulation of tickle.

    c. Conform hand to body contour.

    c. Continuous contact provides therapy to all tissues.

    d. Shift body weight between back and front feet (rocking motion) to achieve stroking force, rhythm and rate. Face patient's head; keep your outside foot forward.

    d. Rhythmic rubbing of body tissues is soothing; force is applied in the direction of motion.

    e. Start stroking with medium upward force and light downward force, increasing to firm upward stroke and medium downward stroke.

    e. Use of body weight produces efficient force; use of strong leg muscles rather than weaker arm and back muscles decreases energy use and avoids injury; massage in the direction of venous return (toward heart) supports venous circulation and total circulation; firm pressure reduces tickle sensation. Assess patient response to determine desired pressure.

    f. Apply firm stroke from base of buttocks parallel to vertebrae; change to thumb strokes at cervical vertebrae continuing up to occipital area (see Fig. 27–20A); return down to base of cervical vertebrae. Next, compress, squeeze and lift trapezius muscle (see Fig. 27–20B).

    f. Squeezing muscle belly increases circulation and reduces tension. Assess muscle tension; repeat motions until relaxation is obtained.

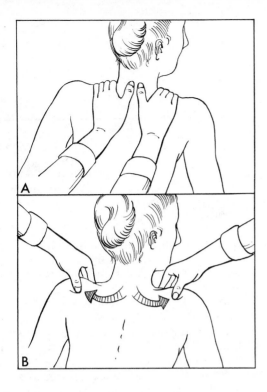

Figure 27-20. Stroking, squeezing, and lifting movements during back massage.

SUGGESTED STEPS	RATIONALE/DISCUSSION
5. Maintain skin contact with back of one hand while adding lubricant and distributing lubricant between hands.	5. Nonverbally informs patient you have not completed massage or that it will not end suddenly.

> *Assess tissue condition and avoid damaged tissue throughout procedure.*

6. Kneading

    a. Knead one-half of back and upper arm, starting at buttocks and moving up to shoulder; include deltoid and upper arm. Knead down or stroke down. Repeat on other half of body.

    a. Kneading and squeezing at right angles to muscle fibers increases circulation to muscles.

    b. Knead by using palmar pressure with thumb abducted; pick up tissue between thumb and fingers and release before pinching or twisting of skin (see Fig. 27-21).

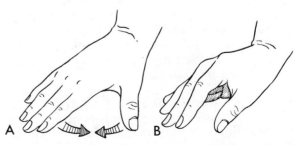

Figure 27-21. Kneading motion using palmar pressure during back massage.

Procedure continued on the following page

SUGGESTED STEPS	RATIONALE/DISCUSSION

SUGGESTED STEPS

c. Achieve force, rhythm and rate by shifting weight between right and left foot with feet perpendicular to patient's body.

d. Begin kneading motion with other hand before release of first hand, rhythmically alternating hands.

7. Use *friction* by exerting pressure in small circular motion *around* skin lesions and bony prominences. Exert gentle pressure with tips of second and third fingers.

8. Throughout massage, maintain contact with skin and rhythmically proceed from *stroking,* to *kneading,* to *friction.* Rapidity of rhythm varies with purpose of procedure, e.g., slow for sedative massage, fast for stimulating massage.

9. End massage with *long stroking movements.* Signal end of massage with light tap on patient's shoulder.

B. *Side-lying position (alternative method)*

1. Position patient on left side to massage right half of back. Turn patient to right side to massage left half of back.

2. If unable to turn patient, support uppermost side with one hand and massage lowermost side with other hand. Use forward-backward motion for all one-handed massage movements.

3. Flex at hips, with trunk rotated slightly toward patient, to accomplish stroking and kneading movements. Place feet in forward-backward stance, advancing forward foot gradually. Maintain comfortable position with good body alignment.

RATIONALE/DISCUSSION

c. Apply force in direction of movement; shift in body weight produces an efficient force; rhythmic massage is soothing.

d. Continuous contact with skin is soothing. Assess muscle tension, and repeat motion until relaxation is obtained.

7. Assess skin for indications of tissue injury. Assess color of skin and response to friction (duration of redness, response of blanched or red skin). Healthy tissue blanches upon pressure and returns to normal color following release of pressure. Inadequate circulation is characterized by white, bluish or reddened skin that responds sluggishly to pressure or does not change.

8. Sedative effect is achieved by slow massage movements and is enhanced by reduction of environmental stimuli, e.g., subdued lighting and reduction of sound, including conversation (unless patient needs to verbalize concerns). Stimulation effect is achieved by rapid massage movements, conversation and frequent change of position.

9. Long stroking is the most soothing massage movement. Nonverbal communication (e.g., tap) avoids conversation.

1. Turning patient exposes all skin surfaces and enables effective massage.

2. Permits best body mechanics for worker.

3. See steps *d* and *e* in A, 4. Increased pressure can be obtained by applying force to massaging hand; i.e., place one hand flat over the other.

SUGGESTED STEPS	RATIONALE/DISCUSSION
4. Proceed with massage, stroking, kneading and friction as outlined above. Avoid skin lesions.	4. Visualize area to avoid pressure over damaged tissue.

C. *Supine position (alternative method)*

SUGGESTED STEPS	RATIONALE/DISCUSSION
1. With patient lying in center of bed, massage one half of back at a time. To accomplish this, the worker moves from one side of the bed to the other.	1. Reduces strain on nurse's back. When possible move patient from one edge of bed to the other to minimize reaching.
2. Lower bed level to comfortable working height.	2. Helps worker maintain straight back while leaning forward, thus avoiding hyperextension of her back.
3. Fist of worker's near arm depresses mattress while other hand massages closer half of back area. Stroking and kneading massage movements are accomplished with the outside foot forward; force is supplied with forward-backward movements.	3. Stroking movement is not possible if patient cannot be positioned to clear the bed.
4. Bilateral massage of cervical areas, trapezius, and deltoid is accomplished with fingers of both hands stroking up and down cervical region. Lift and squeeze trapezius and deltoid muscles with thumb in front and fingers in back.	
5. Face patient in forward-backward stance and shift weight to obtain additional force.	5. Shift weight to obtain additional force.

POST-PROCEDURE ACTIVITIES

Wipe excess lubricant from back with bath towel; tie or replace gown; change patient's position if indicated for comfort; cover patient and remove bath blanket.

Aftercare of Equipment.   Place lubricant in bedside stand; fold bath blanket and bath towel or discard in laundry; store unnecessary pillows; put unit in order.

Final Patient Assessment.   Determine patient's general response to massage (e.g., relaxed, stimulated); assess condition of skin following massage (e.g., presence of blanched or reddened areas or lesions). *Chart/report* procedure, final assessment data, and individual patient-family teaching.

HAIR CARE

Novice nurses are often unfamiliar with methods of caring for hair of a different texture and style from their own; the opposite sex; or someone who is unable to do self-care. Therefore, the novice nurse may neglect hair care of the patient. If the nurse is truly concerned about the patient as a total person, then hair care is included as part of hygiene care. Not only does clean, well-groomed hair prevent skin irritation and infections, it also affects the patient's self-image. The appearance of the patient's hair can influence how others respond to him. For example, the patient with dirty, unkempt hair may be viewed as slovenly. This person normally may be meticulous about hygiene, but because of illness he may be unable to do self-care. The patient with unkempt, dirty hair usually reflects neglect of this aspect of care by the nursing staff. A knowledge of various hair care practices (e.g., care of the black person's hair) and methods of caring for patients who are unable to do self-care should encourage you to be sensitive to the need for including hair care as a routine part of hygiene care.

Anatomy and Physiology of Hair

Most of the body is covered by hair. As part of the integumentary system, hair serves as body insulation and acts as an organ receptor for the sense of touch. A specialized muscle (arrector muscle) contracts at times of stress and with changes in temperature. This muscle action causes the epidermis to be depressed so that hair stands on end (goose bumps). Most hair follicles are associated with sebaceous glands, and some sweat gland ducts open into hair follicles. The arrector muscle presses on sebaceous glands to aid in discharge of sebaceous gland secretion. For these reasons the scalp becomes moist and oily, particularly in a hot environment.

Hair Growth and Loss.   Hair grows in a cyclic pattern from clusters of epithelial cells at the base of the hair follicle. The cyclic pattern consists of growth, atrophy and rest phases. This partly accounts for varying rates of hair growth and loss. The scalp has about 100,000 hair follicles, and in general, about 50 hairs are lost per day.[10] Hair growth in some areas is affected by hormones or hereditary factors. Hormones influence hair growth on the trunk of the body as well as the nasal and facial areas. Hair growth at the scalp is not affected by hormones but stems from factors such as heredity and nutrition. Other areas not influenced by hormones include eyebrows and eyelashes. Hair on most other areas of the body is under several mechanisms of control. One may see hereditary baldness or changes in facial and body hair growth at puberty and after menopause. The presence of body hair generally decreases with the aging process.

ALOPECIA.   Alopecia is the loss of hair, often in round patches, resulting in a mosaic appearance. The etiology is not known. Sometimes trauma to hair in an area gives the same appearance. For example, a small child who constantly rubs his head on the sheet will develop bald patches.

EXCESSIVE HAIR LOSS.   Excessive hair loss may be seen at times of hormonal changes; stress; poor nutrition; and secondary to drug therapies, e.g., some drugs used in the treatment of cancer. Most often this condition improves when the underlying cause is corrected.

Purposes of Hair Care

The purposes of hair care are as follows: (a) promote hair growth; (b) prevent hair loss; (c) prevent infection; (d) maintain the condition of skin surrounding the hair; (e) promote circulation/nutrition to hair follicles; (f) remove dirt and old oils; (g) distribute oils along hair shaft; and (h) enhance the patient's appearance. To fulfill these purposes, hair care must involve shampooing to remove dirt, dead cells and old oils; brushing and combing to distribute oil along hair shaft, prevent accumulation of dirt and harboring organisms; avoiding trauma to the scalp and hair; shaving and styling hair.

Assessment and Nursing Judgment of Need for Hair Care

Assessment of the Hair and Scalp.   The condition of the hair and surrounding skin reflects general health. If a patient complains of itching or is seen scratching, ask him about the duration of the problem and examine the area for lice (pediculi), dryness, scaly patches, lesions or rashes, abrasion, and excoriation. Note whether hair is straight or extent of curliness. Also observe hair for distribution, length, cleanliness, thinness or thickness, texture (coarse, fine), gloss or dullness, color, matting and tangles. The condition of the scalp is easiest to examine while doing hair care.

Assessment of the Need for Assistance with Hair Care. Most patients are able to care for their own hair, but some will need encouragement for self-care. A patient who is depressed or disoriented may show little interest in hygiene. Likewise, patients with limited joint mobility, decreased muscle strength or poor coordination (e.g., a patient with arthritis or stroke) may neglect hair care because extra energy is required to perform self-care. Most bedridden patients require some assistance with hair care.

Some patients ask family members to provide hair care because the family is familiar with the patient's preferences. Self-care or having a family member provide hair care for the patient is therapeutic and should be encouraged. While self-care provides greater range of motion and fosters less dependency, hygiene care by a family member allows physical contact and provides a means for demonstrating care and concern.

Hair care involves cleansing, grooming and shaving. Some facilities have a beautician or barber available for assisting with other than basic hair care, e.g., cutting and shampoo. Regardless of the situation, it is the nurse's responsibility to ensure that hair care is provided for the patient.

Nursing Judgment of Need for Hair Care. The type of hair care required depends on the assessed condition of the hair and surrounding skin, need for cleansing and styling, patient's cultural practices and preferences, and self-care abilities. Each of these factors may be influenced by the length and texture of hair, length of hospitalization, imposed mobility (e.g., bed rest, arm cast) and the patient's overall state of health. Patients who are hospitalized for short periods usually require only basic hair care.

Basic Hair Care

Hair care should be provided at least daily. This may be done in conjunction with morning care so that the patient can feel refreshed and appear well groomed before starting daily activities. For the patient's psychologic and social well-being, it is important that he be well groomed prior to receiving visitors. Routine daily hair care consists of brushing and/or combing and styling hair.

Assisting the Patient with Hair Care. Assist the patient in collecting hair care items: comb, brush, towel and grooming aids. When possible, have the patient sit in a bedside chair. Whether the patient is totally capable of self-care or needs assistance, sitting is easier for care. To protect the patient's clothing from becoming soiled, place a towel over the patient's shoulders to catch loose hair and dirt. Fowler's position is best for most bedridden patients. When the patient is in bed, provide complete hair care before changing the pillow case or protect the bottom sheet and pillow case with a towel.

Brushing/Combing and Scalp Massage. Examine the brush and comb for cleanliness. Excess hair is easily removed from the brush by sliding the comb through the bristles. Remove excess dirt and oil by soaking the brush in ammonia or use *hot* water and soap. Patients should be encouraged to purchase blunt-toothed combs and brushes with firm (but not sharp) bristles. These prevent scratching of the scalp and unnecessary broken hairs. Patients who have coarse and curly hair need wide-toothed combs.

Brushing fosters better massage of scalp and distribution of oil along hair shaft than combing the hair. The worker's fingertips also can be used for scalp massage. If hair is *not* matted, tangled or crinkly, start at the scalp and comb/brush toward ends of hair. If the scalp is irritated or very sensitive to touch, be gentle to avoid trauma and discomfort.

GROOMING HAIR IN BED. First brush or comb the sides, and then have the patient turn his face away from the worker for doing the back portion. If unable to reach all areas, have the patient turn his face toward you for completing brushing/combing. Style the patient's hair in a manner that prevents excessive matting and tangling.

PROBLEMS WITH HAIR AND SCALP. If the patient has excessive flaking of the scalp, work the dry patches loose with your fingertips and brush toward ends of hair. Conditioners such as petroleum jelly or various oils sometimes help to decrease itching and flaking. If the hair appears clean but oiliness is causing skin irritation on the forehead at the scalp line, the forehead may be cleansed with alcohol or another drying agent.

Special Considerations

Hair texture and curliness as well as preferred styles vary among patients. Hair may be fine and soft, thick and coarse, straight or tightly curled. For naturally straight or permanently straightened hair, grooming, shampooing and styling is similar to that for straight hair. For the patient whose hair has been pressed or straightened with a hot comb, shampooing returns the hair to its natural curly state.

Very Curly Hair. When the patient has very curly, coarse hair, allow more time for hair care in order to effectively remove tangles. Ask the patient what equipment is needed and the style preferred. Usually a wide-toothed comb and a brush with firm bristles are needed. If a conditioner is needed and none is brought from home, petroleum jelly can be used to oil the hair.

Various methods can be used in caring for very curly hair. One suggested method is presented here. First *divide the hair into small sections,* and *brush before combing* to remove some tangles and tightness. (This is important for both males and females.) Each section of hair is then combed separately. *Comb* first at ends of hair to remove tangles, then from middle of hair shaft to the ends and finally by stroking from the scalp to ends of hair. If the hair appears dry, *oil* is applied at the scalp. Many black patients tend to have dry hair and require oil application during basic care and after shampooing. Shampooing removes old oil, which needs replacing to condition the hair and make it easy to manage (see Fig. 27–22).

Styling. When the natural, Afro, or brush style is desired, *picking* is done with a pick comb. The hair is lifted gently from scalp outward (see Fig. 27–23). The hair is then patted gently to achieve an overall smooth contour. To prevent matting and tangling, some female patients may desire to have their hair braided.

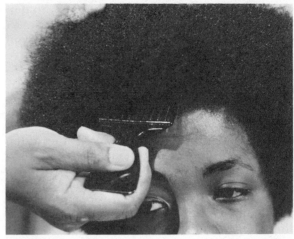

Figure 27–23. "Picking" used with Afro/brush styling. (Courtesy of George McNeal.)

Other females may request to have their hair set on regular rollers for later styling.

Wigs. If a wig is worn, the patient's natural hair needs daily basic care before the wig is put on. Wigs prevent exposure of scalp and hair to the air, altering the natural environment. If the wig is not removed periodically to allow the scalp and hair to "breathe," the patient can develop hair and scalp problems. Many patients use a wig because of difficulty styling hair while ill. When wearing a wig improves the patient's self-image, she should be encouraged to wear the wig. This is particularly true when illness or drug therapy has caused balding. Wigs can be helpful in preventing tangling for patients with long hair, and many black females prefer a wig for this reason. Wigs also need hair care. Ask the patient about the appropriate type of care. Never apply any solution to the wig without specific instructions from the patient. To prepare natural hair before donning the wig, brush the patient's natural hair toward top of the head. Some patients use bobby pins to hold natural hair in place. Caution patients not to place pins in areas where they can cause pressure, which can lead to scalp irritation and discomfort. Natural hair also can be braided before donning the wig. Most black patients' hair requires braiding to prevent tangles.

Special Problems

Excessively Tangled or Matted Hair. Patients who remain in bed frequently have a problem with excessively matted or tangled hair. This is particularly true for patients with long or curly hair. This problem usually can be prevented by thorough daily hair care. Water

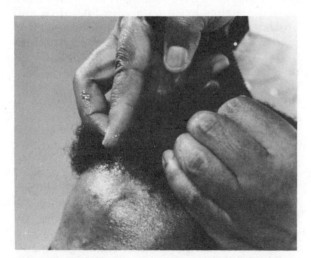

Figure 27–22. Applying oil to scalp hair. (Courtesy of George McNeal.)

with alcohol or vinegar can be applied to hair to help remove matting and tangles. Section the hair, and firmly hold the hair between index finger and thumb. Brush/comb in similar manner as with curly hair. Start at ends, with the worker's hand just above the snarled area, and gently remove snarls. Unless the patient is fully advised of the consequences, *never cut* hair to remove blood, matting or tangles. This should not be necessary if alcohol or vinegar is applied and the worker is persistent. This approach effectively removes matting and tangles without causing unnecessary discomfort from pulling on the hair.

Braiding hair may be indicated in order to prevent future problems with matting and tangles. Braiding also can be used to keep hair off the neck for those who perspire heavily (e.g., during fever). These patients frequently develop rashes, as a result of hair continually rubbing and irritating the moist skin. If the worker is unfamiliar with how to braid hair, check with other nursing personnel for directions. Poorly braided hair can easily tangle. Use two or more braids, as one braid at the back of the patient's head can cause pressure from the patient's head lying on the mattress. This can lead to scalp irritation at the site of the braid. Be careful not to get braids too tight, causing impaired circulation and discomfort. At least daily the braids are undone and basic hair care is provided before rebraiding hair.

Pediculosis. Pediculosis (infestation with lice) may be present on the head (pediculosis capitis), the body (pediculosis corporis), and the perineal area, eyebrows, eyelashes and beard (pediculosis pubis). This problem is associated with poor hygiene, crowded living conditions and exposure to other individuals with pediculosis. The lice live on the skin and attach their eggs (nits) to the hair. Lice bite the skin, subsequently causing itching and scratching. Lice are difficult to remove because the nits are attached to the hair by an adhesive substance.

For the patient with *pediculosis corporis*, complete bathing and clean clothing may be sufficient because these lice cling to clothing while feeding on the host. When the patient has *pediculosis capitis,* the hair and scalp are vigorously massaged with gamma benzene hexachloride. *Pediculosis pubis* may be more difficult to treat because the nits are difficult to remove from areas with heavy hair growth. Apply the medication to the involved area and leave it on the body 12 to 24 hours. Then bathe the person thoroughly with soap and water.

Whenever lice are discovered, remove and bag clothing and linen to prevent spreading the lice. Counsel the patient on the need for good personal hygiene and clean clothing. If crab lice *(Pediculus pubis)* are found, emphasize the need for treatment of sexual partners.

Shampoo

The method of shampooing hair depends on the patient's general condition and patient's preference. Safety is a primary consideration.

Shampooing with Bath/Shower. If the patient is ambulatory, shampooing may be done during the shower or tub bath. However, for some ambulatory patients this can be a safety hazard. The patient can become overly tired from the added time and energy required for shampooing hair, or he may fall while reaching for shampoo. Shampoo items need to be available within easy reach. When safety seems a question, have the ambulatory patient sit for shampooing hair.

Shampooing in Sitting Position. Most patients who are allowed to sit at the bedside can be shampooed in a sitting position. Three methods are possible: (1) shower chair; (2) sitting in chair at sink; (3) sitting in bedside chair with overbed table across the patient's lap for holding the wash basin. When using any of these methods, have shampoo items within easy reach, place a towel over the patient's shoulders and direct water away from face and shoulders. If the *shower chair* is used, have the patient seated and facing away from shower with head and neck hyperextended. If the patient is *assisted* with shampooing at a *sink*, have the patient sit facing away from the sink with his head hyperextended and resting comfortably on the sink. A towel can be placed over the edge of the sink for added comfort. When shampooing at the *bedside* have the patient lean forward with his head over the wash basin.

Shampooing on Stretcher. For the patient who is unable to sit but can be moved from bed, transfer the patient to a stretcher and transport him to a sink or shower equipped with a handheld shower nozzle. Lock stretcher brakes to keep stretcher from moving. Place a pillow under the patient's shoulders to allow hyperextension of the patient's head and neck. Use plastic over the end of the stretcher and have the patient's head extended slightly over the end of the stretcher to allow water to flow away from the patient.

Shampooing in Bed. Most patients can be shampooed using one of the previously mentioned methods, but shampooing can also be done effectively in bed. Unless contraindicated, move the patient's head and shoulders to the edge of the bed nearest you. Position the patient diagonally to the bed in good alignment and remove pillow.

A linen protection device is placed under the patient's head and neck and across the bed. Most facilities have a plastic tray with raised sides, which acts as a trough to drain off water. This device is frequently referred to as a "bed rinser." If this device is not available, an improvised trough can be made out of plastic or rubber and newspapers: roll the newspapers into a horseshoe shape, place the plastic or rubber flat on the bed, and position the rolled newspapers to form a rim on the trough. Roll edges of the plastic or rubber over the newspaper rim to facilitate drainage of water (see Fig. 27–24). Either device is positioned with the open flat end toward the side of the bed to allow water to drain over the side of the bed and into a receptacle. The patient's wash basin can be placed on the overbed table or bedside chair close to the side of the bed. The height of the receptacle should allow water to drain down without splattering.

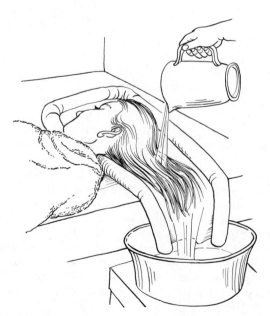

Figure 27–24. Improvised trough for shampooing in bed.

Shampooing in bed usually is not done immediately after bathing, since many patients who require this method will need a rest period before being involved in another procedure. If the bed linen is to be changed, this is done after completing the shampoo and grooming the hair.

Shampoo Equipment and Supplies. Regardless of the method used for the shampoo procedure, have the following items available: two bath towels; washcloth or face towel for protecting eyes from splattering soap; shampoo; hair conditioner, if necessary, comb and brush; and hair dryer, if available. Some patients will bring shampoo from home. If the patient does not have the shampoo in the bedside stand, most facilities have small packets (for one-time use) of a mild liquid soap. Septi Soft solution also can be used to cleanse and condition the hair.

If the patient is receiving a shampoo in *bed* or on a *stretcher*, provide some type of waterproof linen protector. To shampoo a patient in *bed* or a *bedside chair*, the worker needs one or two water pitchers and a water receptacle. For shampooing at the *sink*, a cup or pitcher usually is needed for pouring water, as water from the faucet may only reach a small portion of the hair.

General Procedure for Shampooing. After positioning the patient, providing water-proof covering, and assembling all needed items, you are ready to shampoo the patient. Water is applied to hair until it is thoroughly wet. Maintain water temperature at 43 to 44°C. (109.4 to 111.2°F.). Although warmer water may be desired by the patient, remember that the scalp is easily burned. Once the hair is wet, apply a small amount of shampoo and work up a lather.

Start cleansing at the hair line, working toward the back of the head. While cleansing the hair, vigorously massage all portions of the scalp by applying pressure with your fingertips. Long nails make it difficult to massage without scratching the patient's scalp. Add water as needed to keep a generous lather of soap. *Rinse thoroughly* to remove all residue from the scalp. Repeat washing and rinsing until hair squeaks when it is stroked between your fingers. Squeeze excess water from the hair; then wrap a bath towel around the patient's head, and use the cloth that was protecting the patient's eyes to dry his face. Briskly rub hair and scalp with the bath towel. Once the towel is saturated with water, remove it; use a second towel or hair dryer to *thoroughly dry* scalp and hair. Check the hair dryer for electrical hazards and use caution not to burn the patient.

Although a dry shampoo can occasionally be provided by using a powder preparation, some of these preparations are irritating to the scalp and do not clean the hair adequately.

After completing the shampoo, apply hair conditioner as appropriate, groom, and style the patient's hair. Check that the patient's clothing is dry.

Care of Mustache and Beard

Mustaches and beards vary in length, texture and curliness, as does other hair on the head. Keeping these areas clean and dry is important. Since food can easily collect on the hair growth, offer the patient an opportunity to wash the area after eating. Ask the patient how he usually cares for his mustache or beard. Combing is usually required at least daily. A mustache also requires periodic trimming. Both mustache and beard will need shampooing. Use a mild, non-drying shampoo, as the skin tends to become dry and flaky. Dry the area thoroughly after the shampoo.

Shaving

Shaving is most frequently done for removal of male facial hair. Many women, because of cultural practices, will request shaving of armpits (axillae) and legs. Prior to some types of surgery, the operative site is shaved. This prevents hair from contaminating an open wound. For patients with heavy long hair growth on arms, the area may be shaved prior to starting an IV infusion. The site is shaved to prevent the discomfort of pulling hair when tape is removed at completion of the infusion.

When shaving any area of the body, use *caution not to cut the skin*. This is especially important for patients who are *prone to bleed*, e.g., patients on Coumadin, heparin or high doses of aspirin. An electric razor is safer for such patients. Check electric razors for frayed cords and other electrical hazards.

When using a *razor blade*, soften the skin before shaving. Shaving the *axillae* and *legs* is best done immediately following the bath, while the skin is soft. Apply lathered soap or shaving cream for easy removal of hair. For removing *male facial hair*, soak the patient's face with a warm-hot washcloth (be careful not to burn the face). Allow the cloth to remain on the patient's face until the beard is soft. Then apply thick lathered soap or shaving cream. To shave the area, pull the skin taut and use short, firm but gentle strokes in the direction in which the hair grows. This approach decreases skin irritation and prevents ingrown hairs.

ADDITIONAL GROOMING MEASURES

For most people, grooming has social ramifications, i.e., "looking good" to others. Grooming aids, such as cosmetics, have psychologic effects on one's self-image, but their physical effects are seldom considered. Their use is based on personal preference and sociocultural practices.

In some cultures no deodorants are used. Americans seldom go without a daily application of a *deodorant* to prevent them from "smelling bad." Some antiperspirants/deodorants completely eliminate sweat and odor, yet in warm climates some degree of perspiring is physiologically beneficial. Many deodorants contain chemicals that are irritating to skin. Feminine hygiene sprays used to decrease perineal odor can be *very* irritating to skin and mucosa. In some situations bacteriostatic deodorant soaps eliminate odor at the expense of removing natural flora that protects the skin against fungal overgrowth.

Various *eye* and *facial* makeups may have a drying effect and may cause skin irritation. *Nail polish* and *nail polish removers* tend to dry nails, causing splitting and breaking. Both *hair sprays* and *permanents*, when frequently used, tend to make hair dry and brittle or can irritate the scalp. Depilatory creams that are used to remove hair from underarms, legs and face can also be irritating to skin. Various agents are purported to stimulate hair growth. Contrary to advertising claims, these preparations are not effective. Most balding is hereditary or is due to some underlying physiologic imbalance.

Patient Teaching. Patients should be encouraged to consider the social implications and physical effects of using various grooming aids. However, the nurse must remember that a tactful approach is imperative in attempting to encourage or discourage the use of grooming aids.

COMFORT AND CLEANLINESS IN BED

For the patient who spends many hours in bed, a clean and comfortable bed is an important aspect of care and can have a beneficial psychologic and physical influence on a patient. Frequent tightening or smoothing of the wrinkled bottom sheet adds greatly to a patient's comfort. For the ambulatory patient, returning to bed after undergoing various tests can be refreshing. The patient confined to bed may be hesitant to complain or may be unable to communicate to inform the nurse of discomfort caused by wrinkled sheets. Wrinkled sheets and moist linen can cause skin irritation and can contribute to the formation of decubitus ulcers. Replacing wet linen and loosening top linen over the patient's feet can help to eliminate frustration and discomfort for the patient.

The nurse must be able to assess the patient's need for linen change, be familiar with types of bed linens and beds, and utilize bedmaking procedures that promote the maximum comfort for patients. Bedmaking requires an understanding of asepsis, an appreciation for the patient's need for self-help, an awareness of safety, application of body mechanics, and effective work organization and use of energy. The basic procedure included in this section employs all of the above factors and principles for the comfort and safety of the patient and nurse.

Bed Linens

Need for Linen Change. For many years all bed linens were routinely changed daily. Currently, most health care facilities have decreased the frequency of complete linen change and provide only partial linen change daily or less often in some cases. Partial linen change may refer to replacing only soiled linen, or it may mean reusing top linen and replacing bottom linen and pillow case. Linen change based on assessed need is more economical. In 1975, Rizzo reported that in a 300-bed hospital operating at 90 per cent capacity, the difference between using one sheet versus two sheets per patient per day approximates $30,000 per year.[14] Laundry expenses should stem from need, not ritual. Monies saved by reducing unnecessary laundering can be applied to other areas of care.

Linen may be changed in conjunction with morning hygiene care and at other times of the day, as linen becomes soiled or damp. In addition to changing, linen often requires tightening to keep it wrinkle-free. For the restless patient, linen may need tightening several times a day. Straightening linen at bedtime is one means of promoting a comfortable night's sleep.

FULL SHEETS. Regular full-length flat sheets or contour sheets can be used as a bottom sheet. Sometimes full-length flat bed sheets are confused with stretcher sheets, which have the same appearance but are slightly shorter and more narrow. Some health care facilities have contour bed sheets available. While the bed is easier made with a contour sheet and it usually remains wrinkle-free, contour sheets tend to tear on the ends and sometimes are more expensive. If flat full-length sheets are used, the top sheet, which usually has fewer wrinkles, is rotated to the bottom and a clean sheet placed on top.

DRAW SHEET. In addition to regular sheets, the hospital bed may have a draw sheet made of rubber, plastic or linen. A draw sheet is about half the size of a regular sheet and is placed across the middle section of the bed. In the past, rubber or plastic draw sheets were used to protect the mattress and/or the bottom sheet from becoming wet; those sheets were always covered with a linen draw sheet to protect the patient's skin and to absorb moisture. Most health care facilities no longer use rubber or plastic draw sheets because mattresses are plasticized and several types of disposable linen protectors are available to serve the same purpose.

Today, the linen draw sheet is used primarily for lifting ("pull sheet"). When the draw sheet is used for this purpose, it may be left folded smoothly under the patient rather than being tucked over and under the sides of the bed. However, when left folded on the bed, the draw sheet frequently becomes wrinkled. Application of a linen draw sheet is included in Procedure 9 for situations in which it may be needed, but it is *not* "routinely" placed on the bed. A linen draw sheet should not be used unless it serves a specific purpose, such as lifting or individualizing care for patient comfort. Occasionally a patient will request a linen draw sheet because he has a problem with excessive perspiration from the plasticized mattress. A pad covering the length of the mattress can also be used for this purpose.

MATTRESS PADS. Mattress pads are usually made of thick, soft cotton and have bound edges. The pad, with or without contour corners, is placed lengthwise on the bed between the mattress and sheet. This decreases movement of the sheet, reduces heat generated between the plasticized mattress and the patient's body, and absorbs moisture, all of which aid in the patient's comfort. For accomplishing these same purposes, a bath blanket can be used in place of the mattress pad. Mattress pads are changed only when excessively wrinkled, damp or soiled.

BLANKETS. Several types of bed blankets may be available, including a *bath blanket,* which is made of soft, thin cotton. The bath blanket is used as a water-absorbent linen, often during bed bath. This type of blanket also may be used for added warmth. It is lightweight, smooth against the patient's skin and comforting. A *bed* blanket of a wool, cotton or synthetic material may be used as top linen covering for warmth. *Thermal* bed blankets are used in many facilities. These are made of a porous, synthetic material and have the advantage of being relatively lightweight yet warm. The bed blanket is usually *not* changed during a patient's length of stay unless it becomes soiled or wet.

BEDSPREADS. Bedspreads usually are made of lightweight cotton or synthetic material. This is removed and folded neatly over the back of the bedside chair during linen changes. The bedspread is changed only when it becomes soiled, wet or excessively wrinkled.

PILLOW CASE. The standard pillow case is one of the most frequently changed bed linens. For the bedridden patient, the pillow case becomes soiled from oily hair and wrinkled from movements. One means of decreasing the need for a clean pillow case is to turn the pillow over and tighten the case around the pillow with a tuck. A clean, smooth pillow case can be very refreshing for the patient.

PROBLEMS. The following problems can occur with bed linens.

▶ Skin irritation from dyes and bleaches used in laundering linens

▶ Abraded skin from rubbing heels on seam edges of linen

▶ Decubitus ulcers from lying on wrinkled sheets

▶ Patient's extremities can become entangled in linens during bedmaking procedure

▶ Tears in linen, which can be a source of skin irritation and patient discomfort

Types of Beds and Side Rails

There are three types of standard hospital beds: manual, hydraulic and electric. Each type has its advantages and disadvantages. *Manually* operated beds require the most energy from the worker but usually are the most economical. This type of bed poses few safety hazards unless workers neglect to retract hand cranks at the foot of the bed.

> *Hand cranks should always be in the retracted position when not in use. This prevents injury to people walking by the foot of the bed.*

Hydraulic beds are relatively lightweight for easy movement of the bed. Some hydraulic beds are free of metallic structures; this allows taking x-rays with the patient lying in bed. Many hydraulic beds have a special nylon coating to decrease exposed conductive surfaces. This makes the hydraulic bed safe to use with various types of electrical equipment. The hydraulic bed is more expensive than the manually operated bed and may require an outlet for compressed air.

Electric beds require the least amount of energy for the worker to operate. Because most electric beds have control panels that the patient can operate, patients can be more independent in this type of bed. A primary safety hazard of electric beds is the possibility of plugs or wiring becoming frayed. These beds also can leak electric current and thus may act as conductors of electricity. This can be a hazard, especially if the other electrical equipment is used near the patient.

Side Rails. While side rails do not come as part of the bed, they are applied to most beds. Side rails are raised and lowered by levers or buttons or by sliding the rail. They are used primarily to prevent a patient from falling out of bed and may be used by the patient as an aid in turning. Side rails are available for partial or full length of the bed. Short side rails do not provide as much protection from falls but can be used by the patient in reaching a sitting position or getting out of bed. Some patients object to side rails because they feel "penned in." If the nurse appreciates the value of side rails for safety and provides an explanation that conveys her concern for the patient, most patients will accept side rails.

Side rails are kept up for patients who are disoriented or heavily sedated and when the bed is elevated from the floor and unattended. They are frequently used when the patient is sleeping. Even if the patient was alert before going to sleep, he can become disoriented in a strange environment and fall from the bed.

Bed Positions

Before attempting to change the position of the bed, (a) know how to correctly operate the bed; (b) assess the patient's condition in the present position; (c) determine if the patient has any motility limitations, e.g., check the patient's chart or nursing care plan for diagnosis, activity orders; and (d) know the purposes and contraindications for various positions. Although a patient may request repositioning, which he believes may increase comfort, the desired position actually may be detrimental; e.g., some orthopedic conditions are made worse if the patient does not remain flat. As you approach a patient's bedside, notice if he appears to be in distress; e.g., if a patient has difficulty in breathing and is lying flat, do not wait for him to request a change in position. Use nursing judgment as to whether the patient needs a position change. In most situations, a frequent change in position is therapeutic: it increases comfort, promotes good circulation and prevents skin breakdown.

To facilitate position change, many standard hospital beds are designed so that the entire foot section can be raised or the head section can be lowered below the flat position. Also, most beds have a metal bar attached at the foot of the bed. When the metal bar is retracted, it lies flush with the bedsprings. The metal bar should be pulled upright (perpendicular to bedsprings) to keep the mattress from sliding off the foot end of the bedsprings. This helps to prevent the patient's feet from becoming cramped against the end of the bed.

Several bed positions are possible, but only three of the most common positions will be discussed here:

Contour Position. The patient is positioned with head, knees and feet slightly elevated. This is used for general comfort.

Fowler's Position (see Fig. 27–25). The head of the bed is elevated 30 to 90 degrees, and the knees may or may not be flexed. Depending on the degree of head elevation, the position is referred to as "low," "semi" or "high" Fowler's position. Fowler's position reduces the work of the heart and promotes

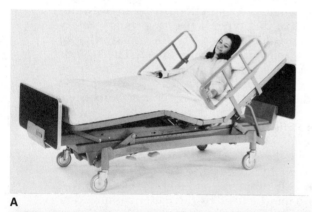

A

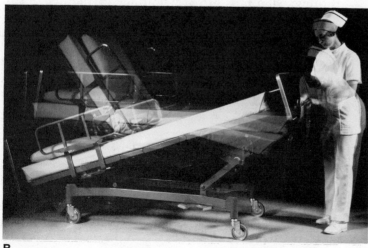

B

Figure 27–25. Electric bed positions. *A*, Fowler's position. *B*, Bed being changed from a head up position to a head down–foot up (Trendelenburg) position. (From Hill-Rom Company, Inc., Batesville, IN.)

better lung expansion, thereby allowing the patient to breathe easier. High Fowler's position is used primarily for patients with orthopnea (difficulty in breathing while lying flat) and dyspnea (difficulty in breathing). If elevation is not needed for improving heart and lung function, high Fowler's position is discouraged because of the shearing force (kinking of vessels between superficial and deep tissues). When using Fowler's position, be sure the metal bar at the foot is upright. In addition, a slight knee gatch is helpful for keeping the patient from sliding toward the foot of the bed. The term "gatch" is often used to indicate flexing the knees by bending the middle part of the lower section of the bed upward.

> Use of high "knee gatch" is discouraged because it produces pressure behind the knees (popliteal area), which can impair circulation, resulting in formation of dangerous blood clots.

Trendelenburg Position (see Fig. 27–25). The foot of the bed is elevated and the head is lowered. This position (a) facilitates return of blood from lower extremities to the heart and (b) helps move lung secretions upward from the bases of lungs, facilitating removal of lung secretions by coughing or suctioning.

Special Types of Beds

The special types of beds discussed here are used as aids for patients with severe restrictions of mobility.

> Before attempting to operate any special type of bed, read the manufacturer's directions and/or the institution's procedure manual and obtain assistance from other nursing personnel.

CircOlectric Bed (see Fig. 27–26). This type of bed is maneuvered in a circular manner by electrical controls. The CircOlectric bed permits (a) easy turning of the patient from supine to prone position; (b) tilting the patient to an upright position; and (c) easy access for taking care of a patient's elimination needs when moving is contraindicated.

Making the CircOlectric bed: The bottom section, which is used when the patient is supine, has an opening in the center. This allows use of the bedpan. Special sheets that are available have a hole in the middle and have elastic bands that fasten to the corners of the mattress. If this type of sheet is not available, two draw sheets can be used. One draw sheet is secured over the head section, and the other is placed over the foot section. The solid part of the bed is used when the patient is prone. A regular sheet is secured in a manner similar to making the base (bottom) of a regular bed. Top linen to cover the patient, whether supine or prone, is placed and secured in the usual manner.

Stryker or Foster Frame (see Fig. 27–26). These two beds are similar in that they both allow the patient's position to be changed

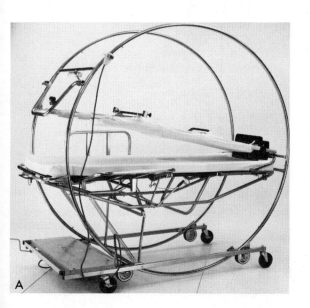

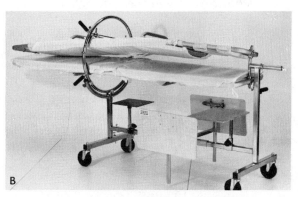

Figure 27–26. Special types of beds. *A,* CircOlectric bed. *B,* Stryker's wedge turning frame. (From Stryker Corporation, Kalamazoo, MI.)

from supine to prone when rolling or lifting maneuvers are contraindicated (e.g., in cases of spinal injury). The frame is narrow and is manually operated on a pivoting device at the head and foot of the bed, where it is held in place by large "pins." The frame is in two sections: anterior and posterior. The posterior frame has an opening in the canvas similar to the CircOlectric bed.

Making the Stryker or Foster frame bed: To make the base of the bed, use the method discussed for the CircOlectric bed. Since the frame is narrow, stretcher sheets fit better than regular full sheets. The linen is secured over the end of the canvas and around the pivoting device as neatly as feasible.

Bedmaking

An effective technique is easy to achieve, and with practice bedmaking can be completed within 5 to 15 minutes. Whenever possible, the patient is encouraged to get out of bed while the nurse changes the bed linens. Some patients must remain in bed because they are weak or have mobility restrictions. For these patients the nurse changes the linens while the patient remains in bed (see Procedure 9).

The nurse should understand the following concepts, principles and activities, which are associated with bedmaking.

Asepsis. Prevent spread of microorganisms by handwashing prior to collecting linen; keeping linen away from your uniform; not touching your hair; minimal shaking of linen; and keeping linen off the floor.

Body mechanics. Prevent tiredness and back problems by facing in the direction of movement; having your center of gravity close to your base of support; using arm and leg muscles as a force with wide base of support; keeping back straight and knees flexed; and having bed at easy work height. Novice nurses have the most difficulty with body mechanics and work organization. Use of poor body mechanics can contribute to chronic back problems. Back problems are common in the general population and frequently a cause of disability for health care workers.

Work organization. Use the least expenditure of time and energy by assessing supplies available in patient's unit; collecting linen in reverse order of use; moving furniture (e.g., bedside stand and overbed table) away from bed; having bedside chair and laundry hamper within easy reach; working at a normal rate of speed; employing a systematic method and rhythmic movements throughout bedmaking.

Individuality. Provide privacy and comfort for the patient by assessing need for linen change and keeping the patient covered.

Safety. Prevent falls and injuries by appropriate use of side rails; keeping call signal within reach of patient; retracting bed cranks on manual bed; and checking beds for malfunction.

9. MAKING OCCUPIED BED

Definition and Purpose.   *This method enables the nurse to change linen while the patient remains in bed.* The purpose is to provide a comfortable and clean bed.

Contraindications and Cautions.   Whenever a patient's condition permits, he should be encouraged to get out of bed for linen change. Keep side rail up on side away from worker to aid in turning and prevent patient from falling. Assess all patients for limitations in movement. Use special caution when turning patients who have burns, peripheral vascular disorders or orthopedic problems. Frequently, for patients in traction, weights must be maintained continuously. Sterile sheets are necessary for some burn patients. Avoid shaking linen to decrease spread of organisms. Report malfunctioning beds.

Patient-Family Teaching Points.   Provide patient and family with the following information: (a) amount of patient participation that is therapeutic; (b) if patient is confined to bed to conserve energy, explain how energy conservation is related to patient's condition; (c) upon discharge, if patient is to be confined to bed at home, explain how procedure can conserve time and energy and promote safety; provide information about renting hospital beds.

PRE-PROCEDURE ACTIVITIES

PRELIMINARY ASSESSMENT/PLANNING

- ▶ check linen available in patient unit
- ▶ assess items of clean linen needed
- ▶ assess additional special need items, e.g., whether patient prefers extra blanket for warmth, need for linen protectors under drainage sites
- ▶ check activity order and specific precautions in movement or positioning
- ▶ assess patient's physical capability for assisting
- ▶ assess patient's ability to comprehend directions
- ▶ wash hands prior to collecting linen
- ▶ wipe bedside chair before placing linen on it
- ▶ place laundry bag over back of bedside chair or on linen hamper

PREPARATION OF PATIENT AND UNIT

- ▶ explain how patient can assist
- ▶ explain sequence of procedure
- ▶ move furniture (e.g., bedside stand) away from bed
- ▶ move bed away from wall
- ▶ remove call signal if attached to bed linens
- ▶ raise side rails
- ▶ adjust bed to comfortable working height
- ▶ position patient supine or as flat as possible
- ▶ place linen and laundry bag within easy reach
- ▶ pull curtain for privacy

EQUIPMENT

For complete linen change (collect linen in reverse order of use):
- ▶ pillow case (place over your arm first)
- ▶ bedspread
- ▶ blanket
- ▶ top sheet
- ▶ draw sheet
- ▶ bottom sheet
- ▶ mattress pad
- ▶ bath blanket
- ▶ laundry bag
- ▶ dust cloth (last item on top of pile)
- ▶ linen hamper
- ▶ bedside chair for placing linen in order of use

PROCEDURE

SUGGESTED STEPS	RATIONALE/DISCUSSION
A. Remove *top* linen.	
1. Loosen linen at foot on both sides.	1. Allows easy removal of linen and prevents tearing.
2. Lower side rail on side of worker.	
3. Remove spread and blanket separately.	3. Method of folding facilitates replacement and prevents wrinkles.

Procedure continued on the following page

SUGGESTED STEPS	RATIONALE/DISCUSSION
a. Fold top edge to bottom.	
b. Fold far side to near side.	
c. Fold again top to bottom.	
d. Place linen over back of chair.	
4. Leave top sheet over patient or remove and cover patient with bath blanket.	4. Provides warmth and privacy (see Procedure 7, A).
B. Move *mattress* to head of bed.	B. Mattress slides toward foot when head is raised, making it difficult to tuck linen and uncomfortable for patient.
1. Stand at side, facing head of bed, and grasp mattress at handles or each end.	
2. With outside leg forward, shift weight and bend knees.	2. Use leg muscles as force. To encourage self-help, have patient grasp head of bed and instruct when to pull. This also saves your energy.
3. Pull metal bar at foot of springs to perpendicular position.	3. Decreases mattress sliding.
C. *Position* patient on his side on far side of bed, facing away from worker. Reposition pillow under head.	C. Provides space to place clean linen. Have patient use side rail for turning. Assess for comfort, ease of breathing and alignment.
D. Prepare *base* (bottom linen) of bed.	*For maximum work efficiency, complete one side of bed before beginning other side.*
1. Loosen bottom linens, moving from head to foot of bed.	
2. Fan-fold bottom linens as close to patient as possible. First fan-fold draw sheet, then bottom sheet.	2. Provides maximum work area and greater comfort when patient later rolls back over linens.
3. If mattress pad is changed, fan-fold to middle of bed.	3. Change only if soiled or heavily wrinkled.
E. Make *base* on one side of bed.	
1. Smooth wrinkles from reused mattress pad or place clean mattress pad with center fold at middle of bed and fan-fold top layer to patient.	
2. Place clean *bottom* sheet even with end	2. For maximum efficiency work from foot

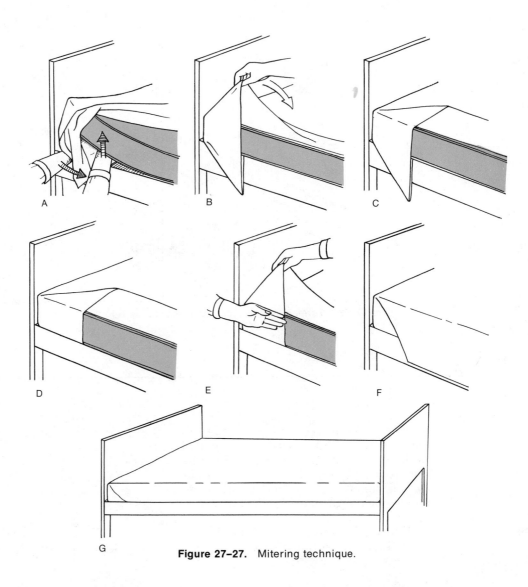

Figure 27–27. Mitering technique.

SUGGESTED STEPS	RATIONALE/DISCUSSION
of mattress with center fold in middle of bed. Open sheet lengthwise, moving from foot to head of bed. Fan-fold top layer to middle of bed, moving from head to foot of bed.	to head and back to foot. Place sheet with hem smooth side up.
3. Miter *bottom sheet* at head of bed (see Fig. 27–27).	3. *Mitering* is used to hold linen firmly in place by folding at equal angles to allow linen to fit corners.
a. Face head of bed diagonally. Place near arm under mattress corner and lift. Use other arm to pull excess sheet over and under head of mattress (Fig. 27–27A).	

Procedure continued on the following page

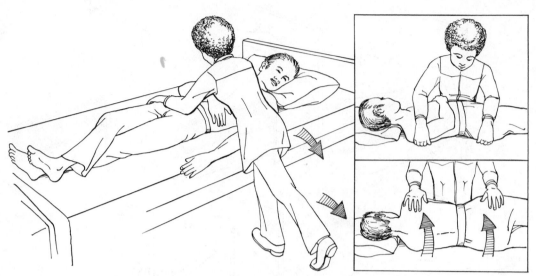

Figure 27–28. Turning incapacitated patient onto his side.

SUGGESTED STEPS	RATIONALE/DISCUSSION
b. Face side of bed. Lift side edge of sheet so that it forms a triangle to head of bed with side edge hanging perpendicular to bed (Fig. 27–27B). Lay upper part of sheet back on bed by creasing along top edge of mattress (Fig. 27–27C).	b. Holds linen firmly in place.
c. Continue facing side of bed; tuck lower hanging portion of sheet smoothly under mattress (Fig. 27–27D).	c. Work with palms down to protect knuckles from bedsprings.
d. Place back side of one hand (with thumb down on palm) firmly against sheet to hold sheet against mattress. With other hand pick up corner of sheet lying on bed and bring it down over the hand holding sheet against mattress edge (Fig. 27–27E and F).	d. Position elbow toward head of bed to allow easy removal of worker's arm while maintaining position of linen.
4. Face side of bed; tuck side edge of sheet under mattress (Fig. 27–27C).	4. While tucking linen under mattress use both hands with palms down. Move smoothly from miter at head to foot of bed.
5. Place *draw sheet*.	
a. Identify center fold. Stand away from bed and open draw sheet so that it folds in half.	

SUGGESTED STEPS	RATIONALE/DISCUSSION
b. Walk to bed and lay center fold of draw sheet along middle of bed.	b. While placing draw sheet, face side of bed, keep arms widely separated to grasp top and bottom edges of draw sheet at center fold and lean across bed, bending at waist with knees flexed and back straight.
c. Position draw sheet so that it lays under patient's torso (shoulders to knees).	c. This placement permits its use as a lifting sheet under heaviest part of body.
d. Fan-fold top layer toward patient.	d. For asepsis, place cleanest part of soiled linen next to new linen.
e. Tuck excess draw sheet smoothly under side of mattress. Work from center to edges.	e. Use both hands while facing side of bed.
F. Help patient roll back onto his side, facing worker (see Fig. 27–28).	F. Lift bath blanket and sheet to keep patient from becoming encased in top linen.
1. After patient is in side-lying position, lean patient toward worker and reach over to push fan-folded linen away from patient. Reposition pillow.	1. If fan-folded linens have been placed to middle of bed, patient will have smooth surface on which to lie. Pushing linens away from patient and moving pillow provide maximum patient comfort.
2. Raise side rail.	2. Promotes safety and security.
G. Move *chair* with remaining clean linen to other side of bed within reach.	
H. Make *other* side of base.	
1. Lower side rail.	
2. Loosen base linens.	
3. Roll soiled draw sheet into bundle and place at foot of bed.	3. Look for objects (e.g., eyeglasses) that might be in linen. Leave draw sheet at foot of bed until removing bottom sheet. This saves time and energy.
4. Remove bottom sheet by rolling into bundle from head to foot. Place draw sheet and bottom sheet in laundry bag together.	4. Draw sheet and bottom sheet are rolled separately so that it is easier to find objects accidentally left in linens. Rolling linen into bundles decreases spread of organisms.
5. Move fan-folded linen to edge of mattress. Inform patient that he may roll back into supine position. Reposition pillow as needed.	5. Position patient supine now or just before placing top linens.

Procedure continued on the following page

SUGGESTED STEPS	RATIONALE/DISCUSSION
6. Miter second side of *bottom sheet*.	
a. Lift mattress as on other side and pull sheet under mattress and toward worker.	a. Maintain tension on linen for maximum tightness.
b. Follow mitering steps in E, 3b–3d.	
c. Gather excess linen in hands with knuckles up.	
d. Facing side of bed, lean back and pull down to tuck excess linen under mattress.	
7. To tighten bottom sheet, grasp sheet edge with knuckles up and gather to top ridge of mattress. Lean back, pull sheet over side and tuck. Work from miter to foot, tucking excess linen as you go.	7. To keep sheet free of wrinkles, do not allow slack in linen.

> Remember: *Bottom sheet is mitered only at head of bed.*

SUGGESTED STEPS	RATIONALE/DISCUSSION
8. Tighten *draw sheet*.	
a. Smooth draw sheet with palms.	
b. Gather excess linen in hands with knuckles up. Tighten and tuck middle then top and bottom of draw sheet.	b. When tightening middle, face side of bed and lean back. Face foot of bed diagonally, lean back and tighten shoulder edge of draw sheet. Face head of bed diagonally for tightening knee edge of draw sheet.
I. *Top* linen.	
1. Place top *sheet* with center fold in middle of bed. Open sheet head to foot. Then unfold sheet across patient.	1. Leave enough linen to make a cuff at patient's shoulder height.
2. Ask patient to hold clean top sheet or tuck around patient's shoulders.	2. Prevents patient exposure. Encourages patient assistance.
3. Stand at foot of bed to remove soiled linen. Grasp soiled sheet and bath blanket under clean top sheet. Roll soiled linen into bundle toward worker.	
4. Place folded *bed blanket* on patient at midchest. Open blanket across patient, then from head to foot.	4. Allow foot end of linens to hang freely over foot of bed.
5. Place *spread* as done with blanket. Cuff spread under blanket; then bring top sheet over spread as second cuff.	5. Leave enough spread to cuff under blanket at patient's shoulder height.

SUGGESTED STEPS	RATIONALE/DISCUSSION
6. Face diagonally to opposite corner of foot of bed; lift mattress corner with near arm and use other arm to pull all three layers of linen under mattress.	6. For ease of lifting, have patient flex knees to decrease weight on mattress. All three layers of linen are tucked at once for work organization (sheet, blanket, spread).
7. Ask patient to flex ankles and point toes up (dorsiflex) before tightening top linen.	7. Provides room for free movement of feet. Tight top linens can lead to foot drop.
8. Miter all three layers of linen at once. Miter while facing diagonally toward foot of bed.	8. Follow steps for mitering only through step E, 3. This allows top linens to hang neatly over side of bed.
9. Raise side rail.	

10. Move to *other side* of bed and lower side rail. Repeat steps 6 through 8 for this side of top linen. Complete cuff on this side as in step 5.

J. Change *pillow case.*

1. Remove soiled linen case and place in laundry bag.

2. Grasp closed end of clean pillow case at center with one hand (see Fig. 27–29A). Next, maintaining grasp, use other hand to grasp open end of case (Fig. 27–29B). Invert case over hand and forearm (at closed end) by pulling open end of case back over hand at closed end. Maintain grasp at closed end.

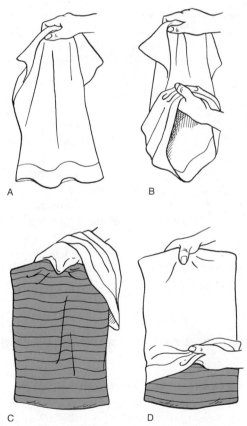

Figure 27–29. Applying pillow case.

3. Grasp end of pillow with hand holding case (Fig. 27–29C). While maintaining this grasp, use other hand to pull case down over pillow (Fig. 27–29D).	3. If a zippered plastic covering is over pillow, grasp zippered end of pillow.

4. Support patient's head, lift and place pillow under head with closed end toward door (see Fig. 27–30).

Procedure continued on the following page

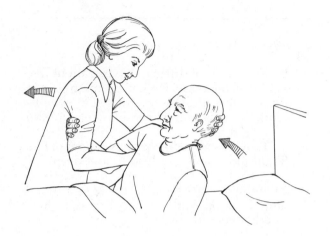

Figure 27–30. Providing support to patient's head while raising him from sitting position.

POST-PROCEDURE ACTIVITIES

For safety, replace call signal; raise side rails as appropriate; lower bed to floor level. If *manual* bed, put hand cranks in; if *electric* bed, be sure plug is flush with wall socket and cord is free of tension.

Care of Equipment.   Replace bedside stand and overbed table within easy reach of patient; take laundry bag containing soiled linen to dirty utility room or linen chute. Do *not* return unused clean linen to linen cart, as it is now considered contaminated. Check institutional policy concerning use or disposal of this linen.

Final Patient Assessment.   Check patient for correct body alignment. Leave patient in position that provides comfort, maximum ease of breathing and good circulation. Evaluate patient's mental and emotional status before deciding to leave side rails down. Place linen protector under drainage sites.

Final Assessment of Condition of Bed Linens.   Is bottom linen taut and wrinkle free? Are top linens off the floor? Can patient move his toes freely under top linen?

Assessment during Bedmaking

Bedmaking, like other aspects of hygiene care, affords the nurse opportunities to assess the patient. During bedmaking, remember to note the following:

▶ Respiratory and/or motor difficulty with movement

▶ Irritated areas of exposed skin, which may be secondary to sheet burns from rubbing on linens

▶ Self-help abilities and limitations

▶ Patient requests for additional covering (may indicate circulatory insufficiency or a need for alteration of room temperature)

Before learning techniques for bedmaking, become familiar with the operation of various beds and additional bed equipment and how to safely position patients as well as when patient movement is contraindicated.

> *When making modifications in the bedmaking procedure, always consider the rationale for the variations. Instead of following a set ritualistic procedure, the adaptive nurse individualizes bedmaking according to patient's preferences and needs and the policies of the institution.*

Unoccupied Bed. When changing linen without a patient in the bed, follow the principles and basic procedures used in making an occupied bed. The differences between the two bedmaking procedures are presented in Table 27–2.

Additional Bed Equipment. Additional equipment may be placed on a bed, as indicated by the patient's condition, to prevent skin problems, promote comfort, facilitate circulation and/or maintain good body alignment.

BED BOARDS. A bed board is placed between the mattress and the bedsprings to provide an extra firm surface for general comfort or back problems. Bed boards are available in several varieties: one solid piece of wood, two pieces of wood hinged together, or slats of wood encased in heavy cloth. The type of bed board used is determined by the amount of bed movement desired and its availability in the health care facility. A solid piece of wood can be used only if the bed remains flat.

When a bed board is initially placed on the bed, be sure it is centered. When *making the bed with a bed board,* the bottom sheet is tucked in the usual manner. It may be somewhat difficult to slide the linen under the mattress, and the nurse needs to be careful to prevent hand injury.

FOOTBOARDS. A footboard can be a piece of wood or some other firm surface placed at the foot of the mattress. The main purpose of the footboard is to maintain the patient's feet at right angles to the legs in order to prevent foot drop (flexion of the foot). When feet are allowed to "drop" into a flexed position for a period of time, muscles at the back of the leg and ankle shorten, and contracture of the Achilles tendon develops. The footboard also can be used to keep the patient from sliding off the end of the mattress or to keep linens off the patient's feet.

The patient's feet must rest firmly against the footboard to maintain foot alignment. Remember to adjust the footboard to the height of the patient so that the feet are kept in an extended position. Some commercially made boards are adjustable. If the board is not adjustable, use a folded bath blanket, sand bag or similar device for filling the space between the patient's feet and the board. All footboards must be covered with linen to protect the patient's feet from the rough surface of the board.

Making the bed with a footboard: Cover the footboard with a draw sheet or other linen and secure linen with tape. Bring top linen *over* the board and then miter. The sides of the miter may need to be tucked in to prevent chilling.

TRACTION AND TRAPEZE. Various traction devices can be attached to the head or foot of the bed. Traction devices may restrict the patient's ability to turn or move about in bed during the bedmaking procedure. If a traction device is attached to the foot of the bed, modify placement of the top linen so that it fits around the device and provides warmth. A *trapeze* bar, suspended over the head of the bed, allows the patient to roll or lift himself off the mattress, making it possible for the nurse to easily place and tighten linens or for the patient to use a bedpan. A trapeze also permits the patient to shift his weight periodically during other times of the day.

Protective Bed Items. Some equipment and supplies are placed on the bed to protect patients who are prone to skin breakdown problems, and other items are used to protect the bed linens from becoming soiled.

OVERBED CRADLE (HOOP; "ANDERSON FRAME"). This wire frame (see Fig. 27–31) is placed over the patient to keep the top linen from resting upon his body. The cradle may be necessary for the patient with burns or other wounds, or if the patient is unable to tolerate the weight of the bed linen. Secure the cradle in place to maintain protection of the appropriate area of the body and to prevent the cradle from collapsing. One method of securing a cradle is to attach one end of a piece of gauze or similar material to the sides of the cradle and

TABLE 27–2. DIFFERENCES IN BEDMAKING PROCEDURES

OCCUPIED BED	UNOCCUPIED BED
Loosen linen base on *one* side. Remain on that side of bed, fan-fold soiled linen to middle of mattress against patient.	Loosen base linen on *both* sides. Remove all soiled base linen.
Complete base *before* top linen is applied.	Complete base *and* top on one side *before* completing bedmaking on second side.

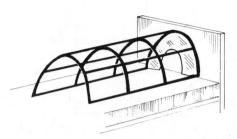

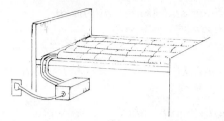

Figure 27–32. Alternating pressure mattress on bed, attached to electrical outlet. (From Wood, L. A., and Rambo, B. J. (eds.): *Nursing Skills for Allied Health Services,* 2nd ed. Vol. 1. Philadelphia, W. B. Saunders Co., 1977, p. 110.)

Figure 27–31. Overbed cradle. *Note:* When placed over a patient the cradle should always be secured to the bed to prevent collapse. Also, the cradle is covered with a full sheet. (From Wood, L. A., and Rambo, B. J. (eds.): *Nursing Skills for Allied Health Services,* 2nd ed. Vol. 1. Philadelphia, W. B. Saunders Co., 1977, p. 110.)

the other end to the bedsprings. When *making a bed with a cradle,* place the top linen over the cradle. Pull the excess linen around the foot of the mattress. Bring the side edge of the sheet perpendicular to the mattress and tuck excess sheet under the mattress (as for the regular mitered corner). Complete the "modified" mitered corner by tucking the side under at the corner to prevent chilling.

ALTERNATING PRESSURE PAD (MATTRESS). This vinyl pad is an electrically inflated double-coiled air mattress that alternates pressure under pressure-bearing areas of the body (see Fig. 27–32). It is used for patients who are prone to develop skin problems (see Chap. 33 for a discussion of immobility). The vinyl pad has numerous sections running the length of the mattress; these sections alternately inflate and deflate. Air is circulated by a motor that is attached to the mattress by way of hoses.

Making the bed with an alternating pressure mattress: First, place a mattress pad over the regular mattress to prevent friction. Then, put the air mattress on top of the mattress pad. The bottom sheet is arranged in the usual manner, except that the miter on the side with the hoses is modified to prevent kinking of the air hoses. Do *not* use a new draw sheet because it counteracts the beneficial effect of the alternating air pressure.

> *Avoid puncturing the plastic pad with pins and other sharp objects, and check for kinks in coil and hoses. Also, examine the air mattress for proper functioning by observing the emptying and filling of the sectioned coils.*

SHEEPSKINS. A sheepskin is placed over the bottom sheet to prevent skin irritation. They are available in several sizes. The most commonly used size extends from the patient's shoulders to his buttocks. To maintain a sheepskin in good condition, have it laundered when it becomes matted or soiled. To decrease problems with matting, fluff the sheepskin by brushing it.

CELLU-COTTON PADS (CHUX OR "BLUE" PADS). These small disposable pads are placed over the bottom sheet. The absorbent side is placed next to the patient and the water-repellent side is placed next to the sheet. They can be used for incontinence or under drainage sites. These pads provide added comfort for the patient and save linen changes.

SUMMARY

When providing any aspect of hygiene care, the excellent nurse:

▶ Assesses the need for hygiene care

▶ Determines the purposes and goals to be accomplished by hygiene care

▶ Assesses the patient's overall status; condition of his oral cavity, sense organs, skin, hair and nails; and various systems of the body such as the respiratory, circulatory and neurologic systems *before* and *during* care

▶ Communicates with the patient to gather information about his mental and emotional status and social and cultural background for planning care and establishing a therapeutic nurse-patient relationship

▶ Adapts hygiene care to the individual patient's needs, based on scientific principles and facts

▶ Evaluates the effects of the hygiene care for use in planning future care

1. Bates, B.: *A Guide to Physical Examination.* Philadelphia, J. B. Lippincott Co., 1974, p. 9.
2. Bibby, B. G.: The cariogenicity of snack foods and confections. *Journal of the American Dental Association, 90*:121, Jan. 1975.
2a. Block, P. L.: Dental health in hospitalized patients. *American Journal of Nursing, 76*:1162–1164, July 1976.
3. Carbary, L.: Foot problems. *Nursing Care, 8*:10, June 1975.
4. Christensen, D. L.: When nails are ingrown, injured, or infected. *Patient Care, 8*:168, Oct. 15, 1974.
4a. Davis, M.: Getting to the root of the problem: hair-grooming techniques for black patients. *Nursing '77, 7*:60, Apr. 1977.
5. *Dorland's Illustrated Medical Dictionary,* 25th ed. Philadelphia, W. B. Saunders Co., 1974, pp. 1164–65.
5a. Dyer, E. D., Monson, M. A., and Cope M. J.: Dental health in adults. *American Journal of Nursing, 76*:1156–1159, July 1976.
6. Freudenthal, N.: What nursing expects of the laundry. *Supervisor Nurse, 4*:19, Nov. 1973.
6a. Greenwood, A. H.: Dental care for the elderly poses special problems. *Geriatrics, 31*:103, May 1976.
6b. Grier, M. E.: Hair care for the black patient. *American Journal of Nursing, 76*:1781, Nov. 1976.
6c. Hogan, R.: Mr. O'Brien's beard. *American Journal of Nursing, 77*:61, Jan. 1977.
6d. Jabaley, M. E., Clement, R. L., and Bryant, W. M.: Recognizing oral lesions. *American Family Physician, 13*:60–64, May 1976.
7. Kinssies, K., et al.: Comparative Study of the Traditional Bed Bath and Towel Bath. Seattle, WA, 1974 (unpublished report).
8. Kreitzman, S. N.: Nutrition in the process of dental caries. *Dental Clinics of North America, 20*:499, July 1976.

9. Levine, P., and Grayson, B. H.: Safeguarding your patient against periodontal disease. *RN, 36*:38–39, July 1973.
10. Luckmann, J., and Sorensen, K.: *Medical-Surgical Nursing: A Psychophysiologic Approach.* Philadelphia, W. B. Saunders Co., 1974, p. 1251.
11. McBean, L.D., and Speckmann, E. W.: A review: the importance of nutrition in oral health. *Journal of The American Dental Association, 89*:109, July 1974.
12. McBean, L. D., and Speckmann, E. W.: A review: the importance of nutrition in oral health. *Journal of the American Dental Association, 89*:112, July 1974.
13. Maurer, J.: Providing optimal oral health. *Nursing Clinics of North America, 12*:671, Dec. 1977.
13a. Michelsen, D.: How to Give a Good Back Rub. *American Journal of Nursing, 78*:1197–1199, July 1978.
14. Rizzo, D. R.: Nursing and the efficient use of linens. *Hospitals, 49*:92, June 16, 1975.
14a. Parish, L. C. and Witkowski, J. A.: Lice Can Happen to Anyone. *Consultant, 18*:34–40. Sep. 1978.
15. Roach, L. B.: Color changes in dark skin. *Nursing '77, 7*:49, Jan. 1977.
15a. Sister Kenny Institute, *Nursing Care of the Skin,* Rehabilitation Publication, Number 711. Revised edition, 1975.
15b. Slattery, J.: Dental health in children. *American Journal of Nursing, 76*:1159–1161, July 1976.
16. Wilkins, E. M.: *Clinical Practice of the Dental Hygienist.* Philadelphia, Lea & Febiger, 1976, p. 237.
17. Zucnick, M.: Care of an artificial eye. *American Journal of Nursing, 75*:835, May 1975.

CHAPTER 28

MONITORING BODY TEMPERATURE AND UNDERSTANDING ITS SIGNIFICANCE

By Mary X. Britten, R.N., Ed.D.

INTRODUCTION AND STUDY GUIDE

In order for the nurse to monitor body temperature intelligently, a basic understanding of the human thermoregulatory mechanisms is necessary. Evaluation of a fever requires knowledge of the mechanisms of temperature control and the way in which control can be supported, maintained or adjusted.

This chapter presents a discussion of what constitutes body temperature, the factors involved in the regulation of body temperature and the ways in which heat is produced, conserved or dissipated. Included in the discussion are those variables that affect body temperature and those which influence heat production and loss.

The chapter begins the exploration of alterations in body temperature that result from changes in environmental temperature and those that occur as a result of medical therapy. Temperature changes caused by illness will be touched upon, but for greater depth, the student must consult medical-surgical nursing texts. Ultimately the purpose of this chapter is to prepare the student for the nursing responsibilities, both independent and interdependent, that are *necessary in monitoring body temperature*.

Nursing assessment, nursing decisions and nursing measures for individuals in relation to body temperature will be discussed.

The following study guide will assist the student in gaining greater knowledge about the subject. Some of the questions refer you to your prior studies, whereas others require you to apply the knowledge you have gained. Still others ask you to explore your personal feelings and to consider and anticipate your actions in certain situations.

1. Either prior to or while reading this chapter,

review your notes from chemistry or physics courses on:

radiation
convection
evaporation
conduction
energy
kinetic energy
basal metabolism
calories
kilocalories

2. Become familiar with and be able to use the following terms:

antipyretic
Celsius
circadian rhythm
convulsion
delirium
diaphoresis
Fahrenheit
febrile
homeothermia
hyperpyrexia
hyperthermia
hypothermia
intermittent temperature
lysis
poikilothermic
pyrexia
pyrogen
recrudescent temperature
recurrent or relapsing fever
remittent temperature
rigor
sudomotor
thermogenesis

thermolysis
vasoconstriction
vasodilation

3. Convert the following temperature readings from one scale to the other: 34°C., 103°F., 110°F., 42°C.

4. Describe in your own words how the human body normally produces heat.

5. Cite internal and external variables that influence and change body temperature.

6. Describe how the body adjusts to or compensates for variation in external temperatures.

7. List the observations the nurse would make of individuals with normal temperatures and of those with altered temperatures.

8. What are the differences in the physiologic mechanisms leading to fever of heat stroke and those leading to the fever seen with a bacterial sore throat? Are there any differences in the treatments of these two conditions?

9. What beneficial effects can you ascribe to elevated body temperatures? Are fevers induced as a form of medical therapy? If so, for which condition?

10. What is a fever of unknown origin? What can you say about the cause of fever of unknown origin?

11. If you suspect that a patient has artificially elevated his temperature reading, what would you do?

12. What medications are commonly administered to lower the temperature of febrile patients?

13. What side effects should the nurse anticipate when administering drugs to patients to induce hypothermia?

14. How does atropine affect thermoregulation? Why is it important for the nurse to know this?

15. You have been informed that oral temperatures with mercury-in-glass thermometers take 9 to 10 minutes to register. Why do you think so few nurses use this knowledge? Consider your actions if a patient says to you, "Why do you take so long? Everyone else takes my temperature for 3 minutes."

INTRODUCTION

Regulation of body temperature in man is an exceedingly complex process that involves the functioning of many organ systems. A constant exchange of energy takes place between compartments within the body and between man and the environment. This exchange involves both chemical and physical transfer of heat. In addition, heat is continually produced in the body and lost from it. The direction of the exchange of heat energy is influenced by sensory impulses from different regions of the body. The thermoregulatory system contains various thermoreceptors or sensors, multiple feedback loops and multiple outputs. In general, unless a strain is placed on the system, man is unaware of the thermoregulatory adjustments taking place.

In spite of extreme variations in environmental temperature, in a healthy individual the temperature of the body deviates little from 36 to 38°C. (96.8 to 100.4°F.). Body temperature is controlled by both conscious and unconscious actions that enable man to live in arctic or tropical regions for extended periods of time with little change in internal temperature. Acclimatization to either extreme does occur, but this change takes time and is not permanent if the person returns to a neutral environmental temperature. Even when wearing little or no clothing in the presence of ambient temperatures fluctuating between 13 and 66°C. (55.4 and 150.8°F.), man is able to maintain his normal temperature.[29]

Man is referred to as *homoiothermic* (homeothermic) because he is "warm-blooded" and maintains a relatively constant temperature independent of the environment. Animals which assume the temperature of their environment are referred to as *poikilothermic*, or "cold-blooded." For the body temperature to remain constant, a balance must exist between heat produced in the body and heat lost to the environment.[29] Heat is produced by the body metabolism, and the rate of heat production is called the metabolic rate. The metabolic rate may be increased by muscular activity (exercise or shivering), increased sympathetic stimulation, an increase in thyroxine, oxidation of food and an increase in body temperature itself, which effects an increase in metabolism.[29, 32] Many of these factors are not subject to voluntary control. On the other hand, the amount of heat lost depends on environmental conditions and may be influenced by man. If an excessive amount of heat exists, the body exchanges heat first within itself and then with the environment, primarily by sweating.

The body's thermoregulatory system functions smoothly and in certain conditions may work at the expense and detriment of other organs. In cold weather, heat loss cannot be turned off, and although a lowered body temperature would conserve energy, man will maintain his temperature, even during periods of starvation. In a hot environment, man may continue to sweat even when the resulting dehydration is so severe that the blood pressure may not be maintained.[34]

Man maintains his homeothermic state (temperature deviation of less than 2 degrees Cel-

TABLE 28–1.   CELSIUS AND FAHRENHEIT
EQUIVALENTS

sius, or 3.6 degrees Fahrenheit, despite large fluctuations in ambient temperature) by the peripheral and central nervous systems, which detect changes and stimulate appropriate actions based on negative feedback loops. Thermal sensors pick up temperature changes and send signals or stimuli to the hypothalamus, where they are integrated. Sensed deviations stimulate the following actions: if cold is felt, internal heat will be preserved by alterations in the flow and distribution of blood and by an increase in heat production. To conserve heat, the individual may change his body position, put on more clothes, increase the temperature of the environment or commence to shiver. If undue heat is felt, *internal measures* for increasing heat dissipation include (1) augmentation of the rate and flow of blood to the periphery and (2) stimulation of the sweat glands to promote evaporation. *External adjustment measures* include a decrease in the amount of insulation or clothing worn, a change in the humidity and temperature of the environment if possible and a change in position. There is a limit to the adaptability of the thermoregulatory system, and extreme stress may result in deviations in body temperature.

The cells, tissues and organs of the body seem to function best between 36 and 38°C. (96.8 and 100.4°F.), although for short periods of time, temperatures as high as 40 to 41°C. (104 to 106°F.), as a result of fever or strenuous exercise, may be tolerated.[32, 33] Cases of patients surviving fevers of 46°C. (114.8°F.) have been reported but are rare. At high temperatures, tissue is damaged, cellular proteins are denatured or inactivated, and most enzyme functions are impaired. Tissues may be irreversibly damaged when they reach a temperature of 50°C. (122°F.).[32, 33] Low body temperatures are also poorly tolerated by man. In the presence of continuing freezing temperatures, cell membranes are damaged and dehydration occurs as a result of changes in capillary and cell permeability. Crystal formation may evolve, further damaging the tissue. For short periods of time, hypothermia (lowered body temperature) of 24 to 27°C. (75.2 to 80.6°F.) may be tolerated, but, unless it occurs under careful medical supervision with adequate support systems, this is usually incompatible with life.[33]

Table 28–1 shows the conversion of temperatures between Celsius and Fahrenheit, which will help you in reading this chapter.

Definitions.   Customarily it is said. that tem-

°C.	=	°F.
−10		14.0
− 5		23.0
0	←Freezing point of water→	32.0
1		33.8
10		50.0
13		55.4
18		64.4
20		68.0
21		69.8
24		75.2
27		80.6
28		82.4
30		86.0
34		93.2
35		95.0
36		96.8
37		98.6
38		100.4
39		102.2
40		104.0
41		105.8
42		107.6
43		109.4
44		111.2
45		113.0
46		114.8
50		122.0
55		131.0
60		140.0
65		149.0
70		158.0
75		167.0
80		176.0
85		185.0
90		194.0
95		203.0
100	←Boiling point of water→	212.0

Interval Equivalents		
a change of 0.5°C. =	*a change of* 0.9°F.
1.0°C. =	1.8°F.
2.0°C. =	3.6°F.
5.0°C. =	9.0°F.
10.0°C. =	18.0°F.

perature is a measure of hotness or coldness. The precision and utility of the concept stems from the definition of a standard system, a thermometer, against which all other systems are judged. Heat content, H, and temperature T, of a body volume, V, and specific heat, C, are related by the equation

$$H = CVT$$

It should be noted that two different bodies at the same temperature may contain quite different amounts of heat depending on differences in volume and specific heat.

Heat is usually measured in terms of the calorie (the amount of heat required to raise the temperature of one gram of water 1°C.) or the kilocalorie (1000 calories). Often the kilocalorie is written as a calorie with a capital C a convention inevitably leading to confusion with the smaller calorie, written without a capital. Reader beware!

In the body, heat is produced mainly by the chemical reactions of metabolism. The metabolic rate is the rate at which heat is produced by these reactions. "Basal" metabolic rate refers to the metabolic rate under a set of standard conditions. A man resting in a sitting position in a neutral environment (basal conditions) produces approximately 40 kcal./hr./m.² of total body surface. For a man with a surface area of 1.8 m.², the heat produced is about 70 kcal./hr.[33] However, muscular activity, external temperature, the availability and digestion of food and the amount of clothing worn all influence body metabolism and inherently the body temperature as well.

Normal Range of Body Temperature. It is not accurate to say that 37°C. (98.6°F.) represents or is the "normal" body temperature. Rather, over a 24-hour period the temperature of the body varies and is not constant. If one were to measure the temperature simultaneously of different tissues and organs of the body, it would be apparent that the temperature is not uniform. A range of temperature that is relatively constant from day to day is a more realistic concept. Body temperature refers to the temperature of the interior of the body—the *core* temperature. The core temperature is the temperature in the thoracic and abdominal cavities and in the central nervous system. This is closely regulated and deviates less than 1°C.[29] The *surface* or skin temperature fluctuates widely, depending upon surrounding conditions. Peripheral tissue, muscle, skin and subcutaneous tissue are generally cooler than core tissue. Skin temperature is usually 5 to 8°C. cooler than interior temperature but recordings ranging from 30 to 40°C. (86 to 104°F.) may also occur.[32] The calf muscle is usually lower (by about 3°C.) than core temperature and the bone marrow may be even cooler (3.5°C. lower). The warmest organs of the body are the liver and brain, which average 1°C. higher than other organs. The temperature of the blood varies as it courses through the body. In a study conducted in a thermally neutral environment, temperatures were 36 to 37°C. (96.8 to 98.6°F.) in the brachial artery and 35.5 to 36.6°C. (95.9 to 97.7°F.) in the radial artery. On exposure to cold, the temperature was 31.1°C. (88°F.) in the brachial artery and 21.5°C. (70.7°F.) in the radial artery.[3, 5, 32] While this dramatic change occurred the subject did not feel cold, nor was there any change in rectal temperature.[32] In general, the skin of the face, trunk, arms and legs is warmer than that of the hands, feet, ears and nose. Proximal portions of the body are warmer than distal areas.

FACTORS AFFECTING BODY TEMPERATURE

External Temperature. Certain factors induce changes in body temperature, but in these conditions, the altered temperatures are considered "normal." External temperatures may affect the internal body temperature. A warm room or a hot day may increase the body temperature by 1°C. In a cold environment, there is usually little change in body temperature, although in infants and older persons, a drop may occur.

Age. Body temperature is generally observed to be lower in the aged, especially if the environment is cold. Since metabolism affects heat and the metabolic rate of the newborn is greater than that of the elderly, infants and young children have body temperatures slightly higher than 37°C. (98.6°F.). In the infant, the thermoregulatory mechanisms are not fully developed and marked temperature fluctuations occur in relation to external conditions. Babies do not tolerate excessive heat or cold and must be protected from them. Until puberty, temperature regulation is quite labile.[3]

Circadian or Diurnal Rhythm. The core temperature in man on a regular sleep-work schedule fluctuates over a 24-hour period between 0.5 and 1.5°C.,[7] being highest with activity and lowest with rest. For most individuals, the lowest temperature is in the early morning between midnight and 6 AM, whereas the highest point is in the late afternoon and early evening between 4 and 8 PM. A few individuals have their highest temperature in the morning,[32] so it is critical that the nurse know the norm for each individual. This information should be obtained while the nursing history is collected. The circadian thermal rhythm is not present at birth but develops gradually during the first years of life.[13] The cause of the temperature fluctuation in relation to the circadian rhythm is unknown, but it is postulated to be hormonal.[32] The temperature change does not depend on environmental temperature and occurs in people on bed rest and in those who do not eat.[32] An appropriate shift occurs when air travel places one in a new time zone,[34] and an inverted shift takes place in the majority of individuals who work during night hours, although it takes 1 to 3 weeks for this to occur.

Stress. Psychologic and physiologic stressors are known to influence body temperature, usually producing an increase by neural and hormonal action. Sympathetic stimulation, with the secretion of epinephrine and norepinephrine, increases metabolic activity, thereby increasing body temperature.

Sleep. In sleep, body temperature tends to be lowered. This follows from decreased heat production, decreased metabolic rate and muscular activity and increased heat loss. In early sleep, sweating occurs at temperatures lower than those required when awake. The thermoregulatory system is normal, but the body temperature is still lower in sleep.[34]

Hormonal Effect. In women, a periodic fluctuation in temperature exists in relation to the menstrual cycle. This appears to be the result of the cyclic rise in progesterone, which increases the body temperature. Immediately prior to the onset of menstruation, the temperature falls 0.2 to 0.5°C. from its previous level. This low level remains until the time of ovulation, when a rise in temperature of 0.2 to 0.5°C. occurs that persists until just prior to the next menstrual period. The degree of change may be higher in some people. During the first trimester of pregnancy a slight rise in temperature is evident, but this gradually decreases as pregnancy continues.[3, 34]

Large amounts of thyroid and growth hormone stimulate and increase body metabolism, which may be reflected by a rise in temperature. Ingestion and digestion, of proteins in particular but other foods as well, affect the metabolic rate and may affect body temperature, but the increase in temperature is usually temporary.

Exercise. Muscular work and exercise generate heat and cause considerable elevations in temperature. The increase depends upon the intensity and amount of work accomplished and is independent of environmental temperatures. The increase is thought to occur as a result of an overload of heat produced, a "load error." After strenuous exercise, athletes have registered rectal temperatures as high as 41.1°C. (106°F.), and temperatures of 39°C. (102°F.) are not unusual. The temperature usually returns to normal within 30 minutes after the exercise has been completed.[3, 34]

Figure 28–1 depicts the range of body temperature in a healthy individual.

REGULATION OF BODY TEMPERATURE

There are two thermoregulatory control systems that maintain body temperature in the presence of environmental extremes. One system, which allows greater individual flexibility and freedom, relies on *behavioral control* of body temperature. In this system, man consciously controls his actions and manipulates his environment. In the other system, known as *physiologic regulation*, the responses are involuntary and, within a limited range of environmental temperature, provide fine control of body temperature.[32, 33]

Behavioral Regulation

Behavioral regulation operates in environmental extremes and is very important. Conscious sensations serve as a warning system and initiate defense actions before the central temperature is changed.[8] Behavioral regulation occurs as a result of sensations of warmth or cold on the skin, which are perceived as comfort or discomfort depending upon the thermal environment and the emotional state of the individual at the time. Marked discomfort from cold does not appear until the ambient temperature is consistently below 21°C. (70°F.).[33] The sensation of cold itself does not change particularly even though the environmental temperature may change from 18 to 13°C. (64.4 to 55.4°F.), but cold is sensed when the skin temperature drops.[33]

Sensory detection alone is not sufficient. Motivation and the means to control or manipulate the environment and exposure must also exist.[33] Today, with the scientific knowledge and technology that is available, we are able to adjust environmental temperatures and humidity as well as design special clothing for thermal control.

Physiologic Regulation

Physiologic regulation refers to the body's involuntary responses that act to maintain a

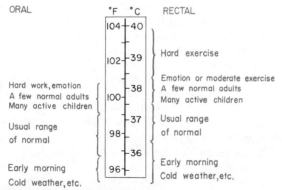

Figure 28–1. Estimated range of body temperature in normal persons. (From DuBois, E. F.: *Fever.* Springfield, IL, Charles C Thomas, 1948.)

constant temperature. This thermal control takes place automatically and may be thought of as providing the "fine tuning" that behavioral modification lacks.[33] Guided by central thermoreceptors, the response to changes in body temperature is *swift and vigorous*.[8] Changes as small as 0.01°C. effect thermoregulatory changes.[8] The response to cold is slower and less vigorous than that to warmth and requires a larger variation within internal temperatures before action is instituted.

Hypothalamus

Neural signals that reflect temperature sensation from both internal and superficial structures converge in a central integrator thought to be in the hypothalamus.[74] The hypothalamus is probably the controller of physical and chemical thermoregulation.[37] Peripheral signals, signals from other deep thermal receptors and those from within the hypothalamus itself are all integrated within the central structure, but sensory areas are able to operate independently of each other.[74] The hypothalamus has a neural representation of something which approaches mean body temperature. It appears to act as if it has within it some ideal temperature, which has been called a temperature setpoint. If the mean body temperature is in excess of this reference point, control effector signals are sent out for action to reduce the body temperature by increasing the peripheral blood flow, decreasing metabolic heat production and increasing evaporative heat loss. If the temperature of blood circulating through the hypothalamus is greater than the setpoint, the following physiologic actions occur:

$$\begin{array}{ccc} \text{T} & \text{T} & \text{Dissipation of heat} \\ \text{circulating} > \text{setpoint} \Rightarrow & \text{Vasodilation} \\ \text{blood} & & \text{Sweating} \end{array}$$

If the blood circulating through the hypothalamus is lower than the setpoint, the action leads to an increase in metabolic heat production, a decrease in peripheral blood flow and shivering:

$$\begin{array}{ccc} \text{T} & \text{T} & \text{Heat conservation} \\ \text{circulating} < \text{setpoint} \Rightarrow & \text{Vasoconstriction} \\ \text{blood} & & \text{Heat generation} \\ & & \text{Shivering} \end{array}$$

The temperatures at which the various actions are stimulated, such as shivering, sweating or motor activity, need not be the same.[34] For example, warmth sensors which activate heat loss mechanisms may operate at lower temperatures than heat-producing mechanisms stimulated by cold sensors.[34]

Anterior Hypothalamus. The anterior hypothalamus is concerned with protecting the body from hyperthermia (high temperatures). Special heat-sensitive neurons increase their output as the body temperature rises, and decrease it when the temperature falls. With an increase in body temperature of 10°C. (18°F.), the firing rate will increase tenfold.[29] Their firing initiates an *increase in heat dissipation*, by vasodilation of peripheral and cutaneous vessels, increased sweat gland activity and decreased muscular and metabolic activity. Warming this part of the brain also stimulates these responses.[34]

Posterior Hypothalamus. This part of the brain is concerned with protecting the body against hypothermia (lower body temperature). The action initiated is largely mediated through the sympathetic nervous system.[5, 29, 34] Heat loss is decreased and more heat is produced. Hypothalamic cooling activates *vasoconstriction*, *shivering* and *metabolic increase*. There is also decreased sweat gland activity. Connections exist between both portions of the hypothalamus, and activity in one area inhibits action in the other. Under normal conditions, their actions are balanced and in harmony.

Temperature Sensors. Thermoregulation is dependent upon the body's ability to detect temperature differences and the ability to transmit this information to an integrator where interpretation and comparison of the data will produce the appropriate action. Nerve receptors for heat and cold exist throughout the skin and provide the information used in physiologic and behavioral regulation.[29] They send impulses to the hypothalamus and also elicit local cord reflexes that affect skin blood flow and sweat gland activity. Man is able to discriminate heat from cold and qualities of heat and cold, and to interpret whether these are pleasant or unpleasant. Heat pain occurs at temperatures of 45°C. (113°F.) and is characterized as sharp, burning and localized in the outermost layer of the skin.[34] Cold pain is sensed at temperatures below 17°C. (62.6°F.), is dull and poorly localized and radiates to surrounding areas. Blood vessel spasm from the cold contributes to the dull pain that is felt.[34] (These sensors are nociceptors and not thermoreceptors.) The threshold and intensity of thermal sensations depend on the area of stimulation. Sensors can detect temperatures of the skin at the site of the receptor and can pick up the rate of temperature change. Though the internal core temperature may be constant or decreasing, warming the skin can activate heat loss mechanisms.[34] Skin temperature also contributes thermal information that controls sweating.

Thermal receptors exist in the deep visceral organs (Auerbach plexus), the spinal cord, the mesencephalic reticular formation, the hypothalamus and the preoptic region of the brain stem. Temperature-sensitive cells exist in the tongue, the respiratory tract, the medulla, the motor cortex and the muscle spindles. Other sensations may initiate thermal responses, for instance, those felt after eating curry or other hot spicy foods.[32, 34]

Temperature directly affects effector organs and can facilitate actions that have been initiated from central signals.[32] Local skin temperatures influence cutaneous blood flow and sweat secretion and modify the effect of centrally stimulated sympathetic impulses.[34] Skin temperature influences central as well as local thermoregulation. Skin changes do not alter internal temperature markedly, but their sensations stimulate heat-losing or heat-producing activities and thereby assist in temperature control.[29] Local skin reflexes exist, but their intensity is centrally controlled.[32, 34]

Research on paraplegic patients shows that some integration of thermal information occurs at the spinal level. Thermosensitive structures exist in the spinal region, and the cord possesses mechanisms to produce shivering. Body temperature regulation is impaired if the spinal cord is severed in the lower cervical region, but more function is preserved if the cord is cut in the thoracic region. A person is hypothermic if the cord is severed between C4 and C6. If the cord is severed between T3 and T8, there is slight thermal sweating as a result of cord reflex action.[31, 33]

Thermal Homeostasis

Balance. Thermoregulation depends on the balance between heat production and heat loss. To an extent, the balance is maintained by control of the amount of heat produced, but more of the regulation is effected by control of the amount of heat lost.[5] Heat produced in the body is balanced by heat lost to the environment. The heat balance equation may be summarized as:

$$\text{rate of heat storage} =$$
$$\text{rate of heat production} - \text{rate of heat loss}$$

HEAT PRODUCTION AND HEAT CONSERVATION

Although some heat comes from sources such as radiation from the sun or heating fixtures or by conduction from heating pads or from ingestion of hot foods and liquids, the principal source of heat is from combustion of food in the body. During rest, most heat is produced in the body core, which represents one-third of the body mass. Respiration and circulation contribute one-tenth of the heat production, and the brain and muscle metabolism each contribute two-tenths. The liver primarily and other abdominal viscera contribute one half.[3] During active physical work, the major focus for heat production shifts to the muscles. Maximum muscle exercise can increase heat production to 20 times normal for a few minutes.[29] During strenuous exercise, as much as 500 kcal./m.²/hr. of heat may be produced.[72]

Hypothalamic Cooling

When the hypothalamus detects a temperature below 37°C. (98.6°F.), various processes occur that are directed at preserving body heat and increasing the rate of heat produced.

Vasomotor Control. Thermoregulation involves adjustment in peripheral blood flow, which may vary according to region. One region includes the extremities, meaning the hands, feet, ears, lips and nose. Another region is the head and brow, while the final one is the trunk and proximal limbs. The flow of blood is controlled by noradrenergic sympathetic fibers. An increase in sympathetic stimulation and tone leads to *vasoconstriction and a decrease in vasodilation.*[34] Vasoconstriction can result in almost total shutdown of blood flow to the arm, leg and skin vessels. Intense adrenergic vasoconstriction occurs throughout the body and prevents heat loss from the skin by reducing the venous surface area. This also lessens the transfer of heat from the central portion of the body to the surface area, ultimately conserving heat.[29, 34] Body heat from the core is lost slowly by conduction through muscles and fatty tissue because they are good insulators. With vasoconstriction, the skin will be cool, maybe even cold, to the touch and will look pale. Digits of the extremities appear cyanotic or purple and the skin may have a mottled appearance. The skin is often dry and may itch and become chapped; these are conditions the nurse should note and correct.

Shivering. The primary motor center for shivering is in the posterior hypothalamus, which transmits impulses to anterior motor neurons to increase the tone of skeletal muscles and the muscle metabolism. This in turn increases the rate of heat production. Even before shivering starts, there is a rise in heat production. Beyond a critical muscle tone level, shivering (rigor) commences—rapid involuntary muscle contractions, usually beginning in the pectoral and masseter muscles. The teeth may chatter because of shivering of the jaw muscles. With shivering, heat production may increase as much as 200 to 400 per cent of normal.[29] Shivering is efficient as a method of heat production because 50 per cent of the heat produced in this manner is retained in the body.[31] All these changes may usually be seen with the onset of fever when the shivering becomes part of a chill. It is important for the nurse to identify and time a chill so that the resultant increase in body temperature can be assessed and measures can be taken to alleviate the discomfort.

Piloerection.   Another result of hypothalamic cooling is *piloerection*, in which the "hair stands on end," commonly referred to as "goose bumps." Because of the absence of significant amounts of hair in man, this has no physiologic effect. In animals, when the hair stands upright, a thick layer of air is entrapped, providing insulation next to the skin and significantly decreasing the transfer of heat to surrounding areas.

Hormone Release.   Chemical excitation, hormonal secretion and sympathetic stimulation increase chemical thermogenesis and result in increased cellular metabolism. Catecholamine release provides for more oxidation of food materials. In a cool environment, acclimatized animals respond by a 100 to 200 per cent increase in metabolism, but the figure in man is closer to 50 per cent.[29] Hypothalamic cooling increases the production of thyrotropin, leading to an increased output of thyroxine from the thyroid gland. Thyroxine stimulates the rate of cellular metabolism, and it appears that increased thyroxine secretion is responsible for the increased basal metabolic rate seen in people living in cold climates.[29]

Exercise and Heat Production.   Exercise is an effective method for producing heat. In muscular exercise, the rate and the degree of work and metabolic heat production increase linearly, and exercise results in a rise in body temperature. Rectal temperatures recorded on athletes register linear increases with oxygen consumption.[63] The rise in temperature is independent of environmental temperatures, and is assumed to be beneficial for muscle performance,[63] a fact utilized by athletes when engaging in "warm-up periods." Within limits, it appears that the higher the body temperature, the more efficient the metabolic reactions. The muscles perform better, and the physiologic adjustments lead to greater efficiency.

HEAT LOSS FROM THE BODY

Thermoregulation would be incomplete unless the heat produced and stored in the body can be eliminated when indicated. The exchange of heat occurs through four modes: (1) radiation, (2) conduction, (3) convection and (4) evaporation. The effectiveness of each of these modes depends upon the amount of heat to be lost and the environmental conditions. The ambient temperature, humidity, wind velocity and air currents each influence heat exchange. The amount of clothing worn influences heat exchange as well as the body position in reference to available surface area. In general, in the physiologic temperature range, the rate of heat lost from a hotter object to a colder object will be proportional to the temperature difference between the objects (Newton's law).

Radiation.   Heat is lost by radiation in the form of infrared rays. The flow of heat is direct and occurs even through a vacuum. At rest, at normal room temperature, 50 to 70 per cent of heat loss occurs by radiation. In a warm environment, the amount of heat lost by radiation decreases and can even reverse.[3, 29, 31]

If one stands in front of an oven, the oven heat is radiated to the surface of the body, which absorbs the heat rays. Dark skin absorbs more solar heat from light rays than white skin. To a limited degree, we are able to control the surface area of our bodies available for heat loss by radiation. A person standing with arms and legs extended has a radiating area of 75 per cent of total, but this drops to 50 per cent when the fetal position is assumed.[32] Other variables that influence heat loss by radiation include the skin or surface temperature, the effective surface area, the reflective power of the skin and clothing, the radiant temperature and the nature of the environment.[31]

Conduction.   Conduction refers to the flow of heat from one object to another with which it is in direct contact. No material is transferred between the two objects, however. Conduction takes place in solids, gases and liquids. In the body, heat is conducted from the warm internal tissues to the skin surface. Heat is conducted from the skin to any cooler object touching it through the thin layer of air that is adherent to the skin. Hot objects conduct heat back to the body. Some objects are better conductors than others; e.g., metal conducts better than wool or air. Muscle and fat are poor conductors and thus are considered good insulators, since they provide resistance to heat flow. Layers of clothing or feathers provide good insulation. The larger layer of subcutaneous fat women have is an advantage in preventing heat loss.

In general, because an object quickly assumes the temperature of the body touching it, only small quantities of heat are lost by conduction. Heat loss by conduction to air represents a greater proportion (12 per cent) of body heat loss, but unless air currents are present, this too is self-limiting.[29, 31, 32]

Convection. Heat loss by convection is the exchange of heat between hot and cold objects by physical transfer to circulating liquid or gas molecules with which the objects are in contact.[29, 31] Heat is conducted from the body to the air and then is carried away by convection. Convection depends upon the existence of a fluid medium between warm and cold objects and upon streaming movement of warm molecules. *Natural convection* refers to warm air rising from the skin and moving to cooler areas. *Forced convection* refers to air currents produced by artificial means, such as electric fans or other machines. The air layers next to the skin, often referred to as "private climate," adhere to it and do not move. However, air molecules beyond this climate move freely and quickly. Heat must be conducted through the private climate. Forced convection and increased wind velocity can decrease this layer.[32]

The rate of heat loss by convection depends on skin and air temperature as well as air velocity. If the individual is at rest, most heat loss occurs by natural convection. However, if the individual is exercising and running, forced convection plays a larger role. If the wind velocity is high, cold is felt to be more penetrating because heat is lost more rapidly. The transfer of heat by the bloodstream to the skin is important. The body can lose roughly 1 kcal. of heat per hour for each liter of blood at 37°C. (98.6°F.) that flows to the skin and returns to the body core at 36°C. (96.8°F.). In cold, vasoconstriction prevents heat loss by convection. The converse is true in heat or during exercise, when vasodilation can increase heat flow almost ten times, proving an efficient avenue for heat transfer.[32] Convective heat transfer assumes greater importance during increased muscular activity.

Heat exchange occurs not only at the skin surface. When warm blood in the arteries comes in contact with cooler venous blood returning from the skin and peripheral tissues heat in the arteries is transferred to the cooler venous blood. This exchange is referred to as *countercurrent exchange*. It can reduce convective heat transfer and helps maintain a constant body temperature even when the extremities may be quite cold. This mechanism is particularly well developed in wading birds, allowing them to stand for long periods in cold water.

Evaporation. In the change of water from a liquid to a gaseous state, thermal energy is required. For each gram of water evaporated from the skin, 0.58 kcal. of heat is lost.[29] Without active sweating (i.e., from the insensible water loss from the lungs and skin, some 600 ml./day), man loses approximately 10 kcal./m.²/hr.[33] Insensible water loss constitutes the only evaporative heat loss for temperatures below 28°C. (82.4°F.).[33] Decreases in body temperatures below 37°C. (98.6°F.) inhibit sweating, and cooling by evaporation ceases except for insensible water loss.[29] Evaporation of water (sweat) is an efficient way to lose heat in a warm environment. Excess insensible losses from evaporation, even in a cold environment, cause dry itchy skin and nasal and pharyngeal irritation and disturbances. (Humidifiers are often needed to correct this situation.) This method of heat loss accounts for 25 per cent of total heat loss.[3, 29, 32] Above 30°C. (86°F.) as sweating is initiated, evaporative heat loss increases linearly as temperatures increase. This corrects for the decreasing heat loss from radiation and convection. When skin and environmental temperatures are equal, all metabolic heat must be lost by evaporation. Evaporation, which depends upon sweat secretion, is considered a chief protective mechanism of the body against overheating.

Sweat Glands. The number of sweat glands in man is prodigious—close to 2.5 million.[32] They are controlled by the central nervous system via sympathetic innervation. Secretion of sweat occurs as a result of thermal stimuli, muscular activity and emotional or mental stress. Stress in particular triggers sweat glands in the palms of the hands and soles of the feet. Thermal sweat, in response to heat stimuli, is chiefly produced by the eccrine glands. The motor nerves acting on these glands are sympathetic, but the glands are innervated by cholinergic fibers though they are also stimulated by epinephrine and norepinephrine circulating in the blood.[29] The activation of sweating in situations of stress and forms of circulatory shock accounts for the cold clammy skin that is observed in these conditions.

In cold weather, sweat production is minimal, but it can increase to 4 L./hr. in a person maximally acclimatized to heat,[29] and heat loss can increase to 110 kcal./m.²/hr.[33] Sweating can be initiated by either high skin temperature or high internal temperature; as each increases, sweating increases. If the heat stress is moderate, sweating can continue indefinitely, but the ability to sweat at high rates declines during long exposure to severe heat stress.[33] Sweating is particularly evident on the forehead and lower extremities. A person exposed for several weeks to hot climates, as a result of increased sweat gland capability, sweats progressively more profusely.[29] Sweat contains sodium; therefore, sodium depletion may occur. With acclimatization, however, sweat contains less sodium. Initial losses of sodium may be as high as 10 to 15 Gm./day but even as the amount of sweat increases, the sodium loss drops to 3 to 5 Gm./day.[29] In the presence of high humidity, evaporative heat loss will decrease. If the skin is very wet, sweat gland function is inhibited, while the reverse occurs if the skin is dried. With high humidity, the individual continues to sweat, but it becomes more difficult to lose body heat because the sweat remains in the fluid state. Convection by air currents increases evaporative heat loss; therefore fans and dehumidifiers aid in heat dissipation.

An important mechanism in the body for heat loss is vasodilatation, which occurs in response to stimuli from warm sensors. This brings heat to the surface and allows for removal by radiation, convection, conduction and evaporation. In fact, sweating and the resultant loss of heat occur only if a supply of heat is brought to the skin surface. By vasodilation, body heat conductance can increase seven times over the basal rate if there is heat stress, be it external or internal. An increase as little as 0.3°C. in the hypothalamic temperature initiates vasodilation; rapid vasodilation occurs with an increase

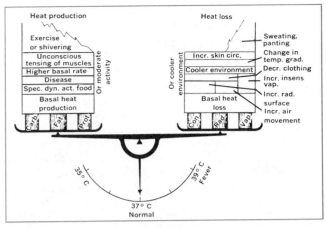

Figure 28–3. Balance between factors increasing heat production and heat loss. (From DuBois, E. F.: *Fever and the Regulation of Body Temperature.* Springfield, IL, Charles C Thomas, 1948.)

in temperature of 0.8°C.[8] Peripheral circulation therefore increases with temperature increase, and the skin generally appears flushed or pink in color and is warm to touch.

Figure 28–2 diagrammatically summarizes the human thermoregulatory system. The heavy lines indicate energy transfer and the thin lines refer to information that is transferred.

Figure 28–3 describes not only the balance between heat production and heat loss but the methods by which these occur and the factors that influence the system.

MODIFICATION AND ALTERATION OF BODY TEMPERATURE REGULATION

Age and Thermoregulation

As a person grows older, the mean body temperature lowers. This is especially noticeable in a cool or cold environment. Though the older person often feels "cold" (prefers added layers of clothing and a warm room), sensitivity to cold may be decreased.

Thermoregulation of the Newborn. The thermoregulating capacity of newborn infants is immature. This is especially true of premature infants. Nurses in neonatal units have a vital responsibility to protect the infants from wide variations in environmental temperatures. Alterations in body temperature place unnecessary stress on newborns and adversely

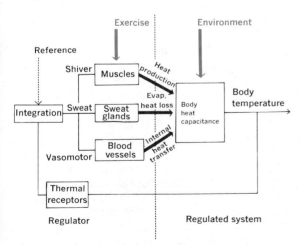

Figure 28–2. Simplified block diagram of human thermoregulatory system. (From Stolwijk, J. A.: Mathematical model of thermoregulation. *In* Hendy, J. D., et al.: *Physiological and Behavioral Temperature Regulation.* Springfield, IL, Charles C Thomas, 1970.)

influence respiratory effort, nutritional status, acid-base balance and the infant's feeling of security. Premature infants with lowered temperatures have a greater chance of dying than those protected against heat loss.[47, 52, 53] A warm environment promotes growth, preserves energy stores and enhances survival.

Premature infants and very small infants respond rapidly to changes in environmental temperature. Premature babies and infants during the first month are unable to shiver. Compared to adults, they have a larger surface area for heat loss. Muscle mass to produce heat is small, and their mechanisms for producing heat are limited. Premature infants have little subcutaneous fat for insulation and the blood vessels that are close to the skin further augment heat loss.[52] Thermogenesis in infants relies little on muscle contraction; instead, chemical thermogenesis is of greater importance.

The source for thermogenesis is considered to be the fat, or *brown adipose tissue*, which is rich in energy-producing mitochondria. This tissue contributes 10 per cent of an infant's body weight and is present behind the sternum, in the neck, between the shoulder blades and surrounding the kidneys and adrenal glands. This tissue is located near vital organs and major vessels where the produced heat can be most effective.[73] If the infant is continually stressed by cold, this tissue is rapidly used up.

At birth, a *wet* newborn loses approximately 200 cal. of body heat/kg. of body weight/minute.[52] Therefore, in order to maintain a temperature of 37°C. (98.6°F.), it is important to dry and clothe the infant quickly and to then place the infant in a radiant warmer or Isolette. The temperature should be monitored frequently until stable.[52] Axillary temperatures may be taken in premature infants since the difference between axillary temperatures and those taken rectally has been shown to be only 0.05°C. (95 per cent of the axillary temperatures in one study had stabilized within 4 minutes when taken with a conventional mercury-in-glass thermometer).[76] During the warming period of a neonate following birth, the infant must be carefully observed for apnea, which may ensue if the warming is too rapid.[47] Controversy still exists as to how rapidly a neonate should be warmed, but in any case, care and close supervision are warranted. There is some evidence that brain development may be adversely affected by a period of low energy input and increased heat loss immediately following birth. Data suggest that it is important that infants be fed and nursed in thermally neutral comfortable environments.[35]

Fever

A fever is conventionally defined as an elevation in body temperature beyond that which is usual for an individual. Such elevation in body temperature most often stems from either inadequate heat loss or what appears to be an elevated setpoint with an intact thermoregulatory mechanism. Fever is generally considered to be the latter, i.e., when there is an elevated temperature in a resting individual greater than 37°C. (98.6°F.) related to an elevated setpoint. This fever may indicate a disease process. Except in the elderly, a temperature below 36°C. (96.8°F.) is generally considered *low* or *hypothermic*. A consistently elevated temperature beyond 37.1°C. but below 38.2°C. is considered a *low-grade fever*. A temperature above 38.2°C. is considered *high-grade fever*. *Hyperpyrexia* or *hyperthermia* is used to describe fevers greater than 40.5°C.[66]

An *intermittent*, or *quotidian*, fever has a pattern whereby the temperature alternates each day or every few days between an elevation and one that is normal. If the fever is *remittent*, the temperature remains elevated, above normal, but there is marked daily variation in its level. In a *relapsing* fever, febrile periods are interspersed with normal periods that last from one to several days. A *hectic* fever refers to an intermittent one that is characterized by *marked* changes in temperature elevations.[23, 45] Fever accompanies many different conditions and disease states. The nurse encounters fevers in patients with varied disabilities: neoplastic disorders, injuries, infections, cerebrovascular accidents, drug reactions and transfusion reactions.

Postulated Hypothesis for the Etiology of Fever. A *pyrogen* is an agent that causes a rise in temperature. In man there exists a substance known as *endogenous pyrogen*, derived from polymorphonuclear leukocytes.[3] It is released when leukocytes are damaged and causes an immediate rise in body temperature by seeming to elevate the temperature setpoint. Many other substances, called *exogenous pyrogens*, act by damaging polymorphonuclear leukocytes and causing release of endogenous pyrogen. Examples of exogenous pyrogens include bacterial toxins, chemical toxins and transfused blood. The exact mechanism by which endogenous pyrogen elevates the temperature setpoint is unknown. Myers et al. suggest that pyrogens change the ratio of sodium and calcium ions in the tissue fluid of the posterior hypothalamus. The ratio appears to determine the discharge rate of the thermoregulatory neurons within the hypothalamus, and leukocyte pyrogen removes the inhibitory influence of calcium ions on the permeability of these neurons to sodium.[4, 8, 26, 34] It is thought that this might displace the "apparent" setpoint.

It should be remembered that not all elevated temperatures are "fevers" in the sense we are using the term. In fever, the balance between heat production and heat loss still exists, but the setpoint is higher. Salicylates do not inhibit heat production, but act to reset the setpoint of the hypothalamus to a normal temperature. Salicylates may antagonize the action of the pyrogen within the hypothalamus, and current research implicates prostaglandins as being involved in the mechanisms of temperature control. Salicylates may reduce temperature by inhibiting prostaglandin synthesis.[26, 34] The mechanism of the other major antipyretic drugs such as acetaminophen (Tylenol, Datril) is unknown.

Signs, Symptoms and Complications of Fever.
Increased heat production accompanies fever and for a short time the increase may be as much as 600 per cent, with abrupt temperature elevations caused by shaking chills.[66] Increased body metabolism and metabolic activity accompany elevations in body temperature and may be as high as 10 to 13 per cent for each 1°C. increase. This increased metabolism places a demand on oxygen consumption. In addition, during shivering and shaking chills, the need for oxygen may increase 400 per cent. There is an increase in oxygen requirement of 13 per cent for each degree Celsius increase.[4] Patients with respiratory and cardiac difficulties may be severely compromised by fever.

Febrile patients reveal various signs and symptoms which must be assessed by the nurse. An individual may or may not know and sense that his temperature is elevated. Initially, the person may feel cold and seek more clothing, blankets, electric blankets, heating pads and/or get into a heat-conserving position. The skin is at first cool and looks pale. In some cases the onset of fever is signaled by shaking chills. The skin will have goose bumps, and there may be severe paroxysms of shaking with chattering teeth. The nurse should note the onset and duration of a chill (which generally lasts 10 to 30 minutes). At this time the nurse's aim is to provide comfort and protection. It is acceptable to provide warmth during the chill; however, *it is contraindicated when shivering ceases.* The nurse may take the temperature during the chill (not orally lest the glass thermometer be broken between chattering teeth) to determine the low point and high point. However, it is vitally important that the *temperature be taken after the chill has ceased*, for it is at this time the temperature will be increased as a result of the increased heat production from muscle activity and shivering. If a hospitalized person is experiencing a chill, the temperature *elevation should be confirmed* and the physician should be notified so that appropriate diagnostic procedures may be instituted (e.g., blood cultures, malarial smears).

Other signs and symptoms to be assessed include the degree of restlessness, whether or not the face is flushed, whether the skin is warm, hot or dry to the touch, and the color and condition of the mucous membranes. The person may complain of thirst and may show other signs of dehydration. Febrile patients often complain of gastrointestinal disorders: anorexia, vomiting, diarrhea or constipation. Some complain of headache, photophobia, general malaise and muscle aches. Delirium may occur in the presence of high fever (39 to 40°C., 102.2 to 104°F.), but in the elderly may be present at lower temperatures. In children, convulsions may be prevalent with high fever. In adults with elevations to 41°C. (105.8°F.), convulsions may also be anticipated. Disturbed levels of consciousness may be observed and irreversible brain damage may result from temperatures higher than 42.2°C. (107.6°F.).[66] In children, the onset of a very high fever may be abrupt and the course of the fever hectic, but the return to normal may be equally dramatic and sudden.

Since most fevers are cyclic to an extent and a return to normal temperature is effected largely by sweating (evaporation), fluid and electrolyte depletion may occur in prolonged febrile illness. Unless contraindicated, fluids should be *increased* and forced. *Intake and output should be measured* and recorded, including specific gravity determination. In acutely ill patients, central venous pressures may assist the nurse in evaluating and correcting fluid balance. If the patient is diaphoretic, clothing and bed sheets should be kept dry, not only for comfort but also to aid in heat dissipation.

In febrile individuals, a mild metabolic acidosis is often present. It is not unusual to see fever blisters on the mouth (herpes simplex), and albuminuria may be evident.[3, 32] In addition to noting body temperature, it is important to note the pulse and respirations. Since an increase in pulse of 10 to 15 beats per minute is not unusual for each 1°C. rise in temperature, the pulse may be rapid and either full or weak.[4, 32] A tachycardia of 130 beats/minute is less significant in a patient with a temperature of 40°C. (104°F.) than in one with a temperature of 37°C. (98.6°F.). Because of the increased oxygen demand, the respiratory rate also increases.

Heat Stroke

Heat stroke is a serious condition manifested by *high internal temperatures*, hot dry skin, delirium or coma and low blood pressure. It may be preceded by weakness, nausea, vomiting, lethargy, headache and visual disturbances. The pulse is rapid; the muscles are weak and flaccid. For reasons that are not well understood, *thermoregulatory mechanisms are altered* and the *sweating and other mechanisms of heat loss* fail. Increased probability of heat stroke should be anticipated when the humidity is 100 per cent and environmental temperature is high in the 30's C. (90's F.). If the individual has been strenuously exercising under similar conditions of humidity, the critical environmental temperature for heat stroke may be about 27 to 30°C. (80's F.). People taking high doses of atropine may be more susceptible, as well as those who suddenly exercise without prior conditioning. Therapy is directed at rapid restoration to normal temperature by immersion in cold (ice water) baths and by supporting blood pressure with IV fluids. Fans increasing the amount of forced convection will accelerate heat dissipation. Friction and massage to the skin and body is necessary to prevent dermal stasis. Gastric lavage with ice saline may be performed or iced saline enemas administered. Approximately 4000 Americans die annually of heat stroke; the mortality rate is as high as 80 per cent, and 80 per cent of the deaths occur in people over 50. However, in high school students, heat stroke is the second most common cause of death.[25]

A related condition which may occur when exposure to severe environmental heat stress places strain on the thermoregulatory system is called *heat exhaustion* (prostration). This ensues from *failure of the cardiovascular system* and results in dyspnea and syncope. Heat cramps may or may not be present. The skin feels cool and clammy and appears pale. *The body temperature may be increased, normal or slightly decreased.* Nursing care includes placing the individual in a supine position out of the sun, in the coolest place possible, and arranging for medical attention.

Malignant Hyperthermia (Anesthesia Hyperthermia)

Anesthesia hyperthermia is a lethal condition associated with the administration of a general anesthetic. Fortunately it is rare. It is hypothesized that as a result of anesthesia, the thermoregulatory reflexes for hyperthermia are suppressed and that excessive heat from increased muscle activity leads to increased body temperature. Succinylcholine is one of the agents implicated, but other drugs are being studied, and there have been cases of anesthesia hyperthermia in which succinylcholine was not used. Once the process has begun, termination of anesthesia does not reverse the hyperthermia. When malignant hyperthermia occurs, there is a sudden and rapid rise in body temperature that continues and is accompanied by cardiac arrhythmias and tachycardia. A rise of 2 to 3°C. in 1 hour is not unusual. Drastic measures are used to lower the temperature. If these are successful, there is no further tendency for the hyperthermia to recur.[32]

HYPOTHERMIA

Hypothermia refers to a core body temperature that is consistently below normal; it varies in degree from mild to deep.

Etiologies. Hypothermia may be either accidental, spontaneous or induced.[75] *Accidental hypothermia* occurs in the elderly, who may not perceive cold; the debilitated; alcoholics, who may lose excess heat from vasodilation in cold climates; and mountain climbers with inadequate experience, preparation or clothing. *Spontaneous hypothermia* may occur in pathologic conditions such as cerebrovascular disease, acute alcoholic intoxication, drug toxicity (especially barbiturates or phenothiazines), severe infections, liver or renal failure, and certain endocrine disorders (e.g., myxedema). Hypothermia is a serious sign and may indicate a poor prognosis in septic shock and cirrhosis. Some individuals run subnormal temperatures for a few days following high fevers. *Induced hypothermia* refers to that instituted for therapeutic purposes. Cold applications have been used for years to reduce swelling, to alleviate fever and pain or increase muscle tone in physical therapy. More recently, cold has been used in the treatment of burns and gastrointestinal bleeding and for neurologic or cardiac surgery. Hypothermia decreases bleeding during surgery as a result of vessel constriction. A further purpose of hypothermia is to decrease the body cells' requirement for oxygen. The need for oxygen may be reduced by 50 per cent if the temperature of the tissue is reduced to 30°C. (80°F.).[7] (Or a reduction of body temperature of 1°C. reduces the metabolism by approximately 12 per cent.[42]) As a form of therapy, mild hypothermia generally is used for neurologic patients and refers to a body temperature of 30 to 35°C. (86 to 95°F.). In moderate hypothermia, the temperature is between 24 and 30°C. (75.2 and 86°F.). Deep hypothermia refers to temperatures below 24°C. (75.2°F.). Moderate or deep hypothermia sometimes is used as an adjunct to surgery, and the degree and duration are strictly controlled.[36]

Signs and Symptoms of Hypothermia. Hypothermia has many effects on the functioning of the body. Some of these effects are desired and are the reason for the induction of hypothermia, e.g., reduction of cerebral edema and high cerebral spinal fluid pressure. Others are untoward but occur, and their presence must be assessed. The blood pressure falls and the respiratory rate slows as a result of hypothermia. At 28°C. (82.4°F.) the respirations generally cease. Bradycardia occurs and the pulse becomes weak. At 30°C. (86°F.) atrial fibrillation is common; at 24°C. (75.2°F.) the blood pressure is low and ventricular fibrillation may occur, with cardiac arrest. Changing levels of consciousness occur with decreasing temperature; amnesia and somnolence are likely at 34°C. (93.2°F.). At 27°C. (80.6°F.) or below, there is little voluntary movement and the individual is unable to speak and is usually comatose. Reflex movement disappears at about 24°C. (75.2°F.). Glomerular filtration decreases with falling temperature and oliguria is evident. Electrolyte disturbances are common and metabolic acidosis is usually present. The clotting time is increased.[4, 7, 32, 36] "Goose bumps" may or may not be present and the skin is pale and mottled. Chills occur as hypothermia is initiated and the individual feels cold and is uncomfortable. As hypothermia progresses, the extremities become numb and a loss of sensation occurs.[4, 7, 32, 35] Some individuals show allergic phenomena in the presence of cold.

Induction of Hypothermia. Various external or internal methods are used to induce hypothermia. *Internal methods* include the use of drugs that alter the thermoregulatory mechanism of the body. They may be used alone or in conjunction with other methods. Chlorpromazine is used to cause vasodilation, to reduce shivering and for sedation. It exerts a direct effect on the hypothalamus and in high doses abolishes the thermoregulatory mechanisms. Promethazine is used to control shivering, and meperidine for sedation. Together they are referred to as the "lytic cocktail" and may reduce the temperature 2°C.[26, 36]

In the operating room during cardiac surgery, direct cooling of the blood by the use of a heat exchanger during extracorporeal circulation is efficient and rapid.

Induced hypothermia by external methods, or surface cooling, includes the use of cool baths, ice packs, cool sponges, iced saline lavages or enemas, and electrically controlled thermal blankets or mattresses. Heat may be lost rapidly if the person is placed in a cool bath, because the thin layer of air that adheres to the skin and acts as an insulator is displaced. Artificially cooled mattresses are used more frequently than cool baths and sponge baths today, and a great amount of heat can be lost by conduction. During hypothermia induction, the person will feel colder than when the temperature has stabilized at the desired lower temperature. Shivering must be prevented and controlled; otherwise it counteracts the desired effect. Obese individuals take longer to cool.

Nursing Responsibilities with Hypothermia. A patient undergoing hypothermia requires constant nursing supervision. The procedure must be carefully explained to the patient without causing undue alarm, which would increase the incidence of shivering. The nurse should closely observe the patient for shivering, which can be detected by an increased muscle tone and quivering movements of the face and pectoral muscles that occur prior to frank shaking chills.[1] *Shivering must be controlled to prevent increases in intracranial pressure.* Shivering also increases the need for oxygen, generates heat and prevents heat dissipation. Chlorpromazine, 25 mg., may be ordered, and if ordered p.r.n. should be administered.

The temperature should be checked frequently; most thermal blanket machines come with rectal probes for monitoring purposes. (Checking is done every 15 to 30 minutes, initially, and then every hour when the temperature is stabilized.[36]) Cooling measures should be stopped 1 to 2°C. above the desired temperatures because temperatures usually drift downward for an additional degree or two after cessation of active cooling. During induction, apical pulse and blood pressure should be monitored every 5 to 15 minutes and every hour thereafter.[36] Cardiac arrhythmias should be anticipated by the nurse and ECG monitoring is desirable. During induction, the patient should be supine to provide a large surface area for heat dissipation. Once the desired temperature is attained, a position of comfort is permitted. If hypothermia is to be prolonged, the skin should be protected from drying by the application of lanolin, cold cream or mineral oil. This also allows for better contact between the skin and the cooling mattress by decreasing the layer of insulating air adherent to the skin. It also protects the skin from cold burns or frostbite.[7] In frostbite, there is blood vessel damage and circulation in the area ceases; the tissue is frozen, and cell aggregates and thrombi result.[66]

All patients should be turned at least every 2 hours and skin care given. The skin should be observed for decubiti, cold burns and fat necrosis. Fat necrosis is consolidated subcutaneous fat which feels hard to the touch. If the person is comatose, eye care and mouth care must be instituted and respiratory assistance may be indicated. Careful monitoring of intake and output is also necessary. Because the absorption, metabolism and excretion of drugs may be altered, the patient must be carefully evaluated for drug side effects.

Rewarming. Warming shock may occur as a result of cardiovascular collapse from vasodilation when patients are warmed. Cardiac arrhythmias may also occur; therefore monitoring of cardiac status and the vital signs is necessary. The health team must be prepared to institute resuscitative measures. *Passive rewarming* may be ordered. This refers to the patient being exposed to normal room temperatures in order to increase body temperature slowly, i.e., 1°C. an hour. *Active rewarming* uses artificial heating devices and warm baths. The temperature of the latter should be around 43.5°C. (110.3°F.). If the temperature of the bath water is lower, it is ineffective because the heat returned to the body is inadequate and is lost by countercurrents.[32] If it is higher, skin damage may occur from an inadequate blood supply.

MEASUREMENT OF BODY TEMPERATURE

Frequently the nurse has the responsibility of taking vital signs. Measurement of body temperature is one component and provides the health team with important data. Body temperature is one of the oldest and most frequently used indicators of whether an individual is healthy or ill. Unfortunately the procedure is often "ritualistic" and follows the routine of an agency rather than being instituted when indicated. Research data reveal that what is recorded and reported may be inaccurate. In one study, only 37 per cent of readings by nursing personnel were identical with those taken by the researchers. For normal or elevated temperatures, 66 per cent of the readings recorded were lower than actual patient temperatures; 61 per cent of the subnormal temperatures were recorded inaccurately at a higher degree.[77]

If temperatures are to be taken, *they must be taken with care and reported and recorded accurately.* If you question the temperature obtained, repeat the procedure with the same or a different thermometer. Temperature monitoring is a serial process providing the data to establish a base against which a person's health status is compared and his progress evaluated. For those reasons, systematic collection and evaluation of data are important.[18, 38]

Thermal Monitoring Devices

Body temperatures have been recorded since the 16th century, when a precursor of the modern glass thermometer was developed. Until recently, the most frequently used thermometer has been the mercury-in-glass thermometer, which operates on the property of thermal expansion—whereby a substance expands as it is heated and contracts as it is cooled. The mercury thermometer consists of a capillary tube that is sealed at one end and has an enlarged cylindrical bulb filled with mercury at the other. Other types of thermometers are thermosensitive probes, thermocouples and thermistors. These operate on one of two principles: heat alters contact voltages or heat changes the resistance of a conductor to electric current. Measurements of the change in voltage (thermocouples) or the change in resistance (thermistors) provide the measure of temperature.

Electronic thermometers are now being used more frequently. The initial problems of accuracy, bulk, cost, servicing and calibrating have been corrected. The new solid-state electronic thermometers are convenient to use, accurate, safe and remarkably quick in registering temperature (usually 30 seconds). Their disposable covers save time and work and prevent contamination.

Thermometers are calibrated in degrees Celsius or Fahrenheit. The Celsius scale (also known as centigrade) is named after Anders Celsius, who originally devised it. In this scale 0°C. is the point at which water freezes and 100°C. is the point at which water boils. The distance between the two points is divided into 100 equal parts, each corresponding to one degree Celsius. In the Fahrenheit scale, water freezes at 32° and boils at 212°. To convert Fahrenheit measurements to Celsius, subtract 32 and multiply by 5/9. To convert Celsius measurements to Fahrenheit, multiply by 9/5 and add 32.

Hazards of Thermometers. Any glass thermometer poses the risk of breaking. If a patient is coughing or has shaking chills, he may inadvertently break the thermometer by biting it. In small infants, rectal thermometers may perforate the colon and rectal wall. When this occurs, the mortality rate has been reported to be high, close to 70 per cent.[48]

Temperature Monitoring Methods

Many agencies in which nurses work stipulate the route and frequency with which temperatures should be taken and recorded, yet nurses should and do exercise considerable discretion and judgment in monitoring temperatures. Temperature measurement should be performed in a manner that is accurate, practical, safe, convenient and efficient.[38] The condition of the patient or individual influences the decision of the nurse in the selection of route and the frequency with which the temperature should be taken.

10. USE OF MERCURY-IN-GLASS THERMOMETERS

By Jean Saxon, R.N., M.N.

Definition and Purposes. *Measurement of the average body core temperature by means of a glass-enclosed tube of mercury calibrated on a Celsius or Fahrenheit scale.* Body temperature is used in conjunction with the other vital signs (respiration, pulse and blood pressure) to assess the patient's present condition.

Contraindications and Cautions. *Oral temperatures* with clinical thermometers should not be taken on children below 4 to 5 years of age (danger of injury to mucosa, inaccurate if mouth open and danger of biting thermometer); patients who can't open or close their mouths because of facial handicaps or injuries or nasal obstruction due to tubes, surgery or injuries; patients with oral infections (e.g., abscessed tooth); and patients who are unconscious or who cannot follow directions. Oral temperature determinations must be delayed for 15 minutes after smoking, taking hot or cold food/fluids, or chewing gum; until a shaking chill ceases; until patient has become acclimated to room temperature after exposure to heat or cold. *Rectal temperatures* should not be taken with clinical thermometers in patients with rectal disorders, e.g., thrombosed hemorrhoids or rectal or perineal injury or surgery. Rectal thermometers must be lubricated and inserted gently and with caution to prevent damage to the mucosa or perforation of the anus or rectum. They must constantly be held in place to prevent progression into the rectum, breaking, or false readings from repeated contractions of the rectal muscles. Some physicians believe that repeated anal stimulation from rectal thermometers produces gastrointestinal and anal irritation in infants. Consequently, nurseries and children's hospitals take rectal temperatures only when especially ordered. Rectal temperatures are not taken routinely on patients with heart attacks (myocardial infarction) because of the theory that anal stimulation can produce bradycardia (slow pulse) due to stimulation of the vagus nerve. *Axillary thermometers* must be held in place to maintain accurate position.

> *Children or adults who are not responsible should* never *be left alone with a thermometer.*

Patient-Family Teaching Points.   Provide the patient and family with the following information as appropriate: (a) explain why the patient's body temperature is being measured; (b) explain the body temperature measurement in terms of "normals"; (c) teach about types of thermometers and how to shake down, read and care for thermometers; (d) explain therapy in terms of patient's temperature and other vital signs, e.g., more fluids, medications; (e) explain factors that influence choice of route for measuring body temperatures: and (f) emphasize temperature readings that should be investigated further.

PRE-PROCEDURE ACTIVITIES

PRELIMINARY ASSESSMENT

Includes determination of
- diagnosis
- date and type of surgery
- ability to follow directions
- presence of oxygen, nasogastric tube, rectal tubes or dressings
- previous method of temperature determination
- last measurement and range of temperatures
- present need to measure temperature

EQUIPMENT

- thermometer (pear, stubby or long mercury bulb as appropriate)
- paper and pencil or pen
- plastic covers for thermometer
- toilet or facial tissue
- thermometer tray, bedside thermometer holder, or plastic box for thermometer and plastic covers
- for rectal temperature taking, also obtain water-soluble lubricant and disposable glove

PRELIMINARY PLANNING

- Includes determination of method of temperature to be taken—oral, rectal or axillary
- location of equipment in health agency, e.g., thermometer tray, plastic box in bedside stand, individual thermometer in holder on wall or counter with or without a disinfectant

PREPARATION OF PATIENT

- Explain to patient that his temperature will be taken, even if patient is not responsive
- Tell patient not to eat, drink, smoke or chew gum 15 minutes prior to oral temperature
- Explain to patient how he will assist in temperature determination
- Wash hands to protect patient

PROCEDURE

SUGGESTED STEPS	RATIONALE/DISCUSSION

Oral Temperature

A. *Oral temperature* for individuals over 4 or 5 years of age, able to follow directions, close lips and breathe through nose, and with healthy nose and throat

A. Generally the most accurate, convenient measurement of core temperature. Normal range 36.5°C. to 37.5°C. (97.6°F. to 99.4°F.). A long, pear or stubby bulb *oral* thermometer is used.

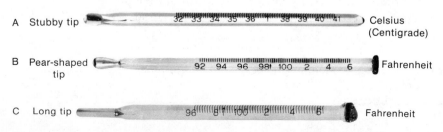

A Stubby tip ... Celsius (Centigrade)

B Pear-shaped tip ... Fahrenheit

C Long tip ... Fahrenheit

Figure 28–4. Oral thermometers have stubby *(A)*, pear-shaped *(B)* or long *(C)* tips; those with stubby or pear-shaped tips are also used as rectal and axillary thermometers. All designs are available in the Celsius (centigrade) scale *(a)* or the Fahrenheit scale *(B* and *C)*. (Courtesy of Becton, Dickinson and Company, Rutherford, NJ 07070.)

SUGGESTED STEPS	RATIONALE/DISCUSSION

Oral Temperature (Continued)

1. Hold thermometer at end opposite bulb.	1. Prevents touching bulb end which will be placed in patient's mouth.
2. Rinse in *cold* water if thermometer has been soaked in disinfectant. Dry with clean tissue, from bulb end to fingers.	2. Hot water, over 41°C. (106°F.), will break mercury thermometers. Avoid dripping water on floor or furniture. Maintains asepsis of bulb end.
3. Read level of mercury in good light.	3. Heat expands mercury in thermometer, causing it to rise in the stem. Constriction in mercury tube prevents mercury from dropping back into bulb unless thermometer is shaken.
a. Hold thermometer with fingertips of right hand horizontal to floor with bulb to your left at eye level (or below head for individuals with bifocals).	a. Numbers would be upside down if held in left hand.
b. Rotate thermometer with hand until numbers and long and short lines can be seen simultaneously.	b. Note that each small line measures 0.1°C on Celsius thermometer and 0.2°F on Fahrenheit thermometer (Fig. 28–4).
c. Very slowly rotate the thermometer back and forth until flat silver mercury line comes into view.	c. Mercury is colored red by some manufacturers.
d. Read measurement to the nearest line.	
4. Shake down thermometer if mercury above 35.0°C. or 95.0°F.	4. Thermometer measures heat; reading must be below actual temperature of the patient before use.
a. Grasp the thermometer securely at upper end.	a. Maintains asepsis of bulb end.
b. Stand away from walls, furniture and equipment.	b. Avoids striking thermometer and breaking it.
c. Flex wrist and give snapping movement of hand, as in cracking a whip.	c. Produces centrifugal force needed to move mercury past constriction and into bulb.
5. Place plastic cover on thermometer.	5. Maintains asepsis of patient's personal thermometer. Decreases contamination, therefore decreases cleaning time of common-use thermometer.
6. Moisten thermometer in cold water and/or ask patient to moisten lips.	6. A dry thermometer will adhere to dry mucous membranes. Danger of tearing tissue when thermometer removed.

Procedure continued on the following page

SUGGESTED STEPS	RATIONALE/DISCUSSION

Oral Temperature (Continued)

7. Place bulb of thermometer *under* patient's tongue in the anterior sublingual area. This area is a pocket formed by the frenulum of the tongue, base of the tongue and floor of the mouth on the right or left side.

7. The "heat pocket" at posterior base of the tongue adjacent to the molars is more accurate, but the thermometer easily moves from the correct position. The anterior sublingual area is used by most helpers; therefore comparison of serial measurements is more meaningful.

8. Tell patient to close lips around thermometer, but not to bite with teeth.

Caution: *Thermometer can break if bitten. Danger of suffering cuts of mouth or lips or lacerations of gastrointestinal tract if swallowed.*

9. Leave in place 9 to 10 minutes. (Other vital signs can be taken during this time.)

9. Research studies show that clinical thermometers require this length of time. If patient opens mouth, count time again.

10. Grasp end of thermometer and ask patient to open his mouth.

10. Allows for visualization of area before thermometer is removed.

11. Lift the thermometer from mouth carefully. Moisten mouth with cool water if thermometer adheres to lips or mouth.

11. Prevents injury to mucous membranes.

12. Push off plastic cover by grasping at finger end, or use a tissue to wipe off secretions with back and forth rotary friction motion from fingers to bulb end.

12. Allows for visualization of thermometer markings and mercury. Pushing off plastic cover or wiping away from fingers protects helper from contamination. Friction removes mucus from grooves in thermometer markings.

13. Read thermometer measurement. (See 3 above.)

Caution: *Studies have shown careless readings are a large source of error.*

14. Record temperature on paper.

14. Celsius is recorded in nearest one tenth of a degree. Fahrenheit is recorded in nearest two tenths of a degree.

15. Care for thermometer according to agency policy.

15. Oral clinical glass thermometers are a source of oral contamination.

a. Place thermometer in common receptacle for processing in central supply, or

b. Return thermometer to plastic box with plastic covers after shaking down, or

c. If thermometer is left in a holder with or without disinfectant, cleanse thermometer with cold running water,

c. Studies have shown that disinfectant in thermometer holders quickly becomes a reservoir for bacterial growth

SUGGESTED STEPS	RATIONALE/DISCUSSION
using back and forth rotary friction with a tissue, shake down.	unless disinfectant is changed daily and thermometers are washed after each use.
16. Wash hands upon leaving patient.	16. Protects helper and others.

Rectal Temperature

B. *Rectal temperature* for individuals who are not able to have an oral temperature taken, who have healthy perineal tissue, and for whom axillary method is too difficult to use.	B. Normal range of rectal temperature 37.0°C. to 38.0°C. (98.6°F. to 100.4°F.). A pear or stubby bulb *rectal* thermometer is used.
1. Follow steps 1 to 5 in A above.	
2. Draw curtains, close door.	2. Prevents patient's embarrassment due to exposure.
3. Tell patient to turn on his side, with upper leg flexed, or assist him as necessary. Infant should be placed on side if possible.	3. Places patient in position which allows visualization of anus and placement of thermometer at correct angle.
4. Fold back bed clothes to expose anus.	4. Exposes anus, but maintains warmth and privacy as much as possible.
5. Put on disposable glove if taking temperature of adult patient.	5. Protects helper's fingers from contamination from skin in area of patient's anus.
6. Lubricate thermometer at bulb end with water-soluble jelly for distance of 1 cm. (½ inch) for infant, 7.5 cm. (3 inches) for adult.	6. Prevents friction and adherence of thermometer to mucosa of anus and rectum.
7. Lift upper buttock to expose anus. If orifice difficult to visualize, ask patient to bear down as when moving his bowels.	7. Allows for better visualization if skin tags or hemorrhoids obscure orifice.
8. Insert bulb end of thermometer into anal orifice in the direction of patient's umbilicus to depth of 1 cm. (½ inch) for infants and 7.5 cm. (3 inches) for adult. Slide thermometer along wall of rectum.	8. Direction of insertion conforms to anatomy of rectum.

> Caution: *Do not use pressure or force to insert thermometer. Thermometer may break or perforation of anus or rectum can occur.*

Maintaining same depth of thermometer insertion enables more accurate comparisons of serial readings. Keeping thermometer on rectal wall measures temperature of blood in hemorrhoidal artery and not the possibly higher temperature of feces.

Procedure continued on the following page

Rectal Temperature (Continued)

9. *Hold* in place for 2 to 4 minutes. (Respiration and pulse may be obtained during this time.)	9. Some studies recommend 2½ minutes, others 3 minutes. Holding ensures accurate reading and prevents displacement of thermometer, prevents injury to tissue or loss of thermometer into rectum or bed.
10. Remove thermometer in the same direction inserted.	10. Prevents injury to rectum and anus.
11. Wipe thermometer with toilet tissue from fingers to bulb end using twisting motion or push off plastic cover.	11. Cleans thermometer. Protects helper's fingers and provides for visualization of mercury.
12. Discard used tissue on several thicknesses of toilet tissue and place thermometer on toilet tissue (or in plastic box or container if not contaminated).	12. Prevents spreading bacterial contamination from tissue and thermometer. Do not place tissue in patient's waste container or in his bedside waste sack.
13. Wipe patient's anal area to remove lubricant and feces.	13. Lubricant feels wet and uncomfortable.
14. Cover patient and assist him to a comfortable position.	14. Assess patient's comfort and safety.
15. Read thermometer measurement.	15. See A-3 above.
16. Care for thermometer according to agency policy.	
a. Place in common rectal receptacle for processing in central supply, or	a. Rectal thermometers are separated from oral thermometers for esthetic reasons.
b. Shake down thermometer after removing plastic sheath and glove and return thermometer to plastic box, or	b. Removing glove prior to handling thermometer protects thermometer from contamination.
c. If thermometer is to be left in holder with or without disinfectant, cleanse thermometer with soap on tissue and cold running water, using back and forth rotary friction. Dry and shake down.	c. Gloved hand protects helper's hand from contamination.
17. Pick up soiled tissue in gloved hand and pull glove off wrist, turning inside out. Discard glove in soiled utility room with tissue inside glove.	17. Prevents spreading bacteria and protects helper from gross contamination.
18. Wash hands.	18. Prevents spreading contamination.
19. Record temperature on paper, with "R" to indicate rectal route.	19. Record Celsius readings to nearest tenth and Fahrenheit to nearest two-tenths of a degree. Record route when not oral. Delayed recording requires memorizing temperature until hands are clean.

SUGGESTED STEPS	RATIONALE/DISCUSSION

Axillary Temperature

C. *Axillary temperature* for infants or others who cannot have an oral temperature taken. Axilla must be accessible and tissue healthy.

C. Axillary temperature is the best method for infants. The axilla is a hygienic, accessible site. Some patients may be unable to maintain the necessary position for 10 minutes. Normal range 36.0°C. to 37.0°C. (96.6°F. to 98.4°F.). A pear or stubby tipped oral thermometer is used. (Danger of injury to tissues with long bulb.)

1. Repeat steps 1 to 5 of A above.

2. Ask patient to lie down in bed.

   2. Prevents danger of dropping thermometer on floor.

3. Ask patient to remove arm from sleeve of gown; assist as necessary.

   3. Prevents displacement of thermometer by tight clothing; exposes axilla.

4. Dry axilla by patting gently with a tissue.

   4. Friction is not used because of heat produced. Moisture cools skin.

5. Ask patient to place hand over chest and lift elbow; assist as necessary.

   5. This "wing-like" position provides the largest axillary "pocket."

6. Place bulb of thermometer in axilla with bulb end pointed toward patient's head. Ask patient to lower elbow to bed keeping hand in contact with chest; assist as necessary.

   6. Provides airtight pocket, with bulb in contact with skin over axillary artery.

7. Leave in place for 11 minutes (4 minutes for premature infants).

   7. If thermometer moves from area or air is introduced, count time again.

8. Hold exposed end of thermometer and maintain position of patient's arm if patient is unable to follow directions. Always hold for infants and children.

   8. Prevents an inaccurate measurement due to displacement of thermometer or exposure to air. Prevents danger of breaking thermometer.

9. Grasp end of thermometer and raise patient's elbow.

   9. Raising elbow prevents tissue injury from friction of thermometer on skin.

10. Push off plastic cover or wipe thermometer dry with tissue.

10. Allows for visualization of thermometer markings and mercury level.

11. Read thermometer measurement.

11. See A-3 above.

12. Record temperature on paper, with "A" to indicate axillary route.

12. Record Celsius to nearest tenth and Fahrenheit to nearest two-tenths degree. Label route other than oral.

13. Assist patient with placing arm in gown and to a comfortable position.

13. Assess comfort and safety of patient.

Procedure continued on the following page

SUGGESTED STEPS	RATIONALE/DISCUSSION

Axillary Temperature (Continued)

14. Care for thermometer according to agency policy. Axillary thermometers are handled with oral thermometers. (See A-15 above.)	14. Axillary thermometers are less of a contamination hazard than oral or rectal thermometers. Intact skin is the body's first line of defense.
15. Wash hands upon leaving patient.	15. Protects self and others.

POST-PROCEDURE ACTIVITIES

Tell patient and family the patient's temperature if appropriate. Ensure patient's comfort and safety. Provide oral fluids if indicated.

Aftercare of Equipment. Follow agency policy. Give individual thermometer unit to patient and family on discharge if unit has been billed to the patient.

Final Patient Assessment. Evaluate patient's temperature in comparison to behavior, appearance and other vital signs. Recheck temperature with another thermometer and/or another route if temperature measurement not reasonable. *Chart/report* temperature on TPR "Day Sheet," bedside vital signs sheet or graph and/or "Graphic Sheet" in chart. Write "A" for axillary route or "R" for rectal route. Immediately report deviations from normal to team leader, charge nurse and/or physician as appropriate.

11. USE OF ELECTRONIC AND DISPOSABLE ORAL THERMOMETERS

By Jean Saxon, R.N., M.N.

Definition and Purposes. *Predictive measurement or measurement as close as possible to arterial blood temperature (approximate core temperature) by means of an electronic sensor probe or heat-fired disposable chemical probe. Instruments are calibrated in Celsius or Fahrenheit (or both) scales. Oral thermometers measure temperature in the "heat pocket" (junction of base of tongue and floor of mouth at level of the right or left lower molar teeth), an area which has a rich lingual artery blood supply and is near the carotid arteries. Electronic instruments are predictive in 2 to 60 seconds on a digital readout, dial or scale. Chemical dot thermometers contain chemical units which change color at specific temperatures in 45 seconds. Single temperature measurement provides data for assessing a patient's present condition; serial temperature measurements provide data for assessing the course of a patient's condition. Temperature data are always evaluated in conjunction with other vital signs data.*

Contraindications and Cautions. Follow manufacturer's directions exactly to avoid errors. Check calibration and accuracy according to directions. Oral determinations should not be taken on patients who cannot open mouth because of facial handicaps or injuries, follow directions, or maintain tongue in position long enough for instrument to register. Remove lower dentures or removable bridges. Delay temperature determinations for 15 minutes after smoking, taking hot or cold food or fluids, chewing gum or exposure to cold atmosphere. *Note:* Some instruments are calibrated for temperature registration with mouth closed and some with mouth open. Follow directions of manufacturer for rectal or axillary determinations when unable to use oral route.

Patient-Family Teaching Points. Provide the patient and family with the following information as appropriate: (a) explain that properly used electronic and chemical thermometers are as accurate as mercury-in-glass clinical thermometers; (b) explain why the patient's body temperature is being monitored; (c) explain the body temperature "normals"; and (d) explain how patient's temperature and other vital signs affect his therapy, e.g., fluids, medications, activity.

PRE-PROCEDURE ACTIVITIES

PRELIMINARY ASSESSMENT

Includes determination of:
- diagnosis
- date and type of surgery
- ability to follow directions
- ability to open mouth (and close if necessary)
- previous measurement and range of temperatures

PRELIMINARY PLANNING

- Determine feasibility of oral route
- Locate equipment and inspect for proper function: *electronic*—functioning batteries, correct calibration, rolling cart if needed, oral probe attachment and probe covers; *chemical*—box of thermometers open less than 3 days and stored at 15 to 30°C. with 30 to 70 per cent relative humidity; intact individual dispenser case

EQUIPMENT

- Electronic thermometer oral probe and probe covers (see Fig. 28–5A to C) or chemical thermometer (see Fig. 28–6)
- Paper and pencil

PREPARATION OF PATIENT

- Explain to patient that his temperature will be taken
- Tell patient not to eat, drink, smoke or chew gum 15 minutes prior to temperature determination
- Ask patient to remove lower denture or removable bridge
- Wash hands to protect patient

PROCEDURE

SUGGESTED STEPS

A. Electronic oral thermometers

1. Check that *oral* probe is plugged into electronic unit.

RATIONALE/DISCUSSION

A. As accurate as clinical mercury-in-glass thermometers, *provided* manufacturer's directions for care and operation are followed.

1. Some units, such as LaBarge Model 12, have separate circuitry for various probes (oral, rectal and continuous). Incorrect probe may give a false high or low reading.

Procedure continued on page 651

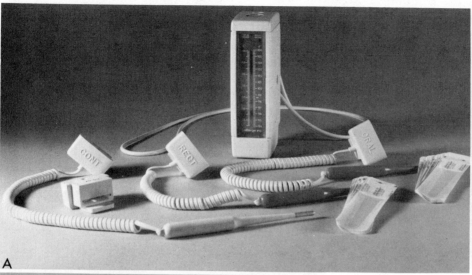

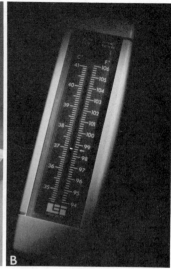

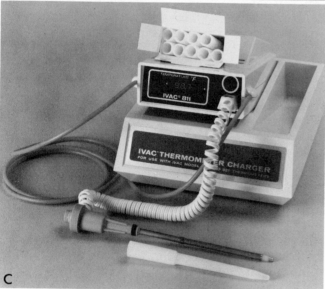

Figure 28–5. *A,* LaBarge Model 12 electronic thermometer, probes and probe covers. *B,* LaBarge Model 12 "DIGILOG" temperature readout. *C,* IVAC Model 811 electronic thermometer with digital readout, oral probe and probe covers. (*A* and *B* courtesy of LaBarge, Inc., St. Louis, MO 63102. *C* courtesy of IVAC Corporation, San Diego, CA 92121.)

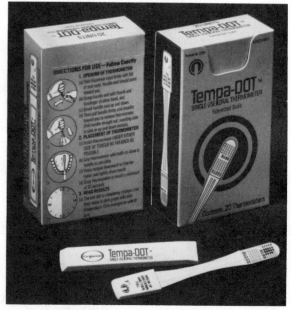

Figure 28–6. Tempa-DOT chemical disposable thermometers. (Courtesy of Organon Pharmaceuticals, West Orange, NJ.)

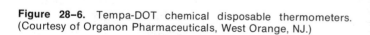

SUGGESTED STEPS	RATIONALE/DISCUSSION
2. Check for adequate power source.	2. Some units contain rechargeable batteries and others replaceable batteries.
3. Insert probe into disposable probe cover; tip touching end of cover.	3. Use probe cover and probe designed for the unit. Correct temperature reading requires use of instrument as designed by manufacturer.
4. Ask patient to open mouth and lift tongue. Place probe tip in "heat pocket" at posterior base of tongue on right or left side. Ask patient to lower tongue.	4. Worker holds probe in place because displacement from "heat pocket" will give lower, incorrect reading. Probe tip must be in contact with tissue in "heat pocket." See Figure 28–7.

> Caution: *Incorrect placement of tip of electronic thermometer probe results in misleading readings. Highest oral temperature reading is not under the anterior part of tongue but is at posterior base of tongue.*

SUGGESTED STEPS	RATIONALE/DISCUSSION
5. Ask patient to close mouth if indicated.	5. Units are designed differently; for mouth open or closed. If not stated in directions, ask patient to close mouth if possible, to decrease time of measurement.
6. Maintain position of probe for 2 to 60 seconds (according to manufacturer's direction) and obtain reading on digital readout, e.g., IVAC; dial; or scale, e.g., LaBarge, Model 12 "Digilog." (See Fig. 28–5.)	6. Some models, such as LaBarge Model 12, require disposal of probe cover and reactivation of unit by returning probe to probe holder if probe tip is displaced from heat pocket during temperature taking. Models differ in signal given to indicate unit has recorded the temperature, e.g., audible tone, flashing or steady light.

Figure 28–7. Heat pocket (A) gives the highest reading—36.9°C. (98.4°F.). Traditional site under tongue at front of mouth gives lowest reading—36°C. (96.8°F.). (Adapted from LaBarge, Inc., poster and *The Guthrie Bulletin, 43*:173, April 1974.)

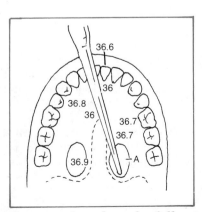

Procedure continued on the following page

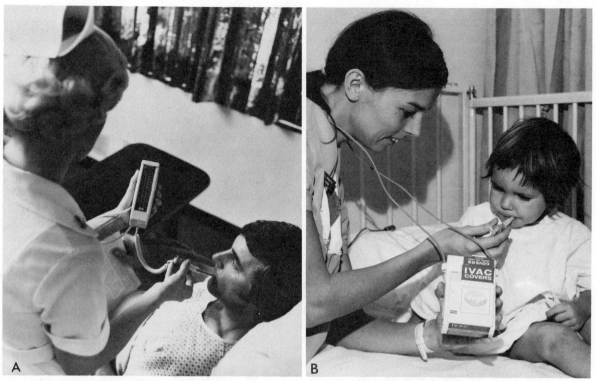

Figure 28–8. *A,* The LaBarge Model 12 electronic thermometer provides simultaneous readings in Fahrenheit and Celsius in less than 30 seconds. (Courtesy of LaBarge, Inc.) *B,* IVAC covers are useful for taking a child's temperature. (Courtesy IVAC Corporation.)

SUGGESTED STEPS	RATIONALE/DISCUSSION
7. Ask patient to open mouth; remove probe.	7. Allows helper to recheck position of probe.
8. Discard probe cover according to manufacturer directions.	8. Protects helper's hands from contamination by oral secretions.
9. Return probe to holder.	9. Turns off power and resets unit for next temperature determination in some units (LaBarge Model 12). Provides protection to sensor probe.
10. Record reading in scale (Celsius or Fahrenheit) of electronic unit. If both scales are displayed, record measurement in scale used in facility.	10. Recording at bedside assists in preventing error.
B. *Chemical Disposable Thermometers.* Tempa-DOT and BMS Single Use Thermometers (Figs. 28–9 and 28–10).	B. As accurate as clinical mercury-in-glass thermometers, provided manufacturer's directions are followed *exactly* for shipping, storage and use of thermometers.
1. Take "Single Use Oral Thermometer" to bedside in dispenser case.	1. Unit must remain sealed until ready to use.

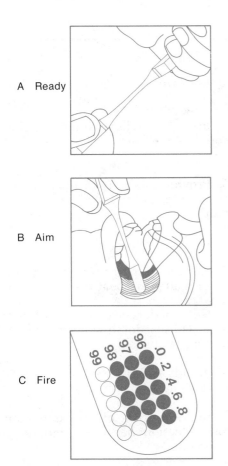

A Ready

B Aim

C Fire

Figure 28–9. Use of the Tempa-DOT disposable oral thermometer. (Courtesy of Organon Pharmaceuticals.)

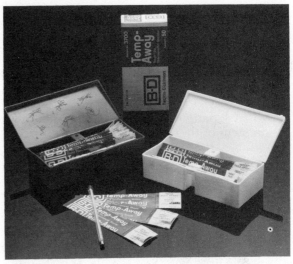

Figure 28–10. Oral and rectal single-use thermometers. (Courtesy of Becton, Dickinson and Company.)

Suggested Steps	Rationale/Discussion
2. Open thermometer.	2. Removes thermometer unit from protective plastic case and activates the dye dots (see Fig. 28–9A).
a. Hold dispenser case firmly in nondominant hand. Point handle toward you.	
b. Grasp handle end with thumb and forefinger of dominant hand.	
c. Break seal by moving handle up and down.	
d. Pull handle straight out with a firm steady pull.	Caution: *Avoid up-and-down or side-to-side motion. Straight pull removes a barrier-film and pressure from a pressure-roller produces contact of dye-impregnated paper and each dot's solid solution.*

Procedure continued on the following page

SUGGESTED STEPS	RATIONALE/DISCUSSION
3. Ask patient to open mouth and lift tongue.	3. Allows worker to visualize "heat pocket."
4. Place thermometer tip in "heat pocket" on right or left side. (See Figs. 28–7 and 28–9B.)	4. Provides oral measurement closest to "core" temperature.
5. Ask patient to lower tongue, bite down on stem of thermometer and close lips.	5. Provides stability of placement of the sensor units and reduces cooling influence of air currents.
6. Leave thermometer in place for a *minimum* of *45 seconds*.	
7. Ask patient to open mouth and lift tongue.	7. Allows helper to verify position of sensor matrix in "heat pocket."
8. Read *highest* measurement of completely fired dot. (See Fig. 28–9C, showing temperature of 98.6°F.)	8. Color of dots change from white to dark green. The last dot showing green is the correct temperature.
9. Record the temperature on paper.	9. Avoids error by recording with labeled dot in sight.
10. Discard thermometer and plastic case in waste container.	10. Reduces risk of contamination and cross infection because complete unit is disposable.

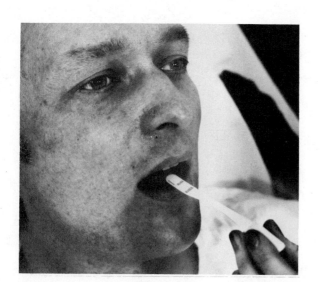

Figure 28–11. Use of the Tempa-DOT oral disposable thermometer. (Courtesy of Organon Pharmaceuticals.)

POST-PROCEDURE ACTIVITIES

Tell patient and family the patient's temperature if appropriate. Ensure patient's comfort and safety, remove or add covers, adjust air currents and room temperature according to patient's temperature. Provide oral fluids if indicated. Worker washes her hands if she has touched patient.

POST-PROCEDURE ACTIVITIES

Aftercare of Equipment. Follow agency policy. Recharge batteries according to schedule recommended by manufacturer. Store electronic unit in a safe, dry area. Wipe off unit as necessary to remove dust or contamination according to manufacturer's directions. Notify appropriate individual for repair or maintenance if electronic unit dropped, damaged or malfunctioning. Store chemical thermometers at room temperature. Once opened, 20 unit box of chemical thermometers should be used within 3 days.

Final Patient Assessment. Evaluate patient's temperature in comparison to behavior, appearance and other vital signs. Recheck temperature with another instrument and/or another route if temperature not reasonable. *Chart/report* temperature on TPR "Day Sheet," bedside vital signs sheet, or graph and/or Graphic Sheet in chart. Immediately report deviations from normal to team leader, charge nurse and/or physician as appropriate.

Rectal Temperatures. Rectal temperatures are believed to be more accurate. They are used in infants, children to the age of 5, delirious patients or those who are unconscious or critically ill. They are also used in patients recovering from oral surgery, or in patients with respiratory difficulty and in individuals who must keep their mouths open or who have had their jaws wired together. However, a rectal temperature is not necessarily more accurate or desirable. It may better reflect the temperature of peripheral blood returning from the legs than the temperature of the core. The temperature registered depends upon the proximity of the thermometer to a major artery and the location of the artery itself; the thermometer must be carefully placed. Contrary to common belief, the rectal temperature is not necessarily 1°F. higher than the simultaneous oral temperature. In fact, studies reveal that it may be the same or higher or lower. Most subjects had rectal readings within 0.2 to 2.8°F. higher than their oral temperatures (67 per cent of the rectal temperatures were less than 1°F. higher and in 22 per cent it was greater than 1°F.). In one study, the difference between oral and axillary temperatures ranged between 0 and 4.2°F.[57] What is important is that when a site is selected, it be used consistently and not changed when subsequent temperature readings are taken.[53] Avoid the trap of comparing temperatures at one site with those from another site on the same patient. For conventional ranges, see procedures.

Tympanic Membrane Monitoring. Monitoring body temperature by the placement of a thermocouple touching the tympanic membrane is indicated if accurate core temperature is desired. Branches of the external carotid artery supply the membrane and the temperature registered reflects that of the thermoregulatory centers of the brain. Tympanic membrane monitoring registers temperature changes that occur with the ingestion of hot or cold foods.[15] These changes are not detected in the rectal temperature.[8, 15]

Oral Temperatures. Oral temperatures are accurate if the thermometers are placed next to a major artery sublingually. The placement is easy, convenient and more acceptable to patients than that for rectal thermometers. Taking temperatures orally is generally safe and reliable; however, it is time-consuming. Oral temperatures may be taken in patients with nasogastric tubes in place. Studies show that they are not contraindicated in patients receiving nasal oxygen.[18, 27, 41] Some agencies require oral temperatures in cardiac patients in order to prevent cardiac arrhythmias from vagal stimulation that may result from rectal stimulation. This danger is minimal, but it is advisable to know the agency policy and to follow your clinical judgment.

Axillary Temperatures. Axillary temperatures may be taken when there are contraindications to the other routes. They are usually considered to be less accurate and more easily influenced by environmental and other variables.

Frequency of Temperature Monitoring. The frequency with which temperatures are taken depends on the situation and institutional policy. The nurse must take a temperature if there is reason to suspect a deviation. Do not wait until the "next scheduled time," even if it is soon. To detect deviations, hospitals routinely require nurses to take temperatures twice a day. Nursing research indicates that once a day is sufficient.[6, 13, 70, 77] Most elevations will be discerned if the temperatures taken in the hospital coincide with the diurnal shift. Therefore, temperatures may be taken in the evening between 4 and 8 PM, preferably closer to 7 or 8 PM. The temperature should be taken more frequently for febrile patients, postoperative patients and those undergoing various diagnostic and therapeutic measures. A chill indicates that the temperature should be taken.

Time Required for the Thermometer to Register the Temperature. The time required for the thermometer to register the temperature depends on the site, the age of the person, the environmental temperature and the type of instrument. Nichols et al. have extensively researched this subject. In an environmental temperature of 20 to 24°C. (68 to 75.2°F.), the optimal placement time for oral thermometers in adults is 9 to 10 minutes. Oral temperatures in children aged 7 to 12 years require 10 minutes. Rectal temperatures require 2 to 4 minutes in adults and 4 minutes in children to register. Axillary temperatures require 11 minutes.[55-62] Other conclusions regarding the time required appear in the literature, but the methodology of the studies is not included so there is no way to evaluate the findings. Following the ingestion of hot or cold foods or liquids, smoking or chewing gum, it is necessary to wait 15 minutes for an accurate temperature.[22]

Nursing Measures in Temperature Regulation

In order to take appropriate action, the nurse interprets and evaluates the temperature data. The normal range for the individual must be known to the nurse. Some individuals routinely run low temperatures whereas others have higher ones. Some individuals easily develop fevers and others do not. This information should be acquired while obtaining the nursing history. Other factors considered by the nurse in interpreting the findings include the environmental temperature, the age of the person, the site used to obtain the temperature, the diagnosis and any emotional stress. (One study on healthy subjects revealed that those who perceived themselves as having to make a greater number of daily life adjustments for examinations, sports and movies also had higher mean temperature ranges.[11]) Especially in children the amount of physical activity should be noted.

A febrile patient should be made comfortable, and the thermoregulatory mechanisms of the body supported. Except during a chill, the person should be lightly covered by a sheet and blanket. Patient clothing and bed sheets should be dry. Intake and output should be monitored and adequate fluid intake maintained. Antipyretic medications should be administered if ordered or such orders obtained. Cooling blankets should be turned on and off as indicated; to minimize electrical hazards, the nurse must check that the particular machine is grounded. The use of fans in the patient's unit may be helpful. The room temperature and humidity should be controlled, if possible. Exposing the skin surface area to air, thereby increasing heat loss, may be desirable if the temperature is very elevated, by removing sheet and blanket. Placing febrile children in tepid baths is also an effective method of lowering the temperature.

Alcohol Sponges. Another method used to lower body temperature is the administration of "alcohol sponges." Though used today less frequently than in the past, alcohol sponges may still be ordered. The method is more likely to be used in the home, since most hospitals use cooling mattresses, which are more effective. It is also used if placing a patient in tepid water is not feasible. After baseline vital signs are taken, alcohol sponges may be applied. Tepid water (20 to 30°C.) [68 to 82.4°F.], is used to increase vasodilation. (Ice or cold water will result in vasoconstriction, which defeats the purpose.) Sometimes some alcohol is added to the water. Evaporation increases heat loss, and as alcohol evaporates (vaporizes) at a lower temperature it is thought to remove the heat from the skin more rapidly. Cold compresses on the forehead or a hot water bottle at the feet may make the patient feel more comfortable. The hot water bottle may also make the patient feel less cold and thus may reduce the incidence of shivering.

Cool sponges over large vessels in the groin and in the axillae may increase heat loss. Each extremity is sponged for 5 minutes and the back, abdomen and trunk each for 5 minutes. An alcohol sponge generally takes 30 minutes. If the patient starts to shiver and other symptoms of cold appear, sponging is stopped. Vital signs are checked upon completion of the alcohol sponge and again in 30 minutes. Forced

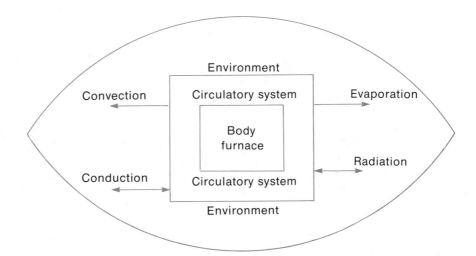

Figure 28–12. Representation of the thermoregulatory system.

convection by electric fans will aid in heat dissipation.

If you use alcohol sponges with children, have an emesis basin ready because the vaporizations of the alcohol may induce vomiting. This may be prevented by good air circulation in the room.

After the sponging, cover the patient lightly.

All temperature readings that are taken should be recorded, but any unusual findings or significant changes are reported immediately. Because certain fever patterns correlate with disease states, and this augments the data base, the nurse looks for fever patterns or trends. Other symptoms noted by the nurse should be recorded and reported. In the presence of an infection, the nurse must consider the complete blood count, the erythrocyte sedimentation rate, and bacteriologic findings in order to evaluate the patient's condition and response to therapy. A low temperature in the presence of active infection is not necessarily a good sign unless it is expected and confirmed as the response to the therapy instituted.

SUMMARY

This chapter has been concerned with the nursing care related to body temperature. The physiologic mechanisms by which man maintains a relatively constant internal body temperature in spite of wide fluctuations in environmental temperature were explored. In a warm environment, body temperature is controlled primarily by varying heat loss, while in a cold environment control depends principally on variation in heat production. In behavioral regulation, man actively manipulates environmental temperature, clothing and humidity based on conscious sensations of heat and cold. Thermal receptors from many parts of the body all provide input to the coordinating center, which interprets and activates effector organs to either conserve, produce or dissipate heat.

Perhaps it will be helpful to think of the thermoregulatory system in the following manner. The body can be represented as a furnace on the inside surrounded by a "fluid jacket" or the circulatory system, which can distribute heat and/or act with other tissues as an insulator system subject to internal adjustments to maintain a constant core temperature.

Alterations in temperature occur as a result of either disturbances in control function (furnace), in heat production (furnace) or from disturbances in distribution (circulatory system) and/or dissipation of heat (circulatory system and environment). Nursing care and medical therapy are directed at supporting thermoregulation and/or at detecting and correcting the underlying disorder.

In order to care for individuals with abnormal temperatures, the nurse needs an understanding of the physiology of thermal regulation. But this understanding is incomplete without knowledge of the physical factors which influence and act on the system; hence they were presented. Finally the nursing responsibilities were outlined. The study guide at the beginning of the chapter and the bibliography that follows will assist you in gaining greater understanding of this complex topic. As you progress in the nursing program, you will learn much more in relation to temperature in disease states and the inherent nursing care.

BIBLIOGRAPHY

1. Abbey, J. C.: The world of work—the world of client: a general systems approach to physiological nursing research. *In* Werley, H. H., et al. (eds.): *Health Research: The Systems Approach*. New York, Springer Publishing Co., 1976, pp. 211–214.
2. Alderson, M. J.: Effect of increased body temperature in the perception of time. *Nursing Research, 23*:42–49, Jan.–Feb. 1974.
3. Atkins, E.: Fever. *In* MacBryde, C. M., and Blacklow, R. J. (eds.): *Signs and Symptoms*, 5th ed. Philadelphia, J. B. Lippincott Co., 1970.
4. Auld, M. E.: Body temperature status. *In* Mitchell, P. H.: *Concepts Basic to Nursing*. New York, McGraw-Hill Book Co., 1973, Ch. 17, pp. 390–409.
5. Bazett, H. C.: The regulation of body temperature. *In* Newburgh, L. H. (ed.): *Physiology of Heat Regulation and the Science of Clothing*. New York, Hafner Publishing Co., 1968, pp. 109–192.
6. Bell, S.: Early morning temperatures. *American Journal of Nursing, 69*:764–766, April 1969.
7. Beland, F. L., and Passos, J.: *Clinical Nursing: Pathophysiological and Psychosocial Approaches*, 3rd ed. New York, Macmillan Publishing Co., 1975.
8. Benzinger, T. H.: Heat regulation: homeostasis of central temperature in man. *Physiological Reviews, 49*:671–759, Oct. 1969.
9. Benzinger, T. H.: The human thermostat. *Scientific American, 204*:134–147, Jan. 1961.
10. Blainey, C. G.: Site selection in taking body temperature. *American Journal of Nursing, 74*:1859–1861, Oct. 1974.
11. Cassidy, C. A.: The relationship between daily life changes, physical symptoms, and body temperature range. *Image, 8*:30–35, June 1976.
12. Cena, K.: Radiative heat loss from animals and man. *In* Monteith, J. L. (ed.): *Heat Loss from Animals and Man: Assessment and Control*. London, Butterworths, 1974, pp. 33–58.
13. DeRisi, L.: Body temperature measurement in relation to circadian rhythmicity in hospitalized male patients. *ANA Clinical Sessions*, New York, Appleton-Century-Crofts, 1968.
14. Devney, A. M., and Kingsbury, B. A.: Hypothermia in fact and fantasy. *American Journal of Nursing, 72*:1424–1425, Aug. 1972.
15. Dickey, W. T., et al.: Body temperature monitoring via the tympanic membrane. *Surgery, 67*:981–984, June 1970.
16. Duffy, T. P.: Hypothermia and hyperthermia. *In* Harvey, A. M., et al. (eds.): *The Principles and Practice of Medicine*, 19th ed. New York, Appleton-Century-Crofts, 1976, pp. 1734–1735.
17. Dyer, E. D., and Bagnell, H. K.: Local tissue and general temperature changes in dogs produced by temperature applications. *Nursing Research, 19*:37–41, Jan.–Feb. 1975.
18. Erikson, R., and Storlie, F.: Taking temperatures: oral, rectal, and when? *Nursing '73, 3*:51–53, April 1973.
19. Everall, M.: Cold therapy. *Nursing Times, 72*:144–145, Jan. 29, 1976.
20. Felton, G.: Effect of time cycle change on blood pressure, temperature in young women. *Nursing Research, 19*:48–58, Jan.–Feb. 1970.
21. Felton, G.: Rhythmic correlates of shift work. *In* Batey, M. V. (ed.): *Communicating Nursing Research: Collaboration and Competition*. Boulder, Western Interstate Commission for Higher Education, 1973, pp. 73–89.
22. Foster, B., et al.: Duration of effects of drinking iced water on oral temperature. *Nursing Research, 19*:169–170, March–April 1970.
23. Fuerst, E. V., et al.: *Fundamentals of Nursing*, 5th ed. Philadelphia, J. B. Lippincott Co., 1974.
24. Gibson, T. C.: A reappraisal of fever in acute MI. *RN, 38*:3–11, May 1975.
25. Goldfrank, L., and Osborn, H.: Heat stroke. *Hospital Physician*, Aug. 1977, pp. 14–18.
26. Goodman, L. S., and Gilman, A. (eds.): *The Pharmacological Basis of Therapeutics*, 5th ed. New York, Macmillan Publishing Co., 1975.
27. Graas, S.: Thermometer sites and oxygen. *American Journal of Nursing, 74*:1862–1863, Oct. 1974.
28. Gragg, S. H., and Rees, O. M.: *Scientific Principles in Nursing*, 7th ed. St. Louis, The C. V. Mosby Co., 1974.
29. Guyton, A. C.: *Textbook of Medical Physiology*, 5th ed. Philadelphia, W. B. Saunders Co., 1976, pp. 955–969.
30. Hardy, J. D., Gagge, A. P., and Stolwijk, J. A. J. (eds.): *Physiological and Behavioral Temperature Regulation*. Springfield, IL, Charles C Thomas, Publisher, 1970.
31. Hardy, J. D.: Heat transfer. *In* Newburgh, L. H. (ed.): *Physiology of Heat Regulation and the Science of Clothing*. New York, Hafner Publishing Co., 1968, pp. 78–108.
32. Hardy, J. D., and Bard, P.: Body temperature regulation. *In* Montcastle, V. B. (ed.): *Medical Physiology*, Vol. 2. St. Louis, The C. V. Mosby Co., 1974.
33. Hardy, T. D., et al.: Man. *In* Whittow, G. C. (ed.): *Comparative Physiology of Thermoregulation*, Vol. 2. New York, Academic Press, 1971, pp. 327–380.
33a. Heineman, H. S.: What to do for the patient with fever. *Consultant, 18*:21, June 1978.
34. Hensel, H.: Neural processes in thermoregulation. *Physiological Reviews, 53*:948–1017, Oct. 1973.
35. Hey, E. N.: Physiological control over body temperature. *In* Monteith, J. L. (ed.): *Heat Loss from Animals and Man*. London, Butterworths, 1974, pp. 77–95.
36. Hickey, M. C.: Hypothermia. *American Journal of Nursing, 65*:116–122, Jan. 1965.
37. Huckaba, C. E., and Downey, J. A.: Overview of human thermoregulation. *In* Iberall, A. S. and Guyton, A. C. (eds.): *Regulation and Control in Physiological Systems*. Dusseldorf, International Federation of Automatic Control, 1973, pp. 212–216.
38. Jarvis, C. M.: Vital signs, how to take them more accurately and understand them more fully. *Nursing '76, 6*:31–37, April 1976.
39. Johnson, B. A., et al.: Research in nursing practice: the problem of uncontrolled situation variables. *Nursing Research, 19*:337–342, July–Aug. 1970.
40. Kalmus, H., and Wilkins, B. R.: Physiological control systems. *In* Kalmus, H. (ed.): *Regulation and Control in Living Systems*. New York, John Wiley & Sons, 1966, pp. 81–136.
41. Kintzel, K. C.: Recognition of clinical problems requiring investigation: a comparative study of oral and rectal temperatures in patients receiving two forms of oxygen therapy. *ANA Clinical Sessions*, held in San Francisco, 1966, pp. 99–103. New York, Appleton-Century-Crofts, 1967.
42. Klingensmith, W.: Inadvertent hypothermia during surgery. *RN, 35*:4–12, March 1972.
43. Kotchek, L. D.: Numbers in nursing. *Nursing Outlook, 19*:653–655, Oct. 1971.
44. Levine, M. E.: *Introduction to Clinical Nursing*. Philadelphia, F. A. Davis Co., 1969.

45. Lewis, L. W.: *Fundamental Skills in Patient Care.* New York, J. B. Lippincott Co., 1976.

46. Luckmann, J., and Sorensen, K. C.: *Medical-Surgical Nursing: A Psychophyciologic Approach.* Philadelphia, W. B. Saunders Co., 1974.

47. Lutz, L., and Perlstein, P. H.: Temperature control in newborn babies. *Nursing Clinics of North America,* 6:15–23, March 1971.

48. Merenstein, G. B.: Rectal perforation by thermometer. *The Lancet, 1:*1007, May 9, 1970.

49. Monteith, J. L., and Mount, L. E. (eds.): *Heat Loss from Animals and Man.* London, Butterworths, 1974.

50. Moorat, D. S.: The cost of taking temperatures. *Nursing Times,* 72:767–770, May 20, 1976.

51. Myers, R. D., and Tytell, M.: Fever: reciprocal shift in brain sodium to calcium ratio as the setpoint temperature rises. *Science,* 1972, pp. 178 and 765–767.

52. Nalepka, C. D.: Understanding thermoregulation in newborns. *Journal of Gynecologic Nursing,* 5:17–19, Nov.–Dec. 1976.

53. Neal, M. V., and Nauen, C. M.: Ability of premature infant to maintain his own body temperature. *Nursing Research,* 17:396–402, Sept.–Oct. 1968.

54. Newburgh, L. H. (ed.): *Physiology of Heat Regulation and the Science of Clothing.* New York, Hafner Publishing Co., 1968.

55. Nichols, G. A.: A replication of rectal thermometer placement studies. *Nursing Research,* 17:360, July–Aug. 1968.

56. Nichols, G. A.: Measuring oral and rectal temperatures for febrile children. *Nursing Research,* 21:261–264, May–June 1972.

57. Nichols, G. A., et al.: Oral, axillary and rectal temperature determination and relationships. *Nursing Research,* 15:307–310, Fall 1966.

58. Nichols, G. A., et al.: Placement times for oral thermometers: a nursing study replication. *Nursing Research,* 17:159–161, March–April 1968.

59. Nichols, G. A., et al.: Rectal thermometer placement times for febrile adults. *Nursing Research,* 21:76–77, Jan.–Feb. 1972.

60. Nichols, G. A.: Taking adult temperature rectal measurements. *American Journal of Nursing,* 72:1090–1093, June 1972.

61. Nichols, G. A.: Time analyses of afebrile and febrile temperature readings. *Nursing Research,* 21:46, Sept.–Oct. 1972.

62. Nichols, G. A., and Verhonick, P. J.: Time and temperature. *American Journal of Nursing,* 67:2304–2306, Nov. 1967.

63. Nielsen, M.: Heat production and body temperature during rest and work. *In* Hardy, J. D., et al. (eds.): *Physiological-Behavioral Temperature Regulation.* Springfield, IL, Charles C Thomas, Publisher, 1970, pp. 205–214.

64. Nielsen, B.: Heat production and heat transfer in negative work. *In* Hardy, J. D., et al. (eds.): *Physiological and Behavioral Temperature Regulation.* Springfield, IL, Charles C Thomas Publisher, 1970, pp. 215–223.

65. Nordmark, M. T., and Rohweder, A. W.: *Scientific Foundations of Nursing,* 3rd ed. Philadelphia, J. B. Lippincott Co., 1975.

66. Petersdorf, R. G.: Alteration in body temperature. *In* Wintrobe, M. N., et al. (eds.): *Harrison's Principles of Internal Medicine,* 7th ed. New York, McGraw-Hill Book Co., 1974, pp. 48–63.

67. Petrello, J. N.: Temperature maintenance of hot moist compresses. *American Journal of Nursing,* 73:1050–1051, June 1973.

68. Riggs, D. S.: *Control Theory and Physiological Feedback Mechanisms.* Baltimore, Williams & Wilkins Co., 1970, pp. 383–400 (Regulation of body temperature).

69. Rowell, L. B.: Human cardiovascular adjustments in exercise and thermal stress. *Physiological Reviews.* 54:75–159, Jan. 1974.

70. Schmidt, A. J.: TPR's: an old habit or a significant routine? *Hospitals,* 46:57–60, Dec. 16, 1972.

71. Scipien, G. M., et al.: *Comprehensive Pediatric Nursing.* New York, McGraw-Hill Book Co., 1975.

72. Spealman, C. R.: Physiologic adjustments to cold. *In* Newburgh, L. H. (ed.): *Physiology of Heat Regulation and the Science of Clothing.* New York, Hafner Publishing Co., 1968, pp. 232–239.

73. Stokes, T. M.: Non-shivering thermogenesis. *Nursing Mirror, 143:*75, Dec. 2, 1976.

74. Stolwijk, J. A. J., and Nadel, E. R.: Sweating response in human thermoregulation. *In* A. S. Iberall and A. C. Guyton (eds.): *Regulation and Control in Physiological Systems.* Dusseldorf, International Federation of Automatic Control, 1973, pp. 221–225.

75. Tolman, K. G.: Why is hypothermia overlooked? *Canadian Nurse,* 67:35–37, Sept. 1971.

76. Torrance, J. T.: Temperature readings of premature infants. *Nursing Research,* 17:312–320, July–Aug. 1968.

77. Walker, V. H., and Selmanoff, E. D.: A note on the accuracy of the temperature, pulse and respiration procedure. *Nursing Research, 14:*72–77, Winter 1965.

78. Whitner, W. M., and Thompson, M. C.: The influence of bathing on the newborn infant's body temperature. *Nursing Research,* 19:30–36, Jan.–Feb. 1970.

CHAPTER 29

MONITORING THE PULSE, RESPIRATION AND BLOOD PRESSURE AND UNDERSTANDING THEIR SIGNIFICANCE

By Carolyn Mueller Jarvis, R.N., M.S.N.

OVERVIEW AND STUDY GUIDE

The pulse, respiration and blood pressure are the *vital signs;** they are indispensable guideposts to the patient's current state of health. They are assessed during a *basic screening physical examination* and upon *admission to the hospital* to establish baseline data from which to judge the significance of any fluctuation. Continued *routine assessment* is necessary because the vital signs are critical indices of a change in the patient's physical or psychologic condition. If such a change occurs, the vital signs are *monitored closely* to aid in planning interventions and to assess the patient's response.

Monitoring of vital signs is an important skill. You will measure vital signs thousands of times during your nursing practice. The technique will flow smoothly as you gain experience, but do not be fooled into performing this assessment hastily or haphazardly. Measuring vital signs is a basic skill upon which your assessment prowess can build. It is the cornerstone for sophisticated problem solving. Although electronic machinery is used in selected situations to help in gathering data, the nurse is irreplaceable in interpreting the data.

For clarity, each vital sign is described separately in this chapter, but every attempt is made to show how they relate to one another and to the patient as a whole. The vital signs are not isolated numbers. They are grouped data that reflect interrelated physiologic systems. From the beginning of your practice, let vital signs aid in your *holistic* appraisal of each patient.

The purposes of this chapter are as follows:

1. To present the physiologic basis for pulse, respiration and blood pressure.

2. To define the normal range of each vital sign as it applies to age, sex, physical state or emotional condition.

3. To describe the technique for measuring vital signs and the underlying principles.

4. To define clinical examples of abnormal vital signs.

Read the following study guide and look for the answers to these questions as you read the chapter. What are the roles of the cardiovascular system and respiratory system in the homeostatic functioning of the human body? How is each system controlled? How does each system respond to external and internal influences? How do the two systems relate to one another?

Familiarize yourself with the following terms:
Pulse:

systole	pulse deficit
diastole	weak thready pulse
cardiac output	pulsus alternans
stroke volume	bigeminy
rate	paradoxical pulse
rhythm	*Respirations:*
PMI	inspiration
tachycardia	expiration
bradycardia	ventilation
cardiac pacemaker	perfusion
arrhythmia	hypoxemia
apical-radial pulse	hypoxia

*Another vital sign, temperature, was discussed in Chapter 28.

hypercarbia
chronic obstructive pulmonary disease (COPD)
dyspnea
stertor
stridor
wheeze
sigh
bronchovesicular
vesicular
rales
rhonchi
tidal volume
tachypnea
bradypnea
hypoventilation
apnea
hyperventilation
Cheyne-Stokes
Biot's
Kussmaul's

apneustic
orthopnea
pallor
cyanosis
Blood pressure:
systolic pressure
diastolic pressure
pulse pressure
Korotkoff sounds
peripheral vascular resistance
mercury and aneroid sphygmomanometers
auscultatory gap
flush method
hypotension
hypertension
coarctation
paradoxical blood pressure

Upon completion of this chapter, you should be able to:

1. Describe internal and external factors which influence vital signs.

2. State the normal values of pulse, respiration and blood pressure, including the normal variation with age, sex, time of day, activity.

3. Perform the techniques of measuring vital signs accurately, including appropriate explanation to patient and family.

4. Distinguish normal from abnormal vital sign data, considering patient's individual characteristics and current physical and emotional state.

5. Interpret data as it fits into each patient's clinical picture, validating when necessary, and communicating results to appropriate persons.

6. Use vital sign data in the assessment step of the nursing process and plan appropriate interventions.

ROUTINE VITAL SIGNS

"Routine" vital signs is a misnomer; rather than a rote task performed automatically so many times per day, the accurate assessment of vital signs is important and crucial for patient care. The nurse must know how to take vital signs, how to interpret the data, communicate it to others, and plan nursing interventions appropriately. Thus taking vital signs is a part of the nursing process.

As you recall, the nursing process (assessment, planning, implementing, evaluating) is a deliberate problem-solving approach to patient care. The first step, assessment, is defined by McCain as ". . . an orderly and precise collection of data about the physiological, psychological, and social behavior of a patient."[28] Assessment is a systematic way of collecting data; it determines nursing judgments, and is the base for development of the nursing care plan. *Taking vital signs means gathering data for the data base.* The more knowledge one has about vital signs, the more enriched the data base will be.

Keep these general guidelines in mind while assessing vital signs:

1. Routine vital signs should be taken by the *person caring for the patient* during that shift—*not* by one person assigned to take vital signs for the whole floor. The former method is actually the most efficient because the staff member who knows the patient best is the one gathering the data and assessing how it fits into the patient's whole health picture.

2. Know the *normal range* of each vital sign.

3. Know the *baseline data* for each patient,

i.e., know what is normal *for him* and know his vital signs from the previous shift. What is "normal" for one patient may differ from the standard range that is typical for his age and physical condition.

4. Know the patient's *diagnosis* and what *treatments* and *medications* he is receiving; these factors may alter the vital sign results.

5. Take the vital signs in a *systematic manner.* Set up a process for yourself and do not vary it or you could omit an important step. Compare the data bilaterally (on corresponding sides on the patient's body) when appropriate.

6. During the shift, gather vital signs as often as you think necessary. Do not wait for the next routine time if you suspect a trend developing. Assessing vital signs is a *serial* process, not a one-time affair. The establishment of trends or the comparison of changes is much more meaningful than stating one-time statistics. For example, after a postoperative patient returns to his room, the order reads, "Check vital signs q 15 min. × 1 hr., then q 1 hr. × 4, then QID." If you note a rapid thready pulse and a B/P significantly below the patient's recovery room value, do not wait for another 15 minutes to elapse. Remain with the patient, check his vital signs at least every 5 minutes, inspect him for signs of hemorrhage, and notify the physician. Your prompt intervention will forestall serious, perhaps fatal, consequences.

7. *Recheck* the vital signs on a *newly admitted patient* at least twice during the first 8 hours of admission. O'Dell suggests pulse and B/P measurement obtained on admission may not be reliable baseline data from which to interpret the patient's subsequent physiologic

status.[32] O'Dell measured the vital signs of 60 adults on admission and at 3 hours and 6 hours after admission. This study showed a significant decrease in systolic blood pressure and pulse rate over the 6-hour period. Diastolic pressure declined too, but not significantly. Temperature and respiration values stayed the same. It was suggested that *anxiety associated with hospital admission* may affect initial readings.

8. At the bedside, be aware of your *nonverbal communication.* If your facial expression and body movements contradict your verbal message, the patient will believe the nonverbal message more than spoken words.[29] That is, assuring a patient he is fine and his vital signs are normal is meaningless if you take the blood pressure three or four times in a row, your brow is furrowed in a concerned fashion, and you call in another staff member to check your findings. The patient will feel much more confident in your skill and in his future if you state the truth, "Your blood pressure is slightly elevated, so I am going to check it a few more times."

9. After collecting the vital signs, put this information together with other data collected about the patient. *Analyze the data* in terms of the patient's complete health status. What *relationships* exist among the data; are any *trends* evolving? Also, consider any *environmental factors* that may influence the data, such as room temperature, humidity, or noise.

Once the data have been collected, analysis leads to the next step, planning the nursing intervention. In order to analyze the data, you must know the physiology behind each of the vital signs, the variations that are normal, and the implications of abnormal vital signs. Let us now review individually the pulse, respirations, and the blood pressure.

PULSE

Introductory Concepts

The heart is a pulsatile pump that regularly ejects blood into the arteries. Sixty to 100 times a minute, specialized cells in the sinoatrial (SA) node initiate an electrical impulse. The current flows in an orderly sequence to all parts of the heart, causing it to contract. This contraction is *systole;* it occupies one-third of the cardiac cycle. *Diastole* (or relaxation) is the resting phase and the time for the ventricles to fill with blood.

This ventricular filling phase constitutes two-thirds of the cardiac cycle. During systole, the heart pumps blood to the pulmonary and systemic circulation simultaneously. The left ventricle pumps an amount of blood into the already full aorta, which greatly increases aortic pressure. This pressure increase expands the wall of the aorta and generates a fluid wave which is felt at a peripheral artery as the *pulse.*

The heart normally beats about 70 times per minute to send 5 L. of blood (the cardiac output) throughout the body. This is expressed as

$$CO = SV \times R$$

That is, the cardiac output (CO) equals the amount of blood in each left ventricular systole (SV) times the heart rate (R) per minute. When internal or external stressors alter either component on the right side of the equation, the other component compensates in order to keep the cardiac output constant. For example, when the stroke volume decreases (as in shock), the heart compensates by increasing its rate; the goal is to maintain a constant cardiac output perfused to the cells.

To determine how efficiently the heart maintains its output, the nurse counts the number of beats per minute and judges rhythm and quality of the pulse. The skills used to assess the pulse include *inspection* and *palpation; auscultation* is used to assess the apical heartbeat if the peripheral pulse is abnormal in some way.

First the patient is inspected for any obvious pulsations. Pulsations may normally be seen in the neck of a recumbent patient and may reflect either the brisk localized carotid artery pulsation or the diffuse undulant pulsation of the jugular veins. The carotid artery lies in the groove between the trachea and the muscles at the side of the neck. Jugular vein pulsations may be seen in the sternal notch and lateral to the neck muscles. The *venous* pulsations normally disappear as the patient is elevated to a sitting position, usually at 45 degrees. Maintenance of distended pulsating neck veins at a sitting position indicates increased central venous pressure, as in heart failure.

A normal pulsation in the left anterior chest is the *point of maximal impulse* (PMI). This is the thrust of the ventricles onto the chest wall during systole. It is located at the fourth or fifth intercostal space in the left midclavicular line (halfway between the sternum and the side of the chest). It may be visible in children and thin adults. When the heart is enlarged (as in congenital heart disease, valvular heart disease, or heart failure), an abnormal pulsation may be seen or palpated over a larger area than that of the PMI. This sustained forceful impulse (known as a *heave* or *lift*) may be seen at the left sternal border, or below and to the left of the normal PMI area.

Pulse Sites

The pulse is palpated over arterial sites that lie close to the skin and are backed by bone or other firm structures. The most common sites for routine assessment are the *radial* in adults and children and the *apical* in infants. Various pathologic states call for assessment of other pulse points (Fig. 29–1).

The *radial* artery is usually the most accessi-

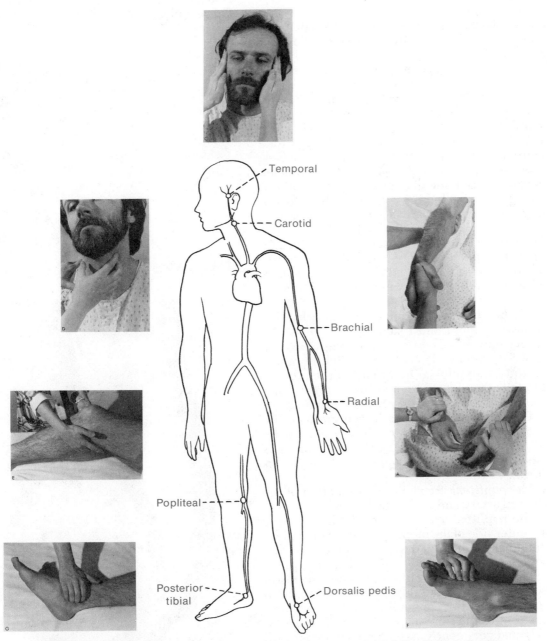

Figure 29–1. Commonly used arterial pulse points. *A*, Posterior tibial. *B*, Popliteal. *C*, Carotid. *D*, Temporal. *E*, Brachial. *F*, Radial. *G*, Dorsalis pedis. (Photographs reprinted with permission from Jarvis, C. M.: Perfecting physical assessment. Parts 1 to 3, *Nursing '77*, 7:28–37 (May), 38–45 (June), and 44–53 (July), 1977. Further reproduction in whole or part without permission expressly prohibited by law.)

ble for *routine* vital signs. It lies along the radius bone below the thumb on the inner wrist (the flexor side).

The *apical* pulse is auscultated over the apex of the patient's heart, the fifth intercostal space at the left midclavicular line.

The *temporal* artery lies between the eye and the hairline just above the zygomatic bone (cheekbone). It is a useful pulse site in *children* and *infants*.

The *carotid* artery runs between the trachea and the sternocleidomastoid muscle at the side of the neck. If a patient collapses, this pulse is palpated to determine if the heart has stopped (*cardiac arrest*). The carotid is a central artery, so pulsations may persist there when the stroke volume is too low to feel the peripheral pulses. The carotid artery is palpated in emergencies because it is immediately accessible without taking off any clothing and it is close to the location where the nurse would perform cardiopulmonary resuscitation (CPR) if necessary. The carotid should be felt gently, one side at a time. Too much pressure could slow down the rate of impulse formation in the heart and block impulse conduction between the atria and ventricles.

The *brachial* pulse is felt by "shaking hands" with the patient and reaching around for the groove between the biceps and triceps muscles above the elbow. It is also felt slightly below the antecubital fossa (inner part of the elbow). This site is palpated to determine *stethoscope placement for the blood pressure reading.*

The *femoral* artery lies in the groin in the femoral "triangle," bordered by muscles on the sides and the inguinal ligament above. It is used to evaluate the *adequacy of perfusion during CPR.*

The *popliteal* artery is a continuation of the femoral artery and is the hardest to locate. It is in the popliteal fossa (back of the knee) along the outer side of the medial tendon. The patient should bend his knee slightly, or roll on his abdomen and flex the knee 45 degrees.

The *dorsalis pedis* pulse runs along the top of the foot (dorsum), lateral to the extensor tendon of the big toe. It is congenitally absent in 8 to 10 per cent of the normal population. It must be palpated very gently, as too much pressure will obliterate it.

The *posterior tibial* pulse is behind the medial malleolus (inner ankle bone).

All superficial pulses must be assessed in the patient having surgery, particularly for open-heart or peripheral vascular operations, and for such procedures as cardiac catheterization. Preoperative baseline information should be charted regarding the bilateral dorsalis pedis, posterior tibial, popliteal, femoral, radial, and brachial pulses. This information is important to nurses in the OR, recovery room and intensive care units (ICU) because it can be used as a standard against which to compare changes in vital signs following the above procedures. These pulses also should be assessed in the

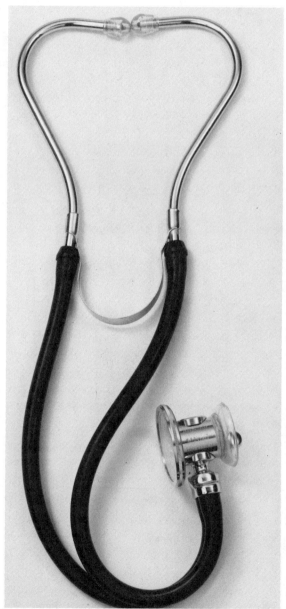

Figure 29–2. Stethoscope with bell (on right) and diaphragm (on left) end pieces.

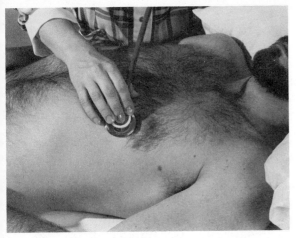

Figure 29-3. Auscultating the apical pulse.

beat has two components, called the first and second heart sounds, or S_1 and S_2. These sounds are caused by events surrounding the closure of the valves in the heart. S_1 occurs with the closure of the mitral and tricuspid valves which separate the atria and ventricles. They close right before systole so that the ventricular contraction will not regurgitate blood back up into the atria. Thus S_1 signals the beginning of systole. At the end of systole the ventricles have ejected their contents, and the aortic and pulmonic valves (located between the ventricles and arteries) close. This produces S_2 and signals the start of diastole. Because systole is normally only one third of the whole cardiac cycle, S_1 and S_2 sound close together, and the worker hears "lub-dup, lub-dup." The apical pulse is best heard in the fifth intercostal space at the left midclavicular line (halfway between the sternum and the side of the chest). Because these are relatively high-pitched sounds, the diaphragm endpiece of the stethoscope is used (Figs. 29-2 and 29-3).

medical patient entering the hospital for diabetes or arterial occlusive conditions such as atherosclerosis, Raynaud's disease, Buerger's disease, and aortic aneurysm.

The *apical* pulse is auscultated to count the pulse rate on *infants*. It is used for adults when there is an *abnormality of the peripheral pulse*, and to assess *heart sounds*. Every normal heart

12. ASSESSING THE PULSE

Definition and Purpose.   *To count pulse rate per minute and assess pulse characteristics.* The number of beats per minute and the quality of arterial pulsation indicates cardiac workload and cardiac efficiency. The presence and quality of peripheral pulses indicates status of the peripheral vascular system, i.e., blood vessels in extremities. Take *radial* pulse for routine assessment of vital signs (T, P, R, B/P) on the adult. Listen to the *apical* pulse when counting pulse rate in an infant, when the pulse is irregular, before giving cardiac medications, or to assess heart sounds. Palpate the *pedal* pulse for presence and quality when the patient has peripheral vascular disease, or undergoes surgery involving the heart or extremities. Palpate the *femoral* pulse during cardiac emergencies to determine how well the heart pumps blood throughout the body, and for heart or peripheral vascular surgery.

Contraindications.   None.

Patient-Family Teaching Points.   Provide patient and family with the following information as appropriate: (a) describe procedure to patient, no matter what his state of consciousness; (b) as a part of discharge planning, teach patient to take his own pulse if he is on certain cardiac medications or if he has a cardiac pacemaker; (c) if stethoscope will be used, ask patient and family to remain quiet during procedure so worker can hear.

PRE-PROCEDURE ACTIVITIES

PRELIMINARY PLANNING/ASSESSMENT

▶ Schedule frequency of obtaining pulse as determined by patient's condition and physician's order
▶ Know previous reported pulse rates
▶ Know purpose for obtaining pulse rate, e.g., routine vital signs, post cardiac catheterization care
▶ Choose site for obtaining pulse rate: for routine vital signs in adults, the *radial* artery is the most accessible; take *apical* rate on infant; for older child, use radial or *temporal* site.
▶ Obtain pulse rate of children prior to other vital signs. If child cries when temperature is taken, crying distorts vital sign data.
▶ Postpone assessing pulse rate for a few minutes if patient has just ambulated or seems very angry or anxious.

PREPARATION OF PATIENT

▶ Identify patient
▶ Explain procedure and reason for obtaining pulse
▶ Position patient appropriately for the site used

EQUIPMENT

▶ Stethoscope (for taking apical pulse)
▶ Alcohol wipes (for cleaning ear tips)

PROCEDURE

SUGGESTED STEPS

A. *Radial Pulse*

1. Wash hands

2. Position patient. In *supine* position, place patient's forearm across his chest with wrist extended, palm down. If patient is *sitting*, bend his elbow 90 degrees and support it on arm rest; extend wrist, palm down.

3. Place your first three fingers along patient's superficial radial artery and gently press artery against radius.

4. Rest your thenar eminence (*not* your thumb) on patient's wrist.

5. Obliterate pulsation, then gradually release pressure just until pulse is again palpable.

RATIONALE/ASSESSMENT

1. Decrease chance of nosocomial infection.

2. These positions are comfortable for most patients and convenient for worker. A painful position for patient may influence his heart rate; an awkward position for worker makes it difficult to concentrate on data being collected.

3. Pulsation is felt over bony prominence and is due to systolic thrust of heart's left ventricle.

4. Thenar eminence is the padded mound on the palm at base of thumb. If thumb is used, worker may feel own pulse, confusing it with patient's pulse.

5. Moderate pressure is desired. Too much pressure occludes pulse; with too little pressure pulse cannot be felt. Obliterating and releasing the pulse tells worker just how much pressure is indicated for accuracy.

SUGGESTED STEPS	RATIONALE/DISCUSSION
6. While observing a watch with a second hand, start to count the rate with "zero" then "one, two", etc.	6. Zero begins the time interval, and the *next* pulse felt is "one" of the sequence.[16]
7. If *pulse is regular*, count number of pulsations in 15 sec. and multiply by 4.	7. Adequate for accurate result, *if* the rate is regular.
8. If *pulse is irregular*, count rate for one full minute.	8. Minimum time needed to accurately determine rate of irregular pulse.
9. Continue palpation to assess pulse volume, arterial elasticity, and type of pulse irregularity, if present.	9. See text for discussion of assessment of these factors.
10. If pulse is irregular, use stethoscope to auscultate the apical beat.	10. Auscultation of the apical pulse and palpation of the radial pulse are done simultaneously to determine the pulse deficit.

1. Take an *apical* pulse rate for one full minute before giving digitalis preparations.

2. Know previous data on pulse rate and rhythm for individual patient.

3. Note pulse rate and rhythm. If very rapid (over 100 per minute), very slow (*below* 60), or *regularly*-irregular (every other or every third beat comes early), hold the drug *and* notify the physician.

NOTE: (a) A rate of 100 or more may *also* mean the patient needs the drug to slow down the rapid rate; (b) A pulse rate of 60 may *also* indicate the drug is doing its job and should be given, or that the patient has been very quiet and metabolism is decreased; (c) an *irregularly*-irregular pulse rhythm may also mean the patient has atrial fibrillation and needs the drug for that.

Thus, you must put pulse data together with individual patient's clinical picture. Never withhold the drug without also notifying the physician.[45]

B. *Apical Pulse*

1. Wash hands.	1. Decrease chance of nosocomial infection.
2. Position patient: supine (preferred) or sitting.	
3. Expose nipple area of left anterior (front or belly surface of body) chest by raising patient gown to shoulders and lowering sheet.	3. Keeping shoulders covered maintains privacy and warmth.

Procedure continued on the following page

SUGGESTED STEPS	RATIONALE/DISCUSSION
4. Inspect the precordium (the region over the heart) for obvious pulsations and palpate* the *point of maximal impulse* (PMI).	4. The PMI is the systolic thrust of the left ventricle, located at the fourth *or* fifth intercostal space in the midclavicular line. It normally may be visible in thin adults. When abnormal, the pulsation appears as a sustained forceful impulse (a *heave* or *lift*) and indicates an enlarged heart. The abnormal pulsation may be seen at the left sternal border, or below and to the left of the normal PMI area.
5. Wipe diaphragm and earpiece tips of stethoscope with alcohol sponges.	5. Prevents spread of microorganisms between patients and workers.
6. Rub diaphragm endpiece in palm of hand.	6. Friction from rubbing warms endpiece. Placement of cold endpiece on patient's chest is uncomfortable and startling, thus momentarily increasing heartrate.
7. Insert earpiece tips in your ears with bend of tips pointing forward.	7. This placement matches forward slope of external auditory canal, so sound is transmitted clearly to eardrum.
8. Place diaphragm over patient's apical area (fifth intercostal space at the left midclavicular line).	8. Apical pulse is best heard in this area because heart is close to chest wall. Use diaphragm endpiece for high-pitched sounds like the apical beat.
9. Listen for "lub-dup" heart sounds.	9. There is a first (*lub*) and second (*dup*) heart sound for each systole.
10. Count the rate and note regularity, as in Steps 6, 7, 8 above.	
11. Again, wipe diaphragm and earpiece tips of stethoscope with alcohol sponges.	11. Prevents spread of microorganisms between patients and workers.

C. *Femoral Pulse*

1. Wash hands	1. Decrease chance of nosocomial infection.
2. Place patient in supine position. Drape sheet to expose one leg at a time from groin area down.	2. Keep rest of body and genital area covered to preserve privacy.
3. Locate femoral arterial pulse in femoral triangle.	3. "Femoral triangle" lies in groin between thigh and trunk of body. It is bordered by muscles in the sides and the inguinal ligament above.

*See Chap. 16 for discussion of palpation.

SUGGESTED STEPS	RATIONALE/DISCUSSION
4. Gently pressing over femoral artery with tips of first three fingers, obliterate pulse, then gradually release pressure until pulse is again palpable.	4. See step A.5 above.
5. Note rhythm, volume, and elasticity, as in steps A.6, 7, 8 and 9 above.	
6. Compare results with findings on the contralateral pulse (on the opposite side).	6. Comparison of pulses on both sides of body indicates range of normal for individual patient.

D. *Pedal Pulse*

1. Wash hands.	1. Decrease chance of nosocomial infection.
2. Lift sheet to expose dorsum (upper surface, opposite the sole) of foot.	
3. With tips of first three fingers, *gently* locate pulse just lateral to the extensor tendon of the great toe. (Have patient dorsiflex foot, i.e., upward flexion, to locate tendon).	3. Palpate lightly; moderate pressure will occlude this pulse.
4. Note presence or absence of pulse. Note volume, as in steps A.6, 7, 8, and 9 above. Also note condition, color and temperature of skin, and any lesions.	4. Pedal pulse is congenitally absent in 8 to 10 per cent of the normal population. If coupled with other abnormal signs, an absent pedal pulse indicates peripheral vascular disease.
5. Compare results with findings on the opposite foot.	
6. If pedal pulses are difficult to find, mark their location with a felt pen.	6. Promotes accuracy in subsequent pedal data collection.

Post-Procedure Activities.   Assess pulse findings in view of patient's overall clinical picture. Record findings. If data show a significant change in patient's condition, take indicated actions, e.g., communicate findings to appropriate persons.

Pulse Rate

Before assessing the pulse, the nurse must know normal parameters of rate, rhythm and quality.

> *The normal rate in the resting adult is 60 to 100 beats per minute, although the American Heart Association accepts 50 to 100 as a normal range.*

Women have a slightly faster rate than men. The heart rate normally is higher in infants and children, gradually decreases toward adulthood, and increases slightly in old age. The range in infants up to 1 year old is 80 to 180 beats/minute, with 120 to 130 as average. At 4 years the range is 80 to 120/minute; at 10 years it is 70 to 110/minute; and over 14 it is 50 to 100/minute.

The peripheral pulse is counted for 15 seconds and multiplied by 4. If any irregularities are detected, the pulse is counted for at least 1 full minute. Some texts differ and recommend counting for 30 or 60 seconds. However, the common clinical use of the 15-second interval is supported in research by Jones.[19] She compared the accuracy of pulse rates counted for 15-, 30-, and 60-second intervals in adults to rates obtained simultaneously by an electrocardiogram. She found that with normal rates, the use of the 15-second interval gave the most accurate results. A tendency to lose count was suggested as the reason for inaccuracy during the longer intervals. At rapid rates, Jones found gross inaccuracy in all counting intervals as compared to the EKG count. She concludes:

Based on the findings of this study it would appear that there is no accuracy advantage to be gained by counting the pulse for the longer intervals of 30 to 60 seconds. Selection of the counting interval should be made after consideration of the quality of the pulse, its rhythm, and the possible effect of medication. . . . Methods other than radial palpation may be indicated, particularly in the determination of the rapid heart rate.

An *increased* heart rate, or *tachycardia,* is a rate *over 100 beats per minute.* It occurs with conditions that stimulate the sympathetic nervous system. This is seen when a patient is in pain. Tachycardia occurs with exercise or fever to increase the cardiac output and meet the body's need for increased metabolism. Thus an increased rate is expected after the patient is ambulated. Tachycardia is a major compensatory mechanism of the heart. Thus an increased pulse is seen with hypoxemia (decreased O_2 in the blood) and congestive heart failure (the heart fails as a pump and blood "backs up"). Because less oxygen reaches the cells, the heart compensates by increasing its rate. Anger, fear, and anxiety also increase the heart rate; if these emotions are suspected, check the pulse rate later to insure validity. Also, crying in infants and children increases

the pulse. For this reason the apical pulse rate is always counted on infants *prior* to taking the other vital signs. If the temperature is taken first and the child cries, the pulse rate increases and it will be harder to hear the heart sounds. Tachycardia also occurs when the blood pressure falls (as in shock); the pulse increases in an attempt to maintain a stable cardiac output. Finally, even psychosocial interactions can affect the heart function. Research studies in patients in coronary-care units describe alterations in rate and rhythm that occur from the nurse comforting a patient, holding his hand, or taking his pulse.[27, 40]

Stimulation of the parasympathetic nervous system causes a *decreased* pulse rate. Thus a *bradycardia* (below 60 beats per minute) may be seen in patients on digitalis, which stimulates the vagus nerves of the parasympathetic system. The apical rate should be auscultated for one full minute before giving a patient digitalis. (See box in Procedure 12.) Bradycardia may be seen in other conditions that stimulate the vagus nerves, such as vomiting or tracheal suctioning. Bradycardia occurs with heart block, in which the impulse conduction pathway is partially or completely blocked. The patient with heart block may have a *cardiac pacemaker.* This is a small electrode implanted inside the heart and attached to a pulse generator that initiates an electrical impulse when the heart fails to do so. The patient with increased intracranial pressure from tumor or hemorrhage may have bradycardia. Finally, a bradycardia may occur normally, as in the well-conditioned athlete. In athletes, each stroke volume is large due to well-developed heart muscle, and thus the rate decreases.

Pulse Rhythm

Pulse rhythm should be regular. However, two irregularities may occur normally. First, *sinus arrhythmia* is a pulse rate that varies with respiration, increasing at the peak of inspiration and decreasing with expiration. It is common in children and young adults. The mechanism of sinus arrhythmia is as follows: with inspiration, there is an increased amount of blood trapped in the lungs, which momentarily decreases the amount returned to the left side of the heart, and the stroke volume falls. By the equation discussed above ($CO = SV \times R$), the rate increases in order to maintain a stable cardiac output. Expiration collapses the lungs, blood return to the heart increases, the stroke volume increases, so the pulse slows down.

The second irregularity is an occasional *premature beat.* This arrhythmia occurs when a pacemaker other than the usual SA node fires prematurely and initiates an early systole. There is a decreased stroke volume with the premature beat because of reduced filling time, so you feel a pause in the rhythm. Everyone has an occasional sensation of their heart "skipping a beat." Frequent premature beats, however, may indicate hypoxia, cardiac irritability, drug overdose (digitalis), electrolyte imbalance, or may be the danger sign of more serious arrhythmias. When frequent, the patient may complain of "palpitations" or of feeling faint or dizzy.

> *If an irregularity is present, the pulse should be counted for one full minute.*

The nature of the irregularity is important: cyclic with the breathing, occasionally skipping a beat, or "irregularly-irregular." No intervention is necessary with the cyclic pattern. If premature beats are noted, the number per minute should be charted and communicated to the appropriate persons. The term "irregularly-irregular" should be charted when noticed. This is the rhythm of *atrial fibrillation,* where there are so many electrical impulses in the heart (500 to 800/minute) that the ventricles respond and contract at random.

When any irregularity is noted, the stethoscope is used to auscultate the apical beat. In addition, auscultation and palpation of the radial pulse are done simultaneously to determine the *pulse deficit;* that is, a radial pulse rate lower than the apical rate. Two workers are positioned on either side of the patient, one auscultating the apical beat, and the other palpating the radial pulse. A watch is placed so that both nurses determine the count during the same time interval (Fig. 29–4). The count is taken for one full minute, and any difference is reported.

A pulse deficit signals an inefficient contraction; with an irregular pulse, there is not enough time for the ventricles to fill with blood between all beats. Thus some systoles will not eject enough blood to produce a palpable peripheral pulse. This occurs with atrial fibrillation and with premature beats.

Research findings support the use of the *serial measurement* (one after the other) of apical beat and radial pulse to determine pulse deficit.[9] No significant difference was found between the use of this method by one worker and the use of the simultaneous method by two workers. However, it was found that *one* serial pulse deficit reading may not be accurate. Determining the average of several serial measurements was suggested.

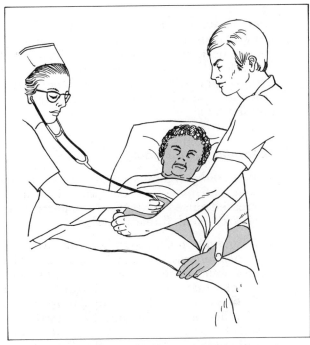

Figure 29–4.   Assessing the apical-radial pulse.

Pulse Force or Quality

Pulse force or quality reflects the strength of the pulse pressure (the difference between systolic and diastolic pressure). If the stroke volume increases as with exercise, anxiety, or alcohol intake, the pulse pressure widens; this is felt peripherally as an increased force. This extremely *bounding* pulse also is felt in pathologic conditions (see section on abnormal findings below).

The quality of the pulse is assessed and may be noted on a three point scale: 3+ is a bounding pulse, 2+ a normal pulse, 1+ indicates a weak thready pulse, and 0 an absent pulse. Some institutions use a different scale, so all staff members must be consistent. This assessment is subjective, and requires clinical experience to make the distinction.

Elasticity of Arterial Wall

This is the expansibility, or springy property, of the normal arterial wall. Practice is necessary to assess this, but the flexible, straight artery of the normal patient easily can be distinguished from the hard, cord-like, tortuous ("S" shaped), artery of atherosclerosis. Elasticity of the arterial wall does not affect the pulse rate per se. It does indicate the general status of the peripheral arterial network. If a hardened tortuous artery is noted, the nurse should be alert for other signs of atherosclerosis (e.g., high blood pressure).

Abnormal Pulse Findings

▶ *Weak pulse* signifies a *decreased stroke volume* and may be accompanied by an increased pulse rate. It is seen in hemorrhagic shock ("weak thready" pulse).

▶ *Bounding pulse* signifies an *increased stroke volume.* It is seen in exercise, anxiety, and with pathology such as complete heart block, anemia, hepatic failure, and the "water-hammer" (Corrigan's) pulse of aortic insufficiency. In the latter, the aortic valve fails to snap shut in diastole, and the diastolic pressure decreases, thereby widening the pulse pressure. With the increased stroke volume, the pulse is felt to slap against the palpating fingers, then collapse abruptly.

▶ *Pulsus Alternans.* The rhythm is regular, but the volume has an alternating strong and weak character. This may be noticed with left-sided heart failure (e.g., after a myocardial infarction), heart block or digitalis toxicity.

▶ *Bigeminal pulse* is an irregular rhythm where every other beat comes early. The second (or premature) beat feels weak, due to inadequate filling time of the ventricle between the two beats. It may be so weak that it fails to produce a palpable peripheral pulse (pulse deficit). The greater the pulse deficit, the more serious is the arrhythmia; a bigeminal pulse is much more significant than an occasional premature beat. This is seen when the heart muscle is irritable after a myocardial infarction, and with drug toxicity (e.g., digitalis).

▶ *Paradoxical pulse.* In this case, the rhythm may be regular but the force or strength of the pulse wave varies, feeling weaker when the patient takes in a breath. The mechanism is similar to that of sinus arrhythmia discussed above. That is, inspiration traps more blood in the lungs, decreases return to

the left side of the heart, decreases the stroke volume, and therefore decreases the strength of the pulse. This may occur normally, but if pronounced may indicate cardiac tamponade. This is a rupture of the heart or a coronary vessel causing blood to collect in the heart's outer lining (pericardium), thus compressing the heart.

RESPIRATIONS

Pulmonary Ventilation and Gas Exchange

The function of the lungs is to maintain homeostasis of arterial blood. By supplying O_2 and taking off excess CO_2, respiration maintains the pH of the blood, thus protecting vital tissues and nourishing the cells. Respiration is thus the most fundamental of body mechanisms; all other processes depend on adequate gas exchange.

The term respiration refers to two processes: external respiration and internal respiration. *External respiration* is the act of breathing; air rushes into the lungs as the chest rises (inspiration or inhalation) and is expelled from the lungs as the chest falls (expiration, or exhalation).

External respiration has four components: (1) *ventilation,* or the mechanical movement of air in and out of the lungs, (2) *distribution* of the air throughout the bronchial tree, (3) *diffusion* of the gases (O_2 and CO_2) across the respiratory membrane and (4) *perfusion,* or the movement of the blood through the lungs.

Any disease state that interferes with these steps will result in *hypoxemia,* or a decreased level of O_2 in the arterial blood. For example, a collapse or an obstruction of a lung section interferes with ventilation of those alveoli. Some diseases (pneumonia, pulmonary edema, emphysema) involve the structure of the respiratory membrane and thus block alveolar-capillary diffusion. Or, the alveoli may be ventilated but not perfused with blood, as in hemorrhage, obstruction of a blood vessel by pulmonary embolism, or inadequate pulmonary blood flow from congenital heart defects or even anesthesia.

Gravity affects pulmonary blood flow and alveolar ventilation too; a healthy adult in a standing position does not have a high enough pulmonary blood pressure to keep all the capillaries open at the apices (tops) of his lungs.[47] This normally occurring imbalance of the ventilation-perfusion ratio is asymptomatic and is relieved by lying down. Similarly, not all of the alveoli are expanded when the body is asleep or resting. These few less ventilated alveoli are re-expanded by the occasional sighs that normally punctuate our breathing.

The quality of the circulating blood is important too. When the number of red blood cells is decreased (anemia) or when the hemoglobin prefers to bind with a substance other than oxygen (e.g., carbon monoxide), the result may be inadequate oxygen delivered to the cells and tissue *hypoxia*.

From the lungs the oxygenated blood goes to the left side of the heart, where it is pumped to every cell in the body. *Internal respiration* occurs at the cellular level; O_2 diffuses from the hemoglobin in the red blood cell to the body cell for use in production of heat and energy, and CO_2 is given off from the body cell as a waste by-product of metabolism.

The pH is an expression of the acid-base balance of the blood. The body tissues are bathed by blood that normally has a very narrow range of pH. Although a number of compensatory mechanisms regulate acid-base balance, the lungs help maintain the homeostasis of blood by adjusting the level of CO_2. Hypoventilation (slow, shallow breathing) causes CO_2 to build up in the blood, and hyperventilation (increased rate and depth) causes CO_2 to be blown off.

Control of Respiration

The act of breathing is automatic and involuntary, but it can be influenced by a person's voluntary control and activities. The involuntary control of respirations is mediated by the *respiratory center* in the brain stem (pons and medulla). The medulla has a basic rhythmicity that can produce repetitive inspiration and expiration, although not in a very smooth pattern. The pattern of breathing is smoothed and the rate of alveolar ventilation to meet the body's demands is adjusted through several feedback mechanisms.

The major feedback loop is *humoral* regulation, or the change in CO_2 and O_2 levels in the blood (and to a lesser extent, hydrogen ion level). Carbon dioxide acts *directly* on the respiratory center, and O_2 acts *indirectly* through the peripheral chemoreceptors (carotid and aortic bodies) in the arteries. The normal stimulus to breathe is an increase of CO_2 in the blood, or *hypercarbia*. The peripheral chemoreceptors react to diminished levels of oxygen in the blood, and in turn stimulate the respiratory center to take more breaths. Under normal conditions, this feedback system is not needed, and most of us breathe as a result of direct CO_2 stimulation to the brain. However, some diseases (e.g., emphysema) cause a gradual increase over the years in the level of CO_2 in the blood. A person with such a disease slowly becomes immune to the CO_2 stimulus and depends on the diminished O_2 level for his respiratory stimulus (called the *hypoxic drive*).

Another involuntary stimulus is the stretch receptors in the lung parenchyma (tissue). When stretched, they send an impulse to the brain through the autonomic nervous system to stop the breath and prevent further inflation. This is called the *Hering-Breuer inflation reflex*.

Blood pressure and respiratory rates are related. It is thought that the respiratory center interacts with the vasomotor center that controls blood pressure; factors exciting one have a parallel effect on the other.[15]

Voluntary controls on respirations include the emotions, such as fear, rage or anxiety. Sudden stressful conditions may alter the respiratory rate, as the body prepares for "fight or flight."[7] Chronic emotional disturbances may affect respirations, e.g., hysteria increases the rate and depression produces frequent sighs.

Voluntary activities may alter the respiratory rate. Impulses from peripheral sensory receptors in the skin run through nerves in the spinal cord and stimulate the respiratory center. Thus breathing is changed by a sudden external temperature change (a jump into a cold shower) or by pain (a slap on the skin). A change in altitude also affects respirations. A person first encountering the lower oxygen content at high altitudes may feel tired, weak, short of breath and complain of "palpitations" (an awareness of heart beat). He compensates by increasing the respiratory rate and the tidal volume (ml. of air inspired).[8] Physical exercise increases the rate of metabolism and thus increases the oxygen requirements of the cells. The respiratory rate and depth is adjusted depending on the level of exercise. Finally, we willfully can adjust our respiratory pattern to augment activities like speaking, singing, crying, laughing, swallowing or defecating.

Assessing Respiratory Status

Of all the vital signs, the respiratory rate is the most vulnerable to sloppy technique. Studies indicate nurses' measurements are not particularly reliable. Eisman studied 48 registered nurses and found that half of the medical nurses really counted the respiratory rate and the others estimated it.[10] Of surgical nurses, twice as many counted as estimated, perhaps due to the belief that the surgical patient's status is more subject to change. Most of the nurses who estimated the rate said they made this judgment based on a general impression of the patient's appearance. Another study by Kory revealed that nurses consistently made inaccurate counts of patients' respiratory rates, when compared with researchers' observations made moments later.[22]

One reason for these findings is that physicians' lack of interest in respiratory rates has led to apathy by nurses toward accurate measurement.[22] Kory studied 200 patient records and found that routine measurement of respiratory rate was clinically useful in less than 5 per cent of those patients' days in the hospital. Also in this study, 40 physicians were encouraged to list all of their patients for whom the measurement of respiratory rate might have the slightest usefulness; approximately 50 patients out of 1000 were chosen. Interestingly, when this same question was asked of the nurses in Eisman's study, 56 per cent of the patients were judged to need an accurate count of respiratory rate. Eisman suggests that since nurses are in more constant attendance of patients, they perceive respiratory rate to be a more important parameter of change in status than physicians do.

Kory suggests "routine" measurement of rate on all hospital patients be eliminated. In patients where it *is* indicated, the character of breathing should be considered equally important and be recorded with the rate. Eisman suggests a similar system; nurses could chart "no abnormality noted" rather than estimating a number. Nurses in her study were using their own judgment anyway about when an accurate rate was needed. Thus the emphasis on *routine* respirations could be replaced by a knowledgeable nursing assessment of the whole patient.

Once established, traditions are hard to change, and many hospitals do have a policy of routine assessment of respiratory rate on all patients. The respiratory rate, while important, is only one parameter of the entire ventilatory status. Other objective and subjective data must be gathered to make a valid judgment. Frequent assessment should be made in patients with acute or chronic pulmonary disease, acute heart disease, shock, neurologic disease, or on any patient who suddenly complains of difficulty breathing. You should know the purpose for assessing respirations for each individual patient, the results of previous assessment, and the patient's current physical condition. In addition to counting the rate accurately (Table 29–1), notice also the quality, depth, pattern and any significant physical characteristics.

Assess the respirations along with other vital signs. Do not tell either the child or adult patient that you will be counting his breathing rate because such an awareness may alter the results. Instead, describe the procedure for taking the other vital signs, and unobtrusively as-

TABLE 29–1.   ASSESSING RESPIRATIONS

SUGGESTED STEPS	RATIONALE/ASSESSMENT
1. Keep fingers in place after assessing radial pulse; observe respirations. (See Procedure 12, Assessing the Pulse.)	1. Maneuver avoids calling patient's attention to his breathing, which could alter the rate.
2. Observe complete respiratory cycle (inspiration and expiration), while observing for symmetrical chest expansion, breathing sounds, use of accessory muscles, bulging or retracting of interspaces, skin color, facial expression, level of consciousness, nasal flaring and/or sternal retraction in the child.	2. Note indications of acute or chronic respiratory problems.
3. For adults and older children, count number of respirations in 30 seconds and multiply by 2.	3. Counting for only 15 sec. gives a result that can vary ± 4, which is significant when working with such small numbers.
4. Count infant respirations for one full minute.	4. It is normal for infants to vary their respiratory rate and pattern.
5. If respirations are abnormal, count rate for one full minute and note patterns, if any.	5. Minimum time necessary to assess abnormal respirations.
6. Note depth and rhythm of respirations.	6. For complete assessment, the character of respirations is noted as well as rate.

sess the respirations. A good time to do this is after obtaining the radial pulse rate, while the patient's forearm lies across his chest. On an infant or young child, obtain the respiratory rate prior to taking the temperature. Many babies cry when a rectal temperature is taken, thus altering accurate respiratory data.

Quality of Respirations

Normal relaxed breathing is effortless, automatic, regular and even, and produces no noise. To determine the quality of respirations, uncover the patient's chest, maintaining modesty, and inspect. Does the chest expand symmetrically with inspiration? Unequal chest expansion occurs when part of a lung is obstructed or collapsed, with pneumonia, and postoperatively when a patient "guards" his operative side to avoid incisional pain from breathing.

Notice the intercostal spaces between the ribs. Is there retraction of the interspaces on inspiration? This suggests obstruction of the respiratory tract or increased inspiratory effort, as is needed with atelectasis. In children, this is accompanied by sternal retraction and nasal flaring. Bulging of the interspaces indicates trapped air, as in the forced expiration associated with emphysema or asthma.

Notice if the respirations are *diaphragmatic* or *costal*. The diaphragm is the major muscle of normal breathing in both males and females, although women may appear to move the chest wall more than men. The diaphragm flattens during inspiration to enlarge the size of the thoracic cage, thus the abdominal contents are pushed out. Costal respirations may be noticed on some women who have been reared to hold their stomach in and their chest out while breathing.

Also notice the use of accessory muscles to augment respiratory effort. In heavy exercise, inspiration is enhanced by the use of the accessory neck muscles (scalene, sternocleidomastoid, trapezius). Accessory muscles are used in acute airway obstruction and massive atelectasis but they still may not improve ventilation and the extra effort may be exhausting. The abdominal rectus and internal intercostal muscles are used to force expiration in chronic obstructive pulmonary disease (COPD). Such patients have increased air-way resistance from collapse of the bronchioles and have difficulty getting the air out. This leaves the lungs hyperinflated and flattens the diaphragm, making it useless as a respiratory muscle. Therefore these patients forcefully contract the stomach muscles, which pushes the abdominal contents against the diaphragm and makes it dome up.

Dyspnea is difficult, labored, or painful breathing. The patient verbalizes a feeling of air hunger, of not getting enough air. His face appears anxious and tired from the exertion, the nostrils flare with the increased inspiratory effort, his color may be dusky, and he has tachycardia. Charting that the patient is dyspneic does not communicate much. Include how much exertion it takes to produce the dyspnea. Does it result from walking to the bathroom, or is he short of breath just talking, pausing every few sentences to rest?

Another noteworthy change in the quality is sound. Normal relaxed breathing produces no noise. Recovery room nurses recognize this and have a maxim, "any noisy breathing is obstructed breathing." The following conditions may be noted:

▶ *Stertor:* noisy respirations (e.g., snoring) produced by secretions in the trachea and large bronchi. Watch for this in patients who have lost their cough reflex and their ability to handle secretions, e.g., neurologic or comatose patients.

▶ *Stridor:* the harsh, inspiratory crowing sound that occurs with upper airway obstruction in laryngitis, the lodging of a foreign body, or croup in children.

▶ *Wheeze:* the high-pitched, musical, whistling sound that occurs with partial obstruction in the smaller bronchi and bronchioles as in emphysema or asthma.

▶ *Sigh:* a very deep inspiration followed by a prolonged expiration which occasionally punctuates the regular breathing pattern. Occasional sighs are normal and purposeful to expand alveoli. Frequent sighs may indicate emotional tension.

The sounds listed above are heard with the ear alone. Nurses may auscultate the lungs with a stethoscope to more accurately assess effectiveness of medication or treatment, determine the need for tracheal suctioning, or confirm suspicions of pathology, such as pneumonia, atelectasis, or congestive heart failure. Normal breath sounds are soft rustling sounds that are termed *bronchovesicular* over the major airways and *vesicular* over the peripheral lung fields. Abnormal breath sounds include *decreased* or *absent* breath sounds that occur with atelectasis or obstruction, and *bronchial* breath sounds. The latter are harsh, loud, blowing sounds that occur when there is consolidated or compressed lung tissue that transmits sound to a greater extent, for example, with pneumonia.

Adventitious sounds are added-on sounds that are *not* normally heard in the lungs. They are caused by moving air colliding with secretions in the tracheobronchial passageways. Sources differ as to the clarification and nomenclature of these sounds.[18] *Rales* and *rhonchi* are terms that are commonly used by most clinicians. Rales are discontinuous, discrete, crackling sounds that are heard more on inspiration. Rhonchi are continuous, coarse, musical sounds heard all through the respiratory cycle, but more on expiration. Tutored practice and detailed study are essential to accurately categorize breath sounds.[18, 34, 41]

Type of Respirations

Rate and depth measure the type of respirations. The normal rate is 12 to 18 breaths per minute in adults. However, in a study of the influence of different surgical procedures on breathing patterns, Zikria et al. noted that nursing personnel commonly believed 20 breaths per minute to be the normal value and results often were charted at this figure.[46] His study showed a normal adult rate of 14 ± 4 breaths per minute and showed that rates of 25 to 30/minute may indicate a significant change in respiratory status. Thus consistent estimates of 20/minute for a normal rate gives a falsely elevated reading and may be misleading when a true increase does occur.

An earlier study of 58 patients showed that nursing personnel made consistently inaccurate observations. They charted a rate of 20 breaths per minute on 40 of the 58 patients, and a rate between 18 and 22 for 57 of the patients.[22] Measurements by the researcher minutes later showed a *true* range of 11 to 33 breaths per minute, with only 5 patients having a rate of exactly 20.

More rapid rates are normal in infants and children: 30 to 60/minute for newborns, 20 to 30/minute for 2-year-old children, and 18 to 26/minute for children 6 to 10 years old. The ratio of pulse to respirations is fairly constant, about 4:1. Both values increase as a normal response to exercise, fear or anxiety.

The depth is the volume of air moving in and out with each respiration. This *tidal volume* is normally about 500 ml. in the adult and should be constant with each breath. A portable spirometer is needed to measure the tidal volume precisely. A gross assessment of depth is made by placing the back of your hand close to patient's nose and mouth and feeling exhaled air and observing adequate symmetrical chest expansion. This is only a rough estimate of tidal volume.

In addition to dyspnea, the following terms describe alterations in respiratory rate. If everyone in your clinical situation is familiar with these terms, use them. If not, describe the specific character.

▶ *Tachypnea.* An increased respiratory rate (>24 breaths/minute), e.g., in fever, as the body tries to rid itself of excess heat. Respirations increase by about 4 breaths per minute for every 1-degree rise in temperature above normal. Respirations also increase with pneumonia, alkalosis, respiratory insufficiency, lesions in the pons of the brain stem, and fear.

▶ *Bradypnea.* A decreased but regular respiratory rate (<10 breaths/minute), such as the depression of the respiratory center in the medulla by opiate narcotics or brain tumor.

▶ *Hypoventilation.* Prolonged depression of the respiratory center alters the pattern (irregular or slow) and the depth (shallow). This is caused by overdosage of narcotics and by anesthetics. It also occurs with bedrest or conscious "splinting" of one side of the chest to avoid postoperative pain. This causes excess CO_2 to be retained in the blood (acidosis).

▶ *Apnea.* Total cessation of breathing. This may be periodic (see *Cheyne-Stokes* below). Continued apnea is incompatible with life and is called "respiratory arrest." This may be caused by a mechanical airway obstruction (mucous plug, blood, vomitus, foreign body) or by damage or depression of the respiratory center in the brain (head trauma, stroke, narcotic or anesthetic overdose, hypercarbia).

▶ *Hyperpnea.* Increased depth of respirations (increased tidal volume). This occurs normally after strenuous exercise.

▶ *Hyperventilation.* An increase both in rate and in depth of respirations. This is seen with extreme exertion, fear and anxiety, fever, diabetic ketoacidosis (Kussmaul's respirations), hepatic coma, salicylate or aspirin overdose (producing a respiratory alkalosis to compensate for the metabolic acidosis), lesions of the midbrain in the brain stem, and alteration in blood gas concentration (either increased CO_2 or decreased O_2). Hyperventilation blows off CO_2, causing a decreased level of CO_2 in the blood (alkalosis).

Pattern of Respirations

Breathing pattern is normally regular and consists of inspiration, pause, longer expiration, and another pause. This may be altered by some disease conditions (Fig. 29–5).

▶ *Cheyne-Stokes.* A cycle where respirations gradually wax and wane in a regular pattern. They increase in rate and depth and then decrease, lasting 30 to 45 seconds. Periods of apnea (20 seconds) alternate the cycles. The most common cause of this periodic breathing is severe congestive heart failure; other causes include renal failure, meningitis, drug overdose, and increased intracranial pressure.

▶ *Biot's.* Similar to Cheyne-Stokes, except that each breath is of the same depth. A series of normal respirations (3 to 4 or more) is followed by a period of apnea. The cycle length is variable, lasting anywhere from 10 seconds to 1 minute. This may be seen with spinal meningitis, encephalitis, head trauma, brain abscess, and heat stroke.

▶ *Kussmaul's (air hunger).* Increased depth and increased rate (more than 20/minute). This dyspnea occurs in metabolic acidosis (diabetic coma) or renal failure.

▶ *Apneustic.* Prolonged, gasping inspiration, followed by extremely short inefficient expiration, seen in lesions of the pons in the midbrain.

Significant Physical Characteristics

Many aspects of a patient's body shape and appearance indicate the respiratory status. For example, persons with emphysema have an anterior-posterior chest diameter as big as their transverse diameter, because of the hyperinflation of their lungs. Similarly, their ribs are horizontal instead of having the normal downward slope. This is called "barrel chest."

Any skeletal deformity should be noted, as it could limit excursion of the thoracic cage and thus interfere with respiration. *Scoliosis* is an S-shaped curvature of the thoracic and lumbar regions of the spine. *Lordosis* (swayback) is an anterior curvature of the lumbar spine, causing the thoracic spine to be displaced in a backward position. *Kyphosis* (humpback) is an exaggerated posterior curvature of the thoracic spine. A markedly sunken sternum is called *pectus excavatum* (funnel breast). It occurs congenitally and with rickets, a vitamin deficiency disease. *Pectus carinatum* (pigeon breast) is a forward protrusion of the sternum, with the ribs sloping back at either side. It is seen often with active rickets.

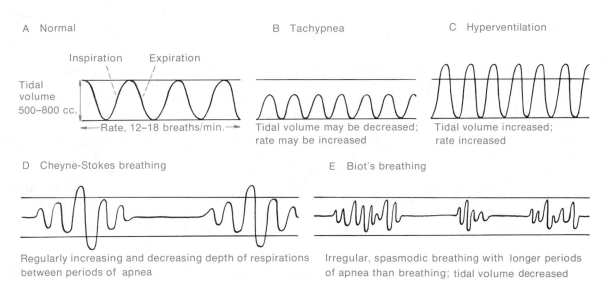

Figure 29–5. Normal and abnormal breathing patterns.

Note the position the patient takes to breathe; for example, persons with chronic obstructive pulmonary disease (COPD) sit leaning forward, with their arms braced against their knees, chair or bed. This gives them leverage so that their abdominal rectus, intercostal, and accessory neck muscles can all aid to force expiration. Such persons also may purse their lips in a whistling position. This technique is taught to patients with COPD. By exhaling slowly and against a narrow opening, the pressure in the bronchial tree remains positive and fewer airways collapse. *Orthopnea* is the inability to breathe except when sitting in an upright position. For accuracy, chart the number of pillows the patient uses, e.g., "two-pillow orthopnea" or "three-pillow orthopnea."

The skin should be observed for *pallor* or *cyanosis*, especially of sudden onset. Lips and nailbeds vary with the person's skin color and are not always accurate parameters. Instead look under the tongue, in the buccal mucosa, or in the conjunctiva around the eyes. However, these signs are relatively unreliable indices of respiratory status.

The normal pink color of mucous membranes is due to oxygenated hemoglobin in the red blood cells. Pallor indicates a diminished amount of red blood cells, or *anemia*. It is best seen in the conjunctiva and mucous membranes, although skin pallor is always a gross estimate of adequate tissue oxygenation. A more definitive indicator is a laboratory analysis of complete blood count.

Cyanosis is a bluish mottled color that signifies a decrease in adequate tissue perfusion of oxygenated blood. It is caused by an increased amount of reduced hemoglobin* in the superficial blood vessels. (That is the reason fingers, nose or ears look blue when coming in out of the cold; the cold temperature makes the blood flow sluggish in exposed areas so there is more time for O_2 to be taken up by the cells, thus more *reduced* hemoglobin.)

Like pallor, cyanosis is a nonspecific sign. Peripheral blood flow may be unrelated to the adequacy of respiration. A patient who is anemic could die of hypoxia without ever looking blue, because he does not have enough hemoglobin

---

*Hemoglobin (the oxygen-carrying pigment of the red blood cells) is referred to as "reduced" when it is not combined with oxygen.

(either oxygenated *or* reduced) to color the skin. On the other hand, a patient with polycythemia (too many red blood cells) will look ruddy-blue at all times and not necessarily be hypoxic. This patient just is unable to fully oxygenate the massive numbers of red blood cells. In a patient with chronic lung disease, cyanosis will be of little diagnostic value because it appears so late. However, cyanosis of *sudden onset* always indicates *hypoxia* (inadequate tissue oxygenation) and will be accompanied by mental confusion, impaired motor function, increased pulse, increased respiration, and increased blood pressure. If the hypoxia is prolonged, the patient may be diaphoretic and lose consciousness, and eventually his blood pressure falls.

One of the most important criteria of adequate ventilation is neurologic status. A *change in the previous level of consciousness* may be the first indication of cerebral hypoxia. With progressive pulmonary decompensation, a previously alert patient becomes anxious and restless, then irritable, then excessively drowsy, and finally comatose. Or a patient who was calm and cooperative may suddenly become combative. Alert nursing observations will pick up even subtle personality changes and lead to appropriate interventions.

BLOOD PRESSURE

The arterial blood pressure is an important parameter of the cardiovascular system and the status of fluid balance. Recorded blood pressure readings have been part of patient assessment since the first decade of this century, although preliminary developments occurred long before. William Harvey first described the circulation of blood in 1628, but he could not explain *why* it circulated. In 1733 Stephen Hales discovered that blood was under pressure by inserting a 9-foot tube into the carotid artery of a horse. Blood rushed up the tube and then oscillated with the animal's heart beat. This crude experiment marked the discovery of blood pressure and its measurement by the *direct* method (i.e., through the wall of an artery).

Indirect measure of blood pressure began in 1855 when Vierordt used the principle of estimating the amount of counterpressure necessary to obliterate the peripheral arterial pulse. Forerunners of today's equipment and technique came when von Basch devised a sphygmomanometer in 1876 and Riva-Rocci introduced the blood pressure cuff in 1896.

Early readings of *maximal* or *systolic* blood pressure were taken by the palpatory method introduced by Riva-Rocci. That is, a pressure cuff is inflated until it obliterates the distal artery pulsation. Then pressure is lowered gradually and the point when the arterial pulsation returns is noted. In 1905 a Russian surgeon named Korotkoff described sounds heard over an artery just distal to the pressure cuff. This *auscultatory* method was superior in identifying the maximal and minimal pressures and gradually replaced the palpatory technique. Later divided into five phases, these still are known as the *Korotkoff sounds*.

Physiology of the Arterial Blood Pressure

Blood pressure is the "... force exerted by the blood against any unit area of the vessel wall."[15] Expressed in millimeters of mercury, it means that pressure in the artery would push a column of mercury up a corresponding number of millimeters. The objective of the measurement is to obtain the *systolic* pressure (the maximum pressure exerted on the arteries with the left ventricular systole), the *diastolic* pressure (the elastic recoil pressure constantly present on the arterial walls), and the *pulse* pressure (difference between the systolic and diastolic).

Blood pressure is a product of the *cardiac output* (stroke volume × heart rate) times the impedance to blood flow through the vessels, or the *peripheral vascular resistance*. This is expressed as:

$$P = CO \times R$$

While other factors do contribute to the level of arterial blood pressure, changes in cardiac output and vascular resistance are relatively more important because they are occurring constantly and quickly. Other determinants of blood pressure (circulating blood volume, viscosity, and elasticity of the arterial walls), are usually of lesser importance but may become primary determinants of blood pressure in certain disease states.[5]

Factors that increase either the cardiac output or the vascular resistance will increase pressure. An increase in cardiac output is a normal response to meet the metabolic demands when a person engages in heavy exertion. Thus an increased B/P is expected after running or hopping. The B/P also reflects the efficiency of the heart as a *pump*. When the cardiac output is decreased due to weak pumping action of the heart (e.g., after a myocardial infarction or in shock), the B/P falls. Vascular tone or peripheral vascular resistance also influences the B/P, especially the diastolic reading. The smaller the caliber of vessel through which the blood flows, the greater the pressure necessary to push it. When resistance is increased (vasoconstriction), the same volume of blood is being pumped into a smaller compartment, hence the B/P increases. A fall in B/P is expected with vasodilation because the blood occupies a larger space and less pressure is exerted on the arterial wall.

The blood *volume* of a normal adult is about 5000 ml. This is relatively constant. The B/P reflects how tightly the blood is packed into the arterial system. Conditions causing blood volume to vary will affect blood pressure: the B/P decreases when the volume is low, as in hemorrhage; the B/P increases when vigorous intravenous infusions of fluid are administered. Blood *viscosity* refers to "thickness" as determined by its formed elements. Blood pressure is higher when the blood is more viscous, as in conditions that produce increased numbers of red blood cells (polycythemia) or plasma proteins. Viscosity rises markedly when the hematocrit is above 50 per cent (the percentage of whole blood that is the cells), thus elevating the B/P.[5] Finally, B/P reflects the *elasticity* or distensibility of the arterial walls. Atherosclerosis hardens the arteries, causing them to lose their ability to stretch. The heart has to pump against a greater resistance, so the B/P elevates.

As mentioned above, the B/P is regulated mainly by the cardiac output and the peripheral vascular resistance. Regulation also is mediated by the *vasomotor center* in the brainstem. It receives sensory impulses from baroreceptors and chemoreceptors in the heart, aortic arch, carotid arteries, lungs and blood vessels, and from the hypothalamus and cerebral cortex. The vasomotor center sends its adjusting impulses back through the autonomic nervous system to the heart and blood vessels so that B/P is correlated to circulatory need.

Range of Normal Blood Pressure

The average B/P in the young adult is 120/80, although this varies normally with many factors. There is a slow, steady rise during childhood growth and with increasing age. Pressure readings are labile in children, but average values include: 80 mm. Hg systolic for a 1-month-old infant; 90 mm. Hg systolic in a 6 year old; and 110/70 at puberty, or close to the adult value. Pressure gradually increases until 45 to 50 years, after which it accelerates sharply.[5]

There is no difference in B/P values between boys and girls until puberty. After that, females usually have a lower B/P than males of the same age, until menopause when their pressure readings increase over men's. Body weight makes a difference; B/P consistently is higher in overweight persons than in normal weight persons of the same age, making obesity a serious health problem. Weight reduction usually will decrease the blood pressure.

Blood pressure varies with race, though the reasons for this are complex and involve such factors as heredity, climate, diet and disease, as well as measuring techniques in different countries. In the United States, Negroes have higher B/P readings than do Caucasians of the same age. Climate can make a difference; pressure norms are lower in tropical climates than temperate and are highest in polar climates.[5]

In all persons, the B/P is usually lowest in the early morning, rises throughout the day to a peak in the late afternoon or early evening, and then starts to decline. This same cyclic variation occurs every day. Thus blood pressure is an example of a *circadian rhythm,* from the Latin *circa dies* meaning "about a day." Body temperature is another internal biological function that peaks and dips in a daily pattern. In a study of these biological rhythms, Felton concludes that we should be mindful of the daily peak and trough of the circadian cycle when evaluating normalcy of each pressure reading.[12]

Blood pressure increases with exercise; it rises in proportion to the amount of activity, and returns to resting levels within 5 minutes after cessation of activity.[5] It also increases with anger, fear or pain. Blood pressure is more likely to increase in persons who live in stressful urban environments or who have jobs with constant mental tension, than in persons leading relaxed tranquil lives.

Sources vary as to the effect of change in position on blood pressure. It is often stated that B/P is lower when lying down than when sitting or standing,[42] yet it may stay the same or may even decrease upon standing. The latter is called *orthostatic hypotension* and is noted particularly as a side effect of antihypertensive medications or when a person first arises after a period of prolonged bedrest. Blood pressure varies with different recumbent positions. Foley noted that a fall in pressure normally occurs in the uppermost arm when a person is turned onto his side, and that it returns to the original level when the person is again supine.[13] About one fourth of the population has a difference in B/P between the right and left arm, usually higher in the right arm. This difference is usually transient, quite variable; it may reach 10 to 20 mm. Hg. Finally, the B/P is slightly higher in the lower extremities than in the arms.[5]

Blood Pressure Equipment

The standard instrument used to measure the blood presure is a *sphygmomanometer.* It consists of a pressure manometer, an occlusive cuff containing an inflatable rubber bladder, and a pressure bulb with a release valve to pump up the cuff. There are two types of pressure manometers, mercury and aneroid (Fig. 29–6). Both give accurate readings when they are functioning properly.

In the *mercury manometer,* pressure in the compression cuff offsets the constant gravitational pull on the mercury and pushes it up the calibrated glass column. To be accurate, the mercury column should have no "zero error" (i.e., mercury level should rest at zero before pressure is applied), and it should fall freely as cuff pressure is released. Mercury manometers are accurate, reliable, and do not require periodic recalibration. Disadvantages are breakable glass parts, the need to be vertical for correct reading, and greater size and bulk than the aneroid.

The *aneroid manometer* has a metal bellows inside the gauge that expands and collapses in response to pressure variations in the compression cuff. Movement of the bellows bounces an indicator needle across a calibrated dial. Elastic properties of the metal parts make the aneroid gauge subject to drift and therefore somewhat less reliable than the mercury gauge. A needle resting at zero when the cuff is flat is no guarantee that the reading will be accurate throughout cuff deflation. Perlman et al. studied the accuracy of 335 sphygmomanometers and found almost one third (31.6 per cent) of the aneroid models deviated from the standard by more than ±3 mm. Hg.[33] All mercury models were within ±3 mm. Hg of the standard. The variance of the aneroids was usually below the value of the control model, thus these instruments gave a falsely low reading. Such errors could be significant when making clinical decisions on critically ill patients, in screening of patients with hypertension, or drawing conclusions on clinical research that uses B/P as an outcome measurement. This study found that accuracy of aneroid manometers depended on the agency's maintenance procedure; more instruments were inaccurate when used heavily and rarely calibrated. The aneroid should be recalibrated against a perfectly working mercury manometer at least once a year, or more often if errors are suspected. The advantages of

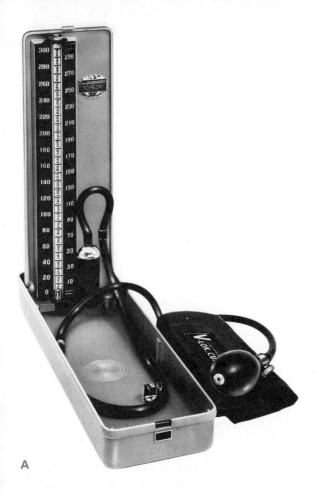

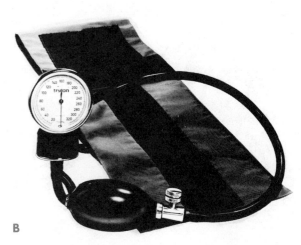

Figure 29–6. Portable mercury *(A)* and aneroid *(B)* sphygmomano-meters. (*A* courtesy of W. A. Baum Co., Inc., Copiague, NY 11726; *B* courtesy of Aloe Medical Division, Sherwood Medical Industries, St. Louis, MO 63103.)

the aneroid gauge are that it is portable and that it can be used in any position as long as the nurse faces it.

The width of the cuff bladder should be 20 per cent greater than the diameter of the extremity on which it will be used; it should be long enough to encircle the extremity completely. Cuffs are available in at least six standard sizes, from newborn to extra-large adult. Use of the proper size cuff is necessary or results may be off by as much as 25 mm. Hg.[2] If the cuff is too narrow, the results will be erroneously high because extra pressure is needed to compress the artery. A cuff that is too wide for the extremity yields a falsely low reading. (Steinfeld suggests that for true accuracy we develop individually sized "prescriptions" for compression cuffs, just as we would tailor antiembolism hose or eyeglasses to each patient's specification.[38]) Further, the cloth cover for the bladder should be nonstretchable so that pressure can be distributed uniformly over the arm. The control valve on the pressure bulb must be clean and free from leaks or sticking so that the cuff can be deflated evenly.

Blood Pressure Technique

Assessment of the blood pressure combines the skills of inspection, palpation and auscultation. Whether you obtain a sitting or supine B/P, the patient should be in a stable relaxed position for 5 to 10 minutes. Try to avoid or control any factors which could influence the B/P: meals, smoking, exercise, pain, anxiety, or even the patient's need to urinate. The room should be a comfortable temperature, and it must be quiet, for noise could disturb the patient, elevate his B/P, and also make it hard to hear through the stethoscope. Have the patient comfortably seated, arm slightly flexed and unconstricted by clothing, with the forearm supported at the level of the heart. Position yourself directly in front of the manometer, not more than 3 feet away. Make sure your eyes are level with the mercury manometer to avoid errors of parallax (Fig. 29–7).

Make certain your own affect is relaxed and unhurried. The patient and family will watch you carefully and will be quick to pick up any sign that all is not well. Explain the procedure

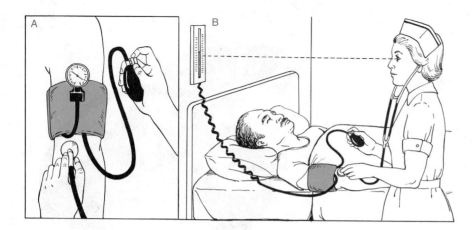

Figure 29–7. Correct positioning for patient, nurse and equipment for obtaining blood pressure reading.

to them. If the patient asks you his B/P reading, respond honestly. First ask his usual blood pressure, so that you will have an idea of his level of knowledge. Then you might say, "It is 118/70 now, which is within normal limits for you," or "It is 140/90 now, which is a little higher than your usual reading. This might be from your walk down the hall, so I'll check it again in 10 minutes." Every person should know his normal range of blood pressure, just as he knows his blood type. This knowledge is an important impetus to control hypertension and encourages the patient to be *part* of the health team and not merely the object of the team's efforts. However, stating a precise number might alarm the patient in some situations, such as a sudden dramatic increase or decrease in pressure. Judgment is necessary to determine how much information to give the patient then.

Auscultatory Method. Locate the brachial artery in the medial side of the antecubital fossa. Place the center of the deflated cuff over the brachial artery, with the lower margin 1 inch above it, and wrap the cuff evenly. Palpate the radial artery, inflate the cuff until the radial pulsation disappears and then 20 to 30 mm. Hg beyond that point. Cuff inflation compresses the tissue around the brachial artery. When that pressure exceeds the heart's systolic pressure, the brachial artery collapses and blood flow is occluded. Place the diaphragm of your stethoscope snugly but lightly over the brachial artery, forming an airtight seal. Avoid producing any artefact from contact of the stethoscope with clothing or the cuff. Do not push the stethoscope too hard, as excess pressure will distort the artery and you will

continue to hear sounds below the true diastolic pressure. Release the pressure valve at a rate of 2 mm. Hg per heartbeat. This lowers pressure in the arm tissues. When the pressure inside the brachial artery equals that in the compression cuff, the artery opens, a small amount of blood is pumped through with each cardiac systole, and Korotkoff's sounds are heard. As the pressure falls, note the following sounds:

▶ The *systolic* pressure (phase I Korotkoff) is the first reappearance of clear tapping sounds. Note the figure at which you hear the tapping sound for at least *two* consecutive beats; then the sounds increase in intensity. Occasionally, the palpatory systolic pressure is higher and should be accepted and recorded as the systolic pressure.

▶ The *diastolic* pressure (phase IV Korotkoff) is the abrupt muffling or damping of sound to a soft, blowing, murmurlike quality. The sound changes in quality, rather than intensity. The American Heart Association feels this to be the most accurate index of diastolic pressure.[21]

▶ Many institutions accept the *final disappearance of sound* (phase V Korotkoff) as the diastolic pressure. It is important to be consistent with the policy of your institution. However, diastolic readings taken at this point may vary with the quality of the stethoscope, its optimal placement over the artery, and the hearing acuity of the nurse. Frequently both the fourth and fifth phases will be noted and recorded as: 138/80/76.

13. MEASURING BLOOD PRESSURE

Definition and Purpose.   *To measure systolic and diastolic blood pressure.* The blood pressure is a parameter which reflects circulating blood volume, peripheral vascular resistance, the efficiency of the heart as a pump, viscosity of the blood, and elasticity of the arterial walls.

Contraindications.   Do not take a blood pressure reading on a patient's arm (a) if the arm has intravenous fluid infusing in it; (b) if the arm is injured or diseased; (c) on the same side of the body where a female patient has had a radical mastectomy; (d) if the arm has a shunt or fistula for renal dialysis.

Patient-Family Teaching Points.   Provide patient and family with the following information: (a) describe the procedure to the patient, no matter what his state of consciousness; (b) explain that the inflated cuff will feel temporarily uncomfortable; and (c) instruct the patient and family to remain quiet during procedure so worker can hear through stethoscope.

PRE-PROCEDURE ACTIVITIES

PRELIMINARY PLANNING/ASSESSMENT

▶ Schedule frequency of obtaining blood pressure as determined by patient's condition and physician's orders.

▶ Know reason for taking B/P on *this* patient (routine vital signs, postoperative care, etc.).
▶ Know latest series of B/P readings on this patient and his position when they were obtained.
▶ Postpone B/P reading for 10 min. on a patient who is angry, anxious, or who has just ambulated.
▶ Postpone B/P reading on a crying infant or child: it may be necessary to take it when he is asleep.

EQUIPMENT

▶ Stethoscope
▶ Mercury or aneroid sphygmomanometer
▶ Cuff of appropriate size for patient.

PREPARATION OF PATIENT

▶ Patient should be in a stable, relaxed, sitting or standing position for 5 to 10 minutes prior to taking B/P.
▶ Permit a child to handle the B/P equipment prior to using it on him, to help reduce his fears.

PROCEDURE

SUGGESTED STEPS

1. Whether patient is sitting or lying, position his arm at level of heart, palm up.

2. Position yourself no more than 3 feet away from sphygmomanometer; directly in front of aneroid model and at eye level with meniscus of mercury model. On a portable model, have mercury column vertical.

RATIONALE/ASSESSMENT

1. Arm above level of heart produces falsely *low* reading.

2. A position more than 3 feet away produces inaccuracies. Looking up at meniscus gives a *falsely high* reading. Looking down on the meniscus gives a *falsely low* reading. If a portable mercury model is tilted on bed, reading is falsely high.

Procedure continued on the following page

SUGGESTED STEPS	RATIONALE/DISCUSSION
3. On a mercury manometer, the level of mercury must be at zero before cuff inflation.	3. No "zero error" assures proper calibration and an accurate reading.
4. Choose a bladder cuff size 20 per cent wider than diameter of extremity.	4. A too narrow cuff gives *falsely elevated* reading because excessively high amount of pressure is needed to occlude brachial artery.
5. Center the arrow marking on the cuff over brachial artery, located at the medial side of the antecubital fossa (inner aspect of the elbow).	5. Cuff pressure must be applied directly to artery.
6. Expel any air in cuff, wrap cuff evenly, with lower edge 1 to 2 inches above maximal brachial artery pulsation. Avoid contact with clothing.	6. An uneven or too loose cuff gives a *falsely high* reading because excessive amount of pressure is needed to occlude brachial artery. Cuff edge should be high enough to avoid covering stethoscope. Accidental contact with clothing or tubing produces confusing extraneous noises.
7. Palpate radial artery (on flexor surface of wrist) and inflate cuff 20 to 30 mm. Hg above point at which radial pulsation disappears.	7. Principle of counter pressure; cuff pressure occludes blood flow and systolic pressure is estimated to be point where radial pulsation is no longer felt. If cuff not inflated high enough, true systolic pressure may be missed. Especially significant if patient has an *auscultatory gap*, i.e., the tapping sounds fade out for 10 to 40 mm. Hg and then return. Inflating the cuff too high causes unnecessary pain and may produce vasospasm, which distorts pressure reading.[1]
8. Place stethoscope diaphragm over brachial artery. Listen carefully, and release cuff pressure at an even rate of 2 mm. Hg per heartbeat.	8. Deflating cuff too slowly produces venous congestion, which *falsely elevates* diastolic pressure. Deflating cuff too rapidly invites guessing at exact pressure, especially important when pulse irregular, as in atrial fibrillation.
9. Note manometer number at which sound first begins (first Korotkoff phase).	9. First sound is made when blood begins to flow through brachial artery again. This is called the *systolic pressure*.
10. Continue to release cuff pressure evenly and note a "muffling" or "damping" of sound (fourth Korotkoff phase).	10. American Heart Association states this sound is the most accurate index of *diastolic pressure*.
11. Note the final disappearance of sound (fifth Korotkoff phase).	11. Many institutions use this as the index of *diastolic pressure*.
12. Deflate cuff completely to zero and wait 30 to 60 sec. before taking B/P again. Repeat the reading if you are unsure of accuracy.	12. Occlusion of blood during pressure reading causes venous congestion in the forearm. Venous blood must be allowed to drain or it will *falsely elevate* succeeding B/P readings.

SUGGESTED STEPS	RATIONALE/DISCUSSION
13. If unable to determine B/P due to feeble sounds, elevate patient's arm and then inflate the cuff. Then lower arm, deflate cuff and listen.	13. Decreases venous pressure and should make the sounds louder.
14. If still unable to hear, note the *palpatory systolic pressure* by feeling for reappearance of radial pulse. (See step 7.)	14. B/P by palpation is a few mm. Hg lower than by auscultation, but will still be meaningful as long as subsequent measurements are made in the same way.

Post-Procedure Activities.   Assess B/P findings in view of patient's overall clinical picture. Record findings (including patient's position) on chart. If data show a significant change in patient's condition take indicated actions, e.g., communicate findings to appropriate persons.

Occasionally you may notice an *auscultatory gap*, especially in patients with hypertension. In this instance, the sound initially appears at a high value, then fades out completely and reappears 10 to 40 mm. Hg later.[21] The pulse is palpable during this period of abnormal silence. If you do not pump the cuff high enough, you will miss the top sound and seriously underestimate the systolic pressure. To avoid this, palpate the radial artery while pumping the cuff. Five per cent of patients with hypertension may be unrecognized if the palpatory pressure is not checked against the auscultatory findings.[1]

When all sounds disappear, deflate the cuff rapidly. Wait 30 to 60 seconds before repeating the reading, as venous congestion in the arm will falsely elevate subsequent diastolic pressure values. If you are unsure of the value, repeat the procedure.

Palpatory Method.   The stethoscope is omitted, and the point at which the radial artery pulsation is *first palpated* during cuff deflation is taken for the systolic pressure. This method is useful clinically when a patient is in shock and has a greatly reduced cardiac output. Although the pulsations may be too feeble to auscultate, they may be palpable even when the radial pulse is rapid and thready. The systolic reading is usually a few mm. Hg lower by palpation than by auscultation.[21] The diastolic reading is difficult to determine by palpation and usually is not done. Enselberg describes the sensation when the diastolic pressure is

reached as a thin, abrupt snapping vibration felt over the brachial artery.[11] This method of diastolic determination is subjective, and is not recommended for clinical use. With a critically ill patient, blood pressure readings by palpation will not be as accurate as the *direct method* by use of an arterial line.

Thigh Pressure.   Blood pressure readings are taken in the lower extremities to compare values with arm readings or when the arms are injured or otherwise unavailable. Position the patient on his abdomen, apply the cuff to the thigh centered over the popliteal artery located in the back of the knee. Perform the procedure as detailed above, auscultating at the popliteal artery. If the patient is unable to lie on his abdomen, place him supine with the knee bent slightly. The systolic pressure will be 10 to 40 mm. Hg higher in the thigh than in the arms, and the diastolic pressure will be the same in both sites.

Blood Pressure Readings in Children and Infants

For children, use the procedure as described above. The most common source of error is inappropriate cuff size. On children, the cuff should cover two-thirds of the arm above the elbow.[21] Make sure the child or infant has been quiet for 5 to 10 minutes before the reading; crying can elevate the systolic reading 30 to 50 mm. Hg.[21]

An infant under one year may have such small extremities that it is impossible to hear auscultatory sounds. In this situation, the *flush method* gives a mean systolic-diastolic pressure. Make sure the baby is quiet; if necessary use a bottle or pacifier. The room must be well-lighted, and the manometer gauge placed close to the extremity so both can be seen at the same time. Apply the appropriate neonatal cuff around the arm or leg. Elevate the extremity and squeeze the part distal to the cuff with your hand or wrap it tightly with an elastic bandage. These maneuvers will blanch the extremity. Pump the manometer to 120 to 140 mm. Hg and lower the extremity. Release the pressure of your hand or bandage, at the same time that you deflate the cuff at a rate not more than 5 mm. Hg per second. The point at which the baby's arm or leg flushes is the mean systolic-diastolic pressure. A normal reading is 30 to 60 mm. Hg for infants weighing more than 6.5 lbs.[43]

Measurement Errors

Since many nursing judgments are based on the results of blood pressure determination, it is crucial to avoid errors in the measurement (Table 29–2). Mitchell and Van Meter documented errors in a study comparing B/P readings obtained by nursing personnel, who were unaware that they were being studied, with readings obtained by the investigators.[30] They found an average difference of 7 mm. Hg or less between the two groups; a difference of more than 10 mm. Hg in 37 to 46 per cent of the readings; and a difference of more than 15 mm. Hg in 21 to 27 per cent of the readings. Nursing personnel consistently recorded higher pressures than the investigators. Among the levels of nursing personnel, RNs varied the most with the investigators. This may be due to their knowledge of previous readings, their preconceived idea of what the B/P should be, or that RNs were busier due to their other responsibilities and thus prone to haste.

Haste or subconscious bias are important examples of observer error. The preconceived idea of pressure means that the observer may be influenced subconsciously by the patient's age or weight and may "hear" a value in line with what is expected for that group. Another example is "digit preference," where the observer hears more values that end in zero (e.g., 140/80) than would be expected by chance alone.[21] Other sources of error are listed in Table 29–2.

When such errors—defective equipment, poor technique, haste—are eliminated, the results are reliable. Glor et al. studied three groups of workers (professional nurses, nursing students, and nonprofessional nursing personnel) and found no significant difference in systolic or diastolic measurements among the groups' B/P results.[14] They conclude that standardization of the procedure contributed to the elimination of observer error.

TABLE 29–2.   COMMON SOURCES OF ERROR IN BLOOD PRESSURE MEASUREMENT

Errors that produce a falsely **high** reading

▶ Failure to use the appropriate cuff size; a too narrow cuff gives a higher reading.
▶ Wrapping the cuff too loosely or unevenly (cuff pressure must be exceedingly high to compress the brachial artery).
▶ Recording the B/P just after a meal, with smoking, or while patient's bladder is distended.
▶ Failure to have the mercury column vertical.
▶ Deflating the cuff too slowly: this produces venous congestion in the extremity which falsely elevates the diastolic pressure.

Errors that produce a falsely **low** reading

▶ Having the patient's arm above the level of the heart (effect of hydrostatic pressure can give an error up to 10 mm. Hg in systolic and diastolic pressure).[21]
▶ Failure to notice an auscultatory gap.
▶ Diminished hearing acuity of the worker.
▶ Stethoscope that is too small, too large, or has tubing that is too long.
▶ Inability to hear feeble Korotkoff sounds.

Errors that produce *either* falsely **high** or **low** readings

▶ Inaccurately calibrated manometer.
▶ Defective equipment (valve, connections).
▶ Failure to have meniscus of mercury at eye level.
▶ Performing the technique too quickly, with too little attention given to details.

Technique and equipment must be well controlled to produce accurate and reliable results. "No data is better than wrong data!"[5]

Abnormal Findings

Blood pressure determination is a part of every screening physical examination both in the hospital and in ambulatory settings. Certain groups of patients require more frequent monitoring. These include patients with heart disease (such as myocardial infarction), patients having surgery, those with hypertension or taking antihypertensive medications, and patients with neurologic disorders (e.g., increased intracranial pressure). Following are categories of abnormal B/P results.

Hypotension in adults is a B/P below 95/60. However, in the healthy adult, a persistent systolic pressure of 90 to 100 with no accompanying symptoms is not clinically significant. Remember that a normally hypertensive patient experiences hypotension at a much higher level. It is important to know the average vital signs for your patient before you attach significance to one isolated figure. Hypotension occurs with Addison's disease (hypofunction of the adrenal glands), hemorrhage as the total blood volume is decreased, and vasodilation as the peripheral resistance decreases. Expect a small drop in B/P when you apply blankets to warm up a postoperative patient who is vasoconstricted from the cool OR environment. The drop is not significant if the pulse remains stable. Should the drop continue and the patient become diaphoretic and the pulse increase, inspect the patient for signs of hemorrhage and notify the physician.

Hypotension also occurs with conditions of decreased cardiac output, such as an acute MI or shock. Here the patient has an increased pulse, dizziness, diaphoresis, confusion and blurred vision. The skin feels cool and clammy as vasoconstriction attempts to shunt blood to the vital organs. A patient having an acute MI may also complain of crushing substernal chest pain, high epigastric pain, and shoulder or jaw pain.

The World Health Organization gives the following definition of *hypertension*:

> *Hypertension is a persistent elevation of the systolic blood pressure above 140 mm. Hg and of the diastolic pressure above 90 mm. Hg.*

This occurs with kidney disease, pheochromocytoma (tumor of adrenal medulla), coarctation of the aorta, and essential hypertension (i.e., of no known cause). There is a strong familial tendency for hypertension, and the patient may also have nosebleeds, severe headaches, and irritability. Also classified as hypertension are conditions of increased systolic pressure while the diastolic remains normal, as in anemia, hyperthyroidism, aortic insufficiency, and atherosclerosis in the older patient.

Elevated blood pressure is a danger sign of increased intracranial pressure in the patient having neurosurgery or brain trauma. An increasing hematoma in the brain increases the intracranial pressure and decreases blood flow. The vasomotor center in the medulla responds to the decreased O_2 and causes vasoconstriction throughout the body in an attempt to increase perfusion. The pulse rate decreases, and the respirations are Cheyne-Stokes or may cease altogether. Unfortunately these vital signs are *late* consequences of increased intracranial pressure. Earlier warning signs are clouding of consciousness, changes in movement (hemiparesis, positive Babinski's sign), and pupil inequality (one suddenly dilated nonreactive pupil).

You may notice other alterations in blood pressure in your practice. A surprisingly high blood pressure in the arms of the young adult or teenager may suggest *coarctation* (congenital narrowing) of the aorta. Pressure increases as the heart works harder to pump blood through the narrowed opening. Right arm pressure always increases with coarctation; elevation of left arm pressure depends on the location of the stricture.[5] Blood pressure in the legs is much lower than normal as the blood supply to the legs is below the constriction in the aorta.

Another noteworthy alteration is *paradoxical blood pressure*. The audible sound varies with the patient's respirations, fading out with inspiration and becoming stronger with expiration. The mechanism is similar to that of paradoxical pulse discussed above. Paradoxical blood pressure occurs normally with very deep breathing, but if pronounced it may signify cardiac tamponade in some patients.

Communicating the Findings

Analysis of the data gathered during the taking of routine vital signs enables you to make your nursing judgments and plan your interventions. Integrate the data into the patient's overall clinical picture. Record the numerical

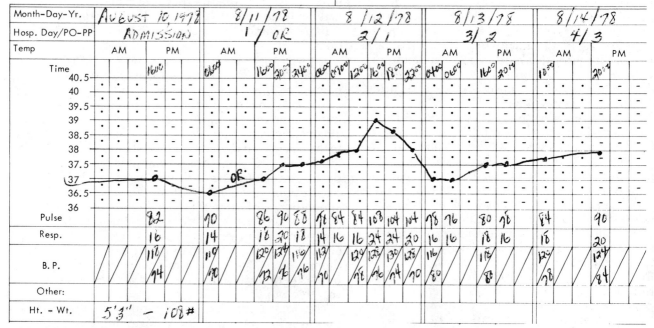

Figure 29–8. Sample form of a vital signs "graphic" sheet. Notice all the vital signs when this patient "spikes a temp" on her first "post-op" day. Also notice the increased frequency of measurement as the nurse suspects a developing trend. (Courtesy of University of Missouri–Columbia, Medical Center, Nursing Service Department, Columbia, MO 65201.)

data in the appropriate place on the patient's graphic sheet (Fig. 29–8). Further significant data should be charted in the progress notes. For example, charting about a rapid thready pulse on a patient who has had surgery also should include B/P reading, skin temperature and moistness, skin color, level of consciousness, and any sign of blood loss. Similarly, charting about respiratory status would include the following: rate, pattern of respirations, subjective feeling, and mental status.

If the data indicates a significant change, communicate the results and your interventions to the appropriate persons. To make the message meaningful, you must communicate all vital signs, how they have changed from previous values, how they fit into the patient's entire clinical picture, and any interventions you have planned or have made already. Aberrant vital signs lead to countless interventions, both in partnership with others on the health care team and as independent nursing measures. Detailed knowledge of vital signs gives you a broad base for planning patient care.

ELECTRONIC MONITORING

Advances in technology make it possible to constantly and accurately monitor the vital signs of critically ill patients. Such equipment includes the cardiac monitor, photocell, Doppler ultrasonic flowmeter, arterial line for direct B/P measurement, central venous pressure (CVP) catheter, and temperature probe (Fig. 29–9).

Electronic equipment may be necessary to monitor a very irregular or a very weak pulse. A patient prone to *arrhythmias* (any variation from the normal heart rhythm) requires a continuous electrocardiogram (EKG) monitor. Electrodes pasted on the patient's chest sense

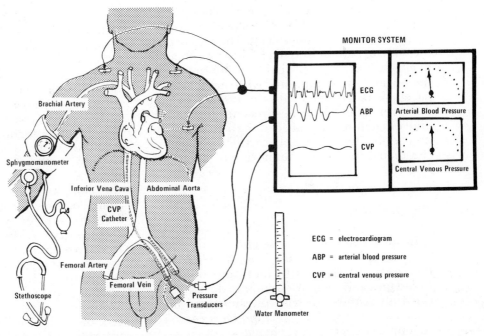

Figure 29-9. Monitoring the vital signs of a critically ill patient. (Courtesy of Judy Taylor, R.N., University of Missouri Medical Center.)

the conduction pathway that the impulse takes through the heart and transmits this pattern to a viewing screening or oscilloscope. Nurses skilled in determining arrhythmia patterns watch the patient and his cardiac monitor for signs and symptoms of irregular heartbeats. Patients having a myocardial infarction are particularly prone to arrhythmias that could be fatal if not noticed immediately and treated.

Although electronic monitoring is painless, it communicates nonverbally to the patient that he must be sick indeed to require such intricate machinery. Psychologic support is paramount for this patient. Reassure him that the cardiac monitor is a preventive measure; it aids the health care team in treating a possible problem before it becomes serious. The patient and family may watch the screen anxiously and may confuse a harmless wandering of the pattern (called artifact or mechanical interference) with a serious arrhythmia. Teach them that the sensitive electrodes pick up electrical impulses from the skeletal muscles as well as from the heart, so the pattern will change whenever the patient moves around in bed. Help the family understand that the nurses are skilled in differentiating the meaning of these patterns.

The *photocell* monitors perfusion of each

cardiac systole to the peripheral parts of the body. Attached to the helix of the ear, it senses blood flow by bouncing light off the moving red blood cells (Fig. 29-10). This is transformed to a waveform, which is displayed on a bedside oscilloscope. When displayed right below the EKG pattern, the nurse can determine if every

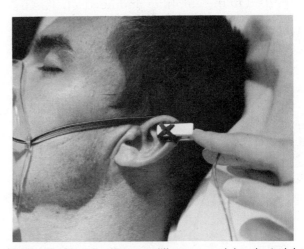

Figure 29-10. The "photocell" senses peripheral arterial pulsations and transmits them to a viewing screen. (Courtesy of Judy Taylor, R.N., University of Missouri Medical Center.)

heartbeat is being perfused by noting the height of each photocell wave. When stroke volume is decreased, the photocell records a diminished wave or none at all. The photocell is useful with patients having multiple premature heartbeats where ventricular filling time is reduced and with patients who have cardiac pacemakers for whom it is important to note that every paced heartbeat reaches the peripheral circulation. Because it is a noninvasive procedure, the photocell carries less patient risk than direct pulse monitoring by an arterial line.

The Doppler

In some conditions, pulse and B/P data must be obtained by use of the *Doppler Ultrasonic flowmeter*. This small electronic device is based on a variation of a principle described by the 19th century Austrian physicist and mathematician, Christina Johann Doppler. The "Doppler effect" is the change in pitch as the distance between a sound source and a listener are rapidly varied.[3]

A transducer the size of a pencil is placed gently on the skin over an arterial pulse covered with conducting gel. The transducer has two crystals. One transmits ultrasound produced in the Doppler and beams it against the artery. The energy from the moving red blood cells backscatters (bounces back) the sound at a slightly different frequency than the original. The second crystal receives the sound and sends it to the amplifier and headset. The frequency change is the change in pitch noted by the listener through the earphones (Fig. 29–11). Because cardiac systole moves the cells

through the artery in a rhythmic fashion, the listener hears a *pulsatile* beat. The sound has a swishing, wooshing quality, rather than the tapping heard through a stethoscope. The advantages of this system are that it is portable, reliable, technically easy to master, relatively inexpensive, and noninvasive (i.e., there is no trauma to the vessel wall as there would be if a measuring catheter were placed *directly* into the artery).[20]

The use of the Doppler allows the operator to obtain both quantitative and qualitative data (presence or absence of pulse and its characteristics) for a variety of clinical situations.[20] The Doppler technician can determine the patency of veins when the patient has venous disease, such as varicose veins, venous stasis ulcers, or phlebothrombosis. During surgery, the Doppler is used to check success of vein grafts before the surgical incision is closed. Continued patency of these grafts is monitored by the nurses in the recovery room and surgical intensive care unit. When an artery to an extremity is plugged by a thrombus or an embolus (a moving clot), the Doppler allows the operator to locate the site of occlusion. The Doppler is used to screen patients under high risk of stroke, by determining patency of the arteries that supply the brain. In persons undergoing hemodialysis, the Doppler is used to verify the patency of the vascular shunt used to connect the patient to the dialysis machine. The Doppler also is used to ascertain whether blood flow to and from an organ transplant (e.g., the kidney) is normal. The Doppler can be used to evaluate blood flow to extremities after trauma, such as gunshot or knife wounds or auto accidents. Also, Doppler is used to monitor B/P in lower limbs when upper ones normally used for B/P readings are involved in trauma. Studies show that ankle pressure equals arm pressure ±10 mm. Hg.[24] The Doppler also is used to monitor blood pressure in patients who are difficult to check in the usual manner, such

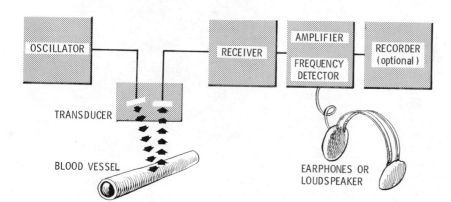

Figure 29–11. The components of the Doppler ultrasound system. (From Scherr, D. D., Lichti, E. L., and Lambert, K. L.: Tissue-viability assessment with the Doppler ultrasonic flowmeter in acute injuries of extremities. *Journal of Bone and Joint Surgery,* 55A:157–161, Jan. 1973.)

as newborn or premature babies and obese patients. In an obese patient, the layers of fat muffle Korotkoff's sounds, making them difficult or impossible to hear accurately. Also, an obese upper arm is conical shaped, which makes it difficult to apply the armcuff smoothly. To obtain a blood pressure reading in the obese patient, the Doppler probe is held over the radial artery and the cuff is placed below the elbow. Studies show the pressure reading with cuff placement below the elbow equals that obtained when the cuff is in the normal position above the elbow if there are no abnormalities (such as occlusion) of the artery.[23]

The Arterial Line

Direct monitoring of B/P via a catheter placed *within* an artery is indicated in critically ill patients, e.g., after open-heart or other major surgery when moment-to-moment changes are anticipated, or in low pressure states such as congestive heart failure and shock, where cardiac output is decreased greatly and peripheral vascular resistance is increased. The increased resistance impedes the already low blood flow into the arms, thus diminishing Korotkoff sounds. The only accurate method of B/P determination is via the direct route, called an *arterial line.*

A plastic catheter is inserted into the radial or femoral artery and anchored. It is filled with heparinized fluid to prevent clotting and attached by tubing to an electronic pressure sensor, the transducer. This transforms mechanical energy from the pulsating blood into electrical energy. The electrical pattern is transmitted as a waveform and is displayed continuously on a bedside oscilloscope (see Fig. 29–9). The electronic equipment also may display numerical systolic and diastolic pressure values.

Values obtained by direct B/P monitoring are higher than the indirect or auscultatory method.[21] The readings are continuous and are accurate when equipment is working properly. Sources of error are in the nurse's technique and in the calibration of the equipment. The nurse must be skilled in operating this complex and expensive equipment.

Although the arterial line may aid in prompt lifesaving interventions, it also carries some risk to the patient. Because the artery has been invaded, there are dangers of hematoma, thrombus formation, and infection. Improper technique carries the hazards of injecting air into the artery, or rapid blood loss if the system comes apart.

Patient anxiety due to the arterial line *itself* is comparatively small, and many patients are unable to distinguish it from the other intravenous lines.[31] However, since patients who require an arterial line are seriously ill, nurses must try to allay anxiety from the overall crisis situation.

Other equipment frequently used with critically ill patients includes a central venous pressure (CVP) catheter. The CVP reflects the pressure of the blood in the right atrium of the heart as measured by a catheter threaded through a vein into the superior or inferior vena cava (see Fig. 29–9). The CVP reading indicates the amount of circulating blood volume, the efficiency of the heart in pumping the blood, and the vascular tone. The CVP will increase with vigorous intravenous fluid infusion, when the heart fails as a pump and blood becomes congested, and with peripheral vasoconstriction. A low CVP is expected with hemorrhage or vasodilation.

BIBLIOGRAPHY

1. Askey, J. M.: The auscultatory gap in sphygmomanometry. *Annals Internal Medicine,* 80:94–97, Jan. 1974.
2. Beaumont, E.: Blood pressure equipment. *Nursing '75,* 75:56–62, Jan. 1975.
3. Beene, T. K., et al.: The ultrasonic flowmeter. An aid for blood pressure determinations during cardiopulmonary bypass. *Journal of Thoracic and Cardiovascular Surgery,* 66:12–15, July 1973.
4. Broughton, J. O.: Chest physical diagnosis for nurses and respiratory therapists. *Heart and Lung,* 1:200–206, March–April 1972.
5. Burch, G. E., and DePasquale, N. P.: *Primer of Clinical Measurement of Blood Pressure.* St. Louis, The C. V. Mosby Company, 1962.
6. Butler, E. K.: Dyspnea in the patient with cardiopulmonary disease. *Heart and Lung,* 4:599–606, July–Aug. 1975.
7. Cannon, U. B.: *The Wisdom of the Body.* New York, W. W. Norton and Company, 1939.
8. Comroe, J. H.: *The Physiology of Respiration: An Introductory Text,* 2nd ed. Chicago, Year Book Medical Publishers, Inc., 1974.
9. Doyle, M. P., and Jordan, L. E.: A comparison of pulse deficit reading by serial and simultaneous measurement. *Nursing Research,* 17:460, Sep.–Oct. 1968.
10. Eisman, R.: *Criteria Registered Nurses Reportedly Use in Making Decisions Regarding the Observation of Respiratory Behavior of Patients.* Unpublished master's thesis, University of Washington, Seattle, 1970.
11. Enselberg, C. D.: Measurement of diastolic blood pressure by palpation. *New England Journal of Medicine,* 265:272–274, Aug. 1961.
12. Felton, G.: Effect of time cycle change on blood pressure and temperature in young women. *Nursing Research,* 19:48–58, Jan.–Feb. 1970.
13. Foley, M. F.: Variations in blood pressure in the lateral recumbent position. *Nursing Research,* 20:64–69, Jan.–Feb. 1971.

14. Glor, B. A., et al.: Reproducibility of blood pressure measurements: a replication. *Nursing Research,* 19:170–172, March–April 1970.
15. Guyton, A. C.: *A Textbook of Medical Physiology,* 6th ed. Philadelphia, W. B. Saunders Company, 1976.
16. Hargest, T. S.: Start your count with zero. *American Journal of Nursing,* 74:887, May 1974.
17. Jarvis, C. M.: Vital signs—how to take them more accurately and understand them more fully. *Nursing '76,* 76:31–37, April 1976.
18. Joint Committee on Pulmonary Nomenclature, American College of Chest Physicians and American Thoracic Society: Pulmonary terms and symbols. *Chest,* 67:583–593, 1975.
19. Jones, M. L.: Accuracy of pulse rates counted for fifteen, thirty and sixty seconds. *Military Medicine,* 135:1127, Dec. 1970.
20. Keitzer, W. F., and Lichti, E. L.: Applications of the Doppler—common and unusual situations. *Angiology,* 26:172–185, Feb. 1975.
21. Kirkendall, W. M., et al.: Committee of the American Heart Association: Recommendations for human blood pressure determination by sphygmomanometers. *Circulation,* 36:980–988, Dec. 1967.
22. Kory, Ross C.: Routine measurement of respiratory rate: an expensive tribute to tradition. *Journal of the American Medical Association,* 165:448–450, Oct. 1957.
23. Lichti, E. L.: Use of the Doppler ultrasonic flowmeter to monitor blood pressure during ileal loop bypass for extreme obesity. *The American Surgeon,* 40:398–399, July 1974.
24. Lichti, E. L., et al.: Atraumatic evaluation of peripheral vascular disease in older patients. *Geriatrics,* 26:80–85, 1971.
25. Lovell, S., and Dugdale, A. E.: The history of pulse taking. *Australian Nurses' Journal,* 3:32–33, April 1974.
26. Luckmann, J., and Sorensen, K. C.: *Medical-Surgical Nursing-A Psychophysiologic Approach.* Philadelphia, W. B. Saunders Co., 1974.
27. Lynch, J. J., et al.: The effects of pulse taking on the cardiac function of patients in a coronary-care unit. *Psychophysiology,* 10:200, 1973 (Abstract).
28. McCain, F.: Nursing by assessment–not intuition. *American Journal of Nursing,* 65:82, April 1965.
29. Marsden, A., and Sana, J. M.: Nurse–patient communication and relationship in the physical appraisal process. *In* Sana, J. M., and Judge, R. D. (eds.): *Physical Appraisal Methods in Nursing Practice.* Boston, Little, Brown and Company, 1975.
30. Mitchell, P. W., and Van Meter, M.: Reproducibility of blood pressures recorded on patients' records by nursing personnel. *Nursing Research,* 20:348–352, July–Aug. 1971.
31. Nielsen, Mary A.: Intra-arterial monitoring of blood pressure. *American Journal of Nursing,* 74:48–53, Jan. 1974.
32. O'Dell, M. L.: Are routine admission signs really reliable? *RN,* 38:23, April 1975 (Condensed from O'Dell, M. L.: Vital signs of surgical patients on routine admission to the hospital and three and six hours post-admission. *Military Medicine,* 139:719–721, Sep. 1974.
33. Perlman, L. W., et al.: Accuracy of sphygmomanometers in hospital practice. *Archives Internal Medicine,* 125:1000–1003, June 1970.
34. Pinney, S. M.: Physical appraisal of respiratory system function. *In* Sana, S. M. and Judge, R. D. (eds.): *Physical Appraisal Methods in Nursing Practice.* Boston, Little, Brown and Company, 1975.
35. Shapiro, B. A., et al.: *Clinical Application of Respiratory Care.* Chicago, Year Book Medical Publishers, Inc., 1975.
36. Skidmore, E., and Marshall, A.: Towards a more accurate mesurement of blood pressure. *Nursing Times,* 72:376–378, March 1976.
37. Sparks, C.: Peripheral pulses. *American Journal of Nursing,* 75:1132–1133, July 1975.
38. Steinfeld, L., et al.: Needed: better techniques for reading blood pressure. *RN,* 37:1CU-1, May 1974.
38a. Stright, P. A., and Soukup, S. M.: How to hear it right: Evaluating and choosing a stethoscope. *American Journal of Nursing,* 77:1477, Sep. 1977.
39. Sweetwood, H.: Bedside assessment of respirations. *Nursing '73,* 3:50–51, Sep. 1973.
40. Thomas, S. A., et al.: Psychosocial influences on heart rhythm in the coronary-unit. *Heart and Lung,* 4:746, Sep.–Oct. 1975.
41. Traver, G. A.: Assessment of thorax and lungs. *American Journal of Nursing,* 73:466–471, March 1973.
42. Ward, R. J., et al.: Cardiovascular effects of change in posture. *Aerospace Medicine,* 37:257–259, March 1966.
43. Warren, F. M.: Blood pressure readings—getting them quickly on an infant. *Nursing '75,* 5:13, April 1975.
44. West, J. B.: *Respiratory Physiology: The Essentials.* Baltimore, The Williams & Wilkins Company, 1974.
45. Winslow, E. H.: Digitalis. *American Journal of Nursing,* 74:1062–1065, June 1974.
46. Zikria, B. A., et al.: Alterations in ventilatory function and breathing patterns following surgical trauma. *Annals of Surgery,* 179:1–7, Jan. 1974.
47. Zuck, D.: Life, metabolism and hypoxia 1. *Nursing Times,* 64:1680–1681, Dec. 1968.

CHAPTER 30

MAINTAINING BOWEL AND KIDNEY FUNCTIONS

By Barbara S. Innes, R.N., M.S.

INTRODUCTION AND STUDY GUIDE

One of the body's basic physiologic needs is to rid itself of wastes. The three main routes for accomplishing this are the respiratory tract, gastrointestinal tract, and urinary tract. The skin is a more minor route of elimination—by secretion. Since elimination of wastes is a first-level need for survival, the body sets high priority on maintaining optimal functioning of these systems.

People frequently need assistance from health professionals in order to safely and effectively meet their elimination needs. This chapter discusses bowel and kidney elimination. Since stress in any form has a definite impact on these two systems and people in contact with health professionals are often under stress, health professionals have to deal with bowel and kidney elimination problems many times. This chapter will discuss how to (a) help people maintain their normal elimination function, (b) identify existing and potential problems with normal bowel and kidney function, and (c) plan and implement nursing actions designed to prevent or resolve elimination problems.

After completing this chapter, the student should be able to:

1. Define the following terms:

anuria	enuresis
bacteriuria	fecal impaction
clean-catch specimen	feces
constipation	flatulence
defecation	flatus
diarrhea	fractional
dysuria	guaiac
hematuria	peristalsis
hemorrhoid	pyuria
incontinence	retention
ketone bodies	retention with overflow
melena	specific gravity
micturition	stool
nocturia	suppository
occult blood	void
oliguria	

2. Discuss normal anatomy and physiology of the lower gastrointestinal and urinary tracts.

3. Describe in detail the act of defecation and factors that influence it.

4. Describe in detail the act of micturition and factors that influence it.

5. List data needed to make a complete assessment of a person's bowel and kidney status.

6. Discuss independent nursing measures to aid patients in maintaining normal bowel and kidney elimination.

7. Discuss the following common problems of bowel and kidney function and the modes of treatment for these problems: constipation, fecal impaction, diarrhea, flatulence, hemorrhoids, incontinence, urinary retention, retention with overflow, urinary tract infection, urinary stones, and established fecal and urinary diversion.

8. Discuss how to collect fecal and urine specimens.

9. Describe how to perform selected tests on urine and feces.

BOWEL FUNCTION

Normal Anatomy and Physiology

The gastrointestinal tract, or alimentary canal, is a hollow, muscular tube which runs from the mouth to the anus. The main functions of this tube are to receive fluids and nutrients, digest and absorb them, and eliminate waste products from the body. This description portrays the anatomy and physiology of the gastrointestinal tract in the simplest terms. Actually the processes described require a number of ancillary organs and anatomic structures, chemical substances, and physiologic processes. We will briefly consider these as they relate to the elimination process. For more in-depth study, the reader is referred to any standard anatomy and physiology text.

Although in our discussion of waste elimination, we are mainly interested in the lower part of the gastrointestinal tract—the large intestine terminating in the rectum and anus—we must be aware of the influence of the upper part of the tract. As food is taken in through the mouth, the process of digestion is begun. Mastication, or chewing, starts the mechanical and chemical breakdown of food. The bolus of food is swallowed and moves through the esophagus into the stomach.

Food moves through the esophagus, and indeed through the entire gastrointestinal tract, by a process called *peristalsis*. Peristalsis is a propulsive movement in which there is a wave of smooth muscle contraction moving forward along a tube, forcing contents of the tube ahead of it. Although the direction of the force may be in either direction, the movement in the gastrointestinal tract is usually toward the anus. This peristaltic movement is essential to the digestive and elimination functions of the alimentary canal, and if it stops for any reason, the tract cannot fulfill its intended activities.

The stomach is mainly a storage chamber, in which food is further broken down into a semifluid state called "chyme" and is readied to be slowly passed into the small intestine. As chyme travels through the small intestine, the digestive processes are completed and absorption of nutrients takes place. The chyme then passes through the ileocecal sphincter into the large intestine, which is about 1.5 m. (5 ft.) long.

Figure 30–1 details the anatomy of the lower gastrointestinal tract. Refer to Chapter 40, Figures 40–1 and 40–2, to review how the pelvic organs are positioned in relation to each other. In addition to passing waste materials out of the body, the colon has the function of absorbing water, sodium, and chlorides. As the chyme travels through the ascending, transverse, and descending colon segments into the sigmoid, it becomes concentrated into a more solid mass. The longer the fecal material stays in the colon, the more water is absorbed from it.

Movement of the *feces*, or excrement, through the large intestine is accomplished by peristalsis, segmental contractions, and haustral churning, as in other portions of the gas-

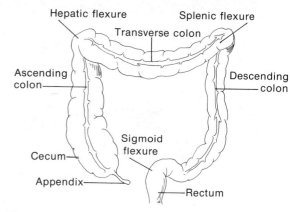

Figure 30–1. Anatomy of the lower gastrointestinal tract.

trointestinal tract. In addition, periods of mass peristalsis occur two or three times a day, usually following meals. This movement pushes the contents along the intestine for some distance. These massive contractions are stimulated by two reflexes that are very important to bowel elimination and that occur most strongly when a person eats following a period of fasting, such as breakfast after a night's sleep. The *gastrocolic reflex* occurs when the bolus of food enters the stomach and stimulates peristalsis throughout the entire gastrointestinal tract; the *duodenocolic reflex* acts in a similar manner, but is the weaker of the two reflexes.

The fecal material moves into the sigmoid portion of the colon, where it is stored until being passed out of the body. Transit time through the gastrointestinal tract is affected by such things as rate of motility, amount of dietary residue, and the presence or absence of irritating substances in the colon. However, it usually takes from 6 to 8 hours for the contents to travel from the stomach to the sigmoid colon.

Another substance which must be removed from the gastrointestinal tract is gas, or *flatus*. This gas is formed partially from the fermentation processes in the bowel and partially from air taken in through the mouth.

Act of Defecation

To complete passage from the body, the feces and gas move through the rectum, anal canal, and anus during the act of *defecation*. The act is also referred to as "having a bowel movement" and is under both voluntary and involuntary control.

The rectum, which is about 10 to 15 cm. (4 to 6 inches) long, usually remains empty until just before and during defecation. When the fecal mass or gas moves from the sigmoid colon into the rectum, the defecation reflex begins. Feces enter the rectum either as a result of a mass propulsive movement in the colon or voluntarily, through increase of the intra-abdominal pressure by contraction of the abdominal muscles and forced expiration with a closed glottis, which forces the diaphragm downward. Distention of the rectum causes increased intrarectal pressure and the perceived desire or urge to evacuate the bowel.

The anal canal has two sphincters. The internal sphincter is smooth muscle and is innervated through the autonomic nervous system. Distention of the rectum causes it to involuntarily relax in order to allow passage of the feces. The external sphincter at the anus consists of striated muscle and is under voluntary control. At the same time that the internal sphincter is being stimulated to relax by descending feces or *stool*, so is the external sphincter. However, a person, after a successful period of toilet-training, can voluntarily control this sphincter, and if the time is not right, the act of defecation can be delayed by constriction of the anus. Contraction of the levator ani muscle reinforces the voluntary constriction of the anus. If the act of defecation is stopped, the stool in the rectum remains there until the defecation reflex is again stimulated.

Factors Affecting Normal Defecation

Defecation is normally a painless process, which can be affected by many factors—both psychologic and physiologic. Many of these become the bases for independent and dependent nursing interventions.

Psychological Factors. The relationship between alteration of a normal defecation pattern and the psyche has been clearly shown, although sometimes it is difficult to determine which came first—the gastrointestinal disturbance or emotional condition.[12] Selye has demonstrated that stress is manifested in measurable changes in organ function—and one of the organs frequently affected is the gastrointestinal tract.[97] Several disease processes with severe gastrointestinal disturbances—diarrhea, gaseous distention—as part of their symptomatology are considered to have a significant psychologic overlay; examples include ulcerative colitis and Crohn's disease. Mental depression slows all bodily activities, and constipation may be the presenting symptom. You have probably experienced some kind of gastrointestinal disturbance when faced with a high-anxiety situation, such as a public speaking engagement or a blind date. When a patient develops a gastrointestinal problem, the nurse must carefully determine whether a psychologic concern is precipitating or supporting it.

Toilet-Training Experiences. Experiences linked with toilet-training during childhood can have long-lasting effects. A person's negative or positive attitudes toward bowel elimination sometimes can be traced back to this developmental period. Rewards, or reinforcement for positive behavior, tend to result in continued problem-free elimination patterns. On the other hand, a person who received punishment as the primary motivator during toilet-training may carry over into his adult life feelings of guilt and anxiety that are manifested in gastrointestinal problems. In addition, use or nonuse of the toilet for defecation may be a means by which some children reward or punish their parents, and this behavior may have an effect on their own adult life. Much has been written to help parents guide their children through this learning process.

Cultural Teachings. Cultural teachings have a great influence on a person's defecation habits. In American society, we are taught strict rules about when and under what conditions defecation can take place. Failure to follow these rules results in social censure and even isolation if behavior strays too far from the established mores. In the United States, the act of defecation is generally a very personal, private matter and we go to great lengths to build special rooms with locked doors to ensure this privacy. For many people, bowel activity is a topic not to be discussed. Therefore, when a person must seek out a health professional regarding problems with bowel elimination or finds himself in a situation where he is no longer able to meet his elimination needs in his accustomed manner, there is conflict with his cultural and personal practices. This conflict leads to embarrassment and anxiety.

The inability to maintain privacy regarding bowel function and the resulting psychologic reactions affect both the patient and the nurse. The patient is the pivotal person since it is he who must personally face the reactions of others when he is unable to privately take care of his own elimination needs. In the hospital setting especially, there are numerous invasions of privacy. Even if the patient's primary problem has nothing to do with the gastrointestinal tract, he is (or should be) questioned carefully about his bowel patterns before and during his period of hospitalization. If he is very lucky, he will have a private bathroom; more often, at best, he will share a bathroom with one or more strangers. At worst, he will be in a multiple-bed room and will have to use a commode or bedpan for the act of defecation, with its accompanying sounds and odors—during visiting hours. Empathetically, place yourself in your patient's position. If you had diarrhea, wouldn't you rather be in your own home with your own bathroom? Because of the lack of privacy, many people will deliberately avoid having a bowel movement; this only results in problems, such as constipation, which require intervention and focus even more attention on the patient and his elimination.

The nurse is also subject to feelings of embarrassment and anxiety when dealing with patients' elimination needs, particularly at the beginning of her career. The student brings to the clinical unit her own cultural background and personal experiences, and if these emphasized privacy, there will be conflict between expectations and feelings. The student will be required to discuss elimination patterns openly with patients, to identify elimination needs and to plan and implement actions designed to prevent and resolve elimination problems. Because elimination is a first-level, basic need of all people, the nurse will be required to take on this responsibility very early—often in the first or second meeting with a patient. The nurse's embarrassment and anxiety are easily transmitted to the patient, often aggravating the feelings that the patient is already having. The student is reassured by others that these feelings will diminish with experience; discussing these feelings with peers and instructors hastens the socialization process.

Indeed, the nursing student will gain the ability to deal with patients' elimination needs in a matter-of-fact fashion. However, even this development can be detrimental to the patient. What is matter-of-fact to the nurse may not be so to the patient. The nurse must continually remain sensitive to patients' feelings of embarrassment and anxiety about elimination needs. We in the nursing profession often forget this.

It must also be mentioned that not all patients will be embarrassed or reluctant to discuss bowel habits. Americans tend to be very bowel-conscious, a fact which is amplified by advertising in the mass media. Some elderly persons have a particular tendency to be concerned about their bowels and actively pursue measures that will continue their established patterns. In essence, the nurse must carefully assess each patient's willingness to discuss his bowel function and potential problems with it.

Personal Habits. In addition to the psychologic influences on defecation, there are many physical factors that may affect a person's elimination patterns. An individual's habits regarding bowel function are very important. As will be discussed later, the bowel can be trained to evacuate at a certain time, and if this pattern is followed (and all other variables remain constant), the bowel will continue to empty regularly. On the other hand, if the person continually ignores the urge to defecate, no rhythmical pattern will be established. Travel, which usually disrupts a person's normal schedule, is a well-known villain, often leading to constipation and sometimes diarrhea.

Along with timing, many people have other established components of their habit pattern, e.g., drinking warm or cold water, having a cup of coffee, smoking a cigarette, reading. Continuing these activities may trigger conscious mental stimulation of the defecation reflex.

Diet. Dietary intake has a great influence. The fiber, or undigestible residue in the diet, provides the bulk in the fecal material. Bulk assists peristalsis and increases the intensity of stimulation of the defecation reflex. A low-fiber, high-carbohydrate diet tends to diminish the reflex stimulation. Reduction of overall intake also directly reduces the amount of bulk present. Gas-producing foods may stimulate peristalsis by distention of the intestinal walls.

Individual gastrointestinal tracts react differently to foods. For instance, while chocolate has no effect on many people, it causes constipation in some and diarrhea in others. Milk and milk products are considered by some to be constipating. However, this certainly isn't universally true, as has been demonstrated by studies on lactose intolerance. This syndrome of flatulence, diarrhea, and vague abdominal pain is the direct result of milk ingestion. Children with this condition gradually lose the ability to make lactase, the enzyme needed to break down lactose. Although people of all races develop lactose intolerance, those at highest risk are blacks, orientals, and Native Americans.[1, 110] Other foods can also adversely affect defecation patterns. The nurse must attempt to determine what foods affect her patients so that they can be avoided.

Timing of the intake is also important in regard to taking advantage of the gastrocolic and duodenocolic reflexes. These, as you remember, stimulate defecation.

Fluid Intake. The amount of water in the fecal mass dictates the consistency of the stool, and the harder the mass, the more difficult it is to pass it through the anus. As mentioned above, one of the main functions of the large intestine is to absorb water from the feces. Absorption of water also occurs in the small intestine. If the patient is fluid depleted, more fluid will be absorbed from the gastrointestinal tract in order to regain and maintain adequate hydration at the cellular level of the tissues. This can result in constipation. Therefore, the adequacy of fluid intake plays a role in maintaining bowel patterns.

Muscle Tone.   The degree of muscle tone affects not only the activity of the intestinal musculature itself but also the ability of the supporting skeletal muscles to aid the process of defecation. Weak or atrophied abdominal or pelvic floor muscles will be ineffective in increasing intra-abdominal pressure or assisting the anus to voluntarily control defecation. This inadequate musculature may result from lack of exercise, such as may occur in bedrest, or neurological impairment.

Medications.   There are a variety of medications that can be given to prevent or reverse constipation and diarrhea. If the dose is too large, the medication may cause the opposite disorder; for example, a drug to prevent constipation may cause diarrhea and vice versa. Overuse of laxatives leads to physiologic dependence on them.

Many medications given for other purposes have side effects that alter bowel patterns. Examples include narcotics (especially codeine and morphine sulfate), which are potent constipators; antibiotics, which may cause diarrhea as they destroy the normal bacterial flora of the intestine; antacids, which may result in either constipation or diarrhea depending on their chemical formula. General anesthetics depress central nervous system activity, thus slowing peristalsis and making postoperative patients susceptible to gastrointestinal disturbance. The list could mention many other agents.

Irritants.   Irritants within the gastrointestinal tract usually stimulate peristalsis by local reflex stimulation, thereby affecting bowel function. Common sources of these irritants include spicy foods, poisons, and bacterial toxins.

Surgical Procedures.   Surgical procedures tend to contribute to constipation. Direct handling of the bowel itself causes a temporary stoppage of peristalsis called "paralytic ileus." Any procedure done in the perineal area, such as rectal or gynecological surgery, can affect the defecation pattern both through the obstructing effects of postoperative edema and through pain that defecation may cause because of traumatized tissues and nerve endings. If defecation is at all painful, the patient has an overwhelming tendency to avoid bowel evacuation.

Diagnostic Tests.   Diagnostic tests can have a profound effect on defecation patterns. Many tests of the gastrointestinal tract involve direct or x-ray visualization of the intestine. For these examinations to be successful, the bowel must be cleared of solid and gaseous contents. Bowel preparation involves reducing oral intake and using laxatives and enemas to clean out the bowel. This type of preparation, also often done before surgery or delivery of a baby, reduces the amount of fecal material present in the bowel and thus eliminates the need for evacuation temporarily.

If barium is used as the contrast media for x-ray studies, whether it is administered orally or rectally, measures must be taken to assure its complete evacuation. Otherwise it will harden and may cause an impaction or bowel obstruction. After the x-ray study is completed, the patient is usually given a large dose of a cathartic; he must then be instructed to watch carefully for passage of the barium through the rectum. If it does not pass, the patient should seek medical advice. If the patient is incapable of taking care of this need, the nurse or the patient's family must watch for the evacuation of the barium.

Age.   Age plays a role in establishing habit patterns. For instance, before acquiring bowel control through toilet-training, defecation occurs whenever the rectum is stimulated by entering stool. Vulnerability to gastrointestinal disturbances increases with age: malignancies are more frequent, decreased gut resiliency increases healing time, motor and neurological disturbances are more prevalent, and diverticulosis (an out-pouching in the intestinal wall) occurs almost exclusively after the age of 40. Psychosomatic disorders are also increasingly significant; in one study of 300 patients over 65 years old, only 56 per cent of gastrointestinal disorders were found to be functional.[115]

Motor and Sensory Disturbance.   Any motor or sensory disturbance also affects defecation. Spinal cord injuries, head injuries, stroke, neurological disease, and any condition causing immobility or otherwise interfering with the patient's motor activity may diminish the sensory stimulation required for defecation or the patient's ability to actively and appropriately respond to the urge to defecate. For instance, fecal incontinence, or soiling, may really be the direct result of the patient's being unable to reach the call bell and summon help.

Characteristics of Feces

Fecal material is composed of food residues, bacteria, leukocytes, epithelial cells, intestinal secretions, and water. Several characteristics aid the nurse in identifying problems within the gastrointestinal tract.

Frequency.   Frequency of stool passage is an individual thing; the normal range is from two to three times per day to one to three times per week for an adult. A small infant often has 3 to 5 stools per day. The frequency of bowel movements is very important to many people. Because of advertising and inadequate health knowledge, many people think that a daily bowel movement is essential to healthy living and become very distraught if this goal is not achieved. This area of health education is fertile ground for nurses. Stools more than three times a day or less than once a week may indicate a problem in regards to frequency.

Amount.   The amount of stool varies with the amount and type of food ingested, fluid intake and frequency of bowel evacuation. It is normally about 150 grams per day. Because of the high percentage of the feces that is not dietary in origin, the nurse must remember that the patient with no oral intake will still be expected to pass stool. Also it may take several days for any given bolus of food to transit the entire intestine and be evacuated. Thus the colon is not often empty of all food material. The patient may need to be informed of these facts to motivate him to follow preventive measures.

Color.   The normal brown color is produced by bile pigments in the stool. Absence of bile causes the stool to be white or clay colored and may indicate biliary obstruction or lack of bile production. Pale stools, mixed with observable fat and mucus, indicate malabsorption of fats and are called steatorrhic stools. Black stools may be the result of supplemental iron intake or may indicate bleeding in the upper gastrointestinal tract, especially if they have a tar-like consistency. This tarry, black stool is called *melena*. In infants, the first stools, called *meconium*, are normally black and tarry due to ingested amniotic fluid, epithelial cells, and bile. Red-colored stools may be caused by the ingestion of beets or may be the result of bleeding in the lower gastrointestinal tract, where the red blood cells have not been hemolyzed by digestive processes in the intestine. If this red color is smeared on the surface of the fecal mass, hemorrhoids may be the source, while red blood mixed in with the stool comes from a point higher in the colon. Large amounts of ingested chlorophyll may result in green stool.

Consistency.   The consistency of the stool is the most significant factor in determining the presence of constipation or diarrhea. The consistency ranges from liquid to soft, unformed to soft, formed to hard and is a direct reflection of the water content. Very hard stool is often described as "rock-like," "marbles," or "pellets."

Shape.   The shape of the stool normally resembles that of the rectum. An abnormal finding would be that of a consistently narrowed, pencil-shaped stool. This usually indicates obstruction of the distal portion of the large intestine, as might occur with carcinoma.

Odor.   Odor of the stool is characteristically pungent and is produced by bacterial action in the colon. It is normally affected by the type of bacterial flora present and by the food and medications ingested. Blood or infection in the gastrointestinal tract causes detectable noxious changes in the normal odor.

Assessment of the Bowel Status

A detailed assessment of the patient's bowel status will assist the nurse to accurately identify current and potential problems with gastrointestinal function and to intervene appropriately. A complete data base includes the following information:

► Usual *patterns* of defecation. Frequency? Time of day? Any aids used, e.g., drinking warm prune juice, medications, smoking? Does patient ever have problems with diarrhea or constipation? If so, what does he usually do to relieve them?

► *Changes* in usual patterns resulting from current illness or stress.

► Presence of *artificial orifices*—colostomy, ileostomy. If present, how is it usually managed?

► *Character of stool.* Color? Consistency? Amount? Odor? Shape? Any unusual constituents, e.g., blood, mucus, pus, undigested food, worms, foreign bodies?

► Relevant *medications*, e.g., is patient taking laxatives, antacids, iron supplement, analgesics?

► Current *disease processes* or *surgical procedures* which may influence defecation pattern or be influenced by it, e.g., cardiac disease, ulcerative colitis, neuromuscular problems, intra-abdominal surgery, hemorrhoidectomy.

▶ *Dietary intake.* Amount and kind of food intake? Times of food intake? What kinds of food affect defecation pattern?

▶ *Fluid status.* Amount and kind of fluid intake? State of hydration, e.g., dry skin, dry mucous membranes, edema; intake and output determination?

▶ *Level of activity.* Muscle tone? Amount and kind of activity? Will patient use toilet, commode, or bedpan? What assistance with mobility does patient need?

▶ *Emotional state*, e.g., depression, anxiety, embarrassment.

▶ Results of relevant *diagnostic tests*, e.g., barium x-ray studies, colonfiberoscopy, sigmoidoscopy, occult blood, ova and parasites.

▶ Quality of *bowel sounds* obtained by auscultation with a stethoscope. Presence or absence? Frequency? Pitch?

▶ Presence of *gaseous distention.* Distended abdomen? Measurement of abdominal girth with measuring tape at level of umbilicus? Changes in girth? Respiratory distress may indicate an elevated diaphragm.

▶ Results of *abdominal percussion.*

▶ Results of *abdominal palpation.* Masses? Tenderness?

▶ *Pain.* Cramping pain of gas? Any pain on defecation?

▶ Results of *digital examination* of the rectum, if appropriate. Use caution with patients with cardiac disease; anal stretching causes vagal nerve stimulation, which may lead to cardiac arrhythmias.

▶ Presence of *hemorrhoids* or other *rectal* or *perineal* trauma.

▶ *Level of development.* Toilet-trained? Mental ability?

▶ *Level of knowledge* regarding bowel function.

Collecting this information will require some time. However, the more complete your data base, the more effective your care planning process will be.

Independent Nursing Measures to Aid Normal Defecation

Nursing personnel take full responsibility for the majority of their patients' bowel elimination needs. Many of these needs can be met through independent nursing measures. Independent nursing actions are those that require no physician's order but can be initiated by the nurse, based on an appropriate assessment of the situation and application of relevant scientific rationale.

In aiding patients to attain and maintain suitable defecation patterns, the nurse has a wide assortment of independent nursing measures available. These include patient teaching, providing for relaxation and privacy, supporting normal habit patterns, timing, positioning, diet, fluids, and exercise. If these actions are not effective, the nurse may want to administer laxatives, suppositories or enemas. These latter measures are dependent nursing actions, requiring a physician's order, and will be discussed below.

Patient Teaching. Patient teaching is the most fundamental intervention in helping patients with their elimination needs. In the first place, even people assumed by the nurse to be knowledgeable may possess many misconceptions about defecation. We have already considered the belief held by many people that it is necessary to defecate every day. If a daily bowel movement does not happen naturally, these people freely make use of over-the-counter laxatives, suppositories and even enemas to reach their goal. As will be described later, continued use of these medications begins a cycle that leads to physical dependence on them. There are many other misunderstandings about the normal characteristics of defecation, and it is the nurse's responsibility to help patients gain accurate information about this normal body function.

Secondly, patients will be more likely to comply with care plans if they understand the reasons behind suggestions from health professionals. Patients have the right to know what will help them maintain healthy bowel habits and what will be detrimental. Given this information about what to do and what not to do and why, patients can then decide what to do for themselves intelligently.

Therefore, the area of bowel function provides excellent teaching opportunities for nurses. It is a prime example of how patient education can be a vital part of health promotion as well as illness intervention.

Diet. The addition of fiber to the diet is probably the single most important element in stimulating good bowel function. The action of fiber on the colon was discussed earlier. Bass demonstrated that increasing the fiber content of the diets of elderly persons greatly diminished their established need for laxatives and enemas.[4] Other people have reported that supplementing diets with bran, whole grain cereals, and raw fruits and vegetables has been effective in resolving elimination problems. If you are suggesting that a patient add bran to his diet in appreciable amounts, warn him that he may feel bloated at first, but that this feeling will usually disappear in 2 to 3 weeks.[115]

It is also being hypothesized that high-fiber diets can prevent the development of diverticular disease. When the muscular rings of the colon contract during peristalsis, the diameter of the lumen decreases, causing high intraluminal pressures around the site of the temporary occlusion. This pressure transmitted to weakened walls of the intestine may cause herniation, or pouching, of the colon wall. It is estimated that by the age of 80, 70 per cent of the American population has this disease.[115] The theory is that a high-fiber diet produces bulkier feces, resulting in a larger diameter colonic lumen. Thus, occlusion does not occur during peristalsis and the high intraluminal pressures are avoided.[19]

The patient must also be helped to identify and avoid foods that cause disruption in his bowel pattern. If there are several suspect foods, the patient should eliminate all of them from his diet and then add one at a time with several days, or longer if necessary, between each introduction to see exactly which ones cause the problem. A dietician can help the patient plan his diet to exclude the problem foods.

Fluids.   We know the importance of a good state of hydration to the formation of a stool that is of a consistency easy to pass through the anus. Although authorities differ on the amount of fluid intake necessary to maintain an adequate state of hydration, the recommended baseline for adults is about 1200 to 1500 ml. of measurable fluid per day. If the patient is subjected to internal or external environmental conditions requiring significant fluid replacement, this intake should be correspondingly increased. Situations that require increased fluid intake include hot, humid weather; physical exertion; fever; vomiting; diarrhea; or increased losses through the respiratory tract. Immobility calls for increased fluid intake since one of the normal aids to defecation—exercise—is greatly limited. Before instituting a plan for increased fluid intake, however, the nurse must be certain that the patient has no condition in which increased fluids would be detrimental, e.g., cardiac or renal disease or head injury.

Review Unit VII for discussion of fluid balance and suggestions on how to help the patient establish an adequate state of hydration within his own body. The nurse may need to use some creative approaches to motivate the patient to take in adequate fluids.

Although the amount of fluids taken in is the crucial element, the kind of fluids might also be considered. Some liquids, such as milk, may be constipating; fruit juice is often beneficial to defecation. Prune juice is a natural laxative for most people, and many people claim that other juices, such as apricot, lemonade, cranberry, and orange, help them maintain regular bowel activity.

Exercise.   Exercise improves general muscle tone and specifically can be used to strengthen the muscles directly concerned with defecation. The patient should be encouraged and assisted as necessary to take part in whatever physical activity he is capable of doing. Walking is an excellent body toner. The nurse should help the patient plan into his daily routine some periods of physical exercise. Elderly persons and persons with sedentary jobs may particularly need this assistance.

In addition to general exercise, the patient can be instructed in exercises specifically designed to strengthen the abdominal and pelvic floor muscles. Probably the most effective are isometric exercises in which these muscles are contracted, or tightened, as much as possible for about 10 seconds and then relaxed. This pattern of contraction and relaxation should be repeated 5 to 10 times each session. Exercises should be done at least four times a day, and results may be even better if the patient does the exercises every 1 or 2 hours. These exercises are appropriate for use by immobilized patients. Isometric exercises, however, do raise the blood pressure and may cause coronary ischemia (deficient blood flow to the cardiac muscle) in persons with underlying cardiac disease. Caution must be used with these patients and the patient's physician should be consulted before instituting an exercise program.

Normal Habit Patterns.   Establishing consistent habit patterns around the act of defecation is a great adjunct to normal bowel elimination. As described in the following pages, the bowel can be trained to react to a variety of physical and mental stimuli producing successful bowel evacuation.

Although defecation can occur at any time, the best physiologic time is that linked with activation of the gastrocolic reflex. As described earlier, the reflex is strongest after a meal eaten following a period of fasting. Therefore, attempts to have a bowel movement after break-fast are likely to be the most successful. However, other factors in the patient's life-style have great influence on the designated time, e.g., availability of the bathroom, family responsibilities, the need to get to work. Also, of course, not all people work during the day and sleep at night. The nurse must assess the patient's daily routine before suggesting any given time to the patient.

The nurse can help the patient select a time during the day when he can take a few minutes to attend to his bowel needs. The time chosen will depend totally on the patient's life-style and the other activities in his daily routine. However, once decided on, the patient should be encouraged to make this habit a rather strict part of his daily routine. If the time selected is inappropriate, it can be altered until a suitable one is found. People who have little routine to their daily lives will be a particular challenge.

Other parts of a person's system of actions that stimulate defecation are very much individualized matters, established over the years. The nurse's responsibility is to discover what the patient's habit pattern is and then to help the patient maintain it. Unfortunately, the hospital routine sometimes makes this very difficult.

Relaxation and Privacy. Relaxation at the time of attempted bowel evacuation is critical. Since mental concentration assists nervous stimulation of the defecation reflex, anything that disrupts the person's focus of attention will interfere with adequate bowel elimination. Also, anxiety causes tension in the voluntary musculature. Therefore, because the levator ani muscle and the external sphincter at the anus function to intentionally suppress the act of defecation, it is essential that these muscles be relaxed.

Probably the most important factor in achieving relaxation is privacy. Since the act of defecation is culturally a nonpublic affair and since the odors and sounds that naturally accompany this normal body function are so easily communicated to others, providing privacy for the patient greatly helps normal defecation. Privacy is not always easy to obtain, especially in an in-patient setting. Patients often cannot use the bathroom, but must use a commode or bedpan. There may well be other people in the room, and the patient may never feel certain that someone will not walk in on him. Physicians seem to have a particular knack for making rounds just when the patient is meeting his elimination needs!

The nurse should create as private an environment as feasible and ensure that it will be preserved as long as the patient needs it. If the patient is using the bathroom, make sure that other people will know that the room is occupied; this is especially important when a bathroom has two doors opening into adjacent rooms. If the patient must use the bedpan or commode in the room, several measures can help the situation: pull the bed curtains around the patient for visual privacy, ask visitors or staff to leave the room to reduce the number of people present, open the window if this is appropriate, and turn on the television or radio to mask the sounds if this is feasible. Room deodorizers can be used to reduce the odor.

In all cases, be sure that the patient has a way to summon the nurse when he is finished or needs help. Fainting in the bathroom is a rather frequent occurrence. Bathrooms are notoriously warm and stuffy and when a weakened patient strains to have a bowel movement, the cardiovascular system may not be able to maintain sufficient blood flow to the brain. Ways to manage a fainting patient are discussed in Chapters 21 and 43.

In addition to providing a call bell or light, the nurse should also assure the patient that he can have as much time as he needs. Relaxation is disrupted when the nurse is constantly popping in to ask the patient if he is finished. This is especially a problem if the nurse is waiting outside the door or curtain. Soon the patient gets the idea that he is detaining the nurse from other, more important duties and he does not adequately complete bowel evacuation. On the other hand, the nurse must keep careful watch on any patient who is at risk of fainting or any other problem. You must use your tact and good sense to reach a happy medium.

Physical comfort is needed for relaxation. Positioning is one important element. Whether the patient is using the toilet, commode, or bedpan, he should be made as comfortable as possible through use of padding, supports, and body positioning (see Chap. 27). The patient may also need pain relief. However, if narcotic analgesics are used, the nurse must plan carefully. Since narcotics depress central nervous system function, timing is very important so that the patient can attempt defecation when pain has been relieved, but before he gets too sleepy.

Positioning. In addition to being comfortable, the patient's position should take advantage of gravity to aid defecation and should enlist the help of increased intra-abdominal pressure. Since squatting is the most suitable position for defecation, the nurse should position the patient as near this posture as possible.

When the patient is using a bedpan, this can be achieved by rolling the head of the bed up into a high-Fowler's position, if this position is not contraindicated by the patient's condition. The commode and toilet allow for this position naturally. External pressure on the abdomen can be increased by having the patient lean forward.

If the patient is short, a footstool or other appropriate device can be placed under his feet at the toilet, to increase hip flexion. Caution must be used, however, with patients who have had hip surgery, especially total hip replacements. These patients must avoid hip flexion beyond 90 degrees, to reduce the chance of dislocating the prosthesis. They can use the toilet only when a device is attached that raises the height of the seat to decrease the degree of hip flexion; they must also be instructed not to lean forward.

In summary, the nurse has a large variety of independent nursing actions available. Motivating patients to follow these suggestions will resolve most of the problems they have with bowel function.

Common Problems with Defecation and Modes of Treatment

There are several problems with defecation that the nurse will frequently encounter. Although sometimes these problems are the primary reason the patient is seeking professional help, more commonly they accompany other disorders. Most of these problems are treated by intensification of the independent nursing measures to aid normal defecation plus the addition of dependent measures, such as medications. The common problems we discuss include constipation, fecal impaction, diarrhea, flatulence, hemorrhoids, incontinence, and fecal diversion.

CONSTIPATION

Many people will claim to be constipated if they have not had a bowel movement for a day or so. Although time may be a consideration, the primary characteristic of constipation is the consistency of the stool. *Constipation* is defined as the passage of dry, hard stool requiring much use of the supporting voluntary muscles. Patients also describe accompanying symptoms, such as headache, lethargy, anorexia, halitosis, furry tongue, and a bloated feeling. These discomforts are considered to be due to reflexes resulting from prolonged distention of the rectum.

Causes of constipation are many. Common sources include no established habit pattern, especially regarding timing; inadequate diet, fluids, and exercise; emotional upset; and medications. Immobilizing a patient for any reason heightens the risk of developing constipation. Overuse of laxatives, suppositories, and enemas contributes to the problem. Systemic disorders such as cancer, adhesions, heart failure, and interruptions in neuromuscular activity in the colon can lead to constipation, as can hemorrhoids and other lesions in the anal region.

Besides being uncomfortable, constipation can actually be hazardous for many people. In order to pass a constipated stool, the person usually employs *Valsalva's maneuver*. As the person strains, he forces air out against a closed glottis, which increases the intrathoracic pressure. The increased pressure within the chest cavity causes decreased venous return to the heart and an increase in the heart rate, as the heart attempts to overcome the obstruction to blood flow. When the person stops straining, the intrathoracic pressure drops precipitously and bradycardia (slow heart rate) develops. A healthy cardiovascular system can tolerate these changes, but a weakened one cannot. This maneuver may result in angina pectoris (paroxysmal chest pain) or even sudden death. Because of the increased pressure throughout the venous system caused by the Valsalva maneuver, it may also be detrimental to patients with head injuries, respiratory disease, and thromboembolic disorders. Exhaling through the mouth during straining will reduce the chances of increasing the intrathoracic pressure, but the best precaution is to avoid constipation.

Straining to pass a stool can be detrimental in other ways. If the patient has had recent bowel surgery, straining might disrupt the suture line. The rectum and perineal area require some time to heal after surgical treatment. As a precaution, these patients are often given enemas preoperatively to eliminate the need for a bowel movement for several days after surgery.

The treatment of constipation requires, first of all, intensification of all the preventive measures mentioned: patient teaching, diet, fluids, exercise, following established habit patterns, relaxation, and positioning. However, by the time true constipation has developed, dependent measures are usually required to solve the problem. These require a physician's order.

Laxatives. Laxatives and cathartics are drugs used to induce emptying of the bowel. The two terms are often used interchangeably, although cathartics have a stronger action than laxatives. There are four categories of laxatives: stimulants, lubricants, bulk-forming agents, and saline agents. The *stimulants* are probably the most frequently used. They work directly on the nerves innervating the intestine or by local irritation of the mucosa to stimulate peristalsis. Examples of stimulants include cascara, castor oil, senna, and bisacodyl. If the patient is taking drugs containing phenolphthalein, as do many of the proprietary preparations, he should be alerted to the possibility that his urine may turn pink or red; this occurs if the urine is alkaline. Some drugs in this category can be transmitted through breast milk, causing diarrhea in the nursing infant.

Lubricants do not stimulate peristalsis, but instead act directly on the stool bulk to increase the moisture content and make the outer surface slippery so that it can more easily pass through the gastrointestinal tract. Mineral oil actually penetrates the fecal mass to soften it and also coats the outside to reduce fluid absorption from the feces by the colon. It is suggested that this medication not be given close to mealtime since it may interfere with absorption of fat-soluble vitamins, especially vitamin K. Mineral oil itself is not very palatable, and the nurse may seek to mask the oily aftertaste by mixing it with orange juice or root beer. Dioctyl sodium sulfosuccinate and dioctyl calcium sulfosuccinate are stool softeners frequently given prophylactically to patients who are at high risk for developing constipation. They act like detergents, reducing the surface tension of the fecal mass and allowing water to penetrate. The calcium preparation is preferred for patients with a sodium retention problem.

The *bulk-forming* laxatives use synthetic or natural polysaccharides and cellulose derivatives that absorb water and add bulk to the stool. This increased volume stretches the intestinal wall, thus stimulating peristalsis. Common examples are psyllium, agar, and methylcellulose or sodium carboxymethylcellulose. Drugs in this classification are the most natural and least irritating and are frequently used to wean laxative-dependent patients from their need. It is essential that patients take this type of laxative with plenty of fluid, to avoid obstruction of the gastrointestinal tract. The agent should be mixed with water and followed by more fluid to make sure that none of the substance is left in the esophagus. A high fluid intake also helps the medication work more effectively, since its main function is to absorb moisture.

Saline cathartics contain sodium sulfate and other poorly absorbed salts, such as magnesium sulfate and citrate, which, through their osmotic activity, draw water into the intestine where it increases the bulk of and lubricates the fecal mass. Milk of magnesia is a saline cathartic. These drugs usually act within 1 to 3 hours and are often used as *purgatives* to completely empty the bowel. Because of the salts used and the severity of their action, saline cathartics are usually contraindicated in patients with renal or cardiac disease or inflammatory bowel disease.[11, 21, 31, 109]

Laxatives are one of the most widely used and misused types of drugs available over the counter. There are approximately 700 brand names, and in 1969, consumers spent $192 million for these products.[11] Most of this abuse of laxatives is the result of advertising that supports the public's misconceptions about the need for a daily bowel movement. As mentioned above, the consistent use of laxatives leads to physical dependence on them. The mechanism for this is as follows: the laxative causes defecation and complete emptying of the bowel; the colon then requires several days to collect enough fecal bulk to stimulate normal defecation; in the meantime, the person becomes so anxious about the lack of another bowel movement that he takes another laxative and so on. Since the colon's normal defecation reflexes are not called on to function normally, the reflexes diminish; the colon becomes dilated and atonic and is capable of responding only to the strong stimulation of a laxative, suppository or enema.

Use of laxatives should also be avoided in other instances. Patients should be warned never to take them in the presence of undiagnosed abdominal pain or cramps, nausea or vomiting, or diarrhea, since these symptoms may indicate appendicitis, inflammatory bowel disease, or obstruction.

Suppositories. Suppositories are solid, cone- or oval-shaped masses that melt at body temperature. In order to stimulate defecation, medicated suppositories are inserted into the rectum, where they release their active ingredients as the suppository melts. There are several varieties of suppositories available. The most frequently used are glycerine and bisacodyl. Glycerine acts as a local irritant which stimulates secretion by the mucosa, while bisacodyl acts directly on the nerve endings, stimulating peristalsis. Fecal softeners may be given by suppository to moisten and lubricate the fecal mass. Carbon dioxide suppositories release about 200 ml. of carbon dioxide as they melt, which distends the rectum and stimulates defecation.

Some suppositories should be kept refrigerated to facilitate insertion since they become mushy as they melt; others do not require this. The nurse should check the label on the container. Once it is established that the patient needs a suppository, the procedure and his part in it should be explained to him. The patient may be positioned on his back, abdomen, or either side; the requirement is that the rectum be easily accessible. Since the nurse will be inserting a finger into the rectum, a glove or finger cot is usually worn. The suppository is removed from its package and generously lubricated, preferably with a water-soluble lubricant. Exposing the anus with one hand, the nurse gently inserts the suppository with the other, using the forefinger to advance it once it has passed through the anus. Since anything in the anal canal is reflexly expelled, the suppository must be inserted beyond the internal sphincter; otherwise, the suppository will not be effective in causing defecation. If the intended action of the medication is on the intestinal wall, the nurse must be sure that the suppository is positioned to the side of the rectum against the mucosa rather than into the fecal mass itself, where it will be ineffective. Once the suppository is in place and the anal area has been cleaned of the lubricant material, the patient should be instructed to retain the suppository as long as is comfortable—at least 20 to 30 minutes or longer. When the urge to defecate is very strong, the patient may heed it.

Enemas. An *enema* is the injection of fluid into the rectum, usually for the purpose of stimulating defecation. Because enemas have been used since ancient times and because this treatment is frequently administered in the home by persons who have had no formal instruction in the procedure, enemas are often considered a harmless, necessary treatment for constipation. Some people even use a daily enema to prevent constipation. We have already discussed more appropriate ways to promote proper defecation. However, in the case of true constipation and in certain other cases, it may become necessary to administer an enema to a patient. In order to achieve the safest and most effective results, the nurse must fully understand and apply the scientific principles underlying the procedure for enema administration.

Enemas may be given for several purposes, the most frequent being to stimulate defecation. The *cleansing* enema may be used (a) to treat constipation or fecal impaction; (b) to clean out the bowel prior to x-ray studies, direct visualization of the bowel by optic instruments, surgery, or delivery of a baby or (c) to help establish regular bowel function during a bowel training program. A *retention* enema, which must be retained in the bowel over a prolonged period of time, is usually used to lubricate or soften with oil a hard fecal mass, thus facilitating its expulsion through the anus. Less frequently, a retention enema may be given to administer medications, to protect and soothe the mucous membrane of the intestine, to destroy intestinal parasites *(antihelmintic),* to relieve distention *(carminative),* or to administer fluids and nutrition *(nutritive).* The third kind of enema, the *return flow* enema, is used to relieve gaseous distention. It is sometimes called a *Harris flush* and is discussed later under the heading "Flatulence."

The cleansing effect of enemas is accomplished through distention of the bowel and/or irritation of the mucosal wall, both of which stimulate peristalsis. Bowel distention results from filling the colon with fluid either by administering a *volume enema,* which injects large amounts of fluid into the rectum from an external source, or a small-volume enema, which draws internal fluid into the bowel.

The concepts of osmosis and concentration gradient are important in understanding the action of many enema solutions. Briefly, *osmosis* refers to the passage of water through a semipermeable membrane in order to approximately equalize the concentration of nondiffusable molecules on both sides of the membrane. Although water will continuously flow back and forth across the membrane, when there are solutions of different concentrations on either side of the semipermeable membrane, the major *net flow* of water will be toward the solution with the higher concentration of nondiffusable molecules, in order to achieve equilibrium. Thus the *concentration gradient* is toward the higher concentration. Readers needing more explanation of these concepts should consult any basic physiology text.

Cleansing enemas utilize hypotonic, isotonic, or hypertonic solutions to distend the bowel and induce defecation. Figure 30–2 shows how solutions of different tonicity affect the net flow of water into or out of the colon. *Hypotonic* solutions have a lower osmotic pressure than the fluid in the interstitial tissues, so the net flow of water is out of the bowel into the tissues. Tap water is the basic hypotonic solution and is frequently used. The net flow occurs slowly, and defecation is usually stimulated before any appreciable fluid is absorbed into the body.

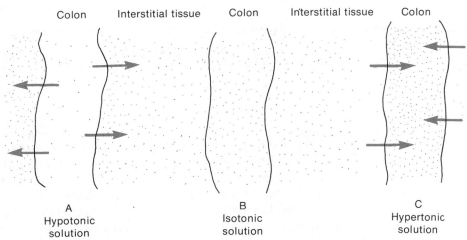

| Colon | Interstitial tissue | Colon | Interstitial tissue | Colon |

A
Hypotonic
solution

B
Isotonic
solution

C
Hypertonic
solution

Figure 30–2. Concentration gradients across a semipermeable membrane. *A, Hypotonic solution:* Concentration is greater in interstitial tissues, so net water flow is out of colon. *B, Isotonic solution:* Concentration is the same on both sides of membrane, so there is no net water flow. *C, Hypertonic solution:* Concentration is greater inside colon, so net water flow is into colon.

Exceptions to this may be when the patient is fluid depleted or repeated enemas are given, i.e., "enemas until clear"; then the net water flow may be significant. *Isotonic* solutions have equal concentrations on both sides of the semipermeable membrane; consequently, no net water flow occurs. Physiologic saline is the isotonic enema solution. *Hypertonic* solutions are of higher concentration than the interstitial fluid, so that when these solutions are used in an enema, the net water flow is into the colon, leading to distention. These commercially prepared enemas contain about 120 ml. of sodium phosphate or sodium biphosphate solution. They draw water into the colon and irritate the mucosal wall to stimulate the defecation reflex.

Soapsuds may be added to either tap water or saline solution to augment the effect of distention by irritating the intestinal mucosa. The recommended formula is 5 ml. of castile soap per one liter of solution. Other available soaps may have untoward effects: household detergents are too harsh; bar soaps used for washing may harbor organisms; soft soaps, such as green soap, are more irritating to the intestinal mucosa than hard soaps;[59] and some hexachlorophene soaps may cause blood dyscrasias.[123] As you might suspect, the use of soapsuds enemas is highly controversial and the detrimental effects will be discussed with the other hazards of enemas.

There are a variety of other enema solutions reported in the literature, e.g., milk and molasses, vegetable oils, hydrogen peroxide, and champagne. However, these are rarely used. Various medications and nutritive formulas may also be used depending on the patient's needs.

Equipment needed for an enema depends on the type of enema to be given, the patient's condition, and the surrounding environment. Basically, the list includes (a) reservoir—a plastic or metal container or funnel, (b) solution, (c) administration tip—rubber or plastic tubing or small catheter, (d) lubricant—prelubricated tip or any standard grease or oil, (e) protector pad to keep linen clean, (f) recovery container—bedpan, commode, or toilet. If the patient will have difficulty retaining the enema solution, a baby bottle nipple may be prepared to fit around the administration tube. (See Fig. 30–8.) The nipple can then be pushed snugly against the anus to form a watertight seal. An alternative to the nipple is to administer the enema with a Foley catheter having a 30 ml. bag. Once the catheter is inserted into the rectum, the balloon is inflated and the catheter gently pulled back against the internal sphincter to form an internal seal. When the patient is about to expel the enema, the nipple or the catheter with the deflated balloon is removed.

Procedure 14 describes in detail the *technique* for administering a normal saline enema. This same procedure is used for any volume enema by making the necessary changes in solution preparation.

14.   NORMAL SALINE ENEMA (N.S.E.)

By Jean Saxon, R.N., M.N.

Definition and Purpose.   *Injection of 500 to 750 ml. of normal (physiologic) saline (salt) solution into the large intestine (bowel) by means of a tube inserted into the anus. Fluid breaks up fecal material and stimulates peristalsis and the urge to defecate by distending the bowel.* Used to: treat constipation; empty the colon of fecal material and gas prior to surgery, delivery, radiographic studies, proctoscopy or colonoscopy; cleanse the bowel following diagnostic injection or ingestion of barium; relieve gas pains; and establish bowel evacuation pattern during bowel training program.

Contraindications and Cautions.   Patients with congestive heart failure or other sodium-retaining conditions may absorb sodium from the enema fluid, thus disrupting fluid-electrolyte balance. Vaso-vagal reflexes produced by distention of the rectum may cause myocardial infarction or other severe cardiac disturbances. Therefore, enemas should be avoided or given with caution to patients who are elderly and who have known heart disease. Frequent enemas may cause potassium depletion or irritation of mucosa, particularly in the presence of disorders which inflame mucosa, e.g., colitis or diverticulitis. Abrasions or perforations of the anterior rectal wall can occur: (a) if rectal tip is inserted too deeply; (b) if fluid is inserted under excessively high pressure; (c) if enema tip is inserted while patient is in sitting position. Anal injuries can occur when edema, hemorrhoids or inflammation make it difficult to visualize the anus. Diseases, especially infectious hepatitis, can be transmitted by contaminated enema equipment. (Used equipment should never be stored with patient's clothing or hygiene equipment.) Fluid inserted under excessive pressure or amounts may force bacteria in colon past the ileocecal valve into the small intestine or rupture colon. Bulb syringes are dangerous because amount of pressure cannot be controlled. If pain is produced during attempt to insert enema tip, do not give enema since there may be a stricture, abscess or other lesion of anus or rectum.

Patient-Family Teaching Points.   Provide the patient and family with the following information as appropriate: (a) explain why the enema is to be given; (b) explain that an enema is not administered when on the toilet because abrasions or perforations of the anterior rectal wall may occur; (c) explain that enema solution should be given slowly, under low pressure (no bulb syringes), at a lukewarm temperature, and should not cause pain or cramping; (d) teach how to prepare a physiologic saline enema and explain that it is the safest, least damaging solution; (e) teach how breathing through the mouth relaxes patient's abdominal muscles and helps avoid cramps; (f) teach how to avoid constipation by exercise, diet modifications (especially increasing bulk), and adequate fluid intake and explain the need for taking adequate time for defecation; (g) teach when enema should be used at home and how to care for equipment; and (h) teach how to recognize constipation and the variance in "normal" periods between bowel evacuations.

PRE-PROCEDURE ACTIVITIES

PRELIMINARY ASSESSMENT

Includes determination of:
- diagnosis and activity orders
- date and type of surgery or tests
- medical order for cleansing enema or saline enema (N.S.E.)
- abilities and limitations concerning movement
- presence of skin, muscle, bone, perineal or rectal lesions
- medical order for fecal specimen for tests
- time and character of previous stools
- ability to retain enema solution

PRELIMINARY PLANNING

- Locate equipment. If enema is one of series, e.g., ordered "N.S.E. until clear," patient's enema equipment may be labeled and stored in lavatory or soiled utility room for future use.
- Determine comfort and safety needs of patient, e.g., need for assistant to move patient to commode or toilet, adequate covers.

PREPARATION OF PATIENT

- Explain that an enema will be given and why, even if patient is unresponsive
- Explain that patient is not to flush toilet or allow other personnel to empty commode or bedpan until helper checks enema returns
- Explain patient's part in obtaining specimen if ordered, e.g., use of commode or specimen collection vessel under toilet seat

EQUIPMENT

- Enema reservoir, i.e., fluid holder
- Rectal tube and tubing if not attached to reservoir
- Lubricant—water soluble
- Table salt and tap water—40.5°C. (105°F.) (or prepared physiologic saline solution if table salt not available)
- Waterproof pad

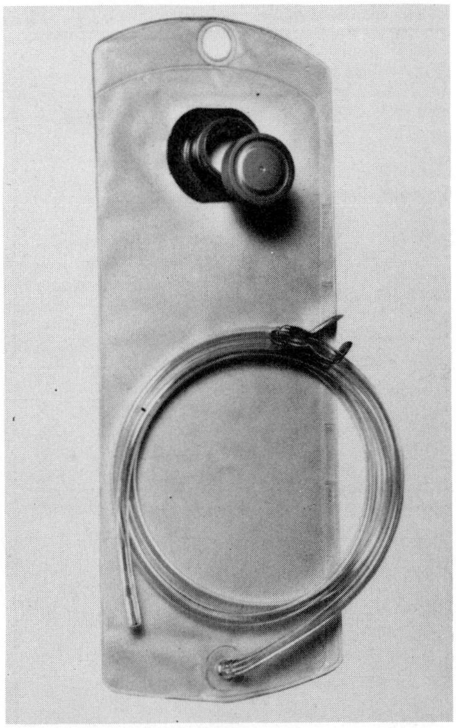

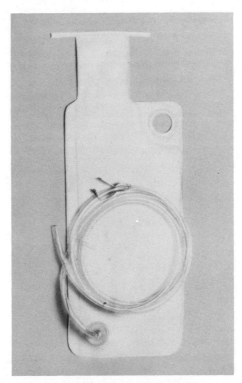

Figure 30–3. Bard disposable enema bag with a screw cap; tubing with enema tip attached. (Courtesy of C. R. Bard, Inc., Murray Hill, NJ 07974.)

Figure 30–4. Bardic enema administration unit with foil top closure; tubing with enema tip attached. (Courtesy C. R. Bard, Inc., Murray Hill, NJ 07974.)

Procedure continued on page 709

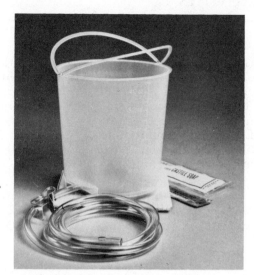

Figure 30–5.   Bardic enema administration unit with bucket; tubing with enema tip separate. (Courtesy C. R. Bard, Inc., Murray Hill, NJ 07974.)

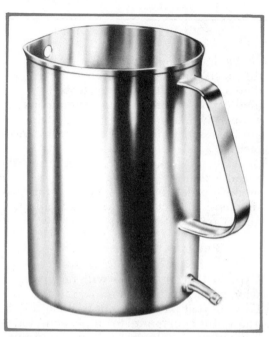

Figure 30–6.   Vollrath stainless steel irrigating can. (Courtesy of the Vollrath Company.)

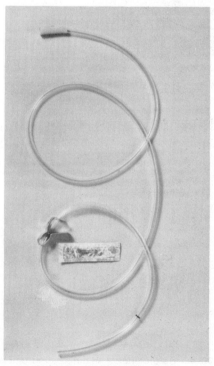

Figure 30–7.   Disposable tubing with enema tip. (Courtesy C. R. Bard, Inc., Murray Hill, NJ 07974.)

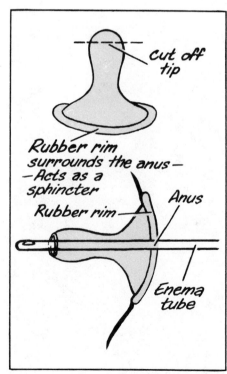

Figure 30–8.   Nipple guard for rectal tube. (From Chisholm, R.: *Nursing '74, 4*(1):68, 1974.)

PREPARATION OF PATIENT

▶ Ask patient if he has difficulty retaining enema fluid
▶ Ask patient which bed lying position is most comfortable, e.g., cardiac patients are often uncomfortable when lying on left side
▶ Explain that enema fluid should be retained for about 15 min. after enema is given
▶ Provide privacy, draw curtains, close door
▶ Cover patient with bath blanket and fan fold top covers to foot of bed
▶ Remove pajama bottoms
▶ Place bed at working height
▶ Adjust IV pole or overbed table to hold enema reservoirs

EQUIPMENT

▶ Bedpan (warm a metal pan with hot water)
▶ Commode if indicated
▶ Baby nipple or Foley catheter with 30 ml. bag and 30 ml. syringe if patient unable to retain fluid
▶ Plastic disposable unsterile gloves
▶ Bath blanket
▶ Toilet tissue
▶ Patient's robe and slippers
▶ Containers for collecting specimen, if indicated
▶ Teaspoon or disposable plastic or glass medicine measuring container
▶ Overbed table or IV pole
▶ Tubing clamp or hemostat (if clamp not attached)
▶ Remove packet of castile soap from commercial units (save for shampoos!)

PROCEDURE

SUGGESTED STEPS	RATIONALE/DISCUSSION
Preparation of Saline Enema	
A. *Preparation of saline enema:* at patient's room sink or, if equipment contaminated, in soiled utility room.	A. Physiologic saline is solution of choice for cleansing enema unless patient has sodium retention condition. Normal fecal flora contains pathogens. Previously used equipment would contaminate sink for patient and personnel.
1. Attach tubing and rectal tube to reservoir (bucket, can) after moistening ends (see Figs. 30–5, 30–6, and 30–7).	1. Moistening ends of reservoir opening and tube decreases friction (lubricates), facilitating connection.
2. Apply clamp or hemostat to tubing approximately 30 cm. (12 in.) from rectal tube tip. Close clamp or hemostat.	2. Closing lumen of tubing prevents accidental loss of fluid. Places clamp or hemostat within easy reach during enema administration.
3. Rinse metal reservoir with hot water (see Fig. 30–6).	3. Warms cold metal. Prevents excessive cooling of solution.
4. Prepare physiologic saline solution:	
a. Adjust water flow at sink to lukewarm, 40.5°C. (105°F.).	a. Use utility thermometer if not able to ascertain correct temperature on inner aspect of wrist. Temperatures *above* 43°C. (110°F.) may injure the tissues, and temperatures *below* 21°C. (70°F.) may produce severe cramping.

Procedure continued on the following page

Preparation of Enema (Continued)

Suggested Steps	Rationale/Discussion
b. Add 1000 ml. (32 oz. or 1 quart) water and 2 teaspoons table salt to reservoir for adult. For infants or children, prepare 500 ml. (16 oz. or 1 pint) water and 1 teaspoon of table salt.	b. Isotonic saline or physiologic salt solution is approximately 0.9 per cent salt in water. Only 500 to 750 ml. (16 to 24 oz. or 1 to 1.5 pints) will be used for adult. Additional amount is ready in case of loss during administration. Smaller amounts are used for infants' and children's enemas, 15 to 250 ml. Unneeded amount is discarded.
c. Alternative to steps 4a and 4b: Place *commercially prepared* flask of normal saline solution in a basin of hot water. Add lukewarm solution to reservoir.	c. This method is more expensive, and it is difficult and time consuming to bring solution to desired temperature.
5. Seal reservoir containers (see Figs. 30–3 and 30–4).	5. Prevents spillage from collapsible plastic bags.
6. If patient has difficulty holding solution, place baby bottle nipple with small amount of tip cut off on tubing (see Fig. 30–8).	6. Provides mechanical obstruction of anal canal around the rectal tube when nipple is pushed up against anal sphincter to form "seal." See text for discussion.
Or attach Foley catheter with 30 ml. bag to rectal tube or to connector (if rectal tube not present).	Foley catheter is used as rectal tube. See text for discussion.
7. Hang reservoir on IV pole or place on overbed table. Hang or stabilize tubing and rectal tube to prevent falling to floor.	7. Places enema equipment in position for use. Enema equipment must be kept clean, free of pathogens before use.

Administration of Enema

B. *Administration of enema*

Suggested Steps	Rationale/Discussion
1. Place waterproof pad under patient by turning him from side to side.	1. Protects bed from possible moisture or soilage.
2. Tell patient to turn to side most comfortable for him to receive enema. Assist patient as necessary. (Patient may be rolled onto bedpan after step 9, below.)	2. Patient's position does not affect flow of fluid enough to be a factor in administration of enema. Enema may be given on bedpan with patient in supine position if he is anxious or unresponsive.
3. Expose anus by draping bath blanket.	3. Bath blanket maintains warmth and prevents unnecessary exposure.
4. Adjust IV pole or overbed table so that top of fluid in reservoir is 45 cm. (18 inches) above anus for optimum pressure (Fig. 30–9).	4. Height of column of fluid produces hydrostatic pressure. A 46 cm. column of fluid produces sufficient pressure for fluid to reach cecum in 2 to 5 minutes. Increasing column height above this produces increased pressure and more rapid dilation of bowel. This causes pain and the urge to defecate immediately. It also presents the danger of carrying colon contents past ileocecal valve and the danger of rupturing the colon.

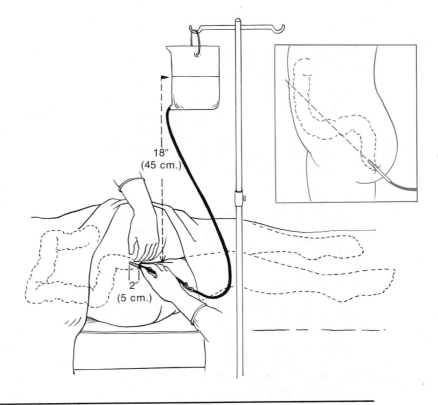

Figure 30–9. Administering an enema. Note that nurse has adjusted IV pole so that the top of the fluid in the reservoir is 18 inches above the patient's anus. The rectal tube tip has been inserted 5 cm. (2 inches) into the patient's rectum and is pointed upward in the direction of the patient's umbilicus.

SUGGESTED STEPS	RATIONALE/DISCUSSION

Administration of Enema (Continued)

5. Put on clean plastic gloves.

5. Protects helper's hands from contamination.

6. Place bedpan on bed behind patient below level of fluid in reservoir. Hold enema tip inside bedpan, open clamp (hemostat) and allow small amount of fluid to flow. Reclamp tubing.

6. Eliminates air in tubing. Not critical, but air seems to stimulate defecation impulse more than fluid. Avoids spillage from enema tip end and side openings (tip eyes).

7. Lubricate rectal tube from tip to 5 cm. (2 inches) above tip with water-soluble lubricant.

7. Prevents abrasion of tissues of anal canal. Petroleum jelly (Vaseline) may be used at home.

8. Separate the patient's buttocks to clearly visualize anus. Hold rectal tip against anus pointing in direction of umbilicus (see Fig. 30–9). After anal sphincter relaxes, *gently* insert tip 5 cm. (2 inches).

8. Stimulation of anal canal produces a protective reflex which contracts the anal sphincter. Relaxation of sphincter usually follows initial reflex contraction. Other methods to open or relax anal sphincter may be used, e.g., ask patient to bear down "as if moving your bowels," ask him to "pant like a dog" or gently insert tube while he exhales a deep breath. Forceful insertion of tip may injure anal or rectal tissue.

Procedure continued on the following page

Administration of Enema (Continued)

9. *Hold enema tube in place throughout procedure.* If Foley catheter used instead of rectal tube, advance catheter 5 cm. beyond collapsed balloon. Next, inflate balloon with 30 ml. water and maintain gentle tension on catheter to pull balloon against internal anal sphincter. If special baby nipple used, hold rectal tube tip in anal canal, maintaining constant pressure against nipple.

9. Presence of enema tube in anus distends anal sphincter. This causes bowel contractions, which tend to push tube out of anus. Holding tube prevents displacement. Balloon inflation of Foley catheter *inside* anal canal, along with maintenance of gentle tension on catheter, prevents solution leakage from bowel. *External* placement of special baby nipple against anus also prevents leakage from bowel.

10. Read level of fluid in reservoir before beginning fluid administration. This is the first step in calculating amount of fluid administered.

10. Remember, some solution has been used to flush air from tubing.

11. Open clamp (hemostat). Level of fluid in reservoir should fall slowly. If fluid level does not fall, briefly raise reservoir to 50 cm. (20 inches) or slightly higher to increase pressure. Patient is usually unable to feel fluid until distention occurs because solution is near body temperature by the time it is administered.

11. Temporarily increasing pressure opens lumen of rectal tube if blocked by feces. If blockage is not relieved, clamp tubing, remove rectal tube and clean lumen of tube with toilet tissue. Fluid administered near body temperature (37–39°C. or 98.6–102°F.) is not usually felt by the patient.

12. Gradually adjust height of reservoir to compensate for falling level of fluid. Goal is to keep fluid level in reservoir 46 cm. (18 inches) above anus.

12. Maintains desired hydrostatic pressure.

13. Administer solution *slowly.* (750 ml. should take 10 min. to administer.) Remember: goal is to give adult 500 to 750 ml. of solution.

13. Saline enema works by causing distention of bowel (or mechanical irritation), resulting in contractions. Rapid administration of solution causes contractions of colon before desired amount is given, making retention of solution difficult.

14. Temporarily stop solution administration and follow step 15 until symptoms subside if:

14. Stop flow of solution by kinking or folding tubing to obliterate lumen. This method stops flow more quickly than trying to close clamp or use hemostat with one hand.

    a. Patient has urge to *defecate* or has *abdominal cramps.*

    a. Distention of bowels causes discomfort; rapid closing of tube is desirable.

    b. Patient begins to *expel solution* around rectal tube or if *solution level rises* in reservoir. Turn bedpan on end, placing open lip of pan below anus to catch fluid. *Do not* remove rectal tube. Reassure patient that changing bed is no trouble; estimate amount of fluid lost.

    b. Removal of rectal tube stimulates defecation impulse. Anxiety increases peristalsis. Amount of fluid lost is subtracted from total to determine volume retained.

SUGGESTED STEPS   RATIONALE/DISCUSSION

Administration of Enema (Continued)

15. During solution administration ask patient to open mouth and "pant like a dog" for short periods of time. Avoid hyperventilation.

15. Breathing with mouth open relaxes abdominal muscles, decreasing pressure on colon. Also, distracts patient enough to relax abdominal muscles.

> Caution: *Do not allow patient to hyperventilate for long periods or he will lose consciousness.*

16. Administer 500 to 750 ml. of solution, repeating steps 14 and 15 as necessary. Do not give desired amount if patient is uncomfortable.

16. Normal adult colon holds 750 ml. comfortably. Large amount of feces in colon decreases volume of solution retained comfortably.

17. Clamp tubing. Gently remove enema tip by pulling it through 5 to 10 layers of toilet tissue. Hold tissues around tube and firmly against anus. During removal continue to point tip toward umbilicus.

17. Toilet tissue: (a) cleanses feces from tube and (b) helps patient maintain anal sphincter control. Maintaining correct direction during withdrawal of tip avoids stimulation and damage of anal canal.

18. Discard soiled toilet tissue in bedpan. Coil rectal tip and tubing inside reservoir or place rectal tip in empty package from disposable set. Remove gloves.

18. Avoids contamination of environment by soiled articles. Inside of reservoir is already contaminated by solution back-flow from colon during administration.

19. Ask patient to retain fluid while lying quietly in bed for 15 minutes if possible. Encourage slow breathing through open mouth for relaxation. Give patient pad of 5 to 10 layers of toilet tissue to hold over anus. Place patient in comfortable position.

19. Enema is most effective if solution retained for 15 minutes. Patient may be positioned on bedpan, commode or toilet if apprehensive; anxiety stimulates peristalsis. Pressure over anus helps patient maintain anal sphincter control.

20. Assist patient onto toilet, commode or bedpan.

20. Sitting position and privacy encourage maximally effective defecation.

21. Give call signal to patient and leave him alone if safe. Remind patient not to flush toilet or to allow results of enema to be discarded.

21. Sense of privacy enhances act of defecation. Patients under stress often forget instructions.

22. Explain to patient that during the next hour or so he may need to evacuate bowels several more times.

22. Slow distention of colon delays onset of strong peristalsis, resulting in delayed expulsion of solution and feces.

23. Observe enema results, noting color, consistency and amount. Obtain specimen for tests if ordered.

23. Use disposable tongue blades to lift formed fecal material into specimen container. If no formed feces passed, pour sample of returned enema solution into specimen container.

Procedure continued on the following page

Post-Procedure Activities.   Assist patient to cleanse rectal area with toilet tissue as necessary. Remove patient from toilet, commode or bedpan. Nurse washes her hands. Tell patient the results or effectiveness of enema. Ask patient if he expelled gas (flatus), feels dizzy or lightheaded, has abdominal cramps, nausea or rectal discomfort and if he feels he has emptied his bowel. Tell him if additional enemas are to be given. Wash perineum and buttocks with soap and water. Provide for washing of patient's hands. Ensure patient's comfort and safety, remove bath blanket, replace covers, lower bed, clean contaminated surfaces, air room as necessary. Immediately send specimen to laboratory.

Aftercare of Equipment.   Discard disposable equipment. Empty unused solution into toilet. Place reusable tubing, enema tube and stainless steel reservoir in soiled utility room to be reprocessed (cleansed with soap and water and autoclaved). If series of enemas is ordered, label reservoir with patient's name, place in patient's bathroom or soiled utility room for his reuse. Do not store used enema equipment in bedside stand with hygiene or personal articles. Return IV pole to storage area. Cleanse commode and bedpan and store as appropriate.

Final Patient Assessment.   Evaluate patient's condition and comfort. Take vital signs if patient is pale, diaphoretic (perspiring), etc. If patient is pale, diaphoretic, has rectal bleeding or pain, immediately place him in supine position, take vital signs and obtain assistance. *Chart/Report:* Time of day and amount of saline enema given; color, consistency, amount and time(s) of evacuation; patient's reaction to administration and evacuation of enema; time specimen sent to laboratory. Immediately report any untoward effects or results, e.g., pain, failure to expel fluid, blood or tissue expelled, change in vital signs. Record N.S.E. on Graphic Sheet and/or Day Sheet.

Administration of a hypertonic enema requires several deviations from the process described above, mainly because the solution comes prepackaged and ready to inject. The solution does not need to be warmed, but should be at least room temperature to prevent intestinal cramps. The patient may be in any position to receive this enema; some authorities recommend the knee-chest position to more fully distribute the solution throughout the colon. The kit comes with a prelubricated tip, and once it is inserted into the rectum, the collapsible reservoir is steadily squeezed or rolled until the solution is gone. The patient is instructed to retain the enema until the urge to defecate is felt very strongly. Patients can easily be taught to self-administer a hypertonic enema, and they are frequently advised to administer one at home before x-ray studies or proctologic examination.

The procedure for administering a retention enema is very similar to that for a normal saline enema, except that the main goal is for the solution to be retained over a prolonged period of time. The minimum retention time is one hour; some enemas, e.g., medicated or nutritive, should never be evacuated. The method of solution preparation depends on what is to be used. A smaller administration tip is used, usually a No. 14 to No. 20 Fr. catheter for adults, to diminish stimulation of the defecation reflex by stretching the sphincters (the French scale is briefly discussed in Chapter 40). The reservoir is elevated above the anus only far enough to allow the solution to slowly run into the rectum. Administration under higher pressure will distend the rectum, causing defecation. Finally, provision for expulsion of the solution is not needed, although the bed linen should be well protected in case the patient cannot retain the enema.

Enema administration is not without its *hazards*. These include fluid and electrolyte imbalances, tissue trauma, vagal nerve stimulaion in susceptible persons, and dependence. Fluid imbalances usually occur because of the tonicity of the enema solution. Water is absorbed by the body from hypotonic solutions. Usually this causes no significant problem. However, if tap water enemas are repeated or in patients susceptible to fluid changes, e.g., infants or patients with decompensated cardiac or kidney reserve, water intoxication can occur. Symptoms of this condition include weakness, dizziness, pallor, sweating, and respiratory difficulties. Signs of congestive heart failure or cerebral edema may be present. On the other hand, hypertonic solutions, because they draw fluid from the interstitial tissues, can lead to fluid depletion, especially with children and others susceptible to dehydration. Davis and associates report occurrences of dehydration in children following administration of a single hypertonic enema.[28] These enemas should not be given repeatedly to any patient.

Electrolyte imbalances may also occur. Usually, normal saline is the safest enema solution to use because of its isotonicity. However, if the patient has a problem with sodium retention, e.g., congestive heart failure or cirrhosis of the liver, he will absorb the sodium from the saline enema. This will lead to further fluid and electrolyte imbalance. Therefore, these patients should not receive saline solutions. Potassium depletion may occur as a result of enema administration. Other electrolyte imbalances have been reported, e.g., hypocalcemia and hyperphosphatemia, following small-volume phosphate enemas.[28] Consequently, enemas must be used with great caution in persons vulnerable to these problems.

Tissue trauma can come from three main sources: the administration tip, the solution, and peristalsis itself. If a hard tip is used and it has any chips or broken areas, it may mechanically lacerate or abrade the mucosa. The intestinal wall may be ruptured by either the administration tip or the injection of solution under too high a pressure. Because sensory innervation stops at the pectinate line, there may be no pain at the time of perforation; the first indication of rupture may be signs of developing peritonitis (inflammation of the peritoneum). These hazards can be avoided by following proper procedure. Tissue trauma resulting from peristalsis occurs in patients with inflammatory bowel disease; increased motility enhances their symptoms of cramping, bleeding, etc. Enemas should be avoided in people with these problems.

As indicated above, the use of soapsuds enemas has been under fire for some time, and yet they are frequently ordered. The solution acts by virtue of chemical irritation of the mucosa. This irritation frequently leads to rectal inflammation and colitis, sometimes lasting up to 3 weeks after the enema. The higher the concentration of soap in the solution, the greater its inflammatory results. This problem is somewhat alleviated if standardized packages of castile soap are used, but is especially intensified if any other reservoir of soap solution is used. The practice of swirling a bar of soap or soap pieces in the enema reservoir is highly dangerous since no determination of the concentration can be made. The use of this enema solution requires more research to scientifically establish its efficacy.[100, 103, 106]

Vagal nerve stimulation occurs with stretching of the anal sphincters and distention of the bowel. This activity is particularly hazardous to patients with cardiac disease. Pais reported that 25 per cent of a group of patients over the age of 60 developed cardiac arrhythmias during and after barium enema studies; 90 per cent of these patients had had cardiac problems before the x-rays.[103] Patients have been known to develop myocardial infarctions as a direct result of enema administration.

As with laxatives and suppositories, patients can develop physical and psychologic dependence on enemas. The mechanism is the same: The enema cleans the bowel so that it takes 2 or more days for enough fecal mass to collect again to stimulate defecation. In the meantime, the patient becomes anxious because he does not have a bowel movement when he thinks he should. He then takes another enema, thus beginning the cycle. The bowel becomes less and less sensitive to normal defecation reflex stimuli, and the patient is truly physically dependent on bowel aids.

FECAL IMPACTION

A *fecal impaction* is actually an extension of constipation. It is a collection of putty-like or hardened feces in the rectum, which usually prevents the passage of a normal stool. As feces remains in the rectum, more and more water is absorbed from it by the colon and additional fecal material is added to the mass as it moves down from the sigmoid colon. Eventually, the mass becomes so hard and large that it cannot physically pass through the anal canal and anus.

The first symptom arousing suspicion of an impaction is the inability to pass a normal stool. However, probably the most definitive symptom is the seepage from the anus of liquid stool, which is the only thing that can get around the impaction. Usually this liquid appears in small amounts, which helps differentiate it from true diarrhea, but sometimes because of bacterial action on the fecal mass, copious amounts of liquid stool are produced. This seepage of stool is usually uncontrolled, because the anus has become less competent in containing the stool because of prolonged stimulation of the defecation reflex by the hardened mass.

Other symptoms indicating impaction include an almost continuous urge to defecate that is unfulfilled, rectal pain and abdominal fullness. If an impaction is suspected, a digital examination of the rectum should be done. To do this, the nurse dons a glove and liberally lubricates the forefinger. The finger is then inserted through the anus into the rectum. If the hard fecal mass is felt, diagnosis of an impaction is certain. However, if a mass is not felt, but the symptoms are present, the mass may be higher up in the colon, out of reach.

The goal of treatment for a fecal impaction is removal of the mass from the rectum. Oral laxatives or cathartics may be used to moisten and lubricate the fecal mass, although their action may be too slow if the patient is in much distress. A program of enemas may be instituted, starting with the administration of an oil retention enema. A commercially prepared oil solution or 100 to 200 ml. of mineral oil or olive oil is injected into the rectum under very low pressure to avoid stimulation of the defecation reflex. The oil solution must be retained until it has had time to perform its function. It should be kept in the rectum at least 60 min. and is often left overnight. The retention enema is usually followed by a volume cleansing enema. These two enemas may need to be repeated.

If the fecal mass is extremely large or the enemas are ineffective in expelling it, the impaction will have to be digitally removed. To do this, a gloved finger, which has been heavily lubricated, is inserted into the rectum and the mass is mechanically broken up. Pieces may be manually removed so a bedpan should be conveniently placed to receive them. At best, this procedure is very uncomfortable for the patient—and embarrassing. And the pressure of the hard stool against the mucosa causes laceration and bleeding. Gentleness may help, but prevention is the best treatment.

DIARRHEA

Diarrhea is the passage of liquid or unformed stool. As with constipation, some consider the frequency of defecation as part of the definition, but consistency of the stool is the primary component. In general, diarrhea indicates that intestinal motility has been greatly increased, so that the gastrointestinal contents are rapidly moved through the tract. Because of the rapid transit time, the normal amounts of water are not removed from the feces. In addition, irritation of the mucosal walls may stimulate increased secretions, which add moisture to the fecal mass. Therefore, when the feces reaches the rectum, it is still in its liquid state and is passed out through the anus in this form.

The causes of diarrhea are numerous. Emotional states, especially anxiety, frequently cause diarrhea. Infectious organisms, most frequently staphylococci and streptococci, release irritating toxins. Irritating foods are an individualized matter, but fried, greasy, and spicy foods are common factors. Medications, e.g., iron, thyroid agents, some antacids, laxatives, and antibiotics, may cause diarrhea. Travelers often develop diarrhea a day or two after beginning their trip. Usually, this is from the change in bacteria in the water; however, it may be caused by any bacteria, virus or parasite to which the person has no immunity and may occur in spite of proper precautions about food and water.

Accompanying symptoms may include abdominal cramps, distention, flatus, nausea and vomiting, bleeding, anorexia, urgency, fever, malaise, and symptoms of fluid imbalance. Continuing diarrhea can lead to severe fluid and electrolyte imbalance, since water, sodium and potassium are not reabsorbed by the body. There is also nonabsorption of all other nutrients, leading to a starvation syndrome. Diarrhea stool is usually acidic and contains digestive enzymes, and if it comes in prolonged or frequent contact with the skin, anal excoriation occurs; this is made worse by frequent wiping with toilet paper.

The treatment for diarrhea is to slow down peristalsis. The precipitating factors must be removed, then the diarrhea itself stopped. If necessary, all oral intake should be eliminated so as to avoid stimulating peristalsis. Commonly used antidiarrheal drugs are the adsorbents, such as kaolin and pectin. These medications bind and remove irritants from the gastrointestinal tract and form a soothing, protective coating on the mucosa. Sometimes, the bulk-forming laxatives are used to hold water in the gastrointestinal tract and thus reduce the fluid imbalance problem. In cases of severe diarrhea, opiates, such as paregoric and codeine, or anticholinergic drugs may be needed to slow down the transit time. Normal intestinal bacterial flora can be re-established by giving the patient yogurt, buttermilk, or bacillus-containing medications.[9, 109]

While these measures are stopping the

diarrhea, treatment of the accompanying problems must be instituted. The most crucial is the potential for fluid and electrolyte imbalance. Those elements being lost by the body must be replaced. Infants and debilitated persons are especially susceptible to these losses. If the patient cannot tolerate oral fluids, parenteral therapy must be started. If necessary, the patient must be assured that decreasing his fluid intake will not stop the diarrhea! Ventura describes a way by which travelers with diarrhea can replace fluids and electrolytes lost in diarrhea stool. She suggests preparing two glasses, the first one to contain 240 ml. of orange, apple, or other potassium-rich juice; 2.5 ml. of honey, corn syrup, or table sugar, which is necessary for absorption of the salts; and one pinch of table salt. The second glass should contain 240 ml. of carbonated or boiled water and 1.25 ml. baking soda. The patient should drink from the glasses alternately and supplement his fluid intake with carbonated beverages.[127] Although this procedure was designed for travelers, it would also be appropriate for use in the home.

The perianal skin must be protected. Providing the patient with soft material for wiping after each stool will reduce the mechanical irritation, and washing with soap and water after each stool will reduce the time that the acidic feces and digestive enzymes are in contact with the skin. The outer tissue may also be protected from these chemicals by the application of petroleum jelly, zinc oxide, or other protective ointments.

The frequency and urgency of bowel movements also causes the patient much fatigue and embarrassment. One way to reduce these factors is to make sure that the patient has quick and easy access to the bathroom, commode, or bedpan. The call bell should be placed conveniently near the patient at all times. Also, provision for privacy and odor control are greatly appreciated by the patient.

FLATULENCE

Gas is normally found in the gastrointestinal tract, some of it being swallowed and some produced by the fermentation processes in the intestine and part from diffusion of gases from the bloodstream. *Flatulence,* or gaseous distention, is the presence of abnormal amounts of gas within the gastrointestinal tract. Symptoms include a bloated feeling, abdominal distention, cramping pains, and excessive passage of gas from the mouth *(eructation)* or from the anus *(flatus).* Respiratory distress may also occur if the distention pushes on the diaphragm. Percussion of the abdomen produces a tympanic sound.

As with other gastrointestinal disturbances, causes are numerous. Probably the most common predisposing factor in flatulence is excessive air swallowing, which may result from various activities: chewing gum, drinking carbonated beverages, eating rapidly, or sucking through straws. Anxiety states and postnasal drip can also lead to air swallowing. Some people intentionally swallow air so as to cause belching of the gas already in the stomach; however, this is ineffective since the burp expels less air than was swallowed.[134]

Other causes of gaseous distention include constipation; slowed intestinal motility, such as may occur after abdominal surgery; bowel obstruction; medications which decrease peristalsis; and decreased activity. A number of foods are reputed to be gas-formers; the most common ones are beans, cabbage, radishes, onions, cauliflower and cucumbers.

Treatment is aimed at removing the gas from the gastrointestinal tract. Initially, the patient must be helped to avoid the situations and substances that precipitate the flatulence. The most effective, natural way to expel the flatus is by exercise. Walking is the best method, but if this is not possible, moving around in bed will help. Exercise stimulates peristalsis, which speeds the transit time of the gas through the colon.

Rectal Tube. A *rectal tube* inserted into the rectum provides a ready passage out of the body for the gas. A rubber or plastic rectal tube, from No. 22 to No. 32 Fr. for adults, is lubricated and inserted about 10 cm. (4 inches) into the rectum. The distal end of the tube is placed into a collecting receptacle to catch any feces that may be expelled through it. The tube is taped into place and left for not more than 20 min. Longer periods of insertion reduce the responsiveness of the sphincters and can lead to permanent sphincter damage. The tube can be reinserted every 2 to 3 hours if necessary. Other types of gastrointestinal tubes may also be used (see Chap. 41).

Return Flow Enema. A *return flow enema* can be used to relieve flatulence, although use of this intervention is controversial due to reports of intestinal trauma resulting from it. With this enema, the intestine is alternately filled and drained so as to help remove flatus and to stimulate peristalsis to move the gas down the gastrointestinal tract. The patient, equipment, and solution (tap water or saline) are prepared as in Procedure 14. After the rectal tube has been inserted, approximately 200 to 300 ml. of fluid is allowed to run into the colon. Then the solution container is lowered 45 cm. (18 inches) below the level of the anus to allow the solution, with gas, to drain back into the reservoir. Gas being expelled will bubble up through the solution in the container. When the return flow has ceased, the reservoir is again raised 45 cm. above the anus and 200 to 300 ml. is allowed to flow in. This process is repeated until the return of gas is minimal. After the procedure is completed, the reservoir and tubing must be carefully washed out if they are being stored for reuse since the inside surfaces are contaminated with fecal material and will develop odor if allowed to stand.

Several medications may be helpful in relieving flatulence. Although it is highly controversial because of the intensity of its action and its many side effects, some physicians order neostigmine to be given intramuscularly about 20 min. before using a rectal tube or return flow enema. This medication increases gastrointestinal motility and facilitates downward movement of the gas. If the patient's air swallowing problem is the result of postnasal drip, a decongestant or antihistamine may eliminate this cause. Simethicone-containing medications may be helpful. It is claimed that this substance causes gas bubbles to coalesce, making them easier to expel.[109]

HEMORRHOIDS

Also called piles, *hemorrhoids* are dilated veins found around the anal area. They are classified as internal or external, depending on where they are in relation to the anal canal. The main cause is increased pressure on the portal venous system, such as may occur with straining to have a bowel movement, pregnancy, or chronic liver disease. While hemorrhoids often present no problem to the patient, other patients complain of pain, itching, and bleeding. Quiescent hemorrhoids may develop complications, such as infection or thrombosis, and incontinence can be the result of sphincter damage from them. The nurse, faced with massive hemorrhoids, may have difficulty finding the anus with a finger or rectal tube. Gentleness is the key. Gently manipulating the tissue flaps until the anus is located and generous lubrication will avoid tissue trauma.

Although surgical intervention may be necessary, most hemorrhoids are treated conservatively. Medications may be used to soften the stools, thereby reducing trauma during defecation. Local treatments to the hemorrhoidal tissue might include local anesthetics for pain relief (this is particularly effective before a bowel movement), vasoconstrictors to decrease the bleeding from traumatized tissue, antiseptics to prevent infection, and astringents to shrink the tissues.[10] These medications are usually applied by suppository or ointments. Sitz baths are also effective in increasing blood flow to the area and relieving pain.

INCONTINENCE

Fecal incontinence is the inability of the patient to voluntarily control passage of feces and gas through the anus. Bowel evacuation usually occurs whenever the defecation reflex is stimulated. Lack of control is accepted during infancy and toddlerhood until primary toilet training has occurred. From that point on, continence is the norm and any deviation meets with both personal and social disapproval. Incontinence causes much embarrassment for the patient and he arranges his life so as to conceal his problem from other people.

Causes of fecal incontinence are both physical and psychologic in origin. Anything interfering with the integrity of sphincter function—hemorrhoids, tumors, lacerations, fistulas, or loss of sensory innervation—will likely lead to incontinence. Patients with explosive diarrhea may find the urge to defecate too overwhelming for the anus to control. Incontinence may simply be a matter of no one answering the patient's call light in time. Psychologically, incontinence may be the result of an emotional state—as well as the cause of various emotional problems. *Encopresis* is the passage of a normal stool in an abnormal place; it is believed to occur because of an emotional disturbance or delay in the maturational process.[17] Sometimes a formerly continent child will become incontinent as a means to gain attention or to express anger; this may also happen with adults. The development of incontinence may be a sign of "giving up." This is frequently seen with institutionalized elderly persons; in fact, the personnel often encourage this behavior by expecting it and accepting it as inevitable.

Probably the most important consequence of incontinence is the loss of self-respect, which can easily be intensified by the reactions of other significant people in the patient's environment—family, friends, nurses. Besides this, the other problems incontinence causes for the patient are skin irritation and breakdown and soiling of clothes and linen.

The skin is relatively easy to care for, although it may be a time-consuming task. The main goal is to prevent prolonged contact between the skin and fecal material, which may lead to excoriation and breakdown. Washing the perianal area with soap and water and drying it well after each stool will keep the skin in good condition and control fecal odor. Powders and creams must be used with great caution since they may actually add to the potential for skin breakdown. If plastic or rubber sheeting is used to protect the bed linen, make sure that it does not contact the patient's skin, since these substances often cause skin irritation. Disposable pads can be used as a protective barrier. If the patient's incontinence is severe, he may need to wear waterproof undergarments to protect his clothing. Diapering an incontinent patient makes him feel like a baby and actually gives him "permission" to be incontinent; thus this practice should be avoided at all costs.

The best way to reduce the psychologic impact of incontinence is to re-establish bowel control. If this is not possible, the intervention available to the nurse and family is a positive, supportive attitude.

Bowel Training Program. Bowel training programs have been very effective in helping patients re-establish bowel control. They do require time, patience, and commitment from the nursing personnel and the patient, but the positive results are well worth the effort.

First, the factors causing the incontinence must be eradicated if possible. Then the nurse discusses the planned program with the patient and his family. Together they decide on the routine to be established. This is based on previous bowel habits and changes that have occurred because of the illness or trauma. It may be helpful to note when the patient is most likely to be incontinent during the day, although this information does not necessarily play a part in planning the patient's routine.

All bowel training programs include some of the independent nursing measures used to aid normal defecation: diet, fluids, exercise as possible, maintenance of habit patterns. Probably the most crucial element of the program is the timing. The time for defecation must be carefully determined and then adhered to strictly. If at all possible, the patient should be positioned on the commode or toilet to take advantage of gravity.

Other than these general guidelines, bowel programs are individualized, although there are many common factors. Most contain provision for the patient to receive fecal softeners to facilitate easy passage of the stool. This is especially important with spinal cord–injured or otherwise debilitated patients, since they often do not have the ability to perform abdominal straining. Suppositories are frequently used every 1 to 3 days to stimulate evacuation. With spinal cord–injured patients especially, the suppository may be followed in 20 to 30 minutes by digital stimulation of the anal sphincter to augment stimulation of the defecation reflex. Health care personnel have developed a number of hand appliances which help the paralyzed patient do this for himself. In some programs, enemas are used in place of the suppositories.

The patient's program may need to be altered until a successful routine is found. Cornell suggests that a patient be kept on a particular program for at least three days before it is changed. This allows the nurse to be sure that modification is indeed necessary.[22]

Other Methods. Other methods of treating incontinence are available. Surgical intervention to create new tissue sphincters has been tried. Electrical stimulation of sphincter control has met with some success. Work has been done on a ball valve mechanism that can be inserted into the rectum, where it can function as an artificial sphincter.[122] More work is needed to perfect these methods.

FECAL DIVERSION

Fecal diversion involves channeling the intestinal contents out of the body at a site other than the anus. This involves an *ileostomy*, which is a surgically created opening in the ileum, or a *colostomy*, which is a surgically created opening in the large intestine. These surgical procedures establish a *stoma*, or opening, on the abdominal wall through which the fecal material passes at the point of the ostomy.

Psychological Impact. Ostomies may be either permanent or temporary. All cause great emotional stress for the patient and his family. Initially, ostomates must go through a period of grieving over the loss of a normal body function. They are hypersensitive to the reactions of those around them. They may become very depressed and feel themselves to be unclean and undesirable to others; they usually feel that they can no longer lead a normal life. Sexual activity is almost universally affected. Even though these initial feelings may be resolved, psychologic problems may occur as the patient meets new and trying situations.

The best way to achieve psychologic stability is for the patient to learn how to care for his ostomy and to resume his previous life-style. The nurse can be an excellent source of strength and support for the patient. However, there are other resources that can be utilized in implementing a care plan for the patient. Almost every city has an ostomy club—a voluntary organization of ostomates who meet together to help each other live with their ostomies. One of their major functions is to meet new and potential ostomates. They can set a good example for the patient and help him with the practical aspects of caring for his ostomy. They are an excellent resource for the patient and his family.

Enterostomal therapy is a field that a growing group of nurses specializes in. These clinical therapists help the patient by providing technical care of and information about his ostomy, by providing psychologic support, by teaching him self-management of his ostomy, and by helping him re-establish his previous life in relation to his family, occupation and recreation.[81] In addition to in-patient therapy, stoma rehabilitation clinics are being established to provide ongoing preventive maintenance and crisis intervention.

In terms of physical care, this section will deal only with the established ostomy. For information about the new ostomy and more information about the ostomy patient at any stage of his rehabilitation process, the reader should consult a medical-surgical nursing text and some of the articles cited at the end of this chapter.

Ileostomy.   An ileostomy may be performed because of cancer, congenital defect, or trauma, but by far the most frequent reasons are ulcerative colitis or regional ileitis (Crohn's disease). Because of the placement of the stoma in the small intestine, the flow of fecal material is, in most cases, constant and cannot be regulated. Isler does describe a surgical technique in which a continent ileostomy is formed by creating an internal pouch with a nipple valve that can be emptied at the patient's convenience.[62] However, most ileostomy patients have not had this procedure.

The ileostomy patient's major problems are obstruction, diarrhea, and skin irritation. Obstruction may be prevented by chewing food very well and can usually be relieved by massaging the abdomen around the stoma or by gentle lavage (washing out) of the stoma with a catheter. Diarrhea is treated as described in the previous section. The ileostomy patient is particularly susceptible to fluid and electrolyte imbalances, so must take vigorous steps to avoid them. Skin irritation is best treated by prevention through proper bagging. If irritation does occur, the skin should be kept clean and dry and a protective skin barrier used between the pouch faceplate and the skin. Topical medications may be needed to treat severe irritation.

Because the ileostomy, except for the continent ileostomy, is continually draining fecal material, a bag must be worn at all times. The pouch is emptied through the bottom whenever necessary; the patient often does it whenever he urinates. After healing of the stoma is complete, the patient is fitted with a reuseable appliance. Your patient will likely be very knowledgeable about changing this appliance. If not, Jensen[65] provides an excellent guide to help you with this task. Odor control, which can be a distressing problem, can be achieved by carefully washing the appliance after use, by placing a deodorizing agent in the pouch, or by internal medications, such as bismuth subgallate.

Colostomy.   Colostomies are performed because of trauma, intestinal obstruction, birth defect, or cancer. They may be done in the ascending (rarely), transverse, descending or sigmoid colon. The further down the intestine the stoma is placed, the better the chances of regulating the bowel. Some patients develop such reliable bowel control that they do not wear a bag, only a small dressing to protect the stoma from irritation by the clothes.

Like the ileostomy patients, many people with colostomies wear a pouch that must be changed periodically. If the reader needs help with this procedure, Jensen[64] is a good resource. The main thing is to attach the pouch firmly, so as to avoid spilling of the intestinal contents onto the patient's skin and clothing.

Traditionally, daily irrigation has been considered an integral part of colostomy care. Some now argue that this is not always necessary. The main reason for performing the irrigation is to avoid fecal spillage through the day; the colostomy will physically function adequately without the irrigation. The irrigating process is a time-consuming and somewhat involved one and some patients are not well suited to learning it, e.g., those with poor eyesight or manual dexterity, inability to learn new techniques, excessive fear, previous inflammatory bowel disease, or those who are unwilling to spend the time each day.[131] These patients simply need to wear a pouch at all times and care for it much as an ileostomy patient would.

If the decision has been made that the patient's colostomy needs to be irrigated, the nurse may have to help the patient. Since we are discussing the patient with an established colostomy, we will assume that the irrigation is being done with the patient in the bathroom.

Alterations in the process can easily be made for other circumstances.

Irrigation of a colostomy is very similar to the administration of a normal saline enema. The major difference is that the patient will be unable to control the expulsion of the solution and fecal material, so some variations in equipment and technique are necessary. An irrigation sleeve is used to channel the expelled contents into the toilet; the sleeve is a plastic tunnel that fits around the stoma and is held in place by a belt around the patient's waist. The irrigating solution and enema equipment are prepared as for any volume enema. The rectal tube can be placed through a baby bottle nipple as in Figure 30–8, or there are cone-shaped irrigating tips available that reduce the danger of bowel perforation. The nipple and cone seal off the stoma so that the irrigating fluid cannot leak out. The nurse should be positive of the location of the stoma before inserting the catheter or cone. If a catheter is used, it should be inserted very gently about 7.5 to 10 cm. (3 to 4 inches). Administer the solution as in Procedure 14.

When you are about ready to remove the administration tip, be sure the irrigating sleeve is well in front of the stoma, since the initial drainage may gush out. Close the top of the sleeve with clips, and allow most of the contents to be expelled. This will usually take about 10 to 15 minutes. Odor control can be achieved by occasionally rinsing the sleeve with water and flushing the toilet. When the primary returns are finished, the patient can dry the end of the sleeve, clip the bottom end to the top, and go about his daily activities. There is often another bowel evacuation within 30 to 45 minutes. When the patient is sure that the irrigation returns have finished, he may remove the irrigation sleeve, clean the peristomal skin and apply either a clean pouch or a dressing.[64]

For the patient who wears a pouch, as with the ileostomy patient, odor control is an ongoing problem. As mentioned before, careful washing, deodorizers in the pouch, and medications may be used. The patient should also avoid gas-forming foods. Cabbage, cauliflower, onions, and turnips often increase fecal odor, while yogurt, buttermilk, parsley, and green, leafy vegetables may reduce fecal odor. Some people advocate placing crushed aspirin tablets in the pouch, but others advise against it because of the potential chemical irritation of the stoma.[6]

Collection of Specimens

A stool specimen is collected in a sterile or a clean bedpan or some other receptacle depending on the requirement of the test. If the patient is using the toilet, a bedpan can be placed in the toilet under the seat. The fecal specimen should be kept uncontaminated by urine if at all possible. Once the specimen has been deposited in the larger container, the necessary amount of it can be transferred to a covered specimen container with one or two tongue depressors. The lid is put on the container, and the specimen is properly labeled and sent to the laboratory.

The nurse must be aware of the conditions necessary to facilitate accurate test results. For instance, a stool specimen to be tested for ova and parasites should be examined immediately since the organisms will slowly die if they cool below body temperature; however, artificial heat hastens their death. These specimens must also be free of any oil, barium, or bismuth. Specimens for culture should be sent to the laboratory immediately or placed in a proper medium to avoid overgrowth of the bacterial population.[95]

A specimen is collected from the anal region to check for pinworms. A strip of nonfrosted cellophane tape is pressed sticky-side down over the anus. It is removed immediately, placed on a glass slide, and sent to the laboratory for microscopic examination. This specimen must be collected in the early morning before the patient has either a bath or a bowel movement. The worms hatch at night and crawl out through the anus in the morning.

Diagnostic Tests Performed by the Nurse

The most common diagnostic test performed on a stool specimen by the nurse is for occult blood (hidden blood). This is also called a *guaiac test*. The chief process involved in this test is exposing the stool specimen to certain chemical reagents and observing for a color change; with most procedures, a blue color indicates a positive result—the presence of blood. There are a variety of materials and methods available for performing this test. The main thing for the nurse to do is to read the directions carefully before beginning the test and to follow them explicitly.

KIDNEY FUNCTION

Normal Anatomy and Physiology

The urinary system functions to (a) remove waste products from the body and (b) regulate the fluid, electrolyte, and acid-base balances and the osmotic pressure within the body. Failure of the urinary tract is incompatible with life unless medical intervention can compensate for the loss.

The urinary tract has four major anatomical structures with which to accomplish its functions: the kidneys, which perform the selection processes necessary to maintain a healthy internal environment, and three components whose only task is to transport urine from the kidney out of the body—ureters, bladder, and urethra. Figure 30–10 illustrates the anatomy of the urinary tract. See Figures 40–1 and 40–2 to review how the urinary tract structures relate anatomically to other pelvic organs. The male reproductive system is closely allied with the urinary tract since both share the same passageway from the body. However, this chapter will consider only those factors regarding urinary tract function.

KIDNEYS

The kidneys are located retroperitoneally along the thoracolumbar spine, with the left kidney usually a little higher than the right. They are supported by a mass of adipose tissue

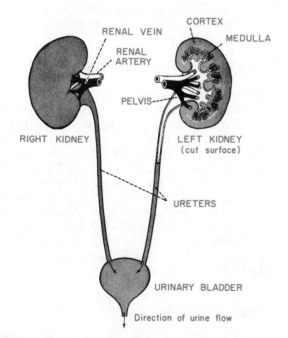

Figure 30–10. Anatomy of the urinary tract. (From Guyton, A. C.: *Function of the Human Body,* 4th ed. Philadelphia, W. B. Saunders Co., 1974.)

and the renal fascia. Each kidney is enclosed in a fibrous capsule and consists of three general areas: pelvis, medulla, and cortex. The *nephron* is the functioning unit of the kidney. There are at least 1.5 million of these units in each kidney. Each one consists of two major parts: the *glomerulus*, which is a cluster of capillaries surrounded by a capsule (Bowman's capsule), and a system of *tubules*.

The main function of the kidney is to form urine, by which it accomplishes the rest of its roles. Blood supply for the kidney comes from the renal artery, which branches from the abdominal aorta. An estimated 1700 liters of blood per day is received by the kidneys. The blood comes to the kidney under high pressure and is channeled through dividing vessels until it reaches the glomerulus. Here, as the result of filtration pressure, a plasma-like fluid without any substantial amount of protein is filtered out of the blood at a rate of about 125 to 130 ml. per minute. This filtrate enters Bowman's capsule and then the tubule system, where reabsorption of the substances needed by the body takes place. As the filtrate travels through the proximal convoluted tubule, the loop of Henle, and the distal convoluted tubule, water, sodium chloride and other electrolytes, creatinine, glucose, lactate, amino acids, and vitamin C are absorbed according to the body's demands. By the time the filtrate reaches the collecting tubules that transport it to the renal pelvis, about 98 per cent of it has been reabsorbed, so that actual urine production is about 1 to 2 ml. per minute. The kidney tubules also have the ability to actively secrete substances, but this plays a very minor role in the overall function of the kidney.

The urine is deposited into the renal pelvis, from which it is carried into the lower urinary tract through the ureters. The nephron is very susceptible to external pressure, so if urine remains in the renal pelvis and pressure builds up, kidney damage occurs.

URETERS, BLADDER, URETHRA

For review of the anatomy of the ureters, bladder, and urethra, the reader is referred to Chapter 40.

Act of Micturition

Micturition is the process of emptying the urinary bladder. Synonyms for this function are *urination* and *voiding*. It is a necessary physiologic function, under both voluntary and involuntary control, by which the waste products filtered by the kidneys are finally removed from the body.

The urine enters the bladder from the ureters. The bladder acts as a storage vessel so that urine does not continually dribble from the body. The bladder slowly fills with urine. Until there are 150 to 500 ml. in the bladder, the detrusor muscle slowly accommodates to the increased volume and the intravesicular pressure rises very little. The ability to store urine without stimulation of the micturition reflex depends on the person's normal habit patterns, although trauma and disease processes can interfere with proper reflex activity.

As the amount of accumulated urine continues to increase, the intravesicular pressure rises and the stretch receptors in the bladder wall are stimulated. These impulses are sent to the spinal cord, where the micturition reflex is initiated, causing the bladder to contract and the sphincters to open involuntarily. The external sphincter, however, is under voluntary control after a period of successful toilet training and in the absence of disease. The impulses initiating micturition are also sent to the cerebral cortex and, if the environmental conditions are not right for urination, the external sphincter is contracted to stop the flow of urine. Contraction of the perineal muscles aids the tightening of the external sphincter. If urination is to occur, the external sphincter opens, the perineal muscles relax, and voiding occurs. Increasing intra-abdominal pressure also aids micturition by providing increased external pressure on the bladder.

Factors Affecting Normal Micturition

The act of micturition can be affected by several factors. Some of these can lead to problems within the urinary tract, and many are the foundation for nursing intervention.

Psychological Factors.   Probably the most important effect the psyche has on micturition is a result of the mind's tremendous susceptibility to the power of suggestion. The various sensory areas of the brain have associated fibers connecting with the micturition control center in the cortex, and micturition can be initiated by any number of auditory, visual, or somesthetic stimuli. Many of these are described below under independent nursing measures. In fact, it would not be unusual for you to have to make a trip to the bathroom at some time while reading this chapter.

Anxiety states definitely affect the micturition pattern by either initiating or hindering it. The most noticeable effect is that of frequency and urgency. Very commonly, when facing a stressful situation, the person has a strong urge to void, even though he may have voided just moments ago.

Conversely, anxiety characterized by generalized muscle tension can interfere with urination since relaxation of the perineal muscles is absolutely essential to completing the act of micturition. Therefore, anything that interferes with perineal relaxation may lead to retention of urine in the bladder.

Toilet Training Experiences.   As with defecation, the life-long effects of experiences during the toilet-training period in childhood may affect a person's micturition pattern in adult life. One example of this may be prolonged *enuresis* (involuntary discharge of urine, usually during sleep at night); however, this problem is complex and surrounded by controversy regarding its etiology. The reader will find more discussion of enuresis below.

Cultural Teachings.   The purpose of cultural teachings is to pass on the rules and regulations for living within a given society. Inability to follow the prescribed course of action usually causes stress and distress for the person involved.

The most important cultural rule for micturition affected by illness and hospitalization is that requiring privacy. For most Americans, privacy is very important to successful urination. As was discussed under bowel function, this component affects both the patient and the nurse.

Personal Habits.   Although usually less complex than the routine surrounding defecation, some people have developed an individualized set of behaviors to help stimulate the micturition reflex. Because of the vulnerability to suggestion, often nothing more is needed than placing oneself in the appropriate environment. Some people may employ additional relaxation techniques, such as reading.

Fluid Intake.   Undoubtedly the most important physical factor affecting micturition is the patient's fluid status. One of the kidney's main functions is the maintenance of fluid balance within the body, and the amount of urine produced depends greatly on the body's need to retain or excrete water in order to preserve this balance.

If all other variables of fluid balance remain constant, the amount of urine produced is in direct correlation to the amount of fluid taken in. And the amount of urine produced has direct influence on the frequency of urination. The kind of fluid ingested may be important, since some beverages are reported to have a *diuretic* (increased secretion of urine) effect on some people. Examples include coffee, tea and alcoholic beverages. In addition to the amount and kind of measurable fluids taken in, some foods, e.g., fruits and vegetables, have a higher fluid content than others and so affect the patient's total fluid intake. Highly salted foods and beverages may cause the person to retain fluids so that less urine is produced.

Timing of fluid intake may also determine or interfere with normal micturition habits. For instance, people do not normally awaken at night to urinate. However, if a person drinks a large amount of fluid just before retiring, the need to urinate will likely awaken him before the alarm clock goes off.

Medications. Several medications have a direct effect on the act of micturition. Diuretic drugs increase the amount of urine being produced, mainly by interfering with tubular reabsorption of sodium and thus water. Cholinergic drugs stimulate contraction of the detrusor muscle resulting in micturition, while cholinergic-blocking agents may be used to stop bladder spasms. Any medications, such as analgesics and tranquilizers, which suppress the central nervous system will also interfere with micturition by diminishing the effectiveness of the neural reflex.

Muscle Tone. A lack of muscle tone means that the abdominal musculature may not be able to effectively contract in order to increase intra-abdominal pressure. Increasing this pressure aids bladder contraction. Weakened pelvic musculature also reduces the external sphincter's ability to hold back the flow of urine. This may result in involuntary discharge of urine from the bladder. Immobility strongly fosters development of decreasing muscle tone.

On the other hand, as discussed above, too much muscle tone in the pelvic region inhibits the micturition reflex. For instance, straining to void doesn't work; instead, the person must concentrate on relaxing. Straining actually can produce detrimental effects in the lower urinary tract since it aids the contraction of the bladder and yet helps block passage of urine out through the meatus. Increased pressures are built up in the urinary structures.

Since the bladder is itself a muscle, its tone also affects the act of micturition. Its ability to function properly depends on alternate filling and emptying and periodic activation of the micturition reflex. If it is kept continually emptied, as with straight catheter drainage, it loses its tone like any unused muscle and may not function properly when the catheter is removed. Likewise, if it is continually distended, it becomes insensitive to micturition stimuli and again loses its tone. Hypertonus, in the form of bladder spasms, may cause frequency and premature bladder emptying.

Surgery and Other Trauma; Obstruction. The surgical experience affects the act of micturition in several ways. Initially, most patients are in a state of fluid depletion at the start of the surgical procedure and more fluid is lost during surgery, so the amount of urine produced is diminished. Anesthetics and narcotics used during surgery reduce the glomerular filtration rate and interfere with the sensory and motor pathways necessary for the micturition reflex. One study of 840 surgical patients showed that 13.3 per cent of them had some degree of postoperative urinary retention. Patients having spinal anesthesia either alone or in combination with other anesthetic agents were at particularly high risk.[63] Hormonal changes caused by the stress of surgery initially decrease the amount of urine produced and then cause diuresis to occur.

The surgical procedure itself, or any other trauma, may interfere with micturition if it results in damage to the urinary structures or surrounding tissues. Edema formation can obstruct the passageways and mucosal irritation causes pain. Pain produces increased muscle tension and thereby inhibits urination.

In addition to edema, obstruction may also be caused by tumors or scar formation. Another common obstructive process occurs in males. The prostate gland normally surrounds the urethra just below the bladder neck. Many men develop benign prostatic hypertrophy and the enlarging prostate gland slowly squeezes off the urethra. These patients often complain of dribbling of urine, difficulty starting the stream, and a feeling that the bladder does not empty with each voiding.

Diagnostic Tests. Diagnostic tests may affect the patient's fluid balance, since many examinations require that the patient have nothing by mouth for a period of time. Also direct visualization of the urinary tract, i.e., cystoscopy, may cause edema formation and discomfort, which interferes with micturition.

Motor and Sensory Disturbances. As with defecation, any disturbance that interferes with the patient's motor or sensory abilities affects the act of micturition. Factors which impede sensory impulses centrally or peripherally may result in a bladder that does not empty effectively, or empties totally outside the conscious awareness of the patient. Motor difficulties mean that the patient cannot independently meet his kidney elimination needs.

Other Factors. *Hormonal changes* within the body affect urination patterns. A common influence concerns the hormonal changes involved in the menstrual cycle. Premenstrually, many women retain fluid, which decreases urine production, and then after the start of menstruation, have a period of diuresis.

Pregnancy affects a woman's micturition pattern because of both the hormonal changes and the anatomic changes that occur in her body. At various times during the pregnancy, the weight of the growing fetus pushes on the bladder, causing increased frequency of voiding.

Age affects the micturition reflex mainly in terms of voluntary control being gained through toilet training. Other age-related changes that occur are really the result of anatomic and physiologic alterations described before.

This extensive list of factors that influence the act of micturition serves to demonstrate the potential problems in kidney elimination. Thus, the nurse needs to remain observant.

Characteristics of Urine

Urine is normally composed of water, urea, sodium chloride, phosphoric acid, sulfuric acid, uric acid, ammonia, hippuric acid, creatinine, and several other substances. Being familiar with the normal characteristics of urine helps the nurse identify potential or actual problems. Laboratory findings of *glycosuria* (glucose in the urine), *bacteriuria* (bacteria in the urine), *pyuria* (pus in the urine), *hematuria* (blood in the urine), and *albuminuria* (albumin in the urine) are all indications of possible disease. There are also several observable characteristics that can be assessed.

Frequency of Urination. The frequency of urination is very individualized. It depends on the person's bladder capacity, fluid intake, and availability of toilet facilities, etc. Some people void every 2 hours and some only two or three times per day. Looking at the extreme boundaries, if the patient voids more than every 1.5 hours or less often than every 12 hours, more investigation may be indicated.

Amount. The amount of urine, in terms of both total volume each day and the volume of each voiding, depends on a number of factors: fluid intake, losses from other routes, presence of fever, environmental temperature, age of person (a child excretes proportionately more than an adult), ingestion of a high-protein diet which produces more urine, or diuretic drugs. Daily averages for an adult are 1200 to 1700 ml. Concern is greatest if the amount gets too low. The kidneys usually produce 30 to 50 ml. of urine per hour. So, if the urine formation falls below 25 ml. per hour or 500 ml. in a day, the patient's physician should be notified. *Oliguria* is the term used to indicate scanty urine production and *anuria* means no urine production by the kidneys. On the other hand, *polyuria,* or excessive urine production, may also indicate disease.

The amount per voiding normally depends on the patient's bladder capacity; 250 to 500 ml. is an average normal voiding. Amounts far less or much greater than this normal range should be brought to the physician's attention.

pH. The normal pH of the urine is between 4.5 and 7.5. Deviations may indicate systemic acid-base imbalances. However, many foods and medications, e.g., ascorbic acid, meat, vegetables, and cranberry juice, can change the normal pH. Altering the urine pH may be done intentionally to inhibit bacterial growth or to facilitate therapeutic activity of certain medications.

Color. The normal color of urine is pale, straw-colored to amber, depending on its concentration. When there is bleeding in the upper urinary tract, the urine may be dark red, or *smoky;* bleeding in the lower urinary tract is seen as *red* urine. Foods that may turn the urine red are rhubarb, beets, blackberries, and red dyes. Dark *yellow* urine may indicate the presence of urobilin or bilirubin, while bright yellow urine comes from ingesting large amounts of carotene. A number of common medications will cause color changes in the urine. Examples include anthraquinone laxatives—reddish brown in acid urine, red in alkaline; chloroquine—rusty yellow; chlorzoxanzone—orange or purple-red; methylene blue—green; phenazopyridine—orange-brown, orange-red, or red; phenolphthalein—pink-red in alkaline urine; and rifampin—bright orange-red.[33]

Opacity. Urine is usually transparent when freshly voided. It turns cloudy on standing. Fresh urine that does not look clear may indicate bacteriuria or an inflammatory process within the urinary tract.

Odor. The normal odor of urine is specifically aromatic. Concentrated urine usually smells stronger than dilute urine. When urine stands, it may develop an ammonia smell due to bacterial action; this is frequently noted with babies in diapers or with incontinent patients. Certain foods, such as asparagus, cause characteristic odor changes. Inflammatory reactions also alter the normal odor.

Specific Gravity. The normal range for the specific gravity of urine is 1.010 to 1.025. This measurement indicates the concentration of the urine, and deviations from the normal range may indicate systemic fluid imbalance or an inability of the kidney to dilute or concentrate urine, indicating some degree of renal failure.

Assessment of Kidney Status

As with any body system, in order for the nurse to effectively identify problems in the urinary tract and take the appropriate course of action, a complete and accurate data base is needed. To have an adequate assessment of the patient's kidney status, the following information is needed:

▶ *Usual patterns* of micturition. Frequency? Times of day? Behavior pattern used to stimulate urination?

▶ *Changes* in usual pattern resulting from current illness or stress.

▶ Presence of *artificial orifice.* If present, how is it usually managed?

▶ *Characteristics of urine.* Amount? Color? pH? Specific gravity? Odor? Opacity? Any unusual constituents, e.g., mucus shreds, tissue, stones, foreign bodies?

▶ *Relevant medications,* e.g., diuretics, phenazopyridine, antibiotics.

▶ Results of relevant *diagnostic tests,* e.g., urinalysis, culture and sensitivity, white blood count, x-ray studies, cystoscopy.

▶ *Fluid status.* Amount and kind of fluid intake? State of hydration, e.g., intake and output determination, dry skin, dry mucous membranes, thirst?

▶ *Level of activity.* Muscle tone? Amount and kind of activity? Will patient use toilet, commode, or bedpan? What assistance with mobility will patient need?

▶ *Surgery* or other *trauma* in perineal area, e.g., amount of edema.

▶ Presence of *catheter* or *external drainage device.* Kind? Type of drainage system? Length of presence? Reason for presence? Functioning properly? Irrigation being done?

▶ *Pain* on urination. Severity? Kind? Duration? Location? When during the act of micturition does it occur?

▶ Feeling of *urgency.*

▶ *Incontinence.* Amount? Frequency? Constant dribbling? Occurs with what kind of stress? Duration of problem? What does patient normally do about it?

▶ *Difficulty starting stream.*

▶ Does patient feel like he is *emptying bladder?*

▶ History of *urinary tract infection.*

▶ History of *prostatic hypertrophy.*

▶ *Residual urine,* as determined by catheterization.

▶ Presence of *fever.*

▶ Condition of *urinary meatus.*

▶ Results of *bladder percussion.*

▶ *Level of development.* Toilet trained? Mental ability?

▶ *Level of knowledge* regarding kidney function.

Independent Nursing Measures to Aid Normal Micturition

Most of the assistance patients need in reestablishing and maintaining normal micturition can be provided by independent nursing measures. These include patient teaching, fluids, exercise, maintaining normal habit patterns, relaxation and privacy, positioning, and use of the power of suggestion. Sometimes medications or catheterization, which require a physician's order, may be needed. Further medical or surgical intervention may also be necessary.

Patient Teaching. The lay public usually has fewer misconceptions about kidney function than about bowel elimination. Nevertheless, the nurse must be sure that the patient correctly understands how the urinary tract functions, what he can do to help maintain normal elimination patterns, and why he should do it. A patient will be much more likely to follow your advice to increase his fluid intake if he knows why it is necessary.

Be careful to determine the patient's level of knowledge before starting a teaching plan. Many a patient has been annoyed, for instance, when nursing personnel have repeatedly explained why the patient should increase his fluid intake without finding out whether he already knows the reason. Many patients feel harassed by this and may actually "punish" the nurses by reducing their fluid intake.

Fluids. Increasing fluid intake is probably the primary nursing measure available to the nurse. Increasing fluid intake increases urine production, which increases the stimulation of the micturition reflex. An average daily intake of 1200 to 1500 ml. of measurable fluid is recommended, with additional amounts if there are increased demands on the body's fluid stores, e.g., fever, hot and humid weather, or abnormal losses from other routes. Immobilized patients must maintain dilute urine to offset their high risk for urinary stones and urinary tract infection; for them a fluid intake of 2000 to 2500 ml. daily is recommended if there is no contraindication. Foods with high fluid content can be encouraged to further supplement the measurable fluids.

Unit VII dealt with the ways in which the nurse can plan and implement an appropriate fluid intake program for the patient. Caution must be used with patients who have a fluid restriction order or who should otherwise avoid large amounts of fluid intake.

Exercise. The benefits of exercise, both as a general body toner and specifically to strengthen the abdominal and perineal muscles, were discussed in the section regarding independent measures to aid normal defecation. As with defecation, the abdominal musculature can assist micturition and the pelvic muscles will help prevent urinary incontinence. The isometric exercises described in that section can also be used to aid micturition.

Maintaining Normal Habit Patterns. As mentioned above, some patients have developed a system of behaviors which help trigger the micturition reflex. One of the common ones involves the usual times for voiding. Most people usually urinate at particular times in their daily routine, e.g., on arising, after lunch, upon getting home from work, before going to bed. Although the hospital routine sometimes makes it difficult, the nurse should support the patient's habit pattern as much as possible, since micturition is such a conditioned reflex.

Relaxation and Privacy. As we have discussed, relaxation is crucial to urination. Providing the patient with privacy is one element in promoting relaxation. Nurses also need to avoid pressuring the patient to void. Many times nurses accentuate the patient's difficulties by continually asking him if he needs to void yet, threatening him with a catheter, and telling him that a specimen is needed "right now." These situations are not at all conducive to relaxation techniques.

Physical discomfort must be relieved, since pain causes increased muscle tension and reduces the mental concentration possible on the act of urination. A cold bedpan causes instant muscle tension. If the patient is still unable to relax, he may be taught relaxation techniques.

Positioning. The normal positions for voiding are the squat position for females and the standing position for males. Trying to void while lying flat on your back is very difficult, since two normal aids are lacking: gravity and increased intra-abdominal pressure. Helping a male patient to stand, even if it requires two assistants to help him stay upright, is often the only intervention needed to produce micturition. In either the squat or standing position, leaning forward or pushing on the abdomen with the hands or arms may help the patient void.

Use of Power of Suggestion. As we have described, micturition is very much a conditioned response. There are a number of nursing measures that have been used for years that do not necessarily have sound physiologic rationale. However, they do succeed, likely through the power of suggestion. Probably the most effective is running water within hearing of the patient, or flushing the toilet. This technique not only suggests flowing water, but also masks the sound of voiding if the patient finds the sound embarrassing. Dabbling the patient's hands in water sometimes works. Pouring warm water over the perineum or sitting in a warm bath not only appeals to the power of suggestion but also promotes muscle relaxation. Stroking the inner thigh with light pressure or applying ice to the inner thigh may also stimulate trigger points which activate the micturition reflex.

The nurse has a large repertoire of nursing actions to help the patient maintain normal micturition before dependent measures must be employed. The overriding requirement is that the nurse maintain a positive attitude. If the nurse is confident that the actions followed will work, the patient will also be more apt to expect success.

Common Problems with Micturition and Modes of Treatment

There are several common problems that occur with kidney elimination. The ones that are discussed here are urinary retention; retention with overflow; incontinence, including enuresis; urinary tract infections; urinary stones; and, very briefly, urinary diversion. Treatment for most of these problems involves intensification of the independent nursing measures described above and sometimes the addition of dependent measures.

URINARY RETENTION

Urinary retention means that the urine is retained in the bladder. Urine production continues, but accumulated urine is not released from the bladder. Retention may be the result of urethral obstruction, decreased sensory input to and from the bladder, emotional anxiety, and muscle tension. There have been cases where fecal impaction has caused urinary retention in children probably because of pressure on the bladder outlet and neurological impairment to the detrusor muscle.[45] Poor fluid intake may lead to retention. Very slow urine production fills the bladder just as slowly; this may allow the detrusor muscle to accommodate the increased volume in such a manner that the stretch receptors are never activated. Once the detrusor muscle fibers are stretched beyond a certain point, they become incapable of contracting at all, so micturition never occurs.

As the bladder fills, it rises above the level of the symphysis pubis. In women who have just delivered a baby, the distended uterus may push the bladder over to the side of the abdomen. As it increases in size, the bladder can be palpated as a tense, very sensitive area and percussion over it reveals a "kettle-drum" sound. The patient may complain of increasing discomfort and need to urinate and may become increasingly restless and diaphoretic. The cardinal sign is the absence of voided urine.

Initial treatment requires implementation of the independent measures described above, especially promoting relaxation, positioning, and utilizing the power of suggestion. If these actions are not successful, a cholinergic drug, bethanechol or neostigmine, may be used. These drugs stimulate bladder contraction and must never be used if mechanical obstruction is present. In this instance, intravesicular pressure is increased against an obstructed outlet, which could result in reflux of accumulated urine into the kidney or possibly a ruptured bladder.

If all other measures fail to effect urination, the bladder needs to be catheterized. Procedures 28 and 29 in Chapter 40 describe the technique for insertion of a bladder catheter, and Chapter 40 also discusses care of the patient with a catheter.

RETENTION WITH OVERFLOW

Retention with overflow is an extension of urinary retention. As the bladder continues filling, the intravesicular pressure rises. At some point, this pressure overcomes the restraining ability of the sphincter. Enough urine flows out of the bladder to reduce the intravesicular pressure to the level at which the external sphincter can again control the flow of urine. Then the bladder starts filling again, and the cycle is repeated over and over. The amount of urine expelled each time is usually 25 to 50 ml.

The definitive sign of this condition is frequent (more often than once an hour) voiding of small amounts of urine in the presence of a distended bladder. The patient may also complain of a feeling of urgency. Treatment is the same as for urinary retention, although the likelihood of catheterization is much greater.

INCONTINENCE

Urinary incontinence is the inability of the urinary sphincters to control passage of the urine from the bladder. Complete incontinence indicates total emptying of the bladder, while partial incontinence refers to dribbling of urine without total drainage of the bladder. Whatever its form, this condition is highly embarrassing to the patient, destroys his self-esteem, and can become the overwhelming force controlling his life.

Incontinence can be caused by anything that interferes with sphincter control. Examples include intake of narcotics, sedatives, and alcohol, which decrease sensation of the need to void; sphincter damage; weak perineal muscles; tumor; urinary tract infection; strictures; fecal impaction; and neurological conditions. As with defecation, incontinence may be a sign of "giving up" or may be a matter of no one answering the patient's call light.

Two specific kinds of incontinence are stress incontinence and urge incontinence. *Stress incontinence* usually affects women, although men with prostatic hypertrophy may also have this problem. Any kind of physical stress, such as coughing, sneezing, or laughing causes dribbling of urine. Women with this problem may put toilet paper or rags in their undergarments or wear sanitary napkins to protect their clothing. This condition often occurs because of displacement of the bladder, as may occur after hysterectomy or delivery of several babies, which interferes with normal functioning of the bladder neck. Closely allied to stress incontinence is *urge incontinence* in which the patient has to void so urgently that he simply cannot get to the bathroom in time. This results from inflammation of the lower urinary tract, neurologic bladder, or bladder spasms.[88, 108]

Treatment, initially, must involve medical or surgical correction of the causative factors if possible, e.g., treatment of urinary tract infections, correction of anatomic problems, relief of bladder spasms, reduction of predisposing medications. Electrical stimulation has been successful in aiding sphincter control, and some work has been done with artificial sphincter development.

Bladder Training Program. Nursing intervention can be very effective. Overall, the patient must be given a feeling of hope that something, indeed, can be done about his incontinence problem. Then the planned program is discussed with the patient and his family.

A bladder training program centers around implementation of the independent nursing measures discussed above. Fluid intake is maintained at 2000 to 2500 ml. if the patient's condition permits. Incontinent patients have often reduced their fluid intake because they believe that if they do not drink anything, there will be no urine to void. Actually, adequate urine production is necessary to stimulate the micturition reflex. In a bladder training program, fluids are carefully spaced through the day and are limited before bedtime so that urine production is reduced during the night. An exercise program is instituted to strengthen involved muscles. Some people institute a program of behavior modification in which only positive results by the patient are rewarded. This requires careful coordination of all the staff and the family.

In the meantime, the patient is placed on the commode or toilet every 1 to 2 hours and aided to void. This time span may be even less at first, depending on how frequently the bladder empties; the intervals are lengthened as the program progresses. Although the patient's clothing and bed linen may be padded during this time to protect them from getting wet, actual diapering of the patient should be avoided. Diapering further demeans the patient and gives him "permission" to be incontinent.

Chapter 40 describes bladder training programs involving use of the bladder catheter, i.e., intermittent catheterization. It also discusses one of the serious complications that can occur, especially with spinal cord–injured patients—a nervous system crisis called autonomic hyperreflexia.

Skin Care. Besides the embarrassment, odor, and laundry problems, the major physical problem caused by incontinence is skin irritation and breakdown. Skin that is constantly bathed in moisture becomes macerated, and urine allowed to stand breaks down into ammonia, which is very irritating to the skin. Mothers know this condition very well; it is commonly called diaper rash. This skin irritation can be very painful and easily breaks down into pressure sores.

Treatment involves prevention by keeping the skin clean and dry. Washing with soap and water and exposing the skin to the air are excellent ways of preventing this complication of incontinence. Various creams and ointments are sold for diaper rash, but clean, dry skin is the best means of prevention and treatment.

External Drainage. For the male patient whose incontinence cannot be controlled, an external drainage appliance called a *condom catheter* can be used. Figure 30–11 illustrates this device. It consists of a plastic or rubber sheath that is placed over the penis; drainage tubing at the bottom of the condom attaches to a leg bag or Foley catheter drainage bag. The chief problem with a condom is to attach it securely, so that it stays on, but in a way that

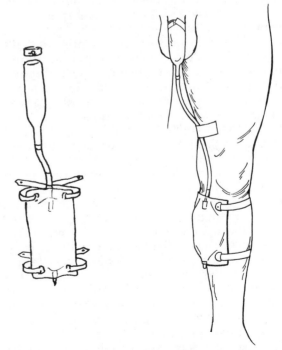

Figure 30–11. Condom drainage and leg bag. Leg bag may be attached to calf of leg, as shown, or to thigh.

does not impair circulation to the distal penis or damage the skin. The most effective attaching substances are surgical adhesive and elastic tape.

Prepare the patient's skin by washing with soap and water and drying well. If there is excess pubic hair, it may be shaved off. Wiping the shaft of the penis with alcohol removes skin oils. Apply the surgical adhesive if it is being used. Roll the condom sheath onto the penis leaving a one-half-inch gap between the distal end of the penis and the closed end of the sheath. Apply the elastic tape in a spiral; never completely encircle the penis because, if swelling occurs, circulation will be impeded. If there is excess rolled rubber or plastic after the sheath is in place, cut it off; otherwise it will constrict the penis like a rubber band.

The condom must be removed at least daily so that the penis can be washed and exposed to the air. The sheath must be checked to see that it does not twist around on itself, which would block drainage of the urine.[136]

Enuresis. Enuresis is a special kind of incontinence, usually occurring with children, although it can extend into adulthood. The incidence of adult enuresis is estimated at 1 to 3 per cent.[18] *Enuresis* involves incontinence of urine, usually at night, and presents a major problem for the patient and his family. *Primary* enuresis means that there has never been a dry period; and *secondary* enuresis is a resumption of night incontinence after a successful period of dryness. There are several theories regarding the etiology of enuresis. These include delayed development, parental failure, genetics, sleep arousal disorder, toilet-training difficulties, food allergies, and behavior problems. Only 10 per cent of children with enuresis are found to have neurologic or urinary disease.[18]

Treatment of enuresis follows two main paths: psychotherapy or physical treatment, depending on the causative theory accepted by the practitioner. Behavior modification programs and operant conditioning (using alarm systems in the bed) have met with success. Components of physical programs include correction of physical problems, restriction of bedtime fluids, getting the child up to void in the night, and keeping the bedroom warm. Tricyclic drugs may relax the detrusor muscle and increase sphincter muscle tone or they may alter sleep patterns. The parents will need supportive teaching to help them handle the problem effectively.[3, 120]

Urinary tract infections are a very common problem. Because of the anatomy of the female urethra, woman are more affected than men, and sexually active or pregnant women are the most vulnerable. The most common causative organisms are *Escherichia coli*, *Klebsiella aerobacter*, *Proteus*, and *Pseudomonas*, and the source of most of these organisms is the patient's own colon.

Lapides has postulated that many urinary tract infections are the result of bladder distention. As the bladder wall overdistends, blood flow to the tissue decreases. The ischemic tissue is now more vulnerable to invading organisms. Infection can occur from the patient's own gut via the hematogenous or lymphogenous route.[79]

There are a number of predisposing factors. Sexual intercourse predisposes women to development of urinary tract infection, because of the resultant inflammation of the urethra; this can lead to strictures which lead to urinary stasis and pools of good growth medium.[69] Bubble baths often cause irritation of the lower urinary tract.[90] Any anatomic abnormalities that interfere with free flow of urine increase the patient's susceptibility to infection. Previous urinary tract infection makes the patient more vulnerable to recurrent infections. The convalescent bladder is less resistant to bacterial invasion, and studies show that this period of susceptibility increases in length with each successive infection.[77] The role of bladder catheters in the development of urinary tract infections is discussed in Chapter 40.

The cardinal symptoms of urinary tract infection are burning on urination, urgency, and frequency. Other symptoms include hematuria, abdominal pain, malaise, chills, nausea and vomiting, fever, and flank pain. The final diagnosis is based on the results of urine cultures.

Treatment is multifaceted. The principal component is an antibiotic specific to the causative organisms. The antibiotic therapy must be continued for some time after the symptoms subside to ensure elimination of the organisms. Vulnerable women may take post-intercourse antibiotics for a prolonged time. Strictures and other anatomic abnormalities should be corrected by surgical intervention. Increased fluid intake keeps the urine dilute and facilitates its movement through the urinary tract and out of the body. At the same time, patients are encouraged to void at least every 2 hours during the day and one or two times at night to prevent bladder distention. Altering the pH of the urine with cranberry juice, ascorbic acid, or an acid-ash diet (see Chap. 40) makes the urine less supportive of bacterial growth. Women should avoid underpants made of synthetic materials, which keep moisture in the perineal area. These are the major components of a treatment program for urinary tract infection.

URINARY TRACT STONES

Although urinary tract stones may occur at any time, this discussion mainly deals with the potential for stone formation as the result of immobility. Bedrest increases the patient's tendency to form urinary stones. Predisposing factors are (1) urinary stasis in the kidney and bladder, which increases the tendency for solutes in the urine to settle out, (2) alkaline urine caused by the lack of acid end-products from muscle activity, (3) concentrated urine, and (4) demineralization of bones, which increases the amount of circulating calcium and thus the amount of calcium being excreted in the urine. Calcium is the constituent of 90 per cent of all urinary stones; other elements are oxalate, uric acid, and cystine.

Symptoms of ureteral stones include severe flank pain, nausea and vomiting, diaphoresis, pallor with possible fever, and hematuria. Stones in the bladder usually cause no problem until they are passed into the urethra. Problems caused by stones are mucosal trauma and obstruction of urine flow. If it is suspected that a patient has urinary stones, the nurse may be asked to strain the urine for stones. To do this, the nurse pours all urine voided through at least four layers of gauze pads and inspects the pads carefully for any stones filtered from the urine. The patient must be reminded not to use the toilet.

Treatment of existing stones involves surgical removal if the stones are not passed. However, the key is prevention. The patient's calcium intake should be reduced to 200 to 300 mg. per day, and he should avoid excessive vitamin D in foods. Fluid intake should be 3000 to 4000 ml. per day, and nocturnal diuresis is just as important as daytime diuresis—the urine must be kept dilute.[101] The urine can be acidified by ingesting cranberry juice, ascorbic acid, and an acid-ash diet.

URINARY DIVERSION

Urinary diversion, or the drainage of urine from the body at a site other than the perineal meatus or tip of the penis, can be either congenital or surgically induced. *Hypospadias* is an example of a congenital diversion; in this case, the urethra opens on the underside of the penis or inside the vagina. Surgical diversion is done because of cancer, birth defects, obstruction, or neurogenic bladder. There are a large variety of surgical procedures used to effect urinary diversion, but the most common is the ileal conduit, also called ileal loop and ileal bladder. With this technique, the ureters are attached to a dissected piece of ileum; the ileal bladder is attached to the internal abdominal wall, and a stoma to the outside is surgically created.

Since the urine drains continuously from this stoma, the patient must wear a collection bag at all times. This pouch may be self-contained or may be attached to a leg drainage bag. The patient usually attaches the bag to a Foley catheter drainage system at night so that he does not have to wake up to empty it. The collection bag must not be allowed to get too full since the weight of it may break the seal at the skin. The bag needs to be changed at least every day; this should be done in the early morning or after some other period of limited fluid intake so that less urine is being produced.

As with colostomies and ileostomies, the ongoing physical problems of a patient with an ileal conduit are potential skin irritation and odor control. The urine is usually not as corrosive as the enzymes in fecal drainage, so the main skin problems are maceration and yeast infections. Use of a skin barrier and proper fit of the pouch help prevent these problems. If a yeast infection occurs, appropriate medications may have to be used. Odor control is achieved by washing the appliance well with soap and water, soaking it in white vinegar when necessary, and putting commercial deodorizers in the pouch. Keeping the urine acid will also help to reduce the odor.

Collecting Specimens

There are several types of urine specimens collected by nursing personnel: random, midstream, catheter, 24-hour, and double-void. If the specimen is not obtained properly, the ensuing tests may give false findings, resulting in wrong diagnoses and improper treatment. One of the biggest problems in diagnosing urinary tract infections is the rather high percentage of false negatives and false positives on urine cultures because of improper urine specimen collection. Nurses must consistently be strict in their technique. A study done by Chavigny and Nunnally showed that carefully instructed patients in a clinic contaminated fewer urine specimens than did the nurses studied.[15]

Random Specimen. Most urine tests can be done on a *random* specimen, which means that the specimen can be collected any time. The routine urinalysis done as a screening test is the most common example of this type. The random specimen is collected in any clean container, often with no physical preparation of the patient. However, the female patient may be asked to wash the perineal area to clean away any collected debris. There is no special instruction needed by the patient as to cleaning since this type of specimen is not used for a culture.

Clean-catch (Midstream) Specimen. If the urine is to be cultured, a *clean-catch*, or *midstream*, specimen is usually required. These two terms are often used interchangeably. This collection procedure is designed to reduce as much as possible the potential contamination of the specimen by external organisms.

The first step of the procedure involves meticulously cleansing the penis or perineal area. The cleansing agent may be soap and water, benzalkonium chloride, hexachlorophene, or iodine preparations. Studies show that iodine is the most effective.[15, 96] It is important that the agent be completely removed at the end of the cleansing process, since contamination of the specimen by the agent may sterilize the urine. With a female patient, the labia are separated for the cleansing and kept apart until the urine has been collected. If a male patient is uncircumcised, the foreskin is retracted before cleansing the penis and is returned to its original position after the urine has been obtained.

The patient then voids directly into a sterile container. If necessary, a sterile bedpan or urinal can be used and the urine transferred to the specimen container. If a midstream specimen is needed, the patient begins voiding into the toilet, commode, or bedpan. Then the patient stops the stream of urine, the sterile container is positioned as necessary, and the patient continues voiding into the container. When enough urine has been voided for the specimen, the patient stops the stream again, the container is removed, and then he finishes voiding in the original receptacle. If the patient is unable to stop the stream, the person holding the sterile container may want to wear a glove as she places and removes the sterile container while the patient is voiding. It is felt that this procedure flushes out the organisms usually present at the meatus so that an accurate picture of the bladder urine can be obtained.

Catheter Specimen. Sometimes a specimen for culture is to be obtained by catheterizing the patient. Because of the risk of introducing microorganisms during the catheterization procedure, this method is not used very frequently. The procedure for obtaining this type of specimen is described in Procedures 28 and 29 in Chapter 40.

24-Hour Specimen. Some diagnostic tests require a 24-hour collection of urine. This urine may be collected in one container for each voiding or dumped together in one large container. Before beginning the collection, the nurse must find out from the laboratory whether or not a preservative is needed in the container. If there is a preservative in the bottle, the patient should not void directly into the container. Many of the preservatives are acid, and if this splashes up onto the patient, it will cause burns.

To start the specimen collection, the patient is instructed to void and the time noted; this voiding is discarded so that urine formed prior to the noted time is not included in the specimen. All urine voided for the next 24 hours is kept; 24 hours from the time the first voiding was discarded, the patient is instructed to void and this urine is added to the specimen. This procedure assures that all urine formed during the collection period is included in the specimen. Successful collection requires careful communication with all persons who may be involved. Notices put on the patient's bed, in the bathroom, in the utility room, and on the nursing care plan help. If, at any time during the 24 hours, the patient voids in the toilet or someone discards a specimen, the entire collection process must be begun again.

Double-Void Specimen. If a diabetic patient's urine is being tested for glucose and ketones, a *double-void* specimen is needed. This assures that the urine being tested reflects the current status of these two substances being filtered from the blood. The patient empties his bladder, but this first specimen may or may not be tested. In some agencies, this urine is tested and if it is found to be negative, no further specimen is obtained; in some agencies, it is tested in case a second specimen is not obtained; in some agencies, it is discarded without being tested at all. If a second specimen is needed, the patient waits 20 to 30 minutes after he empties his bladder and voids again. The patient may be given water to drink to help form enough urine, but the test requires as little as six drops. The specimen is collected in a clean container as with a random specimen.

The nurse frequently performs tests on urine. This section will not discuss the laboratory and microscopic examinations that a nurse might perform while working in an out-patient clinic, but will include those tests most often done on the clinical unit: fractionals, specific gravity, and various dip sticks. The key to accurate test results is to read and follow the manufacturer's directions explicitly. Williams observed 122 nursing personnel at all levels doing fractionals and found a 36 per cent incidence of error. Most of these errors occurred at the higher concentrations of glucose and acetone, leading to increased chance of erroneous insulin dosage.[137] Use your watch to calculate elapsed time. If color changes are to be calibrated, compare the specimen very carefully against the manufacturer's color chart. Do not guess! Color charts are not interchangeable between different products. Check expiration dates before beginning the test, and keep bottles capped tightly.

Fractionals. A *fractional* involves testing the urine for glucose and ketone bodies. The test may also be called a Clinitest or checking for sugar and acetone. Whenever the urine is tested for glucose, the test for acetone should also be done. The procedure is done on a double-void specimen as described above.

Testing for glucose may be done by one of two methods: copper reduction, e.g., Clinitest, or the enzyme glucose oxidase, e.g., Testape, Clinistix, Ketodiastix. Nursing mothers and pregnant women in their third trimester have lactose in their urine, which will give a false positive if the copper reduction method is used; they should use the enzyme method. Ascorbic acid (from natural as well as chemical sources) and aspirin in doses of seven or more tablets per day may cause false results, as can levodopa, cephalosporins, nalidixic acid, probenecid, methyldopa, and other substances. Be sure to check drug information.[114] The method used for testing depends on agency policy and what the patient has been or will be using at home. The prime concern is that the agent chosen be used consistently, since results from the two different methods are not necessarily interchangeable.

The usual method for the copper reduction test (Clinitest) is the five-drop method. Materials needed for this test are a small test tube, a medicine dropper, urine, tap water, watch, paper towel, and the reagent tablet. The tablet should be speckled robin's egg blue; if it is white with dark blue patches, it is unreliable and should be discarded. Five drops of urine are placed in the test tube with the medicine dropper, then ten drops of water. The Clinitest tablet is manipulated from its bottle into the bottle cap and dumped onto a dry paper towel. The tablet is poured from the towel into the test tube. Do not touch the tablet with your hands; it is very caustic and even the perspiration on your hand may start its chemical reaction, causing severe burns. If you do not have a test tube rack and must hold the tube, hold it at the top, since the bottom will get very hot. Do not agitate the tube until the reaction is over. Observe the reaction from the beginning to the end in case the pass-through phenomenon occurs. Pass-through occurs when the color change goes through orange to greenish-brown and indicates a glucose content over 2 per cent or 4+; if this phenomenon occurs and is not observed, the final color may be falsely identified as a lesser concentration. Fifteen seconds after the boiling has stopped in the tube, compare the solution with the appropriate color chart. Results are usually reported as negative, trace, or 1 to 4+, as indicated on the chart.

If the pass-through phenomenon occurs, the test should be repeated using the two-drop or one-drop method. These alternatives measure glucose content up to 5 per cent and 10 per cent, respectively. The procedure is exactly the same as the five-drop method except that the ratios change: 2 drops urine in 10 drops water and 1 drop urine in 10 drops water. Be sure to use the two-drop color chart or the one-drop chart as appropriate.[93]

If the glucose oxidase method is to be used, the process is essentially the same as used with any dip stick. The procedure for using this material is discussed below.

Testing for acetone or ketone bodies may be done with a dip stick as described below or with a reagent tablet. If a tablet is used, it is removed from its bottle and put on a clean paper towel or tissue. One drop of urine is placed in the middle of the tablet with a medicine dropper, and one minute later the color of the exposed tablet is compared to the appropriate color chart. Ketoacidosis may be found with such conditions as diabetes, pregnancy, lactation, fasting, vomiting, and diarrhea.

Specific Gravity. Specific gravity indicates the degree of concentration of the urine and is a good measure of the patient's state of hydration if the patient has normal renal function. Equipment needed includes a urinometer (Fig. 30–12), a urinometer cylinder, and a urine

spinning, it must be spun again; it must be floating free. When the urinometer has stopped spinning, the line above the bottom of the fluid meniscus is determined. It is reported as 1.0–1.0, e.g., 1.010, 1.022.

Dip Sticks. Dip sticks are pieces of treated paper or plastic strips with treated pads attached to them. Various ones can be used to test pH and for numerous substances: glucose, bile, blood, ketones, protein and others. Use of a dip stick to test for microorganisms has been successful.[85]

The general procedure for using dip sticks is to dip the stick into the urine, remove the stick and tap it gently on the side of the specimen container to remove excess urine. Wait the specified time and compare the color changes to the appropriate charts. Some of the dip sticks have seven or more test pads, so the nurse must be careful to follow instructions, meet the time requirements, remember the readings, and record them accurately.

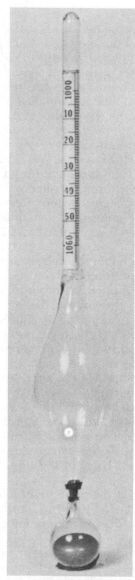

Figure 30–12. The urinometer is used to measure specific gravity. The more concentrated the solution, the more the urinometer is displaced upward. (From Metheny, N. M., and Snively, W. D.: *Nurses' Handbook of Fluid Balance,* 2nd ed. Philadelphia, J. B. Lippincott Co., 1974, p. 70.)

specimen. The urine specimen, which should be at room temperature, is mixed by swirling its container. The urine is then poured into the cylinder so that when the urinometer is placed in the cylinder, the line above the meniscus of the fluid can be easily seen. The urinometer is placed in the cylinder and spun between the thumb and forefinger. If the urinometer is touching the side of the cylinder when it stops

BIBLIOGRAPHY

1. Add milk to your GI suspect list. *Patient Care, 10:*116, Feb. 1976.
2. Anderson, E.: Women and cystitis. *Nursing '77, 7:*50, April 1977.
3. Arnold, S., and Ginsburg, A.: Understanding and managing enuresis in children. *Postgraduate Medicine,* 58:73, Nov. 1975.
4. Bass, L.: More fiber—less constipation. *American Journal of Nursing,* 77:254, Feb. 1977.
5. Belinsky, I., et al.: Colonfiberoscopy: technique in colon examination. *American Journal of Nursing,* 73:306, Feb. 1973.
6. Bosten, A., and Litman, L.: Controlling colostomy odor. *American Journal of Nursing,* 77:444, March 1977.
7. Bowles, W.: When hematuria means cancer. *Consultant, 13:*133, Nov. 1973.
8. Brocklehurst, J.: Incontinence in the elderly. *Nursing Mirror and Midwives Journal,* 136:30, June 1973.
9. Brown, M.: Over-the-counter gastro-intestinal drugs: antidiarrheal drugs. *Nurse Practitioner, 2:*23, Sep.–Oct. 1976.
10. Brown, M.: Over-the-counter gastro-intestinal drugs: anti-hemorrhoids medications. *Nurse Practitioner, 2:*17, Nov.–Dec. 1976.
11. Brown, M.: Over-the-counter gastro-intestinal drugs: laxatives. *Nurse Practitioner, 1:*15, July–Aug. 1976.
12. Buchan, D.: Mind-body relationships in gastrointestinal disease. *Canadian Nurse,* 67:35, March 1971.
13. Burnum, J.: Adverse reactions to enemas. *Journal of the American Medical Association,* 235:476, Feb. 1976.
14. Caldwell, K.: Sphincter stimulators to prevent incontinence. *Nursing Times,* 69:1524, Nov. 1973.
15. Chavigny, K., and Nunnally, D.: A comparison of methods for collecting clean-catch urine specimens in a clinic population of obstetric patients. *American Journal of Obstetrics and Gynecology,* 122:34, May 1975.
16. Chezem, J.: Urinary diversion: select aspects of nursing management. *Nursing Clinics of North America, 11:*445, Sep. 1976.

17. Clayden, G.: Constipation and soiling in childhood. *British Medical Journal*, 1:515, Feb. 1976.

18. Cline, F.: Enuresis: a frequent problem with multiple causation and generally manageable. *Nurse Practitioner*, 1:36, July–Aug. 1976.

19. Connell, A.: Dietary fiber and diverticular disease. *Hospital Practice*, 11:119, March 1976.

20. Connors, M.: Ostomy care: a personal approach. *American Journal of Nursing*, 74:1422, Aug. 1974.

21. Corman, M., et al.: Cathartics. *American Journal of Nursing*, 75:273, Feb. 1975.

22. Cornell, S., et al.: Comparison of 3 bowel management programs during rehabilitation of spinal cord injured patients. *Nursing Research*, 22:321, July–Aug. 1973.

23. Cosper, B.: Physiological colostomy. *American Journal of Nursing*, 75:2014, Nov. 1975.

24. Cox, C., and Hinman, F.: Experiments with induced bacteriuria, vesical emptying and bacterial growth on the mechanism of bladder defense to infection. *Journal of Urology*, 86:739, Dec. 1961.

25. Cressy, M.: Psychiatric nursing intervention with a colostomy patient. *Perspectives of Psychiatric Care*, 10:69, No. 2, 1972.

26. Crouch, J.: *Functional Human Anatomy*. Philadelphia, Lea and Febiger, 1972.

27. Curtis, C.: Colonoscopy: the nurse's role. *American Journal of Nursing*, 75:430, March 1975.

28. Davis, R., et al.: Hypocalcemia, hyperphosphatemia, and dehydration following a single hypertonic phosphate enema. *Journal of Pediatrics*, 90:484, March 1977.

29. Delehanty, L., and Stravine, V.: Achieving bladder control. *American Journal of Nursing*, 70:312, Feb. 1970.

30. Dericks, V.: The psychological hurdles of new ostomates: helping them up . . . and over. *Nursing '74*, 4:52, Oct. 1974.

31. Derezin, M.: Laxatives and fecal modifiers. *American Family Physician*, 10:126, July 1974.

32. Derr, S.: Testing for glycosuria. *American Journal of Nursing*, 70:1513, July 1970.

33. DiPalmo, J.: Drugs that induce changes in urine color. *RN*, 40:34, Jan. 1977.

34. Donovan, W., et al.: A finger device for obtaining satisfactory voiding in spinal cord-injured patients. *American Journal of Occupational Therapy*, 31:107, Feb. 1977.

35. Dowd, J.: Methods of urinary diversion. *AORN Journal*, 23:37, Jan. 1976.

36. Doyle, P.: Enuresis—causes and treatment. *Nursing Times*, 71:424, March 1975.

37. Doyle, P.: Urinary incontinence: diagnosis and treatment. *Nursing Times*, 69:1521, Nov. 1973.

38. Drake, W.: Bladder decompensation in cancer, cardiac disease and stroke. *Journal of the Medical Society of New Jersey*, 68:884, Nov. 1971.

39. Dysuria: UTI may not be the cause. *Patient Care*, 8:134, Feb. 1974.

40. Eckstein, H.: Treatment of incontinence by electrical stimulation. *Nursing Times*, 71:1423, Sep. 1975.

41. Evans, P.: The Treatment of Enuresis in Childhood. *Nursing Mirror and Midwives Journal*, 142:62, March 1976.

42. Feustel, D.: Autonomic Hyperreflexia. *American Journal of Nursing*, 76:228, Feb. 1976.

42a. Fisher, L. A., et al.: Collection of a clean voided urine specimen: A comparison among spoken, written, and computer-based instruction. *American Journal of Public Health*, 67:640, July 1977.

43. Flower, M., et al.: Serratia: how we tracked it down. *RN*, 39:ICU-8, Sep. 1976.

44. Gallagher, A.: Body image changes in the patient with a colostomy. *Nursing Clinics of North America*, 7:669, Dec. 1972.

45. Gallo, D., and Presman, D.: Urinary retention due to fecal impaction in children. *Pediatrics*, 45:292, Feb. 1970.

46. Gardner, K.: Diagnosis: urinary tract infection. *Consultant*, 14:83, Jan. 1974.

47. Gibbs, G., and White, M.: Stomal care. *American Journal of Nursing*, 72:268, Feb. 1972.

48. Goldstein, F.: Normal physiology of the digestive tract. *Consultant*, 13:69, Feb. 1973.

49. Greenfiels, S., et al.: Protocol management of dysuria, urinary frequency, and vaginal discharge. *Annals of Internal Medicine*, 81:452, Oct. 1974.

50. Gross, L.: Ostomy care: a letter to parents. *American Journal of Nursing*, 74:1427, Aug. 1974.

51. Grubb, R., and Blake, R.: Emotional trauma in ostomy patients. *AORN Journal*, 23:52, Jan. 1976.

52. Gutowski, F.: Ostomy procedure: nursing care before and after. *American Journal of Nursing*, 72:262, Feb. 1972.

53. Habeeb, M., and Kallstrom, M.: Bowel program for institutionalized adults. *American Journal of Nursing*, 76:606, April 1976.

54. Hatcher, J.: The history of urine testing. *Nursing Mirror and Midwives Journal*, 142:65, April 1976.

55. Heffernan, E.: What to do about irritable colon. *Consultant*, 13:132, April 1973.

56. Hodgkinson, A.: The changing pattern of urinary tract stone disease. *Nursing Mirror and Midwives Journal*, 142:58, April 1976.

57. Hogstel, M.: How to give a safe and successful cleansing enema. *American Journal of Nursing*, 77:816, May 1977.

58. Hutch, J.: *Anatomy and Physiology of the Bladder, Trigone and Urethra*. New York, Appleton-Century-Crofts, 1972.

59. Ince, L., et al.: Conditioning bladder responses in patients with spinal cord lesions. *Archives of Physical Medicine and Rehabilitation*, 58:59, Feb. 1977.

60. Incontinent women. *Lancet*, 1:521, March 1977.

61. Innes, B., and Bruya, M.: Post-operative voiding patterns and related contributing factors. *Washington State Journal of Nursing*, 49:13, Summer/Fall, 1977.

62. Isler, C.: If the ileostomy is continent, the benefits are obvious. *RN*, 40:39, April 1977.

63. Is that GI complaint "a bug going around"? *Patient Care*, 8:20, April 1974.

64. Jensen, V.: Better techniques for bagging stomas: colostomies. *Nursing '74*, 4:30, Aug. 1974.

65. Jensen, V.: Better techniques for bagging stomas: ileostomies. *Nursing '74*, 4:60, Sept. 1974.

66. Jensen, V.: Better techniques for bagging stomas: urinary ostomies. *Nursing '74*, 4:60, July 1974.

67. Johnson, S.: Understanding hyperuricemia: nursing implications. *Nursing Clinics of North America*, 7:399, June 1972.

68. Kahn, H., et al.: Effect of cranberry juice on urine. *Journal of the American Dietetic Association*, 51:251, Sep. 1967.

69. Kellogg, C.: Female urethral strictures and recurrent urinary tract infections: how to break the cycle. *Journal of Practical Nursing*, 25:18, June 1975.

70. Khan, A., and Pryles, C.: Urinary tract infection in children. *American Journal of Nursing*, 73:1340, Aug. 1973.

71. Kick, E.: Rx for incontinence. *ANA Clinical Sessions*, New York, Appleton-Century-Crofts, 1973.

72. Kimble, M.: Diabetes. *Nursing Digest*, 2:113, Nov.–Dec. 1974.

73. Koppel, A.: A device to free the legs from pressure of rubber urinary drainage bags. *Journal of Urology*, 106:765, Nov. 1971.

74. Kunin, C.: *Detection, Prevention and Management of Urinary Tract Infections*. Philadelphia, Lea and Febiger, 1972.

75. Kunin, C.: Urinary tract infections in children. *Hospital Practice*, 11:91, March 1976.

76. Lamanske, J.: Helping the ileostomy patient to help himself. *Nursing '77*, 7:34, Jan. 1977.

77. Landes, R.: Urinary tract infection—more than a one-time thing. *Consultant*, 15:32, Feb. 1975.

78. Lapides, J.: Urinary tract infections in women. *Journal of Practical Nursing*, 25:19, Dec. 1975.

79. Lapides, J., et al.: Clean, intermittent self-catheterization in the treatment of urinary tract disease. *Journal of Urology*, 107:458, March 1972.

80. Lapides, J., et al.: Followup on unsterile intermittent self-catheterization. *Journal of Urology*, 111:184, Feb. 1972.

81. Lenneberg, E.: The role of the enterostomal therapists and stomal rehabilitation clinics: a second look. *Cancer*, 34:977, Sep. 1974.

82. Levy, S.: Fecal flora in recurrent urinary-tract infection. *New England Journal of Medicine*, 296:813, April 1977.

83. Lewin, D.: Care of the constipated patient. *Nursing Times*, 72:444, March 1976.

84. Lewis, J., and Alexander, J.: The urine culture revisited. *Southern Medical Journal*, 70:15, Jan. 1977.

85. Litvak, A., et al.: A clinical evaluation of a secondary screening device (Microstix) for urinary tract infection. *Southern Medical Journal*, 69:1418, Nov. 1976.

86. Lowthian, P.: Enuresis in the home—protecting the bed. *Nursing Times*, 69:408, March 1973.

87. Lowthian, P.: Portable urinals for women. *Nursing Times*, 71:1739, Oct. 1975.

88. Managing Urinary Incontinence. *Patient Care*, 7:70, Feb. 1973.

89. Maney, J.: A behavioral therapy approach to bladder retraining. *Nursing Clinics of North America*, 11:179, March 1976.

90. Marshall, S.: The effect of bubble bath on the urinary tract. *Journal of Urology*, 93:112, Jan. 1965.

91. McCarthy, R.: Postoperative patterns of voiding in patients with spinal anesthesia. *In Communicating Nursing Research: The Many Sources of Nursing Knowledge*. Boulder, Colorado, WICHE, 1972.

92. McDonogh, M.: Is operant conditioning effective in reducing enuresis and encopresis in children? *Perspectives in Psychiatric Care*, 9:17, No. 1, 1971.

93. McFarlane, J., and Nickerson, D.: Two-drop and one-drop test for glycosuria. *American Journal of Nursing*, 72:939, May 1972.

94. McGuckin, M.: Microbiologic studies: urine cultures—key to diagnosing urinary tract infections. *Nursing '75*, 5:10, Dec. 1975.

95. McGuckin, M.: What you should know about collecting stool culture specimens. *Nursing '76*, 6:22, March 1976.

96. Moore, D., and Bauer, C.: Effect of Prepodyne as a perineal cleansing agent for clean catch specimens. *Nursing Research*, 25:259, July–Aug. 1976.

97. Mowchenko, G.: Care of patients with G.I. diseases that have a psychological component. *Canadian Nurse*, 67:38, March 1971.

98. Murray, B.: The patient has an ileal conduit. *American Journal of Nursing*, 71:1560, Aug. 1971.

99. Nickey, K.: An investigation of the urine pH of selected subjects on prescribed regimens of cranberry juice and ascorbic acid. Unpublished Master's Thesis, University of Washington, Seattle, Washington, 1973.

100. No soap. *Emergency Medicine*, 3:151, Nov. 1971.

101. Oyama, J.: Kidney stones? Diet can help. *Consultant*, 13:35, March 1973.

102. Padilla, G., and Baker, V.: Variables affecting the preparation of the bowel for radiologic examination. *Nursing Research*, 21:305, July–Aug. 1972.

103. Pais, J.: GI x-rays, some other complications. *Emergency Medicine*, 7:247, April 1975.

104. Patterson, D., and Schuster, P.: Artificial urinary sphincter. *Canadian Nurse*, 71:27, Nov. 1975.

105. Phillpotts, E., et al.: The continent colostomy. *Nursing Mirror and Midwives Journal*, 142:53, May 1976.

106. Pike, B., et al.: Soap colitis. *New England Journal of Medicine*, 285:217, July 1971.

107. Plourde, M.: Reflections on urinary diversion. *AORN Journal*, 23:45, Jan. 1976.

108. Presman, D.: Urinary incontinence: therapy begins with a complete workup. *Consultant*, 15:212, Nov. 1975.

109. Rodman, M., and Smith, D.: *Clinical Pharmacology in Nursing*. Philadelphia, J. B. Lippincott Company, 1974.

110. Rosenberg, F.: Lactose intolerance. *American Journal of Nursing*, 77:823, May 1977.

111. Rowbotham, J.: Advances in rehabilitation of stoma patients. *Cancer*, 36:702, Aug. 1975.

112. Scharli, A., and Kresewetter, W.: Defecation and continence: some new concepts. *Diseases of the Colon and Rectum*, 13:81, March–April 1970.

113. Schauder, M.: Ostomy care: cone irrigation. *American Journal of Nursing*, 74:1424, Aug. 1974.

114. Schuman, D.: Tips for improving urine testing techniques. *Nursing '76*, 6:23, Feb. 1976.

115. Schuster, M.: Disorders of the aging GI system. *Hospital Practice*, 11:95, Sep. 1976.

116. Shapbell, N., and Sweigart, J.: A urinary device for patients with problem stomas. *Nursing Clinics of North America*, 9:383, June 1974.

117. Sheridan, J.: Obstructions of the intestinal tract. *Nursing Clinics of North America*, 10:147, March 1975.

118. Shipley, S., and Wrye, S.: Myoglobinuria. *Heart and Lung*, 5:950, Nov.–Dec. 1976.

119. Sill, A.: Bulb-syringe technique for colonic stoma irrigation. *American Journal of Nursing*, 70:536, March 1970.

120. Simonds, J.: Enuresis. *Clinical Pediatrics*, 16:79, Jan. 1977.

121. Sotiropoulos, A., et al.: Management of urinary incontinence with electronic stimulation: observations and results. *Journal of Urology*, 116:747, Dec. 1976.

122. Stanley, T.: Artificial control of fecal incontinence. *Surgery*, 68:852, Nov. 1970.

123. Tillery, B., and Bates, B.: Enemas. *American Journal of Nursing*, 66:534, March 1966.

124. Todd, J.: Urinary tract infections in children and adolescents. *Postgraduate Medicine*, 60:225, Nov. 1976.

125. Trimethoprim sulfamethoxazole. *Nursing '74*, 4:59, Feb. 1974.

126. Tudor, L.: Bladder and bowel retraining. *American Journal of Nursing*, 70:2391, Nov. 1970.

127. Ventura, J.: The international traveler's health guide. *American Journal of Nursing*, 77:968, June 1977.

128. Watson, E.: Clinical laboratory procedures. *Canadian Nurse*, 70:25, Feb. 1974.

129. Watson, P., et al.: Comprehensive care of the ileostomy patient. *Nursing Clinics of North America,* 11:427, Sep. 1976.
130. Watt, R.: Colostomy irrigation—yes or no? *American Journal of Nursing,* 77:442, March 1977.
131. Watt, R.: Urinary diversion. *American Journal of Nursing,* 74:1806, Oct. 1974.
132. Wentworth, A., and Cox, B.: Nursing the patient with a continent ileostomy. *American Journal of Nursing,* 76:1424, Sep. 1976.
133. What does that high uric acid mean? *Patient Care,* 8:164, Aug. 1974.
134. When the problem is intestinal gas. *Patient Care,* 7:81, March 1973.
135. When the patient is spilling protein. *Patient Care,* 9:18, March 1975.
136. Whyte, J., and Thistle, N.: Male incontinence: The inside story of external collection. *Nursing '76,* 6:66, Sep. 1976.
137. Williams, S.: Diabetic urine testing by hospital nursing personnel. *Nursing Research,* 20:444, Sep.–Oct. 1971.
138. Willington, F.: Incontinence: psychological and psychogenic aspects. *Nursing Times,* 71:422, March 13, 1975.
139. Willington, F.: Incontinence: the nursing component in diagnosis and treatment. *Nursing Times,* 71:464, March 29, 1975.
140. Willington, F.: Incontinence: the prevention of soiling. *Nursing Times,* 71:545, April 3, 1975.
141. Willington, F.: Incontinence: training and retraining for continence. *Nursing Times,* 71:500, March 27, 1975.
142. Willington, F.: Problems in the aetiology of urinary incontinence. *Nursing Times,* 71:378, March 6, 1975.
143. Willington, F.: Significance of incompetence of personal sanitary habits. *Nursing Times,* 71:340, Feb. 1975.
144. Wilson, M.: Bladder training for the chronically ill. *RN,* 38:36, June 1975.
145. Yahle, M.: An ostomy information clinic: a community clinic. *Nursing Clinics of North America,* 11:457, Sep. 1976.

CHAPTER 31

MEDICATION PRINCIPLES AND ORAL ADMINISTRATION

By Margaret Auld Bruya, R.N., M.N.

OVERVIEW AND STUDY GUIDE

In practically every health care setting, the nurse is responsible for administration of medications. In most instances,* before the nurse can administer any medication, the medication must be ordered by a physician (M.D. or D.O.) or a dentist (D.D.S.). In all instances, the nurse is responsible for ensuring that the "Five Rights of Giving Medications" are followed.

Be sure that the:

1. *Right drug*
2. *Right dose*
3. *Right route*
4. *Right time*
5. *Right patient*

are all given equal consideration before the medication is given

---

In this chapter, we discuss the purposes of medication administration and present the theories and techniques of safe and accurate administration. General drug classifications are explored, as are sources of medication information, abbreviations common to medication administration, and the legal and ethical responsibilities of the nurse's relationships with other members of the health team. Patient assessment techniques and patient interview forms for medication administration are presented.

The nursing student must appreciate the responsibilities assumed in the administration of medications. The conscientious nurse is knowledgeable regarding: (a) the *pharmacology* of medications given, (b) the *legal implications* involved in the preparation and administration of medications and (c) the *tech-*

niques of safe and accurate medication preparation, transport and administration. All of this knowledge must be correlated with the patient's diagnosis or suspected diagnosis and incorporated into the patient's care plan.

In addition, if the nurse is to safely administer medications, she must have the mathematical skills necessary to verify that dosages have been correctly calculated. While the physician or dentist is responsible for the *prescription* of dosages, the nurse is responsible for *checking* dosages. Moreover, the nurse must be able not only to check dosages but also to *calculate* them, using the metric system and using the hodgepodge of weights and measures that are common in the United States today.

While the emphasis in health care delivery systems is on the use of the metric system (i.e., measurements in milligrams, grams, milliliters and liters), medication orders are still usually written in the apothecaries' system (i.e., measurements in grains, drams, ounces, minims, fluidrams, and pints) or in household measures (e.g., teaspoons and tablespoons). To add to the confusion, medication dosages are typically calculated on the basis of the patient's weight in kilograms (metric system) rather than in pounds (apothecaries' system). Because most scales give the patient's weight in pounds, the nurse must first be able to convert pounds to kilograms to compute dosages. Figure 31–1A provides conversion factors for changing to metric measurements; Figure 31–1B shows how to do the reverse—change *from* metric measurements *to* inches, pounds, etc. The chance for errors in calculations as one converts from system to system is evident in the variety of conversion factors.

Because both the metric and apothecaries' systems are still currently being used, it is important to be able to use both systems with ease. The *apothecaries' system* was historically based on familiar anatomic and domestic concepts: an inch was originally defined as the length of "three barleycorns, round and dry and a foot was the length

---

*In some instances, specially educated nurses can prescribe medications. However, this is not a function of a beginning practitioner.

of a man's foot; a yard, the distance from the tip of the nose to the tip of the finger."[61] Standardization using arbitrary units was established, but convenience in changing between units was not improved. To deal with volume, for instance, you must be aware of teaspoons, tablespoons, ounces, cups, pints, quarts, etc.

The *metric system*, on the other hand, is easy to work with because it is based on the decimal system. (We are all familiar with it because it underlies the monetary system of the United States.) In the metric system, there is only one basic unit of measurement for length, area, mass, liquid and temperature, and so the chance for errors in calculations is reduced. If the student is hesitant about the use of the metric system, it would be wise to review some of the basic calculations and the following vocabulary: meter, centimeter, millimeter, gram, kilogram, milliliter, liter and Celsius degrees. Until we learn to *think* in metric terms, a chart such as "All You Will Need to Know About Metric" from the National Bureau of Standards can help us understand the basic units of the metric system (p. 740).

Because the administration of medications carries so much responsibility, it raises many questions about the legal and ethical position of the nurse. Some relevant questions are as follows:

1. In what ways can the nurse verify that the medications ordered for her patients are both therapeutic and safe?

2. What are some of the safeguards that the nurse can utilize when preparing and dispensing medications, and recording their administration?

3. What current research is being done in pharmacology that will have an impact on the practice of nursing?

4. What are legal limitations the nurse must consider when administering medications?

5. What is the desired therapeutic effect of each medication given, and how can the nurse best augment this effect?

6. What is the nurse's responsibility in relation to patient and family education in the hospital and in the home and community?

In order to answer these questions, this chapter will focus on the following areas:

▶ general pharmacology overview

▶ historical, ethical and legal aspects of medication administration

▶ roles and responsibilities of the health team members

▶ rights and responsibilities of patients receiving medications

▶ medication administration systems, and factors essential to carrying out responsibilities

▶ patient assessment

This chapter deals particularly with medications that are given orally. Chapters 32 and 38 will discuss the administration of medications topically and by injection, respectively.

1. Upon completion of this chapter, you should be

METRIC CONVERSION FACTORS

Approximate Conversions to Metric Measures

Symbol	When You Know	Multiply by	To Find	Symbol
LENGTH				
in	inches	2.5	centimeters	cm
ft	feet	30	centimeters	cm
yd	yards	0.9	meters	m
mi	miles	1.6	kilometers	km
AREA				
in²	square inches	6.5	square centimeters	cm²
ft²	square feet	0.09	square meters	m²
yd²	square yards	0.8	square meters	m²
mi²	square miles	2.6	square kilometers	km²
	acres	0.4	hectares	ha
MASS (weight)				
oz	ounces	28	grams	g
lb	pounds	0.45	kilograms	kg
	short tons (2000 lb)	0.9	metric ton	t
VOLUME				
tsp	teaspoons	5	milliliters	mL
Tbsp	tablespoons	15	milliliters	mL
in³	cubic inches	16	milliliters	mL
fl oz	fluid ounces	30	milliliters	mL
c	cups	0.24	liters	L
pt	pints	0.47	liters	L
qt	quarts	0.95	liters	L
gal	gallons	3.8	liters	L
ft³	cubic feet	0.03	cubic meters	m³
yd³	cubic yards	0.76	cubic meters	m³
TEMPERATURE (exact)				
°F	degrees Fahrenheit	5/9 (after subtracting 32)	degrees Celsius	°C

A

Approximate Conversions from Metric Measures

Symbol	When You Know	Multiply by	To Find	Symbol
LENGTH				
mm	millimeters	0.04	inches	in
cm	centimeters	0.4	inches	in
m	meters	3.3	feet	ft
m	meters	1.1	yards	yd
km	kilometers	0.6	miles	mi
AREA				
cm²	square centimeters	0.16	square inches	in²
m²	square meters	1.2	square yards	yd²
km²	square kilometers	0.4	square miles	mi²
ha	hectares (10 000 m²)	2.5	acres	
MASS (weight)				
g	grams	0.035	ounces	oz
kg	kilograms	2.2	pounds	lb
t	metric ton (1000 kg)	1.1	short tons	
VOLUME				
mL	milliliters	0.03	fluid ounces	fl oz
mL	milliliters	0.06	cubic inches	in³
L	liters	2.1	pints	pt
L	liters	1.06	quarts	qt
L	liters	0.26	gallons	gal
m³	cubic meters	35	cubic feet	ft³
m³	cubic meters	1.3	cubic yards	yd³
TEMPERATURE (exact)				
°C	degrees Celsius	9/5 (then add 32)	degrees Fahrenheit	°F

B

Figure 31–1. Metric conversion factors. (From National Bureau of Standards Publication LC 1051.)

All You Will Need to Know About Metric
(For Your Everyday Life)

10

Metric is based on Decimal system

The metric system is simple to learn. For use in your everyday life you will need to know only ten units. You will also need to get used to a few new temperatures. Of course, there are other units which most persons will not need to learn. There are even some metric units with which you are already familiar: those for time and electricity are the same as you use now.

BASIC UNITS

METER: a little longer than a yard (about 1.1 yards)
LITER: a little larger than a quart (about 1.06 quarts)
GRAM: a little more than the weight of a paper clip

(comparative sizes are shown)

1 METER

1 YARD

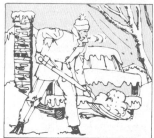

25 DEGREES FAHRENHEIT

COMMON PREFIXES
(to be used with basic units)

milli: one-thousandth (0.001)
centi: one-hundredth (0.01)
kilo: one-thousand times (1000)

For example:
1000 millimeters = 1 meter
100 centimeters = 1 meter
1000 meters   = 1 kilometer

1 LITER 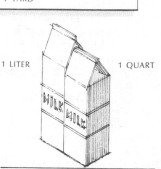 1 QUART

OTHER COMMONLY USED UNITS

millimeter:	0.001 meter	diameter of paper clip wire
centimeter:	0.01 meter	a little more than the width of a paper clip (about 0.4 inch)
kilometer:	1000 meters	somewhat further than ½ mile (about 0.6 mile)
kilogram:	1000 grams	a little more than 2 pounds (about 2.2 pounds)
milliliter:	0.001 liter	five of them make a teaspoon

OTHER USEFUL UNITS

hectare: about 2½ acres
metric ton: about one ton

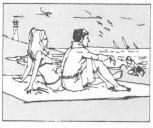

25 DEGREES CELSIUS

WEATHER UNITS:

FOR TEMPERATURE
degrees Celsius

FOR PRESSURE
kilopascals are used
100 kilopascals = 29.5 inches of Hg (14.5 psi)

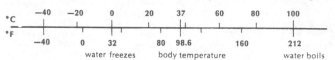

°C	−40	−20	0	20	37	60	80	100
°F	−40	0	32	80	98.6		160	212

water freezes   body temperature   water boils

1 POUND

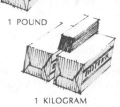

1 KILOGRAM

U.S. DEPARTMENT OF COMMERCE
National Bureau of Standards
Washington, D.C. 20234

Letter Circular 1052
February 1976

TABLE 31–1. COMMON ABBREVIATIONS FOR PRESCRIBING AND ADMINISTERING MEDICATIONS

ABBREVIATIONS	MEANING
a.a.	of
a.c.	before meals (30 min.)
ad lib	freely
aq.	water
$\bar{c}$	with
$\bar{s}$	without
q.	every
ID	intradermal
IM	intramuscular
IV	intravenous
SQ or SC	subcutaneous
OD	right eye
OS	left eye
OU	both eyes
p.r.n.	at nurse's discretion
p.o.	by mouth
stat.	immediately
t.	tincture
HS	hour of sleep

able to define the terms listed below and be able to use them in your nursing practice:

formulary	medication card
physician's order	incident report
written order	tablet
verbal order	enteric-coated
telephone order	capsules
standing order	effervescence
prn	powder
stat	pill
topical	lozenge
drug	analgesic
medication	syrup
therapeutic effect	solution
side effect	suspension
toxic effect	hydroalcoholic
synergistic effect	meniscus
controlled substance	elixir
unit dose system	magma
stock supply system	emulsion
self-medication	tincture

TABLE 31–2. APPROXIMATE EQUIVALENTS

VALUE	APPROXIMATE EQUIVALENT
1 gr.	60 mg.
$1/60$ gr.	1 mg.
15 gr.	1 gram
1 oz.	30 ml.
15 minims	1 ml.
8 fl. oz.	250 ml.
1 pint	500 ml.
1 quart	1000 ml.
1 kg.	2.2 lb.

2. In order to safely understand and transcribe orders, administer medications and evaluate their effects, you must be aware of the meanings of the abbreviations in Table 31–1.

3. To accurately calculate and measure medication dosages, it is important to be familiar with the approximate equivalents listed in Table 31–2.

After you finish this chapter, you should understand facts and principles that guide the nurse in the preparation and administration of medications and be able to apply these facts and principles to patient care situations. You should also understand the health professional's legal and ethical responsibilities in the preparation and administration of medication, understand the essential techniques necessary to safely pour and administer medications, be aware of sources of information about medications and understand the complementary roles of the members of the health team in the safe delivery of all types of medications. You should know the rights and responsibilities of patients receiving medications, be aware of the need for patient education, be familiar with the different systems for medication delivery in health care settings, and be able to do a patient assessment for a patient receiving medications.

GENERAL PHARMACOLOGICAL OVERVIEW

Aids for Studying Pharmacology

A minimum of information regarding the safe delivery of pharmacologic agents is presented in this section. It is suggested that the student also make a habit of consulting a basic reference on pharmacology. In addition, the student needs to be able to obtain information about the medications she administers from these sources: pharmacology textbooks, the *American Hospital Formulary*, the particular formulary used at the student's clinical facility, the *Physician's Desk Reference* (PDR), the inserts

provided with packaged medications, nursing literature, and pharmacists.

The student's pharmacology textbook should include basic information about medications, e.g., actions and uses, dosage, range, toxic effects and side effects. Additionally, nursing implications and observations are frequently given. The *American Hospital Formulary* gives a full description and rationale for the use of each therapeutic agent. The *individual hospital formulary* should give information regarding medications used in that institution.

The *PDR* is an annual publication that compiles information provided by drug manufacturers. An important feature of the PDR is the section of colored illustrations of a variety of medications, designed to aid the health care worker to identify medications by sight. Inserts from manufacturers are included in boxes used to package medications. Read inserts thoroughly when you are unsure of detailed information. For parenteral medications (those given by routes other than oral), the manufacturer will give information as to dilution and speed of delivery. *Nursing literature,* particularly the *American Journal of Nursing, Nursing* and *RN,* have helpful monthly updates on medications.

Finally, one of the best, most up-to-date and reliable sources of information about medications will be the *pharmacist.* He should be consulted whenever a question of dosage, compatibility or incompatibility, rate and route of excretion, side effects and interaction, or rationale for administration needs to be answered.

Once the student has obtained information about a medication from the above sources, it is very helpful to write that information on a medication reference card like the one pictured in Figure 31–2 for her own use while in the health care agency.

The nurse must be proficient in the use of pharmacologic weights and measures in order to safely prepare and administer medications. The student is referred to Tables 31–3, 31–4, and 31–5 to review weights and measures.

Similarly, the nurse needs to be fluent in "pharmacologic language." In order to interpret orders and act appropriately when working with medications, knowledge of the common abbreviations and symbols is essential. The student is referred to Tables 31–1 and 31–2. If you have difficulty remembering the meaning of the abbreviations and symbols, you may find it helpful to make a set of flash cards, with the abbreviation or symbol on one side and the definition on the other, to use in memorizing these terms.

TABLE 31–3.   METRIC WEIGHTS AND APOTHECARY EQUIVALENTS

METRIC	APOTHECARY EQUIVALENT
0.1 mg.	$1/600$ gr.
0.15 mg.	$1/400$ gr.
0.20 mg.	$1/300$ gr.
0.4 mg.	$1/150$ gr.
1.0 mg.	$1/60$ gr.
2.0 mg.	$1/30$ gr.
10.0 mg.	$1/6$ gr.
15.0 mg.	¼ gr.
30.0 mg.	½ gr.
60.0 mg.	1 gr.
75.0 mg.	1¼ gr.
0.1 Gm.	1½ gr.
0.3 Gm.	5 gr.
0.6 Gm.	10 gr.
1.0 Gm.	15 gr.
3.0 Gm.	45 gr.
30.0 Gm.	1 oz.

DRUG: Valium (diazepam)
DOSE ORDERED: 5 mg po TID
USUAL DOSE/RANGE: 2–10 mg. BID or QID po
    May give IM or IV (caution—low dose in children or elderly)
DESIRED ACTION
    a. GENERAL: Symptomatic relief of anxiety & tension, apprehension. Adjunct to anticonvulsive agents. Pregastroscopy & esophagoscopy. (IM or IV muscle spasm, status epilepticus & recurrent convulsive seizures)
    b. FOR THIS PATIENT: Alleviate apprehension associated with myocardial infarct (heart attack).
SIDE EFFECTS: Drowsiness, fatigue & ataxia.
    Caution in hazardous tasks & driving, lightheadedness, vertigo, weakness, nausea, vomiting, epigastric distress.
TOXIC/UNDESIRED EFFECTS: Constipation, syncope, headache, double vision, dry mouth, psychic dependence or addiction esp. in alcoholics. Prompt withdrawal after prolonged administration of high dosage may result in epileptiform seizures and death.

Figure 31–2.   Completed medication reference card.

TABLE 31–4.   UNITS OF LIQUID VOLUME

METRIC UNITS OF LIQUID VOLUME

1 liter (L) = 1000 milliliters (ml.), or
                    1000 cubic centimeters (cc.)
    0.001 L = 1 ml. or 1 cc.

APOTHECARY UNITS OF LIQUID VOLUME

60 minims (♏ or min) = 1 fluidram ($f\mathbf{3}$)
                    8 $f\mathbf{3}$ = 1 fluidounce ($f\mathbf{3}$)
                    16 $f\mathbf{3}$ = 1 pint (pt.)
                    2 pt. = 1 quart (qt.)
                    4 qt. = 1 gallon (gal.)

(Adapted from Pecherer, A. R. and Vertuno, S. L.: *How to Calculate Drug Dosages.* Oradell, N. J., Medical Economics Co., 1978.)

HOUSEHOLD UNITS OF MEASUREMENT

60 drops (gtt.) = 1 teaspoon (tsp.)
3 tsp. = 1 tablespoon (tbs.)
6 tsp. = 1 ounce (oz.)
2 tbs. = 1 oz.
6 oz. = 1 teacup
8 oz. = 1 glass
8 oz. = 1 measuring cup

APPROXIMATE HOUSEHOLD EQUIVALENTS

Household		Apothecary
1 drop (gt.)	=	1 minim (η or min.)
15 drops (gtt.)	=	15 min.
1 teaspoon (tsp.)	=	1 fluidram ($f\,\bar{3}$) [60 min.]
1 tablespoon (tbs.)	=	$4\,f\,\bar{3}$
2 tbs.	=	1 fluidounce ($f\,\bar{3}$)
1 ounce (oz.)	=	$1\,f\,\bar{3}$
1 teacup	=	$6\,f\,\bar{3}$
1 glass	=	$8\,f\,\bar{3}$
1 measuring cup	=	$8\,f\,\bar{3}$
2 measuring cups	=	1 pint (pt.)

Household		Metric
1 drop (gt.)	=	.06 milliliter (ml.)
15 drops (gtt.)	=	1 ml. [1 cc.]
1 teaspoon (tsp.)	=	5 (4) ml.*
1 tablespoon (tbs.)	=	15 ml.
2 tbs.	=	30 ml.
1 ounce (oz.)	=	30 ml.
1 teacup	=	180 ml.
1 glass	=	240 ml.
1 measuring cup	=	240 ml.
2 measuring cups	=	500 ml.

*The American standard teaspoon is accepted as 5 ml., but you may use 4 ml. as the equivalent if it provides a more accurate calculation.
(From Pecherer, A. R. and Vertuno, S. L.: How to Calculate Drug Dosages. Oradell, N.J., Medical Economics Co., 1978.)

Basic Facts About Medications

You will recall that a *drug* is any substance taken that can modify or change the organism's function, while a *medication* is a drug which is administered with therapeutic intent, i.e., to helpfully modify or change the organism to some degree. There are many types and classifications of medications. The following table includes *general drug classifications* and *drug actions* and the names of common medications the student may encounter in her nursing practice. Table 31-6 can be used for review, but you will need to consult a pharmacology book for more detailed information on each drug and information on the physiology of the system each affects.

Medications can be administered to the patient in many different ways. The most common dosage form is oral. For oral administration, tablets, capsules, elixirs and syrups are frequently used. *Topical* (to the surface) agents can be applied in the form of sprays, paints, ointments, irrigations and instillations (see Chap. 32). *Parenteral* (by needle) routes of administration are considered in Chap. 38.

Medications have many effects, some beneficial and some undesirable or even toxic. Some important *therapeutic effects* are as follows: (a) promotion of health, such as might be provided by vitamin supplements, (b) the prevention of disease, as provided by vaccinations and serums, (c) the alleviation of discomfort or pain, by narcotics or analgesics and (d) cure or control of disease processes through the use of antimicrobials, hormones or antineoplastic agents.[50] Medications may also have *side* and/or *toxic effects*. Many side and toxic effects are known and documented in the literature. The nurse has the responsibility to know of and be observant for those effects. As some of the side or toxic effects of medications may be dangerous or even fatal, it is imperative that the nurse be alert. When you suspect an abnormal reaction, consult the physician. It will be his decision to continue or discontinue the medication.

Medications also have local and systemic effects. The nurse may expect *local effects* of medications, particularly when they are applied topically to skin or mucous membranes. The injection of medications may cause an erythematous (reddish) reaction if the injected medication is irritating, and the nurse should be aware of this potential reaction.

Systemic effects are expected from administration of most orally ingested or injected medications. That is, the various organ systems in the body are affected by the medication even though the target organ (the organ or system for which the medication was administered) shows the greatest response. For example, consider the ingestion of a penicillin tablet for an infection of the hand. While the penicillin is bactericidal for the organism, penicillin also circulates throughout the blood and other fluids of the body, thus creating systemic effects. Synergism, or a *synergistic effect*, occurs when a combination of medications are given. This effect is seen when one medication compounds or heightens the effect of another. Synergism may be a desired therapeutic effect or an undesirable complication. The pharmacist should be consulted when the patient is receiving multiple therapeutic agents, as his knowledge may prevent complications.

TABLE 31–6. GENERAL DRUG CLASSIFICATION AND ACTION*

CLASSIFICATION*	ACTION
1. Autonomic nervous system	Regulate the body's physiologic tasks essential for homeostasis, repair and emergency
a. Catecholamines (epinephrine, isoproterenol)	A wide variety of physiologic responses
b. Direct and indirect alpha and beta stimulants (ephedrine, Neo-Synephrine, Aramine)	Indirect action Sympathomimetic amines
c. Alpha blocking agents (Dibenzyline)	Compete with catecholamines at receptor sites
d. Beta blocking agents (Inderal)	Compete with catecholamines at effector site
e. Cholinergic (Urecholine)	Chemically related to acetylcholine (important in nerve transmission)
f. Anticholinesterase (neostigmine)	Act as cholinergic agents by inactivating or inhibiting enzyme cholinesterase
g. Anticholinergic (atropine)	Act selectively on postganglionic sites Relax smooth muscle, inhibit duct gland secretion Prevent or reduce action of acetylcholine
2. Cardiovascular system	
a. Cardiac glycosides (digitalis)	Increase myocardial contractility Slow atrioventricular conduction
b. Antiarrhythmic (quinidine, lidocaine)	Prevent and treat disorders of cardiac rhythm by reversing electrophysiologic abnormalities
c. Vasodilator	Relax smooth muscles of body resulting in reduction in decreased work load and blood pressure
d. Antihypertensives	Inhibit sympathetic nervous system function (reserpine) Vasodilation of vascular smooth muscle (Apresoline) Ganglionic blocking agent Amine oxidase inhibitor Thiazides
e. Vasoconstrictors (angiotensin amide)	Contraction of muscle fibers in blood vessels
f. Antianemic (hemopathetic) (Imferon, iron)	Provide essential constituents for blood formation
g. Whole blood and constituents	Provide cells and restore blood volume
h. Affect coagulation	
(1) Hemostatics (Gelfoam)	Act as a tampon, liberate thromboplastin
(2) Anticoagulants (heparin)	Decrease blood coagulability
i. Antilipemic	Unknown, most thought to inhibit synthesis of lipids
3. Central nervous system	
a. Depressants	
(1) Pain relievers (morphine, codeine, aspirin)	Relieve pain without loss of consciousness
(2) Hypnotics and sedatives (barbiturates)	Produce sleep
(3) Alcohol	Depresses vasomotor center in the medulla; action similar to general anesthetics
(4) Anticonvulsants (Dilantin)	Suppression of seizure center
b. Stimulants	Stimulate central nervous system
4. Psychotropic drugs	
a. Major tranquilizers (Mellaril, Trilafon)	Increase rate of dopamine turnover, and block transmission
b. Tranquilizers (antianxiety agents) (Vistaril, Valium)	Depressive effect on polysynaptic reflexes
c. Antidepressants (Tofranil, Elavil)	Action is not known
5. Anesthetics	
a. General anesthetics (ether, cyclopropane)	No one theory of action is acceptable to all
b. Local anesthetics (Xylocaine, benzocaine)	Act by stabilizing or elevating the threshold of excitation of nerve cell membrane
6. Skeletal muscle relaxants/antagonists	
a. Neuromuscular blocking agents (curare, pancuronium bromide)	Prevent stimulation of muscle fibers
b. Centrally acting: skeletal muscle relaxants (Robaxin)	Unknown
c. Direct acting skeletal muscle relaxant (Dantrium)	Inhibits release of calcium from sarcoplasmic reticulum resulting in decreased muscle response
d. Curariform antagonists	Anticholinesterase agent
e. Antiparkinsonism (L-dopa)	Replenish dopamine levels and enhance dopaminergic mechanism

*Adapted from Bergersen, B. S.: *Pharmacology in Nursing*, 13th ed. St. Louis, C. V. Mosby Co. 1976.

TABLE 31–6. GENERAL DRUG CLASSIFICATION AND ACTION (*Continued*)

CLASSIFICATION	ACTION
7. Respiratory system	
a. Therapeutic gases (O_2)	Replenish gas lack
b. Bronchodilators (Isuprel)	Relax smooth muscle of tracheobronchial tree
c. Mucolytic agents (Mucomyst)	Reduce thickness and stickiness of purulent and non-purulent pulmonary secretions
d. Respiratory stimulants (Dopram)	Blockage of inhibition at the presynaptic or postsynaptic area
e. Respiratory depressants	Depress respiratory center
(1) Antitussives (Romilar)	Inhibit ciliary activity of respiratory tree
(2) Demulcents (honey, hard candy)	Coat lining of respiratory tract to prevent contact with air
(3) Expectorants	Clear mucus from bronchial tubes
8. Histamine and antihistaminics	
a. Histamine	Contraction of smooth muscle
	Dilatation of capillaries
	Promotion of gastric acid secretion
b. Antihistaminics (Benadryl)	Prevents physiologic action of histamine
9. Diuretics	
a. Proximal tubule action (Lasix)	Increase flow of urine
b. Distal tubule action (Diuril)	May depress proximal tubular resorption of sodium and chloride
10. Antimicrobial	
a. Bacteriocidal (penicillin)	Cause cell death and lysis
b. Bacteriostatic (sulfonamides)	Inhibit bacterial growth
c. Antiviral (gamma globulin)	Prophylactic action of specific virus; interfere with viral penetration into host cell
d. Antifungals (amphotericin)	Fungiostatic and fungicidal
11. Parasitic disease chemotherapy	
a. Antiprotozoan	Rid body of protozoa
b. Anthelmintics (Povan)	Rid body of worms
c. Amebicides	Rid body of amebae
12. Antiseptics and disinfectants	
a. Phenol	Denaturation (not to be ingested)
	Lowers surface tension of cell, which allows greater permeability
b. Dyes (gentian violet)	Interfere with some metabolic products
c. Heavy metals (mercurochrome)	Bacteriostatic
d. Halogens:	
Iodine	Unknown action
Chlorine	Antibacterial
e. Oxidizing agents (H_2O_2)	Active germicide when liberates oxygen
f. Surface acting agents (benzalkonium chloride)	Lower surface tension and aid in mechanical removal of bacteria and soil
13. Serums and vaccines	
a. Immune serums (gamma globulin)	From humans with antibodies to act upon disease microorganism
b. Vaccines (pertussis)	Killed or attenuated microorganisms given so the body makes antibodies toward infecting agent
c. Cutaneous tests for immunity (PPD)	Diagnostic tests
14. Antineoplastic	Toxicity to cells (non-selective)
a. Alkylating agents	Interfere with cancer cell division; results in cell death
b. Antimetabolites (methotrexate)	Inhibits folic acid reductase, interfering with a coenzyme necessary for DNA synthesis
c. Plant alkaloids (Velban)	Metaphase arrest
d. Antibiotics (actinomycin D)	Inhibit synthesis of RNA
e. Radioisotopes (ionizing radiation)	Cytotoxic effects not well understood
15. Hormones	
a. Endocrine	Work to maintain physiologic balance in body, control protein synthesis, AMP and membrane permeability
b. Sex (estrogen, testosterone)	Bring about changes in females and males which lead to puberty and sexual maturity

Table continued on the following page

TABLE 31–6. GENERAL DRUG CLASSIFICATION AND ACTION (*Continued*)

CLASSIFICATION	ACTION
16. Enzymes (Varidase)	Catalysis (accelerators) to chemical reactions that occur in living cells
17. Ocular agents	Action dependent upon therapeutic necessity
18. Dermatologic agents	
a. Emollients (lanolin)	Soften or smooth irritated skin and mucous membrane
b. Antiseptics, antibiotics (parasiticedes)	Treat or prevent microbial infection of skin and mucous membranes
c. Stimulants, irritants (tar)	Produce mild irritation to slough inflammatory exudates
d. Keratolytics (salicylic acid)	Soften scales
e. Antipruritics	Allay itching
f. Protectives (collodion)	Form film on skin
g. Cleansers (bath soaps)	Cleanse skin
19. Gastrointestinal agents	Action on smooth muscle, gland cells, indirectly on autonomic nervous system
a. Mouth (mouthwashes, gargles)	Cleansing; local therapy
b. Stomach:	Symptomatic relief of nausea and vomiting
Antacids	Reduce amount of acid
Digestants	Promote process of digestion
Emetics	Produce vomiting
Antiemetics	Symptomatic relief of nausea and vomiting
c. Intestines	
(1) Cathartics (mineral oil, cascara)	Produce defecation
(2) Antidiarrheics	Prevent hypermotility of bowel
(3) Carminatives	Increase GI motility

Computation of Medication Dosages

Computation of medication dosages has traditionally been the "undoing" of many nurses. Problems typically arise because nurses are either unable to solve math problems related to medication administration or they cannot remember conversion factors. Because the nurse is often called upon to compute dosages quickly and accurately, she must be able to solve math problems "on the spot." Nursing educators have been concerned with providing learners and practitioners with an easy, reliable and fail-safe method for such computation. Carr et al. in the *American Journal of Nursing* for December 1976 presented a technique to solve dosage problems for such diverse nursing tasks as calculating IV drip rates, calculating cubic centimeters of a liquid drug to obtain the ordered amount in milligrams, converting kilograms to pounds, and converting Fahrenheit to Celsius temperature.[7] The student may wish to consult this article. (Calculation of IV rates is discussed in Chapter 24.)

In addition to being able to calculate adult dosages, the student should also be able to calculate *pediatric dosages*.

Particular caution needs to be exercised in the determination of pediatric dosages because (owing to a child's small body size), overdoses can result in serious or even fatal consequences.

Because infants and children have special needs in relation to dosages, the determination of a pediatric dosage should preferably be made by referring to the manufacturers' guidelines or the hospital formulary. However, when a therapeutic dosage has yet to be determined for a child, the physician and pharmacist must calculate a pediatric dose as a fraction of the adult dose. There are three basic ways to calculate pediatric dosages: (1) on the basis of age, (2) on the basis of body weight and (3) on the basis of the square meters of body surface area.

Three commonly used formulas on the basis of *age* are: Young's and Cowling's (for children over 2 years of age) and Fried's (for children less than 1 year of age).

Young's rule:

$$\frac{age}{age + 12} \times adult\ dose = child's\ dose$$

Cowling's rule:

$$\frac{\text{age of child on next birthday}}{24} \times \text{adult dose} = \text{child's dose}$$

Fried's law:

$$\frac{\text{age in months}}{150} \times \text{adult dose} = \text{infant's dose}$$

Calculation on the basis of *body weight* is more accurate than on the basis of age. *Clark's rule* is used to estimate dosage on the *basis of weight:*

$$\frac{\text{weight in pounds of child}}{150} \times \text{adult dose} = \text{child's dose}$$

However, the problem in attempting to calculate dosages on the basis of body weight should be immediately apparent: the normal weight in any age group is highly variable and is not really subject to standardization in terms of therapeutic doses. For this reason, calculation on the basis of *body surface area* (BSA) is perhaps the most accurate.

For calculations derived from BSA, the formula is based on a 100 per cent adult dose for an individual weighing 140 pounds, who has a BSA of 1.7 m². BSA of the child can be estimated from a height and weight nomogram (see Fig. 31–3).

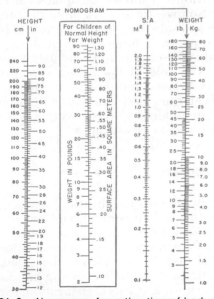

Figure 31–3. Nomogram for estimation of body surface area. A straight edge is placed from the patient's height in the left column to his weight in the right column, and this intersect on the body surface area column (S. A.) indicates his body surface area. For children of average build, the body surface area may be estimated from the weight alone by referring to the enclosed area in left center of the figure. This nomogram was prepared by C. D. West and is from Shirkey, H. C.: Table of drugs. *In* Vaughan, V. C., and McKay, J. R.: *Nelson Textbook of Pediatrics,* 10th ed. Philadelphia, W. B. Saunders Co., 1975, p. 1713.

$$\frac{\text{BSA in. m}^2 \text{ of child}}{1.7} \times \text{usual adult dose} = \text{child's dose}$$

The calculation of dosages must be performed with absolute accuracy. If a student believes that her mathematics skills are deficient, some remedial work must be undertaken. Attention should be directed towards decimals, fractions, percentages and ratio and proportion.

HISTORICAL, ETHICAL AND LEGAL ASPECTS OF MEDICATION ADMINISTRATION

Historical Aspects

Historically, medications were often the domain of the herbal healer or of certain old men and women of the community who were knowledgeable about the various medicinal properties of botanical agents. For example, these persons knew that "dropsy" (congestive heart failure) responded to the administration of a concoction formulated from the purple foxglove plant, a substance that we now know as digitalis. Such folk mixtures, when tested by modern research chemists, laid the groundwork for modern-day pharmaceutical preparations.

While most people in industrialized countries utilize medications chemically formulated by pharmaceutical companies, there are many who continue to use herbal preparations given to them by their local healer. One can walk into an herbal "drug" store in San Francisco or New York and purchase any number of "therapeutic agents." We suggest that nurses be aware that while a patient may be taking medications prescribed by his doctor, he may also be taking medication prescribed by such a healer.

Ethical Issues

There are a number of ethical issues that the nurse must consider when working with medications. One issue is the problem of *drug addiction*. Because of increased use and abuse of over-the-counter (OTC) and street drugs (e.g., amphetamines, heroin, cocaine), the nurse often encounters hospitalized individuals who are addicted to medications. Addicted individuals have social, medical and psychologic problems that complicate their course of recovery and their response to medically ordered therapeutics. The nurse must be aware of her own personal reactions to "abusers" but must also recall that the nurse's role is a helping one, rather than a judgmental or punitive one. Nursing care planning must, however, include preventing abuse and assisting the patient to curtail use.

A second ethical issue that the nurse faces is that of self-medication and the *illegal dispensing of drugs*. Because the health care provider has relatively free access to a variety of drugs, there may be a temptation to experiment with self-medication. Also, friends and relatives may ask doctors and nurses to obtain medications illegally for them. Your moral and ethical position in regard to medications must be established early in your career, and deviation from this position must be avoided.

The nurse's role in giving *experimental drugs* constitutes a third ethical problem. When giving experimental medications, one responsibility of the nurse is to make certain that the patient's rights are not violated. Use of human subjects in experiments is a controversial and emotional issue; there are now very strict guidelines for human experimentation. The federal government regulates many of the research projects which involve human experimentation. Such government agencies as The National Commission for the Protection of Human Subjects of Biomedical and Behavioral Research; the Department of Health, Education and Welfare (DHEW); and the Federal Food and Drug Administration (FDA) are involved in the legal control of the majority of experimental medical programs. In addition, ethical considerations involving the rights of human experimental subjects have been clearly outlined by the American Hospital Association's "Statement on a Patient's Bill of Rights" (1073) (see Chapter 20). Also, the American Nurses' Association (ANA) has stated the nurse's responsibilities in preserving the rights of patients who serve as research subjects in "The Nurse in Research: ANA Guidelines on Ethical Values (1968)" and "Human Rights Guidelines for Nurses in Clinical and Other Research" (1975).[9a]

When involved in an experimental drug program, the nurse has a legal obligation to be fully informed about any investigational medication which she will be administering to a patient.[50a] In addition, prior to administering an experimental drug, the nurse must witness that her patient has received a complete explanation of the investigational drug (benefits, side effects, toxic effects) and has signed a consent form allowing administration of the medication.[51a]

The nurse can assist in the evaluation of an experimental drug by observing and recording deviances or nuances in patient behavior, coordination and body functioning that might indicate side, toxic or local effects of the medication. The nurse must keep in mind that significant risks as well as potential benefits are involved in the use of experimental medications.

The Federal Food and Drug Administration (FDA) maintains strict control of all drugs proposed for human use in the United States. Because of this, persons promoting a new drug must submit their proposal through the FDA, and until the efficacy of the drug is demonstrated, its use is limited. Because of the FDA policy, frequently certain medications are available in Europe, Mexico or Canada—but not in the United States. For example, in the 1960's, the FDA prohibited distribution of thalidomide, a drug that caused numerous children in Europe to be born with defects. Thus, the FDA offers vital protection from possibly dangerous drugs to American consumers.

A final ethical consideration centers around the distribution and use of "quack" drugs. The FDA also investigates and prohibits the distribution and sale of such medications. This control, however, is often insufficient to prevent individuals from obtaining and using worthless items. The role of the health care provider, then, is to alert individuals to the potential harm both from use of the quack item and from lack of treatment for an illness that is treatable with legitimate medications.

Legal Aspects

Legally, the responsibilities associated with preparation, administration and evaluation of medications are immense. First of all, the nurse must be *knowledgeable* about medications. It is essential that she keep up to date about new medications. Also, before giving any medication, she must know its classification, expected action, significant side effects and the reason for its administration. In addition, the nurse's legal responsibility includes *prevention of medication errors* by observing the "Five Rights of Giving Medications" that we discussed earlier: right drug, right dose, right route, right time and right patient. Also, the nurse can prevent medication errors by mixing and giving only compatible medications and by always checking with patients concerning allergies before administering any medication to which the patient might be allergic. (Penicillin and codeine are two medications that are known to cause allergic reactions.) Charting the administration of medication or its omission is the legal responsibility of the person who gives the medication. Because observing and reporting untoward effects or errors is a nursing responsibility, the nurse must observe and record observations in the patient's permanent record.

Furthermore, it is essential that the nurse know what is and what is *not* included in the state nurse practice act and follow all state rulings explicitly.

The nurse must know what is and what is not acceptable practice in her institution. For example: leaving medications or IV fluids at the patient's bedside is strictly prohibited in some institutions; in others, certain medications (e.g., nitroglycerin) may be left at the patient's bedside with written permission of the physician. In some hospitals mixed or labeled IV bottles, ready for the next hanging, can be left at the bedside.

In summary, because the nurse is independently licensed, she must take full responsibility for her knowledge base and for her activities.

> *No matter what a physician orders, if the nurse questions the order, she has the right and responsibility to decline to give a medication and to report this to her immediate superior. The nurse has an independent license, and she must act according to her education and the scope of the nurse practice act.*

ROLES OF HEALTH TEAM MEMBERS IN REGARD TO MEDICATION ADMINISTRATION

The Physician's Role

In the United States, the physician is the individual who is usually responsible for taking the patient's history, performing the physical examination, diagnosing the symptoms and prescribing the medicinal therapy. (In some instances, a nurse or paramedic with special education can prescribe a limited variety of medications.) The physician uses his knowledge base of disease and treatment as well as a careful review of a patient's medication history and appropriate laboratory tests before prescribing any agent.[41]

When writing a prescription for a patient to have filled at a pharmacy, certain information is essential. This information includes: the medi-

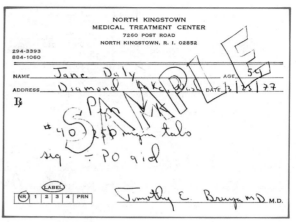

Figure 31–4. Sample prescription.

cation, the dosage, times to be given and duration. The physician's signature is also required. A sample prescription is shown in Figure 31–4.

Because medications are prescribed (ordered) in health care agencies in various forms, the nurse needs to be familiar with the various kinds of orders and her responsibility for each.

The most common types of orders include the following:

PRN: a directive to be followed at the nurse's discretion.

Single: a directive to be followed one time.

Standing: a directive to be carried out until cancelled by the physician or by agency policy.

Stat: a directive to be carried out immediately.

Basically, physician's orders may be written or verbal. A *written order* is written in the patient's chart and is signed by the physician at the time of the writing. *Verbal orders* include telephone orders (T.O.) as well as emergency verbal orders (V.O.). Because of the problems associated with verbal communication, verbal orders are discouraged in most institutions for the protection of the patient, physician and nurse. If a verbal order is accepted, the registered nurse must record the date, time, medication, dosage, route and frequency of administration, as well as T.O. or V.O. and the physician's name, and she must sign her name. At the physician's earliest convenience, the order must be countersigned by him (Fig. 31–5).

Standing Orders are used in patient care areas where patients receive very similar kinds of care. Such patient areas might be in the labor and delivery room or in coronary care units. An example is shown in Figure 31–6.

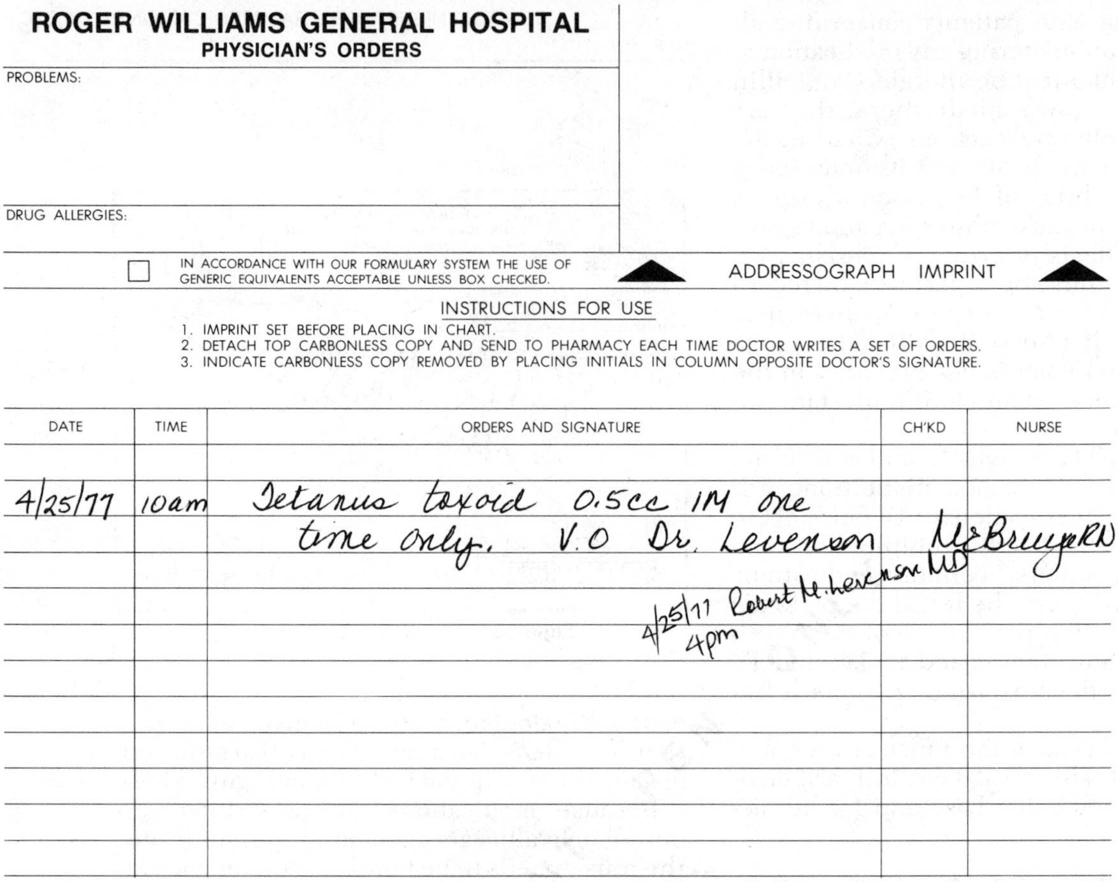

ROGER WILLIAMS GENERAL HOSPITAL
PHYSICIAN'S ORDERS

PROBLEMS:

DRUG ALLERGIES:

☐ IN ACCORDANCE WITH OUR FORMULARY SYSTEM THE USE OF GENERIC EQUIVALENTS ACCEPTABLE UNLESS BOX CHECKED.

ADDRESSOGRAPH IMPRINT

INSTRUCTIONS FOR USE
1. IMPRINT SET BEFORE PLACING IN CHART.
2. DETACH TOP CARBONLESS COPY AND SEND TO PHARMACY EACH TIME DOCTOR WRITES A SET OF ORDERS.
3. INDICATE CARBONLESS COPY REMOVED BY PLACING INITIALS IN COLUMN OPPOSITE DOCTOR'S SIGNATURE.

DATE	TIME	ORDERS AND SIGNATURE	CH'KD	NURSE
4/25/77	10am	Tetanus toxoid 0.5cc IM one		
		time only. V.O Dr. Levenson		McBrueyRN
		4/25/77 4pm Robert M. Levenson MD		

Figure 31–5. Sample verbal order. (Courtesy of Roger Williams General Hospital, Providence, RI.)

Stat medication orders are usually given in emergency situations or when the patient's condition warrants immediate attention. Medication given during a cardiopulmonary arrest or during an acute attack of asthma would probably be ordered "Stat." The Stat order can be verbal or written. If verbal, the physician again has the responsibility to sign the order sheet as soon as practical. If written, the chart is "flagged" by placing a brightly colored tag on the patient's record. Also, the charge nurse can be notified that the medication needs to be administered immediately.

> *The administration of "Stat" orders should take first priority over almost any other nursing activity.*

When PRN orders are written, the nurse must use her discretion and judgment to determine whether to give or to withhold the ordered medication. For a beginning practitioner, this determination is somewhat difficult, and the student should consult her instructor or the charge nurse. Examples of patient situations in which PRN orders are appropriate are for incisional pain following surgery, for sleep while in the hospital or for angina pain.

When the patient's condition changes, the physician is responsible for changing his medication order to reflect this change. The route (PO, IM), dosage or times of administration may be changed, and additions to or deletion from the order may be made. These new orders are written on the physician's order sheet, just as are all other orders.

Physicians also have the responsibility for educating the patient, the patient's representative (parent or guardian) and the staff regarding medication therapy. This aspect of the physician's responsibility is frequently delegated to the professional nurse in the hospital or institutional setting. However, delegating should not result in an abrogation of the physician's responsibility.

The Pharmacist's Role

The pharmacist is thought of by some as a person who merely dispenses medication upon receipt of a prescription. This concept is very narrow and does not begin to cover the actions and responsibilities of the modern pharmacist.

While compounding medications was once done by local pharmacists, currently the majority of medications are compounded by pharmaceutical companies and then distributed to consumers through the pharmacist. Thus, pharmacists spend the majority of their time *filling prescriptions* for medications that are either phoned in by the physician or brought into the pharmacy by the patient. Pharmacists, at the time they "fill" a prescription, may offer advice (and are required to in some states) about taking the medication (e.g., timing in relation to meals); contraindications; and significant side effects to be aware of and to notify the physician of.

In addition to simply dispensing medications, pharmacists in some areas are also acting as *outreach paramedics*, e.g., when they refill an order for antihypertensive medications, they take the patient's blood pressure. This has been the result of an effort by pharmacists to make their services more useful and valuable to the community they serve.

In the agency (hospital or other institution), the pharmacist's role is greatly expanded, although many of the same services are provided as in a local pharmacy. The pharmacy and pharmacists are responsible for *medication control*. Not only are pharmacists responsible for the controlled substances (e.g., narcotics), they are also responsible for stocking, checking for outdated medications and ensuring return of unused medications to the pharmacy. They also normally work as *educators* on committees with nurses and physicians to disseminate pertinent information. In some health care agencies, pharmacists add *all additives to intravenous solutions*. However, in most agencies, the nurse still retains the responsibility for mixing additives for IV solutions. (This procedure will be discussed in Chapter 38.)

Pharmacists are also heavily involved today in the *unit dose method of medication administration* (discussed in detail later in this chapter). Unit dose systems have been replacing the traditional methods of giving medications in some agencies. In this system, each patient is assigned a drawer in a special medication chest of drawers, which contains the medication that his physician ordered for him. His drawer is theoretically stocked with each day's medications by the pharmacist in the pharmacy and the medication is delivered to the patient's bedside either by the floor nurse or by a pharmacist responsible for that floor's medications. This method of delivery seems to promise: (a) fewer problems with medication control, (b) use of fewer outdated medications, (c) less chance of synergistic or antagonistic medications being given simultaneously, since the pharmacist keeps a "drug profile" for each patient and has the specialized knowledge to prevent such errors, (d) a closer, more intimate relationship among pharmacists, patients and staff and (e) greater opportunities for the pharmacist to educate patients, physicians and nurses concerning medications.

It has greatly helped doctors and nurses to have clinical pharmacists on the hospital unit. Since the whole health team is ultimately responsible for optimum health care delivery, it is essential that all team members work cooperatively, realizing that each has special expertise and skills to contribute to the care of the patient.

The Nurse's Role

The nurse's role in medication preparation and administration is complex and involves a number of important areas and a multitude of exacting tasks. First, the nurse must have *up-to-date knowledge* about the medications that she administers, e.g., indications for their use, routes and means of administration; range of dosages, side or toxic effects, and incompatibilities with other medications.

A second major area of the nurse's role involves *skills*. For example, nurses need specific skills in the correct methods of giving an IM injection, starting an IV, and other techniques. The nurse must also develop supervisory and teaching skills, because nurses are often responsible for: (a) instructing patients in self-medication techniques and (b) in states where it is legal, teaching licensed practical nurses to give medications.

Third, nurses are responsible for the *assessment* of patients who are or who will be taking medications. Because it is most frequently the nurse who gives medication to the patient, it is her job to obtain a medication history, even if such a history has already been taken by someone else (e.g., a clinical pharmacist). A typical medication history form is shown in Figure 31–7. Basically, a medication history is a component of the nursing assessment process. It should be completed during the initial interview with the patient and before any medica-

Text continued on page 755

ROGER WILLIAMS GENERAL HOSPITAL
PHYSICIAN'S ORDERS

PROBLEMS:

DRUG ALLERGIES:

☐ IN ACCORDANCE WITH OUR FORMULARY SYSTEM THE USE OF
GENERIC EQUIVALENTS ACCEPTABLE UNLESS BOX CHECKED.   ▲ ◀ ADDRESSOGRAPH IMPRINT ▶ ▲

INSTRUCTIONS FOR USE
1. IMPRINT SET BEFORE PLACING IN CHART.
2. DETACH TOP CARBONLESS COPY AND SEND TO PHARMACY EACH TIME DOCTOR WRITES A SET OF ORDERS.
3. INDICATE CARBONLESS COPY REMOVED BY PLACING INITIALS IN COLUMN OPPOSITE DOCTOR'S SIGNATURE.

DATE	TIME	ORDERS AND SIGNATURE	CH'KD	NURSE
		CCU ROUTINE ORDERS:		
		To be done in order written:		
		1. Start O_2 @ 4-6 L/min. via cannula or 8 L/m via mask.		
		2. Start IV of 500 5% D/W. Run at 20-30 micro gtts/m (20-30cc hr.) use Soluset.		
		3. Attach to cardiac monitor.		
		4. Temperatures 6^A - 10^A - 2^P - 10^P, BP & R q. 15' until stable for 1 hour then q. 2°.		
		5. Demerol 75 mg sc Stat if patient complaining of pain and was not medicated prior to admission to CCU; then sc q. 4° prn.		
		6. EKG Stat unless done in E.R., then daily X 2 days.		
		7. If EKG or monitor pattern at any time shows 5 pvc's or more per min., or R on T pvc start Xylocaine routine as follows:		
		a) Give Bolus of 50 mg. (2 1/2 cc 1% Xylocaine in 10cc through Soluset.		
		b) Attach 500cc D5W with Xylocaine 2% gm. to IV via 3 way stopcock.		
		c) Unless otherwise ordered, start at 30 micro gtts/min.; increase as necessary to eliminate pvc's. Must notify physician in order to raise rate up to 60 micro gtts/min.		
		Laboratory work to include:		
		8. CBC, PT, APTT, Chemistry Profile, Serology.		
		(continued on reverse side)		

Figure 31-6. Standing orders. (Courtesy of Roger Williams General Hospital.)

ROGER WILLIAMS GENERAL HOSPITAL
PHYSICIAN'S ORDERS

PROBLEMS:

DRUG ALLERGIES:

☐ IN ACCORDANCE WITH OUR FORMULARY SYSTEM THE USE OF GENERIC EQUIVALENTS ACCEPTABLE UNLESS BOX CHECKED.   ▲ ADDRESSOGRAPH IMPRINT ▲

INSTRUCTIONS FOR USE
1. IMPRINT SET BEFORE PLACING IN CHART.
2. DETACH TOP CARBONLESS COPY AND SEND TO PHARMACY EACH TIME DOCTOR WRITES A SET OF ORDERS.
3. INDICATE CARBONLESS COPY REMOVED BY PLACING INITIALS IN COLUMN OPPOSITE DOCTOR'S SIGNATURE.

DATE	TIME	ORDERS AND SIGNATURE	CH'KD	NURSE
		<u>CCU ROUTINE ORDERS (CONTINUED)</u>		
		9. SGOT, LDH, CPK on admission then daily X 2 days.		
		10. Portable chest X-ray on admission.		
		11. Strict coronary precautions:		
		a) absolute bed rest		
		b) feed, do not turn		
		c) when patient's condition is stable, may turn, feed and use commode.		
		12. Strict I & O.		
		13. Liquid diet — no iced drinks. When patient's condition stable advance to 1200 calorie, 2 gm na LO cholesterol soft diet, or other therapeutic diet as ordered by physician.		
		14. Urinalysis.		
		15. If admission is after last routine laboratory rounds, do stat CBC, BS, BUN, Electrolytes, SGOT, LDH & CPK.		
		16. If ventricular Fibrillation is observed on ECG tracing the trained registered nurse should proceed as follows if no physician immediately available.		
		a) hit patient hard on sternum with closed fist		
		b) call Code Blue		
		c) continue resuscitative procedures until physician arrives.		
		Signature:		
		Revised 11/25/75		

Figure 31-6 Continued

MEDICATION HISTORY

Name_____ Phone_____Age_____Weight_____

Occupation_____ Chief complaint_____

Clinical problems
(requiring drug therapy)

Known allergies (food, pollens, vaccines and drugs). Explain fully_____

1._____

2._____

3._____ Previous adverse drug reactions_____

4._____

5._____

Prescription drugs prior to admission

Name of drug	Dose	Duration of therapy	Reason for therapy

Non prescription drugs	No	Yes	Please Explain		**General**	No	Yes
Do you take sleep medications					Do you smoke		
Iron tonic or iron tablets					Do you drive a car regularly		
Vitamins			If yes, what kind		Do you work around machinery		
Eye drops					Have you had a blood transfusion in the past year		
Home remedies							
What do you take for pain					Have you been exposed to solvents or pesticides for long periods of time		
Headache							
Constipation					How often do you drink		
Diarrhea					How many drinks do you have		
Earaches							
Colds					**Diet**		
Heartburn					Do any foods upset your stomach		
Upset Stomach					Are you on a diet—low calorie		
Menstrual Pain					Low salt/sodium		
Do you carry any drugs with you					Low cholesterol		

Figure 31–7. Sample medication history form. (From Parker, W. A.: Medication histories. *American Journal of Nursing, 76*:1969, Dec. 1976.)

ions are given. After taking a drug history, the nurse alerts all who are involved in his medication therapy in order to protect the patient from medications to which he might be allergic. Once the patient starts his medication regimen, the nurse is responsible for assessing the patient's need for and responses to medications.

The fourth area of the nurse's role in medication is *recording* the medications that she administers, as well as recording the patient's reactions to them. Figure 31–8 provides examples of two types of medication records. Because the medication record is a legal document and a permanent part of the patient's chart, the nurse should write in an accurate, concise and legible way. It is vital that the nurse clearly indicate which medications were given and which medications were withheld, along with the reasons for withholding medication.

The *safeguarding, storage* and *care* of medications constitutes the fifth aspect of the nurse's role. For example, the nurse is responsible for making certain that the labels on medication bottles are clear and easily readable. It is also her job to store medications properly, to discard old medications (those that have passed their expiration date), to order stock medications (e.g., aspirin), to keep refrigerated medications at the proper temperature, etc.

In addition, the nurse must safeguard "controlled substances," of which narcotics and their synthetic derivatives are an example. The federal "Controlled Substance Act" (May 1971) controls the importation, production, compounding, selling, dealing in, dispensing and distribution of certain drugs of varying degrees of abuse potential.[46] Within the hospital, nurses are answerable to the Federal government for the day-to-day control of all narcotics and other controlled substances (e.g., barbiturates and amphetamines). The nurse must count, record, and sign for the quantity of controlled substances in her charge at the end of her shift. The procedure by which the "count" is done varies from institution to institution. However, in all institutions, controlled substances *must* be counted and signed for at each change of shift, in order to protect both the nurses who are leaving and the nurses coming on duty.

In addition, the nurse is accountable for the safe storage of narcotics on her floor or ward. Narcotics *must* be stored in a locked cupboard at all times, and the key to the cupboard must be kept by the charge person. Because of the potential for abuse of narcotics by both lay and professional persons, the responsibility for the storage and administration of narcotics is a grave one.

A sixth aspect of the nurse's role is to act as *role model* for the public, neighbors and friends and the patient. Thus, in regard to medications, nurses must practice what they preach. A nurse should avoid taking (a) any medications unless absolutely necessary, (b) most nonprescription drugs, (c) medications that are potentially addicting, (d) all nonprescription drugs if pregnancy is suspected or confirmed and (e) any other person's medications.

A final aspect of the nurse's role is to act as *patient advocate* and thus to protect the rights of patients to whom she administers medications. The rights of patients receiving medications are considered below.

RIGHTS AND RESPONSIBILITIES OF PATIENTS RECEIVING MEDICATIONS

Patients' rights have been a subject of great interest and concern in the past decade (see Chap. 20). Clearly, there are certain patient rights that must be kept in mind when administering medications.

Remember: patients receiving medications have the right to

▶ have drug history and allergies properly assessed by skilled practitioners

▶ be asked to give written consent before taking experimental medication

▶ be informed of drug name, actions and possible side effects

▶ receive medications safely and comfortably

▶ receive labeled medications

▶ avoid unnecessary medications

▶ refuse medications

While patients have rights, they also have important responsibilities as members of the health team. The major responsibilities of patients and family members regarding medications are as follows:

▶ to understand the therapy and to question, *to the best of their ability*, what they do not understand. (*Remember:* It is the professional's absolute responsibility to make certain that the patient or family understands his therapy.)

ROGER WILLIAMS GENERAL HOSPITAL
MEDICATION RECORD A

(Continuous Medications)

Name Plate

Medication	Freq. Dose Route	Hour 8am to 7pm	Due 8pm to 7am	8am to 7pm	8pm to 7am	8am to 7pm	8pm to 7am	8am to 7pm	8pm to 7am	8am to 7pm	8pm to 7am	8am to 7pm	8pm to 7am	8am to 7pm	8pm to 7am	8am to 7pm	8pm to 7am	8am to 7pm	8pm to 7am	8am to 7pm	8pm to 7am	8am to 7pm	8pm to 7am	8am to 7pm	8pm to 7am	8am to 7pm	8pm to 7am	8am to 7pm	8pm to 7am	8am to 7pm	8pm to 7am
Pen. G		8	8																												
	1,000,000 u	12	12																												
q 4°	IV	4	4																												

Initial Legend

MA	MEQuld RN

Room # 437   Name: Burnett, Karolyn   Allergic To: ∅   Diagnosis: R/o Meningitis

Figure 31–8. Medication record. (Courtesy of Roger Williams General Hospital.)

ROGER WILLIAMS GENERAL HOSPITAL

MEDICATION RECORD B

(Preliminary, Once Only, Prn, Stat Medications)

Name Plate

Medication	Dose Route	Frequency Date & Time due	AM	PM	AM	PM	AM	PM	AM	PM	AM	PM	AM	PM	AM	PM	AM	PM	AM	PM	AM	PM	AM	PM	AM	PM	AM	PM	AM	PM
Tylenol supp prn T > 103.6°F	300mg																													

Once only, Stat Medications

Due Date	Time Due	R.N. Init.	Medication	Given Time	Given Signature	Due Date	Time Due	R.N. Init.	Medication	Given Time	Given Signature

Figure 31–8 Continued

▶ to understand the ways in which patient or family will participate in the medical and pharmacologic therapy

▶ to comply with the regimen, e.g., take medication at correct times and in correct amounts for as long a time as prescribed, unless significant changes occur that warrant reassessment

▶ to notify the doctor or nurse of untoward effects instead of stopping the medication or continuing it without reporting the effects

▶ to refrain from asking for unneeded medication

▶ to refrain from "sharing" medications with others—friends, neighbors, children, relatives

▶ to discard old or unlabeled medication

It is the nurse's task to inform patients of their rights in regard to medications and to instruct patients and families about their responsibilities.

ASPECTS OF MEDICATION ADMINISTRATION

Systems for Giving Medications

Methods for giving medications in the hospital have gradually evolved over a number of years. Medication systems have been developed with three goals in mind: (1) reducing medication errors as much as possible, (2) reducing time and motion on the part of nurses and pharmacists and (3) maintaining cost within reasonable limits.

The four major kinds of medication systems in current use are: (a) the stock supply system, in which medications are stored in bulk for all the patients on a particular hospital floor or ward; (b) the individual cubicle system, which requires each patient to have his own cubicle in the medicine room that contains medications ordered specifically for him; (c) the unit dose system in which medications come from the manufacturer, in most instances, labeled as to generic name, trade name, dose warnings, recommendation for storage, and expiration date and (d) self-medication, in which the patient, after proper instruction, takes his own correctly labeled medications.

The use of the *stock supply system* is common in many agencies. Some advantages of this system are as follows: (a) many medications are constantly available, (b) no request slip or calls need to be made to the pharmacist for medication and (c) the medication regimen can be changed without having to return unused medications to the pharmacy.

Unfortunately, the disadvantages are many, e.g., (a) the nurse frequently has to order stock and fill shelves, (b) medications may be outdated, (c) costs may rise owing to the loss or misplacement of medications, (d) medication errors may increase owing to the numerous medications stocked on the shelves and (e) drugs may be stocked in a limited selection of strengths, requiring complicated dose calculations.

Many institutions use a system in which each patient has his own drawer, whether in the "med room" or in a rolling cart that can be moved from room to room. This system has the following advantages: (a) there is no loss of medication, (b) each patient pays for the medication used and should receive credit for unused, returned medications, (c) the pharmacist can provide medications that are not outdated and (d) the nurses' time is not spent ordering and stocking medications, as pharmacy aides are responsible for this task. Disadvantages include handling of numerous individual orders and charge slips.

The *unit dose packaging system* has been utilized for the control of narcotics for a number of years. The pharmacist's role in this system was discussed earlier. Recently, the most frequently ordered medications have been made available packaged in unit dosage form. Cost to the patient is less due to reduction in waste, since medication does not become contaminated. For the person administering the dose, the medication is completely labeled until opened at the patient's bedside. An unplanned advantage for the nurse can be the teaching associated with administration. For example, the medication can be identified by name, shape and color. Also, the nurse can point out the basic warnings, which are usually printed on the medication package.

Self-medication in agencies is not common except for those medications that patients take in emergencies, e.g., nitroglycerin, taken for chest pain due to cardiac disease. However, for selected patients, particularly those whose rehabilitation goals include independence, self-administration is being tried. While legal issues regarding controlled substances limit leaving these medications at the bedside, most other medications can be left in limited amounts for the patient who is learning self-care techniques. The health care team must work together to ensure that such a plan is workable, and each member of the team (including the patient) must understand his role and responsibility. Teaching opportunities arise frequently regarding the appropriate time, the right amount and the need for medications. The nurse should be aware of and utilize such opportunities.

The Timing of Medication Administration

The timing of medication administration involves (a) the number of doses the physician orders to be given each day, (b) the possible interaction of a medication with foods or fluids, (c) the number and kinds of other medications to be given and (d) the diagnostic and therapeutic examinations scheduled for the patient. Although the physician prescribes the number of times a day a medication is to be given, it is frequently the nurse who decides when the medication is *actually* given. She must make that decision in relation to (a) the standard times used by her agency or unit and (b) the goal of therapy. For example, if a physician writes an order for an antibiotic four times a day, the medication could be given at:

$$9a - 1p - 5p - 9p$$

or

$$6a - 12p - 6p - 12a$$

While both schedules read "four times a day," each schedule will provide the patient with a different circulating blood level of antibiotic over a 24-hour period. If the patient receives the antibiotic at $9a - 1p - 5p - 9p$, his blood level of the antibiotic will drop during the 12 hours between $9p$ and $9a$. On the other hand, if the patient is placed on a $6a - 12p - 6p - 12a$ schedule, his circulating blood level of antibiotic will remain fairly constant over the 24 hours. Unfortunately, the latter schedule requires that the nurse awaken the patient during the night, which interferes with his much needed rest. The nurse must know the effect of the specific drug and schedule the drug for the most therapeutic effect. If necessary, she should check with a pharmacist to determine which modifications of schedule will offer the patient the most therapeutic effect. If the medication interferes with the patient's needed sleep, the order should be clarified with the physician.

As apparent in the discussion above, there are other factors in addition to the physician's order that the nurse must consider when timing medication administration. For example, some medications should never be given with meals; others always. Certain medications are very dangerous—possibly even fatal—when ad-

ministered in combination with each other (see Table 16–10 for a listing of drugs in combination); other medication mixtures are completely compatible. Some medications must be withheld before diagnostic tests; other medications cannot be withheld safely. Until the nurse has sufficient clinical experience to make such decisions, she should consult with the physician and pharmacist.

Some researchers are studying the timing of medication administration in relation to biologic or circadian rhythms (see Chap. 3). As you recall, the application of theories concerning biologic rhythms to clinical medicine and nursing is still in its early stages. However, it is possible that within our lifetimes, medications will be administered at times that correlate with the patient's individual rhythms.

Safety Measures Pertinent to Medication Administration

Safety in medication administration is paramount. Through the years, procedures and policies have been developed to ensure that the patient receives the right medication in the right dosage at the right time and by the right route. There are three types of safety measures that must be observed when working with medications: (1) clear and verifiable communications concerning medications, (2) safeguarding the medications and (3) safeguarding the patient. Procedure 15 provides details about these measures.

Clear and Verifiable Communications. In a hospital setting, certain communications are essential to order, obtain, and safely deliver the medication to the patient. Generally, the physician or dentist writes an order (Fig. 31–9), which can be transcribed by a clerk or nurse by hand or a carbon copy of which can be forwarded to the pharmacy. Medication cards (Fig. 31–10) are made out according to the agency policy; the medication name, dosage, route and time are transferred to a medication Kardex (Fig. 31–11), chart or other patient record and/or a computer printout generated by the pharmacy. Before a medication can be safely administered to a patient, it is essential to check the medication card: (a) against the original order (when the medication is to be given for the first time) and (b) against the Kardex each time a medication is administered. If the person checking the medication cards notes an

ROGER WILLIAMS GENERAL HOSPITAL
PHYSICIAN'S ORDERS

PROBLEMS:

Burnett, Karolyn
321-76-0001

DRUG ALLERGIES:

☐ IN ACCORDANCE WITH OUR FORMULARY SYSTEM THE USE OF
GENERIC EQUIVALENTS ACCEPTABLE UNLESS BOX CHECKED.   ADDRESSOGRAPH   IMPRINT

INSTRUCTIONS FOR USE
1. IMPRINT SET BEFORE PLACING IN CHART.
2. DETACH TOP CARBONLESS COPY AND SEND TO PHARMACY EACH TIME DOCTOR WRITES A SET OF ORDERS.
3. INDICATE CARBONLESS COPY REMOVED BY PLACING INITIALS IN COLUMN OPPOSITE DOCTOR'S SIGNATURE.

DATE	TIME	ORDERS AND SIGNATURE	CH'KD	NURSE
5-8-77	4³⁰p	1. Admit: Dx r/o meningitis		
		2. Isolation precautions		
		3. Lab work: CBC, differential	✓	
		SGOT	✓	
		blood cultures x3	✓	
		chest x-ray	✓	
		4. Spinal tap ✓ done		
		5. Diet NPO	✓	
		6 IV's #1 1000cc D₅NS 8hr	up	
		#2 1000cc D₅NS + MVI 10hr		
		#3 1000cc D₅NS + MVI 10hr		
		7. Vital signs q 2 hr	✓	
		T > 103.6°F Tylenol Supp 300mg		
		8. Medications		
		Pen G IV 1,000,000 u q 4 hours		P. Kane RN
		9. Activity: bed rest		
		C. Charles, MD		

DOCTOR: DO NOT WRITE NEW ORDERS ON THIS FORM IF NO CARBONLESS
COPIES REMAIN AS INDICATED IN WINDOW AT RIGHT; PLEASE
START A NEW FORM.

136164 (REV. 10/74)

NUMBER OF CARBONLESS
COPIES REMAINING IN SET.   ▶ 1

SEND TO DEPARTMENT OF PHARMACY

Figure 31–9. Physician's orders. (Courtesy of Roger Williams General Hospital.)

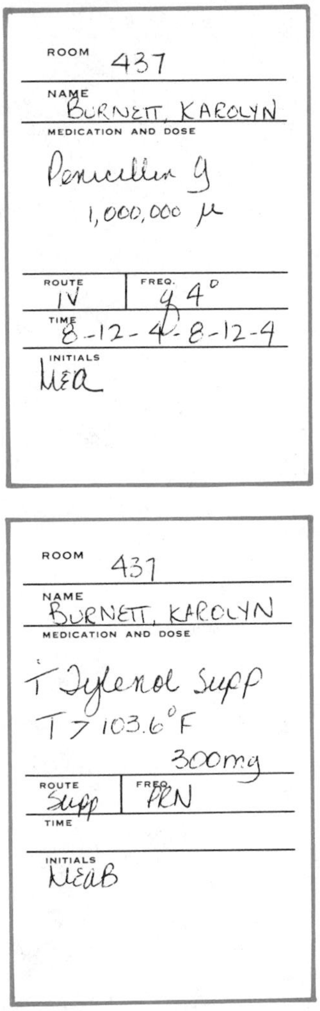

Figure 31-10. Medication cards.

rolling cart until they are delivered to the patient. It is essential that labels be clean and easily readable. Medications that need to be refrigerated should be dated and kept at the recommended temperature. Medications that have an expiration date printed on them must be returned to the pharmacy or discarded (according to agency policy) as their date approaches.

> *At no time should an outdated medication be given to a patient: the therapeutic effect may be less than desired, or totally lacking.*

When a tray is being used to deliver medications to the patient, it should not be left unattended at any time.

Narcotics and other controlled substances should be counted before and after a medication is poured and signed for by the nurse responsible for the key or by her designate. Controlled substances are counted at the end of each shift by the out-going and on-coming nurses, as described previously.

Safeguarding the Patient. The patient should be safeguarded by a system that ensures his receiving the medications that have been ordered for him. All efforts must be directed at the prevention of errors. Most established medication procedures, if conscientiously followed, will prevent the majority of errors, e.g., checking the patient's arm band and calling him by name before giving him medication, making certain that the patient swallows the medication, etc.

Unfortunately, because doctors and nurses are human and thus not perfect, medication errors do occur. To account for errors in medications given (i.e., wrong medication, dosage, route, time or patient), all agencies have a special form for reporting errors called an *incident report* (Fig. 31–12). The report includes patient identifying data and the nurse's narrative regarding the events of the incident. In addition to making out an incident report, the nurse or appropriate person should notify the patient's physician of the error. It is particularly important to call the physician immediately if the medication error involved giving the *wrong drug* to the patient or giving a *higher dosage* than the physician ordered. The physician will then decide what action to take to counteract the medication error.

error on either the card or the Kardex, it must be reported to the appropriate person at once. In addition, any order that the nurse thinks questionable should be checked with the physician. Legitimate questions will ultimately lead to safe patient care.

> Remember:
> *Because of the number of people involved in the ordering and administration of medications (doctors, pharmacists, nurses), the possibility of human error in the interpretation of orders is ever present. Errors are significantly reduced if communications concerning medication orders are checked and double-checked before a medication is given to the patient.*

Safeguarding Medications. Medications are carefully monitored by the pharmacy. They should be kept in a locked cabinet or locked

006242-A

PATIENT CARE PLAN

GOAL

Init., Date & Shift	PATIENT NEED / PROBLEMS	NURSING APPROACH	PATIENT RESPONSE

Date	NURSING PROCEDURES	Date	MEDICATIONS
		5/8	Pen G 1,000,000 μ IV q 4°
		5/8	Tylenol Supp prn ① > 103.6 °F (300mg)

Room 437   Name BURNETT, K.   Nurse's Interview (When completed) ☐

Figure 31–11. Medication Kardex. (Courtesy of Roger Williams General Hospital.)

Psychologic Factors in Medication Administration

Psychologic factors are important in both the administration of and the patient's compliance with the medication regimen. One's *past experiences* with medications can lead to either a positive or a negative attitude toward the effect expected or toward the actual effect. *Motivational factors* need to be considered also when giving medications. For example, some persons believe that "more medicines" will lead to quicker recovery or immediate relief of symptoms. Life-threatening illnesses such as diabetes may prompt one person to conscientiously take a medication while another person, in denial of the illness, omits dosages. Another example of a highly motivated individual would be a woman who diligently takes her birth control medications

Roger Williams General Hospital, Providence, R.I.   **PATIENT INCIDENT REPORT**

PATIENT

PATIENTS LAST NAME	FIRST NAME	MIDDLE INITIAL	ROOM NO.	AGE	SEX ☐ MALE ☐ FEMALE

ADMITTING DIAGNOSIS	ATTENDING PHYSICIAN

UNIT OR AREA (INJURY) (INCIDENT) OCCURRED IN	DATE (INJURY) (INCIDENT) OCCURRED	TIME OF OCCURENCE ☐ AM ☐ PM	CHARGE NURSE

APPARENT CONDITION BEFORE INCIDENT ☐ ORIENTED ☐ DISORIENTED | TYPE OF MEDICATION WITHIN PAST 6 HOURS ☐ SEDATIVE ☐ TRANQUILIZER ☐ NARCOTIC ☐ OTHER (SPECIFY) | ACTIVITY ORDERS (INDICATE)

TYPE OF INCIDENT
☐ FALL ☐ MEDICATION ☐ PROCEDURE ☐ TREATMENT ☐ BURN ☐ OTHER (Specify)

BED RAIL ORDERED BY PHYSICIAN ☐ YES ☐ NO	BED RAIL IN POSITION ☐ YES ☐ NO	BED POSITION ☐ HIGH ☐ LOW	SIGNAL CORD NEAR ☐ YES ☐ NO

GENERAL

WITNESS LAST NAME	FIRST NAME	MIDDLE INITIAL	HOME PHONE	R.W.G.H. EMPLOYEE ☐ YES ☐ NO

ADDRESS — NUMBER AND STREET	CITY	STATE	ZIP CODE

EXAMINING PHYSICIAN'S NAME	DATE OF EXAMINATION	TIME OF EXAMINATION ☐ AM ☐ PM	X-RAY ORDER ☐ YES ☐ NO

SUPERVISOR NOTIFIED ☐ YES ☐ NO	TIME	☐ AM ☐ PM	ATTENDING PHYSICIAN NOTIFIED ☐ YES ☐ NO	TIME	☐ AM ☐ PM

INJURY INCIDENT

TO BE FILLED IN BY CHARGE NURSE OR ADMIN. NURSING SUPERVISOR   DESCRIBE THE (INJURY) (INCIDENT) AND CIRCUMSTANCES LEADING TO IT . . . INCLUDE ALL PERTINENT INFORMATION (use additional paper if necessary).

SIGNATURE OF CHARGE NURSE OR SUPERVISOR

MEDICAL FINDINGS

TO BE FILLED IN BY PHYSICIAN   PHYSICIAN'S FINDINGS IN DETAIL

SIGNATURE OF EXAMINING PHYSICIAN

PREVENTION

TO BE FILLED IN BY CHARGE NURSE OR ADMIN. NURSING SUPERVISOR   REMEDY (AS A SUPERVISOR, WHAT ACTION HAVE YOU TAKEN OR PROPOSE TO TAKE TO PREVENT RECURRENCE?)

SIGNATURE OF CHARGE NURSE OR SUPERVISOR

REMARKS

ADDITIONAL INFORMATION AND SAFETY COMMITTEE COMMENTS

SUPERVISOR'S SIGNATURE	TITLE	DATE
SIGNATURE OF NURSING DIRECTOR		
SIGNATURE OF HOSPITAL FIRE/SAFETY DIRECTOR		

White — Insurance Company   Pink — Nursing Admin. Copy
Yellow — Safety Committee   Goldenrod — Hospital Admin. Copy   *N.C.R. PAPER — USE BALL POINT PEN — PRESS HARD

Figure 31–12. Patient incident report. (Courtesy of Roger Williams General Hospital.)

as prescribed in order to avoid an unwanted pregnancy.

If a nurse finds that her patient is not complying with the medication regimen, she needs to examine the situation. *Compliance* and *noncompliance* have been investigated by many nurse researchers. Some of the reasons for noncompliance have been linked to forgetting, thinking one is "better," feeling that the cure is worse than the disease, and not having enough money to fill or refill prescriptions. Individuals with chronic disease may have high percentages of forgetting; persons with neurological diseases may be unable to self-administer medications or to remember if medications were taken.

Another important psychologic factor is the tendency toward *drug abuse* among many patients and some professional people. Unfortunately, narcotics and barbiturates are not the only drugs abused; frequently over-the-counter drugs are indiscriminately purchased by an unknowing public. More informative labeling, public education campaigns and certain limitations on mass advertising are designed to eliminate many of the abuses. Every person is different, and therefore, when the nurse encounters a problem of drug abuse she must investigate the individual situation. The nurse has an obligation to prevent abuses of medications; this can be done through role-modeling, through education of patient groups and the general public and through judicious use of "prn" medications.

Assessing the Patient Receiving Medications

The nurse is vitally involved in the assessment of the patient receiving medications. She assesses both the patient's need for medications and the effectiveness of the medications. Assessment begins during the taking of the *nursing history*, when the nurse inquires about the patient's use and need for medications as well as previous response to therapy. The *medication history* was mentioned earlier (see Fig. 31–7). The nursing history should be a written document, preferably included in the nursing notes of the patient's agency chart. Critical information, such as previous allergies or adverse reactions to medications, should be noted on the patient's arm band and in a conspicuous place on the cover of the patient's chart, as well

as in the nursing care plan Kardex. Suggested questions in a nursing history form are listed below. Specialized agencies would require more specific information, e.g., a diabetic clinic or an oncology (cancer) clinic, and the questions can be elaborated and adapted as necessary.

1. Are you currently taking any medication?
2. What medications do you take?
3. What are they for?
4. Have you ever experienced an adverse reaction to any medications (e.g., penicillin, sulfa drugs, anesthetics, novocaine)?
5. How did you react?
6. If you take insulin, are you able to give your own injection?
7. Do you have any difficulty with vision, strength or swallowing that the nurses should know about to help you while you are in the hospital?
8. If you have been hospitalized before, did you require a sleeping medication?
9. *Nurses' observations*
   a. Note if the following are normal or abnormal. If abnormal, describe the difficulty.
     Vision
     Hearing
     Swallowing
     Language problem (foreign language or comprehension difficulty)
     Level of consciousness
     Condition of skin, veins, muscles
     Strength in extremities
   b. Does patient have the following:
     (1) Knowledge of own history?
     (2) Family or friend to assist at home?
     (3) Desire to assist in therapy?
   c. Does patient understand the medication regimen?
   d. Has patient experienced hospitalization before? Does he understand distribution system for regular and prn medications?
10. Additional Comments

It is the physician's responsibility to assess and prescribe medications for the patient, based on the clinical, laboratory and physical examination findings. After this has been completed, he delegates responsibility to the nurse, patient and family to carry out the regimen. When a medication is ordered "prn" (give as necessary), it is essential that the purpose of the medication is clearly understood, as well as the limitations of dosage and frequency. (The order *prn* does not mean that the patient must ask for the medication.) In the hospital, most narcotics are written to be given every 3 to 4 hours as necessary (q. 3–4 hrs. prn), and sleeping capsules are prescribed for bedtime and may repeat once (e.g., Seconal 100 mg. prn H.S. may repeat × 1). The nurse's clinical judgment is important in determining the need for and the response to medications. Clinical judgment is learned, and until such time as the student or new graduate nurse feels competent, a more experienced nurse should be consulted before a prn medication is administered.

The effectiveness of medications can be judged in several ways: clinical observation, measurement and determination of body fluids and observation and use of monitoring systems.

Clinical observation takes into consideration both objective and subjective data. Objective data can include such data as desirable changes in pulse, temperature and respiration. Subjective data can include statements made by the patient that indicate a response to the medication, such as "My cough is less severe since I took the cough syrup."

Blood serum level determinations can assist the physician in deciding whether to increase or decrease dosages and in identifying overdosage (intentional or unintentional). Gas chromatography can also be used in assessment of medication levels. The patient's serum is chemically analyzed and fractionally extracted or absorbed on a porous solid. The laboratory can then evaluate the level as therapeutic or not by analyzing the resultant "picture."

Urine can also be analyzed to determine the effectiveness of some medications. Urine levels are checked when there is some question about the reliability of the patient taking the medication or when urinary clearance is questioned.

Other body fluids, exudates and transudates can be chemically analyzed to determine medication effectiveness. While these procedures are not routinely done, the nurse may be asked to assist in obtaining specimens from wounds, drains or spinal column fluid for this purpose.

Monitoring systems can be helpful in assessing the patient's response to therapy. Monitoring is particularly useful in coronary care units when a patient may have experienced an arrhythmia (abnormal heart rhythm) and is receiving a medication to diminish or counteract the abnormal rhythm. A nurse working on a coronary care unit has special education and skills to evaluate the effectiveness of the medications. New nurses should not be asked to monitor patients for medication effectiveness, as life-threatening rhythm disturbances may occur without their cognizance.

The nurse is also responsible for assessing the need for revising or terminating a medication regimen. Again, this kind of clinical judgment is learned, but knowledge about the ex-

pected effects of medications will assist the nurse in developing these skills. When the nurse recognizes a need for revision or termination of a medication regimen, it is *not* her responsibility to alter or stop the medication. She should consult with the physician. Together, their observations and expectations can result in the best possible care for the patient.

An example of a situation in which a nursing assessment led to revision of a medication regimen follows:

Ms. K. Townsend was admitted to the hospital complaining of a severe cough, fever and pleuritic pain. Her diagnosis was pneumonococcal pneumonia. A sample of her sputum was taken and sent to the laboratory for culture and sensitivity determination. Without awaiting the laboratory results, the physician prescribed intramuscular penicillin to counteract the bacteria. The patient's nursing and medication histories did not reveal any medication allergies or sensitivities.

Thirty minutes following the first intramuscular injection, Ms. Townsend developed urticaria (raised, pale wheals) of her thighs. The nurse contacted the physician immediately. He prescribed an antihistaminic and changed the patient's prescription to another antibacterial preparation.

As allergic reactions may occur within minutes of intramuscular or intravenous administration of medication, it is important to observe the patient carefully for adverse side effects. Even patients who have no history of sensitivities may have an untoward reaction.

Patients with Special Needs

The nurse often encounters patients who need special assistance in taking medications. *Children* pose particular difficulties for the medication nurse. One problem may be the need for *special dosages.* You will recall that dosage calculations for children are weight related or age related. While drug companies have developed pediatric dosages for many medications, the nurse is still responsible for checking all dosages and sometimes for calculating dosages. A second problem that arises is that most children object to *ingesting substances that are bitter or unpalatable.* Fortunately, pharmaceutical houses produce many medications in the form of sugar syrups to disguise their taste and thus facilitate administration to children. If the medication does not come in a syrup form, the nurse must crush the medication and place it in a medium such as ice cream, custards, or applesauce in order to make it palatable to the child who cannot swallow a capsule or tablet. A third difficulty the nurse may encounter is that most children *fear needles and injections.* Depending upon the age of the child and his previous experience with injections, the nurse should alter her approach to the medication administration. It can be generally stated that the injection should be quickly but safely administered and that the child, if at all possible, should be held and comforted by a parent or nurse after the procedure. Some children's hospitals have a program of role-playing in which a child is given a syringe and a doll and allowed and encouraged to vent his frustrations by giving "shots" to the doll. While not uniformly successful, this approach could be used for desensitization and as a safe outlet for aggressions.

Some *geriatric* patients may have special needs when taking medications. It is the nurse's responsibility to assess what those needs are and to assist elderly individuals to take their medications in the manner easiest for them. Some common problems relate to the *neurosensory system.* For example, blind diabetic persons may have difficulty drawing the right dosage of insulin into a syringe; blind and deaf patients may have difficulty implementing instructions given to them; confused patients may or may not know if they have taken a medication.

Unconscious patients may also present the nurse with problems. Oral medications may need to be given through a nasogastric tube after they are crushed and put in a fluid medium. Medications for unconscious patients can also be administered via the veins or into the muscle until such time as the patient's symptoms are controlled or he regains consciousness (see Chap. 38). However, an altered route of administration requires a written change of order by the physician.

Another commonly encountered problem is the patient with *impaired* sensation of the oropharynx and concomitant *impaired swallowing.* For the patient with unilateral (one-sided) impaired sensation or motor ability, the nurse can administer the medications, often crushed and mixed with ice cream or applesauce, by placing the medication in the patient's mouth on the unaffected side and laterally flexing his head to the unaffected side. The patient can then safely swallow. For patients with severely impaired swallowing ability, it is not safe to give medications orally. Aspiration (drawing into the lungs) may occur, which can result in an aspiration pneumonia. Until the swallowing abilities return, it is preferable to give medications intramuscularly, intravenously or through a nasogastric or gastrostomy tube.

Patients always have a right to refuse treatment, including medications. While it does not happen very often, a nurse will sometimes meet a patient who does refuse to take medications. Such patients present the nurse with a real challenge. The excellent nurse would discuss the situation with the patient in a quiet and nonjudgmental way. She would try to understand the patient's point of view, and she would explain the therapeutic rationale for the prescribed medication. In this way, a satisfactory conclusion is usually reached and effective patient care is achieved. Either the patient agrees to the medication as prescribed or the nurse advocates for the patient with the doctor and/or pharmacist and an alternate medical regimen is established.

For the patient with tendencies toward *abuse of drugs,* it should be the nurse's obligation to see that medications are controlled and the patient does not have inordinate opportunities for abuse.

The nurse may encounter a patient with *chronic, long-term pain,* unrelieved by multiple medical, surgical or psychiatric maneuvers. Behavior modification programs are being used successfully to ablate the pain behavior. One successful maneuver has been to have the patient participate in developing a "contract" (similar to a legal document), which allows certain privileges for non–pain related behavior. Other programs do this but in addition have developed a "pain cocktail," which is given every 4 hours around-the-clock. Therefore, the medication is not contingent on pain behavior. Initially, the pain cocktail consists of a certain dosage of an analgesic in a syrup solution. Over a 6-to-8 week period, the physician orders a gradual reduction of the dosage of the analgesic. While the patient *knows* the analgesic is being reduced, he does not know *when or how much.* This contract allows the patient to be gradually "weaned" from the analgesic while learning acceptable coping behavior for the pain. The underlying theory is that as behavior is learned, it can also be unlearned and new, socially acceptable behavior can be learned. This plan has been most successful when the patient is an active participant in the contract negotiation. The nurse must ignore pain behavior and not ask the patient about the quality, intensity, etc., of his pain when the patient is on a behavior modification program.

Basically there are two forms of oral medications: solid and liquid. The administration of each of these forms carries with it distinct nursing responsibilities.

Administration of Solid Forms of Oral Medication

The most commonly used solid forms of medication include tablets, capsules, powders, pills and lozenges.

Tablets can be *prolonged acting,* which means that the medication has been specially formulated for absorption at various times or places in the gastrointestinal tract. Some prolonged action tablets need to be spaced between meals for maximum therapeutic effect. Others are unaffected by the presence of food or the process of digestion. *Enteric-coated* tablets are medications that have been coated with a hard surface that impedes their absorption until the tablet has left the stomach. Tablets of this sort should *never* be chewed or broken or crushed for ease of administration, because they have an irritating effect on the stomach mucosa. Dosages that require the nurse to divide these tablets must be reviewed with the doctor before the medication is given. Conversely, there are tablets that are intended to be chewed for maximum therapeutic effect. The nurse should endeavor to teach the patient the appropriate means of taking these medications.

Capsules are made of hard or soft gelatin. They contain medications that are powdered, semiliquid or granular. The capsule is used as a vehicle to ease administration. Capsules are not to be chewed, but swallowed whole. If the patient has a nasogastric tube in his stomach for feeding purposes, the nurse can open the gelatin capsule and mix the medication in another solution for administration through the tube. Hard capsules should not be broken for oral administration because the medication that they contain is irritating to the mouth and esophagus. Soft capsules may be opened and mixed with jelly or other food to disguise their taste.

Medications that come in forms to be mixed with liquids (water or juices) prior to administration are called *powders.* Powders come in three basic forms: bulk, effervescent powders and effervescent tablets. *Bulk powders* are frequently utilized on nursing units. Because they must be mixed by the nurse prior to administration, dosages and solution must be accurately calculated and measured. As some powders turn into gelatinous solutions within minutes of the mixing, often the powder and the water or juice must be mixed at the patient's bedside immediately prior to administration. Dosages need to be carefully determined, either by weight or volume. *Medicated effervescent powders* and *tablets* are intended to be mixed immediately prior to administration and to be swallowed immediately after dissolution of the powder or tablet. The effervescence is a mechanism by which unpleasant medications are made more palatable. Because of the unpleasant taste, it is essential that the medication be swallowed quickly. Some patients claim that holding their nostrils shut while they swallow helps to overcome the unpleasant taste. Iced fluid also helps mask the taste. Manufacturers have tried to make effervescent medications palatable and to eliminate bitter after-tastes by using citrus flavorings. In some of the medications, the gaseous bubbles that form are a part of the therapy, and therefore, the patient should *not* drink a large amount of water afterwards to mask the taste. The nurse is reminded to read manufacturers' recommendations carefully.

Pills are an infrequent dosage form. Nevertheless, the public as well as the health professions often call all oral medications "pills." A "pill" is a mixture of medication(s) with a cohesive material. The mixture is then molded into shapes and sizes suitable to swallow.

Lozenges are a solid form of a liquid, which should be sucked, not chewed, until completely dissolved: Some medications are destroyed by the acid media of the stomach, and absorption takes place in the oral mucosa; for some medications, there is a desired local therapeutic effect which would be lost if the lozenge were chewed and swallowed. Lozenges available in over-the-counter forms for coughs and "ticklish" throats often contain medicational properties that, if taken in excess, over-medicate or mask the important symptoms of the individual. The nurse should caution persons to use any over-the-counter products judiciously.

Administration of Liquid Forms of Oral Medication

The other common form of oral medication is the various types of liquids: syrup, solution, suspension, and alcohol-water. *Syrups* are a blend of medication in a sugared or fruit-based liquid. The taste of the medication is effectively masked in most situations. Syrups can be used for (a) *coughs,* in which case they should not be followed by liquid of any sort, as the medicating effect is local and would be thus washed away, (b) *pain cocktails,* in which various dosages of opiates and tranquilizers are mixed to allow the patient freedom from injections and (c) *infant medications,* because they are easily administered by the use of a dropper, the taste is acceptable and infant acceptance is good.

Solutions are homogeneous mixtures of a liquid and a solid medication form, similar to syrups. They may be swallowed as prepared by the manufacturer or may require further dilution in another medium to prevent oral irritation or to dilute the taste.

Suspensions are mixtures of two or more substances which settle out upon standing. Because they do settle, gels, magmas (thick, milky suspensions of an inorganic substance) and emulsions (suspensions of fine droplets of oil) must be shaken prior to each administration or improper dosages will be given. Whether or not the patient may follow the dosage with water or juice to clear his mouth depends on the desired effect of the medication.

Elixirs are drug preparations in a solvent medium of alcohol and water (a *hydroalcoholic* medium) plus sugar. Because of their composition, elixirs are slightly sweet-tasting, inoffensive smelling medications that are relatively pleasant to ingest. Common examples of elixirs include elixir of terpin hydrate, which is a cough medicine, and elixir of phenobarbital, which is a sedative.

Tinctures are preparations derived from animal or plant drugs or from chemical substances which are dissolved in a hydroalcoholic medium. Tinctures range in strength from 10 per cent to 20 per cent. Common tinctures include tincture of belladonna (a smooth muscle relaxer), tincture of iodine (a topical antiseptic) and tincture of opium (an intestinal sedative).

Emulsions are pharmaceutical mixtures characterized by the suspension of fats, oils, or petrolatum in water. Examples of oily liquids are mineral oil, which is a lubricating laxative and stool softener, and codliver oil, which is an important source of vitamins A and D. Some emulsions contain particles that tend to join together and settle to the bottom of the bottle, e.g., milk of magnesia. Such emulsions must always be thoroughly shaken before they are poured into a cup and administered to the patient.

The procedure for administering oral medications, whether solid or liquid, is generally the same. The principles and steps for the administration of oral medications are discussed in Procedure 15.

15. ADMINISTERING ORAL MEDICATIONS

Definition and Purposes.   *Methods for preparing, transporting, administering and recording oral medications to patients safely and accurately.* Oral medications are administered for their therapeutic effects upon the body, e.g., alleviation of pain, correction of imbalances, etc.

Contraindications and Cautions.   Oral medications should not be given to persons (a) who have impaired swallowing, (b) who are unconscious or (c) who refuse to take medications orally. In such cases, discuss the situation with the patient, doctor and pharmacist as appropriate. An alternative regimen may be decided on, e.g., stopping medication, prescribing medication in a more acceptable form or by an alternate route (injection, nasogastric tube). Oral medications that are highly irritating to the gastric mucosa may need to be diluted in a fluid or given with meals. The nurse should employ all safety measures possible, e.g., have knowledge of medication, double-check calculations for correct dosage, etc. Medications should never be left unlocked or unattended. Also, the nurse should: (a) develop safe and effective habit patterns to reduce errors, (b) use clean techniques, (c) report and record accurately and (d) be knowledgeable about steps to take when medication error occurs.

Patient-Family Teaching Points.   Provide the patient and family with the following information as appropriate: (a) tell the patient the name of the medication and how it works, (b) explain the need for the medication, (c) explain how often the medication is to be given, (d) teach the necessity for following the prescription, (e) explain the side effects to be expected, as well as those that should be reported, (f) point out the relationship or interaction of the medication with activities, rest, food and fluid intake and (g) emphasize the need to take the medication for the duration of the prescribed time.

PRE-PROCEDURE ACTIVITIES

PRELIMINARY PATIENT ASSESSMENT

Includes determination of:
- diagnosis
- age
- abilities and limitations in swallowing
- presence of nausea or vomiting
- presence of oral or esophageal lesions
- comfort of patient
- prior experience with medications; i.e., does patient find medication objectionable in any way

EQUIPMENT
- Medication cards
- Medication tray
- Souffle cups
- Plastic measuring cups
- Drinking water, juice
- Drinking straws
- Adequate lighting (if necessary, a flashlight for evening and night duty)

PREPARATION OF PATIENT

- Discuss need for medication with patient
- Provide information about medication
- Assist to sitting position
- Moisten mouth prior to giving medications
- Offer each medication separately
- Offer fluid as necessary to aid in absorption of medication

PROCEDURE

SUGGESTED STEPS

A. Gather medication cards or form containing medication orders and Kardex (or medication sheet).

RATIONALE/DISCUSSION

A. Medication cards are a device for convenience, but may be misplaced or lost. The *Kardex* is also written from original order but is a more reliable source. The physician's order on the chart is the only legal source.

> *Remember: When giving medications for first time, check medication cards and Kardex against original order in chart.*

Procedure continued on the following page

SUGGESTED STEPS	RATIONALE/DISCUSSION
1. Systematically check medication cards (or record) against Kardex (or medication sheet) for completeness, accuracy and expiration date.	1. Helps identify errors made when medication orders were transcribed from chart to: (a) Kardex (or medication sheet) and (b) medication cards. Identifies missing medication cards, verifies medication cards.
2. Notify appropriate staff member of errors or omissions on cards or Kardex.	2. Initiates action to rectify or alleviate error. Appropriate individual must initiate "Incident Report" (see discussion in text) if error is found.
3. Correct cards, Kardex and/or records if they do not comply with physician's order, with guidance of appropriate individual.	3. Reduces potential errors and promotes patient's safety. Previous errors in medication or dose must remain in chart as given.
B. Pull your own medication reference card for each medication to be given. Card contains this information: (a) medication name, (b) route, (c) dosage, (d) time and (e) stop date on some medications. If you do not have personal reference cards, look up medication in agency references.	B. Knowledge concerning medications is basic to determining appropriate action. It is the nurse's responsibility to correlate information from reliable drug sources for optimum therapeutic effect.
C. Know patient's diagnosis, the purpose of the medication and its intended therapeutic effect.	C. This information helps nurse determine if patient is receiving intended therapeutic effect from medication.
D. Wash hands.	D. Bacterial contamination of skin may contaminate medication and/or equipment; increases risk of transfer of organisms.
E. Obtain key and unlock medicine drawer or cart.	E. Medications are safeguarded when kept in locked cupboard or cart.

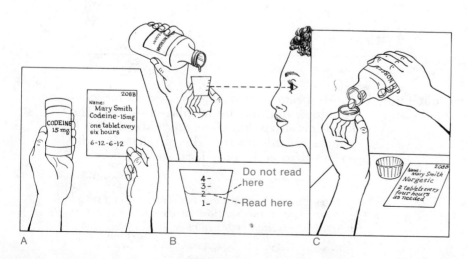

Figure 31–13. Pouring medication. *A* demonstrates the nurse comparing the medication to the medication bottle. *B* shows the nurse properly pouring and measuring liquid medications. Note that a liquid is poured at eye level. The nurse's thumb nail indicates proper fill mark. To check dosage, set on level surface and read fluid level at bottom of meniscus. Proper pouring of tablets and capsules is shown in *C*. With medication card in sight, pour medication first into cap, and then into souffle cup. In this way, if too many are poured, extras can be returned to original bottle. *Do not handle medications with fingers.*

SUGGESTED STEPS	RATIONALE/DISCUSSION
F. Assemble appropriate equipment or supplies. Arrange cards *purposefully*, basically by location of each patient. Keep all medications for one patient together.	F. Organization and planning result in safe practices as well as in economy of time and effort.
G. Prepare medication.	G. Pour one medication at a time to ensure accuracy and prevent errors.
1. Obtain medication from drawer or closet, compare with medication card. *First safety check.* (Fig. 31–13.)	1. Use of one medication card at a time, comparing with drug to be poured, reduces possibility of pouring the wrong medication. Remember to read the entire label, including expiration date.
2. Measure medication. (Calculate dose if necessary.)	2. Use paper and pencil to calculate dose. Request supervision from appropriate individual until absolutely certain of accuracy.
a. Pour solid medications (tablets, capsules, etc.) into cap first, then into souffle cup (Fig. 31–13). To prevent accidental mixing of medications, never pour back extra tablets from souffle cup. Discard extra tablets.	a. Shaking medications into cap while holding bottle and cap together makes obtaining desired number of medication easier. Extra tablets are in contact with bottle, not with souffle cup.
b. Pour liquids from side of bottle into plastic measuring cup. Place thumb nail at correct measurement mark. Read plastic measuring cup at bottom of meniscus for liquids (Fig. 31–13). If too much is poured, pour excess in sink. Hold measuring cup at eye level for accuracy in measurement. Wipe lip of bottle with paper.	b. Pouring from side of bottle prevents obliteration of label. Placing thumb nail at correct measurement maintains location of correct dose since some medications obliterate the markings. "Palming label" maintains legible label. To prevent contamination, never pour medication back into bottle. Wiping maintains clean bottle that seals easily.
c. If unit dose, leave medication in wrapper to be opened at patient's bedside.	c. Maintains individual label of medication for an additional safety check.
3. Recheck medication bottle with card. *Second safety check.* (Fig. 31–13.)	3. Guards against error. Make certain dose has been calculated and measured accurately.
4. Return medication bottle to storage, reading label. Check card again. *Third safety check.*	
H. Place card with medication on tray.	H. Proper identification of each medication assures accurate administration of correct medication to correct patient.

Procedure continued on the following page

SUGGESTED STEPS	RATIONALE/DISCUSSION
I. Repeat steps G and H for preparation of each medication. Pour each medication into a separate container.	I. Mixing medications in a single container is hazardous. If medication spills, patient refuses one or more, or one medication must be withheld, nurse is dependent on knowing color and shape of each of the medications in order to replace or record omission.
J. Lock medicine cabinet or room.	J. Safety of medications is protected when locked cupboard is provided.
K. Take medications to patient at correct time.	K. Medications should be given on time to maximize therapeutic effect. (Within 20 minutes before and 20 minutes after the designated time is accepted as "on time.")
L. Identify patient with medication card or medication record. Methods available are:	L. Responsibility for proper identification is the nurse's. Agency policy often requires use of three methods of identification.
1. Address by name in a questioning voice.	1. Requires a response from patient. Confused patients may answer to another name. If you are in doubt, ask patient to state his name.
2. Read name at door or bedside.	2. Not infallible, for patients have been known to crawl into another patient's bed.
3. Read name on I.D. band.	3. Most accurate identification. Make sure missing name bands are replaced!
4. Verify identification with staff member who knows patient.	
M. Assess patient for appropriateness of medication administration (i.e., take apical pulse for patient receiving digitalis preparation).	M. Clinical assessment should precede administration.
N. Administer medication.	
1. Assist patient to sitting position if possible.	1. Swallowing is easier in sitting position.
2. Administer medication in accord with patient's comfort and needs.	2. Individuals differ in style of taking medications. Illness may require modification.
a. Allow patient to take tablets, capsules all at once or one at a time; place in patient's hand or use souffle cup.	a. Patients should be encouraged to identify their medications and report any deviation from usual appearance or number.

SUGGESTED STEPS	RATIONALE/DISCUSSION
b. Place tablets, capsules in patient's mouth using your clean fingers if patient unable to do so.	b. Assists in placement of medication for ease in swallowing.
c. If patient has difficulty swallowing medications, give small amount of fluid to moisten mouth, place pill on back of tongue, slightly flex head, give a mouthful of fluid and instruct to "swallow."	c. Patients who have difficulty in swallowing "pills" usually make the error of throwing back their heads (hyperextension), making swallowing very difficult. Remember, artificial respiration uses the head back position to *open the airway*.
3. Administer medication properly (e.g., dilute drugs that stain teeth and give through straw). Remind patient to allow buccal tablets or lozenges to melt in cheek or mouth.	3. Do not give fluids after cough syrup or medications to be melted in mouth.
4. Disguise ill-tasting or objectionable medications: Some should be well diluted, others iced or disguised in food or juice.	4. Use judgment about disguises: prevent overhydration or development of aversion to food used as disguise. Iced fluids may numb taste buds and be less aromatic.
5. Encourage consumption of fresh cold fluid unless patient is on limited fluids.	5. Chart liquids given with medication: for Intake and Output and/or individual preference. Patients on limited fluids usually have a stated volume that can be taken with medication.
O. Check patient's mouth when indicated to verify that medications are swallowed. Do not leave medications at bedside for patient to take later unless there is an order to do so.	O. Ask patient if medication went down. Patient usually opens his mouth for inspection. Unless nurse has seen patient swallow drug, she should not record that drug was administered. Patient may not take dose or he may save doses and harm himself by taking them at one time.
P. *Modification for Narcotics:* Verify count in container, remove dose, count again. Immediately record required information on narcotics record.	P. Narcotics require precise counts and must be recorded when removed from supply. (Charting of *administration* is done immediately *after* the medication is given.)

Post-Procedure Activities.   Provide for patient comfort and safety. Nurse washes hands. Use medication card to record medications given or omitted.

Aftercare of Equipment and Medications.   Return medication cards to storage area or give to appropriate person. Throw away disposables (cups, straws). Return tray to storage area, cleanse with disinfectant if contaminated.

Procedure continued on the following page

Final Patient Assessment.   Return to patient to observe for expected as well as unexpected reactions. *Report/Record:* Immediately on leaving patient's bedside, record medications given and omitted on medication sheet; record reason for omission of medication and desired or untoward reactions observed on nursing notes. Report to the appropriate person immediately any errors, problems, omissions and untoward reactions. (See step P for recording Narcotics.)

BIBLIOGRAPHY

The references for Chapter 31 can be found at the end of Chapter 32, p. 784.

ADMINISTERING TOPICAL MEDICATIONS

By Margaret Auld Bruya, R.N., M.N.

INTRODUCTION AND STUDY GUIDE

Topical medications are applied directly to the skin and mucous membranes. Topical medications act directly on the site to which they are applied, e.g., lotions soften rough skin, powders help dry a draining area, etc. In addition, some topical preparations have a systemic effect, e.g., steroid creams. As with any other type of medication, a physician's order is *essential* before the nurse can administer topical drugs to a patient. Also, it is imperative that the nurse:

▶ be knowledgeable about the anatomy and physiology of the sites to which topical agents are applied, e.g., skin, vagina, ear, eye, nose

▶ know and observe the general procedures and precautions for medication administration

▶ be aware of the desired effects and the side and toxic effects of topical agents

▶ know local and systemic effects and *observe* for these effects

▶ determine if clean or sterile technique is essential for safe applicaton

▶ be alert to outdated preparations and discard such preparations

▶ understand the necessity for adhering to pre-

scribed dosages and manufacturer's printed instructions

Upon completion of this chapter, you should be able to do the following:

1. Define these terms and be able to use them in your nursing practice:

topical	irrigation
asepsis	zygomatic arch
lotion	aspiration pneumonia
ointment	sterile cavity
aerosol	nonsterile cavity
insertion	inhalation
buccal	volatile
sublingual	nonvolatile
suppository	douche
cot	ampule
instillation	vaporization
canthus	atomization
conjunctival sac	nebulization

2. Differentiate between sterile and nonsterile cavities and carry out appropriate and safe nursing practices for each.

3. Describe (a) the types of topical medications used, (b) the techniques of application and (c) the safety considerations involved for each of the following: the skin, mucous membranes, vagina, rectum, eye, nose, ear, and respiratory tract.

ADMINISTRATION OF TOPICAL MEDICATIONS TO THE SKIN

Nursing care of the skin is of vital importance to the patient's general well-being. The skin is truly a barometer of the body's condition, reflecting the general health of the individual. Ill health can inhibit the normal physiologic processes, including the functions of the skin, so that the ill person's appearance and sense of well-being are affected even more. A healthy skin is characterized by the terms "glowing," "clean" and "clear." Because the skin is the first line of defense against infection and as such is subject to constant environmental abuses, the nurse must knowledgeably use appropriate measures for promoting its integrity. Skin problems can affect a person's self-concept, social life, and sense of well-being. Thus, when skin disorders are observed, the conscientious nurse investigates with the physician the various products and treatments available for skin care, diagnoses the problem, and plans therapy to alleviate or counteract the condition. The nursing care plan would include patient and family teaching regarding diet, hygiene, and proper use of medications as prescribed by the physician.

When applying topical medications to the skin, the desired effect is usually *local* (cleaning, soothing or disinfecting) rather than *systemic*, although systemic effects occur with some medications, e.g., nitroglycerin. Various methods of administration have been devised for the different types of skin preparations. Some medications, such as tincture of benzoin, are "painted on." The nurse applies these preparations to the patient's dry skin with a cotton ball, gauze or an applicator.

If treating a wound, the nurse applies surgical asepsis principles, i.e., "painting" from the wound *outward* to avoid contamination (see Chap. 42). With a multiple-use container, one guiding principle is always to be followed:

> *Once an applicator has touched the skin, it is never to be placed back in the original bottle as contamination of the entire bottle will occur.*

While the temptation to break this principle when treating one patient may be great, micro-organisms may colonize in the container and recontaminate your patient. Do not be tempted.

After the medication is applied, the skin is allowed to dry before a dressing is applied. If the nurse is using cotton balls or a gauze, she should wear gloves for two reasons: to maintain asepsis and to prevent unwanted effects on her own skin.

Lotions and Ointments

Medications are placed in an oil or fat base to facilitate absorption through the sebaceous glands. The slight absorption that will occur can best be facilitated by applying the lotion or ointment to clean skin in which the blood ves-

sels have been dilated by a warm bath or by application of warm packs. The one most important nursing care activity before the application of an ointment is *cleaning* the skin. The nurse also can instruct patients to thoroughly cleanse their skin before applying a prescribed medication.

Lotions and *ointments* are difficult to apply by "painting," so a process of "patting" or "rubbing in" is used to achieve a therapeutic effect. A lotion should be shaken well first, then patted onto clean skin and allowed to dry. Because lotions tend to flake and fall off, they have to be reapplied as necessary. Whether or not the lotion or ointment should be completely removed before reapplication is variable: the nurse should consult the package insert. The nurse should assess for local skin irritation. She should discontinue any lotion she identifies as causing irritation and notify the physician. *Ointments* are thicker than lotions and need to be rubbed into the skin. The nurse should do so with either a sterile or a clean glove, depending upon the condition and integrity of the patient's skin. A thin coating of ointment is preferable to a thick layer, both for economy of medication and for efficacy.

The nurse must use a glove for two reasons: (1) to avoid self-treatment and (2) to avoid picking up organisms on her hand from the patient, which increases the risk of transferring them to other patients, particularly patients who have impaired dermatologic systems.

Ointments frequently come from large "stock" jars on nursing units; it is important to prevent contamination of the stock jar. Remove the necessary quantity with a tongue blade and take the smaller portion to the patient's bedside.

> *Take only sufficient medication for one application to the patient's unit. Any other use will cause wastage.*

If a patient has his own jar of prescribed medication, it may be left at his bedside if clearly labeled. If dermatologic problems occur frequently, e.g., as with psoriasis or eczema, the nurse should instruct the patient in therapeutic self-care.

The nurse needs to apply ointments cautiously over draining tissue, proceeding carefully so as not to impede drainage or cause unwanted systemic effects. Again, the nurse should use sterile or clean gloves to prevent ointment from getting on her hands.

Some liquid and powder medications come in *aerosol* and *spray* forms. These agents can be applied directly to the clean, dry skin without the nurse having to touch the medication. To protect the nurse's and patient's respiratory systems, precautions should be taken to prevent the inadvertent inhalation of aerosols and sprays. Turn the patient's face away from the direct force of the spray. If the spray is directed toward the patient's head or neck, protect the patient's nose and mouth from inhalation of the particles by providing him with a cloth or gauze and asking him to exhale during the procedure. Reapplication should be made on clean, dry skin. *Therapeutic tub baths or soaks* can be given for patients whose entire skin surface requires therapy or who need local therapy to a limb (see Chap. 27). As with any bath, the nurse must consider patient comfort and safety, i.e., control the temperature of the bath water, position the patient in the tub properly, and either stay with the patient, if he requires it, or check on him frequently. Patient privacy during this procedure should be guaranteed. *Wet dressings* can be used for smaller areas of the body when an immersion bath is impossible. The dressing can be soaked in a warm solution ordered by the physician, and either removed after cooling, or allowed to dry in place and then removed. (Wet dressings are discussed in Chap. 42.)

ADMINISTRATION OF TOPICAL MEDICATIONS TO MUCOUS MEMBRANES

Many of the same techniques that are used to apply topical medications to the skin are used when treating mucous membranes. The mucous membranes most frequently treated with topical preparations are those of the mouth, vagina, rectum, bladder, and respiratory tree. While not a mucous membrane, the ear is considered in this section because it is often treated in the same manner as a mucous membrane.

Therapeutic agents can be painted or brushed on to mucous membranes with a technique similar to that used on skin. Asepsis, prevention of contamination, and education against patient self-diagnosis and treatment are nursing responsibilities. Aerosol or hand-pumped sprays can be directed at the throat and other mucous membranes.

Insertion

Dosages of medication can be placed into an area of mucous membrane requiring local treatment; this method is called *insertion*. *Buccal* tablets placed in the cheek pouch or *sublingual* tablets placed under the tongue are forms of insertion commonly used. It is a nursing responsibility to be sure that the patient understands that these types of tablets are not to be chewed. Their action depends upon absorption through the blood vessels in the sublingual area and cheek pouches. Chewing and swallowing such tablets reduces the effectiveness of the prescribed medication or drug.

Suppositories. Other common forms of medications to be inserted are suppositories, drugs with a base such as lanolin, glycerin or gelatin that are solid at room temperature but melt at body temperature. *Rectal suppositories* can be inserted by either the patient or nurse. By inserting the suppository past the internal sphincter, inadvertent expulsion of the suppository is prevented, and maximum effect is realized. The suppository is inserted in a manner similar to the insertion of a rectal thermometer. Good visualization is essential, as well as a knowledge of anatomy. The suppository should be placed along the wall of the rectum, in the direction of the umbilicus, avoiding a fecal mass.

A nurse should always wear a rubber finger covering (cot) or glove for insertion to prevent contamination of her finger. While it is desirable for a patient to protect his own finger from contamination, he can insert rectal suppositories without a finger covering if he is properly instructed in (a) correct placement of the suppository within the rectum and (b) proper handwashing technique following rectal insertion.

Vaginal suppositories and medicated creams usually come with an inserter that allows the patient (or nurse) to place the suppository or cream high in the vaginal vault for maximum effect. Vaginal suppositories come in conical, cylindrical and globular shapes, and if not supplied with an applicator, should be placed in the vagina with a gloved finger. Although the vagina is normally not considered sterile, good nursing practice emphasizes hygienic measures and use of a gloved hand. The nurse assesses patient understanding and learning abilities to ascertain comprehension of self-therapy, Patient position (supine), placement (a down and backward direction), perineal care (front to back cleansing), and handwashing (before and after) should all be covered by the nurse in a teaching situation. Also, the nurse should warn the patient that some suppositories and medicated creams stain undergarments. An external sanitary pad should be used to protect clothing. The thin pads that adhere to undergarments by adhesive strips are good to use. They can absorb small amounts, are easily changed to maintain cleanliness, and prevent fabric staining. Tampons should be avoided as they may (a) irritate local tissue and (b) prevent drainage of fluids and exudates. Also, if tampons are not changed frequently (e.g., every 1–2 hours) they may harbor harmful microorganisms, which can increase the danger of infection.

If at all possible, the patient should remain horizontal for maximum therapeutic effect; otherwise, as the medication melts it tends to run out of the vagina.

Instillation and Irrigation

Instillation is the process by which a liquid is introduced into a cavity drop by drop. The three most common sites are the nose, eyes, and ears. *Irrigations*, another topical procedure, use a greater volume of therapeutic agent, in a washing or flushing out procedure (bladder irrigation will be discussed in Chap. 40).

Nasal Passages.   The nose is not considered a sterile cavity, therefore clean technique is deemed appropriate unless the sinus cavities are involved. The patient can be in either a supine or a sitting position, with his head resting back on a pillow. Any other position would allow the drop to flow out of the anterior nares before the therapeutic result was achieved.

Sufficient solution is drawn up in the dropper, the dropper is placed just inside the nares, and the prescribed solution is instilled. The patient is instructed to keep his head tilted back to maximize therapy. Since the nasal passages drain into the back of the mouth and throat, the taste of the medication may be disagreeable and cause the patient discomfort and a desire to expectorate. Provide the patient with tissues in which to do so. Small children may lustily resist therapy owing both to the enforced position as well as the taste. *Carefully* instill the drops into the nares to prevent injury. Using soft droppers may help prevent injury.

Also, because of the risk of aspiration, oily solutions, such as mineral oil, or any drug not absorbed by the nasal tissues should be prohibited. Aspiration pneumonia or abscesses occur when the oily solution passes from nose to larynx to lung and the body initiates an inflammatory response to remove or isolate the solution.

Nasal irrigations (washing out nasal cavity by a stream of liquid) are infrequently attempted, owing to dangers of forcing purulent material into the sinuses. This procedure, if attempted, is usually carried out by a physician. Patient cooperation is essential and is achieved through careful and complete directions prior to the procedure.

Eyes.   Although the eye is not a sterile organ, health professionals advocate sterile technique when treating the eye. Sterile technique is preferable because of the sensitive nature of the tissue as well as the value of sight. Most professionals advocate treating each eye separately, having separate solutions and equipment for each eye.

The position of the patient is important for placement of eye drops (or ointment). The patient can sit up or lie down, but his head must be tilted slightly backward. To instill eye drops or ointment first wipe away any secretions on the lid and/or lashes with a sterile cottonball, always wiping from inner to outer canthus. Discard the cotton ball. Hold the dropper or

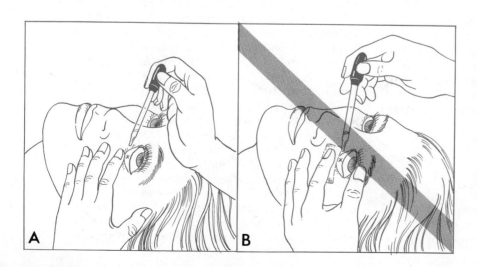

Figure 32–1. Administering eye drops. *A* shows the *correct* method. Note that the nurse's hand rests on the patient's forehead. If the patient moves, the nurse's hand will tend to move also, thereby diminishing the chance that the dropper might strike the eye. The incorrect method (*B*) could result in injury to the patient's eye if she suddenly moved her head. The gauze, in *B*, is not necessary.

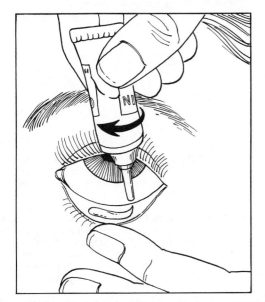

Figure 32–2. Administering ointment to the eye. With the nurse's hand resting on forehead for support to prevent eye damage, the ointment is squeezed into the conjunctival sac. About a ½-inch line of the medication is squeezed into the sac; with a twisting motion, the ointment tube is withdrawn. The nurse releases the conjunctival sac, and the patient closes and "rolls" his eye. The ointment melts and treats the eye. Disoriented patients and young children may need to have their hands temporarily restrained during the administration of eye ointment.

ointment in your right hand; rest your right hand on the patient's forehead. Place your left hand on the zygomatic arch (cheek bone) and expose the lower conjunctival sac by pulling down gently. Another method is to pick up a small bit of tissue below the eye between thumb and forefinger and gently pull out: this creates a "well" for medication deposit. Either method is acceptable as long as the nurse is competent and patient cooperation is gained. Figure 32–1 shows proper administration of eye drops using the method of pulling down the lower conjunctival sac; Figure 32–2 demonstrates the placement of eye ointment.

Ask the patient to "look up" and then deposit the medication. The reason for asking the patient to "look up" is to reduce the corneal reflex, which could cause injury to the eye as the patient startles and jerks away. The drop is placed in the conjunctival space, and the lid is allowed to close, distributing the medication over the eye.

Several cautions are necessary when dealing with eye care and medications:

▶ Use sterile technique

▶ Use separate equipment for each eye

▶ Draw up only amount of medication to be used; excess cannot be returned to bottle

▶ *Never* drop medication on cornea

▶ Provide patient with tissue to wipe cheek following instillation

▶ *Never* share one patient's eye medications with another patient

An eye irrigation is done to wash the conjunctival sac or sclera with a stream of liquid. The purposes of an eye irrigation are: (1) cleansing, (2) removal of a foreign substance and (3) application of therapeutic solution for treatment of an existing eye condition.

As for any eye therapy, all equipment and solutions that come into contact with the eye during an irrigation should be sterile. Physiologic saline is commonly used for cleansing and mechanical removal of debris from the eye. Other solutions are ordered by the physician.

Position the patient so that the eye to be treated is inclined to the side. This position allows drainage, foreign bodies or secretions to be flushed in a direction away from the other eye. Potential contamination is thus prevented. Provide the patient with a basin to catch the solution and a towel to absorb any excess moisture. Provide adequate lighting, but remember not to shine the light directly into the patient's eye. Expose the conjunctival sac with a technique similar to that for eye instillation. Direct the irrigation from the inner canthus toward the outer angle. If the patient has an eye infection, the nurse needs to protect her own eyes from splatters.

A sterile intravenous bag of solution and tubing hung on an adjustable height rolling stand is useful when the eye needs to be irrigated with copious amounts of fluid. Another method is the use of a hand held bulb syringe, gently squeezing the solution from the bulb into the conjunctival sac.

Ears.   To instill drops or irrigate the external auditory canal, the nurse needs to recall structural differences between the infant and adult ear. The infant has an external auditory canal that is mostly cartilaginous and nearly straight. To place medication and fluids within the external auditory canal, it is necessary to draw the auricle down and backward to effectively separate the walls of the canal. Because the adult canal is longer and composed mostly of bone, a different angle of pull is necessary to straighten the external auditory canal. For an adult, the operator pulls the auricle upward and backward. Figure 32–3 shows the difference between correct and incorrect methods of administering ear drops to an adult.

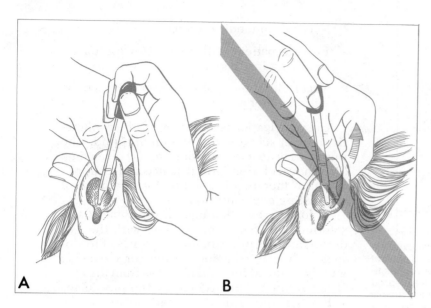

Figure 32–3. Administering ear drops to an adult. *A* shows the *correct* method. Nurse pulls patient's ear *up* and *back* to straighten canal. Hand rests on head; should the patient move, the hand and dropper will move with his head and there is less chance that the dropper will enter and damage the ear. The method shown in *B* is dangerous, as the hand is not supported on the patient's head. If the patient suddenly jerks his head, the dropper could be forced deep into the ear canal.

To place drops or to do an irrigation, the patient's head is tilted to the side, placing the ear to be treated uppermost. The solution is ordered by the physician and should be sterile if any doubt exists about the integrity of the tympanic membrane. The ear and external auditory canal are not considered sterile cavities. A solution at body temperature will be the most comfortable for the patient. Solutions and drops should be directed towards the canal, not the eardrum. Dropping or squirting solution on the eardrum will be uncomfortable and startling for

the patient. The solution should be allowed to drain from the ear unless the physician has ordered a cotton pledget to be loosely placed in the external auditory canal. Clean and dry the outer ear and assist the patient back to a comfortable position.

A review of the key points in nose, eye and ear care is given in Table 32–1.

Vagina. Because vaginal douches are very common in care agencies, as well as at home, the technique for a vaginal douche is presented in Procedure 16.

TABLE 32–1.   COMPARISON OF TECHNIQUES USED IN NOSE, EYE AND EAR
INSTILLATION AND IRRIGATION

	NOSE	EYE	EAR
Technique and Solution	Clean technique; sterile if sinus involved.	Sterile procedure. Separate equipment for each eye.	Sterile solution if eardrum (tympanic membrane) is torn or broken.
Insertion (Using Dropper Technique for Instillation)	Patient supine—head tipped back. Drop placed in affected nostril. Do not use oily solution (aspiration pneumonia may result).	Lower conjunctival sac. See Figs. 32–1, 32–2.	*In adult:* straighten ear canal by pulling auricle upward and backward. See Fig. 32–3. *In children:* pull auricle down and backward.
Irrigation	Dangerous. Should be avoided or carried out by physician.	Inner canthus toward outer angle—Sclera or conjunctival sac.	Stream directed toward wall of canal (not eardrum)

16.   VAGINAL IRRIGATION (DOUCHE)

Definition and Purposes.   *A stream of tap water or medicinal solution directed into vaginal cavity.* Used to cleanse, apply heat and/or apply a medicated solution to the vaginal mucosa and cervix of the uterus.

Contraindications and Cautions.   The condition of the vaginal tissues determines whether sterile technique is necessary or if medical asepsis (clean technique) is sufficient. If an open wound is present in or around the vagina, sterile technique is essential. If vaginal tissues are intact, medical asepsis is adequate. Exudate debris around labia and vulva should be washed off first to avoid introducing it into the vagina, which could cause infection. The normal vagina is self-lubricating and self-cleansing. For women without discharge or pathology, douching is not necessary. Douching can be dangerous if the level of solution in the douche bag is higher than 60 cm. (23⅝ inches) above hips, for infectious material could be forced into the uterus. Use of an acidified, physiologic solution is best for vaginal tissues. No douching should be done during menstruation, late stage pregnancy or during the post partum period. There is a danger in using a solution that is too hot: delicate mucous membrane tissue can be easily burned. Body temperature is suggested for the solution. Examine nozzle of douche for chips, breaks or cracks that might cause injury. Postcoital douching is *not* a method of birth control; discuss alternative methods if the patient expresses this need. Postcoital douching is not necessary for cleanliness.

Patient Teaching Points.   Provide the patient with the following information as appropriate: (a) explain the reason for administering the vaginal douche; (b) explain the frequency of the procedure; (c) explain the steps of the procedure as well as the rationale for the steps; (d) explain the contraindications (pregnancy, post-delivery); (e) teach safe home douche techniques and the reason for using a luke-warm weak vinegar solution (2 tbsp. to 1 quart of water is recommended); (f) emphasize the fact that the normal vagina is self-cleansing and self-lubricating and that douching is unnecessary unless the physician orders it; and (g) point out that douching is not an effective birth control method.

PRE-PROCEDURE ACTIVITIES

PRELIMINARY PATIENT ASSESSMENT

▶ Diagnosis
▶ Level of consciousness
▶ Presence/absence of breaks in vaginal mucosa
▶ Understanding of procedure
▶ Previous experience with vaginal instrumentation

PREPARATION OF PATIENT AND UNIT

▶ Discuss with patient the procedure and how she may cooperate
▶ Prepare unit to avoid drafts, provide privacy
▶ Fan-fold linen to foot of bed
▶ Instruct patient to void prior to procedure
▶ Remove pajama bottoms or roll gown to waist
▶ Adjust bed to working height

Procedure continued on the following page

PRELIMINARY PLANNING

▶ Provide for continuing privacy throughout procedure
▶ Provide clean bed linen and gown if necessary
▶ Provide for comfort and safety of patient
▶ If patient can do procedure herself, or at home, instructions are the same, but may lie in a bathtub

EQUIPMENT

▶ Commercial douche kit containing prep solution (to be ordered by physician): normal saline, antiseptic, medication, or acetic acid
▶ If not using commercial kit:
    Cotton balls
    Prep solution, as described above
    Irrigating set with douche nozzles
    Gloves (sterile or clean)
▶ Basin of water, prep solution
▶ Bed protector
▶ Bath blanket for drape
▶ Bedpan
▶ IV pole or overbed table
▶ Towel
▶ Toilet tissue

PROCEDURE

SUGGESTED STEPS	RATIONALE/DISCUSSION
1. Help patient assume dorsal recumbent position, with buttocks on bedpan. Place bed protector under pan.	1. Dorsal recumbent position will allow maximum tissue exposure; solution will not run in and out without cleansing all tissue.
2. Drape patient as for gynecologic exam and arrange bed gown to provide maximum exposure of perineum.	2. Provides for patient modesty while insuring proper exposure of vaginal orifice.
3. Cleanse external genitalia prior to treatment, using cotton balls and prep solution. Use one downward stroke with each cotton ball. Discard cotton balls.	3. Prevents infection. Cleansing the perineal area from front to back prevents fecal contamination of the vagina and urinary meatus. Or pour warm water over vagina.
4. Elevate bag containing fluid, approximately 30–46 cm. above patient's hips.	4. Gravity causes solution to flow into vagina from douche bag and to drain out into bedpan. Correct height of bag prevents solution from entering vagina with too much force.
5. Inspect douche nozzle carefully for any imperfection.	5. Prevents possibility of injury to vaginal mucous membrane.
6. Have solution run through nozzle over genitalia opening prior to insertion.	6. Provides lubrication of nozzle; prevents mucus and other materials present on genitalia from being pushed into vagina.
7. Gently insert nozzle into vagina directing it backward and slightly downward.	7. When the patient is in the dorsal recumbent position, anatomically vagina is directed downward and backward.
8. Rotate nozzle gently during treatment.	8. Rotating motion helps direct solution to all folds of mucous membranes.

SUGGESTED STEPS	RATIONALE/DISCUSSION
9. When treatment is complete, clamp tubing and gently remove nozzle from vagina.	9. Prevents air from entering vagina; prevents tissue damage.
10. Place douche container in original box for disposal at later time.	
11. Assist patient to sit up on bedpan if possible.	11. Allows remaining solution to drain from vaginal canal.
12. Have patient lie down. Dry external genitalia with toilet tissue and place tissue in bedpan.	12. Provides for patient comfort.
13. Assist patient to side lying position and remove bedpan.	
14. Dry anal region with toilet tissue.	14. Provides for patient comfort.
15. Replace covers.	15. Provides for continuing patient comfort.
16. Remove and clean bedpan and replace patient's stand.	

Post-Procedure Activities.   Check patient for comfort; clean and dry perineum if necessary; provide dry linen and bed clothes; position comfortably; check that call light is handy.

Aftercare of Equipment.   Most hospitals use disposable douche equipment; if equipment is reusable, follow central services directions for preparing equipment for sterilization.

Chart/Report.   Time of day, type and amount of solution, amount and type of vaginal discharge (if present) and patient's reaction to administration of douche.

Inhalation

The mucous membrane of the respiratory tract can be treated by inhalation of *volatile* or *nonvolatile* preparations. Inhalation should be considered a clean procedure, preceded and followed by complete handwashing.

Three methods of administration of *volatile* drugs for systemic effect are (1) inhalation of a gas or vapor, (2) inhalation of a drug embedded in an inert substance and (3) inhalation of fumes. Inhalation of a *gas* or *vapor* is achieved by breaking an ampule (a small, sealed glass container) or other wrapped container to release the medication. The most common use of this method is to revive the fainting patient. A "pearl" of ammonia is broken and held close to the person's nostril. Since the fumes may be irritating to the patient's eyes, care must be taken to shield them from the fumes. The second method—inhaling a medication embedded in an *inert substance*—is based on the principle that the uncapped medication will vaporize, and the vapor will be drawn into the respiratory tract by deep inhalation. However, two problems emerge: (a) the patient must be able to inspire deeply to benefit from the medication and (b) uncapped or open vials of medication quickly lose their potency. Inhalation of fumes is achieved by burning a therapeutic substance in fireproof vessels and having the person inhale the fumes. Patient safety considerations are paramount.

Nonvolatile methods are also available for therapy to the respiratory tract. Moist or steam vaporization, atomization, nebulization and aerosol therapy are all used for nonvolatile therapy.

Vaporization is a process whereby a medication is carried in steam. When heated vaporization is used, several benefits can be expected from the moisture, drug and heat. In care agencies, vaporization equipment is electrically operated and is usually safe and convenient if used properly. Electrically operated vaporizers are available for home use, but vaporizers can also be improvised from equipment already in the home (probably the most convenient is breathing steam from a hot wash cloth). The medication and duration of therapy for patients receiving vaporization therapy is ordered by the physician. Nursing care includes (a) comfortable positioning, (b) maintenance of dry bed and personal linen to prevent chilling and (c) prevention of burns and scalds from overheated water vapor. Nursing assessment is essential to prevent the complication of overhydration.

Atomization and *nebulization* are done by mechanical devices that separate a solution into fine droplets and mist that can be inhaled. Electrically operated and hand operated equipment is available. Atomization produces larger droplets than does nebulization; thus nebulization is used when therapy is directed towards the alveoli or other small areas of the lung. The patient must be taught to inhale deeply to achieve maximum therapeutic effect (and also to avoid swallowing drug). Equipment must be kept clean to prevent development of nosocomial infections. The reader is referred to Chapter 36 for a discussion of *aerosolized medication* application to the respiratory tract.

The nursing responsibility for application of topical medications includes assessing the need, giving the therapy and recording the data in the appropriate place. Other responsibilities include appropriate patient and family teaching about administration of topical preparations, care of the skin and mucous membranes, side and toxic effects of medication and nursing care particular to the medication in use.

BIBLIOGRAPHY (Chapters 31 and 32)

1. Bentz, P. M., and Deliganis, S. G.: Protocol: patient medication education. *Northwest Medical Journal,* 1(3):33–40, March 1974.
2. Bergersen, S.: *Pharmacology in Nursing,* 13th ed. St. Louis, C. V. Mosby Co., 1976.
3. Blackwell, B.: Drug therapy: patient compliance. *New England Journal of Medicine,* 289:249–252, Aug. 1973.
4. Budd, R.: We changed to unit-dose system. *Nursing Outlook,* 19(2):116–117, Feb. 1971.
5. Burnette, G. M.: The unit dose system. *Supervisor Nurse,* 2:72–74, Oct. 1971.
6. Byers, J. F.: To douche or not to douche. *American Family Physician,* 10(3):135–138, Sep. 1974.
7. Carr, J. J., et al.: How to solve dosage problems in one easy lesson. *American Journal of Nursing,* 76:1934–1937, Dec. 1976.
8. Cockerham, M. F.: Self-medication. *Hospitals JAHA,* 44:57–58, Jan. 1970.
9. Conway, B., et al.: The seventh right. *American Journal of Nursing,* 70:1040–1043, May 1970.
9a. Creighton, H.: Legal concerns of nursing research. *Nursing Research,* 26:337, Sep. through Oct. 1977.
10. Crossland, J.: Human experimentation: drugs. *Nursing Digest,* 3:33–35, May–June 1975.
11. Curtis, T. M.: Medication errors in hospitals. *Northwest Medical Journal,* 1(2):5–11, Feb. 1974.
12. Daylight on prescription prices. *Nursing Forum,* 11(4):346–355, 1972.
13. Deberry, P., et al.: Teaching cardiac patients to manage medications. *American Journal of Nursing,* 75(12):2191–2193, Dec. 1975.
14. DelBueno, D. J.: Verifying the nurse's knowledge of pharmacology. *Nursing Outlook,* 20:462–463, July 1972.
15. Dickey, F. F., et al.: Pharmacist counseling increases drug regimen compliance. *Hospitals JAHA.,* 49:85–89, May 1975.
16. Eckel, F. M.: Improving system didn't help—but change to unit dose did. *Modern Nursing Home,* 27:10, Sep. 1971.
16a. Gabriel, M., et al.: Improved patient compliance through use of a daily drug reminder chart. *American Journal of Public Health,* 67:968, Oct. 1977.
17. Garb, S.: Narcotics addiction in nurses and doctors. *Nursing Outlook,* 13:30–34, Nov. 1965.
18. Getting ready for a metric America. *RN,* 37:40–41, Jan. 1974.
19. Greenblat, D. J., and Miller, R. R.: Rational use of hypnotic drugs. *Nursing Digest,* 3:32, July–Aug. 1975.
20. Hayes, M. H.: Pharmacists need nurses, nurses need pharmacists, patients need both. *American Journal of Nursing,* 72(4):723–726, April 1972.
21. Hershey, N.: Question that drug order. *American Journal of Nursing,* 63:96–97, Jan. 1963.
22. Hussar, D. A.: When giving medications. *Nursing,* 75:10, June 1975.
23. Isler, C.: For severe pain: self-medication on demand. *RN,* 38:51–59, May 1975.
24. Jeffrey, L. P.: Pharmacy: drug administration, unit dose, hospital pharmacist's role. *Hospitals JAHA,* 46:155, April 1972.
25. Kelly, S. P.: An experiment in self-medication for older people. *The Canadian Nurse,* 68:41–43, Feb. 1972.
26. Lambert, M. L.: Drugs and diet interactions. *American Journal of Nursing,* 75(3):402–406, March 1975.
27. Laugharne, E.: Insulin goes metric: a time for review. *Canadian Nurse,* 71:22–24, Feb. 1975.
28. LaVerde, S.: Evaluation of drug history program. *Hospitals JAHA,* 74:106–111, Aug. 1973.

29. Leary, J. J. A., et al.: Self-administered medications. *American Journal of Nursing, 71*(6):1193–1194, June 1971.

30. Levine, M. E.: Breaking through the medications mystique. *American Journal of Nursing, 70*(4):799–803, April 1970.

31. Levine, M.: This I believe . . . about patient-centered care. *Nursing Outlook, 15*:53–55, July 1967.

32. Lewis, L. W.: *Fundamental Skills in Patient Care.* Philadelphia, J. B. Lippincott Company, 1976.

33. Lowenthal, W.: Factors affecting drug absorption: programed instructions. *American Journal of Nursing, 73*:1391–1408, Aug. 1973.

34. MacPherson, D. D., et al.: Function-structure relationships and unit-dose dispensing: a time study. *American Journal Hospital Pharmacy, 30*:1034–1037, Nov. 1973.

34a. Matus, N. R. (Consultant): Topical therapy: choosing and using the proper vehicle. *Nursing '77, 7*:8, Nov. 1977.

35. Mead, W. B.: Unit-dose drug packaging. *Hospitals JAHA, 44*:85–87, Jan. 1970.

36. Moggach, B. B.: Drug administration times should be re-examined. *Canadian Nurse, 71*:17–19, Jan. 1975.

37. Mohney, S.: Some important clues to drug reaction. *RN, 36*:48–49, March 1973.

38. Nudleman, P.: New patient information regulation in Washington. *Northwest Medical Journal, 1*(1):29–35, Jan. 1974.

39. Odom, J. V.: Going metric. *American Journal of Nursing, 74*:1078–1081, June 1974.

40. O'Reilly, W. J.: Drug interactions. *Canadian Nurse, 37*:47–50, April 1972.

41. Parker, W. A.: Medication histories. *American Journal of Nursing, 76*:1069–1071, Dec. 1976.

42. Pearson, R. E., et al.: Regional drug information network—part III: utilization of information received from a drug information center. *American Journal of Hospital Pharmacy, 29*:229–234, March 1972.

43. Pitlick, W. H., and Plein, E. M.: Evaluation of clinical pharmacy by nurses. *Nursing Research, 22*(5):434–437, Sep.–Oct. 1973.

44. Pharmacists and nurses discuss mutual problems. *Hospitals JAHA, 44*:116–117, Jan. 1970.

45. Platiau, P. B., et al.: Computer stores total drug data. *Hospitals JAHA, 47*:66–69, Aug. 1973.

46. Plein, J. B., and Plein, E. M.: *Fundamentals of Medications.* Hamilton, IL, Drug Intelligence Publications, 1974.

47. Regan, W. A.: You and experimental medicine. *RN, 29*:75–81, July 1966.

48. Robinson, D. S.: Pharmacokinetic mechanisms of drug interactions. *Postgraduate Medicine, 57*(2):55–62, Feb. 1975.

49. Rodman, M. J.: Adjusting medications for the need of the elderly. *RN, 38*:65, May 1975.

50. Rodman, M. J.: Dangers of unsupervised medications. *RN, 37*:51–68, July 1974.

50a. Rodman, M. J., and Smith, D. W.: *Clinical Pharmacology in Nursing.* Philadelphia, J. B. Lippincott Co., 1972.

51. Rodman, M. J., and Smith, D. W.: *Pharmacology and Drug Therapy in Nursing.* Philadelphia, J. B. Lippincott Company, 1968.

51a. Rozovsky, L. E.: Answers to the IV legal questions nurses usually ask. *Nursing '78, 8*:73, July 1978.

52. Saxon, J.: Administration of medications. *In Nursing Process I Syllabus.* Seattle, University of Washington, Summer 1975.

53. Saxon, J.: Medications: drugs and solutions. *In Nursing Process I Syllabus.* Seattle, University of Washington, Summer 1975.

54. Shiery, S.: Insight into the delicate art of eye care. *Nursing '75, 5*(6):50–56, June 1975.

55. Sholtz, S. M., et al.: Medication errors reduced by unit-dose. *Hospitals JAHA, 47*:106–112, March 1973.

56. Smith, H.: Drug information service for health care professionals. *Northwest Medical Journal, 1*:37–39, Jan. 1974.

57. Smith, M. D.: Drugs of the future and the future of drug distribution. *Nursing Digest, 3*:36–38, July–Aug. 1975.

57a. Snipes, F. L.: Putting zip in prescription writing: a proposal. *Post Graduate Medicine, 63*:185, Jan. 1978.

58. Stimson, G. V.: Obeying doctor's orders. *Social Science and Medicine, 8*:97–104, 1974.

59. Sutton, A. L.: *Bedside Nursing Techniques*, 2nd ed., Philadelphia, W. B. Saunders Co., 1969.

60. Swift, R. G.: Semiautomated, centralized unit-dose. *Hospitals JAHA, 48*:72–76, Aug. 1975.

61. Tobey, L. E., and Covington, T. R.: Antimicrobial drug interaction. *American Journal of Nursing, 75*:1470–1473, Sep. 1975.

62. Unit-dose system: the successful failure. *Hospitals JAHA, 47*:138–146, July 1975.

63. Wiley, L. (ed.): How many of your patients are taking their medications? *Nursing '73, 3*:16, April 1973.

63a. Wilson, B. S.: Medication error policy. *Supervisor Nurse, 9*:53, May 1978.

64. Wood, L. A.: Nursing Skills for Allied Health Services, Vol. 3. Philadelphia, W. B. Saunders Co., 1975.

CHAPTER 33*

MINIMIZING THE HAZARDS OF IMMOBILITY

INTRODUCTION AND STUDY GUIDE

The patient who lies in bed day after day with little reason to move, little appetite to eat, and little capacity for hope is a vulnerable person. While he lies "resting" and inert, such a patient (especially if he is aged and weak) is susceptible to many dangerous conditions, e.g., thrombosis, decubitus ulcers, pneumonia, renal calculi, osteoporosis, contractures, footdrop, and mental disturbances.

The benefits of rest for such an individual are obviously negated if he develops any one of these immobilization disabilities—disabilities which can usually be prevented by foresight and by careful planning on the part of the nursing and medical staffs. For example, consider the following description of Mr. R. Jones, an elderly bedridden man of 71, whose condition has deteriorated as a result of oversights and misconceptions on the part of the hospital staff.

Mr. Jones lies in his bed on the top floor of the city hospital, which is the geriatric division. On this floor patients sometimes wait for months to be transferred to a rest home where they will live out what remains of their lives.

The ward has 16 beds crowded closely together; two overworked aides care for the patients as best they can. The entire geriatric floor consists of four wards like Mr. Jones' and is supervised by one RN who rarely has time to leave her desk because of excessive paperwork; as a result of inadequate supervision, there is little organized planning of patient care.

Mr. Jones has been on this ward for two weeks following a massive stroke which left him paralyzed and unable to turn himself. He spends the greatest portion of his time in bed with the side rails up. He is turned twice during the night, once during the afternoon and again in the evening. In the morning, following breakfast, Mr. Jones, along with other patients, is lifted from bed and placed into a wheelchair by his bed where he remains until two in the afternoon. Sitting for hours in his wheelchair, Mr. Jones usually slumps and sleeps. The aides believe that getting Mr. Jones up and into a chair every day will prevent the development of pressure sores. Thus, today, the aides were shocked to discover the beginning of a decubitus ulcer on Mr. Jones' sacrum—an ulcer which was actually produced by sitting for long hours, immobile, in a wheelchair.

Decubitus ulcers are not Mr. Jones' only problem. He is dehydrated, malnourished, and severely constipated. His joints are getting stiffer daily, and he is developing a noticeable footdrop.

Mr. Jones' mental state has also deteriorated. Although he was once a jovial and talkative person, this patient has gradually withdrawn into himself. To whom, after all, can he talk? The patient on the right side of his bed lies silent and coiled into the fetal position; the patient on his left seems incoherent, muttering to himself all day long; the patient across the ward is dying; the aides are hurried and impersonal; the nurses and doctors are busy and seldom in his room; and his relatives come only rarely as he upsets them by crying throughout their visit.

Mr. Jones will soon be transferred to a nursing home where his condition may continue to deteriorate. Even if he should be cared for by an interested and motivated nursing staff in the nursing home, Mr. Jones' present immobilization disabilities would be extremely difficult and expensive to correct. The tragedy is that Mr. Jones' disabilities could generally have been *prevented.* Intelligent, conscientious care on the part of the nursing staff might have made the last period of Mr. Jones' life comfortable, active, and meaningful.

It is the purpose of this chapter to discuss the patient on bed rest, the helpful and hazardous effects of bed rest and immobility upon the patient, and the major nursing actions that help to prevent the complications of bed rest from developing. Our discussion will briefly cover the following areas:

- ▶ The problem of defining bed rest
- ▶ The beneficial and untoward effects of bed rest
- ▶ The responses of the body to bed rest and immobilization.

More specifically, we shall review the responses of the skin, the musculoskeletal system, the cardiovas-

*Rosemarian Berni, R.N., M.N., critically reviewed and assisted with the revision of this chapter.

cular system, the respiratory system, the renal system, the gastrointestinal tract, the metabolic system, and the psyche to prolonged "rest."

As an aid to your study of this chapter, we urge you to make use of the following brief study guide.

Upon completion of this chapter, you should be able to do the following:
1. Define generally the following terms:
   bed rest
   immobilization disability
   decubitus ulcer
   shearing force
   disuse atrophy
   contracture
   disuse osteoporosis
   orthostatic hypotension
   venous thrombosis
   embolism
   Valsalva maneuver
   urinary stasis
   renal calculi

2. Discuss generally the following:
   a. The major benefits of bed rest.
   b. The pathologic effects of bed rest upon every major system of the body.
   c. Which groups of patients are most prone to the development of the complications of bed rest.
3. Perform the following nursing actions when caring for patients:
   a. Identify among patients assigned to you those who are most susceptible to the complications of bed rest.
   b. Assess patients on bed rest in order to prevent the possible complications of immobilization.
   c. Draw up a specific plan of care for patients on bed rest and put the plan into action.

THE PROBLEM OF DEFINING BED REST

In general terms, "bed rest" is an activity status which specifies that the patient be put to bed for the purpose of "rest." Bed rest is either specifically prescribed for a patient by his physician, or it is simply assigned to a patient by the staff on the basis of that patient's inability to walk, move, and perform activities for himself. In clinical practice you will find that the status of bed rest is actually a hazy concept and that few doctors and staff members define bed rest in precisely the same way.

For example, when a doctor prescribes bed rest for a patient, he may *assume* that the staff will allow the patient to perform certain simple activities such as using a bedside commode, washing his face and hands, and feeding himself. To his dismay, the physician may discover that his patient has been almost totally immobilized by the hospital staff, because the head nurse views bed rest as meaning complete confinement for the patient, with no self-care activities allowed on his part. As a result of such confusion in defining bed rest, the physician may become angry, the staff may be upset, and the patient may actually develop potentially fatal complications owing to his total immobilization. This type of confusing and dangerous situation is all too common in hospital settings. Thus, it is important that *all* members of a hospital staff, from the doctor to the aide, agree upon a definition of bed rest, upon the amount of activity a patient on bed rest is to be allowed, and upon the exact means by which the complications of bed rest are to be prevented.

THE BENEFICIAL AND UNTOWARD EFFECTS OF BED REST

Beneficial Effects

While the emphasis in this chapter is upon the complications and the development of disabilities consequent to bed rest, we wish to emphasize that there are many benefits to be derived from bed rest. Some of its beneficial aspects and some important indications for its use are as follows:

▶ To *relieve pain* due to coronary ischemia, surgical procedures, trauma, fractures, and wounds. Rest, by decreasing movement, prevents excessive irritation of injured tissues, and it reduces the oxygen demands of such vital organs as the heart muscle, thereby easing discomfort.

▶ To *promote healing and repair* of injured tissues by reducing the metabolic need of tissues and by preserving the fibrin barriers that prevent the migration of microorganisms from sick tissues into healthy tissues.

▶ To *relieve ankle edema and venous congestion* by placing the patient in bed and elevating his legs on a continuous body plane.

▶ To *give support* to the weak, exhausted, perhaps febrile patient who, because of illness, is simply unable to remain standing and active, e.g., patients debilitated by carcinoma or by severely incapacitating neurologic diseases.

To be of any benefit to a patient, bed rest must, of course, *be restful*—physiologically and psy-

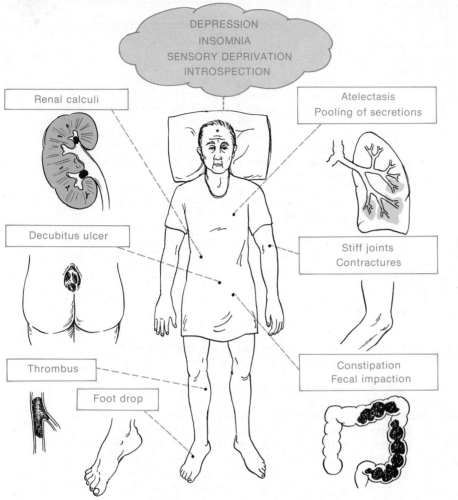

Figure 33–1. Major complications of bed rest.

TABLE 33–1. IMMOBILIZATION DISABILITIES AND THEIR CONSEQUENCES

ORGAN SYSTEM	MOBILIZATION DISABILITY	CONSEQUENCE
Skin	Decubitus ulcers	Osteomyelitis
Musculoskeletal system	Muscle weakness, increased immobilization, backache, muscle atrophy, joint stiffness	Contractures, deformities
	Disuse osteoporosis	Pathologic fractures, renal calculi, deformities, osteoarthropathy
Cardiovascular system	Increased workload of the heart	
	Increased use of the Valsalva maneuver	Tachycardia, cardiac arrest
	Orthostatic hypotension	Pulmonary embolism
	Thrombus formation	Thrombophlebitis
Respiratory system	Decreased chest expansion, stasis of secretions, CO_2 narcosis, respiratory acidosis	Hypostatic bronchopneumonia
Renal system	Difficult micturition, urinary stasis, renal calculi	Urinary infection, urinary incontinence, urinary obstruction
Gastrointestinal system	Anorexia, negative nitrogen balance, constipation	Fecal impaction, bowel obstruction
Metabolic system	Decreased production of adrenocortical hormones, increased protein breakdown	Regulatory system breakdown
Psyche	Depression, boredom, increased introspection	Insomnia, disorientation, decreased self-worth

chologically. This vital requirement, which sounds so simple to achieve, is commonly overlooked by nurses and doctors alike. How often we order a patient who is beset with worry, harassed by pain, and panicked from fear "to rest." Such a patient may be in bed quietly enough, but his mind may be churning and his emotions in a state of flux; in other cases, the patient may become bored, depressed, and withdrawn. If the patient is truly to benefit from rest, his pain must be eased, his concerns and fears must be allowed open discussion, and his interests in life and in his surroundings must be kept alive.

Untoward Effects

Even when properly prescribed, defined, and carried out, bed rest like any treatment has its hazards as well as its benefits. The complications of bed rest are sometimes called *dependent disabilities* or *immobilization disabilities*. Such complications constitute the *iatrogenic* consequences of rest in bed. The bulk of the information in this chapter pertains to these disabilities and their prevention.

Briefly, immobilization disabilities affect every system and major organ in the body, i.e., the skin, muscles, bones, heart, brain, kidneys, and lungs. The most important immobilization disabilities and their consequences according to physiologic systems are summarized in Table 33–1. In addition, major complications of bedrest are depicted in Fig. 33–1.

These disabilities mainly affect patients who are elderly, malnourished, critically ill, quadriplegic, and/or comatose. Prevention of the complications of bed rest is one of the major goals in nursing today.

RESPONSES OF THE BODY TO BED REST AND IMMOBILITY

Each system responds in its own way to prolonged bed rest and immobility. In this chapter we briefly investigate the major responses of each system to bed rest, the major complications of bed rest, and the planned prevention of disabilities.

The Effects of Prolonged Bed Rest upon the Skin

Intense pressure for a brief period of time, or the continuous pressure resulting from lying on a bed mattress, or sitting on a chair seat (e.g., wheelchair seat) for a prolonged period of time may produce a "pressure sore" or *decubitus ulcer* on those areas of the skin subjected to the greatest amounts of pressure. In these areas of pressure, the compressed skin and underlying tissue become necrotic (i.e., the cells die) be-

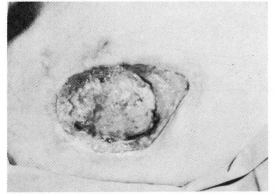

Figure 33–2. Sacral-trochanteric decubiti. (From Isler, C.: Decubitus/Old truths and some new ideas. *RN, 35*:43, July 1972.)

cause of ischemia (deficiency of blood circulation) produced by the pressure. A decubitus ulcer can thus be defined simply as "an area of cellular necrosis which is produced from a lack of blood flow." (See Fig. 33–2.)

Areas of the body which are commonly *susceptible to the development of pressure sores* (often called "bed sores" by lay persons) include: the back of the head, the spines of the scapulae, the heels, the malleoli, the palms of the hands, the iliac crests, the ischia, the greater trochanters, and the lower sacrum. Areas such as these are particularly vulnerable to pressure damage because: (1) the skin lies over bony prominences; (2) these areas are not adapted, as are our feet, to the bearing of large amounts of weight for prolonged periods; and (3) the patient's weight, when lying supine, is borne *specifically* by many of these sites rather than by the total posterior of the body.

> *Areas of the body subject to pressure breakdown* must *be thoroughly and frequently inspected when caring for a bedridden person, or a person who sits immobile in a chair for prolonged periods. Commonly these inspections need to be made* at least *every 2 hours. They must be made more frequently for high-risk patients.*

Figure 33–3 illustrates the points of pressure that occur in the supine, side lying and prone positions. Study this figure carefully so that you can make appropriate inspections of *all* pressure points as you provide patient care.

Prolonged or intense pressure *simultaneously* produces ischemic changes and degeneration of the entire tissue segment (at *all* levels) between a bony prominence and the

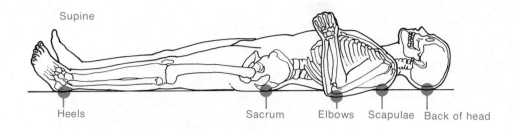

Supine

Heels Sacrum Elbows Scapulae Back of head

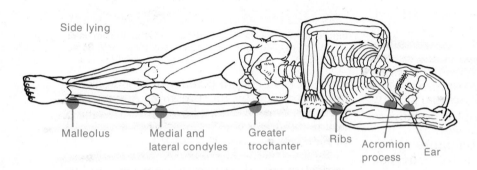

Side lying

Malleolus Medial and lateral condyles Greater trochanter Ribs Acromion process Ear

Figure 33–3. Pressure points in various positions. (From Gruis, M. L., and Innes, B.: Assessment: essential to prevent pressure sores. *American Journal of Nursing,* Nov. 1976.)

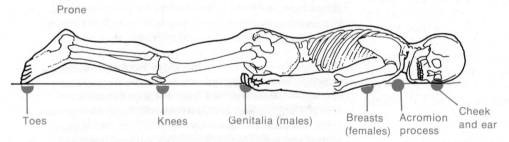

Prone

Toes Knees Genitalia (males) Breasts (females) Acromion process Cheek and ear

skin surface. Deep necrosis thus often occurs *prior to* or at the time that skin breakdown is initially observed.

Groups of patients who are particularly susceptible to the development of pressure sores include:

▶ Patients whose general condition is *rapidly deteriorating.* Such patients may have: sudden loss of appetite, dehydration, development of urinary or fecal incontinence or both, increasing confusion, a sudden elevation in temperature, the onset of diarrhea or constipation, and/or new complaints of pain. When any of these signs appear suddenly in a bedridden patient not previously bothered by them, that patient must be actively managed for the prevention of pressure sore development.

▶ *Newly admitted patients* whose condition prior to admission has so deteriorated that it is necessary for them to come to the hospital and be placed on bed rest. One investigator discovered from a study of 250 elderly patients admitted to the hospital that of the 59 patients who developed ulcerations, 70 per cent did so within the first two weeks after admission and 34 per cent did so within the first week.[46]

▶ *Elderly* bedridden patients who make few spontaneous bodily movements.[31, 34]

▶ *Obese* patients whose extra weight creates additional pressure over weight-bearing areas.

▶ Very *thin* emaciated patients whose skin lies in a thin layer over the body's bony prominences.

▶ *Sedated* patients who are taking large doses of tranquilizers or sleeping pills and who consequently are not moving readily.

▶ *Agitated* patients in *restraints*.

▶ *Paralyzed* patients who have suffered spinal cord injuries (e.g., paraplegics and quadriplegics).

▶ *Neurologic* patients with diseases of the central nervous system such as disseminated sclerosis and Parkinson's disease and patients in coma due to cerebral vascular accidents, trauma, and so forth.

▶ *Edematous* patients, especially those with edema of the sacrum and buttocks.

▶ *Malnourished* patients with protein and vitamin deficiencies.

Superficial skin breakdown may occur from various causes, e.g., friction, maceration, toxins. We will examine several physiologic factors that contribute to the development of pressure sores. They are: (1) severe elevations in the capillary pressure; (2) prolonged pressure on a body tissue; (3) decreases in the number of spontaneous bodily movements, and (4) an increase in the shearing force.

Landis, who studied the capillary pressure in ischemic areas, was one of the first investigators to attempt to explain the etiology of decubitus ulcers. In his studies he found that the blood pressure in capillaries normally ranges from 16 to 33 mm. Hg. He theorized that *prolonged tissue ischemia* causes extremely *high elevations of the external capillary pressure*, resulting in death of cells in the ischemic area and in ulceration. Landis found that a person sitting on a wooden chair without padding would have, over his ischial tuberosities, a capillary pressure of up to 300 mm. of mercury! However, when he experimented with an alternating pressure pad, Landis discovered that pressure in all body positions was reduced toward more normal limits.[51]

In similar studies Rudd emphasized the factor of *time* in the development of pressure sores. From his investigations, Rudd concluded that *less pressure over a prolonged period* of time contributes more to the possible formation of pressure sores than more pressure over a short period of time. Thus, patients who are acutely or chronically ill, heavily sedated, or unconscious are all in grave danger of developing pressure sores because they cannot readily move themselves, and therefore tend to lie in one position for long periods.[51]

Any decrease in the number of spontaneous bodily movements that a patient makes during the night will result in an increase in the potential for decubitus ulcer formation. Investigators discovered that: (1) normal people made as many as 400 spontaneous movements of some kind during an eight-hour night, (2) elderly patients who made 25 to 225 movements during

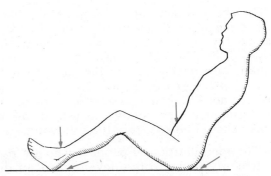

Figure 33–4. The shearing force exerts a downward and forward pressure. (After Norton, *Nursing Times*, March 27, 1964.)

the night did not develop pressure sores, and (3) patients with a nightly average of less than 25 movements *all* developed tissue damage.[46]

Another important etiologic factor contributing to the formation of decubitus ulcers is a "pushing" pressure described in clinical literature as the *shearing force*. This force is in play when the head of a patient's bed is raised or when a patient is allowed to assume a slumped sitting position. Because a *pushing* force is being exerted on the tissues, tissues tend to tear, producing deep and serious pressure sores. Ulcers created by the shearing force most often develop upon the sacrum and heels (Fig. 33–4).

There are four major stages in the progression of a deep penetrating pressure sore: (1) *irritation* of the skin with a resultant redness, (2) *edema* and swelling due to the leakage of fluid from dilated damaged blood vessels, (3) *tissue necrosis* with the result that the reddened area turns bluish and then black (the dead skin, at this point, separates from the necrotic tissue; this exposed area of necrosis is called the slough), and (4) *healing by second intention*, which can easily break down again. During this stage, granulation takes place, and the area finally becomes fibrotic and scarred. The scar tissue which develops is not so strong as normal tissue, and, with pressure, the area can easily become ulcerated once more. Often tissue necrosis develops in underlying tissues near the bone *before* ulceration of the skin appears. Nursing staff, observing intact skin, may thus not suspect the deeper tissue damage. Increasingly prolonged periods of skin redness are possible indications of underlying tissue damage. However, such underlying damage may be present *without* any indications on the skin surface, e.g., between periods of skin redness.

PREVENTION OF DECUBITUS

The above described unfortunate sequence of pathologic events leading to the development of severe ulcerations can be prevented by means of intelligent observation, planning, and patient care on the part of the nursing staff. Indeed, it is far easier to prevent the development of decubitus than to treat it. Some of the most important preventive measures, all of which should be used, are the following:

▶ The identification of patients who are particularly prone to the development of decubitus ulcers, e.g., patients with a deteriorating general condition, emaciated patients, and patients without mobility and/or without sensation.

▶ *Daily examination* of decubitus-prone patients for redness, discoloration, or a blistering of their back, buttocks, or heels.

▶ The immediate institution of a *preventive regimen* for any patient who is liable to develop pressure sores or whose condition is rapidly deteriorating.

Such a preventive regimen may include the following:

▶ The use of an *alternating-pressure pad or mattress*. This is a pneumatic mattress, electrically operated, with air strips that cyclically inflate and deflate alternately, at three- to five-minute intervals. As a result of this device, no one area of the body is exposed to pressure for more than a few minutes at a time. In many hospitals, nurses can use this mattress without a doctor's order.

In caring for patients on an alternating-pressure mattress, remember the following points:

---

1. *Place only a bottom sheet over the mattress and tuck this sheet in lightly. Do not use draw sheets or incontinence pads, because these added layers of linen decrease the efficiency of the mattress.*

2. *Make certain that the air input tube does not become kinked.*

3. *Never insert a pin into the mattress for any reason.*

4. *Place a sign on the patient's bed which informs the staff that the patient is on an alternating-pressure mattress, and which warns them not to use pins or added linens.*

5. *Inspect the mattress at least twice daily to make certain that it is working properly.*

If an alternating-pressure mattress develops any defect, however small, it *must* be replaced at once as it will no longer provide the patient with maximum protection.

It is important to realize that skin breakdown can occur even though an alternating pressure mattress is functioning correctly. This is because the mattress is plastic and because debilitated patients may perspire a lot. Maceration of the skin (i.e., skin damage due to prolonged moisture) may thus develop, leading to skin breakdown. Therefore, instead of using an alternating pressure mattress, some patients are managed better by: (1) placing *covered foam rubber cushions* in such a manner that the patient is suspended or *"bridged"* over an air space created between the patient and the mattress (Fig. 33–5) and/or (2) using moisture-absorbent artificial or real *sheepskins* between the patient and the mattress.

▶ *Turn patient* a minimum of once every 2 hours from the prone to the supine to the side-lying positions. Sometimes a *Foster* or *Stryker* frame is used to facilitate the turning of paralyzed patients. It is important to post a precise turning schedule both on the patient's bed and in the Kardex. The times for turning and the positions in which the patient should be placed need to be clearly noted. Turning the helpless patient is discussed in Chap. 21. Remember to use good body mechanics while turning patients and remember to leave the patient in a position of proper alignment with appropriate body support. Foster and Stryker frames are discussed in Chap 43. The prone (flat face-lying) position is presented in Procedure 17.

While a strict turning schedule is of real value, the skillful nurse does not rely *exclusively* upon turning a patient to prevent pressure sores. It is recommended that, in addition to turning, the nurse also use other preventive methods as discussed in this chapter.

▶ Keep the decubitus-prone patient in *positions that avoid the problem of shearing force* and the deep and dangerous ulcerations that this force can produce. Such positions may include: (a) placing the patient on a low, hand-operated stretcher for prone lying and to increase mobilization, (b) placing the patient on a tilt table for periods of time or (c) placing the patient at home on padded lawn furniture, e.g., lounge chair. In each of these situations the sitting position is avoided.

When the patient is in bed his position should be flat. However, if it is necessary for the patient to be rolled up in bed (e.g., due to severe dyspnea, heart disease or pulmonary edema) be sure to support the soles of the

If a patient has a pressure sore on the back of his heel, support his calves with a cushion or pad and see that his feet are supported in good alignment.

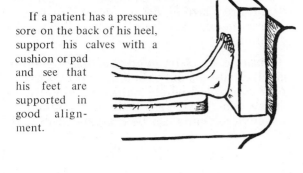

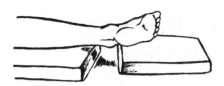

A pressure sore on the ankle can be bridged by supporting the foot and the calf.

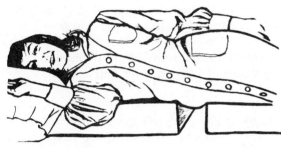

When a patient has tissue damage over the trochanter, the side-lying position can be used if the area is relieved of pressure by elevating the trunk and lower extremities.

Figure 33–5. "Bridging" for the prevention or treatment of decubiti. (From Bergstrom, D., and Coles, H. C.: *Basic Positioning Procedures.* Minneapolis, Sister Kenny Institute, 1971, p. 13.)

patient's feet with an added *footboard*, thereby counteracting the shearing force to some extent. When using a footboard, be certain that the patient's heels are not touching the bed. To prevent a sacral decubitus from developing when a patient is sitting up in bed, try rolling the bed up to a 90-degree angle and use a pressure-distributing cushion under the patient.

► Use a *bed cradle* to keep the weight of the bed blankets off the patient's feet. This device, along with the use of an alternating-

pressure mattress, helps to prevent the development of heel sores, and it keeps the patient more comfortable.

► *Bed socks or elbow or heel pads* made of foam rubber or sheepskin help to reduce friction between the patient's heels or elbows and the bedding, thus reducing the incidence of pressure sores. However, remember that such devices do cause some skin pressure and thus cannot be relied upon exclusively for prevention. Frequent skin checks and appropriate skin care are essential when protective devices are being used. Also, use caution when applying protective pads to make certain that you are not applying them too tightly.

► *Avoid* the use of *doughnuts* and *rubber rings* since these devices compress the area of skin beneath them, decreasing blood supply around points of pressure. As a result, doughnuts and rubber rings can actually cause large decubiti to form around the very area that they are designed to protect, thus enlarging the ulcer.

► *Avoid* the use of *rubbing alcohol* for back rubs; alcohol dries the patient's skin and makes it more prone to breakdown.

► *Avoid* the overuse of *sedatives* and *tranquilizers,* as these drugs tend to reduce the patient's desire to move and turn.

► Provide the patient with adequate *fluids* and with a *nutritious diet* that is high in protein and vitamin C—nutrients that encourage tissue build-up and repair. *Note:* Merely *providing* a nutritious and fluid balanced diet is often not sufficient therapy. The nurse needs to ensure that the patient is actually *consuming* the food and fluids that are provided. (See Unit VII.)

► Keep the patient's *skin clean, dry and well lubricated.* However:

> *Skin care* alone, *including the use of special soaps, silicone preparations, and zinc oxide, will* not *prevent the development of pressure sores.*

► *Teach* patients and their relatives the value of frequent turning and movement. Also, alert patients can be taught to examine their own skin on a daily basis for the slightest signs of pressure. Finally, the patient confined to a wheelchair can be taught to lift his buttocks off the seat of the wheelchair by pressing down with his hands on the arms of the chair. This maneuver, if done at least twice an hour, reduces the shearing force. Paraplegics, in particular, benefit from learn-

ing to perform this technique. Some patients who are particularly prone to skin breakdown need to do their "pushups" every 15 minutes.

Continue to assist even the most severely disabled patients out of bed for short intervals. Voice controlled wheelchairs give mobility to persons who have very little motor function. These wheelchairs can be operated with very little energy output.

17. PRONE (FLAT FACE-LYING) POSITION FOR BED PATIENTS

By Jean Saxon, R.N., M.N.

Definition and Purposes.   *Lying horizontal on abdomen.* Used to: provide comfort by relieving pressure on bony prominences of back and sides and relaxing muscles; prevent or treat decubitus ulcers or draining wounds on back, heels, ankles and elbows; prevent joint stiffness, muscle weakness; provide range of motion (ROM) for head, shoulder, hips, knees and ankles; expand lungs and provide postural drainage; and prevent or treat foot drop. Also used to overcome effects of stroke, e.g., flexion of neck, elbow, wrist and fingers; flexion, adduction and internal rotation of shoulder. Nurse modifies procedure to utilize patient's capabilities and achieve objective.

Contraindications and Cautions.   Patients with artificial airway (tracheostomy), unstable vertebral fractures, recent spinal surgery, or conditions which would make torsion of the neck dangerous should be turned by mechanical aids, e.g., turning frames (Stryker or Foster) or CircOlectric bed. Patients with recent strokes, dyspnea (difficult breathing), congestive heart failure or respiratory problems do not tolerate the prone position. Patients who exhibit respiratory distress in prone position should immediately be turned out of this position. Provide call signal that can be activated in prone position for patients who cannot turn alone.

Patient-Family Teaching Points.   Provide the patient and family with the following information as appropriate: (a) encourage patients who can move themselves to do so, thereby maintaining and strengthening their muscles; (b) explain to patient how the move is to be accomplished even if he appears to be unconscious and how long the prone position will be maintained; (c) explain reason why patient is to be in prone position; (d) emphasize to helper that correct body mechanics will prevent injury; (e) emphasize that pads under body hollows maintain patient's body alignment and relieve pressure on bony prominences; (f) teach helper to check for pressure by feeling under ear, face, shoulders, anterior superior iliac spines, knees and toes; (g) explain how deep breathing and coughing while in prone position expands lungs and promotes postural drainage; (h) explain that proper prone position resembles normal standing alignment (however, postural drainage may require flexion of the lumbar vertebrae with base of lungs higher than head); (i) encourage patient to remain in prone position for up to two hours and (j) explain to patient that position of his arms, head and legs can be adjusted for comfort and that he will be turned if he becomes uncomfortable or has difficulty breathing.

PRE-PROCEDURE ACTIVITIES

PRELIMINARY PATIENT ASSESSMENT

Includes determination of:
- Diagnosis
- Level of consciousness
- Abilities and limitations concerning movement
- Date and type of surgery
- Ability to follow directions
- Catheter, IV or other attachments
- Order for postural drainage
- Schedule for prone position
- Previous prone positioning method

PRELIMINARY PLANNING

- Determine number of personnel required to safely move patient and ways personnel can participate
- Provide pillows, pads and bolsters as needed (check patient's supply)
- Provide bed linens or gown if needed
- Plan moves to be made for comfort and safety of patient
- Determine movement and positioning of IV, bladder drainage and other attachments

EQUIPMENT

- Firm bed with mattress at head of bed (allows space for toes at foot of bed)
- Two 6 mm. vinyl plastic sheets 4 ft. × 4 ft. (for heavy patient)
- Two folded draw sheets or pull sheets (for heavy patient)
- Side rails, footboard
- Pillows (3–4); flat pillow or pad for head
- Foam rubber or linen pads for shoulders
- Bath blanket
- Sputum container and facial tissues
- IV pole

PREPARATION OF PATIENT

- Discuss move with patient and helpers
- Avoid drafts, provide privacy
- Fan-fold top linen on top of footboard or remove top linen
- Cover patient with bath blanket
- Remove pillows or other positioning aids
- Level bed; adjust bed to working height, and lower side rails
- Place vinyl plastic and pull sheet under heavy patient
- Move IV, bladder drainage and other attachments as necessary

PROCEDURE

SUGGESTED STEPS	RATIONALE/ASSESSMENT

Prone Position for Helpless Patient

A. *Prone position for helpless patient.* One or two assistants necessary for heavy patients.

1. Move patient's body diagonally in sections *down* in bed so that heels and ankles are off end of the mattress. (See Procedure 1, Steps A, B and C, Chap. 21.) Omit this step if there is not enough room for patient's feet between end of mattress and footboard or foot of bed.

2. Move patient to the side edge of bed. (See Procedure 1, Step D.)

3. Place head pillow with side of pillow under head so patient will be off of pillow when turned.

4. Raise side rail next to patient; go around bed.

A. Helpless patient is vulnerable to decubiti. Adequate help prevents friction on patient's skin.

1. Remember, to move patient down in bed, his head and shoulders are moved first, then hips, and last legs. Provides for extension of feet with pressure on soles of feet against footboard or firm pillow; prevents plantar flexion.

2. Provides space on bed for patient when turned.

3. Avoids hyperextension of neck and smothering.

4. Protects patient from falling.

Procedure continued on the following page

SUGGESTED STEPS	RATIONALE/ASSESSMENT

Prone Position for Helpless Patient (Continued)

5. Place second vinyl plastic and pull sheet on bed next to heavy patient.	5. After the turn, heavy patients usually need to be moved toward center of bed in prone position to provide room for arms.
6. Place pillows on bed next to patient in line with his body hollows as follows:	6. Provides support of body hollows and simulates standing body alignment in prone position.
a. Lower chest and abdomen for woman patient; from waist to symphysis pubis for men. Use large pillow if no space at end of mattress.	a. Protects breasts and reduces lumbar curve; protects scrotum and reduces lumbar curve.
b. Lower legs, below knees and above ankles (Fig. 33–6). One pillow at thighs and two pillows at lower legs if it is not possible to place feet over edge of bed (Fig. 33–7).	b. Provides slight flexion of knees; prevents hyperextension of knees and lumbar vertebrae.
7. Fan-fold bath blanket to far side of patient; adjust gown or pajama top so is smooth over chest, loose at neck and shoulder.	7. Prevents catching bath blanket under patient. Provides smooth surface under patient; provides loose garment at neck and axillae.
8. Place patient's near arm (arm on which he will be turned) flat against his body with palm next to his thigh.	8. Prevents injury to patient's hand and arm; prevents catching patient's arm under his body.
9. Tuck edge of abdominal pillow and leg pillow(s) under patient.	9. Holds pillows in place during turn.
10. Flex far leg and place over near leg. Omit this step if spine and/or hips must remain extended.	10. Provides for easier turn. Remember to tell patient before moving leg.

Caution: "Log rolling" using two or three helpers must be used to prevent flexion of hips and spine.

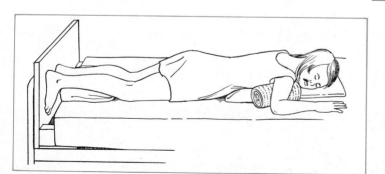

Figure 33–6. Patient supported in prone position with toes over end of mattress. Correct prone position is similar to standing posture: neck extended; spine straight, with reduced lumbar curve, hips extended; slight flexion of knees; feet at right angles (90 degrees) to body. *Note:* footboard should be covered for patient use.

Figure 33–7. Correct prone positioning when it is not possible to place patient's toes over end of mattress. Pillows under lower legs *and* thighs reduce knee flexion and remove knee pressure. Larger abdominal and head pillows are needed than for patient in Figure 33–6, to prevent hyperextension of hips and to maintain hip alignment. Shoulder rolls must also be larger to provide adequate support.

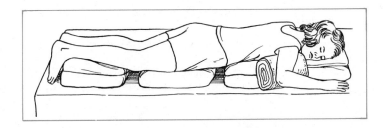

SUGGESTED STEPS	RATIONALE/ASSESSMENT

Prone Position for Helpless Patient (Continued)

11. Place patient's far arm with palm against his thigh.	11. Prevents patient's arm from getting caught under his body during turn.
12. Assume a forward-backward stance at patient's side. Hold patient's far shoulder and hip (securing patient's arm with your hand) or grasp vinyl and pull sheet for heavy patient. If additional assistants are needed, they should support patient's head, shoulder and hip, and far leg.	12. Provides for safe body mechanics for helper(s) and patient. Patients fear smothering with face in bed while in prone position. One assistant supports head and turns head to one side. Second assistant lifts far leg by holding under ankle and knee.
13. Signal by count of "1, 2, 3" and pull when count of "3" is stated. If assistants are used, all must move patient's body sections in unison.	*Remember: Patient must be warned of turn even if he appears unresponsive.* Assistants provide support to patient's body sections simultaneously to maintain spinal or hip alignment. (Do *not* use this method if cervical spinal alignment is necessary).
14. Smoothly turn patient to abdomen. Reach across patient; move his arm away from body (abduct shoulder) and place palm up (internal rotation of shoulder and arm).	14. Prevents jarring and/or frightening patient; prevents injury to arm and provides range of motion to shoulder, arm and hand.
15. *Immediately check patient's nose and mouth to make certain he can breathe.* Turn head if necessary and/or place flat pillow or pad under cheek and head. Remove large head pillow and cover patient with bath blanket.	15. Prevents respiratory distress or airway obstruction caused by nose and mouth pressing into mattress.
16. If patient is heavy, two assistants return to other side of bed, lower side rail and pull patient to middle of bed. Remove vinyl and pull sheet from patient's back.	16. Prevents injury to patient's arm and leg, which could fall over edge bed.
17. Feel under patient's knees, heels and toes for pressure. Adjust footboard and pillow support to relieve pressure as necessary.	17. Prevents pressure that may cause decubiti. Footboard pressure on heels can produce decubiti.

Procedure continued on the following page

SUGGESTED STEPS	RATIONALE/ASSESSMENT

Prone Position for Helpless Patient (Continued)

18. Place rolls of linen or sponge rubber at angle between lateral clavicle and armpit.	18. "Shoulder rolls" provide support to upper chest and facilitate chest expansion; reduces lateral flexion of neck and pressure on ear; and removes pressure on anterior shoulders.
19. Feel under patient's anterior superior iliac spines for pressure. Adjust abdominal pillow support to relieve pressure.	19. Prevents pressure which may cause decubiti.
20. Position near arm above patient's head, with forearm at head level or with arm extended at side. Use hand roll if indicated. Check under shoulder and elbow for pressure. Adjust shoulder roll and/or provide pads above and below elbow to relieve pressure.	20. Provides change of position of arm, range of motion of shoulder, elbow, lower arm, wrist and fingers. Prevents pressure which may cause decubiti.
21. Raise side rail.	21. Provides patient safety.
22. Observe patient from side and foot of bed for correct body alignment. Make adjustments to correct spinal alignment by pulling body sections. (See Procedure 1, step D.)	22. Assess for "normal standing position" from lateral and posterior view.
23. Following adjustments in position, recheck body alignment, airway, and pressure areas. Check IV, bladder drainage and other attachments for proper functioning. Observe for relaxation; ask patient if he is comfortable.	23. Even if the patient is unresponsive, he appears relaxed and comfortable when properly positioned. Remember, pressure can be determined by feeling under ear, shoulders, anterior superior iliac spines, knees, heels and toes.
24. Cover patient with top covers, place signal, and raise side rail.	24. Provides physical and psychologic comfort and safety.
25. Periodically change position of patient's arms, and encourage deep breathing and coughing while prone position maintained.	25. Provides comfort; increases range of motion and lung expansion; prevents joint stiffness and muscle weakness.
26. To return patient to supine position, reverse procedure, using only head pillow. If feet over edge of bed, move footboard away from feet and guide feet during turn. Observe male for scrotal edema.	26. Removes patient from pillow supports by turning him off them. Report scrotal edema, which may result from dependent edema associated with medical conditions or pressure which obstructs circulation.

Caution: Injuries to toes, heels and ankles can occur from footboard, scratches from patient's toenails and/or pressure on ankle bones (malleoli).

SUGGESTED STEPS	RATIONALE/ASSESSMENT

Prone Position for Patient Who Can Use Arms

B. *Prone position for patient who has use of upper extremities and can follow directions.*	B. May be used for patient who: needs to strengthen muscles and increase range of joint motion, is paraplegic (paralyzed lower extremities) and/or has amputation above or below knee.
1. Tell patient to move down in bed if there is room for his feet at end of mattress.	1. Patient may be able to sit up, flex knees, and lift buttocks down in bed. Assist only as necessary.
2. Tell patient to move to edge of bed. Tell patient with unilateral amputation to move toward unaffected side.	2. Teach patient to move his body in sections.
3. Tell patient to place abdominal pillow and leg pillows in line with body parts on bed; tuck edges of pillow under body. (See A6 above).	3. Paraplegic patients must learn to avoid pressure at knees and toes, since they cannot feel pressure and are vulnerable to decubiti. Amputees must avoid hip flexion and excessive knee flexion.
4. Tell patient to lift leg at edge of bed over other leg, onto leg pillows.	4. Provides long lever pull toward the turn-to-prone position.
5. Tell patient to raise head and chest by pushing up on elbows.	5. Increases strength of upper extremities.
6. Tell patient to turn onto pillows by reaching across bed with arm which was on edge of bed and elevating chest with weight on other elbow.	6. Arm at edge of bed serves as a long lever to turn body.
7. If patient unable to raise head and chest on elbows, tell him to place arm on which he will turn to the side of his body (see A8 above), use other arm to reach across bed to opposite mattress edge or grasp opposite side rail.	7. Arm at edge serves as a long lever to turn body. Protects injury to arm on which patient turns.
8. Tell patient to place "shoulder rolls" and flat head pillow as desired.	8. Assist only as necessary.
9. Tell patient to correct his alignment by pulling head, chest and abdomen in line with legs.	9. Assess for "standing posture" and teach patient how to assess. Amputees must learn to assess for maintaining extension of hip and only slight flexion of knee.
10. Teach patient to reverse procedure to assume supine position, except:	10. Returning to supine position is more difficult to learn. Assist patient as necessary until strength increases.

Procedure continued on the following page

SUGGESTED STEPS

RATIONALE/ASSESSMENT

Prone Position for Patient Who Can Use Arms (Continued)

a. Tell weak patient and/or amputee to push with far knee and hand, also with elbow of other arm.

a. Arm and leg become long levers to complete turn after gaining momentum with push off.

b. Tell paraplegic to push with far hand and elbow. Tell patient to uncross legs.

b. Turning force is provided by upper extremities; as trunk is turned, legs follow.

Post-Procedure Activities.   Assist patient to a comfortable position. Provide oral hygiene if expectoration has occurred. Provide call signal; lower bed. Raise side rails if needed. Ask patient how he feels and for his suggestions for additions or modifications to increase his comfort.

Aftercare of Equipment.   Discard soiled linen; store pillows, pads, shoulder rolls, vinyl and turning sheets in patient's unit.

Chart/Report.   Time of day; length of time in prone position; how tolerated; problems encountered; method and equipment used; suggested modifications (from helper and patient); patient's ability to deep breathe, cough and expectorate (measured or estimated amount, color and consistency); treatment given while patient in prone position, e.g., therapy to treat or prevent decubiti. Immediately report respiratory distress or untoward results, e.g., red pressure areas or tissue abrasions, scrotal edema.

TREATMENT OF DECUBITUS

Despite the conscientious use of the preventive measures just listed, certain patients, because of their extremely debilitated condition, *do* develop pressure sores. Also, you may be assigned patients who have pressure sores that they developed before admission to the hospital. When a pressure sore is present, what are some of the treatment measures that you can take?

Because decubitus ulcers are extremely difficult to treat, numerous methods of treatment have evolved over time. Some of these treatments (e.g., flotation therapy) are based on strictly scientific principles, while others, such as the pouring of granulated sugar into the wound, are derived from folk medicine. Below are listed some methods of treatment, both new and old, that are being employed today.

Covered Foam Rubber Supports or Pillows. Firm cushions are used to provide the "bridging" of pressure prone areas of the skin from contact with other surfaces. Refer back to Figures 33–3 and 33–5. Foam cushions are also used to support the body in good alignment and to free an entire body surface from pressure as in Figure 33–8.

Special Mattresses.   Special mattresses such

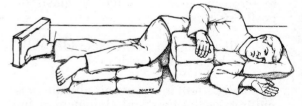

SIDE LYING   Support upper extremities on firm, double pillows to prevent overstretching shoulder and hip muscles. Place lower leg in slight hyperextension, flat on bed, with foot supported at right angle to leg, and malleolus protected. Usually, no back support is needed if the patient has been correctly postured.

Suggested by Nicholas F. Saverine, L.P.N., New Jersey

Figure 33–8. Posturing a patient in a side-lying position to prevent or treat decubitus ulcers. (From Larrabee, J. H.: The person with spinal cord injury: physical care during early recovery. *American Journal of Nursing,* 77:1327, Aug. 1977.)

as the alternating-pressure mattress and special *turning devices* such as the Foster and Stryker frames are used not only as preventive measures against the development of decubiti, but are employed in treatment as well.

Flotation Therapy. Flotation therapy is a sophisticated form of therapy in which the patient is placed upon a plastic tarpaulin which, in turn, floats upon water. Flotation therapy is based upon Archimedes' principle that when a body is partially submerged in water, it gives up its weight. Thus, when a patient with a decubitus ulcer is allowed to float upon water, his body displaces some of the liquid which fills the "water bed." As a result, the patient's body becomes lighter and the pressure exerted against the patient's skin by the "water mattress" is far less than that which would be exerted by an ordinary mattress. This form of therapy is highly successful with paralyzed patients and with burn victims. In these cases, the "water bed" definitely seems to promote healing of the ulcer. Another advantage of flotation therapy is that the routine constant turning and positioning normally required by paralyzed patients is not necessary and can be virtually discontinued; as a result, these individuals receive more rest.

Unfortunately not all patients can tolerate weightlessness. Individuals with serious emotional problems sometimes experience hallucinations and nightmares; others become emotionally isolated and withdrawn. Also, because flotation therapy reduces the need for turning, some patients on "water beds" have developed contractures and other immobilization disabilities. To prevent these iatrogenic problems, nurses must put patients on flotation therapy through range-of-motion exercises at least two or three times a day. Also, the nursing staff must constantly observe for the signs of thrombus formation, renal calculi, anorexia, and constipation.

Air-fluidized Bed. The air-fluidized bed is another method for preventing decubitus ulcers. The patient who lies upon this special device floats upon a loose polyester filter sheet placed over a bed filled with fine sterile glass beads. Air, which is delivered by a blower, continuously flows upward through the beads (Fig. 33–9). As a result of the constant airflow, the patient's body is supported and his weight is evenly distributed. This form of therapy has proved to be of special value in the care of paraplegics with ulcerations of the chest wall, sacrum, and the ischial tuberosities. With this treatment, hallucinations and other mental disturbances have not been reported to date.

The Screen Box. Griffin describes a simple gauze-covered device that has been demonstrated as an aid to decubitus healing (Fig. 33–

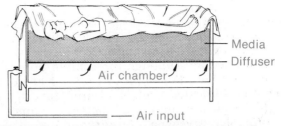

Figure 33–9. Air-fluidized bed. (From Harvin, J. F., and Hargest, T. S.: The air-fluidized bed: a new concept in the treatment of decubitus ulcers. *Nursing Clinics of N. A.,* 5:181, March 1970.)

10). For construction details for this device refer to the original report.[26]

Local Therapeutic Measures. Numerous different types of local therapeutic measures (i.e., therapies that are applied directly to the ulcerated area) are used, despite the fact that many of these therapies are without a known scientific basis. Some of the more common local treatment measures are listed below. All these "therapies" are applied directly to the pressure sore.

> Karaya products
> Gelfoam
> granulated sugar
> Elase ointment
> A and D ointment
> salt solutions
> irrigations
> desloughing agents
> exposure to the air
> exposure to ultraviolet light
> mixtures of tincture of benzoin and mineral oil
> sheepskins
> yeast

Anabolic Steroids. Anabolic steroids are sometimes given to promote the retention of nitrogen. The rationale for this use is to counteract the state of negative nitrogen balance which seems to characterize most patients with decubiti.

Application of Insulin. Van Ort describes the following procedure: "10 units of U-40 regular insulin (USP) twice daily immediately following breakfast and the evening meal. The insulin

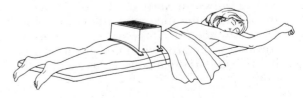

Figure 33–10. The screen box. (From Griffin, A.: The screen box. *Nursing '75, 5*:25, March 1975.)

was dropped from a syringe from which the needle had been removed. The decubitus ulcer was then exposed to the air to dry. No dressing was applied.''[60] Although the sample population was small, the improved rate of healing resulting indicated a need for further investigation of topical insulin as a treatment regimen.

Surgical Intervention. Surgical intervention is sometimes used when the decubitus ulcer is healing very slowly, thereby leaving the patient open to infection and increasing disability, owing to loss of serum and protein from the draining sore. In surgery, the ulcer is usually debrided and then closed. In some cases, skin must be grafted over the ulcerated site.

The doctor may choose any one of the treatment measures just listed. However, no matter which treatment is instituted, it is important that the nurse carry out the following:

▶ Institute immediately a program containing the vital preventive measures discussed earlier (i.e., patient teaching, ordering of nutritious diet, placing the patient on a special mattress). Whenever possible, prevent pressure on the decubitus by placing the patient on firm pillows or foam cushions so that the bony prominences do not touch the bed.[3, 28] The nurse should reach under the patient and feel with her hand to be certain that no pressure is over bony prominences.[3, 28, 44]

▶ Give the patient firm psychologic support. Remember that this patient faces the additional trauma of seeing and smelling a draining, foul sore that is actually eroding *his* body. Also, the sick individual who develops a pressure sore will now be confined for a longer period because of his new affliction.

▶ Prevent the ulcerated area from becoming infected. Infection will retard healing of the ulcer and may eventually result in *osteomyelitis*—a condition characterized by inflammation of the bone marrow. Patients with a pressure sore in the early stages should have the ulcerated site cultured for the presence of *Staphylococcus aureus*. Antibiotic therapy will need to be started immediately if organisms are present in the drainage.

Tepperman's[57] overview of the problem of pressure sores provides a useful summary (Tables 33–2 through 33–5).

TABLE 33–2.   MAJOR AND SECONDARY SITES OF PRESSURE SORES*

MAJOR
Sacrum or coccyx
Ischial tuberosity
Greater trochanter
Medial condyle of tibia
Head of fibula
Malleolus
Heel
Olecranon
Lateral condyle of humerus

SECONDARY
Acromion
Spine of scapula
Occipital prominence
Mastoid
Ear
Lower cervical or upper or middle thoracic spine (apex of kyphosis)
Anterior iliac crest

*From Tepperman, P. S., et al.: Pressure sore: prevention and step-up management. *Postgraduate Medicine*, 62:86, Sep. 1977.

The Effects of Prolonged Bed Rest upon the Musculoskeletal System

While relief from the stress of activity is helpful in certain orthopedic conditions, immobilization of the body's bones, muscles, and joints can result in severe and permanent disabilities. Major musculoskeletal problems created by bed rest are: (1) weakness; (2) backache; (3) muscle or disease atrophy, joint stiffness, and contractures; and (4) disuse osteoporosis. Figure 33–11 depicts the poor positioning which many patients tend to assume as they lie in bed with the back rest elevated.

Weakness. Any person who has been

TABLE 33–3.   FACTORS INFLUENCING THE RISK OF PRESSURE SORE DEVELOPMENT*

INTRINSIC
Degree of mobility
Nutritional status
Age
Mental status
Cardiovascular status
Presence of anemia or blood dyscrasia
Presence of tissue fragility
Presence of motor or sensory deficit (diabetic, orthopedic, neurologic, rheumatologic, neoplastic)

EXTRINSIC
Positioning
Turning
Passive mobilization
Condition of bedclothes
Skin care

*From Tepperman, P. S., et al.: Pressure sore: prevention and step-up management. *Postgraduate Medicine*, 62:86, Sep. 1977.

TABLE 33–4.   AIDS TO PRESSURE SORE MANAGEMENT*

MATTRESSES FOR RECUMBENT PATIENTS
Cube (foam)
T foam (Temper foam)
Air (Roho, alternating ripple)
Water (do not overinflate)

CUSHIONS FOR SEATED PATIENTS
Foam rubber (might be used with plywood cutout)
Cube (foam)
T foam (Temper foam)
Sculptured foam
Gel
Air (Roho, Adaptive)
Water
Back support

OTHER AIDS
Pillows of various size to help maintain position
Blankets (cellular and flannel) to help maintain position
   and decrease friction
Sheepskin mats, boots, elbows
Bed cradles to improve ventilation and to decrease friction
   and pressure

*From Tepperman, P. S., et al.: Pressure sore: prevention
and step-up management. *Postgraduate Medicine*, 62:86,
Sep. 1977.

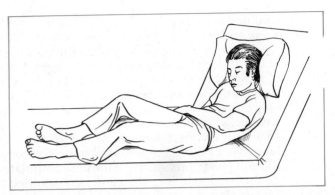

Figure 33–11.   Poor position often assumed by a patient in bed with back rest elevated. *Note:* flexion of neck, curve of back, compression of chest, external rotation of hips and foot and wrist drop. Also observe the areas of the body bearing the patient's weight, thus being prone to development of pressure sores.

TABLE 33–5.   STEP-UP MANAGEMENT OF PRESSURE SORES*

MEASURES	STAGE 1 OR 2 (BLANCHING OR NONBLANCHING HYPEREMIA)	STAGE 3 (CLOSED BLISTER OR ESCHAR)	STAGE 4 OR 5 (CLEAN OR INFECTED ULCER)
Surface agents	Silicone spray, cornstarch	Not indicated	Antiseptic (physiologic or hypertonic saline solution, Hygeol,† brown soap)
Thermal agents	Cool pack for five to eight minutes three times a day	Not indicated	Contraindicated
Exposure	To air (fan or cool blower may be used)	Same	Same; dry nonstick dressing if necessary
Positioning	Turn patient every two hours, keep pressure off affected area until redness is gone (minimum of four hours in stage 1, average 48 hours in stage 2)	Same; keep pressure off area >48 hours in blister stage or until eschar has healed	Same; keep pressure off area until ulcer is healed and skin toughened
Ultraviolet light	Not indicated	Not indicated	May be indicated
Pressure redistribution (aids and devices)	Sheepskins, pillows, folded cellular blankets, bed cradles, plus (in stage 2) pressure-distributing cushions and mattresses (air, gel, foam)	Same	Same
Other	None	None	Surgical débridement, excision, closure, grafting, placement of rotating flap, and (in stage 5) systemic antibiotic therapy

*From Tepperman, P. S., et al.: Pressure sore: prevention and step-up management. *Postgraduate Medicine*, 62:86,
Sep. 1977.
†Marketed in Canada by Wampole Laboratories. The US equivalent is a stabilized solution of sodium hypochlorite,
Zonite (Dunbar Laboratories).

confined to bed for even three or four days feels weak and wobbly when he first gets up. This weakness upon ambulation is attributable both to the underlying illness and to the weakening of antigravity muscles, i.e., those muscles that support the body while standing, walking, and balancing movements. To prevent excessive weakness, patients should be ambulated as soon as it can be tolerated. Also, patients who have been bedridden will feel more comfortable and less apprehensive if they are ambulated gradually, first being "dangled," then guided to a chair placed near the bed, and then walked to the bathroom or day room where they can remain for a longer period of time each day. By means of a planned program of ambulation, bedridden patients will slowly regain confidence concerning their ability to walk and to balance themselves. The longer a patient has remained in bed, the longer it will take him to regain his strength, balance, and coordination. Remember:

> *It takes a patient three or four days to recover from a short period of immobilization, but four to six weeks to recover from six weeks of immobilization.*

Backache. Patients confined to bed for a period of time often complain of backache. Backaches may result from poor posture, awkward alignment of the patient's body when in bed, and/or a soft mattress that gives poor support to the patient's back. To combat backache, the following measures are helpful: (1) scheduled position changes, (2) a firm mattress and/or bedboards placed under the mattress, (3) frequent back rubs, (4) a daily exercise program, and (5) physiotherapy.

Muscle Atrophy, Joint Stiffness, and Contractures. For the body's muscles and joints to remain healthy and mobile, they must be subjected to a certain amount of daily stress and strain and they must be put through a normal range of movements. Without daily strain and movement, muscles quickly weaken, atrophy, and shorten, and joints become stiff and immobile. Indeed, when muscles are not sufficiently exercised and joints are allowed to remain immobilized in one position for a prolonged time, *contractures* result that can doom the patient to permanent crippling deformities that resist all attempts at treatment!

A *contracture* is defined as a permanent contraction of a muscle in which the muscle is fixed, shortened, and resists stretching. Contractures can result from: (1) lack of exercise, (2) muscle spasticity, (3) prolonged joint immobilization, (4) pain that prevents movement, and (5) edema and swelling which can splint an area and thereby limit muscular activity. Three of the most common deformities that result from prolonged bed rest are footdrop, wrist drop, and external rotation of the hip.

Contractures are an extremely difficult disability to treat once they form; indeed, the treatment of a contracture involves extensive physiotherapy and may even require surgery. Thus, as with all immobilization disabilities, it is best to *prevent* contractures from developing in the first place. Some important preventive measures are the following:

▶ Group exercises as appropriate for all patients in the same room or setting.

▶ Frequent scheduled position changes and *individualized* exercise programs. Individualized exercise programs have demonstrated an improvement in appetite and reductions in constipation, skin breakdown and use of narcotics among immobilized patients.

▶ The use of bedboards and a firm mattress ensures better alignment of the patient's body.

▶ A padded footboard placed *firmly* against the patient's feet helps to prevent footdrop.

▶ A trapeze over the patient's bed will encourage him to move and turn himself and to perform self-care activities. *Note:* At times the trapeze is removed to reinforce "pushing" rather than "pulling" activities, thus preparing the patient to transfer himself, e.g., from bed to wheelchair, from commode to bed.

▶ Handrolls help to maintain the patient's hand in a position of function.

▶ A soft foam-rubber sponge for the patient to squeeze helps to prevent finger flexion contractures, particularly at the metacarpophalangeal joint.

▶ A trochanter roll (made by folding a bath-towel or bath blanket into thirds lengthwise and then in half) can be tucked under the patient's thigh and hip and then rolled firmly under itself to prevent external rotation of the hip.

▶ Avoidance of the use of the knee-gatch bed position helps to prevent hip and knee flexion contractures.

▶ Range-of-motion exercises in which each joint is put through as complete a range of motion as possible without producing pain. Each range-of-motion exercise should be done six times during each of three periods scheduled throughout the day. Range-of-motion exercises are presented in Procedure 18.

▶ Isometric exercises during which the patient, at first, need not move his joints but can simply contract his various limb and trunk muscles. Later the patient may exercise against resistance by pushing against a weight or sandbag.

▶ Shoulders, in particular, must be put through a full range of motion several times daily.

> *Elderly patients who are receiving intravenous infusions, and whose arms are immobilized for even an hour a day, may develop a "frozen shoulder" if their arms are not exercised.*

18. RANGE-OF-MOTION PASSIVE EXERCISES

By Jean Saxon, R.N., M.N.

Definition and Purposes.   *The movement of a patient's joints through their complete range-of-motion (ROM) when the patient is unable to use these muscles that normally move the joint. Persons who perform this activity may be: the patient, using his strong side to move his paralyzed side; nurse or other helper; physical therapist; occupational therapist; family member or friend.* Used to: *maintain* joint mobility; *prevent* adaptive shortening of muscles and tendons, ligaments and joint capsule, which can lead to stiffness and limitation of motion and result in ankylosis (fixation of a joint) and contractures (limitation of joint motion because of shortening of the muscles); prevent adaptive stretching or lengthening of connective tissue around joints; prevent deformities that limit function (ankylosis and contracture); *stimulate* circulation and sensory nerve endings; and *restore* loss of joint function. Nurse obtains physician's orders for passive ROM exercises if pathologic conditions are present, alerts physicians of early functional deficits, and independently carries out regular daily passive ROM exercises on normal joints that a patient cannot move.

Contraindications and Cautions.   Do not give passive ROM to joints with pathologic conditions, e.g., acute arthritis, fractures, torn ligaments, joint dislocation. A physician's order is required before starting passive ROM following recovery and for acute cardiac conditions. You can injure a joint by moving it beyond the point of pain, spasm or tremor, spasticity or by stretching a contracted muscle or ligament. Obtain guidance of physician, occupational therapist or physical therapist when muscle spasms are due to central nervous system damage. Stop passive ROM exercises when patient exhibits pain, resistance or fatigue. Individuals vary widely in range of joint motion, so check range of opposite extremity if feasible; otherwise, check motion on yourself and observe for resistance or pain. During passive ROM exercises, movement of joints should be slow, rhythmical and supported (controlled).

> *An immobilized joint will begin to exhibit connective tissue changes in as short a time as 4 days, therefore preventive passive ROM exercises must be started as soon as possible.*

Patient-Family Teaching Points. Provide the patient and family with the following information as appropriate: (a) explain why ROM exercises are being given; (b) explain that exercises must be given daily, preferably three times a day; (c) explain that passive exercises given correctly will maintain joint mobility, but will not preserve muscle mass or bone mineralization (since there is no voluntary contraction and lengthening of muscles or tension on bones); (d) teach how to perform movement of joints through their complete range of motion; (e) teach how to protect joints during exercise and symptoms to look for indicating injury, e.g., pain, spasm; (f) explain how positioning which provides change of joint alignment can contribute to joint mobility; (g) explain how poor body positioning can damage joints; (h) teach patient how to give passive ROM to a paralyzed extremity by using a good extremity, including use of pulley and bicycle and (i) explain the importance of progression from passive to assistive to active ROM exercises as soon as possible.

PRE-PROCEDURE ACTIVITIES

PRELIMINARY ASSESSMENT

Includes determination of:
- Diagnosis
- Activity orders
- Physician's order for passive ROM of joints with pathologic conditions, e.g., red, swollen joints, subluxation of shoulder (dislocation), fractures, pulled or torn ligaments
- Nursing orders for passive ROM exercises
- Ability to follow directions
- Abilities and limitations of joint movement

PRELIMINARY PLANNING

- Determine joints to be exercised and patient positions to be used
- Review normal movements of joints to be exercised, e.g., flexion, extension, hyperextension, rotation, etc.
- Determine goal of exercise, e.g., maintain current function, prevent loss or further loss of function, or restore function
- Assess need for additional helper if patient's extremities heavy
- Provide for comfort and safety of patient, e.g., cover for warmth and prevention of exposure of genitalia, pillows for positioning, siderails
- Arrange unit to provide space for helper's use of correct body mechanics

EQUIPMENT

- Firm bed (hi-low if possible)
- Bath blanket
- Crotch cover, shorts
- Pulley for arm or leg exercise if indicated
- Mitt, strap and/or sling for pulley if indicated
- Bicycle for leg exercise if indicated
- Gown, robe, shoes and socks as appropriate
- Wheelchair or chair if indicated

PREPARATION OF PATIENT

- Explain that passive exercises will be carried out and how (even if patient is not responsive)
- Explain that exercise should not be painful or fatiguing and instruct patient to tell helper if it is
- Discuss with patient how he is to assist
- Level bed and raise to working height; lock bed wheels
- Transfer patient to chair or wheelchair if appropriate
- Fan-fold top linen to foot of bed
- Cover patient with bath blanket
- Dress patient in shorts or crotch cover or in robe, shoes, socks if appropriate

PROCEDURE

SUGGESTED STEPS	RATIONALE/DISCUSSION
A. *General considerations* for performance of passive ROM exercises.	Caution: *Do not move inflamed joints. Acute cardiac patients tolerate passive ROM better than isometric exercises, but a physician's order is necessary for any exercise.*

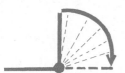
EXTENSION
Straightening a
flexed or bent joint

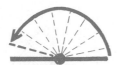
FLEXION
Bending a joint to
form an acute angle

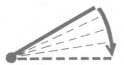
ADDUCTION
Moving arm, leg, or
finger toward normal
resting position

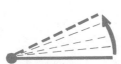
ABDUCTION
Moving arm, leg, or
finger away from
normal position

ROTATION
Turning on axis

Figure 33–12. Extension, flexion, adduction, abduction, and rotation. (From Drury, J. H.: Handbook of range-of-motion exercises. *Nursing '72, 2*:19, April 1972.)

SUGGESTED STEPS	RATIONALE/DISCUSSION
1. Maintain good posture, facing direction of movement and in a position to watch patient's face. Use shifting body weight and strong leg muscles when lifting patient's heavy arms or legs.	1. Provides efficient body movement and good body mechanics for helper. Allows helper to observe patient's reaction to movements.
2. Place patient in normal alignment for exercises if possible.	2. Medical orders for position or deformities may limit positions. Normal body alignment of patient provides reference for movement of joints.

> Caution: *Individuals vary in their normal range of motion.*

3. Move specific joint in normal direction of movement as far as it normally moves (Fig. 33–12). Ask physician, occupational therapist or physical therapist for guidance if in doubt.

Comparison of both sides of the body sometimes gives clues to the patient's normal joint movement. Prevents injury to joint.

> Caution: *Stop movement at point of pain, resistance or fatigue to prevent injury.*

a. Move the joint to point of: (1) *pain,* (2) *spasm* (sudden involuntary muscle contraction), (3) *tremor* (involuntary trembling or quivering of muscle, (4) *spasticity* (continuous hypertonicity or increase in tension and resistance in muscle) or (5) *contracture.* If spasm due to central nervous system damage, seek guidance of physician, physical or occupational therapist.

Fear of pain or exposure of genitalia may produce these reactions. Careful explanations, gentle manner, prior warm bath, massage, or analgesic may reduce these reactions. Experienced specialist can provide instruction for individual patient.

b. Support joint to be moved at joint unless joint is tender, e.g., arthritis, then support above and below joint.

b. Bed provides support when joint rests on bed, otherwise helper supports joint with one hand.

c. Support body part distal to joint to be moved when moving extremities by (1) cupping in hand(s) (see Fig. 33–13) or (2) cradling in arm (see Fig. 33–14).

c. Allows for controlled movement of joint.

Procedure continued on the following page

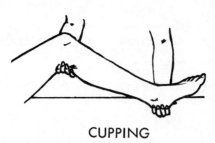

CUPPING

Figure 33–13. Support of leg by cupping. (From *Rehabilitative Aspects of Nursing;* Part 1, Physical Therapeutic Nursing Measures; Unit 2, Range of Joint Motion, National League for Nursing, Code Number 19-1277, 1967, p. 132.)

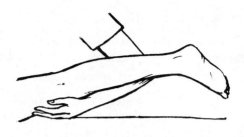

CRADLING

Figure 33–14. Support of leg by cradling. (From *Rehabilitative Aspects of Nursing;* Part I, Physical Therapeutic Nursing Measures; Unit 2, Range of Joint Motion, National League for Nursing, Code Number 19–1277, 1967, p. 131.)

SUGGESTED STEPS	RATIONALE/DISCUSSION
d. Move the joint in all its movements (flexion, extension, etc., see Fig. 33–12) six times slowly, rhythmically and with control.	d. Studies have shown that six movements of each range of motion once a day will maintain mobility of the joint; however, up to three times a day is recommended. Slow, rhythmical and supported movements prevent injury and complications, e.g., pain, spasm, etc.
4. Teach patient to perform passive exercise to paralyzed extremity with good arm or leg by one or more of these:	4. Provides active ROM to maintain muscle strength, mineralization of bone and ROM of noninvolved extremities.
a. Holding arm and hand with strong hand	
b. Supporting leg with strong foot or leg	
c. Using pulley for arm or leg	
d. Using bicycle exerciser for leg	
5. Utilize opportunities to prevent injury and provide passive ROM during personal care, turning and positioning:	5. Remember to move joints with support, slowly and rhythmically.
a. Wash, rinse and dry extremities with joints in two or three different positions, e.g., flexion, extension, abduction of shoulder.	a. Conserves nursing time while giving additional passive range-of-motion exercise.
b. Position joints in different positions every two hours, when patient's position is changed.	b. Prevents limitation of joint motion which can occur in perfect anatomical alignment.
c. Support parts with pillows or other bolsters to prevent stress on joint.	c. Prevents injuries from adaptive stretching and lengthening of joint connective tissue.

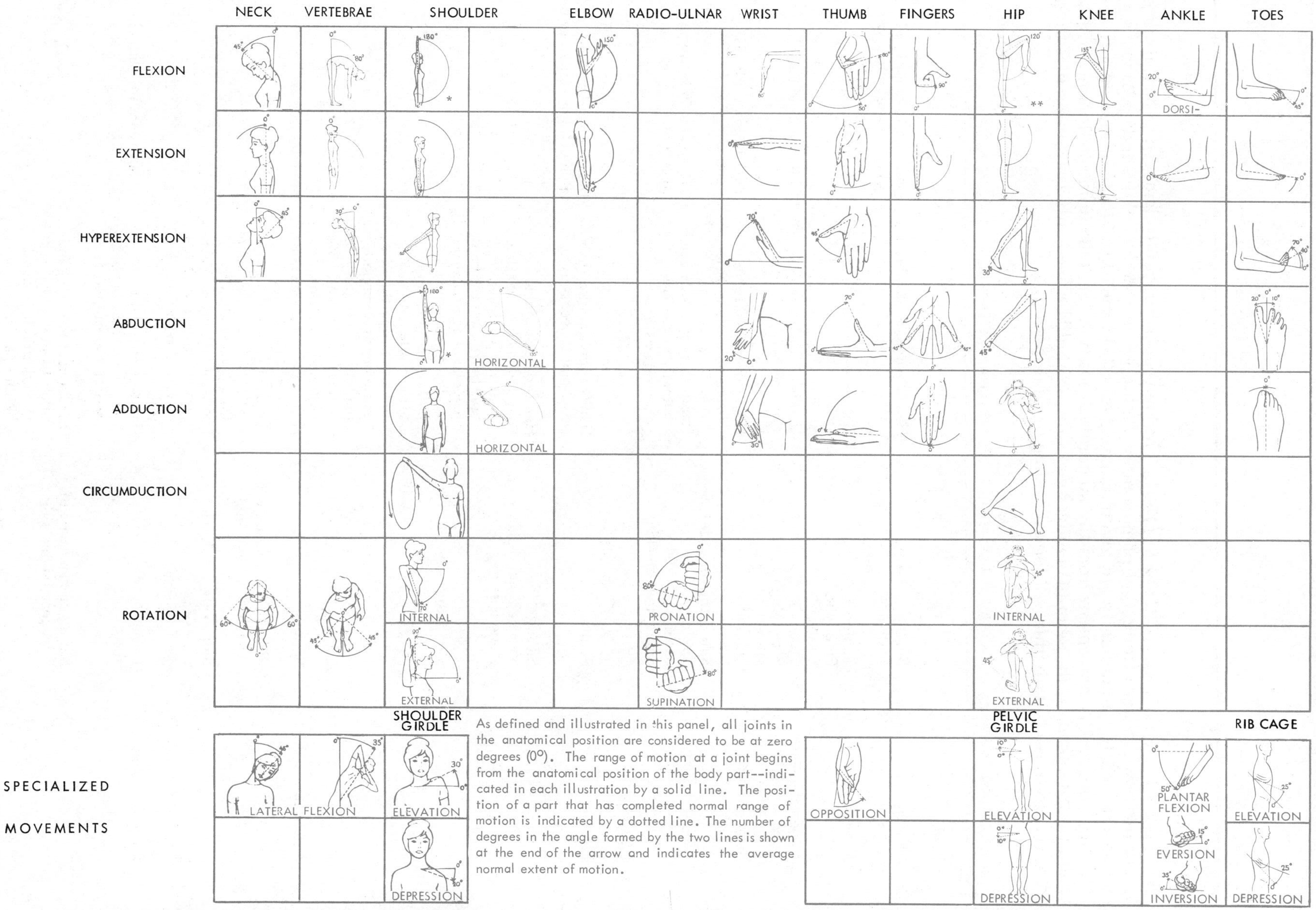

Figure 33–15. Movements of joints. *Notes:* *Shoulder abduction and flexion to 180° includes motion of the scapula (it represents combined glenohumeral and scapulothoracic motion).** Hip flexion to 120° is normal only with the knee flexed. (From Rehabilitative Aspects of Nursing, Part 1. Physical Therapeutic Nursing Measures. Unit 2. Range of Joint Motion. National League for Nursing, 1967.)

B.   *Table of Passive Range-of-Motion of Joints.* The joints most frequently damaged by lack of movement are shown. Name of joint, type of movement, method of support by helper, and terms that may be used to teach patient/family are given. See Figure 33–15 for illustrations of movements and "normal" degrees of movement from the anatomical position (patient supine with arms to side, palms up). *Remember:* the amount of movement shown should be used only as a guide, since there is variation in each individual's "normal" range of joint motion.

JOINT AND MOVEMENT	BODY POSITION	SUPPORT BY HELPERS	INSTRUCTIONS TO PATIENT/FAMILY
1. Neck			
Flexion	Supine Sitting	Hands over ears; flex head.	"Chin down; bend head forward, as motioning 'yes'."
Extension	Supine Side lying Sitting	Hands over ears; extend head.	"Straighten head."
Hyperextension	Prone Side lying Sitting	Hands over ears; hyperextend head.	"Chin up; head back."
Rotation	Supine Sitting Side lying (up side)	Hands over ears; rotate head, one side to other.	"Turn head to side, as motioning 'no'."
Lateral flexion	Supine Sitting Side lying (up side)	Hands over ears; flex head laterally to one side, then other side.	"Tip head to side, toward shoulder."
2. Vertebrae			
Flexion	Supine	Hands over scapulae (use assistant if necessary).	"Bend forward at waist, as if to touch knees/toes, or tie shoe laces."
	Sitting Standing with balance on one leg	Hands over scapulae. Foot and knee to stabilize patient's paralyzed leg; hold belt to provide trunk movement and balance.	
	Side lying	Use of pull maneuver to pull trunk down and toward side, one hand and arm supporting head and other arm supporting lower chest. (Support hollows at head and waist with pads or pillows.)	
Extension	Supine	Hands under body sections, use pull maneuver.	"Straighten back."
	Sitting and standing with balance on one side	Hands at far shoulder to pull trunk into alignment from paralyzed side.	
	Side lying	Use of pull maneuver. (Support of hollows at waist and head with pads or pillows.)	
Hyperextension	Prone	Hands over collar bone (clavicle). (May need assistant to support head at forehead.)	"Bend backward with chin up."
	Sitting or standing with balance on one side	One hand at forehead and other hand at paralyzed shoulder (helper stands behind patient).	
	Side lying	Use of pull maneuver from back of patient.	

JOINT AND MOVEMENT	BODY POSITION	SUPPORT BY HELPERS	INSTRUCTIONS TO PATIENT/FAMILY
Rotation	Supine	Hands under scapula and lower chest; pull as if to turn to side lying. (Place under arm next to body.)	"Twist one shoulder forward and one backward, then change to other side."
	Prone	Hands under shoulder and lower chest—same as supine procedure.	
	Sitting and standing	Hands at patient's shoulders; pull one shoulder forward, other back.	
3. Shoulder			
Flexion (If 180 degrees, includes motion of scapula, combined glenohumeral and scapulothoracic motion)	Supine Side lying Sitting Standing	Hands at wrist and elbow; flex arm over head. (Bend elbow if not adequate room for arm at head of bed.)	"Raise straight arm in front of your body until even with your head." (Use pulley in front of you to pull weak arm up with strong.)
Extension	Supine	Hands at wrist and elbow; extend arm to side. If elbow bent, straighten at side.	"Bring arm down to side in front of your body." (Use pulley to lower arm.)
	Side lying Sitting Standing	Hands at *shoulder* and wrist.	
Hyperextension	Prone	Hands at wrist and elbow; hyperextend arm.	"Bring arm straight back behind your back." (Use pulley behind you.)
	Side lying Sitting Standing	Hands at *shoulder* and wrist; hyperextend arm.	
Abduction (If 180 degrees includes motion of scapula, combined glenohumeral and scapulothoracic motion)	Supine Prone Side lying Sitting Standing	Hands at wrist (with patient's palm facing forward) and elbow; abduct arm. Hands at *shoulder* and wrist (palm facing forward); abduct arm.	"Bring your straight arm up over your head to the side of your body with palm in front of you, as if reaching to the side." (Use pulley to side of your body.)
Adduction	Supine Prone	Hands at wrist (with patient's palm facing forward) and elbow; adduct arm.	"Lower your straight arm, as if reaching to the side with palm facing forward." (Use pulley to side of your body.)
	Side lying Sitting Standing	Hands at *shoulder* and wrist (palm facing forward); adduct arm.	
Horizontal abduction	Supine (incomplete)	Hands at wrist and elbow with patient's arm extended; abduct arm at shoulder level.	"Move your straight arm at shoulder level behind your back."
	Side lying (incomplete) Sitting Standing	Hands at *shoulder* and wrist with patient's arm extended at shoulder; abduct arm.	
Horizontal adduction	Supine (incomplete)	Hands at wrist and elbow with patient's arm extended at shoulder; adduct arm.	"Move your straight arm at shoulder level toward your other shoulder."
	Side lying (incomplete) Sitting Standing	Hands at *shoulder* and wrist.	

Procedure continued on the following page

JOINT AND MOVEMENT	BODY POSITION	SUPPORT BY HELPERS	INSTRUCTIONS TO PATIENT/FAMILY
Circumduction	Supine Prone with shoulder off edge of bed. Side lying Sitting Standing	Hands at *shoulder* and wrist with elbow extended; circumduct shoulder.	"Make a big circle with your arm straight."
Internal rotation	Supine	Hands at wrist and upper arm (holding upper arm against bed); internally rotate by moving forearm toward bed.	"With your arm out from body at shoulder and with elbow bent, move hand down next to side of body." (Use pulley to side of body.)
	Side lying Sitting Standing	Hands at wrist and supporting upper arm in abduction; internally rotate by moving forearm.	
External rotation	Supine	Hands at wrist and upper arm (holding upper arm against bed); externally rotate by moving forearm toward head.	"With your arm out from body at shoulder and with elbow bent, move hand up next to your head." (Use pulley to side of body.)
	Side lying Sitting Standing	Hands at wrist and supporting upper arm in abduction; externally rotate by moving forearm.	
4. Shoulder Girdle			
Elevation	Supine Prone Sitting Standing Side lying	Hands at flexed elbows (or elbow and wrist of extended arm); move toward head. (Move on inspiration to increase lung expansion.)	"Shrug your shoulders as you take a deep breath." (Use pulley.)
Depression	Supine Prone Sitting Standing Side lying	Hands at shoulders; move toward feet. (Exert pressure during expiration to increase exhalation.)	"Pull down your shoulders as you breathe out."
5. Elbow			
Flexion	Supine Side lying Sitting Standing	Hands at elbow and wrist; flex extended arm at elbow toward shoulder.	"Bend your arm and touch your shoulder." (Use pulley.)
Extension	Supine Side lying Sitting Standing	Hands at elbow and wrist; extend arm.	"Straighten your arm." (Use pulley.)
6. Radio-Ulnar			
Pronation	All positions	Hand in patient's hand (as if shaking hands) with forefinger at patient's wrist and elbow; pronate hand.	Turn your palm down."
Supination	All positions	Hand in patient's hand (as in shaking hands) with forefinger at patient's wrist and elbow; supinate hand.	"Turn your palm up."

JOINT AND MOVEMENT	BODY POSITION	SUPPORT BY HELPERS	INSTRUCTIONS TO PATIENT/FAMILY
7. Wrist			
Flexion	All positions	Hands at wrist and grasping dorsum of hand and fingers; flex hand.	"Bend your hand down."
Extension	All positions	Hands at wrist and grasping palmar surface of hand and fingers; extend hand.	"Straighten your hand." (Use pulley.)
Hyperextension	All positions	Hands at wrist and grasping palmar surface of hand and finger; hyperextend hand.	"Bend your hand back."
Abduction (radial deviation)	All positions	Hands at wrist and grasping dorsum of hand and fingers; abduct hand.	"Turn your hand toward your thumb."
Adduction (ulnar deviation)	All positions	Hands at wrist and grasping dorsum of hand and fingers; adduct hand.	"Turn your hand toward your little finger."
8. Thumb			
Flexion	All positions	Hands at dorsum of patient's hand and grasping patient's thumb with fingers of your other hand; flex thumb.	"Bend thumb into your hand."
Extension	All positions	Hands same as flexion to extend thumb.	"Straighten thumb next to your forefinger."
Hyperextension	All positions	Hands same as flexion to hyperextend thumb.	"Move thumb out to side of your fingers."
Abduction	All positions	Hands same as flexion; abduct thumb.	"Move thumb out from inner part of your forefinger."
Adduction	All positions	Hands same as flexion; adduct thumb from abduction position.	"Move thumb back (after doing above) to position next to your forefinger."
Opposition	All positions	Hands same as flexion; oppose each of patient's fingers.	"Touch each finger tip with your thumb."
Rotation (not pictured in Fig. 33–15).	All positions	Hands same as flexion, rotate thumb.	"Make a circle with your thumb."
9. Fingers			
Flexion	All positions	Hands at wrist—hand holding palmar surface of patient's hand in extension or hyperextension; curl fingers of other hand around patient's fingers to flex fingers.	"Make a fist."
Extension	All positions	Hands at wrist—hand holding dorsal surface of patient's hand in extension (or flexion if difficult to move) to extend fingers.	"Straighten your fingers."
Abduction	All positions	Hand at wrist and other hand's fingers interlaced in patient's fingers to abduct (or separate) each two fingers individually.	"Separate your fingers or move fingers apart."
Adduction	All positions	Hands at wrist and around patient's fingers (or put each two fingers together individually).	"Put your fingers together."

Procedure continued on the following page

Joint and Movement	Body Position	Support by Helpers	Instructions to Patient/Family
10. Pelvic girdle			
Elevation Depression (alternate sides)	Supine Prone	Hands under patient's hips; use pull maneuver after moving legs, as if moving down then up in bed. (See Procedure 2, Chapter 21.)	"Tilt your pelvis up, then down."
	Standing	Hands at slightly flexed knee and hip; alternately move pelvis toward head and toward feet.	
11. Hip			
Flexion (To 120 degrees is normal only with knees flexed)	Supine Standing	Hands under knee and ankle; flex knee and hip.	"Bend your knee and hip." (Bicycle provides some flexion.)
	Side lying	One hand and arm cradles lower part of leg, other hand at hip; flex hip and knee.	
Extension	Supine (incomplete on bed mattress) Prone (with feet over mattress end) Standing	Hands under knee and ankle; extend leg.	"Straighten your leg." (Bicycle provides some extension.)
Hyperextension	Prone Standing Side lying	Hands under knee and ankle; hyperextend leg. One hand and arm cradle leg, other hand at hip; hyperextend leg.	"Move your leg back."
Abduction	Supine Prone Standing Side lying	Hands under knee and ankle; lift leg (or pull) to abduct. One hand and arm cradles lower part of leg, other hand at hip; abduct leg.	"Move your leg to the side of your body."
Adduction	Supine Prone Standing Side lying	Hands under knee and ankle; lift leg over other leg, adduct leg. One hand and arm cradles lower part of leg, other hand at hip; lower leg in front of or behind other leg.	"Move your leg over the other leg."
Circumduction	Side lying	One hand and arm cradles lower part of leg, other hand at hip; circumduct leg.	"Move your straight leg in a circle."
	Standing	Hands at knee and ankle; circumduct leg.	
Internal rotation	Supine Standing	Hands above ankle and above knee; roll leg inward to internally rotate hip.	"Roll your foot inward."
	Sitting	Hands at flexed knee and ankle; move knee toward other knee with lower leg abducted.	"Bend your knee and move it over other knee with foot to side."
External rotation	Supine Standing	Hands above ankle and above knee; roll leg outward to externally rotate hip.	"Roll your foot outward."

Joint and Movement	Body Position	Support by Helpers	Instructions to Patient/Family
	Sitting	Hands at flexed knee and ankle; move knee outward and foot toward other knee to externally rotate.	"Bend your knee and turn it outward with foot on leg near knee."
12. Knee			
Flexion	Prone Standing Side lying Supine	Hands under knees and ankles; flex knee. (Allows 135-degree flexion.) *See hip flexion supine position.*	"Bend your knee."
	Sitting	Hands on knee and under heel; flex knee. (Approximately 90 degrees.)	
Extension	Prone (with foot over end of mattress) All other positions	Hands over knees and under ankles; extend knee.	"Straighten your knee."
13. Ankle			
Dorsiflexion	Supine Sitting Side lying	Hands under foot and at ankle *or* hand on heel with foot on wrist and other hand on ankle; dorsi-flex.	"Turn your foot toward your head."
	Standing	Patient's heel on floor; lift forefoot up.	"Heel down and toes up."
Extension	Supine Sitting Side lying	Hands under foot and at ankle; extend foot.	"Straighten your foot, as if standing in bare feet."
	Standing	Hands under knee and heel; guide foot to extended position.	"Place foot flat on floor."
Plantar flexion	Supine Prone Sitting Side lying	Hands over dorsum of foot and under heel and/or ankle (ankle for prone); plantar flex.	"Turn foot down or point toes
	Standing	Hands at knee (to elevate foot) and dorsum of foot; plantar flex.	
Eversion (ankle abduction)	All positions	Hands under heel and ankle (ankle for prone) and over dorsum; evert foot.	"Turn outside of foot up and inside down."
Inversion (ankle adduction)	All positions	Hands under heel and ankle (ankle for prone) and over dorsum of foot; invert foot.	"Turn inside of foot up and outside down."
14. Toes			
Flexion	All positions	Hands under plantar surface of foot and over toes; flex toes.	"Curl your toes."
Extension	All positions	Hands under plantar surface of foot and under toes; extend toes.	"Straighten toes."
Hyperextension	All positions	Hands as in extension (above); hyperextend toes.	"Turn up your toes."
Abduction	All positions	Hands separate each of two toes individually; abduct toes.	"Separate your toes."
Adduction	All positions	Hands over dorsum of foot and around toes; adduct toes.	"Pull your toes together."

Post-Procedure Activities.   Check patient's pulse and observe reaction to activity. Ensure patient's comfort and safety: remove crotch cover, position in correct alignment, replace bed covers, raise side rails, lower bed level and place call bell for patient's use.

Aftercare of Equipment.   Place unit in order, discard crotch cover and bath blanket in laundry if soiled or store in patient's unit, store wheelchair and patient's clothing appropriately.

Final Patient Assessment.   Determine patient's tolerance to activity, his comfort and safety. *Chart/Report:* Number of times, joint movements and joints exercised; evidence of stiffness, pain, spasm or other untoward effects; patient/family teaching; and recommendations for additional exercises and/or progression to assisted or active ROM if indicated. Enter in Kardex or Exercise Work Sheet; schedule modifications, reductions or increases in passive ROM exercises.

Learning Reinforcement with Exercises.   Patient teaching intervention includes the development of human environmental factors and material environmental factors which lead to the probability that what is demonstrated by the patient will be maintained by the patient. An example in Figure 33–16 illustrates a registered nurse's plan for teaching a patient self range-of-motion exercises and the plan for *reinforcing the learning* for the purpose of learning maintenance. The stars are the reinforcers for activity. The example documents the plan and the patient's response to the plan. As you can see, the patient's response progressed from *refusal* to *observation* to *actual self range-of-motion exercises* with the help of a starting cue from the nurse and positive reinforcement from the health care team. Positive reinforcement was given in the form of a star and staff praise. Figure 33–16 illustrates a universal flow sheet which enables a nurse to organize and follow a plan of care for the purpose of preventing one of the serious complications of immobility, joint contracture. The first column on the flow sheet identifies the day the activity takes place. The second column identifies one of the patient's problems: #1, Left Cerebral Vascular Accident (L. CVA), with right upper and lower extremity paralysis. The nursing order instructs the nursing assistant to perform passive range-of-motion (PROM) to Ms. Doe's right upper and lower extremity (R. U&LE) at 9 AM and 8 PM every day according to the in-house procedure book. The nursing assistants and the student nurses did the treatment successfully for 15 days. The third column describes the patient teaching nursing order, "Teach Mr. and Ms.

Doe to do Ms. Doe's passive range-of-motion exercises at the time of the evening exercises every 8 PM plus record the patient's and husband's response to the teaching." In the example, the teaching instructions were also noted to be included in the procedure book, starting on page 25. According to the flow sheet, Ms. Doe first refused to take any interest in the exercises for her own right leg. Then she actively observed the teaching and by the third evening she was able to do her own PROM to her right lower extremity, (R.L.E.). Ms. Doe learned to do her own PROM on her elbow and forearm but had some difficulty with her shoulder. Finally she was able to do her total right ROM with cues to start. Column 4 shows that the staff checked that the footboard was functional every evening. Column 5 illustrates the rewards of praise and a star for "well behaviors" performed by Ms. Doe. The order reads, "A star equals a good practice by Ms. Doe, but praise her for listening each session." Column 6 illustrates that the care plan has been changed to a simple procedure of reminding Ms. Doe to start her exercises and to continue to reinforce her success by utilizing Column 5. Columns 2 and 3 are no longer current and have been discontinued. In the "Comments" column is the order for discontinuing nursing orders in Columns 2, 3 and 4. The registered nurse makes an entry in the patient's chart when the care plan is changed.

Disuse Osteoporosis.   This painful, crippling condition is the most frequently seen metabolic bone disease in the United States. The word "osteoporosis" means *porosity of bone*. The increased bone porosity is caused by a substantial loss of bone calcium, phosphorus, and matrix. These losses result from an increase in the rate of bone destruction, which *exceeds* the rate of bone production.

While osteoporosis can be caused by several different factors, *disuse* osteoporosis develops because the musculoskeletal system is immobilized and is not being used. This condition is very common among paraplegics and severe arthritics, and it affects *all* immobilized patients on bed rest. Because some degree of osteoporosis always occurs in the immobilized patient, osteoporosis is actually a *physiologic* reaction to bed rest rather than a pathologic one.

While disuse osteoporosis inevitably affects the bedridden, one must nevertheless make every effort to prevent the occurrence of a severe degree of osteoporosis, along with its attendant complications, namely:

▶ Renal calculi due to the draining of calcium from the patient's bones.

▶ Pathologic fractures due to the bone's lack of structural firmness.

▶ Deformities due to the bone's soft sponginess.

▶ Osteoarthropathy due to the deposit of calcium in the joints.

To prevent disuse osteoporosis, authorities recommend that patients be allowed to stand and to bear weight as soon as possible. The paralyzed patient can obtain the effect of weight bearing by being placed for a period each day on a tilt table or oscillating bed, either of which is raised and locked into a standing position. Patients who can ambulate to some extent can learn to stand or walk between parallel bars. All patients need to exercise and to contract their muscles daily, particularly against resistance. While a nutritious diet is essential, increasing calcium intake definitely does *not* prevent osteoporosis; indeed, additional calcium in the diet simply adds to the large load of minerals that the patient is already excreting.

The Effects of Prolonged Bed Rest upon the Heart and Vascular System

There are four major effects that prolonged bed rest has upon the heart: (1) an increased load of work upon the heart, (2) the development of orthostatic hypotension, (3) an increased use of the Valsalva maneuver, and (4) an increased incidence of thrombus formation and pulmonary embolism.

WORKLOAD OF THE HEART

Bed rest may rest a person's muscles and bones, but it definitely does *not* rest his heart. Indeed, when one lies down there is a 25–30 per cent increase in cardiac output, a 40 per cent increase in the stroke volume (amount of blood that the heart puts out at each beat), and a 30 per cent increase in the total work of the heart. According to one study by Deitrick et al., four normal, healthy subjects, at the end of a six-week period of immobilization, had an average increase in their heart rates of 3.8 beats per minute.[16] This progressively increasing heartbeat indicates that prolonged immobilization produces a decline in cardiovascular function.

Another investigator reports that in the supine position, the heart works 30 per cent harder than in a sitting position.[13, 50] Thus, a patient whose heart needs rest should actually be nursed in a sitting position rather than supine for the best results.

Despite the fact that bed rest does cause the heart to work harder, there is no evidence that bed rest harms the heart. Indeed, with prescribed rest, large hearts do become smaller, since the general stresses and muscular strains to which ambulatory patients are subjected are reduced. Rest in an armchair is an alternative that protects the patient both from the stresses of active ambulation and from the increased cardiac output stimulated by rest in bed.

THE VALSALVA MANEUVER

When a person uses his arm and upper trunk muscles to move in bed or when he strains to defecate, he performs the Valsalva maneuver. In other words, the individual fixes his thorax and holds his breath, which is consequently forced up against his closed glottis. As a result, the patient's intrathoracic pressure increases, his pulse decreases, blood flow to the heart slows, and venous pressure rises. As a result bradycardia develops. When the patient finishes moving or straining, he lets his breath out, which, in turn, causes his intrathoracic pressure to decrease and his pulse to increase. In the vulnerable heart, angina and even sudden death due to cardiac arrest may ensue.

Patients on bed rest have been shown to perform the Valsalva maneuver 10 to 20 times per hour. Because of the danger of cardiac arrest,

1	2	3	4	5	6	7
PROBLEM	#1 L.CVA	#1	#1	#1	#1	COMMENTS
DATE	PROM R U&LE q̄ 9A/8P Book p 25	Teach PROM R U&LE to Mr. & Ms. Doe q̄ 8P Record Response (Book p 25)	Padded foot-board Check q̄ PM	⋆ = Ms. Doe + practice, but praise p̄ @ class for PROM 8 PM	PROM U&LE/ self c̄ cue to start Monitor BID bk p. 25	
11/8/77	8P OK/AB	Mr. Doe = OK/RLE Ms. Doe = Refused 8P/AB	In place 8P/AB	– 8P/AB		
11/9	9A OK/RT 8P OK/AB	Mr. Doe = OK/RLE Ms. Doe = Observed only 8P/AB	OK 8P/AB	– 8P/AB		
11/10	9A OK/RT 8P OK/AB	Mr. Doe = OK/RLE Ms. Doe = OK/RLE 8P/AB	OK 8P/AB	⋆ 8P/AB		
11/11	9A OK/RT 8P OK/AB	Mr. Doe = OK/RUE Ms. Doe = Observed 8P/AB	OK 8P/AB	– 8P/AB		
11/12	9A OK/RT 8P OK/AB	Mr. Doe = OK/RUE Ms. Doe = Observed 8P/AB	OK 8P/AB	– 8P/AB		
11/13	9A OK/DO 8P OK/RJ	Mr. Doe = OK/RUE Ms. Doe = Observed 8P/RJ	OK 8P/RJ	– 8P/RJ		
11/14	9A OK/DO 8P OK/RJ	Mr. Doe = OK/RUE Ms. Doe = OK/R. Elbow 8P/RJ	OK 8P/RJ	⋆ 8P/RJ		
11/15	9A OK/RT 8P OK/AB	Mr. D = OK/RUE Ms. D = OK/R. Forearm 8P/AB	OK 8P/AB	⋆ 8P/AB		

Figure 33–16. Universal flow sheet used to document increased mobility treatment and response (prepared by Rosemarian Berni, R.N., M.N.).

1	2	3	4	5	6	7
11/16	9A OK/RT 8P OK/AB	Mr. D. = OK/RUE Ms. D = OK/RUE but shoulder 8P/AB	OK 8P/AB	★ 8P/AB		
11/17	9A OK/RT 8P OK/AB	Mr. D = OK/RUE Ms. D = OK/RUE but shoulder 8P/AB	OK 8P/AB	★ 8P/AB		
11/18	9A OK/RT 8P OK/AB	Mr. D = OK/RUE Ms. D = OK/RUE c̄ cue to start 8P/AB	OK 8P/AB	★ 8P/AB		
11/19	9A OK/RT 8P OK/AB	Mr. D = Absent Ms. D = OK/RUE cue to start 8P/AB	OK 8P/AB	★ 8P/AB		
11/20	9A OK/DO 8P OK/RJ	Mr. D = Absent Ms. D = OK/RUE c̄ cue to start 8P/RJ	OK 8P/RJ	★ 8P/RJ		
11/21	9A OK/DO 8P OK/TT	Mr. D = Observed Ms. D = OK/RUE c̄ cue to start 8P/TT	OK 8P/TT	★ 8P/TT	OK 9A/RT OK 8P/AB	
11/22	9A OK/RT D.C.	D.C. D.C./RB	OK 8P/AB	★ 8P/AB	OK 9A/RT OK 8P/AB	11/22/77 D.C. PROM by NA PROM/self c̄ cue to start Monitor BID RB/RN
11/23			OK 8P/AB	★ 8P/AB	OK 9A/RT OK 8P/AB	

Flow Sheet/Progress Notes
Key:

RJ = Ruth Jensen LPN
TT = Tam Taylor NA
DO = Donna Olson NA
RT = Rose Tall, Student Nurse

AB = Amy Blaze, Student Nurse
MS = May Sun RN
SS = Sue Smith NA
RB = Ruth Brown RN
MM = Mary Miles NA

Name
JANE DOE

Number
67-89-10

coronary patients on bed rest must be taught not to strain while defecating. It is preferable that these individuals use a bedside commode for defecation rather than a bedpan, because the commode allows the patient to assume a normal sitting position, which reduces the need to strain. Of course, every effort must be made to prevent constipation in the heart patient.

ORTHOSTATIC HYPOTENSION

As we stated earlier, all patients when they first get up after a period of bed rest feel weak, wobbly, and dizzy. The dizziness and faintness are due, in part, to muscular weakness; however, faintness also results from hypotension or a low blood pressure which is caused, not by cardiac disease, but by a failure of arteriolar vasoconstriction upon assuming an erect position.

The exact etiology of orthostatic hypotension is still somewhat obscure. Evidently when a patient is in bed for a prolonged period of time, the parts of his circulatory system that respond to changes in posture (i.e., going from the supine to the erect position or vice versa) deteriorate in their ability to function. Thus, upon rising after a prolonged period in bed, the splanchnic and muscle arterioles do not constrict but dilate; blood pools in the abdominal viscera and muscles, and the patient faints. Exactly why vasoconstriction fails is not known. Browse[8] hypothesizes that, since the nervous system is intact, the problem of orthostatic hypotension must result from a *local* failure of the blood vessels. He believes that the patient's vessels have become habituated to the bed rest state, in which they generally remain somewhat dilated. Consequently, when the patient suddenly stands up, these "habituated" vessels are unable to constrict appropriately in response to nervous stimuli, and the blood pressure drops. Other authorities suggest that because muscle tone generally decreases during bed rest, there is a decrease in the efficiency of those muscles that press against the veins, thereby aiding venous return to the heart. When this factor, known as the "vasopressor mechanism" is diminished, venous blood pools in the lower parts of the body rather than being propelled through the heart and out into the arterial circulation.

The problem of orthostatic hypotension cannot be completely prevented. Some suggestions for lessening the severity of the problem are:

▶ Try to have the patient ambulate as soon as permissible.

▶ Get the patient up very gradually. At first only raise the head of the bed and let the patient become accustomed to that position. Slowly increase his period of ambulation each day.

▶ Place pressure bandages on the patient's legs. This will aid venous return to the heart and augment the vasopressor mechanism. An abdominal binder may also aid venous return.

THROMBUS FORMATION AND PULMONARY EMBOLISM

Deep vein thrombosis (i.e., the formation of a blood clot within the deep veins) is unfortunately a common complication of bed rest that seems to be related to the *length of time* the patient is in bed. However, bed rest is not an absolute necessity for the development of thrombi, for blood clots sometimes form in the veins of normal, healthy individuals. In either case, the major danger from thrombus formation is *pulmonary embolism*, in which the clot breaks loose from the vein wall and is carried to the lungs where it blocks off the blood supply to a portion of the lung tissue. If the embolus is a small one, damage may be minimal; if damage is extensive, the patient may die.

Three factors contribute to the formation of thrombi and potential emboli: (1) increased blood coagulability, (2) venous stasis, and (3) damage to the vein wall's intima. Let us briefly examine each factor.

An Increase in Blood Coagulability. In general medical patients on bed rest there apparently are no changes in the blood due to immobility other than an increase in plasma volume which, in turn, decreases the viscosity of the blood. However, in post-trauma cases (following either surgery or an accident) there tends to be an increase in blood viscosity, platelet count, platelet stickiness, and prothrombin time—all of which increase blood coagulability. Also, if the bedfast patient is dehydrated, his blood will be more viscous and thus more prone to clot formation. While these changes may not actually cause thrombi to form, they possibly *accelerate* their formation.

Venous Stasis. A slowing of the flow of blood in the veins can result from a lack of muscular contraction in the legs. Evidently venous stasis alone will not cause thrombosis. However, venous stasis *in addition* to another factor, such as hypercoagulability or damage to the intima of the vein, can cause thrombosis.

Damage to the Intima of the Vein Wall. When the intima or inner coat of a vessel is damaged, platelets quickly cover the defect and intimal cells grow over the platelets, thereby restoring

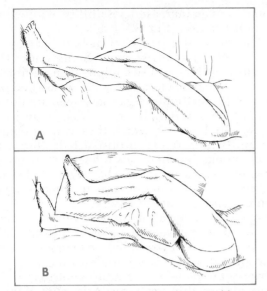

Figure 33–17. *A,* The lateral recumbent position as an etiologic factor in venous thrombosis. *Note:* weight of upper leg resting on lower leg. *B,* Correct positioning will prevent thrombosis. (After Browse, *The Physiology and Pathology of Bedrest.* Springfield, IL, Charles C Thomas, 1965.)

the vessel wall. Generally the process of healing terminates at this point; however, in some cases, the plaque of platelets continues to grow and a thrombus develops.

How do vein walls become damaged during bed rest? Several factors are known to promote damage. One is the use of the *lateral recumbent position,* especially following anesthesia or when the patient is heavily sedated. In this position the tibia of the lower leg is compressed by the calf of the upper leg; moreover, the femoral vein of the upper leg is squeezed and possibly damaged as it presses against the lower leg. To correct this uncomfortable, potentially dangerous position, the upper leg should be lifted off the lower leg and placed so that its total length and weight rest upon a pillow (Fig. 33–17). A second factor promoting intimal damage is the use of the Fowler position, in which the knees are flexed over a bent-knee gatch. Third, the placing of pillows directly under the patient's knees may lead to blood clot formation.

Prevention of Thrombus and Embolism. Because of the danger of pulmonary embolism, it is naturally most important to prevent thrombus formation. Some important preventive measures are:

► Encourage patient to move his legs throughout the day.

► Set up a definite program of complete range-of-motion exercises three times daily.

► Encourage the ingestion of fluids to decrease the viscosity of the blood.

► Use pressure bandages to augment venous return to the heart.

► Never rub the patient's legs, as you can dislodge a clot that may have formed, thereby releasing an embolus into the circulation.

► Avoid the use of the knee gatch, pillows beneath the knees, and the lateral recumbent position.

The Effect of Prolonged Bed Rest upon the Respiratory System*

Prolonged bed rest apparently has little direct effect upon pulmonary function, once the patient's lungs have made certain adjustments to the supine position. However, respiratory problems secondary to immobilization may develop. For example, the general muscle weakness that results from bed rest may cause respiratory difficulties, since greater effort is required to breathe while lying down.

Under certain conditions, prolonged bed rest can result in respiratory problems that can lead to such grave complications as bronchopneumonia and carbon dioxide narcosis. These are brought on by: (1) decreased chest expansion and decreased chest movements, (2) stasis of secretions and pooling of mucus, and (3) CO_2 narcosis and respiratory acidosis.

DECREASED CHEST EXPANSION AND DECREASED CHEST MOVEMENTS

The prolonged pressure of a bed mattress against a patient's chest will tend to decrease the expansion of his chest cage. Decreased chest expansion and weakness of the muscles of respiration cause a decrease in ventilation. This, in turn, results in a decrease in the oxygenation of the blood and an inadequate expiration of CO_2. Factors that contribute to a limited chest expansion and that must be controlled or avoided are: heavy sedation and narcotics, which depress the respiratory center in the medulla; and tight abdominal or chest binders, and abdominal distention due to ascites, feces, or flatus, which interfere with the normal descent of the diaphragm. To encourage maximum chest expansion, the patient on bed rest must periodically breathe deeply.

STASIS AND POOLING OF SECRETIONS

When secretions and mucus begin to pool in the bronchi and lungs of the bedridden patient,

*See also Chap. 36, Supporting Respiratory Function.

the patient becomes highly susceptible to the development of *hypostatic bronchopneumonia*. Major factors leading to the stasis and pooling of secretions and thus to bronchopneumonia are:

The patient's *underlying weakness,* which results in reduced bodily movements and a decrease in the efficiency of the cough reflex. This weakness is usually due both to the disease condition requiring bed rest (e.g., cancer, heart disease, recent surgery, burns, accident trauma) as well as to prolonged immobilization itself.

While a normal healthy person will move around in bed and will cough up any secretions that pool in his bronchi during the night, a sick, weakened individual may not have the strength to do so. Thus, the bedridden are prone to pooling of mucus, bacterial invasion, and atelectasis (collapse of a portion of lung) as a result of the obstruction of bronchi. If the patient on bed rest is also taking *narcotics or sedatives,* his muscle strength is further weakened and his chest expansion further decreased.

The supine position causes *disturbance of the normal distribution of mucus around the bronchi*. Normally mucus is spread out rather evenly around the bronchial tubules. However, in the supine position, mucus tends to pool on the dependent sides of the bronchi while the upper surfaces may become very dry. Both the pooling of mucus and the drying of the upper bronchial walls interferes with adequate functioning of the cilia (whose job it is to sweep excess mucus up and out of the bronchi). As a result, there is an even greater pooling of

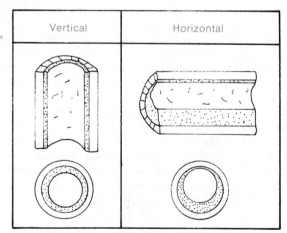

Figure 33–18. Gravity's effect upon mucus distribution within a bronchial tube. (After Browse, *The Physiology and Pathology of Bedrest.* Springfield, IL, Charles C Thomas, 1965.)

mucus and an increased possibility of infection and obstruction (Fig. 33–18).

The mucus that pools during bed rest may be *abnormal in consistency.* Sometimes the mucus is watery and so copious in amount that it cannot be expectorated by the weakened patient. Other patients, e.g., those who are dehydrated or on anticholinergic drugs, may have heavy, thick mucus which they cannot cough up and which tends to obstruct the bronchi. Such mucus is sometimes referred to as being "ropey" or "stringy" in character. If the secretions are very thick or copious, suctioning of the patient may be necessary.

When caring for a patient who seems too weak to cough up his secretions or to turn himself, make certain that you help him to move, cough, and deep-breathe at scheduled times. As you observe the patient's respiratory rate, carefully note his breathing patterns. Ask yourself these questions as you evaluate his pulmonary function:

▶ Are the patient's respirations shallow rather than full and deep? If so, the patient's chest expansion may be seriously restricted by one of the factors that we just discussed.

▶ Does he have to labor to get his breath? Labored breathing may indicate hypoxia and clogged respiratory passages due to mucus secretions.

▶ Do his respirations sound moist or wet? If so, the patient may be developing a hypostatic bronchopneumonia.

▶ Is the patient trying to cough up mucus? Is the mucus thick or thin in consistency, white or greenish yellow in color, copious or sparse in amount? Ropey thick mucus might indicate that the patient is dehydrated and needs fluids. Thin, copious mucus indicates that the patient may need suctioning if he is very weak. Greenish yellow mucus is one diagnostic sign of hypostatic bronchopneumonia.

▶ Is the pulse rapid? A rapid pulse is one of the *first* indications of oxygen lack.

▶ Is the patient's temperature elevated? If so, the patient may be developing bronchitis or bronchopneumonia.

▶ Does the patient seem irritable, confused, or disoriented? If so, the patient may need oxygen.

▶ Is the patient using his neck muscles to breathe rather than his abdominal muscles? The use of the axillary neck muscles to breathe is a *late* sign of severe respiratory disability.

▶ Are cyanosis and severe dyspnea present? These are the *late* signs of hypoxia and must be reported at once.

Finally, you and the physician must observe the patient for the following *specific* signs of hypostatic bronchopneumonia: cough, fever, pain on breathing, leukocytosis, greenish yellow sputum, and patchy infiltration of the lung on x-ray. If hypostatic pneumonia is present, antibiotics and vigorous coughing are the treatment measures of choice.

CARBON DIOXIDE NARCOSIS AND RESPIRATORY ACIDOSIS

When a patient's respiratory movements decrease and his cough reflex diminishes, the oxygen-carbon dioxide exchange in his lungs is severely affected. As a result, CO_2 accumulates in his blood; at the same time the oxygen tension of the blood decreases and tissue hypoxia develops.

At first, the increase in plasma CO_2 stimulates the respiratory center in the medulla with the result that respirations increase. At the same time the lowered oxygen tension of the blood stimulates the aortic and carotid bodies, which also stimulate the respirations. These compensatory changes, however, are only *temporary*. The medulla soon refuses to respond to the rising CO_2 blood level. Carbon dioxide continues to build up in the blood, and CO_2 narcosis develops. At the same time, the responses of the carotid and aortic bodies are weakened, and the oxygen levels of the blood continue to drop. Without prompt treatment, such patients can rapidly progress to states of respiratory acidosis, respiratory and cardiac failure, coma, and death. Chapter 35 discusses provision of immediate life support for persons in respiratory and cardiac failure.

The Effect of Prolonged Bed Rest upon Metabolism

Prolonged bed rest has the following effects upon metabolism.

▶ The basal metabolic rate (BMR) tends to fall slightly; however, it returns to normal within three weeks following the patient's return to ambulatory status.

▶ Muscle mass decreases; however, the patient's total body weight tends to remain stable.

▶ A state of negative nitrogen balance develops within four days following the patient's immobilization. By the tenth day of bed rest, the state of negative nitrogen bal-

ance reaches its peak; then gradually the patient returns to a normal state of balance.

▶ There is a decreased production of adrenocortical hormones—"stress hormones."

To counteract these changes in metabolic function, make certain that the patient receives a diet that is adequate in protein. Also, to reduce the problem of muscle atrophy, encourage active and/or passive exercises and movement.

The Effect of Prolonged Bed Rest upon the Gastrointestinal Tract

Immobility has little effect upon the functional activities of the gastrointestinal tract. Thus, both digestive and bowel function remain relatively unchanged during bed rest; however, as the energy requirements of the patient's cells are lessened, appetite may decrease. Also bowel habits may change as a result of shifts in the patient's routine and environment.

ADVERSE EFFECTS UPON INGESTION

Anorexia may develop due to the patient's underlying malady as well as from the general weakness, worry, and boredom accompanying immobility. *Hypoproteinemia* is a common problem in the bedridden patient. Lowered blood protein levels are due to anorexia; to some disease conditions, e.g., cancer and tuberculosis; and to the increased catabolic activity that immobilization causes.

To *prevent* patients on bed rest from becoming seriously malnourished, the following suggestions may prove useful: (1) help the patient to select foods that have high nutritional value; (2) encourage the patient to eat foods that are high in protein, e.g., cheese, milk, meat, fish, and eggs; (3) serve small, frequent feedings; (4) ask the dietitian to visit the patient to determine his food preferences and dislikes; (5) chart carefully exactly how much the patient eats and which foods he leaves on his tray; and (6) notify the physician if the patient has a poor appetite and is refusing his meals. (See Unit VII: Providing Food and Fluids.)

ADVERSE EFFECTS UPON ELIMINATION*

Constipation is a frequent complication for patients on bed rest. Many factors can contrib-

---

*See Chap. 30, Maintaining Bowel and Kidney Function.

ute to its development. First of all, patients who are sick enough to be on bed rest experience changes in their diet, changes in their daily schedule and routine, and a decrease in their general level of activity—all of which can lead to a change in bowel habits. Second, patients often feel embarrassed to use a bedpan and they find bedpans uncomfortable; consequently, patients frequently suppress their desire to defecate. Many patients on bed rest who have the desire to defecate find that they simply cannot do so in this unnatural position. Finally, the general muscle weakness that characterizes the immobilized patient also extends to those muscles that are involved in the act of defecation, e.g., the abdominal muscles, the diaphragm, and the levator ani. Particularly in the elderly, muscle weakness and poor sphincter tone often contribute to problems with constipation.

In sum, the immobilized patient, his diet and routine changed, and his natural desire to defecate inhibited by embarrassment, discomfort, and muscle weakness, gradually neglects his body's urgings. In time, owing to habitual neglect, the patient loses even his *desire* to defecate. As a result, his rectum becomes chronically distended and the patient becomes severely constipated. Malaise, headache, dizziness, loss of appetite, and abdominal distention often accompany constipation.

Fecal impactions will develop if the patient's severe constipation is not treated conscientiously. A fecal impaction is a hardened or putty-like stool that remains in the rectum or colon; it must often be removed manually or even surgically. Impactions can be diagnosed by (1) the presence of a distended abdomen; (2) in some cases watery diarrhea (which passes around the impacted stool); and (3) the identification of a hard mass in the rectum or colon upon digital examination or sigmoidoscopy. Without proper intervention, a fecal impaction can lead to a mechanical bowel obstruction.

It is of prime importance to prevent fecal impactions from developing in immobilized patients with heart disease, in those who have suffered a cerebral vascular accident, and in postoperative patients who have undergone eye surgery. When patients with these particular conditions develop a fecal impaction, they often try to expel the hardened stool by excessive straining. Straining, in turn, may lead to such complications as cardiac arrest, additional cardiovascular accidents, and serious damage to the operated eye.

Careful observation is very important in the *prevention* of constipation and the development of fecal impactions. Note the frequency, color, consistency, amount, and shape of the patient's stools. The absence of stools for over three or four days, frequent stools (three or more per day), hard dry stools, watery stools, blood-tinged stools, and thin ribbon-like stools (indicating a possible bowel obstruction) should be charted and reported to the doctor.

If you suspect the development of a fecal impaction, digitally examine the patient's rectum for the presence of a hard mass and examine his abdomen for distention.

In addition to careful observation and reporting, constipation can be prevented by placing the immobilized patient upon a regimen that encourages good bowel habits. If possible, get the patient up to the bathroom or to the bedside commode each day at the same time. For best results, identify the time of day during which the patient normally has a bowel movement. Encourage the patient to drink ample fluids, to eat fruits and vegetables, and to drink a glass of prune juice whenever his bowels fail to move for a few days; discourage him from becoming dependent upon laxatives and enemas. Use of local suppositories and rectal massage, as part of a planned regimen, usually prevents the need for laxatives and enemas. Also, help the immobilized patient to exercise his abdominal muscles daily since this will help him to strengthen those muscles used in defecation.

The *treatment* of constipation and fecal impactions will probably require the use of stool softeners, mineral oil, enemas, and digital removal of the stool. For more complete instructions concerning the treatment of constipation, see Chapter 30.

The Effect of Prolonged Bed Rest upon Renal Function*

Prolonged bed rest has relatively little direct effect upon the work of the kidney nephron; however, when a patient is *first* immobilized, his renal functioning is almost immediately affected by the supine position in the following ways: (1) renal blood flow greatly increases, in turn increasing the cardiac output; and (2) blood volume increases by 10 to 15 per cent owing to both a slight increase in capillary filtration and a large increase in the volume of tissue fluid being reabsorbed into the plasma. This increase in blood volume creates a temporary increase in urinary excretion.

---

*See also Chap. 30, Maintaining Bowel and Kidney Function.

After the patient has adjusted to the state of bed rest (this usually takes around 3 weeks) the immediate increase in blood volume described above is followed by, first, a slow decrease in blood volume and then a slow increase.

Although immobility has no ill effects upon the functioning of the kidney nephron itself, the patient on prolonged bed rest may experience the following adverse effects upon his urinary excretory functions: difficulty in urinating, urinary stasis, and the formation of renal calculi.

DIFFICULTY IN URINATION

To urinate normally it is necessary to have integrated action of the internal urethral sphincter, the external urethral sphincter, and the detrusor muscle of the bladder wall. When the bladder fills with urine its walls are stretched and the individual experiences a sensation of bladder fullness or pressure. Urination can occur by voluntarily relaxing the perineal muscles and the external sphincter. Relaxation of the external sphincter, in turn, initiates the micturition reflex (an autonomic nervous system reflex) in which the detrusor muscle contracts. Upon contraction of the bladder wall, intrabladder pressure increases, the internal sphincter relaxes, and urine flows out through the urethra.

When patients are immobilized, they continue to experience normal sensations of bladder fullness. However, despite their desire to void, most bed patients experience difficulty in actually passing their urine. Common causes for difficult micturition are as follows:

▶ Hypertrophy of the prostate gland is a common cause of difficult micturition among elderly males. The enlarged prostate acts as a mechanical obstruction to urine flow, and it frequently causes such acute urinary retention that catheterization is required.

▶ Embarrassment may inhibit a patient from asking for the bedpan or urinal.

▶ The use of a bedpan or urinal, while in bed, makes the act of urination both uncomfortable and awkward. In the supine position it is difficult to relax the perineal muscles or to consciously bear down, as one normally does, to raise the intrabladder pressure. When these voluntary actions are not carried out, detrusor muscle contraction cannot be initiated.

When patients have difficulty in urination, because of any of the above causes, their bladders tend to become overly distended. Bladder distention results in an excessive stretching of the detrusor muscle, which, over a period of time, results in a decrease in the sensation of bladder fullness. The patient, consequently, has little desire to void even though he needs to do so. As pressure from urine in the bladder builds up, the patient may experience an overflow incontinence. Catheterization may be necessary to gradually relieve bladder distention. Without catheterization, back pressure from the bladder distention may become so great that it actually damages the kidney nephron. However, the catheterization procedure itself is always hazardous because it can lead to serious urinary tract infections. Because of the dangers inherent in catheterization, emphasis should be placed on preventing bladder distention.

To *prevent bladder distention* due to difficulty with micturition, the nurse must first make careful observations. She needs to note and chart: (1) how frequently the patient voids, (2) the amount of urine that the patient passes with each voiding, (3) urinary incontinence, (4) any pain or difficulty that the patient experiences while voiding, and (5) the presence of bladder distention. If the patient has not voided for over eight hours despite adequate fluid intake or if he "dribbles" urine continuously and if his bladder is distended, you will need to try various appropriate measures to help the patient void. Some of the fundamental methods are: (1) allowing the male patient to stand beside his bed to void and the female patient to sit on a bedside commode, (2) running water, the sound of which may help the patient to relax his perineal muscles, (3) pouring warm water over the perineum itself, and (4) placing gentle manual pressure on the lower abdomen. If these methods fail, you should request an order for catheterization or for intermittent catheterization. Clean intermittent catheterizations can be performed in the home by many patients. (Catheterization is discussed in Chap. 40.)

URINARY STASIS AND RENAL CALCULI

When human beings stand in their normal erect position, the force of gravity enables urine to flow freely from the renal pelvis and out through the ureter. However, when they are lying supine, gravity no longer aids the flow of urine and it tends to collect and to *stagnate* in the renal pelvis (Fig. 33–19).

As the urine stagnates, various tiny particles and crystals in the urine also remain in the

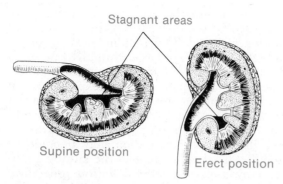

Stagnant areas

Supine position

Erect position

Figure 33–19. The effect of gravity upon renal flow out of the renal pelvis. (After Olson and Schroeder: *American Journal of Nursing,* April, 1967.)

stagnant pools of the renal pelvis where they may form the nuclei of renal calculi.

Renal calculi, sometimes called "kidney stones" or "recumbency stones," occur in 15 to 30 per cent of all immobilized patients. Most commonly, calculi develop after at least 14 to 21 days following the initial immobilization; they may develop sooner in patients with diseases characterized by elevated urine calcium concentration.

Major factors contributing to the formation of renal stones in patients on bed rest are:

▶ Urinary stasis.

▶ A slightly alkaline urine (which is common in patients on bed rest).

▶ Urinary tract infection.

▶ Elevated calcium concentrations in the urine. The amount of urine calcium can triple after only two weeks in bed. This increase is due to the draining of calcium from the bones as a result of disuse osteoporosis.

▶ Elevated phosphorus owing to disuse osteoporosis.

▶ A decrease in the *ratio* of citric acid to calcium in the urine. Citric acid normally acts to keep calcium in solution.

When the above factors are present, the patient in the supine position develops renal stones within his bladder and renal pelvis. These stones, which are composed mainly of calcium salts, can cause bleeding (hematuria), severe pain (renal colic), backache, nausea, and vomiting.

To *prevent* renal calculi, it is important to (1)

combat urinary stasis by ambulating the patient as soon as permissible and by scheduling passive and active exercises; (2) keep the urine diluted by increasing fluid intake; (3) in some cases, lower the urinary pH by means of an acid-ash diet that includes cereals, poultry, meat, and fish; and (4) eliminate possible urinary infection by avoiding catheterization unless absolutely necessary.

The Effect of Prolonged Bed Rest upon the Mental State

Persons on prolonged bed rest often feel lethargic, lonely, and depressed. Removed from their usual routine of work and play, bedfast patients may also suffer from acute anxiety and insomnia as they worry about their homes, families, jobs, and finances. Moreover, immobilized patients with neurotic or psychotic tendencies may tend to become emotionally disturbed. Some may act in hostile, belligerent ways; others may become severely withdrawn; still others may become disoriented, losing track of time and place.

To help patients adjust emotionally to bed rest, consider the following suggestions:

▶ If possible, place the immobilized patient in a room with patients who are oriented and interested in their surroundings. Contact with such individuals may help the bedridden patient to feel less isolated and less out of touch with the world. Strive to help the patient's significant others to feel comfortable with the patient and encourage them to take part in the patient's activities of daily living.

▶ Attempt to bring the outside world to the patient by having a bedside telephone and radio and a television with remote controls.

▶ Allow the patient, as much as possible, to help in the planning of his own care. This will help the patient feel that he is an active participant in his own program of care and rehabilitation.

▶ Identify patients with exaggerated or inappropriate emotional responses and report your observations to the physician so that a psychiatric consultation can be arranged if necessary.

▶ Reinforce the patient's "well" behaviors of activity, e.g., the nurse gives *special* attention to the patient when the patient is doing self–range-of-motion exercises, as illustrated previously in Figure 33–16.

▶ Allow patients on bed rest to openly discuss with you their anxieties and worries. Such discussion, while momentarily taxing, may serve to ease the patient's mind enough so that he can truly rest—both physically and mentally.

BIBLIOGRAPHY

1. Anderson, E., Anderson, T. P., and Kottke, F. J.: Stroke rehabilitation: maintenance of achieved gains. *Archives of Physical Medicine and Rehabilitation*, 58(8):345–352, Aug. 1977.
2. Asher, R. A. J.: The dangers of going to bed. *British Medical Journal*, Oct. 1947, p. 967.
3. Bergstrom, D., and Coles, C. H.: *Basic Positioning Procedures*. Sister Kenny Institute, Minneapolis, 1971.
4. Berni, R., and Fordyce, W.: *Behavior Modification and the Nursing Process*, 2nd ed. St. Louis, C. V. Mosby Co., 1977.
4a. Beverley, E. V.: An assortment of fitness programs for the unconditioned retiree. *Geriatrics*, 31:122, Feb. 1976.
4b. Beverley, E. V.: The mechanics of putting those little-used muscles in motion. *Geriatrics*, 31:132, Jan. 1976.
5. Bliss, M. R., and McLaren, R.: Preventing pressure sores in geriatric patients. *Nursing Mirror*, 123:379, Jan. 1967.
6. Bliss, M. R., and McLaren, R.: Preventing pressure sores in geriatric patients. *Nursing Mirror*, 123:405, Feb. 1967.
7. Brower, P., and Hicks, D.: Maintaining muscle function in patients on bed rest. *American Journal of Nursing*, 72:1250, July 1972.
8. Browse, N. L.: *The Physiology and Pathology of Bedrest*. Springfield, IL, Charles C Thomas, 1965.
9. Burnside, I. M.: Reality testing: an important concept. *Journal of the Association of Rehabilitation Nurses*, 2(3):3–4, May–June 1977.
10. Cardenas, D. D., Stolov, W. C., and Hardy, R.: Elongation and collapse of the parallelogram structure. *Archives of Physical Medicine and Rehabilitation*, 58(10):423–426, Oct. 1977.
11. Carnevali, D., and Brueckner, S.: Immobilization: reassessment of a concept. *American Journal of Nursing*, 70(7):1502–1507, July 1970.
11a. Ciuca, R., et al.: Active range-of-motion exercises: a handbook. *Nursing '78*, 8:45, Aug. 1978.
12. Clark, J. A., and Roemer, R. B.: Voice controlled wheel-chair. *Archives of Physical Medicine and Rehabilitation*, 58(4):169–175, April 1977.
13. Coe, S. W.: Cardiac work and the chair treatment of acute coronary thrombosis. *Annals of Internal Medicine*, 40:42, Jan. 1954.
14. Dayhoff, N.: Re-thinking stroke. Soft or hard devices to position hands? *American Journal of Nursing*, 75(7):1142, July 1975.
15. DeLateur, B. J., et al.: Wheelchair cushions designed to prevent pressure sores: an evaluation. *Archives of Physical Medicine and Rehabilitation*, 57:129–135, March 1976.
16. Deitrick, J. E., et al.: Effects of immobilization upon various metabolic and physiologic functions of normal men. *American Journal of Medicine*, 4:3, Jan. 1948.
17. Downs, F. S.: Bed rest and sensory disturbances. *American Journal of Nursing*, 74(3):434–438, March 1974.
18. Drury, J. H.: Handbook of range-of-motion exercises. *Nursing '72*, 2:19, April 1972.
19. Edberg, E. L.: Prevention and treatment of pressure sores. *Physical Therapy*, 53:246, March 1973.
20. Ford, J. R., and Duckworth, B.: Moving a dependent patient safely, comfortably: part 1—positioning. *Nursing '76*, 6(1):27–36, Jan. 1976.
21. Germain, C. P.: Exercise makes the heart grow stronger. *American Journal of Nursing*, 72(12):2169–2173, Dec. 1972.
22. Gilstone, A.: Bedsore of the ear. *Lancet*, 2:1313, Dec. 1972.
23. Goldstrom, D. K.: Cardiac rest: bed or chair? *American Journal of Nursing*, 72:1812, Oct. 1972.
23a. Gordon, M.: Assessing activity tolerance. *American Journal of Nursing*, 76:72, Jan. 1976.
24. Gosnell, D. J.: An assessment tool to identify pressure sores. *Nursing Research*, 22:55, Jan.–Feb. 1973.
25. Greene, R.: Ostomy skin barriers for decubitus ulcers. *The Canadian Nurse*, 71:34–35, Feb. 1975.
26. Griffin, A.: The screen box. *Nursing '75*, 5:25, March 1975.
27. Griffin, W., Anderson, S. J., and Passos, J. Y.: Group exercise for patients with limited motion. *American Journal of Nursing*, 71(9):1742–1743, Sep. 1971.
28. Gruis, M. L., and Innes, B.: Assessment: essential to prevent pressure sores. *American Journal of Nursing*, 76(11):1762–1764, Nov. 1976.
29. Harvin, J. S., and Hargest, T. S.: The air-fluidized bed: a new concept in the treatment of decubitus ulcers. *Nursing Clinics of North America*, 5:181, March 1970.
30. Hirschberg, G., Lewis, L., and Vaughan, P.: Promoting patient mobility. *Nursing '77*, 7:42, May 1977.
31. Hodkinson, M. A.: Clinical problems of geriatric nursing. *Nursing Clinics of North America*, 3(4):675–686, Dec. 1968.
32. Hrobsky, A.: The patient on a CircOlectric bed. *American Journal of Nursing*, 71(12):2353, Dec. 1971.
33. Isler, C.: Decubitus: old truths and some new ideas. *RN*, 35:42, July 1972.
34. Johnson, M. L.: Problems involved in the prevention of pressure sores. *Nursing Mirror*, 135:37, July 1972.
35. Jungreis, S. W.: Exercises for expediting mobility (and decreasing disability) in bedridden patients. *Nursing '77*, 7:47–51, Aug. 1977.
36. Kavchak-Keyes, M. A.: Four proven steps for preventing decubitus ulcers. *Nursing '77*, 7:58–61, Sep. 1977.
36a. Kavchak-Keyes, M. A.: Treating decubitus ulcers using four proven steps. *Nursing '77*, 7:44, Oct. 1977.
37. Kelly, M. M.: Exercises for bedfast patients. *American Journal of Nursing*, 66:2209, Oct. 1966.
38. Lang, C., and McGrath, A.: Gelfoam for decubitus ulcers. *American Journal of Nursing*, 74(3):460–461.
39. Larrabee, J. H.: The person with spinal cord injury: physical care during early recovery. *American Journal of Nursing*, 77:1319–1329, Aug. 1977.
40. Lavin, M. A.: Bed exercises for acute cardiac patients. *American Journal of Nursing*, 73:122, July 1973.
41. Lehmann, J. F., et al.: Stroke: does rehabilitation affect outcome? *Archives of Physical Medicine and Rehabilitation*, 56:375–382, 1975.
42. Mitchell, P. H.: Motor status. In *Concepts Basic to Nursing*, 2nd ed. New York, McGraw-Hill Book Co., 1977.
43. Moolten, S. E.: Bedsores. *Hospital Medicine*, 13(5):83–103, May 1977.
44. Morley, M. H.: Decubitus ulcer management—a team approach. *The Canadian Nurse*, 69:41–43, Oct. 1973.
45. Mutter, D., et al.: Isometric exercise and the cardiovascular system. *Modern Concepts of Cardiovascular Disease*, 41:11, March 1972.

46. Norton, D.: Breakdown of pressure areas. *Nursing Times,* 60:399, March 1964.

47. How to negotiate the ups and downs, ins and outs of body alignment. *Nursing '74,* 4:46–51, Oct. 1974.

48. Nursing Education Department: *Nursing Care of the Skin,* Rev. Ed. Sister Kenny Institute, Minneapolis, 1975.

49. Olivari, H., et al.: The surgical treatment of bedsores in paraplegics. *Plastic and Reconstructive Surgery,* 50:477, Nov. 1972.

50. Olson, E. V., and Edmonds, R. E.: The hazards of immobility: effects on motor function. *American Journal of Nursing,* 67(4):788, April 1967.

51. Olson, E. V., and Thompson, L. F.: The hazards of immobility: effects on respiratory function. *American Journal of Nursing,* 67(4):783, April 1967.

52. Rantz, M. J., and Courtial, D.: *Lifting, Moving and Transferring Patients. A Manual.* St. Louis, The C. V. Mosby Co., 1977.

53. *Rehabilitative Aspects of Nursing—A Programmed Instruction Series. Part 1, Physical Therapeutic Measures: Unit 1, Concepts and Goals.* National League for Nursing, New York, 1966 (Code #19–1220).

54. *Rehabilitative Aspects of Nursing—A Programmed Instruction Series. Part 1, Physical Therapeutic Measures: Unit 2, Range of Joint Motion.* National League for Nursing, New York, 1967 (Code #19–1277).

55. Rubin, C. F., Dietz, R. R., and Abruzzese, R. S.: Auditing the decubitus ulcer problem. *American Journal of Nursing,* 74(10):1820–1821, Oct. 1974.

55a. Ryan, R.: Thrombophlebitis: assessment and prevention. *American Journal of Nursing,* 76:1634, Oct. 1976.

56. Taylor, J. C.: Decubitus ulcers. *Nursing Science,* 2:293, Aug. 1964.

57. Tepperman, P., et al.: Pressure sores: prevention and step-up management. *Postgraduate Medicine,* 62(3):83–89, Sep. 1977.

58. Toohey, P., and Larson, C. W.: *Range of Motion Exercise: Key to Joint Mobility.* Sister Kenny Institute, Minneapolis, 1977.

59. Torelli, M.: Topical hyperbaric oxygen for decubitus ulcers. *American Journal of Nursing,* 73(3):494, March 1973.

60. Van Ort, S. R., and Gerber, R. M.: Topical application of insulin in the treatment of decubitus ulcers: a pilot study. *Nursing Research,* 25(1):9–12, Jan.–Feb. 1976.

61. Verhonick, P. J., Lewis, D. W., and Goller, H. O.: Thermography in the study of decubitus ulcers. *Nursing Research,* 21(3):233–237, May–June, 1972.

62. Wiley, L. (ed.): The threat of thrombophlebitis. *Nursing '73,* 3:39–43, Nov. 1973.

63. Williams, A.: A study of factors contributing to skin breakdown. *Nursing Research,* 21(3):238–243, May–June 1972.

64. Works, R. F.: Hints on lifting and pulling. *American Journal of Nursing,* 72(2):260, Feb. 1972.

65. Yentzer, M. A.: Conquering those obstinate decubiti: foam leg supports. *Nursing '75,* 5:24, March 1975.

66. Young, C., Sr.: Exercise: how to use it to decrease complications in immobilized patients. *Nursing '75,* 5:81, March 1975.

CHAPTER 34*

PROVIDING PAIN RELIEF

He preaches patience that never knew pain.
PROVERB

INTRODUCTION AND STUDY GUIDE

This chapter provides an introduction to the complex phenomenon of pain and the assessment and nursing care of persons experiencing pain. Detailed discussions of types of pain, theories of pain transmission and the treatment of pain are beyond the scope of this text. The reader interested in these topics is referred to specialized texts and/or more advanced nursing texts, e.g., Luckmann and Sorensen's *Medical-Surgical Nursing: A Psychophysiologic Approach.*

Nurses, because of their prolonged and intimate contacts with patients, are in a unique position for being of assistance to persons in pain. Providing such help is a challenge, a responsibility and a privilege. Surely one of the greatest meanings of "caring" for a patient is realized when one can prevent or relieve pains, or at least make pains more tolerable. The practicing nurse continues throughout her career to gain new knowledge and skills relating to pain prevention and management. The sensitive nurse learns about pain not only from patients, coworkers, and publications, but also from her own inner life experiences with pain.

Because of the importance of understanding the content of this chapter, the student is advised to read the chapter more than once. Also, the student is advised to thoughtfully study this chapter with the aid of the following *study guide*:

▶ Review anatomy, physiology and pharmacology as necessary.

▶ Define "pain" in your own words.

▶ List three ways in which pain can serve as a protective mechanism.

▶ Cite examples of situations in which individuals may *not* experience pain even though a hurtful stimulus is present.

▶ Write out definitions of terms or phrases that are unfamiliar. (You may need to use a medical dictionary to assist with this task). Some of these may be:

noxious	pain reaction
psychic	pain threshold
somatic	pain localization
hyperalgesia	spontaneous pain
causalgia	reflex pain
sympathetic	secondary pain
parasympathetic	referred pain
psychogenic pain	central pain
organic pain	thalamic pain
pain reception	phantom limb pain
pain conduction	visceral pain
pain perception	

▶ Identify the three component parts of the sensation of pain.

▶ List ten factors that can influence an individual's perceptions and meanings of pain. Provide an example for each factor you have listed. (This topic is suitable for group discussion.)

▶ Consider ways in which a nurse's attitude toward pain can enhance or reduce her effectiveness in caring for patients experiencing pain. (This topic is suitable for group discussion.)

▶ Summarize in your own words sociocultural and individual factors that may influence the meanings of pain.

▶ Identify your own attitudes about pain and suffering. How do you expect yourself and others to react to pain? When was the last time you experienced pain? How did you react? How were you wanting others to react to your suffering? What experiences have you had in your past that you think influenced your present attitudes toward pain and your expectations of persons experiencing pain, e.g., childhood experiences, reactions of

*Ruth McCorkle, R.N., Ph.D., and T. Hongladarom, M.D., critically reviewed and assisted with the revision of this chapter.

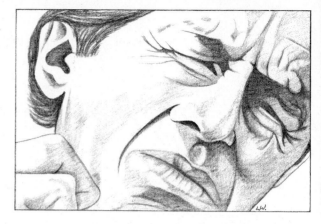

significant others? How do you feel when you are with a person whose reactions to pain are different from yours? (These topics are suitable for group discussion.)

▶ In your clinical practice, work to become increasingly aware of pain experiences. Identify ways in which you can prevent or minimize pains that are the direct result of your actions while administering care. Conduct thorough assessments of patients experiencing pains, following guidelines presented in this chapter. Plan appropriate nursing interventions based upon your assessments and upon the information presented in this chapter.

THE PHENOMENON OF PAIN

If you come to think about it, physical pain has many singularities. Of all human experiences it is, as long as it lasts, the most absorbing; and it is the only human experience which, when it comes to an end, automatically confers a real if not perhaps a very high kind of happiness. It is also the only experience this side of death which is by its nature solitary. But the oddest thing about it is that despite its intensity, despite its unequaled power over mind and body, when it is over you cannot really remember it at all.

Peter Fleming: On Pain from My Aunt's Rhinoceros and Other Reflections

The nurse needs to be aware that pain is a complex phenomenon. Pain, in general, is an unpleasant experience that is primarily associated with tissue damage. There are two distinct types of pain in relation to duration—acute pain and chronic pain. *Acute pain* functions to inform us of noxious stimulation or to warn us to take care of ourselves. It frequently occurs suddenly and leads us to take action to relieve the source of pain. With acute pain, there is every likelihood that relief will be obtained because the cause can be identified and treated. *Chronic pain* may begin as an acute episode or it may be more insidious, making it difficult to describe its onset. Contrary to acute pain, persons cannot give meaning to the chronic pain. When the pain continues over an extended period of time, it is classified as long term. The pain may be continuous or intermittent. It may vary in intensity or remain the same. In some instances the source of pain may be identified but an effective treatment not known, or the source may be uncertain and diagnosis deferred. Chronic pain becomes intractable when treatment is provided without the person obtaining relief or if the pain persists without demonstrable disease.

Bodily pain was regarded for hundreds of years as a means of obtaining religious grace, or as a punishment considered to be God-given and "good for the soul." This acceptance and affirmation of pain as divine retribution underlay all Oriental as well as Western religions. Because of this long-standing attitude toward pain, efforts to control or abolish it were inhibited.

Only recently has medicine been able to bring multiple treatment methods to focus on the goal of pain control. A variety of approaches are found in the pain therapy of today, e.g., drug therapy, electrical stimulation, hypnotism, nerve blocks, open and closed stereotaxic surgery and other surgical approaches, physical therapy, behavior modification techniques, and psychiatric therapies. *Scientifically* pain is currently subjected to the scrutiny of many disciplines. *Philosophically* the problem of pain continues to pose enduring questions such as, "Why must man suffer and be subjected to pain?"

Although major advances have been made within the past few decades in both understanding and alleviating pain, much remains to be learned and many fallacies about pain still exist. The nurse must be able to discriminate between fact and fallacy in this important area of her practice.

FACTS AND FALLACIES ABOUT PAIN

Listed below are some misconceptions about pain as well as a few statements that are generally accepted as accurate—or as facts:

Fallacy	*Fact*
All persons who are critically ill or gravely injured experience intense pain.	Persons who are critically ill, e.g., have terminal cancer, or are gravely injured, do *not* inevitably experience pain. While some persons do have pain at such a time, others may not.

Fallacy	*Fact*
The greater the pain, the greater the amount of tissue damage.	Intensity of pain is *not* directly proportional to the severity or extent of tissue damage.
Pain is symptomatic of *incurable* illnesses, e.g., "If I have pain, it's probably 'too late' for a doctor to help me."	Pain is an important symptom which often indicates that treatment is necessary. Many painful conditions *are* treatable, indeed curable!

THE UNIQUE NATURE OF PAIN

Although much *is* predictable about the pain response, there are aspects of it that remain incomprehensible. In a way, attempting to understand and describe pain is like trying to talk about the wind—*only its effects can be observed*. Thus, with pain we see the grimace, the clenched fist; *the phenomenon itself cannot be seen*, is difficult to describe, and is often hard to recall precisely. "The symptom which most frequently warns the patient of the presence of a pathological condition, and which most often causes him to seek medical advice, is at the same time that about which he remembers least."[81]

Following are some statements about the complex, unique experience of pain:

▶ Pain is mediated by receptors that are chemosensitive.*

▶ Pain is difficult to evaluate because it is an entirely subjective phenomenon. Also, it is especially difficult to differentiate psychologic from organic factors. For example, both *organic pain* (originating essentially from organic, i.e., physical, sources) and *psychogenic pain* (originating essentially from psychologic sources) are called "pain" and are experienced in the same way even though there are differences in how they develop.

▶ Whereas slight wounds may be quite painful, it is also possible to have extensive wounds that are painless. Under certain stressful conditions, even severe wounds may not be painful.

▶ Pain does not indicate the seriousness or the amount of tissue damage, but rather it is generally indicative of the *rate* of tissue damage. Pain, thus, indicates that tissue damage is in progress.

▶ Pain patterns (e.g., intensity, duration, rhythmicity) vary, depending upon the etiology or the organ system involved.

▶ Individuals vary in their ability to withstand the same pain. The same stimulus may produce varying results in various persons and even in the same person if conditions are altered. The female is generally conceded to be able to withstand pain better than the male.

▶ Pain intensity (conduction and perception, not response) has a definite ceiling or maximum. Studies with heat demonstrate that even though the rate of pain stimulation and tissue damage continues to increase, there is a point at which pain intensity fails to increase. In fact, pain can disappear if pain sensitive structures are destroyed, as with third degree burns.

▶ The word "pain" is often inaccurately used to refer to feelings (both physical and mental) that are actually not painful. For example, feelings of "pressure" may be confused with feelings of "pain."

▶ There are distinguishable qualities of pain (e.g., burn, prick, sharp, dull) and distinguishable intensities (e.g., minor, slight, excruciating).

▶ Interpretations of the pain sensation vary: It is debatable whether pain is always an "uncomfortable" experience. For example, some believe that pain is not an unpleasant sensation to persons with masochistic tendencies or to persons who have had leukotomy (prefrontal lobotomy).

▶ Pain originating from bodily disorders is believed to differ from pain that is experimentally produced. Also, pain that is self-inflicted is believed to be experienced differently from pain that has its source outside of oneself.[67]

▶ Pain may be present in the absence of demonstrable bodily disease, injury or noxious (hurtful) stimulation. For example, with *phantom limb pain* the individual experiences pain as though it is arising in a limb even though the limb has been amputated.

DEFINITIONS OF PAIN

An accurate definition of the term "pain" is difficult to arrive at. One dictionary defines

---

*Chemosensitive means sensitive to changes that occur in chemical composition.

pain as "a feeling of distress, suffering or agony, caused by stimulation of specialized nerve endings." Pain cannot be satisfactorily defined in other than subjective terms.[69] W. K. Livingston, a pioneer in the study of pain, writes: "I am unwilling to call anything pain unless it is perceived as such."[54] Thus, if a person has what appears to be a "painful" injury but experiences no pain himself, the injury cannot accurately be called painful.

It has been said simply that "Pain is what the subject says hurts."[69] *Pain is ultimately defined by every individual introspectively in terms of his own experience and the "meaning" that pain holds for him.*

PAIN AS A PROTECTIVE MECHANISM

Pain is an important warning of danger to man; however, it is not essential for biologic adjustment, since persons who have pain pathways surgically or pathologically interrupted, and those persons born without the ability to experience pain, can adjust themselves to their environment. Nevertheless, the loss or absence of the ability to feel and respond to pain predisposes an individual to repeated bodily injury.

Let us examine more closely the function of pain and how some of man's defenses against injury are related to one another.[54]

▶ The *withdrawal reflex* is the simplest and the most familiar defense, e.g., pulling away from something hot. These reflexes are violent and irrepressible when the threat is great. The muscular reflexes act as a *first* line of defense against injury and often effectively help us to break contact with an offending stimulus by causing us to pull away from it. In order to reduce the length of contact with the stimulus to a minimum—and thus to reduce or prevent tissue damage to the body—the withdrawal reflex occurs with fantastic speed. The impulses race over the shortest possible route from the injury site to the spinal cord and back again to the musculature in the area of injury.

▶ *Visceral reflexes* involving the glands of internal secretion act as a *second* line of defense against bodily injury. Be preparing us for "fight or flight" such reflexes can give us the almost superhuman agility and strength needed in a crisis to save us from real danger.

▶ *Voluntary responses* to a situation (those responses that we willfully or consciously decide to perform) are a *third* line of defense. Once a hurtful stimulus is translated by the brain into perceived pain, the individual, having felt pain, can locate its source and decide, on the basis of his past experience, what he should do.

These three lines of defense are intimately related, and all are activated by the same hurtful stimuli. Because reflex responses occur much faster than voluntary ones, they give better protection against injury. However, reflexes are always stereotyped and may be totally inappropriate to a situation, but they occur whether or not they will serve any useful purpose. Thus, if injury or pain is sustained or repeated, these reflexes may actually waste and deplete bodily resources to the extent that new stresses or infection cannot be withstood. Livingston points out: "As a matter of fact, actual tissue injury need not be present to cause this exhaustion. Fear can do exactly the same thing. Often the threat of pain does a person more harm than the injuries that taught him to fear it."[54]

In sum, while pain is protective in some situations, it is useless and can be detrimental to health in others. For example, pain serves a useful function when abdominal tenderness shields an inflamed gallbladder; however, reflex pain can become detrimental and the pain associated with a phantom limb apparently has no protective value.

THE "COMPONENTS" OF PAIN

The entire pain experience is complex in nature, involving an interplay of perception, physiology, feeling states or emotions, and other reactions. Thus, pain is evidently linked to a group of complex experiences rather than to a single sensation produced by a specific stimulus.

> *Pain is a complex "mind-body" experience involving the total person rather than only the mind or only the body. Indeed, the mental (psychic) and physical (somatic) experiences of pain are inseparable.*

Therefore, although we shall discuss pain in terms of its *"component parts"* (e.g., perception, reaction), the reader is asked to bear in mind that this is done only for purposes of discussion and has no basis in actual experience.

The sensation of pain may be said to have three component parts: (1) *reception* of the pain stimulus by the pain receptors (free nerve end-

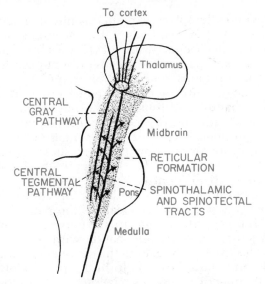

Figure 34–1. Transmission of pain signals into the hindbrain, thalamus, and cortex through multiple diffuse pathways. (From Guyton, A. C.: *Textbook of Medical Physiology.* 4th ed., Philadelphia, W. B. Saunders, 1971.)

ings in the skin and certain other tissues) and *conduction* of the pain impulses by nerves; (2) *perception* of pain in the higher centers of the brain (e.g., thalamus and cerebral cortex [Fig. 34–1]); and (3) *reactions* to pain, which are physical, emotional, and psychologic in nature.[59]

The *perception* of pain is a neurophysiologic process that can be modified by drugs and psychic factors. It can subsequently be completely prevented after the conduction of pain is interrupted by surgical or chemical procedures (e.g., surgery or nerve blocks).

The *reaction* to pain is a complex physiopsychologic process involving the cognitive functions (e.g., awareness, reasoning). Reactions to pain are highly individualistic and may vary for a given individual from one time to another in his life. Reactions may be *anticipatory*, occurring prior to the pain-producing stimulus and in expectation of it, or they may occur *after* pain perception as a response to it.

Physiologic and emotional reactions contribute to every individual's unique perception of his pain; many factors influence this perception.* For example, it was observed that some soldiers severely wounded in battle during World War II said that they felt no pain and wanted no pain-relieving drugs. Because they had lived through battle, and believed that being wounded meant that they would be sent home, they experienced no pain, but rather felt relief. Therefore, these men did not perceive their wounds as terrible, painful experiences, but rather as a means of relief and escape from an intolerable situation.[8] Other examples are known of soldiers failing to perceive pain from their wounds because they were under the influence of rage or of the exaltation of battle.[23]

On the other hand, it has been observed[6] that victims of automobile or industrial accidents (whose ages and types of wounds were similar to those of wounded soldiers) overwhelmingly sought relief by medication from what they experienced as excruciating pain. These wounds, to accident victims, *meant* a sudden deterioration from an existing acceptable situation into an impossible one, the consequences of which would be loss of income, unexpected expenses, and mutilation.

Some factors that influence the perception and meaning of pain and the reactions to pain are: (1) attitude toward pain; (2) past experience with pain; (3) value judgment, e.g., pain is "good" or "bad"; (4) mood; (5) emotional status, e.g., stable or unstable; (6) will and self-control; (7) state of the nervous system and the various cerebral processes, e.g., fatigue, disease; (8) situational and environmental components; (9) social, cultural, and economic elements; and (10) the presence or absence of anxiety.

Mental faculties may play a definite part in how persons react to pain, but they should not be used as an indicator to predict response. It has been observed,[81] for example, that: (1) patients with *severe, chronic painful conditions* gradually become free of pain with a decrease in mental capabilities, e.g., with senility; (2) patients with *moderate mental deficiency*, e.g., due to retardation, may react abnormally strongly to painful stimuli because they lack the intelligence to reason out beforehand the extent of the discomfort that will be produced by the noxious stimuli. In addition, *personality defects*, as well as level of intelligence, are evidently factors in the pain reaction. "Those persons who display an abnormal mental reaction to pain will frequently display corresponding mental instability on other occasions."[81] Emotionally unstable individuals seem extraordinarily prone to develop pain.[77]

THE PAIN THRESHOLD

The pain threshold is the smallest perceivable pain, i.e., "the lowest perceptible intensity

---

*Students desiring to read further about the psychologic and interpersonal functions of pain are referred to Engel[32] and Szasz.[89] For a discussion of the symbolic and communicative aspects of pain read Szasz.[89]

of pain."[95] Various factors may alter the pain threshold. For example, inflammation or injury of tissues near the nerve endings which subserve pain may *lower* the threshold for pain. This means that stimuli which ordinarily are nonpain-producing (i.e., "non-noxious") may induce pain; also, stimuli which previously produced mild pain may now produce a more intense pain. Such situations are referred to as *hyperalgesia*, meaning a state of excessive sensitiveness to pain.

Wolff and Wolf[95] report that all persons having healthy body structures have approximately the same *capacity* for perceiving pain, that is, the threshold for the perception of pain is approximately the same in all normal subjects. Recently, researchers have begun to distinguish between two levels of pain threshold. The first is a *sensation threshold,* the lowest noxious stimulus intensity at which a sensation such as warmth or pressure is first noted. This is the threshold that seems to be relatively constant among people with healthy and intact neurological structures.[64] The second is a *pain perception threshold,* "the lowest stimulus level at which a person reports feeling pain."[64] This threshold is influenced by many factors, as presented in the previous section, and varies from person to person.

Beecher[7] and subsequent investigators have separated the pain experience into two areas: the *pain sensation* and the *pain reaction. Pain sensation* is sometimes equated with pain threshold. *Pain reaction* is considered in terms of the patient's tolerance for pain. The threshold for reaction to pain varies between wide limits for given individuals and for the same person under differing circumstances.

The intensity of two pains that exist separately, but at the same time, is no greater than that of the more intense of the two. It has long been observed that the existence of one pain may actually raise the threshold for perception of another; thus, the person in intense pain may bite his lip or squeeze his fingernails into the palms of his hand and, by creating this "counter pain," lessen the intensity of the original pain.

THE LOCALIZATION OF PAIN

The cerebral cortex of the brain functions to localize the sensation of pain. There have been several attempts to explain this phenomenon.* According to Holmes,[43] the accuracy with which this occurs varies with (1) the abundance or sparseness of sense organs present in various bodily regions and (2) the frequency with which the entire sensory circuit is utilized. The lips, hands, and tongue are diffusely impregnated with sensory nerve endings and have proportionate cortical representation in the cerebrum in relation to other sense organs. These parts of the body are frequently employed to identify objects. As the sensory nerve endings are stimulated, the cortex precisely and accurately localizes the pain.

It is possible to compare the nerve endings of the tongue, eyes, and hands with fire alarm boxes in a building. Both the nerve endings and the fire alarm boxes help in the process of localizing disturbances. Nerve endings will signal the brain about an area of pain (on the tongue, for example) just as the fire alarm boxes will signal the firehouse about a fire in a building. Moreover, if the signal relay system, e.g., from the alarm box to the fire station (or from the nerve ending to the brain), is maintained in working order, then each part of the system, or each member of the team, knows what functions need to be performed and operates smoothly and rapidly, thus reducing difficulty in the transmission of the signal.

In contrast to the areas of the tongue, lips, and hands, visceral† pain is usually poorly localized because of: (1) the relative paucity of nerve endings, (2) the relative lack of use of this sensory pathway, and (3) the lack of a reference point. One possible explanation is that there is a relative absence of cortical training in the brain in the process of identifying the area affected. However, those deeper structures that are subject to more frequent stimulation by contacts giving rise to sensory impulses may have more clearly localized pain sensations; for example, muscles and periosteum of bones near the body surface.

Pain-producing stimuli almost invariably excite *other forms of sensation:* a pinprick thus usually evokes sensations of touch or pressure and of penetration of the skin; a bruise produces feelings of pressure; and a burn is accompanied by a sensation of heat. These sensations, which are evoked at the same time as pain, probably also provide a basis for localizing and discriminating painful experiences.[43]

---

*Students desiring to read further about the psychophysiology of pain for a detailed explanation of the evolution of pain theories are referred to Melzack and Wall.[63]

†Viscera are the large organs located in the three great body cavities, particularly the abdomen.

The patient is the expert in localizing his pain. Both qualitative and quantitative aspects must be determined by him because he is the only one who really knows what he is experiencing. Unfortunately, in the past, professionals have treated and judged patients according to their own biases and previous experiences. Conversely, it is more important to stress the individuality of pain perception and response. Professionals need to learn to help patients to identify factors contributing to their pain and deal constructively with them.

ASSESSMENT OF PAIN AND OF PATIENTS EXPERIENCING PAIN

The evaluation of pain so that it can be treated adequately is made difficult by its being an entirely subjective phenomenon. It is especially difficult to differentiate organic from psychic factors. The problem is further complicated because in most, if not all, patients, both factors contribute to the final expression of the pain. Furthermore, the proportion of contributions by the somatic and psychic spheres changes constantly.[33]

The assessment of pain and of patients experiencing pain is an activity that nurses perform frequently. As we have demonstrated, pain is difficult to assess because it is a highly personalized, subjective experience which is manifested uniquely in each patient and which stems from diverse etiologies.

THE NURSE; THE PATIENT

Important areas in the assessment of a patient experiencing pain are: (1) the nurse's understanding of the patient's personality; and (2) her impression of herself as she is reflected in the patient's response to her.[27]

Does one ever become accustomed to witnessing pain in others? It is hoped that a nurse never becomes "hardened" to the presence of pain. And, certainly she must build a constructive attitude toward pain if she is to encounter and help to alleviate suffering.

To form such a constructive attitude, the professional nurse strives to clarify her own feelings about suffering. For example, a nurse will not be able to help a patient to find meaning in his pain-filled life if she does not truly believe that his life is meaningful; a nurse cannot hope to clarify the "nightmare" of pain for a patient if she is not willing to look at the nightmare herself; and she cannot help a patient to break out of his shell of isolation if she, because of her anxiety, encloses herself in a shell. The helpful nurse comes to the realization that pain,

though subjective, is also a very real and universal experience, and that to understand pain, and hopefully to alleviate it, is one of nursing's greatest challenges.

Before planning specific care, consider your own feelings about a patient in pain—your attitudes toward the patient as a person and toward pain and suffering generally. If you possess the attitude that *pain is not inevitable, intolerable, and unmanageable,* you will be in a position to be helpful to patients who are afraid that they will have pain, as well as to those who currently have it. *Thoughtful, intelligent nursing care can prevent, reduce, make bearable, and control pain.* An optimistic, informed attitude toward pain control can bring to the fore each patient's strengths in responding to pain and help each to achieve a more realistic view of his situation.[10]

Because a patient's pain has special meanings *to him,* he may expect that those caring for him will, intuitively, understand his individual view of his situation and will respond appropriately. If your view of a patient's pain fails to coincide with *his* view of it, problems ensue.

Consider how you think the patient having pain perceives you. For example, does he act toward you as if you are there to help him, or as if you are there to inflict further pain and add to his misery? Does he seem to think that you believe what he is telling you about his pain and will act to help him, or as if he thinks you doubt what he says and will dismiss it without seeking relief for him? Does he view you as interested and concerned, or bored and unimpressed with his situation?

Further discussion of ways in which a nurse can help the patient having pain, by means of her interaction with him, is presented further on. The individual personalities of both patient and nurse are important determining factors in the specific process of interaction. The meanings that both nurse and patient assign to pain are also important and must be considered. (See also Chap. 3, Therapeutic Nurse-Patient Relationship.)

ASSESSING THE MEANINGS OF PAIN

The alleviation of pain on a professional level does not take place in a social vacuum. It takes place in a social situation. The patient in pain reacts diffusely to painful experiences and to the efforts of those who are trying to help him. The efforts expended on his behalf, as well as the pain itself, have meaning for the patient. Existing potentialities for alleviating pain can be fully exploited only when the meaning to the patient is given careful consideration.[27]

Sociocultural Factors

As we have previously demonstrated, the experience of pain cannot be explained in purely physiologic or biologic terms; cultural and social aspects of pain must also be considered. For example, as a result of cultural influences, manifest (i.e., observable) behavior in pain experiences will vary. Some patients will quietly accept intense pain, whereas others quake, wail, and show other obvious signs of distress at the thought of a small needle prick.

Zborowski[96] points out that cultural influences may affect attitudes concerning *pain expectancy* (i.e., the anticipation of pain viewed as unavoidable in certain situations) and *pain acceptance* (i.e., the willingness to experience pain). For example, while pain may be "expected" as a part of medical treatment, some patients will be less willing to "accept" the pain than others.

> *Pain expectancy influences the perception of pain.*

Thus, in a person who has a morbid fear of cancer, every pain he develops may be intensified because to him it suggests the onset of cancer, which the individual "expects" he will develop. Expectations of pain are often out of proportion to the actual situation. For example, not all persons with cancer experience pain; however, most people with cancer "expect" that they will have pain. Such expectations can cause people to misinterpret other discomforts, such as pressure, for pain. Postoperative pain represents another situation in which pain expectations are important. Not all postoperative patients have pain.

In addition to pain expectancy and pain acceptance, other factors that may culturally vary are *pain apprehension* and *pain anxiety*. Pain apprehension is related to the tendency to avoid pain. Pain anxiety refers to the state of anxiety that the pain experience provokes; it mainly focuses on the cause of pain, the meaning of pain, and its significance for the welfare

of the individual. Several factors have been identified as contributing to the anxiety of the patient experiencing pain. Some of these are: the element of the unknown; the loneliness of pain, and the helplessness engendered by pain; and the threat to the self or body image.[10, 27, 52]

Past experiences with pain, and past observations of others in pain, markedly affect individual perceptions of pain-producing situations. Therefore, learning and experience *condition* one's reactions to pain and add to the meaning that pain has for each different individual.

The pain that a child experiences is often conditioned by the fears, attitudes and afflictions of his parents. Indeed, parental influences may be decisive factors in determining the amount of pain their children will suffer from minor injuries throughout the rest of their lives.[54]

Zborowski[96] concludes that there are ethnic variations in attitudes toward pain. In each culture, parents' approval or disapproval of their children's responses to pain promotes in the children specific acceptable forms of behavior in reaction to pain. When the responses to pain of three ethnic groups were studied it was observed that: (1) the model "Italian" patient responded to pain by *complaints* of discomfort caused by the pain as such; (2) the model "Jewish" patient mainly worried about the extent to which the pain indicated a *threat* to himself; and (3) the model "Old American" tended to avoid complaining and provoking pity and *minimized* his pain.

The Old American group provides the dominant values and attitudes in the United States, and thus represents those attitudes toward pain which many patients, doctors, and nurses have in this country. In his survey, Zborowski observed that the Italian and Jewish subjects manifested suffering and admitted to pain more readily than the Old Americans. Thus, depending on their culture, some persons will readily say that they are in pain whereas others are hesitant to mention it.

Moreover, it has been noted that pain occurring in culturally "unacceptable" body areas, e.g., areas embarrassing to the patient like the rectum, anus, genitalia, or buttocks, appears to be underreported compared with pain in more "acceptable" areas.

In striving to accept various cultural differences in response to pain, the nurse needs to realize that the responses to pain of persons of cultural groups that differ from her own are as valid as her own responses to pain would be. Obviously, one must be cautious in judging how severe another person's pain may be.

At certain moments my body is illuminated. . . .
It is very curious. Suddenly I see into myself. . . . I
can make out the depth of the layers of my flesh; and
I feel zones of pain, rings, poles, plumes of pain. Do
you see these living figures, this geometry of my
suffering? Some of these flashes are exactly like
ideas. They make me understand—from here, to
there. . . . And yet they leave me *uncertain.*
  Paul Valéry: Monsieur Teste (tr. by J. Mathews)

In addition to those cultural factors that affect
reactions to pain, the nurse assessing pain also
considers the variety of individual meanings
which pain may hold for different patients.

> *Pain is a concept with wide connotations and
> with multiple meanings which often are
> difficult to identify since they derive from
> peoples' individual experiences.*

Because of its central importance, the
superior nurse attempts to understand how
pain is viewed by each patient and what meanings it may have for him. It is also important to
identify a patient's level of *anxiety* in response
to these meanings. *As anxiety increases, so
does suffering; anxiety increases a patient's
estimation of the intensity of his pain and his
emotional responses to it.* Uncertainty or fear of
the meaning or significance of pain also exag-
gerates responses.

Emotional states and the *observable behavior* related to them reflect, as a rule, the meaning or significance of the pain to an individual.[56]
Thus, observations should include watching
for indications of depression, anger, fear, excitement, weeping, and so forth. Because
people in pain are suffering, they may be
jumpy, cross, bitter, fearful, depressed,
childlike, and so on. Acceptance of such behavior and an understanding of its origin will lessen the strain on the patient.[10]

In addition to observing a patient's behavior
you can also obtain some idea of the meaning of
pain to the patient by *listening* carefully to what
he says. Perhaps he views his pain as deserved
punishment; he may think that pain means he is
getting worse. Many other meanings are possible. Patients who have had severe pain may be
fearful of going to sleep and of relaxing because
they are afraid their pain will return or that the
pain means that they may die because the condition is critical.[10] By appreciating the meanings pain has for a particular patient, the excellent nurse can plan care that meets the
patient's needs more effectively.

For example, if a patient perceives of himself
as being trapped and helpless in his painful
state, the nurse can alleviate some of these perceptions by planning with the patient what she
and he can both do to reduce or prevent his
pain. For example, *together* they can decide:
how to best position the patient; how he can
help to move himself; and how often to change
his position. Also, they can determine activities
the patient can do by himself to prevent or to
reduce his pain, e.g., slow deep breathing
through open mouth when pain increases, or
exercises in bed to maintain and strengthen
muscle tone. By identifying together ways to
reduce or to prevent pain, both patient and
nurse will feel less helpless against pain and
will become more effective in pain prevention
and pain management.

Important pain-conditioning experiences
take place during childhood. A nurse sees in
patients the results of such experiences. "A
child learns many of his responses from his
family during his early formative years. A
mother, by belittling, or, conversely, by comforting and cajoling, may implant in her small
son the basis of the reaction the nurse meets
when the son, grown to manhood, recovers
from anesthesia following a surgical operation."[47] Pain can cause some adults to *regress* to
childlike behavior patterns, since basic patterns
of responding to pain were learned then. Patients' expectations of how they should be
treated when they are in pain vary from individual to individual. A patient can often be
made more comfortable if the nurse responds to
him in a manner that he feels is appropriate and
helpful to him.

When the nurse cares for the patient who
regresses, she may respond with sympathy to
his needs but she must *never* treat such a patient with pity. LeShan[52] observes that pity is an
extremely corrosive emotion. Pity for a person
who is already unsure of his status and uncertain of the meaning of his life only confirms his
uncertainty. Pity enforces regression because it
carries with it a sense of condescension. It
confirms the patient's feeling of childish
helplessness and loss of dignity and status.
Consequently, the nurse needs to strive to treat
patients as equals and as adults who are worthy
of her esteem and her respect. Only thus can a
nurse halt regression and help patients to rebuild self-images equal to their former stature.

Finally, in assessing the individual meanings
of pain, recall that in some situations, pain actually *benefits* a patient psychologically. While
this is not usually so, it may be the case in some
psychogenic pain or secondary pain. Also,
under some conditions, pain may be a welcome

sign of improvement and, as such, may be associated with pleasurable emotion, e.g., pains such as those that occur upon the return of sensation or feeling to a previously analgetic paralyzed limb.[55]

Psychogenic Factors

Perhaps the most obscure meanings of pains are those attached to psychogenic pains. Psychogenic pains have highly individualized meanings that are generally imperceptible to observers. The dualistic "mind-body" assumption, which permeates much of our medical philosophy as well as our language, is a major cause of confusion in thinking about pain. "When pain is regarded as a psycho-physiological phenomenon it becomes easier to talk and write about, but more difficult to understand."[67]

We have said that pain is always accompanied by some psychologic or emotional meaning. And yet, because such meanings are difficult to identify and verbalize, patients will rarely discuss their painful feelings in psychologic or emotional terms and instead use medical, somatic, or physical terms.

One physician writes, "No matter what the patient's problem, he often feels that he must speak to his doctor in medical terms. . . . The patient wants to be accepted and understood by his doctor; therefore, he talks of somatic pain rather than of painful emotional experiences. The doctor, on the other hand, because of his limited time and his own emotional needs, often would rather hear and discuss somatic pains than . . . complicated emotional pains."[78]

Psychogenic pain raises, in an acute form, the problem of communication. Many people find it difficult to believe that pain in the absence of discoverable organic disease is the same kind of sensation that is felt when organic disease is present.[20]

ASSESSING PAIN

The Nature of Pain

Numerous factors, joined together, contribute to the "nature" of various pains. Some general factors that influence the nature of pains are:[55]

▶ *The integrity of the patient's nervous system.* If the nervous system is impaired so that it cannot maintain normal functioning, then a patient's responses to pain-producing situations are altered, e.g., an increase in causalgia. If the nervous system is faulty, the patient cannot be expected to have typical reactions to pain or, at times, even to feel pain.

▶ *The patient's state of consciousness.* The meaning of pain depends upon the state of consciousness, since past and present experiences have symbolic meanings that influence perception of a sensation.

▶ *Previous experience, training, or conditioning.* Depending on the person and the previous pain experiences, the reactions may be either increased or decreased. For example, one individual suffering extremely severe pain may at first bear it stoically, but, with repetition of the experience, become so fearful of additional pain that anticipation of it alone causes vomiting, fainting, or other physical-emotional reactions. Another person, in a similar situation, may develop fortitude or resignation in response to repetition of painful experiences and progressively show a decrease in psychologic reactions.

▶ *The patient's racial or ethnic background.* In general, Anglo-Saxon or Nordic individuals are relatively less sensitive or less reactive to pain, whereas Jews and Latins are more sensitive and more reactive.

▶ *The patient's age.* Sensitivity to pain varies with age, since learned emotional attitudes alter greatly the perception of pain. Infants are less sensitive to pain than adults. Repeated studies demonstrate that in any one individual sensitivity is learned as an infant, it increases as the person grows to adulthood, and then gradually diminishes with advancing age. In fact, the intensity of pain in the elderly may be of such low quality that it may be *overlooked* or its significance discovered later than is desirable.

▶ *Fatigue, debility,* and *repeated painful procedures* can all reduce the ability to tolerate pain. Likewise, *worry, lack of sleep,* and *prolonged suffering* (e.g., nausea, vomiting, diarrhea) can reduce a patient's ability to tolerate pain and, thus, increase his magnification of it. The exhausted patient's powers of self-control and resistance may become so depleted that one more pain becomes unbearable. In such conditions, a hypodermic injection may precipitate extreme psychologic responses, and the patient may weep uncontrollably, cry out, or attempt to flee or withdraw. On the other hand, some patients become so weary that their attention is withdrawn from their injuries and they almost apathetically accept any painful experience directed at them.

Detailed information concerning the nature of any pain is essential for accurate diagnosis and treatment. For example, to make a diagnosis of organic pain, medical personnel must be able to document clear objective changes in the nature of the pain or to recognize the extent to which the pain conforms to a known syndrome.

In formulating a complete clinical picture of any pain it is helpful to consider the following factors about the nature of the pain.

Assessment of the Nature of Pain

1. *History* of the origin and occurrence of pain.
   a. When did it begin?
   b. Has it interfered with sleep, other vital functions, or the performance of duties?
   c. Is it a factor in litigation or could it be related to malingering?
2. *Localization* of the pain in the body.
   a. In what area or areas of the body is the pain felt? Do the areas of pain differ under differing circumstances?
   b. If several parts of the body are painful, do the pains occur simultaneously and are they dependent on one another?
   c. Is the pain unilateral or bilateral? If bilateral, is it present in identical areas on the two sides of the body? (Pain such as thalamic pain can be localized to the whole of one side of the body.)
3. *Extension, radiation, and depth:* A description of the "size and shape" of the pain.
   a. Does it extend diffusely over a large area or can it be pinpointed? Is the area poorly or well defined?
   b. Does the pain originate in a definite area and then radiate to other areas? Both the point at which the pain starts and its radiation are important in diagnosis and treatment.
   c. Can the pain be described in terms of three dimensions, e.g., width, length, and depth? Generally, the patient is able only to determine whether the pain is localized to the skin or to deeper structures. Usually it is not possible for him to give a more exact description of depth localization.
4. *Duration:* How the pain occurs in time or its time-relations. Often separate paroxysms of pain are assembled in series. When a patient speaks of the "duration of an attack" he usually means the duration or length of such a series.
   a. How long does the pain last?
   b. Is it paroxysmal, intermittent, steady or continuous, rhythmic, throbbing or pulsating? These are some terms commonly used to describe the nature of pain.
5. *Onset or pattern:* Occurrence and character of the attack as a whole.
   a. What time did the pain begin? Is it seasonal? (For example, peptic ulcer pain tends to recur in the spring and fall, possibly due to changes in diet.)
   b. Do any events, activities, or persons precipitate the pain? Can times or patterns be identified when pain is anticipated to occur? Is a stimulus, precipitating factor, or trigger zone identifiable? Is pain associated with changes in position or the weather?
   c. What factors alter the character of the pain, increase, reduce, or otherwise modify it?
   d. Does an attack begin gradually or acutely? Does the pain reach a "peak" and then rapidly diminish after reaching maximum? Does the pain have a "plateau" at which it remains at a constant intensity for a period of time? Between attacks is the patient without pain or other symptoms, or does he have mild pain, paresthesia, or other symptoms?
   e. Have changes occurred in the pain pattern or in the patient's life, e.g., weight loss, stress, working conditions, or way of life?
6. *Day pains.* Some pains usually occur during the day since they are made worse by mental or physical activities. Examples are: locomotor pains such as rheumatism, sciatica, and flat foot; eye pain; and morning sinus pain caused by no chance for sinuses to drain at night.
7. *Night pains.* Pains occurring at night, particularly if they awaken the patient, are typically characteristic of organic disease (as opposed to psychogenic pains). However, some psychogenic pains may occur at night if the patient has insomnia and if, freed from the distractions of the day, he becomes fearful and anxious. Colic and ulcer pains typically occur at night, since at night our bodies are largely governed by autonomic nerve control, and, therefore, it is

the time of vagus and parasympathetic activity. Also, because relaxation of protective muscle contraction occurs at night, involuntary movements occur. Thus, the pains of joint disease are mainly nocturnal. The patient whom the nurse finds sleeping well or resting quietly is not likely to be having pain.

8. *Character or quality* of the pain: Is it dull, sharp, shooting? Often the character of pain is dependent on both its localization and its duration. It is not unusual for the character of a pain to alter during its course. The character of pain is often used in the classification of painful conditions, and particular types of pain are associated with special types of attack, e.g., some pains occur in attacks of paroxysms of pain while other pains are dull, constant and boring.

MacBryde[55] lists the following conditions and bodily areas and the quality of the pain associated with each:

Aneurysmal erosion: boring, pounding
Bones: deep, aching, boring
Muscles: sore, aching
Colic: twisting, griping, clamping
Angina: compression, constriction, comes on with exertion, great weight, agonizing, impending death
Pleuritis: stabbing, knifelike, with each breath
Peptic ulcer: burning, sharp, associated with hunger
Tabes: lightning-like, shooting, stabbing
Neuritis: burning, stinging
Neuralgia: sharp, cutting, paroxysmal, intermittent
Causalgia: burning, peculiar stinging
Burns, blisters, superficial skin lesions: burning, smarting, stinging, hot

9. *Intensity* of the pain must be determined to delineate proper therapy; e.g., morphine would not be given for a *mild* headache. Because of variable, individual psychologic factors it is often difficult to determine the intensity of pain. Some idea of the intensity can be obtained by noting the patient's physical appearance and whether the pain interferes with his activities.
   a. Does the patient describe his pain as mild, moderate, intense, severe, or excruciating? Such terms indicate intensity.
   b. What is the patient's physical appearance, e.g., grimacing, curled up in bed?
   c. Does the pain interfere with sleep, employment, eating, conversation, and so forth? Does the patient have to go to bed or stay in bed because of his pain?
10. *Cessation* of a pain is important to note.
    a. When did it stop?
    b. Did it stop suddenly or gradually?
    c. Was anything done to stop it or did it stop spontaneously?
11. *Associated symptoms* should be assessed. For example: skin changes (e.g., glossy skin); sensory changes (e.g., numbness); vomiting; photophobia (visual intolerance of light); fever; abnormal glandular secretions (e.g., excessive sweating); and fever.
12. *Presumptive etiologic factors.* Most patients have a definite opinion about what is causing their pain, and their views about the etiology should always be noted. Hereditary conditions should also be considered.

The cause *of a pain should always be sought, since pain is a symptom, not a disease itself.*

When a patient's pain stops suddenly, changes in character, or appears in a new or unexpected area, it should be noted and, if the change seems to be highly significant, reported to the physician. Also, a point to remember in the assessment of a patient following injury (a car accident, for example) is that *pain may initially be absent following sudden trauma.* Thus, such a patient requires ongoing reassessment, since pain may begin to appear some time after the accident, heralding the discovery of previously undetected injuries.

The nurse assessing pain will want to recall that patients may have pain even though no adequate organic cause can be found. She should also keep in mind that patients with a primarily psychiatric disorder may have pain arising from some associated physical disease. For example, a patient with a psychiatric disorder may also have a peptic ulcer that causes him pain.

Recognizing Psychogenic Pain

Many authorities believe it is futile to attempt to tell the difference between physical and psychogenic pains;[67] however, such a differential diagnosis is commonly necessary. The implications of such diagnoses are important. For example, the diagnosis may determine whether or not a patient should have surgical intervention. A physician attempts to correctly diagnose physical illness and also to recognize psychologic illness and provide suitable treatments. A nurse's careful observations may be helpful in deciding whether a pain is believed to be psychogenic in origin.

The following are some factors of importance in identifying psychogenic pain:

▶ Pain symptoms do not fit into any known anatomic pattern.

▶ Pains recur at precise intervals or under conditions of emotional disturbance.

▶ Pain symptoms are not relieved by ordinary analgesic measures.

▶ Pain symptoms cannot be explained by the presence of demonstrable organic disease or structural abnormalities.

▶ Evidence exists of psychiatric illness that is sufficient to account for the development of the pain symptoms.

▶ Pain tends to be located centrally in the head and trunk, or, where lateral, tends to occur on the left.

▶ Pain occurs continuously from day to day, without disturbing sleep.

▶ Pain arises at irregular times for no apparent reason and lasts for a few hours.

When some of these factors begin to appear together, there is a strong presumption that the psychologic aspects of the pain problem are important. Grounds for a psychogenic diagnosis must always be found by means of psychiatric investigation. Painful conditions should never be considered as psychogenic merely because no explanation for the symptoms have been found.[81]

Physiologic Bases of Pain

Although innumerable conditions can give rise to pain, the actual factors leading to the excitation of pain fibers can be reduced to simple proportions. Some pathophysiologic processes that stimulate pain are:

▶ Direct irritation of nerve endings, e.g., by mechanical factors operating in exposed tissues.

▶ Chemical substances, e.g., those occurring in acute inflammations (globulin, bradykinin, histamine, serotonin).

▶ Certain pathologic processes, e.g., some forms of ulceration and new growth.

▶ Irritation of peripheral nerves or of nerve roots, e.g., from a foreign body, displaced bone, or from local pressure caused by a neoplasm or inflammatory products in a confined space.

▶ Muscle spasm, e.g., from myocardial ischemia, or cramps from Buerger's disease.

▶ Overstretching, e.g., from acutely distended viscus or the passage of a calculus through a narrow duct.

Although such classifications are not all inclusive (e.g., central pains do not fit into the above outline) and are oversimplifications, they are nevertheless useful guides for evaluating the more common causes of pain and thus make it easier to clearly identify the measures necessary to bring relief. Therefore, in evaluating a patient's pain the nurse should try to identify the cause of the pain anatomically and physiologically so that she can give the patient appropriate help.

Covert and Overt Signs and Symptoms of Pain

It is possible to divide the *signs* and *symptoms* of pain into two groups:[27] (1) those that are essentially of sympathetic origin and (2) those primarily of parasympathetic origin. This division is presented in Table 34–1 along with other signs of pain.

Characteristically, pain sets off protective reactions within the body which may include occlusion of nasal passages with or without lacrimation, cardiospasm, cardiac arrhythmias, disturbances of gastric and colonic function, and elevation of arterial pressure. If such body changes are sustained, they may themselves lead to a significant impairment of function or perhaps to actual tissue damage. Shock and even death may be caused by severe pain.

A patient malingering or pretending to have pain cannot imitate the facial expression of true pain, e.g., the pallor, pinched features, knotted brow, clammy skin, and dilated pupils.[59]

Since some patients hesitate to say that they have pain, you will need to observe carefully for the physiologic signs of discomfort; on the other hand, it is equally important to observe

TABLE 34–1.   OBSERVABLE SIGNS AND SYMPTOMS OF PAIN

SYMPATHETIC IN ORIGIN (VITAL FUNCTIONS ARE STIMULATED)	PARASYMPATHETIC IN ORIGIN (VITAL FUNCTIONS ARE DEPRESSED)
A basically sympathetic response occurs with pain of low to moderate intensity or superficial pain. Observable signs and symptoms are: pallor, elevated blood pressure, dilated pupils, skeletal muscular tension, increased respiratory rate, increased heart rate	A basically parasympathetic response occurs with pain of severe intensity or deep pain. Observable signs and symptoms are: pallor, decreased blood pressure, decreased heart rate, nausea and vomiting, weakness and fainting, prostration, possible loss of consciousness
The body prepares to act by either overcoming or fleeing from an external threat as epinephrine output is increased. Bodily defenses are mobilized.	The body tries to minimize the effects of an internal threat. Bodily defenses may collapse.

OTHER SIGNS OF PAIN

Patient assumes a posture or position that will minimize his pain, i.e., draws up knees or lies rigidly.
Patient may moan or make other sounds indicating his discomfort and may blink rapidly.
Patient may cry and appear frightened or restless; or, may lie quietly, afraid to move, withdrawing from being touched.
Patient may grimace and clench jaw or fists; his face may have a drawn expression and muscles may twitch.
Patient may perspire profusely (have diaphoresis).
Patient may hold or protect the painful area with his hands; the physical attitude may thus indicate pain and its location, e.g., holding head, pressing on abdomen.

---

the patient's reactions, since physiologic signs may not be helpful.

The Patient's Statements About Pain

Not only degrees of Pain, but its existence, in any degree, must be taken upon the testimony of the patient.
Peter Mere Latham: *Diseases of the Heart, Lect. XI*

It is not always accurate to conclude that a patient who does not mention pain is comfortable. He may have severe pain but may not say that he does. (Note: Patients' reports of pain are often referred to by staff as "complaints" of pain. Possibly it would be more accurate to simply state that the patient *reports* pain instead of conveying the impression that the patient is "complaining.") As previously mentioned, complete descriptions of pain are an aid to accurate diagnosis and the effective treatment of pain syndromes. Because pain is subjective, the nurse's assessment should include *listening* to what a patient says about how he feels as well as watching for observable indications of pain.

Communication about pain is often a problem. When we deal with patients, we encounter the double difficulty of first defining an experience and then of communicating it: "The patient must find a word to describe the pain, and we must then understand it. Communication implies translating the patient's experience into one of our own."[20] Often it is hard to be sure of what is happening; the patient may be trying to explain an experience we may not have had, e.g., referred pain, spontaneous pain, or phantom pain. Because of these factors it is helpful to:

▸ Have the patient who states he has pain point to the area of pain and describe it in his own words. Avoid using leading questions that could result in the patient's giving misleading information[10] and avoid opening up new areas for worry or arousing false hopes.[27]

▸ In charting, use the patient's own words about his pain, e.g., "Patient states: 'I feel like I have a tight band around my head,' or, 'It feels pricking.'" Patients often have difficulty finding words to describe what a pain is like. Nevertheless, the words that they use should be charted.

▸ Help the patient to talk objectively about his pain, to describe it as accurately as possible, and to distinguish between pain and other unpleasant bodily feelings, e.g., pressure, soreness, itching.

▶ Clarify what a patient means when he says he is "miserable," "uncomfortable," "suffering," etc.; do not assume that he means he is "in *pain*." Perhaps he feels nauseated, dizzy, and so forth.

Mettler[69] believes that it is not justifiable to neglect a patient's *own* estimation of his pain, since few people complain of pain who are not, in fact, miserable. Because of its subjective nature, a nurse must be guided by what a patient tells her about pain; however, a patient's description of pain (for example, its severity) must be accepted without assessing many other factors, since he may consciously or unconsciously minimize or exaggerate his symptoms. Remember:

A patient's description of his pain is influenced by his perception of the pain and what the pain means to him.

NURSING CARE OF PATIENTS EXPERIENCING PAIN

> Divine is the work of subduing pain.
> —*Hippocrates*

Caring appropriately for a patient experiencing pain calls for a high level of nursing acumen, sensitivity, and skill. One nursing leader summarizes this as follows:

Nursing the patient in pain demands all the imagination, all the knowledge and skill and all the humanity the nurse has at her command. It is a mature kind of seasoned thoughtful nursing that the patient requires whether he knows it or not.[41]

If you observe a skilled nurse caring for patients having pain, you will see in practice what is described above. Watch the experienced nurse at work as she cares for numerous patients who are having a variety of pains; you will see that she has learned, in the hard school of clinical practice, to evaluate and respond to both the physical and emotional aspects of pain. Versed in both the art and science of nursing, she patiently appraises these patients' personalities, analyzes the physical and behavioral evidence that they present, and strives to constantly cultivate deeper insight into their characters and problems. Alert for changes, she constantly reevaluates her assessments and actions. All successful nurses are good psychologists in a sense, and all are multidisciplinary in their practice.

The clinical care of any patient experiencing pain, whether acute or chronic, must be based upon an understanding of: the pain *being treated; the* individual *being treated; and the* mode *of treatment.*

Appropriate professional nursing intervention in caring for patients having acute or chronic pain is a complex activity requiring many skills on the nurse's part. In order to perform adequately, the nurse must have some knowledge of: the nature of pain and how it is experienced; the anatomy and physiology of pain; types of pain and the problems created when awareness of pain is absent; evaluation of pain; and medical, surgical, and nursing measures that can be taken to reduce or prevent suffering. Appropriate professional nursing intervention in caring for patients having pain obviously involves far more than merely giving a medication. Some additional factors involved in this clinical area are:[27]

▶ Concern with the physiologic, environmental, sociocultural and psycho-emotional components of pain.

▶ Awareness of both the nurse's and the patient's perceptions of pain, as well as reactions to pain.

▶ Consideration of the individual as a person as well as a member of a social unit, e.g., a family.

▶ Dedication to the prevention of pain as well as to its alleviation.

As with other nursing activities, the clinical care of the patient in pain begins with the nurse's assessment or evaluation of the patient's condition. On the basis of her observations, the nurse next decides on the course of action that she believes is appropriate. In addition to trying to prevent or alleviate pain, the nurse relieves and comforts the patient by giving him hope and strength, even though it may be possible to achieve only limited goals in some situations.[27] The final step in the nurse's plan of care is to reevaluate her actions to determine the accuracy of her judgments and the effectiveness of her course of action. In actual practice these steps do not occur separately from one another but are part of an ongoing process. (Chap. 17 discusses the nursing process.)

THE NURSE: AN AGENT OF PAIN PRODUCTION AND PAIN RELIEF

The nurse acts as both an agent who produces pain and an agent who relieves patients' pains. She cares for many patients whose medical or surgical therapies are pain-producing; such pains are thus added to pains that may already be present from disease. Persons who are made to suffer, as patients must often be, frequently experience feelings of fear and anger directed at those who cause the suffering. This may be so even though the patient's best interests are being followed. It is naturally essential that you carry out pain-producing procedures as gently and skillfully as possible, and that you administer them while giving the patient emotional support and recognition of his discomfort.

Because the nurse can, within the sanctions of society and the realm of her responsibility, produce pain in others, she is in a position of power over patients and must be aware of the psychologic impact that this fact has upon them. The production of pain or discomfort in patients should never result from an intention to punish. It is a nurse's obligation to consciously evaluate her behavior so that a patient can in no way interpret what she is doing to him as punishment. Because medical, surgical, and nursing therapies may produce pain, the nurse needs to give constant support and encouragement to those in her care, so that they will not refuse treatments that are in their best interests. However, remember always that:

> *It is the right of a rational person to refuse treatment. Far too many patients refuse treatment because they have not received the mental preparation and support that would enable them to receive the care they need.*

Broadly speaking, the nurse works to prevent, alleviate, or remove the cause of pain and also strives to reduce the patient's perception of pain. Her clinical care encompases three broad areas: (1) psychologic, (2) physical, and (3) pharmacologic or medical. The nurse's practice involves all these areas in an integrated manner, although at one moment she may emphasize one aspect of care and then shift to concentrate on another as she works to prevent, palliate, and attenuate or remove pain.

General Aspects of Care

Earlier in this chapter we reviewed details to be considered in evaluating the patient experiencing pain. As we emphasized, the nurse evaluates many factors: the patient's statements, his personality, the nurse's own personality and view of pain, the source of noxious stimulation, and the types of pains. She carefully surveys the patient to determine the extent of his suffering, realizing that there are wide variations in the physiologic manifestations of pain. She also knows that, due to the diversity of psychosocial responses and the various threats that pain poses, all patients do not manifestly express pain to the same extent.

Before you do anything to try to relieve a patient's pain, talk with him to find out as precisely as possible what the problem is. Rather than assuming that you know how a patient feels, *find out from him* how he feels. For example, a patient who is only 12 hours postoperative may tell you he has pain; do not assume that he means pain in the area of the surgical procedure. He may have a headache, perhaps severe chest pain, or pain in the calf of his leg. Therefore:

> *Assess a patient's pain prior to taking any action to relieve it.*

Also, ascertain whether he is actually in *pain* or whether he is uncomfortable. For example, a patient may say he is in pain when he actually has a feeling of pressure from flatus (gas).

On the basis of her assessment, the nurse decides whether the patient is having pain, and, if it *is* present, whether it is of such intensity that it requires relief. Next she decides the appropriate method of providing relief and plans her care.

The following general statements about the clinical care of patients experiencing pain are important to consider as you begin to formulate a plan of nursing care:

▶ Pain is a *"cry for help"* that the able clinician will recognize and attempt to eliminate, whether the cause is physical or mental.[2]

▶ Pain should be respected and treated as pain, *regardless of its origin*. There is no subjective difference between psychogenic pain and organic pain. Psychogenic pain exists; it is not "imaginary."

▶ The *entire patient*—as a whole—should receive attention and care, rather than just the patient's pain symptom.

▶ *Specific therapy,* directed at the *cause* of the pain, must be used to treat pain whenever possible. For example, if a patient has pain caused by a broken bone, it would not be sound therapy to give analgesics to reduce the pain while neglecting to give specific treatment directed at setting the broken bone. Try to *identify the source* of discomfort or pain and then take *appropriate action* to reduce it, e.g., padding, positioning, turning, medication.

▶ *Ancillary problems,* which contribute to discomfort or aggravate pain, require treatment as well as the major pain problem. Examples of ancillary problems are: constipation, diarrhea, cough, anorexia, and frequent urination.

▶ *Plan with the patient, listen to his suggestions, encourage his help,* and *let him know if something is going to be painful.* Plan with the patient what you will be doing for him so that he feels a part of his treatment rather than like an object that is constantly having something done to it. Listen to his suggestions about how something might be done, such as moving him. He knows what hurts; you don't. With the patient's help, you can identify situations, movements, and so forth, that cause pain, and those measures that bring the greatest relief. Always forewarn a patient if a procedure is expected to be painful. Help him to understand what to expect as well as what will be done to minimize the pain. Such information may make the pain more bearable.

▶ While *palliation* is not a substitute for treating the source of pain, it may be: (1) employed as a relief-giving measure in situations in which the source of pain cannot be treated or removed; (2) used as a temporary measure until the source of the pain can be established; or (3) utilized as a supplement to other measures in the treatment process.[27]

Skill should be developed in administering all nursing procedures. A sympathetic approach and the careful use of preventive measures should help each patient to realize that he will not be hurt through clumsiness, thoughtlessness, or a hurried approach.

Balme[4] points out that even so ordinary a procedure as the giving of hypodermic or intramuscular injections can be robbed of its terrors for the nervous patient if scrupulous attention is paid to details such as: the site of injection, the sharpness of the needle, the complete relaxation of the part to be injected, the use of a stabbing motion rather than a slow push, the avoidance of injecting a hypodermic solution into the skin, the realization that an intramuscular injection contains irritants to subcutaneous nerves and must therefore be deposited in the muscular layers, and avoidance of injecting too rapidly.

Psychologic Aspects of Care

Broadly speaking, there are three major areas of psychologic care to be considered in providing relief from pain; these are (1) relieving anxiety, (2) utilizing distraction and diversion, and (3) combating anticipatory fears.

RELIEVING ANXIETY

Excessive anxiety, which pain or the threat of pain often produces, must be reduced or attenuated, since it can lower a patient's pain reaction threshold and trigger systemic responses that make pain harder to combat. Generally, the more severe a patient's anxiety is, the greater will be his overreaction to pain stimulation. Thus, fear of pain and conditions that promote anxiety must be controlled.[12]

Just as anxiety can cause physical illness that may result in pain, so can pain produce anxiety. A few ways to diminish a patient's anxiety are to: let him talk; rub his back; stay with him for a while or at least do not appear rushed during the time you are with him; communicate your empathy; and help the patient to deal with situations that are stressful to him. Unless a patient can be helped to reduce excessive fears and anxieties, he is likely to become caught in the vicious circle depicted in Figure 34–2.

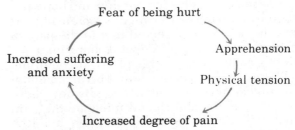

Figure 34–2. A vicious cycle of suffering which the nurse strives to break.

Much pain can be prevented by lessening a patient's fearful attitude toward pain. This can be accomplished in part by: (1) trying to determine the meaning that pain has for the patient, how fearful he is about experiencing pain, and what his reactions to pain are, e.g., physical tension, weeping, silent suffering; (2) helping the patient to describe accurately how he feels and to distinguish between pain and other sources of discomfort, e.g., between a feeling of pressure and one of pain and (3) talking with the patient about his pain so that he realizes he can communicate with others about it rather than having to suffer alone.

> *Help the patient to gain some sense of control over the situation he is in.*

A patient's fearful attitude toward pain can also be reduced by helping him to realize that his pain will not necessarily get worse, become as severe as he might have anticipated, or remain as intense as it may be at the moment. Reassurance that everything possible will be done to *prevent* pain and to *lessen* pain when it does occur can be most comforting. Another way to reduce the patient's fear of pain is to let him know that he is *not completely helpless* as far as his pain is concerned; he can do a variety of things to help to prevent or lessen his pain, e.g., splint his incision when coughing. Also, he can tell the nurses how best to move him, or he can decide how to move himself in the least painful manner. A patient can also prevent some pain by not waiting until the pain is intense before requesting help for it.

> *Reassurance and hope increase tolerance for pain.*

The nurse can give reassurance and hope and thereby help to keep a patient's morale high. It has, in fact, been observed that in the pain of cancer, the pain may depend more on a patient's morale than on his physical condition. "There can be no pain without involvement of the higher nervous centers and it is how these centers handle, absorb and integrate the pain that will determine its perception and the ability to resist it."[52]

The conversion of a sensation into a painful experience is mainly an emotional reaction or a psychologic phenomenon. Reaction to pain, unlike perception of it, is a complex physiologic and psychologic response involving the highest cognitive mechanisms. In general, the intensity of suffering depends upon the extent to which pain is allowed to dominate the conscious mind.[12] "The use of drugs to alleviate suffering makes us all aware of the relationship between pain and the state of consciousness."[54] *Since pain perception is a conscious process, the nurse can reduce pain perception if she can reduce a patient's conscious awareness of his pain.*

Focusing a patient's attention on a painful procedure may increase his pain; conversely, distracting him may reduce his suffering. There are times when it is necessary for a patient's well-being to focus his attention on his pain, e.g., telling a patient he will have pain or other sensations associated with a procedure you are performing, such as an injection; and when making a thorough evaluation of the pain and of the helpfulness of measures that have been taken to reduce the pain. However, it is never advisable to excessively focus a patient's attention on what is being done to him or on the pain he is having. Skillful nursing is a combined effort to keep the patient informed and to turn his attention away from himself and his suffering.

Diversion must be carried out with sensitivity on the nurse's part. Attempts at distraction are not as successful in severe pain as in pain that is milder. Appropriate timing and a sincere manner are necessary, or the patient may feel that his pain is being minimized or that it is viewed as "all in his mind" and not real. Distraction maneuvers, therefore, call for skill, subtlety, and planning so that the patient's attention will be diverted to an area of interest and benefit to him. Individualized activities in occupational therapy or vocational rehabilitation may beneficially redirect a patient's concern and attention. Conversation, reading, and television watching are other types of distraction. Small talk (idle chatter), however, is not a satisfactory diversion; rather it is likely to increase the patient's tenseness and discomfort. Likewise, excessive noise is tiring rather than being helpfully distracting. While one patient in pain may want his radio on, another may prefer as quiet an atmosphere as possible. Sensitivity to patients' individual preferences during painful experiences is essential.

On the basis of one's individual nature and his past experiences with pain, as well as other life experiences that he has had, each person selects certain patterns of behavior in response to pain that may help to divert his attention from the pain. For example, pacing the floor may reduce one patient's pain, while another clenches his fist, holds his breath, or grasps a bed rail. Frustration ensues if these usual patterns of response are blocked, as they may be by a patient's physical, mental, or environmental circumstances. A patient confined to bed cannot pace the floor, for example, or a patient paralyzed from stroke cannot clench his fist. In situations such as this, the nurse will need to help the patient to identify new ways of coping with his painful situation;[27] he must learn new distractions.

Both *physical activities* and *mental activities* may serve as ways of attenuating or removing pain. In severe pain, *self-hypnosis* and *autosuggestion* may raise the pain threshold and may thus be a source of comfort to a patient. Also, it is possible to distract a patient from his pain by involving him actively with things he can do physically to help himself, e.g., "move your legs," "hold onto the siderail and roll onto your side," "breathe through your mouth."

Patients differ from one another concerning whether they want company if they are having pain. Some patients who are in pain feel most comfortable if they are left by themselves and not disturbed; others desire companionship at such a time and want the nurse to stop by frequently or to have a friend or relative at the bedside. Your awareness of these wishes and your accommodation to them will be appreciated by the patient.[27]

As distractions are reduced, a patient's attention may focus more completely on himself and his pain. Thus, pain often seems worse at night or in the early morning hours when the activities of the daytime are absent.

COMBATING ANTICIPATORY FEARS

As stated earlier, pain is a combination of reception, perception, and reaction. *Reactions* may be *anticipatory*, occurring prior to the pain-producing stimulus and in expectation of it, or they may occur *after* the perception of pain and as a response to it.

The nurse is in an excellent position to help to combat fearful anticipatory reactions, since she is often with a patient when he undergoes painful treatments and because she, herself, may be instrumental in producing some pain. An important nursing service is, thus, to help to prepare a patient to meet the pains that he will have by talking with him about the pain that he fears.[27] Talking about what the patient may expect to happen can help him to relax and to reduce muscle resistance that could be pain-producing; also, the nurse can help a patient to assume correct body alignment and positioning, which can help him to more comfortably tolerate a painful procedure.

It is helpful to patients if they can try to reason out beforehand the extent of discomfort that will be caused by a particular stimulus, e.g., a needle. Thus, it is beneficial to discuss procedures in advance so the patient will have some idea of what to expect. Prior to catheterization, for example, a patient may be told: "You will feel pressure as I insert the tube. It will probably not be painful although it may be uncomfortable."

Johnson has demonstrated that when patients are given information about the procedures and sensations to be experienced, their anticipatory distress will be reduced. In addition, patients receiving a description of the sensations experienced during a procedure were less tense than those patients who only received a description of the procedure.[46]

Mental preparation of a patient preoperatively can help to allay fears of uncontrolled postoperative pain. One common fear about pain is that it will not be controlled or minimized. The preoperative suggestion that medications *will* help to alleviate much postoperative discomfort and that they *will* be given as needed can help a patient to benefit more from his postoperative medications.

The preoperative teaching of ways in which postoperative discomforts can be minimized or prevented is of great value. "In the fight to control pain, the valuable minutes before the pain commences—when the patient can give his full attention to learning how to cope with it—are indeed too precious not to be fully exploited. In any situation in which a patient could have been taught how to deal with his pain and has not been, a valuable opportunity has been wasted."[27]

The power of suggestion is a useful agent in combating fears of pain—an agent that can serve as the nurse's constant ally in her efforts to prevent or reduce pain. If a patient *believes* that a measure that is taken to reduce his pain *will indeed* reduce his pain, then the measure will often be successful.

It has long been recognized that the personality of a person (e.g., nurse) who is administering a treatment, and that person's verbal and nonverbal suggestions to a patient about the effectiveness of the treatment, play a powerful part in determining the ultimate therapeutic effect. Because this suggestive element is present in clinical care, it should be utilized whenever possible. Thus, a patient who is being given a medication to reduce his pain should enthusiastically and sincerely be told that the medication *will* help to relieve his pain and about when it should begin to be effective.

> *Gaining the patient's* trust *and* confidence *is of vital importance in pain therapy.*[82]

A *fear of future pain,* rather than present discomfort, may prompt some requests for medications; i.e., some patients will request analgesics on the basis of fear that pain will begin rather than the actual presence of pain. Evaluate whether the fear seems out of proportion to the patient's physical condition.[83] Try to prevent the use of analgesics *in anticipation* of pain rather than for relief of pain. Related to this is the fact that patients may occasionally want more medication than they need for pain relief because they *want to be "knocked out"* so that they can become oblivious to reality.[83] It is not in the long-term best interests of patients to give them more medication than they actually require. If drug usage is controlled, patients having long-term pain are less likely to reach a point at which they cannot obtain relief. Persons experiencing long-term pain need reassurance that their medications are being regulated carefully for their well-being and that every attempt will be made to keep them as comfortable as possible.

All patients with chronically painful conditions live in dread, partly of the pain increasing in intensity, and partly of the knowledge that there is no effective therapy.[81]

This fear can be greatly reduced for patients with chronic conditions with proper drug management. Initially when drug therapy is instituted, whether narcotics or nonnarcotics are needed, a larger dose of the maintenance drug should be used in order to obtain the confidence of the patient that control will be achieved. Once control is obtained, the drug is reduced to a maintenance level. In the past, physicians have started analgesics at a minimal dose and increased them until relief was obtained. Consequently, many patients developed a lack of confidence in their physician and in the ability of the drug to control their pain.[73]

In sum, everything possible should be done to give the patient the feeling that he will be protected from pain and spared pain in all possible ways. Gentleness, patience, and tolerance are essential qualities for the nurse to project when she is caring for the patient in pain. A lack of these will create fear and tension in the patient, causing increased pain and distress, and resistance in cooperation. The patient who is aware that the nurse is trying to do everything possible to prevent pain will typically be able to relax more readily and thus will have less pain than if he were tense and fearful.

Physical Aspects of Care

General supportive nursing care is directed at minimizing or relieving any irritations that could lower the patient's pain tolerance. The patient is thus kept warm, dry, and comfortable. Backrubs and exercise are also of importance.

In attempting to prevent pain and complications the nurse strives to *protect the patient from pain-producing situations* such as: local irritation or inflammation; muscle spasm or muscle strain; interference with local blood supply or venous and lymphatic drainage; and distention of hollow visceral organs. Specifically, the nurse evaluates each patient to see how she might prevent such painful complications as: infection, thrombophlebitis, decubitus ulcers, contractures, muscle strain, muscle spasm, pulmonary congestion, impaired circulation, bladder and bowel distention, and other painful conditions. (See Chap. 33 for discussion of minimizing the hazards of immobility.) Moreover, nursing care is planned to avoid further damage to traumatized tissue.[27]

All injured tissue should be handled gently! Lacerated tissue is more sensitive than intact skin and should not have anything dragged across it, e.g., bedcovers, or have adhesive substances, such as dressings, pulled off. Anything adhering to an open wound should be bathed with warm sterile water to soak it off, rather than being pulled off. Open wounds should never have irritating antiseptics, e.g., surgical spirit or tincture of iodine, applied to them. Protective dressings may prevent pain.

Painful dressing changes or pain-producing manipulations, such as bed change, can be planned to be carried out at a time when pain-relieving medications will be having their greatest effect on the patient. Not only do patients need to be medicated prior to painful dressing changes, but draining and ulcerative wounds that must be dressed daily or more often should always be done by staff members working in pairs. When there are at least two staff members on each shift that know how such procedures are done for an individual patient, then the patient does not have to use his energies to teach and re-teach staff. This permits the procedure to be carried out quickly and efficiently with minimal focusing on the discomfort of the procedure. In addition, many open wounds can become distasteful in appearance and odor, causing staff to dread the procedure. The "buddy system" enables the staff to support each other and vent their feelings about their shared experience.[61]

To prevent pain or complications from *drainage tubes*, periodically check the tubes to be certain that they are not caught, stretched, or pulled; that they are patent and not kinked, looped, or higher or lower than they should be in relationship to the patient's body plane; and that they are properly in place.

Fatigue can lower tolerance to pain. All activities (including visits from family and friends) should be structured by the nurse and patient together so that the patient will not become overly tired. Planned periods of rest can greatly reduce discomfort and should, thus, follow periods of activity.

Immobilization may reduce pain caused by inflammatory lesions as well as pain caused by the interruption of blood supply to some local bodily area. With pain due to inflammation, immobilization reduces the pain that would be caused by local pressure or mechanical friction. When pain is due to interruption of a local blood supply, immobilization acts therapeutically by: (1) reducing the oxygen requirements of the tissue that is deprived of its arterial blood supply and (2) reducing the formation of metabolic wastes that would build up in the area as a result of circulation that is impaired and inadequate to carry wastes away.

Elevation of a swollen part uses the force of gravity to reduce painful swelling. Edematous and casted limbs should be elevated, since increased tissue fluid can produce pain. Elevation facilitates the drainage of fluid by way of the lymph channels and also reduces the production of fluid in the area of inflammation. Also, a sitting position helps to alleviate the pains of cervical lymphadenitis, tonsillitis, and acute sinusitis.

A *position of semiflexion* reduces the pains of those painful joint disorders, e.g., arthritis, in which an increase in pressure within the joint cavity increases the severity of pain. When a joint is partly flexed, the capacity of the joint cavity is greatest, and thus the pressure of synovial fluid is at a minimum.

A *change of position* may help to relieve pain by relieving muscle spasm and reducing muscle strain. Frequent position changes and keeping the patient in good body alignment pre-

vents painful muscle contractions. The patient should be told that his position is being changed to lessen pain. For some patients it is desirable to have a schedule of times posted for position changes as well as suggested positions for each time. The time of position change, the type of position the patient was placed in, and the patient's apparent comfort or discomfort in the position should be charted.

The patient in pain may avoid *movement*, since movement usually increases pain. Explain why certain movements are necessary, e.g., to prevent complications or to ultimately increase comfort. Demonstrate to the patient that future discomfort can be prevented by procedures carried on in the present. When movement is important following a painful procedure, such as following surgery, do patient teaching whenever possible in advance of the procedure so that the patient will expect to move and will know how to do so most comfortably.

The following points are helpful to recall when moving a patient:

▶ Tell the patient what you are going to do, why the move is necessary, and what he can do to help.

▶ Listen to the patient's suggestions about the move and do not hurry; give him time to think about the move.

▶ Let the patient move himself as much as possible since he knows what hurts and you don't. He can protect himself from unnecessary pain better than you can protect him.

▶ Consider and maintain body alignment and support in preparing for the move and in moving the patient. (See Chaps. 21 and 33.) Utilize knowledge of correct anatomic position and normal range-of-motion of bodily parts. Remember that some painful parts may be fixed by muscular spasms or have range of movements restricted.

▶ Hold injured limbs firmly but do not squeeze them. Support extremities from underneath, cradling them on the flat of your hand and arm rather than grasping them from above in pinching fashion.

▶ Have the patient keep his spine stiff and move his body or body parts as a unit. Limbs should be moved as a whole, as support is given to the joints. Never allow a part of a limb to drag while other parts are being moved. While supporting the injured part and letting the patient help, accomplish the move slowly and steadily, stopping if the patient requests you to, and pausing if muscular resistance is incurred.

▶ If the patient needs help to move, make certain you have adequate help available. Before lifting or moving the patient, appoint yourself or another person as leader and tell each helper and the patient what each person is to do, so that everyone will work together as a team. The leader should direct the activities out loud, e.g., "When I count to three we will all move smoothly together. You support Mrs. Jones' head and shoulders and I will lift her legs and buttocks. Mrs. Jones, you try to keep your spine stiff as we move you. Now. Ready? One, two, three." Always have several people help to move a patient with bone and joint problems (e.g., bone cancer) regardless of the patient's size, since these conditions are most painful.

Pillows, braces, casts or splints may be necessary for the support of painful body parts during movement or for purposes of immobilization. "Splinting" may also be accomplished by manually supporting an area during movement. For example, painful incisions may be splinted with the hands, a folded towel, or a small pillow during periods of postoperative movements, coughing, sneezing, and so forth. Abdominal binders are also a splinting device that may be used postoperatively to give added support to the incisional area during periods of stress.

Following a move, *arrange pillows* so that they support and relax all muscles acting on an injured part and so that proper alignment is maintained. Also, combine gentle traction with the support of an injured limb.

The accumulation of toxic substances in muscles can be a cause of muscle pain. *Massage* can relieve such pain since it increases the flow of blood to the area. This, in turn, relieves hypoxemia and carries off some of the toxins that have accumulated. However, remember:

Never *massage the calf of the leg!* Since blood clots may form in that area, massage could break loose the clots and possibly cause a fatal embolism.

Hot and cold applications, e.g., wet compresses or dry heat, are useful in relieving some pains by: (1) altering the rate and volume of regional blood flow; (2) decreasing pain sensitivity; and (3) relieving muscle spasm. Heat acts, generally, by producing a depressing action on the central nervous system; cold produces a local anesthetic effect. The specific actions of hot and cold applications are outlined below:*

Hot Applications

Dilate local superficial blood vessels.
Increase blood flow (perhaps more than doubling the flow).
Increase capillary pressure, thus causing more transudation of fluid through capillary walls with increased lymph formation and accelerated lymph flow.
Reduce painful muscle spasm by causing muscle to relax.
Increase peristaltic movement in intestines if the abdominal wall is heated. (This is important in treating painful abdominal distention caused by paralytic ileus of the bowel.)

Cold Applications

Constrict local superficial blood vessels.
Decrease blood flow.
Produce temporary reduction of inflammatory swelling which, in turn, reduces pain.
Reduce pain sensitivity, since marked chilling acts as a local anesthetic.
Decrease peristaltic movement in intestines if the abdominal wall is cooled. (This is important in the treatment of inflammatory disorders in the peritoneal cavity, since intestinal immobilization slows down spread of infection.)
Decrease muscle spasm.

Pharmacologic Aspects of Care

Before a nurse is qualified to administer analgesic agents, she should possess knowledge not only of the medications she is using but also of the nature of pain and the processes through which it is mediated. Additionally, in order to effectively administer pain medications, the nurse will need to familiarize herself with expected patterns of pain. For example, the intensity of postoperative pain is related to the type of anesthetic used as well as to the patient and his operation.

The aim of giving pain medications should be to control the pain while preserving the patient's personality and maintaining his morale.

---

*See also Chapter 44, Caring for Persons Receiving Applications of Heat and Cold.

Also, these goals should be attained ideally without upsetting the patient's clarity of vision, his digestion, bowel function, or balance.

GUIDELINES

As you administer analgesic medications you may find the following guidelines helpful to recall:

▶ Just as people vary in their responses to pain, they vary in their sensitivity to pain and to pain-relieving drugs.

▶ Individual patients may require different doses of an analgesic, and the same patient may also, at different times, have a variable requirement.

▶ Pain relief should provide comfort without producing harm as a result of the medications administered.

▶ Use potent narcotics wisely by avoiding excessive or unnecessary administration. Avoid administering narcotics on a "routine" basis in the absence of actual need; but once needed, do not be afraid of narcotic drugs.[91]

▶ Use non-narcotic drugs, rather than narcotics, if they will relieve symptoms.

▶ Know the basic actions, doses, routes of administration, side effects, and precautions for use of analgesic agents prior to their administration.

▶ Chart the apparent effectiveness of the analgesic, and chart and report any apparent side effects, e.g., drug dependency, respiratory depression.

▶ Opiates should be used with extreme caution in patients with increased intracranial pressure, hepatic insufficiency, severe CNS depression, myxedema, acute alcoholism, delirium tremens, convulsive disorders, and Addison's disease.

▶ When patients are being treated with several medications simultaneously, patterns of drug interactions must be considered in selecting narcotic analgesics. For example, severe adverse reactions have been reported in patients receiving monoamine oxidase inhibitors who were given meperidine for pain. (Reactions of this nature have not been reported for morphine.) Similarly, chlorpromazine may intensify and prolong the respiratory depression produced by meperidine.

> Timing *is as important to successful pain drug therapy as is drug or dose or interval.*

Early, adequate relief is an important principle in pain therapy, because if pain can be treated effectively soon after its onset, it is relatively easier to control. The longer a patient suffers, the greater his apprehension becomes and, consequently, the more difficult it becomes to achieve pain relief with medications.[48]

It is *not* considered to be good practice to administer analgesic agents *routinely*. Too often one finds "routine" pre- and postoperative medication orders. As we have emphasized, reactivity to pain is highly variable from one individual to another. A "routine" approach to pain therapy ignores individual patient variability and can thereby result in either overuse or underuse of analgesics. This results in either: (1) a negation of the potential strength of the analgesic, with consequent inadequate pain relief, or (2) "snowing" the patient and increasing the incidence of undesirable side effects. Analgesic agents of appropriate strength need to be utilized for the varying degrees of pain that individual patients are experiencing. As the pain increases so must the potency of the drug; the opposite is also true. *Both the prescription and the administration of a drug should be tailored to meet each patient's individual needs.*

Only a very incomplete idea of the intensity of pain can be obtained from the *quantity* of drugs that patients may require. It has been observed that patients with pain that is constant and of moderate intensity have a far greater drug requirement than those with transient, intense pain.[81]

WORKING WITH THE PHYSICIAN

Physician and nurse must coordinate their efforts to provide pain relief.

In some situations analgesics are withheld until diagnosis of the patient's condition is established. Analgesics may be contraindicated for a period of time because they may mask or confuse the diagnosis. However, once the diagnosis is made, appropriate pain relief is in order.[37]

> *Because pain often is an important diagnostic aid (e.g., abdominal pain), it is frequently hazardous to administer analgesics before the cause of pain is reliably determined.*

Generally for temporary and acute conditions analgesic medications are ordered on a *p.r.n. basis*, with specific directions concerning the drug, the dose, and the time interval between doses. However, the actual administration of the drug or its timing is left to the nurse's discretion. Sound nursing judgment is called for when pain-relieving medications and treatments are ordered p.r.n.

Physicians may leave more than one analgesic order for a patient, and it is up to the nurse to decide which medication to administer at the appropriate time. Moreover, at times more than one dosage may be ordered, so that the nurse must decide which she should administer. Such flexibility of orders permits the patient to receive medication that is appropriate to meet his variable needs. Thus, pain relief can be made adequate while avoiding overmedication or inadequate medication. A system of this nature is obviously advantageous; however, at the same time it requires that the nurse make informed decisions based on numerous facts about analgesics, such as their: benefits; side effects; indications; contraindications; duration and onset of action; typical doses; routes of administration; mixing properties with other medications; and the type of pain they most effectively relieve.

The effectiveness of medications given for the relief of pain should be *charted*. The nurse should check patients regularly and especially within 20 to 30 minutes after they receive analgesics. The effects of the analgesic should be charted as well as the duration of pain relief. From such charting, doctors and other nurses will be able to discern which medications are most effective, and in what doses. Information about *which drugs* are effective and *how much* medicine is used can be helpful to the physician in diagnosing the etiology of a patient's pain. By knowing how much medicine is used the doctor can also form an opinion of the patient's general condition, especially with regard to his renal function. When a patient's drug requirement is high, it must be determined whether his pain is great enough to require such high doses of medications or whether alterations need to be made.

Changes in the patient's acknowledgment of his pain can be quickly assessed by asking the patient to rate his pain on a scale of one to ten. The number one represents no pain and ten represents pain that is no longer bearable and the patient would prefer to die rather than continue to live. Patients can be asked to rate their pain prior to interventions and afterwards to measure their effectiveness. Patients informed of the purpose of monitoring their pain usually are cooperative in reporting changes because they soon realize that the staff is interested in lessening their pain.

At times the nurse may *plan with the patient* when he may need medication; at other times the nurse will make such a decision on the basis of her own judgment. Obviously the administration of ordered medications for the relief of pain must be based on the nurse's anticipation of the patient's needs, as well as on her own observations of the signs and symptoms of pain.

As previously mentioned, it is well recognized that the efficiency of drug therapy is not solely dependent upon the nature of the drugs. Therefore, even though pain in severe physical disease has a physiologic basis, psychologic mechanisms greatly influence a patient's reaction.[15] Such *psychologic factors* need consideration in planning care. The nurse administering medications for purposes of pain relief should always make use of the augmentative effect on drug therapy that the *situation*, the *personality* and *attitude of the person administering the drug*, and the *patient's suggestibility* have on the results achieved.[27]

The very presence of the nurse should indicate to the patient her willingness to help. This is an important first step in pain therapy.[17] "Giving a medication" involves both the process of "giving" and "the medication" itself. The two are inseparable, but often the nurse's manner or attitude in giving medications does not receive sufficient attention. As we have previously indicated, the power of suggestion is strong and is a power that should be used in administering medications. Thus, when a medication is being given for pain relief, the patient might experience greater relief if he is told, "This medication will help to relieve your pain. I'll check back with you in a little while to see how you are feeling."

Prior to administering an analgesic, place the patient in a *comfortable position* and attend to other activities that will help the patient to relax generally, e.g., open the window and draw the curtain. Plan your care and the activities of others (e.g., other staff members, visitors) so that once the medication is given the patient will not be disturbed further.

Following administration of an analgesic allow the patient to rest so that the medication's helpful effects can provide maximum relief. With most narcotics dizziness and vomiting are observed more often in ambulatory patients than in those who are in bed. *Patients receiving narcotics should remain in bed, have siderails up, and be transported by stretcher.*

Chronic, Intractable Pain

GENERAL CONSIDERATIONS[31, 44, 47, 52]

There are some individuals whose pains become chronic and intractable in nature. When such pains cannot be relieved by physical means, the nurse may find some of the following suggestions and insights helpful.

After working for 10 years with patients suffering chronic pain from neoplastic conditions, LeShan reached the following philosophic conclusions about chronic pain and the world of the patient in pain of long duration:[52]

▶ The patient in chronic, intractable pain lives during his waking moments in the cosmos of a nightmare. There are three basic similarities between the terror dream and the universe of the patient in chronic pain: (1) terrible things are being done to the person and worse are threatened; (2) others, or outside forces are in control and the will is helpless; and (3) there is no time limit set and one can, therefore, not predict when it will end.

▶ The above factors give rise to fearful feelings of helplessness and uncertainty, leading to a sense of futility. The patient's futility is made worse by the fact that his pain seems to serve no purpose in his life—it is meaningless and inexplicable.

▶ Meaningless and purposeless suffering is much harder for a person to accept and resist than pain that the subject can place in a coherent frame of reference.

▶ Chronic pain indicates only a state of existence; it does not warn or tell us what to do, in the way that acute pain does. It does not help us to act. Instead, it may be so severe that it disrupts potentially useful habits and activities.

▶ It is important to ourselves that we *respond* to strong stimuli, that we are connected to and react to our environment. However, this is difficult with chronic pain, since we are pushed toward suffering rather than reacting. Thus, one cannot act, one can only bear.

▶ When filled with pain, a patient is pulled to the immediate present, and goals for the future are lost. Pain forces personal existence to continue with little assistance from one's usual orientations, defenses, safeguards, and associations.

We should not leave the chronically suffering individual alone and suspended in his pain-filled existence. First we must determine the significance and meaning that pain has for the individual as the duration of the pain is extended. It is important not to assume the patient's meaning, but to validate our assumptions and observations. What may be suffering to one individual may be a reminder to another that he is still alive. For the patient experiencing intractable pain, it is important to identify some actions that can be taken to lessen suffering through effective clinical care.

One of the hardest basic tasks of a nurse is to help a patient experiencing intractable pain to formulate for himself suitable meanings for his pain that are not based on old guilts, fears, and anxieties. Each patient must be helped to find a meaning that makes sense to *him*, whether or not it makes sense to the nurse. For example, if the patient is from a different cultural or social background than the nurse, it is important for the nurse to realize that this patient may have an entirely different set of values from her own. Instead of imposing her values on the patient, the nurse helps the patient to reaffirm his own values and rediscover his own meaning in life.

Emphasis can helpfully be placed upon the patient's ability to find purpose and meaning in his life in spite of his difficult circumstances and his hopeless feelings about the future. The fact may be emphasized that no one, sick or well, knows the future. We, as human beings, can only hope that we shall live to have a future, but there is no guarantee. Such insecurity about future time is a universal human condition, the reality of which must be accepted. When a patient having chronic pain has lost interest in the present and has lost hope in the future, he needs the nurse's encouragement to turn his energies outward from the pain to other activities and to establish new goals. LeShan points out that the therapist must avoid being too gentle with the patient who needs such direction. High demands imply high respect, and consequently give strength to the patient.[52]

When a nurse helps a patient to set up new goals, she must remember that these goals are for the patient who is an individual; consequently, the goals must suit the individual patient's needs rather than the nurse's needs.

A sense of loneliness is said to haunt sufferers of chronic pain, since the patient in pain cannot share his feelings of pain with others so that others may realize his suffering. He can only try to express his feelings in words or actions that frequently are not structured to fully communicate the depth of his pain or despair. In such a situation the nurse must make every attempt, even in minor ways, to let the patient know that she is attempting to understand him, uncritically accepts him, and has an appreciation for what he is enduring.

The nurse who realizes that she is not concerned with a sensation (pain) but rather with a human being experiencing a sensation will make a conscious effort to bring a sense of companionship to even the most lonely sufferer. "The nurse may decide that in a particular situation the most appropriate ministration is not a *doing* but a *being*. Just being there as a nonverbal comforter or a listener may help the patient to drain off psychic pressure which has translated itself into physical pain."[47]

We have said that the patient in chronic pain has been described as living in a nightmare—a terrible and timeless cosmos in which the patient feels helpless and alone. How can a patient who lives in such a waking state be helped? Hundreds of years ago Spinoza wrote, "Suffering ceases to be suffering as soon as we form a clear and precise picture of it." This statement implies that knowledge of precisely what is happening to cause suffering may help to abate the suffering. The patient must be helped to *reach conscious awareness* of the "nightmare" in which he lives, so that he can better understand it and accept it. If the doctor and nurse can help to clarify for a patient why he has pain, and why he is afraid of the pain, they may help to relieve much of the nightmare quality of the patient's existence.

Also, it may help some persons having chronic pain to realize that the experience of pain, though unique to each individual, is also a *universal* experience, touching all people at some time in their lives. Albert Schweitzer wrote eloquently of "a fellowship of pain" in which human beings all over the world are united by the desire to be free from pain. The individual sufferer who realizes that he has a common bond and shares a common problem with all people who suffer pain may, through his identification with mankind, lose some of his sense of hopeless isolation in a nightmare.

One final insight concerning chronic, intractable pain is this: Remember that for some individuals, *pain serves positive functions* as: (1) a form of communication, an attempt to say something that words alone cannot convey and (2) a means of adaptation to the world. Pain, thus, for some persons, fills an inner need and acts to maintain the psychodynamic structure of the person. LeShan observes that "our cultural orientation towards pain that it is evil and must be immediately relieved is so strong that, in spite of our knowledge of the cases when chronic pain has been relieved, to be followed immediately by emotional breakdown or suicide, we often ignore this problem."[52]

LONG-TERM PAIN DRUG THERAPY

In treating patients having severe *chronic pain* of *nonmalignant* origin, narcotic analgesics must be given judiciously. The development of addiction can ultimately cause a patient greater distress than his momentary pain. Only during episodes of severe pain should one of the potentially less addicting narcotics (e.g., codeine) be used for a brief period along with large doses of non-narcotic analgesics.[91]

> *While addiction poses potential problems, the nurse must guard against withholding necessary medication for fear that addiction will occur.*

If a patient is in need of a narcotic, has it ordered, and shows no toxic effects, then the nurse should not indiscriminately prolong the interval between narcotics or withhold them. Signs of tolerance to narcotics should, of course, be observed for and reported, but it is ultimately the physician's decision whether the medication regimen should be changed. Patients in pain whose analgesics are indiscriminately withheld by the nurse will become fearful, panic-stricken, and angry. They will lose confidence in staff members and in the ability of their medications to lessen their pains. Moreover, their pain may increase to an intolerable intensity, taxing the limits of human suffering.

Narcotics should be avoided as an initial medication for controlling pain in *chronic* pain syndromes. When chronic pain occurs (e.g., with terminal malignant disease), it is impossible to predict when it will end. It may well go on getting worse. It may appear to be utterly meaningless and causes intense suffering. Narcotics may be the only way to obtain relief from this type of pain. When narcotics are used, their usage must be individually prescribed for the patient. Great skill is needed to find the right drug, at the proper dosage, administered in sequential increments.

> *The goal is to control moderate pain and to prevent severe pain.*

To treat excruciating pain, a higher dose of narcotic is needed, followed by sequential decrements until analgesia without sedation is achieved,[90] as illustrated in Figure 34–3. Successful pain control is best achieved by altering doses at intervals of 48 to 72 hours. If the patient is on more than one drug, it is important to change only one variable at a time and observe its effects. Initiation of narcotics may produce transient sedation lasting 1 to 2 days. It is helpful to reassure the patient that pain can be controlled and that the initial drowsiness is temporary. The patient's confidence that pain control will be achieved will promote analgesia.

> *Adequate therapy for pain, particularly when the pain is expected to continue for some time, brings with it the problems of increasing requirements, by the patient, of the narcotic medication prescribed, with ultimate tolerance, dependence, and addiction.[49]*

One means of trying to avoid (or at least to prolong the occurrence of) the above problems is to utilize other agents, nonanalgesic in themselves, to potentiate the action of the analgesics by sedation and tranquilization of the patient. Therapy of this nature is an attempt to reduce the patient's discomfort to what might be considered a baseline, in order for treatment with minimal but adequate doses of narcotic agents to be as effective as possible.[49]

Pain tends to be worse when it occurs at night; it interferes with sleep and consequently makes a patient tense and exhausted during the day. The sedative hypnotic drugs are useful adjuncts to pain therapy. Sleeplessness is, in itself, a difficult clinical problem to manage, since habituation, tolerance, and addiction to sedatives are potential problems. As a general rule, the nonbarbiturate hypnotics are useful since they are typically faster acting than barbiturates (usually acting within 15 or 20 minutes) and they are short-acting, thereby causing relatively little feeling of "hangover."[82]

With prolonged pain drug therapy the development of toxic manifestations may preclude the use of many excellent analgesics unless frequent, careful observations of the patient are made. Particularly in treating chronic pain, it is necessary that laboratory work and physical follow-up examinations be done periodically. When these details are attended to conscientiously, it is possible to prevent iatrogenic diseases that might be caused by prolonged analgesic usage. Some of the more common side effects to be anticipated are those affecting the hematologic, renal, hepatic, and dermatologic systems.[49] Thus, in situations of prolonged pain management the physician usually tries to prescribe adequate dosages of medication that will control pain. An attempt is also made to use nonnarcotic drugs first, with an understanding that narcotics will be prescribed in conjunction with other drugs, e.g., phenothiazines, when needed.

Progressive Pain

In the previous section, we presented material about the management of severe chronic pain of nonmalignant origin. Pain associated with *progressive malignant diseases* requires a different philosophical approach to management. The nurse must become skilled at differentiating between the two distinct types of pain in relation to duration—acute pain and chronic pain. In both instances if a cancer process continues to grow and/or metastasize, the pain may become progressive, involving one or more parts of the pain pathway. Determining the significance and meaning that pain has for the individual becomes increasingly important as

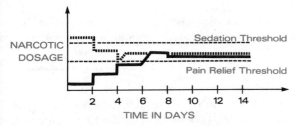

Figure 34–3. Alternative methods of adjusting the dosage of narcotic and phenothiazine (Brompton mixture). Pain relief in the absence of sedation may be achieved with sequential increments in narcotic dose at intervals of 2 days (━━━). In a few cases the severity of the pain will require an initially high dose, followed by sequential decrements until the pain reappears (■ ■ ■). A slight increase in dose provides analgesia without sedation (- - - -). (From Mount, B. M., et al.: Use of the Brompton mixture in treating the chronic pain of malignant disease. Canadian Medical Journal, *115*:112, July 1976.)

the duration of the pain is extended and progression of disease occurs.

Pain associated with disseminated cancer varies according to many factors, e.g., integrity of the central nervous system, level of consciousness, previous experience. Pain caused by cancer is different from that of other diseases because it is associated with painful agonizing ways of dying. Certainly, not all patients with progressive cancer have pain; but for those in whom pain does occur, it can be devastating to the patient, family, and staff if relief is not achieved. In the past, physicians and nurses have been reluctant to use effective narcotic agents at the proper strengths and time intervals to relieve distress. Cancer victims have been unduly penalized for progressively deteriorating. Their pain medications have been ordered on a p.r.n. basis, which often require the patients to ask for relief; and each and every time they ask, they are reminded that their distress has reached a point where they can no longer bear it. We, as professionals, ask the cancer patient to be the most assertive (i.e., to ask for pain relief) at the exact time when he is most vulnerable. It is at these times that the nurse must learn to intervene for the cancer patient with progressive pain due to his disease process.

We as nurses must learn to apply the same principles of management to patients with progressive pain of malignant origin that we practice with other declining diseases, such as heart disease and diabetes. For example, the patient with heart disease is taught to take his vasodilator at specific time intervals. Great efforts are made by physicians to find the correct medication to relieve the patient's symptoms once the disease process is understood. Similarly, diabetics are monitored for control, and varying amounts of insulin are given at specific intervals. Physicians may need to persuade patients with heart disease and diabetes to take prescribed medications to control their symptoms in order to allow these patients to perform their everyday activities. The same is true for patients with progressive pain of malignant origin.

If regular doses of a narcotic at consistent time intervals are needed to control a patient's symptom of pain related to cancer, then the patient has a right to be managed medically in this manner. Just as a diabetic takes his insulin to *prevent* his symptoms, so also a patient with cancer may need his pain medication to *prevent* unbearable pain. It is not easy to convince

patients to take narcotics because of prevalent fears of addiction. However, a patient experiencing pain associated with widespread cancer is no more addicted to his narcotic than a patient with heart disease is to his vasodilator. The time has come to stop persecution of patients with malignant progressive pain. Such patients must be allowed to be as free of their symptoms as possible.

A nurse soon learns that medications alone are not the answer to managing progressive pain, and learns that a blend of therapeutic approaches and human contact is needed instead. Frequently, once pain control is maintained and providers consistently see the patient, narcotics can be reduced and in some instances eliminated.[60]

Absence of Pain

While the nurse is most frequently involved with caring for patients experiencing chronic and acute pains, she will also have patients in her care who *lack* the ability to experience pain. Such persons lack the sensory coordination that is necessary for the perception and interpretation of pain. A few persons are *born with* this deficit, but it occurs more commonly as a result of *injury*, e.g., traumatic severance of the spinal cord; *disease* process, e.g., tabes dorsalis; or *therapy*, e.g., neurolytic nerve block or surgical severance of sensory branches of nerves.

Persons lacking the protective mechanism of pain are handicapped in some ways and are less perfectly equipped to withstand the hazards of the environment. As a result, traumatic incidents leading to severe tissue damage may occur without a patient's awareness when pain is absent.

> *A prime goal of nursing therapy for patients who lack awareness of pain is to prevent injury and to teach the patient how he can prevent injury.*

Without awareness of heat, pressure, and pain it is difficult to realize when tissue is injured. Thus, if tissue is in contact with injurious agents, is exposed to noxious agents for a dangerous length of time, or is exposed to them in dangerous amounts, unnoticed injury will result. Both patient and nurse must learn to think *ahead* to prevent injury by protecting and frequently inspecting affected areas for signs of injury that may already have occurred.

▶ Prevent burns from radiators, hot water, heating pads, electric elements, cigarettes.

▶ Prevent cuts, scrapes and bruises, e.g., from wheelchairs.

▶ Prevent pressure sores. Use alternating pressure mattress, sheepskin, cradle; keep bed free from wrinkles and crumbs.

▶ Teach patient to change his position, lift himself up, smooth his clothing and bed linens, and inspect his skin at least every two hours for redness or blanching. Perform these activities for patients who cannot help themselves.

BIBLIOGRAPHY

1. Adler, R., and Lomazzi, F.: Psychological factors and the relationship between perceptual style and pain tolerance. *Psychotherapy and Psychosomatics*, 22: 347, 1973.
2. Alling, C. C., III, et al. (eds.): *Facial Pain.* Philadelphia, Lea & Febiger, 1968.
3. Analgesics: The special challenge of chronic pain. *Patient Care*, 6:135, March 1972.
4. Balme, H.: Principles of treatment. *In* Ogilvie, W., and Thomson, W. (eds.): *Pain and Its Problems.* London, Eyre and Spottiswoode, 1950.
5. Bandler, R. J., Jr., et al.: Self-observation as a source of pain perception. *Journal of Personality and Social Psychology* (Washington), 9:205, July 1968.
6. Beecher, H. K.: Pain in men wounded in battle. *Bulletin U.S. Army Medical Department*, 5:445, 1946.
7. Beecher, H. K.: *Measurement of Subjective Responses.* New York, Oxford University Press, 1959, p. 158.
8. Beecher, H. K.: An inspection of our working hypotheses in the study of pain and other subjective responses in man. *In* Keele, C. A., and Smith, R. (eds.): *International Symposium on the Assessment of Pain in Man and Animals.* Edinburgh, E. and S. Livingstone, Ltd., 1962.
9. Beecher, H. K.: Anxiety and pain. *J.A.M.A.*, 209:1080, Aug. 1969.
10. Beland, I. L.: *Clinical Nursing: Pathophysiological and Psychosocial Approaches.* 2nd ed. New York, The Macmillan Co., 1970.
11. Bellville, J. W., et al.: Influence of age on pain relief from analgesics. A study of postoperative patients. *J.A.M.A.*, 217:1835, Sep. 1971.
12. Blaylock, J.: The pathological and cultural influences on the reaction to pain: A review of the literature. *Nursing Forum*, 7:263, 1968.
13. Bobey, M. J., et al.: Psychological factors affecting pain tolerance. *Journal of Pscyhosomatic Research*, 14:371, Dec. 1970.
14. Boehm, G.: At last—A nonaddicting substitute for morphine. *Today's Health*, 46:69, April 1968.
15. Bond, M. R., and Pilowsky, I.: Subjective assessment of pain and its relationship to the administration of analgesics in patients with advanced cancer. *Journal of Psychosomatic Research*, 10:203, Sep. 1966.
16. Bond, M. R.: Personality studies in patients with pain secondary to organic disease. *Journal of Psychosomatic Research*, 17:257, 1973.
17. Bonica, J. J.: *Clinical Applications of Diagnostic and Therapeutic Nerve Blocks.* Springfield, IL, Charles C Thomas, 1959.
18. Bonica, J. J.: Pain—basic principles of management. *Northwest Medicine*, 69:567, Aug. 1970.
19. Boucher, J. D.: Facial displays of fear, sadness, and pain. *Perceptual and Motor Skills*, 28:239, Feb. 1969.
20. Brain, L.: Presidential address. *In* Keele, C. A., and Smith, R. (eds.): *International Symposium on the Assessment of Pain in Man and Animals.* Edinburgh, E. and S. Livingstone, Ltd., 1962.
21. Bruegel, M. A.: Relationship of preoperative anxiety to perception of postoperative pain. *Nursing Research*, 20:26, Jan.–Feb. 1970.
22. Brunner, L. S., et al.: *Textbook of Medical-Surgical Nursing*, 2nd ed. Philadelphia, J. B. Lippincott Co., 1970.
23. Cahn, J., and Herold, M.: Pain and psychotropic drugs. *In* Soulairac, A., Cahn, J., and Charpentier, J. (eds.): *Pain.* New York, Academic Press, Inc., 1968.
24. Carini, E., and Owens, G.: *Neurological and Neurosurgical Nursing*, 5th ed. St. Louis, C. V. Mosby Co., 1970.
25. Chambers, W. G., and Price, G. G.: Influence of nurse upon effects of analgesics administered. *Nursing Research*, 16:228, Summer 1967.
26. Copple, D.: What can a nurse do to relieve pain without resort to drugs? *Nursing Times*, 68:584, May 1972.
27. Crowley, D. M.: *Pain and Its Alleviation.* Los Angeles, UCLA School of Nursing, 1962.
28. Donovan, M. I., and Pierce, S. G.: *Cancer Care Nursing.* New York, Appleton-Century-Crofts, 1976.
29. Dorsey, J. M.: Problems with pain in a general surgical practice. *Medical Clinics of North America*, 52:103, Jan. 1968.
30. Dundee, J. W.: Management of chronic pain. *Transactions of the Medical Society of London*, 85:153, 1969.
31. Engel, G.: Psychogenic pain and the pain-prone patient. *American Journal of Medicine*, 26:899, June 1959.
32. Engel, G.: Psychogenic pain. *Journal of Occupational Medicine*, 3:249, 1961.
33. Finneson, B.: *Diagnosis and Management of Pain Syndromes*, 2nd ed. Philadelphia, W. B. Saunders Co., 1969.
34. Fordyce, W. E.: Operant conditioning as a treatment method in the management of selected chronic pain problems. *Northwest Medicine*, 69:580, Aug. 1970.
35. Garland, D.: The care of the dying. *Nursing Times*, 64:355, March 1968.
36. Gildea, J.: The relief of postoperative pain. *Medical Clinics of North America*, 52:81, Jan. 1968.
37. Grollman, A.: Use of drugs in relief of pain. *In* Finneson, B.: *Diagnosis and Management of Pain Syndromes*, 2nd ed. Philadelphia, W. B. Saunders Co., 1969.
38. Guyton, A. C.: *Textbook of Medical Physiology*, 5th ed. Philadelphia, W. B. Saunders Co., 1976.
39. Hackett, T. P.: Pain and prejudice. Why do we doubt that the patient is in pain? *Medical Times*, 99:130, Feb. 1971.
40. Halpern, L. M.: Treating pain with drugs. *Minnesota Medicine*, 57:176, March 1974.
41. Hassenplug, L. W.: Introduction. *In* Crowley, D. M.: *Pain and Its Alleviation.* Los Angeles, UCLA School of Nursing, 1962.
42. Hilgard, E. R.: Pain as a puzzle for psychology and physiology. *American Psychologist*, 24:103, Feb. 1969.
43. Holmes, G.: Some clinical aspects of pain. *In* Ogilvie, W., and Thomson, W. (eds.): *Pain and Its Problems.* London, Eyre and Spottiswoode, 1950.
44. Hunter, J.: The mark of pain. *American Journal of Nursing*, 61:96, Oct. 1961.

45. Jacox, A. K. (ed.): *Pain: A Source Book for Nurses and Other Health Professionals*. Boston, Little, Brown & Co., 1977.

46. Johnson, J. E.: Effects of structuring patients' expectations on their reactions to threatening events. *Nursing Research*, 21:489, 1972.

47. Kaufman, M. A., and Brown, D. E.: Pain wears many faces. *American Journal of Nursing*, 61:48, Jan. 1961.

48. Keats, A. S.: Use of analgetics at the bedside. *In* Way, E. L. (ed.): *New Concepts in Pain and Its Clinical Management*. Philadelphia, F. A. Davis Company, 1967.

49. Kolodny, A. L., and McLoughlin, P. T.: *Comprehensive Approach to the Therapy of Pain*. Springfield, IL, Charles C Thomas, 1966.

50. Lauer, J. W.: Hypnosis in the relief of pain. *Medical Clinics of North America*, 52:217, Jan. 1968.

51. Leake, C. D.: Introduction. *In* Way, E. L. (ed.): *New Concepts in Pain and Its Clinical Management*. Philadelphia, F. A. Davis Co., 1967.

52. LeShan, L.: The world of the patient in severe pain of long duration. *Journal of Chronic Diseases*, 17:119, 1964.

53. Lim, R. K. S.: Sites of action of narcotic and nonnarcotic analgesics: Mechanism of pain and analgesia. *Headache*, 7:103, Oct. 1967.

54. Livingston, W. K.: What is pain? Reprinted from *Scientific American*, March, 1953. San Francisco, W. H. Freeman and Co., 1953.

55. MacBryde, C. (ed.): *Signs and Symptoms: Applied Pathologic Physiology and Clinical Interpretation*, 4th ed. Philadelphia, J. B. Lippincott Co., 1964.

56. Markham, M. M.: The relief of pain. *Nursing Times*, 66:1579, Dec. 1970.

57. McBride, M. D.: The additive to the analgesic. *American Journal of Nursing*, 69:974, May 1969.

58. McCaffery, M.: *Nursing Management of the Patient with Pain*. Philadelphia, J. B. Lippincott Co., 1972.

59. McCaffery, M., and Moss, F.: Nursing intervention for bodily pain. *American Journal of Nursing*, 67:1224, June 1967.

60. McCorkle, R.: The advanced cancer patient: how he will live and die. *Nursing '76*, 6:46, Oct. 1976.

61. McCorkle, R.: Hospices: a British reality and an American dream. *In* Kellogg and Sullivan: *Current Practice in Oncology Nursing*, Volume II. St. Louis, C. V. Mosby Co., 1978, pp. 125–131.

62. Meares, A.: *Relief Without Drugs: The Self-Management of Tension, Anxiety, and Pain*. Garden City, New York, Doubleday, 1967.

63. Melzack, R., and Wall, P. D.: Psychophysiology of pain. *The International Anesthesiology Clinics*, 8:3, 1970.

64. Melzack, R.: *The Puzzle of Pain*. New York, Basic Books, Inc., 1973.

65. Merskey, H.: Psychologic aspects of pain. *Postgraduate Medical Journal*, 44:297, April 1968.

66. Merskey, H.: Pain. *Nursing Times*, 67:988, Aug. 1971.

67. Merskey, H., and Spear, F. G.: *Pain: Psychological and Psychiatric Aspects*. London, Baillière, Tindall and Cassell, 1967.

68. Merskey, H., et al.: The concept of pain. *Journal of Psychosomatic Research*, 11:59, June 1967.

69. Mettler, F. A.: Pain, I: What is it? *The Journal of the Medical Society of New Jersey*, 61:10, Jan. 1964.

70. Moertel, C. G., et al.: Relief of pain by oral medications. *Journal of American Medical Association*, 229:55, July 1974.

71. Moran, Lord: The meaning and measurement of pain. *In* Ogilvie, W., and Thomson, W. (eds.): *Pain and Its Problems*. London, Eyre and Spottiswoode, 1950.

72. Moss, F. T.: The effect of a nursing intervention on pain relief. *ANA Regional Clinical Conferences*, 1967. New York, Appleton-Century-Crofts, 1968, p. 247.

73. Mount, B. M., et al.: Use of the Brompton Mixture in treating the chronic pain of malignant disease. *Canadian Medical Journal*, 115:112, July 1976.

74. Murray, J. B.: Psychology of the pain experience. *Journal of Psychology*, 78:193, July 1971.

75. Ogilvie, W. H., and Thomson, W. A. R. (eds.): *Pain and Its Problems*. London, Eyre and Spottiswoode, 1950.

76. Pennmann, J.: Pain as an old friend. *Lancet*, 1:633, 1954.

77. Petrie, A.: *Individuality in Pain and Suffering*. Chicago, University of Chicago Press, 1967.

78. Pilling, L. F.: Psychosomatic aspects of facial pain. *In* Alling, C. C., III, et al. (eds.): *Facial Pain*. Philadelphia, Lea & Febiger, 1968.

79. Poswillo, D. E.: Pharmacodynamics of pain relief. *In* Alling, C. C., III, et al. (eds.): *Facial Pain*. Philadelphia, Lea & Febiger, 1968.

80. Raney, J. O.: Pain, emotion and a rationale for therapy. *Northwest Medicine*, 69:659, Sep. 1970.

81. Rasmussen, P.: *Facial Pain*. Copenhagen, Ejnar Munksgaard, 1965.

82. Sadove, M. S., and Albrecht, R.: Sedatives and tranquilizers in the treatment of pain. *Medical Clinics of North America*, 52:47, Jan. 1968.

83. Sharp, D.: Lessons from a dying patient. *American Journal of Nursing*, 68:1517, July 1968.

84. Smith, D. W., Germain, C. P., and Gips, C.: *Care of the Adult Patient*, 3rd ed. Philadelphia, J. B. Lippincott Company, 1971.

85. Soulairac, A., Cahn, J., and Charpentier, J. (eds.): *Pain*. Proceedings of the International Symposium on Pain. April 11–13, 1967. New York, Academic Press, Inc., 1968.

86. Stephen, C. R.: Complications of analgetic therapy. *In* Way, E. L. (ed.): *New Concepts in Pain and Its Clinical Management*. Philadelphia, F. A. Davis Co., 1967.

87. Sternbach, R. A.: *Pain; A Psychophysiological Analysis*. New York, Academic Press, Inc., 1968.

88. Szasz, T. S.: The nature of pain. *Archives of Neurology and Psychiatry* (Chicago), 74:174, 1955.

89. Szasz, T. S.: *Pain and Pleasure: A Study of Bodily Feelings*. New York, Basic Books, 1957.

90. Twycross, R. G.: Principles and practice of the relief of pain in terminal cancer. *Update*, July 1972.

91. Wang, R. I. H.: Control of pain. *The American Journal of the Medical Sciences*, 246:112, Nov. 1963.

92. Weddell, G.: The relationship between pain sensibility and peripheral nerve fibers. *In* Knighton, R., and Dumke, P. (eds.): *Pain*. Boston, Little, Brown & Company, 1966.

93. Weisenberg, M. (ed.): *Pain—Clinical and Experimental Perspectives*. St. Louis, The C. V. Mosby Company, 1975.

94. White, J. C.: Foreword. *In* Knighton, R., and Dumke, P. (eds.): *Pain: International Symposium on Pain*. Henry Ford Hospital. Boston, Little, Brown & Company, 1966.

95. Wolff, H. G., and Wolf, S.: *Pain*. Springfield, IL, Charles C Thomas, 1958.

96. Zborowski, M.: Cultural components in responses to pain. *Journal of Social Issues*, 8:16, 1952.

97. Zborowski, M.: *People in Pain*. San Francisco, Jossey-Bass, Inc., 1969.

UNIT
IX
ADVANCED CLINICAL CONSIDERATIONS

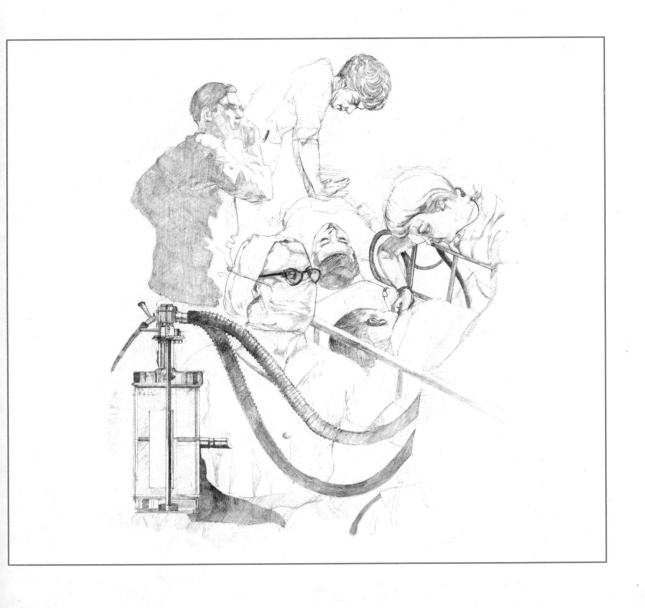

CHAPTER 35

PROVIDING IMMEDIATE LIFE SUPPORT

By Martha L. Tyler, R.N., M.N., R.R.T.

OVERVIEW AND STUDY GUIDE

The main purpose of this chapter is to help you learn how to recognize a patient who requires immediate life support. Temporarily providing breath and circulation for a patient is one of the most dramatic and vital services one person ever provides for another. To prevent a natural tendency to panic in this situation, actions and skills must be learned in advance. Recognition of cardiopulmonary (heart-lung) arrest is not difficult, but it must be done quickly and accurately as immediate action must be taken to prevent death or the complications associated with prolonged lack of oxygen (hypoxemia).

Second, you should be aware of the pathophysiologic changes that occur during cardiopulmonary arrest. The pathologic changes due to brain tissue hypoxia that occur in the central nervous system help the nurse identify cardiopulmonary arrest. For example, cerebral hypoxia results in unconsciousness and loss of muscle tone.

A third purpose of this chapter is to present the methods used in basic life support. These are simple actions based on knowledge of the anatomy and physiology of the heart and lungs. Learning the reasons for the various steps in cardiopulmonary resuscitation (CPR) and why they are done in the order outlined makes it easier for you to remember the "what and how" of CPR when immediate action must be taken.

A final purpose is to review the complications and performance problems that can occur during basic life support and to suggest methods for prevention and treatment.

1. To guide your learning while reading this chapter, be thinking about the following questions:

What have I already learned about CPR? How does my previous learning compare with what I've read in this chapter?
How do I think I will react in a crisis?[15]
Will I feel guilty if the patient doesn't revive?[10]

How do I feel about "No Codes"?[13, 14] ("No Code" is a term used to indicate patients who will not be resuscitated if cardiac arrest occurs.)
Can I talk to a patient who requests "No Code"? In other words, will I be able to talk to a patient about his impending death?

2. As you read this chapter, be sure you know the definitions of these terms:

clinical death	aspiration
biological death	grand mal seizure
cardiac arrest	fit
respiratory arrest	intubation
rescue breathing	precordial thump
artificial circulation	acrocyanosis
artificial ventilation	alveoli
compression to venti-	acidemia
lation ratio	anaerobic metabolism
cardiac output	aerobic metabolism
tidal volume	ischemia
hypoxia	asystole
hypoxemia	bradycardia

3. At the end of the chapter you will be ready to practice with a mannikin. You should also be able to answer the following questions:
   a. What are the signs of respiratory arrest?
   b. What are the signs of cardiac arrest?
   c. What is done first in cardiopulmonary arrest?
   d. What is done in a *witnessed* cardiac arrest that is not done in an unwitnessed arrest?
   e. What is the basic method of artificial ventilation?
   f. Where are the hands placed during external cardiac compression?
   g. What does pupil size indicate about success/failure of CPR?
   h. Where are the two major sites used to assess pulse?

PATHOPHYSIOLOGY OF CARDIOPULMONARY ARREST

Overview

The function of the respiratory system is to provide the body with the oxygen required for the normal function of every cell in the body. The lungs also eliminate the carbon dioxide produced during the course of cellular metabolism.[23] Therefore, as oxygen is going into the blood, carbon dioxide is coming out. This process is descriptively called *gas exchange* or *respiration*. Gas exchange occurs in the alveolar capillaries of the lung. In the normal lung it is a very efficient operation. All that is required is that ventilation take place. *Ventilation* is the movement of air in and out of the lungs. It is necessary for normal gas exchange but does not guarantee that gas exchange will occur. For instance, gas exchange may not take place if the lung tissue is diseased, despite the movement of air in and out of the lung.

Gas exchange occurs not only in the lung's alveoli but also in the cells of the body. There, oxygen and carbon dioxide exchange occurs in directions opposite from those in the lung. In the cells, *internal respiration* occurs, with oxygen moving from the blood into the cell (for aerobic metabolism) while carbon dioxide leaves the cell and enters the blood to be carried back to the lungs.

Normal Cardiovascular Function.   To get oxygen from the lungs to the cells and to carry carbon dioxide from the cells to the lungs, a *gas transport system* is needed. The cardiovascular system serves as this gas transport system. The heart acts as "pump"; the arteries, capillaries and veins are the "conducting pathways."

The two systems (respiratory and cardiovascular) are interdependent. The heart consumes more oxygen per minute than any other organ of the body; consequently, when the lungs fail the heart fails. Conversely, ventilation stops soon after the heart stops or soon after the central nervous system's blood flow is blocked. Cessation of ventilation occurs because the respiratory centers in the medulla cannot function without the continuous supply of oxygen that is normally transported to them by the cardiovascular system.

Acute and Chronic Respiratory Failure.   *Acute failure* of the respiratory system is marked by "hypoxemia," a sudden fall in the arterial oxygen tension (PaO_2), and is often accompanied by "hypercapnea," a rise in the arterial carbon dioxide tension ($PaCO_2$). An abrupt rise in $PaCO_2$ results in "respiratory acidosis," causing a fall in blood pH and acidemia. Acidemia, or "acid blood," occurs when there is a disturbance in the acid-base balance of the blood, in which the blood becomes more acid than normal. In this case, it is due to the rapid accumulation of respiratory acids. *Chronic respiratory* failure can also occur; but in chronic respiratory failure there is time for the respiratory acids to be buffered, so the blood pH and acid-base balance may be near normal. The PaO_2 will remain low, however, unless treated by oxygen therapy. Causes of acute and chronic respiratory failure and treatment measures are discussed in Chapter 36. See also the discussion of fluid-electrolyte imbalance in Chapter 24.

Of major importance in either acute or chronic respiratory failure is the PaO_2. If there is insufficient pressure of oxygen in the blood to load the hemoglobin molecules with oxygen, the content of oxygen (ml. of oxygen/100 ml. of blood) falls. Every 100 ml. of blood passing through the heart normally carries 20 ml. of oxygen. The heart typically consumes 15 ml. of this 20 ml. This oxygen consumption is much higher than the consumption of other body tissues. The heart has very little reserve compared to the body as a whole, which uses, overall, only about 5 ml. of oxygen of the 20 ml. available in each 100 ml. of blood. The heart uses more oxygen because it is constantly beating. This heart action requires much more oxygen than skin metabolism, for instance. When the heart fails to get an adequate supply of oxygen, orderly conduction of the electrical signal that causes the cardiac muscle fibers to contract is disrupted and arrhythmias occur. If hypoxemia is severe enough, *cardiac standstill* (also called *cardiac arrest* and *asystole*) eventually develops.

At the same time, hypoxemia is also affecting all the other tissues of the body. This often causes symptoms that are noticeable earlier than cardiac arrhythmias. For example, confusion and disorientation are indications of cerebral hypoxia. This is because the *brain* is even less tolerant of hypoxia than the heart. While the brain uses less oxygen per minute than the heart, the brain is capable of only very limited anaerobic metabolism. Consequently, thought processes are altered with only *moderate* hypoxemia and unconsciousness occurs precipitously when hypoxemia is *severe*. When severe hypoxemia remains untreated, the brain tissue itself begins to deteriorate. If too much damage to the cellular structure of the brain occurs before hypoxemia is corrected, brain function will never again be normal.

Peripheral tissues such as skeletal muscles and organs (e.g., kidneys) are much more tolerant than heart and brain of hypoxemia. However, pyruvic and lactic acid is produced when there is insufficient oxygen for normal aerobic metabolism in peripheral tissues and organs. Thus *metabolic acidosis* is added to the (usually) already present respiratory acidosis, further compromising homeostasis.

Failure of the Cardiovascular System

Sudden Cardiac Arrest. When the heart suddenly stops beating due to causes other than hypoxemia (e.g., arteriosclerotic heart disease[12] or electrical shock), the oxygen content of the blood may be entirely normal at first. Normal blood levels of oxygen do not last long, however. Because cellular activity continues throughout the body, the 20 ml. of oxygen in every 100 ml. of blood is soon gone and abrupt unconsciousness occurs due to cerebral hypoxia. Peripheral cells continue to metabolize but without oxygen. This is called *anaerobic metabolism*. Metabolic acidosis soon follows because the waste products of anaerobic metabolism are lactic and pyruvic acid.

If cardiac arrest ("heart beat stoppage") is identified very quickly and CPR started immediately, *respiratory arrest* ("breathing stoppage") may not occur. The respiratory center is less sensitive to hypoxia than the cerebral cortex. For instance, hypoxia of the cerebral cortex causes unconsciousness, but loss of consciousness can occur without respiratory arrest.[6] Whether respiratory arrest occurs following cardiac arrest depends on how fast oxygen delivery is restored to the respiratory center. If restoration of circulation is delayed, respiratory arrest occurs and is followed promptly by respiratory acidosis, as carbon dioxide is no longer eliminated by the lungs.

Obviously, failure in one system (cardiovascular or respiratory) is soon apparent in the other, so great is their interdependence. But more important is the result of failure of either system on the brain, as it is more sensitive than the systems that support it. The respiratory and cardiovascular systems have been discussed separately because indications of impending arrest are different depending on which system is failing first. Failure of the respiratory system is often accompanied by a prodrome of confusion and delirium due to hypoxemia. If this is recognized and treated promptly, it is often possible to prevent the sequence of events described above. Too often, abnormal or confused behavior is dismissed without checking the status of the patient's respiratory function (by drawing arterial blood gases). Frequently, only the *symptom* of abnormal or confused behavior is treated by giving sedatives or tranquilizers without investigation of the underlying cause of the symptoms. Often, oxygen therapy is the treatment that is really needed (see Chapter 36).

Coronary artery disease, the most frequent cause of cardiac arrest,[8, 12, 14] is also associated with a recognizable early symptom. Angina pectoris is chest pain produced by heart tissue that is hypoxic. Most often in angina pectoris the hypoxia is localized to the heart tissue itself. It is due to insufficient blood flow through narrowed or clogged vessels rather than generalized hypoxemia (low blood oxygen tension) due to respiratory failure. Pain is not often ignored by the patient; consequently, the nurse does not ignore pain as she might ignore the abnormal behavior of respiratory failure. However, treatment of coronary artery disease is not as straightforward as it often is in hypoxemia caused by respiratory failure.

Clinical Versus Biologic Death

Safar, one of the early exponents and teachers of CPR, describes the change from life to clinical death as a "bridge from life to death."[17] The term bridge is used because although it spans a large gap, it is possible to come back across the bridge from clinical death. *Clinical death* occurs with cessation of blood flow and/or respiratory arrest. It is manifested by *reversible* loss of consciousness. Biologic death, however, is *irreversible* destruction of brain tissue.[15] Preventing biologic death is the goal of CPR. It is dependent on the prompt recognition of clinical death and the provision of immediate and skilled support of the respiratory and cardiovascular systems.

> *Only 3 to 4 minutes of cerebral ischemia results in brain damage; 5 to 6 minutes of cerebral ischemia results in biologic death—and no return across the bridge to life.*

RECOGNITION OF CARDIOPULMONARY ARREST

The Unconscious Patient

A patient may be unconscious for many reasons; however, *sudden* and *unexpected* unconsciousness is often caused by cardiopulmonary arrest. Resuscitation will not hurt[6] a patient who is suddenly unconscious for reasons other than cardiopulmonary arrest. On the other hand, delay in starting CPR when the reason for unconsciousness is arrest is a major cause of failure of CPR. Failure to promptly initiate CPR is also associated with residual brain damage after recovery from arrest.[6, 8, 11]

Examination for Signs of Cardiopulmonary Arrest. A very brief shout or shake to verify unconsciousness in a patient suspected of arrest should be followed immediately by placing a hand under the patient's neck and lifting up (or grasping the patient's jaw and lifting it forward) while tilting the head back to open the airway. Roll the patient on his back first, if necessary, to facilitate these actions. At the same time bend over the patient and place your ear next to his mouth to listen for or feel breaths. Turn your head towards the patient's chest while doing this so that you can observe the chest to see if it is moving. Push the patient's gown out of the way so that you can clearly see his chest. Simply opening the airway may restore respirations. If not, you must immediately start rescue breathing (technique described later). As you give these first breaths, begin feeling for the carotid artery to determine if there is a pulse. Do not bother with attempting to check the radial artery. The location of the radial artery may be more familiar to you, but it is peripheral and thus a pulse is often absent when a central (carotid or femoral) pulse can still be felt. Besides, you are already positioned at the head of the patient, so the carotid artery is easily reached. When present, a carotid pulse is palpable by gentle pressure over the depression between the trachea and the sternocleidomastoid muscle about on a level with the Adam's apple. If the carotid pulse is absent, you must immediately begin external cardiac compressions (described in detail later).

> *If you are alone, you should be calling for "HELP" while doing the above. CPR is much more effective with two rescuers instead of one. Also, most hospitals have well-organized and skilled CPR teams. However, the team won't come unless you SHOUT or signal your need with an emergency button.*

Secondary Signs of Cardiopulmonary Arrest. Other physical findings or signs that develop soon after arrest may include dilated pupils, occasionally grand mal seizure (sometimes called a "fit"), complete loss of muscle tone and acrocyanosis (symmetrical blue and/or red-tinged mottling of extremities). Examination of the pupils for size is not mandatory (pupil size can be quite variable during an arrest) according to Gilston.[6] Nevertheless, their reaction is often used to judge the length of time since arrest, and later, the success of CPR. Widely dilated and nonreactive pupils indicate cerebral hypoxia has been present for approximately 2 minutes.[15] For these reasons, the time you discover the unconscious patient or witness the arrest, and the size of the pupils, should be noted (mentally) if possible. However, do not delay starting CPR to make these observations if you are alone.

Witnessed Cardiopulmonary Arrest

Agonal gasps and clutching at the chest are often noted just prior to cardiopulmonary ar-

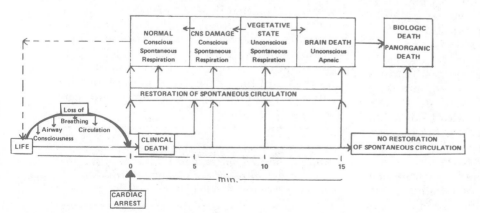

Figure 35–1. Bridge from life to death and reverse pathways with resuscitation. (From Safar, P., et al.: Teaching and organizing cardiopulmonary resuscitation. *Clinical Anesthesia,* 10:163, 1974.)

rest. Agonal gasps are large irregular sighs or breaths. The alert nurse will recognize these premonitory signs and call for help before apnea or pulselessness. When the arrest is witnessed, a slightly altered sequence in the steps of CPR is taken. A precordial thump (for technique, see below) is given after an absent pulse is noted, but before ventilation and external cardiac compression are begun.[19]

IMMEDIATE LIFE SUPPORT

Basic Life Support

Cardiopulmonary resuscitation techniques are divided into two categories or levels.[19] These are *basic* and *advanced* life support techniques. In this chapter we are concerned primarily with basic life support, which is the "first aid" of cardiac or respiratory arrest (see Procedure 19). Figure 35–2 illustrates the relationship between basic and advanced life support.

Safar described "mouth to mouth" resuscitation in 1956[16] and the successful use of external heart compression was reported by Kouwenhoven et al. in 1960.[11] Over the years, the techniques of CPR have been formalized and ritualized as more and more experience has been gained. The whole of basic life support has been reduced to a deceptively simple "A-B-C" sequence.[19] While formalization of technique sometimes stifles change and perhaps even inhibits improvement in techniques,[7] it also provides a framework for remembering *what to do when* and allows people who have never worked together before to function together more smoothly and effectively.

Sequence of CPR

"A-B-C" stands for *Airway, Breathing* and *Circulation*. This is the order in which basic life support actions (cardiopulmonary resuscitation) are taken in the majority of arrests. In other words, the airway is established first, then breathing is assisted and finally circulation is assisted. (Exceptions are monitored patients and witnessed arrests, which will be discussed below.) The A-B-C sequence is carried out in this order because it is felt by many CPR experts that it does no good to pump severely hypoxemic blood to the brain.[8, 15, 21] They feel that air must be gotten into the lungs first so that it is available to provide oxygen for the newly re-established or artificially supported circulation to pick up as it passes through the lung. Other authors advocate CPR technique in which cardiac compressions are started before artificial ventilation.[2, 6] They feel that, except in cases of acute hypoxemia or asphyxiation, the lungs contain sufficient oxygen to saturate the blood for approximately 30 seconds. The difficulty of determining the presence and magnitude of hypoxemia, particularly in unwitnessed arrests, resulted in the recommendation of the A-B-C sequence by the National Conference on Standards for Cardiopulmonary Resuscitation (CPR) and Emergency Cardiac Care (ECC).[19] This is the sequence most commonly used in the United States; however, starting cardiac compressions before ventilation is popular in the United Kingdom and European countries. The A-B-C method is described in this chapter to conform with standard practice in this country. Also, the author feels that two rescuers can initiate compression and ventilation almost simultaneously, eliminating the need for deciding what to do first. One rescuer is hampered, but if she works speedily and decisively, cardiac and pulmonary resuscitation should both be underway within 30 seconds.

A: Airway

During cardiac arrest all the muscles of the body are relaxed, including the jaw muscles. This relaxation causes the tongue to fall back and obstruct the airway. Sometimes this obstruction is noticeable if the patient is still making respiratory efforts. In such situations, retractions of the soft tissue of the chest wall will be seen in the suprasternal, supraclavicular and intercostal areas. If food or vomitus is obviously obstructing the airway, scoop it out with two fingers, with the patient turned on his side. If the airway is not obstructed by food or vomitus it is opened by (a) turning the patient to his back, (b) removing any pillows and (c) tilting the head back by lifting behind the neck with one hand while pushing down on the forehead with the other. This hyperextended position of the head and neck is maintained throughout CPR. Holding the jaw forward is sometimes required in addition to the head tilt to open the airway. To accomplish this, the rescuer's fingers are placed behind the angle of the jaw and it is lifted forward.

B: Breathing

If opening the airway is not promptly followed by spontaneous breathing (get your cheek close to the patient's mouth so that you can feel his breath and watch his chest), you must start artificial ventilation.

Mouth-to-Mouth. The simplest and fastest way to re-establish ventilation is to use mouth-to-mouth respiration. Waiting while someone goes for a self-inflating bag (bag-mask resuscitator) wastes valuable time. Lost time can be

lethal to a patient who is not breathing. If you are alone, you *cannot* handle the bag *and* give external heart compressions: so, it is best to consider this an item to be used only when a skilled CPR team arrives.[3]

While maintaining the head tilt and supporting the jaw, the patient's nose is pinched and the rescuer blows a big breath into the patient's mouth. Figure 35–3 illustrates the proper mouth-to-mouth technique. A tight seal must be formed between the mouth of the victim and your mouth during the breath. Then the seal is broken to allow the air to escape. It is easier to make the seal if the patient's dentures are left in

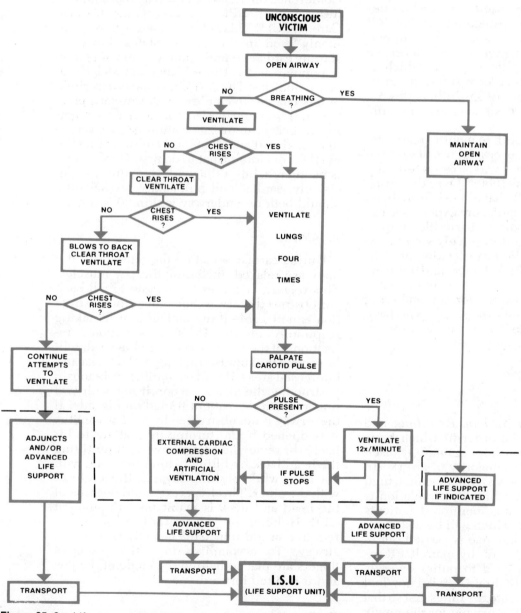

Figure 35–2. Life support decision tree (unwitnessed arrest). The sequence of basic life support decisions and actions. The dotted line separates basic life support from advanced life support. (Reprinted from the Supplement to Journal of the American Medical Assoc. Feb. 18, 1974. Copyright, 1974, The American Medical Assoc. Reprinted with permission of the American Heart Assoc.)

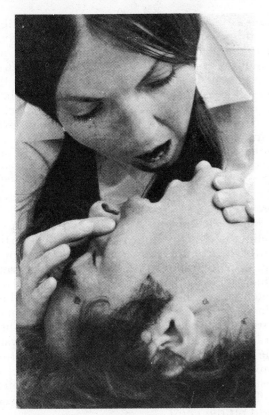

Figure 35–3. The quickest way to establish ventilation is to use mouth-to-mouth ventilation. The rescuer pinches the victim's nose, supports his head to maintain an open airway and breathes directly into the victim's mouth. No time is lost in getting a resuscitation bag or fitting the mask. (From Pribble, A. H., and Tyler, M. L.: Emergency! Part 1: On-the-spot cardiopulmonary resuscitation. *Nursing '75*, 5:48, Feb. 1975.)

place, although some authors advocate their removal because they may slip out of place.[2] Obviously if they are causing obstruction, they will have to be removed.

> *Artificial ventilation is successful if you can (a) see the victim's chest rise, (b) feel the compliance of his lungs as they fill with air and (c) feel the victim exhale air.*

Other Rescue Breathing Methods. Variations on basic mouth-to-mouth resuscitation are mouth-to-nose, mouth-to-stoma and mouth-to-tracheostomy tube. Mouth-to-nose resuscitation is used when it is impossible to get a tight seal around the victim's mouth or when his mouth cannot be opened. In mouth-to-nose ventilation, the victim's mouth is held closed by a hand under the jaw, if necessary, and the breath is given with rescuer's mouth tight over the patient's nose. Mouth-to-stoma breathing is done when a patient has had a laryngectomy. A stoma is a permanent opening in the neck

through which the patient breathes following the removal of the larynx (laryngectomy). The upper airway is separated from the trachea during this operation so there is no passageway for air from the patient's nose (or mouth) to his trachea; therefore, the rescuer's mouth is placed directly over the stoma during ventilation. A patient with a tracheostomy tube is ventilated similarly. Neither mouth-to-stoma nor mouth-to-tracheostomy tube resuscitation requires the head tilt as the airway is opened below the tongue. However, the mouth and nose of the patient with a tracheostomy tube may need to be held closed to prevent escape of the rescuer's breath if the tube does not have an inflatable cuff.

Rate and Size of Breaths. Initially, four breaths are given in rapid succession without waiting for full expiration. The rescuer must always give large breaths, as some air leak is inevitable. But more importantly, exhaled air (i.e., the air you are breathing into the patient) contains only about 16 per cent oxygen compared to the 21 per cent oxygen available during normal breathing, so minute ventilation will have to be higher than normal to make up this deficit. *Minute ventilation* is the product of the size of the breath (tidal volume) times the frequency (rate) of respiration. Minute ventilation can be increased by either increasing the rate of breathing *or* the size of the breath. During CPR, however, the frequency of respiration is limited by the need to give cardiac compressions. Therefore, the necessary overall increase in minute ventilation (to make up the oxygen deficit) must come from an increase in the size of the breath given by the rescuer to the patient. The big breaths may also produce a respiratory alkalosis in the patient, by eliminating carbon dioxide faster than it is produced. This is a possible advantage to the patient, as it may partially compensate for any metabolic acidosis that is present.

When you are the only rescuer and cardiac compressions must be started, give two breaths in succession after every 15 compressions of the heart. The ratio for two rescuers is 5:1, i.e., five cardiac compressions followed by one breath. (Compression of the heart is discussed in *Circulation*, below.)

In some cases, opening the airway and giving artificial ventilation (at 12 to 15 breaths per minute) will be all that is necessary to restore consciousness. This is because the blood, although hypoxemic, is still circulating. If hypoxemia is reversed (by opening the airway and/or giving artificial ventilation) and the myocardium is reoxygenated, effective pumping action resumes before cardiac arrest occurs.

C: Circulation

While opening the victim's airway and giving the first breaths, the rescuer also feels for the victim's carotid pulse. If the pulse is absent or questionable, external heart compressions are started, i.e., artificial circulation.

> *The patient must be flat on his back on a hard surface for external cardiac compression to be effective.*

Artificial circulation is possible because the heart lies between the sternum and the vertebrae. Pressure on the pliable sternum "squeezes" the heart against the spine, forcing blood out of the heart into the aorta. The cross-section view of the chest in Figure 35–4 illustrates the anatomic location of the heart in relation to the spine and the sternum. If the patient sinks into a soft mattress (instead of being correctly placed on a hard surface), it is difficult to evaluate the amount of sternal depression ob-

tained during each compression. The patient must be horizontal because the blood pressure generated by external compression is not adequate to pump blood up to the head (when the patient is seated). Slide the victim to the floor if he is in a chair. If the victim is on a bed quickly look for a large, firm and flat object to slip under his thorax. A food tray often serves as a temporary board. If nothing is at hand, do not delay. Begin heart compressions promptly, and observe the chest carefully during compression to see that the sternum is actually being depressed about 1½ to 2 inches with each compression.

Hand Placement. Artificial circulation is maintained by rhythmic pressure applied to the lower third of the victim's sternum but not over the xiphoid process. Locate the xiphoid by running your lower hand up along the last rib to the notch where the ribs meet the sternum. Then place the heel of the other hand on the chest parallel to the long axis of the sternum, about 1 to 1½ inches above the palpating hand (toward the patient's head) (Fig. 35–5). The palpating hand is then placed on top of the hand which is resting on the sternum. The fingers are interlocked as shown in Figure 35–6 or otherwise held off the chest.

The force of the compression must be delivered directly below the heel of the hand for effective compression. If the fingers (or palm of the hand) are resting on the chest, the force is dissipated. Each cardiac compression must be applied quickly and released immediately and completely following sternal depression. This allows time for the heart to fill with blood before the next compression. Incorrect hand position is associated with an increased incidence of rib fractures. Lacerations of liver, spleen, and stomach by the xiphoid have also been reported.[5]

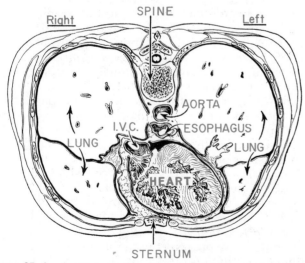

Figure 35–4. A cross section at the level of the lower sternum showing the location of the heart in relation to the sternum and the spine. (From Jude, J. R., et al.: Cardiac arrest. *Journal of the American Medical Association*, 178:1064, Dec. 1973.)

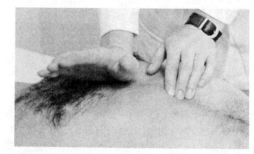

Figure 35–5. Locating correct position of hands for cardiac compression. The rescuer locates the xiphoid process first, then places the heel of the other hand on the victim's sternum 1 to 1½ inches above the xiphoid process. (From Pribble, A. H., and Tyler, M. L.: Emergency! Part 1: On-the-spot cardiopulmonary resuscitation. *Nursing '75, 5*:49, Feb. 1975.)

Correct hand placement is important. Too low, and the xiphoid process may be fractured and driven into the upper abdomen. Too high, and compressions are not effective because the upper sternum is rigid and very difficult to depress.

Position yourself as pictured in Figure 35–6, with your shoulders directly over the patient's chest. Most of the force of the compression can then be developed by the weight of your body as you rock forward, keeping your arms fully extended. If the rescuer is small, kneeling on the bed beside the victim is necessary, in addition to the addition of some muscular effort from the shoulders to depress the sternum sufficiently. The lower arms are not strong

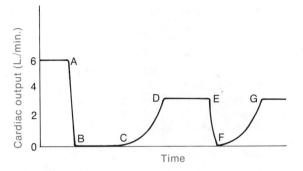

Figure 35–7. Effect of interrupted cardiac compression on cardiac output. At point A, ventricular fibrillation or asystole occurs and cardiac output falls to zero (B). Chest compressions begin at C, but several compressions are needed before cardiac output reaches a life-supporting level (D). Interruption of cardiac massage for ventilation at E results in immediate cessation of flow (F), and again, several compressions are needed to regain adequate cardiac output (G).

enough to keep up effective compression for long when flexion and extension of the elbow is used to depress the sternum. This technique is thus not advisable.

Rate of Compressions. When you are the only rescuer, give cardiac compressions at a rate of 80 per minute. In other words, one compression is given every 0.75 second. Interrupt the compressions after every 15 compressions to give two quick, deep lung inflations. This results in a cardiac compression–to–ventilation ratio of 15:2. Dölp has found that a 15:2 ratio given at a rate of 80 cardiac compressions per minute equals a "real work rate" of 53 compressions and 7 ventilations per minute.[4] The "real work rate" is lower than you might expect, but remember that time is lost with each change from cardiac compression to ventilation. Figure 35–7 illustrates the effect on cardiac output of interrupting cardiac compressions to ventilate the patient. It takes about five heart compressions to achieve an adequate level of cardiac output. The 80 per minute cardiac compression rate helps to make up for cardiac output lost during ventilation and thus must be maintained. This rate is difficult for a single rescuer to keep up for long. You should get help as soon as possible. In this situation, it is all right to *shout* for help in the normally "quiet" setting of the hospital.

When there are two rescuers, position yourselves as illustrated in Figure 35–8. Working on opposite sides of the victim keeps you out of

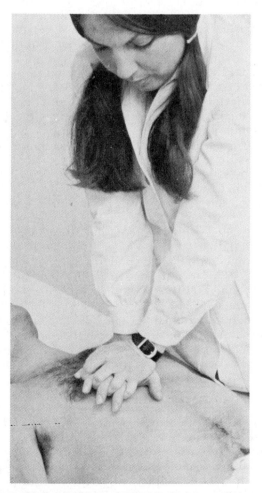

Figure 35–6. Position of rescuer during cardiac compression. The rescuer's shoulders and arms are directly over the victim's chest. This position provides the best mechanical advantage and is the least tiring for the rescuer during external cardiac compression. (From Pribble, A. H., and Tyler, M. L.: Emergency! Part 1: On-the-spot cardiopulmonary resuscitation. *Nursing '75, 5:*49, Feb. 1975.)

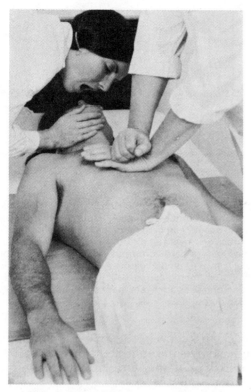

Figure 35–8. Cardiopulmonary resuscitation: two rescuers. When two rescuers are available, they position themselves on opposite sides of the patient so that they can switch from ventilating to cardiac compression without losing a beat. (From Pribble, A. H., and Tyler, M. L.: Emergency! Part 1: On-the-spot cardiopulmonary resuscitation. *Nursing '75, 5*:50, Feb. 1975.)

each other's way and facilitates the change from acting as "ventilator" to being "compressor." When two rescuers are available, one rescuer does external cardiac compression while the other does artificial ventilation. The compression to ventilation ratio is 5:1, i.e., five cardiac compressions to one ventilation. Compressions are given at a rate of 60 per minute. Breaths are given *between* cardiac compressions without interrupting or slowing the rate of compressions. Because no time is lost in changing from compression to ventilation, the "real work rate" equals 60 cardiac compressions and 12 ventilations per minute.[4] This coordinated effort obviously provides better maintenance of blood flow than the interrupted pattern of cardiac compression necessary when there is only one rescuer.

Switching from "compressor" to "ventilator" is accomplished in the following manner when the compressor tires. The "ventilator" gives a breath as usual after the fifth cardiac compression. Next, the "ventilator" starts counting out loud with the "compressor" and places her hands in the air next to the "compressor," in preparation for taking over the cardiac compressions. At about the third compression, the switch is made and the new person ventilating gets ready to give the next breath.

Assess Patient's Pulse and Pupils. If there are two rescuers, the person giving the artificial ventilation will have time to assess and partially confirm the adequacy of the cardiac compressions by palpating the carotid pulse. This should be done every couple of minutes and particularly after a new rescuer begins cardiac compressions.[19]

The pulse wave palpated at the carotid is actually a shock wave produced by cardiac compression and does not definitely confirm blood flow. However, without such a "shock wave" there is no possibility of blood flow. The carotid pulse is thus only a crude (although important) estimate of blood flow. Even feeling a "wave" of good volume does not confirm the effectiveness of the artificial circulation. Vigorous CPR can produce systolic blood pressures of more than 200 mm. Hg (the shock wave), but the diastolic pressure is always zero. Therefore, the mean arterial pressure, which is the true driving power of the circulation, is usually low.[6] (See Chapter 29 for a discussion of blood pressure.)

If you were able to check the size of the patient's pupils initially, a comparative change from dilated, fixed pupils to smaller or reactive pupils during CPR is a reassuring indication of adequate cerebral circulation. However, continued dilation of the pupils may be the result of some brain damage due to a delayed onset of CPR. This occurrence may be unavoidable, e.g., when CPR is started upon discovery of a patient who has been unconscious for an unknown amount of time. The brain damage is not necessarily permanent. Generally, CPR efforts are not terminated on the basis of continued fixed dilation of the pupils alone.

WITNESSED CARDIAC ARREST

If you happen to be *present* when a patient suddenly collapses, use the following technique. It is only slightly different from the usual A-B-C method of cardiopulmonary resuscitation. This "witnessed arrest" technique is also used in coronary or intensive care units where asystole (cardiac standstill) or ventricular fibrillation can be observed on bedside cardiac monitors. Ventricular fibrillation is an ineffectual quivering of the ventricles, which is incapable of circulating blood.

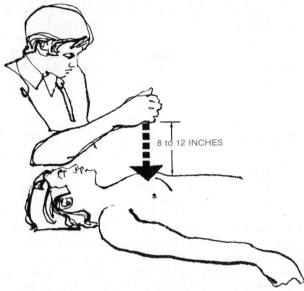

8 to 12 INCHES

Figure 35–9. Precordial thump. A precordial thump is used only in a witnessed or monitored arrest. The blow sometimes restores the heart beat if the myocardium is not anoxic. (Reprinted from the Supplement to Journal of the American Medical Assoc., Feb. 18, 1974. Copyright, 1974, The American Medical Assoc. Reprinted with permission of the American Heart Assoc.)

As usual, the first step is opening the patient's airway, using the head-tilt method described previously. Simultaneously, the carotid pulse is palpated; if absent, give a *single* precordial thump (described below). Next, if the patient is not breathing, give four quick breaths. If these three actions do not restore carotid pulse and breathing *immediately*, start cardiac compression and artificial ventilation at the rates and ratios already described, depending on the presence of one or two rescuers.

The precordial thump is a sharp blow delivered to the patient's midsternum by the rescuer's fist. Strike chest from a height of 8 to 12 inches with the fleshy part of the fist, as illustrated in Figure 35–9. To be effective, the blow must be delivered *within a minute of cardiac arrest*. It is used in a witnessed arrest because it is hoped that the blow will stimulate cardiac activity (restart normal heart beat) in a heart that has not yet become anoxic. The blow generates a small electrical impulse in a reactive (oxygenated) heart that may restore heart beat in ventricular asystole or may organize the chaotic beat in ventricular fibrillation. In an *anoxic* but still *beating* heart, however, a precordial thump may do the opposite and actually precipitate ventricular fibrillation.[19, 22] Therefore, the precordial thump is not advised when the length of time since cardiac arrest is unknown (unwitnessed arrest). The precordial thump is not a substitute for cardiac compression. If a single blow is not effective, CPR must not be delayed.

PERFORMANCE ERRORS AND PROBLEMS IN CPR

Each step of the A-B-C sequence is associated with potential problems and/or errors in performance. Practice can eliminate most performance errors. In addition, knowledge of the type of problems frequently encountered during CPR is helpful in anticipating and preventing problems before they develop.

Continued Airway Obstruction

Extreme resistance to ventilation or failure of the patient's chest to rise during artificial ventilation often indicates airway obstruction. Carefully check the victim's head and jaw position; his tongue may still be obstructing the airway. Remember to lift the jaw in addition to the head-tilt maneuver if you are having trouble. If these actions fail to solve the problem, inspect the oropharynx for food, vomitus or foreign bodies. If any of these materials are observed, turn the patient to the side and use one or two fingers to scoop material out of the airway, then quickly try another breath. If ventilation is still inadequate, try a blow to the middle of the victim's back with the patient turned towards you. The blow may dislodge a laryngeal obstruction (often a piece of food) that was not visible during your inspection. Repeated rapid attempts to ventilate and clear the airway must be made, as it is vital to establish ventilation.

When oxygen is immediately available, it should be administered to the patient when mouth-to-mouth ventilation is unsuccessful. If the airway is not completely blocked, oxygen may be able to get into the lung (and eventually the blood) by the process of diffusion rather than by being carried in by ventilation.[1] Cardiac compression must be continued, of course, to circulate the blood. The expert help of a skilled CPR team and possibly tracheal intubation (a technique of advanced life support) are better solutions.

Failure of Chest to Rise

Obstruction of the upper airway may be the cause of failure of the patient's chest to rise during artificial ventilation; however, there are other possible causes.

Be sure your mouth is forming a good seal with the victim's mouth, and that most of the air is not escaping. The usual cause of inadequate seal is squeamishness. Remember, while the tight mouth-to-mouth contact may be uncomfortable for you, lack of it may be fatal to the patient. As you work to improve the seal, check the size of your rescue breaths. You will have to take larger than normal breaths yourself to be able to give the patient the big breath he needs. However, don't continue to take large breaths after you have delivered the patient's breath(s). You may become dizzy due to hyperventilation. Breathe normally between giving rescue breaths.

Occasionally, a patient will have "stiff" lungs that are very resistive to ventilation. In fact, this may be the underlying cause of the patient's respiratory and cardiac failures. Examples of conditions resulting in stiff lungs are: (a) asthma attacks characterized by very severe bronchospasm (constriction of the bronchi due to muscle spasm), (b) pulmonary edema (fluid in the interstitial spaces of the lung) or (c) pulmonary fibrosis (scarring of the connective tissue framework of the lung). All of these conditions result in lungs that are very difficult to ventilate. The rescuer will have to blow very hard. In fact, it may be impossible to ventilate such a patient without a cuffed endotracheal tube in place.

Failure to Feel Carotid Pulse

Insufficient cardiac compression is a common cause for failing to detect carotid pulse waves. Is the sternum actually being depressed 1½ to 2 inches? Are your hands too high on the sternum or are you just not using enough force? The small rescuer will have to get squarely over the victim and use back and shoulder muscle in addition to body weight. Be sure to practice cardiac compressions with a training mannikin. Practice gives you the "feel" of the compression force necessary to provide adequate artificial circulation.

Sometimes the carotid pulse wave is dampened because the pressure of the cardiac compression is not completely relaxed between compressions. This restricts cardiac filling and decreases the amount of blood that is ejected with each subsequent compression. Incomplete release of pressure on the chest is most likely to occur as the rescuer tires. When tired, there is a tendency to lean on the patient between compressions. The general rule is that

it is best not to remove the rescuer's hands from the chest after locating the correct hand placement position. However, some CPR experts feel that a sudden, total removal of the hands from the chest wall enhances cardiac filling by assuring complete release of pressure on the heart.[15]

Exhaustion of Rescuer

Errors in performing the various steps of CPR are the most frequent cause of rescuer exhaustion during CPR. Some examples of performance errors are (a) flexing and extending the lower arms during cardiac compression, (b) continued deep breathing between rescue breaths resulting in self-induced hyperventilation, (c) failure to kneel on the bed so that your shoulders are directly over the patient and (d) working on too soft a surface, which means extra effort must be expended in depressing the patient's sternum. All these errors increase the work of the rescuer during CPR and lead to premature exhaustion.

COMPLICATIONS OF CPR

When a patient has had a recent neck injury, hyperextension of his head during airway management is contraindicated. Hyperextension of the neck may *damage the spinal cord* by dislodging an unstable vertebrae or vetebral fragment. A strong jaw-thrust is substituted to open the victim's airway. However, this maneuver requires two rescuers, as it is impossible for a single rescuer to keep the victim's jaw in place while compressing the chest. Therefore, you must get help to perform CPR effectively on a patient with a recent neck injury.

Gastric distention with air is a significant problem during CPR for several reasons: (a) it can result in rupture of the patient's stomach (gastric rupture); (b) it often triggers *vomiting;* (c) if severe, it can impede movements of the diaphragm thus compromising ventilation and (d) gastric dilatation is associated with increased vagal tone, which can cause reflex *bradycardia* (slow heart beat) and *hypotension.* Severe gastric distention that needs to be treated can be observed as a bulge in the patient's abdomen just below the rib cage. Gentle abdominal pressure applied by the rescuer over the patient's stomach may cause the air to "belch" out. However, be careful because gastric rupture or vomiting can also occur.

Gastric distention occurs most often when a patient's lungs are difficult to ventilate. It can also occur when cardiac compressions and ventilation are mistimed and occur simultaneously. The esophagus and cardiac sphincter open when a pressure above 15 to 20 cm. H_2O is applied.[18] This pressure is often exceeded during artificial ventilation. If the victim's lungs are stiff with bronchospasm, or worse yet (because it is preventable), if the patient's tongue has fallen back blocking his glottis, this pressure is easily exceeded. In both of these situations, it is easier for the air to go into the stomach than the lungs. The stomach fills with air and the chest fails to rise.

Aspiration is a likely complication if vomiting occurs during CPR, because the patient is without gag reflex or cough. In addition, he is positioned flat on his back. Aspiration of gastric contents may cause immediate problems with *mechanical blockage of the patient's upper or lower airways* and/or later problem of *aspiration pneumonia*, particularly if the gastric contents have a low pH.

Incorrect hand placement during CPR increases the incidence of *rib* and *xiphoid fractures*. While the fractures in themselves are often not serious, the damage the fractured pieces can inflict is often very serious. For example, *intrathoracic or intra-abdominal hemorrhage* or *pneumothorax* (air trapped in pleural space) from lacerations caused by a fractured xiphoid process or rib is not uncommon.

Myocardial contusion (bruising of heart muscle), *hemopericardium* (blood in the pericardial sac) and *myocardial rupture* (rupture of the heart muscle) have also been reported.[5] However, fear of inflicting these injuries should not prevent you from following established guidelines and carrying out CPR to the best of your ability. A complication-free patient may be a dead victim of cardiopulmonary arrest.

Termination of Basic Life Support

Most often, your primary responsibility for the A-B-C of basic life support will end at the arrival of more skilled help or the CPR team. You may feel "let-down"; however, you can still help by relaying to the team the time sequence and events occurring before their arrival. Often, you will also continue to help by keeping records for the rest of the CPR episode.

Another terminating event is the restoration of *spontaneous respiration and/or circulation*. Signs of restored ventilation or circulation are (a) struggling movements (although these may also occur during effective CPR), (b) decrease in pupil size, (c) improved color, (d) change in the quality of the pulse and (e) the return of systemic blood pressure.

If you are entirely alone (seldom the case in the hospital setting), *complete exhaustion* may of necessity cause you to stop CPR. You

will probably have some feelings of guilt if this occurs, but these feelings should not be exaggerated.[10] You will have the satisfaction of knowing you tried. You should realize that two large studies have shown that only 16 to 17 per cent of patients requiring CPR are discharged home.[20, 22] Jude[9] reported a 24 per cent cardiac arrest survival rate while another, smaller, study had a 28 per cent discharge rate.[14] This latter study also looked at the CPR success rates for victims in Intensive Care Units (ICU) (47 per cent) versus those on regular nursing care floors (39 per cent). The influence of the time of day or night that the arrest occurred on CPR success was also examined with the following results: 7 AM to 3 PM (40 per cent), 3 PM to 11 PM (31 per cent), and 11 PM to 7 AM (45 per cent). Obviously, ICU units (lots of sophisticated equipment) and daylight (more people available) are not necessary for successful CPR.

On occasion, a medical decision to stop CPR without going on to advanced life support techniques is made due to the *nature of the patient's underlying disease or condition*. Often these decisions are made beforehand by patient and family in consultation with the physician; however, there is disagreement about the legal advisability of making a notation of a plan not to resuscitate on the chart.[13, 14] The student nurse is often not a party to these tacit agreements and so is ethically and legally bound to initiate CPR on discovery or witness of sudden and (to the student) unforeseen cardiac or respiratory arrest.

ADVANCED LIFE SUPPORT

Advanced life support includes: (a) basic life support, (b) use of special equipment such as bag-mask resuscitators and endotracheal tubes, (c) cardiac monitoring, (d) cardiac defibrillation, (e) establishing intravenous lines, (f) definitive therapy of acidosis, cardiac rhythm and circulation and (g) general stabilization of the patient's condition.[19] The role of the nursing student during administration of advanced life support may be, as noted above, to be timekeeper and note taker. The details of advanced life support may be read about in *Fundamentals of Cardiopulmonary Resuscitation* by Jude and Elam,[8] *Cardio-respiratory Resuscitation* by Gilston and Resnekov[6] and in *Standards for Cardiopulmonary Resuscitation (CPR) and Emergency Cardiac Care (ECC)*.[19]

In addition, many of the references cited at the end of the chapter contain material about advanced life support techniques.

HELPING THE PATIENT'S SIGNIFICANT OTHERS

One of the most significant contributions the nurse can make, after being relieved of the basic life support role, is to talk to the patient's significant others. Explain to them what is going on, without giving false hope, and encourage expression of their feelings. These feelings may include fear and anxiety and perhaps indignation at having been "pushed aside" at this most crucial time. The patient's significant others may also feel guilty about not having called for help or not having brought the patient to the hospital sooner. Guilt may also be expressed over not seeking medical advice "soon enough." Your natural tendency is to want to absolve these feelings of guilt, but often you will have too little information to do so with confidence. The family members will know this, and you will lose their confidence if you say empty comforting words. Reflective techniques of drawing out feelings without comment or judgment are best used at this time, with "absolution" left to the physician (if it is appropriate). (See Chap. 3 for discussion of the therapeutic nurse-patient relationship.)

19. BASIC CARDIOPULMONARY RESUSCITATION (CPR)

Definition and Purpose.   *First aid procedures, including recognition and treatment of circulatory or respiratory arrest, capable of maintaining life until advanced life support is available.* Used to provide artificial ventilation and artificial circulation to the victim of cardiac and/or respiratory arrest. Nurse modifies procedure depending on the presence of one or two rescuers and the nature of the arrest, e.g., respiratory arrest (without circulatory arrest) or witnessed cardiac arrest.

Contraindications.   Patient should not be resuscitated when a medical decision not to resuscitate has been *noted* in the patient's chart.

Patient-Family Teaching Points.   Because of the emergency nature of this procedure, the nurse will seldom have the opportunity to explain the procedure to the patient prior to its use. The family, however, will need to be provided with the following information as appropriate. If the family is present at the time of the arrest explain: (a) why the patient is receiving such apparently "rough" treatment, e.g., being put on the floor; (b) the necessity of having a hard surface under the patient's thorax; (c) the expected results of artificial ventilation and circulation; (d) why the rescuers are counting together; (e) why it is necessary to push "so hard" on the sternum; (f) emphasize that struggling motions made by the victim are a good sign but that they do not necessarily indicate that the emergency is over; (g) tell the family that they were asked to leave the room because the rescuers need room to work and to lessen the distraction and (h) family members may be taught CPR if living with a person who may arrest.

PRE-PROCEDURE ACTIVITIES

PRELIMINARY PLANNING	PRELIMINARY ASSESSMENT
▶ Know the code words for cardiopulmonary arrest used in the setting in which you work, e.g., "Code 99"	Includes determining if patient has: diagnosis frequently associated with sudden cardiac arrest or respiratory failure or previous history of cardiac arrest.

PRELIMINARY PLANNING

▶ Note the locations of emergency buzzers, e.g., in patient rooms, bathrooms
▶ Know the special telephone number for reaching the operator who calls the CPR team
▶ Periodically practice CPR technique with a training mannikin and skilled instructor
▶ Clarify with nursing team members whether specific patients in your care are or are not to have CPR if sudden cardiac or respiratory arrest occurs

EQUIPMENT

▶ No equipment is *absolutely* required for effective performance of cardiopulmonary resuscitation (CPR).
▶ Cardiac arrest board desirable if patient is in bed or on other soft surface.

PREPARATION OF PATIENT

Not possible due to sudden nature of cardiopulmonary arrest.

PROCEDURE FOR UNWITNESSED CARDIOPULMONARY ARREST

SUGGESTED STEPS

I. Diagnostic Actions

To rapidly determine presence of cardiopulmonary arrest in patient who suddenly collapses or is unexpectedly found unconscious.

1. Shake patient and call name loudly.

2. Check the patient for the following signs confirming cardiopulmonary arrest:

a. Absent or inadequate respiratory motions.

▶ Remove or push aside clothing over patient's chest.
▶ Place your cheek close to patient's nose and mouth.
▶ Observe patient's chest and upper abdomen for respiratory motions.
▶ Check for retraction of soft tissues in patient's suprasternal and intercostal spaces.

b. Absence of major pulses (carotid or femoral).

▶ Palpate for carotid or femoral pulses.

RATIONALE/ASSESSMENT

I. Diagnostic Rationale

The success of CPR depends largely on the speed with which basic life support measures are effectively initiated.

1. To assess state of consciousness. Do this quickly and only once while you move into position for further assessment.

2. Prompt treatment is based on rapid, accurate recognition of respiratory or cardiac arrest.

a. Assess ventilation first. Correction of respiratory arrest may prevent subsequent cardiac arrest.

▶ Must have unobstructed view for proper assessment.
▶ To "feel" patient's exhalations—if present.
▶ Absence of motion confirms *respiratory arrest.*
▶ Retractions indicate airway obstruction.

b. Central pulses, i.e., the pulses in large arteries close to the heart, are palpable when more peripheral pulses, e.g., radial artery, are no longer palpable.

Procedure continued on the following page

SUGGESTED STEPS	RATIONALE/ASSESSMENT

Unwitnessed Arrest—Diagnosis (Continued)

▶ Preferably check carotid pulse.	▶ Carotid pulse is most easily checked because rescuer is already at patient's head (having just checked patient's breathing). Also, patient's clothing does not need to be removed to check carotid pulse. Tight clothing at patient's neck should be loosened, however. ▶ Absence of pulse indicates cardiac arrest.
c. Dilated pupils	c. Cerebral hypoxia (lack of O_2 to brain) causes loss of muscle control in entire body, including eyes.
▶ Raise patient's eyelids and observe pupil sizes and reactivity to light.	▶ Pupils that are dilated and do not react to light (fixed) indicate that brain centers controlling motion of the iris of the eye are not receiving enough O_2 to cause normal (constricting) response of the iris to light.

II. Treatment Actions—One Rescuer

II. Treatment Rationale—One Rescuer

1. Call loudly for help as soon as you confirm or even strongly suspect either respiratory or cardiac arrest.

1. CPR is much more efficient with two rescuers. Other assistants can summon expert help, which you may not be able to do from your position by the patient.

2. Roll victim flat onto his back.

2. The victim must be in this position for airway management and external cardiac compressions.

3. Remove pillows from under victim's head and neck.

3. Flexion of neck may cause or add to upper airway obstruction.

A – Airway

4. Open airway by tilting victim's head backwards as far as possible by: (a) lifting under back of his neck with one hand while (b) pressing down on his forehead with your other hand.

4. Relaxed muscle tone present in cardiopulmonary arrest: (a) causes slack jaw muscles and (b) allows the tongue to fall to the back of the throat and obstruct the airway. Correction of airway obstruction may restore spontaneous respiration and prevent subsequent cardiac arrest.

▶ Assess patient to see if ventilation has been restored. Can you feel victim's breath on your cheek or see his chest rise, or (if patient was making respiratory motions) have chest retractions decreased?

SUGGESTED STEPS   RATIONALE/ASSESSMENT

Unwitnessed Arrest—One Rescuer (Continued)

▶ Clear airway of obvious foreign matter, e.g., vomitus, *only if obstruction has not been relieved* by the above maneuvers. You may be wasting valuable time unnecessarily.

5. Pull victim's jaw forward with hand previously used to lift neck.

5. *Necessary only if retractions continue* following head tilt or if the victim is difficult to ventilate.

a. The fingers are placed under the lower jaw on the bony part near the chin; the thumb is used only to depress the lower lip, not to lift the chin. The jaw should be lifted so that the teeth are nearly brought together.

B – Breathing

6. Begin artificial ventilation *immediately* by appropriate route (see below) if respirations are absent or inadequate.

6. Lack of ventilation rapidly leads to severe hypoxemia (and hypercapnea), which in turn may result in brain damage, cardiac arrest and death. Rescuer's expired air supplies the ventilation needed to support victim's oxygen requirements and carbon dioxide elimination needs.

a. *Mouth-to-mouth ventilation*

a. *Mouth-to-mouth ventilation*

▶ Maintain victim's head tilt.
▶ Take in a *large* breath, about 1000 to 1500 ml.

▶ To keep airway open.
▶ You will breathe this air back into victim's lungs. Your exhaled air doesn't contain as much oxygen as normal inhaled breaths; thus you need to breathe into patient a breath two to three times larger than he would normally breathe in.
▶ To prevent air leaks.

▶ Place your mouth *tightly* over the victim's mouth and *pinch* his nostrils.
▶ Blow air from your lungs into victim's lung, then remove your mouth to allow air to escape. (Thus you permit patient to artificially inhale and exhale.)

▶ Assess adequacy of artificial ventilation by: (a) watching chest rise, (b) feeling in your lung compliance or "give" of victim's lungs as they open and (c) feeling the air exhaling from the victim.

b. *Mouth-to-nose ventilation*

b. *Mouth-to-nose ventilation*

Used when victim's mouth cannot be opened or seal cannot be made for mouth-to-mouth ventilation.
▶ Maintain victim's head tilt.
▶ To keep airway open.

Procedure continued on the following page

SUGGESTED STEPS	RATIONALE/ASSESSMENT

Unwitnessed Arrest—One Rescuer (Continued)

▶ Place your mouth tightly over victim's nose while holding his mouth closed if necessary.	▶ To prevent air leaks. All other steps are the same as in mouth-to-mouth ventilation.
c. *Mouth-to-stoma ventilation*	c. *Mouth-to-stoma ventilation* Occasionally a victim will have had surgery removing the larynx ("voice box"). He will have a permanent opening in the neck, called a *stoma*. Ventilation must be applied directly into this opening as the upper airway (via nose and mouth) is no longer connected to the lower airway (i.e., tracheobronchial tree and lungs).
d. *Mouth-to-tracheostomy tube ventilation*	d. *Mouth-to-tracheostomy tube ventilation* A tracheostomy tube also must be ventilated directly, as it bypasses the upper airway.
▶ Hold the victim's mouth and nose closed when ventilating through an uncuffed tracheostomy tube.	▶ Air will escape from victim's nose or mouth unless upper airway is sealed off by inflated cuff.
7. Give the victim *four rapid breaths*.	7. To rapidly reoxygenate blood prior to starting artificial circulation. Do not wait for complete exhalation of each breath. It is vital to begin external cardiac compressions as soon as possible.
8. Continue artificial ventilation at rate of 12 to 15 breaths per minute if respiratory arrest is only problem.	8. This rate is maintained only if external cardiac compression is not needed. Continue to assess pulse while ventilating.
9. If pulse cannot be felt, begin external cardiac compression.	9. Compression will help circulate the blood.

C – Circulation

10. Begin external cardiac compression immediately following initial four rapid breaths.	10. Tissue hypoxia will cause irreversible brain damage if adequate circulation is not restored within 3 to 4 minutes.
a. With the middle and index fingers of the lower hand, locate the lower margin of the victim's rib cage on the side next to you. Then run your fingers up along the rib cage to the notch where the ribs meet the sternum in the center of the lower chest. (If the patient is obese and the ribs cannot be felt, you should locate the xiphoid	a. Sternum is flexible here and heart lies directly below. (See Figure 35–4.)

SUGGESTED STEPS

RATIONALE/ASSESSMENT

Unwitnessed Arrest—One Rescuer (*Continued*)

process and continue as follows.) With one finger on the notch, the other finger is placed next to it on the lower end of the sternum.

b. Place the heel of the other hand on the lower half of the sternum above the finger of the palpating hand. Keep fingers and palm off the chest and apply force only with the heel of the hand.

c. Remove the first hand and place it on top of the hand on the sternum. Both hands should be parallel and aimed away from you. The fingers may be extended or interlaced as long as they are kept off the chest.

▶ To provide added strength.
▶ If the whole hand is flat on the chest, the force of the compression is dissipated to the ribs instead of being applied directly below to the heart.
▶ Note hand position in Figure 35–6.

d. Straighten your arms by locking your elbows. Lean forward until your shoulders are directly over your hands; in this way the weight of the back adds pressure for chest compression. Applying pressure with both hands, depress patient's sternum 1½ to 2 inches with each compression.

d. Circulation is maintained as blood is squeezed from the heart with each compression.

e. Release pressure on sternum *quickly* and *completely* following each compression.

e. Allows time for the heart to fill with blood before next compression.

11. Continue external cardiac compressions at a rate of 80 per minute, giving 2 quick, full breaths following every 15 compressions.

11. A single rescuer must provide both artificial ventilation and circulation and must therefore work very rapidly.

12. Periodically assess victim's status.

12. Assessing circulation is difficult for one rescuer. Improvement of color and return of spontaneous motion are the only observations possible in this situation.

III. Treatment Actions—Two Rescuers

III. Treatment Rationale—Two Rescuers

1. Cardiac compressions are given at a rate of 60 per minute, with no interruption for ventilation.

1. Uninterrupted cardiac compression provides victim with more even flow of blood (see Figure 35–7).

2. Ventilation is provided by the second rescuer. One breath is given to the victim following every fifth cardiac compression.

2. The breath is given quickly, between compressions.

Procedure continued on the following page

SUGGESTED STEPS	RATIONALE/ASSESSMENT

Unwitnessed Arrest—Two Rescuers (Continued)

3. Periodically assess victim's status.	3. Assessment of the victim's status is done by the person ventilating, who periodically checks the carotid pulse and the pupils.
4. Continue artificial ventilation and external cardiac compression as necessary.	4. CPR is continued until: (a) effective spontaneous ventilation and circulation are restored; (b) CPR team takes over basic life support and/or begins advanced life support actions; or (c) rescuer is exhausted and unable to continue resuscitation.

Post-Procedure Activities.   Change over smoothly to compression and ventilation by the CPR team when they arrive. Or, discontinue CPR if spontaneous ventilation and circulation return. In this case the patient will require close observation and frequent assessment.

Charting/Reporting.   Includes: (a) time victim discovered, (b) type of arrest (respiratory and/or cardiac), (c) any complications during CPR, e.g., vomiting, (d) time CPR team arrived, (e) time spontaneous ventilation or pulse returned, (f) time CPR discontinued if rescuer became exhausted or (g) time decision was made to stop CPR because it was futile.

PROCEDURE FOR WITNESSED CARDIAC ARREST

SUGGESTED STEPS	RATIONALE/ASSESSMENT
A "witnessed" cardiac arrest, as the name implies, is an arrest that occurs in your presence.	Cardiac arrest is suspected whenever a patient suddenly collapses or becomes unconscious. Cardiac standstill or ventricular fibrillation causes almost immediate unconsciousness. Respiratory arrest follows unconsciousness if circulation is not quickly restored.
A. *Sequence of actions* for CPR for victim whose cardiac arrest was witnessed.	A. The sequence of resuscitative actions is altered in witnessed cardiac arrest because witnessing the arrest allows you to take action before the heart muscle becomes anoxic.

   1. Open airway (technique previously described)

   2. Assess carotid pulse.

   3. Give one precordial thump if carotid pulse absent.

   4. Reassess carotid pulse and respirations.

   5. Start CPR immediately if carotid pulse and respirations still absent.

SUGGESTED STEPS	RATIONALE/ASSESSMENT

Precordial Thump Technique

B. *Precordial thump technique*

B. See Figure 35–9 for illustration of this technique.

1. Deliver a sharp, quick single blow to victim's midsternum, using the fleshy portion of your fist.

1. The precordial thump generates a small current of electricity which sometimes "shocks" the myocardium into: (a) beating again following cardiac asystole or (b) "reorganizing" the chaotic beat of ventricular fibrillation. In either case (asystole or fibrillation) when a precordial thump is successful adequate cardiac pumping action is restored and blood circulation resumes.

2. Assess response to precordial thump immediately.

2. Carotid pulse should be palpable immediately if blow was successful.

3. If victim's heart beat and respirations are not restored immediately, *do not* repeat the blow. Begin CPR (as previously described) without delay.

3. Only one attempt is made to stimulate cardiac activity with the precordial thump because the myocardium rapidly becomes anoxic when circulation is inadequate, and consequently, the myocardium becomes less and less responsive to the blow. Circulation and respiration must be re-established using standard CPR methods without further delay.

4. Continue artificial ventilation and external cardiac compression as necessary.

4. CPR is continued until: (a) effective spontaneous ventilation and circulation is restored; (b) CPR team takes over basic life support and/or begins advanced life support actions or (c) rescuer is exhausted and unable to continue resuscitation.

Post-Procedure Activities. Change over smoothly to compression and ventilation by the CPR team when they arrive. Or, discontinue CPR if spontaneous ventilation and circulation return. In this case, the patient will require close observation and frequent assessment.

Charting/Reporting. Includes: (a) time victim discovered, (b) type of arrest (respiratory and/or cardiac), (c) any complications during CPR, e.g., vomiting, (d) time CPR team arrived, (e) time spontaneous ventilation or pulse returned, (f) time CPR discontinued if rescuer became exhausted or (g) time decision was made to stop CPR because it was futile.

BIBLIOGRAPHY

a. Add cerebral to CPR. *Emergency Medicine*, 9:159, June 1977.

b. Advanced life support. *American Journal of Nursing*, 75:242, Feb. 1975.

c. Allcock, M., and Wilson, S.: "Code 66." From anxious "amateurs" to smooth-working code team. *Nursing '75*, 5:7, Nov. 1975.

d. Ask an expert: IV bicarb before defibrillation? *Emergency Medicine*, 9:115, Feb. 1977.

1. Bartlett, R. G., Jr., Brubach, H. F., and Specht, H.: Demonstration of aventilatory mass flow during ventilation and apnea in man. *Journal of Applied Physiology*, 14:97, 1959.

2. Bradley, D.: Cardiac and respiratory arrest. *Nursing Times*, 71:1367, Aug. 1975.

3. Carden, E., and Hughes, T.: An evaluation of manually operated self-inflating resuscitation bags. *Anesthesia and Analgesia*, 54:133, Jan.–Feb. 1975.

3a. Coodley, E. L. (ed.): Therapeutic conference. Problem: cardiac and respiratory arrest. *Emergency Medicine*, 10:166, May 1978.

3b. Davis, A. J.: Code 45. *American Journal of Nursing*, 77:627, April 1977.

3c. DeLaurentis, D. A.: Resuscitation in the injured patient: do's and dont's. *Hospital Medicine*, 14:82, June 1978.

4. Dölp, F., et al.: Cardiopulmonary resuscitation techniques: experimental tests related to clinical recommendations. *Resuscitation*, 3:95, Feb. 1974.

5. Enarson, D. A., and Gracey, D. R.: Complications of cardiopulmonary resuscitation. *Heart and Lung*, 5:805, Sep.–Oct. 1976.

5a. Geolot, D., et al.: Cardiopulmonary resuscitation. *Nurse Practitioner*, 3:24, May–June 1978.

6. Gilston, A., and Resnekov, L.: *Cardio-respiratory Resuscitation*. Philadelphia, F. A. Davis Co., 1971.

7. Harken, D. E.: *In* letters to the editor. *Heart and Lung*, 4:972, Nov.–Dec. 1975.

8. Jude, J. R., and Elam, J. O.: *Fundamentals of Cardiopulmonary Resuscitation*. Philadelphia, F. A. Davis Co., 1965.

9. Jude, J. R., Kouwenhoven, W. B., and Knickerbocker, G. G.: Cardiac arrest. *Journal of the American Medical Association*, 178:1063, Dec. 1973.

10. Klute, C. G.: I can't quit now! *Canadian Nurse*, 71:38, March 1975.

11. Kouwenhoven, W. B., et al.: Closed-chest cardiac massage. *Journal of the American Medical Association*, 173:1064, July 1960.

11a. Lee, A.: The Lazarus syndrome: caring for patients who've "returned from the dead." *RN*, 41:53, June 1978.

12. Loeb, J. S.: Cardiac arrest. *Journal of the American Medical Association*, 238:845, May 1975.

13. McCarthy, D.: The use and abuse of cardiopulmonary resuscitation. *Hospital Progress*, 56:64, April 1975.

13a. Noone, R. B.: The airway in the injured patient: guide to emergency management. *Hospital Medicine*, 12:94, April 1976.

13b. Palen, C. S.: The passage. *American Journal of Nursing*, 75:2004, Nov. 1975.

14. Parson, W. R.: An evaluation of emergency cardiopulmonary resuscitation procedures in a teaching hospital. *American Surgeon*, 41:546, Sep. 1975.

14a. Patterson, A.: Keeping in trim for "Code Blue." *Supervisor Nurse*, 7:12–14, May 1976.

15. Pribble, A. H., and Tyler, M. L.: Emergency! Part 1: on-the-spot cardiopulmonary resuscitation. *Nursing '75*, 5:45, Feb. 1975.

15a. Resuscitation, Houston style. *Emergency Medicine*, 9:223, May 1977.

16. Safar, P., et al.: A comparison of mouth-to-mouth and mouth-to-airway methods of artificial respiration with the chest pressure arm-lift methods. *New England Journal of Medicine*, 258:671, April 1958.

17. Safar, P., et al.: Teaching and organizing cardiopulmonary resuscitation. *Clinical Anesthesia*, 10:161, 1974.

18. Spence, A. A., Moir, D. D., and Finlay, W. E. I.: Observations on intragastric pressure. *Anaesthesia*, 22:249, 1967.

19. Standards for cardiopulmonary resuscitation (CPR) and emergency cardiac care (ECC). *Journal of the American Medical Association*, 227 Suppl.:833, Feb. 1974.

19a. Stanley, L.: The near drowning victim: CPR is not enough. *RN*, 41:41–44, June 1978.

20. Stephenson, H. E.: *Cardiac Arrest and Resuscitation*. St. Louis, C. V. Mosby Co., 1969.

21. Ungvarski, P. J., Argondizzo, N. T., and Boos, P. K.: CPR: current practice revised. *American Journal of Nursing*, 75:236, Feb. 1975.

22. Vijay, N. K., and Schoonmaker, F. W.: Cardiopulmonary arrest and resuscitation. *American Family Physician*, 12:85, Aug. 1975.

23. West, J. B.: *Respiratory Physiology: The Essentials*. Baltimore, Williams and Wilkins Co., 1974.

CHAPTER 36

SUPPORTING RESPIRATORY FUNCTION

By Rosemary Jo Craig, B.S., R.N., C.R.T.T., R.R.T.

INTRODUCTION AND STUDY GUIDE

The respiratory system and the cardiovascular system work together to nourish the body with oxygen and remove the waste products of metabolism (e.g., carbon dioxide). Everyone is affected with some form of respiratory dysfunction at some time in his life. For many persons, this only means "acute upper respiratory infections"—usually common colds. Other persons are afflicted with more serious types of acute or chronic respiratory dysfunction. For detailed discussions of respiratory disorders, you can refer to many texts* that deal in depth with respiratory dysfunctions, their prevention and treatment. This chapter deals with the respiratory dysfunctions and therapeutic modalities the nurse commonly encounters in non-critical care situations. Respiratory dysfunction is found in patients in all types of patient care facilities. The directions in which the care of these patients are moving are exciting and promise many changes.

In the past, the care of patients with respiratory dysfunctions was delegated solely to the nursing staff. As medicine developed more awareness of respiratory disorders and as mechanical means of therapy were developed, nurses often delegated the operation of respiratory equipment to orderlies or aides. These persons were typically called "Oxygen Orderlies" or "Oxygen Therapists" and spent much of their time moving heavy cylinders of oxygen and giving breathing treatments with the newly marketed and somewhat mysterious respirators.

The advent of aviation medicine and polio outbreak of the early 1950's accelerated the production of advanced types of respirators and other respiratory equipment. Since that time, the paramedical specialty known as *Respiratory Therapy* has developed.

Nurses continue to care for patients with respiratory disorders. However, the care of such patients is often shared with persons who have advanced specialized training in Respiratory Therapy. Currently a variety of health care personnel participate in the specialized field of Respiratory Therapy. Some Registered Nurses, Licensed Practical Nurses and Physical Therapists have taken advanced training and are recognized by the National Board for Respiratory Therapy (NBRT) as either *Registered Respiratory Therapists* (RRT) or *Certified Respiratory Therapy Technicians* (CRTT). The background and experience of these respiratory specialists is valuable to other members of the health care team in providing the best possible care for their patients with dysfunctions of the respiratory system.

This chapter discusses the causes of respiratory system dysfunction and the basic forms of therapy the nurse must be aware of—mobilization maneuvers, hydration, oxygen administration, medication, positive pressure breathing treatments, suctioning of the airways, and respiratory exercises. Detailed *Procedures* are presented for oxygen administration and tracheobronchial suctioning.

The field of pulmonary medicine, like all other specialties, has many terms and symbols specific to its specialty. As you read this chapter you should become aware of the following terms:

ventilation	perfusion
P_{O_2}	hypoventilation
P_{CO_2}	hydration
arterial	humidification
alveolar	nebulization
hypoxia	IPPB
hypercapnia	COPD
hypoxemia	cyanosis
dyspnea	sputum
hypoxic drive	arterial blood gas
inspiration	nasal airway
inhalation	oral airway
exhalation	aspiration
expiration	rales
diaphragm	rhonchi
tidal volume	wheeze

---

*For example, refer to Luckmann, J., and Sorensen, K. C.: *Medical-Surgical Nursing: A Psychophysiologic Approach.* Philadelphia, W. B. Saunders Co.

hyperinflation
bronchospasm
sustained maximal
    inflation

postural drainage
chest physiotherapy

Upon completion of this chapter, you should be able to:

1. Discuss the importance of adequate lung function.

2. Describe primary and secondary stimuli to ventilation.

3. Describe the reason for caution in administering oxygen to a patient with a "hypoxic drive."

4. List the causes of respiratory dysfunction.

5. List the signs of hypoxemia.

6. List the physical clues of chronic respiratory dysfunction.

7. Understand reasons for administering oxygen.

8. List at least seven safety considerations in oxygen administration.

9. Define cyanosis and understand the relationship of this symptom to hypoxemia.

10. Describe five methods of therapeutic oxygen administration.

11. Understand how objective and subjective assessments of oxygen therapy are made.

12. Discuss methods of liquefying thick tracheobronchial secretions to enhance removal.

13. Compare the uses of incentive respiratory devices with Intermittent Positive Pressure Breathing.

14. Be able to demonstrate and teach: effective coughing techniques and the procedure for a sustained maximal inflation.

15. Undertake supervised practice of aspiration (suctioning) of the tracheobronchial tree, based upon knowledge of: (a) how to assess the need for suctioning and the effectiveness of suctioning, (b) the techniques of suctioning and (c) the complications and side effects of suctioning and how to prevent them.

16. Recognize the need for uninterrupted oxygen administration for patients requiring oxygen therapy.

DYSFUNCTIONS OF THE RESPIRATORY SYSTEM

Causes of Sudden/Acute Respiratory Dysfunction

Sudden/acute respiratory dysfunctions may occur from conditions affecting the integrity of the upper airway, which begins at the nose and extends to the end of the trachea (Fig. 36–1). Causes of upper airway dysfunctions include the following:

1. Obstruction in the upper airway from foreign material, e.g., choking on food and having it lodge in the trachea

2. Laryngospasm and laryngeal edema, i.e., a swelling and closure of the larynx due to trauma or infection, which may close off the airway and prevent adequate ventilation

3. Tumors, polyps, enlarged tonsils

4. Bilateral vocal cord paralysis

5. An enlargement of the thyroid gland

Sudden/acute dysfunction occurring elsewhere in the respiratory system includes conditions affecting the lower airway, from the main bronchi to the alveolar level (see Fig. 36–1). Causes include the following:

1. Obstruction of the airway from aspiration of foreign material into the lower airway, e.g., aspiration of vomitus

2. Pneumothorax, i.e., a collapse of the lung from air or blood collection in the pleural space

3. Trauma to the chest

4. Acute bronchospasm, i.e., a constricting of the smooth muscle of the airway—a swelling of the mucosa and vasculature leading to a narrowing of the airways. Causes include allergic response; response to foreign particles, chemi-

cals and other substances; and a response to stress, both physical and emotional.

5. Acute infections

6. Pulmonary edema, i.e., fluid from the circulating blood volume that is drawn into the alveoli from the capillaries

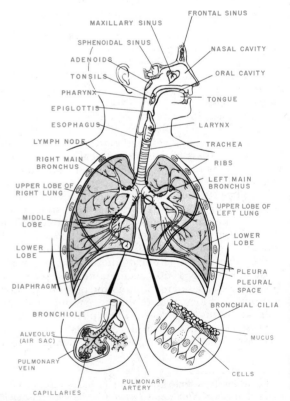

Figure 36–1. Anatomy of the respiratory system. (From *What You Can Do About Breathing.* New York, American Lung Association, 1974.)

7. Pulmonary infarction and emboli, i.e., blood clots in the blood vessels of the pulmonary system

8. Cardiac arrest, i.e., a cessation of cardiac and respiratory function. No oxygen is being exchanged and no blood is being circulated in the body. Without oxygen, the brain will cease to be viable in 4 to 6 minutes.

Causes of Chronic Respiratory Dysfunction

Many names and abbreviations are used to designate chronic respiratory dysfunction ("chronic lung disease"). Some of these terms or categories are (a) chronic airway obstruction (CAO), (b) chronic obstructive pulmonary disease (COPD), (c) chronic obstructive lung disease (COLD) and (d) chronic obstructive respiratory disease (CORD). These terms are frequently used in the literature of respiratory therapy. They all basically refer to progressive diseases that destroy lung tissue or impair the function of the lungs on a permanent basis. These disorders may be divided into obstructive lung diseases and restrictive lung diseases.

Obstructive Lung Disease. These diseases are commonly associated with chronic airway disease, such as emphysema, chronic bronchitis, bronchiectasis, asthma and cystic fibrosis. These all cause destruction of lung tissue and interfere with the movement of air out of the lungs.

Restrictive Lung Disease. Restrictive lung diseases decrease the volume of air that can be taken into the lung without decreasing the rate of flow of the air out of the lungs.

There are four categories of restrictive lung disease:

1. *Thoracic changes.* Either structural changes or reduced thoracic flexibility, such as in kyphoscoliosis—a condition in which the spine curves and distorts the thorax and decreases the volume of air that may be taken into the lungs.

2. *Intrathoracic (nonpulmonary) changes.* Found in diseases which impede lung expansion, e.g., a pleural effusion, in which fluid collects in the pleura and prevents the lung from fully expanding.

3. *Pulmonary causes.* For example, fibrosis or scarring of the lung, which prevents the normal stretch of the lungs.

4. *Abdominal causes.* Postoperative pain and splinting, fluid collection in the abdomen and distention of the abdomen all impede the full expansion of the lungs.

Assessment of the Respiratory Patient

The observations and studies performed by many departments within the hospital provide the physician with information that aids in the diagnosis and treatment of the patient with a respiratory disorder.

Physical and Historical Assessment. Persons with chronic respiratory disorders often show physical changes that can be observed during assessment by physician, nurse, or other health care workers. Many respiratory disorders are caused by specific circumstances in a patient's life, such as smoking or occupational exposure to certain substances; these circumstances may be discovered during a historical assessment.

Laboratory Assessment. The most frequently performed laboratory studies include (1) arterial blood gas analysis; (2) examination of the sputum for bacteria, foreign material, and abnormal cellular structure; (3) skin tests to determine the presence of antibodies to various substances and disease; (4) pulmonary function studies and (5) exercise tolerance tests.

Other Diagnostic Studies. Other examples of studies performed to aid in the diagnosis or evaluation of respiratory disorders include (1) radiologic procedures; (2) direct visualization of the tracheobronchial tree by flexible fiberoptic bronchoscopy; (3) biopsy of the lung parenchyma; and (4) thoracentesis.

BASIC THERAPEUTIC MEASURES

Respiratory therapy is concerned with the repair, maintenance and/or prevention of complications in the respiratory system. Therapy should be individualized and goal oriented. For example, one goal of therapy may be to assist a patient in clearing his congested airways; another common goal of therapy is postoperative prevention of atelectasis.

The overall goal of all respiratory therapy is to maintain lung function sufficient to support life.

Respiratory therapy modalities have been divided into general categories. These activities may be used singly or in combination to achieve the desired goals of therapy. The following treatment modalities are discussed in detail in this chapter:

▶ *Mobilization Maneuvers.* Coughing, turning, deep breathing and early ambulation are techniques employed by the nurse to prevent the complications of secretion retention and to promote spontaneous secretion removal.

▶ *Hydration/Humidification/Nebulization.* *Hydration* is best defined as the addition of water, and the maintenance and restoration of a proper level of hydration is one of the most important concepts in the care of patients with respiratory dysfunction. Hydration may be done systemically, by oral or parenteral means, and through the respiratory system. A wide variety of modes of hydration are employed to hydrate the lungs.

▶ *Oxygen Administration.* Oxygen administration is the most frequently used form of respiratory therapy. When a patient cannot effectively oxygenate himself, he must be given oxygen to meet his physiologic requirements in order to maintain life and a state of health. You must learn the methods of administering oxygen. Oxygen is a drug and must not be administered casually, but when needed, it must be administered swiftly, safely, and effectively.

▶ *Aerosol Administration of Medications.* Medications which are active on the respiratory system may be given via aerosol to: (a) open the airways (bronchodilators and decongestants); (b) mobilize and liquefy pulmonary secretions; (c) prevent or treat allergic activity and response and (d) topically treat pulmonary infections.

▶ *Intermittent Positive Pressure Breathing Treatments.* This form of therapy is usually called by its abbreviation, IPPB, and involves mechanically inflating the lungs with a pressure higher than ambient pressure. When IPPB is administered correctly, "deep breaths" may be given to the patient. In the recent past, IPPB was the mainstay of respiratory therapy and as somewhat of a panacea and a means to show that "something was being done for the patient." Currently IPPB is of controversial value. No doubt it has been overused, but it does have a place in treating the patient who is unable to: (a) spontaneously deep breathe, (b) cough effectively, (c)

raise secretions effectively and/or (d) coordinate his respiratory efforts to cooperate with other forms of therapy.

Breathing with positive pressure is also used to assist the ventilation of patients unable to maintain their own ventilation. When this is required, *Continuous Mechanical Ventilation* is used. Patients requiring continuous mechanical ventilation must be cared for in a critical care setting.

▶ *Suctioning—Airway Management. Suctioning* is the mechanical removal of retained tracheobronchial secretions, using vacuum pressures to pull the secretions through a suction catheter inserted into the airway. This form of therapy is employed when a patient's cough is ineffective, to maintain a patent airway or to obtain a special specimen of sputum for laboratory analysis. Safe, effective suctioning requires knowledge and skill; the technique is discussed in detail in this chapter.

▶ *Respiratory Exercises.* There are two general categories of respiratory exercises; both modalities aim to promote deep breathing. (1) *Expiratory resistance exercises*, such as those performed with blow bottles, have now generally been abandoned because they promoted atelectasis and airway collapse. (2) *Incentive device exercises* have replaced expiratory resistance exercises. Incentive devices utilize the principle of a *voluntary sustained maximal inflation* to promote deep breathing (like a "sigh"). This increases intrathoracic pressures, thus reducing and preventing airway collapse and atelectasis.

▶ *Postural Drainage and Chest Physiotherapy. Postural drainage* is the technique of positioning a patient so that gravity and positional changes assist with the drainage of secretions out of the lungs. One postural drainage position is depicted in Figure 36–2. *Chest physiotherapy* is performed with the patient in postural drainage positions. Chest physiotherapy consists of the manual application of *vibration* and *clapping* over the affected areas of the lung. The clapping and vibration help dislodge retained mucus from the airways.

▶ *Breathing Retraining and Education.* These techniques encompass a variety of teaching activities: (a) educate a patient about his disease, (b) teach a patient how to deal with his disease in relation to activities of daily living, (c) identify and correct a patient's incorrect breathing habits and (d) establish activity and exercise programs which allow a patient to live as near normal a life as possible.

▶ *Artificial Airways.* In conditions where a patient is unable to maintain a patent airway and insure adequate ventilation of the lungs, an artificial (manmade) airway may be inserted into the trachea. This procedure is termed *intubation.* The artificial airway may be placed into the trachea through either the nose (nasotracheal intubation); the mouth (oraltracheal intubation); or through a surgical incision in the trachea (tracheostomy).

MOBILIZATION MANEUVERS

The nurse can encourage certain activities to assist the patient in preventing the retention of secretions in his lungs and to assist the spontaneous removal of retained secretions. These activities include mobilization, turning, deep breathing and coughing.

Mobilization should be one of the first objectives in the care of any patient. Unless the condition of the patient strictly prohibits an increase in his activity, the transition from bed rest to full ambulation should be of primary concern. Other mobilization activities include *turning the patient confined to bed,* encouraging him to *deep breathe frequently* to expand his lungs, and teaching him to *cough effectively.*

> *Mobilization (a) stimulates deep breathing, (b) helps the redistribution of air and blood flow, (c) aids in drainage of secretions, (d) may promote a cough and (e) aids in recirculation of blood.*

Turning a patient, encouraging his deep breathing and assisting him in ambulation and physical mobilization require teaching the patient and family, providing encouragement, and skillfully eliciting the patient's cooperation. Teaching effective, expulsive coughing also requires skill and ingenuity; instruction, demonstration and often "coughing tricks" need to be used.

Effects of Immobility

The effects of immobility may be seen in every system of the body (see Chap. 33). The respiratory system is no exception. The effects of gravity combined with immobility lead to *pooling of secretions* in the gravity-dependent areas of the lung. Immobility will cause the

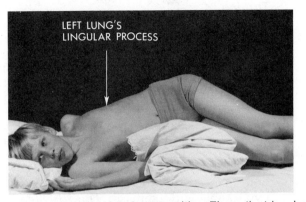

Figure 36-2. A postural drainage position. The patient has been placed on his right side with his left side in the upper position and his torso rotated one quarter turn backward. The foot of the bed has been elevated 14 inches, or 15 degrees. This position will aid in drainage of the left upper lobe—the lingular segment. (From Hospai Medical Corporation, Littleton, CO 80122.)

closure of some of the small airways and may also *interfere with the normal pattern of ventilation.* This may lead to inadequate tidal volumes and inadequate sigh volumes. When any of these factors are present, respiratory dysfunction is either created or furthered. Hypoxemia is the end result of immobility, gravitational pooling of secretions and a diminished ventilation pattern.

Many patients with chronic lung disease have a predisposition to *venous stasis.* Prolonged inactivity may potentiate the stasis of blood in the dependent limbs. The risk of *pulmonary emboli* increases with inactivity. Patients with a history of pulmonary disease should wear anti-embolic stockings, move their toes and feet frequently and always sit with their legs elevated to promote venous return.

The importance of mobilization activities for patients with respiratory dysfunction is obvious. However, such patients may resist physical mobilization because of the fear that movement may cause them additional shortness of breath. Such fears are understandable in persons who often are fighting an exhausting battle for every breath. It takes a skillful nurse to be supportive of the patient while ensuring that essential mobilization activities are carried out. It is extremely important that patients receiving oxygen continue to receive the oxygen during mobilization maneuvers.

Turning

Frequent turning of the patient confined to bed aids the treatment of respiratory dysfunction by (a) assisting redistribution of pulmonary blood flow and ventilation, (b) promoting drainage of the upper lung fields and (c) preventing pooling of secretions. However, turning can be hazardous in the patient with *consolidation of a lung.* Such patients must never be positioned on the affected side. If this is done, blood flow (due to gravitational effects) will increase to the unventilated area, and hypoxemia will increase. *The affected lung should always be in the "up" position.*

Effective Coughing

A cough is one of the most important protective reflexes of the respiratory system. An effective cough is essential to good respiratory care. There are many nerve endings in the trachea. Impulses pass through the vagus nerve to the medulla of the brain. The mechanism of a cough occurs when impulses from the brain stimulate the appropriate muscles to begin a cough.

A cough clears the tracheobronchial tree of excessive secretions, particulate matter and possibly even large pieces of debris, e.g., food particles. When normal airway defense mechanisms are functioning, bronchopulmonary debris and secretions are propelled upward by ciliary action to the upper trachea. Then they are swallowed or readily expectorated. When conditions exist that result in retained secretions and/or impairment of the "mucociliary escalator," the cough becomes less effective. Ineffective coughing may significantly increase a patient's energy expenditure as he works to clear his airway. Many patients are afraid to cough. Their reluctance may be from fear of pain or from fear of increasing their level of dyspnea by ineffective coughing. Other patients are unable to cough due to the effects of disease or medications.

1

A cough can be induced voluntarally or caused by an irritation.

2

The beginning of a cough starts with a deep inspiration. This distends the trachea and hyperinflates the lungs.

Figure 36–3. Anatomy of a cough. (From Cherniack, R. M., Cherniack, L., and Naimark, A.: *Respiration in Health and Disease,* 2nd ed. Philadelphia, W. B. Saunders Co., 1972, p. 169.)

3

After inspiration, the glottis closes quickly and tightly while the expiratory intercostal and abdominal muscles contract forcibly. This is called the "COMPRESSIVE" phase because of the rise in intrathoracic and intra-abdominal pressures.

4

After the intrathoracic pressure has reached a high level, the glottis opens slightly. Since intra-abdominal pressure is now higher than that in the thoracic cavity, the diaphram is pushed up producing a violent, explosive movement of air.

An effective cough occurs in the following sequence (Fig. 36–3):

1. A deep inspiration to distend the trachea and hyperinflate the lungs.

2. A quick tight closure of the glottis to build up thoracic pressure. This is called the *Valsalva maneuver*. It involves closing the glottis to increase intrathoracic and intra-abdominal pressures. An adequate force must be created to expel the bolus of mucus and debris.

3. A contraction of the intercostal and abdominal muscles. In this phase there is a compression of the thoracic and abdominal cavities.

4. When the intrathoracic pressure has reached a high level, the glottis opens.

5. With the glottis open, the intra-abdominal pressure is higher than the intrathoracic pressure. This pushes the diaphragm upward.

6. The diaphragmatic motion produces a violent, explosive movement of air through the trachea. This is often called a "pillar of air." The patient's vital capacity must be great enough to ensure an adequate "pillar of air" behind the material to be expectorated.

Coughing is associated with two hazards that the nurse must be aware of. Patients with thin-walled alveoli, or *blebs* (found in some forms of chronic lung disease), may rupture them with a forceful cough and produce a pneumothorax. Forceful coughing also may increase the strain on both the cardiac and cerebral functions. These patients must be observed and cautioned to avoid forced coughing.

There are certain *nursing actions* that may be employed to assist the patient in effective coughing. In order for the cough to be effective in removal of secretions, the airway must be well hydrated (hydration is discussed in the next section of this chapter). An expectorant aids in the removal of secretions by aiding the cough. The best expectorants are oral and parenteral fluids and bland medical solutions (water, saline and 0.25 to 0.45 per cent saline) delivered directly to the airway by mechanical means such as a nebulizer. There are also expectorant drugs on the market that help raise the mucus and clear the airway. If secretions are produced, observe them closely. The mucus removed by coughing is called *sputum*. If sputum is produced with the cough, note its color, consistency, odor and quantity.

Another factor in producing an effective cough is the patient's position. He must be in a position that allows him to relax his abdominal and thoracic muscles to dispel the explosive "pillar of air." Sitting is the best position, as forward flexion motion is required. This is impossible to perform if lying flat.

The patient must be instructed in the step-by-step progression of a cough (Table 36–1) and the instructions repeated as often as necessary.

Merely telling a patient to cough is not enough. The therapeutic nurse carefully teaches and supervises the patient as he learns to cough effectively.

The nurse encourages the patient to relax and not to tire himself with hacking, ineffective coughing. It may be necessary to alleviate operative site pain in order to have a patient cough effectively. However, *oversedation must be avoided, as this would further impair the clearance of any retained secretions by depressing the cough reflex.*

Sometimes it becomes necessary to modify or augment coughing techniques. Some "coughing tricks" a nurse might use to assist an effective cough are:

1. *Changing positions.* Position so that patient is comfortable; roll the patient from one side to the other side to move secretions into the large airways from the periphery of the tracheobronchial tree.

TABLE 36–1. BASIC PROCEDURE FOR ASSISTING A PATIENT TO COUGH

1. Position the patient in a sitting position (or position the bed in a semi to moderately high Fowler's position), with his head flexed, shoulders relaxed and slightly rolled forward, and his feet supported against a firm surface or pillow.
2. If possible, position the patient so that his feet can be pushed against a solid object during the expulsive stage of the cough.
3. Splint the abdomen or chest with pillows or your hands so that support is given to the abdominal or chest muscles. If the patient has an incision, support the incision also.
4. Instruct the patient on "how to" cough prior to his attempt.
5. Stress that the cough must be explosive and deep. The phrase "cough from your boots" is descriptive and often gets your point across to the patient.
6. If a sudden, deep inspiration is difficult for the patient, have him build a pyramid of air *behind* the mucus by taking three to four "stacked" breaths. (A "stacked breath" is an inspiration, only partially exhaled, with an additional inspiration taken in on top of the first breath.) This allows a greater force of air to expel the material. The key words to stress are: *pillar of air behind the mucus.*
7. Have the patient repeat a slow deep breath three or four times to fill the bases of the lungs with air and get air behind the mucus. Next, have him take a comfortable deep breath with his shoulders relaxed while his lower chest expands.
8. Finally, have the patient bend forward and contract the thorax and abdomen. Produce a forceful, expulsive cough sufficient to propel the mucus without collapsing the airways. Push with the abdominal muscles. (The force of the expulsion may have a velocity or flow rate of 200 to 300 liters per minute.)

Note: If the patient has a diagnosis of chronic lung disease, encourage slow, controlled exhalation during the expiration phase of the cough. This will help prevent air trapping and over-distention of the alveoli.

2. *Increasing the patient's level of activity.* Place patient in a chair; ambulate the patient. Encourage deep breathing and slow exhalation during ambulation.

3. *Prolonging exhalation.* Have the patient breathe in through his nose slowly and then exhale slowly and completely through pursed lips. Have him continue to exhale until secretions are moved to one of the cough reflex centers and a cough is stimulated.

4. *Vibrations/end expiratory assist.* Place your hands on the patient's lower thorax and "vibrate" with a firm, upward movement during his exhalation. This often helps the patient achieve enough expulsive expiratory force to expel the secretions.

5. *Sips of water.* A few sips of water may stimulate a cough.

6. *Discussing with the patient about alternatives to coughing*, e.g., suctioning.

7. *Manually stimulated cough.* Give the patient a deep breath with a self-inflating resuscitation bag or an anesthesia bag. This may mobilize secretions and promote a cough.

8. *Splinting.* Place a pillow against the patient or maintain firm contact with your hands on the abdomen and thorax. In both surgical and non-surgical patients, this often aids in producing the necessary "assist" to the expulsive expiratory force required for an effective cough.

HYDRATION

The human body has specific fluid requirements; part of the total amount of body water is used by the respiratory system to warm and humidify inspired air. Body water is also contained in large amounts in the mucus layer of the tracheobronchial tree. Many disorders affecting the respiratory system are tied directly to adequate fluid maintenance of the patient. In other words, the patient's condition will worsen if he is dehydrated. The pulmonary system (together with skin losses) utilizes approximately 1000 ml. of water per day. When physical conditions (e.g., fever, diaphoresis) or other conditions affecting the balance of fluid in the body are present, a readjustment and supplementation of fluids must be made to maintain fluid balance.[24] If the airway becomes dehydrated, secretions dry and an increase in airway resistance develops.

The supplemental administration of fluids is termed *hydration.* Hydration may be accomplished by oral (systemic) fluid administration, parenteral (intravenous) fluid administration, and topical fluid administration.

This section deals primarily with methods of *topical hydration.* The nurse must also consider the oral and parenteral methods of hydration, for it is she who is primarily responsible for the administration and documentation of these forms of hydration. These topics are discussed in Chapters 24 and 38. The respiratory therapist is most often the person who administers the topical forms of hydration to the patient. It is important that both the nurse and the therapist understand and look for the positive as well as the negative effects of the therapy and communicate them to the physician and to each other. As with any therapy, a clear cut goal for hydration therapy is essential. Without establishing a *therapeutic goal*, there is no definite means to assess the effectiveness of a particular therapy.

Means of Topical Hydration

The methods of topical hydration include (a) increasing the relative humidity, e.g., with an oxygen room humidifier, and (b) creating an aerosol, such as with heated nebulizers, ultrasonic nebulizers and nebulizers utilizing other principles. Some of the methods for hydration are more appropriate for home care of the patient with respiratory dysfunction than for acute care in the hospital. The more sophisticated methods of topical hydration should only be used in the hospital setting unless adequate instruction and maintenance are available in the home.

Humidifiers. Humidifiers add water vapor to the inspired air, which increases the relative humidity of the air. Equipment may use and deliver water that is at room temperature, heated to body temperature or slightly above body temperature. *Heated air is able to carry more moisture.*

A *humidifier* is the mechanical device that delivers humidity. One type is the *bubble-diffusion humidifier* used in oxygen administration. Another type, the *pass-over humidifier*, simply passes air over a water reservoir. Water in the reservoir may either be heated or cold. Water vapor is added to the air through evaporation; this type of humidification is employed by many mechanical ventilators. A third type is the *impeller humidifier*, which actually produces particles of water. These particles are too large to penetrate deeply into the tracheobronchial tree. The room humidifier used in many homes for upper respiratory infections, especially in children, is the most common example of this type.

Other examples of humidification devices are baby bottle warmers, a steaming tea kettle, a facial sauna, and pans of water on a radiator. All of these devices increase the relative humidity of the inspired air.

Aerosolization. An "aerosol" is a fine suspension of a liquid or a powder carried on a stream of gas. Aerosols may be large in volume (for hydration) or may be produced in small amounts, such as dry aerosols that deliver medications topically into the airway. Devices which produce an aerosol are called aerosol generators. In order to enter the tracheobronchial tree, the particle of liquid produced by an aerosol generator must be 1 to 3 microns in size (one micron is equal to 3.937×10^{-5} inches).

Nebulizers. Nebulizers produce aerosol particles of uniform size. The more effective the nebulizer the better the system of baffles employed by the nebulizer to deliver a volume of uniform sized particles. Nebulizers may be classified as follows:

1. *Small volume nebulizers* are for short term or intermittent therapy and the administration of medications.

2. *Large reservoir nebulizers* can potentially run on a continuous basis. They deliver a dense, large volume of water (or other bland liquid) on a large volume of gas. The large volume of gas plus the dense aerosol significantly helps to hydrate the tracheobronchial tree.

Many nebuilizers also utilize the *Venturi principle*. This allows the nebulizer system to entrain air from the room to aid in delivery of the aerosol particles and to increase further the total liter flow of gas delivered to the patient.

Hazards of Hydration

Bacterial Contamination. All methods of topical hydration carry the risk of microbiological contamination, because all of the devices include a water reservoir. There is always the possibility that bacteria and other organisms may grow in this reservoir. If this occurs, the mechanical device becomes contaminated and bacteria may be deposited in the patient's respiratory system along with the water particles. This hazard may be reduced or eliminated by use of sterile solutions in the water reservoir and by decontaminating or maybe sterilizing the nebulizer and the tubing system leading to the patient frequently (usually every 24 hours or less). If sterilization is required, it is usually done by means of cold (chemical solution) or ethylene oxide (gas) sterilization.

Bronchospasm and Shortness of Breath. The lungs respond to irritation by constricting the smooth muscle lining the airways. This is called *bronchospasm*. Bronchospasm also leads to mucosal edema. *During the administration of any inhaled substance, the lungs may react adversely and go into a bronchospasm.* This may occur with any of the inhaled liquids designed to improve the level of pulmonary hydration.

> *When any patient receiving topical administration of inhaled hydration develops sudden shortness of breath (dyspnea), cough, or audible wheeze, the therapy should be stopped and the incident documented and reported to the physician.*

Removal of the source of irritation may reverse the bronchospasm. If not, it may be necessary to administer bronchodilating agents to relieve the bronchospasm. *The most common agent used for hydration* is sterile distilled water. Saline (0.9 per cent) and 0.45 per cent saline are also used. Bronchospasm produced by distilled water is partially reversed by bronchodilating agents. Bronchospasm produced by saline (0.9 per cent) is not as responsive to bronchodilators. The cause of these reactions is still disputed. The optimal solution for hydration therapy where actual particles of solution are inhaled is 0.25 to 0.45 per cent saline (0.9 per cent is normal saline). The airway resistance and bronchospasm from the one-half to one-quarter strength saline is partially responsive to bronchodilation agents.[16]

Overhydration. If large volumes of fluid are delivered into the tracheobronchial tree, there is danger of overloading the airways and body with fluid. Overhydration is less critical in adults, as the fluid is absorbed by the lungs and excess fluid is usually carried off by the lymphatic system and drained into the circulatory system. In pediatric therapy, the balance of fluids is more critical and pulmonary system fluid overload is a greater hazard.

OXYGEN ADMINISTRATION

The administration of oxygen is the most common form of therapy for patients with respiratory dysfunction. Oxygen is a drug. It is widely used and has at times been abused. It is important to have an appreciation and respect for oxygen. This section deals with: (a) the drug

TABLE 36-2.   LEVELS OF HYPOXEMIA AND
ASSOCIATED SYMPTOMS

Moderate Hypoxemia
1. Tachycardia
2. Mental confusion
3. Restlessness
4. Increased respiratory rate
5. Air hunger
6. Tunnel vision, visual disturbances
7. Sweating

Severe Hypoxemia
1. Lethargy
2. Somnolence
3. Bradycardia
4. Slowing respiratory rate
5. Gasping respiratory pattern—agonal respiration
6. Cyanosis

Grave Hypoxemia
1. Shock
2. Coma
3. Death

oxygen, (b) oxygen administration techniques and safety considerations, (c) benefits of oxygen and (d) hazards and precautions to consider during oxygen administration.

Purpose of Oxygen Therapy. The body requires oxygen to maintain health and life. Oxygen is administered to relieve *hypoxemia*—the condition present when the amount of oxygen in the blood is below normal. The "normal" amount of oxygen in the arterial blood should be in the range of 80 to 100 mm. Hg. If the arterial oxygen tension (PaO_2) is allowed to fall below 55 to 60 mm. Hg, irreversible physiologic effects may occur.

Hypoxemia may cause irreversible tissue damage. Thus, it is urgent to correct hypoxemia promptly. Once hypoxemia is relieved by the administration of oxygen, the condition causing the hypoxemia must be determined and treated. *Oxygen administration treats the effect (hypoxemia) of the underlying pathology, but it does not treat the pathology itself.*

Determining the Presence of Hypoxemia. Hypoxemia may be assessed by objective or subjective means. Objectively, the presence of hypoxemia is determined by an arterial blood gas analysis. The arterial blood gas evaluation is the only "sure" means of determining the presence of hypoxemia. Subjectively, the hypoxemia can be suspected by the presence of the symptoms listed in Table 36–2.

Cyanosis is defined as a bluish color of the skin, nail beds, and mucous membranes when there is a decreased amount of oxygen in the hemoglobin of the blood. Unoxygenated hemoglobin is purple; oxygenated hemoglobin is red. Cyanosis may occur with respiratory and cardiac disorders. Cyanosis is generally not observable in the presence of mild or moderate hypoxemia. It is only regularly noted when severe hypoxemia exists.

> *Cyanosis is* not *a reliable indicator of hypoxemia.*

The detection of cyanosis is a subjective clinical observation that cannot be correlated to the level of hypoxemia. Patients who are anemic may never appear cyanotic simply because all of their available hemoglobin may be saturated with oxygen. However, the amount of oxygen available to the tissues may be inadequate and hypoxemia will exist even though the saturation of hemoglobin is "normal" and no clinical evidence of cyanosis is present.

The clinical recognition of cyanosis is highly variable, depending upon factors such as: (a) skin thickness, (b) skin pigments, (c) available light in the room, (d) color of the surroundings and (e) the judgment of the observer.

> *The goal of oxygen therapy is to achieve an optimal arterial oxygen tension for an individual patient by giving the lowest possible, most effective dose of oxygen—while avoiding the toxic effects of oxygen.*

Goal of Oxygen Therapy. The goal of oxygen therapy is to keep the arterial PO_2 above 55 to 60 mm. Hg. The PO_2 must be kept at physiologic levels. The administration of oxygen should not cause the PCO_2 to rise above 45 mm. Hg. The exception to this is a patient with chronic lung disease. Such a person normally retains carbon dioxide and thus has a chronic elevation of the PCO_2 (above 45 mm. Hg). This patient's drive to respiration is his low oxygen blood level. Thus, he cannot tolerate doses of oxygen as high as those given to patients who do not have a chronic lung disease with retention of carbon dioxide. It is very important to assess the arterial blood gas status of the patient prior to beginning oxygen therapy, to determine if the patient has chronic carbon dioxide retention.

Oxygen administration by itself may not be successful in maintaining an acceptable PO_2. More intensive therapy, e.g., a mechanical ventilator, may be required to maintain the arterial blood gases within physiologic limits.

If the lack of oxygen threatens the immediate survival of the patient, administer oxygen without delay. Laboratory assessment of blood gases must be made after the oxygen administration has been started.

Effect of Oxygen. The administration of oxygen will (a) increase the *alveolar* oxygen tension—it may or may not increase the *arterial* oxygen tension, depending upon the underlying cause of the hypoxemia, (b) reduce the work of breathing and associated fatigue and (c) decrease the work of the heart and vascular system. The cardiovascular system increases its work load in an attempt to compensate for hypoxemia in certain conditions, e.g., hemorrhagic shock.

Table 36–3 lists some of the commonly observed symptoms of hypoxemia and the observable response with oxygen administration. This is not a complete list, but rather one that includes the more obvious and frequently observed signs of hypoxemia.

The effect of the oxygen therapy must be assessed both by arterial blood gas analysis and by observation of the patient for improvement in the clinical symptoms of hypoxemia.

Continuous Oxygen Administration. Oxygen is not stored in the body. Oxygen must, therefore, be administered continuously when acute hypoxemia is present. The tissue needs for oxygen must be met at all times. *Oxygen administration must never be stopped until those factors that caused the hypoxemia are reversed.* During all phases of care, when a patient is to receive continuous oxygen administration, the oxygen source must *never* be removed. Sudden withdrawal of oxygen may lead to more severe hypoxemia and result in serious, possibly life-threatening cardiovascular and cerebral hypoxic effects.

Intermittent Oxygen Therapy. The use of oxygen on an intermittent basis is, at times, of questionable value. Random "doses" of oxygen will not maintain the constant physiologic oxygen requirement of the body. The following are three circumstances in which intermittent oxygen therapy may be used:

1. To relieve psychologically induced breathlessness, chest pain or other cardiopulmonary symptoms.

2. To treat exercise-induced breathlessness or hypoxemia. Many patients with chronic lung disease may maintain marginally satisfactory arterial oxygen tensions while they are at rest or while performing mild activities of daily living.

TABLE 36–3. COMMONLY OBSERVED SYMPTOMS OF HYPOXEMIA AND FAVORABLE RESPONSES TO OXYGEN ADMINISTRATION

SYMPTOM OF HYPOXEMIA	FAVORABLE RESPONSE FOLLOWING OXYGEN ADMINISTRATION
1. Tachycardia	1. Return to normal rate
2. Cardiac arrhythmias	2. Decrease or elimination of irregularities
3. Increase respiratory rate and increase in work of breathing (WOB)	3. Return to normal rate, pattern of ventilation and reduction of excess work of breathing
4. Breathlessness, shortness of breath; air hunger	4. Return of quiet respirations that do not require conscious effort
5. Confusion, hallucinations, restlessness	5. Improved mental status
6. Cyanosis	6. Return of healthy pink color to skin, nailbeds, and mucous membranes

However, when these patients exercise, their cardiopulmonary compensatory mechanisms are typically unable to maintain an adequate oxygen tension in the arterial blood. Administration of intermittent supplemental oxygen allows the patient to exercise.

3. To treat pulmonary hypertension. Such therapy frequently includes 12 to 18 hours of continuous oxygen administration out of every 24-hour period.

Oxygen Dosage. The amount of oxygen to be administered is determined by considering the desired clinical effect, the patient's medical history, and the results of the arterial blood gas analysis. Oxygen delivery systems measure the dose as either *liters per minute* (LPM) or the *percentage of oxygen* (%). The dose of oxygen is prescribed according to the appliance to be used and the method of measurement. For example, a prescription for oxygen might state: "Oxygen per nasal cannula at 3 LPM continuously." This means the patient is to be given oxygen continuously at a rate of 3 liters per minute through a nasal cannula.

Previously it was thought that a patient breathing through his mouth while receiving oxygen via nasal cannula was not actually receiving oxygen. It is now known that the anatomy of the upper respiratory passages (nose, mouth and oral and nasal pharynges) creates an anatomic reservoir for the momentary "storage" (not to be confused with storing oxygen for physiologic use) of oxygen before it is inhaled into the tracheobronchial tree. This "anatomic reservoir" has a capacity for about 6 liters of gas.

This gas may be used as a portion of the total inspired gas volume. When the patient inhales, air is inhaled from both the oxygen administration device and from the room. Therefore, oxygen is still being received by the patient and the same variables apply to the percentage of oxygen delivered by the appliance: the patient's respiratory rate, the pattern of ventilation and the tidal volume of each breath.[25]

> *The desired clinical effect of the dose of oxygen must be monitored by observing the patient for indications of:*
> *1. Improved oxygen status*
> *2. Development of undesired effects, e.g., depression of the respiratory centers with subsequent depression of respiration and a build-up of carbon dioxide.*
> *3. The presence of arterial blood gas imbalances, e.g., continued hypoxemia or the development of a sudden elevation of the P_{CO_2}*

The adjustment of the dose of oxygen depends upon the disease state, the degree of hypoxia present and the presence of unwanted side effects. The physician decides adjustments in the dosage of oxygen.

Safety Considerations

Certain safety considerations are mandatory when oxygen is being administered. The nurse must make certain that she and other workers are aware of and practice the following:

▶ Recognize that oxygen is a drug that has beneficial effects as well as undesirable side effects.

▶ Know that oxygen *supports* combustion. It must not be administered in the presence of fire, smoke, or sparks from electrical equipment. Special precautions, e.g., hospital-grade plugs, are necessary to ensure that electrical appliances are safe for use in oxygen-rich environments.

▶ Perform arterial blood gas measurements to determine the effectiveness of therapy. In persons with chronic lung disease such measurements must be made before beginning oxygen therapy as well as periodically during therapy.

▶ Observe the patient for signs of undesired effects of oxygen therapy, e.g., somnolence, increased lethargy.

▶ Always check the dose (flow rate or percentage of oxygen) to make certain the correct amount of oxygen is being administered.

▶ Never remove the oxygen source from a patient receiving continuous oxygen therapy. Continuous oxygen must be supplied at all times, for all activities.

▶ Do not fear that the patient will develop a psychologic dependence on oxygen. For patients with proven hypoxemia, the need for oxygen becomes a *physiologic dependence*.

▶ Administer oxygen cautiously when it is prescribed for patients with chronic lung disease. Excessive administration of oxygen to such patients may actually cause them to stop breathing (apnea).

▶ Humidify oxygen during administration, to prevent drying of mucous membranes and mucosal irritation (except when venturi masks are used).

▶ Analyze the percentage of O_2 delivered by all types of oxygen administration devices by using an oxygen analyzer.

Humidification. Humidification of oxygen is necessary to prevent irritation and encrusting of the airways and to maintain an optimal environment for the normal function of the mucociliary blanket. *Humidification* is the addition of water vapor to a dry gas. The addition of water vapor reduces the drying effect of the oxygen on the patient's mucous membranes, thus making the administration of oxygen more comfortable.

> *Oxygen is a dry gas. Prolonged exposure to the drying effects of oxygen may cause irritation and damage to the mucous membranes of the oral and nasal pharyngeal area.*

The type of humidification device most often used with oxygen administration is the *bubble-diffusion humidifier* (Fig. 36–4). The gas (oxygen) is bubbled through water. The bubbling of the oxygen through the water allows the molecules of oxygen to pick up molecules of water vapor.

Oxygen Delivery Systems

The devices used to deliver oxygen may be divided into two broad categories: low flow systems and high flow systems. A *high flow system*

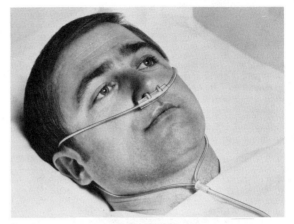

Figure 36–5. A nasal cannula (nasal prongs). This is the most frequently used appliance for oxygen administration. (Courtesy of Hudson Oxygen Therapy Sales Co., Temecula, Cal. 92390.)

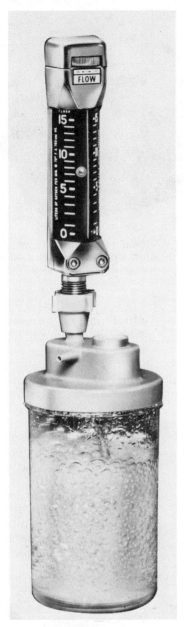

Figure 36–4. A bubble-diffusion humidifier for use in oxygen administration with low flow oxygen administration devices. (Courtesy of Hudson Oxygen Therapy Sales Co., Temecula, Cal. 92390.)

delivers a flow of gas that exceeds the volume of air required for the patient's minute ventilation. *Low flow systems* deliver oxygen at variable flows designed to add to, but not meet, the total air volume requirements. As a result, oxygen percentages in low flow systems are variable and not as consistent as the percentages in the high flow system. In a low flow system, the percentage of oxygen delivered to the tracheobronchial tree is determined by: (1) the patient's respiratory rate, (2) the tidal volume and (3) the pattern of ventilation (deep, fast, shallow, irregular, etc.).

LOW FLOW SYSTEMS

Oxygen may be administered via low flow systems in the following ways: (a) nasal cannula (prongs), (b) nasal catheter, (c) standard mask or (d) oxygen mask with reservoir bag (nonrebreathing).

Nasal Cannula (Prongs) (Fig. 36–5)

Description:	Two ⅝ inch projections that fit into the entry to the nasal passages.
Liter flows:	1 to 6 LPM
Percentage of Oxygen:	Variable—dependent upon the liter flow, respiratory rate, or pattern of respiration. The range is 22 to 40 per cent.
Comments:	Most common device used. Relatively comfortable; allows continuation of activities, e.g., eating, talking; disposable. May be easily dislodged by restless or disoriented patients. Nasal passages must be patent.

Nasal Catheter (Fig. 36–6)

Description:	A disposable plastic tube available in French sizes 10, 12, and 14 with a number of small holes at the patient end. It is passed through the nose just to the

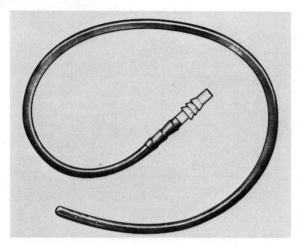

Figure 36–6. Nasal oxygen catheter. (Courtesy of Hudson Oxygen Sales Co., Temecula, Cal. 92390.)

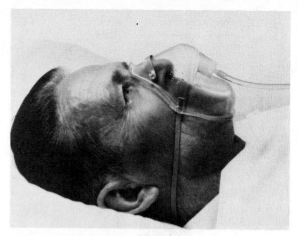

Figure 36–7. A standard oxygen mask, which is used to administer moderate ranges of oxygen. (Courtesy of Hudson Oxygen Sales Co., Temecula, Cal. 92390.)

uvula—the tip of the catheter should be just out of sight and visible only when the uvula lifts.

Liter flows: 1 to 6 LPM

Percentage of Oxygen: Variable for same reasons stated for the nasal cannula. May achieve slightly higher percentage of oxygen than cannula but not higher enough to outweigh its disadvantages.

Comments: Uncomfortable; must be changed every 4 to 6 hours due to mucus collection at catheter tip; irritating. Dangerous if inserted too far into pharynx and if liter flows over 6 LPM are used—may cause dilation of gastric cardiac sphincter and lead to abdominal distention and rupture.

Standard Mask (Fig. 36–7)

Description: A clear plastic appliance that encompasses the oral and nasal cavity and creates an additional area for collection of oxygen (a reservoir). Exhaled air passes out small holes in the sides of the mask. The small holes also allow entrainment of room air to add to the inspired oxygen flow rate to meet the patient's each breath tidal volume needs.

Liter flow: *Must not be administered at flow rates under 6 LPM. Range of 6 to 12 LPM.*

Percentage of Oxygen: Variable; dependent upon the same factors listed for cannula. Range: 40 to 65 per cent (moderate range).

Comments: May cause the patient to have a feeling of confinement or claustrophobia. Must be used with caution on patients who may be unable to maintain an unobstructed, patent airway, or patients who may vomit easily and be unable to turn onto their side to prevent aspiration of gastric

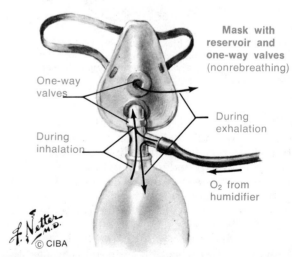

Mask with reservoir and one-way valves (nonrebreathing)

One-way valves

During exhalation

During inhalation

O₂ from humidifier

Figure 36–8. Oxygen mask with nonrebreathing bag, for short-term high concentration of oxygen. (From *Ciba Clinical Symposia, Bronchial Asthma,* Vo. 27, Nos. 1 and 2, 1975. Ciba Pharmaceutical Co., Summit, NJ 07901.)

contents. The mask must be replaced with nasal prongs during eating. This will cause a reduction in the inspired oxygen concentration. The mask must be repositioned immediately at the finish of the meal.

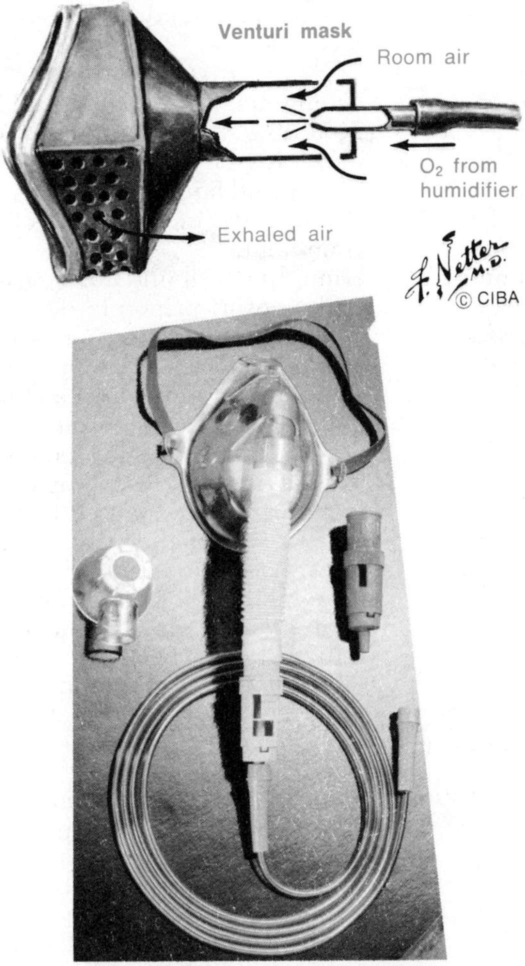

Oxygen Mask with Reservoir Bag–Non-rebreathing (Fig. 36–8)

Description:
: A standard mask with a reservoir bag designed to give high oxygen concentrations. A one-way valve between the reservoir bag and the patient permits inspired air to come only from the reservoir bag. Exhaled air exits through one-way valves at the sides of the mask.

Liter flows:
: As required to keep the reservoir bag inflated at least one third full during inspiration. Ranges of flow rates vary: 6 to 15 LPM.

Percentage of Oxygen:
: Variable, due to respiratory rate, ventilatory pattern, and the minute ventilation along with the liter flow of oxygen required to keep the bag inflated. Range: 60 to 90 per cent.

Comments:
: Useful for short-term, high concentrations of oxygen. Same hazards as standard oxygen mask. The fullness of the bag must be monitored as the bag must never completely collapse with each inspiration. The liter flow must be increased if this occurs.

HIGH FLOW SYSTEMS

Venturi Mask (Fig. 36–9)

Description:
: A mask engineered to utilize the venturi principle of High Air Flow Oxygen Enrichment (HAFOE). Oxygen moves through the connecting tube to a channel in the mask that has one diameter on the distal side and a smaller diameter on the proximal side. Oxygen flows through this passage. At the point of exit, a pressure drop occurs and creates a suction or entrainment effect. This entrainment has

Figure 36–9. The Venturi mask, a means of administering specific and more consistent doses of oxygen. A high flow oxygen administration device, it uses the HAFOE principle. (*A* from *Ciba Clinical Symposia, Bronchial Asthma. B* from McGaw Respiratory Therapy Division of American Hospital Supply, Irvine, Cal. 92714.)

been engineered to give specific doses (percentage) of oxygen. The venturi action allows a large volume of oxygen and room air to be mixed and delivered to the airway so that all ventilation needs are met.

Useful for specific dose (%) requirements. Useful for patients with irregular and inconsistent volumes and patterns of ventilation *as long as the patient's total minute ventilation does not exceed the liter flow delivered by the venturi system.*

Liter flows: As recommended by the manufacturer.

Percentage   Commercially available in 24%,
of Oxygen: 28%, 35% and 40%. Other masks may provide concentrations of 45, 50, and 55 per cent by using the same principles of air entrainment.

Comments: Humidifiers should *not* be used with venturi principle devices. They create a restriction to flow that will decrease the amount of air entrained and deliver a higher than desired concentration of O_2. The patient's supplemental oxygen requirements must be met during eating and other activities where the mask interferes. A cannula is used at this time. Many other types of equipment, such as nebulizers, utilize the HAFOE or venturi effect of air entrainment.

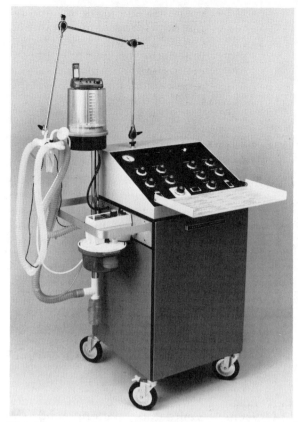

Figure 36–10.   A volume ventilator. The MA-I is a machine capable of supporting a patient's ventilation. It is used in critical respiratory care. (From The Puritan Bennett Corp., Kansas City, Mo. 64106.)

Volume Ventilator (Fig. 36–10)

Description: A machine capable of totally taking over a patient's ventilation, including the administration of specific oxygen percents, ventilatory flow rates, respiratory rate, tidal volume, etc. Used in intensive critical care settings where support of ventilation is required. Refer to critical respiratory care texts for discussion.

20. ADMINISTERING OXYGEN

Definition and Purpose.   The drug oxygen is administered for the treatment of hypoxemia. Hypoxemia may be caused by: breathing low concentrations (partial pressures) of oxygen, e.g., at high elevation; inadequate ventilation (hypoventilation) with an inadequate amount of oxygen supplied to the alveoli; diseases or conditions in the alveoli that interfere with the exchange (diffusion) of oxygen across the alveolar-capillary membrane; inadequate amounts of hemoglobin (anemia) resulting in insufficient amounts of oxygen circulated to the tissues; chemicals that alter the tissue's ability to accept oxygen (cyanide); and diseases or conditions that cause an imbalance in the ratio of ventilation to blood flow (perfusion) in the alveolus, resulting in atelectasis. Oxygen administration keeps the human machine functioning and treats the effects of hypoxemia to prevent the irreversible results of hypoxemia (brain damage). Oxygen will decrease the work of breathing; it may increase the arterial oxygen level; it will aid in the maintenance of a state of homeostasis. Oxygen administration will not treat the pathology of the underlying disease. The goal of oxygen administration is to maintain the P_{O_2} of the arterial blood in the minimum range of 55 to 60 mm. Hg (or to 100 mm. Hg) without causing the efficiency of ventilation to be impaired (the hypoxic drive or secondary respiratory stimulus for respiration), with the resulting elevation of CO_2.

Contraindications and Cautions.   Oxygen itself is not strictly contraindicated. Caution must be observed if the patient's drive for ventilation is due to a chronic low arterial oxygen tension (the hypoxic drive). Generally, the arterial P_{O_2} on 21 per cent oxygen (room air) will be below 50 mm. Hg and the arterial P_{CO_2} will be above the 45 to 50 mm. Hg range if the patient has a secondary hypoxic drive to stimulate respiration. It must be remembered that if hypoxemia is allowed to persist, the lethal effects of oxygen lack may occur. Oxygen administration may require the addition of more complex forms of respiratory therapy such as mechanically assisted ventilation to maintain physiologic oxygen and carbon dioxide tensions. High doses of oxygen (above 50 per cent) given for long periods of time may lead to oxygen toxicity or other hazards of therapy. Oxygen administration must always be preceded with pretherapy measurement of arterial blood gases. Subsequent arterial blood gas analysis must be made to note the progression of effectiveness of therapy. However, the hazards of oxygen therapy must never prevent the administration of oxygen to a patient in an acute emergency situation in which the rapid administration of oxygen is required to maintain life.

Patient-Family Teaching Points.   (a) The patient, visitors and staff must not smoke, use combustibles or spark-producing appliances or equipment in an oxygen-enriched environment; (b) oxygen must be administered only as prescribed and doses must not be randomly changed; (c) oxygen must be administered continuously, as it cannot be stored in the body; (d) when tanks are being used, they must be secured to prevent them from falling; (e) instruct the patient and family to observe for the signs of hypercapnia (elevated P_{CO_2}) such as tremors, increased lethargy, somnolence and headache; and signs associated with increasing hypoxemia, such as a change in pulse rate, degree of breathlessness, change in color.

PRE-PROCEDURE ACTIVITIES

PRELIMINARY ASSESSMENT/PLANNING

▶ Check the results of the arterial blood gas analysis
▶ Check the chart to determine the liter flow, delivery device, reason for therapy, further assessment required
▶ Note any significant pulmonary history
▶ Observe patient for physical signs of chronic respiratory dysfunction
▶ Observe for clinical signs of hypoxemia so that reversal may then be noted and effectiveness of therapy determined

PREPARATION OF PATIENT AND UNIT

▶ Ensure that electrical appliances have hospital-grade plugs and that equipment is safe for use in oxygen rich environment.

EQUIPMENT

▶ "No Smoking" sign
▶ Oxygen flowmeter
▶ Oxygen connecting tube
▶ Oxygen delivery device
▶ Humidifier (optional and dependent upon the delivery device)
▶ Distilled water if humidifier used
▶ Oxygen analyzer if applicable

Procedure continued on the following page

▶ Post "No Smoking" sign on the door and above head of patient's bed
▶ Announce to others in the room that no smoking is allowed when the oxygen is running
▶ Remove cigarettes, matches and other smoking equipment from the room
▶ Compare the patient's identification band with the requisition
▶ Place the patient in a comfortable position

PROCEDURE

SUGGESTED STEPS	RATIONALE/DISCUSSION
A. Assemble equipment at bedside	
1. Fill humidifier with sterile distilled water.	1. Humidifier adds water vapor to the dry gas (O_2) to reduce the drying and irritating effects.
2. If HAFOE mask (Venturi style) is used, do not add humidifier.	2. With the HAFOE mask, the humidifier acts as a resistance to the efficiency of air entrainment so that higher than desired O_2 per cent is delivered.
3. Plug in flowmeter to outlet or turn on tank valve.	3. Determine if system is functioning.
B. Adjust liter flow as ordered by physician or as required by the delivery device.	B. HAFOE masks have a specific liter flow for each per cent of O_2 delivered. The venturi portion of the mask entrains a specific amount of air to mix with the O_2 so that high total liter flows of air and O_2 are delivered to the patient. Any other O_2 liter flow may be insufficient to meet the inspired ventilation needs of the patient so that the percentage of O_2 remains constant. Determine that the liter flow prescribed is within acceptable range to achieve the goal of therapy.
C. Apply the cannula, mask, etc., to the patient; connect the oxygen connecting tubing to the humidifier or to flowmeter adapter if humidifier not used.	C. The device must be applied correctly to prevent hazards and discomfort and to insure accurate flow rates of O_2.
1. Make certain patient is not lying on connecting tube.	1. Flow will be restricted or obstructed; humidifier will not bubble. A characteristic audible noise might be heard depending upon brand of humidifier.
D. Note the effects of O_2 on the patient.	D. Symptoms of hypoxemia should improve or disappear. Observe for signs of hypercapnia, e.g., tremors, lethargy, somnolence.

SUGGESTED STEPS	RATIONALE/DISCUSSION
E. Do not remove the oxygen unless ordered by physician and arterial blood gases show return to normal.	E. O_2 is not stored by the body; it must be administered continuously during all activities, e.g., eating, sitting in a chair, being transported to other departments.

Post-Procedure Activities.   While O_2 is flowing, continue to evaluate the effects of oxygen therapy; periodically look at the flowmeter to check the flowrate; continue to provide oxygen for all activities. If patient is confused, raise side-rails; if necessary, safely restrain patient to prevent him from tampering with equipment or harming himself. Provide other forms of therapy to correct the cause of hypoxemia if the process is treatable (see Table 36–3).

Aftercare of Equipment.   Change the delivery device, humidifier and water reservoir daily. Discard disposable equipment as it is discontinued. Reusable equipment must be decontaminated and stored dry.

Final Assessment.   Continue to observe for the effects of the therapy; chart the liter flow, device used, and the effects of therapy. Recheck liter flow and device. Arrange for follow-up arterial blood gas assessment.

Chart/Report.   Results of oxygen administration. Report on positive effects of therapy, e.g., respiratory rate decreased to normal, heart rate returned to normal, breathing pattern improved and distress relieved; or negative effects such as increased confusion, lethargy or other signs of CO_2 retention. Chart and report the results of all arterial blood gas measurements immediately to the physician; enter arterial gases on a flow sheet to provide visualization of the trends of therapy at a glance. The flow sheet should include: Date and time; pH; PCO_2; HCO_3^-; SaO_2; liter flow or percentage of oxygen; brief narrative of effects of therapy and assessment of patient reaction to therapy.

Undesirable Effects of Oxygen Therapy

The undesired effects of oxygen therapy include: (a) oxygen-induced hypoventilation, (b) oxygen toxicity, (c) retrolental fibroplasia and (d) atelectasis. The following paragraphs describe the etiology of these undesired effects and some nursing actions to reduce or eliminate their occurrence.

Oxygen-induced Hypoventilation. Patients with chronically elevated levels of CO_2 may hypoventilate when O_2 is administered. This happens because the administration of O_2 removes the hypoxic drive to breathe that these patients have. If oxygen is administered to the patient with chronic CO_2 elevation and chronic hypoxemia, the stimulus to breathe (the hypoxemia) may be eliminated. The result of the elimination of the hypoxic drive is apnea (a cessation of respirations).

The following *nursing actions* and observations may alert the nurse to the presence of chronic lung disease and potential chronic CO_2 retention. They may also provide a guide to preventing oxygen-induced hypoventilation.

1. Look for indications of existing chronic pulmonary disease, including the following:
   a. Clubbing of the fingers and toes
   b. Pursed-lip exhalation breathing pattern
   c. Use of accessory muscles to assist with ventilation
   d. Obvious dyspnea
   e. Increased anteroposterior (AP) diameter of the chest
   f. Characteristic body positions used to increase the capacity of the thorax, e.g., sit-

ting leaning forward with elbows propped and shoulders elevated

g. Nicotine stains on fingers and teeth. Persons with chronic pulmonary disease usually are (or have been) heavy smokers.

2. Always request base-line arterial blood gas analysis *prior to* the administration of oxygen. This is especially important in patients whom you suspect of having chronic lung disease. Evaluate the P_{CO_2}. If it is elevated, observe for signs of respiratory depression during the oxygen administration, e.g., increased lethargy and disorientation. Promptly report such observations to the physician.

3. Limit the liter flow to 2 LPM if O_2 must be started before base-line arterial blood gases can be obtained.

4. Request arterial blood gases 20 to 30 minutes after the initiation of oxygen. Observe for an elevation of the P_{CO_2}.

5. Maintain a flow sheet to record arterial blood gas results, respiratory rate and pattern and other observations.

6. Monitor the patient carefully during the oxygen administration to assess the therapeutic effectiveness of the therapy. Observe the following:

a. Respiratory rate. If rapid prior to therapy, does it return to the patient's normal range of breaths per minute? (See Chap. 29.)

b. Respiratory pattern. If irregular prior to oxygen administration, does the pattern resume a normal inspiratory and expiratory pattern? (See Chap. 29.)

c. Level of consciousness. If patient is confused prior to therapy, does he become less confused and more rational?

d. Presence of tremors. This may indicate that even if physiologic oxygen requirements are met, the patient may be developing an elevation of CO_2. Other types of therapy would need to be instituted in order to meet oxygen requirements without causing CO_2 retention.

7. Report any undesired effects immediately.

8. Follow the guidelines for use of oxygen delivery systems and observe safety precautions.

The fear of oxygen-induced hypoventilation in persons with suspected chronic pulmonary disease should not prevent the administration of oxygen in life-threatening and emergency situations.

Oxygen Toxicity. *Oxygen toxicity is a medically induced disease*, characterized by alterations in the pulmonary parenchyma, e.g., thickened, hemorrhagic alveolar walls. Oxygen toxicity occurs when oxygen is administered in high dosages for prolonged periods of time. Generally, oxygen toxicity in its acute, lethal form does not occur with concentrations of oxygen less than 50 per cent. Pulmonary changes do not appear until the high dose of oxygen has been administered for 24 hours or more.

The development of oxygen toxicity is often difficult to recognize. However, any patient receiving long-term high-dose oxygen therapy should be carefully observed. The most common symptoms are:

(a) substernal distress—an ache or burning sensation behind the sternum

(b) increase in the amount of respiratory distress

(c) nausea and vomiting

(d) restlessness

(e) dry hacking cough

The specific clinical indication of oxygen toxicity development is: *An inability of the patient to maintain his arterial oxygen tensions in a physiologic normal range while the percentage of inspired oxygen is progressively increased.*

The nurse is encouraged to take the following *nursing actions* to reduce the potential risk of the development of oxygen toxicity:

▶ Always check the dose of oxygen and maintain the liter flow or percentage of oxygen at the prescribed dose.

▶ Analyze the percentage of oxygen delivered by all types of oxygen administration devices by using an oxygen analyzer.

▶ Request frequent assessment of the patient's oxygen status by arterial blood gas analysis. *Arterial blood gas analysis must accompany all changes in oxygen dosage.* Evaluate the results of these tests, especially the P_{O_2}. Notify the physician immediately if a trend of increasing high inspired oxygen percentage yields a diminishing P_{O_2}. Remember, as stated earlier: The goal of oxygen therapy is to *achieve an optimal arterial oxygen tension for the individual patient by delivering the lowest, most effective dose of oxygen.*

The fear of causing oxygen toxicity should not prevent a nurse from administering oxygen when it is needed to maintain life and prevent the undesirable and potentially lethal effects of hypoxemia. However, oxygen must always be administered cautiously and under carefully supervised conditions.

Retrolental Fibroplasia. In the 1950's,

numerous infants who were cared for in oxygenated isolettes developed retrolental fibroplasia (RLF). In this condition, blood vessels in the retina of the eye constrict and the retina becomes fibrotic (thickened). Irreversible blindness develops. It was determined that this tragedy was caused by high oxygen tensions in the infant's arterial circulation. Recently oxygen-induced blindness has been reported in adults following prolonged arterial oxygen tensions above 250 mm. Hg.[12]

An important consideration in retrolental fibroplasia is that the causative factor is the patient's arterial oxygen tension level, rather than the inspired oxygen tension. If the patient's arterial oxygen tension can be maintained in the range of 50 to 80 mm. Hg., the risks of RLF are decreased. However, there is no magic number, as premature infants of low birth weight run the greatest risk of developing RLF and RLF has developed in infants even breathing room air (21 per cent O_2).

The care of the infant should include the following *nursing actions* to prevent the development of retrolental fibroplasia:

▶ Analyze the inspired oxygen tension with an oxygen analyzer.

▶ Document the recorded oxygen tension on the chart.

▶ Arrange for arterial blood gas analysis before instituting oxygen therapy in the isolette or oxygen therapy by other means. Re-analyze the arterial oxygen tension after placing the infant in the oxygen-rich environment.

▶ Have the eyes of the infant examined for fibrotic changes if his care involved oxygen therapy.

Atelectasis. "Atelectasis" is the name for a condition in which lung tissue (alveoli) collapse, either due to compression of the lung tissue or due to absorption of the "filler" gas, nitrogen. The absorption of the nitrogen may occur as a result of unmonitored oxygen administration. If oxygen is administered in high doses (80 per cent or more), the normal mixture of oxygen and nitrogen in the alveolar units is altered. The oxygen "washes out" the nitrogen, and the once expanded alveoli collapse. This same absorption occurs when secretions plug the airways. The result of the absorption of nitrogen is collapse of the alveoli.

Atelectasis is frequently seen in postanesthesia patients. When a surgical procedure requires long-term anesthesia and ventilation with oxygen, much of the patient's nitrogen becomes replaced with the oxygen and many alveoli may collapse. Immobile patients, especially those with shallow tidal volumes and few or no "sigh" breaths, also develop atelectasis. Obstruction of the airway by mucus or foreign material also leads to atelectasis of the lung in positions beyond the obstruction.

The following *nursing actions* may prevent atelectasis:

▶ Encouraging deep breathing with an end-inspiratory pause as soon as the patient is able to follow directions.

▶ Positional changes to facilitate aeration of the lungs and prevent pooling of secretions.

▶ Early mobilization to stimulate deep breathing and coughing.

Determination of Effective Oxygen Therapy

Oxygen therapy, like other forms of drug therapy, must be evaluated frequently. The effectiveness of oxygen therapy may be measured objectively and subjectively. *Objectively*, the effectiveness of oxygen therapy is evaluated by arterial blood gas analysis to determine: (a) that the PO_2 is between 60 and 80 mm. Hg (in chronic CO_2 retention, a PO_2 between 55 and 60 mm. Hg may be satisfactory) and (b) that as hypoxemia is relieved, hypercapnia has not been produced or aggravated.

Subjectively, the effectiveness of oxygen therapy is assessed by making the following observations:

(a) Pulse rate. Has the rate and rhythm of the pulse returned to "normal"?

(b) Blood pressure. Is the blood pressure in a "normal" range?

(c) Level of mentation. Have confusion, restlessness and other central nervous system impairments returned to a more stable or "normal" level?

(d) Skin temperature and condition. The skin should feel normally warm and dry and not cold, clammy or sweaty

(e) Respiratory rate and pattern of breathing. Is the rate within the normal range, with a normal pattern of breathing established (e.g., no shortness of breath)?

If your objective and subjective assessments determine that the patient's physiologic oxygen needs are being met, you know that therapy is appropriate. If any of the symptoms of hypoxemia are still present, alterations in the therapy are indicated. The correction of hypoxemia is important; it must be corrected before irreversible effects occur. *The oxygen source must not be withdrawn until both laboratory and clinical verification of adequate oxygenation has been obtained.* Therapy must be continued until the underlying disease process has cleared. In chronic conditions, supplemental oxygen is often required for the patient's lifetime.

A nurse is responsible for knowing blood-gas "normals" and informing the physician of all results, both normal and abnormal. The nurse should not stop oxygen without a physician's order. It is the physician's responsibility to order changes. Some physicians may leave an order to discontinue oxygen if certain laboratory results are reported. If this is the case, a nurse may stop oxygen. Oxygen may be started and stopped by a qualified nurse in certain areas of the hospital (e.g., post-anesthesia room, labor room, and some critical care areas) depending upon hospital policy.

Oxygen and Exercise

Normally when we increase our level of activity, we increase our oxygen requirements, and at the same time, we increase the level of ventilation to meet the increased oxygen requirement. Patients who have chronic respiratory dysfunction may not be able to meet their increased ventilation requirements as they increase their level of activity. The destruction and dysfunction of tissue in the lungs may be so great that hypoxemia exists even "at rest." When this is true, the additional oxygen needs demanded by exercise cannot be met. When the rate of oxygen consumption is raised but no additional oxygen is available to the tissues, anaerobic (without oxygen) metabolism occurs in the body.

For patients with chronic "resting" hypoxemia or those with "exercise-induced" hypoxemia, supplemental oxygen is essential. The flow rate of oxygen must be prescribed to maintain the PO_2 at a level of 55 to 60 mm. Hg or better without a significant elevation in the PCO_2. If oxygen is prescribed for use "at rest," then it most certainly must be given during exercise. Often the physician prescribes a resting liter flow of oxygen and a different liter flow to be used during exercise. *Strict attention must be given to ensuring that the correct liter flow of oxygen is administered at all times.*

MEDICATIONS FOR THE PATIENT WITH RESPIRATORY DYSFUNCTION

Medications are administered into the respiratory system by aerosolization. As discussed in the section on hydration, an *aerosol* consists of solid or liquid particles suspended in a stream of gas. Medications are aerosolized with a *nebulizer*, a device which breaks up liquids or powders into uniform particles with a system of baffles to eliminate the large particles. Aerosolized administration of medications may have either systemic or topical effects.

> Remember:
> *Medications that are injected into the blood stream produce the most rapid effects. The second most rapid effects are obtained through absorption in the pulmonary system.*

Drugs that are aerosolized and delivered to the respiratory system by inhalation can be classified as either "potent" or "bland" drugs. Generally, medications aerosolized in large-volume nebulizers are considered *bland* and act to hydrate and liquefy secretions to aid in the removal of secretions. Saline, distilled water, and one-quarter to one-half strength normal saline are examples of bland aerosol drugs. *Potent* drugs generally are aerosolized in small-volume nebulizers and are always given for a short period of time. Potent drugs may be classified in four categories:

1. *Bronchodilators and decongestants.* Bronchodilator drugs open the airways by relaxation of the smooth muscle of the tracheobronchial tree. Decongestants open the airway by reducing swollen, boggy, edematous airways. All bronchodilators must be used with caution in patients with known cardiac disease and hypertension. All bronchodilators may increase the heart rate and may affect the blood pressure. Bronchodilators may increase the level of hypoxemia. Always check the pulse rate before and after administration of bronchodilators. Two frequently used aerosol bronchodilators are isoproterenol hydrochloride and Bronkosol (the bronchodilating component is isoetharine).

2. *Mucolytics/Liquefactants/Detergents.* Drugs in this category aid in the clearance of retained secretions, by chemically altering the mucus, by increasing the water content of the mucus, or by changing the surface tension of the mucus so that it is more easily expectorated. Bronchospasm may be a side effect of the aerosol administration of these drugs. (Bronchospasm may occur any time a foreign substance is inhaled into the airway.) Bronchorrhea may also occur if the cough mechan-

ism is weak and ineffective. Large quantities of mucus may be mobilized by the drug and may cause obstruction of the airway. Some names of drugs in this category are Mucomyst (mucolytic), Dornavac (mucolytic and proteolytic enzymatic), Alevaire (detergent), ethyl alcohol (alters surface tension of secretions).

3. *Anti-inflammatory/Anti-allergenic.* Steroids are potent chemicals known for their anti-inflammatory and antifibrogenic properties. Sometimes steroids are aerosolized for a topical effect, but during acute bronchospasm they must also be administered systemically. The two most common aerosolized steroids are Decadron and Vanceril. Cromolyn sodium (Aarane, Intal) is the drug administered to prevent allergic responses in the airway. It is not a steroid; nor is it a drug used during acute bronchospastic episodes.

4. *Antibiotics.* Antibiotics are at times administered topically to treat pulmonary infections; the topical effects are generally less effective than the effects of antibiotics given systemically.

POSITIVE PRESSURE BREATHING TREATMENTS

Positive pressure breathing treatments are the administration of higher-than-ambient pressures to the airway to cause a flow of gas (oxygen and ambient air) into the airway. Positive pressure is usually abbreviated *IPPB* (intermittent positive pressure breathing) or *IPPV* (intermittent positive pressure ventilation). IPPB is administered via machines called *respirators.* Generally, when the patient initiates an inhalation, the machine cycles on and a flow of gas enters the upper airway through either a plastic mouthpiece or a mask. When a pre-set pressure is reached in the airway, the machine cycles off and the patient is allowed to exhale (Fig. 36–11).

> *IPPB therapy must be given only under the careful supervision of a person trained and skilled in its administration. A poorly given IPPB treatment carries more hazards than no therapy at all.*[33]

There is no one right way to administer IPPB. As with all respiratory therapy, modifications may need to be made to achieve effective therapy. These modifications depend in part on the patient's condition and his level of cooperation. More detailed and specific information may be obtained from respiratory therapy texts.

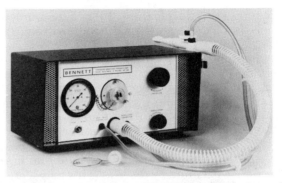

Figure 36–11. The Bennett AP-4 Respirator—a type of IPPB machine. (From The Puritan Bennett Corp., Kansas City, Mo. 64106.)

Uses of IPPB. IPPB may be administered to: (1) stimulate and promote deep breathing in patients with decreased levels of consciousness, (2) mobilize secretions through cough stimulation, (3) produce mechanical bronchodilation, (4) administer aerosol medication, (5) hyperinflate the lungs to prevent atelectasis, (6) control pulmonary edema and pulmonary congestion and/or (7) decrease the work of breathing (temporary effect only).

Precautions in the Use of IPPB. To be effective, an IPPB machine must deliver a volume of air equal to or greater than the patient's normal tidal volume. Inadequate volumes of gas delivered to the airway will result in inadequate ventilation of the lungs. This is termed *alveolar hypoventilation.*

Patients with chronic lung disease who receive IPPB therapy should have the respirators powered with compressed medical air (21 per cent oxygen) to prevent oxygen-induced hypoventilation. IPPB machines may be powered either by a high-pressure source (usually oxygen from a pipe in the wall) or by compressors that create the required driving pressure for the activation of the respirator. If oxygen is used as the driving gas, the range of oxygen percentages delivered to the patient cannot be controlled. The range may unpredictably vary from 35 to 100 per cent O_2.

Side Effects of IPPB. There are six adverse physiologic effects that may be created with IPPB administration: (1) overventilation, (2) decreased venous return, (3) overdistention of alveoli, (4) gastric distention, (5) excessive oxygenation and (6) increased intracranial pressure.

1. *Overventilation* from moving excessive

volumes of air during the IPPB cycles. Dangerously low P_{CO_2}'s may result from overventilation, leading to central nervous system complaints, dizziness, tremors, and decreased cerebral blood flow.

2. *Decreased venous return* of blood to the heart, caused by the positive pressure effects on the great vessels in the thorax. The pulse may increase and the blood pressure may fall.

3. *Overdistention of alveoli* from the positive pressure, which enlarges alveoli that have become weakened by disease. This may lead to rupture of these alveoli, producing a pneumothorax, i.e., air in the pleural space.

The inspiratory phase of breathing (both natural and under positive pressure) produces bronchodilation, in which the airways open wider. If the normal elasticity of the airways is destroyed (e.g., with chronic lung disease), the lung tissue may not sufficiently recoil (decrease in size) to aid in the removal of air during exhalation. The air may then become "trapped." Air trapping also causes overdistention of alveoli. *If the risk of alveolar distention is great, IPPB is contraindicated.*

4. *Gastric distention* (resulting from "air swallowing") may occur with improper administration of IPPB and/or lack of supervision during the therapy. Gastric distention may lead to nausea, vomiting and aspiration of gastric contents into the airway.

5. *Excessive oxygenation* has been discussed above under precautions in the use of IPPB. The uncontrolled oxygen dose may eliminate hypoxic drive in patients with chronic lung disease. For such patients, IPPB should be administered with compressed medical air (21 per cent oxygen).

6. *Increased intracranial pressure* may occur in patients with pre-existing central nervous system damage. The thoracic increase in airway pressure caused by the IPPB is reflected in the cranial cavity. This causes a potential impediment to venous return in the cerebral circulation and pressure on the capillary blood flow to the brain.

Contraindications to the Use of IPPB. Precipitation of any of the side effects of IPPB presented above constitutes a contraindication to further positive pressure therapy. Also, *IPPB is strictly contraindicated in the presence of an untreated pneumothorax.* Active tuberculosis and hemoptysis are no longer considered contraindications to IPPB therapy.

MAINTAINING A PATENT AIRWAY BY TRACHEAL SUCTIONING

Respiratory dysfunctions may interfere with a patient's clearance of tracheobronchial secretions and other defense mechanisms of his respiratory system. As a result, secretions (mucus or pus) are retained, and the normal exchange of gases is impaired. Prolonged retention of secretions may lead to infection and other more severe respiratory dysfunction, such as atelectasis or pneumonia. The secretions need to be removed via either the mouth or the nose by mechanical means (suctioning) when a patient cannot "clear" his own tracheobronchial tree. The term *aspiration* is used interchangeably with the word "suction."

Aspiration of the tracheobronchial tree via a catheter is necessary for the airway management of any patient who is unable to handle his retained secretions. This would include any patient with medical or surgical disorders that prevent him from coughing effectively and raising secretions. Suctioning is frequently required for such patients following position changes, such as being turned from one side to another. Suctioning should only be done on an "as needed" basis because excessive suctioning can be traumatic. Assessment of the need to suction is discussed in a following section.

All patient care areas must be equipped with effective means of clearing an airway. An occluded airway, either from retained secretions or aspirated foreign material, is a potentially life-threatening occurrence. All personnel permitted to suction by hospital or agency policy should be familiar with the types of suction equipment available on the patient care unit, know the location of this equipment and be certain it is always in properly functioning order.

Removal of secretions can be carried out through the oral-pharyngeal route (mouth), the nasopharyngeal route (nose), or through an artificial airway, e.g., endotracheal or tracheostomy tube. (An endotracheal tube is inserted into the trachea through the nose or mouth; a tracheostomy tube is inserted into the trachea through a surgical incision in the trachea.) The choice of the route of suctioning depends upon: (a) the patient's level of consciousness, (b) his level of cooperation and (c) the availability of an artificial airway. The type of material to be suctioned or aspirated must also be considered. The thicker the material, the more difficult it is to aspirate it through the smaller size catheters.

Hydration is one of the most important factors in removal of secretions, because hydration helps to liquefy the secretions. Hydration of tracheobronchial secretions may be accomplished through: (a) parenteral or oral methods, (b) aerosolization of liquid into the tracheobronchial tree to thin the mucus and/or (c) direct instillation of liquefying agents into the tracheobronchial tree. There is a direct relationship between the thickness or viscosity of secretions, the size of the suction catheter, and the amount of vacuum required to remove the secretions. That is, the thicker the secretions, the larger the size of the suction catheter required.

Assessing Need for Suctioning. *Suctioning must be done only when it is needed.* It must not be done unless retained secretions are present and the patient is unable to maintain a patent airway with effective expulsive coughing. The nurse must observe the patient and make a decision to suction based on her assessment in the following ways:

1. *Visual assessment.* A change in the respiratory pattern may be noted when a patient requires suctioning. The rate of respiration may increase and the patient may demonstrate difficult or labored breathing.

2. *Auditory assessment.* Moist, noisy, rattling or gurgling sounds may indicate that airway patency is impaired with secretions.

3. *Tactile assessment.* A term often used in pulmonary assessment is *tactile fremitus.* It refers to the transmission of vibrational impulses through the chest wall. The impulses are created when air moves through the retained secretions. These impulses can be felt directly over the portion of the tracheobronchial tree where the secretions are retained. When the flat palm of the hand is gently placed over the affected area, a rumbling, or vibration-like feeling, is noted. If the tactile fremitus is not felt after the procedure, this would indicate the effectiveness of the suctioning.

4. *Auscultation.* The practice of listening to a patient's breath sounds with a stethoscope before and after the suction procedure is the best clinical tool for determining the need to suction. It is also the best way to determine if you have been successful and effective in your procedure.

The adventitious (abnormal) breath sounds associated with retained secretions and the need to clear the airway are called *rhonchi.* A *rhonchus* is best defined as a continuous and sometimes musical coarse rattling sound or vibration. Such sounds may be high or low pitched and are of longer duration than the other common abnormal breath sound, the *rale.* *Rales* are best defined as a crackling or bubbling sound not heard continuously, but rather discontinuously, during inspiration. They usually are indicative of fluid or fibrosis at the alveolar level. The level of intensity and the quality of the "bubbling" or the "crackling" varies. Rhonchi can usually be cleared with tracheobronchial aspiration. Rales cannot be eliminated with a suction catheter. *Wheezes* are a type of whistling rhonchi usually associated with airway edema and bronchospasm in addition to the retained secretions. The higher the pitch of the wheeze, the further out in the periphery of the airway the wheeze is occurring.

It is more important for the nurse to listen to the chest and describe in her own words the sounds she hears with the stethoscope than it is for her to try to use the "proper" terminology.

Vacuum Pressures. Suctioning of the airway requires a source of vacuum. Most hospitals that have piped oxygen also have a piped-in source of vacuum. When a piping system is not available, portable suction units may be used. Portable units need to be connected to an electrical source to power the suction pump.

Suctioning is accomplished by using *negative* or *vacuum pressures* to aspirate the retained secretions through the catheter and into the collection container. The gauges mounted on the wall in a hospital with a piped-in vacuum system are calibrated in mm. Hg vacuum pressure. The gauges found on portable suction units are generally measured in inches of Hg. The safe range for vacuum pressures for adults is 80 to 140 mm. Hg (2 to 3 inches Hg). If the catheter is too small or the secretions are too thick, excessive (higher than the safe limits) pressures may be required. Additional hydration and tracheal irrigation may also be required to effectively aspirate tenacious secretions.

Suctioning Catheter. A suction catheter must be made of a material that is as non-trauma producing as possible. Many newer brands of suction catheters are designed with a smooth rounded tip and are manufactured from a silicone and polyvinylchloride (PVC) compound, which reduces resistance and friction when the catheter is passed through an artificial airway. The end of the suction catheter should have two to three "vents," i.e., openings. This type of catheter is called the *whistle-tip catheter.* The vents should be spaced along the lower 1½ to 2 inches on alternate sides of the catheter. This prevents the collapse of the catheter if it becomes occluded and high vacuum pressures are created. These vents also help to reduce mucosal trauma by reducing the pull of the catheter against the mucosa.

A suction catheter must be long enough to reach and pass through the bifurcation of the trachea (the carina). The proximal end (i.e., the end closest to you) of the catheter must have a port (opening) which the therapist or nurse can occlude as desired or leave open to the room air. When the port is open, air can pass in and out of the trachea. When this port is occluded, the vacuum pressure is transmitted into the airway and secretions are removed through the catheter to the collection container (Fig. 36–12).

Suction catheters are sized using the French scale. The smaller the French number, the smaller the catheter. Suction catheters generally range in size from 5 French to 18 French. The 12 and 14 French size are most commonly used for suctioning an adult. Smaller catheters not only do not remove the secretions as effectively as larger ones, but they also tend to curl and are more difficult to direct into the airway. An important rule of thumb for catheter size selection is:

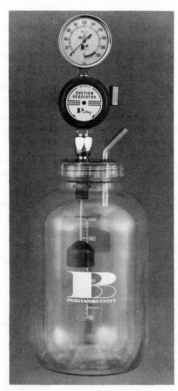

Figure 36–12. Suction gauge and collection bottle for tracheobronchial aspiration. (From The Puritan Bennett Corp., Kansas City, Mo. 64106.)

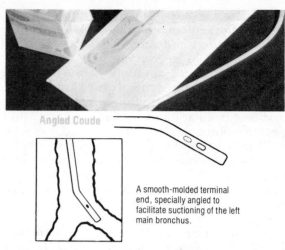

Angled Coude

A smooth-molded terminal end, specially angled to facilitate suctioning of the left main bronchus.

Figure 36–13. A coudé-tip suction catheter is necessary to successfully enter the left main bronchus. (From Portex, Inc., Wilmington, Mass. 01887.)

The size of the suction catheter must never exceed one-half the diameter of the artificial airway or the natural airway it is to enter.

When artificial airways are in place, the size of the catheter is critical. When a catheter is inserted into the airway, atmospheric air must pass through and along side of it, or the patient will suffocate. Remember, as secretions are aspirated, air is also removed from the lungs. *The larger the catheter in relation to the artificial airway, the more air will also be removed from the lungs.*

COUDÉ-TIP SUCTION CATHETER. The standard straight whistle-tip catheter is generally used for suctioning the airway. However, when it is necessary to suction the left main bronchus, an angled coudé-tip catheter is required (Fig. 36–13). A review of the anatomy of the tracheobronchial tree reveals that the trachea divides (bifurcates) into the right and left main bronchi at the point called the carina. The angle of this bifurcation calls for an angled, or coudé-tip catheter, to facilitate entry of the catheter into the left bronchus. The right main bronchus leaves the trachea at a 27-degree angle. The left main bronchus leaves the trachea at a sharp 45-degree angle. Obviously, a suction catheter, or any object for that matter, will more likely enter the right main bronchus than the left.

When a patient has retained secretions on the left side of the tracheobronchial tree, a coudé tip suction catheter is used; when inserted into the airway, it will enter the left main bronchus 45 to 50 per cent of the time. It was once thought that if the patient's head were turned to the right with the chin in line with the right shoulder, a suction catheter would enter the left main bronchus. Recent fluoroscopic studies have shown this technique successful only 10 per cent of the time—the catheter entered the right bronchus in 90 per cent of the attempts no matter how far the head was turned.[15]

Tracheal Suction Procedure.   It is important to remember that sterility must be maintained for any item to be inserted into the airway to prevent the introduction of bacterial contaminants into the tracheobronchial tree. The following points must be considered: (a) the catheter and the rinsing solution must always be kept sterile; (b) the catheter must be guided by a sterile-gloved hand; (c) the catheter must not be allowed to touch the patient or any part of the environment, e.g., the bedclothes; (d) any irrigating solution must be kept sterile; (e) the catheter must be discarded after each suction insertion and a fresh sterile catheter used for each subsequent insertion and (f) collection bottles must be emptied and decontaminated or discarded every 8 to 24 hours.

The procedure for sterile suctioning of the airway follows.

21. SUCTIONING THE TRACHEOBRONCHIAL TREE

Definition.   *The removal of secretions from the tracheobronchial tree by means of applying vacuum (suction) by way of a sterile suction catheter inserted into the airway.* The procedure is carried out through insertion of the catheter through one of three routes: (1) the nasopharyngeal route; (2) through the oral pharynx; or (3) through an artificial airway, e.g., endotracheal or tracheostomy tube.

Purpose.   The purposes of suctioning the tracheobronchial tree are: (a) to maintain a patent airway by removal of retained secretions and foreign material; (b) to prevent the effects of retained secretions, such as infection and atelectasis; (c) to promote improved exchange of oxygen and carbon dioxide; (d) to stimulate or substitute for an effective cough when a patient is unable to cough due to diminished mentation, progressive weakness, etc. and (e) to obtain a tracheal aspirate specimen for laboratory analysis.

Cautions and Contraindications.   Suctioning is an exacting procedure requiring careful training and particular attention to safety considerations. Study the complete discussion in the text of the side effects of suctioning. Care should be directed toward: (a) maintaining a sterile field and sterile procedure to prevent infection; (b) avoiding excessive traumatic vacuum pressures and mechanical trauma induced by suction catheter; (c) ensuring oxygen administration before, during, and after procedure; (d) hyperinflating the lungs with an anesthesia bag or self-inflating type bag before and after each catheter insertion if patient is unable to deep breathe on his own and (e) observing extra caution if the patient has an unstable cardiovascular system.

Suctioning can create hypoxemia and atelectasis; insertion of the catheter into the tracheobronchial tree stimulates the vagus nerve. Vagal stimulation and hypoxemia may cause cardiac arrhythmias, such as ventricular tachycardia, ventricular fibrillation and cardiac arrest.

> *Always use a sterile catheter. Ideally the catheter should be discarded and replaced after each tracheal insertion; however, many hospitals change the catheter only after each series of insertions into the trachea. Never store the suction catheter in any type of solution, including those that are antibacterial in nature.*

Procedure continued on the following page

Never use the same catheter to suction by different routes; discard the catheter and replace with another sterile catheter. The size of the catheter should never be more than one-half the diameter of the airway. Safe vacuum pressures for an adult are 80 to 140 mm. Hg. Apply vacuum only intermittently and only on withdrawal of the catheter. *The length of time to complete the entire insertion and removal of the catheter should not exceed 10 to 15 seconds.*

Patient-Family Teaching Points.   Enlist the patient's cooperation. Tell the patient what you are going to do. Encourage him to cooperate and not "fight" the procedure as this will cause both trauma and potential introduction of a contaminated catheter into the lungs. The family and patient should be reassured that the procedure is essential to maintain an open airway to allow for comfortable, effective breathing, or to obtain a sterile sample of the sputum so that correct antibiotic therapy can be instituted.

PRE-PROCEDURE ACTIVITIES

PRELIMINARY PATIENT ASSESSMENT

Determine the need to suction by:
▶ Visual assessment of respirations
▶ Auditory assessment of respirations
▶ Tactile assessment of respirations by noting if vibrations from secretions are transmitted through chest wall
▶ Auscultate chest to determine need to suction and location in tracheobronchial tree of retained secretions

Determine level of patient cooperation:
▶ Assess need and obtain assistance if needed to restrain patient
▶ Obtain assistance for oxygenating and hyperinflating patient

PRELIMINARY PLANNING

▶ Gather and assemble all equipment at bedside
▶ Wash hands
▶ Test vacuum pressure by pinching off the connecting tube and noting the amount of vacuum recorded on the suction gauge
▶ Determine route of suctioning, and obtain appropriate equipment, i.e., airway and correct size catheter
▶ If manual hyperinflation is not to be done, plan means of delivery of oxygen: The patient must always be preoxygenated as well as oxygenated after each insertion of the suction catheter into the trachea

EQUIPMENT

▶ Vacuum gauge
▶ Collection bottle
▶ Connecting tubing 6 to 10 feet long
▶ Sterile whistle-tip straight catheter, or coudé tip catheter
▶ Sterile glove
▶ Sterile cup for solution
▶ Sterile solution (saline or water) to rinse catheter and connecting tubing
▶ Hyperinflation equipment (anesthesia bag or resuscitation bag)
▶ Oxygen administration equipment (flowmeter, tubing)
▶ Means of delivery of oxygen (cannula, mask, etc.)
▶ Sputum trap if tracheal aspirate specimen needed
▶ Oral airway to facilitate oral pharyngeal suctioning (use only if patient has a diminishing gag reflex)
▶ Nasal airway to facilitate nasal route of entry and reduce trauma to nasal mucosa

PREPARATION OF PATIENT

▶ Explain procedure to patient and/or family
▶ Position patient comfortably; restrain as necessary
▶ Screen patient from view of other patients and visitors

PROCEDURE

SUGGESTED STEPS	RATIONALE/DISCUSSION
A. Prepare patient and suctioning equipment	A. *See Chapter 37 for sterile technique.*
1. Insert nasal or oral airway.	
2. Open bottle of sterile rinsing solution.	2. Use sterile technique for opening bottle.
3. Turn vacuum ON and test vacuum and suction system.	3. Occlude, pinch or bend connecting tubing between index finger and thumb. Observe vacuum pressure on gauge.
4. Aseptically open catheter, glove and cup.	
5. Put on sterile glove (Proc. 23, p. 935).	5. Glove dominant hand.
6. Fill sterile cup with sterile rinsing solution.	6. Remove cap and pour solution with ungloved hand.
7. Attach sterile catheter to connecting tube.	7. Hold catheter with gloved hand and hold connecting tube with ungloved hand.
B. Increase the inspired O_2 concentration to highest possible percentage of oxygen and hyperinflate lungs with manual or spontaneous deep breaths.	B. Best levels of oxygenation and hyperinflation are achieved with 100% O_2 delivered via anesthesia bag or self-inflating bag.
1. Be aware of patient's blood gas and cardiac status, e.g., note PO_2 on blood gas report, check pulse rate.	1. Suctioning can cause cardiac arrhythmias and increase hypoxemia.
	2. Suctioning causes airway collapse, which can increase hypoxemia and lead to atelectasis.
C. Lubricate sterile catheter with sterile rinsing solution and test patency of catheter by placing gloved thumb over vent in catheter.	C. Catheter will enter airway more easily. Pretest assures functioning of system prior to insertion.
D. Remove O_2 source and quickly begin to suction.	D. Oxygen is not stored. It must be supplied on a continual basis. The maximum time oxygen may be interrupted is 10 to 15 seconds.
E. Use gloved hand to insert catheter.	E. Sterile gloved hand necessary to prevent bacterial contamination of airway during procedure.

Suctioning via Oral Route

F. If oral airway in place, slide catheter alongside it and back into pharynx. If airway not in place, guide catheter into posterior oral	F. Oral route is least successful as it is difficult to pass a catheter into the trachea by this route. An oral airway facilitates entrance of catheter

Procedure continued on the following page

SUGGESTED STEPS	RATIONALE/DISCUSSION

Suctioning via Oral Route (Continued)

pharynx as patient sticks out tongue. Insert during inspiration until cough stimulated or catheter resists further insertion, or secretions located.

into trachea. Tongue displaced forward also facilitates catheter entry.

1. *Caution:* Catheter may stimulate gag reflex when inserted into oral pharynx and lead to vomiting and aspiration of gastric contents.

2. Oral route usually used to remove secretions sitting in back of mouth.

Suctioning via Nasal Route

G. Insert and advance catheter during inhalation. Guide the catheter along floor of nares; or pass catheter through nasal airway, if in place, until cough stimulated, catheter resists insertion, or secretions located.

G. During inhalation, the epiglottis is out of the way and airway almost open. A nasal airway not only reduces trauma to nasal mucosa, but facilitates entrance of catheter into trachea.

Suctioning via Artificial Airway

H. Insert catheter into artificial airway during inhalation carefully so as not to touch patient or environment. Continue insertion until cough reflex stimulated, resistance met, or secretions located.

H. Airway diameter larger during inhalation. To prevent contamination of catheter.

1. To cannulate the left bronchus with a suction catheter, a coudé-tip catheter must be used.

I. Do *not* cover thumb control and apply vacuum during insertion of catheter.

I. Application of vacuum during entry dangerously increases hypoxemia and creates more atelectasis.

J. Apply *intermittent* vacuum as catheter withdrawn.

J. Do not force entry of catheter; this would increase trauma. Intermittent vacuum reduces the trauma to mucosal lining of airway. *Never* apply continuous vacuum.

1. Rotate catheter and wind it around gloved index finger during withdrawal.

1. Reduces dragging of catheter along one portion of mucous membrane of airway and controls catheter, thus preventing it from touching bed clothes or patient.

2. Length of time to complete entire insertion and removal of catheter should not exceed 10 to 15 seconds.

2. Longer time would increase the risk of dangerous complications.

SUGGESTED STEPS	RATIONALE/DISCUSSION
K. Discard catheter, glove, cup and solution if changing routes or no more secretions remain in trachea to be aspirated.	K. Never use a catheter to suction more than one route.
L. Re-oxygenate and hyperinflate for minimum of 5 breaths. Allow patient to rest between insertions.	L. Reduces and corrects hypoxemia and re-opens small airways that may have collapsed from vacuum pressures.
M. Assess patient and repeat steps if retained secretions still present.	M. Unnecessary suctioning may increase side effects.
N. Take fresh catheter, glove, cup and solution for each tracheal insertion; or after three repeated tracheal insertions (follow agency policy).	N. To prevent bacterial contamination.
O. Discard catheter, glove, cup, solution if all secretions removed at this time.	O. Catheter and other items are contaminated; never store for re-use.

Post-Procedure Activities.   Reassure patient; auscultate chest and make other assessments to determine effectiveness of procedure; note vital signs, pattern and sound of respirations; return patient to presuctioning oxygen administration appliance; reassure patient and family that procedure is completed until needed again; loosen or remove restraints if appropriate; if secretions were thick, tenacious and difficult to suction, reassess the status of the patient's hydration and bring to physician's attention if hydration inadequate to facilitate secretion removal; note appearance, consistency, and estimate amount of tracheal aspirate; if sputum trap used to collect specimen, take it promptly to the appropriate lab with appropriate lab slip and labeled with the patient's identification information.

Aftercare of Equipment.   Discard catheter, glove, cup, used solution; discard contents of collection bottle; turn off vacuum; coil connecting tubing around gauge to prevent it from falling to the floor; recheck oxygen flow rate; cover hyperinflation bag to keep the equipment clean. Oral or nasal airways may be removed or left in place as patient comfort allows.

Final Patient Assessment.   Recheck breath sounds, pulse, respiratory rate and pattern, and blood pressure; note appearance and amount of aspirate—color, presence of blood, thickness, etc.; note if hypoxemia or arrhythmias created by the procedure; notify physician if aspirate appears infected or abnormal or difficult to remove due to inadequate state of hydration; assess general tolerance of procedure by the patient.

Chart/Report.   Chart time procedure done; route used; pre- and post-procedure vital signs; breath sounds before and after procedure; position of patient prior to suctioning; appearance, quantity and quality of secretions; general patient tolerance including status of oxygenation and cardiac reaction; re-application of pre-procedure oxygen administration appliance. Record whether tracheal aspirate specimen sent to the laboratory and type of laboratory study requested.

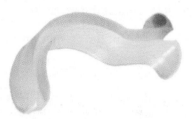

Figure 36–14. Oral-pharyngeal airway. The airway is inserted into the mouth by sliding the airway, on its side, along the tongue. When the curved end of the airway reaches the back of the mouth, the airway is rotated so that the curved end holds the tongue in a forward position. The patient may bite or close his mouth over the flat portion of the airway. (From Portex, Inc., Wilmington, Mass. 01887.)

Use of Airways During Suctioning. Often during loss of consciousness, the muscles of the tongue become relaxed and the tongue falls back into the posterior pharynx and occludes the airway. Placing a proper size *oral airway* in the mouth will hold the tongue in a forward position. This facilitates suctioning and also keeps the airway from becoming occluded by the tongue. If the *oral-pharyngeal* route of suctioning is tried, the placement of an oral pharyngeal airway may allow the passage of the suction catheter into the posterior pharynx (Fig. 36–14).

Nasal airways are similar in appearance to an uncuffed, short endotracheal tube (Fig. 36–15). The external end of the airway is flared to fit against the external nares. A nasal airway, lubricated with an anesthesia jelly, is inserted into the external nares of any patient requiring

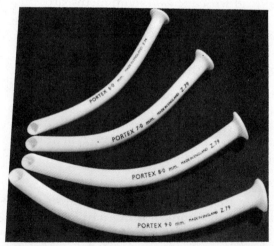

Figure 36–15. Nasal airway. The insertion of the nasal airway into the nares assists the suction catheter in entry into the tracheobronchial tree. It also is less traumatic to the nasal mucosa. (From Portex, Inc., Wilmington, Mass. 01887.)

moderate to frequent nasotracheal suctioning. The nasal airway reduces trauma to the nasal mucosa from frequent introduction of the suction catheter. Also, the nasal airway helps direct the tip of the catheter into the trachea.

Side Effects of Suctioning

The suctioning procedure to remove the retained secretions from the airway can have ill effects, including: (a) hypoxemia, (b) alveolar collapse and atelectasis, (c) vagal stimulation, (d) mucosal trauma, (e) hypotension and (f) paroxysmal episodes of coughing.

Hypoxemia. When vacuum is applied to the airway, not only are secretions removed, but also oxygen is removed. The removal of oxygen may be of critical importance if the patient has a marginal state of oxygenation. In fact, suctioning may cause such a patient to become hypoxemic. Hypoxemia induced by the suctioning procedure may be prevented or corrected by taking the precaution of supplying supplemental oxygen to the patient. If hypoxemia is created, the patient will develop alterations in the heart rate—usually a tachycardia that reverts to the patient's normal rate following oxygenation.

All patients should be given a minimum of five oxygenated breaths prior to each suctioning attempt. This can be done by applying an oxygen appliance such as a cannula or mask on the patient and using the appropriate liter flow of oxygen to achieve the maximal oxygen concentration the appliance is capable of delivering. An alternate method is to manually give the patient five deep breaths with 90 to 100 per cent oxygen using an anesthesia bag or manual resuscitation bag. This is the method used with all patients having an artificial airway.

> Remember, oxygen cannot be stored in the body. It is necessary to re-oxygenate the patient between each suctioning attempt. *Never suction a patient a second time until he has been re-oxygenated for at least five breaths. Suction-induced hypoxemia may lead to fatal complications.*

Alveolar Collapse and Atelectasis. As oxygen is removed during aspiration, so is the filler gas, nitrogen (N_2), which helps maintain the alveoli in an open position. If it is removed, alveoli may collapse and atelectasis will occur. Collapse of alveoli and atelectasis may also occur if the vacuum pressure is too high for the size of the airway.

Atelectasis will further impair the patient's

level of oxygenation. To prevent the collapse of lung tissue, it is important to *sigh* the patient. This is also called *hyperinflation*. Some patients are able to deep breathe (sigh) for themselves. When hyperinflating a patient by mechanical means, e.g., with an anesthesia bag, a deep breath is automatically given at the same time the oxygen is administered. The most important measures used during the suctioning procedure to prevent hypoxemia and atelectasis are:

1. Pre-oxygenation and re-oxygenation
2. Hyperinflation

Vagal Stimulation. The major nerve supplying the tracheobronchial tree is the *vagus nerve*. When it is stimulated, the heart responds by slowing its rate (bradycardia). Bradycardia combined with hypoxemia will lead to cardiac arrhythmias.

If any cardiac irregularities are created by the suctioning, stop immediately *and re-oxygenate and hyperinflate the patient's lungs.*

During any suctioning attempt it is important to assess the reaction of the cardiac system by observing the cardiac monitor or by taking the patient's pulse. If cardiac irritability is allowed to progress, potentially *lethal* cardiac arrhythmias such as ventricular tachycardia, ventricular fibrillation, or cardiac standstill will occur.

Trauma to the Airway Mucosa. Entry of the suction catheter into a patient's natural airway is traumatic to the mucosal lining of the airway. Hemorrhage and edema commonly occur in the airways from the mechanical irritation caused by suctioning. Even with meticulous technique, this damage nearly always occurs. Repeated irritation and mucosal laceration may also increase the incidence of airway infection due to the denuding of the cilia and the mucosal layers of defense, which line the tracheobronchial tree.

As vacuum is applied, the airway mucosa is elevated and is drawn into the holes in the catheter tip. This causes irritation. Eventually, bleeding and erosion of tissue occur at the site of the trauma.

The incidence of trauma during suctioning may be reduced by following a few basic guidelines:

▶ Never apply vacuum during insertion of the catheter.

▶ Apply vacuum *intermittently during withdrawal* of the catheter only.

▶ As the catheter is withdrawn, rotate it 360 degrees to prevent continued trauma to any single area of mucosa.

▶ Lubricate the catheter prior to insertion with either sterile saline or a water-soluble lubricant to reduce trauma induced from friction.

▶ Use a nasal airway to reduce the trauma to the nasal mucosa during nasotracheal suctioning.

▶ If any "grab" or pull is felt through the catheter, immediately release the vacuum.

▶ The suction catheter entry and withdrawal must not exceed a time limit of 10 to 15 seconds, i.e., never keep a suction catheter in the patient for longer than 10 to 15 seconds—counted from the beginning of insertion to the time of complete withdrawal of the catheter.

Hypotension. A drop in the patient's blood pressure may occur following suctioning, either due to profound bradycardia from vagal stimulation or due to prolonged coughing maneuvers during the suction procedure. If this should occur, stop the procedure and administer oxygen to the patient.

Paroxysmal Coughing. A suction catheter may cause a tracheal irritation that may stimulate tracheal and carinal cough reflexes. This results in paroxysmal cough-like maneuvers which interrupt ventilation. These coughing maneuvers may seriously affect the cardiac output and venous return of the blood to the heart. The problem may be avoided by: (a) pre-oxygenation and re-oxygenation with high inspired oxygen concentrations, (b) limiting the suction process to 10 to 15 seconds or less and (c) monitoring the cardiac status during the procedure.

INCENTIVE RESPIRATORY DEVICES

The complexities and costs of IPPB therapy stimulated practitioners of respiratory therapy to find alternate methods of preventing the hypoaeration of the lungs that leads to atelectasis. Many cooperative, motivated patients do not require the "forced" positive pressure breaths given by IPPB. Incentive respiratory devices help such patients to deep breathe voluntarily, reducing the possibility of atelectasis. An *incentive respiratory device* requires the patient to spontaneously take a voluntary deep breath (like a "sigh") and then pause in the inspiratory phase for 3 to 5 seconds to expand the lungs. The beneficial effects of a deep breath are perpetuated by some means of reinforcement if the procedure is performed: This visual reinforcement may be activated by balls rising in a column; lights; or other indicators on the device. Often, the reinforcement is activated even though the maneuver is incorrectly performed. Some supervision is essential to insure effectiveness of therapy.

A sustained deep breath is the most effective means of reducing the hypoaeration so common postoperatively. The principle used by all incentive devices is that of *voluntary sustained maximal inspiration*. The greatest benefit from this therapy is realized when the sustained maximal inflation is maintained for 3 to 5 seconds or more. The added benefit of mechanical bronchodilation is also achieved when a deep breath is taken.

Incentive respiratory devices are useful only in those patients who: (a) do not require mechanically induced deep breaths as with IPPB, (b) are not uncooperative, senile, or uncoordinated in breathing, (c) are motivated and not

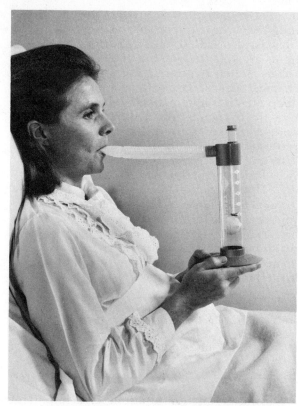

Figure 36–17. Bunn Respirex (incentive respiratory device). A device used to exercise the lungs in a goal-directed approach to stimulate and promote voluntary sustained maximal inflation of the lung. (From John Bunn Co., Buffalo, NY 14209.)

fearful of pain, (d) are not obtunded or oversedated and (e) have sufficient strength to create a sufficient inspiratory flow to *maximally* inflate their lungs.

Those patients who best qualify for incentive respiratory devices in their respiratory care are: (a) previously healthy postoperative patients, (b) patients with minor atelectasis who are alert and motivated and (c) patients who require frequent effective deep breaths as additional therapy to promote airway clearance.

The maximal effect of incentive therapy is achieved when 10 to 20 sustained breaths are taken each hour. The sustained deep breaths must not be performed in rapid succession as the patient's P_{CO_2} may be lowered below normal and dizziness and tremors may result.

Figures 36–16 and 36–17 show two examples of incentive respiratory devices commonly seen in hospitals. These devices are generally left at the patient's bedside. The patient is requested to perform these exercises by using the device on his own with a minimum of supervision by the nursing or respiratory therapy staff. To assist the nurse in giving quality care, the basic steps for performing a *voluntary sustained maximal inflation* are outlined here. The instructions accompanying each device must also be consulted.

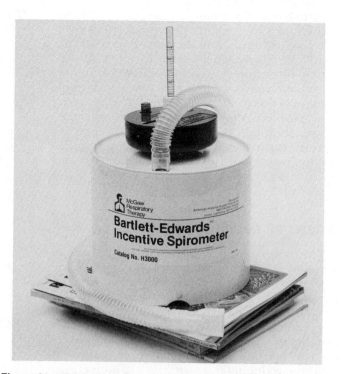

Figure 36–16. Bartlett-Edwards incentive respiratory device. This device is used to promote goal-oriented deep breathing utilizing a sustained maximal inflation. (From McGaw Respiratory Therapy Division of American Hospital Supply, Irvine, Cal.)

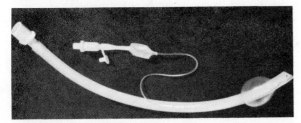

Figure 36-18. Artificial airway. This is an endotracheal tube. It may be inserted either through the mouth or through the nose into the trachea. (From Portex Inc., Wilmington, Mass. 01887.)

Basic Steps for an Effective Incentive Breath

1. Exhale completely
2. Place the mouthpiece between the teeth
3. Take a slow, sustained, deep inspiration
4. When the indicator on the device reaches the pre-set goal, hold the breath in the inspiratory phase for 3 to 5 seconds
5. Exhale slowly
6. Repeat 10 to 20 times per hour

ARTIFICIAL AIRWAYS

An artificial airway may be placed in the trachea when: (a) a patient is unable to maintain his level of ventilation to meet physiologic requirements of oxygenation and carbon dioxide removal; (b) a patient is unable to handle his tracheal secretions and maintain a clear airway or (c) a patient has an obstruction in the airway preventing ventilation. The process of placing an artificial airway into the trachea is called *intubation*. A patient may be "intubated" through (a) the *nose* (nasotracheal intubation), (b) the *mouth* (oral tracheal intubation) or (c) a

surgical procedure in which an opening is made into the *trachea* (tracheostomy) below the larynx into the cricothyroid cartilage and a tube is placed directly into the trachea. The oral and nasal routes of tracheal intubation are used in an emergency when an artificial airway is needed to maintain life or when short term support of ventilation and the airway is required. The tubes used to intubate the nose or the mouth are called *endotracheal tubes* (Fig. 36-18). A tracheostomy is usually an elective procedure and should be considered in an emergency situation only if an endotracheal tube cannot be inserted because the upper airway is obstructed or the larynx is crushed or if there is any other contraindication to use of the oral or nasal routes for intubation. The artificial airway placed directly into the trachea is called a tracheostomy tube (Fig. 36-19).

BIBLIOGRAPHY

a. Affonso, D., and Harris, T.: Continuous positive airway pressure. *American Journal of Nursing*, 76: 570, April 1976.
1. Arnold, V.: *Respiratory Care Laboratory Skills Manual*. Ventura, CA, Respiratory West Co., 1977.
1a. Bakow, E. D.: Sustained maximal inspiration—a rationale for its use. *Respiratory Care*, 22:379, April 1977.
2. Bates, B.: *A Guide to Physical Examination*. Philadelphia, J. B. Lippincott Co., 1974.
3. Brewis, R. A. L.: *Lecture Notes on Respiratory Disease*, 18th ed. Oxford, England, Blackwell Scientific Publications, 1975.
4. Briggs, W. H., Vanatta, J., and Vollmer, V.: *Oxygen Transport, Hypoxia, and Cyanosis*. Bowie, MD, Robert J. Brady Co., 1974.
5. Burrows, B., et al.: Pulmonary terms and symbols, a report of the ACCP-ATS Joint Committee on Pulmonary Nomenclature. *Chest*, 67:5, May 1975.
6. Burrows, B., Kettel, L. J., and Knudson, R. J.: *Respiratory Insufficiency*. Chicago, Year Book Medical Publishers, 1975.
7. Cherniack, R. M., Cherniack, L., and Naimark, A.: *Respiration in Health and Disease*, 2nd ed. Philadelphia, W. B. Saunders Co., 1972.
7a. Chrisman, M.: Dyspnea. *American Journal of Nursing*, 74:643, April 1974.
7b. Chusid, E. L., et al.: When your patient is on respiratory therapy. *Nursing Digest*, 4:43, Summer 1976.
8. Comroe, J. H., et al.: *The Lung, Clinical Physiology and Pulmonary Function Testing*, 2nd ed. Chicago, Year Book Medical Publishers, 1962.
9. Comroe, J. H.: *Physiology of Respiration*. Chicago, Year Book Medical Publishers, 1965.
10. Cotes, J. E.: *Lung Function, Assessment and Application in Medicine*, 3rd ed. Oxford, Blackwell Scientific Publications, 1975.

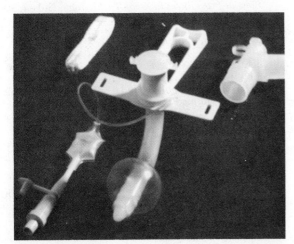

Figure 36-19. Artificial airway. A tracheostomy tube is inserted directly into the trachea through a surgical incision. (Courtesy of Portex, Inc., Wilmington, Mass. 01887.)

10a. Cugell, D. W.: Guide to modern lung function tests. *Hospital Medicine*, 14:57, Jan. 1978.

11. Davenport, H. W.: *The ABC of Acid-Base Chemistry: The Elements of Physiological Blood-Gas Chemistry for Medical Students and Physicians*, 6th ed. Chicago, University of Chicago Press, 1974.

11a. del Bueno, D. J.: A quick review on using blood-gas determinations. *RN*, 41:68, March 1978.

11b. Dines, D. E.: The dyspneic patient. *Hospital Medicine*, 12:6, Jan. 1976.

12. Egan, D. F.: *Fundamentals of Respiratory Therapy*, 2nd ed. St. Louis, C. V. Mosby Co., 1973.

13. Filley, G. F., et al.: *Pulmonary Insufficiency and Respiratory Failure*. Philadelphia, Lea & Febiger, 1967.

13a. From positive to negative. *Emergency Medicine*, 9:213, May 1977.

14. Gaskill, D. V., and Webber, B. A.: *The Brompton Hospital Guide to Chest Physiotherapy*, 2nd ed. Oxford, Blackwell Scientific Publications, 1973.

15. Haberman, P. B., et al.: Determinants of successful selective tracheobronchial suctioning. *New England Journal of Medicine*, 289:1060, Nov. 1973.

16. Harrison, R. A., Shapiro, B. A., and Trout, C. A.: *Clinical Application of Respiratory Care*. Chicago, Year Book Medical Publishers, 1975.

16a. Herron, C., Sr.: Home care for the patient with C.O.L.D. *Nursing '76*, 6:81, April 1976.

16b. Kanto, W. P., Jr.: Dealing with respiratory distress. *Emergency Medicine*, 9:67, Oct. 1977.

16c. Kanto, W. P., Jr., and Calvert, L. J.: Neonatal resuscitation. *American Family Physician*, 16:76, Dec. 1977.

16d. Kanto, W. P., Jr.: Resuscitation comes first. *Emergency Medicine*. 9:31, Oct. 1977.

16e. Kettel, L. J.: Acute respiratory acidosis. *Hospital Medicine*, 12:31, Feb. 1976.

17. Lagerson, J.: The cough—its effectiveness depends on you. *Respiratory Care*, 18:434–448, July–Aug. 1973.

18. Long, J., and Newfield, P.: *Tracheostomy Care Handbook*. Wilmington, ME, Portex Division, Smith Industries, 1976.

18a. Malkus, B. L.: Respiratory care at home. *American Journal of Nursing*, 76:1789, Nov. 1976.

18b. Marcott, M.: There's more to post-op extubation than just pulling out a tube. *RN*, 40:43, Sep. 1977.

18c. Moody, L. E.: Primer for pulmonary hygiene. *American Journal of Nursing*, 77:104, Jan. 1977.

19. Mechner, F.: Patient assessment: examination of the chest and lungs. *American Journal of Nursing*, 76(9):1–23, Sep. 1976.

20. Mitchell, R.: *Synopsis of Clinical Pulmonary Disease*. St. Louis, C. V. Mosby Co., 1974.

20a. On the ready for intubation: *Emergency Medicine*, 9:216, Aug. 1977.

20b. Ostrow, L. S.: Intensive respiratory care: from ICU to home. *American Journal of Nursing*, 76:111, Jan. 1976.

21. Petty, T. L.: *Intensive and Rehabilitative Respiratory Care*, 2nd ed. Philadelphia, Lea & Febiger, 1974.

22. Petty, T. L.: *Postural Drainage*. Littleton, CO, Monaghan, 1974.

22a. Programmed instruction: blood-gas and acid-base concepts in respiratory care. *American Journal of Nursing*, 76:P.I.1–P.I.30, June 1976.

22b. Programmed instruction: patient assessment: examination of chest and lungs. *American Journal of Nursing*, 76:P.I.1–P.I.23, Sep. 1976.

22c. Rau, J., and Rau, M.: To breathe or to be breathed: understanding IPPB. *American Journal of Nursing*, 77:613, April 1977.

23. Ruppel, G.: *Manual of Pulmonary Function Testing*. St. Louis, C. V. Mosby Co., 1975.

23a. Sandham, G., and Reid, B.: Some Q's and A's about suctioning. *Nursing '77*, 7:60, Oct. 1977.

24. Scribner, B. H. (ed.): *University of Washington Teaching Syllabus for the Course on Fluid and Electrolyte Balance*, 7th ed. Seattle, University of Washington School of Medicine, 1969.

25. Shapiro, B. A.: *Clinical Application of Blood Gases*. Chicago, Year Book Medical Publishers, 1973.

25a. Sladen, A.: Maintenance of patent airway. *Hospital Medicine*, 13:56, Aug. 1977.

26. Slonim, N. B.: *Pediatric Respiratory Therapy, an Introductory Text*. Monsey, NY, Glenn Educational Medical Services, 1974.

27. Slonim, N. B., and Hamilton, L. H.: *Respiratory Physiology*, 2nd ed. St. Louis, C. V. Mosby Co., 1971.

27a. Stanley, L.: You really can teach COPD patients to breathe better. *RN*, 41:43, April 1978.

27b. Stone, E. W., and Zuckerman, S.: The esophageal obturator airway. *American Journal of Nursing*, 75:1148, July 1975.

27c. Sweetwood, H.: Acute respiratory insufficiency: how to recognize this emergency. . . . How to treat it. *Nursing '77*, 7:24, Dec. 1977.

27d. Tinker, J. H., and Wehner, R.: The nurse and the ventilator. *American Journal of Nursing*, 74:1276, July 1974.

27e. To ventilate, obturate. *Emergency Medicine*, 9:75, July 1977.

28. Traver, G. (ed.): Symposium on care in respiratory disease. *Nursing Clinics of North America*, 1974.

29. Tucker, S. M.: *Patient Care Standards*. St. Louis, C. V. Mosby Co., 1975.

30. Tyler, M. L.: Artificial airways—suctioning, tubes and cuffs, weaning and extubation. *Nursing '73* (reprint), Feb. 1973.

31. Vennes, C. H., and Watson, J. C.: *Patient Care and Special Procedures in X-ray Technology*, 2nd ed. St. Louis, C. V. Mosby Co., 1964.

31a. White, S. J.: Respiratory drugs: when to give them . . . what to watch for. *RN*, 41:46, June 1978.

31b. Wilson, R. F.: Acute respiratory failure and how to manage it. *Consultant*, 18:25, May 1978.

32. Young, J. A., and Crocker, D.: *Principles and Practice of Respiratory Therapy*, 2nd ed. Chicago, Year Book Medical Publishers, 1976.

32a. Zavala, D. C.: The threat of aspiration pneumonia in the aged. *Geriatrics*, 32:46, March 1977.

33. Ziment, I.: IPPB: correct usage. *Critical Care Update* (reprint), Aug. 1976.

CHAPTER 37

PRACTICING STERILE TECHNIQUE

By Carolyn Ann Livingston, R.N., M.N.

OVERVIEW AND STUDY GUIDE

Sterile technique is another term for *surgical asepsis*, which is defined as *those practices that make and keep objects and areas microorganism free.* Microorganisms are minute living animals or plants found everywhere in our environment. Some are helpful to man, but some cause disease. One of the best means by which disease-producing microorganisms can be controlled is through the use of sterile techniques. It is important that the health care worker understand the need for and the principles of sterile technique so that high standards of practice can be maintained.

This chapter reviews concepts inherent in surgical asepsis—asepsis and medical asepsis—and discusses processes, methods and means by which sterile technique is carried out. Medical asepsis is discussed in greater detail in Chapter 25.

1. Before beginning this chapter, review the following terms:

aerobe—microorganism that requires air to live

anaerobe—microorganism that lives in the absence of air

antiseptic—an agent that hinders the growth of microorganisms

asepsis—free of pathogenic organisms

bacterial agent—an agent that can kill bacteria but not their spores

bacteriostatic agent—an agent that stops the production of bacteria

carrier—an individual or animal harboring specific pathogens who shows no signs of disease, but has the capacity to transmit the disease to others

clean technique—procedures done to help reduce the number of microorganisms and prevent their spread from one place or person to another

contamination—practices that render an item or area unclean

disinfectant—any agent that destroys pathogens

host—an individual or animal that houses microorganisms

medical asepsis—procedures done to help reduce the number of microorganisms and prevent their spread from one place or person to another (clean technique)

microorganism—minute living animals or plants found everywhere in our environment

nonpathogen—microorganisms that do not usually produce illness

nosocomial infection—an infection obtained while in a hospital

pathogenic—microorganisms that are harmful to man

port of entry—entryway for microorganisms to get into a host

reservoir—a collecting place for microorganisms to reproduce and grow

sterile—free of all living organisms

surgical asepsis—those practices that make and keep objects and areas microorganism free

2. The following terms will be defined as you read this chapter:

autoclave	sterile field
cross contamination	sterile forceps
envelope wrap	sterile gloves
gas sterilization	sterile supplies
immunological disorders	sterile technique
	sterilization
sepsis	sterilization indicators
septic state	

3. Keep the following questions in mind as you read:

What is the difference between "clean" technique and "sterile" technique?

Why is sterile technique necessary?

In what situations is sterile technique necessary?

How can you determine if an object is sterile or contaminated?

How does an object lose its sterility?

SURGICAL ASEPSIS

Definitions

As discussed in Chapter 25, microorganisms that have been harmful to man are called *pathogenic* (disease producing). When these organisms multiply within the body, they cause a condition known as *sepsis* (poisoning). A *septic state* means any condition in which pathogenic organisms are present and growing within a system.

In order to combat and control the spread of disease, aseptic procedures must be observed by all health care personnel. *Aseptic* means exactly the opposite of septic. It means free of pathogenic organisms. Aseptic procedures are those activities by which an aseptic condition or relatively germ free state is achieved or maintained. Aseptic procedures fall into two descriptive classifications: *medical asepsis* and *surgical asepsis*.

Remember that in medical asepsis every effort is made to help reduce the number of microorganisms and prevent their spread from one place or person to another. Medical aseptic procedures are sometimes referred to as "clean technique" procedures. An example of a medical aseptic procedure is handwashing.

Earlier we pointed out that *surgical asepsis* is defined as those practices which protect man not only against pathogenic organisms, but against all living organisms in his environment. When all organisms are destroyed, a *sterile*, or *aseptic, state* is created, e.g., when a dressing is sterilized. Any item or area that is not in the state of sterility—is not free of living organisms—is considered to be *contaminated*. Thus, a blanket on a patient's bed is considered to be "clean" in terms of medical asepsis, but since it does have some of the patient's organisms on it, it is considered "contaminated" in terms of surgical asepsis because it is not sterile.

Why Is Sterile Technique Used?

The purpose of sterile technique is to prevent the introduction or spread of disease producing microorganisms from the environment into a person.

When Is Sterile Technique Used?

Sterile technique is employed for (a) certain procedures, (b) for patients with conditions which lower their resistance to infection, and (c) during surgical operations. Some specific examples of procedures during which sterile technique is essential include the following:

▶ *Catheterization*, in order to prevent the introduction of organisms into the sterile bladder

▶ *Injections or IV's* in order to prevent the introduction of organisms through the skin, which is the body's first line of defense

▶ *Dressing changes*, in which sterile technique is required to prevent the introduction of organisms into the wound and/or to prevent spread of organisms from the wound to the health worker

Patients who are more susceptible to infections, and therefore require sterile technique, include:

▶ Patients with *burns*, because the skin's protective covering is broken, leaving them highly prone to invasion by organisms

▶ Patients with *immunological disorders* (i.e., those disorders which are the result of the body's incapacity to ward off invasion by foreign or antigenic substances), because the body's protective immunological defenses are impaired, rendering the patient more susceptible to infections

▶ Patients who are *debilitated* (run-down), e.g., malnourished, dehydrated, or infected with tuberculosis, because body defenses against infection are weakened.

In the *operating room,* strict sterile technique must be used to prevent introduction of infection-producing organisms through the incised (cut) skin or into body cavities.

When Is Sterile Technique Not Necessary?

Nonsurgical procedures involving the mouth, ears, gastrointestinal tract, vagina, and rectum generally do not require sterile technique. Examples of such procedures include: temperature measurement with a thermometer, administration of ear drops, gastric tube feedings, insertion of vaginal suppositories, and administration of enemas. While sterile technique is not maintained during these procedures, the equipment used for these procedures is usually initially sterile. Sterile equipment is selected in order to keep the patient as free from contamination as possible. Equipment used in the above procedures would be oral and rectal thermometers, eardrops and dropper, gastric tube, vaginal suppository and enema set up.

Guidelines for Practicing Sterile Technique

Significant facts and principles relevant to sterile technique are summarized in Table 37–1. Important points for the health care worker to observe while practicing sterile technique are listed, along with the rationale or principles behind each precaution.

STERILIZATION TECHNIQUES

Sterilization means the process by which an object becomes free of ALL microorganisms. There is no such thing as an "almost sterile" or "practically sterile" state. An object is either sterile or not sterile

In most *hospitals* the health care worker does not have to make any decisions about sterilization of equipment. This is taken care of by personnel in central supply or central service areas—where the sterilization actually takes place. On the other hand, the health care worker may be responsible for sterilizing objects in the *home* or *clinic* setting.

Emergency sterilization measures are taken when *time* is of the utmost importance. When

supplies are needed quickly, the recommended period of time for sterilization or disinfection is shortened. This does pose the risk that sterilization has not taken place, and it is only done in cases of extreme emergency.

The sterilization process must insure the destruction of all bacteria and of resistant spores. If bacteria or spores escape destruction during sterilization and enter the human body, they reproduce at a phenomenal rate—possibly causing infection.

Boiling, soaking, baking and steaming have been the traditional methods for sterilizing medical and hospital equipment. A more recent method of sterilizing is the use of ethylene oxide gas. Ultraviolet light is another type of sterilization that is being currently used. Each of these methods will be discussed, as they vary in effectiveness.

> *Sterilization is impossible by boiling, uncertain by soaking, limited in baking, but achievable by steam. In addition to steam, ethylene oxide is a safe and effective sterilizing agent.*

Boiling Water Sterilization

Some bacteria and viruses and all spores are resistant to boiling. Thus *boiling water*, at its maximum sea level temperature of 100°C. (212°F.), does not sterilize. A temperature of 121°C. (249.8°F.) is necessary to destroy bacterial spores; thus, boiling water is not an effective method for sterilizing equipment. Nevertheless, boiling water is commonly used in the home environment for sterilization because other, more sophisticated methods are not available. Objects can be rendered clean but not sterile after being submerged in boiling water for 10 to 20 minutes.

Altitude is an important factor when boiling supplies. At sea level, water boils at a higher temperature than it does at increased altitudes. Thus when the boiling method for sterilization is used in areas substantially higher than sea level, the boiling time must be lengthened (Table 37–2).

Cold Sterilization

Cold sterilization, or *soaking,* is used for (a) objects with plastic or rubber parts that cannot

TABLE 37–1.   PRINCIPLES OF SURGICAL ASEPTIC TECHNIQUE

CORRECT TECHNIQUE	RATIONALE/PRINCIPLE
1. Always face the sterile field. Do not turn your back or side on a sterile field.	1. Sterile objects which are out of the line of vision are considered questionable or their sterility cannot be guaranteed.
2. Keep sterile equipment above your waist level or above table level.	2. Waist level or table level are considered margins of safety which can be uniformly enforced and which promote maximum visibility of the sterile objects.
3. Do not speak, cough, sneeze or laugh over a sterile field. If it is necessary to do any of these, turn your head away from the sterile field.	3. Microorganisms from the oral cavity are spread into the air when a person speaks or coughs and the organisms may drop onto the sterile field.
4. Never reach across the sterile field. Instead (a) move yourself around the field (while continuing to face the field), (b) reach around the edges of the sterile field or (c) cautiously turn the entire sterile field by touching either the edges of the bottom wrapper or by reaching underneath the bottom wrapper.	4. When a non-sterile object is held above a sterile object, gravity causes microorganisms to fall onto the sterile object.
5. Prevent excessive air currents around the sterile area, e.g., move slowly, close doors, minimize flapping of clothes and drapes.	5. Microorganisms are present in and travel in air currents.
6. Keep unsterile objects away from the sterile field.	6. Microorganisms can be transferred whenever a non-sterile object touches a sterile object, thus rendering the sterile object contaminated.
7. Handle liquids cautiously near the sterile field to prevent drapes or wrappers from becoming wet. Do not allow splashing to occur.	7. When a liquid connects a nonsterile surface to a sterile one, microorganisms may be transferred from the unsterile to the sterile area. Consequently, the sterile area becomes contaminated by capillary attraction.
8. Dry sterile objects (e.g., sterile towel) may have one surface that is contaminated and one surface that is sterile.	8. Microorganisms do not pass easily through a dry surface; rather, they tend to slowly move along the surface.
9. Sterile instruments (e.g., forceps or scissors) may be picked up with the bare hand, thus rendering the handle contaminated—but the other end of the instrument is still considered to be sterile.	9. A standard rule is that there is a one-inch margin of safety around a contaminated part of a sterile object.
10. The edge of a sterile field is considered unsterile.	10. Proximity to a contaminated area makes sterility doubtful. A general rule is that there is a one-inch margin of safety around the edge of the field.
11. Never assume that an object is sterile. Always check the sterilization indicators on wrappers of sterile objects.	11. Sterilization indicators are used to demonstrate whether or not an object has been exposed to the sterilization process.
12. Always check the sterility expiration date, which is clearly stated on the package.	12. Sterility expiration date indicates the last possible date upon which the contents of the package can be assumed to be sterile.
13. Do not trust sterility of an object wrapped in paper or muslin for longer than 4 weeks after its sterilization.	13. A standard rule is that the sterility of an object wrapped in paper or muslin becomes doubtful after 4 weeks.
14. Do not trust sterility of an object in a see-through bag for longer than 1 year.	14. Sterility of objects in see-through bags becomes doubtful after 1 year.

TABLE 37-2.   ALTITUDE AND APPROXIMATE
BOILING TIME NECESSARY FOR DISINFECTION

| ALTITUDE | | BOILING POINT OF WATER | | APPROXIMATE BOILING TIME |
(m.)	(ft.)	(C.)	(F.)	(min.)
0	0	100	212	30
500	1,640.4	98.33	208.9	38
1000	3,280.8	96.68	206	47
1500	4,921.3	95.01	203	54
2000	6,561.7	93.34	200	63
3000	9,842.5	90.01	194	77
3500	11,482.9	88.33	190.9	88
4000	13,123.4	86.65	187.9	95
4500	14,763.8	84.98	184.9	103
5000	16,404.2	83.29	181.9	113

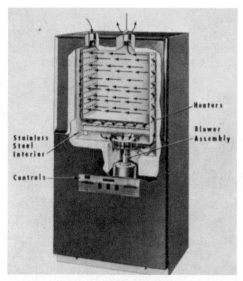

Figure 37-1.   Electrically heated hot air sterilizer. (From Perkins, J. J.: *Principles and Methods of Sterilization in Health Sciences.* Springfield, IL, Charles C Thomas, Publisher, 1969, p. 291.)

tolerate heat or (b) metallic objects prone to corrosion. Germicidal solutions vary in the length of soaking time necessary for sterilization:

Solution	Soaking Time
Alcohol	Uncertain
Aqueous Zephiran	Uncertain
Betadine	Uncertain
Cidex	10 hours

Soaking instruments in any of these germicidal solutions does not kill all spores, and this method is used only when prolonged heat would damage equipment being disinfected. There is also the possibility that patients may experience discomfort or injury when exposed to equipment soaked in strong antiseptic solutions. For example, a rubber face mask may retain a chemical that might cause facial irritation or may have an unpleasant odor. Instruments soaked with germicides must be adequately rinsed with sterile water before being used.

Dry Heat Sterilization

Dry heat sterilization, or *baking,* is restricted in its usage because of the destructively high temperature and long exposure required for sterilization. Compared to steam at the same temperature and pressure, dry heat sterilization takes three times as long or more. Dry heat destroys microorganisms by an oxidation process. Dry heat is used to sterilize instruments with sharp edges, needles, and some glass equipment, to prevent the equipment from rusting or becoming dull as may occur from contact with solutions. The most commonly used dry heat methods for medical equipment are the dry heat sterilizer or an electrically heated hot-air sterilizer. In effect, both of these methods "bake" the equipment. The electrically heated hot-air sterilizer (Fig. 37–1) is the

most reliable and accurate method of dry heat sterilization.

Autoclave Sterilization

Autoclave sterilization, or *steam sterilization,* is the most widely used, the most economical and one of the most effective methods of destroying microorganisms. This method uses high temperature, pressure, and humidity to destroy bacterial life. It is impractical for sterilization of equipment with plastic or rubber parts or with parts sensitive to heat or moisture. In an autoclave, steam is present under pressure to maintain the necessary high temperatures for sterilization (Fig. 37–2). Equipment being sterilized in an autoclave is wrapped in special cloth or paper wrappers. The wrapped packs are placed in the autoclave, and the temperature and pressure of the autoclave is monitored. The five factors that must be taken into consideration when using autoclave sterilization are: (1) type of equipment being sterilized, (2) type of wrapper, (3) method for packing the sterilizer, (4) temperature and pressure used and (5) length of time the wrapped objects are in the sterilizer.

In the home setting, the health care worker will find that a pressure cooker can be used to

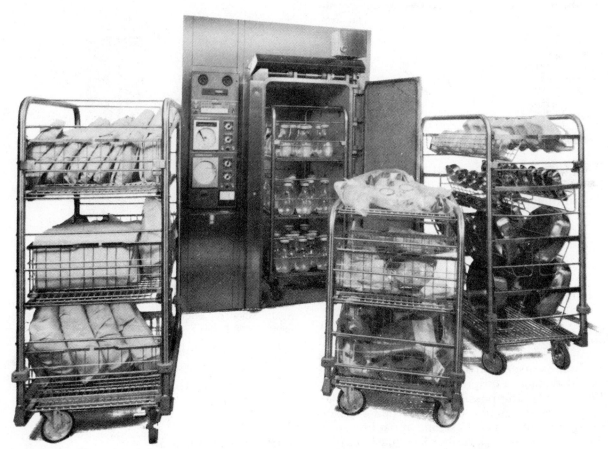

Figure 37–2. Steam autoclave. (From *Infection Control in Central Services.* Rochester, NY, Castle Company, 1976, p. 24.)

sterilize equipment, as it operates on the same principle as an autoclave. Items to be sterilized should be placed on a rack above the water level in the pressure cooker. The closed system and the higher temperature will sterilize items more quickly than boiling water alone.

Gas Sterilization

Gas sterilization kills *all* bacteria by the use of gases. *The most widely used means of gas sterilization is an ethylene oxide gas sterilizer* (Fig. 37–3). Any item may be sterilized in ethylene oxide gas provided the following five variables are correct: (1) gas concentration, (2) temperature, (3) exposure time, (4) humidity and (5) type of wrap. Recommended gas con-

centration is 760 mg. of ethylene oxide per liter of air. (At 60°C. [140°F.] the exposure time is 3 hours; for a higher temperature the time is decreased.) The range of temperature is between 54.4 and 65.4°C. (130 to 150°F.). Exposure time varies from 48 minutes to several hours. Humidity should be held between approximately 30 and 60 per cent in the sterilizer. Ethylene oxide is not effective for items wrapped in foil.

Ethylene oxide sterilization is gradually replacing dry heat and soaking sterilization in hospital settings. "Reports from a wide range of hospital and medical sources indicate that ethylene oxide could be used exclusively, eliminating dry heat sterilization, provided that ample time or enough equipment were available to handle the longer exposure and aeration period needed."[16]

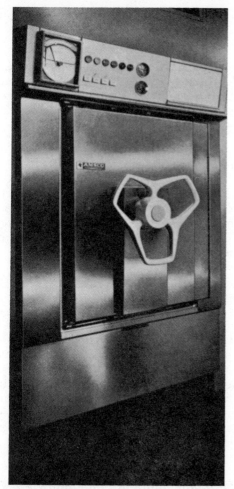

Figure 37–3. Ethylene oxide gas sterilizer. (From Perkins, J. J.: Principles and Methods of Sterilization in Health Sciences. Springfield, IL, Charles C Thomas, Publisher, 1969, p. 525.)

Ultraviolet Light Sterilization

Ultraviolet light sterilization is effective for disinfecting working surfaces and air inside rooms. There are several limitations to the use of this method: (1) ultraviolet light does not penetrate liquids, (2) all surfaces must be exposed to the rays, since areas in a shadow will not be sterilized, (3) adequate time must be allowed, for sterilization is not immediate and (4) prolonged exposure to ultraviolet light may cause injury to workers' eyes, tissues and skin. Ultraviolet lights may be placed in doorways leading into the operating room, patient rooms or elevators. Probably the cheapest form of ultraviolet radiation is obtained free, from the sun.

STERILIZATION INDICATORS

Sterilization indicators are devices placed on wrappers and inside packages to indicate whether or not an object has been exposed to the sterilization process. Indicators allow the health care worker to determine which items have met the conditions of proper temperature, pressure, humidity, etc., to insure that sterilization has taken place. When selecting a sterile item for use, the health care worker must be aware of what indicators are on or in the package to indicate that the contents are indeed sterile. Different items may have different indicators, depending on the type of sterilization.

The four major types of indicators are: (1) paper tape indicators, (2) glass pellet indicators, (3) multi-use bags with indicators, and (4) commercially imprinted indicators.

Paper Tape Indicators

A paper tape indicator is a piece of specially impregnated masking-type tape that is placed on the outside of a package to be sterilized. This tape serves dual purposes: (1) sealing the package and (2) indicating whether sterilization has taken place. The tape is a uniform color before being exposed to conditions sufficient to sterilize. The appearance of the tape changes once the condition for sterilization are obtained, e.g., adequate levels of heat, temperature, pressure, etc. The nature of these changes depends on the method of sterilization used.

When an item has been placed in an *autoclave,* dark diagonal lines appear on the indicator tape. These lines appear as a result of exposure to levels of heat and moisture in the autoclave and indicate sterilization of the contents. This change in the indicator tape differentiates "processed" from "unprocessed" materials. While the appearance of dark lines does not guarantee internal sterility, the health care worker commonly assumes that items on which the indicator tape has changed can be safely used for sterile procedures. (Fig. 37–4 B). The only way to determine positively that a package is sterile is to culture the contents. This is not a practical method to use on all sterilized objects but is done on random samples at periodic intervals in the central supply or sterilizing area of the hospital. Inside each package will be found an internal indicator, described below. This indicator does guarantee sterility if the proper changes have taken place.

The indicator tape used on objects to be sterilized in an *ethylene oxide gas sterilizer* is dark before processing. When the item is ex-

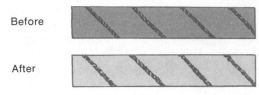

A   Gas sterilization—ethylene oxide indicator

Before

After

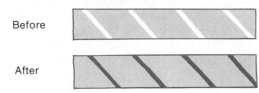

B   Steam sterilization—autoclave indicator

Before

After

Figure 37–4. Indicator tape color change. *A,* When all conditions for the ethylene oxide gas sterilization process have been obtained, the paper tape indicator will become lighter in color. *B,* For items submitted to the steam sterilization process, dark diagonal lines will appear on the paper tape indicator.

posed to ethylene oxide gas, the indicator changes from a dark color (e.g., dark green) to a light color (e.g., light green). The color of the tapes vary from one manufacturer to another but the change is always *from dark to light.* Again, this color change only differentiates "proc-

Multi-use bags with indicators

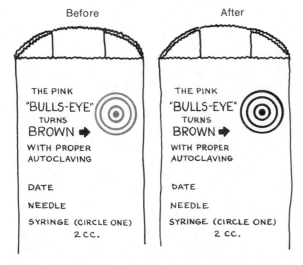

Figure 37–5. Multi-use bags with indicators. When the "bulls-eye" on the bag turns brown, conditions for sterilization have been met, and it is safe to use the item in the bag for sterile procedures.

essed" from "unprocessed" materials. It does not guarantee sterility (Fig. 37–4 *A*).

> *If you find a package in which the indicated color change has not taken place,* do not use this item. Return it to the sterilizing area in your facility.

Glass Pellet Indicators

A glass pellet indicator is a small glass tube that contains a temperature-sensitive pellet that melts and changes color when subjected to heat. This indicator will be found inside each "processed" package.

Multi-Use Bags with Indicators

Sterile items may be hospital wrapped in a variety of plastic or paper bags that have sterility indicators built into the material of the bag. Such bags are used for both autoclave and ethylene oxide gas sterilization. In Figure 37–5, you will note that before the item is sterilized the "bull's eye" is light in color—but after sterilization has taken place, the bull's eye has become darker.

Commercially Imprinted Indicators

Commercially prepared sterile items have the word "STERILE" clearly printed on the front of the package (Fig. 37–6).

MAINTAINING STERILITY

Packaging and Storing Sterile Supplies

Sterile objects are packaged in special *wrappings* in order to insure that their sterility is maintained until they are needed for use. Once objects are sterilized, it is necessary to protect them from contamination. Four factors need to be considered in maintaining the sterility of objects: (a) wrappers used, (b) storage location, (c) shelf time and (d) expiration date.

Contamination of sterile objects can occur by direct or indirect contact. Objects remain sterile only as long as they are in a package with an impervious cover. An "impervious cover" is a specially treated cover that is waterproof. Unless a sterile item has an impervious cover, it becomes contaminated as soon as it is removed from the sterilizer. If the wrapper is torn or tampered with, the object is contaminated.

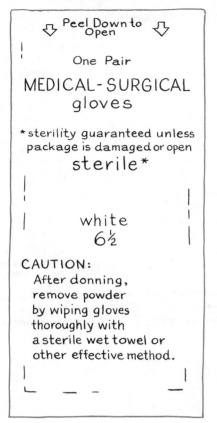

Figure 37–6. Commercially imprinted indicator.

If properly wrapped and then *stored* in a clean, dry, bacteria-free place where they are *not handled excessively* before use, sterile objects remain sterile for an indefinite period. However, this is an ideal situation which rarely exists in the majority of health care agencies.

The *storage time* of sterile objects is commonly referred to as their *shelf life*. No one has researched the question of what is the maximal *storage time* of sterilized objects. There are a few rules of thumb concerning safe storage time. One rule is "don't trust sterility after 4 weeks." Packs wrapped in double muslin wrappers should remain sterile for at least 4 weeks. At the time of sterilization, packs are marked with a date beyond which sterility of the contents cannot be safely assumed. Another storage time rule for sterilized objects is "first in, first out." This means that sterile objects with the earliest expiration dates are used first. With rapid and orderly usage, the maximal storage time is seldom exceeded. However, if a sterile object is found with an expired date, it

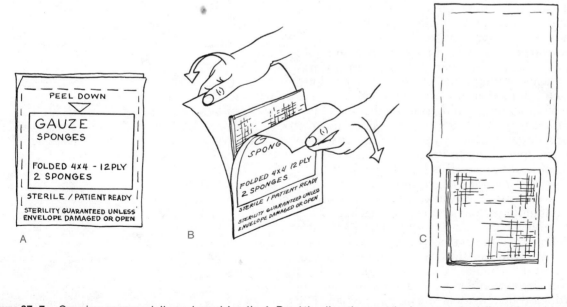

Figure 37–7. Opening commercially packaged 4 × 4's. *A,* Read the directions marked on commercially packaged 4 × 4's. *B,* Follow the directions and grasp the flaps at the top of the package and "peel down." *C,* When you open the package according to the directions, you are assured that the sterility of the 4 × 4's has been maintained.

should be returned to central supply for resterilization.

Before using sterile equipment, check:
1. *Condition of package or wrapper*
2. *Sterilization indicator*
3. *Expiration date*
4. *Internal indicator*

Handling Sterile Supplies

A sterile field is a work surface area prepared with sterile drapes to hold sterile equipment during a procedure that requires sterile technique. The major purpose of a sterile field is to provide an area in which sterility is continually maintained. A sterile field can be any size, depending on the procedure to take place. In the operating room you might find several large tables draped with sterile drapes and having lots of sterile equipment on them. At the patient's bedside you may see one sterile package opened up with the package's inner wrapper being used for a small sterile field.

Once a sterile field is established, the sterility of the field has to be maintained. It is essential that you know how to unwrap both an envelope wrapped sterile item and a commercially wrapped sterile item.

An *envelope-wrapped package* is commonly used for hospital-prepared sterile items. It has one layer of wrapping, either paper or cloth, which is folded around the object with each of the wrapper edges folded across the object in a uniform way. The wrapper, the size, and the shape depend entirely upon the object within the wrapper. Refer to Procedure 22 for the details of how to open this type of package.

Commercially packaged items are packaged in a wide variety of ways. Equipment may be individually packaged or may be packaged in a set, with all the pieces needed to perform a certain procedure. This provides both safety and convenience; thus, the sterile equipment needed to change a dressing or to do a catheterization may be together in one big cardboard box inside a sterile plastic bag. The contents of the package are clearly marked on the outside. Prepackaged items are usually wrapped in a combination of a plastic outer covering with a paper wrap on the inside. The

variations of packaging in the commercial field are limited only by the creativity of the manufacturer and the principles of asepsis. The best way to open commercially packaged items is to read the directions that are clearly marked on the front of each package. Some may say to "pull down," "pop the top," or "snap smartly." *Read and follow the directions.* These items can be dropped directly onto the sterile field if necessary. The inside of any commercially prepared sterile item can be used as a sterile field. See Figure 37–7 for an example of commercially packaged 4 × 4 with directions to "peel down."

Sometimes it may be necessary to add sterile items or sterile liquids to a sterile field. When *adding a sterile item to a sterile field,* use one of these techniques: (1) pick up the item with sterile forceps (the prongs of forceps are sterile) and place it carefully in the central part of the field, (2) put on a sterile glove in order to transfer a sterile item or (3) use the package

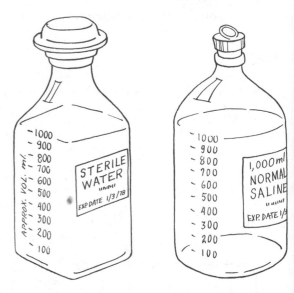

A Sterile water prepared in central supply of hospital

B Normal saline commercially prepared

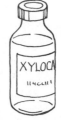

C Commercially prepared solution in vial

Figure 37–8. Sterile liquid containers. *A,* Sterile water in a glass bottle with a rubber cap. *B,* Sterile normal saline in a nonreusable bottle with a flip-top cap. *C,* Vial containing sterile liquid medication has a rubber diaphragm seal and an aluminum lift-off cover over the diaphragm.

wrap around the item as a protection to prevent the clean hand from coming in contact with the sterile item. The details of these techniques are presented in Procedures 22 and 23.

Sterile liquids are often necessary for procedures requiring sterile technique, e.g., a catheter irrigation, in which it is necessary to use a sterile solution so as not to introduce any microorganisms into the sterile bladder. Most liquid medications are commercially prepared in sterile bottles or vials.

Sterile liquids may be packaged either by the hospital or commercially. The hospital-prepared liquids come in glass bottles that are reusable and have a large rubber cap (Fig. 37–8 A). When the lid is lifted off, the health care worker can readily hear that the vacuum is broken. If the vacuum release is not heard, you must assume that the solution is not sterile. Return the bottle to the sterilizing area in the health care agency. Commercially prepared liquids come in nonreusable bottles and have a metal flip-top lid. They are clearly labeled as sterile (Fig. 37–8 B).

It is a standard rule that the *outside* of the bottle and cap are considered clean but that the *inside* of the bottle and cap are considered sterile. Thus, it is essential when handling sterile liquids to observe the following cautions: (1) place the cap so that the top of the cap rests on the table, so as not to contaminate the inside, (2) place your palm over the label so that the contents do not drip on the label and obscure it, (3) pour the liquid so that it does not splash, possibly causing a wicker effect in a paper or cloth barrier being used to separate clean from sterile and (4) do not allow the lip of the bottle to touch a contaminated source.

Some sterile liquids, such as medications for injection, come in vials with rubber diaphragms through which a sterile needle can be pierced in order to withdraw the sterile contents (Fig. 37–8 C).

It is vitally important to keep equipment and solutions sterile until needed for use. Items are packaged so as to facilitate their use once they have been opened.

---

22. HANDLING STERILE SUPPLIES

Definition and Purposes. *Methods of opening and using sterile supplies.* Used in sterile procedures to maintain sterility of equipment, supplies and liquids.

Contraindications and Cautions. There are many ways in which sterile supplies can be *contaminated*, e.g., touching a sterile field with an unsterile object, sneezing onto a sterile field or item, or reaching across a sterile field with a bare hand or arm. Health care workers need to *constantly* keep in mind what is "sterile" and what is "contaminated." Items of questionable sterility should automatically be discarded and replaced with sterile items. Health care workers with infectious diseases or open wounds should not be involved in sterile technique procedures because their microorganisms may spread to the patient.

Patient-Family Teaching Points. Provide the patient and family with the following information as appropriate: (a) meaning of the term "sterile supplies" and reason for their use, (b) techniques of opening and using sterile supplies at home and (c) specific instructions to the patient not to touch the sterile supplies.

PRE-PROCEDURE ACTIVITIES

PRELIMINARY PATIENT ASSESSMENT

Includes determination of:
▶ patient's diagnosis to assess need for sterile technique

PREPARATION OF PATIENT

▶ Explain to patient why sterile supplies are being used
▶ Place patient in comfortable position

Procedure continued on the following page

PRELIMINARY PATIENT ASSESSMENT

▶ physician's and nursing orders
▶ patient's level of consciousness and ability to understand and follow worker's directions
▶ prior amount and type of sterile supplies used

PRELIMINARY PLANNING

▶ Obtain correct equipment
▶ Inspect sterile supplies for intact cover or seal, sterility indicator, date, etc.
▶ Prepare large, clean, dry area to open supplies
▶ Plan work area for convenience of use and maintenance of sterility

PREPARATION OF PATIENT

▶ Adjust the environment (level of bed, placement of bedside stand, position of windows, doors, etc.) as necessary
▶ Provide appropriate patient teaching
▶ Helper washes hands

EQUIPMENT

▶ Varies, depending on procedure to be done

PROCEDURE

SUGGESTED STEPS	RATIONALE/DISCUSSION

A. Opening Envelope Wrapped Sterile Packages

An envelope wrapped package has one layer of wrapping, which is folded around the package with each of the edges folded across the package in a special way. When the sides are totally opened, the inside of this wrap is a sterile field.

1. Remove outer package or tape.	1. Seal provides one check on sterility of contents.
2. Place sterile package in center of working space with first fold away from you (Fig. 37–9 A).	2. Avoids unnecessary handling of package.
3. Open sterile package by grasping the outside top fold of wrapper at edge. Open this portion of wrapper *away* from you, reaching across package (Fig. 37–9 B).	3. Using first motion to open the top cover away from you eliminates need to later reach across sterile field while opening package.
4. Reach to center of package from one side (right or left); grasp folded tip of uppermost layer of wrapper with right (or left) hand and fold open to side (Fig. 37–9 C).	4. Handle only tip of wrapper to decrease chance of contaminating sterile contents. Reaching from side protects contents if wrapper is displaced.
5. Reach to center of package from opposite side (left or right); grasp folded tip of next layer of wrapper with left (or right) hand and fold open to opposite side (Fig. 37–9 D).	5. Same as 4 above.

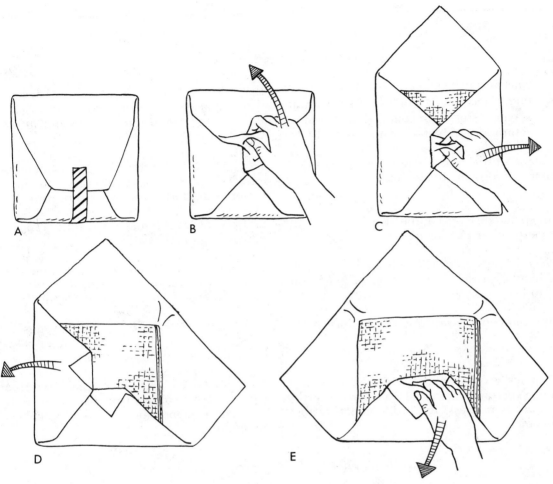

Figure 37–9. Opening envelope wrapped sterile package.

SUGGESTED STEPS	RATIONALE/DISCUSSION

A. Opening Envelope Wrapped Sterile Packages (Continued)

6. Reach from center front, grasp the final tip of wrapping with hand protected by wrap; and pull open toward worker (Fig. 37–9 E).

6. Extreme caution is needed to lift this wrapper as it lies directly over the sterile contents. Prevents reaching over sterile field.

7. Identify sterile field before proceeding with use of sterile tray.

7. Remember areas considered contaminated: 1 inch from edge of wrapper and any part of wrapper which falls below level of working level.

B. Using Sterile Transfer Forceps

Sterile forceps are instruments used to handle sterile supplies so that the supplies do not become contaminated by a worker's bare hands. Forceps are used to

Procedure continued on the following page

SUGGESTED STEPS	RATIONALE/DISCUSSION

B. Using Sterile Transfer Forceps (Continued)

remove sterile objects from their sterile enclosure and to transfer sterile objects from one place to another. New sterile transfer forceps should be obtained for each separate sterile procedure. The transfer forceps are kept in a dry sterile field and are returned to the sterilizing area to be resterilized after use.

1. Obtain sterile transfer forceps in package. Open and maintain sterile field.	1. The handle of the forceps is considered *unsterile* after opening package. If in muslin or paper wrap, follow previous procedure.
2. Grasp forceps by handle. Keep prongs of forceps together by closing ratchets.	2. Prevents accidentally opening prongs, with danger of contamination.
3. Place forceps on sterile field between uses, with handles away from portion of field you want to keep sterile.	3. Maintain sterility of prongs. Remember, if handles are near or on edge of sterile field, that area of sterile field is "contaminated."
4. Open forceps by pushing thumb forward.	4. Disengages ratchets, while prongs under control with thumb and index finger (as when holding a pair of scissors).
5. Transfer forceps can be used to pick up any sterile object and move it to a nearby sterile field, e.g., extra dressings, instruments, swabs, applicators.	5. In order to prevent cross-contamination (spread of microorganisms from one source to another), use one pair of forceps for one patient procedure.

C. Dropping Sterile Items onto Sterile Field

1. Unwrap the sterile package. If item is in an envelope wrap, unwrap as stated in Part A of this procedure. If item is commercially wrapped, follow directions on cover.	
2. Grasp edge of contents with one hand on outside of sterile wrapper.	2. Protects sterility of package contents.
3. Carefully fold each end of wrapper back toward wrist.	3. Sterile wrapper protects hand from sterile contents.
4. While holding edges of sterile wrapper back around wrist, let sterile items fall directly onto sterile field (Fig. 37–10).	4. Hold edges back so they do not accidentally drag across sterile field. Edges are considered unsterile. Remember, 1 inch around sterile field is considered contaminated. If item falls in this area, it is discarded.
5. Arranging of dropped sterile items on a sterile field can be done with (a) use of sterile forceps (see Part B of this procedure) or (b) use of a sterile glove (see Procedure 23).	5. Be careful when arranging sterile items not to let arm pass over sterile field.

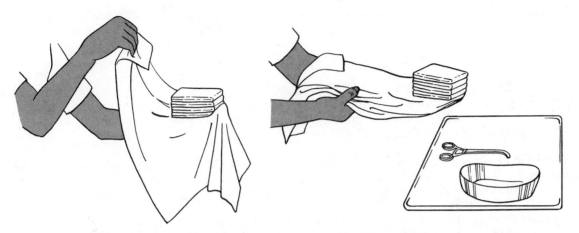

A   Holding sterile package while unwrapping   B   Dropping sterile item onto sterile tray

Figure 37–10.   Dropping sterile items onto sterile field.

SUGGESTED STEPS	RATIONALE/DISCUSSION

D. Pouring Sterile Liquids

1. Unscrew or push up the cap on bottle and place cap on table surface with top of cap resting on table. Be careful not to touch bottle rim or inside of bottle cap (Fig. 37–11, A and B).

1. Bottle rim and inside of cap are considered *sterile*.

2. Hold bottle with label against palm (Fig. 37–11 C).

2. Palming the label protects label from dripping solution. A clean label can easily and safely be read.

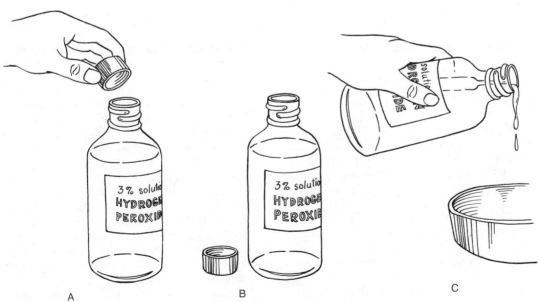

A   B   C

Figure 37–11.   Pouring a sterile liquid.

SUGGESTED STEPS	RATIONALE/DISCUSSION

D. Pouring Sterile Liquids (Continued)

3. Pour liquid into sterile container by holding bottle about 6 inches above container being poured into. To avoid splashing liquid, pour slowly in a steady stream (Fig. 37–11 C).	3. To prevent contamination, do not touch bottle lip against container and do not let your arm pass over sterile field.
4. If container is on a sterile field, the portion of the sterile field over which the bottle was held is considered contaminated.	4. Organisms may drop onto a sterile field. Always pour from area which will create the smallest amount of contaminated field.
5. Replace the cap securely and place date and time on label of vacuum packed liquid. Return the bottle to storage area or discard as appropriate.	5. Vacuum packed sterile liquids can be used for 24 hours if cap reseals bottle.

> *Remember: Do not touch inside of bottle cap or bottle rim. If cap or rim becomes contaminated, discard bottle.*

Post-Procedure Activities.   Provide for patient's comfort and safety, helper washes hands.

Aftercare of Equipment.   Disposable supplies are placed in bag, removed from patient's room and discarded in appropriate covered container. Nondisposable supplies are returned to central supply to be resterilized. Sterile stock liquid bottles are cleansed with disinfectant and returned to proper designated storage area on unit. Remember to label vacuum packed sterile liquids with date and time.

Chart/Report.   Results of procedure as appropriate.

Putting on Sterile Gloves

"Sterile" gloves are not to be confused with *clean (unsterile) gloves.* Clean gloves are made of inexpensive plastic and are worn when it is necessary to protect yourself from contamination and/or contact with disease causing organisms, e.g., when inserting a rectal suppository or handling highly contaminated dressings or body drainage. There is no special procedure for putting on clean gloves; they are packaged separately with one glove per package or in a dispenser box like facial tissues. Read the label carefully before using to be sure that you have clean rather than sterile gloves.

You may find that clean or sterile gloves have a light powder on them. This helps in the ease of donning them, as powder absorbs body moisture and decreases friction.

Sterile gloves are packaged in a paper envelope wrap (see Fig. 37–6). The wrap is labeled "sterile gloves" and gives the size of gloves plus the number of gloves in the package. One or two gloves are in each package. The outside of the sterile glove package is unsterile. The inside, including gloves and wrapper, is sterile. Because of its sterility, the wrapper may be used as an extra sterile field. If the wrapper becomes wet, it is considered contaminated. When two gloves are in the package, the inner wrapper is labeled to indicate left (L) hand and right (R) hand. After opening the outer wrap, be sure to have the cuffs placed closest to you. This is to avoid possible contamination in reaching across the sterile field.

Sterile gloves are used in handling sterile supplies. The *purpose* of sterile gloves is to prevent contamination of the patient. For example, when a patient needs to be catheterized, sterile gloves are worn to prevent the entrance of pathogenic organisms into the sterile bladder cavity. Other times the nurse would use sterile gloves include (a) doing a sterile dressing change, (b) caring for a patient in protective isolation or (c) assisting with surgical procedures.

> *If at any point you feel you have contaminated a sterile glove (when putting the glove on or in the process of using it for a sterile procedure), immediately discard the glove and reglove. Also, reglove if anyone else questions the sterility of your gloves.*

Procedure 23 includes a list of cautions about gloving and the step-by-step sequence of gloving.

23. PUTTING ON STERILE GLOVES

Definition and Purposes.   *Methods of donning sterile gloves without contamination of outside of gloves.* The gloves are worn to prevent contamination of wounds, sterile equipment or supplies (from microorganisms on the worker's hands) and/or to prevent transmission of microorganisms in the environment to a patient.

Contraindications and Cautions.   There are several ways in which sterile gloves can be contaminated, e.g., touching the outside of a sterile glove with an ungloved hand, touching any unsterile object or piece of material with the sterile gloved hand, or tearing or puncturing the sterile glove. Health care workers should keep their fingernails short and avoid wearing rings. Long fingernails and rings both cause increased tension on the sterile glove, which thus becomes more prone to tearing or puncture. Anyone with open wounds on their hands should not be using sterile gloves, due to the increased chance of contamination of the patient if the glove should tear. The health worker is in danger of increased growth of infecting organisms in the moist, warm, dark environment of the gloved hand. Be cautious when handling the wrapped sterile gloves not to spill any liquid on them. Solution spilled on a permeable glove wrapper will contaminate the gloves. Thus the gloves should be considered unsterile and discarded or returned to central supply for reprocessing.

Patient-Family Teaching Points.   Provide the patient and family with the following information as appropriate: (a) meaning of the concept of "sterile technique," (b) why sterile gloves are used, (c) instruct the patient not to touch the worker's gloved hands.

PRE-PROCEDURE ACTIVITIES

PRELIMINARY PATIENT ASSESSMENT

▶ Review patient's diagnosis, type and date of surgery
▶ Determine physician and nursing orders
▶ Determine need for sterile gloves

PREPARATION OF PATIENT

▶ Explain to patient why sterile gloves are being used
▶ Place patient in comfortable position
▶ Assure privacy

Procedure continued on the following page

PRELIMINARY PATIENT ASSESSMENT

▶ Assess level of consciousness to determine if patient can understand directions of how to assist helper with procedure

PRELIMINARY PLANNING

▶ Obtain correct size of sterile gloves
▶ Inspect sterile supplies for sterility
▶ Prepare a large clean dry area to open gloves at bedside
▶ Open other sterile supplies to be used; add sterile medications, fluids

PREPARATION OF PATIENT

▶ Adjust bed linen and level of bed as necessary, close window and doors as necessary
▶ Provide appropriate patient teaching
▶ Wash hands

EQUIPMENT

▶ 1 package of sterile gloves
▶ Equipment for procedure to be done

PROCEDURE

SUGGESTED STEPS	RATIONALE/ASSESSMENT
A. Follow directions on glove package. Peel down outer cover of glove package or open outer envelope wrap; leave on cleared, dry area that will not be disturbed by patient.	A. Commercial packages differ in types of wraps. Remember to keep sterile gloves and sterile equipment in view.
B. Inspect package of gloves and place with cuff facing worker.	B. Gloves are packaged so that right hand glove is on right and left hand glove is on left when cuffs face worker.
C. Open the inner glove wrap by touching the cuffed edges of the wrap and fold open. Fold up the paper cuff at top of wrap, then fold down the paper cuff at bottom of wrap. Uncrease paper folds from bottom or under side of inner wrap to keep package open (Fig. 37–12 A).	C. Opening the inner glove wrap away from you first avoids reaching across the sterile field, which would increase the chance of contamination. The outer edge of the opened wrap is considered contaminated. Paper tends to spring back to original fold, which might produce contamination of glove.
D. Pick up a glove by the folded-back cuff. Be careful to handle just the inside portion of the cuff (Fig. 37–12 B). Stand away from anything which could possibly touch glove.	D. It does not matter whether right or left glove is put on first. The inner surface of the glove, including this part of the cuff, will be in contact with helper's skin. Touching a sterile area with an unsterile object contaminates the sterile area. Remember: exterior of gloves must remain sterile. Worker must avoid touching sterile exterior of glove with ungloved hand.
E. While keeping the fingers of the hand being gloved pointing to the floor, slide your hand into the glove with a firm, easy pull. Keep hands out in front of you and above waist level (Fig. 37–12 C).	E. Keeping fingers apart makes it easier to find glove fingers for each of your fingers. Gravity assists in keeping fingers of glove open. The area below waist level is considered contaminated.

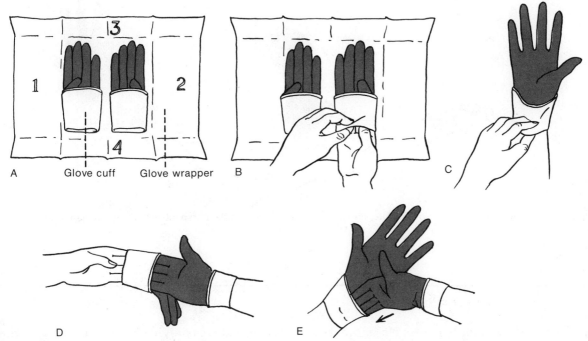

Figure 37-12. Putting on sterile gloves. Note: Illustrations are drawn from perspective of the worker looking *down* on her hands. Fingers in *C* are pointing down, toward floor.

SUGGESTED STEPS	RATIONALE/ASSESSMENT
F. Do not make any adjustments with the glove (fingers or cuff) at this time. Wait until second glove has been put on.	F. Contact of sterile object with unsterile area contaminates the sterile object. Frequently two fingers may enter one glove finger; this can be adjusted after second glove is donned.
G. Pick up second glove by sliding fingers of gloved hand *under cuff* of second glove (Fig. 37–12 *D*).	G. Keeping sterile fingers of gloved hand under cuff of second glove maintains sterility of fingers of gloved hand.
H. Place this second glove on other hand by maintaining a firm and steady pull under the cuff. Be careful not to touch gloved hand to bare hand or wrist (Fig. 37–12 *E*).	H. Thumb of 1st gloved hand is most vulnerable to contamination. Folding thumb in with fingers or extending thumb away from hand helps prevent contamination.
I. Do not attempt to adjust *cuffs* once gloves are pulled on.	I. Attempting to adjust glove cuffs increases chances of contaminating the gloves.
J. Adjust position of fingers in gloves until gloves fit comfortably. Always keep gloved hands in sight and above waist level. Do not touch unsterile objects.	J. Proper fit permits maximum function of hands. Loose glove fingers which are not covering a finger may lead to contamination.

Procedure continued on the following page

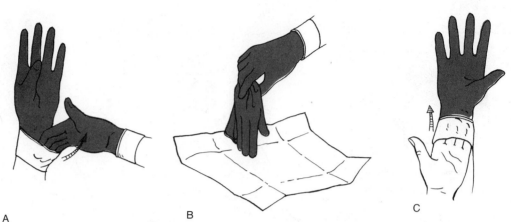

Figure 37–13.   Removing sterile gloves. *Note:* Illustrations are drawn from the perspective of the worker looking *down* on her hands.

SUGGESTED STEPS	RATIONALE/ASSESSMENT
K. If a glove is torn or becomes contaminated, immediately discard and start over.	K. Torn gloves provide an open pathway to the helper's skin, which is considered "contaminated."
L. *To remove gloves,* gloved fingers of one hand are placed under the folded-over cuff of the opposite hand. The glove is inverted as it is removed with a firm steady pull (Fig. 37–13*A*).	L. Remove gloves so that the surface that was sterile does not come in contact with the hands. After being used in sterile procedures, the outer surface of the gloves is considered contaminated.
M. If the cuff is not folded over so that step K can be carried out, then pinch the outside of the glove at heel of hand with other gloved hand and remove with a firm steady pull. Discard glove in paper wrapper (Fig. 37–13 *B*).	M. Gloved fingers must not touch helper's skin.
N. Slip fingers of ungloved hand inside of glove on other hand at wrist and pull glove off without touching exterior of the glove (Fig. 37–13 *C*).	N. Remember: exterior of gloves is now contaminated. Worker thus avoids touching outer surface of glove with ungloved hand.
O. Discard the gloves in trash and wash hands.	O. Wash hands, as organisms multiply rapidly in the warm moist atmosphere of the gloved hand.

Post-Procedure Activities.   Ensure safety and comfort of patient after sterile procedure. Helper washes hands.

Aftercare of Equipment.   Gloves and wrapper are discarded in trash after use. If they are grossly contaminated, discard with other used equipment in the dirty utility room.

Chart/Report: Results of procedure as appropriate.

Maintaining Standards of Practice

The facts and principles of sterile technique plus the methods of sterilization have been discussed. The maintenance and insurance of sterile technique is a vital responsibility of the health care worker. After the process of sterilization has taken place, it is up to the health care worker to ensure strict asepsis by practicing proper procedure based on specific rationale. It is thus necessary that the health care worker be conscientious and honest when applying the principles of sterile technique in the health care setting. The health care worker must be responsible and accountable for professional actions. By knowing and practicing good sterile technique, the health care worker maintains high standards of professional practice.

BIBLIOGRAPHY

1. Boger, W.: A better understanding of ethylene oxide sterilization. *Hospital Topics*, 54:12, Sep.–Oct. 1976.
2. Burgess, R. E.: Aseptic management of disposables. *Hospital Topics*, 48:95, Jan. 1970.
3. Engley, F. B., Jr.: Proper use of ethylene oxide discussed in sterilization and disinfection session. *Hospital Topics*, 49:67, May 1971.
4. Ginsberg, F., and Clarke, B.: When to use disinfectants and which ones not to use. *Modern Hospital*, 119:110, Aug. 1972.
5. Golden, D. L.: Constant monitoring guarantees sterility. *Hospitals, Journal of American Hospital Association*, 46:79, Sep. 1972.
6. Halleck, F. E.: Hazards of ethylene oxide sterilization in hospitals. *Hospital Topics*, 53:45, Nov.–Dec. 1975.
7. Halleck, F. E.: Packaging materials for ethylene oxide gas sterilization. *AORN Journal*, 21:104, Jan. 1975.
8. Huth, M. E.: Principles of asepsis. *AORN Journal*, 24:790, Oct. 1976.
9. Litsky, B. Y.: Standards for packaging needed for improved safety. *AORN Journal*, 23:27, Jan. 1976.
10. MacClelland, D. O.: The evolution of sterilization. *AORN Journal*, 24:37, July 1976.
11. Marinaro, A.: Rationale of sterility, sterilization and sterility testing. *Hospital Topics*, 49:118, Jan. 1971.
12. Mehaffy, N. L.: Rationale for asepsis standards. *AORN Journal*, 21:1213, June 1975.
13. Perkins, J. J.: *Principles and Methods of Sterilization in Health Sciences*, 2nd ed. Springfield, IL, Charles C Thomas, 1969.
14. Porter, K. W.: EO: despite call for FDA action. *Hospitals, Journal of American Hospital Association*, 47:117, Aug. 1973.
15. *Principles and Practice of Autoclave Sterilization.* North Hollywood, CA, Aseptic-Thermo Indicator Company.
16. *Principles and Practice of Ethylene Oxide Sterilization.* North Hollywood, CA, Aseptic-Thermo Indicator Company.
17. Rendell-Baker, L., and Roberts, R. B.: Gas versus steam sterilization: when to use which. *Hospital Topics*, 48:81, Nov. 1970.

ADMINISTERING INJECTABLE MEDICATIONS

By Margaret Auld Bruya, R.N., M.N.

OVERVIEW AND STUDY GUIDE

In this chapter we discuss the principles and practices that the student nurse needs to learn in order to administer injectable medications. Most people in the modern world have had experience with injections ("shots"), and so it is not unreasonable to expect that each student brings to the nursing situation many preconceived notions. Apprehensions may arise; traumatic memories may be recalled.

There have been many recent advances in scientific knowledge applicable to parenteral therapy and technical equipment. Widespread use of "disposables" such as syringes, needles, and intravenous therapy equipment and the advent of premixed and prepackaged medications have greatly facilitated preparation and administration, allowing the nurse more time for other nursing care activities. In addition, cross-contamination and consequent infections have been reduced.

This chapter includes a detailed discussion of the nursing responsibilities associated with equipment selection and parenteral medication preparation. In addition, the major anatomical sites used for intramuscular (IM), subcutaneous (SQ or SC) or hypodermic (H), intradermal (ID), and venipuncture or intravenous (IV) injections are discussed. The special needs of certain patients—children, the elderly, the emaciated, the neurologically impaired, and diabetics—are considered.

This chapter does not discuss intravenous fluids or administration of blood. These topics are discussed in Chapters 24 and 39, respectively.

To safely administer parenteral medications, the nurse needs to review the anatomy and physiology of the areas (skin, muscles, subcutaneous tissues, and veins) used for medication administration. To understand the advantages and disadvantages of the sites available, it is essential to know the depth and size of the muscles and the location of adjacent nerves, bones, joints, arteries and veins.

For intramuscular sites, the student should review these commonly used muscular areas: gluteal area, deltoid area, and the vastus lateralis. For subcutaneous injections, review the anatomy and physiol-

ogy of the skin (dermis) and adjacent tissues (loose areolar connective tissue, fat, deep fascia, aponeurosis and periosteum). Intradermal injections require consideration of the anatomy and physiology of skin. Intravenous sites demand review of the anatomy of the veins and surrounding supporting tissue. Additionally, the nurse must know the anatomy of the hands and arms in relation to the venous system of adults and study the scalp veins in infants.

At the end of this chapter, the student will be able to:

1. Identify factors to be considered in choosing a site for injections of medication
2. Describe the anatomy of the site selected
3. Select appropriate needle gauge and length to use in parenteral therapy, based on medication viscosity and route ordered
4. Discuss techniques that ensure a comfortable injection
5. Identify hazards of parenteral therapy (e.g., nerve and tissue damage, inadvertent IV administration, abscess)
6. Integrate aseptic principles essential for parenteral therapy
7. List indications and contraindications for parenteral medication injections.
8. Begin practicing the preparation and administration of parenteral medications.

To meet the above objectives, you should be able to identify and understand the following terms, and use them in your nursing practice.

abscess	bactericidal
adipose	bacteriostatic
air lock technique	bolus
allergen	colloidal osmotic
ampule	pressure
anaphylactic	deltoid
antibody	dermis
antecubital space	diffusion
antigen	edema
asepsis	epidermis
autoclaving	fibrosis

gluteus minimus
gluteus medius
hub
hydrostatic pressure
hypodermic
indurated
infiltration
inflammation
infusion
interstitial
Intracath
intradermal
intramuscular
intravenous
lipodystrophy
lipohypertrophy

necrotizing
needle
nodular
parenteral
pathogenic
phlebitis
sepsis
septicemia
subcutaneous
syringe
thrombophlebitis
vastus lateralis
ventrogluteal
vial
viscosity
wheal

INDICATIONS AND CONTRAINDICATIONS

The administration of medications parenterally serves many purposes: (1) provides rapid onset of medication effect, although the duration of effect is shorter than for medications given orally; (2) allows the practitioner to provide the needed effect even when the patient is unconscious, unable to swallow due to neurological or surgical alterations affecting the mouth and throat, or uncooperative; (3) assures that total dosage will be administered; (4) allows less total dosage to be used since total absorption is assured and (5) provides the only means of administration for medications that cannot be given orally, e.g., some medications are rendered ineffective in the gastrointestinal tract (e.g., insulin), while others are poorly absorbed, too toxic, or too irritating.

Contraindications to parenteral therapy occur in several disease states in which the administration of IM injections alters serum enzyme levels essential to diagnosis and therapy. When burned, edematous or shock patients need medications, the nurse needs to assess the route as well as the site. Contraindications would also exist when patient's musculature and development prohibit locating a muscle mass large enough to accept the dose.

PHYSIOLOGIC CONSIDERATIONS

Parenteral medications must be absorbed into the circulatory system to be effective; however, a number of factors can delay or hinder absorption. For example, medications deposited in the interstitial fluid are absorbed into the capillaries by the process of diffusion, but if abnormalities of the tissue are present, diffusion is impaired. This is particularly true of patients who are burned or who have tissue

edema. If medication is deposited in edematous tissue the medication will be absorbed slowly, if at all, leaving the patient without therapeutic effect until the edema subsides. Then the medication from multiple injections may be absorbed all at once, causing an inadvertent overdose. In addition, factors such as injection pressure, hydrostatic pressure, colloid osmotic pressure, blood flow and capillary permeability affect diffusion of a medication into the circulatory system.* A change in any of these factors will affect absorption into the circulation. Persons who have changes in any of these parameters need to be evaluated carefully to determine the best method of giving parenteral medications.

The rate of blood flow through a capillary is dependent on the pressure gradient between arterial and venous pressures. Absorption will be diminished in a person who has venous congestion or who has neurogenic, cardiogenic or vasogenic shock.

Skin lesions such as inflammation, excoriation, abrasion, fibrosis, lipodystrophy and lipohypertrophy delay absorption of medications from the injection site. Sites should be rotated at frequent intervals and great care should be given to depositing irritating medications deep into muscles, and avoiding dribbling medications through subcutaneous tissue.

Circulation time of the blood (the amount of time for the blood to make one complete circuit in the body in the venous and arterial systems) is 20 seconds. With such rapidity of circulation, great care must be exercised by the nurse to be sure that correct dosage and medication are given.

SAFETY CONSIDERATIONS

You should recall the five rights of medication administration (from Chapter 31), which are as crucial in parenteral administration as they are in oral administration of medications:
1. right dosage
2. right drug
3. right time
4. right patient
5. right route

*We suggest you review your physiology text to recall these principles.

washing inadequately or (3) using or storing multiple-dose vials improperly.

Route of Administration

Because the structures involved in the various routes are different (vein, muscle, skin), the speed and completeness of absorption vary greatly. Intravenous absorption of parenteral medications is by far the fastest as medication is injected directly into blood vessels and total absorption of the medication occurs. Generally, intramuscular injections are the next fastest route of absorption as muscles are well supplied with blood vessels. The muscle is able to withstand medications which are irritating, painful, or several milliliters in quantity. Total absorption is expected, except in areas of fibrosis from multiple injection trauma.[10] Subcutaneous injections would theoretically have the next greatest absorption. Absorption is less due to the diminished blood supply found in the area. The parenteral structure with the least blood vessels and therefore least absorption is the intradermal area. Figure 38–1 shows the tissues penetrated by each of the above injection techniques.

In addition, to safely administer parenteral medications, the nurse must be knowledgeable about preparation of the medication, site selection, and techniques of a comfortable injection. Because the medication is injected into the intradermal, subcutaneous, muscular or venous system, knowledge of the anatomy and physiology of the affected tissue, as well as knowledge of aseptic technique is essential. Also, because medication effect is potentially immediate (as with IV's) knowledge and practice of accurate medication dosage, proper site selection and rate of injection are critical. Bergersen has said that "an injected drug is irretrievable."[3] Errors in dosage, method, or site of injection are not easily corrected.

> Once a drug is injected, it is irretrievable. Antidotes may be available for particular medications, but the best antidote is prevention: be sure you feel confident in your skills of medication administration.

Geolot and McKinney suggest an expanded assessment of five influences on parenteral administration of medications:
1. the route of administration
2. the patient's age
3. body size
4. diagnosis and presenting condition
5. physical and chemical properties of the drug.[21]

Site

Although there are many sites available, the nurse normally selects a site with the following considerations: (1) the route ordered by the physician, (2) the quantity of medication to be given, (3) the muscular development and condition of the patient, (4) knowledge of the anatomical location of large nerves, and (5) the characteristics of the medication to be given.

Improper choice of *site* could result in (1) nerve damage, (2) inadvertent deposition of medication into an artery or vein, (3) deposition of medication into joints, (4) striking the bone or (4) too large a medication dosage for the site selected.

Asepsis

Sterile aseptic technique must be strictly followed. Strict adherence to technique helps prevent both local and systemic infections, which could potentially be fatal. Faulty technique can cause abscess formation at the site of injection or cause contamination from the skin to enter the puncture site.

Breaks in aseptic technique often occur (1) when the nurse is rushed; (2) when procedures become so routine that little thought is given to the potential seriousness of an error and (3) in emergencies. For patient safety and well being, aseptic technique must be maintained regardless of the situation. The actions that may be the cause of breaks in aseptic technique include: (1) using equipment when its sterility is doubtful, (2) workers not washing their hands or

Diagnosis

The nurse considers the patient's diagnosis when planning parenteral therapy. In some circumstances, the diagnosis contraindicates certain routes, e.g., when a patient's serum creatinine phosphokinase (CPK) is being monitored for diagnostic purposes (such as with a heart attack), intramuscular injections are normally contraindicated. Even the slight local tissue trauma caused by IM injection is thought to contribute to elevation of this en-

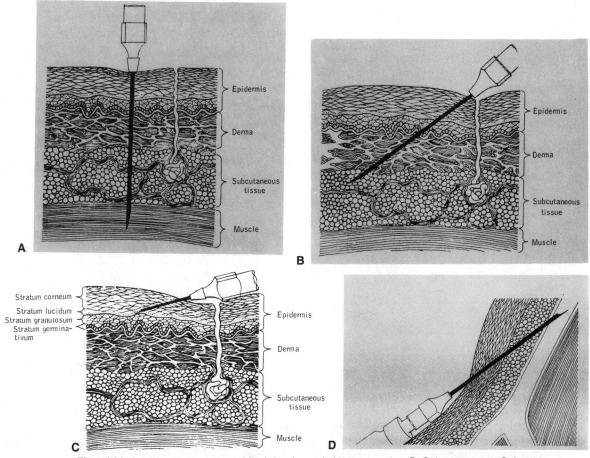

Figure 38-1. Tissues penetrated by injections. *A,* Intramuscular. *B,* Subcutaneous. *C,* Intradermal. *D,* Intravenous. (From Falconer, M. W., et al.: *The Drug, The Nurse, The Patient,* 6th ed. Philadelphia, W. B. Saunders Co., 1978.)

zyme, rendering measurements false for diagnostic purposes.[12] For a patient with conditions known for poor tissue perfusion, e.g., burns, shock and edema, medications should be given in sites and routes in which prediction of absorption can be reliable. For some patients the intravenous route would be best, for others the use of an intact healthy muscle would suffice.

Characteristics of the Medication

As the solutions or suspensions in which medications are mixed are often irritating to tissues (as may be the medications themselves), the nurse should be aware of and follow explicitly the manufacturer's guidelines before administering medications. If irritating IM medications must be given for therapeutic effect, efforts should be made to reduce discom-

fort by: (a) rotating sites, (b) giving medication into deep muscles, (c) using skillful technique and (d) adding a small amount of local anesthetic to the medication.

PRINCIPLES OF ADMINISTRATION

Because of the risks and responsibilities involved with parenteral medication administration, the nurse must understand the principles of skin cleansing and pain reduction, as well as possess the manual and technical skill to administer medications.

Skin Cleansing

Any time the principle "Intact skin is the body's first line of defense" is violated, as in any parenteral therapy, special consideration must be given to skin preparation. If no obvious soil is present, it is common practice to cleanse the skin with a 70 per cent alcohol or a Betadine pledget, using friction to remove surface bacteria, and surgical asepsis principles (going from the center outward). The skin is then considered to be "clean" enough for piercing with a sterile needle. When the skin is obviously soiled, as with drainage or feces, washing with soap (or detergent) and water and thoroughly drying the skin before using the antiseptic pledget is the common nursing practice.

> *For all parenteral therapy, surgical asepsis is essential; any other method should be considered ineffective or inadequate.*

Pain Reduction

Pain is a complex psychobiological phenomenon. We know that with an intact neuromuscular system, individual *pain perception* is relatively uniform among humans. The pain *perception threshold,* however, varies among us and accounts for the varied reactions to pain and the organism's total experience of pain, whether culturally or socially learned.

These three facts about pain are established:

1. There are more pain receptors found in the skin than in any other part of the body.

2. Skin pain receptors are randomly found. There is no way to predict sites which are painless.

3. The speed of insertion of the needle does not alter the pain sensation.[47]

Often, pain reduction can be achieved through *distraction* of the patient. Methods nurses use include involving the patient in conversation, gently slapping adjacent tissue, or pinching another part of the body. *Physical agents* can also be used to reduce pain. Applying ice to the tissue is often effective, as is spraying a local cooling agent, such as ethyl chloride. Some antibiotics cause a great deal of local discomfort when given intramuscularly. In this situation, the physician may order a local anesthetic to be drawn up in the same syringe and given concomitantly.

Most nursing educators and practitioners agree that manual and technical skills in giving an injection can greatly reduce discomfort and alleviate or prevent complications.

▶ The nurse should select equipment appropriate for the therapy:
  (1) Needle sharp, without burrs
  (2) Needle size smallest gauge appropriate for medication
  (3) Needle length appropriate to site and/or muscle mass
  (4) Needle affixed tightly to syringe so that injection pressure will not "blow" off needle

▶ The nurse needs to develop skill to be able to
  (1) Manipulate antiseptic pledget, syringe and needle without hesitation
  (2) Locate site accurately and quickly
  (3) Pierce skin quickly and without hesitation; aspirate for blood before injecting
  (4) Inject medication slowly
  (5) Remove needle quickly
  (6) Use firm pressure to massage
  (7) Ascertain patient response to therapy

▶ The nurse should
  (1) Select site free of abrasion, excoriation, irritation, etc.
  (2) Select site appropriate to volume of therapy
  (3) Rotate sites to allow maximum absorption and minimal tissue irritation. Chart in nursing care plan.
  (4) Cleanse skin according to assessment: if soiled, wash with soap and water first, then antiseptic pledget

▶ To prepare medications, the nurse should
  (1) Use aseptic technique
  (2) Mix IM medications in one syringe, if possible, to reduce number of injections

PREPARATION OF MEDICATIONS AND EQUIPMENT

Needles and Syringes

Needles come in various lengths and gauges, with different sizes of bevels. The common available sizes for subcutaneous, intramuscular, intradermal (also called tuberculin), and insulin injections are presented in Table 38–1.

Needle *gauge* is determined by the lumen of the needle. As the diameter increases, the gauge decreases. For example, a 14-gauge needle is substantially larger in diameter than a

TABLE 38–1.   TYPICAL NEEDLE AND SYRINGE SIZES FOR PARENTERAL THERAPY

TYPE OF INJECTION	SIZE OF SYRINGE	SIZE OF NEEDLE
Subcutaneous	2, 2.5 or 3 ml. Calibrated in 0.1 ml. units	25 gauge ½ or ⅝ inch
Intramuscular	2, 2.5 ml. Calibrated in 0.2 ml. units	18, 20, 22 gauge 1½ inch
	2.0 ml. Calibrated in 0.2 ml. units	18, 20, 22 gauge 1 inch
Intradermal (tuberculin)	1.0 ml. Calibrated in 0.01 ml. units	26 or 27 gauge ⅜ to ⅝ inch
Insulin	1 ml. calibrated in "units" for 100 units per ml.	25 gauge ½ or ⅝ inch
Intravenous	Dosage and kind of medication to be given determine whether syringe and needle or intravenous infusion set is used.	(a) Steel needle with plastic sleeve, which is left in vein—14 to 20 gauge (b) Plastic catheter inside steel needle (c) "Butterfly" steel needle—18 to 21 gauge, 1 inch.

22-gauge needle. The nurse's choice is limited by the equipment purchased by her institution but will be sufficient for her to choose a larger gauge needle when a viscous solution, such as penicillin, is given (Fig. 38–2).

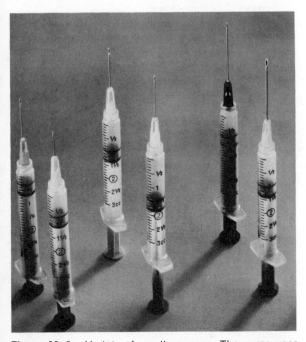

Figure 38–2. Variety of needle gauges. The nurse uses her judgment when choosing a needle gauge depending upon site and viscosity of the medication. (From Becton-Dickinson, Rutherford, NJ.)

The *bevel* of the needle is designed to make a narrow, slit-type opening that closes quickly to prevent seepage of blood, serum and medication. Figure 38–3 shows a regular bevel, and intradermal, short, and huber bevels. Each is designed to achieve a particular result.

A wide variety of syringes is available—glass as well as plastic (Fig. 38–4). Some syringes have a locking mechanism at the needle attachment; others do not.

Needles usually come in sterile, individual packages so that the nurse can select the needle she needs. If the needle is accidentally contaminated, the nurse can change needles without having to discard the syringe. Because of the wide variety of syringe sizes available, syringes also come separately packaged, so that the nurse may select the most suitable one. However, manufacturers do prepackage insulin and tuberculin syringes and some IM syringes with needles attached because the needle length is so standard.

Criteria for Selection. The nurse's discretion must be used in equipment selection. Factors to be considered are: (1) route ordered, (2) viscosity of medication solution, (3) amount of medication to be administered and (4) body size and amount of fat. In addition, the syringe chosen must be marked in units that allow the nurse to accurately measure the dosage ordered (e.g., for skin testing). If, according to the manufacturer's specifications, the medication should

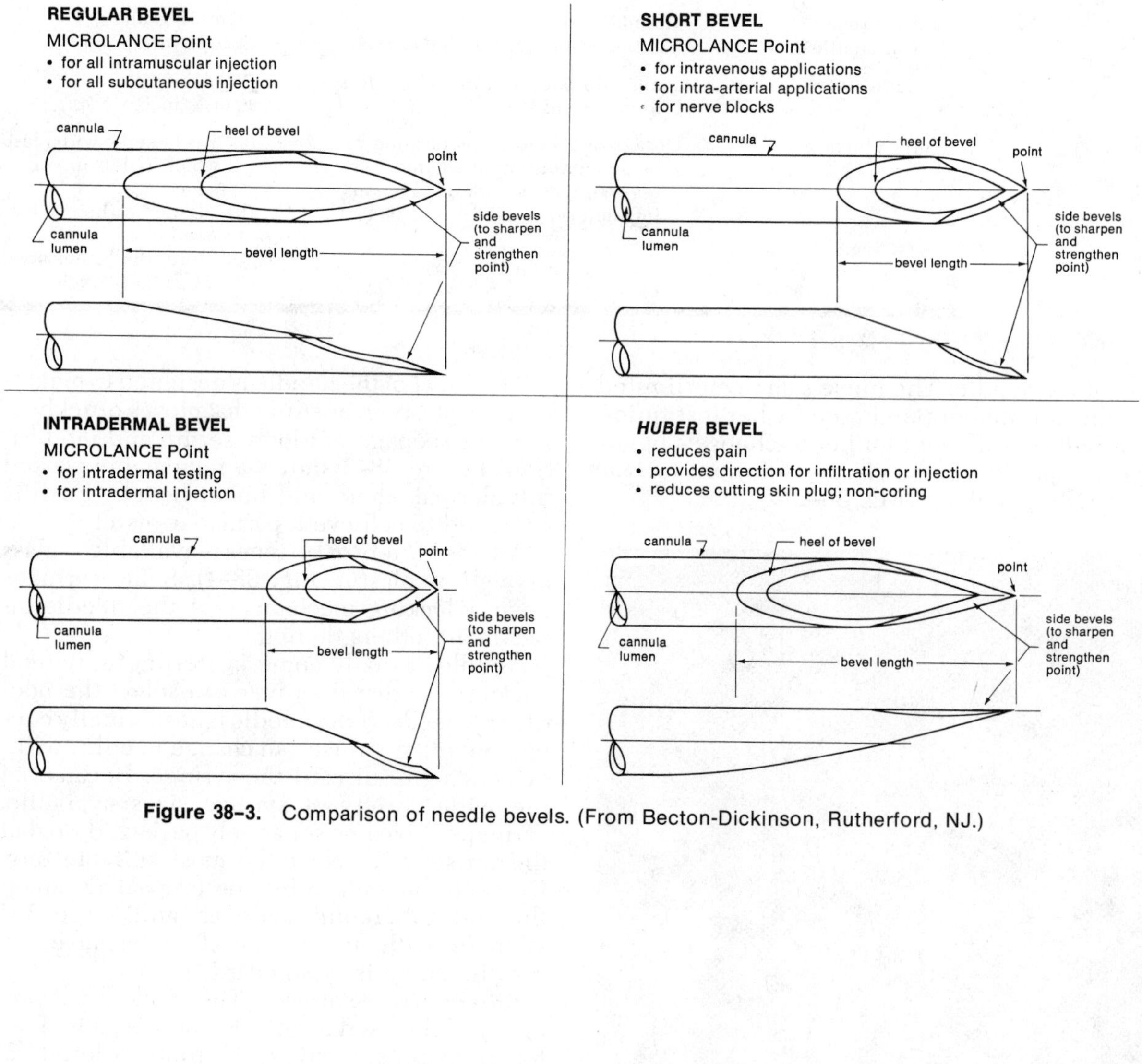
REGULAR BEVEL
MICROLANCE Point
• for all intramuscular injection
• for all subcutaneous injection
cannula
heel of bevel
point
cannula lumen
bevel length
side bevels (to sharpen and strengthen point)
SHORT BEVEL
MICROLANCE Point
• for intravenous applications
• for intra-arterial applications
• for nerve blocks
cannula
heel of bevel
point
cannula lumen
bevel length
side bevels (to sharpen and strengthen point)
INTRADERMAL BEVEL
MICROLANCE Point
• for intradermal testing
• for intradermal injection
cannula
heel of bevel
point
cannula lumen
bevel length
side bevels (to sharpen and strengthen point)
HUBER BEVEL
• reduces pain
• provides direction for infiltration or injection
• reduces cutting skin plug; non-coring
cannula
heel of bevel
point
cannula lumen
bevel length
side bevels (to sharpen and strengthen point)

Figure 38–3. Comparison of needle bevels. (From Becton-Dickinson, Rutherford, NJ.)

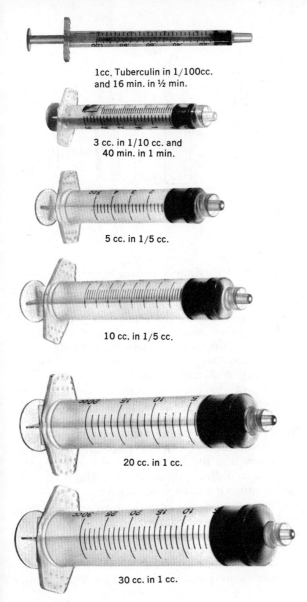

1cc. Tuberculin in 1/100cc. and 16 min. in ½ min.

3 cc. in 1/10 cc. and 40 min. in 1 min.

5 cc. in 1/5 cc.

10 cc. in 1/5 cc.

20 cc. in 1 cc.

30 cc. in 1 cc.

Figure 38–4.   A sampling of the wide variety of syringe sizes available. (From Becton-Dickinson, Rutherford, NJ.)

not be left in a plastic syringe for any length of time prior to administration, it may be preferable to use a glass syringe. Some medications are prefilled by the manufacturer.

Once packages are opened, the nurse must use great caution in handling the syringe and needle in order to preserve their sterility. Fig-

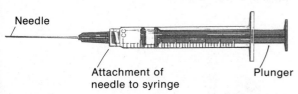

Needle

Attachment of needle to syringe

Plunger

Figure 38–5.   The areas identified are to be kept sterile while preparing and administering parenteral therapy.

ure 38–5 shows the areas of the syringe and needle that must be kept sterile.

> *The nurse should take care to avoid contaminating the shaft of the needle, the area where the needle attaches to the syringe, and the plunger. If these areas are accidentally contaminated, the contaminated needle and/or syringe must be discarded.*

Care and Handling.   Aftercare of needles and syringes has been greatly simplified in recent years. Indeed, in modern health facilities, it is uncommon to find anything but disposable steel needles and plastic syringes for routine patient care. The use of disposable needles and syringes has alleviated the problems of cleaning, autoclaving, sorting and storing equipment. However, some special procedure needles (for example, bone marrow biopsy needles) must be sterilized for reuse, as must the glass syringes that are routinely used by the laboratory for collection of arterial blood.

Syringe and needle controls are essential in health care agencies. The Joint Commission on Hospital Accreditation highly recommends that *all* needles and syringes be kept under locked conditions. The reason for tight security is to prevent theft by those who would abuse drugs. Following use, manufacturers suggest breaking off the needle at the hub, breaking the plunger and discarding all in clearly marked containers. Used needles and syringes should *not* be dropped into patient's bedside bags, waste baskets or the nurse's pocket. The risk of accidental needle puncture by housekeeping personnel as they collect the trash is too great. Putting used needles in a nurse's pocket risks a puncture also, as the needle protector may dislodge and leave an exposed needle.

Preparation of Parenteral Medications

Tablet.   While it is uncommon today to crush a tablet, mix it with a solution, and inject it into the patient's tissue, this awkward procedure is still occasionally done. We recommend that the nurse ask the pharmacist's assistance in obtaining another form of the medication for parenteral therapy. The obvious problem associated with this method is the difficulty in maintaining sterility.

Powder. Because some medications deteriorate when mixed in a solution, the manufacturer may dispense them in powder form in a sterile vial. Each medication has clear directions concerning the kind and amount of solution to mix with the medication. Sterile normal saline, bacteriostatic water, and a solution provided by the manufacturer are the three most commonly used solutions. The nurse must follow the recommendations closely to (1) prevent overdosage or underdosage, (2) prevent local tissue damage from a too concentrated solution and (3) provide the patient with the maximum therapeutic dosage. Michel[40] reported on the proper manner of entering a rubber-stoppered vial to prevent small "cores" of rubber from entering the vial. He suggests that if the needle is inserted bevel side up with two simultaneous pressures exerted as in the diagram (Fig. 38–6), a minimum number of cores would enter the vial.

After the solution is placed in the vial containing the powder, the vial can be gently rotated to allow mixing. Thorough mixing is achieved when the solution is clear and free of clumps of powder. The nurse then aseptically draws up the appropriate dosage and administers it to the patient.

Ampule. An ampule is a glass container of medication in solution (Fig. 38–7). To obtain the medication, the nurse should gently tap the stem, thereby causing the medication to drop into the base. Opening the ampule may require

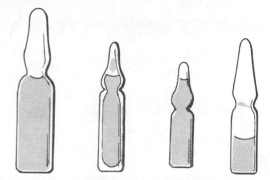

Figure 38–7. A selection of ampules. Note the various shapes of the necks.

a specially designed file or not, depending upon the manufacturer's design and strength of glass. Whether or not to wipe the stem with an alcohol pledget is debated, but we strongly suggest doing so as a preventive measure.

To open the ampule, use of a sterile gauze wrapped around the stem is suggested for the following reasons: (1) to protect the nurse's fingers, (2) to prevent contamination of the medication through contact with a nonsterile material and (3) to prevent flying glass splinters from harming the nurse or anyone else. A glass splinter in the eye is a real possibility, and you must develop the habit of always opening the ampule in a direction away from the body, *but never toward another person.*

Once opened, the ampule is an open system, and the medication should be quickly drawn up in order to minimize airborne contamination. The nurse can withdraw the medication with the base on a flat surface (Fig. 38–8) or with the ampule turned upside down (Fig. 38–9). Great

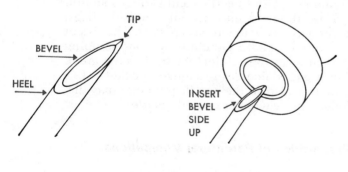

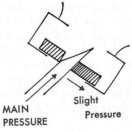

Figure 38–6. One method of entering a rubber-stoppered vial while preventing small "cores" of rubber from entering the vial. (From Michel, F.: The vexing core. *American Journal of Nursing, 71*:768, April 1971.)

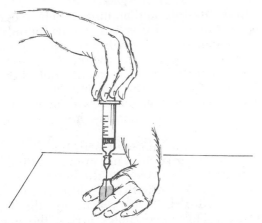

Figure 38-8. Withdrawal of medication from an ampule on a flat surface. Notice that the position of needle is in center of opening to prevent contamination, and needle bevel is in medication to prevent drawing up of air into the syringe.

care must be exercised to avoid touching the edge of the glass ampule, which would contaminate the needle. If you are using the inverted method, keep the needle in the medica-

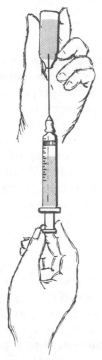

Figure 38-9. An alternate method of withdrawing medication from ampule. Note that to prevent losing medication, the needle must be centered in opening and *never* touch the side. (If the needle touches the side, the capillary forces preventing gravity from pulling out the medication will be broken.) Note position of the hand holding the ampule and the hand holding syringe and needle.

tion at all times or the capillary pressure will be broken and the solution will dribble out onto your hands and the floor and there may not be enough left for the proper dosage. Also, the medication may irritate and/or sensitize your skin. If any medication does splash on your skin, you should wash your hands immediately.

Manufacturers are using the ampule less and less as it is thought that there is a slight chance of administering splinters of glass that might have fallen into the medication.

Vials. Vials are probably the most commonly used form of parenteral medication. They can be single- or multiple-dosage containers. The sterile solution (or powder requiring reconstitution) contained in the vial is protected with a rubber stopper and a soft metal cap, which is taken off before the medication is removed. (The rubber stopper is theoretically sterile; however, it is advisable to cleanse the top with an alcohol pledget. This is particularly true for multiple-dose vials.)

In order to draw the medication into the syringe easily, an amount of air equal to the amount of medication to be drawn up should be injected into the vial first. If medication is to be drawn up from two vials and mixed in one syringe, first inject air into each vial—the total amount injected being equal to the total dosage to be withdrawn. Then withdraw the dosage. If a multiple-dose vial and single-dose vial are used, withdraw the dosage from the multiple-dosage vial first to prevent possible contamination from the single-dose vial.

When injecting air into a multiple-dose vial, care should be taken to inject an amount of air equal to the amount of medication to be withdrawn. If too little is injected, it will be difficult to withdraw a sufficient dosage. If too much air is injected, the syringe plunger may be explosively blown out because of the high pressure in the vial, causing a loss of medication as well as contaminating the equipment.

Multiple-dose vials should be stored according to the manufacturer's directions. Some need to be dated and refrigerated, while others have a preservative that allows them to be stored at room temperature for various lengths of time. It is essential to be aware of the storage requirements for each medication and follow manufacturer's directions explicitly. To do otherwise endangers the patient or causes needless wastage.

Empty glass vials must be disposed of properly. They may be separated from the other burnable disposables and sent to be crushed. They are not playthings.

Tubex. Tubex is a commercial system that has been developed to provide the nurse with a variety of prefilled cartridges. In this system, a reusable syringe holder (1 or 2 ml. size) is selected; the prefilled cartridge is loaded and screwed into place, and the medication is delivered to the patient.

In institutions and on units in which certain medications and dosages are commonly ordered (e.g., on a postoperative unit), the Tubex system can save time for the nurse. Preparation time is cut drastically, narcotic control can be rigorous, waste is minimal, and the medication cartridge is clearly labeled with name, dosage and route of administration—helping to reduce errors.

Problems encountered with the Tubex system usually arise from not understanding how to place the cartridge into the holder properly. Another problem is that if additional medication is ordered, it may not fit into the Tubex syringe. This necessitates giving the patient two injections when one may have sufficed.

24. PREPARING MEDICATIONS FOR INJECTIONS AND CARING FOR EQUIPMENT

Definitions and Purposes. *Preparing medications that are to be given by syringe and needle and caring for used equipment.* Techniques are used to prepare medications for intradermal, subcutaneous, intramuscular and intravenous injection and to dispose of equipment safely.

Contraindications and Cautions. Because medications given by injection act more rapidly than do oral medications and because they may sometimes precipitate irreversible toxic effects, the nurse *must* be accurate when preparing and administering drugs by injection; this is particularly true for medications given by the intravenous route. Also, the nurse must use meticulous sterile technique when working with parenteral injections because the needle pierces the skin (the body's first line of defense against infection) and pathogens can cause serious infections in the tissues or blood (septicemia). The nurse should pay careful attention to washing her hands before and after preparing any medication for injection. Syringes and needles must be properly disposed of to prevent injury to the housekeeping personnel and sanitation workers and to prevent the theft of used needles and syringes by drug abusers.

Patient-Family Teaching Points. *If the patient is to receive an injection,* explain: (a) purpose of the injection; (b) site of injection; (c) amount of discomfort to be expected and (d) methods for relaxing muscles at the site of the IM injection. *If injections are to be administered by the patient and/or family,* explain and demonstrate (a) aseptic technique essential for safe preparation; (b) scientific principles and facts essential to the above; (c) precautions to reduce or eliminate errors; (d) importance of safe practices to prevent injury; (d) where to obtain equipment and what equipment is used and (f) how to destroy used disposable needles and syringes.

PRE-PROCEDURE ACTIVITIES

PRELIMINARY ASSESSMENT

Includes determination of:
- age
- diagnosis
- state of consciousness
- body size
- tissue consistency (presence of scars, tenderness or nodules)
- location of sites available for use; e.g., mid-deltoid site, ventrogluteal site
- site of previous injections
- physician's order for medication and route

PRELIMINARY PLANNING

- Determine appropriate length and gauge of needle to be used, considering viscosity of medication, route to be used and size of patient
- Determine appropriate volume of syringe (e.g., 1 ml., 2 ml.) and type (e.g., insulin, Tubex, etc.)
- Provide for comfort and safety of the patient
- Provide for continuing privacy

EQUIPMENT

- Correct forms of parenteral medication(s) (e.g., powders, multiple vials, tablets, ampules, etc.)
- Solvents (e.g., normal saline, sterile water) if medication is to be reconstituted
- Syringes, Tubex cartridges—appropriate sizes and types of needles, include extras of appropriate lengths and gauges
- Alcohol or Betadine pledgets
- Medication cupboard or cart and refrigerator storage, narcotic storage
- Keys to medication room, cupboards
- Medication tray
- Plastic or water/moisture impervious bag for waste disposal
- Containers for disposal of needles and syringes

PROCEDURE

SUGGESTED STEPS	RATIONALE/DISCUSSION
1. Collect and organize medication cards so that only medication being prepared is visible.	1. Reduces errors.
2. Check medication order on Kardex or original written order.	2. Prevents errors.
a. Ascertain route, time, date and frequency.	
b. Verify that medication card is same as original order (see Procedure 15, Chap. 31).	
3. Wash hands.	3. Reduces bacteria on hands. Maintain medical asepsis in handling medication and equipment.
4. Use quiet place to organize medications.	4. Lack of disruption and interruption helps prevent errors.

Procedure continued on the following page

SUGGESTED STEPS	RATIONALE/DISCUSSION
5. Select appropriate needle and syringe for medication, route, size and position patient will possibly assume.	5. Proper equipment insures a safer and more therapeutic injection.
a. Select needle.	a. Consider needle length, gauge, and bevel sharpness
(1) Needle length: ¼–⅝ inch; 1 inch; 1½ inch.	(1) *Needle length* should be chosen to accommodate patient's muscle size, site selected and route ordered. *Generally,* a 1 inch needle can be used for IM injections on adult deltoid and children's vastus lateralis muscles and 1½ inch needles for adult IM injections into dorsal gluteal and ventral gluteal sites. Needles less than 1 inch long can be used for ID and SC injections.
(2) Needle gauges for standard patient care are: 18, 19, 20, 21, 22, 23, 25, 26, 27.	(2) The *larger* the gauge, the finer the diameter of the needle (see Fig. 38–2). Needle gauge selected depends upon viscosity (thickness) of medication. A small gauge is needed for a viscous medication; a larger gauge for "thin" or "watery" medications.
(3) Needle bevel. *Bevels* of hospital needles are fairly standard (see Fig. 38–3).	
b. Select syringe.	b. Select syringe according to amount of solution and type of medication.
(1) Amount of solution to be given determines size of syringe barrel, whether 1 ml., 3 ml. or larger.	(1) Generally syringe barrel sizes for IM injections are 2 to 2.5 ml. Volumes greater than this may be divided and given in two sites. Always select a syringe that is marked in the units necessary to measure the volume of medication needed.
(2) Type of medication determines whether a glass or plastic syringe should be used. Insulin is given in a special insulin syringe.	(2) Manufacturers' specifications will state whether glass or plastic syringe is essential for medication being used. If not specified, the nurse can use the plastic disposable hospital-type equipment.
6. Obtain carrying tray (Fig. 38–10).	6. Organizes all the equipment necessary for efficient patient care during injections.

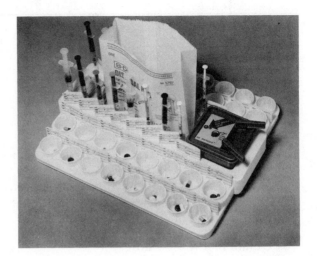

Figure 38–10. Assembled medication tray, ready for delivery to patients. Note organization for orals, parenterals, and disposal bag. (From Becton-Dickinson, Rutherford, NJ.)

Suggested Steps	Rationale/Discussion
7. Obtain alcohol or Betadine pledget.	7. Available in individual, one-time use foil packets to assure sterility and patient safety.
8. Select correct medication (vial, ampule, etc.) from storage area (shelf, refrigerator or cart).	8. See Procedure 15, Chapter 31.
9. Compare selected medication to medication card.	9. Helps diminish errors. *First check.*
10. Read label, determine dosage to be drawn up. If premixed, calculate appropriate dosage, shake or mix solutions, as directed.	10. Proper calculation of dosage diminishes error. Mixing solution assures homogeneity; allows nurse to check solution for clarity.
11. Check expiration date.	11. To ascertain freshness. Do not use after expiration date.
12. Select proper dilutant (solvent) if this is indicated.	12. If necessary for proper mixing, manufacturer specifies type of dilutant to be used. If not specified, normal saline or bacteriostatic water is used.
13. Remove needle and syringe of correct size from packaging. If in paper package, peel apart; if in plastic container, screw off cap and pull unit straight out.	13. Maintain sterility of needle and inner part of syringe.
14. If right handed, hold syringe in left hand, remove needle guard with backward and forward motion of the right hand. If left handed, reverse procedure.	14. Allows control of needle cover; prevents accidental puncture of self with unprotected needle.

Procedure continued on the following page

SUGGESTED STEPS	RATIONALE/DISCUSSION
15. Test the security of the needle.	15. Tighten needle with a one-quarter turn, to ensure that it is attached securely. If you need to change needles, remove attached needle from syringe by backward and forward motion, and replace with new choice. Tighten. Replace needle guard.
16. Cleanse stopper of vial or ampule selected with alcohol or Betadine.	16. Promotes asepsis.
17. Draw up into syringe amount of air equal to dose if to be removed from vial.	
18. Obtain medication dose.	

Vial (Single or Multiple Dose)

a. Holding vial with two fingers and in palm of one hand, guide needle through diaphragm with other hand.

a. Prevents stress on needle which could bend or weaken needle.

b. Inject air into vial.

b. Insert only as much air into vial as you will be removing medication. Too much or too little air will hinder removal.

Note: If medication is to be removed from *two* vials into *one* syringe, inject amount of air into each vial—so that total air injected is equivalent to the total dose to be drawn up. This must be done prior to withdrawing drug from either vial.

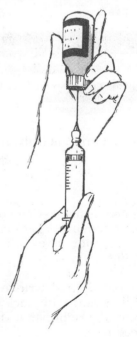

Figure 38–11. Inserting needle through diaphragm of vial.

SUGGESTED STEPS	RATIONALE/DISCUSSION

Vial (Single or Multiple Dose) (Continued)

c. Withdraw prescribed amount of medication into barrel, holding syringe perpendicular (90 degrees) to floor at eye level, with bevel of needle in medication.

c. Bevel of needle must be in medication to withdraw the solution. If air bubbles remain in barrel, withdraw 0.2 to 0.4 ml. medication beyond dose, tap syringe to make bubbles rise to needle end, and expel air and excess dosage into vial. If bubble remains, withdraw and expel medication several times to moisten barrel of syringe.

d. Remove needle from diaphragm. Replace needle guard. Do not allow stress on needle.

e. Check that dosage in syringe and label on vial agree with medication card.

e. Insures accuracy. *Second check.*

f. If multi-dose vial, reconstitute, label with identifying data: patient's name, dosage, strength, date, time and nurse's initials.

g. Return medication to original cabinet or refrigerator if necessary.

g. Proper storage prevents premature deterioration of medication.

Ampule

a. Shake or snap medication into bottom of ampule.

a. Centrifugal force moves medication through narrow neck.

b. Clean neck of ampule with alcohol pledget. Wrap pledget around neck of ampule. Grasp ampule in dominant hand, thumb against bottom, index finger around top. Snap off with pushing pressure away from you.

> *Be sure to snap glass away from your eyes and never toward anyone else. Glass particles may chip off and become flying missiles.*

If any glass particles get into ampule, discard and obtain another. Return to pharmacy.

c. Place ampule upright on flat surface, steady with two fingers or hold it with two fingers. Or turn ampule completely upside down, holding it in palm (Figs. 38–8 and 38–9).

c. Learning to invert the ampule takes practice. Solution will remain in ampule unless broken edges are irregular.

d. Guide needle into opening so as not to touch ampule sides. Withdraw medication dose with bevel submerged in solution. Remove needle from ampule.

d. Do not inject air while removing medication, or air will displace solution and force medication out of ampule. Always remove needle from ampule before ejecting air from syringe.

Procedure continued on the following page

SUGGESTED STEPS	RATIONALE/DISCUSSION

Ampule (Continued)

e. Hold syringe, needle up, perpendicular to floor, tap sides to get air bubbles to rise; expel air and medication to appropriate dose.

e. Expelling air bubbles allows accurate dosages to be determined prior to giving medication.

f. Change needle if irritating substance leaks onto needle.

f. Prevents irritation of patient's tissues when needle is inserted.

g. Replace needle guard.

g. Protects needle and insures sterility.

h. Check dosage with medication card and ampule label. Place on tray with pledget.

h. Promotes accuracy. *Second check.*

i. Discard unused portion of medication in ampule after medication given.

i. Provides additional medication if small amount lost before administration.

Tubex Metal Cartridge System

a. Read manufacturer's directions carefully.

b. If soiled, cleanse reusable part of syringe. Should be cleaned after each use.

b. Prevents cross-contamination between patients.

c. Select correct cartridge of medication and compare label with medication card.

c. Promotes accuracy. *First check.*

d. Select Tubex syringe that is the correct size to accommodate cartridge: 1 ml. syringe for 1 ml. cartridge; 2 ml. syringe for 2 ml. size cartridge.

d. If 1 ml. Tubex syringe is not available, the 2 ml. syringe can be used.

e. Read cartridge carefully for dosage. Compare to written order.

e. Promotes accuracy. *Second check.*

f. Mix solution if necessary by rolling cartridge in palms. Check clarity, homogeneity.

f. Mixes medication.

g. Grasp metal syringe in nondominant hand. Pull plunger back firmly with dominant hand, and swing until plunger is at right angle (90 degrees). It will lock in position (Fig. 38–12).

h. Insert medication cartridge with needle into unit. Tighten screws in needle end by turning needle clockwise in the threads while holding movable rim at needle end of syringe.

h. Locks needle unit into place.

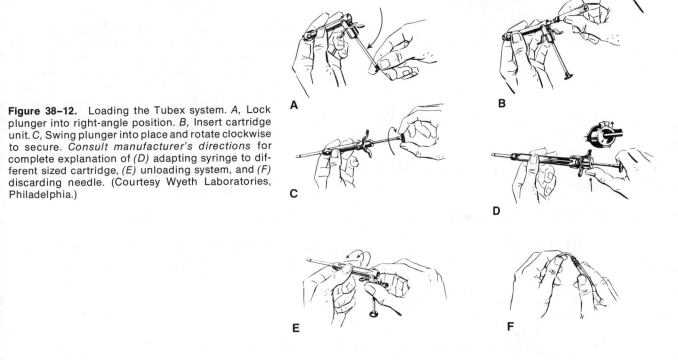

Figure 38–12.   Loading the Tubex system. *A,* Lock plunger into right-angle position. *B,* Insert cartridge unit. *C,* Swing plunger into place and rotate clockwise to secure. *Consult manufacturer's directions* for complete explanation of *(D)* adapting syringe to different sized cartridge, *(E)* unloading system, and *(F)* discarding needle. (Courtesy Wyeth Laboratories, Philadelphia.)

SUGGESTED STEPS	RATIONALE/DISCUSSION

Tubex Metal Cartridge System (Continued)

i. Swing plunger back into position and attach to threaded end of cartridge. Turn end of plunger while holding cartridge in position.	i. Cartridge must be firmly screwed into place to assure proper functioning of system.
j. Remove rubber needle sheath (which covers and protects needle from contamination) and expel excess medication.	j. Compare dosage with medication card. *Third check.*
k. Replace needle sheath. Place unit, medication card and alcohol or Betadine pledget on tray to take to patient bedside.	Caution: *The rubber needle sheath is designed to fit snugly over the needle. To protect needle, completely insert needle into sheath. If sheath is accidentally punctured by needle, discard entire unit because needle is now contaminated.*
19. Wash hands if contaminated with medication, especially antibiotics.	19. Nurse may develop a sensitization to antibiotics.

Procedure continued on the following page

SUGGESTED STEPS	RATIONALE/DISCUSSION
20. Handle narcotics to be given parenterally according to federal law and hospital policy.	20. Narcotics require special handling. They are always kept under lock and must be signed out at the time the medication is drawn up. If patient refuses the narcotic, if the wrong medication is drawn up, or if the medication is inadvertently contaminated, the nurse should discard it down a sink drain *in the presence of* another nurse. Both should sign the narcotic record as "medication wasted."
21. Lock medication room, cupboard or closet upon leaving.	21. Reduces chance of unauthorized access to medications.
22. Carry medication to patient.	

23. Identify patient:
  a. Read identification band
  b. Call by name
  c. Check chart at bedside
  d. Verify identification with a nurse who knows the patient
	23. At least two checks are essential to prevent errors. (See Procedure 15, Chap. 31.)

24. Explain action of medication to patient.	24. To teach and to gain patient cooperation.
25. Screen patient for privacy.	25. Exposure of entire site essential.
26. Select appropriate site.	26. See Procedures 25, 26, and 27 later in this chapter.
27. Check medication dosage against medication card.	27. Safety check.
28. If medication is irritating to subcutaneous tissues, prepare air lock: aspirate 0.2 to 0.3 ml. air for IM medication when indicated.	28. See Procedure 25 for explanation of air lock.
29. Cleanse chosen site with pledget, using surgical asepsis.	29. Removes surface bacteria.
30. Inject medication.	30. See Procedures 25, 26, and 27.
31. Replace cap on needle on syringe.	
32. Return used equipment to medication room. Discard syringes and needles appropriately, rendering them inoperable.	32. The needle and syringe that have been used should be disposed of according to the institution policy (1) to minimize or discourage illegal use of hypodermic equipment, (2) to prevent cross-contamination and (3) to protect housekeeping and sanitation personnel from hurting themselves with needles as they collect the trash. One system for destruction is the "Destru-clip," a mechanical device for cutting needles.

SUGGESTED STEPS	RATIONALE/DISCUSSION
	Other methods to render the equipment inoperable are separating the needle from the syringe and breaking off the needle in the cover at the junction of the hub of the syringe. Needles should not be discarded in patient's overbed table bag or in waste can in the room. Discard needles in marked containers only.
33. Disinfect or wash medication tray if contaminated.	
34. Wash hands.	34. Removes surface bacteria.
35. Chart medication given in appropriate place. See Procedures 25, 26, and 27.	35. Complete record is essential in care of patient.
36. Return cards to storage area.	36. Prevents loss of cards.

Post-Procedure Activities.   Order medication for next 24 hours if appropriate. Put injection preparation area in order; clean if medication spilled. Chart narcotics. Return to patient to see that desired effect is being achieved. Check to see that patient is comfortable and that no undesired effects are being experienced.

Aftercare of Equipment.   Discard used equipment to provide safety for others, discourage drug abuse, and prevent cross contamination. Needles and syringes known to be contaminated with blood-borne disease (e.g., hepatitis) *must* be very carefully discarded in the isolation room in a clearly labeled bottle with cap to avoid infecting another person with hepatitis. When bottle is filled, dispose of it in incinerated trash. If using reusable equipment, rinse with cold water and follow policy of agency for cleaning.

Chart/Report.   Record as in Procedure 15, Chapter 31. Record the site selected according to established system (e.g., in the nurses' notes and on the back of the medication card) for site rotation on a 24-hour basis.

METHODS AND ANATOMICAL SITES FOR ADMINISTRATION

Intramuscular and Z-track Injections

Intramuscular injections are a common nursing therapy. The nurse has several major responsibilities when administering an intramuscular injection. She must (a) be knowledgeable, as with all medications, about the expected results as well as possible side effects of the medication, (b) use aseptic technique when preparing and administering parenteral medications, (c) be knowledgeable concerning the anatomical sites available and the indications for use of each and (d) be confident and masterful in the art of injection. The nurse must recognize that receiving injections—shots—is not a common, everyday experience for most patients, even though giving injections is commonplace for the nurse. Great apprehen-

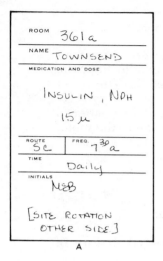

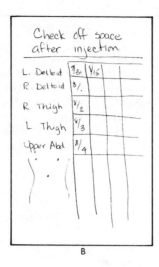

Figure 38–13. Simple tally sheet for site rotation on back of medication card. *A,* Front of medication card. *B,* Example of how the nurse can use the back of card to recall previous site use.

sion can surround injections. IM injection represents an important part of a patient's therapy; it requires a serious approach.

Several sites are available to the nurse for IM injections: the ventrogluteal site, the vastus lateralis site, the dorsogluteal site and the deltoid. Before proceeding with any injection certain factors must be assessed: (a) condition of the tissue, (b) suitability of the site and (c) the patient's state of mind. In assessing the tissue, the nurse should observe whether the skin is intact, free of abrasions, lesions, excoriations, bruises and exudates and/or wound drainage. The subcutaneous fat should be free of nodules (lumps), which may indicate prior parenteral therapy with subsequently poor absorption from the tissue. Ideally, the muscle itself would be free of discomfort from previous IM therapy; if sites have been rotated, this may be the case. The site should be of adequate size for the proposed therapy, or another site should be selected, e.g., it would be inappropriate to inject as much as 5 ml. of fluid into as small a muscle as the deltoid. The quadriceps muscle is more appropriate for large injections. The

patient should be aware of the therapy and participate in it, to the best of his ability. Assessing the patient for undue anxiety should be a standard nursing responsibility. The nurse should approach each patient with the intent to maintain his dignity and privacy; an anxious patient should be given consideration that alleviates his anxiety. One way to alleviate or dispel anxiety is through a skillful and competent manner.

For any intramuscular injection, good lighting is important, as are confidence and manual dexterity. However, the nurse's responsibility does not end as she walks away from the bedside. She must record the injection in the medication administration sheet, and she should establish and communicate a site rotation system, particularly for those patients receiving long-term parenteral therapy. A simple tally on the back of the medication card will suffice; Figure 38–13 demonstrates that elaborate systems are not necessary. To ask the patient to remember the location of his last injection is unwarranted; an individual who is sick cannot be expected to do this—it is the nurse's responsibility.

25.   INTRAMUSCULAR INJECTION INCLUDING AIR LOCK TECHNIQUE

Definition and Purposes.   *Injecting a parenteral medication into the muscle, and using a seal of air.* The technique is used to deposit medication into muscle, where it is absorbed into the blood stream (medications vary in speed of absorption). Some medications that are irritating to subcutaneous tissue may be given into the muscle. Manufacturer states if intramuscular route may be used. Absorption is quicker than subcutaneous route.

Contraindications and Cautions.   Because the nurse is introducing foreign bodies (the needle and medication) into the body tissue, it is essential that strict aseptic technique be employed. Anything but strict aseptic technique may cause infection of the tissue. IM injections of medication eventually lead to nodular and indurated areas, so site rotation is important. Improper technique in drawing up, administering or following through with assessment can lead to further tissue problems. Do not inject medications into scar tissue, because the tissue has a diminished capacity for absorption.

Patient-Family Teaching Points.   Provide the patient and family with the following information as appropriate: (a) explain why the therapeutic results and the safety of the patient must be considered before his modesty or convenience; (b) explain that for this reason the site must be clearly exposed and the muscle selected must be large enough to accommodate the medication; (c) discuss with patient and family the necessity for the route (absorption, blood levels, inactivation by GI tract or rapid effect); (d) discuss need to rotate sites to avoid damage due to repeated injections and (e) explain that a relaxed muscle tissue allows the medication to be deposited easier, producing a less painful injection. Encourage parents of infants to cuddle, rock or speak softly to their baby after the injection. Older children need explanations to the extent that they can comprehend.

PRE-PROCEDURE ACTIVITIES

PRELIMINARY PATIENT ASSESSMENT

Includes determination of:
▶ diagnosis
▶ physician's order for IM injection
▶ amount of medication needed to fill order
▶ muscle mass
▶ quality of muscle (firm, flabby)
▶ neurological/sensory status
▶ level of patient cooperation
▶ previous sites of IM injections that are damaged
▶ areas of poor circulation due to edema or vascular problems
▶ body build, e.g., obese

PREPARATION OF THE PATIENT

▶ Discuss procedure with patient; determine previous experience with IM's
▶ Provide privacy
▶ Position patient for optimum site identification
▶ Identify anatomic landmarks individual on each patient
▶ Cleanse skin thoroughly
▶ Discuss alternate sites

Procedure continued on the following page

PRELIMINARY PLANNING	EQUIPMENT
▶ Determine correct syringe, needle gauge, needle length	▶ Medication
▶ Determine need for assistance if patient uncooperative or infant or child	▶ Medication card
▶ Knowledge of expected medication action	▶ Needle: 18, 20, 21 gauge; 1½ inch 20 gauge; 1 inch
▶ Needle of adequate length	▶ Syringe
	▶ Alcohol pledget
	▶ Restraining device, if necessary
	▶ Bed or stretcher to accommodate prone patient
	▶ Waste disposal containers

PROCEDURE

SUGGESTED STEPS	RATIONALE/DISCUSSION

General Considerations

1. Prepare medication as in Procedure 24.	
2. Identify patient.	2. Essential to prevent errors.
3. Provide privacy, locate sites anatomically, use good light for vision.	3. Patients must be provided with privacy to relax; nurse must have good light to locate anatomical landmarks properly.
4. Check medication dosage against medication card.	4. Safety check.

Air Lock Technique

1. Provide an air lock if medication is irritating to subcutaneous tissues.[47]	1. An air lock (or measured block of 0.2 to 0.3 ml. of air) is essential when administering an IM injection that is irritating to subcutaneous tissue.

> *Highly irritating medications can cause necrosis of subcutaneous tissues.*

The air lock: (a) clears needle of medication, thus preventing tracting of medication through subcutaneous tissues as needle is withdrawn from the muscle and (b) "locks" medication into the muscle site, where it is eventually absorbed. Thereby the air lock prevents leakage of the irritating medication from the muscle into subcutaneous tissues.

2. Draw up 0.5 to 1 ml. of air into syringe. With needle pointed toward ceiling, carefully check amount of medication in syringe and compare with medication card. Push out all of the air	2. Because the air lock is used when administering irritating and potentially toxic drugs, it is mandatory to measure dosage with strict accuracy. Drawing up 0.5 to 1 ml. of air before

SUGGESTED STEPS	RATIONALE/DISCUSSION

Air Lock Technique (Continued)

except for the 0.2 to 0.3 ml. of air required for the air lock. If dosage is inaccurate, draw up more medication or expel the excess medication before preparing air lock.	measuring air lock clears the needle and its hub of excess medication that could make dosage excessive and inaccurate.
3. Inject medication at 90-degree angle to the floor. Position patient either in: (a) the prone position using the dorsal gluteal site or in (b) the sidelying position using either the mid-deltoid or the ventrogluteal sites.	3. The syringe must be held perpendicular to floor if: (a) the bubble of air is to rise to the top of the medication and (b) upon injection, the bubble is to *follow* the medication into the muscle to form the air lock. When a 90-degree angle is not used, air (which is now along the side of the syringe) enters the muscle too soon. As a result, an air lock does not form and medication may leak into subcutaneous tissues.

Position and Site Selection

After locating the appropriate site, the injection procedure is essentially the same for each site. Remember to add air lock if medication is irritating to subcutaneous tissues.

1. Mid-deltoid site.

a. *Position.* Have patient place arm at side, flex elbow to relax muscle. Completely expose muscle.	a. Do not try to give injection with patient's shirt sleeve only rolled up; this does not allow complete visualization. If air lock technique is used with this site, patient must lie on his side (so needle is perpendicular to floor).
b. *Site Selection.* (1) Locate lower edge of acromion process. (2) Form a rectangle (Fig. 38–14).	b. Mid-deltoid site is often chosen for its ease of access. Can be used with patient sitting, standing or lying.
For child, locate densest muscle mass by grasping between fingers.	This site is very limited in children due to shallowness of the muscle. Muscle can accommodate only a very small amount of medication.
c. *Injection*	
(1) *Adults.* Spread tissue between thumb and forefinger (index finger). Inject needle at 90-degree angle to tissue.	(1) Makes tissue taut.
(2) *Children.* (Also for infants and thin adults.) Grasp muscle mass at injection site, compress between thumb and forefinger. Inject needle pointing slightly upward toward shoulder.	(2) Angle of injection ensures deposit of medication in densest portion.

Procedure continued on the following page

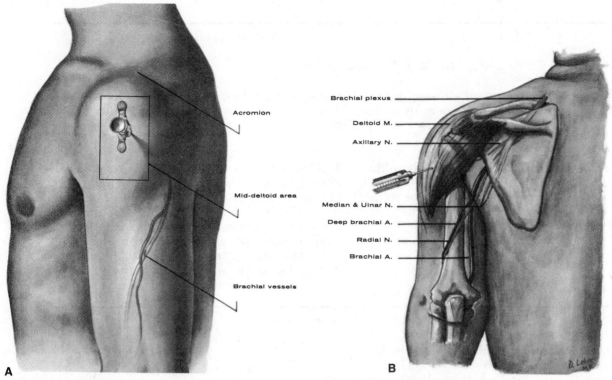

Figure 38–14. Mid-deltoid injection site for adult *(A)* and for a child *(B)*. Refer to procedure for specifics of site location. (From Wyeth Laboratories, Philadelphia.)

SUGGESTED STEPS	RATIONALE/DISCUSSION

Position and Site Selection (Continued)

2. Dorsal gluteal site (gluteus medius muscle)

    a. *Position.* Have the patient lie face down, with toes together and heels everted.

    b. *Site Selection.* Identify greater trochanter of the femur and posterior superior iliac spine. Draw an imaginary line between these two bony landmarks. Site will be the upper outer quadrant of the buttock (Fig. 38–15).

    c. *Injection.* Spread tissue between thumb and forefinger to make skin taut. Needle is inserted perpendicular to (at a 90-degree angle to) the surface on which the patient is lying.

2. Site also called posterior gluteal.

    a. This position allows maximum relaxation of muscles. Avoid side lying or standing position for maximum patient safety, i.e., so you are able to identify anatomical landmarks in order to avoid major nerves and blood vessels. Safety should override modesty.

    b. One of the most commonly used sites for IM injections. Used with extreme caution for small children. When child is walking and has developed good musculature, site is acceptable.

> *Gluteal area is not synonymous with buttock.*

    c. Careful site selection will prevent inadvertent sciatic nerve damage.

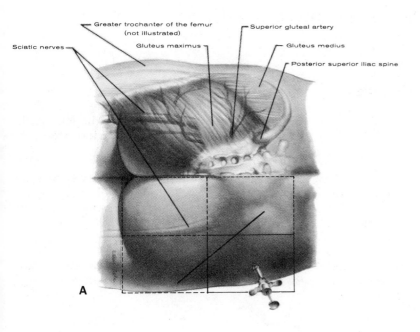

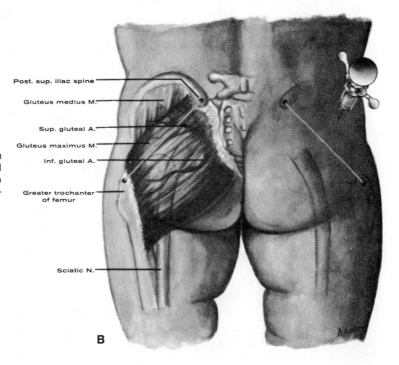

Figure 38–15.   *A,* Anatomic landmarks to be used in gluteus medius injections for adults. *B,* Site for child who has been walking long enough to develop adequate musculature. Refer to procedure for a discussion. (From Wyeth Laboratories. Philadelphia.)

Procedure continued on the following page

SUGGESTED STEPS	RATIONALE/DISCUSSION

Position and Site Selection (Continued)

3. Ventrogluteal site (gluteus medius and minimus muscles)

    a. *Position.* Locate patient on his side with upper knee flexed.

    a. This is a very versatile injection site, and patient can be lying on his side or standing. In order to adequately locate the landmarks for site, patient must be adequately exposed.

    b. *Site Selection.* Place palm on greater trochanter, make a "V" with middle and first fingers on anterior superior iliac spine and iliac crest. Switch finger position for right or left side (Fig. 38–16).

    b. Site is excellent—major nerves, arteries and veins are avoided; muscle very dense. Anatomical landmarks are easily found; site very versatile.

    c. *Injection.* In center of "V" space formed, inject with needle at 75- to 80-degree angle, slightly upward towards head, after spreading tissue between thumb and forefinger.

    c. Angle of injection deposits medication in deepest part of available muscle.

4. Vastus lateralis site

4. Also called lateral femoral site

    a. *Position.* Have adult or child lie on back with knees slightly bent (Fig. 38–17).

    a. Back-lying position preferred. Patient may be sitting, but it is nurse's responsibility to have entire area exposed for anatomical identification.

    b. *Site Selection.* (1) *Adult.* On area between mid-anterior thigh and mid-lateral thigh, measure hand's breadth below greater trochanter at proximal end, hand's breadth above knee at distal end. (2) *Children.* Identify anterior surface of mid-lateral thigh.

    b. Site is relatively free from major nerves and blood vessels.

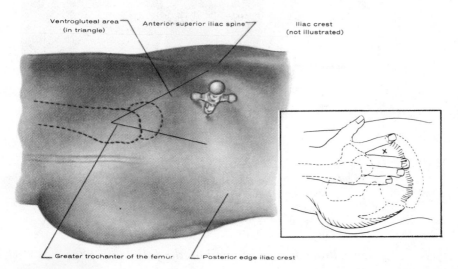

Ventrogluteal area (in triangle)   Anterior superior iliac spine   Iliac crest (not illustrated)

Greater trochanter of the femur   Posterior edge iliac crest

Figure 38–16. Ventrogluteal area in detail. Refer to procedure for specifics. (From Wyeth Laboratories, Philadelphia.)

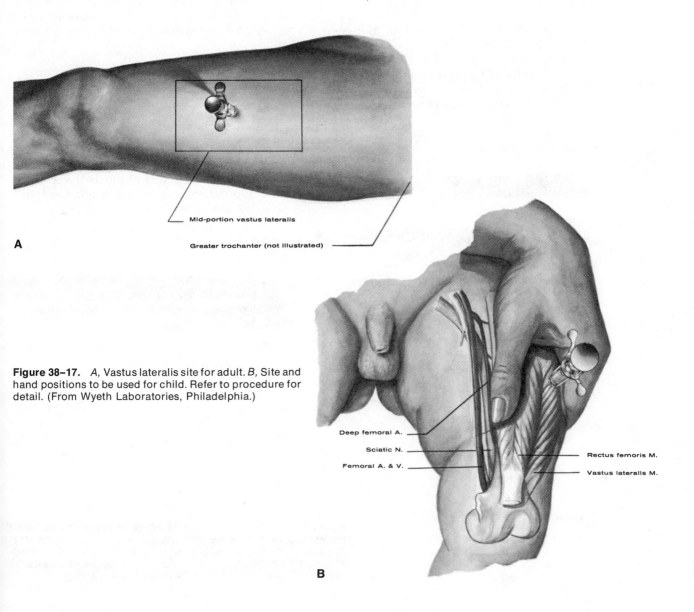

A

Mid-portion vastus lateralis

Greater trochanter (not illustrated)

Figure 38–17.   *A,* Vastus lateralis site for adult. *B,* Site and hand positions to be used for child. Refer to procedure for detail. (From Wyeth Laboratories, Philadelphia.)

Deep femoral A.

Sciatic N.

Femoral A. & V.

Rectus femoris M.

Vastus lateralis M.

B

Procedure continued on the following page

SUGGESTED STEPS	RATIONALE/DISCUSSION

Position and Site Selection (Continued)

c. *Injection*

    (1) *Adult.* Spread tissue taut between thumb and forefinger. Inject needle at 90-degree angle or slightly anteriorly.
(2) *Children.* Compress muscle and/or lift away from femur in infants (to avoid hitting bone). Needle enters tissue at 90-degree angle.

c. Angle of injection will (a) allow medication to be deposited into deep muscle tissue and (b) avoid striking the underlying bone.

5. Z-track Technique

    a. *Position.* Have patient lie prone with toes everted (pointed inward).

a. *Position.* This technique is a variant of the gluteal, or upper outer quadrant; the patient assumes the same position.

    b. *Site Selection.* See ventrogluteal site for anatomical landmarks.

    c. *Prepare air lock*

c. Air lock always necessary when using Z-track technique owing to irritating nature of the medications given by Z-track technique.

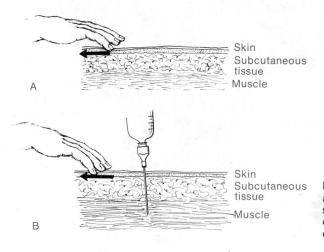

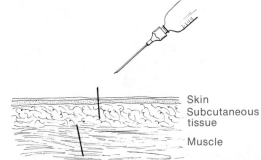

Figure 38–18.   Z-track technique. *A* shows retraction of tissue laterally prior to and during injection. *B* shows needle entry and track. *C* shows needle removed, tissue returned to normal position and track of needle. Note that the track is no longer contiguous, so medication cannot leak out, nor can it cause visible tissue staining.

SUGGESTED STEPS	RATIONALE/DISCUSSION

Position and Site Selection (Continued)

d. *Injection*

(1) Retract tissue laterally (to the side) and downward and hold there throughout time needle is in tissue.

(2) While the tissue is retracted, insert at least a 2-inch needle at an 80- to 90-degree angle to the surface. Aspirate to be sure needle is not in blood vessel. Inject medication slowly; wait 5 to 10 seconds; pull needle straight out.

(3) Release skin and *do not* massage site.

d. This procedure is used to prevent tissue staining with a drug such as Imferon. Staining is prevented by obliterating a straight needle track by which medication could leak out.

(2) The resultant needle track forms a "Z" shape (Fig. 38–18).

(3) Massaging site may spread medication into tissue, causing a stain.

Injection Technique

1. Palpate area for scarring, tenderness, nodules or pain.

1. Patients who receive multiple IM injections into same site may develop all these symptoms. Also, medication deposited into site is poorly absorbed, limiting therapy. Consider other sites if any of these signs found.

2. Check dosage in syringe against medication card. Add 0.2 to 0.3 ml. air if indicated.

2. Last-minute checking prevents errors. Air lock prevents tissue damage from irritating medications.

3. Cleanse skin thoroughly. Let dry. Hold used pledget in dominant hand between fourth and fifth fingers.

3. Cleanse area with an alcohol pledget, using surgical aseptic technique. By working circularly from central to peripheral zone, a clean skin is assured. Skin cannot be rendered *sterile* by this procedure, only clean.

4. Make skin taut by stretching skin between forefinger and thumb.

4. Retain pledget to apply pressure after injection. Taut skin is easier to enter than loose skin.

5. Prepare patient for insertion of needle by diversion.

5. Tell patient he will feel a prick; have him blow a breath out, whistle, look at a spot against surrounding wall; or ask patient a question that will distract his attention.

6. Dart needle quickly into tissue at an angle correct for site.

6. Quick insertion reduces "drag" of needle through tissue and subsequent stimulation of pressure receptors.

7. Release pressure on tissue.

8. Aspirate for blood before injecting. If blood is aspirated into syringe, withdraw needle, remove it from syringe, and destroy it. Replace with sterile needle and repeat steps 4 to 7. If no blood is aspirated continue with steps 9 to 15.

Failure to aspirate for blood before injecting could result in intravascular administration of medication, which could provide patient with unnecessary or undesired therapy.

Procedure continued on the following page

SUGGESTED STEPS	RATIONALE/DISCUSSION

Injection Technique (Continued)

9. Inject medication slowly.	9. Rapid injections cause immediate tissue distention, creating discomfort from pressure.
10. Place alcohol pledget at injection site and remove needle in same direction as injection.	10. Cover wound. Removing needle at same angle prevents tearing of tissue by sharp needle bevel.
11. Apply pressure over site momentarily; if bleeding occurs pressure is maintained for 1 to 2 minutes.	11. Prevents staining of clothes. If bleeding persists, a Band-Aid is necessary.
12. Assist patient to original state; help to dress or position comfortably in bed.	
13. Chart site selection.	13. To plan for rotation of next injection.
14. Record medication administration.	14. Prompt recording prevents another nurse from administering same medication.
15. Dispose of equipment properly.	15. Prevents drug abuse, cross-contamination, and injury to other workers by needles.

Post-Procedure Activities. Assess patient for comfort to see if medication is providing desired effect. Assess area of injection.

Aftercare of Equipment. As in all situations utilizing needles, be sure they are safely discarded.

Chart/Report. Follow Procedure 15, Chapter 31. Also chart/report site used. Keep record of site used on reverse of medication card, or in nurses' notes.

Ventrogluteal Site. The ventrogluteal site is unparalleled in being far removed from major arteries, veins and nerves; it is suitable for both adults and children. The ventrogluteal site is accessible with the patient lying on his back, his side, or his abdomen and even when he is standing. Because of the above, it is probably the most versatile of all deep IM sites available to the nurse. As with any site, the ventrogluteal site must be approached carefully in a combative patient. In a patient who is quadriplegic or paraplegic, the tissue absorption will be slower because of inactivity of the muscle fibers, although any discomfort during the injection procedure is lacking. Caution must be advised also in providing adequate visualization while still providing privacy.

The site is located by locating the greater trochanter, the anterior superior iliac spine and the iliac crest. The palm of the hand is placed over the greater trochanter, with the index and middle fingers spread on the anterior superior iliac spine and iliac crest. A "V" will be formed between the index and middle fingers. The injection is given between the fingers forming the "V." The direction of the needle is slightly cephalad (toward the head), as the deepest portion of the muscle will be found here. In adults, volumes up to 5 ml. may be injected in the site.

Vastus Lateralis Site. The area between the

mid-anterior thigh (on the front of the leg) and the mid-lateral thigh (on the side of the leg) is another site usually recommended because of its safety. Like the ventrogluteal site, the vastus lateralis site is relatively free of blood vessels and nerves in adults as well as in children. The patient can safely assume one of two positions: sitting or lying on his back. The supine position is preferred. In this position, the patient can relax more completely, and if he is anxious, the actual injection can be blocked from his sight. For convenience, this site may be used with a sitting person, once careful site selection is made.

Be cautious when using this site if muscle wasting (atrophy) has occurred. Atrophied muscles (as would be found in patients on prolonged bed rest) do not absorb or transport medication as rapidly; neither is there sufficient muscle mass to accommodate a volume of medication without leaking to the skin surface.

Anatomically, the vastus lateralis site is located in the *adult* by defining an area a hand's breadth above the knee, a hand's breadth below the greater trochanter, and between the mid-anterior and mid-lateral thigh. The needle enters perpendicularly to the skin. For a *child*, grasping the quadriceps femoris muscle group and compressing the muscle laterally will provide an area free of major blood vessels and nerves. A thrashing, struggling pediatric patient can be restrained by holding the restraining arm across the child's pelvis and using the restraining arm hand to locate and grasp the muscle prior to injection.

Gluteal Site. The gluteal site (the gluteus medius) is probably the best known site for IM injections. Lay people consider this site to be the standard site. This area continues to be the "butt" of comic strip and cartoon comedy satire. Anatomically, gluteal injections, if improperly located, can be the source of many patient complaints due to blood vessel and nerve damage. The general prohibition for children less than 2 years old is because of their incompletely developed muscles. When they have been walking for several years, their muscles are better developed and will accommodate IM injections more freely. It is probably better to avoid administering injections into the gluteal site until the child is at least five or six years old.

> *The use of the gluteal site in children under two or in patients who have underdeveloped buttocks from innervation defects or undernourishment is prohibited.*

The nurse must locate appropriate boundaries to avoid the sciatic nerve and the superior gluteal artery (see Procedure 25). To do this, a line of demarcation needs to be established using a diagonal line between the greater trochanter and the posterior superior iliac spine. Other techniques have the nurse "box" off the site by using the buttocks, lateral hip, gluteal fold and posterior spine as boundaries and injecting into the upper outer quadrant of this box. Any technique which aids the nurse in locating a safe site can be employed.

The position of the patient for this site is important. The most recommended position is lying prone with toes "in" (big toes together). Any other position lacks these advantages: (a) best possible relaxation, (b) anatomical landmarks can be clearly discerned and (c) maintenance of maximum modesty. Under no circumstance should the gluteal site be used for a patient who is standing or has only the waist of his pants pulled partially down. The nurse is unable to safely and correctly locate the critical anatomical landmarks. Safe nursing practice is therefore jeopardized.

The volume of fluid given into this site can be up to 5 ml. per injection in an adult if the tissue is in optimum condition. If the tissue is in less than optimum condition, the nurse may elect to administer two separate injections of the medication, or to choose another site.

A variation on an injection given into the upper outer quadrant is the Z-track technique. Used for injecting a tissue-staining iron preparation called Imferon, it is a technique that could be employed whenever medications have been noted to leak from tissue or when complete absorption is critical. Basically, the site selection is the same. The difference is in the lateral retraction of the skin, injection of medication, rapid withdrawal of the needle, and release of skin, sealing the needle tract.

The patient needs to be informed of possible tissue staining. He may assume that the dark areas over his buttocks are bruises and may become alarmed when normal fading does not occur. Alternate buttocks should be used for subsequent injections.

Deltoid Site. The deltoid site has several advantages: (a) accessibility, (b) maintenance of modesty and (c) convenience. The disadvantages are (a) only a small volume (up to 1 ml.) can be accommodated in an adult, (b) the muscle mass is small and (c) the brachial and axillary nerves and blood vessels are close to the site and must be avoided. The safe area is defined as a rectangle bounded by two finger breadths below the acromion process, a line drawn from the axilla (arm pit) and the middle third of the arm. This site should be used with caution on children; a child's muscle is shallow, and only a small volume of fluid can be accommodated.

The technique of injection is to grasp the deltoid muscle, isolating and stabilizing it for the injection. The angle of the needle should be slightly towards the shoulder to maximize the potential for putting the medication in the deepest part of the muscle. In adults, as well as children, this muscle offers limited long term use.

Subcutaneous (Hypodermic) Injections

As with intramuscular injections, the nurse is obliged to assess the condition and quality of the tissue to be used for subcutaneous injections. An area free of inflammation, excoriation, itching, exudate, tenderness, pain, edema, and scar tissue should be chosen. Anatomically, the subcutaneous tissue is below (sub) the skin (cutaneous). Characteristically, subcutaneous tissue is loose areolar tissue lying above the muscle. This tissue is relatively free of pain receptors, and so the only "pain" a patient experiences may occur as the needle pierces the skin.

Subcutaneous tissue is found all over the body, but traditionally the following four sites are used for SQ injections: (a) anterior thigh, (b) abdomen, from below nipples to iliac crests, (c) outer aspect of upper arm and (d) flank. Any site is acceptable if it meets the following criteria: (a) skin and underlying tissue free of abnormalities, (b) not over bony prominences and (c) free of large blood vessels or nerves. Avoiding the midline of the body because of the increased number of nerve endings is suggested by Burke.[6]

As with IM injections, subcutaneous injections should be rotated. For a person on chronic therapy, e.g., a diabetic taking insulin, it is essential that the nurse educate the patient to start and carry through a plan for rotation of sites. Only in this way can the diabetic person assure himself of the maximum absorption by minimizing local tissue inflammatory response. If the nurse is not attentive to this critical point, the patient may assume her lax attitude. In the hospital, the nurse may give the diabetic his insulin injections in sites which are difficult for him to reach, thereby saving the sites he normally uses for "at home" use.

Much controversy exists among nurses about the length of needle and angle of injection appropriate to SC therapy. For each nurse, a method of identifying and locating subcutaneous tissue is essential.

Burke[6] suggests that the controversy and questions over the *angle* and *needle length* for the SQ injection can be answered by the use of a technique which (a) deposits the medication in a fold formed by picking up a layer of skin and fat, (b) uses a needle long enough to go through the fat and (c) inserts the needle at a 20- to 45-degree angle, usually at the base of the fold, almost parallel to the skin (Fig. 38–19).

Again, as with any injection, good lighting is essential for (a) locating the appropriate site, (b) checking the medication dosage on syringe calibrations and (c) observing the patient's reaction. For chronic long-term therapy, a rotating site chart is essential. Figure 38–20 is a suggested chart for abdominal sites; the same kind of charting can be done for the other subcutaneous sites.

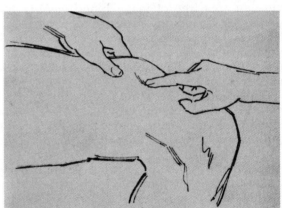
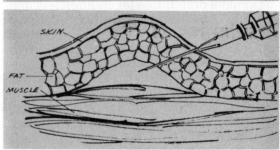

Figure 38–19. Forming a pocket by picking up tissue (skin and fat) and using needle length that will deposit medication in that area. (From Burke, E. L.: Insulin injection: the site and technique. *American Journal of Nursing,* 72:2194–2196, Dec. 1972.)

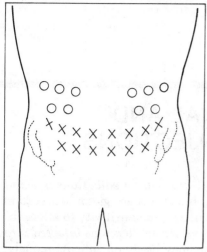

X–Preferred sites

O–May be used if necessary

Figure 38–20.   Chart used to record abdominal sites used for long-term subcutaneous therapy. Rotating-site charts like this can be prepared for all areas used for parenteral therapy. (Courtesy Wyeth Laboratories, Philadelphia.)

Intradermal Injections

Intradermal injections require the same assessment of the condition of the skin and surrounding tissue that IM and SQ injections do. Particular attention needs to be given to (a) the condition of the skin, (b) avoiding any area of previous irritation, discoloration or swelling and (c) avoiding areas where clothing might irritate the skin, because such factors may alter the local tissue reaction.

Anatomically, the injection of a small volume (0.1 to 1.0 ml. fluid) is to be placed in the dermis (Fig. 38–21), between the layers of skin. This route has the slowest absorption rate, allowing adequate time for diagnostic tests such as al-

lergy and tuberculin tests to be completed. If the body has antibodies to a particular allergen (e.g., pollen), the normal response is a histamine-type one, causing redness, itching, wheals, or a palpable nodule beneath the skin. The slow absorption rate is important; if an allergen was given by a more quickly absorbing route, e.g., IM, the patient's histamine response could cause a fatal anaphylactic reaction.

The site normally used for this kind of parenteral therapy is the dorsal forearm; the posterior and lateral aspects of the arm can also be used.

Reporting and recording the date, time, placement and immediate response of the patient to therapy is important. It is common to mark the site of injection with a circle of indelible ink as well as to chart in the nurse's notes the location of the injection. The *exact time* is important, particularly when assessing a person's sensitivity to an allergen. In some situations, a nurse is not allowed to administer intradermal sensitivity tests because of the high risk of anaphylaxis (shock). In all cases, the nurse should know where the emergency cart and epinephrine are located.

Any immediate respiratory rate increase, wheezing or cardiovascular symptoms (such as fast heart beat) due to the intradermal injection must be reported immediately to the physician.

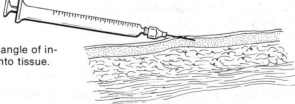

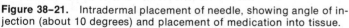

Figure 38–21.   Intradermal placement of needle, showing angle of injection (about 10 degrees) and placement of medication into tissue.

26.   INTRADERMAL AND SUBCUTANEOUS INJECTIONS

Definitions and Purposes.   *Intradermal injections are medications injected "into the skin."* Diagnostic (skin test) intradermal injections are given to ascertain the individual's exposure to diseases (e.g., tuberculosis) or sensitivity to allergens such as grass or medication. *Subcutaneous injections are medications injected into the subcutaneous tissues.* A variety of medications may be given subcutaneously; a common one is insulin. The rate of absorption of medications given by subcutaneous route is *slower* than that of medications given by intravenous or intramuscular routes, but it is *faster* than that of medications given by the oral route.

Contraindications and Cautions.   The skin used for intradermal injections should be free of disease (e.g., psoriasis or eczema), which could be exacerbated or spread by injecting a substance intradermally. Also avoid injections into: (a) hair follicles, (b) areas that have scarring or pustular eruptions and (c) sites which could be irritated by clothing. Rotate repeated subcutaneous injection sites of insulin to prevent lipodystrophy (wasting of subcutaneous fat) and excessive scar tissue. Absorption of medications is delayed with repeated injections near the same site. Do not give any injections into tissues that are tender, painful or "hot" or that appear edematous, red, or diseased. Do not give injections into scar tissue. Air lock technique is not appropriate since medication is to be purposely placed intradermally or subcutaneously.

Patient-Family Teaching Points.   Provide the patient and family with information as appropriate: (a) about allergic reactions or expected reactions resulting from intradermal injections; (b) teach aseptic technique; (c) teach how to read syringe calibrations; (d) teach method for removing medications from a vial; (e) teach location and rotation of appropriate sites; and (f) explain observations pertinent to untoward reactions as well as expected effects.

PRE-PROCEDURE ACTIVITIES

PRELIMINARY PATIENT ASSESSMENT

Includes determination of:
▶ diagnosis
▶ physician's order
▶ body build
▶ sites available
▶ condition of skin
▶ absence/presence of redness, pain, tenderness, disease

PRELIMINARY PLANNING

▶ Type and method of injection
▶ Know location of medication and nursing actions which will counteract untoward reaction

PREPARATION OF PATIENT

▶ Discuss patient's feelings about injections
▶ Discuss expected action of medication
▶ Teach self-injection skill if appropriate
▶ Appropriate site selection
▶ Selection of alternate sites

EQUIPMENT

▶ Syringes, either tuberculin, insulin, or 3 ml.
▶ Needles, usually 25, 26 or 27 gauge ½ to ⅝ inch length, according to particular procedure
▶ Medication card
▶ Medication tray

PRELIMINARY PLANNING	EQUIPMENT
▶ Determine the expected action of the medication and possible untoward side effects	▶ Alcohol or Betadine pledget, sterile dry cotton or 2 × 2 gauze

PROCEDURE

SUGGESTED STEPS	RATIONALE/DISCUSSION

Intradermal Injections

1. Select needle and syringe.

   a. Short bevel; ⅜ to ⅝ inch length; 26 to 27 gauge

     a. *Needles* used for intradermal injections are short (⅜ to ⅝ inch) with a fine gauge (26 to 27). The bevel is at a very different angle from the intramuscular needle (see Fig. 38–22).

   b. Tuberculin (Tbc) syringe

     b. The *syringes* (often called tuberculin syringes) have small volume, and are calibrated in small units, normally 0.01 ml.

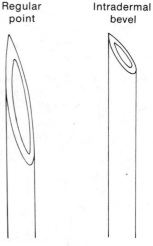

Regular point   Intradermal bevel

Figure 38–22. Note differences in needle bevel. The ID needle is designed to pierce skin to deposit medication just under skin. The regular needle is designed to pierce skin and underlying tissues. (From Becton-Dickinson, Rutherford, NJ.)

2. Draw up medication.

   2. The medication should be drawn up as in Steps 11 to 18 of Procedure 24 (removing medication from single or multiple use vials).

> *Medications given by intradermal injection may cause an anaphylactic reaction. Dosages must be absolutely correct. Do not use air lock technique.*

Procedure continued on the following page

SUGGESTED STEPS	RATIONALE/DISCUSSION

Intradermal Injections (Continued)

3. Identify patient.

4. Position patient with his arm in relaxed position, with inner aspect of arm exposed and elbow flexed. Nurse sits comfortably in front of patient. Grasp middle of patient's forearm from under the forearm, pulling anterior skin taut with your thumb and fingers.

3. See Procedure 15, Chap. 31.

4. Intradermal injections are normally given in the forearm; however, skin testing for allergies can be done on the posterior chest, as well as on the lateral and posterior sides of the arm (Fig. 38–23).

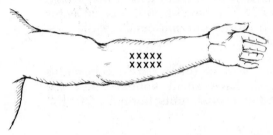

A   Forearm (left inner aspect)

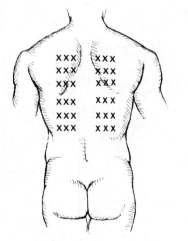

B   Posterior chest

Figure 38–23. Sites used for ID injections. Commonly used are *(A)* forearm, *(B)* posterior chest and *(C)* lateral and posterior sides of arm.

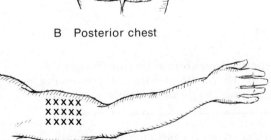

C   Lateral and posterior sides of arm

SUGGESTED STEPS	RATIONALE/DISCUSSION

Intradermal Injections (Continued)

5. Cleanse site with alcohol pledget and allow to air dry.	5. Avoids trailing of alcohol, which may produce false reaction.
6. Check dosage.	
7. With the bevel of needle facing up, insert needle at an angle that allows needle to enter between the layers of the skin (about 10 to 15 degrees to the skin).	7. The nurse should strive to have only the bevel in the skin; the bevel should be practically visible through the skin.
8. Inject medication slowly.	8. A small bleb or raised bubble should appear.
9. Observe patient carefully for drug reaction.	

> *It is very important to observe patient for untoward or unusual reactions. Some patients may need immediate attention. Know how to use and be aware of location of the epinephrine—an emergency drug.*

10. Withdraw needle and cover site with dry cotton or gauze if there is pinpoint bleeding.	
11. Observe injection site for appearance of a *wheal*. Mark the skin around wheal with an indelible pen.	11. When the medication is injected, a wheal (a small circular bump which appears whitened) should be produced.
12. Chart which arm or site was used to inject medication. Give exact time, and note when reaction is to be read.	12. Explain to patient need to chart medication administered.

Subcutaneous Injections

1. Select needle and syringe.

   a. Short bevel; ½ or ⅝ inch length; 25 gauge

   b. Amount of solution to be given determines size of syringe barrel, whether 2, 2.5, or 3 ml.

2. Draw medication up as in Procedure 24.

3. Identify patient.

Procedure continued on the following page

SUGGESTED STEPS	RATIONALE/DISCUSSION

Subcutaneous Injections (Continued)

4. Select injection site.	4. Site selection is based on accessibility, condition of skin and underlying tissue, looseness of fatty tissue, and knowledge of areas with fewest pain receptors. Site rotation must be practiced in long-term therapy for maximum absorption as well as prevention of scar tissue. Avoid lipodystrophy with insulin injections.
a. Anterior and lateral thigh.	a. The area between a hand's breadth below the trochanter and above the knee.
b. Abdomen (avoid 1 inch area around umbilicus and tissue over bone)	b. Anterior surface between waist and anterior superior spine
	Avoid umbilical area, as midline of body seems to be more painful due to increased number of nerve endings.
c. Anterior chest	c. Area over lower ribs.
d. Posterior chest	d. Area over scapulae and lower ribs cannot be used for self-injection, but is satisfactory for nurse to use or for patients who have help at home.
e. Buttocks (if patient is not incontinent), back or any other area where subcutaneous tissue can be lifted from muscle fascia.	e. Avoid buttocks if patient is grossly obese, or if incontinence is a problem.
f. Lateral aspect of upper arm (middle one third)	f. Use dorsal surface.
	If you are having trouble locating the area, have the patient momentarily tense the underlying muscle.
5. Position patient according to site selected.	5. Be sure that entire site is exposed and that underlying muscle is relaxed.
6. Check dosage against medication card.	
7. Cleanse area.	
8. Inject medication safely into appropriate area; follow these steps:	8. Injection must be given in area between muscle and fat.
a. Compress and lift subcutaneous tissue from muscle.	a. Avoid injecting into muscle tissue.

SUGGESTED STEPS	RATIONALE/DISCUSSION
Subcutaneous Injections (Continued)	
b. Insert needle at an angle which will deposit medication well into subcutaneous tissue, and through taut area (60- to 90-degree angle)	b. Angle cannot be prescribed, but must be individualized to amount of subcutaneous tissue. If injection too shallow, injection will be more painful as skin pain endings are compressed.
9. Release pinched skin.	9. Prevents medication from leaking from needle tract. Also reduces pain.
10. Aspirate.	10. Prevents giving medication intravenously.
11. Inject medication into tissue slowly.	
12. Remove needle in the same direction as inserted, apply pressure to limit bleeding.	12. Reduces ecchymosis.

Post-Procedure Activities. Assess patient for any immediate or untoward reaction. Return patient to position of comfort, replace covers or clothes. Assess area of injection.

Aftercare of Equipment. Discard disposables according to hospital safety policy. Reusable glass insulin syringes require special care, e.g., washing, rinsing, and sterilizing by boiling or autoclave.

Final Patient Assessment. Observe patient for reaction to intradermal injection at appropriate times and measure reaction. Observe patient for reaction to medication at appropriate time. *Chart/Report:* Chart and report as for any medication, including site administered. Particularly for intradermal site, it is important to note exact location of injection in chart and to chart reaction.

Venipuncture

In comparison with other techniques we have discussed, venipuncture provides the most rapid absorption of a medication. Any vein that is easily located and accessible through the skin is suitable for medication administration.

GENERAL PRINCIPLES

Any time a needle enters the skin, the body's first line of defense is broken, providing free and potentially unlimited access by opportunistic pathogens to the blood. As you recall from your microbiology class, the blood is an excellent culture medium for bacteria and fungi. Therefore, strict *aseptic technique* is essential in any aspect of intravenous medication administration. Whenever venipuncture is contemplated, attention should be given to thorough handwashing, maintaining strict aseptic technique in preparation and delivery of the medication, and observing the injection sites for untoward effects. Common untoward ef-

> *Because of the almost* immediate effect *to be anticipated from IV medications (recall that circulation time is approximately 20 seconds), incorrect medications or dosages can cause significant untoward or even fatal consequences.*

fects of intravenous medication administration include (a) phlebitis (inflammation of vein), (b) local infiltration of medication into tissue, (c) nodule or abscess formation and/or (d) local tissue infection and inflammation.

A second general consideration to remember is that, while this procedure is common for health care personnel, *patients do not consider this an innocuous procedure.* It is not uncommon for alert patients to be alarmed at venipuncture. Adequate explanation and preparation of the patient should precede the initiation of therapy. Try not to interrupt a patient's daily activity (e.g., bath or meal) to withdraw blood, give IV medication or start an IV infusion. Attend to a patient's discomfort first before starting another irritating procedure.

Intravenous medication therapy has the potential for great good but can also be disastrous.

Examples of significant untoward reactions are as follows: (a) overdosages of narcotics can cause respiratory arrest; (b) a patient may have an anaphylactic response to an antibiotic and enter a state of shock and (c) IV Dilantin may cause heart beat irregularities; therefore, the patient should have his heart beat monitored during therapy. Each of these problems is potentially fatal. Because of complications arising from IV administration of medications, only physicians, registered nurses and students closely supervised by their instructors should give IV medications. Many state nurse practice acts explicitly forbid anyone but registered nurses and physicians from carrying out this procedure.

> *A written physician's order is needed for any IV medication prior to its administration.*

27. VENIPUNCTURE

Definition and Purposes.   *The percutaneous (through the skin) insertion of a needle, either plastic or metal, into a vein.* Venipuncture is used to: (a) withdraw blood, (b) give direct intravenous medication, (c) start an intravenous infusion for fluid, nutrition or blood administration, (d) provide basic nutrition, as with hyperalimentation. Fluids and blood may also be administered intravenously by a cutdown technique in which a surgical incision is made, a vein is directly visualized, and a catheter is placed directly into that vein.

Intravenous medication and fluid administration provides rapid onset and predictable blood levels of medication, as well as rapid or massive replacement of fluids. Individual institutions determine policy for venipuncture performed by a professional nurse.

Contraindications and Cautions.   Patients who have had multiple venipuncture procedures may have "poor" veins that are sclerosed (hardened with scar tissue) or may have multiple bruises from previous venipunctures. Blood cannot be easily withdrawn, nor fluid or medication easily administered, when the vein is in poor condition or when patient is in shock, as his vessels would be collapsed. Surgical asepsis is mandatory in placement of the intravenous needle and in daily care of the site. Significant symptoms of *infection* are (a) pain, (b) redness and (c) swelling of the site and proximal vein. Inflammatory exudate may also be present. Significant symptoms of *infiltration* are (a) discomfort, (b) swelling, (c) whiteness around needle entry site and (d) lack of fluid flowing from the IV bottle. *Thrombosed* veins are (a) swollen, (b) tender, (c) painful and (d) "tight" when felt through the skin.

Patient-Family Teaching Points.   Every patient who is going to have a needle enter his venous system requires an explanation of the following: (a) the purpose of blood withdrawal, administration of medication or other IV therapy, (b) the need for multiple samples of blood if necessary and (c) the importance of compliance with the doctor's order, e.g., the IV infusion solution is ordered by the physician to be given at a certain rate; neither the family nor the patient should alter the established rate. If appropriate, the patient and/or family can be taught to observe and report the following deviations in therapy and request nursing assistance: (a) fluid chamber not dripping, (b) bottle or bag of fluid nearly empty, (c) blood in the IV tubing, (d) inadvertent disconnection of tubing and bottle, (e) (increasing) pain and discomfort at needle site or along vein and (f) swelling of tissue around needle insertion site.

As IV infusion therapy limits the patient's mobility, the nurse should advise the patient/family that: (a) she will attempt to start the IV in the patient's non-dominant hand; (b) his arm/leg may need to be restrained by an arm board or dressing to safeguard the IV; (c) the patient's bathing activity must be modified to keep IV site dry; (d) because IV therapy is based on principles of gravity, the solution source (bag or bottle) must always be kept higher than the patient's extremity (even when ambulating) to allow fluid to flow into the vein and (e) additional restraints may be necessary to remind patient he has an IV or to prevent removal of the IV needle.

PRE-PROCEDURE ACTIVITIES

PRELIMINARY PATIENT ASSESSMENT

Includes determination of:
▶ diagnosis and activity orders
▶ physician's order (legally necessary)
▶ purpose of venipuncture (e.g., blood sample, intravenous infusion, or medication)
▶ condition of skin, vein
▶ presence of bruises or hematomas from previous attempts or therapy
▶ handedness (R or L) of patient
▶ size of vein to accept needle
▶ kind of solution to be given in relation to needle size (e.g., blood administration requires larger gauge needle)
▶ anticipated length of time IV therapy will be required

PRELIMINARY PLANNING

▶ Anticipated length of therapy
▶ Equipment needed
▶ Previous patient experience
▶ Safety measures, such as restraints, that may be necessary

PREPARATION OF PATIENT

▶ Explain to patient purpose of venipuncture
▶ Provide quiet, uninterrupted environment
▶ Adjust working area (bed, arm board) to working height
▶ Protect bed linen from possible blood staining by use of pad under extremity
▶ Discuss nurse's role in IV monitoring
▶ Teach patient/family what they can observe for in monitoring IV fluids
▶ Explain use of restraints to remind patient that he has a needle in his vein
▶ Wash your hands

EQUIPMENT

▶ Tourniquet or sphygmomanometer
▶ Antiseptic solution (Betadine)
▶ Needle
   Steel (butterfly, standard) 14, 16, 18, 20, 21 gauge, 1 or 1½ inch
   Plastic (Angiocath, Intracath) 16, 18, 20, 21 gauge, 1½ inch, 6 and 11 inches
   Heparin lock

Procedure continued on the following page

EQUIPMENT

- ▶ Syringe with medication or vacuum tube or syringe for blood specimen
- ▶ Adhesive or paper tape to secure IV needle
- ▶ Covered arm splint/board
- ▶ Antibiotic ointment if used
- ▶ Sterile gauze pads
- ▶ Band-Aids
- ▶ IV solution—bottle or plastic bags
- ▶ Infusion set includes: tubing, connecting line, drip chamber
- ▶ IV pole
- ▶ Specimen tubes
- ▶ Labels for labeling IV solution

PROCEDURE

SUGGESTED STEPS	RATIONALE/DISCUSSION
A. Assemble equipment for *venipuncture* for giving medication or obtaining blood sample.	A. Syringe equipment depends on volume of blood to be drawn or volume of medication and/or fluid to be given. *Needle size* depends on viscosity of fluid.
1. Syringes large enough to draw sample necessary or deliver medication	
2. Needle (18 to 21 gauge). Usual is 21 gauge, 1½ inch for medications; 20 gauge for blood sample	
3. Laboratory tubes or Vacutainer set (this set includes vacuum tubes and special needle and holder.	
4. Antiseptic pledget	4. For skin cleansing.
5. Band-Aid	5. To cover puncture site until tissue "seals."
6. Sterile gauze pads	6. To apply pressure over wound to promote hemostasis.
7. Medication in syringe according to dose ordered	7. As per physician's order.
B. Assemble equipment for *intravenous infusion*.	B. Intravenous infusions are "into the vein."
1. Intravenous solution.	1. It is the physician's legal responsibility to order IV fluids.
2. Tubing, with attached drip chamber.	2. Essential to establish a line between fluid source and patient.

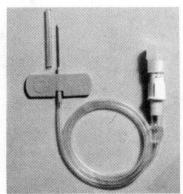

Figure 38–24. Butterfly infusion needle. (From Travenol Lab, Deerfield, Illinois.)

SUGGESTED STEPS	RATIONALE/DISCUSSION
3. Needles	3. Selection depends on purpose of therapy as well as size of vein.
a. Butterfly/scalp vein (Fig. 38–24)	a. A small steel needle that can be used for unstable veins or for difficult insertion. Also used frequently for pediatric purposes.
b. Intracath (Fig. 38–25)	b. Large bore needle that holds a plastic catheter that is threaded into vein following venipuncture. The steel outer needle is removed following venipuncture, leaving the plastic catheter used for prolonged infusion.
c. Angiocath (Fig. 38–26)	c. Plastic tubing covers steel needle. Following venipuncture, the needle is withdrawn, leaving the plastic tubing in the vein. Used for prolonged infusion.
4. Betadine or alcohol pledget	4. Used to cleanse skin prior to insertion, prevents pathogens from entering bloodstream.

Figure 38–25. Intracath infusion set. (From Deseret Pharmaceutical Co., Inc., Sandy, Utah.)

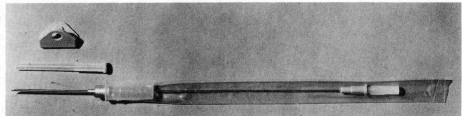

Procedure continued on the following page

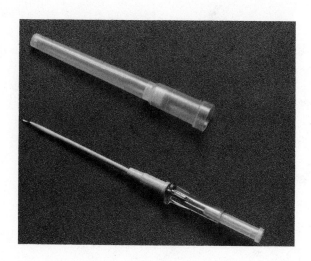

Figure 38–26. Angiocath infusion set. (From Deseret Pharmaceuticals Co., Inc., Sandy, Utah.)

SUGGESTED STEPS	RATIONALE/DISCUSSION
5. Adhesive or paper tape	5. Used to affix needle to skin.
6. Antibiotic treatment if ordered by physician	6. Thought to prevent or reduce bacterial contamination.
7. IV standard	7. Either a rolling stand or fixed to bed to hold fluid at level higher than patient.
8. Arm board and, if necessary, restraints	8. To immobilize arm so infusion site will not be disrupted.
C. Ask the patient's family and visitors to step outside room while performing venipuncture.	C. Removal of family and other distractions will aid in quick and easy insertion of needle. Also, family may become upset by procedure.
D. Select vein appropriate for therapy.	
1. Drawing blood	1. Generally, the *median vein* of the arm is commonly used, but median cubital, cephalic and basilic veins are also used. Other visible or palpable veins are suitable, but are secondary choices.
2. IV Infusion	2. If a patient is to receive long-term therapy, starting at the most distal point usually is best. Hand and forearm, then, must be given first consideration.
a. Attempt to start infusion in non-dominant arm.	a. Using nondominant arm increases patient comfort and mobility.
b. Avoid placing needle over a joint.	b. A needle inserted over a joint obstructs mobility.

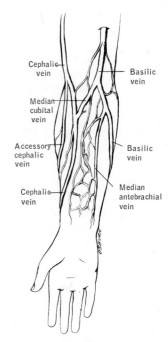

Figure 38–27. Arm veins suitable for drawing blood. (From Sutton, A. L.: *Bedside Nursing Techniques in Medicine and Surgery,* 2nd ed. Philadelphia, W. B. Saunders Co., p. 85.)

SUGGESTED STEPS	RATIONALE/DISCUSSION
E. Position the patient.	E. Position patient so that (a) vein to be used is readily accessible and (b) nurse can work in a comfortable position.

> *Never attempt to draw blood or start IV with patient standing up. If person faints, possibility of injury is greater; also vein might collapse.*

F. Locate vein for venipuncture.

1. Inspect predetermined vein area.

2. Apply tourniquet between site chosen and heart.

    2. Tourniquet must be applied with sufficient pressure to occlude venous return, without occluding arterial flow.

3. Have person clench and unclench hand, if arm is being used.

    3. Activity increases blood flow to area so that adequate visualization and sampling can occur.

4. Palpate vein even if vein can be visualized.

    4. Prevents nurse from accidentally puncturing an artery.

Procedure continued on the following page

SUGGESTED STEPS	RATIONALE/DISCUSSION
G. Venipuncture (arm as model)	
1. Re-apply tourniquet, if necessary	*If locating a vein has taken more than a brief moment, release tourniquet and reapply. Prolonged obstruction causes patient discomfort and may also alter some blood chemistry values.*
2. Scrub area with pledget.	2. Removes surface bacteria. It is not possible to totally decontaminate skin.
3. Dry with sterile gauze.	3. If alcohol enters vein, it can cause reactive vasospasm.
4. Grasp arm distally to point of entry, place left thumb about 1 inch below expected point of entry. Pull skin toward hand.	4. Vein can be "fixed" or held taut in this manner. Taut skin will also help to locate and maintain vein in position.
5. Place needle in line with vein at a 15- to 45-degree angle.	5. Needle will enter and remain in vein.
6. Insert sterile needle assembly into patient's vein.	6. Bevel of needle can be up or down according to operator's choice and preference. Reasons for each position are valid: if the bevel is *up*, it is thought more rapid entry into vein can be accomplished; if bevel is *down*, it is believed that bevel will not come in contact with upper vein wall, thereby diminishing the rate of blood withdrawal.
H. If venipuncture for blood sample, collect venous sample. If for an IV infusion, thread plastic needle into vein, connect pre-assembled IV fluid line.	H. If evacuated tubes (Vacutainer) are being used, follow these steps. With Vacutainer system, a vacuum tube is placed in an outer sleeve and disposable double-needle apparatus. After venipuncture, the tube is advanced so that the other end of the needle pierces the rubber stopper of the tube. By slight vacuum, blood is withdrawn from the vein.
I. Remove tourniquet.	I. Prolonged tourniquet placement will allow leakage from the vein into surrounding tissue, causing bruising.

Post-Venipuncture Procedures

A. Sampling blood	
1. Remove needle gently.	1. Rough removal may cause further vein damage.

SUGGESTED STEPS

RATIONALE/DISCUSSION

Post-Venipuncture Procedures (Continued)

2. Place sterile pledget over site with firm pressure for 3 min.

2. Maintain pressure to aid in hemostasis (clotting). Maintaining a straight arm maximizes pressure contact and is preferable to bending antecubital space, which bends vein and causes it to leak.

3. Once bleeding has stopped, apply Band-Aid.

3. Covers puncture site to prevent contamination.

4. Handle blood sample according to orders or agency policy.

4. Send to laboratory or keep on ward for physician.

5. Remove equipment from patient's bed or room.

6. Dispose of needles appropriately (see Procedure 24).

6. Prevent injury to staff, inadvertent contamination of sterile equipment or misuse.

B. IV infusion

1. Secure IV line in place.

1. Technique of securing cannula and tubing is dependent upon type of equipment used and the position of insertion.

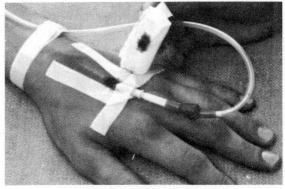

Figure 38–28.   Chevron method of securing Angiocath or any other infusion set. (From Travenol Lab, Deerfield, Illinois.)

Procedure continued on the following page

SUGGESTED STEPS	RATIONALE/DISCUSSION

Post-Venipuncture Procedures (Continued)

▶ Angiocath (Fig. 38–28)

    a. Pull out cannula approximately ½ inch and tape to skin with a chevron.

    b. Secure tubing to skin.

    c. Cover site with sterile gauze and tape down.

    d. Secure several inches of tubing.

▶ Scalp vein/butterfly

    a. Apply 2 strips of tape to "wings" of needle parallel to needle.

    a. Secures needle in difficult-to-hold places.

    b. Place tape across previous two pieces, perpendicular to wing tapes.

    b. Holds needle in place.

    c. Secure scalp vein tubing.

    d. Cover entry site with sterile gauze tape.

    d. Prevents environmental contamination.

    e. Secure IV tubing to skin.

    e. Further prevents accidental withdrawal.

▶ Intracath

▶ It is imperative to read manufacturer's instructions.

    a. Pull cannula out of the vein approximately 1 to 1½ inches and secure.

    a. Secure well to skin to prevent inadvertent displacement.

    b. Secure site of connection between tubing and hub of device.

    b. Additional security check.

    c. Tape over needle clamp.

    c. Assures clamp stays in place.

    d. Cover site with sterile gauze and tape.

    e. Secure length of tubing to allow "give" in system.

2. Use arm board if antecubital space used, or if position of needle is tenuous.

2. Arm board reduces mobility of arm, thereby preventing dislodging of needle.

SUGGESTED STEPS	RATIONALE/DISCUSSION

Post-Venipuncture Procedures (Continued)

3. Maintain fluid flow rate.

3. Fluid flow rate is to be ordered by physician and maintained by registered nurse. Must be maintained at rate ordered. If too fast, the patient's cardiovascular system may not be able to handle the additional fluid; eventually pulmonary edema may result. If too slow, the patient may experience fluid volume deficit and display the symptoms of shock.

4. Remove equipment from patient's room.

C. Care of IV site

C. The intravenous route for administering medication and fluid breaks the integrity of the skin. Because of this, the patient is at risk for iatrogenically induced problems such as: (a) nosocomial infection, local and/or systemic, (b) infiltration and (c) inflammation.

1. Review agency policy.

1. Each agency has specific guidelines for patient care; consult the procedure/policy manual. Only general guidelines can be presented here.

2. Assemble equipment.

a. Sterile 4 × 4 and 2 × 2 inch gauze pads

a. To cleanse the entry site of the needle (4 × 4) and to cover entry site for new dressing (2 × 2).

b. Betadine solution

b. Removes, by friction, microorganisms present and leaves an antiseptic film on the skin.

c. Adhesive or paper tape

c. To re-affix needle and tubing. Check for patient allergies to adhesive tape.

d. Antibiotic ointment if ordered by physician, or if included in agency policy.

d. Thought to prevent or reduce bacterial contamination.

e. Sterile drape

e. For placement of sterile supplies.

f. Waste receptacle impervious to moisture

f. For disposal of soiled dressing.

g. Sterile applicators

g. To place antibiotic on needle entry site.

Procedure continued on the following page

SUGGESTED STEPS	RATIONALE/DISCUSSION

Post-Venipuncture Procedures (Continued)

3. Change dressing

3. Agency policies usually recommend daily (every 24 hours) changes or whenever dressing is wet or soiled.

a. Nurse washes hands.

b. Bring equipment to patient; arrange for nurse's ease of reaching supplies.

c. Position patient comfortably. Nurse sits, if possible.

d. Remove tape and dressing.

d. Pull tape towards needle entry site, otherwise tension on tape may unintentionally dislodge needle.

> *Remove dressing carefully so as not to dislodge or remove needle from the vein. A patient who has few usable veins needs to be treated particularly gently.*

e. Note any discharge/drainage from needle entry site on dressing.

e. Important to detect inflammatory or infectious problems early for initiation of therapy.

f. Discard dressing and tape in waste receptacle.

f. Be careful not to contaminate hands. If so, rewash hands.

g. Inspect entry site for redness, induration, exudate. Question patient regarding discomfort or pain.

g. See step e. above.

h. Pour small amount Betadine on 4 × 4 pad. Cleanse needle entry site in circular motion, outward. Discard pad. Repeat two times, or until site is clean.

h. Always use surgical asepsis to prevent contamination of site by normal skin flora or opportunistic pathogens.

> *Never bring used pad across site after cleansing. Use pad once and discard.*

i. Squeeze about ⅛-inch of antibiotic onto sterile gauze. Discard.

i. Discarding ⅛ inch helps prevent inadvertent bacterial contamination.

j. Squeeze ¼-inch ointment on sterile gauze. Apply to needle entry site with sterile applicator.

j. Steps i and j are to be done only if ordered.

k. Apply sterile 2 × 2 gauze pad to needle entry site.

SUGGESTED STEPS	RATIONALE/DISCUSSION

Post-Venipuncture Procedures (Continued)

l. Secure IV in place. Use as appropriate.

m. On separate tape, write date, time and signature of nurse who did dressing change. Place tape over sterile dressing.

m. To indicate when, how often and who changed dressing.

n. Remove equipment from room.

o. Nurse washes hands.

p. Chart: (1) appearance of site, noting any abnormalities; (2) antibiotic used, if ordered; (3) date; (4) time and (5) signature.

Post-Procedure Activities.   Check to see that (a) all equipment used for venipuncture has been properly discarded, (b) patient is safe and comfortable and (c) the safety of the operator and other staff has been assured. Assess patient for an unwarranted reaction: fainting, lightheadedness, irritation at needle site, signs of fluid overload, allergic reactions, infiltration of fluid and dislodging of needle.

Aftercare of Equipment.   Dispose of equipment properly; label collection and IV fluids appropriately.

Chart/Report.   If blood sample drawn, indicate on appropriate form. If IV, chart site, time, solution needle used. Oncoming staff will need to be informed of the progress of the IV therapy: how much remains to be administered, and what fluids, if any, are ordered to follow the fluid currently hanging.

ASSESSMENT AND CARE OF PATIENTS RECEIVING INTRAVENOUS MEDICATIONS

Assessment of a patient receiving IV medications should focus on: (a) the purpose, response and effectiveness of the medication being given; (b) the condition of the vein(s) being used as well as the tissue surrounding the injection site and (c) the patient's physical as well as psychological responses to the therapy.

The nurse is expected to assess the *purpose, response and effectiveness* of the medication being given. Planning intervention from the assessment would be the next nursing activity; if the therapy is effective, continue the IV as ordered; if not, work with the physician to alter the therapy according to clinical and diagnostic findings.

Assessment of the vein and surrounding tissues is a second important nursing activity. Sepsis (infection) is always a problem if rigorous aseptic techniques are not maintained. It cannot be overstressed: simple, vigorous handwashing by the nurse must precede venipuncture. Inflammatory responses are characterized by hot, tense, tender areas surrounding venous entry site. This inflammation is called "phlebitis." If the inflammatory response is extended, the entire vein should be palpated for a cord-like feel, which would indicate more extensive involvement of the vein. The appropriate nursing action would be to (a) pull out any indwelling IV line, (b) apply warm packs to area, (c) notify physician and (d) *if qualified*, re-start IV infusion line.

Thrombus formation is also a common side effect of IV therapy if an irritating substance is being administered. The etiology may be a clot forming at the tip of the needle or at the point the needle enters the vein. Signs and symptoms are frequently the same as for infections. Eventual obliteration of the vein and embolism are to be avoided.

Assessment of the patient's physical and psychological response to IV therapy requires detailed knowledge of the following: (a) the patient's previous experience, (b) his awareness of the therapy, (c) his view of how the therapy will affect the course of his disease and (d) the approaches used by health care personnel in caring for and maintaining the IV line.

Care of the patient must revolve around (a) maximizing the therapeutic effect of the medication, (b) observing and acting upon the observations and (c) *preventing harm from occurring as a result of the therapy.*

While much of the material presented in this chapter is applicable to the discussion of intravenous fluid and blood administration, the reader is referred to Chapters 24 and 39 for the detailed discussion.

PATIENTS REQUIRING SPECIAL CONSIDERATION

While we discuss several patient groups who may have particular problems with parenteral therapy—children, the elderly, the emaciated, the neurologically impaired, and the diabetic—it cannot be stressed enough that individual assessment is important for every situation. While the principles of parenteral therapy are the same for all patients, anatomical differences must be evaluated to ensure safety in administration.

Children

Parenteral medication administration for children requires that the nurse have two valuable clinical skills: (a) the technical expertise to administer safe parenteral (IM, SQ, ID, IV) therapy and (b) the ability to put the principles of normal growth and development to use in this clinical setting.

Brandt's article[6] is an excellent discussion of both of these areas in relation to intramuscular injections for children. Her premise could be summarized as: the nurse must be cognizant of the predictable outcomes of inflicting pain on children (by IM injection) in relation to their social as well as biological age. It is suggested that the student read this article carefully if she is to perform IM injections in children.

Some children require restraining for their own best interest and safety during these procedures. Restraints should be judiciously used, and removed at the earliest possible time. Restraints must never interfere with adequate visualization of the injection site.

Consideration should be given to the child's and adolescent's body image. Small children can respond to needle punctures as a threat to their integrity and may require a Band-Aid to keep the "body" from flowing out the needle hole. Adolescents, who are striving for identity, may be ambivalent about injection. On one hand, they may wish to resist and cry out during the parenteral procedure, but they recognize that a "mature" person would be able to view parenteral therapy objectively.

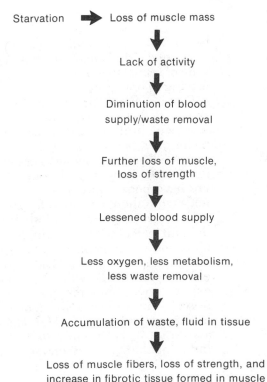

Starvation → Loss of muscle mass

↓

Lack of activity

↓

Diminution of blood
supply/waste removal

↓

Further loss of muscle,
loss of strength

↓

Lessened blood supply

↓

Less oxygen, less metabolism,
less waste removal

↓

Accumulation of waste, fluid in tissue

↓

Loss of muscle fibers, loss of strength, and
increase in fibrotic tissue formed in muscle

Figure 38–29. Disuse syndrome affecting muscle mass and medication absorption.

Of utmost importance in giving safe injections to children and young adults is the identification of sites. Knowledge of anatomical landmarks, evaluation of skin and muscle tissue for appropriateness and adequate size, and assessment of the developmental stage of the child are mandatory.

Emaciated Patients

Patients who are emaciated (thin) because of starvation—either the cause or result of illness—often provide a nursing challenge in locating a muscle mass of sufficient size to accommodate "normal" volumes of IM injections (e.g., up to 5 ml. for the gluteal site). In addition, a person who is emaciated may have several other compounding problems. Disuse atrophy often accompanies emaciation. This syndrome is diagrammed in Figure 38–29.

From Figure 38–1, one can surmise that medication, if deposited in emaciated muscle, is not as likely to be absorbed as it would in normal muscle. Inadequate therapeutic effect could be expected.

Nursing action would be to work with the physician to establish another route (e.g., IV) for medication administration if little effect can be achieved from the IM route.

Another problem frequently encountered is that of inadvertently striking the bone of the emaciated patient. The sound of metal striking bone may startle the nurse, but more serious, the patient may experience additional, unnecessary pain, as the periosteum has many nerve endings and would be irritated even further.

Elderly Patients

Elderly patients who are receiving parenteral therapy should be individually assessed for (a) general physical health, (b) muscle mass, (c) skin tone and turgor, (d) bleeding tendencies, (e) mental status, and (f) previous experience with parenteral therapy. It is not possible to generalize about nursing actions that would be applicable to all elderly persons, but remember that previous general physical health affects all aspects of parenteral therapy.

For example, an elderly man who has been used to daily walks around the block will have better muscle tone and capillary beds than the emaciated elderly man who has been living in a state of semistarvation in his walkup flat, never leaving to obtain exercise.

Disease states also affect the person's response to therapy, e.g., a person with liver disease will bruise easily regardless of skillful techniques because some liver abnormalities cause reduced production of essential elements for clotting. Patients with congestive heart failure have poor circulation and, therefore, will not absorb the medication as predicted.

Confused, combative elderly persons may be difficult to deal with; nevertheless, the nurse is obligated to maintain safe, aseptic technique and a high level of technical skill. A confused elderly person who will not cooperate is difficult to inject, and the nurse, knowing that nerve, vein and muscle damage may occur, undergoes additional mental stress. Therefore, *assistance in restraining the patient* prior to initiating therapy is essential.

Neurologically Impaired Patients

The guiding principle when the nurse is dealing with persons who have neurological defects is to recall that the neurologic system is the body's main regulator of motor (movement) and sensory apparatus. Any condition which interferes with the motor or sensory apparatus of the body has far reaching effects. For example, a person who has had a cerebral vascular accident (stroke) may have residual motor and sensory losses, with diminished motor function, muscle atrophy and all its attendant problems.

Medication deposited in muscles with decreased or absent innervation will be incompletely absorbed due to poor tissue circulation. Limbs with sensory loss may seem ideal for parenteral therapy, as the patient experiences little discomfort. While this argument seems sensible, the patient has concomitantly lost a protective mechanism and may not be able to alert a nurse to potential problems. An example would be of a dislodged needle causing local tissue trauma, the pain of which cannot be appreciated by the patient. Pain is the body's means of alerting individuals to a problem.

Without its appreciation, great damage can occur before intervention is initiated.

Blind persons are neurologically impaired. While this may seem of little concern to the nurse administering parenteral therapy, it can assume importance when the nurse is trying to teach a visually impaired person about his disease and treatment. When dealing with sighted persons, the explanation of an anticipated procedure may be clarified with visual aids, hand movements and facial expressions. This cannot occur with the blind. The nurse, then, is obliged to have the explanation of the procedure clearly formulated, without ambiguous terms. Allowing the person to handle the equipment is also appropriate. Even the most independent blind persons can be very apprehensive about hospitalization and the various therapies. Full explanations are a necessity. In dealing with a blind diabetic who must learn self-administration of insulin, the nurse's teaching skills may be challenged to the fullest. Assistance may be necessary from family and community agencies.

Para- and quadriplegic persons may have both motor and sensory losses, necessitating an evaluation of the need for giving the medication parenterally as well as the route of parenteral therapy. Again, while it may seem "kind" to give an IM into muscle below the level of the injury (and therefore muscle without innervation), absorption is unpredictable. Therefore, the patient may not receive his full therapy. Again, assessment of the route must be made.

Diabetes Mellitus Patients

The hospitalized diabetic person always presents a challenge to the nurse. Whether the patient has been newly diagnosed or has had diabetes mellitus for some time, teaching opportunities frequently occur. It can be in this role that the professional nurse can provide the client with the most personalized service.

Apprehension of *self-injection* is a common concern to most newly diagnosed patients. Frequently, other aspects of disease therapy will go unheeded or unheard until mastering of self-injection techniques has been achieved. Keeping that in mind, a nurse may choose to focus on injections first. As with any teaching situation, assessments must be made, goals and objectives written in conjunction with the learner, and evaluative methods must be designated prior to initiation of the teaching plan.

Techniques of subcutaneous injections must be taught step-by-step. See Procedure 26 for details. Written instructions are helpful in remembering each step of the procedure until sufficient practice allows internalization of the procedure. Site selection, rotational patterns and evaluation of the tissue can all be a part of the educational process of the SQ procedure.

BIBLIOGRAPHY

1. Anthony, C. P.: What makes fluids flow. *American Journal of Nursing,* 56:1256–1258, Oct. 1956.
2. Bahruh, A.: Keeping track of injection sites. *Nursing '73,* 3:51, June 1973.
3. Bergersen, B. S.: *Pharmacology in Nursing,* 13th ed. St. Louis, C. V. Mosby Co., 1976.
4. Brandt, P. A., et al.: IM injections in children. *American Journal of Nursing,* 72:1402–1406, Aug. 1972.
5. Brown, B. A.: Sciatic injection neuropathy. *California Medicine, 116:*13–15. May 1972.
6. Burke, E. L.: Insulin injection: the site and technique. *American Journal of Nursing,* 72:2194–2196, Dec. 1972.
7. Butters, A. G.: Intramuscular injections. *British Medical Journal, 11:*1362, Nov. 1961.
8. Chezem, J. L.: Consultation: aspirating before IM injections. *Nursing '74,* 4:87, Sep. 1974.
9. Chezem, J. L.: Locating the best thigh injection site. *Nursing '73,* 3:20–21, Dec. 1973.
10. Chezem, J. L.: Multiple intramuscular injection. *Nursing Research,* 22(2):130–143, March–April 1973.
11. Chojnacki, R., and Rubini, M. E.: Parenteral nutrition. *In* Maxwell, M. H., and Kleeman, C. (eds.): *Clinical Disorders of Fluid and Electrolyte Metabolism.* New York, McGraw-Hill Book Co., 1972.
12. Cohen, L., and Morgan, J.: Enzymatic and immunologic detection of myocardial injury. *Medical Clinics of North America,* 57:106, Jan. 1973.
13. Craft, F.: Aspirating before IM injections. *Nursing '74,* 87:68, Sep. 1974.
14. Creighton, H.: Nurses' adding drug to IVs. *Supervisor Nurse,* 4:62–64, March 1973.
15. Dann, T. C.: Routine skin preparation before injection—is it necessary? *Nursing Times,* 62:1121–1122, Aug. 1966.
16. Dudrick, S. J.: Rational intravenous therapy. *American Journal of Hospital Pharmacy,* 28:82–91, Feb. 1971.
17. Dugas, B.: *Introduction to Patient Care,* 3rd ed. Philadelphia, W. B. Saunders Co., 1977.
18. Evans, E. F.: Medications injected in upper arm reach blood stream fastest. *RN,* 38:ICU–12, July 1975.
19. Feld, L. G.: The nurse's liability for faulty injections. *Nursing Care,* 7:25, April 1974.
20. Galton, L.: Drugs and the elderly. *Nursing '76,* 6(8):38–43, Aug. 1976.
21. Geolot, D. H., and McKinney, N. P.: Administering parenteral drugs. *American Journal of Nursing,* 75:788–793, May 1975.
22. Grant, J. N.: Parenteral hyperalimentation. *American Journal of Nursing,* 69:2392–2395, Nov. 1969.
23. Hanson, D. J.: Intramuscular injection injuries and complications. *GP,* 27:109–115, Jan. 1963.
24. Hanson, R. L.: A Comparative Study of Heparin-Lock and Keep-Open Intravenouses for Emergency or Intermittent IV Medications: An In-Process Research Report. ANA Council of Advanced Practitioners in Medical-Surgical Nursing. Memphis, Tenn. December 17, 1974.
25. Hays, D.: Do it yourself the Z-track way. *American Journal of Nursing,* 74:1070–1071, June 1974.
26. Herbst, S. F.: A new approach to parenteral drug administration. *American Journal of Nursing,* 75(8):1345, Aug. 1975.
27. Howard-Jones, N.: A critical study of the origins and early development of hypodermic medication. *Journal of Historical Medicine,* 2:201–249, 1974.
28. How to give an intramuscular injection. *Pfizer Laboratory,* 1967. (From up-dating and revision of the original article: The importance of site selection in intramuscular injection. *Spectrum,* Dec. 1960).
29. Inniss, C. N., and Kohns, L.: Disposable syringe hazard. *American Journal of Nursing,* 68:2678, Dec. 1968.
30. Intravenous Techniques. Pfizer Laboratories, Professional Service Dept., 235 East 42nd St., NY 10017, 1967.
31. Isler, C.: The hidden dangers of IV therapy. *RN,* 36(10):23–37, Oct. 1973.
32. Kozma, M. T., and Newton, D. W.: Nursing guidelines for in-syringe mixtures. *Supervisor Nurse,* 6(8):26–33, Aug. 1975.
33. Lewis, L. W.: *Fundamental Skills in Patient Care.* Philadelphia, J. B. Lippincott Co., 1976.
34. Livingston, C.: Assisting with intravenous therapy. *Nursing Process II Syllabus.* Seattle, University of Washington School of Nursing, 1975.
35. Maki, D. G., et al.: Infection control in intravenous therapy. *Annals of Internal Medicine,* 79:867–887, 1973.
36. Martin, E. W.: *Techniques of Medication.* Philadelphia, J. B. Lippincott Co., 1969.
37. McArthur, B. J., et al.: Stopcock contamination in an ICU. *American Journal of Nursing,* Jan. 1975.
38. McDonald, D. E., et al.: Prefilling syringes in the hospital pharmacy. *American Journal of Hospital Pharmacy,* 29:223–228, March 1972.
39. Metheny, N., and Snively, W.: *Nurses' Handbook of Fluid Balance.* Philadelphia, J. B. Lippincott Co., 1967.
39a. Michael, S. L.: Home I.V. Therapy. *American Journal of Nursing,* 78:1223, July 1978.
40. Michel, F.: The vexing core. *American Journal of Nursing,* 71:768, April 1971.
41. Miller, F. F., and Keane, C. B.: *Encyclopedia and Dictionary of Medicine and Nursing,* 2nd ed. Philadelphia, W. B. Saunders Co., 1978.
42. Payne, J. E., and Kaplan, H. M.: Alternative techniques for venipuncture. *American Journal of Nursing,* April 1972.
43. Pitel, M.: The subcutaneous injection. *The Canadian Nurse,* 67:54–57, May 1971.
44. Plein, J. B., and Plein, E. M.: *Fundamentals of Medications,* 2nd ed. Hamilton, IL, Drug Intelligence Publications, 1974.
45. Rauch, P. A.: The prevention of sciatic nerve injuries. *Journal of Neurosurgical Nursing,* 3:45–50, July 1971.
46. Rodman, M. J., and Smith, D. W.: *Pharmacology and Drug Therapy in Nursing.* Philadelphia, J. B. Lippincott Co., 1968.

46a. Rowland, S. A.: A first step in treating injection injuries. *Consultant, 17:*208, Oct. 1977.

47. Saxon, J.: Administration of medications by injection. *Nursing Process II Syllabus.* Seattle, University of Washington School of Nursing, 1975.

48. Snider, M. A.: Helpful hints on IV's. *American Journal of Nursing, 74:*1978–1980, Nov. 1974.

49. Sutton, A. L.: *Bedside Nursing Techniques in Medicine and Surgery,* 2nd ed. Philadelphia, W. B. Saunders Co., 1969.

50. Ungvarski, P. J.: Parenteral therapy. *American Journal of Nursing, 76:*1974–1977, Dec. 1976.

51. Voda, A. M.: Body water dynamics: a clinical application. *American Journal of Nursing, 70:*2594–2601, Dec. 1970.

52. Wempe, B. M.: The new and the old intramuscular injection sites. *American Journal of Nursing, 61:*56–57, Sep. 1961.

53. Wilmore, D. W.: The future of intravenous therapy. *American Journal of Nursing, 71:*2334–2338, Dec. 1971.

54. Wood, L. A.: *Nursing Skills for Allied Health Services,* Vol. 3. Philadelphia, W. B. Saunders Co., 1975.

CHAPTER 39*

ADMINISTERING BLOOD

INTRODUCTION AND STUDY GUIDE

The administration of blood and blood products is one of the most challenging responsibilities of the nurse. Blood transfusions are of great value in correcting many clinical problems (e.g., blood loss, shock, severe anemia), but they must be administered to the patient with full recognition of the dangers and complications involved. In this chapter, we provide basic information concerning blood transfusion activities and blood transfusion reactions. More specifically, we discuss the following concepts:

▶ Blood functions, composition, characteristics and organs of origin

▶ Types and purposes of blood transfusions

▶ Blood group systems (ABO and Rh blood systems)

▶ Blood procurement

▶ Blood typing and crossmatching

▶ Blood administration

▶ Blood transfusion reactions and other complications

▶ The nurse's role in blood administration

The study of blood and blood administration involves many new terms and definitions. The following basic terms are defined here to help you in studying this chapter:

Donor: A person, 18 to 65 years old, with a negative medical history, capable of passing the required physical examination, who wishes to donate (have withdrawn) one unit (450 ml.) of whole blood, to be transfused to another person

Recipient: A person requiring the infusion of blood or blood components from one or more donors

Agglutination: The clumping together of red cells

Antigen (agglutinogen): A chemical substance present on the red cell membrane, which can stimulate antibody production and combine with that specific antibody, resulting in agglutination

Antibody (agglutinin): An immunoglobulin (protein) molecule having a configuration such that it will combine with a specific antigen, resulting in agglutination

Hemolysis: The destruction (lysis) of red cells by the combination of the antigen on the red cell with a specific antibody in the serum

Blood group systems (ABO, Rh): Name given to certain genes that occupy a specific locus or linked loci on a specific chromosome and that confer given antigenic properties upon the red cell

Transfusion: Administration of whole blood or blood components directly into the blood stream

Compatibility testing: A series of procedures performed by the blood bank before transfusion to ensure proper selection of blood for the recipient, including: ABO grouping, Rh typing, antibody screening on donor unit and recipient, followed by crossmatching

Blood transfusion reaction: Any unfavorable event occurring in a patient (recipient) during or following transfusion of blood or blood components

Crossmatching: Testing of recipient serum with donor cells *(major crossmatch)* and donor serum with recipient cells *(minor crossmatch)*, using several mediums and incubation temperatures

The study of this chapter will enable you to familiarize yourself with the exacting procedures underlying safe blood administration and will help you develop skill in assessing patients for signs of blood transfusion reactions and other complications.

*Helene A. Stith, R.N., B.S.N., C.R.N.A., critically reviewed and assisted with the revision of this chapter. Ms. Stith expresses her gratitude to Eloise R. Giblett, M.D., Associate Director, Puget Sound Blood Center, Seattle, Washington, and James C. Detter, M.D., Head, Divisions of Hematology and Genetics, Department of Laboratory Medicine, University of Washington, Seattle, Washington, for their assistance in manuscript preparation.

Upon completion of this chapter, you should be able to discuss the following points:

1. Indications for blood transfusion therapy
2. Five types of transfusions and the purpose of each
3. Characteristics of the ABO blood group system
4. Characteristics of the Rh blood group system
5. The selection process for blood donors
6. The information that must be written on the label of each blood donor unit; of each recipient blood sample
7. Methods for storing blood
8. The procedure as described in this chapter (and in the health care facility in which you are working) for (a) handling recipient blood samples and donor blood units and (b) administering donor blood
9. Eight modes or routes of blood transfusion
10. The hazards of transfusing blood or blood products and the safeguards employed to reduce these hazards
11. Persons who are authorized to (a) initiate blood transfusions and (b) add blood units once transfusion therapy or intravenous therapy has been initiated
12. The causes, signs, symptoms and clinical care of the following complications: (a) hemolytic transfusion reactions, (b) pyrogenic reactions, (c) allergic reactions, (d) nonhemolytic febrile reactions, (e) circulatory overload, (f) massive transfusion complications, (g) anaphylactic reactions, (h) infectious diseases and (i) air embolism

BLOOD: DEFINITION, COMPOSITION, FUNCTIONS, CHARACTERISTICS, AND FORMATION

Chapter 24 states that the total body water is divided into intracellular fluid and extracellular fluid. The extracellular fluid, in turn, is divided into *interstitial fluid* and *plasma.* Interstitial fluid occupies the tissue spaces, whereas plasma occupies the vascular space. Plasma, when mixed with blood cells, is called *blood.* Plasma makes up 55 per cent of blood; solid suspended particles (erythrocytes, leukocytes and thrombocytes), comprise the other 45 per cent of blood.

Plasma, in other words, is the liquid portion of the blood. It is a straw-colored watery substance composed of:

▶ 92 per cent water

▶ 7 per cent proteins which include: (1) serum albumin, necessary for exerting colloid osmotic pressure (see Chapter 24); (2) fibrinogen, essential for hemostasis (blood coagulation); and (3) gamma globulin, which plays a vital role in the body's defense against microorganisms

▶ Less than 1 per cent antibodies, nutrients, metabolic wastes, respiratory gases, enzymes, and inorganic salts

The major *function* of plasma is the maintenance of blood volume within the vascular compartment.

The *particles* which travel suspended in the plasma include erythrocytes (red blood cells), leukocytes (white blood cells) and thrombocytes (platelets). Erythrocytes are principally involved in oxygen transport; leukocytes, in the defense of the body against microorganisms; and thrombocytes, in hemostasis.

Blood circulates continuously through the heart and vascular system. As the blood is propelled through the body by the heart's pumping action it performs many vital functions: It transports oxygen to the cells and carries carbon dioxide from the cells to the lungs for removal from the body. The blood also carries absorbed food products from the gastrointestinal tract to the tissues; at the same time, it removes metabolic wastes from tissues and carries them to the kidney, skin and lungs for excretion. In addition, various hormones are conveyed by the blood from the endocrine glands (where they originate) to other parts of the body. Also, the blood protects the body from dangerous microorganisms by conveying leukocytes to the site of infection, injury or inflammation. Finally, the blood is instrumental in regulating body temperature by transferring heat from within the body to the small vessels supplying the skin, from which it can be released into the surrounding atmosphere.

Major characteristics of blood are as follows:

▶ *Color: Arterial* blood is bright red because of the mixture of oxygen with hemoglobin within the red blood cells. *Venous* blood is dark red because of loss of oxygen from the hemoglobin.

▶ *Viscosity:* Blood is three to four times more viscous than water.

▶ *Reaction:* Blood has a slightly salty taste and a slightly alkaline reaction of pH 7.35 to 7.40.

▶ *Volume:* An adult has approximately 70 to 75 ml. of blood per kg. of body weight; thus, the average adult body contains around 5 to 6 liters of blood.

The organs of origin of blood and its constituent cellular elements are the bone marrow, spleen, liver and lymph nodes. Cells produced by these organs include erythrocytes, leukocytes, thrombocytes, plasma cells and reticuloendothelial cells.

TYPES OF BLOOD TRANSFUSIONS AND THEIR PURPOSES

A blood transfusion is the introduction of whole blood or blood components (packed red cells, plasma, proteins and other fractions) directly into the circulation for therapeutic purposes, e.g., quickly restoring blood volume following hemorrhage, burns or injuries; combating shock; treating severe anemia. Initiating and supervising blood transfusion therapy is an enormous responsibility because blood transfusions can precipitate dangerous and sometimes lethal reactions.

As Wintrobe et al.[48] state:

Blood transfusion must be regarded as a rather dangerous and potentially lethal form of therapy and clear indications for its use must therefore exist. The physician must consciously and deliberately weigh the potential benefits against the known risks. . . . When transfusion seems indicated, the physician must also decide whether the patient needs whole blood or blood components and how much needs to be given.

Whole blood transfusions may be used to : (1) restore blood volume following hemorrhage, trauma, or extensive burns or (2) in unusual instances, to treat certain types of anemia by maintaining an adequate concentration of circulating hemoglobin.

Packed red cells (i.e., red cell concentrate or whole blood *minus* most of the plasma) are transfused to increase the oxygen-carrying capacity of the blood in persons with various types of acute and chronic anemias, either primary disorders or secondary anemias due to leukemia, lymphoma and other diseases affecting blood production or destruction. In certain circumstances, packed red cells are used instead of whole blood for two reasons: (1) to decrease the risk of transfusing incompatible antibodies which may react with the patient's red cells and (2) to lessen the possibility of circulatory overload or electrolyte imbalance.

Fresh pooled plasma transfusions have been used in the past to expand volume in cases of burns or other acute traumatic shock; however, they showed a high hepatitis carrier rate.

Therefore, commercially prepared solutions such as Ringer's lactate, plasma protein fraction, and albumin are currently used. These solutions may also be used in treating protein-losing disorders such as nephrosis and certain diseases of the gastrointestinal tract.

Patients who have been pregnant or have received whole blood on multiple occasions tend to form antibodies against white cells and are candidates for transfusion of *red cells from which the white cells have been largely removed.* This type of transfusion is called *leuko-poor packed red cells.* White cells are removed from the packed red cells by means of a special laboratory procedure.

Fresh frozen plasma or a frozen and thawed fraction thereof (cryoprecipitate) is transfused to patients with deficiencies of specific clotting factors—namely factor VIII and fibrinogen.

Commercially prepared specific *Rh immune globulin* (RhoGAM or Gamulin) is administered intramuscularly to block the primary immune response of an Rh negative mother to her Rh positive infant within 72 hours of birth or abortion.

Platelets are transfused to counter thrombocytopenia due to: (1) a temporary loss resulting from dilution with multiple blood transfusions; (2) decreased platelet production due to certain hematologic diseases such as aplastic anemia,[48] leukemia, lymphoma or infection and in patients on certain drugs[34] or undergoing anti-neoplastic chemotherapy or (3) increased destruction, as with consumptive coagulopathy or immune destruction.

BLOOD GROUP SYSTEMS

The individual who gives his blood to a blood bank, hospital or specific patient is called the *donor,* while the person who receives whole blood or a component is called the *recipient.*

> *It is mandatory that the donor's blood and the recipient's blood belong to compatible blood groups.*

If the donor and recipient belong to incompatible blood groups, antibodies in the recipient's plasma may agglutinate and lyse the donor's erythrocytes. When such an antigen-antibody reaction occurs during a blood transfusion, it is called a *hemolytic transfusion reaction.*

ABO Blood Group System

The ABO blood type is inherited as an autosomal trait, as are eye color, hair color, and other features. The four major blood types of clinical importance in this genetic system are *A, B, AB* and *O*, as extended from the original observation by Karl Landsteiner in 1900.*

Blood typing is based upon the type of *antigens (agglutinogens)* present on the erythrocytes as well as the type of *antibodies (agglutinins)* in the serum. Two major antigens have been identified within the ABO blood group system: antigen A and antigen B (Table 39–1). Thus persons with A type blood have A antigens on their red cells; those with B type blood have B antigens. Persons with AB blood have both A and B antigens, while those with O type blood do not have either A or B antigens on their red cells.

There are also two "naturally occurring" antibodies in the ABO system: anti-A and anti-B (Table 39–1). When a blood specimen contains one or the other antigen, it does not contain that specific antibody. For example, an individual with A type blood does not have anti-A in his serum; if he did, his blood cells would be destroyed. Instead, persons with A type blood have anti-B antibody; those with B type blood have anti-A antibody; those with AB type blood have neither anti-A nor anti-B in their serum; and those with O type blood have both anti-A

---

*Researchers have identified over 300 blood group antigens in addition to those of the ABO classification. Fortunately, most have relatively low immunogenicity. Otherwise, finding acceptably matched blood would be very difficult if not impossible. For more technical information on blood groups, consult a hematology textbook, medical laboratory manual, genetics textbook or source in physical anthropology.

and anti-B antibodies. The source of these "naturally occurring" antibodies is unknown.

Currently, it is not acceptable medical practice to transfuse type A, B or AB blood to patients whose red cells lack those same antigens, since their plasma will contain incompatible antibodies. However, it is acceptable whenever necessary to give A or B blood (preferably as packed red cells with plasma removed) to AB recipients.

Refer again to Table 39–1. Observe that persons with A type blood can receive blood only from persons with the same blood type or, in an extreme emergency, from persons with O type blood either as packed red cells or as whole blood shown not to have anti-A or anti-B in a titer greater than 1:50.[2] If a person with A type blood accidentally receives a transfusion of B or AB type blood, the anti-B antibodies present in his (the recipient's) serum rapidly agglutinate or hemolyse the donor's red cells and a hemolytic transfusion reaction may occur. For the same reasons, persons with B type blood should not receive a transfusion of A or AB type blood. The person with AB blood can receive A, B or O blood if the plasma has been removed. However, individuals with O type blood should receive blood only from other persons with O type blood because their serum contains both anti-A and anti-B antibodies, which will agglutinate A, B and AB red cells.

Rh System

In addition to having one of the ABO blood types, about 85 per cent of Caucasian individuals inherit the antigen "D" (or Rh_0) of the Rh blood group system, and thereby are classified as *Rh positive*. Those individuals who do not inherit "D" are classified as *Rh negative*. The Rh phenomenon was described by Landsteiner and Wiener in 1940 and obtained the name "Rh factor" from the rhesus monkeys used in the experiments.

The Rh blood groups are of equal importance

TABLE 39–1. SUMMARY OF INFORMATION: ABO BLOOD GROUPS[17, 18, 19]

BLOOD TYPE	FREQUENCIES IN POPULATION* (PER CENT)			ANTIBODY IN SERUM	INCOMPATIBLE DONOR BLOOD	COMPATIBLE DONOR BLOOD
	White	*Black*	*Oriental*			
A	45	29	35	Anti-B	B, AB	A
B	8	17	23	Anti-A	A, AB	B
AB	4	4	12	None	None	A, B, AB
O	43	50	30	Anti-A, Anti-B	A, B, AB	O

*These frequencies are representative of American blood donors classified into three quite heterogeneous ethnic groups on the basis of such criteria as color and name.

with the ABO groups because of their relation to hemolytic disease of the newborn and their significance in blood transfusion. The subject is quite complex, and different systems of terminology are in use.

The Fisher CDE nomenclature will be used in these discussions; other Rh nomenclatures are reviewed in standard transfusion texts. The Rh blood groups are determined by a series of three closely linked genes—*C, D* and *E*, with allelic forms *c, d* and *e*. The d has no corresponding antigen or antibody and therefore is simply the absence of D. The D antigen is the strongest and of the greatest clinical significance. By agreement among blood banking experts, the presence or absence of the D antigen determines whether a person is Rh positive or Rh negative. For example, persons with haplotypes such as *CDe, cDE* or *CDE* are all Rh positive, whereas those genotypes *cde/cde, Cde/cde* or *cdE/cde* are Rh negative. Among Caucasians, approximately 85 per cent of the population is Rh positive (the most common gene combinations being *CDe* and *cDE*), while the remaining 15 per cent is Rh negative. The incidence of Rh antigens varies widely among various populations. The frequency of Rh negative (D negative) varies from 20 to 40 per cent among the Basques of the Pyrenees to 0 per cent in the Japanese, Chinese, Burmese, Indonesians, Maoris and Eskimos.[35]

As in the case of the ABO blood types, persons who are Rh positive (i.e., whose erythrocytes carry the Rh_0 or D antigen) do not have anti-Rh_0 (anti-D) antibodies in their serum. However, in contrast to the ABO blood type, persons who are Rh negative develop anti-Rh antibodies only after exposure to Rh positive blood, either by transfusion or by transplacental passage of red cells from an Rh positive fetus. For example, if a person with Rh negative blood is accidentally transfused for the first time with Rh positive blood he will not have a transfusion reaction because his blood will not yet contain anti-Rh antibodies. However, about 50 per cent of such transfused persons become sensitized to the Rh antigen and develop antibodies against the D antigen. Should this sensitized person receive a second transfusion of Rh positive blood at a later date, some degree of reaction due to red cell destruction will occur. A similar situation arises when an Rh negative mother is "sensitized" by red cells from an Rh positive fetus. The maternal IgG (immunoglobulin) anti-Rh is capable of crossing the placenta and destroying fetal red cells. This usually occurs during a second or third pregnancy with an Rh positive fetus. Severe fetal anemia and fetal intrauterine death may occur unless therapeutic intervention such as intrauterine fetal transfusion or early delivery is undertaken. This problem has been largely prevented by prophylactic administration of anti-Rh (brand names: RhoGAM or Gamulin) to the susceptible Rh negative mother within 72 hours of delivering an Rh positive child or following abortion, when Rh of fetus cannot be determined. To protect *subsequent* children, Rhogam must be given (a) after *every* pregnancy—whether delivered or aborted and (b) when there is a question of abortion in an Rh negative mother.

Although anti-D is the most common Rh antibody, others, either alone or in combination, may cause transfusion problems. One quite important variant of the Rh system is the D^u antigen. This peculiar antigen gives a positive result with some anti-D sera and not others. D^u is relatively common among blacks but uncommon among Caucasians.[35] The important aspect in these patients is that they must be transfused as Rh negative recipients but considered Rh positive donors (see Rh Typing, p. 1004).

BLOOD PROCUREMENT

Federal controls on blood banking practices effective December 1975[36] require that all blood banks—in-hospital or regional centers—meet and maintain certain standards regarding donor qualifications, blood drawing, blood testing and storage, component preparation, labelling, records, inspection and handling, and in some cases blood administration. Many of these institutions use the American Association of Blood Banks (AABB) Technical Methods and Procedures[2] as well as the AABB Standards for Blood Banks and Transfusion Services[3] as general guidelines. The Joint Commission on Accreditation of Hospitals (JCAH) also has established requirements for hospitals to meet and maintain accreditation.[28]

Donor Selection

Rigid criteria for donor selection have been established: donor shall be free of disease of the heart, kidneys, lungs, liver, etc.; have no history of cancer, jaundice, hepatitis, tuberculosis, allergies, or any transmissible disease; and have not donated within the previous 90 days. A physical examination shall include general appearance, age, temperature, hemoglobin or hematocrit determination, pulse, blood pressure and weight. Donors are disqualified who have a history of recent pregnancies, dental surgery or major surgery, receipt of blood or blood components, immunizations or vaccinations, use of narcotics or drug abuse, therapeutic bleeding, and all oral medications, with the exception of birth control pills and occasional aspirins.

When a potential donor has met or passed the above qualifications, the drawing and collection of blood from the donor must meet equally stringent regulations. Following donation, the donor must be cared for in a supervised setting, and all necessary equipment must be available should the donor have an adverse reaction.

Currently, donor blood is drawn into one of two anticoagulant solutions in a sterile container, usually plastic. Although ACD (acid-citrate-dextrose) or CPD (citrate-phosphate-dextrose) are both currently used as the anticoagulants, CPD permits the maintenance of a greater level of 2,3 DPG (Diphosphoglycerate), an intraerythrocytic glycolytic intermediate which affects the oxygen-releasing capacity of the red blood cells. CPD is therefore usually the solution of choice. In the near future another substance, adenine, will also be added. This purine base increases red cell viability by maintaining the level of ATP (adenosine triphosphate), thus extending the shelf-life of a donor unit from the current 21 days to 35 days.

Adenine has passed FDA (Federal Drug Administration) standards and will soon be available to laboratories within the United States.

Identification of Donor Blood[2, 3, 36]

Each donor unit must be properly labelled in clear, readable letters bearing the following important information to be verified at the time of administration: name of blood product or component, name and number of donor, expiration date, ABO and Rh types, results of tests for hepatitis and syphilis, and the name and address of the blood bank drawing the unit. Precautions to be displayed on the label include warnings to administer only to a recipient who has been shown to be compatible by crossmatch, to use a filter, to add no medications to the blood prior to or during administration, and to dispense only with a prescription (written order).

Storage and Transportation[2, 3, 28, 36]

Immediately after being drawn, the donor unit should be placed in storage at a temperature of 1 to 6°C. If platelets are to be harvested, the unit should remain at room temperature for a period not to exceed 4 hours and then be returned to proper refrigeration after removal of the platelets.

All refrigerators, in blood banks or hospitals, used to store blood should: contain *only* whole blood and blood products, have adequate circulating air, be equipped with a verified recording thermometer, and be inspected daily for temperature maintenance. The proper functioning of the refrigerator must be constantly confirmed by a system of audible and visible alarms that are either battery-operated or powered by a different circuit from that of the refrigerator. Stored blood shall be inspected for evidence of hemolysis or bacterial contamination daily and prior to use.

Intra-hospital transport of whole blood or packed red cells should be limited to 30 minutes, since the temperature of a refrigerated unit will rise to above the allowable 10°C. in about that period of time. Precooled, insulated bags may be used to extend this time limit (by 15 to 30 minutes) for transport to remote areas.

Inter-hospital transport of whole blood or packed red cells should be done using insulated containers that have been verified for temperature maintenance so that at no time does the temperature exceed 10°C.

Fresh frozen plasma must be stored below −20°C. and therefore must be transported in

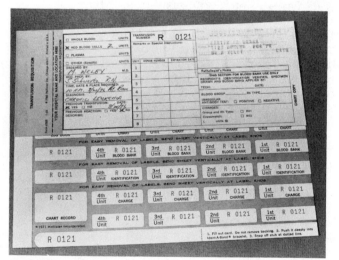

Figure 39–1. Requisition to initiate order and control number that will correlate entire transfusion procedure. (Courtesy of Ident-A-Blood, Hollister, Inc., Chicago 60611.)

containers using dry ice to maintain this temperature.

Platelets harvested from freshly drawn donor units must be maintained at 22°C. on a constantly moving platform. If "pooled" prior to administration, their expiration time is 2 hours "post-pooling" in order to insure viable platelets and minimize bacterial growth.

Cryoprecipitate (Factor VIII, used in treating hemophiliacs) is prepared from freshly drawn donor units and must be maintained at below −20°C. If thawed and pooled prior to administration, the expiration time is 6 hours "post-pooling" in order to minimize bacterial growth.

TYPING AND CROSSMATCHING[2, 3, 28, 36]

Collection of Sample

The recipient blood sample for typing and crossmatching *must be labelled immediately at the bedside* with the following identifying information obtained from the wristband: hospital; recipient's name, last name first; hospital number; date; and in many cases the signature of the person drawing the sample. To assure positive identity of the recipient, several companies have introduced banding procedures (Figs. 39–1 to 39–3), which are also very suitable for the unconscious patient or disaster or ac-

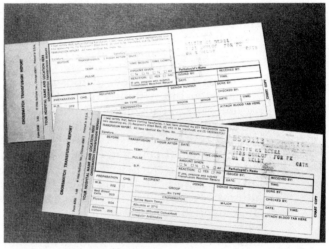

Figure 39–2. Crossmatch Report Form—one for each unit ordered correlated by application of numbered label from requisition. Becomes actual transfusion record for chart and includes space for signatures of persons performing final identification and administration. (Courtesy of Ident-A-Blood.)

cident victim. For detailed information regarding one such system refer to reference 12.

Preferably the sample should be drawn from a fresh venipuncture site, although intravenous tubing or a heparin lock may be used if it is thoroughly flushed and the first 5 ml. of blood withdrawn is discarded. Fresh samples, less than 48 hours old, must be used for typing and crossmatching.

A blood request form should accompany the specimen and should contain: hospital name; recipient's name, last name first; hospital number; date; requesting physician; exact amount of blood or component requested; diagnosis; and date and time desired. *Accuracy* and *legibility* are of prime importance in preparing both the tube label and the request form.

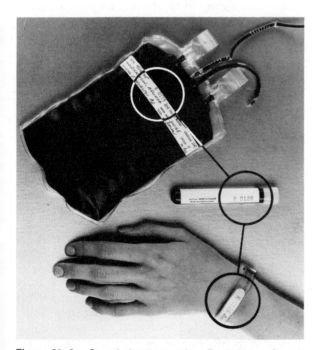

Figure 39–3. Correlation by number. Recipient → Specimen → Unit of blood. Positive identification that unit was crossmatched to specimen drawn from correct patient. (Courtesy of Ident-A-Blood.)

COMPATIBILITY TESTING

▶ *Recipient Typing.* The first step in compatibility testing is to determine the ABO type of the recipient. This is done by placing the recipient's red cells in tubes containing known anti-A and anti-B serum and is referred to as "forward typing." To verify the recipient cell typing, another method is used, "reverse" or back typing. This is performed on the recipient serum using known type A and B cells. Both tests must match exactly in order to determine the recipient's true ABO type.

Discrepancies in forward and reverse typing may result from the following: (a) technical errors, (b) the presence of unusually weak antigens on the patient's red cells, (c) the presence of cold agglutinins in the patient's serum, (d) rouleau formation (abnormal red cell stacking due to diseases such as multiple myeloma or collagen diseases and volume expanders such as Dextran), (e) low levels of gamma globulin (group O, A or B individuals who may lack expected anti-A and/or anti-B, usually found in newborns who do not exhibit any passively acquired antibodies) and (f) mixed fields where more than one cell population is present, for example, a group A patient who has been transfused with type O blood.[17, 19]

▶ *Rh Typing.* Rh typing is performed on the recipient's red cells using a high-protein anti-D serum. If the recipient's red cells are agglutinated by this anti-D serum, the recipient is considered Rh positive. If there is no agglutination, the recipient is considered to be Rh negative. Testing of the donor, but not the recipient, by the antiglobulin technique is necessary to establish the presence of the D^u type.*The anti–human globulin technique is very useful in the detection of a variety of antibodies that are incapable of producing direct agglutination. A relatively common problem related to the use of the antiglobulin test is the interpretation of a positive result when the patient is taking the antihypertensive alpha methyldopa (Aldomet), since this drug induces production of antibodies against red cells in 10 to 20 per cent of patients, simulating autoimmune hemolytic anemia. In rare cases, increased red cell destruction does occur.

---

*The test for D^u employs incubation of the donor's red cells with incomplete anti-D (obtained from Rh negative subjects known to have been sensitized to Rh positive blood) and, after thorough washing to remove immunoglobulins, the addition of anti–human globulin (Coombs) serum. This antiserum is produced in another species (usually rabbits) by injecting human immunoglobulin or serum fractions to produce specific anti–human antibodies. When the anti–human gamma globulin antibodies, which were produced in the rabbit, come in contact with the red cells coated with human globulin, agglutination occurs (the incomplete anti-D is incapable of producing agglutination by itself).

▶ *Crossmatching with Potential Donor.* After the recipient's ABO and Rh groups have been ascertained, donor blood of the appropriate ABO and Rh types is selected and testing may proceed. This consists of determining compatibility of the recipient's serum and the donor's red cells (sometimes referred to as the "major" crossmatch) as evidenced by lack of agglutination or clumping using a high protein and an antiglobulin technique (described above). In some institutions, a "minor" crossmatch is also performed, using the recipient's red cells and the donor's serum. However, this test is usually accomplished in advance by screening the donor serum for antibodies against a pool of selected red cells.

Compatible units are then properly identified with a Report of Crossmatch and dispatched as requested.

The serum of multiply-transfused recipients may contain antibodies of one or more specificities which must be individually identified. Finding compatible blood under these circumstances may be extremely difficult.

The recipient's sample and samples of each transfused unit are retained by the crossmatching facility for at least 7 days for further testing in the event of an adverse reaction. Thorough documentation of all steps in typing and crossmatching is mandatory under federal regulations. This enables laboratory personnel to retrace each step in the typing and crossmatching process for possible errors should an adverse reaction occur during or following transfusion.

ADMINISTRATION OF BLOOD AND BLOOD PRODUCTS[2, 3, 28, 36]

Modes or Routes of Blood Transfusion

1. *Indirect transfusion:* A random donor, usually a volunteer, donates a unit of blood to be used by any compatible recipient. This procedure encompasses the majority of all hospital transfusions.

2. *Intrauterine* transfusion is performed on the fetus when the level of maternal antibodies against the fetal red cells is high enough to cause severe fetal anemia. In this type of transfusion, the red cells used are compatible with the mother's serum and are re-suspended in plasma devoid of maternal antibodies.

3. *Neonatal exchange transfusion* is employed when fetal red cells are prematurely destroyed by maternal antibodies that have crossed the placenta, causing erythroblastosis

fetalis, also called hemolytic disease of the newborn (HDN). Since such premature red cell destruction can cause anemia, two things must be considered: loss of oxygen-carrying capacity due to decreased numbers of red cells, and an increased amount of free-circulating unbound bilirubin (a product of the heme constituent of hemoglobin), which may cause kernicterus. The result may be mental retardation, convulsions, or even death in those infants severely affected. Anti-D is the most common cause of HDN, although other antibodies occasionally cause HDN. Maternal IgM antibodies do not cause HDN because they are incapable of passing the placental barrier. Blood used for exchange transfusions may be ABO specific with the infant and compatible with the mother's serum. In some cases, type O blood with low titered anti-A or B is used. Small amounts of the infant's blood are removed, usually from the umbilical vein, and an equal volume of the filtered, compatible blood is infused. Careful monitoring of the baby's venous pressure dictates the actual volume of blood injected. This procedure may be repeated as necessary until the infant has stabilized.

4. *Autotransfusion* (autologous) refers to self-transfusion. This form of transfusion may be used (a) in patients with rare antibodies for whom compatible blood is thereby very difficult to obtain; in the case of a planned surgical procedure the patient may deposit one unit of whole blood within a week prior to surgery for use as necessary; (b) in bone marrow transplants; the marrow donor may donate one unit of whole blood to be re-infused after aspiration of his bone marrow and (c) in cases of religious or moral objections to the infusion of blood from unknown donors.[7]

5. *HLA-matched donor* transfusion most frequently refers to platelet transfusion from a specific donor who has the same HLA antigens (human leukocyte or white cell antigens) as the recipient. When possible, regular platelet transfusions should be ABO and Rh type-specific, since it is impossible to remove all the red cells from the plasma-suspended platelets. Foreign antigens on random donor platelets very frequently stimulate the multi-transfused recipient to produce platelet antibodies. When such antibodies have developed, transfusions of platelets containing the corresponding antigens are no longer effective in raising the platelet count, and HLA-matched donors are necessary for continued therapy. Numerous potential donors must be screened to obtain one matched donor. Family members, especially siblings, provide the most useful platelet donors.

6. *Extra-corporeal* transfusion is employed on patients undergoing open heart surgery using the heart-lung (bypass) machine.

Intra-arterial and *intra-peritoneal* transfusions have been used by some physicians but generally are no longer employed.

Procedures for Blood Administration

When blood is ordered for a patient, the nurse is largely responsible for its safe administration. This is a grave responsibility because the transfusion of blood and blood products is fraught with hazards that can be fatal. Therefore, it is essential that the physician *write* all orders for typing and crossmatching and for the administration of all blood or blood products.

> *Verbal orders from physicians should be accepted by a registered nurse only in extreme emergencies and should be written as soon as circumstances permit.*

Full documentation of each transfusion event must be kept, not only in the laboratory, but also in the patient's chart. An acceptable record system should make it possible to trace a unit of any blood or blood product from donor to recipient; and to recheck all the laboratory records applying to a specific product.[3, 20]

Although Federal regulations[36] and the Joint Commission on Accreditation of Hospitals (JCAH)[28] have set guidelines for the administration of blood and blood products, the American Medical Association[4] and the American Association of Blood Banks[3] have suggested more specific guidelines or criteria. Many individual hospitals use a House Staff Manual[47] to assist their staff in following proper procedures. Other hospitals have specific procedure manuals designed to guide hospital personnel in their own internal policies and procedures, such as the one published by the University Hospital, University of Michigan.[16] The major difference between these two types of manuals is that many hospitals maintain their own internal blood bank,[16] while others obtain blood and blood products from blood centers, some of which perform all of the testing prior to issuing the product.[47] Basically all internal policies for the ordering, handling and administration of blood and blood products are similar and follow the guidelines of the Federal regulations and the JCAH.

Identifying the Patient

> *The most important consideration in transfusion is to be absolutely certain the correct blood product is administered to the proper patient. Misidentification of the patient causes most of the errors that result in major adverse reactions.*

Elaborate procedures have been established to insure the identity of the recipient. When blood or a blood product is to be administered it is recommended that *two* registered nurses, or a physician and a registered nurse (in some cases licensed practical nurses), should independently verify all identifying information on the Report of Crossmatch, unit label and patient wristband (patient name, hospital number, blood type of patient and of unit, unit number and donor name). In many hospitals the signatures of the nurses, physician and/or practical nurse are required to document that accurate identification has been completed prior to transfusion (see Fig. 39–2). Should there be any discrepancy, the unit should be returned to the blood bank immediately. Following transfusion the Report of Crossmatch should be placed in the patient's chart and retained as a part of his permanent record.

Initiating Blood Transfusion. Who is actually responsible for initiating and continuing blood transfusion therapy? While state laws and institutional policies vary, typical rules for administration of blood and blood products are as follows:

1. If venipuncture is required, the *physician* must perform the venipuncture and hang the first unit of blood or blood products.

2. Upon a physician's order, registered nurses (and in some institutions, specially trained practical nurses) may add further units of blood and blood products once blood transfusion therapy is in process.

3. If venipuncture was performed earlier (e.g., for giving intravenous fluids), registered nurses may themselves initiate transfusions of blood and blood products with a physician's order.

Administering Blood. All blood and blood products should be administered through an appropriate sterile, pyrogen-free transfusion set containing a *filter* (Fig. 39–4), which will remove clots and larger aggregates of leuko-

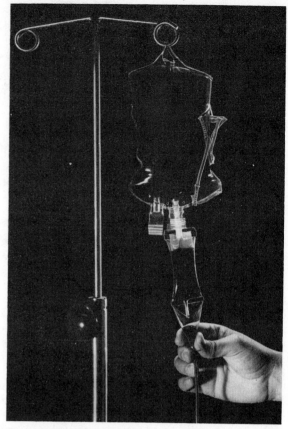

Figure 39–4. Unit of whole blood with administration set properly in place. Note that set has two chambers; upper filter chamber and lower drip-rate chamber. (Courtesy of Fenwall Laboratories, Division of Travenol Laboratories, Inc., Deerfield, IL 60015.)

cytes and platelets. Due care should be taken when inserting the filter to prevent puncture of the plastic blood bag and to avoid the introduction of air into the system, which may result in an air embolus. Studies are being undertaken to determine the need for, and efficiency of, microfilters. This type of filter is not now used routinely in most hospitals.

It is generally recommended that an *18-gauge needle*, or larger, be used for infusion, to prevent damage to the red cells and provide an adequate rate of flow. *No medications* (antibiotics, anesthetic agents, muscle relaxants, vitamins, etc.) should be added to the unit of blood or administered through the same intravenous system, as they may injure the red cells. Where permissible, and when the patient is not on salt restriction, a 0.9 per cent saline solution is recommended for administering blood via a Y-type infusion set or through the medication injection site of a straight infusion set. To increase the flow rate of packed red cells, 50 ml. of 0.9 per cent normal saline may be added to reduce viscosity. Solutions containing dextrose should be avoided as they can cause red cell hemolysis. Other solutions containing calcium, such as Ringer's lactate, may cause clotting.[43] When the transfusion has been initiated, the infusion site should be stabilized in a manner comfortable to the patient, using an armboard or other device to prevent dislodging of the needle. However, the site should not be completely covered, since constant observation for possible infiltration is necessary. If the infusion does infiltrate into the patient's tissues, the transfusion should be discontinued and restarted at another site. (Intravenous therapy is discussed in detail in Chapter 38.)

Prior to administration the patient's vital signs must be recorded to provide a baseline for further observation. The *initial* flow rate (for approximately 15 minutes) should be slow (1 ml. per kg. of body weight per hour) so that any immediate reaction will be observed. (Transfusion reactions and their signs, symptoms, causes and treatment are discussed in the next section.)

> *The usual rate of infusion is from 80 to 100 drops per minute. The subsequent flow rate depends on the condition of the patient and the need for rapid infusion.*

For patients in shock it is possible to infuse a unit within 5 to 8 minutes by squeezing the bag. A much slower rate is essential if the patient has impaired cardiac status.

A pressure cuff may be applied to a unit of whole blood to increase the rate of flow, but care should be taken not to exceed 200 mm. Hg. Higher pressures cause the filter to be ejected from the plastic bag.

Many authorities advocate that a unit of whole blood or packed red cells be infused within 4 hours, and that all tubing used for transfusion be changed every 24 hours to minimize bacterial contamination.

Temperature of Blood for Administration. Whole blood and packed red cells should be administered *cold,* having been taken directly from proper refrigeration. However, in cases of massive transfusion where cardiac arrhythmias might occur, the use of a special monitored warming device may be warranted. These types of devices must be carefully monitored to assure that the temperature does not rise above 37°C. Two major disadvantages resulting from the use of a blood-warmer are the slow rate of flow due to the length of coiled tubing in the warming device and the increased destruction of red cells. These disadvantages should be considered prior to using any blood warming device. Microwave warming of blood should be avoided, as the temperature is

difficult to maintain and excessive warming causes red cell hemolysis.[30]

Storage and Handling of Blood Products. Fresh frozen plasma should be thawed in its protective package, using a water bath carefully monitored to remain below 37°C. A standard blood infusion set should be used for administration.

Platelet concentrates stored in individual plastic bags are normally pooled by the laboratory prior to issue and must be administered within a 2 hour period to insure viability and minimize bacterial growth. Many transfusion services and blood banks recommend using a platelet infusion set equipped with a special type of filter to permit passage of the platelets. It is necessary to "flush" the filter with approximately 20 ml. of sterile 0.9 per cent normal saline to insure that all of the product reaches the patient and that none is trapped in the filter and tubing.

Cryoprecipitated factor VIII (for hemophiliacs) is stored frozen in individual plastic bags; in many blood banks it will be thawed and pooled prior to issue. This product should be administered using a standard blood infusion set within 6 hours of pooling to insure viability and minimize bacterial growth.

TRANSFUSION REACTIONS AND OTHER COMPLICATIONS OF TRANSFUSION THERAPY

Many types of transfusion reactions may occur during administration or in the following hours or days. It is estimated that approximately 5 per cent of all transfusions are associated with some type of adverse reaction, generally falling into the following categories: hemolytic, pyrogenic, allergic and non-hemolytic febrile. Other complications may include circulatory overload, citrate toxicosis, electrolytic imbalance, anaphylactic response, infectious diseases, hemosiderosis and air embolism.

As this list of complications indicates, blood and blood component transfusion is dangerous and should be undertaken only when absolutely necessary. It is particularly risky to give blood to an *unconscious* patient, to any individual who is anesthetized or heavily sedated, to a young child or to any adult who is unable to communicate. Because of their depressed consciousness, such persons are unable to complain of symptoms (e.g., dyspnea, cough, chills, headache) should they develop a transfusion reaction. Unless observable symptoms are noticed by the nurse, such persons could receive an entire unit of incompatible blood and, as a result, die from hemolysis and shock. Patients who are unable to communicate may require continuous monitoring of: (a) blood pressure via a direct arterial line or (b) central venous pressure via a catheter which has been threaded through a vein into the superior vena cava (see Chap. 29).

While it is difficult to observe a reaction in the unconscious patient, it is also difficult to evaluate whether symptoms experienced by *any* patient during a transfusion are due to the *blood* he is receiving or to his *illness*. Many symptoms of transfusion reactions (dyspnea, apprehension, headache, vomiting) are the same as the symptoms caused by common disorders. Because it is the nurse who usually detects the first signs and symptoms of a potential transfusion reaction, she must pause for a moment and carefully evaluate the "total" situation before stopping the flow of the transfusion and summoning the physician. The physician, upon assessing the status of the patient, will determine if the transfusion must be terminated.

> *Should an adverse reaction occur, stop the flow of blood or blood product and notify the physician immediately.*

Do not remove the needle but use an acceptable solution to keep the needle patent.

The specific nursing actions in the clinical care of patients with hemolytic transfusion reactions, pyrogenic transfusion reactions, allergic transfusion reactions and circulatory overload are detailed in Table 39–2, p. 1009.

Hemolytic Transfusion Reactions*

A hemolytic transfusion reaction may be classified as either intravascular or extravascular. *Intravascular hemolysis* is the rupture of circulating red cells with the release of free hemoglobin. It is most commonly caused by ABO incompatibility with complement fixa-

---

*Further information may be obtained in references 3, 13, 19, 22, 29, 34, and 48.

tion. It may also be due to other antibodies or to improper storage of blood (uncontrolled refrigeration resulting in freezing; storage beyond the 21 day limit; warming of blood above 40°C. prior to transfusion), or by exposure of the red cells to dextrose solutions.

Signs and symptoms of acute intravascular hemolysis due to an immune mechanism may include anxiety, restlessness, nausea and vomiting, heat along the vein into which the blood is being transfused, flushing, chest and/or lumbar pain, tachypnea, tachycardia, chill followed by fever, cyanosis, hemoglobinemia and hemoglobinuria. These symptoms may progress to shock, with a resultant drop in blood pressure. Oliguria followed by anuria may signal renal failure. If the patient is under anesthesia or in a coma, the first signs noted may be a sudden drop in blood pressure and the oozing of blood from the operative site or mucous membranes.

Treatment of a patient with intravascular hemolytic transfusion reaction should include: (a) discontinuing the transfusion, notifying the physician and initiating fluid therapy such as plasma; (b) diuresis using the osmotic diuretic mannitol; (c) vasopressors to maintain blood pressure; (d) oxygen and (e) hemodialysis, if necessary, for complete renal failure. The use of steroids should be avoided. Intravascular coagulopathy, evidenced by oozing, may be controlled by the administration of appropriate coagulation factors and/or platelets. If recognized early and particularly when 500 ml. or more of known incompatible blood has been transfused, exchange transfusions with compatible blood may be beneficial in rare instances.

Extravascular hemolysis occurs outside the circulatory system in the reticuloendothelial cells and is most commonly caused by antibodies in the Rh system, notably anti-D, anti-C and E. The free hemoglobin is converted into bilirubin, which circulates to the liver and after further degradation is passed through the gastrointestinal tract. The signs and symptoms are much milder than those of intravascular hemolysis and may include malaise, fever and hyperbilirubinemia, but shock and renal failure rarely occur. This type of reaction may not occur until one week or more after the transfusion and usually represents an anamnestic (systemic recall) response due to prior sensitization by one or more antigens on red cells received by prior transfusion or pregnancy.

The treatment of patients with extravascular hemolysis is conservative. Further transfusions are avoided unless the patient's life is threatened.

Immediate laboratory investigation of all hemolytic transfusion reactions is imperative.

A fresh blood sample should be carefully drawn from the recipient to be observed for hemolysis, and a second tube sent to the laboratory to repeat the initial crossmatch with the donor "pilot tube." Clerical errors and the administration of blood to the wrong patient are the most common causes; a thorough follow-up and documentation of all steps taken are essential.

Pyrogenic Reactions

Pyrogenic reactions, in the past, most frequently resulted from pyrogenic substances in the transfusion tubing after sterilization. How-

TABLE 39–2. CARE IN TRANSFUSION REACTIONS

CARE IN HEMOLYTIC TRANSFUSION REACTION

*Drugs and Treatments Used to Counteract Reaction**	*Nursing Actions*
1. Intravenous infusions of dextrose in water or Ringer's lactate to counteract shock and promote diuresis.	1. Discontinue blood flow immediately.
2. Oxygen and epinephrine to treat dyspnea and wheezing.	2. Notify physician and laboratory.
3. Sedation to counteract restlessness and apprehension.	3. Return blood and fresh sample of patient's blood to laboratory for repeat crossmatch.
4. Indwelling catheter to accurately evaluate urine output.	4. Administer ordered IV fluids using new sterile tubing and connect directly to the needle to keep needle patent. (Do *not* remove the needle.)
5. Mannitol (an osmotic diuretic) to counteract oliguria.	7. Start intake and output record; observe for oliguria or anuria.
6. Blood transfusion (with properly matched blood) to control shock.	8. Insert Foley catheter and measure urine hourly.
7. Vasopressor drugs in event of severe shock.	9. Allay patient's anxiety.
	10. Observe for effects of vasopressor drugs.
	11. Attempt to reduce patient's anxiety

CARE IN PYROGENIC TRANSFUSION REACTION

*Drugs and Treatments Used to Counteract Reaction**	*Nursing Actions*
1. Intravenous infusions of dextrose in water or Ringer's lactate to counteract shock and promote diuresis.	1. Discontinue blood flow and notify physician.
2. Vasopressor drugs to maintain systolic blood pressure above 100 mm. Hg.	2. Return blood and fresh sample of patient's blood to laboratory for culture and sensitivity tests.
3. Corticosteroids to abate inflammatory reaction.	3. Take vital signs every 15 to 30 minutes despite patient's "rosy" coloring; observe for hypotension and shock.
4. Broad spectrum antibiotics in high dosages.	4. Administer IV fluids and medications as ordered.
5. Indwelling catheter to properly evaluate urine output.	5. Insert Foley catheter; record intake and output.
6. Blood (properly tested for contaminants) to counteract shock.	6. Take temperature every hour; start cooling measures (alcohol rubs, cool sponge or cooling blankets) if temperature is elevated above 101°F.
	7. Keep patient comfortable.

CARE IN ALLERGIC TRANSFUSION REACTION

*Drugs and Treatments Used to Counteract Reactions**	*Nursing Actions*
1. *Mild reactions:* antihistamines and antipyretics given directly to patient and *not* into the blood transfusion.	1. *Slow* blood flow if *mild* reaction; *stop* blood flow if *severe* reaction and initiate appropriate intravenous fluids.
2. *Severe reactions:* epinephrine, vasopressors and corticosteroids.	2. Notify physician.
3. Appropriate *respiratory therapy.*	3. Administer medications to patient as ordered.
	4. Allay patient's anxiety.

CARE IN CIRCULATORY OVERLOAD

*Drugs and Treatments Used to Counteract Reactions**	*Nursing Actions*
1. Digitalis to counteract congestive heart failure.	1. Stop blood flow and notify physician.
2. Venesection and phlebotomy or rotating tourniquets to remove excess fluid from the general circulation.	2. Administer digitalis as ordered.
	3. Set up for venesection and phlebotomy or rotating tourniquets.
	4. Provide emotional support to patient and significant others.

*Per physician's orders.

coagulant that is routinely used for preserving blood samples for blood count determinations, etc.

ever, bacterial contamination of donor blood may occur from improper preparation of the donor phlebotomy site or from improper refrigeration. The reaction may be profound—with hypotension, abdominal pain, vomiting, diarrhea, shock and renal failure—in which case the outlook is poor. Pseudomonas is one of the most common bacteria found (although coliforms and achromobacters bacteria may also be involved), utilizing the citrate as nourishment and surviving in the cold 4 to 8°C. storage temperature. Antibiotics are of little value and the differential diagnosis may be made by a gram stain of the remaining blood in the unit as well as by noting the absence of the other signs of a hemolytic reaction. Multiple cultures should be taken of the donor pilot sample, pre- and post-transfusion samples from the patient, and the unit itself. This type of transfusion reaction is becoming less common owing to proper screening of donors, improved phlebotomy site preparation and use of disposable, sterile, pyrogen-free transfusion sets. Supportive therapy may be used as necessary.

Allergic Reactions

Allergic reactions usually are first recognized by hives, rash (urticaria) and itching and occur in about 1 per cent of all transfusions.[22] This form of reaction may become more severe, with laryngeal edema and bronchial spasm. The most common causes are sensitivity of the donor to such materials as milk, eggs, chocolate or pollens (hay fever). In order to reduce this type of reaction, potential donors who are under therapy for allergies are normally refused. Treatment normally consists of an injection of an antihistamine such as Benadryl and the initiation of a different unit of blood. If the same transfusion unit must be continued in a severely sensitized patient, the additional administration of epinephrine and corticosteroids may be necessary.

Since these same symptoms may appear with other types of suspected transfusion reactions, a thorough investigation should be undertaken including (a) drawing one tube of blood in EDTA solution, to be spun and the serum checked for hemolysis and (b) sending a second tube of clotted blood to the blood bank to verify the initial crossmatch. EDTA (ethylene diamine tetra-acetic acid) is a common anti-

Nonhemolytic Febrile Reactions

Nonhemolytic febrile reactions have been reported in 3 to 4 per cent of patients in some transfusion centers.[48] This type of reaction is usually caused by sensitization to white cell, platelet or plasma antigens, especially in patients who have received multiple transfusions. Usually this type of reaction is first noted when the patient complains of a chill, followed by a fever within about an hour after the transfusion. Headache, nausea, vomiting and back or leg pain may also occur. Initial actions include the discontinuation of the transfusion and the drawing of specimens from the patient as previously described to check for hemolysis and to verify the crossmatch. Antihistamines are frequently administered both pre- and post-transfusion, and analgesics are administered to relieve muscular discomfort. If this type of reaction continues, the patient should be transfused with packed red cells from which the majority of white cells and plasma have been removed.

Other Complications

CIRCULATORY OVERLOAD

Circulatory overload is a type of reaction likely to develop in patients with cardiac or renal impairment. Excessive amounts of fluid may overload the capacity of a weakened heart and cause circulatory failure and pulmonary edema. The first indications are usually a dry cough, precordial and back pain, dyspnea and cyanosis, followed by a productive cough.

> *Circulatory overload demands* immediate *treatment and consists of slowing the infusion rate and administration of oxygen and diuretics.*

The use of exchange transfusion—withdrawing the patient's whole blood, spinning down and discarding the plasma, and reinfusing the packed red cells—may be indicated. The prevention of circulatory overload includes establishing a central venous pressure monitoring system, infusing packed red cells at a slow rate (not to exceed 50 drops or 2 ml. per minute), and placing the patient in a sitting position to aid breathing. Should symptoms become severe, phlebotomy may be required.

This type of reaction may also result from the infusion of hypertonic or high protein solutions, causing fluid from the tissue to return to general circulation. Continuous observation of the patient is required, with frequent recording of the vital signs.

MASSIVE TRANSFUSION COMPLICATIONS

Massive transfusions of blood are warranted for patients who have extensive blood loss due to severe trauma and/or the severance of a major blood vessel. Unfortunately, massive transfusion of stored whole blood frequently results in several complications, none of which are transfusion reactions per se. One type of complication is due to the *build-up of citrate,* used as one of the preservatives. Citrate is rapidly metabolized and seldom reaches a toxic level unless large amounts of citrated blood are transfused rapidly or the patient has impaired liver function. Muscular twitching and spasm may be noted and the electrocardiogram shows prolongation of the QT interval.[48] Still higher levels of citrate can cause cardiac arrest. Treatment consists of intravenous administration of calcium gluconate to prevent or eliminate this toxic effect by neutralizing the acidosis and restoring the cellular calcium levels. Subsequent to the initial transfusions, which give rise to metabolic acidosis, a period of metabolic alkalosis may follow owing to the breakdown of sodium citrate.

A second problem involves *elevation of the serum potassium (hyperkalemia)* owing to increased levels of potassium in the plasma of stored blood. This is especially likely to occur in infants undergoing exchange transfusion, especially when ACD blood stored for over 4 days is used.

Patients with liver disease may be adversely affected by the *increased amount of ammonia* that occurs in the plasma of stored blood.

Another problem of massive transfusions is a type of *hemorrhagic reaction* apparently due to dilution of circulating, effective platelets and clotting factors by use of banked blood low in platelets and coagulation factors. Treatment consists of administration of platelet concentrate and/or clotting factors as indicated.

ANAPHYLACTIC REACTIONS

Anaphylactic reactions are rare and usually occur in patients who have antibodies against IgA immunoglobulins. They may occur in patients who have had no history of previous transfusion or pregnancy, but are more common in multitransfused patients. Symptoms occur with the administration of only a few milliliters of blood and consist of generalized flushing, bronchospasm with labored breathing, substernal pain, laryngeal edema and collapse.[34] Some patients experience severe gastrointestinal distress, with vomiting and diarrhea. These reactions are usually quite serious and potentially fatal.[13] Treatment consists of supportive care; should further transfusions be required, frozen washed cells or blood from other subjects lacking IgA are the products of choice. A special register of IgA-deficient donors has been established at the Irwin Memorial Blood Bank of San Francisco Medical Society,[2] and by the American Association of Blood Banks Rare Donor File.[13]

INFECTIOUS DISEASES

Among infectious diseases that may be transmitted by transfusion are hepatitis, malaria, syphilis, cytomegalovirus, toxoplasmosis and brucellosis.

Of major concern are donors who have had any *jaundice related to hepatitis.* Although all donor blood must now be tested, by radioimmunoassay, for hepatitis B surface antigen (HB_sAg), this test does not detect carriers of other viruses causing hepatitis. Thus, blood from volunteer donors is preferable to blood from paid donors, since the latter are less likely to give a reliable history. After transfusion, the development of hepatitis may not be seen for several weeks to months. The patient may complain of fatigue and general malaise, followed by jaundice. Laboratory testing is necessary to confirm the diagnosis and the blood bank should be notified immediately. Prolonged convalescence is not infrequent and in some patients total liver failure and death ensue. Supportive therapy is instituted as necessary.

Donors who have had *malaria* are now acceptable as donors, as are persons who have been in malarial areas or have taken antimalarial medications. These persons may donate blood three years after their last illness, return from the malarial area, or discontinuation of medication.

The routine screening of donor units for *syphilis* has virtually eliminated transmission of this disease by transfusion. However, donors in the late primary or early secondary stages occasionally have a negative test and still may transmit the disease. Fortunately, the causative agent *(Treponema pallidum)* does not usually survive storage in a temperature of 4 to 6°C.

beyond 96 hours. Again, the use of volunteer donors has aided in decreasing this problem.

Cytomegalovirus infection is usually transmitted by fresh whole blood, since the causative virus does not usually survive in 4°C. beyond 48 hours. Symptoms include fever and an influenza-like illness and occur 3 to 5 weeks after transfusion. Although this mononucleosis-like syndrome is rarely fatal, it may have an adverse effect on the recovery of the patient.

Toxoplasmosis, brucellosis, and viral encephalitis have reportedly been transmitted by transfusion but are rarely encountered.[22, 48]

TRANSFUSION HEMOSIDEROSIS

Transfusion hemosiderosis is not a problem in patients who require repeated transfusions when they are actively bleeding. However, in patients with aplastic or hemolytic anemia and continued transfusion, excessive amounts of iron from the red cells are stored in almost all body tissue, especially liver, heart and skin (the last resulting in brown discoloration). Death may occur owing to the increased amount of iron in the liver and cardiac muscle. Treatment consists of medications to cause excretion of the excess iron and keeping further transfusions to a minimum.

AIR EMBOLISM

Air embolism results from the accidental introduction of air into the circulation and may occur when changing or adding units to an infusion or while transporting a patient with a transfusion in progress. The patient may suddenly become cyanotic, followed by circulatory collapse. Treatment consists of placing the patient on his left side in a head-down position.[2] Because air embolism is potentially lethal, it is mandatory to prevent this problem.

> Remember: *To prevent air embolism, do not allow air to move past the filter into the tubing.*

Fortunately, air embolism is now rare, owing to the use of plastic blood containers instead of the glass bottles of the past. At one time, air embolism was more common because the staff, under emergency circumstances, would sometimes force air into the bottle to increase the rate of transfusion administration.

Warning!

> *Blood or blood products should be administered only when absolutely necessary and only when definite indications exist. Absolute accuracy—from the drawing and proper labelling of the patient sample, through testing and crossmatching, to double-checking before administration—is essential to prevent catastrophic results.*

BIBLIOGRAPHY

1. Allen, J. G.: Problems in liability for transfusion. *Journal of the American Medical Association, 215*:1329 Feb. 1971.
2. American Association of Blood Banks: *Technical Methods and Procedures of the American Association of Blood Banks,* 6th ed. Washington, D.C., 1974.
3. American Association of Blood Banks, Committee on Standards: *Standards for Blood Banks and Transfusion Services,* 7th ed. Chicago, Gunthorp-Warren Printing Co., 1974.
4. American Medical Association, Editorial Board for the Committee on Transfusion and Transplantation: *General Principles of Blood Transfusion.* Chicago, revised edition, 1973.
5. American Medical Association, Editorial Board for the Committee on Transfusion and Transplantation: *General Principles of Blood Transfusion.* Chicago, 1970.
6. Baxter, C. R., Marvin, J. A., and Curreri, P. W.: Early management of thermal burns. *Postgraduate Medicine, 55*:131, Jan. 1974.
7. Blake, M. V.: Autotransfusion: a better way? *Medical Laboratory Observer,* Dec. 1976, p. 77.
8. Buchholz, D. H., and Bove, J. R.: Unusual response to ABO incompatible blood transfusion. *Transfusion, 15*:577, Nov.–Dec. 1975.
9. Button, L. N., Orlina, A. R., Kevy, S. B., and Josephson, A. M.: The quality of over- and undercollected blood for transfusion. *Transfusion, 16*:148, March–April 1976.
10. Byrne, J. P., Jr., and Dixon, J. A.: Pulmonary edema following blood transfusion reaction. *Archives of Surgery, 102*:91, Feb. 1971.
11. Collins, J. A.: Clinical review/problems associated with the massive transfusion of stored blood. *Surgery, 75*:274, Feb. 1974.
12. Crosson, J. T., and Anderson, M. M. T.: A positive blood recipient identification system in a general hospital. *Laboratory Medicine, 8*:9, June 1977.
13. DADE Division American Hospital Supply Corporation: *Blood Group Immunology; Theoretical and Practical Concepts.* Miami, 1976.
14. Djaldetti, M., et al.: Haemorrhagic diathesis following transfusion of incompatible blood. *Scand. Journal of Haematology, 10*:197, 1973.
15. Elin, R. J., Lundberg, W. B., and Schmidt, P. J.: Evaluation of bacterial contamination in blood processing. *Transfusion, 15*:260, May–June 1975.
16. Friedman, B. A.: *Blood Transfusion Policies and Standard Practices.* Ann Arbor, University Hospital, University of Michigan, Revised April 1976. (Copies available on request.)
17. Giblett, E. R.: Erythrocyte antigens and antibodies. *In* Williams, W. J., et al.: *Hematology,* 2nd ed. New York, McGraw-Hill Book Co., 1977.

18. Giblett, E. R.: *Genetic Markers in Human Blood.* Oxford, Blackwell Scientific Publications, 1969.

19. Giblett, E. R.: Blood groups and blood transfusions. *In* Thorn, G. W. (ed.): *Harrison's Principles of Internal Medicine,* 8th ed. New York, McGraw-Hill Book Co., 1977.

20. Gleason, D. E.: Blood transfusion records, an asset or a liability? *Medical Record News,* No. 54, April 1969, American Medical Record Association, Chicago, 1971.

21. Greenwalt, T. J., and Goldsmith, K. L. G.: Delayed haemolytic transfusion reaction with renal failure. *The Lancet,* 1:327, Feb. 1972.

22. Hardisty, R. M., and Weatherall, D. J.: *Blood and Its Disorders.* Oxford, Blackwell Scientific Publications, 1974.

23. Harker, L. A.: *Hemostasis Manual.* Seattle, University of Washington Press, 1970.

24. Hillman, R. S., and Finch, C. A.: *Red Cell Manual,* 4th ed. Philadelphia, F. A. Davis Co., 1974.

25. Issitt, P. D., and Issitt, C.: *Applied Blood Group Serology.* Oxnard, CA, Becton, Dickinson and Company, 1975.

26. Jarvis, S., and Jarvis, B. W.: Beyond the blood bank; transfusion liability. *Laboratory Medicine,* Sep. 1975, p. 701.

27. Jenkins, G., Banks, A., and Manhelm, A.: A review of transfusion complications. *Journal of the American Association of Nurse Anesthetists,* Aug. 1975, p. 369.

28. Joint Commission on Accreditation of Hospitals: *Accreditation Manual for Hospitals.* April 1976, p. 140.

29. Kimmell, R. A.: Blood transfusion: report. *The American Journal of I. V. Therapy,* Aug.–Sep. 1975, p. 34.

30. Lippmann, M., and Myhre, B. A.: Hazards of massive transfusion. *Journal of the American Association of Nurse Anesthetists,* June 1975, p. 269.

31. McCredie, K. B.: Platelet and granulocyte transfusion therapy. *Postgraduate Medicine,* 62:151, Aug. 1977.

32. McCurdy, P. R.: Blood component therapy. *Postgraduate Medicine,* 62:143, Aug. 1977.

33. Miale, J. B.: *Laboratory Medicine: Hematology,* 4th ed. St. Louis, C. V. Mosby Company, 1972.

34. Mollison, P. L.: *Blood Transfusion In Clinical Medicine,* 5th ed. Oxford, Blackwell Scientific Publications, 1972.

35. Mourant, A. E., Kopec, A. C., and Domaniewska-Sobczak, K.: *The Distribution of the Human Blood Groups and Other Polymorphisms,* 2nd ed. London, Oxford University Press, 1976.

36. Office of the Federal Register, National Archives and Records Service, General Services Administration: *CODE OF FEDERAL REGULATIONS; #21/*Food and Drugs; Part 600–1299, Title 21, Chapter 1, Revised 4/1/75, U.S. Government Printing Office, Washington, D.C., 1975, *Part 640.

37. Ortho Diagnostics Inc.: *Blood Group Antigens and Antibodies as Applied to Compatibility Testing.* Raritan, NJ, 1967.

38. Ortho Diagnostics Inc.: *Blood Group Antigens and Antibodies as Applied to Hemolytic Disease of the Newborn.* Raritan, NJ, 1968.

39. Ortho Diagnostics Inc.: *Blood Group Antigens and Antibiotics as Applied to the ABO and Rh Systems.* Raritan, NJ, 1969.

39a. Pineda, A. A., Brzica, S. M., and Taswell, H. F.: Hemolytic transfusion reaction—recent experience in a large blood bank. *Mayo Clinical Proceedings,* 53:378–390, 1978.

40. Puget Sound Blood Center: *Circular of Information: Use of Whole Blood (Human) and Red Blood Cells (Human).* Seattle (pamphlet).

41. Race, R. R., and Sanger, R.: *Blood Groups in Man,* 6th ed. Oxford, Blackwell Scientific Publications, 1975.

42. Rudowski, W. J.: Complications associated with blood transfusion. *Progress in Surgery,* 9:78, 1971.

43. Ryden, S. E., and Oberman, H. A.: Compatibility of common intravenous solutions with CPD blood. *Transfusion,* 15:250, May–June 1975.

43a. Scarlato, M. (Consultant): Blood transfusions today: What you should know and should do. *Nursing '78,* 8:68, Feb. 1978.

44. Thorn, G. W., et al.: *Harrison's Principles of Internal Medicine,* 8th ed. New York, McGraw-Hill Book Co., 1977.

45. Tovey, G. H.: Preventing the incompatible blood transfusion. *Hematologia,* 8:389, 1974.

46. Ward, H. N.: Blood grouping tests and transfusions; medicolegal aspects. *Medical Trial Technique Quarterly,* 1972, p. 423.

47. Winterscheid, L. C.: *University Hospital House Staff Manual.* Seattle, University Hospital, 1977.

48. Wintrobe, M. M., et al.: *Clinical Hematology,* 7th ed. Philadelphia, Lea and Febiger, 1974.

CHAPTER 40

CARING FOR PERSONS REQUIRING URINARY CATHETERS

By Barbara Innes, R.N., M.S.

OVERVIEW AND STUDY GUIDE

This chapter discusses the use of urinary catheters. In Chapter 30 you learned about normal micturition and how to help the patient achieve and maintain normal bladder elimination patterns, using such means as fluid intake, exercise, proper positioning and use of the power of positive suggestion. Sometimes, however, these means are not sufficient. Then the use of urinary catheters becomes necessary. In order to help you make safe and efficient use of these catheters, we discuss (a) purposes for and hazards of catheterization; (b) how to select the proper catheter; (c) procedures for inserting and removing a urethral catheter, irrigating a catheter and obtaining a specimen from a urethral catheter and (d) care of the patient who has an indwelling catheter.

As you read this chapter, you need to understand the following terms:

bacteriuria
lumen
patent
bladder atony
catheter clamp
urinary retention
incontinence
residual
nosocomial
meatus
renal calculi

After studying this chapter, you should be able to do the following:

1. List the purposes for which a urinary catheter might be indicated.

2. Describe the variety of catheters available and state possible uses for each.

3. Describe in detail the following procedures: male and female catheterization with a straight catheter and an indwelling catheter; irrigation of a urethral catheter; obtaining a specimen from a catheter; and removal of a urethral catheter.

4. Compare and contrast the lateral position for female catheterization with the dorsal recumbent position.

5. Discuss the techniques and advantages of intermittent self-catheterization.

6. Discuss the common physical and psychological hazards of catheterization.

7. Discuss in detail the nursing care required by a patient with an indwelling catheter.

8. Discuss the needs of patients going home with an indwelling catheter.

Introduction

A *catheter* is defined as a tubular instrument of rubber, plastic, metal or other material, used for draining or injecting fluids or gases through a body passage. *Catheterization* is the process of passing a catheter into a body cavity or channel.

Urinary catheters have been used in medical practice since at least 3000 B.C. The variety of materials used for these first catheters included tin, gold, bronze, wood, iron and plant leaves. It was not until 1730 A.D. that the first flexible catheter was made from woven silk. It is recorded that Benjamin Franklin in 1752 used a catheter made of fine gut. When Goodyear developed the vulcanizing process in the 1800's, rubber catheters soon were produced. This was the advent of catheters as we know them now.[53]

Today the use of urinary catheters is a common medical and nursing intervention, and the care of patients with indwelling catheters is a prevalent nursing activity. Recent years have brought changes in procedure, drainage systems and suggested care of the patient with an indwelling catheter. Numerous studies have been done in this area, often showing contradictory results. Many different recommendations have been made regarding appropriate nursing care. In general, the opinions about urinary catheters are continually fluctuating, with protocols for care varying from agency to agency and even from one person to another. In order to provide quality care, the nurse must be aware of the scientific principles involved and should become familiar with prudent practice in the locale.

The initial factor involved in the consideration of urinary catheters is the decision whether to use a catheter or not. The usual *purposes* for catheterization include the following:

▶ Relief of urinary retention

▶ Preoperative bladder decompression and maintenance of decompression during lower abdominal or pelvic surgery

▶ Lower urinary tract obstruction or paralysis

▶ Splinting of the ureters or urethra to facilitate healing following surgery or other trauma in the region

▶ Instillation of medications into the bladder

▶ Determination of urine residual following voiding

▶ Accurate measurement of urinary output

Until recently, it was considered essential to catheterize the patient in order to obtain a sterile specimen for laboratory analysis. However, it is becoming a much more accepted practice to acquire these specimens by the midstream or "clean catch" method (see Chap. 30). Sometimes the incontinent patient has to be catheterized to achieve a dry environment and prevent skin breakdown, particularly if dressings or skin lesions need to be protected. However, in many cases the catheter is inserted solely for the convenience of the nursing staff and/or the patient's family. Catheterization for the incontinent patient should be used only as a last resort; the

decision to employ this nursing action should be preceded by a concerted effort to achieve continence through careful assessment of the patient's circumstances and a rigorous bladder training program.

There are good reasons not to use the urinary catheter haphazardly. The urinary tract is the most common site of nosocomial infections. Forty per cent of all nosocomial infections reported, involving approximately 400,000 patients in the United States every year, affect the urinary tract; 75 per cent of these patients have undergone urologic instrumentation of some kind.

> *Urinary tract infection is the most frequent complication of catheterization. Elderly, critically ill, and female patients seem to be the most susceptible, and it has been documented that the incidence of bacteriuria increases in direct relationship to the length of time the catheter is left in place.*[8, 64]

Several studies have claimed that the incidence of bacteriuria in catheterized patients ranges from 35 to 95 per cent.[6, 61] Sequelae of these urinary tract infections range from chronic bacteriuria and pyelonephritis through an increasing incidence of gram-negative septicemia.

Other hazards of catheterization include trauma to the lower urinary tract; loss of bladder tone; bladder spasm; and the formation of abscesses, fistulas and skin lesions. These hazards and measures to prevent them are included throughout the rest of the chapter.

ANATOMY OF THE URINARY TRACT

In order to safely perform a catheterization and properly care for the patient subsequently, the nurse must be familiar with the anatomy of the urinary system. The student who feels the need for a more complete review than presented here is encouraged to consult any standard anatomy text.

There are four main anatomical structures in the urinary system: kidneys, ureters, bladder and urethra. The *kidneys* are located retroperitoneally above the iliac crests. Their main function is to filter the blood in order to remove wastes from and regulate fluid and chemical components in the body. Urine excreted from the kidneys travels down the ureters by means of peristaltic action to the bladder. The *ureters* are approximately 25 to 30 centimeters long in adults, begin in the renal pelvis, and enter the bladder obliquely in the pos-

terior portion. At this ureterovesical junction, there is usually an anatomical sphincter that prevents the backward flow, or reflux, of urine into the kidney.

The *urinary bladder* is essentially a holding vessel for the urine. It is a hollow organ with three muscle layers forming its walls. These layers of smooth muscle come together at the base to form the internal sphincter, which is under reflex control from the spinal cord. As the urine enters the bladder from the ureters, the detrusor muscle initially relaxes and the bladder expands. As the bladder distends, it rises above the symphysis pubis and can be palpated and percussed there if it becomes overdistended. Distention continues until there are approximately 150 to 500 ml. of urine in the bladder. At this point, stretch receptors in the detrusor muscle send stimuli to the spinal cord, which returns impulses that cause the internal sphincter to open and urine to flow from the bladder. If the bladder becomes distended with more than 1000 ml., there is danger of resultant loss of bladder tone.

The *urethra* provides the normal channel for expulsion of the urine from the body. It is a simple tube with a mucous membrane lining. The distal end of the urethra includes the external sphincter; it is usually under voluntary cortical control after the toilet-training period in childhood. It is this sphincter which allows continence. The female urethra is approximately 3 to 5 cm. long, and its meatus is normally located in the perineum between the clitoris and the vagina. The male urethra is about 20 cm. long and follows an S-shaped curve from the bladder neck to its meatus on the tip of the penis. The *prostate gland* is an important structure as it relates to the male urinary tract. It is located below the bladder and completely surrounds the proximal urethra. Problems arise when this gland enlarges, as often occurs in older men, to the point that it partially or completely obstructs the urethra. This condition is referred to as benign prostatic hypertrophy and is a common cause of urinary retention in males.

Figures 40–1 and 40–2 diagram the male and female anatomy as it involves the urinary tract. The nurse should be entirely familiar with these anatomical structures before beginning a catheterization procedure.

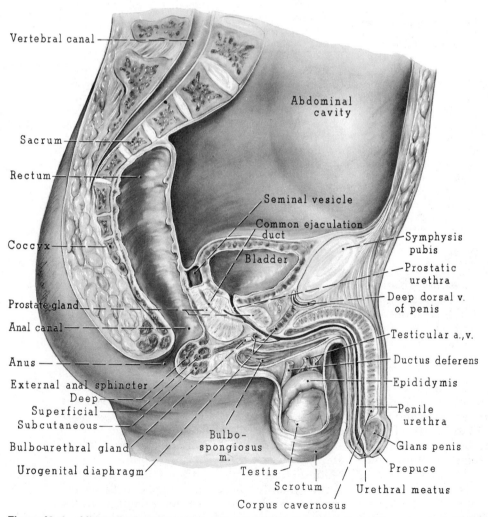

Figure 40–1.   Mid-sagittal section of the male pelvis and external genitalia. (From Jacob, S. W., and Francone, C. A.: *Structure and Function in Man,* 2nd ed. Philadelphia, W. B. Saunders Co., 1970, p. 567.)

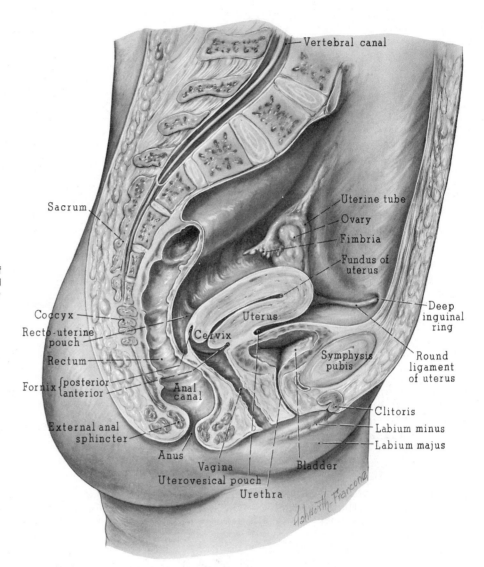

Figure 40–2. Mid-sagittal section of the female pelvis. (From Jacob and Francone: *Structure and Function in Man*, 2nd ed., p. 512.)

Labels in figure: Vertebral canal — Uterine tube — Ovary — Fimbria — Fundus of uterus — Sacrum — Deep inguinal ring — Uterus — Coccyx — Recto-uterine pouch — Cervix — Symphysis pubis — Round ligament of uterus — Rectum — Fornix {posterior, anterior} — Anal canal — Clitoris — Labium minus — Labium majus — External anal sphincter — Anus — Vagina — Bladder — Uterovesical pouch — Urethra

TYPES OF CATHETERS

Materials

Most catheters are currently made of plastic, although some rubber ones are also being used. Glass, metal or woven silk catheters may be used at times during diagnostic or therapeutic procedures or with male patients where attempted insertion of a rubber or plastic catheter has been unsuccessful.

Several studies have been done to determine whether specific catheter materials could reduce the incidence of bacteriuria. Contradictory results have been reported. In some studies, the use of silicone-coated catheters rather than latex seemed to decrease the amount of encrustation that occurred on the catheter itself, presumably due to the reduced adsorption of organic material to the catheter and absorption of it by the catheter. The inert surface seemed to produce less mucosal reaction, with its resultant hemorrhage and edema.[5, 23, 63] However, another study— including 287 patients—showed no significant differences when a polymer-coated catheter was used.[52] These studies also demonstrated contradictory findings regarding the relationship between the duration of catheter placement and the amount of encrustation found.

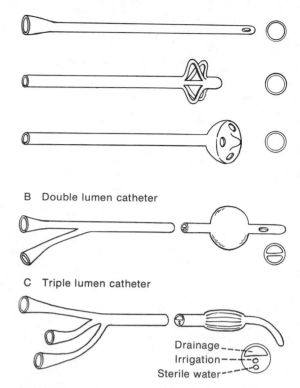

Single lumen catheter

B Double lumen catheter

C Triple lumen catheter

Drainage
Irrigation
Sterile water

Figure 40–3. Catheter configurations. The circles at the right of the figure demonstrate the inner configuration of the tubing. *A,* These catheters are single-lumen catheters for drainage. The straight catheter is to be inserted and removed. The other two catheters are retention catheters. *B,* This is a retention catheter, with an inflatable balloon by which it is retained in the bladder. *C,* This retention catheter is used for closed continuous or intermittent irrigation of the bladder or catheter.

Sizes

Catheters are sized according to the French scale. In this system, each French unit is the equivalent of 1/3 mm. in diameter. Thus an 18 Fr. catheter would be 6 mm. in diameter.

The size of the urethral catheter used depends on the size of the patient. While there is no rule, a general guideline is to use size 8–10 for children, 14–16 for adult females and 18–20 for adult males. If the catheter is *too small,* it is liable to curl up on itself when it meets any kind of obstruction in the urethra. Also, the smaller the catheter diameter, the more likely it is to be obstructed by blood clots or mucus plugs. On the other hand, if the tube is *too large* and causes undue pressure on the meatus or urethra and surrounding structures, it can lead to tissue erosion.

Configuration

Figure 40–3 depicts a variety of catheter configurations. The principal differences in configuration are in the shape of the catheter tip and the number of lumens within the tube. The most commonly used catheter has a rounded tip with either a single or multiple drainage holes, called eyes. The *Coudé* catheter has a curved tip, which allows easier passage around a partial obstruction in the urethra. The variety of *mushroom-tip* catheters provide for single lumen catheters which can be self-retaining, although external immobilization is usually essential.

The number of *lumens* in a catheter refers to the various compartments into which the inside of the catheter tubing is divided. Each compartment has a specific purpose. The urethral catheter usually contains one to three lumens, depending on the number of functions it is meant to perform.

The most commonly utilized catheters are the straight catheter and the indwelling. The *straight* catheter is usually a single- or multi-eyed round-tip tube. It is not intended to be left in the bladder beyond the insertion procedure itself and is used to check for residual urine, obtain a urine specimen, instill medication, and intermittently relieve bladder distention. It can be left in place but requires very careful exterior taping and greatly restricts the movement allowed the patient.

The *indwelling,* or *Foley,* catheter is a reten-

tion catheter, which may be used for all of the above reasons plus for more long-term decompression of the bladder. It is usually connected to drainage tubing and a collection bag so that it can continually drain urine from the bladder. This catheter is usually a single-eyed, round-tip catheter with a double lumen. One lumen provides for drainage of urine while the other lumen leads to a balloon located just above the drainage eye on the catheter. This balloon is deflated during insertion of the catheter, but once the catheter is in place inside the bladder, the balloon is inflated with sterile water through the appropriate lumen. The balloon is then too large to pass into the urethra and so rests on the trigone and keeps the catheter in place as long as desired. Some triple lumen catheters are also used as retention catheters; with these tubes, the third lumen provides a channel for irrigation fluid.

The *condom,* often called the condom catheter, is an external collecting device used with incontinent males. It consists of a plastic or rubber sheath which is placed over the penis and connected to a drainage system. Because it is an entirely external device, it does not fit into the discussion of urinary catheters and was discussed more fully in Chapter 30.

ROUTES OF CATHETERIZATION

There are three routes of catheterization as related to the urinary tract: ureteral, suprapubic and urethral. *Ureteral catheterization* is accomplished by placing small catheters, called ureteral catheters, through the ureters into the renal pelvis. This may be done by threading the catheters through the urethra and the bladder and then entering the ureters or by surgical insertion through the abdominal wall. These catheters are placed to splint the ureters and prevent their obstruction from edema following surgery or other trauma in the area. If the nurse suspects that ureteral catheters are plugged, the doctor should be notified immediately.

> *Since the renal pelvis holds only 3 to 5 ml. before tissue damage due to pressure begins, it is absolutely essential that ureteral catheters be kept patent. They are never clamped for any reason.*

Suprapubic catheterization is one means of achieving bladder drainage. Although in practice it seems to be gaining popularity, not much has been written in the periodical literature about it. Suprapubic catheterizaion may be accomplished in two ways: (1) the mushroom-tip catheter may be placed in the bladder through a small incision in the abdominal wall or (2) the suprapubic catheter may be inserted into the bladder using a trocar. This procedure may be done under general anesthesia if another surgical procedure is being performed; however, it can also be done at the patient's bedside under a local anesthetic agent. The suprapubic catheter may be sutured in place for added security. The retention catheter is then attached to a drainage system as with the urethral catheter. Care of the system is similar to that of the urethral catheter. When the tube is removed, the muscle layers of the bladder immediately contract over the puncture site and the surface wound is small, negating the need for closing sutures. Langley and others feel that this route reduces the incidence of urinary tract infection to about 10 per cent and is much more comfortable and convenient for the patient.[47]

The *urethral route* of catheterization is by far the most commonly used. The catheter is inserted through the external meatus into the urethra beyond the internal sphincter into the bladder. The rest of this chapter is devoted to catheterization by this route.

URETHRAL CATHETERIZATION

Urethral catheterization is not an independent nursing action, but requires a physician's order. Sometimes there is a definite order for catheterization. Frequently, however, a prn order is left, requesting that the patient be catheterized in the event of urinary retention. If this is the case, the nurse must carefully assess the patient in order to make a sound clinical judgment. You learned in Chapter 30 how to assess for the presence of urinary retention. *Retention is a hazardous condition not only because it can lead to loss of bladder tone, but because of its potential role in the development of urinary tract infection and renal calculi.* Lapides states that most cases of urinary bacteriuria are due to tissue ischemia caused by increased intravesical pressure and/or overdistention. Resultant reduced blood flow makes the tissue more susceptible to bacterial invasion from the patient's own colon via either the blood or lymph circulation systems.[48, 49] Urinary retention should be acted on early. However, you are also familiar with some of the potential hazards of catheterization. Therefore you will want to institute catheterization to relieve urinary retention only when it is prudent. Such a decision is highly individualized and is based on careful assessment of each patient.

Once the decision has been made to catheterize the patient, the nurse must carry out a procedure which strictly adheres to principles of surgical asepsis, body mechanics, work organization, and maintenance of effective interpersonal relationships. The procedures offered here are one model. As you observe other nurses, you will see variations, but make sure the procedure you adopt for yourself is based upon sound principles.

The insertion of a straight catheter is done exactly as is the insertion of an indwelling catheter up to the point where the catheter is in the bladder and urine is flowing out. The insertion procedure stops here, since there is no balloon to inflate or drainage system to connect. The catheter is held securely in place until its purpose has been achieved and then is removed as described later in the chapter.

28.   FEMALE URETHRAL CATHETERIZATION: INDWELLING OR STRAIGHT CATHETER

Definition and Purposes.   *This procedure is done to insert a urinary catheter through the urethra into the bladder.* Bladder catheterization is done to drain urine from or instill medication into the bladder or to splint the urethra and prevent edema from obstructing it.

Contraindications and Cautions.   In order to avoid the introduction of bacteria into the urinary system, strict sterile technique must be used throughout this procedure. Equipment must be arranged so that none of the principles of sterile technique are violated during the procedure. The nurse should also review the procedure each time before doing it on a patient, so that the necessary organization will be well in mind.

Often two or more persons are necessary to help with the catheterization. If the patient is restless or otherwise unable to stay still, enough help must be available to assure good visualization of the meatus and to avoid contamination of the sterile field. Also, depending on the lighting available in the room, another person may be necessary to hold a flashlight shining on the perineum.

Patient-Family Teaching Points.   Provide the patient-family with the following information: (a) reason for the catheterization; (b) what the nurse(s) will be doing during the procedure; (c) how the patient can cooperate during the procedure; (d) that the catheterization is not usually painful, but that the patient will probably experience a sensation of pressure; (e) how the catheter and drainage system will be cared for after the insertion; and (f) how the patient can move around with an indwelling catheter.

PRE-PROCEDURE ACTIVITIES

PRELIMINARY ASSESSMENT

▶ Physician's order
▶ Chart for indication of previous catheterization
▶ Signs of urinary retention, if appropriate
▶ Patient's ability to comply with requests
▶ Patient's ability to achieve and maintain desired position
▶ Gross state of cleanliness of perineum
▶ Kind of lighting in room

PREPARATION OF PATIENT

▶ Explain procedure to patient: reason for catheterization; what nurse(s) will be doing; what patient can do to help

EQUIPMENT

▶ Sterile catheterization tray including:
  wrapper to use as sterile field
  gloves
  fenestrated drape
  plastic-coated underpad
  lubricant
  antiseptic cleansing material
  specimen container and lid
  forceps
  straight or retention catheter
  syringe with solution to inflate balloon, if appropriate
  collection basin
▶ Sterile drainage tubing and collection bag, if appropriate

PREPARATION OF PATIENT

▶ Move bed so you can stand on the side which puts your dominant side toward bottom of bed
▶ Clear off overbed table
▶ Provide for continuing privacy
▶ Raise bed to working height; lower side rail
▶ Place overbed table with equipment on it perpendicular to bed on your dominant side
▶ Move patient close to your side of bed
▶ Position patient in either dorsal recumbent or lateral position (Fig. 40–4). (The dorsal recumbent position will be used in this procedure; the lateral position is an alternative.)

EQUIPMENT

▶ Tape, if appropriate
▶ Rubber band and safety pin, if appropriate
▶ Garbage bag—may use plastic cover of catheterization tray if appropriate
▶ Bath blanket or other appropriate draping material
▶ Flashlight or gooseneck lamp if needed
▶ Basin of warm water, soap, washcloth and towel, if needed

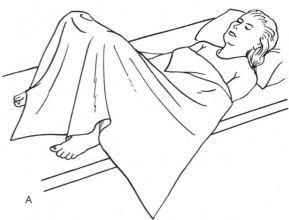

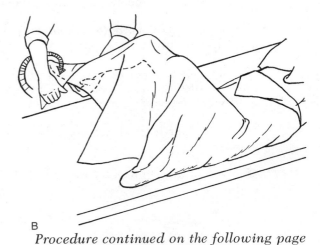

Figure 40–4. Dorsal recumbent positioning and draping for female catheterization. *A*, Bath blanket is placed diamond-fashion over the patient. *B*, One corner is wrapped securely around each foot, leaving the fourth corner draped over the perineum until the procedure is begun.

Procedure continued on the following page

PREPARATION OF PATIENT

▶ Drape patient as shown in Figure 40–4. A bath blanket or sheet is placed diamond-fashion over patient, and two corners are wrapped around each foot respectively. The corner covering the perineum can be lifted out of way just before procedure is begun.
▶ Wash and dry perineum, if necessary
▶ Focus light source correctly. Adjust gooseneck lamp, if appropriate, to shine on perineum. If flashlight being used, position person holding it so light will be effective, but not in the way.

PROCEDURE

SUGGESTED STEPS

1. If you are inserting indwelling catheter which will be connected to *drainage system:*

a. Remove drainage system from its outside container according to directions on package;

b. Attach collection bag to bed frame near bottom of bed;

c. Bring end of drainage tubing up between side rail and mattress;

d. Place end of drainage tubing so it is convenient to reach and will not fall off mattress during catheterization procedure.

2. Open sterile catheterization tray cover according to directions on package.

3. If using the plastic bag as garbage bag, place it so you do not have to pass over sterile field when reaching for it.

4. Open sterile pack as described in Procedure 22.

5. Don sterile gloves as described in Procedure 23.

RATIONALE/ASSESSMENT

a. Be careful not to dislodge cover over end of drainage tubing. This cover assures continued sterility of inside of drainage system.

b. Collection bag must remain below level of bladder to prevent backflow of urine into bladder.

c. Make sure side rail can operate without getting tangled up with or pinching drainage tubing. This helps maintain patency of system.

3. Reaching over sterile area increases risk of contamination.

5. Wearing sterile gloves allows you to handle sterile items without contaminating them.

SUGGESTED STEPS	RATIONALE/ASSESSMENT
6. Pick up solid plastic-coated drape, stand back from table, grasp corner of drape, and allow it to fall open.	6. Standing back from table will prevent drape from becoming contaminated by brushing against table as it opens.
7. Grasping this drape at top, with plastic side away from you, fold top of drape over your gloved hands to make cuff.	7. Be careful not to touch rest of drape with your arm, which would render it unsterile.
8. Place this drape, with plastic side down, on bed between patient's legs. Slip cuffed edge just under edge of patient's buttocks. Pull your hands out, being careful not to touch anything but center of sterile drape itself if it is necessary to straighten drape.	
9. If desired, pick up fenestrated drape (with hole in center) and open it as in Step 5. Then place it over perineum so that hole exposes labia.	9. Although this drape is included in all commercially-prepared catheterization trays, your use of it is optional. Main advantage of this drape is that it provides larger sterile field; however, many people feel that it gets in the way, thereby increasing the chance of contamination. If you decide not to use this drape, pick it out of sterile tray and drop it aside.
10. Place sterile tray on sterile drape between patient's legs.	10. Sterile objects which are out of line of vision may be accidentally contaminated.
11. If you will be obtaining urine specimen, remove lid from specimen container. Place container on end of overbed table. Set lid loosely on container.	11. When you reach point of obtaining specimen, you will have only one hand free. If you won't be needing specimen, pick container out of sterile tray and drop it aside.
12. Lubricate catheter tip with water-soluble lubricant about 3.75 to 5 cm. (1½ to 2 inches). Do not plug drainage hole.	12. Lubrication reduces friction, thereby facilitating insertion of catheter. Some authorities suggest using antimicrobial lubricant to reduce chance of infection.
13. If indwelling catheter being inserted, attach syringe and inflating solution to lumen valve of catheter.	13. Although this can be done later in procedure, you will have only one hand available at that time. Attaching the syringe now is a matter of convenience.
14. Prepare antiseptic cleansing material as directed on package.	
15. Separate labia with nondominant hand to expose meatus. See Figures 40–5 and 40–6.	15. Good visualization of meatus is essential to safe catheterization.
a. Place thumb and forefinger between labia minora.	

Procedure continued on the following page

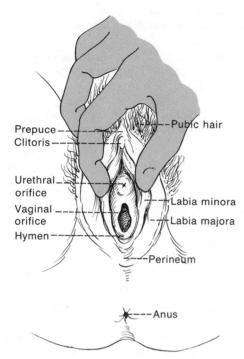

Prepuce
Clitoris
Pubic hair
Urethral orifice
Vaginal orifice
Hymen
Labia minora
Labia majora
Perineum
Anus

Figure 40–5. Anatomic landmarks of importance during female catheterization.

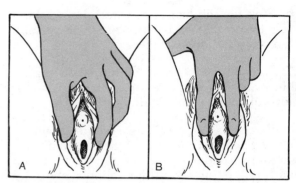

Figure 40–6. Alternate methods of finger placement to separate labia for female catheterization. *A,* Thumb and forefinger. *B,* Forefinger and middle finger.

Suggested Steps	Rationale/Assessment
b. Separate labia and pull up.	b. Pulling up on labia smooths out perineum. If you are catheterizing postpartum patient with episiotomy (incision to enlarge vaginal outlet), stretching outward rather than upward prevents painful pulling on stitches.
c. Maintain this separation throughout insertion procedure.	c. If labia accidentally close over meatus at any time after cleansing process has begun, they must be separated again and procedure restarted with Step 15.

Remember that from this time on, nondominant hand is contaminated and cannot be used to handle any sterile equipment.

16. Cleanse meatal area using cleansing material provided in catheterization tray.	16. Reducing number of microorganisms in area minimizes their introduction into sterile cavity.

SUGGESTED STEPS	RATIONALE/ASSESSMENT
a. Use each cotton ball for only one wipe and then discard in garbage bag.	a. If cotton balls are used, use forceps to handle them. This maintains sterility of glove so it can be used to handle catheter.
b. Wipe from front to back of perineum, i.e., from clitoris toward anus.	b. Moving from cleaner area to dirtier area, prevents introducing new organisms into cleaner area.
c. Cleanse in following order: far labia, near labia, directly over meatus.	c. Downward pull directly over meatus stretches it and makes it more visible. Be sure you have identified meatus before proceeding.
17. Pick up catheter with gloved hand about 7.5 cm. (3 inches) from tip.	17. Be sure drainage end of catheter remains inside collection basin to avoid urine running out over bed. If necessary, move collection basin closer to perineum.
18. Have patient gently bear down as though trying to urinate.	18. Trying to urinate opens sphincters and allows easier passage of catheter.
19. Gently insert catheter about 5 to 7.5 cm. (2 to 3 inches).	19. If urine does not flow, slowly rotate catheter, since drainage hole may be against bladder wall. If catheter is contaminated during procedure, obtain new catheterization tray and begin procedure from Step 2. If catheter enters vagina instead of urethra, leave it in place as landmark until catheterization process is successfully completed.
20. Release labia and hold catheter securely with nondominant hand. Rest hand on patient's pubis for support.	20. Securing catheter will prevent peristaltic action from pushing catheter out into bed. It also prevents contamination from withdrawal and reinsertion of catheter. Maintain this position until catheterization is completed or balloon on indwelling catheter has been inflated.
21. Obtain *specimen* if needed.	
a. Remove lid from specimen container and drop it top down on table.	
b. Place specimen container on bed beside collection basin.	
c. Pinch catheter with nondominant hand to stop flow of urine.	
d. Pick up drainage end of catheter and hold it over specimen container.	
e. Unclamp fingers and allow 30 ml. to drain into specimen container.	

Procedure continued on the following page

SUGGESTED STEPS	RATIONALE/ASSESSMENT
f. Re-pinch catheter and place drainage end into collection basin.	
g. Allow urine flow from bladder to resume.	
h. Place specimen container on overbed table and secure the lid.	
22. Allow urine to continue flowing until bladder empties or until maximum of 1000 ml. has been removed, according to agency's policy.	22. Most textbooks caution against removing more than 1000 ml. from the bladder at any one time. It is theorized that removing more than this will release pressure on pelvic blood vessels, leading to shock syndrome. However, this fact is not substantiated in literature, and very large amounts are often removed from bladders of postpartum women without complication.
23. With straight catheter, when flow decreases, withdraw catheter slowly until urine barely drips. Then remove catheter completely.	
24. If indwelling catheter has been inserted:	
a. Inflate balloon with solution provided in syringe;	a. If patient complains of pain during inflation, balloon may be mispositioned in urethra. Withdraw all solution injected and advance catheter about 1.25 cm. (½ inch). Try again to inflate balloon.
b. Pull gently on catheter to make sure that balloon is inflated enough to retain catheter;	
c. Attach drainage tubing from collection system to catheter without contaminating either end;	
d. Tape catheter to inner thigh;	d. Use nonallergenic tape. Leave enough slack to allow adduction of leg and to avoid pressure on meatus.
e. Coil excess drainage tubing and fasten it to sheet on top surface of mattress with rubber band and safety pin (see text for explanation).	e. Avoiding loops in drainage tubing from top of mattress to collection bag will aid in preventing backflow of urine into bladder.

Post-Procedure Activities. Wash and dry perineum; remove the perineal drapes; return the patient to a supine position; remove the bath blanket or sheet used as a drape and replace the bed covers; lower the bed and raise the side rail if necessary. If the patient has an indwelling catheter, teach her: (a) how to move around without disrupting the drainage system and (b) how the catheter and drainage system will be tended.

Aftercare of Equipment. Discard the disposable equipment; place non-disposable equipment in the appropriate collection area; label and take the urine specimen promptly to the laboratory.

Charting/Recording. Record on the appropriate forms the following information: time, reason for doing the catheterization, type and size of catheter used, amount and characteristics of urine removed, patient's reaction to the catheterization, any problems encountered during the procedure, and whether or not a specimen was taken.

LATERAL POSITION FOR FEMALE CATHETERIZATION

The position utilized in the procedure for female catheterization was the dorsal recumbent. An alternate position is the lateral (Fig. 40–7). In the lateral position, the female patient lies on her side with knees and hips flexed. The upper leg is flexed to a greater degree than the lower leg. The patient's buttocks are placed close to the edge of the bed toward the nurse and the shoulders are angled toward the opposite side of the bed. The patient is thus lying diagonally in the bed. The catheterization procedure is carried out exactly as described in Procedure 28 except that instead of separating the labia with the fingers of one hand, the nurse lifts the upper labia in order to visualize the meatus.[59]

Edman systematically compared the lateral and dorsal recumbent positions during catheterization according to three criteria: patient comfort, meatal visibility and maintenance of exposure. Overall, she determined that the dorsal recumbent position was preferable as measured against these factors.[21] How-

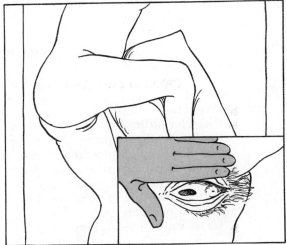

Figure 40–7. Lateral position for female catheterization. Inset demonstrates lifting of upper labia during procedure.

ever, other authors have preferred the lateral position. They felt that the advantages were decreased embarrassment and anxiety, better body mechanics for the nurse, larger working area, and easier maintenance of meatal visibility.[19]

The lateral position is not widely used at this time, but it is certainly an alternative for further investigation.

29. MALE URETHRAL CATHETERIZATION: INDWELLING OR STRAIGHT CATHETER

Definition and Purposes. *This procedure is done to insert a urinary catheter through the urethra into the bladder.* Bladder catheterization is done to drain the urine from or instill medication into the bladder or to splint the urethra and prevent edema from obstructing it.

Contraindications and Cautions. In order to avoid the introduction of bacteria into the urinary system, strict sterile technique must be used throughout this procedure. Equipment must be arranged so that none of the principles of sterile technique are violated during the procedure. The nurse should also review the procedure each time before doing it on a patient so that the necessary organization will be well in mind.

Sometimes, two or more persons may be necessary to help with the catheterization. If the patient is restless or otherwise unable to stay still, enough help must be available to assure good visualization of the meatus and to avoid contamination of the sterile field.

Patient-Family Teaching Points. Provide the patient-family with the following information: (a) reason for the catheterization; (b) what the nurse(s) will be doing during the procedure; (c) how the patient can cooperate during the procedure; (d) that the catheterization is not usually painful, but that the patient will probably experience a sensation of pressure; (e) how the catheter and drainage system will be cared for after insertion; and (f) how the patient can move around with an indwelling catheter.

PRE-PROCEDURE ACTIVITIES

PRELIMINARY ASSESSMENT

▶ Physician's order
▶ Chart for indication of previous catheterization, indication of possible urethral obstruction (i.e., benign prostatic hypertrophy)
▶ Signs of urinary retention, if appropriate
▶ Patient's ability to follow requests
▶ Patient's ability to achieve and maintain desired position
▶ Gross state of cleanliness of perineum

EQUIPMENT

▶ Sterile catheterization tray including:
  wrapper to use as sterile field
  gloves
  fenestrated drape
  plastic-coated underpad
  lubricant
  antiseptic cleansing material
  specimen container and lid
  forceps
  straight or retention catheter

PREPARATION OF PATIENT

▶ Explain procedure to patient: reason for catheterization, what nurse(s) will be doing, what patient can do to help
▶ Move bed so you can stand on side which puts your dominant side toward bottom of bed
▶ Clear off overbed table
▶ Provide for continuing privacy
▶ Raise bed to working height, lower side rail
▶ Place overbed table with equipment on it perpendicular to bed on your dominant side
▶ Move patient to your side of bed
▶ Position patient in supine position
▶ Drape patient as indicated in Figure 40–8. Fold top bed covers back to below perineum. Cover top half of patient with bath blanket for warmth.
▶ Wash and dry perineum, if necessary. If patient uncircumcised, retract foreskin during cleansing.

EQUIPMENT

syringe with solution to inflate balloon, if appropriate
collection basin
▶ Sterile drainage tubing and collection bag, if appropriate
▶ Tape, if appropriate
▶ Rubber band and safety pin, if appropriate
▶ Garbage bag—may use plastic covering of catheterization tray if appropriate
Bath blanket or other draping material
Basin of warm water, soap, washcloth and towel, if needed

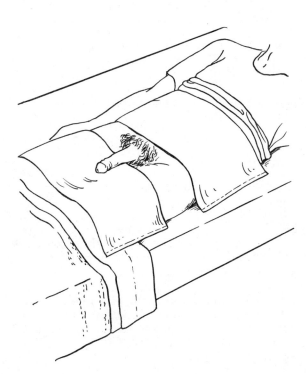

Figure 40–8. Draping for male catheterization.

Procedure continued on the following page

PROCEDURE

SUGGESTED STEPS	RATIONALE/ASSESSMENT
1. If you are inserting indwelling catheter which will be connected to *drainage system:*	
a. Remove drainage system from its outside container according to directions on package;	a. Be careful not to dislodge cover over end of drainage tubing. This cover assures continued sterility of inside of drainage system.
b. Attach collection bag to bed frame near bottom of bed;	b. Collection bag must remain below level of bladder to prevent backflow of urine into bladder.
c. Bring end of drainage tubing up between side rail and mattress;	c. Make sure side rail can operate without getting tangled up with or pinching drainage tubing. This helps maintain patency of system.
d. Place end of drainage tubing so it is convenient to reach and won't fall off mattress during catheterization procedure.	
2. Open sterile catheterization tray according to directions on package.	
3. If using plastic bag as garbage bag, place it so you do not have to reach over sterile field when reaching for it.	3. Reaching over sterile field increases risk of contamination.
4. Open sterile pack as described in Procedure 22, p. 929.	
5. Don sterile gloves as described in Procedure 23, p. 935.	5. Wearing sterile gloves allows you to handle sterile items without contaminating them.
6. Pick up solid plastic-coated drape, stand back from table, grasp corner of drape, and allow it to fall open.	6. Standing back from table will prevent drape from becoming contaminated by brushing against table as it opens.
7. Grasping drape at top, with plastic side away from you, fold top of drape over your gloved hands to make cuff.	7. Be careful not to touch rest of drape with your arm, which would render it unsterile.
8. Place this drape, with plastic side down, on patient's leg below penis. Pull your hands out, being careful not to touch anything but center of sterile drape itself if it is necessary to straighten drape.	
9. Pick up fenestrated drape (with hole in center) and open it as in Step 6. Cuff it over	9. Be careful not to contaminate either of your gloved hands while placing drape. An

SUGGESTED STEPS	RATIONALE/ASSESSMENT
your gloved hands as in Step 7. Then place it so penis goes through hole.	alternative method is to complete Steps 11 to 14 before placing drape. Then nondominant hand can be used to lift penis while dominant hand places drape.
10. If you will be obtaining *urine specimen,* remove lid from specimen container. Place container onto overbed table. Set lid loosely on container.	10. When you reach point of obtaining specimen, you will have only one hand free. If you will not be needing specimen, pick container out of sterile tray and drop it aside.
11. Lubricate catheter tip with water-soluble lubricant about 17.5 cm. (7 inches). Do not plug drainage hole.	11. Lubrication reduces friction, thereby facilitating insertion of catheter. Some authorities suggest using antimicrobial lubricant to reduce chance of infection.
12. If indwelling catheter is being inserted, attach syringe and inflating solution to lumen valve of catheter.	12. Although this can be done later in procedure, you will have only one hand available at that time. Attaching syringe now is a matter of convenience.
13. Prepare antiseptic cleansing material as directed on package.	
14. Bring overbed table with its equipment as close to working area as possible. Place collection basin on patient's legs near base of penis.	14. Sterile objects which are out of line of vision may be accidentally contaminated.
15. Pick up penis with nondominant hand. Retract foreskin and grasp penis directly behind glans and spread urinary meatus between thumb and forefinger.	15. Be sure to grasp penis firmly; otherwise, light stimulation may cause an erection. If erection occurs at any time during catheter insertion, procedure should be discontinued until penis regains non-erectile state. Erection may cause embarrassment for nurse and/or patient; therefore nurse should matter-of-factly tell patient that insertion cannot be done during erection, so procedure will be stopped until erection is gone and then will be started again. If erection disappears immediately, nurse can continue with catheterization. However, nurse may have to leave room for a few minutes; if this is necessary, procedure must begin again with step 2, using new catheterization tray.

> *Remember that from this time on, nondominant hand is contaminated and cannot be used to handle any sterile equipment.*

If penis should be dropped or foreskin released at any time after cleansing process has begun, procedure must begin again with Step 15.

Procedure continued on the following page

SUGGESTED STEPS	RATIONALE/ASSESSMENT
16. Cleanse penis, using circular motion. Start over meatus and work down toward base of glans. Cleanse to just above hand holding penis.	16. Reducing number of organisms in area minimizes their introduction into sterile cavity. Moving from cleaner to dirtier areas prevents the introduction of new organisms into cleaner area.
17. Repeat Step 16 twice more, using new cotton ball or swab each time.	
18. Pick up catheter with forceps about 5 to 7.5 cm. (2 to 3 inches) from tip. Hold distal end of catheter in palm of hand with last three fingers.	18. Catheter is difficult to direct with its long expanse of lubrication.
19. Draw penis upward and forward at 60- to 90-degree angle to patient's legs so that it is as nearly perpendicular to patient's body as possible.	19. Perpendicular position straightens out urethra as much as possible and provides maximum ease for passage of catheter.
20. Have patient gently bear down as though trying to urinate. Insert tip of catheter into urethra. Grasp another 5 to 7.5 cm. (2 to 3 inches) of tubing with forceps and insert until resistance is met.	20. Trying to urinate opens sphincters and allows easier passage of catheter.
21. Gently insert catheter about 17.5 to 20 cm. (7 to 8 inches).	21. If resistance is felt to insertion, stop and wait a few minutes to see if it is temporary spasm of sphincter. Have patient take deep breath; change angle of penis. If there is still resistance, stop procedure and call patient's physician.

Because of the many blind passageways in male urethra, never force catheter.

If urine doesn't flow, slowly rotate catheter since drainage hole may be against bladder wall. If catheter is contaminated during procedure, obtain new catheterization tray and begin procedure from Step 2.

22. Lower penis and hold securely to catheter with nondominant hand. Rest hand on patient's pubis for support. Place end of catheter in collection basin.	22. Securing catheter will prevent peristaltic action from pushing catheter out into bed. It also prevents contamination from withdrawing and reinserting catheter. Maintain this position until catheterization is completed or balloon on indwelling catheter has been inflated.
23. Obtain *specimen* if needed.	

SUGGESTED STEPS	RATIONALE/ASSESSMENT

a. Remove lid from specimen container and lay it, top down, on table.

b. Place specimen container on patient's legs beside collection basin if patient can lie still.

c. Pinch catheter with nondominant hand to stop flow of urine.

d. Pick up drainage end of catheter and hold it over specimen container.

e. Unclamp fingers and allow 30 ml. to drain into specimen container.

f. Re-pinch catheter and place drainage end into collection basin.

g. Allow urine flow from bladder to resume.

h. Place specimen container on overbed table and secure lid.

24. Allow urine to continue flowing until bladder empties or until maximum of 1000 ml. has been removed, according to agency's policy.

24. Most textbooks caution against removing more than 1000 ml. from bladder at any one time. It is theorized that removing more than this will release pressure on pelvic blood vessels, leading to shock syndrome. However, this fact is not substantiated in literature.

25. With straight catheter, when flow of urine decreases, withdraw catheter slowly until urine barely drips. Then remove catheter completely. Replace foreskin.

25. Foreskin is replaced as quickly as possible to avoid constriction at base of glans resulting in edema.

26. If indwelling catheter has been inserted:

a. Inflate balloon with solution provided in syringe;

a. If patient complains of pain during inflation, balloon may be mispositioned in urethra. Withdraw all solution injected and advance catheter about 1.25 cm. (½ inch). Try again to inflate balloon.

b. Pull gently on catheter to make sure that balloon is inflated enough to retain catheter;

c. Attach drainage tubing from collection system to catheter without contaminating end of either;

Procedure continued on the following page

SUGGESTED STEPS	RATIONALE/ASSESSMENT
d. Tape catheter either to inner thigh or abdomen;	d. Use nonallergenic tape. Leave enough slack to allow full range of motion and to avoid pressure on meatus.
e. Coil excess drainage tubing and fasten it to sheet at top surface of mattress with rubber band and safety pin. (See text for explanation.)	e. Avoiding loops in drainage tubing will aid in preventing backflow of urine into bladder.

Post-Procedure Activities.   Immediately report failure to pass catheter or inability to replace foreskin. Wash and dry perineum; replace foreskin over the glans; remove the perineal drapes; remove the bath blanket or sheet used as a drape and replace the bed covers; lower the bed and raise the side rail if necessary. If the patient has an indwelling catheter, teach him (a) how to move around without disrupting the drainage system, and (b) how the catheter and drainage system will be tended.

Aftercare of Equipment.   Discard the disposable equipment, place nondisposable equipment in the appropriate collection area, label and take the urine specimen to the laboratory.

Charting/Recording.   Record on the appropriate forms the following information: time, reason for doing the catheterization, type and size of catheter used, amount and characteristics of urine removed, patient's reaction to the catheterization, any problems encountered during the procedure, and whether or not a specimen was taken.

INTERMITTENT CATHETERIZATION

An alternative to long-term catheters has come about by the development of *intermittent catheterization* protocols. This type of program consists of inserting a straight urethral catheter into the bladder at specified time intervals, draining the urine, and removing the catheter. The purposes of this process are to establish a balanced catheter-free bladder with a reduced incidence of urinary tract infection, for long-term treatment of atonic bladders with a large capacity, and for short-term management of temporary bladder atony.[34] The most frequent participants in intermittent catheterization programs are those patients who have musculo-skeletal and/or neurological deficits which make normal micturition impossible, e.g., spinal cord injury and meningomyelocele.

The catheterization procedure may be done by the patient himself (self-catheterization) or by anyone else in his environment who has been trained appropriately. Patients are encouraged to learn self-catheterization as soon as possible, since it greatly increases their independence and allows for expansion of their environments. Children are taught to do self-catheterization usually at age 6 to 9 years.

Most of the intermittent catheterization procedures described recently in the literature advocate a clean technique rather than a sterile one. The patient is usually away from the hospital, with its high risk of nosocomial infections, and also is more likely to follow the prescribed clean procedure without breaks in technique. Clean technique has not resulted in any increase in the rate of urinary tract infection when compared with sterile technique.[55, 71]

The clean technique used for insertion of the catheter involves some variations from the catheterization technique in Procedures 28 and 29. Gloves are not worn, so good handwashing is essential before the procedure is begun. Treated towelettes may be used if handwashing facilities are not available. Because of the natural lubrication of the female urethra, females use no lubricant on the catheter. Males do use a water-soluble lubricant because of the length of the urethra; they are more susceptible to traumatic urethritis.

The patient's position during self-catheterization may be either sitting or standing. When the female utilizes a standing posture, she usually has one foot on the floor and places the other on a chair or the toilet seat to allow better identification of the meatus. A mirror may be used at first by the female as she is learning to locate the meatus, but she should not be allowed to become dependent upon it since she may frequently find herself in situations without a mirror. The patient is taught, as appropriate, to do the self-catheterization in the various positions he may need to assume. If he wears braces, he must learn to insert the catheter with and without the braces present. The patient must learn to be flexible enough to handle any situation with which he is confronted.

A few authors suggest soaking the catheters in a detergent between catheterizations. However, most advocate washing the catheter with soap and water after the procedure, rinsing and drying, and then storing the catheter in a plastic sandwich bag or other clean container. The catheter may be periodically sterilized by boiling.

Timing is the key factor in the success of intermittent catheterization programs. Catheterizations must be carried out at specified time intervals throughout the entire 24-hour period. If a patient is incapable of adhering to this schedule, he is not an appropriate candidate for the program. The time interval between catheterizations is set for each individual patient according to his degree of continence. For adults, the initial time interval is usually every 4 hours, and for a child, it is every 2½ to 4 hours. This interval is gradually lengthened as the patient progresses.

There is much variety in the amount of fluids allowed. Some programs allow the patient to have fluids as desired, while others restrict fluid intake to varying degrees. This particular aspect of the program needs systematic investigation.

In general, the program seems to be a success. Although not 100 per cent effective with all people, it seems to be successful enough that it is certainly a viable alternative to long-term catheters. Success is measured by two main parameters: catheter-free bladder and absence of bacteriuria. Studies report sterile urine in 39 to 77 per cent of the patients and achievement of a catheter-free bladder in 73 to 90 per cent of the program participants.[34, 49, 55, 66, 71] These results may be due to several factors, including intermittent bladder distention, which stimulates normal micturition reflex and reactivation of the bladder's normal antibacterial properties. The program is not, however, a panacea; and the literature documents cases in which the program was not successful for a variety of reasons.

Problems occur when facilities are not readily available or when a brace's trunk supports press on the bladder. Children sometimes have difficulty interrupting their activities so frequently; this program involves a lot of responsibility on their part. Some patients in the program have developed a silent hydronephrosis secondary to obstruction, infection or reflux due to abnormally high resting bladder pressures. Hydronephrosis involves distention of the renal pelvis with urine and, if allowed to progress, destroys the functioning components of the kidney. This condition is asymptomatic and is only discovered by means of diagnostic intravenous pyelogram and monitoring of renal function, both of which should be done frequently. The problem can be reversed by insertion of an indwelling catheter.[37, 56]

Advantages of the intermittent catheterization programs include increased independence, reduced incidence of complications arising from a retention catheter, better hygiene, ease of sexual relations, decreased cost and less time devoted to bladder care. For many children, it is the first time that they have been able to exert any control over their bladder function.

PHYSICAL HAZARDS OF CATHETERIZATION

Infection

Normally the bladder is inherently resistant to infection. Even though numerous microorganisms reach the bladder, sterility of the urine is usually quickly reestablished. This resistance to infection is probably due to antibacterial properties of the bladder mucosa, and maybe of the urine, and to phagocytosis. The mechanical action of voiding also removes organisms from the lower urinary tract.[13, 40] Placement of a urethral catheter eliminates the washing action of voiding and seems to overpower the other natural defense mechanisms of the urinary tract. As mentioned earlier in the chapter, the incidence of urinary tract infection in the presence of urethral catheters is significantly high.

The most common causative organisms are *Escherichia coli, Proteus, Klebsiella, Aerobacter, Pseudomonas aeruginosa, Streptococcus* and *Staphylococcus*.[46, 60] Most of these organisms are opportunistic from the colon. How these bacteria reach the bladder is a subject of much debate. One factor that has been well-documented is the direct relationship between duration of catheter placement and increased incidence of urinary tract infections. Andriole reports that bacteriuria occurred in 50 per cent of the catheterized patients after 24 hours and increased to 98 to 100 per cent after four days.[2] There seems to be no opposition to the idea that the mere presence of the catheter is the major predisposing factor in the development of bacteriuria.

Potential sources for microbial invasion of the bladder are many. In a classic study, Kass and Schneiderman applied *Serratia marcescens,* an organism thought at the time of the study to be nonpathogenic, to the periurethral epithelium of patients with indwelling catheters. Within 1 to 3 days, large colonies of the organisms were present in the urine of all patients. Even though the exact route of entry into the bladder was not proven, the investigators felt that the organisms moved via the thin layer of fluid and exudate that usually forms around the *exterior* of the *catheter*.[39] Brehmer and Madsen also found in studying 72 patients having prostate gland resection that the bladders of these patients became colonized in 3 to 8 days by organisms ascending along the outside of the catheter.[4] These studies may be supported by others that have cited the normal flora of the urethra as a causative factor. Organisms have been cultured from the distal portion of the urethra in both males and females when the rest of the urethra has been shown to be sterile. The passage of the catheter through this colonized portion of the urethra may mechanically carry organisms into the bladder.[6, 17, 46, 66]

The *inside of the drainage tubing and catheter* is also a major pathway for access to the bladder. Contamination of the system can occur during the catheterization process initially and/or at any time during the care of the patient. Common sites are the junction between the catheter and the drainage tubing and the collection vessel itself. Once these areas are contaminated with pathogens, the organisms may ascend into the bladder either through their own motility or by retrograde flow of urine in the drainage system.

One common source of drainage system contamination may be the *catheter plug units* that are used to protect the exposed ends when the catheter must be separated from the drainage tubing. These two-piece plastic units consist of a plug to fit into the end of the catheter drainage lumen and a cap to cover the proximal end of the drainage tubing. Although these units are sterile initially, they are commonly saved and reused repeatedly. The plugs and urine of 20 patients were cultured and 80 per cent of the patients had the same organisms on the plug and in their urine. Six of these patients also had additional organisms cultured from the plug that were not found in the urine, indicating that the unit reused is certainly not sterile.[3]

Pertinent to bacterial invasion, whether it be by means of the exterior or interior of the catheter, is *cross-contamination between patients.* Maki conducted a study in which part of a patient group with indwelling catheters was colonized with *Serratia marcescens* and part was not. Where a colonized patient shared a room with a noncolonized patient, the latter developed asymptomatic bacteriuria within 48 hours. Noncolonized patients without this shared-room experience remained bacteria-free for up to 14 days. During the study, the investigative team cultured *Serratia* organisms from the hands of the nursing personnel 50 per cent of the time.[50]

Tissue Trauma

Tissue trauma is probably the second most common hazard of urethral catheterization. This damage can occur during the male catheterization process when the catheter is forced against a supposed obstruction in the urethra; the "obstruction" may in fact be one of the diverticula or outpouchings commonly found in the male urethra. Vigorous attempts to get around an actual obstruction may cause the catheter to perforate the urethra. Tissue necrosis is a possibility whenever there is continuous pressure, such as occurs on the meatus when not enough slack is left in the tubing between the meatus and the site of taping on the leg or abdomen. As mentioned before, too large a catheter may lead to tissue damage. There is also a case in the literature where the tip of a long-term catheter eroded through the dome of the bladder.[35]

Even though a retention catheter stays in the bladder, it still has the capability of movement in and out of the urethra at the distal end. This constant friction can cause tissue breakdown and the process is aggravated if encrustation is allowed to form on the outside of the catheter.

Other Hazards

Weinberg has stated that the most common complaint among males with indwelling catheters is *urethral irritation.* Symptoms of this condition include severe burning and pain at the tip of the penis; there may also be a small amount of purulent exudate. Presence of the catheter induces a fibrin reaction and mucus production, and if the process is allowed to progress, it may lead to urinary tract infection and/or the formation of strictures or fistulas.[70]

Muscular spasm may also occur. Bladder spasms themselves may be due to the balloon resting directly on the bladder neck. Sphincter spasticity may occur and, because the urethral and anal sphincters share common innervation from S_{2-3-4}, they may both be involved. This common innervation may also be utilized in the presence of urinary sphincter spasticity to relieve the urethral spasm. Anal dilatation, with the stretch concentrated in a lateral direction, may cause a reflex relaxation of the urethral sphincter.[28]

PSYCHOLOGICAL IMPLICATIONS OF CATHETERIZATION

> *In addition to the physical hazards associated with catheterization, there are also psychological implications: embarrassment, body image change and increased dependency.*

Although these aspects may not be as obvious as the physical hazards, the psychological impact is just as important.

Embarrassment

For the majority of people in the American culture, bladder elimination, especially the act of urination, is a very private and personal matter. It is not usually talked about freely, and numerous measures are taken to achieve privacy during micturition. Thus it is not at all surprising that the process of bladder catheterization is charged with embarrassment—both for the patient and the neophyte nursing student.

Although this chapter deals primarily with the direct concerns of the patient needing catheterization, it is crucial for the nurse to be fully cognizant of any personal embarrassment which might interfere with care being given to the patient. The beginning nursing student comes to clinical practice with the same feelings as the general lay public about bladder elimination. Suddenly this student is required to interview patients about their bladder habits, to physically help people establish normal elimination and then ultimately to catheterize the patient and afterward to care for this catheter. These expectations demand that students talk freely about a topic which may have been very private to them in the past and to otherwise openly confront something that may have always been handled behind closed doors. Embarrassment is the normal human emotion resulting from this conflict. And this embarrassment is very easily transmitted to the patient. Time and experience will diminish these feelings. Soon the student will be able to assess patients' elimination needs and effectively intervene when necessary. However, to facilitate this period of growth, the student needs to be aware of the emotions being felt and to discuss them with peers and others in the teaching-learning environment. Students should also always remember the personal embarrassment originally felt surrounding this area of patient care; this will help them to be more sensitive to the feelings the patient may be having. Sometimes, as experienced nurses, we become so used to dealing with the various aspects of peoples' bodies and lives that we lose sight of the fact that they don't share our frankness.

As mentioned, many patients feel great embarrassment when they find themselves in situations requiring intervention by others in the area of bladder elimination. Look at what happens to the patient from his point of view: he finds himself being asked very personal questions, being placed in a position which exposes the perineum to public view, and having his perineal structures handled both during the catheterization procedure and during the frequent post-catheterization cleansing episodes. Then the patient is left with a drainage system that allows his urine to flow into and be stored in a container readily visible to all others in his environment; he may even have to walk or be wheeled out of his room into more public areas carrying this collection bag in his hand. The causes of his embarrassment are obvious.

It is the nurse's responsibility to alleviate these feelings as much as she can. There are a variety of tools to aid in this. Probably the most vital is *continued sensitivity* on the part of the nurse—only then will the nurse remain aware of the patient's need for help. The patient's *emotions must be openly acknowledged.* The nurse may even be the first one to open the topic for discussion—even before beginning the procedure—by telling the patient that it is not at all unusual to be embarrassed in this situation. By doing this the nurse is giving the patient permission both to feel this way and to openly discuss the emotional aspect of the procedure. Meticulously *telling the patient what you are going to do and what you expect of him* allows him to maintain some self-control and therefore self-dignity by being prepared to cooperate as fully as possible. Thus the patient will not be further embarrassed by his own behavior.

Nonverbal communication is also an important means of reducing embarrassment. A matter-of-fact approach by the nurse conveys to the patient that bladder care is a normal facet of care, that the patient's needs in this area are not uncommon and therefore are no cause for "feeling different." This matter-of-factness also avoids amplifying the patient's feelings through transmission of the nurse's own embarrassment. Conscientiously *preserving the patient's privacy* as much as possible also tells him that you are aware of his potential embarrassment. During the catheterization procedure, curtains around the bed must be pulled, room doors shut to prevent interruptions by other staff and visitors and the patient carefully draped so as to expose the perineal area for as short a time as possible. If there are windows adjacent to the bed, be sure that the shades are closed. When the patient moves from his room with a urine collection bag, make it as inconspicuous as feasible. Be sure that the bag is positioned so that it functions properly to avoid its suddenly becoming the center of attraction in the hallway or waiting room. Although these actions may not totally eliminate the patient's embarrassment, they may help keep the emo-

tion at a level with which the patient can adequately cope.

Body Image Change

Everyone has an image of their own body and how it functions in and relates to its environment (see Chap. 15). This image is developed through life experiences and it allows the person to pattern his behavior in such a way as to achieve his life goals. Most people expect that their urine will flow through the appropriate orifice at the appropriate time and that they will be able to handle this aspect of their care without intervention by others. This is part of their body image. However, people are frequently faced with the fact that they can no longer take care of their urinary elimination needs on either a temporary or permanent basis. In this instance, a change in body image occurs and this change means an alteration in the patient's relationship to his environment. While the patient is adapting to a different body image, many behavioral patterns may be manifested in a whole range of severity. Loss of normal body functions commonly results in grieving and the behaviors usually associated with this process may be observed. Evidence of anger, depression, and withdrawal may be seen. The presence of a catheter may increase a person's level of agitation, especially if he is unable to understand the presence of and need for the catheter. Ways to help the patient effectively deal with this body image change include communicating openly about feelings and accepting them nonjudgmentally, encouraging interaction with other people, and helping the patient be involved in his own care.

Increased Dependency

Closely aligned to body image is the need for independence. As discussed above, bladder elimination is usually an independent activity of daily living. The need for catheterization causes a reduction in independence and a concurrent rise in dependency. The patient is now dependent on other people to help him reestablish emptying of his bladder and is dependent on the drainage system itself, which he needs to drain his bladder. In assisting the patient to cope with this aspect of psychological concern, the nurse should encourage the patient to be as independent as possible both in helping with urinary elimination and in other activities of daily living as well. In addition, the period of catheterization, and therefore the time of dependency, should be kept as short as feasible. Keeping the length of time of dependency on a catheter to a minimum is vital in eliminating all hazards—physical as well as psychological.

CARE OF THE PATIENT WITH AN INDWELLING CATHETER

We have discussed the hazards of catheterization in detail and the psychological care of the patient with an indwelling catheter. Now we look at the care necessitated by the presence of a urethral catheter in order to prevent, or at least minimize, the physical hazards. Table 40–1 summarizes the nursing care needed by patients with indwelling urethral catheters.

The details of the physical care needed by patients with indwelling catheters can vary tremendously depending on who is describing the regimen. Often one person's procedure will contradict another's. This section will discuss a wide variety of care methods. The nurse must select what seems to be the most prudent practice based upon appropriate scientific principles. Physician's orders and agency procedure books will provide additional guidelines.

Maintaining Patency

In order for the catheter and drainage system to perform its intended function, it must be kept patent. Anything that obstructs the flow of urine causes accumulation of urine in the bladder, which can be recognized by a decreased amount of urine in the collection bag and by developing symptoms of urinary retention. Sometimes the patient actually voids around the catheter because of the increased intravesicular pressure.

The nurse can do several things to prevent obstruction in the drainage system. Consideration must be given to both the catheter and the drainage tubing.

Course of the Tubing.   After the drainage tubing is taped to the patient's inner thigh, a decision must be made as to whether the tubing should run under or over the leg. Sources differ in their recommendations and both sides support their views with good rationale. Some say that when the tubing goes over the thigh, it creates a column in which the urine must accumulate until it has reached a volume sufficient enough to push the top of the column over the arc of the thigh (Fig. 40–9). Then the bladder is emptied by siphonage. This may be advantageous if the goal is to maintain some bladder tone but may require special consideration if the patient is very obese. If the bladder must be kept empty at all times, the tubing cannot be put over the leg. On the other hand, running the tubing under the leg may lead to obstruction if the weight of the leg is enough to constrict the lumen of the tubing. If the patient is very obese, a pillow may be placed under the thigh; this causes some flexion of the knee which leaves a space for the tubing. In addition, the

---

TABLE 40–1.   SUMMARY OF PHYSICAL CARE NEEDED BY PATIENTS WITH INDWELLING URETHRAL CATHETERS

Maintaining Patency	*Preventing Infection*
Determine course of drainage tubing	Wash hands before providing care
Avoid pinching drainage tubing in side rail or wheelchair wheels	Separate patients with catheters from each other
Establish adequate irrigation: internal and external	Maintain closed drainage system
Avoid kinking of drainage tubing	Prevent pooling and backflow of urine into bladder
	Empty collection bag
Maintaining Comfort and Safety	Provide for perineal care
	Maintain adequate fluid intake
Teach patients about:	Acidify urine: cranberry juice, ascorbic acid, acid-ash diet
what to expect	Administer systemic and topical medications as ordered
degree of mobility allowed	Change catheter and drainage tubing
patient's role in care program	Instill antimicrobial lubricants into urethra
Apply restraints if necessary	
Tape catheter to thigh or abdomen properly	
Relieve bladder spasms	
Restoring Bladder Tone	
Initiate clamping and releasing routine	

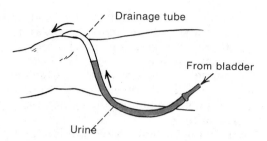

Figure 40-9. Column of urine accumulating in drainage tubing placed over thigh. When the drainage tubing goes over the thigh, urine in the tubing must go over the arc of the thigh before the bladder is siphoned. This is desirable in some instances and not in others (see text).

constant pressure of the tubing on the tissue of the posterior thigh may enhance the formation of pressure sores. One possible solution to the dilemma would be to run the drainage tubing down between the legs, around the patient's foot and over the side of the bed into the collection bag. However, if the patient is very active, this method increases the risk of the patient getting tangled up in the tubing, causing it to become kinked or disconnected. The method of choice depends on the goals of care. However, whatever procedure is followed for positioning the tubing, care must be taken to avoid any kinking of the drainage tubing.

As the tubing goes over the edge of the bed and into the collection bag, it must be clear and free from the operation of the side rails. The tubing should pass between the mattress and the side rail so that it is not pinched in any way as the side rail is raised and lowered. Also if the patient is in a wheelchair, extreme caution must be taken to avoid compressing the tubing in the wheel assembly.

Irrigation. Blood clots and mucus plugs may also partially or completely obstruct the drainage system. Patients who have had surgery of the urinary tract, such as a prostatectomy, are at highest risk for the occurrence of blood clots. Mucus can accumulate anytime, but it is more prevalent in the presence of urinary tract infection. Also, the continued presence of the catheter itself as a foreign object stimulates the production of mucus. The prevention of obstruction resulting from these elements involves irrigation. This "washing-out" action can be achieved through natural internal means or by continuous or intermittent external irrigation. These methods will be discussed in detail later in the chapter.

Clamping the Catheter. The final consideration in maintaining patency of the drainage system involves intentional obstruction of the tubing. A catheter clamp or plug may be used to interrupt the flow of urine through the system as a means of collecting a urine specimen or to facilitate ambulation with some patients.

> *When a catheter is clamped for any reason, it is essential to remember to remove the clamp as soon as the intended purpose is achieved.*

Occasionally after the nurse places the clamp or catheter plug, distractions occur and the patient with the catheter may be forgotten. This is equivalent to putting a cork into the urethra and obviously leads to urinary retention.

Maintaining Comfort and Safety

Patient Teaching. Several problems in the realm of patient comfort and safety can be averted, or at least minimized, through effective intervention. Much of this involves patient education. Patients who have been carefully prepared for and instructed during the catheter care process are usually more relaxed and able to cooperate in their care program. They know what to expect and how they can help to alleviate the physical hazards of catheterization. As an example, many patients experience a constant feeling of urgency for a time immediately after the catheter has been inserted. This discomfort is usually transient and is caused by the continuous stretching of the sphincter. Relief of this discomfort eventually comes as the sphincter adapts to the presence of the catheter and may be hastened by an increased fluid intake. If the patient knows to expect the sensation and knows that it is temporary, he can more easily cope with the stress.

Another example of the need for patient teaching concerns the patient's activity level. Many patients who have been inadequately taught are afraid to move around once the catheter has been taped into place for fear it will come out or be disconnected. You may return to the room some time later and find the patient in precisely the same position as when you left. The patient must be taught how the balloon keeps the catheter in the bladder and how to move without disrupting the functioning of the drainage system. Your teaching plan should include not only telling the patient this information, but asking him to demonstrate how he can move.

Other areas for teaching include the patient's responsibility in (a) taking fluids, (b) providing perineal care, (c) following recommended dietary measures and (d) taking prescribed medications. Another important part of the teaching plan is the realization that teaching once may not be enough. Many things in the hospital situation interfere with the retention of information, e.g., anxiety, medications, other stimuli and organic memory loss. Information may have to be repeated over and over again. Many times this repetitive teaching is at the basic level of telling the patient that there is a catheter present and that it is taking care of the urine in the bladder.

Use of Restraints. Sometimes, even repetitive teaching is inadequate. If the patient is continually pulling at the catheter system, it may be necessary to utilize restraints. This usually requires that restraining devices be placed on both arms and kept short enough that the patient cannot reach the catheter or drainage system. The procedure for applying restraints and the care of the patient with them is discussed in Chapter 43.

Taping of the Catheter. Taping of the catheter is a very important aspect of both the patient's comfort and safety. Usually the catheter is taped to the patient's body in order to prevent constant pressure on the bladder neck by the balloon. Good taping also prevents constant friction on the mucosal walls of the urethra. With the *female* patient, the site for taping is the inner aspect of either thigh. When determining the optimum tautness of the catheter, care must be taken to allow for abduction and extension of the involved thigh. At the same time, continuous pressure on the external meatus by the catheter must be prevented, since this will cause tissue erosion. The literature differs in its recommendation for the taping site on *male* patients. Some sources indicate that the thigh is the location of choice, as with the female. However, most sources are currently suggesting anchoring the catheter to the abdomen, since this more naturally maintains the normal anatomical direction of the urethra and avoids abscess formation at the penoscrotal junction. As with the female patient, care must be taken to avoid undue pressure on the external meatus.

Whatever site is chosen for taping, nonallergenic tape is usually used. Adhesive tape can be applied, although there may be a higher incidence of skin reactions with it. The tape should be left in place as long as it is functioning properly. However, with an indwelling catheter, the tape inadvertently becomes soiled, wet and/or nonadherent. Then it must be changed. It is simply removed and the skin underneath cleansed, dried, and inspected for any reaction to the tape. New tape is then applied as previously. If hair at the site is interfering with the tape's adhesiveness, the area can be shaved.

Bladder Spasms. Bladder spasms were mentioned before as a very uncomfortable side effect of catheterization. Several methods have been cited for relieving them. Manipulation of the catheter to change the position of the balloon on the bladder neck may relieve the spasms. Increased fluid intake may also be helpful. The use of anal dilatation was described above. If none of these measures is effective, the physician may order medications, such as opium and belladonna suppositories. Atropine, antihistaminics or narcotics may be used, and if there is still no relief, a bladder instillation of tetracaine may be done.[20]

Preventing Infection

> *Probably the most important weapon in the prevention of infection is conscientious* hand-washing *by the nursing and medical personnel.*

Also there seems to be strong evidence for *separating patients* with catheters from each other. In addition to these measures, there are a myriad of other suggestions for care discussed in the literature.

Closed Drainage System. A study by Kunin and McCormack found that the use of a closed drainage system significantly reduced the infection rate in 676 patients.[44] This finding has been replicated several times, and as a result, it is now extremely uncommon to find open drainage systems in use. A closed drainage system is one in which the entire system, from the catheter to the collection bag, is closed to the atmosphere. Thus it is protected from microbial invasion from the environment. The only place in the closed system intended to be opened is the emptying spout at the bottom of the collection bag. The constant downflow of urine through this spout prevents microbial access. However, the nurse emptying the bag must be careful not to allow the end of the spout to touch anything that will contaminate it. Any other opening made in the system for whatever the reason diminishes the advantage gained by using a closed drainage system.

Preventing Pooling and Backflow of Urine. Preventing the backflow of urine avoids carrying any bacteria present in the system up through the tubing and catheter into the bladder. One study demonstrated that in 20 of 23 catheterized patients who developed urinary tract infections, the bag urine became infected 1 to 6 days before the bladder urine and the microorganisms were the same in both cultures.[2] One of the most frequent causes of this kind of contamination is raising the collection bag above the level of the patient's bladder. Special care must be taken when the patient is being transferred from bed to cart, from cart to the x-ray table, etc., and when the patient is being ambulated. Always allow gravity to move the urine toward the collection bag. If the bag must be raised above the patient's bladder, kink the tubing with your fingers during the transfer to prevent backflow of urine. This hazard has prompted some manufacturers to put a one-way valve in the drainage tubing as it enters the collection bag. The valve is designed to prevent reflux of urine from the bag. Results of this valve on the incidence of urinary tract infections has so far been inconclusive.

The drainage tubing has enough length to allow patient movement. However, loops in the tubing lead to pooling of urine, which increases the potential for backflow. To facilitate gravity flow, the tubing should be placed so that the urine is in a continuous downhill stream into the collection bag. Earlier we discussed pooling as a disadvantage of running the tubing over the patient's thigh. Another frequent source of pooling occurs when the long drainage tubing loops down over the edge of the mattress, maybe even to the floor, and then up to the collection bag. To prevent this, the extra tubing can be coiled on the top of the mattress. One means of doing this is to make a clove hitch around the tubing with a rubber band and then safety pin the rubber band to the sheet; this securely holds the tubing and yet is safe if the patient moves too far—the rubber band will stretch and break before too much pressure is put on the catheter itself. Finally, when the patient is up walking or in a wheelchair, position the drainage tubing so there are no deep loops in it.

Emptying the Collection Bag. The collection bag needs to be emptied at least every 8 hours, and more frequently if there is a large urine output. Urine left to stand is an excellent growth medium and this opportune environ-ment should not be allowed to remain. Some authorities have suggested using an antimicrobial solution, such as formalin, in the collection bag as a deterrent to microbial growth. However, because of the danger of backflow into the bladder, this practice is not widely accepted.

Sometimes when it is necessary to keep a very close watch on the amount of urine being produced by the kidneys, a special collection device called a *urinometer* is attached to the drainage tubing. The urinometer holds a maximum of 100 ml. of urine and has special markings so that each milliliter of urine can be measured. It is usually emptied every hour to facilitate precise measurement of renal function. However, as the patient's condition improves, intervals between emptying may be increased; if this is occurring, care must be taken to prevent back-up of urine in the drainage system.

Perineal Care. Since one very important route of microbial invasion of the bladder may be from the perineum, perineal care is a crucial aspect of any catheter care program. (See also Chap. 27.) Suggested agents and techniques are numerous, but all do agree on the need for conscientious cleanliness. The main goals for perineal care are to reduce the number of bacteria present and to remove crusts from the catheter itself because they may lead to tissue erosion as the catheter moves in and out of the urethra. Perineal and external catheter cleansing should be done at least twice a day, using soap and water or some other agent, depending on the procedure accepted by the nurse and the agency. Benzalkonium chloride has been used, although now the iodophors, such as povidone-iodine, are being utilized for their broad-spectrum antimicrobial properties.[29] When providing the perineal care for an uncircumcised male, be sure that the foreskin is fully retracted and the area underneath cleaned carefully. Once the perineum has been thoroughly cleansed, it should be rinsed well and dried. Sitz baths may also be used for cleansing.

Some authorities advocate leaving *medicated pads around the catheter* at the meatus between the cleansing treatments to reduce the rate of bacterial growth. Benzalkonium chloride is not effective for this, since it is inactivated by cotton and, after a few hours, becomes a good growth medium.[20] A variety of antimicrobial ointments have been suggested, such as iodophors and Polysporin, as protectors against gram-negative organisms.[20, 46, 61] However, the literature is not conclusive in the reported effects of this preventive measure.

To systematically assess the efficacy of various perineal care regimens, Cleland and associates studied 184 patients who were randomly placed into one of five different care routines:

(1) no care except what the patient did independently without any teaching, (2) care twice a day with a hexachlorophene solution using clean technique, (3) same as routine 2, using sterile technique, (4) bacitracin-neomycin ointment compress applied around the catheter, and (5) a combination of routines 3 and 4. When the data had been analyzed, none of the methods made any significant difference in the incidence of bacteriuria except in the group receiving no care. These patients had a higher rate of urinary tract infections.[11] This study seems to indicate that perineal care is vital, whatever procedure is being carried out.

Fluid Intake. A continuous downward flow of urine through the entire system from the kidneys to the collection bag is thought to impede ascending bacterial invasion. Sanford, while studying simulated urinary tracts, found that flow rates of at least 25 ml. per hour hindered the upward progress of all but 10 per cent of the bacteria.[46] Most sources recommend that in order to achieve this "internal irrigation" of the catheter and drainage system, the patient should maintain a fluid intake high enough to produce at least 50 ml. of urine output per hour. For most people, this requires about 2000 to 2500 ml. of fluid intake every day. Increased fluids also aid in reducing the risk of urinary stone formation. This fluid requirement can get to be very monotonous and requires creativity and gentle persuasion from the nurse.

Acidifying the Urine. Not only is the amount of liquid important, but also the kind of fluid, according to several sources. It has been documented that the pH of the urine has an effect on its ability to support bacterial growth. As the pH moves toward the acid side of the continuum, bacterial multiplication concomitantly decreases. Therefore, the nurse should institute means to decrease the pH of the urine. The most common method used is *cranberry juice.* Cranberries contain rather large amounts of quinic acid, which is not oxidized completely in the metabolic process, resulting in hippuric acid being excreted in the urine. This is unlike other fruits which actually have an alkaline metabolic end reaction—even oranges and lemons. Some sources advocate the use of therapeutic doses of *vitamin C, or ascorbic acid,* as a means of reducing the urine pH. However, there is very little in the literature to help the nurse choose one or the other of these measures or to determine the long-term effect of either. Nickey tested a group of 10 subjects. She tested urine pH on four different fluid regimens: water only, cranberry juice only, cranberry juice with supplemental ascorbic acid, and water with supplemental ascorbic acid. During the cranberry juice periods, the subjects were to drink 1000 ml. per day; ascorbic acid doses were 4 gm. per day. Normal solid diets were maintained during the entire time. Nickey found that both cranberry juice alone and ascorbic acid with water reduced the urine pH almost identically; cranberry juice and ascorbic acid together were the most effective.[54] In terms of longevity of effect, Kahn and associates found in a small study of four patients given cranberry juice that, although they all responded initially with a decreased urine pH, three of the subjects showed only a transient result.[38] More work appears to be indicated here.

Another effective means of acidifying the urine is through an *acid-ash diet.* Foods encouraged in this diet are meats, eggs, cheese, whole grains, cranberries, prunes and plums. These foods metabolize into acid end products that are excreted in the urine. Forbidden foods include carbonated beverages, anything made with baking powder or soda, fruits other than those mentioned above, most vegetables, olives, pickles and nuts other than peanuts.[9] The nurse can help the patient select his diet appropriately.

Systemic and Topical Medications. In addition to ascorbic acid, other systemic medications may be prescribed for the patient with an indwelling catheter. Probably the most frequent of these are the *antibiotics and urinary antiseptics.* There is much controversy over the use of prophylactic antibiotic therapy. Although some sources advocate it strongly, others cite the cost, development of resistant organisms, and possible adverse reactions as reasons not to use these drugs in this way.[64] However, in the event of a documented urinary tract infection, there is almost universal agreement that antibiotic therapy should be started and can be considered a very effective mode of treatment.

Some positive results in preventing urinary tract infections have been obtained by instilling *antimicrobial lubricants into the distal urethra.* The most commonly used lubricant contains polymyxin B sulfate, bacitracin and neomycin, which have a low toxicity when applied topically and are effective against gram-negative bacteria.[8, 51] The lubricant may be instilled into the distal urethra with an irrigating syringe. Kunin and Finkelberg tested several antimicrobial lubricants on 895 patients. They used a lubricating catheter that applied the preparation to the entire urethra. They found that there was no difference between the lubricants used, but that the incidence of urinary tract infections was less in the antimicrobial group as compared to the group who received no lubricant instillation. Therefore, the mechanical action of the lubricant might be the important factor.[45] Another way to apply topical medication to the catheter and/or the bladder is through *irrigation and instillation*. These procedures will be discussed later.

Changing the Catheter.   The final aspect considered in the prevention of infection concerns changing the long-term catheter. Until quite recently it was a common practice to routinely remove and replace these catheters every 1 to 2 weeks. The current literature is suggesting that the decision about when to change an indwelling catheter be individualized for each patient. The catheter can remain in place as long as (a) the urine is sterile, (b) the catheter is soft, and (c) there is no evidence of concretions in the catheter. If there are sandy particles felt when the distal end of the catheter is rolled between the fingers, the catheter needs changing. The collection bag and drainage tubing need replacing only when there is accumulated sediment, a malodor or leakage. Usually it is also changed at the same time as the catheter.[16, 17]

Restoring Bladder Tone

The bladder is a muscle, and as with any muscle, if it is not used, it loses its tone. During the time that the bladder is being continuously drained with an indwelling catheter, the bladder becomes increasingly flaccid. And, as with any muscle, it takes a period of re-use to regain its previous capabilities. If a catheter is removed after a period of time with no preparation of the bladder, the patient is at high risk for developing urine retention due to bladder atony. This may result in the need for reinsertion of the catheter, which is often anxiety-laden for the patient who had expected to be catheter-free.

One way of avoiding this is through a *bladder-training period*. With this program, the catheter is clamped for increasing lengths of time and then released to allow drainage of the urine. Oral fluids are maintained at a high level. By following this regimen, the bladder is alternately stretched and allowed to empty,

thus mimicking normal function. In an individualized period of time, the bladder may be ready to function normally and the catheter may be removed without incident.

One of the complications that may occur with spinal cord injury patients during bladder training programs or if their drainage system becomes obstructed is a medical emergency called *autonomic dysreflexia* or *hyperreflexia*. This condition is the result of an excessive autonomic response to normal stimuli, such as a filling bladder. Common symptoms include excessive blood pressure change, throbbing headache, diaphoresis below the level of the lesion, bradycardia, blurred vision, and nausea. If untreated, the hypertension can lead to seizures and/or stroke. The patient must be taught to recognize the symptoms so he can get help immediately if they occur. Initial treatment includes re-establishing urine flow and making sure the catheter is functioning properly and checking for and removing, if necessary, any fecal impaction. A topical anesthetic inserted into the rectum may be helpful to offset the stimuli occurring from digital examinations. Vital signs should be monitored every five minutes and the head of the bed placed in semi-Fowler's position. Drugs, anesthetic blocks or even surgery may be necessary to relieve the symptoms. This syndrome is a somewhat uncommon incident, but when it does occur, action must be taken promptly.

BLADDER AND CATHETER IRRIGATION AND INSTILLATION

Irrigation of the catheter and/or bladder has been mentioned as one method of maintaining patency of the drainage system and of preventing the development of urinary tract infection. To *irrigate* means to flush out a tube or body part with a liquid. In the case of the urinary catheter, it is usually done to remove blood clots or other debris from the bladder and/or the catheter. Antibacterial solutions are often used to reduce the risk of urinary tract infection. The irrigation may be done using either an intermittent or a continuous procedure.

Open Bladder and Catheter Irrigation

Open irrigation indicates that the closed urinary drainage system must be opened to the environment in order to do the irrigating procedure. Until recently, intermittent open irrigation was often done several times a day prophylactically to prevent the accumulation of debris in the catheter. However, every time the catheter is disconnected from the drainage tubing to do the procedure, there is a great risk of bacterial contamination being introduced into the urinary system. Therefore, it is currently accepted practice to do intermittent open irrigation of the catheter or bladder only when there is a known partial or complete obstruction in the catheter.

Indications for doing a prn bladder and/or catheter irrigation are a reduction or cessation of urine flow through the catheter of a hydrated patient and increasing signs of urinary retention. The signs and symptoms of urinary retention were listed in Chapter 30. When it has been determined that the irrigation is necessary, the nurse checks the physician's order and, if necessary, the agency's procedure book to ascertain the kind and amount of solution to be used and the desired frequency of the procedure.

Equipment for the procedure includes solution at room temperature unless otherwise specified, container for the solution, irrigating syringe, drainage basin, antiseptic sponge and a covering for the drainage tubing. All of this equipment, except the solution, is included in commercially prepared irrigation sets. Any bladder or catheter irrigation is a sterile procedure, although gloves are not usually worn. The parts of the equipment that *must be kept sterile* are the solution, the tip and inside of the irrigating syringe, and the open ends of the catheter and drainage tubing.

As with any procedure, the nurse must first explain the procedure to the patient, gather the necessary equipment, and provide privacy for the patient. Hands are washed before actually beginning the irrigation. Elaborate draping is not necessary. The bed covers can be pulled back from the side of the bed far enough to adequately expose the connection junction of the catheter and drainage tubing.

A suggested procedure for doing a bladder and/or catheter irrigation is as follows:

1. Arrange the equipment so that it can be conveniently used while maintaining sterility. The solution is poured into the solution container. If a tip guard is present, remove it from the irrigating syringe and place the syringe into the solution container.

2. Cleanse the catheter/drainage tubing junction with the appropriate antiseptic as indicated by the agency's policy.

3. Separate the catheter from the drainage tubing, taking care not to contaminate either end. Cover the end of the tubing with a sterile, dry gauze or a sterile plastic cover. Place the tubing so that it does not fall off the bed during the procedure and yet will be easily retrievable when it comes time to reconnect it to the catheter. The end of the catheter is held in the nondominant hand throughout the procedure, with special care taken at all times to avoid contamination of it.

4. Fill the irrigating syringe with the desired amount of solution; 30 to 50 ml. is used each time for a catheter irrigation, while a bladder irrigation uses 90 to 400 ml. of fluid.

5. Insert the tip of the irrigating syringe into the distal end of the catheter, being careful not to contaminate either the tip or the catheter.

6. Slowly inject the solution into the catheter, using either gravity flow or slight pressure from the irrigating syringe. Be sure to hold the catheter and irrigating syringe perpendicular to the floor so that no air is injected into the bladder. It is reported that air in the bladder causes bladder spasms.

7. Usually the irrigating solution is allowed to drain from the catheter by gravity flow. In this case, pinch the catheter with the fingers of the nondominant hand and remove the irrigating syringe from the catheter. Hold the end of the catheter over the collection basin and unclamp the fingers. Keep this position until the flow has stopped. Another method of removing the solution is to leave the irrigating syringe in place and apply suction to the system with the syringe. If this method is employed, care must be taken to avoid the use of too much suction pressure, since it may suck the bladder mucosa into the drainage holes at the tip of the catheter. This amount of suction can cause severe trauma to the bladder mucosa. If the irrigating solution will not return, even with gentle suction and a repeated injection of 30 to 50 ml. of fluid, the procedure should be discontinued and the patient's physician notified.

8. Steps 4 to 6 may be repeated as necessary until the debris is cleared from the lumen of the catheter.

9. When the last of the solution has drained from the catheter, put the irrigating syringe into the catheter and lay them both on the bed. This will help maintain their sterility while you retrieve the drainage tubing and remove its protective covering.

10. Cleanse the end of the catheter with antiseptic. Reconnect the catheter and drainage tubing, taking care to maintain sterility of the two ends. Retape the drainage tubing if necessary.

11. Remove the equipment and discard that which is disposable.

12. Make the patient comfortable.

13. Charting for this procedure should include the reason for initiating the procedure, time, amount and kind of solution used, amount and characteristics of drainage returned, results of the irrigation, and any problems encountered during the procedure. If the patient is on intake and output measurement, be sure to record on that form any fluid retained or urine removed during the procedure.

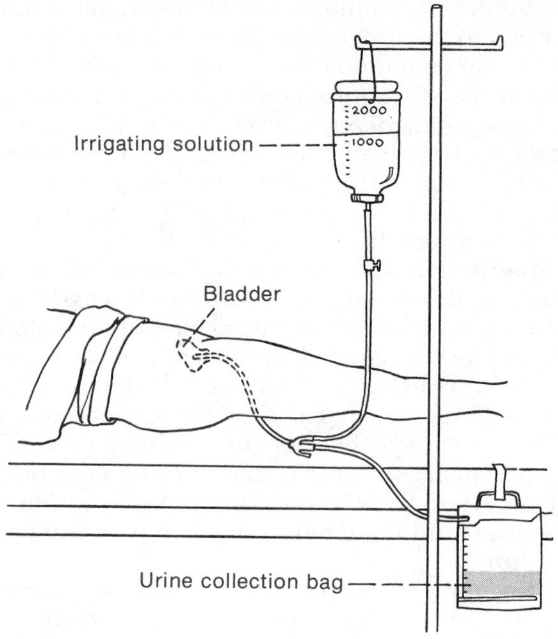

Figure 40–10. Three-way bladder or catheter irrigation set-up.

Closed Bladder and Catheter Irrigation

To avoid the hazard of bacterial contamination present in the open system for bladder irrigation, some patients are set up with a *closed* system. Figure 40–10 illustrates such a system. A three-way irrigating catheter is inserted into the bladder and the irrigating lumen is attached to a bottle of irrigating solution hung above the bed. This solution may be used for either intermittent or continuous irrigation.

In *intermittent* irrigation, there is a clamp on the tubing leading to the catheter, preventing the flow of solution into the bladder. At specified intervals, the bladder drainage tubing is clamped off and the clamp on the tubing from the irrigating container is removed, allowing the ordered amount of solution to flow into the bladder. Then the clamp is reapplied to the irrigation tubing and the drainage system opened. As long as the catheter and drainage systems are patent, the irrigation solution will drain out of the bladder just as the urine is removed.

When *continuous* irrigation is ordered, the irrigating solution is allowed to flow from its bottle at a specified drops per minute rate—similar to an intravenous infusion. As with the intermittent irrigation, the fluid flows into the bladder through the irrigation lumen of the catheter and out through the drainage lumen.

With both of these irrigation set-ups, the nurse should remember that an increased amount of fluid is flowing through the drainage system. Therefore, the collection bag will need to be emptied more frequently to avoid back-up of urine. Also, the amount of irrigating fluid will need to be calculated and subtracted from the total urinary output to determine the exact amount of urine being produced.

Bladder Instillation

A bladder *instillation* is done to medicate the bladder mucosa. Medication is instilled into the bladder through a catheter and is then allowed to remain in place for a specified time in order to achieve its topical effects.

In order for the medication to have its full effect, the bladder must be empty. If a catheter is not already in place, one is inserted and the bladder drained. The medication is injected with an irrigating syringe just the same as irrigating fluid. Then, instead of being drained, the medication is retained in the bladder. If the catheter is to remain in place, it is clamped off for the indicated time and then reconnected to the drainage tubing and the clamp released. However, if, as is usual in an out-patient clinic, the catheter is not needed to drain the bladder, it is removed after instillation of the medication and the patient is instructed not to void for a specified time.

COLLECTING URINE SPECIMENS FROM AN INDWELLING URETHRAL CATHETER

Any kind of urine specimen can be taken from a urethral catheter. A 24-hour specimen can be obtained directly from the collection bag. However, other specimens are not usually taken from the collection bag, but from the catheter itself. Before the specimen is collected, the catheter will probably need to be clamped off for about 15 to 20 minutes to allow for accumulation of urine in the bladder. The traditional way to obtain this specimen is to disconnect the catheter from the drainage tubing as described in the intermittent open catheter irrigation procedure. The urine is allowed to run from the distal end of the catheter into the specimen container. The distal end of the catheter and the proximal end of the drainage tubing, which have not been allowed to touch anything, are reconnected and the specimen is appropriately analyzed.

Because this procedure opens a closed system, another technique for obtaining a specimen from a catheter has been devised. The urine is aspirated from the catheter with a sterile 21 to 25 gauge needle and an appropriate size syringe. The site used is the part of the catheter distal to the sleeve leading to the balloon. After the chosen puncture site is swabbed with an antiseptic solution and allowed to dry, the needle is inserted at an angle to allow for resealing by the catheter when the needle is withdrawn. In order to avoid entering the balloon lumen by mistake, slant the needle down toward the drainage tubing.[15] When the needle is in place, pull back on the plunger of the syringe until the appropriate amount of urine has been obtained. Remove the needle from the catheter. The specimen may be either transported right in the syringe or transferred to a specimen container.

REMOVAL OF AN INDWELLING URETHRAL CATHETER

Planned removal of an indwelling urethral catheter is usually a pain-free process as long as the patient has been informed of the procedure to be done. The main objective of this procedure is to deflate the balloon so that the catheter may be removed with minimal effort. Because the catheters are disposable anyway, many nurses use scissors to cut the end of the balloon sleeve on the catheter. This usually allows the water in the balloon to flow out, until the balloon is empty. However, in some cases partial or total obstruction of the balloon lumen has been known to prevent the release of the solution. Because the end of the sleeve is now gone, it is very difficult to apply any suction or pressure on the lumen. In this circumstance, a physician usually ruptures the balloon by inserting a stylet into the balloon channel or removes the catheter using cystoscopy equipment.

Once the procedure for removing the catheter has been explained to the patient, he can be positioned and draped to allow good visualization of the perineal area. Equipment needed for this procedure includes an appropriately sized syringe, with or without a needle depending on the kind of catheter being used, several paper towels or a small basin, and materials to wash and dry the perineum after the catheter has been removed. When the perineal area is properly exposed, the tape is removed, freeing the catheter. Insert the syringe or needle into the balloon sleeve valve and withdraw all the fluid from the balloon. With one hand, hold the paper towels or small basin near the bottom of the perineum. Have the patient take a deep breath to enhance relaxation; slowly remove the catheter, placing it in the towels or basin as it comes out. Inspect the meatus carefully for signs of infection or edema. After cleansing and drying the perineum, make the patient comfortable and discard all the equipment. Important information to be recorded on the appropriate forms includes the time the catheter was removed, condition of the meatus, and the amount of urine in the collection bag.

Following removal of the catheter, instruct the patient to maintain a good fluid intake. He should not expect to feel the urge to void for several hours, since the bladder was empty when the catheter was removed. However, if he does void earlier, this is also normal. Reassurance of the patient is important to reduce anxiety on his part. The nurse also continues to assess bladder function for approximately 24 hours to assure that urinary retention is not developing.

Sometimes removal of the catheter is not planned. An agitated or confused patient may effect a traumatic removal by forcibly pulling out the catheter without deflation of the balloon. This is especially damaging to the male because of the length of the urethra. Usually there are no permanent sequelae following this kind of catheter removal. It is very painful and some bleeding can be expected. The nurse needs to make follow-up assessment on the amount of bleeding and on bladder function. Sometimes the catheter is replaced, depending on the patient's needs. If this is done, careful measures must be taken to prevent recurrence of the episode.

GOING HOME WITH AN INDWELLING CATHETER

Sometimes the patient must go home with an indwelling catheter. In actuality, discharge with this equipment may be met with mixed emotions on the part of both the patient and his family. While the patient may be very pleased about returning to his home, all the psychological implications of an indwelling catheter —embarrassment, body image change, and dependency—may well be intensified. This is especially true if the patient was not expecting to go home with a catheter in place. The patient's significant others may also have the same feelings as the patient, e.g., embarrassment about the drainage system and concern about how the patient's increased dependency will affect their lives. Both the patient and the people he lives with will probably be concerned about how to take care of the catheter and drainage system and whether or not they will be able to do so properly.

The nurse plays the major role in helping the patient and his significant others adapt to the catheter and its care. Initially, all the people involved must be helped to openly discuss with the nurse and with each other the concerns they are having about the catheter and its drainage system. Only in this way can everyone fully understand the impact of the situation and thus be able to assist each other. The nurse needs to be able to anticipate the questions and concerns the patient and his family may have and to open these topics for discussion if they do not mention them themselves. An accepting, nonjudgmental environment is essential for these discussions.

The nurse's other main function in preparing the patient and his significant others for his discharge from the hospital is to help them learn how to care for the catheter and its drainage system. It is vital for the patient and sometimes for at least one other person to know how to care for this apparatus. And they need to know not only how it is cared for in the hospital, but how to adapt the care to the home environment, i.e., where to keep the equipment, how to clean the equipment with materials available in the home, and how to fit the care into the family's life style and daily activities. An invaluable resource in this process is the community health nurse. As soon as it is known that the patient will be going home with an indwelling catheter, the hospital nurse should discuss with the patient and his physician the option of having a community health nurse continue the supervision of learning in the home. Referrals should be made as soon as possible so that, ideally, the community health nurse can visit the patient in the hospital before discharge and talk to all the people at home who will be involved with his care. This will facilitate even greater continuity of care.

The patient and family member need to know how the catheter and its drainage system work, the physical and psychological hazards of indwelling catheters and how to prevent them, how to care for the catheter and drainage system, how to irrigate the catheter if necessary, where to get supplies, and who and when to call with questions. When it has been determined that the patient will be going home with his catheter, a teaching plan must be developed to include both this content and teaching methods which are appropriate to the learner's needs. Visual aids will be very helpful. The patient must be included as an active participant in his care as early as possible. The significant others involved must also demonstrate the skill and knowledge necessary for providing effective care of the catheter and its drainage system.

Some patients who have long-term catheter drainage use a leg bag as a collection device. A leg bag is a small rubber or plastic bag which is attached to the inner thigh, usually by two adjustable rubber straps. The catheter attaches directly to the top of this bag, and there is a valve in the bottom which allows the urine collected in the bag to be emptied into a toilet or other appropriate receptacle. Because this collection system allows the patient much more freedom and mobility than the conventional drainage system, it can markedly reduce the psychological hazards of catheterization. However, it is not without its physical risks. Because of its small capacity, the bag must be emptied frequently and, at night, the patient usually switches to a conventional drainage system so that he can sleep the night through without emptying the leg bag. All of this requires that the closed drainage system be opened numerous times each day. This increases the chance of infection.

Another set of problems associated with the use of a leg bag is caused by the rubber straps which hold the bag to the thigh. These problems include skin irritation, thrombophlebitis resulting from the stasis of blood and lymph circulation, and ulcer formation. Even if the straps are initially applied loosely, they tend to tighten as the bag fills.[41] Several devices have been developed to help solve these problems, but nothing has yet been standardized. Prevention is the key word. The patient must be taught (a) to remove the bag periodically to allow normalization of the circulation and (b) to take meticulous care of the skin under the bag and straps.

Cleanliness and odor control are also management problems in the use of leg bags. To control odor and the growth of organisms, it is usually recommended that the bag be carefully washed with soap and water, rinsed, and then filled with a 1 per cent acetic acid (vinegar) solution. This should be done after each use (or each night) and the bag should be allowed to soak until it is used again.[15]

Although attempts may be made to wean the patient from the catheter altogether or to get him on an intermittent catheterization program, sometimes the indwelling catheter must remain in place for a prolonged period of time. In this case, the patient and his family must receive continued support and reinforcement teaching.

BIBLIOGRAPHY

1. Altshuler, A., et al.: Even children can learn to do self-catheterization. *American Journal of Nursing*, 77:97, Jan. 1977.
2. Andriole, V.: Hospital acquired urinary infections and the indwelling catheter. *Urology Clinics of North America*, 2:451, Oct. 1975.
2a. Baum, M. E.: I want to be dry! The (almost) carefree way to conquer urinary incontinence. *Nursing '78*, 8:75–78, Feb. 1978.
2b. Bellfy, L. C.: You can improve your catheterized patient's care. *RN*, 40:34–35, April 1977.
3. Birum, L., and Zimmerman, D.: Catheter plugs as a source of infection. *American Journal of Nursing*, 71:2150, Nov. 1971.
4. Brehmer, B., and Madsen, P.: Route and prophylaxis of ascending bladder infection in male patients with indwelling catheters. *Journal of Urology*, 108:719, Nov. 1972.
5. Bruce, A., et al.: The problem of catheter encrustation. *Canadian Medical Association Journal*, 111:238, Aug. 1974.
6. Bultitude, M., and Eykyn, S.: The relationship between the urethral flora and urinary infection in the catheterized male. *British Journal of Urology*, 45:678, Dec. 1973.
7. Champion, V.: Clean technique for intermittent self-catheterization. *Nursing Research*, 25:13, Jan.–Feb. 1976.
8. Chavigny, K.: The use of polymyxin B as a urethral lubricant to reduce the post-instrumental incidence of bacteriuria in females, an exploratory study. *International Journal of Nursing Studies*, 12:33, March 1975.
9. Chezem, J.: Urinary diversion: select aspects of nursing management. *Nursing Clinics of North America*, 11:445, Sep. 1976.
10. Clark, C.: Catheter care in the home. *American Journal of Nursing*, 72:922, May 1972.
11. Cleland, V., et al.: Prevention of bacteriuria in female patients with indwelling catheters. *Nursing Research*, 20:309, July–Aug. 1971.
12. Comarr, A.: Urological management of the traumatic cord bladder. *Clinical Orthopedics and Related Research*, 112:53, Oct. 1975.

13. Cox, C., and Hinman, F.: Experiments with induced bacteriuria, vesical emptying and bacterial growth on the mechanism of bladder defense to infection. *Journal of Urology*, 86:739, Dec. 1961.
14. Dees, J.: The undeflatable Foley catheter. *Southern Medical Journal*, 65:236, Feb. 1972.
15. DeGroot, J.: Catheter-induced urinary tract infections: how can we prevent them? *Nursing '76*, 6:34, Aug. 1976.
16. DeGroot, J., and Kunin, C.: Indwelling catheters. *American Journal of Nursing*, 75:448, March 1975.
17. Desautels, R.: Managing the urinary catheter. *Nursing Digest*, 3:30, Sep.–Oct. 1975.
18. Desaultels, R., et al.: Technical advances in the prevention of urinary tract infection. *Journal of Urology*, 87:487, March 1962.
19. Dobbins, J., and Gleit, C.: Experiences with the lateral position for catheterization. *Nursing Clinics of North America*, 6:373, June 1971.
20. Drake, W.: Bladder decompensation in cancer, cardiac disease and stroke. *Journal of the Medical Society of New Jersey*, 68:884, Nov. 1971.
21. Edman, M.: A comparative study of the dorsal recumbent and lateral positions for female urethral catheterization. Unpublished Master's Thesis, University of Washington, Seattle, 1973.
22. Edwards, L., and Trott, P.: Catheter-induced urethral inflammation. *Journal of Urology*, 110:678, Dec. 1973.
23. Engel, R., et al.: Otis internal urethrotomy with long-term urethral intubation: a comparison of latex and Silastic catheters. *Southern Medical Journal*, 65:55, Jan. 1972.
24. Eppink, H.: Catheterizing the maternity patient. *American Journal of Nursing*, 75:829, May 1975.
25. Feustel, D.: Autonomic hyperreflexia. *American Journal of Nursing*, 76:228, Feb. 1976.
26. Flower, M., et al.: The role of the nurse epidemiologist in infection control and continuing education. *Surgery, Gynecology and Obstetrics*, 141:552, Oct. 1975.
27. Frankel, H.: Intermittent catheterization. *Urology Clinics of North America*, 1:225, Feb. 1974.
28. Gans, B., et al.: Urinary catheterization in severe sphincter spasticity: report of two cases. *Archives of Physical Medicine and Rehabilitation*, 56:498, Nov. 1975.
29. Garner, J.: Urinary catheter care. *Nursing '74*, 4:54, Feb. 1974.
30. Gross, P., et al.: Positive Foley catheter tip cultures—fact or fancy. *Journal of the American Medical Association*, 228:72, April 1974.
31. Gross, P., et al.: The fallacy of cultures of the tips of Foley catheters. *Surgery, Gynecology and Obstetrics*, 139:597, Oct. 1974.
32. Gusfa, A., et al.: Patient teaching: one approach. *Supervisor Nurse*, 6:17, Dec. 1975.
33. Harper, W., and Matz, L.: The effect of chlorhexidine irrigation of the bladder in the rat. *British Journal of Urology*, 47:539, Oct. 1975.
33a. Hartman, N.: Intermittent self-catheterization: Freeing your patient of the Foley. *Nursing '78*, 8:72–75, Nov. 1978.
34. Herr, H.: Intermittent catheterization in neurogenic bladder dysfunction. *Journal of Urology*, 113:477, April 1975.

35. Hughes, J., et al.: Perforation of the bladder: A complication of long-dwelling Foley catheter. *Journal of Urology*, 109:237, Feb. 1973.

36. Hutch, J.: *Anatomy and Physiology of the Bladder, Trigone and Urethra*. New York, Appleton-Century-Crofts, 1972.

37. Intermittent catheterization: A small warning. *Emergency Medicine*, 6:274, April 1974.

37a. Juliani, L.: Assessing renal function. *Nursing '78*, 8:34, Jan. 1978.

38. Kahn H., et al.: Effect of cranberry juice on urine. *Journal of the American Dietetic Association*, 51:251, Sep. 1967.

39. Kass, E., and Schneiderman, L.: Entry of bacteria into urinary tracts of patients with inlying catheters. *New England Journal of Medicine*, 256:556, March 1957.

40. Khan, A., and Pryles, C.: Urinary tract infection in children. *American Journal of Nursing*, 73:1340, Aug. 1973.

41. Koppel, A.: A device to free the legs from pressure of rubber urinary drainage bags. *Journal of Urology*, 106:765, Nov. 1971.

42. Kuhn, H., et al.: Intermittent catheterization as a rehabilitation nursing service. *Archives of Physical Medicine and Rehabilitation*, 55:439, Oct. 1974.

43. Kunin, C.: *Detection, Prevention and Management of Urinary Tract Infections*. Philadelphia, Lea and Febiger, 1972.

44. Kunin, C., and McCormack, R.: Prevention of catheter-induced urinary tract infections by sterile closed drainage. *New England Journal of Medicine*, 274:1156, May 1966.

45. Kunin, C., and Finkelberg, Z.: Evaluation of an intraurethral lubricating catheter in prevention of catheter-induced urinary tract infections. *Journal of Urology*, 106:928, Dec. 1971.

46. Langford, T.: Nursing problem: bacteriuria and the indwelling catheter. *American Journal of Nursing*, 72:113, Jan. 1972.

47. Langley, I.: Suprapubic cystotomy. *Postgraduate Medicine*, 50:171, Oct. 1971.

48. Lapides, J., et al.: Clean, intermittent self-catheterization in the treatment of urinary tract disease. *Journal of Urology*, 107:458, March 1972.

49. Lapides, J., et al.: Follow-up on unsterile intermittent self-catheterization. *Journal of Urology*, 111:184, Feb. 1972.

50. Maki, D., et al.: Prevention of catheter-associated urinary tract infection. *Journal of the American Medical Association*, 221:1270, Sep. 1972.

51. Malek, R., et al.: Urinary tract sterility and indwelling catheters. *Journal of Urology*, 109:84, Jan. 1973.

51a. Marchant, D. J.: Urinary incontinence in the female. *Hospital Medicine*, 13:60, March 1977.

52. Monson, T., and Kunin, C.: Evaluation of a polymer-coated indwelling catheter in prevention of infection. *Journal of Urology*, 111:220, Feb. 1974.

52a. Moolgaoker, R. S.: Management of stress incontinence in women. *Geriatrics*, 31:60, June 1976.

53. Morel, A.: Urethral catheters—an ancient device. *RN*, 35:41, April 1972.

54. Nickey, K.: An investigation of the urine pH of selected subjects on prescribed regimens of cranberry juice and ascorbic acid. Unpublished Master's Thesis, University of Washington, Seattle, 1973.

55. Orikasa, S., et al.: Experiences with non-sterile intermittent self-catheterization. *Journal of Urology*, 115:141, Feb. 1976.

56. Pelosof, H., et al.: Hydronephrosis: silent hazard of intermittent catheterization. *Journal of Urology*, 110:375, Oct. 1973.

57. Poole, P.: Continuous bladder drainage. *Nursing Mirror*, 135:42, Nov. 1972.

57a. Roberts, J. A.: A guide to a urologic examination. *Hospital Medicine*, 12:6, Feb. 1976.

58. Rowan, R.: Catheterization at home. *Consultant*, 13:37, Aug. 1973.

59. Rowson, L.: The lateral position in catheterization. *Nursing Clinics of North America*, 5:189, March 1970.

60. Schneckloth, N.: Indwelling catheter nursing care. *Journal of the Association of Operating Room Nurses*, 21:695, March 1975.

61. Shapiro, S., et al.: Catheter-associated urinary tract infections: incidence and a new approach to prevention. *Journal of Urology*, 112:659, Nov. 1974.

62. Sood, S., and Sahota, H.: Removing obstructed balloon catheter. *British Medical Journal*, 4:735, Dec. 1972.

63. Srinivasan, V., and Clark, S.: Encrustation of catheter materials in vitro. *Journal of Urology*, 108:473, Sep. 1972.

64. Stamm, W.: Guidelines for prevention of catheter-associated urinary tract infections. *Annals of Internal Medicine*, 82:386, March 1975.

65. Stickler, D., et al.: The mode of development of urinary infection in intermittently catheterized male paraplegics. *Paraplegia*, 8:243, Feb. 1971.

66. Stover, S., et al.: Intermittent catheterization in patients previously on indwelling catheter drainage. *Archives of Physical Medicine and Rehabilitation*, 54:25, Jan. 1973.

67. The nurse's guide to safe use of the urethral catheter. *Nursing Update*, 1:16, Dec. 1970.

68. Viant, A., et al.: Improved method for preventing movement of indwelling catheters in female patients. *Lancet*, 1:736, April 1971.

69. Vivian, J., and Bors, E.: Experience with intermittent catheterization in the southwest regional system for treatment of spinal injury. *Paraplegia*, 12:158, Nov. 1974.

70. Weinberg, S., et al.: Evaluation of a catheter-care ointment. *Journal of Urology*, 108:89, July 1972.

71. Zrubecky, G.: Intermittent catheterization with unsterile instruments. *Paraplegia*, 11:179, Aug. 1973.

CHAPTER 41

CARING FOR PERSONS REQUIRING GASTRIC AND INTESTINAL TUBES

By James Bush, R.N., M.N.

INTRODUCTION AND STUDY GUIDE

According to the latest data available on digestive disorders in the United States (1969), they are the leading cause of hospitalization, the second leading cause of days lost from work, and the third leading cause of economic loss (over 8 billion dollars annually). The prevalence of chronic digestive disease in 1969 was 11 per cent.[9, 10, 19]

Symptoms of gastrointestinal disorders may develop in the course of a generalized systemic disease, e.g., patients with the "flu" may vomit. Also, the gastrointestinal tract itself may be diseased, giving rise to gastrointestinal symptoms, e.g., patients with stomach ulcers may vomit. In addition, gastrointestinal symptoms may appear problematic following surgery. Gastrointestinal symptoms are highly varied, ranging from simple anorexia (loss of appetite) to a more complex symptom such as hematemesis (vomiting blood). In any case, the nurse plays a significant role in the care of patients experiencing gastrointestinal symptoms and/or disorders.

Our objective in this chapter is to help you understand the clinical nursing care of patients who require placement of gastric or intestinal tubes, i.e., tubes in the stomach or upper intestinal tract. The purposes of these tubes and their insertion, maintenance and removal are discussed, as are the physiologic and psychologic aspects of caring for intubated patients. This information will help you make sound nursing judgments and provide comprehensive care to patients with disorders requiring gastrointestinal intubation.

As you study this chapter, you should be able to do the following:

1. Reinforce your understanding of the anatomy and physiology of the gastrointestinal tract.

2. List and discuss the five reasons for gastrointestinal intubation.

3. Understand the operation of the three most common methods of applying gastrointestinal suction.

4. Name, describe and recognize the types of gastric tubes.

5. Understand the procedure and be ready to practice the technique of gastric intubation.

6. Understand the procedure and be ready to practice the technique of gastric tube irrigation.

7. Become aware of the patient's physical and psychologic discomfort during gastrointestinal intubation and tube removal and consider the ways in which the nurse can help the patient during these procedures.

8. Discuss the areas of patient care involved with gastric intubation: patient response, tube patency, comfort measures, and monitoring fluid and electrolyte status.

9. Discuss the purposes, types, routes and methods of gastric feedings.

10. Describe the procedure for tube feedings and the nursing care needed by patients receiving tube feedings.

11. Name, discuss and recognize the types of intestinal tubes.

12. Describe the procedure for intestinal intubation and the nursing care needed by these patients.

13. Understand and be able to use in your nursing practice the following terms:

nasogastric tube	esophageal varices
orogastric tube	intubation
intestinal tube	sump
decompression	gastrostomy
compression	gastric aspiration
gavage	patency
lavage	irrigation
gastric analysis	instillation
distention	parotitis
suction	metabolic acidosis

metabolic alkalosis	lactose intolerance
deglutition	regurgitation
anorexia	peristalsis
gastrectomy	intestinal obstruction
jejunostomy	

ANATOMY AND PHYSIOLOGY OF THE GASTROINTESTINAL TRACT: REVIEW

The primary function of the gastrointestinal system is to provide the body with nutrients, fluids and electrolytes in a form that can be used at the cellular level. It must also dispose of the waste products that result from the digestive process. The gastrointestinal system has many functions and comprises the gastrointestinal tract (also referred to as the digestive or alimentary tract) and its accessory organs (Fig. 41–1). The gastrointestinal tract is a continuous tube of mucosa approximately 4.5 m. (15 ft.) in length from mouth to anus. It has specialized functions: (1) ingestion (intake), (2) digestion, (3) absorption and (4) elimination. These four functions have mechanical and chemical components. For example, when food is taken into the mouth, it is chewed *mechanically* (to break it down) and mixed with saliva (to initiate the *chemical* process of digestion).

The gastrointestinal tract is composed of the mouth, pharynx, esophagus, stomach and small and large intestines. The mouth contains the teeth, tongue and salivary glands. The *teeth* grind (masticate, chew) the food with the help of movement of the jaw muscles. The *tongue* is a voluntary muscle covered with mucous membrane. It helps to move food about in the mouth during the processes of chewing and swallowing. *Saliva* is secreted by the parotid, submaxillary and sublingual glands into the mouth. It contains mucus to provide lubrication for swallowing and a starch-splitting enzyme, ptyalin, to begin the digestion of starches and other carbohydrates in the food.

The beginning steps of ingestion and digestion (described above) can be summarized as follows: (a) a bite of food is taken into the mouth, (b) the food is chewed into smaller pieces and mixed with saliva, (c) saliva lubricates the food and starts the process of digestion and (d) the moistened, lubricated food forms a "bolus" and is pushed to the back of the mouth in preparation for swallowing.

The *pharynx* is the next segment of the gastrointestinal tract. It serves as a common pathway for food and air. When its muscular tissue contracts, it directs food and fluid into the esophagus, closing off the entrances to the larynx and nasal cavities.

The *esophagus* is a portion of the gastrointestinal tube which connects the pharynx with the stomach. This muscular, hollow tube is capable of rhythmically expanding and contracting, thus carrying the food down into the stomach. These rhythmic movements are called *peristaltic waves*. The musculature of the pharynx and the upper third of the esophagus is different from that of the rest of the gastrointestinal tract. It is skeletal muscle, controlled directly by vagal and glossopharyngeal nerve impulses from the brain. The remainder of the esophagus and gastrointestinal tract is composed of smooth muscles and is only indirectly controlled by the central nervous system through the effects of the autonomic nervous system on the intramural plexus.

A small portion of the esophagus proximal to the stomach normally remains in a state of tonic contraction. This area of the esophagus is called the "cardiac constrictor" or "esophageal sphincter." It opens ahead of the peristaltic wave and closes behind it, preventing regurgitation.

Like the esophagus, the *stomach* is also a muscular structure. Its function is to continue digestion of food, change the consistency of the food bolus into *chyme*, and store chyme for its gradual release into the small intestine. Chemical changes take place in the stomach as a result of enzymes in the gastric juice. These enzymes act especially on proteins.

The *pyloric sphincter*, the distal opening of the stomach, controls the passage of chyme from the stomach into the *small intestine*. The small intestine is a thin tube which lies suspended by mesentery, coiled in the abdominal cavity, connecting the stomach with the large intestine. While in the small intestine the chyme is (a) churned and mixed with digestive juices from the small intestine, pancreas and liver, and (b) propelled toward the large intestine by peristaltic waves. Within the small intestine, digestive secretions act upon starches, sugars, proteins and fats. Portions of this digestive process are absorbed into the circulation from the small intestine and the remaining products are propelled into the large intestine. Contents at the distal end of the small intestine are of a liquid consistency.

The *large intestine* is composed of the cecum, colon and rectum. The two major functions of the large intestine are: (1) absorption and conservation of water and (2) elimination of digestive wastes. As the liquid chyme enters the large intestine and passes through it,

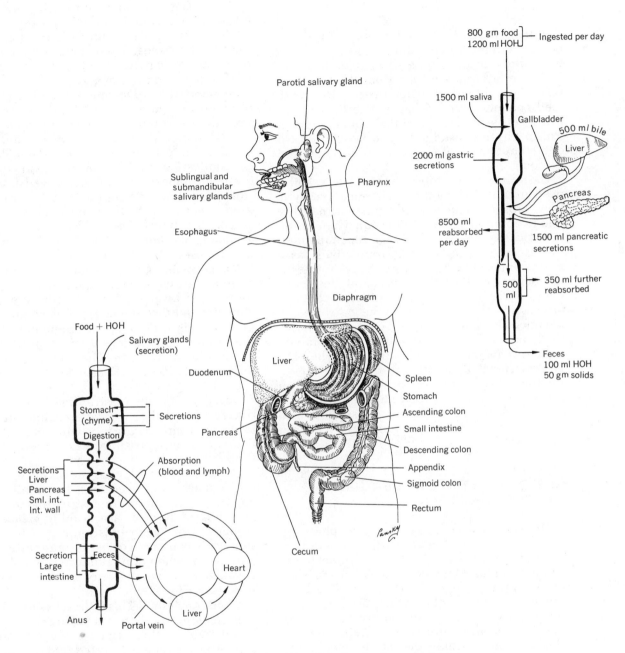

Figure 41–1. Overview of the digestive system. (From Pansky, B.: *Dynamic Anatomy and Physiology*. New York, Macmillan Publishing Co., 1976, p. 412.)

water is reabsorbed and the chyme becomes *feces*, which are normally of a semi-solid or solid consistency. In the large intestine, mucus is secreted. This substance not only facilitates elimination and movement of feces (as they move through the large intestine by massive peristaltic waves), but also helps maintain feces in a formed state. At the distal end of the large intestine, feces pass into the rectum and are eventually eliminated from the body through the anus.[10, 11, 27]

HISTORY OF GASTROINTESTINAL TUBES

The use of nasogastric and intestinal tubes has become so commonplace in the clinical setting that we hardly consider what it was like before their inception. John Hunter was among the earliest to develop a nasogastric tube. In 1869, he fashioned a tube from the skin of a freshly caught eel stretched over a probang to feed a patient with dysphagia (inability to swallow). Ten years later a Philadelphia surgeon, Philip Physick, used a tube to lavage ("wash out") the stomach of a patient who had ingested poison.

Gastrointestinal tubes were successfully used around 1910 for the treatment of paralytic ileus (absent or decreased intestinal motility due to neuromuscular inhibition). Then in the mid-1920's, Matas and Meyer recommended the use of gastric tubes postoperatively as a means of managing persons with gastrointestinal stasis (another term for paralytic ileus). Other surgeons, like Ward, initiated continuous suction of tubes placed in the gastrointestinal tract. However, the use of continuous intestinal suction as a means of managing paralytic ileus was not popularized until 1932, when Dr. Wangensteen demonstrated a method for relieving a simple bowel obstruction: he used an indwelling duodenal tube attached to a mild source of suction.[26] The use of suction with gastric and intestinal tubes is discussed later in this chapter.

GASTROINTESTINAL INTUBATION: OVERVIEW AND USES

Health education places much emphasis on nutrition. Any interference with the integrity of the gastrointestinal system poses a threat to nutritional health. Many conditions—inadequate or excessive intake of food, loss of integrity of the lining, interference with motility or patency or inability to absorb nutrients—can affect the specialized functions of the gastrointestinal system. At times, the interference is secondary to a dysfunction or disease in another part of the body. For example, some disorders of the brain may be manifested first by vomiting or difficulty in swallowing. Complaints of fatigue or shortness of breath that bring a client to seek medical advice may be the signs of primary nutritionally induced anemia. Intubation of the gastrointestinal system may be performed to diagnose the type of disorder, to relieve accumulated digestive secretions and gas,

or to empty the tract in order to allow healing to occur. If a tube is passed through the nose into the stomach, it is called a *nasogastric (NG) tube;* if inserted through the mouth, an *orogastric tube.* If it is advanced further into the small intestine, it is called an *intestinal tube.*

Gastric or intestinal intubation is done for a variety of reasons: decompression, compression, gavage (gastric feeding), lavage (gastric washing), and gastric analysis.

Decompression. Decompression is a process of removing gaseous and liquid substances from the gastrointestinal tract. It is an attempt to relieve pressure caused by an accumulation of gas and intestinal contents because of lack of gastrointestinal motility or an obstruction. If these substances are being removed from the stomach, a short, 125 cm. (50 inch) Levin tube is used (see Fig. 41–5). If, on the other hand, fluid and/or air is being removed from the intestine, a longer, 300 cm. (10 ft.) Miller-Abbott tube may be used (see Fig. 41–22).

Compression. Compression is the process of applying pressure internally, using a specially designed tube placed at a specific site. Probably the most common type of compression procedure is applying pressure on hemorrhaging esophageal varices (veins) at the gastroesophageal junction. The tube used for this purpose is the Sengstaken-Blakemore tube (see Fig. 41–8).

Gavage. Gavage (gastric) feeding is an artificial method of giving patients fluids and nutrients via a nasogastric tube when oral intake is inadequate or impossible. A Levin tube is used for this purpose.

Lavage. Gastric lavage means to wash out the stomach. It is used most frequently as an emergency treatment in gastric dilatation and poisoning. Lavage is also used to cleanse the stomach for gastric surgery. When the stomach's contents consist of undigested food particles or when rapid removal is essential, an Ewald tube (larger diameter than Levin tube) is used (see Fig. 41–9).

Gastric Analysis. This is the laboratory examination of the contents of a fasting stomach and is important in the diagnosis of gastric pathology.[6] A Levin tube is inserted into the stomach to aspirate gastric contents. An increase in gastric acidity usually coincides with the presence of duodenal ulcers. Decreased gastric acidity indicates possible carcinoma or pernicious anemia. Normal fasting contents of the stomach are clear and watery. Gastric contents that are tinged green may indicate a combination of bile and hydrochloric acid. Golden yellow contents may indicate achlorhydria (absence of free hydrochloric acid in the gastric juice).[6]

In order to understand how tube drainage works, several principles of physics related to movement of fluids need to be reviewed.

Flow of Fluids. Liquids flow readily, from an area of higher pressure to an area of lower pressure. Liquid takes the shape of its container and is not compressible; hence it cannot be made to occupy a smaller volume without exerting enormous pressure.

The rate at which a fluid flows depends on the volume of the fluid, pressure difference, viscosity of the fluid, and characteristics of the tube through which it flows—diameter of the tube (size of lumen) and length of the tube. Flow rate is described as the volume of fluid moving in a stated period of time, e.g., ml./hr.; gtt./min.; ml./day.

Pressure Difference. Pressure is equal to the amount of force per unit of area. Pressure difference may be described as the difference in force per unit area on fluid in one area from the force per unit area (or potential force) on the fluid at another area. For example, when a garden hose lies on the ground, water flows out of the open end of the hose because the pressure outside the hose is considerably less than the pressure inside. To restate: fluids flow from an area of high pressure to an area of lower pressure. When fluid is contained within a column, the pressure is determined by the height of the column.

Viscosity. Viscosity refers to the "thickness" or "thinness" of fluid. The more molecules exerting friction against each other in a solution, the "thicker" the fluid and the more resistance to movement.

Diameter of the Tube. The diameter refers to the width of the lumen (inside opening) of the tube. Many tubes used for medical purposes are calibrated on a French (Fr.) scale. The lower the number, the smaller the lumen, i.e., a size 12 Fr. tube has a smaller lumen than a size 18 Fr.

Length of the Tube. Length is the measurement of the tube from one end to the other, usually stated in inches or centimeters. Flow of fluid is slower through a very long tube than through a shorter one (all else being equal), owing to the friction created between molecules of fluid and walls of the tube.[27]

SUCTION

A commonly used method to increase pressure difference and hence vary the flow rate of fluid is called *suction*. Suction is the application of subatmospheric pressure (vacuum negative pressure) to attract fluid or gas and subsequently remove it. When applied to gastrointestinal tubes, suction may be used to prevent or treat postoperative distention (particularly after surgery on the digestive tract); remove fluid and gas accumulation proximal to an obstruction in the gastrointestinal tract; remove dangerous substances (poison) from the stomach following accidental or deliberate ingestion; and to empty the stomach prior to surgery.

When suction is applied to the gastrointestinal tubes, care must be taken to ensure that the amount of subatmospheric pressure created (vacuum) removes accumulated gas and fluid, but that the constant pressure on the tube opening does not produce irritation of mucosal tissue. A single-lumen gastrointestinal tube, attached to apparatus creating suction, poses this danger. The recently developed Andersen and Salem sump tubes seek to combat this problem (see Figs. 41–6 and 41–7). These sump tubings each have a double lumen and are inserted as any other gastrointestinal tube. The larger lumen is then attached to the suction apparatus; the smaller lumen remains unclamped and open. Negative pressure (suction) is applied to the larger lumen, to remove gas and fluid. At the same time the other lumen is open to the atmosphere; therefore, the volume displaced by removal of gas and fluid is replaced by air under atmospheric pressure. Hence, the gastrointestinal tract always contains air to be removed by suction, and the gastrointestinal mucosal lining is less likely to be "sucked" up against the lumen of the tube and become irritated.

Wall-Suction. Some health care facilities now have piped suction with wall outlets. Using different adapters, continuous or intermittent suction is provided (Fig. 41–2).

Wangensteen Suction. One of the first means of providing suction was designed by Dr. Owen Wangensteen and is thus called the Wangensteen suction machine. Figure 41–3 illustrates the main principles of the apparatus. With this setup, suction is promoted by water displacement. The force of the water flowing from the high bottle into the low bottle produces suction. Suction from this method is constant and of low pressure.

Gomco Thermotic Pump. A more recently developed electric apparatus for suction is the Gomco pump. It operates on the principle that air expands and contracts when subjected to

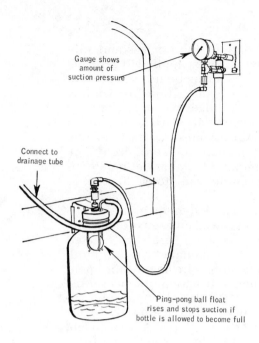

Gauge shows
amount of
suction pressure

Connect to
drainage tube

Ping-pong ball float
rises and stops suction if
bottle is allowed to become full

Figure 41–2.   Wall-suction. (From Sutton, A. L.: *Bedside Nursing Techniques in Medicine and Surgery,* 2nd ed. Philadelphia, W. B. Saunders Co., 1969, p. 159.)

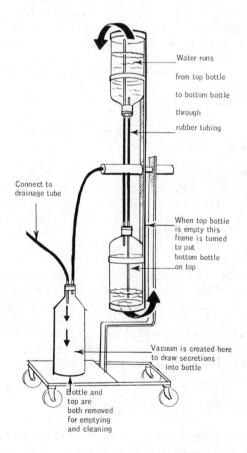

Water runs
from top bottle
to bottom bottle
through
rubber tubing

Connect to
drainage tube

When top bottie
is empty this
frame is turned
to put
bottom bottle
on top

Vacuum is created here
to draw secretions
into bottle

Bottle and
top are
both removed
for emptying
and cleaning

Figure 41–3.   Wangensteen suction. (From Sutton, A. L.: *Bedside Nursing Techniques in Medicine and Surgery.* 2nd ed. Philadelphia, W. B. Saunders Company, 1969, p. 158.)

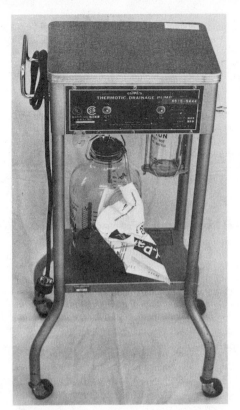

Figure 41–4. Gomco thermotic pump. (Photograph by George H. McNeal, R.N., M.N. (fnp), Ph.C.)

heat variations (see Fig. 41–4). The Gomco pump can produce suction as high as 120 mm. Hg or as low as 90 mm. Hg. of mercury. Charles' and Boyle's laws, which relate volume, pressure, and temperature of gases, are the working principles of the thermotic pump. The volume of gas at a constant pressure varies directly with its temperature. This means that the volume of a given mass of gas increases or decreases as its temperature increases or decreases if its pressure remains constant.[9] In addition, the pressure of a gas increases or decreases as its temperature rises or falls, provided the volume remains constant. This latter statement is the principle at work as the current goes on and off in the thermotic pump. The volume of the chamber does not change. Heating forces some of the confined gas through the outlet valve. Then, as the gas is cooled when the intermittent switch turns the current off, the smaller number of gas molecules in the same area lowers pressure, and suction begins.[9]

The Gomco provides intermittent suction and can be adjusted to high (120 mm. Hg) or low (90 mm. Hg) pressure.

No matter what type of apparatus is used, the worker must monitor the amount, frequency and characteristics of the drainage. Also, the machine must be checked frequently to ensure that it is functioning properly.

TYPES OF GASTRIC TUBES

The specific tube selected for intubation depends on the purpose of the intubation, the effect on the patient, and the personal preference of the one prescribing it. Gastric tubes are "short" tubes, 120 to 150 cm. (48 to 50 inches) in length, some having one or two lumens, others three. Significant facts and characteristics of gastric tubes are summarized in Table 41–1. Intestinal tubes are discussed separately, p. 1079.

Levin. The Levin is the simplest and most widely used tube. It is a single-lumen tube, measuring up to 127 cm. (50 inches) in length. Levin tubes are available in sizes 12 to 16 French (Fig. 41–5). Size 16 French is used most frequently for the adult patient. The Levin tube is made of rubber or plastic and may be inserted via the nostril or mouth into the stomach for decompression, feeding or diagnostic tests. The *rubber* Levin tube should be refrigerated or placed in ice prior to use to stiffen it and make insertion easier. Refrigerated rubber tubing also seems to anesthetize the nerve endings, so that passage of the tube is facilitated. Conversely, a *plastic* Levin tube need not be refrigerated. It becomes excessively stiff when cold and produces more trauma to the mucous membrane when inserted.

Andersen. The Andersen tube measures 120 cm. (48 inches) in length and comes in sizes 12 to 18 French (Fig. 41–6). It is actually two tubes riding beside one another, each having one lumen: a large clear plastic tube used for gastric decompression and a smaller white plastic tube open to the outside to equalize pressure between air in the stomach and atmospheric air.

Salem Sump. The Salem sump tube measures 120 cm. (48 inches) in length and is available in sizes 12 to 18 French (Fig. 41–7). The tube is a double lumen; literally a tube within a tube. There is a large clear lumen for gastric decompression and inside this large primary tube is a smaller, blue "pigtail" tube, which provides an inflow of atmospheric air. Once suction is applied, this airflow controls the suction force at the drainage eyes. Intermittent suction at a high setting (80 to 120 mm. Hg) or continuous suction at a low setting (30 to 40 mm. Hg) is recommended for the Salem sump tube.

Sengstaken-Blakemore. A Sengstaken-Blakemore tube (Fig. 41–8) is 90 cm. (36 inches) long and made of rubber. This tube has three lumens, each with a separate purpose: (1) gastric aspiration, (2) inflation of esophageal balloon, and (3) inflation of gastric balloon. Each lumen

TABLE 41–1. GASTRIC TUBES

Type	Length	Size (French)	Lumen	Uses	Other Characteristics
Levin (Fig. 41–5)	125 cm. (50 in.)	12, 16,* 18	Single	Decompression Gavage-feeding Diagnostic test	Rubber or plastic Inserted via nose or mouth into stomach Taped after insertion Intermittent type suction May need irrigation Rubber tube may need to be iced or refrigerated prior to inspection
Andersen (Fig. 41–6)	120 cm. (48 in.)	12, 14, 18*	Double	Decompression	Plastic Inserted via nose or mouth into stomach Taped after insertion Continuous sump suction
Salem sump (Fig. 41–7)	120 cm. (48 in.)	12, 14, 16, 18*	Double	Decompression	Plastic Inserted via nose or mouth Taped after insertion Continuous sump type suction
Sengstaken-Blakemore (Fig. 41–8)	90 cm. (36 in.)	20	Triple	Compression Decompression	Rubber Inserted via nose into stomach Taped after insertion (with tension) Intermittent type suction
Ewald (Fig. 41–9)	90 cm. (36 in.)	30	Single	Gastric-washing (Lavage) Diagnostic test	Rubber Inserted via mouth into stomach Suction provided by aspirating with Asepto syringe
Pediatric feeding (Fig. 41–10)	105 cm. (42 in.)	8	Single	Feeding-gavage	Plastic Inserted via nose or mouth into stomach Clamped while not in use Water is instilled after feeding
Gastrostomy feeding (Malecot) (Fig. 41–11)	35 cm. (14 in.)	26,* 28	Single	Feeding-gavage	Rubber or latex Inserted directly into stomach through a surgical opening in the abdominal wall Suture to stomach wall Clamped while not in use

*Most commonly used for adults.

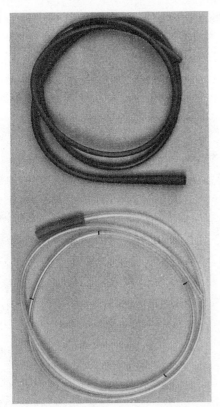

Figure 41–5. Levin tubes.*

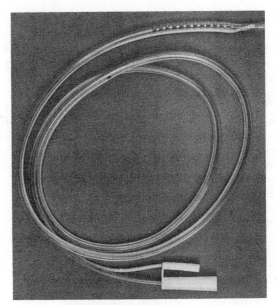

Figure 41–6. Andersen tube.*

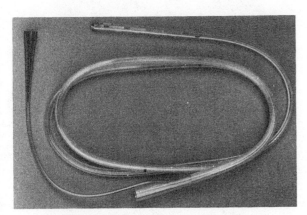

Figure 41–7. Salem sump tube.*

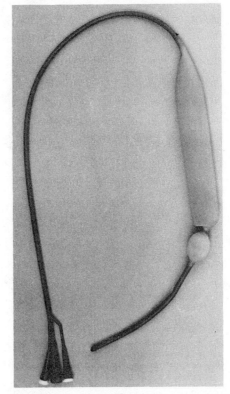

Figure 41–8. Sengstaken-Blakemore tube.*

*Photographs by George H. McNeal, R.N., M.N. (fnp), Ph.C.

is individually marked and identified to prevent accidental deflation or inflation through the wrong lumen. Of all the gastric tubes discussed, the Sengstaken-Blakemore tube is the only one that provides for both *compression* and *decompression*.

Ewald. The Ewald tube is a large-lumen rubber tube passed via the mouth into the stomach to remove unabsorbed stomach contents (Fig. 41–9). If the tube is passed to remove unabsorbed poisons or corrosive agents, extreme caution must be used to avoid inducing vomiting, which could result in aspiration of the agents, and to avoid esophageal or gastric perforation, which could allow the agents to escape into the thorax or abdomen. Escape of stomach contents into the chest cavity would precipitate a type of pneumonia; into the abdominal cavity, a hazardous peritonitis.

Pediatric Feeding. In adult patients who require feeding over a long period of time, the pediatric feeding tube may be inserted. It has characteristics similar to the plastic Levin tube, except that it comes with a self-contained clamp or seal (Fig. 41–10). Because of its size, this

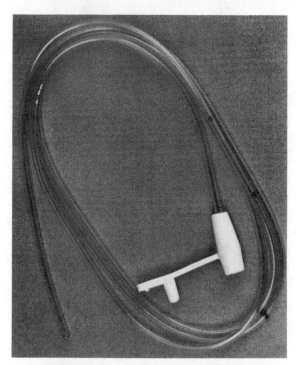

Figure 41–10. Pediatric "feeding" tube.*

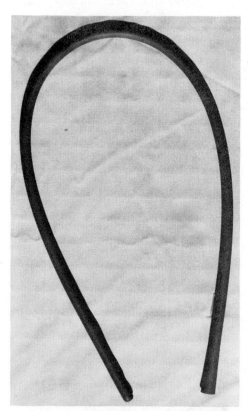

Figure 41–9. Ewald tube.*

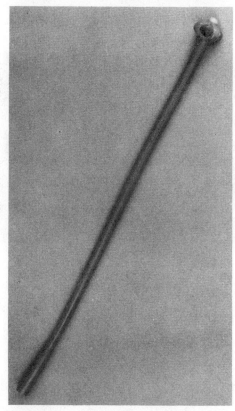

Figure 41–11. Gastrostomy "feeding" tube.*

*Photographs by George H. McNeal, R.N., M.N. (fnp), Ph.C.

plastic tube should be placed in ice at least 10 minutes prior to use to facilitate insertion.

Gastrostomy Feeding. A gastrostomy is a surgical opening into the stomach through the abdominal wall. A large Foley (No. 20 or 22 Fr.) or a Malecot catheter is inserted directly in the stomach and secured by sutures. This procedure is performed for feeding purposes (Fig. 41–11).

PREPARING A PATIENT FOR GASTROINTESTINAL INTUBATION

Gastrointestinal intubation is an unpleasant experience. However, there are physical and psychologic preparations that can make the procedure more tolerable. The equipment used and the positioning is discussed in Procedure 30. First, let us consider the psychologic aspects.

As with any nursing procedure, it is important to assess how much the patient knows about the procedure, his previous experiences, his accuracy in understanding the procedure, and his feelings and expectations about having a tube inserted into his stomach or further into the intestine. Ask the patient, "Have you ever had a tube put down your nose (or mouth) before?" If he answers yes, ask, "How did it go?" or "What kind of experience was it for you?" Assess the patient's verbal and nonverbal response to determine his state of knowledge and his level of anxiety.

Once you have assessed just what the patient knows about and expects from the procedure, you can supplement or correct his conceptions about the purpose of the intubation, the procedure you are going to use, and his participation in the process. Explaining his participation allays anxiety and fear as well as giving the patient some control during the procedure. As the tube is being inserted, you might reinforce his participation by saying "you are doing very well" and making other supportive comments. The amount of fear and anxiety the patient experiences is also related to the degree of competence you project and whether he perceives a caring attitude in you. Reassurance may be helpful; e.g., "I will try to be as gentle as I can."

A variety of information can be given to patients about this procedure. Consequently, there is no reason to assume that different kinds of information will have a common or beneficial effect on the patient's ability to tolerate insertion of a gastrointestinal tube. The nurse's therapeutic use of self, the ability to appropriately *assess, inform* and *allow for patient participation* and the ability to act with *confidence* are the determining factors regarding the patient's response, acceptance and tolerance of the procedure.[15, 16, 17, 18]

GASTRIC INTUBATION FOR DECOMPRESSION

After the patient is physically and psychologically prepared, the purpose for the tube explained and the appropriate tube selected, insertion can be accomplished. Rubber tubes are chilled prior to insertion, reducing friction and lessening irritation to the mucosa and thereby enhancing easy passage.

30. INSERTION OF NASOGASTRIC TUBE

Definition and Purposes. *Method of inserting a tube into the stomach via the nose.* A gastric tube is placed into the stomach for the purpose of instilling food and/or fluids or withdrawing fluids and gas.*

---

*A gastric tube may also be inserted through the mouth. In this case, the procedure is referred to as *insertion of orogastric tube*. The term orogastric is rarely used.

Procedure continued on the following page

Contraindications and Cautions.   A thorough knowledge of the anatomy of upper alimentary tract is essential. Damage to the tissues can result when force is used to pass the tube. Stop the procedure and notify the physician if you meet an obstruction. Avoid introduction of the tube into the respiratory tract. Immediately pull the tube back if respiratory distress is noted, e.g., gasping, coughing or cyanosis. Understand the purpose for inserting the tube in order to give an accurate and honest explanation to the patient.

Patient-Family Teaching Points.   Provide the patient-family with the following information as appropriate: (a) explain the purpose of the tube; (b) explain how the tube will be inserted; (c) tell patient that insertion of the tube is uncomfortable but reassure him that you will be as gentle as possible; (d) show the patient how he can assist with insertion, e.g., drinking fluid through a straw, bending his head forward, swallowing on command, and avoiding touching the tube; (e) inform him how long the tube will be left in place and how it will feel; and (f) explain that patient may experience thirst while intubated and that frequent rinsing of mouth relieves thirst and keeps mouth clean.

PRE-PROCEDURE ACTIVITIES

PRELIMINARY ASSESSMENT

Includes determination of:
- diagnosis to assess the need and purpose of a gastric tube
- physician's or nursing orders
- level of consciousness and ability to understand explanations and direction given by worker
- ability to move, maintain desired positions and follow directions

PRELIMINARY PLANNING

- Obtain correct equipment
- Assurance that accessory equipment functions properly

PREPARATION OF PATIENT

- Explain to patient why the procedure is being performed
- Place patient in a sitting (high-Fowler's) position when not contraindicated
- Adjust the environment (level of bed, placement of bedside stand, good lighting) as necessary
- Provide appropriate patient teaching
- Provide privacy (pull curtains, close door)
- Helper washes hands

EQUIPMENT

- Gastric tube of appropriate size
- Water-soluble lubricant
- Towel and emesis basin
- Glass of cold water and straw
- Suction equipment when appropriate
- Clamp when appropriate
- Equipment for instilling liquids when appropriate
- Basin of ice chips for rubber tube or pediatric feeding tube
- Asepto syringe or Toomey syringe
- Stethoscope
- Tissues

PROCEDURE

SUGGESTED STEPS	RATIONALE/DISCUSSION

1. Place patient in a high-Fowler's position. If not possible, tube may be inserted with patient in side lying or supine position.
  Hand patient a facial tissue.
	1. Facilitates swallowing of water and the movement of the tube downward in digestive tract.
	  Allows patient to mop tears, which are stimulated by intubation.

2. Place a towel or other protective drape over the chest and tuck securely behind shoulder blades.	2. Protects the patient's clothing and top covers.
3. Select a naris which is patent.	3. Trying to introduce a tube into an obstructed naris or previously fractured nose with deviated septum may cause discomfort and unnecessary trauma.
4. Measure distance on tube from the bridge of nose to patient's ear lobe plus the distance from ear lobe to tip of xiphoid process. Mark distance on tubing with adhesive or thread (Fig. 41–12).	4. Rough guide to determine approximate length of tube to reach stomach.
5. Lubricate tube for about 15 to 20 cm. (6 to 8 inches) with water-soluble jelly.	5. Lubrication reduces friction between mucous membrane and tube. *Never use oil product because of danger of aspiration.*
6. Have patient slightly flex head.	6. Facilitates initial insertion of the tube.
7. Twist tube in fingers until downward curve found.	7. Most tubes have a natural curve when held 15 to 20 cm. from tip.

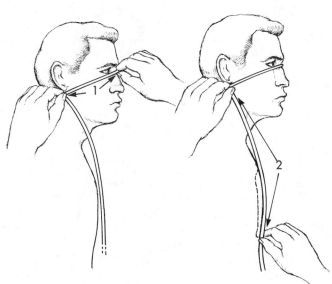

Figure 41–12. Measurement for nasal insertion distance. (Drawing by George H. McNeal, R.N., M.N. (fnp), Ph.C.)

Procedure continued on the following page

SUGGESTED STEPS	RATIONALE/DISCUSSION
8. Following the natural curve of the lubricated tube, gently insert it into naris.	8. Passage of tube is facilitated by natural contours of nasal cavity.
9. Have patient flex head. Advance tube to the nasopharynx (Fig. 41–13A).	9. Flexion of head produces curving passage to esophagus. Momentary resistance may occur as the tube is passed into the nasopharynx (Fig. 41–13B). Withdraw about one quarter of an inch, rotate side to side and gently advance the tube (Fig. 41–13C). *Stop if there is marked resistance. Do not force.*
10. When tube has reached the pharynx, the patient may gag. Allow him to rest for a few moments; tell him to take short "panting" breaths. If gagging persists, inspect posterior oral cavity for coiled tubing. (If necessary, withdraw tubing until straight at pharynx.)	10. Gag reflex is triggered by the presence of the tube. Allowing a brief pause before advancing the tube may prevent vomiting. Panting relaxes the pharynx. Tube cannot be advanced if coiled in pharynx.
11. Have patient take sips of water through a straw and swallow on command. Advance the tube 7.5 to 13 cm. (3 to 5 inches) each time patient swallows.	11. Facilitates passage of tube through the esophageal sphincter. Having patient swallow on command uses physiologic action to assist in the insertion process while the tube is being advanced. Advance at reasonable speed to avoid prolonging process.

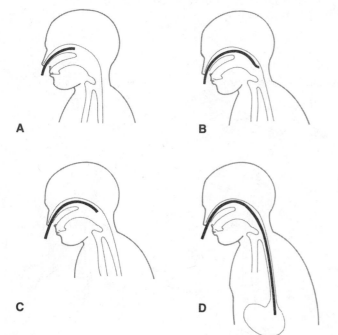

Figure 41–13. Insertion of nasogastric tube. *A,* Head position for initial insertion (slight flexion). *B,* Head flexed, tube may flex at nasopharyngeal junction. *C,* Head flexed, tube partially withdrawn to allow for smooth insertion. *D,* Tube properly positioned in stomach. (Drawing by George H. McNeal, R.N., M.N. (fnp) Ph.C.)

SUGGESTED STEPS	RATIONALE/DISCUSSION
12. Continue to advance tube gently each time patient swallows, until reaching the previously designated mark (Fig. 41–13*D*).	12. Mark indicates the tube might be in the stomach.

> CAUTION: *Excessive gasping or coughing or cyanosis are signs of respiratory distress. Immediately pull back on the tube; it may be in the trachea.*

> CAUTION: *Vapor forming in the tubing may indicate that the tube is in the trachea.*

13. Check placement of tube in stomach.	13. Misplacement is so hazardous, it is well to use at least two tests before concluding that placement is correct.
a. Aspirate for gastric contents with a syringe. (Gastric contents may be noticed in plastic tubing.)	a. Fluid content cannot be freely aspirated from lungs.
b. Place a stethoscope over the stomach, rapidly inject approximately 5 to 10 ml. of air through the tubing. A "swooshing" sound is heard.	b. Since the stomach is a pouch, sound can be heard as air is injected; in lungs, no "swooshing" sound is heard.
c. Place the free end of tube into a glass of water and evaluate rhythm of escaping bubbles (Fig. 41–14).	c. If tube is in bronchi, air bubbles will coincide with expiration of each breath.
d. Ask patient to hum or speak.	d. The tube would separate vocal cords if passed through larynx; hence patient would be unable to hum or speak.

> NOTE: *Accuracy is more assured with the first two procedures.*

14. Aspirate contents for specimen with Asepto syringe if ordered; clamp tube; or attach free end of tubing to the suction machine.	14. Specimen for tests may be single or serial. Avoids spilling of gastric contents through open end of tube if clamped. Begin immediately to withdraw gastric contents (on low intermittent pressure) if this was purpose of intubation.
15. Anchor tube securely with adhesive or thread and nonallergenic tube. (See Figs. 41–15 and 41–16 for methods.)	15. Prevents tube from being displaced. Nonallergenic tape decreases incidence of skin irritation. (Dry skin before applying tape, for better adherence.)

Procedure continued on the following page

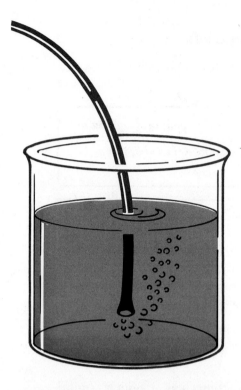

Figure 41–14.   Rhythm of escaping air bubbles in a glass of water. Place end of tube in glass of water as patient exhales. Steady stream of air bubbles indicates tube in respiratory tract. (Modified from Wood, L. A.: *Nursing Skills for Allied Health Services, Volume 3.* Philadelphia, W. B. Saunders Company, 1975. p. 312.)

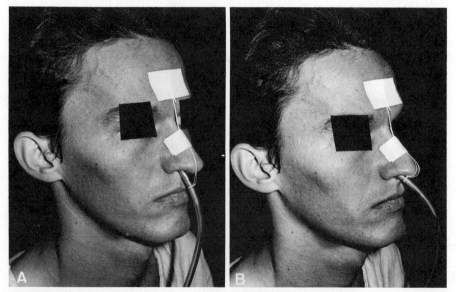

Figure 41–15.   Nasogastric tube stabilized with heavy thread and adhesive tape. *A,* At rest. *B,* During swallowing. (From Sader, A. A.: New ways to stabilize nasogastric tubes. *The American Journal of Surgery, 130*:102, July 1975.)

Figure 41-16. Two methods for securing the Miller-Abbott tube at the nostril. These methods permit advancing the tube as needed without irritation of the skin.

A, For use on beardless patient. *Materials needed:* Two pieces of ½ inch adhesive tape, each about 3¼ inches long. *Procedure:* Fold ¼ inch of the tape back on itself. Punch a hole in the center of end. A piece of string 12 inches long (doubled) is looped through each hole, as shown in *C.* Fasten the tube with a simple knot, with the string from each piece of adhesive. Lay the tube across this knot. Tie another knot, followed by a bow—not so tight as to compress the tube but secure enough to hold tube in place. Open bow knot to advance tube and retie to stabilize it.

B, For use on patients with beard. *Materials needed:* A 1½ inch piece of tape, about 4½ inches long, cut as shown in *C.* The dimensions will vary according to the length of the nose. *Procedure:* Place a piece of adhesive tape on forehead and nose to secure the tube. Fold the small piece of tape "a" back onto the narrow part just below the square so that the tape does not stick on eyebrows if they are bushy. At end of inverted V, strings are fastened through holes as in procedure for beardless patient. Place square portion of tape on forehead with narrow straight part over bridge of the nose. The string ends of the V should be attached to face very close to nose but not high enough to obstruct nostrils. To save adhesive and time, first make a pattern out of paper and fit it to the face. Moleskin is easy to handle and sticks better on the face than ordinary adhesive.

(Procedure and illustration provided by courtesy of Joanne W. Feyock, R.N., M.S.)

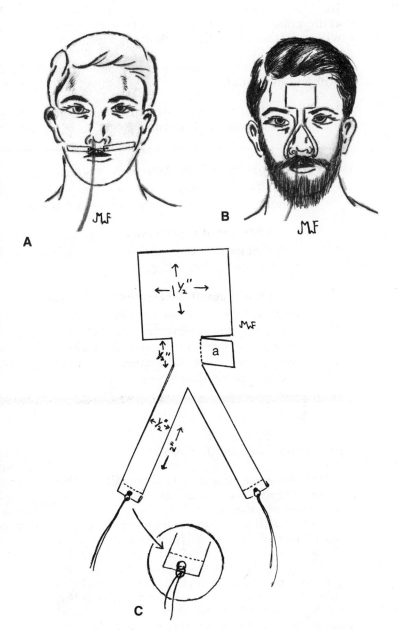

Procedure continued on the following page

SUGGESTED STEPS	RATIONALE/DISCUSSION
16. Place an adhesive tape tab on the tube at the point where attachment of tube to gown will avoid tension on tube. Pin the tab to gown.	16. Affixing tube to gown reduces "pull" and tension on patient's nose. Tape avoids cutting or occlusion of tubing by safety pin.
17. Arrange excess tubing to allow patient to turn and move in bed.	17. Avoid kinks in tubing and occlusion by pressure of body weight.
18. Administer oral hygiene; cleanse tubing at nostrils of lubricant and mucus.	18. Enhances patient's comfort. Avoid crusting of mucus on tube and naris.

Post-Procedure Activities.   Position patient appropriately. Teach patient how to turn and move. Send specimen to laboratory if ordered or indicated. Check connections of suction equipment for airtight seal. Wash hands.

Aftercare of Equipment.   Remove any excess equipment. Used disposables are discarded in dirty utility room trash; reusable supplies are returned to central service for reprocessing.

Final Patient Assessment.   Check naris for signs of pressure and arrangement of tubing; assess patient comfort and safety. Observe for proper functioning of suction equipment and connections. *Chart/Report:* Time of intubation; the patient's response to the procedure; the amount and characteristics of gastric specimen; specimen to laboratory; attachment to suction machine and pressure used; and/or tube feeding given.

Insertion of Orogastric Tube

Oral insertion of a gastric tube follows the same guidelines as nasal insertion, with the following variations:

To assure that the tube reaches the stomach, premeasure the tube from the lips to the base of the sternum. (See Fig. 41–12, Procedure 30.) Place the tube over the center and toward the posterior pharynx. To facilitate passage of the tube, ask the patient to suck on the tube as if it were a straw and swallow at the same time. After inserting the tube 6 inches, move the tube to the left cheek area between the teeth and the cheek to decrease stimulation of the gag reflex.

Advance the tube to the premeasured distance and check for correct placement, using the methods described in Procedure 30. Anchor the tube securely, clamp or connect it, and suction appropriately.

After the tube has been inserted properly, anchored by tape at the cheek and connected to suction, give oral and nasal hygiene to promote patient comfort. Make sure that all connections are airtight and that the movement of drainage through the tubing is apparent. Also, ensure that the patient is able to move freely in bed. Anchor the tubing to the patient's gown as in Procedure 30.

Irrigation of Nasogastric Tube

The principles of the "flow of fluids" were presented on p. 1055, i.e., that fluids flow from an area of higher pressure to an area of lower pressure. The amount of fluid flowing through a tube may be reduced if the texture of the fluid is thick. In this case, periodic irrigation may be needed to assure patency of the tube.

31. IRRIGATION OF GASTRIC TUBE

Definition and Purpose. *The process of instilling and/or flushing a gastric tube with a solution.* Used to maintain or re-establish patency of the tubing when drainage is thick or when drainage is blocked due to obstruction of the tube.

Contraindications and Cautions. Contraindicated for a new gastrectomy. Instilling fluid into gastric tube stimulates stomach to secrete fluids, causing increased loss of electrolytes. Irrigation needs to be carried out gently (under low pressure) when gastric hemorrhage has been a problem. Patient's electrolytes must be monitored when on continuous or intermittent suction and irrigations. Accurate Intake and Output records, which include irrigation fluid and drainage, are imperative.

Patient-Family Teaching Points. Provide the patient-family with the following information as appropriate: (a) explain to the patient that once stomach is emptied, the amount of drainage expected is greatly reduced; (b) explain that irrigation is done if no drainage is observed and patient is feeling gastric discomfort; (c) explain that electrolyte and fluid deficits may occur if he swallows fluids even though they immediately return through suction tube; (d) explain that a mild salt solution (N.S.) is used to irrigate the tubing, to minimize or prevent electrolyte and fluid deficits; and (e) explain why accurate Intake and Output records are maintained.

PRE-PROCEDURE ACTIVITIES

PRELIMINARY PATIENT ASSESSMENT

Includes determination of:
- diagnosis, date of surgery
- type of intubation and reason for use
- fluid and electrolyte status
- physician's order for irrigation and type of irrigant
- reason for irrigation; using nursing judgment as appropriate

PRELIMINARY PLANNING

- Obtain approval of physician for irrigation if indicated
- Assemble equipment for irrigation
- Pour approximately 100 ml. of irrigant into container

EQUIPMENT

- Disposable irrigating tray or assemble: irrigator (Asepto or Toomey syringe) container for irrigation solution protective drape antiseptic swab drainage basin
- Irrigant (usually isotonic saline)

PREPARATION OF PATIENT

- Explain value to patient and what patient might expect to experience
- Provide privacy
- Place bed at working height
- Check tubing for kinks or external pressure
- Helper washes hands

Procedure continued on the following page

PROCEDURE

SUGGESTED STEPS	RATIONALE/ASSESSMENT
1. Place an impervious drape over the area of bed where the tube is to be disconnected and/or irrigant introduced.	1. Prevents spillage of gastric drainage or irrigating solution on bed linen.
2. Determine correct placement of tube in stomach (see Procedure 30).	2. Prevents instillation of fluid into the lungs, which could cause aspiration pneumonia.
3. Clamp the tubing proximal to the drainage system if indicated.	3. Clamping prevents backflow of gastric contents.
a. Clamp Andersen, Pediatric or Levin tube and disconnect.	a. Clamping can be accomplished by a mechanical clamp or folding tubing upon itself.
b. Do not clamp or disconnect Salem sump tube unless ordered. (See Fig. 41–17.)	

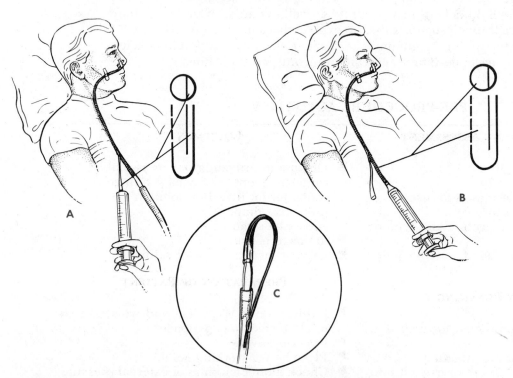

Figure 41–17. Irrigating the Salem sump tube. The Salem sump tube is double-lumened—the larger for gastric decompression (suctioning); the smaller, blue "pigtail," for inflow of atmospheric air. *A,* The tube can be irrigated, without disconnecting from suction, by injecting the solution into the blue "pigtail". Enlarged cross section indicates the tube being irrigated. *B,* The stomach can be irrigated, after disconnecting the suction, by injecting the irrigation solution through the large lumen. Enlarged cross section indicates the tube through which the solution passes into the stomach. (If a "T" connector is used, follow the procedure as illustrated in Figure 41–18.) *C,* When suction is to be interrupted, place the blue "pigtail" over the opening of the larger lumen, as illustrated, eliminating the necessity for a clamp. (Courtesy Sherwood Medical Industries, Inc., St. Louis.)

SUGGESTED STEPS	RATIONALE/ASSESSMENT
c. Maintain clamp on "T" or "Y" tubes. Do not disconnect tubing from "T" or "Y." (See Figs. 41–18 and 41–19.)	
4. Fill the syringe with the amount and kind of solution ordered. (30 to 50 ml. of an isotonic solution is the usual amount.)	4. An isotonic solution maintains osmotic pressure and thus reduces loss of electrolytes from the stomach.

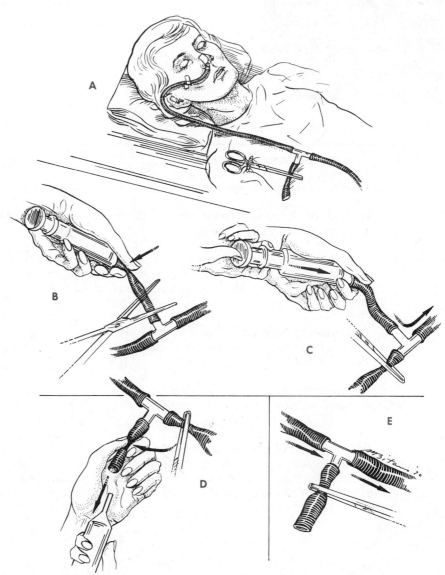

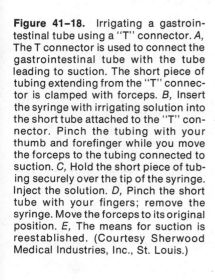

Figure 41–18. Irrigating a gastrointestinal tube using a "T" connector. *A,* The T connector is used to connect the gastrointestinal tube with the tube leading to suction. The short piece of tubing extending from the "T" connector is clamped with forceps. *B,* Insert the syringe with irrigating solution into the short tube attached to the "T" connector. Pinch the tubing with your thumb and forefinger while you move the forceps to the tubing connected to suction. *C,* Hold the short piece of tubing securely over the tip of the syringe. Inject the solution. *D,* Pinch the short tube with your fingers; remove the syringe. Move the forceps to its original position. *E,* The means for suction is reestablished. (Courtesy Sherwood Medical Industries, Inc., St. Louis.)

Procedure continued on the following page

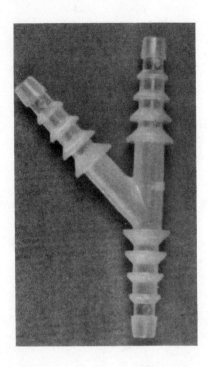

Figure 41–19. Y connector. (Photograph by George H. McNeal, R.N., M.N. (fnp), Ph.C.)

SUGGESTED STEPS	RATIONALE/ASSESSMENT
5. Insert the tip of the syringe into:	
a. End of Andersen, pediatric or Levin tube, and unclamp.	a. Maintains a closed system.
b. Air vent lumen of Salem sump tube (see Fig. 41–17A). If fluid does not flow out after Step 6, disconnect drainage lumen (see Fig. 41–17B) and proceed as in Step 5a.	b. Introduction of fluid is usually adequate. Additional measures are needed if drainage lumen is blocked.
c. Irrigating tube of "Y" or "T" tube. Remove clamp and place on tube leading to drainage bottle (see Figs. 41–18B and C).	c. Maintains a closed system and provides a direct pathway into gastric tube.
6. Holding the syringe perpendicular to the floor, inject solution slowly and gently.	6. Prevents introduction of air; introducing air may cause gastric distention and accompanying pain.
7. If great deal of resistance is found, check tubing again for kinks or mechanical obstruction and have patient turn from side to side. If resistance persists, notify physician.	7. Instilling solution with great deal of force may be hazardous; a sudden forceful injection against tissue that is not healthy may cause injury. Turning patient may change location of "eye" of tube.

SUGGESTED STEPS	RATIONALE/ASSESSMENT
8. Release the bulb (or pull back on plunger if a Toomey syringe is used) to withdraw fluid. With Salem sump tube, observe drainage tube for flow of fluid. With "T" or "Y" connector, maintain pressure on bulb or plunger or pinch tubing below syringe; remove clamp from drainage tubing and place on irrigation tubing (see Figs. 41–18*D* and *E*).	8. Fluids flow from area of greater pressure to area of lesser pressure.
9. If no fluid returns, with syringe still connected to tube, have patient turn from side to side. If still no return, adjust placement of tube a short distance in or out. Notify physician if unable to aspirate or if fluid does not return.	9. "Eye" of tube may be against wall of stomach and turning patient may dislodge it and allow fluid to drain. Adjust by advancing or pulling back on tube.
	Do not cause tube to kink in stomach or come out of stomach by advancing or pulling too far.
10. Collect the aspirated contents in container if appropriate.	10. Allows for later measurement.
11. The process of instilling and withdrawing fluid may be repeated several times until fluid flows freely.	11. Aspiration affirms patency.
	Do not repeat irrigation unless necessary to clear tube. Remember, irrigations further disturb fluid and electrolyte balance. Keep track of amount of solution used.
12. Re-clamp the tubing as in Step 3 above; disconnect tubing from irrigator.	12. Maintains a relatively closed system.
13. Reconnect tubing to suction apparatus and remove clamp if appropriate.	13. Re-establishes suction.
14. Note amount and characteristics of the drainage and the amount of irrigation solution used. Record accurately on Intake/Output sheet.	14. If patient on Intake and Output recording, subtract irrigant volume from returns and chart on *Output*. If irrigant is added to drainage, e.g., Salem sump tube, add amount of irrigant to *Intake*.

Post-Procedure Activities.   Position the patient comfortably. Wash hands.

Aftercare of Equipment.   Clean and tidy the irrigation equipment. Unless it is grossly contaminated or sterile equipment is required, the irrigation equipment is reused. Irrigation solution should be discarded after being open 24 hours.

Procedure continued on the following page

Final Patient Assessment.   Assess patient comfort and safety. Observe for proper functioning of suction equipment and connections, evidence of continuing drainage if appropriate. *Chart/Report:* Time of irrigation, amount and type of solution used; color, odor, consistency, and amount (absence or excess) of drainage. Immediately report inability to irrigate tube and untoward patient reactions.

Nursing Care

Patients who require a tube need to have consistent and competent nursing care. The following guidelines will help you to assess, care for and evaluate patients with gastric tubes.

General Patient Responses. Critically assess the patient, paying particular attention to his responses, both physiologic and psychologic. The nurse should clarify or validate those responses by talking with the patient about his reactions; by reflecting back to the patient the nurse's perceptions of what his nonverbal cues are; and by utilizing the patient's vital signs to determine if there have been any adverse changes. These assessment activities are essential for evaluating the patient's response to the intubation and for preventing untoward effects from the procedure. This permits more participation by the patient and allows the patient to exert some control in the situation.

Tube Patency.   If the tube is used for the purpose of decompression, it will most likely have a suction apparatus attached. Tubes of this nature will be a Levin, Salem sump or Andersen. The Levin is a single-lumen tube and may be connected to suctioning that is low or high; intermittent or continuous. Unless directed otherwise, the suction apparatus is usually set on *low intermittent* suction. An instance in which high continuous suctioning may be indicated—for a short time only—is in a patient with gastric distention due to an obstruction in the gastrointestinal tract. Both the Salem sump tube and the Andersen tube have two lumens; a larger one for suctioning and a smaller "pigtail" one to provide an inflow of atmospheric air. Continuous or intermittent suctioning may be used. If intermittent suction is the method of choice, the machine should be set on "high" (80 to 120 mm. Hg) so that the apparatus will function effectively. Continuous suction should be set first on "low" (30 to 40 mm. Hg), and then the suction slightly increased until fluid flow or bubbling is observed in the larger tube. The tube is functioning properly if a "hissing" sound is heard through the smaller tube, evidence of bubbling and/or drainage in the larger tube. The smaller "pigtail" tube should not be pinched or closed while suction is applied, as this would render sump action inoperative.

The Salem sump and Andersen tubes are designed to maintain effective drainage under most conditions. However, the thickness of the secretions may interrupt the flow. Then irrigation is needed, unless contraindicated. Irrigation is not usually a scheduled procedure, but is done when needed, according to nursing judgment. For proper irrigation, see Procedure 31. To facilitate the irrigation process, a "Y" connection is used, to avoid constant disconnection each time irrigation is necessary.

Functioning of Suctioning Systems.   An important role of the worker is to be observant as to indications of improper functioning of the suction systems. First, make sure the entire system is intact: the machine is plugged in, turned on and functioning properly. Be sure that the tube is free of kinks or external pressure from patient or side rails. Vomiting, distention, and increased abdominal discomfort are indications of improper functioning of the suction system.

Comfort Measures.   It is important to observe the area where the tube has been inserted, because continuous pressure on the area can cause an ulcer. This problem can be avoided by using proper anchor methods (see Procedure 30 and Figs. 41–15 and 41–16). A lubricant applied to the tube will decrease friction and thus decrease the possibility of an ulceration. Allow enough freedom for the patient to turn from side to side without causing any pull on the tubing. In most instances, the patient is NPO, making frequent oral hygiene necessary. Since there is no food to stimulate the salivary glands, parotitis (surgical mumps) may develop. Sucking hard on sour candy at intervals may prevent this problem; however, this aid may be contraindicated for some patients, since having candy in the mouth will stimulate gastric juices, which may promote ulcer formation or further deplete electrolytes.

The patient may complain of a sore throat. This is a result of the constant pressure of the tube against the mucous membranes of the throat, and lozenges or an anesthetic spray may be used to decrease the discomfort. With the tube in the nose, the patient will have a tendency to breathe through the mouth. Thus, he may have dry lips and oral mucosa. Application of petroleum jelly to the lips will help. Oral care, candy, rinsing the mouth with water and/or sucking ice chips (if allowed) may alleviate the dry mouth. (Remember, ice chips must be recorded as intake, the rule being that the fluid recorded is one half the volume of the ice.)

Fluid and Electrolyte Status. * All body fluids contain water and electrolytes. Any disturbance in body functioning that results in a loss of body fluids also results in a reduction of essential electrolytes. Fluid balance can be assured only when intake approximates output. When levels of output exceed levels of intake, disequilibrium occurs, resulting in a cycle of events in which the body attempts to compensate for the loss.

When a patient has a tube inserted for the purpose of decompression, essential fluids and electrolytes are removed. The chief electrolytes in the gastric juice are H^+, Cl^-, K^+ and Mg^{++}. Those of the intestine are HCO_3^-, Na^+, K^+ and Cl^-. *Gastric suctioning* can lead to *metabolic alkalosis* because of a *loss* in HCl and K. Prolonged gastric suctioning without adequate replacement of fluids, nutrients and electrolytes can lead to iatrogenic inanition. In this instance, the body will burn fats for energy, leading to *metabolic acidosis. Intestinal suctioning* can lead to metabolic acidosis if excessive amounts of intestinal and pancreatic secretions, which are normally alkaline, are removed. The excessive base loss results in acidosis. Both gastric and intestinal suctioning can result in extracellular fluid deficit. It is the nurse's responsibility to monitor accurately the fluid and electrolytic status of the patient with gastrointestinal decompression.

Electrolytes may be lost through the process of frequent irrigations. If irrigations are necessary, it is important that an isotonic solution (normal saline) be used to reduce the excessive removal of electrolytes. From time to time, ice chips may be used to satisfy the patient's experience of thirst. However, excessive use of ice chips made of tap water will also induce loss and/or dilution of electrolytes, thus resulting in an imbalance.

Removal of Nasogastric Tube

Removal of a gastric tube may be either a relief to the patient or a cause of anxiety, depending upon why the tube was inserted. If it was inserted for performing a diagnostic test (e.g., gastric analysis), the patient will be relieved to have the tube removed. However, if it was inserted to prevent gastric distention, the patient might fear having to have it reinserted if the problem recurs. It is, therefore, important that the nurse assess the patient's feelings before removing the tube.

There are several steps involved in removing a gastric tube. First, the nurse should identify the patient, evaluate his feelings about the procedure, and then explain the procedure, reassuring the patient as necessary. Place the patient in a high-Fowler's position if possible; although the high-Fowler's position is best, whatever position the patient finds comfortable is acceptable. Turn off the suction apparatus before removing the tube so as not to traumatize the mucous membrane of the gastrointestinal tract. Remove the tape that was used to stabilize the tube and place a towel under the tube. Clamp the tube to prevent drainage within the tube from escaping and being aspirated by the patient. Although using the fingers as a clamp to pinch or bend the tubing upon itself is acceptable, a mechanical clamp is better. The mechanical clamp accomplishes two things: it allows the nurse to use both hands to remove the tube, and it guarantees that the tube will remain clamped during removal. Instruct the patient to take a deep breath and exhale slowly; exhalation helps to prevent aspiration of gastric contents and relaxes the pharynx. While the patient exhales, pull the tube out with one continuous, moderately rapid motion. Wrap the tube in the towel and remove from room and discard it. If the tube is not disposable and is to be reused, return it to Central Supply for cleansing and sterilization. Use a small amount of tape remover solution to remove tape markings from the patient's skin if needed. Wash skin with soap and water to prevent skin irritation. Give oral and nasal hygiene; tidy the linens; position the patient comfortably. Record the time the tube was removed and record the patient's reaction to the procedure, and the amount and appearance of drainage. Remove all equipment from the patient's room.

---

*Fluid balance and imbalances are discussed in detail in Chapter 24.

GASTRIC INTUBATION FOR GASTRIC GAVAGE

Introducing feedings into the stomach is called *gastric gavage*. Patients who have problems with deglutition, extreme anorexia or prolonged unconsciousness may receive their dietary requirements in this manner. The feeding may be given through a tube directly into the stomach without going through the nose; this method is called *gastrostomy feedings*. If the patient has had a total gastrectomy, a tube for the same purpose is inserted through the abdominal wall and into the small intestine.

It is the nurse's responsibility to administer the feeding properly and to assess the patient's nutritional status as a response to this method of feeding.

Tube Feeding—Gastric Gavage

The process of giving liquid nutrients through a tube into the stomach is referred to as tube feeding. It dates back many years, yet only recently have researchers investigated what really constitutes a successful feeding. When oral intake is inadequate or impossible—even though stomach, intestinal passageways, and digestive patterns are normal—gastric feedings may be indicated. This condition may occur when there is an obstruction in the esophagus or after oral or esophageal surgery; when the stomach has been injured by strong alkali solution; after gastrectomy for cancer; or when the patient is recovering from trauma to the head or a cerebral vascular accident. Weakness caused by a chronic debilitating condition, prolonged altered consciousness, or extreme anorexia as a result of serious mental disease may also necessitate feedings through a tube.[2, 6, 8]

Routes.   Routes for tube feeding vary according to patient condition. Feedings can be given via a nasogastric tube, orogastric tube, gastrostomy tube or jejunostomy tube. A gastrostomy tube for an adult is usually an 18 Fr. Foley catheter or Malecot pulled taut and sutured to the abdominal wall (see Fig. 41–11). The tube may be anchored with several purse-string sutures. Complete obstruction of the esophagus due to tumor or scar-tissue contractures from chemical burns (e.g., dishwasher compound, lye) may lead to the necessity for gastrostomy tube feedings. A jejunostomy tube may be used to maintain nutrition if there is obstruction of the superior digestive tract. For an adult, a 12 Fr. red rubber catheter is suitable. It, too, is sutured to the abdominal wall for secure anchoring. The nasogastric tube is used most frequently for adults (see Fig. 41–5). The orogastric tube is used most frequently for infants (see Fig. 41–10).

Types of Feedings.   The physician will prescribe the amount, frequency and kind of tube feeding, as with any other diet. Basically, there are three types of tube feedings: (1) a milk-base solution; (2) a milk-base solution with suspended solids from strained or blenderized foods; and (3) low residue and elemental tube-feedings. Commercial preparations of all types are available.

Protein, carbohydrates, electrolytes, trace metals, fat soluble vitamins and water are included in many tube feedings. The exact proportions of each nutrient vary to meet the nutritional needs of the patient. Most diets lack vitamin K, which is essential for blood clotting; the physician will supplement the diet as necessary.

When milk-base solutions are prescribed, a careful dietary history must be taken in order to ascertain whether the patient has a history of milk lactose malabsorption. Lactose intolerance has been found in 75 per cent of American blacks, 80 per cent of American Indians, 90 to 95 per cent of Asians, and 50 to 55 per cent of Jews and Spanish-Americans. Ensure and Isocal are two commercially prepared feedings that do not have lactose.[1]

Methods of Feeding.   There are basically three ways of administering tube-feeding: gravity flow, drip regulated method and mechanical food pump. All accomplish the same task, but with certain differences.

GRAVITY FLOW.   In this commonly used method, an Asepto syringe (without bulb) is attached directly to the gastric tube and the flow is regulated by the height at which the syringe is held. This method is simple, and the equipment is easy to care for. Its disadvantage is that the flow rate can be only crudely adjusted by raising or lowering the syringe. Also, the syringe usually has to be refilled several times to give the desired amount.

DRIP-REGULATED.   Use of a Murphy drip in conjunction with a Kelly flask (Fig. 41–20); a resterilized IV bottle and disposable IV tubing; or a disposable gastric feeding unit provides better control of the rate of feeding than the gravity flow method. The type of apparatus chosen is hung from an IV stand and connected to the feeding tube. The rate of flow is regulated by a clamp that is opened to increase rate and closed to decrease rate of feeding. The disposable bag has two advantages over the

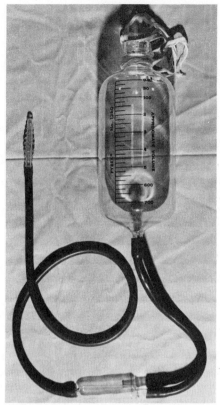

Figure 41–20. Murphy drip. (Photograph by George H. McNeal, R.N., M.N. (fnp), Ph.C.)

once or twice a week. Although less expensive, the Murphy drip uses a resterilized rubber tube, which is difficult to keep free of pathogenic organisms and which also cracks after repeated sterilization.

MECHANICAL PUMP. This method differs from the previous methods in that the feeding is actually pumped by an electric machine. Unlike the other methods, the mechanical pump maintains a continuous flow of feeding at a constant rate, regardless of the patient's position. An example of such a pump is the Barron food pump, which is used to deliver intermittent or continuous feedings (Fig. 41–21). Pulleys, usually on the underside of the pump, control the rate of flow, which is regulated in terms of ml./hour.[22, 31] (1) First speed (very slow)—43 ml./hour; (2) Second speed (slow)—65 ml./hour; (3) Third speed (moderate)—113 ml./hour; (4) Fourth speed (fast)—200 ml./hour.

other two drip-regulated methods: (1) accommodation of both light and heavy fluids, and (2) the convenience and assurance of sterility inherent in disposable equipment. A disadvantage, though, is the cost to the patient, especially when the equipment is changed

Suggested Method of Administration

Ascertain the type of formula, time, frequency, and amount of the feeding as well as specific directions for the individual patient before beginning the procedure. Assemble equipment needed, and obtain formula. Explain the procedure to the patient (even if he does not appear to be responsive) as you place

A   B

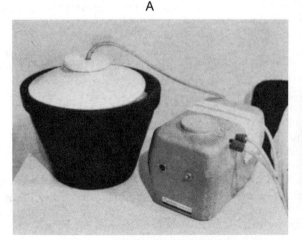 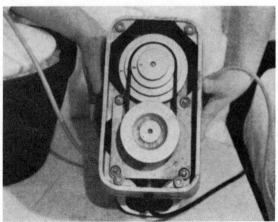

Figure 41–21. The Barron food pump *(A)* consists of the box-like container that houses the mechanism and the insulated container with a bottle (not visible), a cover, and latex tubing. On the other side of the pump *(B)* are the pulleys and belt to control the speed of the motor and, thereby, the rate of feeding. The nurse adjusts the pulley to the prescribed rate. (From Friedrich, H. N.: Oral feeding by food pump. Copyright © 1962, American Journal of Nursing Company. Reproduced with permission from American Journal of Nursing, February, Volume 62, No. 2.)

him in a comfortable, sitting position. Verify the placement of feeding tube by either aspirating gastric or jejunal contents or injecting a small amount of air into the tube and listening for "swoosh" sound with stethoscope over the stomach. (See Procedure 30.) Aspirating gastric contents is the action of choice here, since this not only verifies location of feeding tube, but also indicates the degree of stomach emptying occurring between feedings.

Prepare the formula in the feeding container. Attach feeding apparatus to feeding tube. Allow formula to fill tubing before unclamping, in order to avoid instilling large amounts of air into the feeding tube. (Nerve endings in gut are only sensitive to stretching.) Release clamp and observe the patient carefully for reaction to feeding. (Meal time is traditionally a social time, so this kind of atmosphere should be approximated.) Studies have shown that when patients are first started on tube feedings the infusion rate should not exceed 60 ml. per minute. The patient may experience stomach cramps, and this may indicate a decrease in the infusion rate is necessary. If the feeding container needs to be refilled with formula, clamp the tubing and refill before the container is completely empty; this is done to reduce the amount of air ingested. After formula has been instilled, add the prescribed amount of water to clear tubing of formula, and clamp and detach feeding container from the patient. This reduces the likelihood of the tubing becoming clogged.

After removing feeding container, allow patient to remain in sitting position for at least 30 minutes. If this cannot be tolerated, position the patient on his right side with head of the bed slightly elevated; this position encourages emptying of the stomach and discourages regurgitation and aspiration of stomach contents.

Care for equipment by washing that which will be reused and discarding the disposables. Wash hands. Check again on the comfort of the patient. Provide him with call light or other method of communication. Record time, amount (formula and water), and response to feeding on the patient's chart. Return to check on the patient in at least 30 minutes or before if warranted.

Complications

Although tube feedings have proven to be of immense value, complications can result and warrant ongoing assessment by the nurse. Among these are nausea, vomiting, esophageal reflux, diarrhea, aspiration pneumonia, water deficit, and electrolyte imbalance.

Specific Nursing Care

In order to effectively administer tube feeding, the following nursing care guidelines should be observed:

1. Whatever the setup used for tube feeding, make sure the container is properly cleaned prior to use. Formula is an excellent medium for bacterial growth, which frequently causes diarrhea.

2. Properly store the tube feeding mixture and keep bottles dated.

3. Aspirate the stomach prior to feeding to check for gastric retention as well as correct placement of feeding tube.

4. Let the patient's tolerance determine the amount and rate of feeding. Generally, 2000 ml. is given over a 24 hour period. (This balances the amount of fluid the body loses in a 24 hour period). Divided feedings may be given at intervals of 2, 3 or 4 hours and the amount varied between 150 and 300 ml. The individual feeding should not exceed 400 ml. unless it is given slowly (30 to 60 ml./min.) This minimizes distention, nausea, regurgitation, and excessive peristalsis usually associated with too much and too rapid administration.

5. Eliminate unpleasant stimuli, such as odors, in the environment both before and after feeding. Give oral and nasal hygiene appropriately, both to improve the patient's comfort and to reduce potential for infection for organisms growing in the mouth.

6. Take precautions to avoid introduction of air into the tube during feeding, in order to prevent gastric distention.

7. Follow each feeding with approximately 50 ml. of tap water to flush the remaining mixture from the tube into the stomach. Additional water may be given as needed to maintain water balance.

8. Accurately record amount of feeding and water.

9. Urine output should be monitored and recorded accurately.

10. Monitor fluid and electrolyte balance. Imbalance may be reflected in changes in skin, turgor, thirst, vital signs, intake and output, mucous membrane moisture, level of consciousness, body weight, serum osmolarity, serum sodium and BUN.[21] Sufficient water is especially needed for metabolism. When water intake is inadequate, water will be drawn from the tissues to supply the needed volume for urinary excretion of the increased solute load. Uncorrected dehydration may result in a high fever and disorientation.[4, 18, 20]

When a patient is experiencing gastric discomfort or nausea from the feeding, it might be helpful to place the bed in a reverse Trendelenburg position. This position minimizes compression of the stomach from pressure, which is likely to occur if the patient is in a semi-Fowler's position. In some instances, the drug Mylanta, which has an additive to help relieve gas, has proven helpful in conjunction with this position. Mylanta is administered via the tube as needed, until gastric distress is relieved. If the patient receiving the feeding is semiconscious or unconscious, or in any condition that makes him unable to control the expulsion of vomitus, a suction machine should be available, since vomiting or regurgitation may occur.

Most authorities advise that tube feedings be given at room temperature in order to prevent diarrhea and other untoward effects. Some investigations, however, have demonstrated that the temperature of the tube feedings is not a factor in the incidence of untoward effects.[12] Rather, it is rapid and forced administration of the feedings or intolerance to the lactose content of the feedings that is likely to cause untoward responses.[33] These studies indicate that warming the refrigerated feedings is probably unnecessary.

INTESTINAL INTUBATION

Absence of peristalsis or presence of a bowel obstruction results in an accumulation of gas and liquid material, resulting in distention. Such disorders require inserting a tube through the nose into the stomach and small intestine for the purpose of decompression. Intestinal decompression requires a "long" tube, 6 to 10 feet, which is modified at the distal end to permit easier passage (Table 41–2).

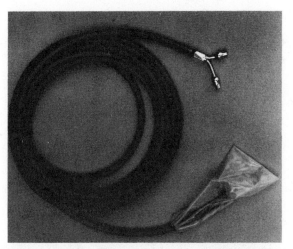

Figure 41–22. Miller-Abbott tube. (Photograph by George H. McNeal, R.N., M.N. (fnp), Ph.C.)

The most commonly used intestinal tubes are the Miller-Abbott and Cantor tubes. The Miller-Abbott tube comes in Fr. sizes 16 and 18, is rubber, 10 feet long, contains two lumens and has a metal tip at the end extending from the patient's nose (see Fig. 41–22). One lumen allows aspiration of fluids and gas from the intestine through perforations in the tube; the other lumen is used to introduce mercury into a balloon at the distal end of the tube. The tube can be mechanically inserted only into the stomach; the mercury-filled balloon assists forward movement by gravity and peristalsis of the intestine. The Cantor tube is a 10-foot long, single lumen tube (Fig. 41–23). A 16 Fr. diameter is most commonly used. It has a mercury-filled bag (that acts like a bolus of food) at the

TABLE 41–2.   INTESTINAL TUBES

Type	Length	Size (French)	Lumen	Uses	Other Characteristics
Miller-Abbott (Fig. 41–22)	300 cm. (10 feet)	16,* 18	Double	Decompression	1. Rubber 2. Inserted via nose into intestine 3. *Not* taped to nose until designated area in gastrointestinal tract is reached 4. Contains mercury bag.
Cantor (Fig. 41–23)	300 cm. (10 feet)	16*	Single	Decompression	1. Rubber 2. Inserted via nose into intestine 3. *Not* taped to nose until designated area in gastrointestinal tract is reached 4. Mercury-weighted

*Most commonly used for adults

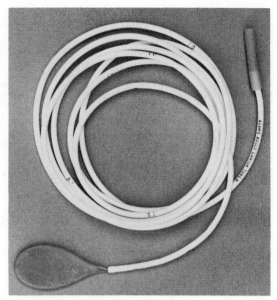

Figure 41–23. Cantor tube. (Photograph by George H. McNeal, R.N., M.N. (fnp), Ph.C.)

end of the rubber tubing to facilitate gravity flow and peristaltic action to propel the tube in the intestines. Usually the physician will insert the intestinal tubes.

Preparation for insertion of an intestinal tube is similar to that described for gastric intubation (see Procedure 30). For specific guidelines regarding insertion and advancement of intestinal tubes, consult a medical-surgical text.

Nursing Care

Basically, the nursing care for patients with a tube in the intestine is similar to that for patients with a tube inserted in the stomach.

After the patient is intubated with an intestinal tube, the tip is in the stomach. Gentle suction is provided via a Wangensteen machine or intermittent low-pressure suction with a Gomco machine or similar machine. Patency of the tube must be ensured to avoid accumulation of fluid and gas and further complications as a result of distention. Repositioning the patient will sometimes facilitate drainage and maintain patency as well as assist in propulsion of the tube. Irrigation with normal saline (usually 30 to 50 ml.) may be necessary at intervals to release accumulation of thick, tenacious secretions.

With intestinal intubation, the patient is placed in right-side lying position to facilitate passage of the tube through the pylorus into the small intestines. It is advanced at specific intervals according to the physician's guidelines. If the tube is advanced too quickly, it will curl and kink in the stomach. The Cantor and Miller-Abbott tubes have markings in centimeters so that their location can be estimated; the location is confirmed by x-ray or fluoroscopy. It is important to remember that tape is not applied to these tubes; they are stabilized with heavy thread (see Fig. 41–15). The thread is tied in a bow in order to release the tube easily for advancing. The *thread is taped* when it reaches the desired area.

Patency of Tubes. Guidelines for maintaining patency of intestinal tubes are similar to those for gastric tubes, p. 1074. Remember: checking for patency involves assessment from the patient to the mechanical apparatus. Determine if irrigation is needed and follow through accordingly.

Comfort Measures. Proper oral and nasal hygiene is extremely important during intestinal intubation. The external naris may become sore from crusted secretions or firm pressure. The tube and naris should be cleansed as needed and a water-soluble lubricant used. The position of the tube in the naris should be changed to relieve pressure. Oral hygiene includes brushing the teeth and tongue to remove debris, stimulate salivation and relieve dryness. These areas of nursing care are frequently missed and can lead to discomfort and unnecessary complications.

BIBLIOGRAPHY

1. Bayless, T., et al.: Lactose and milk intolerance: clinical implication. *New England Journal of Medicine,* 292:1156, 1975.
2. Brunner, L., and Suddarth, D. (eds.): *The Lippincott Manual of Nursing Practice.* Philadelphia, J. B. Lippincott, 1974.
3. Condon, R., and Nyhus, L. (eds.): *Manual of Surgical Therapeutics,* 3rd ed. Boston, Little, Brown & Company, 1975.
4. Friedrich, H. N.: Oral feeding by food pump. *The American Journal of Nursing,* 62(2):63, Feb. 1962.
5. Gault, M. H., et al.: Hypernatremia, azotemia, and dehydration due to high-protein tube feeding. *Annals of Internal Medicine,* 68:778, April 1968.
6. Given, B., and Simmons, S.: *Gastroenterology in Clinical Nursing,* 2nd ed. St. Louis, C. V. Mosby Company, 1975.
7. Goldberger, E.: *A Primer of Water, Electrolyte and Acid-Base Syndromes,* 5th ed. Philadelphia, Lea & Febiger, 1975.
8. Gormican, A., and Liddy, E.: Nasogastric tube feedings. *Postgraduate Medicine,* 53(7):71, June 1973.
9. Greenwood, M. E.: *An Illustrated Approach to Medical Physics,* 2nd ed. Philadelphia, F. A. Davis Co., 1966. (Reprinted by Gomco Surgical Manufacturing Co., 1972.)

10. Grossman, M. I.: Digestive disease as a national problem. *Gastroenterology, 53*(6):821, 1967.
11. Guyton, A.: *Basic Human Physiology: Normal Function and Mechanisms of Disease,* 2nd ed. Philadelphia, W. B. Saunders Co., 1977.
12. Harrison, T. R., et al.: *Principles of Internal Medicine,* 7th ed. McGraw-Hill Book Co., New York, 1974.
13. Hanson, R. L.: A study to determine the difference in effects of administering cold and warmed tube feedings. *In* Batey, M. (ed.): *Communicating Nursing Research, Vol. 6:Collaboration and Competition.* Boulder, Colorado, WICHE, 1973.
14. Hongladarom, G. C., and Russell, M.: An ethnic difference—lactose intolerance. *Nursing Outlook, 24*(12):764, Dec. 1976.
15. Johnson, J. E., et al.: Psychological preparation for an endoscopic examination. *Gastrointestinal Endoscopy, 19*(4):180, 1973.
16. Johnson, J. E., et al.: Easing children's fright during health care procedures. *MCN The American Journal of Maternal Child Nursing,* 206, July–Aug., 1976.
17. Johnson, J. E., et al.: Altering children's distress behavior during orthopedic cast removal. *Nursing Research, 24*(6):404, Nov.–Dec. 1975.
18. Johnson, J. E., et al.: Effects of accurate expectations and behavioral instructions on reactions during a noxious medical examination. *Journal of Personality and Social Psychology, 24:*5:710, 1975.
19. Kaminski, M. V.: Internal hyperalimentation, policy and procedures. *Surgery, Gynecology and Obstetrics, 143*(1):12, July 1976.
20. Kern, F., Jr.: The second conference on digestive disease as a national problem: a brief editorial summary. *Gastroenterology, 66*(2):305, 1974.
21. Kubo, W., et al.: Fluid and electrolyte problems of tube-fed patients. *American Journal of Nursing, 76*(6):912, June 1976.
22. Leininger, M.: *Nursing and Anthropology: Two Worlds to Blend.* John Wiley & Sons, Inc., New York, 1970.
23. Luckmann, J., and Sorensen, K.: *Medical-Surgical Nursing.* Philadelphia, W. B. Saunders Co., 1974.
24. Metheny, N. M., and Snively, W. D., Jr.: *Nurses' Handbook of Fluid Balance,* 2nd ed. Philadelphia, J. B. Lippincott Co., 1974.
25. Mitchell, H., et al.: *Nutrition in Health and Disease,* 16th ed. Philadelphia, J. B. Lippincott Co., 1976.
26. McConnell, E.: All about gastrointestinal intubation. *Nursing '75,* 5:9, Sep. 1975.
27. Nave, C., and Nave, B.: *Physics for the Health Sciences.* Philadelphia, W. B. Saunders Co., 1975.
28. Palmer, E. D.: Duodenal intubation. *JAMA, 233*(7): 818, Aug. 1975.
29. Pansky, B.: *Dynamic Anatomy and Physiology.* New York, Macmillan Publishing Co., Inc., 1975.
30. Reitz, M., and Pope, W.: Mouth care. *American Journal of Nursing,* 73:17, 1973.
30a. Rosenberg, H.: The difficult NG intubation: Tips and techniques. *Emergency Medicine,* 9:235–237, March 1977.
31. Sader, A. A.: New ways to stabilize nasogastric tubes. *The American Journal of Surgery, 130:*102, July 1975.
32. Snyder, J. C., and Wilson, M. F.: Elements of a psychological assessment. *American Journal of Nursing,* 77(2)235, Feb. 1977.
32a. The wandering NG tube. *Emergency Medicine,* 9: 127–128, June 1977.
33. Papper, S. (ed.): *Manual of Medical Care of the Surgical Patient.* Boston, Little, Brown & Company, 1976.
34. Stahlgren, L. H., and Morris, N. W.: Intestinal obstruction. *American Journal of Nursing,* 77(6):999, June 1977.
35. Stroot, V., Lee, C., and Schaper, C. A.: *Fluids and Electrolytes: A Practical Approach,* 2nd ed. Philadelphia, F. A. Davis Company, 1977.
36. Walike, B. C., and Walike, J. W.: Lactose content of tube feeding diets as a cause of diarrhea. *The Laryngoscope,* LXXXIII(7):1109, July 1973.
37. Wallacker, J.: Bowel sounds. *American Journal of Nursing,* 73(12):2100, Dec. 1973.

CHAPTER 42

CARING FOR
PERSONS WITH WOUNDS

By Mary Chelgren, R.N., Ph.D.

OVERVIEW AND STUDY GUIDE

Effective wound care can never be isolated from care of the *person* with the wound. Ideally, the outcome of such care would be not only sound healing of the wound but also the patient's perception of sensitive care. This chapter includes descriptions of wounds; delineation of processes involved in wound healing, along with factors influencing such healing; supportive nursing measures to enhance healing and to assist individuals with self-care of wounds.

Learning about wounds and the care of persons with wounds requires an understanding of many terms referring to types of wounds, complications of wounds, as well as treatment of wounds. Key terms to be defined as you study this chapter include:

abrasion	ecchymosis
abscess	eschar
bruise, contusion	excoriation
cellulitis	exudate, transudate
débridement	fistula
dehiscence, evisceration	gangrene
drainage	hematoma
serous	infection
sanguineous	inflammation
purulent	keloid
serosanguineous	laceration

necrosis	sinus
proud flesh	sutures
scab	wound culture

Upon mastery of the material in this chapter, you should be able to:

1. Describe in your own terms the process of wound healing.

2. Assess a wound for signs of healing or nonhealing.

3. Identify at least four factors influencing wound healing and specific nursing actions that would support each factor.

4. Assess wounds for inflammation or infection, describing signs and symptoms along with appropriate actions to control these processes.

5. Identify systemic responses to infection; prescribe appropriate nursing actions to support those responses considered desirable and reduce those responses considered undesirable.

6. Assess psychological reactions to wounds and plan appropriate intervention.

7. Apply dry sterile dressing.

8. Apply wet sterile dressing.

9. Apply clean dressing.

10. Irrigate an open wound.

INTRODUCTION

Intact skin and mucous membrane support optimal body function, yet disruption of either occurs whenever an applied force is greater than the tissues can withstand. Both intentional and accidental breaking of the skin and mucous membrane happens frequently. You need only to reflect on the ubiquitous nature of wounds (i.e., disruption of tissue continuity with or without opening of skin) to realize that the body has remarkable ability to recover. It is the re-

covery ability of the body as well as measures supporting the healing process that are the focus of this chapter.

Since one function of intact skin and mucous membrane is protection of the internal body environment against invasion by infectious organisms, any wound predisposes the individual to the potential for infection. Hence, much of wound care is directed toward controlling invasive organisms along with giving the body optimal support so that it can combat those organisms that have already entered. In reality, the human organism heals itself; all actions related to healing merely support the process or control interference with the process.

Intact skin and mucous membrane are associated with normal body function. Injury may precipitate altered body function, the degree of which is dependent on the type and extent of the injury. Individual responses differ, both to injury and to treatment. In fact, individual variations must be considered in prescribing therapy as well as in assessing response to care. Repair of broken concrete on a sidewalk requires that certain measures be applied to the break. A wound on a human body requires certain measures but the person having the wound influences the specific measures selected.

PSYCHOLOGICAL RESPONSES TO INJURY

The human organism seeks comfort. When discomfort occurs, much of the energy the organism expends focuses on regaining comfort. In the case of trauma, the injured person needs to cope with the disruption of usual body function produced by the injury as well as with his own sense of wholeness and body integrity and with the fears associated with the change. The fears may seem realistic or unrealistic to the observer (nurse), but always are real to the one injured. Behaviors emanating from the person with the injury will vary, but again, all have meaning to the one behaving—even if mysterious to the observer.

The nurse caring for the injured person anticipates the behavior observed, describing what is seen without ascribing value judgment to it. Labeling the individual as "good" or "bad," "cooperative" or "uncooperative" benefits neither the injured person nor the person in the helping role.

Pain, a frequent accompaniment of injury, in itself evokes many fears. Along with the pain precipitated by the immediate injury, *fear* of pain when having the wound dressed is also common. Observe the child who skins a knee and clasps both hands over it. He needs to have the hands removed before treatment can begin. Subsequent to the immediate reaction, pain or fear of pain may be further elicited during dressing change, irrigation of the wound, or removal of sutures. (Pain is discussed further in Chapter 34.)

Frequently the sight of blood or other drainage precipitates fright. This emotion may be severe enough to even cause fainting. *Embarrassment* may also accompany an injury. The injured person may be embarrassed about the site or cause of injury; he may be embarrassed if the dressing slips and drainage soils his clothes, garments, or he may be embarrassed by the odor of the discharge.

Alteration in body function as well as the sight of *body disfigurement* may also precipitate anxiety and fear in the individual. This may be particularly intense when such changes threaten successful pursuit of vocation or avocation. Finally, the *cost of treatment* whether direct (for care) or indirect (in loss of earning ability) may engender fear.

To the injured there are fears they can name and thus begin to control. In addition, certain anxiety-producing yet *unnamed fears* or threats may be present. These may include the sense of *helplessness*, especially if the trauma necessitates extensive dependency on others. This feeling is furthered as the injured person experiences separation from family and may even lead to a sense of abandonment. During treatment, a sense of *humiliation* may encompass the person. This is especially true if hospital procedures include such things as catheterization, taking of blood samples, or use of the bedpan. When trauma occurs there is subsequent alteration in the person's perception of his physical appearance and hence his *body image*. (See Chapter 15 on body image.) *Loss of consciousness* itself may be a real threat to the severely traumatized person.

In severe trauma, the initial anxiety signals the defense process. The mechanisms of this process lie largely in the unconscious (and are normal), ready to assist as needed in bringing a sense of comfort to the individual. The extent to which the defense mechanisms are used depends upon how long they are needed for support.

Included in these mechanisms are denial, repression, suppression, regression, rationalization, and magical thinking. *Denial* is the unconscious defense preventing one from seeing that which is unpleasant (especially about oneself). *Repression* is considered as unconscious forgetting, while *suppression* includes conscious or deliberate forgetting. Returning to an earlier developmental stage (i.e., the adult taking on childlike behavior at the time of surgery) is described as *regression*. Not accepting responsibility for one's own actions but rather attributing behavior to other persons or causes is called *rationalization*. Finally, the injured person may engage in *magical thinking* and thus attribute to another person, drug, or treatment some impossible power, frequently related to regaining of lost functions.[16] (See also Chapter 11.)

People use these defenses to differing degrees, both when well and when ill. At a time of crisis, though, you can expect to see defenses used to a greater extent than at times of personal equilibrium. The helping person might well remember that the defense will gradually disappear as the need for it decreases.

Into the maze of all or some of these responses comes the nurse or other person in the helping role. The wound or injury itself demands assessment.

> *Nursing assessment of a person with a wound includes not only the wound but also considers the patient's total response to his circumstances.*

As the nurse assesses, she can reduce some fears and threats by careful explanation of each action or expected action either before it is done (if the patient is conscious) or in retrospect (if unconscious). The explanation should not be limited to a single "telling" but rather should include describing and allowing the patient to discuss, ask questions, and/or request clarification. The sense of humiliation may be reduced by providing privacy to the individual so that he may retain his sense of dignity. In addition, allowing the patient some role in decisions relative to his care will reduce the sense of humiliation. The decisions he is capable of making may be limited but should still be allowed. He cannot make some decisions, "Do you or do you not want your wound dressed?" but can have some choices, "Do you want it done now, or would you rather wait 10 minutes?"

Through skillful care, discomfort will be minimized. In addition, use of effective skills along with analgesics will aid in reducing fears.

CLASSIFICATION OF WOUNDS

Wounds, the disruption of continuity in mucous membrane or skin, can be classified in several ways. Classification becomes significant only in so far as it promotes an ordering in the manner of assessing a wound as well as anticipating the reaction to it. The classifications used here are related to continuity of skin covering, cause of wound, type of wound, and presence or absence of pathogenic microorganisms.

A wound may be either closed or open. In a *closed wound*, no break in skin continuity can be observed. A closed wound may be caused by a direct blow with a blunt instrument or by other types of force exerted on the body. Unusual straining, twisting, or sudden deceleration might precipitate a closed wound. An *open wound* is one in which there is disruption of the skin and mucous membrane. This type may be caused by a sharp blow or object. The open wound allows direct loss of fluid from the body and entrance of foreign particles and organisms into the body. Exudate collection with resultant swelling, loss of function and pain accompany both closed and open wound. Inherent in both injuries is the potential for wound complications, discussed later.

Wounds may occur intentionally (surgical) or accidentally (traumatic). When a surgeon operates, there is disruption of skin and mucous membrane. This *intentional* type of wound is usually performed under special conditions, with sharp instruments, and the extent of the wound is related specifically to the purpose of the surgery. The wound thus has smooth, clear edges, readily approximated. An *accidental* wound is unexpected, frequently has jagged edges, and occurs under septic conditions. These factors alter the rate of healing and provide greater potential for complications.

Descriptive terms may also be used in referring to wounds. An *abrasion* is a superficial wound caused by scraping or sliding of skin surface directly over a firm, fixed surface. The floor burn caused by sliding on a sidewalk or floor with skin surface exposed is an abrasion. A *contusion* commonly has no break in the skin surface but underlying damages usually include breaking of blood vessels and swelling. The discoloration caused by the extravasation of blood into tissue is called *ecchymosis*. A *hematoma* may occur if hemorrhaging into the area is localized and significant.

The intentional wound made with a sharp instrument is frequently described as an *incision*. The sharp, clean, smooth, cut edges characteristic of an incision are in direct contrast to the jagged, irregular, torn edges seen in a *laceration*.

An instrument passing through skin and mucous membrane into deeper tissue or organs produces a *penetrating* wound. If the instrument or object both enters and exits from the deeper tissue or organs, it is referred to as a *perforating* wound. A *puncture* (stab) wound is produced by a sharp pointed object piercing deep tissue, leaving a very small opening on the surface. This type of wound commonly bleeds little and seals quickly. It is potentially hazardous, though, because of the anaerobic organisms (*Clostridium tetani* or *Clostridium welchii*) that may enter at the time of the injury.

Finally, wounds may be classified as clean, contaminated, or infected, depending on the presence or absence of pathogenic organisms. Any break in the continuity of the skin or mucous membrane presents a risk from microorganisms entering the wound and multiplying. In addition, any collection of exudate poses a depot for the growth of microorganisms. A *clean wound* contains no pathogenic microorganisms. Because of the aseptic conditions under which surgical incisions are made, these wounds are usually considered clean. A *contaminated* wound is one occurring in a manner in which there is a great likelihood of pathogenic microorganisms invading the wound. An *infected* wound is one in which pathogens have invaded and overcome the body's first line of defense, producing clinical signs of infection. The infected wound may be referred to as a *septic* wound.

PROCESS OF WOUND HEALING

The manner and rate in which healing occurs varies both with the individual involved and the location and type of wounding. If the wound heals without infection or separation of wound edges, the process is called healing by *first* intention (or by primary union). When wound edges are not approximated, granulation tissue fills in the opening prior to healing. This is described as healing by *second* intention. Finally, when there is a combination of the above, namely wound edge initially left open and later approximated or initially sutured and later broken open, healing may be described as occurring by *third* intention (Table 42–1).

This process of healing is orderly and systematic, although individual differences and complications developing during the process lead to variations in the time the process takes. Basically, the process can be divided into four phases: (1) wounding phase, (2) inflammatory phase, (3) proliferative phase and (4) remodeling phase.[15]

The process of healing and the time involved are summarized in Figure 42–1.

Wounding Phase. This is the time of injury—the moment at which tissue disruption occurs. Within minutes there will be loss of organ function, hemorrhage and subsequent blood clotting, bacterial contamination, and foreign body contamination. The extent of the wound, amount of hemorrhage, and degree of contamination by bacteria and foreign bodies directly affects the subsequent phases. As these increase, healing time increases; as these are minimized, healing time is minimized.

Inflammatory Phase. Within hours of the injury, an acute localized inflammatory response occurs. Increased capillary permeability and vasodilation produce local edema from the transudate. The transudate increases in magnitude for approximately 72 hours and contains many of the normal constituents of body fluid. Cells too migrate to the site: primarily white blood cells to control sepsis; macrophages to absorb bacteria and foreign bodies; and plasma cells to produce specific antibodies as needed locally. Finally, bacteria multiply at the site. If the number of bacteria cannot be controlled, sepsis may occur. The exact time the infection occurs may vary, depending on the virulence of the bacteria and resistance of the host, but it can be seen anytime from 48 hours to 4 to 5 days to many weeks after injury.

Proliferative Phase. The so-called "real" work of healing occurs here, beginning 4 to 5 days after wounding (later or earlier depending on the activity described above). The initial scab forms at this time. Fibroblasts, endothelial

TABLE 42–1.   TYPES OF HEALING

Characteristic	First Intention	Second Intention	Third Intention
Wound edges	Approximated	Not approximated	Initially not approximated, later approximated
Infection	Absent	Frequently present	Frequently present
Granulation tissue	Small amount	Large amount	Large amount
Scar	Small	Large	Large
Healing rate	Short	Long	Long
Example	Surgical incision	Decubitus ulcer	Eviscerated surgical wound

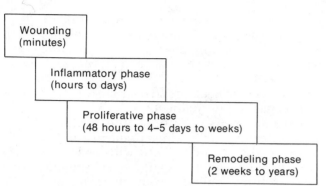

Figure 42–1. The phases of healing and time involved.

cells, and epithelial cells multiply; blood vessels bud; and collagen fibers accumulate. The cells multiply and migrate randomly, following fibrin networks already established. The wound is covered so underlying tissue is protected from contamination, although the strength of the scar is minimal.

Remodeling Phase. Finally, the epithelial covering of the wound becomes multilayered, cell production becomes balanced by cell death and collagen production is balanced by collagen hydrolysis, degradation and absorption. Scar formation occurs and changes. Activity must be resumed in order to avoid adhesions, pain, contractures and loss of function. This phase may continue slowly over a long period of time, even years.

Three terms frequently used to describe particular healing phenomena are eschar, proud flesh and keloid. *Eschar* is the sloughing tissue resulting from gangrene, corrosive trauma or thermal burns. During the healing of large surface wounds, *proud flesh* may develop. This refers to the formation of excessive amounts of edematous, soft granulation tissue. A *keloid* is a progressively enlarging scar which is raised, tumor-like and irregular. This overgrowth of scar tissue results from excessive collagen formation in the skin's dermal layer during the repair of connective tissue.

FACTORS INFLUENCING WOUND HEALING

Although the process of wound healing can be described and the time required analyzed, many factors influence the rate of healing.

The *extent of the injury* obviously influences healing. A small, superficial injury heals more readily than an extensive, deeper wound. When the injury has caused hemorrhage and formation of a hematoma, the healing rate is again prolonged since bleeding increases the dead space to be resolved, provides an excellent culture medium for bacterial growth, and increases the amount of debris to be removed.

The *type of tissue injured* influences both the healing rate and the extent to which the original function is regained. If the type of tissue injured has potential for regeneration, there is no loss of function from the injury. Certain tissues heal by regeneration (assuming underlying structures supporting the tissues are intact): epithelial tissue found on squamous surfaces of skin, interior of mouth, vagina and cervix; lining of salivary glands; vascular epithelium, parts of cornea and kidney, epithelium of digestive and respiratory tracts.[9] The collagenous scar tissue that repairs injured tendons, fascia and connective tissue closely resembles the original structure. The scar tissue mimics the original tissue; thus there is little loss of function of this type tissue. Nerves, myocardial tissue, brain tissue, and renal glomeruli are examples of tissue that does not regenerate. In fact, healing of these tissues results in laying down of nonfunctioning scar tissue. That is, the wound is healed but the scar tissue cannot perform in the same manner as noninjured tissue. For example, scar tissue in the myocardium remains both inelastic and incapable of transmission of electrical impulses, resulting both in altered electrocardiogram and contractile pattern.

The *nutritional* state of the individual influences healing. Healing rate may be retarded and incidence of complications increased in persons with inadequate amounts of protein, vitamins (especially vitamin C), minerals and calories. Deficiencies of these elements occur in the undernourished and underfed individuals but also in the surgical patient who is starved for a period of time just before or just after surgery. Protein is essential for new tissue formation, and its absence predisposes the individual to infections. Vitamin C is essential to the process of collagen formation, and its absence leads to a weak wound. Recent studies suggest that zinc is essential for wound healing and that its absence retards healing. For very poorly nourished individuals, parenteral hyperalimentation may be prescribed as an aid to wound healing.

Oxygen available to the wounded area is significant to healing. All wounds are inherently hypoxic due to blood vessel interruption at the site of the injury. Without oxygen, collagen formation is reduced and slow. Any factors reducing blood supply to the wound area will reduce oxygen available to the site as well as reduce the rate of waste material removal. Causes of reduced blood supply may be hypovolemia (through excessive blood loss), local edema causing constriction of blood vessels, firm bandaging or splinting causing pressure on regional blood vessels; atherosclerotic vascular changes reducing the size of the lumen carrying blood; or myocardial insufficiency. Older persons may experience alteration in healing power due to both reduced blood supply (hence oxygen to the area) and to altered nutritional status.

The presence of *pathogenic organisms* will alter the healing pattern. All open wounds provide direct pathways for pathogens to enter the body. Under aseptic conditions the normal inhabitants of the nasopharynx, skin and gut threaten to enter the wound. Under contaminated conditions, the organisms waiting to enter are myriad. An ubiquitous organism which frequently enters wounds is *Staphylococcus aureus*. In addition to the infectious process this organism creates, additional insult comes to the wound through the coagulase it produces. This coagulase causes thrombosis of blood vessels and hence further hemorrhage at the site, with subsequent necrosis of tissue.

The presence of *concomitant diseases* may also decelerate healing. For example: marked hypertension may lead to hemorrhage and reduced coagulation of blood at the time of wounding; diabetes mellitus may invite greater infection due to the high amount of glucose in body fluids; uremia and renal acidosis will alter the milieu and reduce available oxygen to the site; liver disease and failure affects protein synthesis and hence healing. For optimal healing, the total health of the individual must be assessed and supportive measures offered where appropriate.

Various *chemotherapeutic agents* may also alter the healing rate. Included are anti-inflammatory agents, which are associated with nitrogen and potassium depletion and hence reduced collagen formation (e.g., cortisone); aspirin with its inhibition of platelet aggregation and subsequent capillary oozing; immunosuppressive and cancer drugs that have a depressing effect on bone marrow and hence reduce the available blood cells.

Finally, no injury occurs to an individual without eliciting a *stress response*. This may directly or indirectly effect wound healing. The retained sodium and subsequent fluid, the excretion of potassium and nitrogen—all usual in the stress response—may have varying effects on the process of healing. Both the severity and the extent of the response alter the result.

Remember: *the whole individual must be assessed in evaluating and predicting the healing process. The effective nurse systematically gathers data and utilizes supportive measures to circumvent factors adversely affecting healing.*

ASSESSING PROGRESS IN WOUND HEALING

Just as no two individuals are exactly alike, so healing must be evaluated in an individual manner. When the patient asks, "Am I healing normally?", the perceptive respondent considers all the factors of individual variance as well as the usual pattern of healing. The helpful response might incorporate signs of healing or nonhealing that can be observed rather than a simple "yes" or "no" answer.

In assessing progress in wound healing factors to be considered include the following:

1. *Pain,* a desirable accompaniment of wounding because it alerts the body to a need for care, usually subsides with immobilization and initial treatment of the injury. If pain (hypersensitivity) or tenderness, once nearly gone, suddenly recurs at the site of injury, this needs to be interpreted as a sign of potential complications. Inflammation produces a hypersensitive state and needs to be suspected when pain recurs. The careful nurse queries into type, location and onset of pain before administering an analgesic.

2. *Serum* collection is another accompaniment of injury but needs to be evaluated as to amount, content, and location in assessing wound healing. The fluid collecting may be *serous,* or clear, watery substance; *sanguineous,* or bloody; *serosanguineous,* or watery with some traces of blood; or *purulent,* thick fluid which contains dead or living microorganisms, necrotic debris, and white blood cells (pus). To determine the exact source and content of the fluid, a sample may be sent to the laboratory for analysis. This may be referred to as obtaining a *wound culture.* If bacteria are identified in the culture, further analysis can be made to assist in controlling the organisms.

3. *Hemorrhage* may occur at the time of initial wounding, but may come later if the injury has extended into regional blood vessels. Bleeding may also occur if mobilization of in-

jury occurs too soon and newly budded capillaries are broken. Determining what happened immediately before the onset of frank bleeding is important in finding the source of the blood.

4. Although inflammatory response is characteristic of early healing, it may be prolonged locally or may extend generally and be described as an *infection.* The local signs of infection include heat (calor), redness (rubor), swelling (tumor), pain, and loss of function with involuntary limitation of motion. Physiologic bases for these responses are described above. If the infection precipitates a generalized response, additional signs and symptoms may include: *fever,* with or without chills; increased *pulse* rate; increased *respiratory* rate; *leukocytosis* or increased white blood count; elevated *sedimentation* rate; general *malaise* and lethargy; *headache; anorexia;* and *nausea.*

5. An additional localized complication of wounding is *abscess formation* with subsequent *sinus tract* or *fistula* development. An abscess is simply a "localized collection of pus." It complicates healing by enlarging the dead space which must be filled in (hence predisposing to larger scar area), putting pressure on surrounding blood vessels and other tissues, and necessitating removal of purulent substances and debris by the body. An abscess may be surgically incised and drained, taking care to retain the established boundaries in order to avoid extension of the infection. If the pressure within the abscess is unrelieved, it may cause a weakening at some point on its boundary. An opening between the abscess and the body surface is called a *sinus tract.* If the weakness causes a tract to form between two hollow organs, it is referred to as a *fistula.* In either in-

stance, the patient may describe a "release of pressure" and sense of "feeling better." Whenever an abscess develops, healing is prolonged and occurs by second or third intention rather than by first.

6. If the infection is localized yet not walled in, it may extend to surrounding cells along tissue planes. This is called a *cellulitis* and involves skin, subcutaneous tissue and sometimes deeper tissues.

7. *Necrosis (gangrene)* or death of areas of tissue surrounded by healthy tissue may occur if blood supply is restricted to an area to the point that cell life cannot be maintained. The dead tissue must be debrided (removed) before healing can occur.

8. Finally, a greatly feared complication of wound healing (especially surgical wounds) is wound *dehiscence,* with or without *evisceration.* The appearance of watery pink fluid (serosanguineous) on the dressing frequently precedes separation of wound edges. This separation (dehiscence) may be further accompanied by protrusion of abdominal viscera (evisceration) (Fig. 42–2). The sight of a gaping wound with protruding viscera is frightening to the patient as well as to health personnel. Treatment focuses on prevention of both infection and complex complications. Therefore, covering the protruding viscera with a sterile dressing and calling the physician are appropriate responses to this emergency (see also Chap. 43, p. 1119).

Regular, systematic assessment is very important in care of persons with wounds. The frequency of the assessment depends on the type, extent and recency of the injury. As with all assessments, initially one seeks to establish a baseline, i.e., a level against which to chart change. In injury, this deriving of a baseline may occur as part of preoperative care or as part of the first aid given. Observation of the surgical wound may be focused primarily on the character of the dressing and presence of hemorrhage. Evaluation of the traumatic wound includes

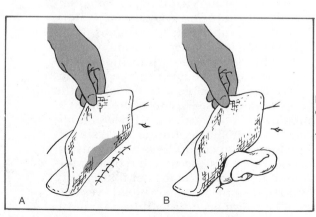

Figure 42–2. *A,* The appearance of watery pink fluid on the dressing frequently precedes wound dehiscence. *B,* Evisceration may follow dehiscence and is a frightening sight to nurse and patient.

TABLE 42–2.   SUMMARY OF WOUND ASSESSMENT

FACTOR TO BE ASSESSED	APPLICABLE TO:	
	Traumatic Wound	*Surgical Wound*
Exudate (drainage); Hemorrhage (type and amount of drainage; number and size of dressings used)	X	X
Proximity of wound edges	X	
Cleanliness of wound	X	
Length of wound	X	
Depth of wound	X	
Necessity for dressing; condition of dressing	X	X
Surrounding tissue injury (extent of injury, in centimeters)	X	X
Limitation of function	X	X
Redness (area covered, in square centimeters)	X	X
Pain (location, action producing pain, action relieving it)	X	X
Sensory perception distal to injury	X	X
Blood pressure	X	X
Pulse rate, rhythm, fullness	X	X
Respiratory rate, depth	X	X
Temperature	X	X
Awareness of time, place, person	X	X

checking for hemorrhage, proximity of wound edges, cleanliness of wound, extent of wound and depth of wound. Subsequent assessment includes the same factors and should be performed regularly. It is done more frequently until findings are stable, indicating the body is reestablishing equilibrium following injury.

In addition to assessing the wound, total body response needs to be evaluated too. This includes blood pressure, pulse rate, respiratory rate, temperature, mental alertness, and complaints of pain.

Regular assessment is needed to observe change. The changes which occur need to be communicated, either in writing, verbally, or both. Communication needs to be precise, using measurable terms whenever possible. It needs also to be thorough. A summary of wound assessment is provided on Table 42–2.

Finally, observations need to be recorded so progress can be noted. When sudden and significant changes occur, immediate notification of appropriate persons is essential in order that proper therapy can be started.

SCIENTIFIC PRINCIPLES WITH RELATED NURSING ACTIONS RELEVANT TO CARE OF WOUNDS

When the nurse understands scientific principles related to specific nursing actions used in wound care, care becomes more deliberate

and the results more predictable. As the scientific basis for nursing care expands, hopefully the application of this knowledge will be accompanied by more effective, less complicated healing. When undesirable developments complicate wound healing, the nurse needs to assess the actions being taken and evaluate whether the proper principles are being followed.

A number of principles specifically relevant to care of persons with wounds have been identified. These are presented on Table 42–3 along with application of the principles to specific nursing actions.

SUPPORTIVE MEASURES TO AID HEALING

Supportive measures directed toward rapid healing, restored function and minimal scarring begin with the initial treatment of the person and wound and continues throughout total healing process. In surgical wounding, the environment establishes a milieu for optimal healing. In accidental wounding, the milieu frequently detracts from optimal healing in varying degrees. In this section, first aid to persons accidentally injured will be discussed first, followed by measures applicable to persons with either surgical or accidental trauma. These measures are wound cleansing and dressing, wound irrigation, wound drains and suction, nutrition, anti-infective agents, im-

TABLE 42–3. SCIENTIFIC PRINCIPLES WITH RELATED NURSING ACTIONS RELEVANT
TO CARE OF WOUNDS

PRINCIPLE	NURSING ACTION
1. A break in the integrity of the skin or mucous membrane provides ready entrance for microorganisms.	1. Plan measures to prevent infections when around persons with wounds: a. Separate persons with wounds from persons with known infections. b. Provide optimal nutrition so body defenses can aid in fighting infection. c. Restrict persons entering room if risk of infection is great.
2. Skin and mucous membrane can be injured by chemical, mechanical, thermal, and microbial agents.	2. Use disinfectants in strengths safe for skin and mucous membrane. When applying heat, keep temperature of solution between 37°C. (98°F.) and 40.5°C. (105°F.) to avoid burning tissue. Keep wound and surrounding area clean. Watch for tape sensitivity, evidenced by itching, redness and blistering under adhesive tape.
3. Skin and mucous membrane normally harbor pathogens.	3. Practice effective handwashing: a. Before and after touching patient, handling dressing or handling bedclothes. b. With soap or other agent (pHisoHex) useful in reducing surface tension and mechanically ridding hands of microbes. Cleaning the wound: consider wound itself cleanest, hence clean over wound first, then area around wound. Discard cleaning swab after one stroke over skin.
4. Microorganisms are present in the air.	4. In clean, primarily closed wounds, a fibrin seal develops within hours after wound closure. These wounds may be left uncovered without risk of airborne organisms penetrating seal. Where dressings are used, removal and replacement should be done when air movement is at minimum. This is especially important in open wounds with known or suspected infection in order to avoid contamination of wound from airborne microbes and of air from infected wound.
5. Respiratory tract harbors microorganisms that can enter wound.	5. When dressing large open wounds, masks may be worn both by patient and health personnel to reduce number of organisms entering wound. When dressing open wounds, avoid talking directly over wound.
6. The ability of pathogens to cause an infection depends on: a. The virulence of the invading organism. b. The blood supply available to the site of invasion. c. The resistance of the host.	6. Extra protective measures are desirable when virulent organisms are known to be in environment. Use of isolation, masks, gloves, and distance all increase barriers to organism. Reduce number of invading organisms by proper handwashing, use of antiseptics, use of disinfectants, and environmental cleanliness. Promote optimal blood supply by nonrestrictive types of bandages. Use gravity to increase blood supply and reduce venous stagnation. Promote high level of resistance in host through good nutrition, proper immunization.

TABLE 42–3. SCIENTIFIC PRINCIPLES WITH RELATED NURSING ACTIONS RELEVANT TO CARE OF WOUNDS *(Continued)*

7. Nutrients and oxygen are carried to the wound via the blood stream and are essential for collagen formation.	7. Avoid constrictive measures when treating a wound. Seek to control edema since pressure from edema may occlude blood vessels. When applying bandage, begin distally and move proximally.
8. Moisture facilitates growth and movement of micro-organisms.	8. Microbes can neither live nor travel without moisture; therefore, keep sterile field dry. A soiled dressing provides bridge for microorganisms to enter and exit wound; therefore keep dressing dry.
9. Fluids flow downward as a result of gravitational pull.	9. Anticipate drainage at lower edge of wound. If wound is being irrigated, instill solution at top of wound and collect it at lower edge.
10. Fluids follow the line of least resistance.	10. Avoid "squeezing pimple" since content of abscess may move along tissue plane rather than through skin surface to outside.
11. Fluids move through materials by capillary action.	11. Cotton between layers of gauze acts as a wick to carry moisture away from wound. This is effective type dressing for draining wound. Penrose drains function by capillary action in removing wound drainage.
12. Obliteration of dead space in a wound aids healing by more closely approximating wound edges.	12. Drains are one method of reducing dead space. Gentle suction with Hemovac removes exudate. External pressure dressings reduce dead space very little but do constrict blood vessels locally.

mobilization, environmental control, and heat and cold.

First Aid

In situations of traumatic injury, responsible action necessitates immediate thorough assessment and treatment. Even before attention can be given to the wound, assessment must be made of the airway, breathing and circulation (see Chap. 35). Treatment of limitations in any of these is followed by wound evaluation and care. The ABC's of first aid on the following page list the immediate actions to be taken.

ABC'S OF FIRST AID

ASSESSMENT	ACTION

A – Airway

If *patent,* air will move freely, in fair quantity, quietly and effortlessly.

If *patent,* move to step B.

If *obstructed,* there will be stridor or wheezing sound, little or no air is felt moving through nose or mouth, patient may be fighting to sit up, and may be using accessory muscles of respiration.

If *obstructed,* use fingers to sweep debris (vomitus, clotted blood, teeth) from throat; extend neck, lift chin, and jaw to extend trachea; insert airway and endotracheal tube to maintain open airway.

B – Breathing

If *unrestricted,* chest movement is equal, bilateral and painless.

If *unrestricted,* move to Step C.

If *restricted,* chest movement is unequal, unilateral, painful.

If *restricted,* check for chest wounds, place clean airtight dressing over sucking wound; splint chest if fracture is suspected, so breathing can be maintained; administer supplemental O_2 or artificial respiration.

C – Circulation

If *adequate,* carotid pulse will be full, regular; skin will be warm; person will be alert mentally.

If *adequate,* inspect for wounds.

If *inadequate,* carotid pulse will be thready, weak, rapid or absent; skin will be cool and moist; there may be mental clouding or confusion.

If *inadequate,* and circulation stopped, use closed cardiac massage; if massive bleeding, apply pressure to control, cover wound site; use supportive measures to control shock, keep warm, flat, quiet.

These first aid actions may be considered as stop-gap measures to maintain life and prevent further injury until more definitive treatment is available. Transporting injured persons carefully is extremely important in order to avoid extension of the wound or predisposing to complications. Once the injured person is in a care center for more definitive treatment, protocol might include:

ASSESSMENT	ACTION

1. Is *bleeding* under control?

If *controlled,* no obvious or hidden blood loss, blood pressure stable, pulse regular and slow, pain limited.

If *controlled,* may replace original dressing with clean, sterile one, remove clotted blood from area (cosmetic effect, reduce scar), and move to next step.

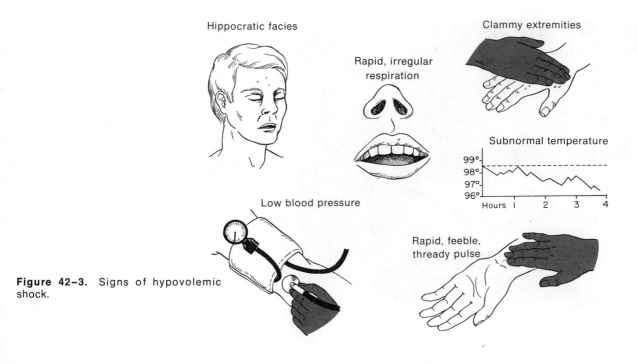

Hippocratic facies

Rapid, irregular respiration

Clammy extremities

Subnormal temperature

Low blood pressure

Rapid, feeble, thready pulse

Figure 42–3. Signs of hypovolemic shock.

ASSESSMENT	ACTION
If *not controlled,* more blood lost, increased pain, and signs of hypovolemic shock. Shock is suspected when there is a rapid, feeble, thready pulse; low arterial pressure; clammy extremities; rapid, irregular respirations; subnormal temperature (Fig. 42–3).	If *not controlled,* may need suturing to control, analgesic for pain, IV fluids, plasma extenders or whole blood to replace lost blood volume.
2. Are *wound edges* approximated?	
If *approximated,* no gaping, no protrusion of underlying contents.	If *approximated,* hold together with Steristrips (butterfly), or simply cover with dressing. (See Fig. 42–4.)
If *not approximated,* wound gaps and interior of wound visible.	If *not approximated,* sutures may be needed to anchor edges, apply dressings and splint as needed.
3. What *general measures* are indicated to support patient through initial shock of trauma?	3. Keep patient quiet until stable; support circulation; support respiration; keep warm; give analgesics.
4. Are there *injuries other than obvious* ones?	4. Make total, systematic head to toe assessment.

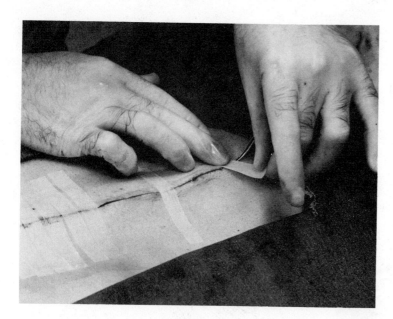

Figure 42–4. Steri-Strip used for holding wound edges together. (Courtesy of the 3M Company.)

Wound Cleansing and Dressing

In caring for the *undressed wound,* actions are based on principles described earlier. It is usually the clean, closed wound, healing by primary intention, which is left uncovered. This type of wound benefits most from "intelligent neglect." That is, the wound is not cleansed (since this may introduce more organisms and mechanically disrupt fibrin seal), but is observed regularly. In some instances, the undressed wound may need to be covered at night (or when friction of clothes would irritate the wound) to avoid unconscious scratching or other disruption of the wound healing. It is the responsibility of the nurse to manage the environment of the patient in such a way that virulent and large amounts of microbes do not come into close proximity of the undressed wound.

A wound is *dressed* for specific reasons, namely, to protect mechanically, to aid in immobilization of the site, to absorb drainage or to retain moisture. A dressing serves as a bacterial barrier only as long as it is dry. Once moist, dressings tend to collect microorganisms and hold them close to the injury. Wounds may be covered with a dry sterile dressing, a wet sterile dressing or a *clean dressing.* Applying a dry sterile dressing is described in Procedure 32. Applying a wet sterile dressing is described in Procedure 33.

A clean dressing would be used to protect the wound from irritation or environmental contaminants or to protect the environment from wound contaminants. Such a dressing provides mechanical protection to the wound and absorbs drainage. When applying a clean dressing, the procedure does not differ from applying a dry sterile dressing except (a) "clean" rather than "sterile" dressings may be used, (b) gloves are worn only if the hands of the nurse need protecting, and (c) a clean rather than sterile field is used for placement of equipment. A clean procedure is most often used in the home since the possibility of introducing an organism foreign to the wound is greatly reduced outside the health care facility.

32.   APPLYING DRY STERILE DRESSING

Definition and Purpose.   *To cover wound with sterile dressing in order to protect wound from environmental contaminants and environment from wound contaminants.* Soiled dressings are replaced (usually with permission of physician) for physical and esthetic comfort of the patient as well as to provide time for personnel to observe the wound, assess healing, and remove moist dressing to reduce potential contamination of wound. Used to protect skin around a wound, support or splint a wound.

Contraindications and Cautions.   A surgeon frequently prefers to change the initial postoperative dressing. Usually subsequent dressings may be changed as needed by nursing personnel. When in doubt, check with the physician. If the dressing is soiled but cannot be changed, it can be reinforced to protect the wound, monitor drainage and maintain patient comfort. Areas around the wound may be hypersensitive to touch, chemicals, and adhesive. Where the individual is known to have specific sensitivities, use of precipitating agents is avoided; at all times observations are made for irritation which may develop during the healing process. Wound drainage may be particularly irritating to the skin. Special measures are taken to reduce the contact of drainage with skin.

Patient-Family Teaching Points.   Providing patient and family information on why dressing change is important may help with the acceptance of the procedure. Fear of pain during the procedure may need to be discussed, along with measures to reduce discomfort. Some individuals may prefer not to see the wound with the dressing removed at the time of the first changing. When the wound is observed by the patient/family, it is helpful to describe what is seen in terms of the healing process. Explanation of the principles of asepsis used during the procedure with emphasis on ways the patient can assist will give him/her a sense of participation. Instruct the patient to keep hands away from wound during dressing change to prevent wound contamination.

PRE-PROCEDURE ACTIVITIES

PRELIMINARY ASSESSMENT/PLANNING

▶ Verify need for dressing change
▶ Check chart for orders relative to dressing change
▶ Note specific preferences of patient from nursing care plan
▶ Schedule change at least disruptive time, e.g., not immediately before or after meals,

EQUIPMENT

▶ Sterile instrument dressing set with:
Forceps
Scissors
Hemostat
4/4 dressing
Cotton tipped applicators
▶ Additional sterile dressings

Procedure continued on the following page

PRELIMINARY ASSESSMENT/PLANNING

not during visiting hours, not late at night, not during other activity in room
▶ Assess size, amount and type dressing used.
▶ Provide privacy
▶ Order room and bedside so clean, dry space available for work.

PREPARATION OF PATIENT

▶ Explain purpose of dressing change, e.g., esthetic value (sight, smell), comfort, prevention of infection.
▶ Assess need for analgesic for comfort during procedure. Allow 15 to 30 min. between time analgesic given parenterally and change of dressing. Allow 30 to 45 min. for oral analgesic to become effective. Note time of previous analgesic before administering.

EQUIPMENT

▶ Ointment if prescribed
▶ Disinfectant or cleansing solution used to clean wound
▶ Tape
▶ Gauze ties if needed
▶ Clean, dry dressing basin/tray
▶ Sterile gloves if appropriate
▶ Unsterile gloves if appropriate
▶ Acetone
▶ 2 sterile towels
▶ Waterproof bag for disposal of used dressing and used equipment

PROCEDURE

SUGGESTED STEPS	RATIONALE/ASSESSMENT
1. Wash hands carefully (see Procedure 6, p. 531).	1. Microorganisms are usual inhabitants of hands and number needs to be reduced to reduce potential contamination of wound.
2. Drape and position patient properly.	2. Provides privacy. Emotional comfort enhances physical comfort. Position patient so he is comfortable yet dressing site is readily and comfortably accessible to worker.
3. Prepare equipment using sterile technique (see Chap. 37).	
a. Spread double thickness of sterile towel on *dry*, flat surface.	a. Microbes require moisture for easy mobility.
b. Open and place sterile supplies and equipment to be used on towel (see Procedure 22, p. 929).	b. Maintains sterility of dressings and equipment.
c. Place sterile bowl beside sterile towel.	c. Metal bowl cannot transport organisms but needs to be nearby for use.
d. Pour small amount of cleansing solution in bowl (if used).	d. Solution is sterile, but outside of bottle is not (see Procedure 22).

SUGGESTED STEPS	RATIONALE/ASSESSMENT
4. Gently fold bedclothes back, exposing dressing.	4. Movement of air disseminates micro-organisms.
5. Loosen tape, beginning at edge of tape distal to center of wound and pull skin away from tape *toward* wound.	5. Avoids tension created by pulling *away* from wound edges which can disrupt newly placed fibrin network. Avoids tearing of skin which occurs when tape pulled from skin.
6. Remove soiled dressing by placing hand inside waterproof bag, grasping dressing and gently rolling it off (observe for adherence of dressing). Then pull bag over dressing. (If dressing large and/or highly contaminated use unsterile gloves to remove individual layers.)	6. Dressing is considered contaminated and organisms can be transmitted to hands of nurse and thence back to wound. Avoids disturbance of fibrin network by not pulling off adhering dressing.
7. If dressing adheres to wound, moisten with sterile water, hydrogen peroxide (3%) at ½ strength, or other appropriate sterile solution until dressing lifts off easily.	7. Forceful removal of the dressing will disrupt healing process.
8. Put on sterile gloves if needed (see Procedure 23, p. 935).	8. Gloves should be used if (a) wound is grossly contaminated; (b) large amount of care is to be given wound; (c) wound is open; or (d) patient's level of resistance is very low and risk of infection catastrophic.
9. Thoroughly assess wound, examining with eyes, nose and gentle palpation.	9. Evaluate for progress in healing and/or complications.

10. Remove adhesive around wound with acetone on swabs. Take care to work gently and with as little acetone as necessary.
  Wash skin with soap and water if acetone used.
	10. Adhesive removal each time reduces potential for skin breakdown and increases comfort.
	  Acetone may cause chemical damage to skin or wound.

11. Use saline (or other cleansing solution) or povidone-iodine (or other disinfectant) to cleanse wound and surrounding skin, discarding swab after each stroke (see Fig. 42–5).	11. Cleanse a wound from center of wound to periphery, discarding the used swab after each stroke, i.e., consider wound line cleaner than skin area even if wound is infected. Skin pathogens would further infect wound. Intact skin around wound provides barrier from infected wound in most cases. (Toxins from staphylococci may cause skin breakdown.)
12. Apply ointment if prescribed, using same technique as for cleansing.	12. Ointments that are difficult to apply to wounds may be applied to the dressing. Avoid covering mesh of gauze, for this occludes drainage.

Procedure continued on the following page

A   Cleansing a linear wound

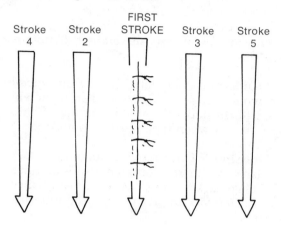

B   Cleansing a circular wound

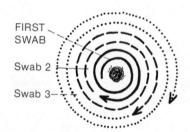

Figure 42-5.   Cleansing a linear and a circular wound.

SUGGESTED STEPS	RATIONALE/ASSESSMENT
13. Remove gloves and discard into bag with used dressing and swabs.	13. Gloves contaminated from use in cleansing skin.
14. Apply sterile dressing, using instruments (Kelly, thumb or hemostat forceps), placing small dressing directly over wound and covering with larger dressing as necessary. Use additional dressings in dependent parts to collect drainage.	14. Once dressing has been placed on patient do not reposition. Sliding the dressing moves contaminants from skin to wound. Contains drainage in dressing.
15. Anchor dressing securely in place.	15. Nonallergenic tape is most desirable since it reduces the risk of skin breakdown. For dressings needing frequent changing, Montgomery straps and ties may be used (Fig. 42-6.)
16. Replace covers over patient and position patient comfortably.	

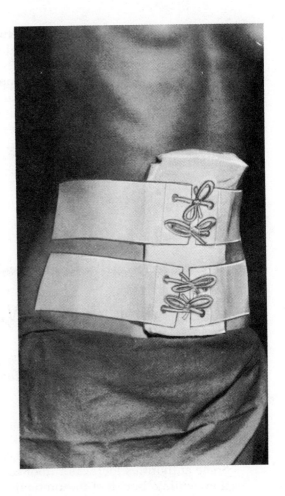

Figure 42-6. Montgomery straps are used when frequent dressing changes are required. (From *Professional Uses of Adhesive Tape,* 3rd ed. Johnson & Johnson, New Brunswick, NJ 08903.)

SUGGESTED STEPS	RATIONALE/ASSESSMENT
17. Collect used equipment for removal to designated place. Discard disposable equipment into waterproof bag. Wrap nondisposable equipment in sterile towel for return to appropriate area.	17. Soiled dressings and used equipment are contaminated. Prevents spread of pathogens to environment.
18. Wash hands thoroughly.	

Post-Procedure Activities.   Assess patient for comfort and safety, making sure bed is in desirable height and position and bedside stand with personal effects within reach. Replace bedrails if indicated.

Final Patient Assessment.   Return to room to assess security and comfort of dressing.

Procedure continued on the following page

Aftercare of Equipment. Return instruments and bowl to Central Service for cleansing and reprocessing; discard towel in laundry.

Chart/Report. Amount (in measurable units), e.g., size of drainage through stated number of layers of dressing and character of drainage, as well as condition of wound and surrounding tissue; patient's response to dressing change including emotional response, local pain, or generalized discomfort. Make notation on nursing care plan of those points of special importance to the patient regarding dressing change.

33. APPLYING WET STERILE DRESSING

Definition and Purposes. *To apply moist sterile dressing to wound in order to increase drainage by wick action thus encouraging healing.* Used to cleanse wound of debris, liquefy drainage.

Caution. Wet sterile dressings need to be alternated with dry sterile ones in order to avoid maceration and breakdown of skin around the wound. There is differing opinion regarding covering wet sterile dressing with sterile waterproof material. Some authorities feel waterproof covering increases the potential for skin maceration, while others feel the protection the covering affords is worth the risk.

Patient-Family Teaching Points. Take time to explicitly explain purpose and goal of wet sterile dressings to gain patient's assistance and cooperation. Explain that this type of dressing can be considered sterile only until applied, for at that point, moist dressing serves as a means of transferring organisms to the air and airborne organisms to the wound. See Procedure 32, *Applying Dry Sterile Dressing*, for additional teaching points.

PRE-PROCEDURE ACTIVITIES

PRELIMINARY ASSESSMENT/PLANNING

See Procedure 32

PREPARATION OF PATIENT

See Procedure 32
► Place waterproof material in manner to protect patient and bed from moisture during procedure

EQUIPMENT

Same as Procedure 32 with following additions:
► sterile container to hold solution
► fine mesh gauze, 4 × 4 (without cottonfill) gauze, or nu gauze
► sterile solution prescribed
► sterile scissors
► waterproof material to protect patient's bed from wet dressing.

PROCEDURE

SUGGESTED STEPS	RATIONALE/ASSESSMENT
Steps 1 to 3d, see Procedure 32.	
3e. Place sterile dressings to be used in sterile bowl and cover with prescribed solution.	
Steps 4 to 13, see Procedure 32.	
14. Apply dressing moistened in prescribed solution to wound, taking care to have dressing moist but not dripping. Use instruments to twist excessive moisture out of dressing or squeeze dry with sterile gloved hands.	14. Moisture dripping from dressing is uncomfortable to patient and makes pathway for organism to travel to wound. Helps to avoid maceration of intact skin.
15. Cover wet sterile dressing with dry sterile sponges and/or sterile waterproof material.	15. Attempt to limit accessibility of organisms since microbes require moisture for easy mobility. Dry dressing enhances wick action.
16. Apply outer dressing.	16. Holds dressing in place.
17. Secure dressing (see Procedure 32).	
18. Collect used equipment and remove (see Procedure 32).	
19. Wash hands thoroughly.	

Post-Procedure Activities.   See Procedure 32.

Proper disposal of soiled dressings is a very important part of any dressing change. The dressings may be odorous and obnoxious to look at as well as contaminated and thus need to be placed in a bag, then directly into an incinerator or in a covered container, usually outside the immediate vicinity of the patient.

When dressing any wound, the nurse should try to control her reaction to the sight of the wound or dressing, especially her facial response to what is obvious. The patient frequently studies the face of the person changing the dressing in order to evaluate the extent of the injury or healing process.

An additional word about *anchoring dressings*. The purpose of this action is to hold the dressing in place without causing further skin breakdown or discomfort. Ideally, an anchor holds dressings securely yet comes off easily when change is necessary. Although it may be a bit more expensive, hypoallergenic tape (sometimes called paper tape) approximates the ideal more closely than the traditional adhesive tape because it is more porous and allows air exchange under the tape.

When dressings are changed frequently, using Montgomery straps will reduce the frequency of removing adhesive and thus decrease the threat to the underlying skin (Fig. 42–6). Indications that the individual may be sensitive to adhesive tape include itching under tape, redness under and around tape, and blisters under tape. When there are large amounts of drainage, adhesive tape may not adhere so other anchors are needed. One effective means may be to use a binder: abdominal or chest for dressings on the torso, perineal for dressings on the perineum, or combinations and variations as the situation warrants. Binders have the additional advantage or disadvantage of splinting the area. This may give added comfort to the patient but needs to be used with caution since limiting activity for too long a period of time may hinder rehabilitation. Firmly applied binders to chest or upper abdomen may also limit lung expansion and predispose to chest complications such as pneumonia. (See Chapter 43 for additional discussion of bandages and binders.)

Finally, *assessment of the dressing procedure* per se by the one performing it as well as peers will enhance the quality of care being given. This assessment asks such questions as:

▶ Is the procedure *safe* for patient, nurse, and environment?

▶ Did the dressing procedure achieve the desired *therapeutic results?* Was wound healing enhanced? Was the wound protected from contamination by microorganisms?

▶ Were both patient and nurse *comfortable* during the procedure? Was the patient in as comfortable position as possible during the procedure? Was the nurse able to avoid strain or muscle stress while performing the procedure? Is the patient comfortable after the procedure?

▶ When procedure was finished, did the *dressing appear neat and orderly?*

▶ Were the *motions* used during the procedure the simplest and most direct possible while still satisfying all other goals of the treatment?

▶ In what ways was the *patient involved* in the procedure? Were personal wishes granted as much as possible? Did patient demonstrate any understanding of the purposes and goals of the procedure? Was the milieu such as to encourage the patient to ask questions and gain insight into actions?

Wound Irrigation

Wounds which are contaminated and/or healing by other than primary intention may need to be irrigated in order to flush out debris collecting between wound edges. Since wound irrigation carries with it potential hazards of wound contamination, wound extension (from too much force or volume of solution used) and spreading of contaminants to other areas from the debris washed out of wound, it is always carried out with a definite purpose and in an effective manner.

Type of solution used in irrigating a wound may vary but those closely approximating intracellular fluid both osmotically and ionically are most desirable. Hypotonic or hypertonic solutions may lead to injury of blood cells contacting the fluid. If the wound is infected, use of a broad-spectrum, poorly absorbed local antibiotic (such as neomycin) may help control the number of microorganisms that the body must fight.

The *volume of solution* used depends on the purpose and method of irrigation. In some instances a liter of fluid may be poured into a wound from a pitcher. In other instances a few ml. of fluid may be carefully instilled into a wound through a needle. This latter technique is sometimes referred to as jet stream irrigation.

When irrigating wounds, *sterile techniques* are desired in order to reduce the potential for introducing additional microorganisms. Also, the patient needs to be protected from the solution and debris draining from the wound. Frequently a small basin is placed at the lower edge of the wound to collect the solution as it drains back. A clean dry dressing may be applied over the wound at the completion of the irrigation in order both to protect the wound and to absorb residual solution.

Wound Drains and Suction

Drains may be used to (a) remove a continuing transudate; (b) provide a vent for unexpected bile, intestinal, or vascular leaks; (c) provide an appropriately situated sinus tract; and (d) to obliterate dead space of an anatomic space, abscess cavity or wound.[15] The drain is placed where collection of fluid is expected. This is frequently in the wound or through a stab wound where fluid depot may occur. The type of drain depends on the purpose (Table 42–4). When drains are in place, anticipate drainage and pad the dressing accordingly. As explained earlier, drainage seeks a low level; therefore the bulk of the dress-

TABLE 42–4. COMMON TYPES AND PURPOSES OF DRAINS

Type of Drain	Purpose	Example
Penrose	Provide sinus tract	After incision and drainage of abscess
Red rubber	Obliterate dead space	Following mastectomy or chest surgery
T-tube	Vent for possible bile leak	Following cholecystectomy
Intercath or pediatric feeding tube	Remove continuing transudate	After paracentesis
Gauze wick, NuGauze, iodoform gauze	Keep sinus open so healing can occur from base	After hemorrhoidectomy

ing should be at the lower edge of the wound. Dressings over wounds with drains need to be changed frequently, and accurate records need to be kept of the amount of fluid lost. The amount of fluid lost may be measured either by recording the number and size of dressings changed or by weighing the dry dressing prior to application and the wet dressing after removal and recording the difference in weight. The drain should be removed as soon as its purpose is achieved.

A drain may be installed with or without *suction* being applied. Hemovac suction may be used when low-pressure suction is desired and the patient is mobile. The Hemovac is a lightweight, self-contained unit composed of a closed collapsible container attached to a drain by a solid rubber or plastic tube. The container is collapsed and tube attached to the drain. As the container expands, it provides suction to the drain. Usually the Hemovac unit is either pinned to the patient's clothing or his bed linen (Fig. 42–7).

When greater pressure (suction) is desired, an electrical pump (Gomco) may be used. If the drain and suction is from a closed cavity where negative pressure is important (such as chest), a water-seal suction (Emerson) arrangement may be used. In all types of suction, it is important that tubes connecting such an apparatus to the wound be unkinked and that the drainage is observed for type as well as volume. In all but the electrical pump suction, the unit must be airtight to function effectively. When emptying suction containers, follow the instructions on the equipment. This is especially important when it is desired to maintain a negative pressure inside the cavity being drained.

Nutrition

The nutritional status of the individual may be a factor in either acceleration or deceleration of wound healing. Optimally, a positive nitrogen balance and caloric balance along with adequate intake of vitamins and minerals improve the rate of healing and reduce the risk of

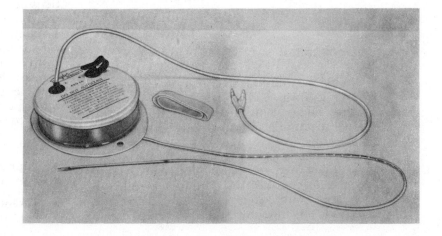

Figure 42–7. The Snyder Hemovac. The parts of a wound suction unit shown here are the evacuator, transparent connector, tubing (perforated along the part that will be placed in the wound), and needle. When you first see the suction device, the wound tubes will already have been placed in the wound and the unit will have been activated by the surgeon. (Courtesy of Zimmer, Inc., Warsaw, Ind.)

infection and other complications. When possible, establish optimal nutritional status prior to surgery. If this could not be done, then nutritional intake after wounding must receive careful attention. Dietary preference, small frequent feedings, and supplemental vitamins and minerals can help the patient reach the desired nutritional state. (See Chapters 22 and 23 for additional discussion of nutrition.)

Anti-infective Agents

Preoperatively, when wound sepsis is anticipated, a systemic broad-spectrum or specific antibiotic may be prescribed. Because of intravascular coagulation, delivery of a systemic antibiotic to the wound after surgery (or wounding) is limited and the drug can be discontinued.[15] If an infection develops, prescribing a specific drug to combat the organism or organisms identified is desired. A poorly absorbed, broad-spectrum antibiotic such as neomycin may be applied directly to an infected wound to reduce the number of microbes the body must fight systemically. Where local agents are applied, using the recommended amount per application is important. Too little may be ineffective and too much wasteful.

In the case of clean wounds, the risk of inducing reactions to antibiotics and the risk of encouraging the growth of attenuated, resistant strains of organisms far outweigh the value of the antibiotic.

When specific powders, solutions or ointments are applied locally, they should be removed daily to avoid crusting and skin irritation.

Immobilization

Immobilization aids the reparative process by allowing fibrin and collagen to form across wound edges with little disruption. Proper immobilization is nonconstrictive and thus enhances blood and oxygen supply to the area and is utilized only as long as necessary for healing to begin. Prolonged immobilization may predispose to contractures, reduced mobility in the area, and overgrowth of scar tissue. Methods of immobilization include use of

casts, splints, slings, and binders as well as dressings (see Chapter 43).

Environmental Control

Whenever possible, exposing the patient with a wound to large concentrations of potentially virulent organisms is to be avoided. Thus, the nurse may need to assume responsibility for (a) limiting the number and movement of persons in the area when dressings are changed, (b) restricting contact with persons who have a known infection, and (c) preventing spread of organisms by not allowing anyone to sit on the patient's bed or use his personal effects. The goal is to establish as many barriers to transmission of organisms as possible in order to reduce the risk of infection.

Use of Heat and Cold

There are times when local application of heat and/or cold may aid both the reparative process and the comfort of the patient. Generally, *heat application* for short periods of time causes vasodilation, with the effect of increasing blood and oxygen supply to the area and removal of waste from the area. Conversely, *cold* for short periods of time causes vasoconstriction with local ischemia ensuing (sometimes desirable to avoid swelling). Prolonged use of either heat or cold causes effects opposite from the desired. As with other measures, heat or cold may aid healing but must be used knowledgeably and with discretion in order to avoid additional injury. (See Chapter 44 for discussion of uses of heat and cold.)

ASSISTING PATIENT IN SELF-CARE OF WOUNDS

Due to length of time required for wound healing, most patients need to take care of their own wounds upon leaving an acute care center. Encouraging patient involvement in wound care throughout hospitalization will give the individual greater confidence in his ability to care for himself upon returning home. Skills, knowledge and understandings the patient (or other person assuming responsibility for care) need to acquire include:

▶ The process of wound healing

▶ Supportive means to aid healing such as preventing infection and good nutrition

▶ Techniques of wound care including cleaning, dressing and irrigating

- Techniques of skin care to prevent further tissue breakdown
- Use of solutions and ointments
- Use of clean vs. sterile dressings
- Control of odor from wound and dressing
- Techniques of anchoring the dressing
- Care of used dressings

When, where and to what degree these are taught will depend on the individual learner. A plan for teaching needs to be developed and a means for evaluating learning established. Without these, preparation for self-care will take on an unstructured form and goals will not be achieved. The patient will go home with the admonition "take care of yourself" and left to figure out exactly how by himself.

Patients who are caring for themselves frequently want guidelines for seeking medical help. They fear something going wrong with their wound, but they do not want to bother the doctor with insignificant details. It can be reassuring to the patient to know the indications for seeking further medical supervision.

Indications for medical consultation include the following:

- An unexplained increase in body temperature
- Unusual redness or tenderness over the wound
- Alteration in type, amount, or quality of drainage from the wound
- Separation of previously approximated wound edges
- Discomfort when performing an activity that caused no discomfort before
- A general sense of "feeling bad" (persisting) although specific explanation cannot be found

Referral to the local public health department will provide assistance to patients and their significant others to adapt teaching to the home situation and provide reports to the physician on the patient's progress. When large amounts of dressings are needed, the public health nurse may provide leads for help in obtaining dressings, such as the local chapter of the American Cancer Society.

CONCLUSION

Wound healing is an orderly process with several phases and much potential for variation. Individual differences must be considered in wound care. The medical team does its best to set the stage for prompt, effective healing but the process itself must be the work of the individual who is wounded.

BIBLIOGRAPHY

1. Altemeier, W. A.: Wound sepsis. *In* Longacre, J. J. (ed.): *The Ultrastructure of Collagen.* Springfield, IL, Charles C Thomas, 1976, p. 5–9.
2. Boericke, P. H.: Emergency: first aid for care of open wounds, severe bleeding, shock. *Nursing '75,* 3:40–46, March 1975.
3. Castle, M.: Wound care, clear-cut ways to speed healing. *Nursing '75,* 5:40–44, Aug. 1975.
4. DuGas, B. W.: *Kozier-DuGas' Introduction to Patient Care.* 3rd ed. Philadelphia, W. B. Saunders Co., 1977, pp. 415–432.
5. Gragg, S. H., and Rees, O. M.: *Scientific Principles in Nursing,* 6th ed. St. Louis, C. V. Mosby Co., 1970, pp. 390–406.
6. Hunt, T. K.: Diagnosis and treatment of wound failure. *Advances in Surgery,* 8:287–309, 1974.
7. Knight, M. R.: A "second skin" for patients with large draining wounds. *Nursing '76,* 6:37, Jan. 1976.
8. Laughlin, V. C.: Stop the constant drip of draining wounds. *Nursing '74,* 4:26–27, Dec. 1974.
9. Luckmann, J., and Sorensen, K. C.: *Medical-Surgical Nursing: A Psychophysiologic Approach.* Philadelphia, W. B. Saunders Co., 1974, pp. 143–163.
10. Madden, J. W.: Wound healing: the biological basis of hand surgery. *Clinics in Plastic Surgery,* 3:3–10, Jan. 1976.
11. Mattsson, E. I.: Psychological Aspects of Severe Physical Injury and Its Treatment. *Journal of Trauma,* 15:217–234, Mar. 1975.
12. Myers, M. B.: Sutures and wound healing. *American Journal of Nursing,* 71:1725–1727, Sept. 1971.
13. Powell, M.: An environment for wound healing. *American Journal of Nursing,* 72:1862–1865, Oct. 1972.
14. Rinear, C. E., and Rinear, E. E.: Emergency bandaging: a wrap-up of better techniques. *Nursing '75,* 5:29–35, Jan. 1975.
15. Schilling, J. A.: Wound Healing. *Surgical Clinics of North America,* 56:859–874, Aug. 1976.
16. Schnaper, N.: The psychological implications of severe trauma: emotional sequelae to unconsciousness. *Journal of Trauma,* 15:94–98, Feb. 1975.
17. Trauma care: expect the unexpected. *Nursing '76,* 6:58–63, June 1976.
18. Wound suction, better drainage with fewer problems. *Nursing '75,* 5:52–55, Oct. 1975.

CHAPTER 43

PROVIDING PHYSICAL PROTECTION AND BODILY SUPPORT

By Margaret M. McMahon, R.N., B.S.N., CCRN

OVERVIEW AND STUDY GUIDE

Providing comfort and support and insuring a safe, therapeutic, and aesthetic environment are major nursing goals. Developing an understanding of the use, limitations and hazards of protective devices assists the nurse in achieving these goals. Throughout the chapter, prevention of complications arising from the use of these aids is emphasized. Attention is focused on nursing assessment and patient-family teaching in the detection of complications. Because nurses frequently need to improvise protective and supportive devices, methods of improvisation are presented. The major topics included in this chapter are:

▶ Chest, abdominal and perineal binders

▶ Roller, tubular and elasticized bandages

▶ Special dressings, gauzes and adhesives

▶ Orthopedic devices including crutches, canes, walkers, cervical collars, splints and slings

▶ Positioning devices, e.g., sandbags, trochanter rolls and footboards

▶ Protective devices such as heel and elbow protectors, bed cradles, sheepskin and air rings

▶ Flotation therapy, air mattresses and turning frames, e.g., Stryker frame, CircOlectric bed, Wedge frame

▶ Linen, leather and environmental restraints

1. As you study this chapter familiarize yourself with the following terms:

ischemia	capillary filling
necrosis	peripheral pulse
denudation	cyanosis
contracture	maceration
edema	dehiscence
compartment syndrome	evisceration

2. As you study this chapter familiarize yourself with aspects of patient's rights and nursing responsibility, accountability and liability relative to each topic discussed.

3. Upon completion of this chapter, you should be able to do the following:

(a) Correctly and safely apply protective and supportive devices to patients when appropriate

(b) Recognize and prevent complications associated with these devices

(c) Identify legal ramifications relative to inappropriate use of each device

(d) Assess patient-family response to protective and supportive devices

(e) Identify and meet patient-family teaching needs specific for each device, with emphasis on the proper application, potential hazards, and effects on the patient's activities of daily living

(f) Record and report nursing activities and observations relative to the use of protective and supportive devices

(g) Evaluate effectiveness of nursing intervention in achieving desired goals

---

BINDERS

Binders are pieces of material applied to large areas of the body, e.g., chest and abdomen. They may be used to immobilize, to provide comfort and support, to secure dressings and to exert pressure. Materials used for binders include heavy cotton, muslin, flannel and synthetics. Disposable paper "T" binders are also available for short-term use.

Key points in the use of binders are:

▶ Binders are applied so that firm, even pressure is exerted.

▶ Binders should not impair neurovascular or pulmonary function.

▶ Since binders are not attached to the skin, they slip out of place easily and may require frequent application.

▶ Wrinkled binders are uncomfortable and may cause tissue damage.

▶ Binders are secured so that there is no movement and friction against underlying skin surfaces.

▶ Pins or knots are placed away from wound edges or tender areas.

▶ Binders are applied with the body part in anatomical alignment and with joints in position of function.

▶ Soiled or moist binders may promote infection if applied over skin surfaces that are not intact.

▶ The skin surfaces underneath a binder should be inspected at frequent intervals.

▶ Neurovascular integrity of areas distal to the binder should be assessed at frequent intervals.

▶ Binders that cause discomfort should be removed and reapplied.

Chest binders may be used to provide support to the chest wall following surgery and to immobilize the ribs in the presence of fractures. They are available as a large rectangular piece of heavy muslin or flannel or as pre-sized commercially made synthetics. Chest binders may be pinned in place or may be secured with self-adhering strips of material. Some chest binders have shoulder straps to keep them in place. *Rib belts* are modifications of chest binders used primarily for patients with rib fractures (Fig. 43–1).

Major concerns in the use of chest binders are: (a) the further impairment of already traumatized lung tissue (respiratory insufficiency) because of restriction of the chest wall; (b) *increased pulmonary secretions* resulting from inadequate lung expansion and inadequate expectoration (coughing up) of secretions and (c) development of pulmonary infections, e.g., pneumonia. Since these binders are frequently prescribed for patients being discharged home, it is important that the patient and family watch for the preceding complications of chest binders and be familiar with removal and reapplication techniques.

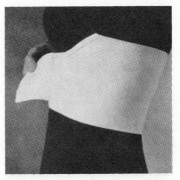

Figure 43–1.   Rib belt commonly used in the treatment of rib fractures. (From Chick Orthopedic *Catalog of Anatomical Supports*, 1973. Chick Orthopedic, Division of Hosmer Dorrance Corp., p. 20.)

The following activities are important when a patient is wearing a chest binder:

▶ Frequently assess excursion of the chest wall by looking directly at the chest and by placing your hands gently on the chest to feel breathing movements. Place hands around posterior portion of chest at the level of the tenth rib and instruct the patient to "take a deep breath."

▶ Frequently assess breath sounds with and without a stethoscope to detect abnormal secretion formation. Listen for rales, rhonchi, wheezes and rubs.

▶ Elicit tactile fremitus to assess presence of pulmonary consolidation.*

Findings which indicate the development of pulmonary infection should be reported promptly, and vigorous pulmonary hygiene measures such as deep breathing, coughing, oral fluids, etc. should be initiated. It should be remembered, however, that these activities are often painful for the patients and pain medication may be indicated to enhance their effectiveness.

Breast binders may be used to apply pressure to the breasts to decrease lactation following childbirth, or to secure dressings. These binders look like sleeveless jackets and are contoured to conform to the chest wall; however, they often need to have tucks pinned in them in order to achieve optimum fit. The patient should be supine when the binder is being

*See Chapter 17 for detailed discussion of assessment.

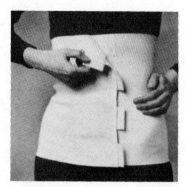

Figure 43–2. Abdominal binder with self-adhering closure strips. (From Chick Orthopedic *Catalog of Anatomical Supports,* 1973, p. 20.)

pinned in order to provide maximum support. The nursing concerns and patient/family teaching requirements are the same as for chest binders.

Straight *abdominal* binders are used primarily to provide support following abdominal surgery and to secure dressings (Fig. 43–2). The binder may be either: (a) a large rectangular piece of heavy cotton, muslin or flannel pinned up the center to fit the patient or (b) a synthetic binder with adhering strips or hooks and eyes. Commercially made binders come in a variety of sizes and may have metal stays to keep the binder in place and wrinkle-free. The abdominal binder is applied with the patient in a supine position and lying on the center of the binder. The binder's lower portion is extended well over the hips, but not so low that it interferes with elimination or ambulation. Attention should be directed at ensuring that the binder does not exert undue pressure on wound edges or interfere with respiration. Abdominal binders may need frequent reapplication because they slip down and become wrinkled.

When an abdominal binder is used postoperatively for support, the length of time it will be required should be estimated, and this estimate should be incorporated into the nursing care plan. Many patients become dependent on the binder and may need encouragement to improve muscle tone. If a patient is so large that the usual sizes will not fit, an abdominal binder may be improvised from a Mayo stand cover (available from the operating room or the laundry). Patients who are being discharged home with binders should have an extra binder to allow for laundering. Recording

of the procedure includes noting the time the binder was applied and removed, whether the skin was cleansed, the condition of the skin, and patient/family teaching completed.

A *scultetus binder* consists of a rectangular piece of strong cloth with many tails attached to the two longer sides. It is most commonly used as an abdominal binder for support of the abdominal musculature, to prevent wound dehiscence (opening of wound edges) and evisceration (protrusion of abdominal contents through the wound edges) following abdominal surgery, and to keep dressings in place.[2] In order to apply a scultetus binder the patient is in a supine position lying on the center of the binder, with the tails equally extended to either side. Powder may be applied to the skin surfaces to decrease friction resulting from the movement of the binder against the skin. *Do not allow powder to get near or into the wound.* Starting at the bottom of the binder, bring each tail across the abdomen, pulling it taut. Overlap

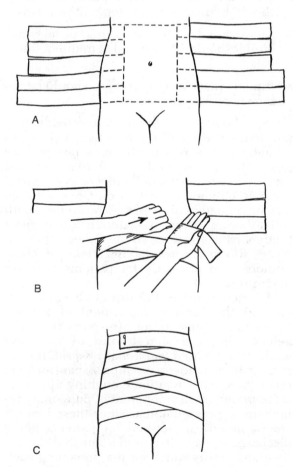

Figure 43–3. Technique for applying a scultetus (many tailed) binder.

each succeeding tail at a slightly upward angle, crossing at the midline (Fig. 43–3). Anchor the end of each tail with your hand until it is secured by the opposite tail. If the tails are too long, they should be folded. The top tails are overlapped along a straight line and pinned in place. When properly applied, there is an even pattern along the midline and a snug fit.

If applied too tightly, chest and abdominal binders may be dangerous devices. The potential complications of chest binders have been previously discussed. Abdominal binders may also inhibit respiratory function if applied too tightly. Furthermore, abdominal binders may compress the vena cava, resulting in hypotension if they are applied with excessive pressure. If respiratory difficulty or hypotension develop, the binder should be removed and reapplied.

A *T binder* is used primarily to secure rectal or perineal dressings (Fig. 43–4). The *double T* binder is used for males and the *single* for females. The single or double T strap is brought between the patient's legs and is pinned to the waist band in front. Patients usually prefer to apply this type of binder themselves, so it is important that the method of application be carefully explained. Most T binders are made of washable material; however, paper binders are available for short-term use. Paper binders fall apart easily and are of limited value. If commercially made T binders are not available, one can improvise by using a sanitary belt and perineal pad or by using wide roller gauze or woven gauze bandage (Kling) and pinning it together to form a "T." T binders are easily soiled and need frequent changing.

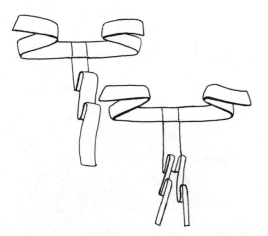

Figure 43–4. Single and double T binders used to secure perineal dressings. The single T binder is used for females and the double T binder for males. (From Leake, M. J.: *A Manual of Simple Nursing Procedures,* 5th ed. Philadelphia, W. B. Saunders Co., 1971, p. 180.)

BANDAGES

Bandaging Materials

A bandage is a length of material applied to fit smaller parts of the body. Bandages are available in a variety of lengths and widths and are softer and more conforming than binders. Bandages have the same functions as binders but are most commonly used to provide pressure and to hold dressings in place.

Materials used for bandages include: straight weave and knit weave cotton gauze (Kling, Kerlix), muslin, flannel, elasticized knit, rubberized self-adhering material (Elastoplast, Coban), elastic net webbing (Surgifix, Surgiflex), ribbed tubular cotton (Stockinet), and knit tubular cotton (Tube-gauz).

Gauze is most commonly used because it is absorbent, yet porous, allowing air to circulate; also, gauze is soft and easily conforms to body contours. Gauze frays when laundered, so it is usually not recycled. *Flannel* is sturdier, withstands repeated washings and keeps the part warm. Both flannel and *muslin* are less flexible than gauze and are used when immobilization and/or pressure are desired.

Elasticized net bandages are available in a variety of sizes and shapes. They may be tubular or may be made in the shape of a shirt or pants. Some elasticized net bandages are designed only to keep dressings in place, while others are more constricting and designed to apply pressure.

Use and Application of Bandages

Key points in the use and application of bandages are:

▶ A bandage is applied from the most distal part toward the trunk.

▶ The area distal to the bandaged part, such as the fingers and toes, should be left exposed whenever possible and observed frequently for color, sensation, temperature and edema. Cyanosis (blue tinge to skin) implies that circulation is impaired. Blood supply is assessed by applying pressure to the nailbed, releasing it, and observing the degree of capillary refill evidenced by the return of color to the nailbed.

▶ Bandages should be bulky enough that they are absorptive and supportive, yet not so large that they interfere with the patient's ability to function.

▶ Bandages applied over wet dressings or draining wounds should be applied more loosely because they may shrink when they dry, causing ischemia (decreased circulation).

▶ Bandages should be applied firmly, with each turn exerting the same amount of pressure. Uneven and unnecessary overlapping is to be avoided.

▶ Bony prominences and hollows should be padded to insure that equal pressure is exerted over all surfaces.

▶ Whenever possible, a bandage is applied with the part held level to or elevated above the trunk, rather than dependent. This will minimize venous congestion and edema.

▶ Bandages should be neat, clean, durable and functional. For both aseptic and aesthetic reasons, bandages should be removed and reapplied when they do not meet these criteria.

> *Bandages that are too tight are not only uncomfortable, they are very dangerous. There are many documented cases of permanent damage resulting from tight bandages.*

With the variety of bandages available, the nurse can use ingenuity in creating an aesthetic, functional bandage if she is familiar with the use and limitations of each of the materials. We discuss separately roller bandages, tubular bandages, the Jones dressing, and elastic stockings.

Roller Bandages

A *roller bandage* is a long strip of material which is wound on itself to form a "roll." The outside end of the roller bandage is the *initial* portion, and the *terminal end* is at the center inside the roll. The roll itself is called the *body.* To apply the bandage, the initial end is held in place with one hand and the body is passed over the part. The bandage is anchored in place by making two turns. Application is then continued by passing the roll from one hand to the other. Equal pressure is exerted with each turn.

This is accomplished by gradually unrolling only small amounts of bandage as needed.

TYPES OF TURNS

There are *several turns* used when applying roller bandages. The type of turn used depends upon the body part to be bandaged and the bandage material.

The *circular turn* is the simplest and most commonly used action in bandaging. It is merely the wrapping of a bandage, used in bandaging circumferential (circular) parts. A circular turn is used when the bandage is to overlap the previous bandage completely and the beginning and termination of the bandage are in the same location. It is used to anchor a bandage when it is started and ended, when starting a figure-of-eight or spiral bandage or when bandaging a small part.

In the *spiral turn* the turn overlaps the previous turn only partially, e.g., from one half to three fourths the width of the bandage. It is used most commonly in bandaging cylindrical parts.

The *spiral reverse turn* involves reversing the bandage halfway through each turn. It is used for bandaging circumferential areas that increase in size, such as the forearm or leg. This turn is required when applying inflexible bandages such as roller gauze. Because of the availability of more adaptable bandages, this turn is rarely used in the hospital setting (Fig. 43–5).

The *figure-of-eight turn* is accomplished by overlapping the turns on the oblique in an alternately ascending and descending fashion. Each turn crosses over the previous turn, so that it resembles a figure-of-eight. This turn is

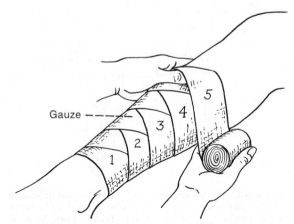

Figure 43–5. Spiral reverse turn is used when bandaging a conical area with nonconforming roller gauze.

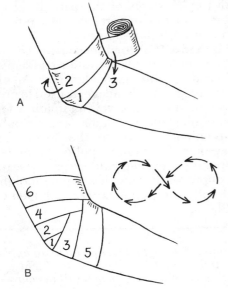

Figure 43–6. Figure-of-eight turn is used when bandaging joints.

tation, the head, and occasionally, the fingers. The bandage is first anchored with a few circular turns, then the bandage is placed in the center of the part to be bandaged, a half turn is made, and the material held with a finger. The body of the bandage is passed back and forth over the tip, from the superior to the inferior surfaces and back again. Each fold is held with a finger to keep it in place. The bandage is overlapped first to one side then to the other, until all parts are covered. The bandage is terminated with several circular turns over the folded bandage and taped or pinned in place. If the area bandaged is large, the turns may be reinforced with adhesive tape strips applied on the oblique (Fig. 43–7).

Turns should be made with equal pressure and tension. Uneven or unnecessary overlapping of turns is undesirable and usually can be prevented by choosing a more appropriate kind or size of bandage. When the bandaging material is to be used again, the bandage is rewound as it is removed. If the material is to be discarded, it is cut along the long axis of the bandaged part, well away from the wound or tender areas.

employed when bandaging joints, especially the knee, ankle and elbow, and is effective in immobilizing the joint. When properly applied, the bandage has a "herring-bone" appearance (Fig. 43–6).

The *spica* is a variation of the figure-of-eight. All turns overlap at a sharp angle and are alternately ascending and descending. This turn is used when bandaging the hip, thigh, groin or thumb.

The *recurrent turn* is used to bandage longer areas, such as the stump remaining after ampu-

TYPES OF ROLLER BANDAGES

Roller bandages are available in a variety of lengths and widths and are made of cotton gauze or rubberized or elasticized material.

Figure 43–7. The recurrent turn is used when bandaging large areas such as the head and amputation stumps.

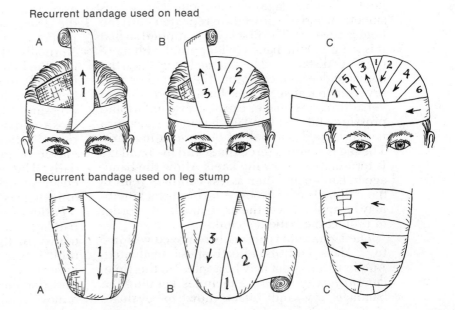

Recurrent bandage used on head

Recurrent bandage used on leg stump

Cotton Gauze Bandages. Types of cotton gauze bandages discussed below are: (1) roller gauze, (2) Kling and Kerlix and (3) Unna boot. *Roller gauze* is one type of cotton gauze bandage. Roller gauze is loose mesh material available in several widths. It is rigid and does not conform well. When bandaging a large area with roller gauze, one must use the spiral reverse turn. Roller gauze is often used temporarily to secure dressings in a "first-aid" setting.[1, 10, 19]

Kling and Kerlix are loose weave or knitted roller gauze bandages which are soft and conform easily. They are used to secure dressings, are highly absorptive, and are appropriate when a bulky dressing is desired. They are applied in a manner similar to other roller bandages; however, they are so flexible that the spiral reverse turn is not needed.

The *Unna boot* is a medication-impregnated cotton gauze bandage containing calamine, glycerine, zinc oxide and gelatin. It is commonly used to provide protection and support to the lower leg and ankle in persons with skin loss due to stasis ulcers or stasis dermatitis, and for patients with strains or sprains. It provides medication to the area while preventing edema and allowing for ambulation. It is packaged as a moist bandage and becomes hard and stiff when dry.

Before applying an Unna boot, the foot and lower leg should be cleansed and dried. The foot is placed at a right angle to the leg. Apply the bandage with a circular turn around the foot and direct the bandage on the oblique, over the heel. The bandage is then cut, the edges smoothed and the procedure repeated until the heel is covered. The first layer is applied so that it is snug and the bandage is applied with more pressure distally and less in the leg.[11] When the bandage does not conform, it is cut rather than reversed because ridges form where the reverse turns are made, causing discomfort and pressure after the bandage hardens. Each turn is overlapped one half of the preceding turn. The leg is covered three times and the bandage is terminated below the knee. Allow the bandage to harden and then assess capillary refill in the nail beds of the toes. A layer of stockinette may be applied over the dry Unna boot in order to protect the patient's clothing.

The Unna boot is normally removed within 5 to 7 days and its effectiveness evaluated. Another Unna boot may be applied at this time. *Patient/family teaching* includes keeping the bandage dry and intact, how to evaluate neurovascular status of the part distal to the bandage and the importance of a return appointment for follow-up care.

Rubberized or Elasticized Bandages. Discussed in this section are elastic roller bandages and elasticized or rubberized adhesives. An elastic roller bandage (Ace bandage) is used to provide support, to minimize swelling in joints following musculoskeletal trauma, and to enhance venous blood return to the heart. Elastic bandages are frequently applied to the legs of postoperative or bed-ridden patients in the hope of preventing the development of thrombophlebitis and pulmonary emboli (see Chapter 33).

Caution: *Elastic bandages which are applied too tightly or which become too tight after "normal application" may result in neurovascular damage. Frequent reassessment of elastic bandages is essential.*

Traditionally, elastic bandages have been applied from the distal part toward the trunk. This is based on the premise that this motion follows the direction of venous circulation, thereby minimizing venous congestion, stasis and edema of the distal part. However, in an interesting study by Guberski and Campbell, leg volumes were compared using the proximal-to-distal and distal-to-proximal elastic bandaging techniques. Their findings indicate that "there is no difference in reduction of leg volume between the two methods of applying elastic bandages to the lower extremity."[8] Their study involved normal volunteers, and the effects may be different in persons with injury and edema. Therefore, it seems reasonable to use either method of bandaging when applying elastic bandages prophylactically, but the distal-to-proximal technique seems appropriate when trauma and edema are present. Normally, the heel of the foot is incorporated into the bandage. The bandage is applied with the body of the bandage held close to the part being bandaged to insure *even* tension and pressure. Elastic bandages frequently become loose and wrinkled and may need frequent reapplication. Even if intact and wrinkle-free, elastic bandages should be removed at least daily. The underlying skin surfaces should be cleansed, dried and assessed for pressure areas or lesions (Fig. 43–8).

Patient/family teaching relative to elastic bandages includes: (a) assessing vascular integrity in the distal part by testing capillary refill in the nail beds, (b) understanding the hazards of a bandage which is too tight, (c) return demonstration of proper application and removal, and (d) how (including a phone

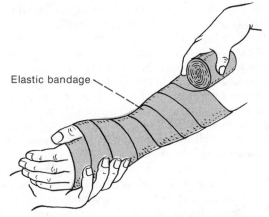

Elastic bandage

Figure 43-8. Application of an elastic bandage.

number) and what to report if complications arise.

It is essential that the use of elastic bandages be documented in the clinical record. Appropriate recording includes when the bandage was removed and reapplied, skin care given and the condition of the skin, and the integrity of the part distal to the bandage. Health teaching done and return demonstrations should also be included. Elastic bandages can be very therapeutic, but they can also be *very dangerous* in the presence of poor application techniques and poor teaching.

Elasticized or rubberized adhesives such as Elastoplast and Coban are conforming, self-clinging roller bandages used when firm, even pressure is desired. They are most commonly applied as an outer dressing wrap over wounds to prevent swelling or promote hemostasis. When applying these adhesives for pressure dressings, relax the tension on the ends of the bandage to prevent the ends from curling.

> *Elasticized or rubberized adhesive bandages applied too tightly can cause* arterial occlusion, *which may result in gangrene. If this occurs, radical surgical procedures, e.g., amputation, may be necessary.*

Tincture of benzoin or other skin adherents are often applied to the skin in order to make elasticized or rubberized adhesives more adherent. Patients who have allergies to perfumes may also have an allergy to benzoin. It is thus important to take a patient history of allergies and do a benzoin skin test as appropriate. Additionally, these bandages should not be applied to the skin of persons who are allergic to rubber. It is imperative that the patient/family understand the hazards of adhesive roller bandages

and be reliable enough to check the area distal to the bandage for signs of impaired circulation.

Tubular Bandages

Elasticized Net. A tubular bandage is a bandage in the shape of a tube. Types of tubular bandage discussed here are elasticized net, stockinette and Tube-gauz. Elasticized net is a highly adaptable net used for a variety of purposes. There are two kinds of elasticized net, and their uses are quite different. One net is used to exert firm, constant pressure in order to decrease edema, prevent scarring and prevent the development of contractures. It is quite constrictive and is commonly employed in the care of patients with burns or in the care of postoperative mastectomy patients, who are prone to develop lymphedema (edema due to interference with lymph drainage). The second kind, Surgifix or Surgiflex, is much more elastic, exerts no pressure at all, and is used to secure dressings, tubes and appliances. It has revolutionized bandaging in that it is useful in applying dressings over difficult areas such as the head, axilla and over joints. It is available in both tubular form or as pre-sized shirts and pants (Fig. 43-9). The pants are especially valuable in securing perineal and buttock dressings. This material is particularly effective for patients who need frequent dressing changes or have excoriation of the skin from repeated removal of adhesives. Holes may be cut in the net without altering the effectiveness of the bandage. Elastic net may also be used to hold IV catheters and tubing, arm boards, splints and ostomy bags in place. It addition to its flexibility and ease of application, it promotes healing by allowing the part to be exposed to air and kept dry. While the initial cost of elastic net may be greater than that of other bandaging materials, it may be more economical for long-term use because it withstands repeated washing and holds its shape well. In order to determine the length of bandage needed, measure the length of the area to be bandaged and allow for any overlap desired. Then, cut the same length of *unstretched* bandage. The hands are placed inside the bandage and it is stretched as it is applied over the part. The net should be washed in warm, soapy water, rinsed well and allowed to drip dry.

Stockinette and Tube-gauz. Stockinette and Tube-gauz are stretchable cotton tubular bandages designed to cover cylindrical parts of

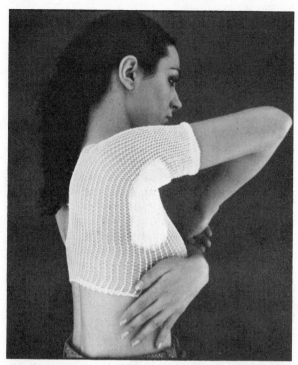

Figure 43–9. Flexible net bandage is used to secure bandages in difficult areas such as the axilla and around joints. (From *Surgifix Catalog,* FRA Surgifix Incorporated, Elmsford, NY 10523.)

the body. Stockinette may also be bias cut and used as a roller bandage. It is available in a variety of sizes and widths. Stockinette is frequently used to protect the skin when casts are applied or as a head cap in postoperative neurosurgical patients. Tube-gauz is used primarily to secure dressings. The desired length is cut from a roll and is pushed onto an applicator. The applicator is placed over the area to be bandaged, and the material is slid off the applicator onto the part and held taut. The entire length of the part is bandaged, as the applicator is gradually rotated. The bandage and applicator are extended beyond the tip of the bandaged part and the applicator is rotated 180 degrees. The applicator is then placed over the part, and the procedure is repeated until the desired thickness of the bandage is achieved. The tubular gauze may then be extended several inches beyond the bandage, cut along the sides, and the tails secured around the joint. This keeps the bandage from slipping off. The ends are tied in a bow rather than a knot so that the bandage can be removed quickly if signs of ischemia develop. In children or confused persons, the bow may be secured with a piece of adhesive tape. If desired, the distal part may be left exposed. When this is done, a small piece of adhesive tape may be applied over the distal folds to keep the bandage from rolling.

Jones Dressing. A Jones dressing is a compression bandage used to immobilize and support an area following musculoskeletal trauma. Although called a dressing, a Jones dressing is actually a splinted bandage. It is effective in decreasing edema or preventing edema from developing and is used in place of a plaster cast in the treatment of fractures or severe sprains. The Jones dressing is left on for several days and often replaced with a plaster cast when the swelling is decreased. The dressing is applied as follows: cotton batting—approximately 30.5 cm. (12 in.) wide and available in large rolls—is wrapped around the area, e.g., toes to knee when the ankle or lower leg is injured. This is followed with application of posterior plaster splints that extend the entire length of the cotton batting. An elastic bandage is then applied from toes to knee, and the final layer of the dressing is 15.3 cm. (6 in.) stockinette, cut on the bias, applied as a roller bandage from toes to knee.[11] Since weight bearing is to be avoided, there is no walking heel incorporated into the dressing. The patient must use crutches until a plaster cast has been applied and is dry. In order to effectively minimize swelling, the patient should elevate the injured area at least 30.5 cm. (12 in.) above the heart.

When doing *patient/family teaching* the nurse should emphasize that: (a) weight bearing is not allowed; (b) the casting material is not sturdy; (c) the Jones dressing is a temporary measure and the patient must return for removal, re-evaluation and possible plaster casting; (d) elevation and application of ice are important for the first 24 hours and (e) it is essential to frequently assess neurovascular integrity in the part distal to the injury and report abnormalities.

Elastic Stockings

Elastic stockings are used to promote venous blood return and prevent pooling of blood, as well as to provide pressure to the legs. They are commonly employed in the care of a patient with varicose veins, impaired circulation, or pregnancy and for the postoperative or bedridden patient as prophylaxis against thrombophlebitis. Elastic stockings are available in different sizes and lengths such as toes-to-knee and toes-to-midthigh.

Remove and reapply elastic stockings at least

twice daily. Once each day the legs are cleansed and the condition of the skin assessed. The stockings should be laundered as needed, but at least twice weekly. Elastic stockings are applied by gathering the material, placing the hands inside the stocking, and pulling the stocking apart while applying it over the foot. It is pulled up using the inside of the fingers and hands since fingernails can tear the material.

Patient and family teaching includes methods of application and removal, assessment of the skin, and laundering techniques. The stockings should be washed with gentle soap, rinsed well and drip dried. Heat drying is avoided since it may weaken the elastic. For long-term use an additional pair of stockings may be desirable. Recording includes: application and removal of the stockings, skin care, condition of the skin and patient-family teaching.

DRESSINGS

Dressings are materials placed directly over wounds or traumatized tissues. Dressings are used to promote comfort, support, antisepsis, immobilization, pressure, débridement, and absorption; to provide a physiologic environment; to provide information; to keep wounds open, and for aesthetic purposes. Since the choice of dressing is often a nursing decision, it is imperative that the nurse understand the uses and limitations of each of the various materials used in dressing wounds.

Components of a Dressing

The components of a dressing used to cover a draining wound are: the contact layer, the intermediate layer, and the outer layer or wrap. The *contact layer,* which is placed directly over the traumatized tissue, should be nonabsorbent and should allow secretions to pass from the wound to the absorbent layer without allowing the contact layer to remain moist.[17] Unless débridement is desired, the contact layer should not adhere to the wound. Normally, the contact layer is made of small mesh gauze. The mesh size should be large enough to promote drainage, yet small enough to prevent granulation tissue from penetrating through the mesh. If granulation tissue penetrates through the mesh, the new tissue will be lost when the dressing is removed. Additionally, dressing removal is usually quite painful.

The *intermediate layer* is an absorbent material, usually made of cotton gauze sponges. The thickness of the intermediate layer is dependent upon the amount of drainage anticipated. A fairly thick layer minimizes the number of times dressing changes are necessary. It also prevents saturation of the outer layer, and helps to prevent contamination of the wound.

The function of the *outer layer* of the dressing is to keep the contact and intermediate layers in close proximity to one another in order to promote drainage of secretions. On circumferential areas such as an extremity, the outer layer is often Kling or Kerlix; adhesive tape serves the same purpose on the trunk. Flexible net may be used on either area. Regardless of what is chosen for the outer wrap, the material should be conforming yet flexible enough to allow for expansion if edema is a concern. Dressings should cling and conform to body contours. Gaps and dead space are to be prevented as they promote the accumulation of secretions and provide an environment for bacterial growth. Dressings are applied using surgical aseptic technique (see Chap. 37). They should be sterile when applied and be dry, aesthetic and functional.

Types of Dressings

There are a variety of dressings available today, and more are being developed. Since the choice of dressing material may directly affect wound healing, the nurse should be familiar with the appropriate use of and indications for each of the following dressings.

Silk is a finely woven material commonly applied over newly sutured wounds. It is also used over wounds which must heal by granulation or secondary intention, e.g., avulsion injuries where there is tissue loss (see Chap. 42). Because the mesh size is so small, silk does not adhere to the wound and is easily removed. *Fine mesh gauze* has a slightly larger mesh size than silk and may promote more drainage. It is commonly used over the donor sites of skin grafts and on avulsion injuries.

Coarse mesh gauze permits drainage but is generally not used on wounds that must heal by secondary intention. This is because the weave is so large that granulation tissue easily penetrates the gauze. This dressing is appropriate when débridement is desired. Gauze sponges made of coarse mesh are commonly used as intermediate layers in many dressings. They are available in several sizes; however, 4 × 4's are the most routinely used. Some gauze sponges have a cottonoid center, which increases the absorbency of the sponge.

Fluffs are coarse mesh sponges that have been fluffed open to make them more absorbent and bulky. They are commonly used when wound drainage is copious and in dressing hand wounds in order to keep the fingers in a position of function.

Abdominal pads, which are also called *ABD's* or *combines,* are multilayer absorbent dressings used primarily for postoperative abdominal incisions. *Burn dressings* are also many-layered pads; they cover very large areas such as the trunk or the entire leg and are commonly used in the emergency management of patients with massive burns. They are highly absorbent and are also helpful in minimizing heat loss through the burn wound.

Dressings that promote drying of the wound are called "hydrophilic" contact dressings, while dressings that are protective and prevent the loss of fluid are "hydrophobic" contact dressings. Hydrophobic dressings are usually coarse mesh gauze impregnated with a petroleum or oil base emulsion. These dressings are used to keep tissues from drying out or to deliver medications. Petroleum gauze, scarlet red ointment dressings, Furacin gauze and Xeroform gauze are examples of hydrophobic contact dressings.

Petroleum (Vaseline) gauze is used to protect tissues from drying; to prevent adherence to the wound; and to create an airtight seal. It is commonly used for nasal packing, over newly sutured wounds, around chest tubes and to seal penetrating ("sucking") chest wounds. *Adaptic,* also coated with petroleum jelly, is a very loose mesh material which is nonadherent and permits wound drainage. *Scarlet red ointment* is nonpermeable and medicated. It is used for protection and to stimulate epithelialization on such areas as abrasions and skin graft donor sites. *Furacin gauze* is an antibacterial impregnated gauze commonly used for minor burns or contaminated wounds. *Xeroform gauzes* are medicated with bismuth tribromphenate and may be hydrophobic or hydrophilic depending on the base. They are deodorizing dressings and may promote epithelialization. *Telfa* is a protective dressing which does not adhere to the wound edges. It should not be used when drying of the wound or drainage are desired, e.g., in abrasions. Fairly new to the list of dressings available is the *Micropad* dressing, which is soft, absorbent and nonadherent. This materi-

al is also being used for burn sheets (linens) for patients with major burns. It absorbs serous drainage, but the patient's wounds do not adhere to the sheet.

Packing consists of thin strips of coarse mesh gauze, which is available in several widths. Packing may be composed of plain gauze or gauze impregnated with Iodoform or Vaseline. Packing may be used to keep wounds open, to permit drainage or to foster healing by secondary intention. It is commonly employed following incision and drainage (I and D) of abscesses or to promote closure of sinus tracts following surgical incision. The use of too much packing may result in ischemia and delayed healing. Since packing is packaged in bottles containing several yards of material, the desired length of packing needed for a single wound must be cut before the instruments are contaminated with drainage from the wound. Each patient should receive his own bottle or container of packing, even though he may not use all of it. Universal jars of packing, used for several patients on a nursing unit, are unsafe. It cannot be assumed that everyone used surgical aseptic technique in removing the packing from the jar. Hence, the packing may be a source of contamination.

Collodian and Resifilm are examples of *chemical sealants* available as liquids or sprays. They are applied directly on the edges of newly sutured wounds in order to create a seal. Use of these agents eliminates the need for other dressings. When dried, they form an occlusive film, impermeable to water. Chemical sealants may be used over small wounds and are quite valuable over head lacerations since they permit washing of the hair. The wound must be completely dry before these agents are applied. The film usually remains intact for 5 to 7 days. Most sealants are easily removed with alcohol or acetone.

Adhesive tape is made from cotton cloth, paper, taffeta, plastic and foam. It is available in several widths. Adhesive tape is used: to secure dressings and splints; to strap joints in the prevention or treatment of athletic injuries (Fig. 43–10), to immobilize or stabilize parts of the body such as the ribs; to provide pressure; and to approximate wound edges or secure skin grafts (Fig. 43–11).

Heavy, cotton-backed adhesive tape has many fibers per square inch and usually has a rubber based adhesive. It is used when strength, support and economy are desired. It is somewhat occlusive and may cause maceration of the skin. Because it adheres well, there may be shearing of the skin when it is removed.

Paper, plastic and acetate taffeta adhesive tapes have an acrylate backing and are used when a great deal of adhesion and support are

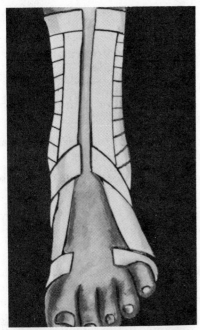

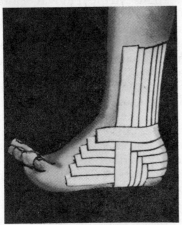

Figure 43–10. Adhesive tape strapping is used for the prevention or treatment of athletic injuries. (From *Professional Uses of Adhesive Tape,* 3rd Ed. Johnson & Johnson, New Brunswick, NJ 08903, p. 87.)

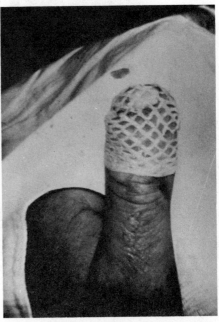

Figure 43–11. Adhesive tape skin closure securing a skin graft. When this adhesive is used sutures are not needed. (Courtesy 3M Company, Surgical Products Division, St. Paul, Minn.)

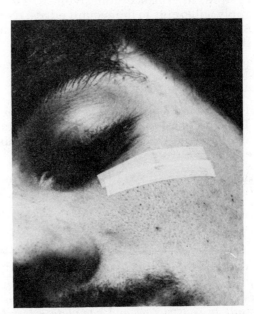

Figure 43–12. Adhesive tape strips may be used to approximate wound edges. (Courtesy 3M Company, Surgical Products Division, St. Paul, Minn.)

not essential. They are slightly more expensive than cotton adhesive tape, but are also more comfortable and cause less skin reaction. Thin strips of paper tape (Steri-Strips, Clearon Skin Closures) are valuable in closing small wounds or supporting wound edges after sutures have been removed (Fig. 43–12).

Plastic tape has small pores which decrease maceration. This tape is transparent, allowing skin surfaces to be visualized. Additionally, plastic tape may have some elasticity and may be used when pressure is desired. Foam adhesive (Microfoam) is a fairly new product designed for use on pressure dressings or as a compression bandage. Foam adhesive has a high degree of stretchability and can be used in much the same way as are rubberized adhesive roller bandages (Fig. 43–13).

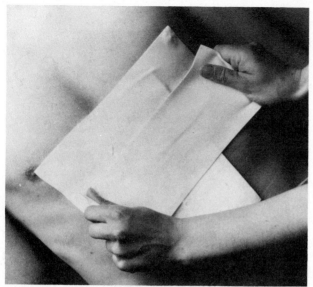

Figure 43–13. Foam adhesive tape is used when pressure is desired. (Courtesy 3M Company, Surgical Products Division, St. Paul, Minn.)

Uses, Application and Removal of Adhesive Tapes

Key points in the application and use of adhesive tapes are:

▶ Clean, dry and shave the area if needed.

▶ Apply a skin adherent such as benzoin if desired, to enhance adhesiveness. Do not apply adherents to the wound edges. (Note: Adherents are not necessary in most circumstances and may increase irritation.)

▶ Tape the body part in a position of function.

▶ Apply tape in strips of equal length.

▶ Tape around wound edges, not over them. This allows air to circulate, promotes drainage and prevents maceration of wound edges.

▶ Assess the area distal to the tape at frequent intervals for signs of ischemia.

▶ Allow the tape to fit the contour of the skin surfaces.

> Caution: *Continuous, circumferential taping of an area with inflexible adhesive tape is dangerous and should not be done. It may result in constriction and complete arterial occlusion. At least 3 cm. (1 in.) of skin surface should be left untaped.*

Key points in the removal of adhesive tape are:

▶ Remove the tape from end-to-end, rather than from side-to-side.

▶ Hold the skin taut and push the skin away from the tape, rather than pulling the tape away from the skin.

▶ Remove tape from the skin in the same direction as the hair grows.

▶ Remove tape by pushing *toward* the wound, not away from the wound.

▶ Use an adhesive solvent, e.g., acetone, to remove any adhesive tape residue left on the skin.

Adhesive tape reactions may be mechanical, allergic or chemical. *Mechanical* irritation may be manifest by either induced vasodilatation or skin stripping. "Induced vasodilatation is a vascular response to the removal of an adhesive tape."[14] It does not indicate trauma to the skin and is characterized by redness of the skin that lasts a very short time. Skin stripping is caused by the removal of cells when the adhesive tape is removed. It is characterized by prolonged (up to 24 hours) redness of the skin and is more commonly associated with occlusive adhesive tapes. *Allergic* reactions are characterized by erythema, edema, vesicles and papules. The allergic reaction may be due to the adhesive itself or due to adherents used to secure the tape. Allergic reactions account for a small proportion of the reactions to adhesive tapes. A patch test can be done to demonstrate true allergy to adhesives. Normally, an allergic response can be elicited within 48 hours. *Chemical* reactions occur when components of the adhesive or backing permeate the tissues. Redness of the skin may be noted. This type of reaction is also associated with the use of occlusive adhesive tapes, which foster overhydration of the cells of the skin. When the cells of the stratum corneum become overhydrated they are more easily penetrated by chemicals in the adhesive tape. Maceration or wrinkling of the skin may be due to an *accumulation of moisture* under the tape and may be prevented by using a more porous tape.

The adhesive material or chemical adherents used to enhance adhesiveness may cause severe allergic reactions in highly sensitive persons. The nurse should question the patient or family carefully regarding allergies to adhesives, adherents, rubber or perfume. If there is question, a skin test may be indicated or an alternative bandage such as elasticized net may be used. The need to frequently evaluate the color, sensation, capillary refill and function of the area distal to the bandage cannot be emphasized enough. The nurse should also carefully record that the assessment was done, the findings, and the patient-family teaching completed.

Postoperative Dressings

Dressings applied during surgery should be assessed frequently in the immediate postoperative period, both in the Recovery Room (Post-Anesthesia Room) and on the regular nursing unit. In order to properly assess a dressing, bed linens and the patient's gown *must be* lifted as appropriate to expose the dressing. The presence of serosanguineous drainage or frank bleeding should be reported immediately, and the dressing reinforced. When assessing for drainage or bleeding, remember to feel underneath the patient, because those fluids will flow downward due to gravity. Frank bleeding or a large amount of serosanguineous drainage may indicate that wound dehiscence or evisceration has occurred. *Dehiscence* is the spontaneous opening of the wound edges. When contents of a cavity protrude through the wound edges, *evisceration* has occurred. Bleeding may also indicate that hemostasis was not achieved or that blood vessel ties may have come loose. All of these problems require *prompt* evaluation and treatment by the surgeon. (See also Chapter 42, p. 1088 and Fig. 42–2.)

When evisceration or dehiscence occurs, the patient often complains of a "ripping" sensation, and some patients understandably become quite upset. Although these wound conditions are also frightening to the nurse, it is imperative that she remain calm, be supportive and provide emergency measures. If dehiscence has occurred, cover the area with a dry sterile dressing and minimize tension on the suture line in order to reduce the potential for extending the dehiscence. When organs are protruding, the major goals are to prevent drying of the mucosa and to prevent the expulsion of more tissues. Cover the area with a large sterile dressing, usually abdominal pads, and moisten the dressing with sterile saline. Do not attempt to replace affected tissues. The patient should be supine and immobile. The knees may be flexed to decrease the tension on the abdominal musculature. Vital signs should be taken and preparations made to return the patient to the operating room. Prepare for the insertion of an intravenous catheter (large bore) for the rapid administration of fluids or anesthetic. It is important, however, that the patient not be left alone if at all possible.

In most agencies, the first postoperative dressing change is done by the surgeon while subsequent dressing changes are usually a nursing responsibility. If an operative dressing becomes soiled with blood or serous drainage, the dressing is reinforced with sterile dressings rather than removed. A record should be kept of the number of times dressing reinforcement is necessary and of the number of dressings used. As previously mentioned, the appearance of bleeding or large amounts of serosanguineous drainage in the immediate postoperative period should be reported promptly.

When patients require frequent dressing changes the nurse may find it valuable to apply *Montgomery straps* rather than using adhesive tape to secure the dressings. (See Figure 42–6.) Montgomery straps are pieces of adhesive tape that have a hole in one end. The end where the hole is has been folded back on itself so that it is not adherent. Tapes or gauze strips are attached through the holes. The Montgomery straps are placed on either side of the wound area, and the gauze is tied over the dressings, keeping them in place. Some nurses prefer to put a large safety pin through each hole and connect the pins to a large rubber band. This holds the dressings in place but has a little "give" as well. When the dressing needs to be changed, the ties are untied and the dressing change done. No additional adhesive tape is needed to secure the dressings. Montgomery straps should be changed when they become soiled. The ties may be changed as needed without removing the straps. Montgomery straps are especially valuable in patients requiring long-term dressings and those with denuded skin from repeated removal of adhesive tape.

Extremity dressings are secured with loose weave or knit roller bandage such as Kling or Kerlix. Occasionally, an elastic (Ace) bandage or cohesive (Coban) bandage is used if pressure is desired to prevent or decrease edema. Whenever there is trauma to soft tissues the nurse should be aware of the potential of "compartment syndrome."[11, 15, 16] Fascial compartments are tissue spaces found in several areas of the body, such as the anterior tibial compartment of the lower leg. Compartment syndrome is due to increased pressure on tissue and results from the accumulation of fluid within the space or from a decrease in the size of the space. A dressing or bandage which is too tight may decrease the size of the space. There may be compression of the nerves and blood vessels, resulting in permanent damage such as wrist drop or foot drop. The symptoms which may indicate the development of compartment syndrome include pain greater than that expected for the injury, tenseness and tenderness of the area, diminished two-point discrimination, pain on passive movement of the extremity, swelling, and possibly, but not always, pallor and decreased sensation in the part distal to the injury.[16] The application of dressings which are initially too constricting or later become too constricting may contribute to the development of compartment syndrome.

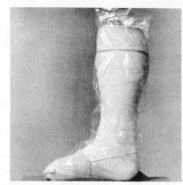

Figure 43–14. Toe caps/shower shields are plastic bags used to protect dressings or casts from moisture. (From Chick Orthopedic *Catalog of Anatomical Supports,* 1973, p. 10.)

> *It is imperative that the area distal to any circumferential dressing be frequently assessed for neurovascular compromise, which may indicate developing compartment syndrome. If compartment syndrome is present,* promptly *loosen the dressing and report the condition.* Do not elevate *the extremity as it is felt that this further* decreases *oxygenation to the area.*

Patient-Family Teaching

The nurse's efforts at providing an appropriate and effective bandage and promoting tissue healing will be completely negated if the aspect of patient-family teaching is ignored. Additionally, failure to provide effective teaching may result in significant liability. In order to insure that the desired outcome is achieved, the nurse should include the following in the *teaching plan:*

1. An explanation of why the dressing is being used.
2. The patient-family responsibility in the care of the dressing, i.e., clean, dry and intact.
3. How to change the dressing.
4. When not to change the dressing, e.g., dressings over avulsed areas or skin grafts are not changed for 10 to 14 days, at which time the patient returns for follow-up care.
5. The kind of dressing material to use and where it may be obtained.
6. How to perform activities of daily living while wearing a bandage, e.g., rubber gloves when washing dishes, covering area with a sturdy plastic bag and securing it above the dressings with ties or a rubber band. Special plastic bags are commercially available (Fig. 43–14).
7. An explanation of wound healing. Wounds often appear more unsightly after the sutures have been removed than they did when first sutured. Scars mature, flatten out and fade over a period of time, usually about 6 months.

Considerations for plastic surgery are not usually made before this time.

8. The signs of infection, both local and systemic, e.g., erythema, edema, pain, drainage, lymphangitis (red streak), lymphadenitis (swollen lymph gland), warmth around area, fever.
9. Application of heat or cold. Cold is used in the first 24 hours to promote vasoconstriction and decrease bleeding, while heat is used after 24 hours to increase the blood supply and aid in removing accumulated fluid.
10. Where and when follow-up care is to be received.
11. *How to assess neurovascular integrity, the importance of doing so, and who to notify or where to go if complications develop.*

In addition to verbal instructions, the patient should also receive written instructions containing the above information. Many agencies require the patient to sign a statement that he has received written instructions, that they have been explained to him and that he understands the information. This statement is retained by the agency and incorporated into the patient's clinical record.

ORTHOPEDIC DEVICES

Crutches

Crutches are devices used to provide support during ambulation and are utilized by persons with both long- and short-term problems. In many institutions the responsibility for teaching crutch walking is assigned to the Physical Therapy Department. However, the nurse must understand the proper use and hazards of crutches to reinforce teaching done by the physical therapist. Additionally, there are many situations (e.g., accidents) in which the need for crutches could not have been anticipated and the teaching responsibility rests solely with the nurse.

When the need for crutches is anticipated, the patient should prepare by performing exercises designed to improve muscle tone of the arms and hands. Such exercises include push-ups to develop the arm and shoulder muscles, and squeezing a rubber ball or using hand grips to prepare the muscles of the hands to bear weight.

Types of Crutches.   Three types of crutches commonly used include axillary crutches, Canadian or Lofstrand crutches and platform crutches. *Axillary crutches* require weight bearing by the hands and are the crutches most frequently used for short-term problems. *Lofstrand crutches* have no axillary support, but rather have metal bands which fit around the forearm to keep them in place (Fig. 43–15). They also require weight bearing on the hands and are commonly used by persons with long-term problems. *Platform crutches* are used when the need for assistance is long-term and the patient is unable to bear weight on the wrists or hands, e.g., patients with arthritis. With platform crutches the elbow is bent and the weight is distributed along the forearm. Since the use of Lofstrand and platform crutches is usually anticipated, and the teach-

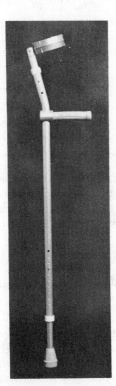

Figure 43–15.   Double adjustable Lofstrand crutch. The metal band fits around the forearm and provides support. (From Chick Orthopedic *Catalog of Anatomical Supports,* 1973, p. 26.)

ing arranged through the Physical Therapy Department, only the use of axillary crutches will be discussed.

Axillary crutches are made of aluminum or wood and may be single or double, with the double being most common. Aluminum crutches are usually adjustable, while wooden crutches may be either adjustable or available in specific lengths. Adjustable crutches are sized "short" through "extra long" for both adults and children.

Proper Crutch Fit.   One of the most important aspects of the use of crutches is proper fit. Measurement for crutches may be made in several ways:

▶ With the patient flat in bed with shoes on, measure from the axillary fold to the heel of the foot and add 5 cm. (2 in.).

▶ Measure from the axilla on the diagonal to a point 15 to 20 cm. (6 to 8 in.) lateral to the heel of the foot, i.e., away from the heel.

▶ Subtract 40.5 cm. (16 in.) from the patient's total height in inches.

The measurement of crutch length includes the axillary pad and the rubber crutch tip.[13, 18, 22]

With the patient standing upright, in sturdy shoes and with the shoulders relaxed, there should be a space of two or three fingers widths between the axillary fold and the top of the crutch. The crutches should extend 15 to 23 cm. (6 to 9 in.) in front of and lateral to the toes (Fig. 43–16). Hand grips should be adjusted so that the patient's elbows are bent while gripping. Adjustments may be necessary when the patient's posture improves and he/she is more skillful in using crutches. Growing children may need frequent crutch adjustments.

Regardless of whether or not adjustments are made in crutches, the nurse is responsible for insuring that the crutches are safe and properly fastened. All bolts should have wing nuts, which must be tight. The crutch tip should be flexible, have adequate groove depth and be securely attached to the end of the crutch. It is wise to tap the crutch end on the floor to correctly position the crutch tip.

Some of the *hazards* associated with crutch use are nerve damage due to pressure on the axilla, contusion of the axilla and palm, falls, and back pain as a result of poor posture or improper crutch fit.

Gaits Used in Crutch Walking.   There are five

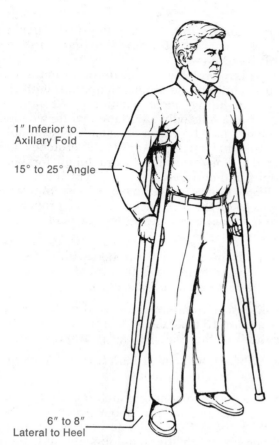

1" Inferior to Axillary Fold

15° to 25° Angle

6" to 8" Lateral to Heel

Figure 43–16. Proper crutch fit. (From Cosgriff, J. H., and Anderson, D. L.: *The Practice of Emergency Nursing.* Philadelphia, J. B. Lippincott Co., 1975.)

gaits commonly used in crutch walking. The gait used depends on the limitations of the patient relative to weight bearing, the patient's preference and the physician's recommendation. The uses and techniques of the major gaits are discussed.

FOUR-POINT ALTERNATING GAIT. This gait is used when weight bearing on both feet is allowed. It is a relatively safe gait because three points are always on the floor to provide support. It is slower and more desirable for older or less stable persons. The technique is:

    Place right crutch down, then
    Place left foot down, then
    Place left crutch down, then
    Place right foot down.

THREE-POINT GAIT. The three-point gait is also called the "orthopedic gait" and is used when complete weight bearing is allowed on one foot and partial or no weight bearing is

allowed on the other foot. It is faster than the four-point gait. The technique is: Both crutches and the non–weight bearing foot are advanced together. Then, the weight bearing foot is moved forward.

TWO-POINT GAIT. A gait similar to walking, this gait is used when weight bearing is permitted on both feet. The technique is: The right crutch and left foot are advanced together; then the left crutch and right foot are advanced together.

SWING-TO-CRUTCH GAIT. This gait involves lifting the body through the crutches and requires good muscle strength in the upper arms. The legs must be capable of bearing some weight. Because this is a very rapid gait, it is commonly adopted by persons having permanent disability. The technique is that the crutches are advanced and then the body is swung forward to the crutches.

SWING-THROUGH-CRUTCH GAIT. This gait has the same requirements as the swing-to-crutch gait, is used by permanently disabled persons, and allows speeds greater than normal walking. The technique is that the crutches are advanced together, then the feet and body are lifted and swung *through* and *beyond* the crutches.

Teaching Crutch Walking Techniques. Before teaching crutch walking the nurse should consider the following points:

▶ The patient must not have an altered level of consciousness or an equilibrium disorder that might interfere with the safe use of crutches.

> *Patients who are intoxicated or who have recently received narcotics, hypnotics or sedatives should not be taught crutch walking.*

▶ There must be no injury or limitation of movement of the hands, arms, shoulders or back that may interfere with the patient's ability to bear weight on hands or mobilize.

▶ The floor surface must be nonslippery and free of obstacles and throw rugs.

▶ The patient should wear sturdy flat shoes, preferably oxford type with nonslip soles. Bedroom slippers are to be avoided.

▶ The patient should wear street clothes that fit well. Bathrobes and night clothes are often loose-fitting and may get caught in the crutches, especially at the axilla. They also interfere with visibility of posture.

▶ The crutches need to be properly adjusted, all bolts tightly fastened, and the crutch tips securely attached.

▶ The limitations of the patient relative to weight bearing and the physician's preference of gait, if any, should be determined.

▶ The practice area used should be sufficiently large and free of traffic and distractions.

▶ A sturdy chair should be available in case the patient becomes fatigued.

It is also helpful if the nurse has a pair of crutches that have been adjusted for her so that she can demonstrate the gait and other techniques. It is invaluable if the nurse has had the opportunity to practice crutch walking, utilizing the various gaits. When you practice crutch walking yourself, you quickly learn the hazards and limitations associated with the use of crutches and can be more effective as a teacher.

When teaching, first demonstrate the appropriate gait, explaining the steps to be used. Emphasize that weight is on the hands, not axilla. Next, assist the patient in standing with crutches. Patients who have never used crutches require a little time to steady themselves. The nurse should stand close by the patient, ready to support him if a fall seems inevitable. If you must support a patient, secure the hips or shoulders. Do not grasp the crutch. A walking belt (see also p. 419) is an excellent aid in that it allows the nurse to have control yet allows independence for the patient. The patient should walk the length of a corridor

several times until he is comfortable and confident. There should be rest periods because crutch walking is very fatiguing to the novice. Once hall walking has been mastered, other techniques can be introduced. Some of the commonly needed maneuvers are discussed below.

In order to *stand from a sitting position* the patient should:

1. Place both crutches together on his weak side, holding them by the handgrips on the inside.

2. Push up with the other hand against the chair.

3. Straighten the strong leg. If the heel of the weak foot is allowed to be placed on the floor, the patient should slide the heel as he rises (Fig. 43–17).

The procedure is reversed when going from a *standing to a sitting position*. The back should be kept straight when changing positions. Most patients find that deep, upholstered chairs are difficult to get out of.

In order to *climb stairs* when there is a railing, the patient places both crutches together under the arm on the side opposite the railing.

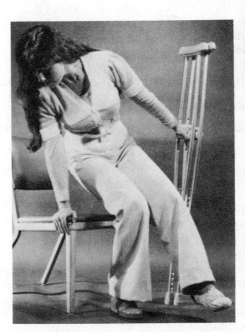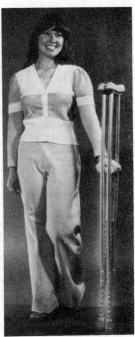

Figure 43–17. Technique of rising from a sitting position while using crutches. (From Swanson, M. A.: *Crutches on the Go.* Bellevue, Washington, Medic Publishing Co., 1974, p. 7.)

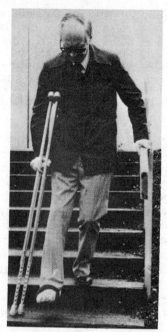

Figure 43–19. Technique for descending steps while on crutches with a railing present. (From Swanson, M. A.: *Crutches on the Go,* p. 11.)

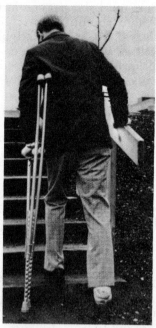

Figure 43–18. Technique for ascending stairs when a railing is present. (From Swanson, M. A.: *Crutches on the Go.* Bellevue, Washington, Medic Publishing Co., 1974, p. 11.)

The crutches can be kept together by holding the inside handgrip with the thumb. The railing is firmly held with the other hand. The crutches are left on the level where the patient is standing. The stronger foot is advanced to the higher step and the weaker leg is dangling behind. The strong leg is then straightened and the crutches advanced. The procedure is repeated until all the stairs have been climbed (Fig. 43–18).

When *descending steps* with a railing present, the crutches are placed on the lower step and the weak foot is extended. Again, the weight is supported evenly between the crutch hand and the railing. The strong foot is advanced to the lower step, and the procedure repeated until descent is completed (Fig. 43–19). Descending stairs while on crutches is dangerous and patients should be encouraged to do so slowly. When there is no railing, the novice crutchwalker may have to sit on each step in order to ascend or descend. If the patient will be confronted with steps immediately after discharge, the nurse should allow him to practice climbing and descent with supervision. Many hospitals have sets of five or six steps designed specifically for this purpose.

There are a variety of other techniques which may be beneficial to the patient, however, space does not permit a more complete discussion. The booklet *Crutches on the Go,*[22] written as a patient-family teaching tool, is an excellent source for a more detailed management of the subject.

Additional Patient-Family Teaching

1. The reason why crutches are being used
2. The hazards associated with inappropriate use of crutches, particularly nerve damage, contusions of the axilla and palms, back pain and falls
3. The need for sturdy shoes with nonslip soles
4. The need to take short, slow steps
5. Keeping the crutches close to the body to avoid catching them on things, e.g., furniture
6. Avoiding highly polished or wet floors, throw rugs, obstacles, plush carpeting, grass or soft ground
7. The need for allowing additional time to get places
8. The use of a backpack or shoulder bag to carry articles
9. The need to check crutch tips for wear and how to obtain replacements
10. The option of crutch rental rather than purchase, especially if crutches will be needed for less than three months, and where rental

crutches may be obtained (most community pharmacies rent crutches)

11. The need to stand erect with the head held level in order to avoid hazards and prevent back pain

12. The need to adjust crutches if changing shoe height

13. The avoidance of crutch walking while using sedating medications or alcohol.

The nurse should include the teaching completed and the gait used in the clinical record. The palms, axilla and inner aspects of the patient's upper arms should be assessed and the findings recorded.

Canes

Canes are hand-gripped devices used as aids to ambulation when complete weight bearing cannot be achieved. Canes are made of wood or aluminum, and some are quite ornate. Wooden canes are sized and are not adjustable, while aluminum ones may be either adjustable or chosen according to length. Canes may be single tipped or four-point (Fig. 43–20). The four-point cane provides more support and is especially valuable on uneven surfaces. Persons who are particularly unsteady or who will require long term use may find the four-point cane more reassuring. It is, however, more expensive than the single tip cane.

When a cane is of proper length (a) the patient's elbow is bent slightly while he bears weight and (b) the patient can hold the hand grip comfortably. Normally, the curve of the hand grip is at the level of the hip. The cane should be held in the hand opposite the impaired leg. As with crutches, the rubber suction tip should be flexible, have deep grooves, be wide based and firmly attached to the end of the cane.

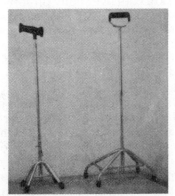

Figure 43–20. Four-point or "quad" cane is used when greater stability is needed. (Taken from Everest and Jennings Co., Los Angeles, Cal.)

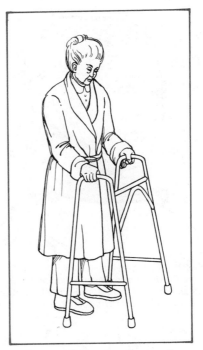

Figure 43–21. Standard walker.

Walkers

Walkers are four-point assist devices used by persons who are unable to bear complete weight on one or both legs, or are unsteady. The *standard walker* is picked up or slid ahead with each step (Fig. 43–21). The orthopedic gait is used with the standard walker. The *reciprocal walker*, which is less commonly used, employs a gait similar to the two-point alternate gait used in crutch walking. One side of the walker is moved when one leg is advanced, and then the opposite side of the walker is moved with the other leg. Modifications of the standard walker may have wheels and a seat. The patient moves along by shuffling his feet.

The walker height is adjusted so that the patient's elbows are flexed at an angle of 30 degrees when the patient grasps the hand grips with his wrists extended. It is important for the patient to relax his shoulders and wear sturdy shoes.[18]

If the need for the walker is short term, the patient should consider renting rather than purchasing the walker. Crutches, canes and walkers are available from health aid stores, pharmacies and charitable organizations.

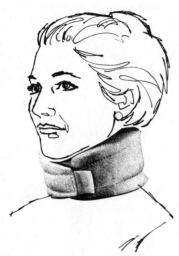

Figure 43–22. Soft cervical collar. (From *Emergency Medical Care Products and Rescue Extrication Equipment for the Sick and Injured.* Rockford Safety Equipment Company, Emergency Medical Products Division. Rockford, Ill., 1975, p. 99.)

Cervical Collars

Cervical collars are supportive appliances applied around the neck. They are commonly used: (a) for immobilization of the neck in suspected cervical spine fractures, (b) to relieve muscle spasm of the neck following trauma and (c) to support the head in degenerative diseases of the cervical vertebrae, following surgery and/or following trauma. Two kinds of cervical collars are frequently prescribed. A *soft collar* (Fig. 43–22) is made of foam or felt padding covered with stockinette. It may be pinned in place or secured with self-adhering strips. It is indicated for short-term use or intermittent use and is relatively inexpensive. The *hard cervical collar* (Fig. 43–23) is made of heavy plastic

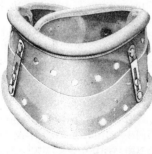

Figure 43–23. Hard cervical collar. (From *Emergency Medical Care Products and Rescue Extrication Equipment for the Sick and Injured.* Rockford Safety Equipment Company, p. 99.)

and/or metal. It is recommended for long-term use or when there is a need for rigid support. This collar has snaps, ties, buckles or adhering strips. A *four-poster cervical collar* is frequently used following hospitalization for a cervical spine fracture. It is called a four-poster because there are four steel rods incorporated into the hard collar. Quite often a prosthetist (a person who makes and fits prosthetic devices) makes the collar specifically for one patient.

The *hazards* of cervical collars include: (a) obstruction of the airway if applied too tightly, (b) ineffective immobilization if applied loosely or positioned improperly and (c) pain, ischemia and necrosis of the tissues of the jaw and inner third of the clavicle. This last problem is seen more with hard collars and may be prevented by padding bony prominences.

Cervical collars are applied with the head erect unless there is suspicion of a cervical spine fracture. When a fracture is believed to be present, the collar is applied with the patient in the position in which he was found. Occasionally, traction may be applied to the head to facilitate application of the collar.

> Caution: *Never move the head of a patient with a suspected cervical spine fracture. Never move the patient unless a cervical collar has been applied and the patient is on a spine or fracture board. The patient's head should be taped to the board before he is transported.*

Some cervical collars are designed to be fastened only in the back of the neck and others only in front. Make sure you know which method the manufacturer recommends in order to achieve maximum support and patient comfort.

Patient and family teaching includes: (a) why the collar is being used, (b) whether it is to be removed, (c) how to remove and reapply the collar, (d) skin care over bony prominences and (e) how to clean the collar. Soft collars are hand washed and allowed to drip dry. Replacement covers are available or one can fashion a cover from stockinette. Hard collars are wiped with a solution of mild soap and water. Excessive heat may damage the plastic.

Recording includes the kind of collar applied, the effectiveness of the collar in relieving pain, and the patient-family teaching completed. Because of the high incidence of litigation associated with injuries to the neck and cervical spine, the nurse is well advised to ensure that recording is accurate, complete and legible with emphasis placed on patient-family teaching done. Patients discharged home with cervical collars should have written as well as verbal instructions.

Splints are used to support or immobilize parts of the musculoskeletal system. They are employed in the management of fractures, sprains, strains, dislocations, lacerations, degenerative disorders or in patients who are unable to maintain a part in position of function, e.g., central or peripheral nervous system disorders.

Key points in the application and use of splints are:

▶ Splints are usually applied with the part in position of function.

▶ Skin surfaces are separated and padded so that maceration of tissues from moisture is avoided.

▶ The joint above and the joint below the involved area are immobilized.

▶ Bony prominences and hollows are padded to prevent necrosis.

▶ The distal part is left exposed whenever possible so that neurovascular integrity can be assessed.

▶ Pulses should be evaluated both before and after splints are applied. Mark the location where the pulse was felt.

▶ Bandages and straps used to secure the splint are applied away from the injured area.

> *A properly applied splint is comfortable and relieves pain. If pain persists or increases, the splint must be removed and reapplied.*

A variety of materials are used for splints, including plastic, aluminum, cardboard, wood, steel, foam rubber, styrofoam and pillows. Splints may be held in place with adhesive tape, gauze, snaps, hooks, self-adhering strips or zippers.

A complete discussion of the many splints available and their application can be found in an orthopedic nursing text. Here we discuss certain splints—air splints and traction splints—that are often applied by nurses and have special considerations.

Air Splints. The *tubular, plastic air splint* is used for emergency immobilization of suspected fractures of an extremity and requires special application techniques. The splint is placed around the nurse's arm like a sleeve. The part to be splinted is supported by the hand of that arm while the splint is slid from the nurse's arm onto the patient's injured area and then is positioned with the nurse's other hand.

The injured area is supported continuously while the splint is inflated *by mouth,* until enough support is provided by the splint. The maximum amount of inflation of an air splint is 30 mm. Hg and this can easily be exceeded if the splint is inflated by a pump device.[10] The nurse removes her hand and inflation is continued until the splint is comfortable and provides sufficient support. The plastic should dent when a thumb is pressed into it. While the air splint is especially valuable in applying pressure to bleeding areas, *it may become too constrictive and occlude the circulation to the extremity.* Capillary refill, color, sensation, warmth and peripheral pulse should be assessed frequently.

The *Thomas (full ring) splint, the Keller-Blake (half ring) splint (often called a Thomas half ring splint)* and the *Hare splint* are traction splints used in the immobilization of suspected or diagnosed fractures of the shaft of the femur. The splint consists of two long rods of lightweight metal, which are joined proximally by a leather covered half or full ring and distally by a cross bar, which is also made of metal. The half ring and Hare splints have a groin strap which is used to secure the splint, and the ring may be turned so that it will fit on either the left or the right leg (Fig. 43–24). The Thomas and Keller-Blake splints are sized short through long and the Hare is adjustable.

Before it is applied, the splint is prepared by attaching slings or towels at various locations on the frame. It is important that a sling be placed on the splint where the fracture site will be located in order to insure that both ends of the bone will be supported. While traction is applied to the foot, and with the fracture site supported, the patient's leg is raised and the splint is positioned under the leg. The ring is placed high in the groin, against the ischial tuberosity. When a half ring is used, the half ring is placed under the patient and a groin strap secured over the anterior thigh. A small amount of padding is applied under the strap in order to prevent compression of blood vessels in the groin. The leg is secured to the frame with tied, pinned or wrapped bandages. Traction is maintained by use of an ankle hitch, which is twisted until enough tension is achieved and the patient experiences relief of muscle spasm. The ends of the ankle hitch are tied to the end of the splint. Two tongue blades taped together and used to twist the hitch are secured to the sides of the frame with adhesive tape. The tongue blades *must* be secured to the

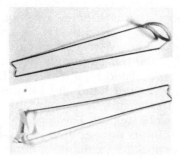

Figure 43–24. Full and half ring traction splints are used in the immobilization of suspected fractures of the femur. (From Chick Orthopedic *Catalog of Anatomical Supports,* 1973.)

splint or the ankle hitch will unwind and traction will be lost (Fig. 43–25). The splint should be elevated so that the patient's heel is not resting on the bed. When the thigh muscles begin to relax, the patient may experience pain and the traction should be increased. Because the ankle hitch may interfere with circulation, it is recommended that foot traction should not be left on longer than 2 hours.[11] Neurovascular integrity of the foot should be assessed at frequent intervals.

Normally, as soon as it is safely possible, a Steinmann pin or Kirschner wire is inserted through the distal femur and skeletal traction is applied. A special attachment called a Pearson attachment is placed on the Thomas splint at this time. Traction is then provided by weights and balanced suspension, and the ankle hitch is removed.

Whenever there is a fracture of the femur the potential for significant blood loss and shock is great. 2000 ml. of blood may be lost when there is a fracture of the femur. In addition to assessing distal pulses, the nurse should also take frequent vital signs in the immediate post-injury period. Because of the proximity of the femoral artery to the femur, arterial lacerations are not uncommon.

> Caution: *A patient with a suspected or confirmed newly fractured femur must never be moved without immobilization and traction on the leg.*

As a result of trauma to the area, there may be spasm of the femoral artery when there is a fracture of the femur. It is difficult initially to

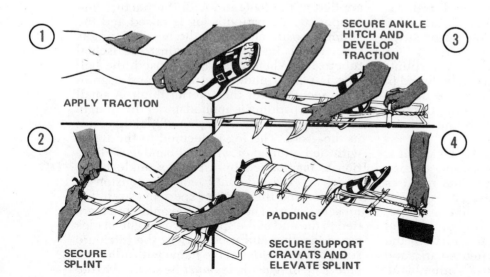

① APPLY TRACTION

② SECURE SPLINT

③ SECURE ANKLE HITCH AND DEVELOP TRACTION

④ PADDING

SECURE SUPPORT CRAVATS AND ELEVATE SPLINT

Figure 43–25. Technique for the application of a half ring traction splint used in the immobilization of suspected fractures of the femur. (From Grant, H., and Murray, R.: *Emergency Care.* Bowie, Md., Robert J. Brady Company, 1971, p. 197.)

assess whether there has been laceration of the artery or spasm of the artery. It is important, therefore, that the distal pulse in the foot (dorsalis pedis) be assessed initially, an "X" marked on the area where the pulse was palpated, and the pulse assessed at least every 30 minutes until the skeletal traction has been applied. Absence of the pulse must be reported *immediately.*

Slings

Slings are used to provide support, immobilization and elevation of the hand, arm or shoulder. They are available as triangular bandages which are pinned and tied according to the size of the patient or as pre-sized, contoured slings adjusted by buckles and straps. Slings are made of cotton, muslin or twill and usually withstand frequent washing. The triangular bandage is highly versatile and can be used for a variety of purposes, especially in first-aid situations.[1, 10, 19]

When an arm sling is applied the patient should be in a comfortable position, preferably sitting (especially if the patient is much taller than the nurse), with the injured arm flexed at the elbow. The point (apex) of the triangle is at the elbow. One tail is placed between the injured arm and the chest and is brought up on the shoulder on the uninjured side. The other tail is brought over the injured arm and chest and placed on the shoulder on the same side as the injury. The anterior tail is brought behind the neck and tied to the other tail with a square knot. The movements to make a square knot are: Left-over-right and under; right-over-left and under. The knot should be positioned to the side of the vertebral column, not midline. If placed over bony areas, the knot may cause pressure and discomfort. The apex of the bandage is folded around the elbow and pinned or tucked in place. The hand and forearm are usually higher than the elbow (Fig. 43–26). Patient comfort is the key to a properly applied sling. The standard size triangular bandage may be folded in half to fit a child. When applying the pre-sized sling, the arm is slid into the sling, and the sling is fitted to the patient by adjusting the straps. Some pre-sized slings have an additional strap which fits around the patient's chest. When this is used, the shoulder is immobilized as well (Fig. 43–27).

Aspects of *patient-family teaching* which should be considered are: (a) proper application and removal of the sling, (b) how to make a square knot (so that the sling can be easily removed), (c) how long the sling will be required and (d) the hazards associated with its use. These hazards include: tissue damage due to poor placement of the knot, edema if the forearm and hand are dependent, and immobility of the elbow joint if the sling is used longer than indicated.

POSITIONING AND PROTECTIVE DEVICES

One of the most difficult and most challenging aspects of nursing is providing care to per-

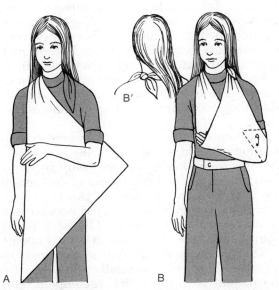

Figure 43–26. Standard sling (triangular bandage). Note that the knot is placed off to the side to avoid pressure to the tissues overlying the vertebrae.

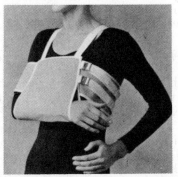

Figure 43–27. Arm sling with shoulder immobilizer. This is commonly called a sling and swathe or velpeaux. (From Chick Orthopedic *Catalog of Anatomical Supports,* 1973, p. 8.)

sons who are critically ill or injured and have little or no control over their own body functions. *While the major nursing goal is directed at life-saving measures, one must be equally as concerned about the consequences of immobility and the potential for permanent disability.* It is a sad, but all too common occurrence, that patients with devastating infirmities are successfully "recovered" only to be left with permanent deformities which should have been prevented.

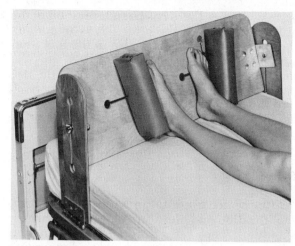

Figure 43–28. Footboard with lateral supports to prevent external rotation of the feet. (From *Posey Guide—Use and Application of Posey Safety Products.* Posey Company, Pasadena, Cal., 1973, p. 8.)

> *Contractures and decubitus ulcers can be prevented. Their presence implies poor nursing care.*

There are a variety of devices available which can be used to prevent such complications from developing, and the nurse must be totally knowledgeable about the use and abuse of these tools. In this section the following are discussed: *positioning devices* such as footboards, trochanter rolls and sand bags, and *protective devices* including bed cradles, special beds, mattresses and frames, heel and elbow protectors, air rings or cushions, and sheepskins.

Positioning Devices for Preventing Contractures

Positioning devices are used for patients with altered levels of consciousness or limited function of body parts. They are used to prevent *contractures*—the freezing and stiffening of joints, usually in flexion. Tendons shorten, normal tissue is replaced with fibrous tissue and the joint cannot be moved. Surgical treatment is usually necessary to restore the joint to some level of function. Contractures develop because the joint is not used and is not put through range-of-motion exercises. The most common contractures seen in the unconscious or immobilized patient are: hip and knee flexion contractures associated with continuous flexion of the knees from elevated bed knee gatches; footdrop from failure to support the sole of the foot and failure to maintain the foot in dorsiflexion; wrist drop due to flexion of the wrist and failure to position the hand and wrist in slight hyperextension; external rotation of the hips with the toes pointing to the side; and contractures of the upper arm and chest mus-

cles due to prolonged adduction of the arms to the side of the chest.[6] (See also Chapter 33.)

Footboards are used to prevent plantar flexion or foot drop. The footboard is adjusted so that the soles of the feet are flush against the board and the ankle joint is 90 degrees. If attention is not paid to this aspect of care, the achilles tendons shorten, become fibrotic and the patient may be unable to walk again without the aid of braces or other devices. Footboards may be padded to prevent the development of pressure areas on the soles of the feet. Some boards are equipped with supports on either side of the foot to prevent external rotation of the leg and foot (Fig. 43–28). If these are not included, the nurse may use *sandbags* on either side of the foot. Footboards are most effective when the patient is supine or prone. When the patient is prone, the feet should extend over the edge of the mattress with the footboard adjusted to provide support. One may wish to elevate the lower legs on a towel or small pillow when the patient is prone. Although footboards are valuable, they do not replace range-of-motion exercises.

Trochanter rolls are used to prevent external rotation of the hips and legs. They extend from the hips to the knees and are easily fashioned from rolled bath blankets. Some institutions use long, tubular sandbags for this purpose.

Sandbags, as previously mentioned, are used to prevent plantar flexion. They are placed against the soles of the feet in such a manner that they keep the feet at 90-degree angles to the legs. Sandbags are especially valuable when the patient is in the lateral recumbent (sidelying) position since a footboard cannot be used. *Pillows* are also used to maintain a body

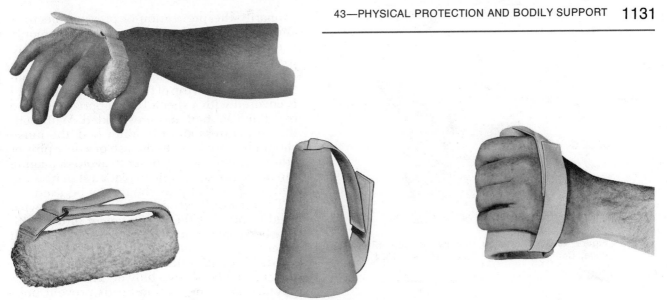

Figure 43–29.   A hand roll is used to prevent contractures of the fingers. Some hand rolls or palm cones can be used to exercise the hand as well. (From *J. T. Posey Company Catalog.* Pasadena, Cal., 1974, pp. 25–26.)

part in proper alignment as well as to pad and protect bony prominences such as the knees when the patient is positioned on his side.

Handrolls are devices which are placed in the palms of the patient's hands to prevent flexion contractures of the fingers and wrist. Although there are a variety of handrolls commercially available (Fig. 43–29), one can improvise by rolling a washcloth and taping it to prevent it from unrolling. Rolls may also be made with ABD's (abdominal pads) which have been folded in half lengthwise and then rolled. These may also be taped or covered with roller gauze to keep them intact. It may be necessary to secure the roll in the patient's hand with roller gauze. However, remember that it is essential to periodically remove the roll, cleanse the area, and put the hand and wrist through range-of-motion exercises.[4] Cockup splints may also be used to promote hyperextension of the wrist.

Bed cradles are used to prevent bed linens from touching an area, especially the feet. They are often used in conjunction with heat lamps to dry an area and promote healing. Cradles are commonly used in patients with decubiti, burns, skin grafts, gout or gangrene. They are usually made of lightweight metal, primarily aluminum. Bed cradles must be secured underneath the mattress and be stable. Bedmaking requires special technique. For home use, bedcradles can be fashioned from cardboard boxes which have been cut out on one side. (See also Chap. 27, p. 623.)

Protective Devices for Preventing Decubitus Ulcers

A second major problem associated with immobility is the development of decubitus ulcers. Decubitus ulcers, or sores, result from sustained pressure to skin surfaces, often over bony prominences, with resultant ischemia. There is "a breakdown in the microcirculation resulting in partial or total occlusion of capillaries by platelet thrombosis."[23] Studies by Barton and Barton at a "Pressure Sore Unit" in England indicate that skin breakdown may occur in 6 to 12 hours, even in a healthy person. Persons who are in shock, or have been in shock in the previous 48 hours, may develop skin breakdown within 2 hours and possibly within 30 minutes. Once skin breakdown has occurred there is rapid enlargement of the ulcerated area and involvement of deeper tissues. Infection of the bone (osteomyelitis) is not uncommon. In addition to the pain and expense they cause and the prolonged treatment required for healing, decubitus ulcers may be a primary source of generalized sepsis and death.[24] Obviously then, the nurse must focus her attention on the area of prevention. There are several beds, frames and mattresses which may be used in the care of patients who are prone to developing decubiti, are difficult to turn, or have injuries which require strict immobilization with continuous traction, e.g., the patient with a cervical spine fracture with Crutchfield tongs and traction. The most commonly used devices are:

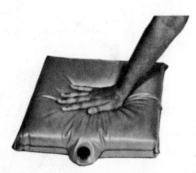

Figure 43–30. Flotation therapy cushion. (From *J. T. Posey Company Catalog.* Pasadena, Cal., 1974, p. 18.)

flotation therapy units, air mattresses, air-fluidized beds, Stryker frames and CircOlectric beds. Some aspects of the use of these devices are presented below; however, the reader is urged to review the manufacturer's instruction booklets and nursing procedure manuals before caring for patients using the Stryker frame, the Stryker Wedge or the CircOlectric bed.

Water-Filled Devices. *Flotation therapy units* are available in the form of cushions (Fig. 43–30) or "water beds." The water bed is composed of a sheet of heavy plastic that rests on water that is encased in a foam-padded shell. The weight of the patient displaces the water, and no pressure is exerted against the patient. These units are particularly valuable for patients who are very decubiti prone and who will probably not ambulate again, such as quadriplegics and persons with crippling diseases such as rheumatoid arthritis. They may not be indicated for use by the patient who will hopefully be restored to normal musculoskeletal function, as it is very difficult to support their joints and prevent flexion deformities because of the movement of the water and of difficulty with positioning. When first placed on the unit, some patients experience nausea and vomiting, similar to sea sickness, because of the rolling motion. An anti-emetic, e.g., Compazine, may be indicated. Some patients experience hallucinations, so it is important that the patient be observed very carefully and reassured as necessary. Flotation therapy cushions are made of a pliable gel-like substance encased in heavy plastic. These cushions are commonly used on the seats of wheelchairs and other chairs.

Air-Filled Devices. *Air mattresses* are used for much the same reasons as water beds,

primarily the prevention of pressure necrosis and decubitus ulcers. The most commonly used mattress is an alternating pressure mattress having segments which alternately expand with air and collapse. Normally, this mattress is placed on top of the regular mattress and is covered with a sheet. It is important that the bed linen be taut and unwrinkled. With both the air mattress and the water bed, the nurse should be careful with the use of safety pins or other sharp objects in order to avoid damaging the units. It is advisable to place a sign near the bed warning that pins should not be used.

The *air-fluidized bed* is an innovative device used to prevent the development of decubiti. The bed consists of a loose polyester filter sheet placed "over a bed filled with sterile glass beads."[9] Air is continually circulated upward through the beads by a blower. The continuous circulation of the air and beads prevent pressure in any one area of the patient.

Stryker Frame. A Stryker frame consists of two narrow frames of lightweight metal that are covered with canvas or other similar materials. The frames are attached to a stand. There are top and bottom frames with openings in the canvas to allow for support of the forehead, elimination, etc. The frames are rotated or "flipped" on the stand to change the patient's position. The patient may be either supine or prone. This frame is commonly used for patients with cervical spine injuries requiring continuous traction. There is a hole in the head of the frame through which the traction rope is passed. When the patient is turned, the rope may rotate slightly, but continuous traction is maintained.

Unlike many of the other devices, the Stryker frame is completely portable. It easily fits into a standard ground ambulance and in a helicopter. A special spring device, which sustains the traction at the prescribed number of pounds, is available for use when transporting a patient on the frame. In general, it is not safe to transport a patient with free-swinging weights, especially in a helicopter or ambulance, because the weights may easily fall off.

When turning a patient on a Stryker frame, the second frame is placed on top of the patient and is *securely* bolted to the frame at each end. The patient is sandwiched between the two frames (Fig. 43–31). A restraining belt is secured around both frames so that the patient will not fall out when the frame is "flipped."

Caution: *When turning a patient on the Stryker frame it is* essential *that a restraint strap be used if the patient is unable to hold on to the top frame.*

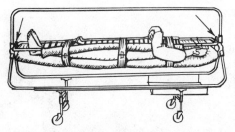

Figure 43–31.   Stryker turning frame. (From Sutton, A. L.: *Bedside Nursing Techniques in Medicine and Surgery,* 2nd ed. Philadelphia, W. B. Saunders Co., 1969, p. 198.)

Before the patient is turned, he should be told in which direction he will be turned. Make sure that drainage tubes and other attachments will not be pulled out when the frame is turned. There are pins at each end of the frame which must be pulled out before the frame will turn. Generally, the frame must be rotated slightly to keep the pins out until you are ready to turn the patient. You *must* hold on to the frames while the pins are out. Although one person can turn a patient on a Stryker frame, it is far easier if two people work together. The patient is informed of the move, and the frames are turned. Turning should be done quickly. When the frames are locked into position, the pins will "click" in, and the frame cannot be rotated. The frame that is now on top of the patient is removed, the patient positioned as necessary, and drainage tubes evaluated for position and function. Any weights should also be checked to make sure they are free-swinging. When patients have cervical traction, the weights often pull the patient to the top of the frame and the weights may be resting on the floor, with the result that no traction is being applied. This problem can be prevented by elevating the head of the frame. Newer models of the frame are adjustable, but it may be necessary to use "shock blocks" to elevate older models. The patient's own body weight then provides countertraction, keeping the weights in place.

A variety of attachments, e.g., footboards, bookholders, etc. are available for use with the Stryker frame. It may be appropriate to have the patient fitted with prism glasses so that he can see more of his environment. Patient's may be anxious when first placed on the frame. They are often concerned about falling off the frame, since it is quite narrow. The use of arm rests and restraining straps may be reassuring, especially at night. Patients are normally turned at a minimum of every 2 hours during the day, and possibly every 4 hours at night. Many of the problems of immobilization, e.g., pneumonia, renal calculi, still remain when a patient is on a Stryker frame. And, although the patient is being turned frequently, remember that pressure areas may still develop. The most common sites are where there are spaces in the canvas, such as at the forehead, the occiput, the chin, and the buttock. Pressure areas may also develop over the iliac crests if the patient is large and those areas are resting on the edge of the frame.

Family members and friends may be alarmed when they see the patient on the frame for the first time. It is helpful if they understand the advantages of the frame and its attachments before they see the patient. Family members may wish to become involved in the care of the patient, and this is to be encouraged. However, family members must never turn the patient without a member of the staff assisting them.

Recording includes the turning schedule, how the turning was tolerated by the patient (especially the first few times), skin care given and the condition of the skin. A well-written nursing care plan is also essential for patients on the Stryker frame. Attention must be paid to the turning schedule, skin care, and the various attachments which are used for the patient.

The CircOlectric Bed.   The *CircOlectric bed* is used for much the same reason as the Stryker frame. It has one distinct advantage in that the patient may be rotated in many positions, not just supine and prone. This aspect is especially valuable in improving the vascular tone of patients, such as paraplegics and quadriplegics, who have lost the nervous innervation to their blood vessels. Because they are unable to vasoconstrict in response to position changes, these patients often develop postural hypotension, which is a fall in the blood pressure due to pooling of blood in the lower part of the body. With the CircOlectric bed, the patient may be gradually moved from a supine position to an upright position. The gradual tilt allows the patient's vascular tree to accommodate, and postural hypotension becomes less of a problem.

When moving a patient from a supine position to an upright position, the footboard is attached to the frame. The patient will be supported by the footboard. The top frame is placed over the patient in much the same manner as with the Stryker frame, and the bolts at either end are tightened. A padded head restraint or head rest is positioned and is secured by clamps to the top frame. The patient should hold on to the turning frame so that his hands will not be caught as the frame rotates. When the patient has been properly positioned, the frame is rotated electrically by a

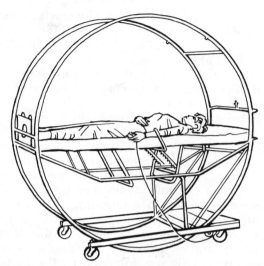

Figure 43–32. CircOlectric bed. (From Sutton, A. L.: *Bedside Nursing Techniques in Medicine and Surgery*, 2nd ed. Philadelphia, W. B. Saunders Co., 1969.)

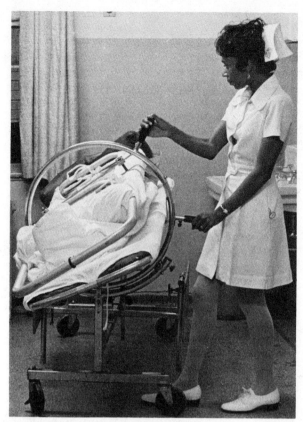

Figure 43–33. Wedge turning frame. (Courtesy Stryker Corporation, Kalamazoo, Mich. 49001)

control switch. (There is also a manual crank which can be used in the event of power failure.) The rotation should be smooth and continuous, without interruption. Once the desired position has been reached, the main mattress is released from the turning frame by removing the bolts. The mattress is on springs that are activated by a release bar. The main mattress is moved away from the patient and locked in place with a catch in the frame (Fig. 43–32).

Patients being turned on the CircOlectric bed must be watched carefully for signs of distress, especially cardiac arrhythmias and cardiac arrest. It is recommended by some that a physician be present for the first few turnings of a patient with neurological damage. Other aspects of care are similar to those of the patient on a Stryker frame.

Stryker Wedge. The Wedge turning frame is a fairly new device that is similar to the Stryker frame. It is commonly used for patients with cervical traction, laminectomy and spinal fusion. Its "wedge" design allows turning of the patient by one person, minimizes the patient's fear of falling, decreases the need for a number of restraining straps and allows elevation of the head of the frame so that proper traction is maintained. Like the Stryker frame, the positions possible are supine and prone (Fig. 43–33).

Heel and Elbow Protectors. Since the heels and elbows are not naturally well padded,

these areas are common sites for the development of decubitus ulcers in the immobilized patient. Heel and elbow protectors are devices used to keep the heel and elbow off the bed and pressure-free. It is not uncommon for skin breakdown to occur merely from the coarseness of bed linen. These devices are commercially available and are made from a variety of materials; however, sheep skin or a synthetic substitute are the most commonly used. Heel protectors not only protect the skin from breakdown, but are also used to prevent plantar flexion and footdrop (Fig. 43–34).

If these are not available, one can improvise by making a "donut" from abdominal pads that have been rolled lengthwise and the ends joined together with adhesive tape. The donut is then covered with roller gauze to make it soft and bulky, and adjusted to fit the patient. The donut is placed over the joint and should be snug enough that it stays in place. It should not, however, apply undue pressure. Donuts may exert pressure themselves and extend the area of skin breakdown; therefore they should be replaced as soon as possible with commercially-made devices. Donuts should be removed with each position change. The area

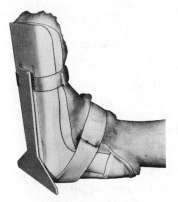

Figure 43-34. Heel protector with foot guard to prevent foot drop and stabilizer bar to prevent external rotation of foot. (From *Posey Guide.* J. T. Posey Company, Pasadena, Cal., 1976, p. 8.)

should be massaged and assessed for signs of pressure. The use of these devices should be recorded in both the clinical record and the nursing care plan.

Air Rings or Cushions. Air rings or cushions are used to relieve pressure on the sacrum, coccyx, rectum or perineum. They may be indicated by the following circumstances: post partum, postoperative hemorrhoidectomy, fracture of the coccyx, perirectal abscesses or decubiti. If improperly used, e.g., if left in place too long, air rings or cushions can *cause* decubiti.

Air rings are rubber and inflated with air. If overinflated, they may be uncomfortable and ineffective. Normally, if inflated properly, the rubber dents when a thumb is pressed into the material. Patient comfort is the best indicator of whether the ring is over or underinflated. Foam rings are not adjustable and are somewhat more conforming than air rings. Both kinds are covered with linen cases designed specifically for this purpose or with a pillow case. Because of the potential for a great deal of contamination, the covers should be removed when soiled and the device should be cleaned well. In most agencies, the foam cushion is sterilized by the use of gas when it becomes soiled and between patients.

Sheepskins. Sheepskins, available primarily as synthetics, are large pieces of material placed between the patient and the bed linen. They are soft, fluffy and somewhat absorbent. Sheepskins are used to prevent pressure areas from developing, to allow ventilation of skin surfaces, and to prevent shearing of skin when the patient is moved. The effectiveness of the sheepskin is minimized if the material becomes damp and matted down. It should be fluffed as necessary and changed when it be-

comes damp or soiled. Patients who use a sheepskin usually have several so that one is always clean. While synthetic sheepskins are expensive, they still cost less than the more expensive natural sheepskin. Since sheepskins are purchased by the patient and will probably be used for a long period of time, they should be marked with the patient's name and handled carefully.

Nursing Care

Since the needs of patients using protective and supportive devices demand constant attention, nursing documentation and reporting is essential. Aspects of care which must be addressed in the clinical record include: devices used; condition of the skin and soft tissues; range-of-motion exercises performed; presence of contractures or decubiti; position changes, including how positioned; and patient response to various positions and devices.

Additionally, there must be a well-developed, current nursing care plan so that all nursing staff will focus their energies on prevention. Written turning schedules are invaluable. It is extremely difficult to reverse the deformity caused by a contracture or to heal a decubitus ulcer. The primary focus must be on prevention. In addition to considering protective and supportive devices used, the nurse should also incorporate aspects of nutrition and the integrity of the skin, soft tissues and vascular supply in developing a comprehensive nursing care plan.

Patients who require protective and supportive devices usually have many other nursing needs as well. The nurse should identify and utilize other resources available to assist with care, especially the family and significant others. Incorporation of the family in the plan of care is not only helpful during the hospitalization period, it is essential if the responsibility for care after discharge is that of the family. In our sterile, controlled hospital environments we often forget that the patient is a family member first and a patient second. By encouraging the family to become *involved in the patient's care*, we can foster a closeness that cannot be achieved by sitting next to the bedside for hours at a time.

In many instances the patient is unconscious and the probability for recovery is minimal. By assisting with the patient's care, the family may be brought to the realization that the patient may not survive. It has been this writer's experience that families who have participated in the care of a terminally ill family member generally are able to handle grief and loss more effectively.

Although the previously discussed devices are very valuable in the prevention of complications in the immobilized patient, they cannot replace very aggressive nursing interventions. The prognosis of the patient is not always a guideline as to whether or not the nurse should actively pursue prevention of complications. This is true especially in the patient with neurological or neurosurgical problems where the ultimate outcome cannot be predicted with absolute certainty. Attention to detail and meticulous nursing care are essential. Above all, remember that the patient is a person who deserves all the care and concern you can give.

RESTRAINTS

Restraints are protectors employed to prevent a patient from harming himself or others, to immobilize and/or to promote a feeling of security in the patient who needs control. Restraints may be made of linen, leather or plastic and include wrist, ankle, chest, waist and total body devices. *Environmental restraint* is achieved through the use of siderails, "quiet" (seclusion) rooms, plastic domes and netting. Included in this section is a discussion of linen, leather and other restraints, seclusion and suicide precautions.

Considerations in the Use of Restraints

The use of restraints is often an emotional issue on the part of patients, families, friends and staff. Many units have nursing philosophies that may guide the nurse in understanding the use and impact of restraints on a particular nursing unit. On some units, restraints are used quite liberally while the personnel on other units may exhaust all possible alternatives before applying restraints. It is helpful if the nurse is familiar with the feelings of the staff in this regard in order to foster harmony and optimum patient care.

The nurse should recognize and anticipate that the patient response to being restrained is rarely submissive. In many instances, patients view the application of restraints as a personal physical assault (and, indeed, it sometimes is),

are frightened, and respond in a normal way by becoming combative. They are fearful of what may happen and are trying to protect their freedom. Patients may feel anger or guilt because what little control they have is being taken away. Patients may also feel guilt if a member of the staff is injured while applying restraint.

When the patient is in panic it is important that a staff member who has developed a good rapport with the patient talk to the patient, constantly reassuring him that the staff is aware of how frightened he is and that they are there to help him.[3, 20] Conversation should be in simple terms that the patient can easily understand.[21] The nurse should speak in a low, calm, reassuring voice and explain to the patient why restraints are being used. It may be necessary to repeat the explanation at frequent intervals, especially if the patient has been medicated with mind-altering drugs or is confused. It is essential that the patient's family and friends understand as well.

When dealing with a patient who is agitated and needs restraining, there are several considerations. There must be adequate personnel to safely and efficiently restrain the patient. One should never attempt to do this alone. Some psychiatric units in general hospitals have either a code number or phrase, e.g., Code 188 or Nursing Services Alert, 7 East, Room 702, which is announced over the hospital paging system. All available personnel from other nursing units go to the unit named to assist in restraining the patient. Hospital security personnel may also be utilized for this purpose if they have been adequately trained in application techniques. When the personnel are gathered they should remain out of the patient's range of vision because a "show of force" serves only to frighten the patient even more. There are several "holds" which the nurse can use to physically control a patient until there is sufficient help to safely restrain the patient (Fig. 43–35).

The second consideration is that the decision to restrain the patient should be made quickly and the procedure carried out promptly and quietly. Indecision on the part of the staff should never be witnessed by the patient; it may be perceived by the patient as the inability of the staff to properly care for him. It also greatly increases the anxiety levels of both patient and staff.

Another consideration is that a strategy must be developed and communicated. It should be perfectly clear to each person involved in the procedure exactly what his job will be. Each person should be assigned a particular task, e.g., restrain right wrist, hold shoulders, etc. Restraints should be prepared in advance, with each person holding the restraint appropriate

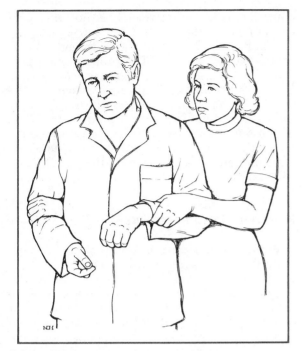

Figure 43–35. Restraining a panicked patient. The nurse grasps the patient's near wrist and far elbow as shown, for maximum control. (From Cosgriff, J. H., and Anderson, D. L.: *The Practice of Emergency Nursing.* Philadelphia, J. B. Lippincott Co., 1974.)

for the part of the body he has been assigned to restrain. It is wise to keep the restraints out of the patient's vision until the patient is in a position to be restrained, such as against a wall and sitting on the floor, or on a bed or stretcher. The team leader should signal to team members that the time to restrain is "now." Restraining combative patients is always stressful to all concerned, but it can be accomplished with a minimum amount of energy and anxiety if there is good preparation and communication.

Patients in restraints should be *observed frequently*. Some psychiatric units utilize *restraint records* to document nursing observations. Restrained patients should be visited at least every half hour. The patient needs to know that the nurse is concerned about his physical and emotional needs and that he is not being "punished." Patients need to know that they have not been abandoned, that they have worth, and that the restraints are a therapeutic tool being used to help them.

Restraints can be dangerous to the patient's welfare. In addition to the detrimental psychological impact, there are significant *legal implications* associated with physical restraint of individuals. The nurse must be knowledgeable of the institutional policy as well as state and local regulations concerning involuntary retention,

imprisonment and restraint. In most agencies a physician's order is required before restraints can be used. Some institutions authorize nursing judgment in the application of linen restraints, but require a physician's order for the application of leather restraints.

Hazards of Restraints

The *hazards* associated with the use of restraints include:

1. Tissue damage under the restraint
2. Damage to other parts of the body, especially shoulder dislocations, if the patient is combative during the application of restraints or has a grand mal seizure while restrained
3. The development of hypostatic pneumonia and pressure areas if the patient is kept restrained for long periods of time and/or does not have frequent position changes
4. Ischemia or nerve damage if restraints are applied too tightly or if they become constrictive after application
5. Wrist drop due to failure to put the joint through range-of-motion exercises
6. Aspiration pneumonia if a patient is restrained in a supine position, has an altered level of consciousness and vomits
7. The use of the restraint by a patient to inflict harm on himself or others
8. The inability to effectively resuscitate a restrained person who has a cardiac arrest because of the amount of time required to remove the restraints in order to place a cardiac arrest board or position the patient supine
9. Injury or death to the helpless restrained person due to fire

The last two problems may occur if restraints are tied in knots rather than bows, and if staff members fail to keep a restraint key on their person at all times.

> *Whenever a patient is placed in locked restraints, all personnel must carry a key to unlock the restraints in the event of a medical or environmental emergency.*

Patients with depressed levels of consciousness may have difficulty handling their secretions or emesis, especially when restrained on their backs. *Aspiration and suffocation are thus potential dangers.*

> Never *restrain a person with a depressed level of consciousness on his back with limbs restrained on either side ("spread eagle"). If the patient vomits while in this position, or if he has copious amounts of secretions, it may be impossible to get him on his side fast enough to prevent aspiration pneumonia. Restraining the patient in a three-quarter prone position is much safer.*

It should be remembered that a patient in restraints is at the mercy of the staff for all activities of daily living, including fluid intake, nutrition, change of position, range-of-motion exercises and elimination. The restrained patient should be in a comfortable position. The head of the bed may be elevated so that the patient may see his environment. This environmental contact may assist in the patient's reorientation and decrease his confusion. If appropriate, the call signal cord may be placed within easy reach.

Re-evaluate the need for restraints at frequent intervals and discontinue restraints as soon as possible. In selected situations it may be appropriate to establish a time limit for the length of the restraint period. Utilize resources such as family and friends instead of using restraints. The use of restraints can have a devastating effect on patients, visitors and staff. Physical restraint is used only when all other alternatives have been exhausted. Restraints should be used therapeutically and are not to be applied as "punishment" for inappropriate behavior.

> *The use of restraints should never be vindictive or merely to "show the patient who's boss."*

Because of the very real possibility of being charged with false imprisonment, documentation in the clinical record is essential. *Recording* should include: (a) the patient behavior which precipitated using restraints, (b) the kind of restraint used, (c) the condition of the skin and skin care given, (d) the frequency of observations and of removal of restraints (at least every 4 hours), (e) the time of restraint application and time of discontinuance and (f) patient response to restraints.

Remember, while patients have a right to be protected from harm, they also have a right not to be restrained against their will unless the court has ruled otherwise. It is no longer acceptable in many states for a nurse to apply restraints merely because she "thought it was for the patient's good." The professional nurse must *know, understand* and *respect* each patient's rights and civil liberties as well as the agency policies in this aspect of care. *The best policy is to avoid restraining patients unless absolutely necessary.* Utilize environmental control or family and friends to provide a safe environment. This is far more therapeutic and humanistic.

Wrist and Ankle Restraints

Wrist and ankle restraints are utilized when it is necessary to significantly restrict motion of the limbs. They may be used for a patient who is potentially harmful to himself or others, to prevent the patient from removing tubes and other appliances, and to immobilize a part so that a procedure may be done, e.g., suturing a wound. These restraints may be leather, linen or plastic (Figs. 43–36 and 43–37). Below are presented some key points in the use of wrist and ankle restraints.

Key Points in the Use of Wrist and Ankle Restraints

▶ Leather restraints must always be locked. A leather belt restraint can be used by a patient as a weapon or as a means of committing suicide by hanging.

▶ When using leather restraints, pad the skin under the restraint well with ABD's to avoid skin irritation and to insure proper fit.

▶ Apply the restraint cuffs snugly around the wrist or ankle, but not too tight.

▶ *Always* carry a restraint key with you when a patient is in leather restraints.

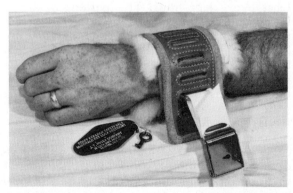

Figure 43–36. Leather limb restraint. (From *Posey Guide.* J. T. Posey Company, Pasadena, Cal., 1973, p. 7.)

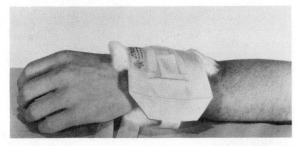

Figure 43–37. Linen wrist restraint. (From *Posey Guide.* J. T. Posey Company, Pasadena, Cal., 1973, p. 6.)

▶ Do *not* tie linen restraints with a regular knot. Such a knot may be difficult to release quickly in the event of any emergency. Use a bow, but place it where the patient cannot easily reach it.

▶ If the linen restraints used are not specifically designed for securing around the wrist or ankle, use a clove hitch knot (Fig. 43–38) to apply the restraint around the limb.

▶ Clean the skin of the wrists and ankles and powder it before applying restraints.

▶ Fasten the restraint to the *bed frame,* not to the siderails. The arms or legs may be injured when the siderails are lowered if the restraint is attached to the siderail. If the bed position is changed the restraints may have too much or too little slack.

▶ Fasten wrist straps below the patient's waist and the ankle straps below his knees.

▶ Wrist restraints must always be used when ankle restraints are used. If this is not done: (a) the patient may be able to take off the ankle restraints if his hands are free or (b) he may also "hang" himself by the heels, either intentionally or accidentally.

▶ Allow enough slack on the straps so that the patient can move his arms and legs if desired.

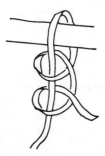

Figure 43–38. Clove hitch knot used in applying restraints. (From *Posey Guide.* J. T. Posey Company, Pasadena, Cal., 1973, p. 30.)

▶ *Never* apply restraints over an IV site.

▶ Ensure that IV and other tubing and equipment lines are not interfered with by the restraints.

▶ Remove and reapply restraints at least every 2 hours during the day and every 4 hours at night. At these times, provide skin care to the areas under the restraints. A moisturizing lotion may be beneficial.

▶ Remove one restraint at a time if you are alone and if the patient is potentially harmful to himself or others.

▶ Change the patient's position at least every 2 hours. Check for color, sensation, temperature, motion and capillary refill in the area distal to the restraint.

▶ Reassess the restrained patient at frequent intervals and provide psychological support.

▶ Assess respiratory status at least every 8 hours in a patient requiring continuous restraint. Respiratory assessment techniques are discussed under chest binders on p. 1107.

Chest or Waist Restraints

Chest or waist restraints are used to prevent a patient from getting or falling out of bed or a chair. When properly applied, they allow the patient full movement of the extremities and permit a fair degree of freedom. A waist restraint is a gentle reminder to the patient, while a chest restraint is more appropriate for the patient who is agitated or more than mildly confused (Fig. 43–39). Chest and waist restraints are made of cotton, muslin or mesh and tolerate repeated washings.

Key Points in the Application and Use of Chest and Waist Restraints

▶ Clean and dry the skin, especially the axilla, prior to applying the restraints.

▶ Ensure that there are no wrinkles or bulges in the restraint that may irritate the skin after application.

▶ Place buckles where the patient cannot reach them, e.g., along the side of the bed, underneath the bed or in back of the chair.

▶ Do not use adhesive tape to secure buckles

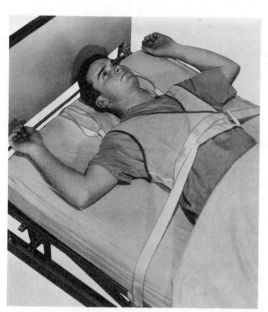
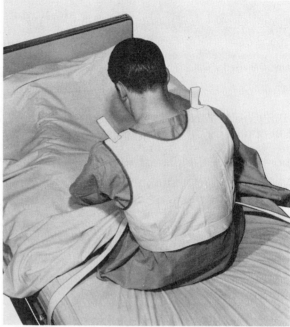

Figure 43–39. Chest restraint. (From *Posey Guide.* J. T. Posey Company, Pasadena, Cal., 1973, p. 4.)

and straps. Tape is very difficult and time consuming to remove in an emergency.

▶ Place buckles face up for easy removal by the staff. Place the straps in buckles or teeth securely. Lock straps that are lockable. Make sure that all personnel have a key to locked restraints or that one is visible in the patient's room.[12]

▶ Assess the patient's respiratory status at least every hour to ensure that the restraint is not interfering with ventilation.

▶ Attach straps to the bed frame, not to the siderails. Patients may be injured if the straps are attached to side rails and the siderails are lowered.

▶ Use a chest restraint rather than a waist restraint when the patient is restrained in a chair or wheelchair. Also, place the back of the chair against a wall to prevent the patient from tipping the chair over. Lock wheelchair wheels.

▶ Remember, patients may develop pressure areas on the sacrum and buttocks from sitting in a chair too long. Use a flotation therapy pad or other cushion on the chair seat when advisable. Do not leave patients restrained in chairs for more than 2 hours at a time.

▶ Select a sturdy, comfortable chair if a patient is to be restrained in a chair. *Never* restrain a patient on a commode or rocking chair. In addition to being hard and very uncomfortable, they are not sturdy and are easily tipped over.

▶ Tie knots in a square knot or with a bow.

Chest restraints made from sheets may be used temporarily as bed restraints. Sheet restraints are unsafe for a patient in a chair. They are either too loose to be effective or too tight to be comfortable.

A sheet restraint for use on a patient on a stretcher can be fashioned from a regular bed sheet. The two long ends of the sheet are grasped by two people and the sheet is twirled until it is a tight roll. The middle of the roll is positioned under the patient's upper back and shoulders. The ends are brought under the axilla, over the anterior shoulders and under the middle portion of the roll. The sheet is applied snugly and the ends are crossed under the bottom of the stretcher at the level of the patient's head. The ends are tied in a square knot. This restraint is designed for temporary use only and is most valuable when the patient is on a stretcher or a narrow frame, e.g., backboard, Stryker frame. Undue pressure on the axilla should be avoided.

Mitt Restraints

Mitts are devices placed over a patient's hands to prevent him: (a) from removing tubes, dressings or appliances, (b) from traumatizing tissue by scratching himself or (c) from undoing restraints. Mitt restraints are available commercially, or they can be fashioned from a variety of materials readily available on most nursing units.[5, 12] Examples of commercially available mitts are pictured in Figure 43–40.

Before applying mitts the patient's hands should be clean and dry. A hand roll may be used to keep the patient's fingers in position of function. Mitts should be removed and reapplied at least every 8 hours, the skin cleansed, and range-of-motion exercises done if necessary. If hand rolls or very constrictive mitts are used, this care should be provided more frequently. Mitts are also available with restraint straps to immobilize the limb. When these are used, the nursing concerns are the same as for wrist restraints.

Body Restraints

Body restraints are utilized when it is necessary to immobilize all or most of the patient's body. They are commonly used for children when performing procedures that require that the patient be motionless, e.g., venipuncture or suturing, and in patients who are combative or hysterical. Body restraints are usually linen or mesh (Fig. 43–41).

Body restraints are usually used for a short time as the problems associated with immobility are so great. Providing nursing care is difficult, and the nursing concerns are the same as those for patients in four-point (wrist and ankle) restraints.

There is often a need to completely restrain children for special procedures; it can be done in several ways. The most readily available restraint is the sheet "mummy." The child is placed on the center of a sheet which has been folded to fit his size. The child's arms are at his sides and the legs are straight. One side of the sheet is brought over the patient's body and

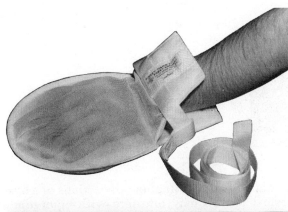

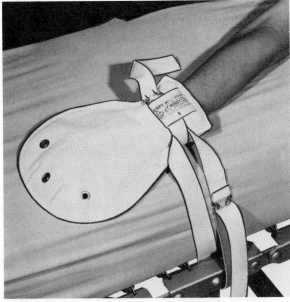

Figure 43–40. Mitt restraints. (From *Posey Guide*. J. T. Posey Company, Pasadena, Cal., 1973, p. 6.)

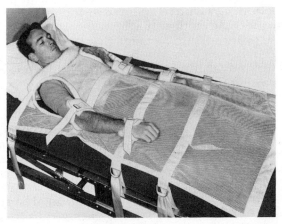

Figure 43–41. Total body restraint. (From *Posey Guide*. J. T. Posey Company, Pasadena, Cal., 1973, p. 5.)

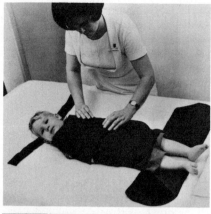
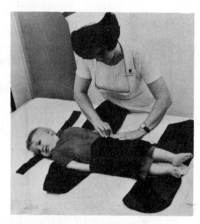
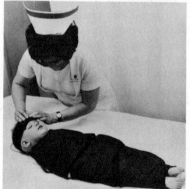
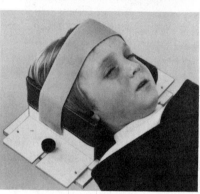

Figure 43–42. Papoose Board with head immobilizer. (Courtesy Olympic Medical Corporation, Seattle, Wash., 98108.)

tucked under his body, encasing the arms and legs securely. The opposite side of the sheet is then brought over the body and tucked underneath the patient. Usually, the weight of the child is all that is needed to keep the sheet taut; however, the sheet may be secured with pins. A commercially made mummying device called a "Papoose Board" is also very effective in immobilizing a child. The linen restraining strips are secured with self-adhering material, and the board is sturdy enough that the child may be transported on the board. There is also a head immobilizer, which is valuable when suturing the face or in the event of a cervical spine injury (Fig. 43–42).

Total body restraint of an adult is somewhat more difficult without special devices designed specifically for that purpose. Applying total body restraints on an adult patient requires at least four people if he is combative and does not have other restraints already in place.

One of the times when immediate total body restraint may be necessary is during a disaster situation where special devices are not readily available. In this situation, the actions of a hysterical person may interfere with emergency care and threaten the lives of others. Temporary restraint may be accomplished by placing the patient on a canvas litter (hand-carried stretcher) and placing a second canvas litter directly on top of him. A litter strap is secured around both litters and the patient is sandwiched in. While this is not an appropriate restraint technique under normal circumstances, it is a quick and effective method when the lives of others are at stake. Needless to say, this restraint must be replaced with proper restraints and/or other therapeutic measures as soon as possible.

Environmental Control or Restraint

Environmental restraint or control is achieved by providing the patient with an environment free of hazards. This is accomplished by the use of siderails, netting, plastic domes, and "quiet" (seclusion) rooms.

Siderails are sturdy metal frames that are attached to both sides of the patient's bed. They may extend the full length of the bed or may extend from the head of the bed to the middle of the bed. Siderails serve as reminders to the patient that he is in a hospital bed and are designed to prevent patients from getting out or falling out of bed. Although the decision to keep siderails raised is usually a nursing decision, some institutions have specific guidelines governing their use. Normally, siderails must be kept raised on the beds of all patients who have altered levels of consciousness, the elderly and children. Many hospitals require that they be raised on the beds of all patients at night, and more and more agencies require that siderails be raised and locked whenever a patient is in bed. Patients may refuse to allow siderails raised on their beds, but usually they are required to sign a form which releases the hospital from liability in the event of an accident that could have been prevented if the siderails were in use.

Siderails themselves can pose a danger to patients. Parts of the patient's body may become caught in the siderails, especially the folding models. Patients who are confused or are unable to get the nurse's attention may climb over the siderails or go over the end of the bed, especially at night. Because of the height from the top of the siderail to the floor, it is sometimes safer to leave siderails down on these patients. Whenever siderails are used, the patient should be informed that it is a hospital policy designed to ensure their safety, especially since hospital beds and stretchers are usually much higher than beds used at home.

Safety straps are used to prevent the patient from falling when on narrow stretchers or tables, e.g., operating room tables. The straps should be placed about 15 cm. (6 in.) above the knees and at waist level. Again, an explanation of why the straps are being used is indicated.

Netting is commonly used over the beds of patients to prevent them from getting out of bed and is most often used on children's cribs. The netting is tied all around the top and sides of the crib and must be secure. There have been instances where children have climbed over the crib sides between the netting and have been caught in the netting, resulting in death from asphyxiation. *It is imperative that all ends of the netting be tied securely to the frame of the bed.*

Plastic domes or bubbles are used for the same reasons that netting is used and are rapidly replacing netting. The domes fit over the top of the crib and allow the child to stand in his crib and see more of his environment. All domes are not adaptable to all cribs currently in use, so it is important that the correct dome be used or the effectiveness will be negated.

Seclusion or "quiet" rooms are rooms specifically designed to be hazard-free and are commonly used for psychiatric patients. Normally, the floor of the room is heated, the walls are padded, any windows are covered with heavy screening, and all electrical outlets or fixtures are inaccessible to the patient. These rooms have no furniture or just a mattress. There may be a drain in the floor for fluids. Seclusion rooms should be located near the nurses station so that the patient will be observed frequently. There is usually a heavy door that can be locked and an observation window.

The use of a quiet room is indicated when patients are agitated, assaultive, suicidal or homicidal. It may also be used when there is a need to minimize the amount of stimuli that the patient is subjected to, e.g., for a patient in a manic state. Many times a quiet room is a temporary measure until medications have taken effect. Some patients elect to go to the quiet room when they feel a need to gain control or desire the security of a locked room.

Patients in seclusion must be visited every half hour. All personnel on duty must carry the key to the room whenever a patient is in locked seclusion because of the potential for a medical or environmental emergency. As with other patients in restraints, the patient in seclusion must have his physical and emotional needs met by the staff. It is often valuable to set a time limit on the length of stay in seclusion, especially if the patient has not been placed there voluntarily. It is essential that the following be recorded: (a) behavior which precipitated the use of seclusion, (b) whether seclusion was voluntary or involuntary, (c) time seclusion started and terminated, (d) accurate account of visits made by staff and patient behavior observed and (e) patient response to seclusion.

Suicide Precautions

"Suicide precautions" is the term given to actions taken by the staff to prevent a patient from harming himself. Although many agencies have specific guidelines identifying what suicide precautions are used, there are some generalizations. Some of these are:

▶ The patient's clothes and effects are searched for dangerous objects, such as glass, weapons, razor blades, scissors, eye glasses, etc., which may be used to inflict harm.

▶ The patient himself is searched for any dangerous objects.

▶ Shoestrings, belts, head bands, scarves, underwear are often used to hang oneself and must be removed from the patient's environment.

▶ Signal light cords and other electrical cords may be removed from the patient's room.

▶ Furniture is heavy or is fastened securely, especially lamps.

▶ Light bulbs from lamps and flashlights can be broken and used to inflict lacerations or can be eaten. Care must be used when the patient is in an examination room with examination lights and flashlights.

▶ All dangerous medical supplies and equipment are locked in a secure place.

▶ Bed linens may be removed in selected cases.

▶ The patient may be restrained, but must be in locked restraints.

▶ The patient is visited and observed at least every 30 minutes.

Suicide precautions are not to be taken lightly. Even with the most diligent efforts by the staff at preventing suicide, some patients may still succeed. The guilt that the staff feels in such situations is tremendous. These feelings may be lessened somewhat if all efforts humanly possible were taken to prevent the suicide. In addition, there are significant legal ramifications if it can be demonstrated that the staff failed to take the appropriate precautions.

SUMMARY

In the care of patients many functions are interdependent; that is, several members of the health care team share responsibility for the same aspects of care. However, the provision of physical protection and bodily support is primarily the responsibility of the nurse. Ensuring that the patient is safe, comfortable, protected from deformities and provided with an aesthetic environment are functions that cannot be negated or delegated. Providing physical protection and bodily support requires the professional nurse to demonstrate responsibility, accountability and true commitment to quality patient care.

BIBLIOGRAPHY

1. American Red Cross: *Advanced First Aid and Emergency Care*. New York, Doubleday and Company, Inc., 1973.
2. Brunner, L. S., et al.: *Textbook of Medical-Surgical Nursing*, 2nd ed. Philadelphia, J. B. Lippincott Company, 1974.
3. Cosgriff, J. H., and Anderson, D. L.: *The Practice of Emergency Nursing*. Philadelphia, J. B. Lippincott Company, 1975.
4. Drury, J. H.: Handbook of range-of-motion exercises. *Nursing '72*, 2:19, April 1972.
5. Feycock, J. M. W.: A do-it-yourself restraint that works. *Nursing '75*, 5:18, Jan. 1975.
6. Foss, G.: The "how to's" of bed positioning. *Nursing '72*, 2:14, Aug. 1972.
7. Gordon, J. E.: CircOlectric beds. *Nursing '77*, 7:42, Feb. 1977.
8. Guberski, T., and Campbell, M. E.: The effects on leg volume of two methods of wrapping elastic bandages. *Nursing Research*, 19:260, May–June 1970.
9. Harvin, J. S., and Hargest, T. S.: The air-fluidized bed: A new concept in the treatment of decubitus ulcers. *Nursing Clinics of North America*, 5:181, March 1970.
10. Henderson, J.: *Emergency Medical Guide*, 2nd ed. New York: McGraw-Hill Book Co., 1969.
11. Iversen, L. D., and Clawson, D. K.: *Manual of Acute Orthopaedic Therapeutics*. Boston, Little, Brown & Company, 1977.
12. Kukuk, H. M.: Safety precautions: Protecting your patients and yourself (part two). *Nursing '76*, 6:49, June 1976.
13. Larson, C. B., and Gould, M.: *Calderwood's Orthopedic Nursing*, 6th ed. St. Louis, C. V. Mosby Co., 1965.
14. Larson, C. B.: *Professional Uses of Adhesive Tape*. New Brunswick, New Jersey: Johnson and Johnson, 1972.
15. Matsen, F. A., III: Compartmental syndromes. *Clinical Orthopedics*, 113:8, 1976.
16. Matsen, F. A., III: Compartmental syndromes: treat now, diagnose later. *Emergency Medicine*, 8:62, May 1976.
17. Noe, J. M., and Kalish, S.: *Wound Care*. Greenwich, CT: Chesebrough-Ponds, Inc., 1975.
18. Ranalls, J.: Crutches and walkers. *Nursing '72*, 2:21, Dec. 1972.
19. Rinear, C. E., and Rinear, E. E.: Emergency bandaging: A wrap-up of better techniques. *Nursing '75*, 5:29, Jan. 1975.
20. Robinson, L.: Coping with psychiatric emergencies. *Nursing '73*, 3:42, July 1973.
21. Rogerson, K. E.: Psychiatric emergencies. *Nursing Clinics of North America*, 8:457, Sep. 1973.
22. Swanson, M. A.: *Crutches on the Go*. Bellevue, WA: Medic Publishing Company, 1974.
23. _____: For decubitus: a new protocol. *Emergency Medicine*, 9:247, April 1977.
24. _____: . . . and a warning. *Emergency Medicine*, 9:250, April 1977.

CHAPTER 44

CARING FOR PERSONS REQUIRING APPLICATIONS OF HEAT AND COLD

By Marylin J. Dodd, R.N., B.Sc.N., M.N.

INTRODUCTION AND STUDY GUIDE

This chapter discusses therapeutic applications of local heat and cold. Knowledge of the physiologic responses of the cutaneous skin circulation upon exposure to heat and cold is the basis for understanding this unit. Factors influencing the effects of heat and cold applications and potential dangers to tissue are discussed. Because patients can receive injuries from heat and cold therapy, this area of practice has enormous potential for law suits. The therapeutic purposes of applications of heat and cold are presented along with specific patient conditions in which these applications are contraindicated, common complications of local applications, and preventive measures. Detailed nursing procedures are provided for the common applications of heat and cold and the equipment used is described and pictured. Nursing assessments to be made and patient teaching required are discussed.

Basic anatomy and physiology of the nerve impulse tracts which transmit the sensations of heat, cold and pain are outlined. You can understand the physiologic effects of heat and cold applications only if you understand the neurological and circulatory structures, including capillary action, that respond to temperature stimuli. You also need to understand some of the basic principles of heat transfer: conduction, convection, evaporation, radiation, conversion. Review these terms before beginning to study the chapter; it will help you understand the principles and procedures presented here.

Upon completion of this chapter, you should be able to:

1. Understand and use these terms
heat
cold
sensory end organs
  cold receptors
  warm receptors
  pain receptors
thermal receptor
  adaptation
hypothalamus
somatic afferent fibers
vasodilation
vasoconstriction
cutaneous
conductor
secondary effect
recovery time
congestion
ischemia
suppuration
phagocytosis
gangrene
necrosis
hypoxia
thrombus
counterirritants
poultice, plaster
consensual response
edema
maceration
pallor
blisters
mottling
diathermy
soaks
débridement
compress
sitz bath
paraffin bath
contrast bath

2. Apply local heat and cold, as ordered for a patient's condition, safely and effectively
3. Name the neurological structures that transmit the cutaneous stimuli to the brain
4. Describe the neurological pathways used in transmitting a stimulus of heat, cold or pain
5. Describe the normal circulatory response after exposure to a hot cutaneous stimulus
6. Describe the normal circulatory response after exposure to a cold cutaneous stimulus
7. Name physiologic disorders that hinder normal transmission of impulses and circulatory response to a hot or cold stimulus
8. List the contraindications to the therapeutic use of heat or cold applications
9. Explain the complications that can result from applications of heat or cold
10. List the essential components of the doctor's orders when applications of heat or cold are prescribed as therapy

11. Describe patient assessments which would lead the nurse to decide to omit heat or cold therapy prior to, during and after an application of heat or cold

12. List the safety measures the nurse should use in handling equipment used for heat and cold applications

13. List the safe temperature and the duration of treatment for each procedure discussed in this chapter

14. Explain the essential patient/family teaching needed in therapeutic applications of heat and cold

OVERVIEW: ANATOMY AND PHYSIOLOGY

Sensory End Organs

Sensory end organs are made up of cold receptors, warm receptors and pain receptors. They are all located in the skin. Sensory end organs are not evenly distributed throughout the body; for instance, cold receptors are more concentrated in the upper trunk and extremities.[5] Cold receptors are more superficial than warm receptors and are eight to ten times more numerous.[5] Minimal to moderate stimulation of the cold or warm receptors produces a sensation of coldness or warmth as interpreted by the brain. Extreme stimulation of the warm receptors produces the sensation of "burning" due to the pain receptors, which are also being stimulated. A widely accepted theory of the functioning of pain receptors states that whenever the stimulation of either the warm or cold receptors is severe enough the pain receptors also become stimulated.[20] Figure 44–1 shows how the three different types of receptors respond at various levels of temperature.

The significance of these levels is demonstrated by the fact all these fibers respond differently at different levels of temperature. For instance, below 12°C. (53.6°F.) the cold receptors cannot be stimulated. If the skin is exposed to a temperature lower than 12°C., the individual will experience the sensation of pain, not cold. This knowledge is useful when assessing patients during an application of cold, as will be discussed on p. 1154.

Thermal Receptor Adaptation

We have all had the experience of getting into a very hot bath only to find in a few minutes that the temperature of the water does not seem hot enough. What happens is that the warm receptors are initially stimulated very strongly, but then these stimuli decrease rapidly. The warm receptors adapt to the warmth of the bath water, and while the water temperature has changed only slightly, our sensation of the warmth is drastically reduced. Often at this point we add more hot water to the bath, probably exceeding the original temperature of the water. This process of thermal receptor adaptation also exists with cold receptor stimulation. There is real danger in this adaptive phenomenon. A person insensitive to the extremes of either the hot or cold stimuli may suffer tissue damage.

Transmission of Sensation

When the skin receptors are stimulated by heat, cold, or pain-producing stimuli, they send impulses via the somatic afferent fibers (the nervous pathway traveled by impulses when skin receptors are stimulated) in the spinothalamic tract (spinal nerve pathway that receives impulses from the somatic afferent fibers and delivers these impulses to the hypothalamus in the brain). The impulses travel up the spinal cord through this tract to the brain's anterior hypothalamus (part of the brain, located in the cranium, that is the body's thermostat). From there the impulses are transmitted to the brain's cerebral cortex, where interpretation of the impulses occurs. In other words, the stimuli are then recognized as hot, cold and/or painful. Although these pathways are long and complex, it takes only a few hundredths of a second for an impulse to ascend to the cortex and for the interpreted message to be sent back to the stimulated skin receptors. Nature has built a "short cut" into even this

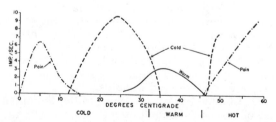

Figure 44–1. Frequencies of discharge of a cold receptor, a warm receptor and a pain nerve fiber at various temperatures. (From Guyton, A. C.: *Textbook of Medical Physiology,* 5th ed. Philadelphia, W. B. Saunders Co., 1976.)

few-hundredths-of-a-second process. When a person exposes a part of his body to a stimulus that severely stimulates his skin receptors, the impulse travels to the spinal cord along a sensory (afferent) neuron. There an association neuron transfers the impulse to a motor (efferent) neuron. The motor neuron carries the impulse to a muscle, which contracts and moves a body part.[14a]

In other words, when the body is threatened, the impulse does not need to travel to the brain for interpretation. You know how quickly you jerk your hand back if you touch a hot stove. The spinal cord reflex withdraws your hand from the noxious (painful) stimuli immediately; the skin's warm receptors are severely stimulated, the impulses travel to the spinal cord, and a reflex action is produced that jerks your hand away. A message does not need to come from the brain to tell you your hand is being burned and you should remove it from the source of damage.

Cutaneous Circulation

The cutaneous circulation, i.e., skin circulation, is made up of a complicated matrix of arterioles and venules. The body has the capacity to either increase (dilate) or decrease (constrict) the lumen diameter of these vessels in response to local or systemic conditions. The volume of blood present in the cutaneous circulation varies and can be from 0 to 30 per cent of the cardiac minute output (the amount of blood expelled from the heart in one minute).[9] Or expressed another way, when the cutaneous vessels are fully dilated, one half to two thirds of the entire body's blood supply can be located there.[8]

Table 44–1 summarizes the local physiologic effects from the application of heat or cold.

TABLE 44–1. LOCAL PHYSIOLOGIC EFFECTS FROM THE APPLICATION OF HEAT AND COLD

Heat	Cold
1. Vasodilation	1. Vasoconstriction
2. Increase capillary permeability	2. Decrease capillary permeability
3. Increase local metabolism	3. Decrease local metabolism
4. Increase oxygen requirement	4. Decrease oxygen requirement
5. Decrease blood viscosity	5. Increase blood viscosity
6. Increase blood flow	6. Decrease blood flow
7. Increase lymph flow	7. Decrease lymph flow
8. Increase motility of leukocytes	8. Decrease motility of leukocytes
9. Decrease muscle tonus	9. Decrease muscle tonus

Ordinarily, cutaneous blood vessels are controlled by sympathetic nervous impulses. These impulses maintain a slightly constricted tonus in the vessels.[9] However, with the application of local heat, the peripheral cutaneous arterioles dilate. Conversely, with the application of local cold the peripheral cutaneous arterioles constrict. The stimulus of heat causes inhibition of the sympathetic vasoconstrictor impulses to the cutaneous arterioles. The stimulus of cold augments the sympathetic vasoconstrictor impulses, thus producing an even more pronounced vasoconstriction.

Peripheral vasodilation also relaxes the capillaries and thereby increases the surface area available for fluid exchange. This increased capillary permeability is not entirely understood. One theory is that, because of the local arteriolar vasodilation, external applications of *heat* briefly cause a greater increase in arteriolar blood flow than in venous blood flow.[19] This causes an increase in the capillary hydrostatic pressure (fluid pressure within the capillary compartment), and the potential then exists for a shift in body fluids from the blood vessels to the tissues. Conversely, the application of *cold* reduces capillary filtration by decreasing the local blood flow, thereby decreasing the capillary hydrostatic pressure.

The sequela of the vasodilation produced by the application of heat goes even further. Because of the vasodilation, the blood's viscosity is reduced and the rate of blood flow and leukocyte motility is increased. The lymph flow increases as well. The application of cold has the opposite effects.

The rate of metabolism and, therefore, of waste production and oxygen consumption, is increased in tissues that are immediately affected by the heat application. As will be discussed later, this is a mixed blessing and the ramifications must always be considered before the therapeutic application of either heat or cold.

It has been believed for some time that since the skin and cutaneous tissues were poor conductors (a substance that permits the passage of forms of energy through it), therapeutic applications of either heat or cold would have only superficial effects. This is not true. In studies conducted by Wise[25] it was found that when an ice bag or a hot-water bag was placed on a person's leg, subcutaneous and intramuscular temperatures were affected strongly (Table 44–2).

TABLE 44–2.   SUBCUTANEOUS AND INTRAMUSCULAR EFFECTS OF HEAT
AND COLD APPLICATION

Cold	
Interior of ice bag	0°C. (32°F.)
Outside of towel covering ice bag	4.4°C. (40°F.)
Decline in temperature:	
Cutaneous in 15 minutes	From 28.9 to 6.1°C. (84 to 40°F.)
Subcutaneous in 1 hour	From 34.4 to 21.1°C. (94 to 70°F.)
Intramuscular in 2 hours	From 36.7 to 26.1°C. (98 to 79°F.)
Heat:	
Interior of hot water bag	56.1°C. (133°F.)
Outside of towel covering hot water bag	50.0°C. (122°F.)
Rise in temperature:	
Cutaneous in 30 minutes	From 32.2 to 43.3°C. (90 to 110°F.)
Subcutaneous in 40 minutes	From 32.9 to 40.9°C. (91.2 to 105.5°F.)
Intramuscular in 50 minutes	From 34.5 to 37.5°C. (94.2 to 99.6°F.)

(Adapted from: Wise, C. S.: Heat and cold. *In* Biermanand, W., and Licht, S. (eds.): *Physical Medicine in General Practice*, 3rd ed. New York, Hoeber, 1955.)

Secondary Effect from Hot or Cold Applications

As noted above, local applications of heat typically result in dilation of peripheral cutaneous arterioles while cold applications result in constriction of these vessels. Some exceptions occur to this general rule; for example, *extreme heat* applied for a short period causes vasoconstriction of local cutaneous arterioles. This vasoconstriction also occurs after 1 hour of continuous application of heat. The phenomenon is called "secondary effect."

Likewise, after 30 minutes to 1 hour of *continuous cold* application, local arteriolar vasodilation occurs for 10 to 15 minutes. This vasodilation after continuous cold is also referred to as "secondary effect" and is the body's defense to prevent damage to the tissue from prolonged ischemia (lack of oxygen to a part of the body). The nursing implications in regard to the possibility of "secondary effect" are obvious:

1. With heat application, the maximal increase in circulation and tissue temperature occurs after 20 to 45 minutes of exposure. After this time the heat application must be discontinued and a recovery time of 1 hour allowed, or the secondary effect (vasoconstriction) will countermand the therapeutic effect of the application.

2. With cold application, the initial exposure must last only 30 minutes to 1 hour. After this time, a recovery time of 1 hour must be allowed or the secondary effect (vasodilation) will occur.

Excessive heat or cold and prolongation of a treatment beyond the prescribed time are definitely contraindicated.

THERAPEUTIC USES OF LOCAL HEAT AND COLD

Heat

A summary of the uses of heat and cold applications is presented in Table 44–3. The physiologic reasons why *heat relieves pain* are based on the etiology of the pain. If pain is caused by ischemic tissue, the vasodilation from a heat application will relieve the pain. If pain originates from muscle spasms, the heat will relax the involved muscles and thereby relieve the pain. This is particularly helpful in poliomyelitis and low back pain. If pain is caused by local congestion (i.e., excess blood in a body part), the application of heat will increase the local circulation and relieve this congestion. Halsell, in her study of 108 abdominal surgical patients, found the application of warm, moist packs to the incision three times a day was helpful in relieving pain and discomfort for the majority (89 per cent) of patients.[10] Use of such packs postoperatively is not a common practice among bedside nurses currently. The full therapeutic potential of these applications has not been realized. A widely

TABLE 44–3.   THERAPEUTIC USES OF LOCAL HEAT OR COLD APPLICATIONS

HEAT	COLD
1. Decrease pain	1. Decrease pain
2. Decrease muscle tonus	2. Decrease muscle tonus
3. Promote healing	3. Decrease oxygen supply to area
4. Promote suppuration (pus formation)	4. Decrease circulation to the area
5. Dilate veins	5. Decrease metabolism
6. Relieve deep congestion	6. Prevent edema (excess fluid between body cells)
	7. Retard bacterial growth

accepted theory about why heat reduces pain is the belief that heat receptors compete with the pain receptors for recognition by the cerebral cortex.[10]

Heat decreases muscle tonus and thereby relaxes the muscle and relieves stiffness. Also, with the increase in blood flow that heat produces, fatigued muscles become rejuvenated. In Halsell's study the surgical patients' muscle spasms were relieved by heat applications to their abdomens.

Heat applications facilitate healing by increasing the supply of leukocytes, antibodies and nutrients to the injury and by removing waste products from the site. This is accomplished by increasing local circulation to the area. The increased circulation also stimulates formation of new tissue. Additionally, heat promotes suppuration (pus formation) and phagocytosis (destruction of bacteria by blood cells) by increasing blood flow to the affected area.

When heat is applied to the skin, vasodilation of the skin's cutaneous arterioles occurs. This superficial increase in blood reduces the blood available for deeper viscera (e.g., abdominal organs). Relief of deep congestion thus occurs. Remember, before using heat to increase blood flow to a part, the nurse must assess whether the patient is able to have a normal vascular response to heat.

Cold

Cold applications relieve pain because nerve impulse conduction decreases with cold temperatures. The intense pain felt during a migraine headache is the result of cerebral arterioles being in spasm; cold reduces this spasm. The pain of a congested body part can be prevented by the application of cold prior to

edema formation. "When cold is applied the cutaneous vessels are squeezed smaller and the fluid in the tissues is reduced, thereby reducing swelling and pain."[12] To apply cold *after* edema is present is counterproductive; at this point the application of heat is appropriate, to increase local circulation and take away the excess interstitial fluid that comprises the edema.

Since cold decreases metabolism of the tissue it can help to prevent gangrene (a form of tissue death). When a patient is burned, cold can decrease the effects of tissue hypoxia (deficiency in oxygen) and thereby decrease toxemia (poison in the blood stream) and delay further necrosis (tissue death) of the tissue.

Cold causes local vasoconstriction and increases blood viscosity in the part of the body touched. These physiologic effects enhance blood coagulation (clotting) and are thus very useful in controlling hemorrhage. However, if circulation to a body part is severely diminished, the continuous application of cold can result in ischemic tissue damage. In an emergency situation, the clinical decision to use cold applications to control hemorrhage is not easily made because of this potential complication. Assessment of the patient's circulatory status and presence of ischemia to the hemorrhaging body part is mandatory.

As pointed out in Table 44–2, the cutaneous application of cold can greatly reduce the underlying tissue temperature. This reduction in tissue temperature makes the environment less favorable for growth of microorganisms within the patient's body.

FACTORS INFLUENCING THE EFFECTS OF HEAT AND COLD APPLICATIONS

The physiologic response of the body to applications of heat or cold is influenced by a variety of factors:

1. The *intensity* of the temperature of a heat or cold application affects the physiologic response.

2. The *prior skin temperature* affects the degree of physiologic response.

3. The *rapidity of the temperature change* determines the degree of receptor organ stimulation (see the description of "thermal receptor adaptation," p. 1146).

To expose the body to extremes in temperature invites tissue damage. For example, an extreme heat stimulus will result in blisters and burns. If a cold stimulus is severe enough, the resulting vasoconstriction might cause anoxic (oxygen deficiency) damage to capillary epithelial cells and increased capillary permeability. Also, dense thrombi (blood clots obstructing blood vessels) may form because of the plasma loss.

4. The *duration* of the application has a direct effect on the response of the body. There is a greater tolerance for extremes of either hot or cold if the exposure is brief.[5] If the duration of exposure is too great, secondary effects (p. 1148) will nullify the therapeutic effect of the application. It goes without saying that no patient should be exposed directly to extremes in temperature as part of a therapeutic procedure.

5. *The environmental temperature* influences the effect of heat or cold applications. If the environment is warm and humid, heat cannot be dissipated through evaporation. When the environmental temperature is greater than or equal to the body temperature, conductive loss is inhibited. Conversely, in a cold dry environment the application of cold will be enhanced since the patient is already losing much heat to the environment.

6. There are *differences in temperature toleration levels* between individuals and within the same individual in different parts of his body. The exposed areas of the body (e.g., parts of the arms and face) have thicker skin and are therefore more tolerant to extremes in temperature. Where the skin is thinner (e.g., eyelids, neck and inner aspect of the forearms), there is less tolerance to heat and cold.

7. Where there has been *traumatic damage to a body surface*, there exists a greater potential for further damage with the application of heat or cold.

8. The amount of *body surface area* involved affects the body's response. The greater the area involved with the application of heat or cold, the less tolerance the patient has to extremes in temperature.[5]

9. If the body surface area affected is large enough, the physiologic effects of local heat or cold can become *generalized systemic responses*. For example, a heat application to an entire leg might result in such extensive local vasodilation of peripheral vessels that the body's blood pressure is lowered. Conversely, a cold application to an entire leg might result in an elevated blood pressure produced by extensive local vasoconstriction. In this instance the widespread application of cold might also cause shivering, which could increase the body's systemic temperature. Heat production within the body may increase to as much as five times normal, thereby negating the therapeutic effects of the cold application. Of course, generalized systemic responses such as shivering and lowered blood pressure are uncomfortable for the patient.

10. The *physiologic condition of the patient* is important to assess. How well will a seriously ill patient, already exposed to many stresses, respond to the further stress of the application? Considering his disease, will the patient have a normal vascular response? In other words, will his blood vessels expand or constrict as expected?

Arteriosclerosis is an excellent example of the differences disease can make in a patient's response to heat and cold. A patient with severe arteriosclerosis (arterial wall thickening) cannot be expected to have a normal vascular response. Because the arterial walls thicken, the small arteries experience a decrease in elasticity and contractility; when heat or cold applications are applied, the arteries do not dilate or constrict adequately. When the arterial walls are markedly thickened, the peripheral blood supply is embarrassed (decreased); if the patient is exposed to a cold application, the blood supply will be decreased further. When this decrease in peripheral blood supply continues over a period of years, the peripheral sensory receptors become less sensitive in detecting dangerous thermal stimuli, so the patient might be unaware that hot applications are causing tissue damage.

Heat or cold applications are rarely prescribed for patients who have severe arteriosclerosis. Patients with a mild or moderate form of the disease may be treated with a modified temperature. When a hot application is ordered, the temperature is reduced; when a cold application is ordered, the temperature used is not as low as that used for a patient without arteriosclerosis.

11. Special considerations must be made for patients with *neurological impairments*, e.g., unconsciousness. The nurse must be in attendance at the patient's bedside during the entire treatment. Unconscious patients sometimes make involuntary movements, and if not observed carefully, they might move too close to the hot or cold appliance. Also, since they cannot report symptoms, the nurse must be totally

responsible for assessing for signs of desired effects and complications.

12. *Impaired perception* may cause a patient to be burned without his realizing it is happening. For example, some patients who have had a cerebral hemorrhage are unable to differentiate the intensity of heat; quadriplegic and paraplegic patients are unable to sense harmful heat stimuli. Precautions utilized for the unconscious patient are essential for these patients also.

13. The very *fatigued patient* will be less sensitive to cutaneous stimulation.

14. *Metabolic disorders* (e.g., diabetes, shock) increase the hazards of tissue damage. Therefore, heat or cold applications must be applied to such patients with caution and frequent assessments are necessary.

15. The *age of the patient* influences the response. At either extreme in age, the very young or very old, there is more danger of tissue damage than in the middle age group. Because the very young and old have thinner skin, they can be burned easier. In the very old person, the sensitivity to pain is decreased; therefore, his "alarm system" is impaired. Infants have limited abilities to adapt to heat and cold because of their immature neurological functioning.

16. *Skin coloring* affects response to heat and cold. Redheads and blonds react more to heat and cold than do brunets, or noncaucasians with deeper skin pigmentation.

Counterirritants. The use of certain drugs to augment the desired effects of heat applications has fallen from popularity in today's nursing practice. Counterirritants (drugs which produce vasodilation in local cutaneous tissues) include mustard, turpentine, capsicum and liniments, e.g., camphor and methyl salicylates. Their actions are twofold: not only do these drugs increase the cutaneous circulation, but in doing this, they also alter the blood supply to deeper organs, thus relieving deep congestion and pain.[7] Of the various types of applications used for their counterirritant effect, the mustard plaster poultice is most commonly used in the home. It is also available commercially. The nurse must teach the patient and family to observe the skin every 5 minutes, to leave the poultice on only 20 minutes, and to recognize the complications of heat applications (p. 1153).

Linseed, bread and milk, and flaxseed poultices are traditional forms of moist heat. Counterirritants and moist heat poultices are seldom used in hospital settings because other, more modern devices produce the same effects more efficiently.

Consensual Response. When the effects of an application of heat or cold are produced in other parts of the body, the response is known as the *consensual response.* Intersegmental or more than one spinal vasomotor reflex is stimulated, resulting in this vascular effect. For example, if a patient receives warm soaks to his right foot, his left foot might also have increased circulation. The patient may notice feelings of congestion or coolness in his left foot. The physiologic reason for this phenomena is that the blood flow to the left foot has increased, but the local metabolism has remained unchanged. Therefore, the vessels dilate in the left foot and relinquish some heat to the environment; the patient feels a cool sensation in his left foot at the same time his right foot feels warm. Likewise, if he receives a cold soak to his right foot, his left foot may feel warm. The patient's sensations resulting from a consensual response usually cannot be assessed objectively by the nurse since the alteration in circulation is not pronounced enough to detect by touch.

Contraindications to the Use of Local Heat

Heat is not used when *malignancies* are present; heat increases the metabolism of both the normal and abnormal cells.

When heat applications involve a large body area the renal, cardiovascular and respiratory status of the patient must be assessed prior to application. The vasodilation of the cutaneous vessels produced by heat might greatly reduce the blood supply to vital internal organs.[2] This reduction may be serious for persons with *impaired kidney, heart, and/or lung function.*

Edema associated with venous or lymphatic disease tends to be aggravated when heat is applied because of the lack of adequate blood outflow. *Diseases or disorders that inhibit the exit of metabolic wastes* contraindicate use of heat applications. For example, arteriosclerosis and atherosclerosis, which are common in diabetic patients, inhibit peripheral blood flow. Patients with these diseases do not have a normal vascular response, so heat should not be used.

Cutaneous injuries such as stomas or scar tissue should be protected when heat is applied. Open wounds require reduced heat. These areas have *limited sensory capabilities* (i.e., impaired "feelings") and limited circulation so damage can occur without the patient's awareness.[2]

Patients who have paralysis (loss of voluntary movement or sensation) or paresthesia (abnormal sensation) may have altered neurological responses when exposed to heat. For example, the degree of vasoconstriction in response to cold or vasodilation in response to heat is not as uniform or as predictable in the paralyzed patient as in the patient with normal vascular response. With either the presence of paralysis or paresthesia, patients may report sensations of numbness or tingling or prickling with exposure to a hot or cold stimulus. Patients' symptoms therefore cannot be relied upon when assessing for tissue damage during a therapeutic application. The altered responses vary depending on the original pathology causing the neurological disorder. If heat is to be used, extreme care must be taken and a lower temperature used.

Heat should not be applied to *acutely inflamed areas* since there may be increased discomfort due to edema formation.

Finally, heat should not be applied to *areas where diffusibility of that heat is limited.* Two examples of contraindicated areas are an abscessed tooth or an inflamed appendix. Heat might cause these areas to rupture, spreading infectious microorganisms into the blood stream and surrounding tissues. Limited heat diffusion is also a problem with embarrassed circulation, e.g., in diabetes, and in neurological conditions such as paraplegia.

Contraindications to the Use of Local Cold

The application of cold is counterproductive after the formation of edema. The decreased blood flow caused by the cold will decrease absorption of the excessive interstitial fluid. Cold may be applied initially to a burn area both to reduce the pain and to decrease the effects of hypoxia and subsequent toxemia. However, the use of cold continued intermittently beyond 24 hours after a burn or a sprain injury retards the healing process. At this time, therapy is focused on the reabsorption of the excessive interstitial fluid, and cold inhibits this process.

With diseases or disorders which have resulted in *impaired circulation,* cold is contraindicated. The tissues already have a diminished nutrient supply and the application of cold would only further accentuate the problem by inducing vasoconstriction of those vessels. Impaired circulation should be anticipated in patients with peripheral vascular disease, arteriosclerosis, diabetes, neurological conditions and edema.

Nursing Judgment

Applications of heat or cold must be very carefully used when the patient is unconscious, anesthetized or otherwise unable to respond to pain stimuli that indicate tissue is being damaged.

The basis for sound nursing judgments concerning heat and cold applications lies in the nurse addressing herself to several questions: Is the patient sensitive to cutaneous stimulation, and if he is, can he *communicate* with me? Does the patient's condition negate a normal physiologic response? If so, is heat or cold application contraindicated? These questions should be answered to your complete satisfaction before administration of heat or cold therapies. You are legally responsible for your own nursing interventions!

PATIENT AND FAMILY EDUCATION

Applications of heat and cold are frequently made at home by lay persons attempting to treat various disorders. Often these persons do not have the knowledge necessary to correctly apply such treatments. At times, patients incorrectly self-prescribe the application of heat or cold. In other instances the treatment is prescribed by a health professional, who fails, however, to adequately explain the correct procedure. Not only can such neglect of patient-family education negate the benefits of the treatment, but it can also jeopardize the patient's well-being. If the appropriate scientific principles are not understood, errors can occur that make the heat and cold applications counterproductive and possibly unsafe. For example, cold may be detrimentally applied to a sprain or contusion after swelling is already present. Or, hot water bottles and heating pads may be applied at dangerously high temperatures for excessive periods of time. The faulty reasoning behind such actions might be "if warm is good, then hot is better" or "if thirty minutes of heat helps, then several hours should help even more."

Such misconceptions may bring patients into conflict with health professionals who are making therapeutic applications of heat or cold. For example, patients may comment that heat applications are not hot enough ("I can stand it hotter") or that the treatments are not long enough ("You can leave this on all day"). Careful explanations of the procedures used in the hospital can help ensure that the patient and family will use correct practices at home.

Comprehensive patient-family education in the application of heat and cold would include the purposes of these treatments, the correct techniques of application, and the warning signs of complications. The patient must know what is relevant to his own disease or disorder: the situations in which heat or cold should not be applied; why wounds, scar tissue, and stomas are especially susceptible to tissue injury; and, for the aged or the family caring for an infant, an explanation of why the very young and aged are more prone to complications. Also the patient should understand the adaptation of thermal receptors, the need for recovery time, and safety considerations, e.g., not lying on or leaning against a heat source and the dangers of safety pins and wetness around electrical heating appliances.

ASSESSMENT OF COMPLICATIONS

Any mention of discomfort or *pain* made by a patient receiving a heat or cold application should be investigated immediately. A cutaneous assessment would include assessing the appearance for the *quality of circulation* and *integrity* of the involved skin.

Maceration (waterlogged skin, which gives a wrinkled effect) can occur with moist hot or cold applications. Since minute fissures of the skin occur with maceration, therapy must be discontinued until the skin returns to normal.

Complications from heat therapy would include redness or *blotchy redness* of the skin with or without the presence of actual *blisters*. *Notable pallor* of the area could indicate vasoconstriction. These reactions demonstrate the body's defenses against tissue damage (see "secondary effects," p. 1148). The appearance of any of these signs requires the immediate removal of the heat application.

Pain occurring during a cold application is caused by *ischemia*. This lack of blood supply produces a very pale, mottled (uneven distribution of circulating blood), or bluish appearance, followed by redness of the skin. This is the result of vasodilation of the ischemic area in an attempt to warm the area with an increased blood supply—another example of the body's defense mechanisms against damage. Cold can produce burns with blisters. All of these complications are indications for the immediate removal of a cold application.

TABLE 44–4. COMPLICATIONS OF HEAT OR COLD APPLICATIONS

HEAT	COLD
1. Pain	1. Pain
2. Burns	2. Blisters and skin breakdown
3. Edema	
4. Vasoconstriction (pallor or mottled redness)	3. Ischemia, mottling (gray or bluish discoloration)
5. Maceration (with moist heat)	4. Vasodilation (redness)
	5. Thrombi
6. Redness which does not blanch with pressure	6. Maceration (with moist cold)

Less common, but nonetheless dangerous, complications of heat or cold applications include the formation of edema with heat and thrombi (blood clots) with cold. One theory of edema formation with heat states that unequal local cutaneous vasodilation of the vessels causes local arterial inflow to be increased more than the venous outflow.[19] Therefore, edema forms owing to an accumulation of fluid in the tissues, increased hydrostatic pressure, and increased capillary permeability. Thrombi also result from a shift in fluid volume. When the vasoconstriction is great enough to cause anoxic damage to the capillary endothelial cells, the capillary permeability will increase. Then, owing to plasma loss and hemoconcentration ("thickening of blood"), thrombi may form.

A summary of the complications of heat and cold applications is presented in Table 44–4.

PHYSICIAN'S ORDERS

The patient's physician initiates the treatment of either hot or cold applications by prescribing the treatment in the physician's orders (usually found in the patient's chart). Essential components of the physician's orders the nurse *always* checks *before* proceeding with a treatment are:

▶ Type of application

▶ Specific body part to be treated

▶ Duration of application

▶ Frequency of application

MEASURES TO PREVENT COMPLICATIONS

Patient Assessment

Comprehensive assessment of the patient receiving heat or cold applications is the ongoing responsibility of the nurse. She is accountable for the complications that develop since she is the one who administers the treatment. Proper assessments must be made before, during and after treatments. Table 44–5 summarizes the patient conditions to assess *before* the treatment. *During* and *after* the treatments the development of any of the complications in Table 44–4 (p. 1153) must be assessed.

Prior to the application of the heat or cold, a good way to assess the patient's level of sensation is to have him close his eyes, then place your fingers over the skin area where the application will be made and ask the patient if he can feel your fingers. Next, lightly trace a letter or number on the patient's skin with one finger and ask the patient what letter or number he feels. Of course, this can only be done with a patient capable of recognizing the alphabet and numbers and able to communicate.

The treatment should be terminated in the event of any medical emergency, for example, a seizure, a heart attack, or unconsciousness. Be sure to remove the source of heat or cold immediately so that it is not overlooked as you deal with the emergency.

Remember, if any of the signs or symptoms of complications occur *during* the application of heat or cold, discontinue the application immediately and report to the appropriate individual. Frequently the occurrence of these complications may be seen immediately *after* the application is completed. If this should occur, report the signs and symptoms to the appropriate individual and carry out any prescribed delegated medical care. Whenever complications occur, ongoing assessment of the affected area is essential.

The "normal" and desired appearance of the skin from the application of heat is an evenly distributed redness. The "normal" and desired appearance of the skin from cold is evenly distributed paleness, followed by a pink blush. Deviations from this appearance must be assessed and reported. Use Table 44–3 to complete assessment for therapeutic effect.

Equipment Assessment

Checking that the equipment functions properly is the responsibility of the nurse. To evaluate each appliance used in heat and cold applications, the nurse must become familiar with many pieces of equipment. If the appliance to be used is unfamiliar to the nurse, she must contact Central Supply and request literature on the equipment *before* she begins the procedure. In the following section the most frequently used appliances for the application of heat and cold are presented. The reader must know how this equipment *should* operate so she can readily recognize when it is malfunctioning.

A general inspection of electrical equipment includes looking for frayed wires and damaged insulation. The electrical appliance should be plugged in and turned on in the clean utility area to determine whether it is functioning before it is taken to the patient's bedside. Assess the appliance for *evenness* of either heat or cold temperature distribution. Uneven temperature distribution indicates malfunctioning. Assess the degree of heat or cold temperatures by exposing the inner aspect of your forearm to the appliance, even with those appliances that include a temperature gauge. Do not assume the temperature gauge reading is always correct.

Commercially prepared chemical compounds that are used for applications of heat or cold come with the manufacturer's instructions attached to the appliance. Follow the directions explicitly and assess for evenness and degree of temperature from the appliance by ex-

TABLE 44–5.   ASSESSMENTS TO MAKE BEFORE HEAT AND COLD APPLICATIONS

CONTRAINDICATIONS

Patient Conditions	Skin Anomalies
Lack of sensation	Scar tissue
Edema (cold contra-indicated)	Stomas

CONDITIONS THAT REQUIRE EXTREME CAUTION IN APPLYING HEAT OR COLD

Peripheral vascular disease
Confusion or unconsciousness
Congestive heart failure
Impaired kidney or lung function
Large area to be treated
Long period of treatment
Very young or elderly
Cold environment during cold therapy
Hot, humid environment during heat therapy
Light skin coloring
Inflamed tissue
Open wounds

posing the inner aspect of your own forearm to the appliance before administering the application to the patient.

Regardless of what equipment is being used for the application of heat or cold, the nurse must carefully examine each appliance for damage to the equipment itself or malfunction.

Safety in Procedures

The safe nurse never begins either a hot or a cold application before she knows what she is supposed to do and how she will proceed with the treatment. She never uses equipment unless she understands its operation. Also, before she exposes the patient to heat or cold, the safe nurse tells him what he can expect to feel during the treatment and urges him to inform her immediately if he experiences a different sensation or any discomfort. Of course, the nurse also supervises the application closely.

With either hot or cold applications, there must be allowance for the recovery time. Continuous applications are detrimental to the health of the tissue (see the discussion of secondary effects, p. 1148). Having the patient, if he is able, watch the clock and/or using an automatic timer can help the busy nurse time the applications accurately.

The safe nurse exposes the patient only to safe temperatures. Different references advise various temperatures. A health agency's procedure manual provides the allowable maximum temperature to be used in that agency. In our discussion of specific procedures below, the most commonly used temperatures are included. All the items discussed under factors influencing the effect of heat and cold applications must be considered when determining safe temperatures for the individual patient's treatments.

The safe nurse does not allow the patient to adjust the temperature control of appliances such as heating pads. Because of thermal receptor adaptation, a heating pad might not feel hot enough to the patient. If he adjusts the controls to a higher temperature, real danger of tissue damage exists.

Always make sure the patient is in a position to remove the application or move himself away from a device if it is causing him discomfort. The patient must have the call button accessible at all times. Special consideration must be given to the safety of those patients who cannot move away from the noxious stimuli or those who are insensitive to cutaneous stimulation and cannot feel themselves being injured. In these cases the nurse stays with the patient during the entire procedure and conducts a continuous assessment of how the patient is tolerating the treatment.

The patient should not lie on a heat appliance. The pressure this creates reduces the air spaces between the patient and the heat application, increasing the likelihood of burns.[8]

Because water is a good conductor of heat, when hot wet packs (cloths used in application of heat or cold) are applied they should be free of excess water and as dry as possible. A thin coat of petroleum jelly or oil should be applied to the skin prior to the application of hot wet packs. This protective layer reduces soaking of the skin and, therefore, maceration.

Do not use electrical appliances close to open oxygen. The smallest spark from frayed wires or exposed wires from worn insulation covers could cause an explosion and fire. Inspect the condition of all appliances used for the application of heat or cold. Badly maintained equipment with signs of deterioration should never be used. Do not use electrical appliances near water or other fluids, or handle with wet hands. Water is a good conductor of electricity and a short circuit may occur, giving you or your patient a shock. Do not use pins to hold an electrical appliance in place. Metal is also a good conductor, and a short circuit may occur.

The practice of placing bedclothes over a heat lamp and the exposed part of the patient, to provide privacy, is ill-advised; this is a tremendous fire hazard and increases the intensity of heat. Privacy for the patient during treatments can be provided in other ways.

CHARTING

Essential components of the patient charting required after each treatment of heat or cold include:

▶ Type of application the patient received

▶ Temperature if appropriate

▶ Specific body part where the treatment was applied

▶ Duration of the treatment, recorded in minutes

▶ Appearance of the patient's skin prior to, during and after the hot or cold application

▶ Patient's subjective reaction to the application

▶ Any complications resulting from the application; whether the presence of any complication necessitated the termination of the application

▶ The effectiveness of the application in terms of the reason for which it was ordered (i.e., is the patient experiencing less pain? Is the edema diminished?)

LEGAL LIABILITY

If tissue injury results from the *incorrect* application of either heat or cold, the nurse who applied that treatment is legally responsible. The doctor who wrote the order or the team leader who directed the nurse to do the treatment is not legally at fault. The nurse must be totally familiar with the procedure and the patient who is to receive the treatment. Malpractice insurance has become a necessity for today's nurses. However, this personal protection does not negate the importance of knowing what you are doing and to whom.

Applications of either heat or cold can be either wet or dry. Examples of *moist* heat include moist hot compresses (gauze dressings) or packs, sitz (hip) bath, hot soaks (immersion of a body part into a solution). Examples of *dry* heat include hot-water bottles, electrical heating pads, chemical heating pads, and heating lamps. Examples of *moist* cold are compresses and soaks. Examples of *dry* cold are ice bags and the Aqua K Pad. Table 44–6 compares the effects of wet and dry applications, using heat as the example.

The terms "hot" and "cold" are relative. The flow of heat is from a hotter area to a less hot area. When heat is to be applied, the source needs to be hotter than the skin surface it will be in contact with. The heat from the hot application will flow toward the skin. When cold is to be applied, the source needs to be colder than the skin surface it is coming in contact with. In this case, the heat from the body surface will flow toward the cold appliance; the body surface gives up heat and is thereby cooled.

Before implementing any therapeutic application of heat or cold, check the patient's chart to ensure that the treatment is not contraindicated by the patient's condition. While review-

TABLE 44–6.   ADVANTAGES AND DISADVANTAGES OF WET AND DRY LOCAL APPLICATIONS (USING HEAT)

ADVANTAGES	DISADVANTAGES
Wet Applications	
1. Wet heat penetrates more deeply than dry heat.	1. Moisture has greater potential for causing skin maceration when exposure is prolonged.
2. Wet heat does not dry skin as much as dry heat.	2. Moist heat applications cool off more rapidly than dry heat, due to evaporation of the moisture from the application.
3. Wet applications cause less loss of body fluid through sweating than dry heat.	3. There is increased potential for burns since moisture is a good conductor of heat.
4. Wet applications conform to body area better.	4. Moist heat is not tolerated as well as dry heat, since the moisture from the application retards evaporation from the skin.
5. Subjective experience of the patient is more favorable.	
Dry Applications	
1. Dry heat is tolerated better than moist heat, since evaporation can occur from the exposed heated skin.	1. Dry applications do not penetrate as deeply as moist applications.
2. Decreased potential for burns since moisture, which is a good conductor of heat, is not involved.	2. Dry applications dry out skin more than moist heat.
3. Dry applications sustain their temperature longer since evaporation of moisture from wet applications does not occur with dry applications.	3. Dry applications cause more body fluid loss due to evaporation of moisture from heated skin area.
4. Decreased occurrence of skin maceration since moisture is not involved in dry applications.	

ing the chart for this information, also check the physician's orders prescribing the application.

Before approaching the patient's bedside, know exactly what you are going to do and how you are going to do it. Confusion and uncertainty at the bedside are very disconcerting to the patient. Of course, wash your hands before handling equipment to be used at the bedside and before coming into direct contact with the patient.

At the bedside, identify the patient by checking his wrist name band and by asking him to say his name. Assess the patient's ability to determine cutaneous sensations and to move away from noxious stimuli. Also assess the condition of the skin which is to receive the application, basing the assessment on the criteria presented in Table 44–5. If there is any evidence of skin injury to the area, seek further clarification from the doctor to determine whether the doctor was aware of the injury and whether he feels the application of heat or cold is contraindicated. If the doctor decides to not discontinue the order even in the presence of skin damage discuss this with the team leader or instructor and then decide whether or not it is safe to apply the heat or cold to the area. If you determine it would not be safe, *do not administer the application.*

Inform the patient of the purpose of the treatment, the duration of the treatment and the sensations typically felt during the treatment. Emphasize appropriate safety factors and encourage the patient to immediately report any discomfort during the procedure.

Maintain the patient's comfort throughout the treatment by keeping his proper body alignment. Provide privacy for the patient by supplying adequate draping and by closing doors or pulling bedside curtains. The immediate environment may need to be modified so that anything the patient might need during the treatment is within easy access and so that drafts are eliminated.

Applications of Dry Heat

In applying dry heat the following principles are important:

▶ Avoid cross infection

▶ Maintain correct temperature for duration of application

▶ Assess the patient prior to, during and after the application

Assessment is made according to the principles previously described (see p. 1154 and Tables 44–4 and 44–5). Charting is done as discussed on p. 1155. Additional charting is listed for each type of application, as needed.

HOT-WATER BOTTLE

Appliances for the application of local heat are used most commonly to increase circulation to a body part and therby enhance suppuration; to relieve edema, ischemia, and muscle spasm; and to warm cold feet.

The use of hot-water bottles has been outlawed in some health care agencies. Burns due to water that is too hot are common.

To assess for leaks in the hot-water bottle before bringing it to the patient, fill the hot-water bottle with hot tap water. Completely secure the stopper, and turn the hot-water bottle upside down. No leakage of the hot tap water should be observed. Remove the stopper and empty the hot tap water from the hot-water bottle.

Then pour warm tap water into a water pitcher. Measure the temperature of this water with a utility thermometer. For children over 2 years old and adults, a safe temperature would be 46 to 52°C. (115–125°F.). A safe temperature for infants under 2 years and elderly persons would be 40.5–46°C. (105–115°F.). While the thermometer is equilibrating, again fill the empty hot-water bottle with hot tap water, to warm the inside rubber of the hot-water bottle. When this hot water is emptied out and water of the correct temperature is added (from the water pitcher), very little heat is lost to warming the rubber and the patient receives the full benefit of the heat application. Before pouring the correct temperature water into the hot-water bottle, fold the hot-water bottle in half, so that the bottle cannot be filled more than one half to two thirds. If the bottle were completely full, it would be too heavy and it would not be flexible enough to mold comfortably to the body to provide even heat. After you have poured the proper temperature water into the hot-water bottle, twist or squeeze the top of the bottle until the water level becomes even with the top of the opening. By doing this you remove all the air inside the hot-water bottle. Air in the bottle prevents it from molding to the body surface and interferes with the transfer of heat to the skin. Turn the screw-top stopper until it is tight or secure the top as appropriate. If you are working with a bottle that has a fold-over seal, note that the various flaps have a number on them; fold in numerical order, then fasten to the pegs provided. Wipe the bottle dry. Place the hot-water bottle in a flannel or disposable cover.

Remember, the thicker the cover used, the more heat the cover will absorb. The cover is used to absorb any moisture, such as the patient's perspiration. Since water is a good conductor of heat, any moisture allowed to accumulate between the hot-water bottle and the patient's skin increases the risk of burns. The bedcovers may be put over the applied hot-water bottle to insulate the heat in the appliance. The hot-water bottle is left on the patient from 20 minutes to 30 minutes. Beyond 45 minutes, the likelihood of secondary effects occurring increases dramatically. When the treatment has been completed, the patient should be dried off if his skin is moist. The cover is discarded in the laundry or trash (if disposable). The bottle is emptied and cleaned with a disinfectant. The sides of the bottle are pulled apart so they do not stick together during drying. In some institutions the bottle is returned to Central Supply for processing.

Be sure to include the temperature of the hot water in the charting.

CHEMICAL HEATING BOTTLES, BAGS, AND PACKS

The purposes of chemical heating devices are the same as those of hot-water bottles. The chemical heating bottles or bags are sealed plastic containers of various sizes containing two different kinds of chemical compounds. This kind of appliance is designed to be used once and discarded, thus greatly diminishing the incidence of cross infection.

Several commercial companies produce these appliances. Although the techniques used to generate heat in the various bottles differ, the principle remains the same. Within each bottle are two compounds, contained in separate compartments. When the heat treatment is to be given, the nurse kneads, strikes or squeezes the bottle vigorously. Because of this action the two compounds mix and produce heat. The actions to be done by the nurse to "activate" the bottle are given in the directions for use on the specific product.

There is no opening to insert a utility thermometer since the plastic container is completely sealed. The temperature must be assessed by the nurse by putting the bottle against the inner aspect of her forearm. The

nurse should experience a sensation of warmth from the appliance, *not* intolerable heat. These bottles are designed to maintain a constant temperature between 40.5 and 46°C. (105 and 115°F.) from 20 to 60 minutes. The duration of the treatment is usually 20 minutes.

> *Do not use pins to secure chemical heating appliances. Leakage of the chemical compound would be injury-producing.*

INFRARED AND ULTRAVIOLET LAMPS

Infrared lamps transmit infrared rays (invisible heat rays beyond the red end of the spectrum). The energy from the transmitted rays is transformed into heat in the superficial layers of the skin. Long-wave infrared rays are emitted from such heat sources as hot-water bottles and electrical heating pads. Short-wave infrared rays are emitted from all incandescent sources, i.e., incandescent lamps.

Ultraviolet lamps transmit ultraviolet rays (beyond the visible spectrum at the violet end). Ultraviolet rays are emitted by very hot bodies and ionized gases.

The use of infrared lamps is usually confined to the physical therapist. The main purpose for the application of infrared lamps is to increase the circulation to a body part and thereby relieve ischemic pain and relax muscle spasms.

Ultraviolet lamps are also confined to the physical therapy department. The main purposes for the application of ultraviolet lamps are pigmentation of the skin, production of vitamin D, and bactericidal effects.

The radiation heat produced by infrared and ultraviolet lamps is more intense than the heat given off from the gooseneck lamp commonly used by the nurse. The physical therapist allows the lamps to warm up (usually for 5 to 10 minutes) before the patient is exposed to the lamp so that the patient receives the full benefit. The patient and therapist must wear protective goggles during the treatment to shut out reflected harmful rays.[3]

The distance an infrared or ultraviolet lamp is placed from the body part being exposed depends on the wattage of the heating element, the skin pigmentation and how well the heat is tolerated. The duration of the treatment is usually 20 to 30 minutes. Careful observation and assessment are essential.

GOOSENECK LAMP

As mentioned earlier, this type of radiation heat source may be used by a nurse at the bed-

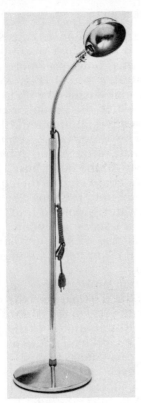

Figure 44-2. Gooseneck lamp. (Courtesy American Hospital Supplies.)

side. The uses of a gooseneck lamp are similar to the uses of an infrared lamp, but the heat from the gooseneck lamp is not as intense as that from the infrared lamp. The flexible-necked lamp is allowed to warm up before the patient is exposed for the treatment. The distance between the exposed body part and the lamp depends on the wattage of the light bulb, the patient's skin pigmentation, and his tolerance of the heat (Fig. 44-2). These are the recommended distances, between the lamp and the body area, with the assumption that there is no cover on the light:[2]

25 watt bulb	....	14 inches
40 watt bulb	....	18 inches
60 watt bulb	....	24–30 inches

During the lamp treatment, scar tissue and stomas should be covered because the lack of sensation in these areas may lead to burning. The practice of putting the bedcovers over the heat lamp and over the body area being treated (to form a "tent") is dangerous. Privacy is important and should be provided, but bedcovers over the lamp are a fire hazard and heat is increased. Drawing the patient's curtains and covering all of the body except for the body part being treated will decrease the sensation of chilling that occurs as the patient's perspiration evaporates from the exposed part. The duration

of this treatment is 20 to 30 minutes, unless complications develop.

In charting, record wattage of the bulb and distance from the skin.

HEAT CRADLE (BAKER)

A heat cradle is made of metal, usually shaped in a half circle or a hutch. Inside the cradle is a light source and a thermometer or thermostat. The purposes for using a heat cradle are similar to the uses of the gooseneck lamp, i.e., improvement of circulation and the promotion of healing. However, the heat cradle is preferred when a large body part is to be treated, e.g., to dry large plaster body casts. It is also used when the patient's condition does not allow covering the skin with gown or sheets, e.g., burns.

A sheet is used to cover the cradle to prevent drafts. The distance between heat source and body part cannot be as easily manipulated with a heat cradle as with a gooseneck lamp, so one or more 25 watt bulbs are used. Lights can be unscrewed to lower temperature, and blankets can be added over the cradle to maintain heat at desired levels. The sheet must not come into contact with the light bulbs. As with all heat source treatments, frequent assessment of the patient's safety and condition is essential.

The duration of a heat cradle treatment is 20 to 30 minutes after the unit has warmed up or it may be used continuously. The low temperature produced by a heat cradle makes continuous use safe.

Care must be taken to store the heat cradle unit safely after a treatment is completed. Because of its size, it is a hazard in small patient units and can easily be bumped into or tripped over. It should be placed out of the way but not on the floor (unless protected from contamination). If the cradle is to be used again by the same patient, it should remain in his unit.

ELECTRIC HEATING PADS

Electric heating pads are composed of an electric coil inside a waterproof rubber covering. The appliance is plugged into an electric socket, and the heat control switch is turned to the desired temperature. Usually the heat control switch consists of three settings: high, medium, and low. As a precautionary measure some hospitals remove the "high" setting on the heat control, thereby preventing the controls from being set at a dangerous temperature, in-

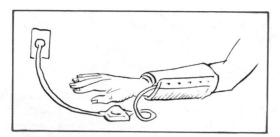

Figure 44–3. Electric heating pad. (From Wood, L. A., and Rambo, B. J.: *Nursing Skills for Allied Health Services, Vol. 2*, 2nd ed. Philadelphia, W. B. Saunders Co., 1977, p. 580.)

advertently or consciously. The "medium" setting provides a temperature of 46 to 52°C. (115 to 126°F.). Electric heating pads come in a variety of sizes; the pad chosen should completely cover the area being treated.

As previously emphasized, all heat appliances must be assessed as to their general condition and operating performance prior to use on a patient. This is especially true for electric heating pads. Short circuiting, electric shock of the patient or the nurse, or fire can result if wires or plug are faulty. The electric coil must be contained in the waterproof cover, for if wetness from the treatment, such as perspiration, or wet hands come in contact with the "live" wires, a short circuit results.

> Never use pins to secure the electric pad! *The metal in pins easily conducts electricity, and a dangerous short circuit will occur.*

An electric heating pad should be covered with a flannel cloth to absorb the patient's perspiration and insulate the pad. No wet dressings should be applied when an electric heating pad is being used. Also, do not apply a heating pad with pressure since the pressure reduces the number of air spaces between the patient and the appliance, increasing the chance for burns (Fig. 44–3).

Instruct the patient not to lie on or lean against the heating pad because the weight of his body compresses the tissue between the heating pad and the body. When the vessels in the tissues become compressed, heat accumulates because the vessels are unable to carry off the excess heat. Burning is thus possible.

In charting, include the heat setting of the heating pad.

An Aqua K pad or module consists of a waterproof pad connected by two rubber hoses to a control unit that houses a small motor and an electric heating element (Fig. 44–4). The inside of the pad is designed with hollow parallel channels in which the heated or cold (depending on the desired application) distilled water circulates. The water passes from the control unit to the pad through one rubber hose and returns by way of the other hose. The two rubber hoses are connected to the control unit by being screwed onto the unit.

Distilled water is poured into the top of the control unit at a screw cap opening. Tap water is not used in the control unit since it would leave mineral deposits in the unit and lead to costly repairs.

The control unit houses a small, low-powered motor. The pad and the rubber hoses that connect the pad to the control unit must be kept level with the motor. If the pad is above the motor, the workload of the motor is greatly increased because it has to push the water *up* to the pad, against the force of gravity. For the best performance, it is suggested that the motor should even be placed *above* the level of the hose and pad.

The rubber hoses must be kept free of kinks. After filling the control unit with distilled water (two thirds full), tilt the unit from side to side with tubing and pad below motor unit to allow any air bubbles to escape. If this is not done, an

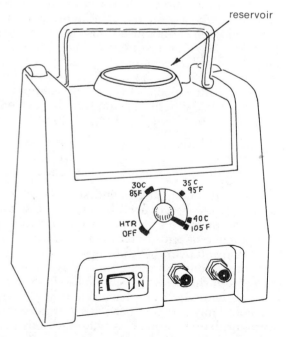

Figure 44–4. Control unit for Aqua K Pad. (From Wood, L. A., and Rambo, B. J.: *Nursing Skills for Allied Health Services, Vol. 2*, 2nd ed., p. 579.)

air lock may develop and stress on the motor will increase as it attempts to propel water past the air lock.

The temperature regulating gauge is located on the control unit. The temperature setting is adjusted by inserting a plastic key (that the manufacturer provides) into the temperature regulator and turning clockwise to increase the temperature of the distilled water or counterclockwise to decrease the temperature. The key can be removed, so once the desired temperature is selected the temperature cannot be altered to nontherapeutic levels. The temperature range can be set between no heat and 40.5°C. (105°F.). The health agency policy may provide limits of heat and may even preset the temperature in Central Supply.

Since the Aqua K pad is an electric device, follow the safety rules that apply to all electric appliances, e.g., check for frayed ends; do not plug in the cord when your hands are wet; position the cord so that it will not be tripped over. After plugging in the unit, allow several minutes for the water to reach the desired temperature. The temperature regulating gauge displays the actual temperature of the distilled water in the control unit through a viewing window located on the gauge.

Aqua K pads come in various sizes; select one to cover just the body area being treated.

> *Do not use pins to secure Aqua K pads/ modules. A puncture of the pad or tubing can cause leakage, which requires repair of pad.*

The pad can be secured with roller gauze, tape or adhesive tape. The pad should be covered with flannel to absorb perspiration.

Because Aqua K units provide constant heat or cold and are so convenient to use, the nurse

must be especially careful to stop treatments at the proper time and to allow adequate recovery time (see p. 1148).

DIATHERMY

Short wave or microwave diathermy [a method of heating that converts electrical or vibrational energy into thermal energy (heat)] is a treatment carried out by physical therapists to provide deep heat within the tissues of the body (Fig. 44–5).

In preparing a patient for diathermy treatment the nurse must remove metal from him; this would include watch, rings and a hearing aid. The electrical or vibrational forms of energy from diathermy must not be directed at any metal within or on the patient's body, e.g., metal pins or prosthesis. Metal exposed to diathermy attains tremendously high temperature levels that *will burn the patient and may even be lethal.* A patient who has a cardiac pacemaker, either implanted or external, must not receive diathermy because it will interfere with the functioning of the pacemaker.

Applications of Moist Heat

WARM SOAKS

Warm soaks are used most commonly to increase circulation to the body part and thereby enhance suppuration and relieve edema, ischemia and muscle spasms. Another specific reason for using warm soaks is to facilitate débridement of a wound.

It may be helpful to have a plastic or rubber sheet underneath the basin to protect bed linen from spillage.

The body part to receive the moist heat application is submerged in a basin of warm water 40.5 to 43°C. (105 to 110°F.).

If medication is to be added to the warm water, make sure it is evenly distributed throughout the water by gently stirring the solution with a spatula. The duration of the treatment is usually 20 minutes. To maintain the desired temperature of the soak the limb and vessel are covered with a bath blanket. If necessary, water is removed and warmer water added after ten minutes. Have the patient remove his limb momentarily from the soak while the cooled water is removed and warmer water [40.5 to 43°C. (105 to 110°F.)] is added. Before

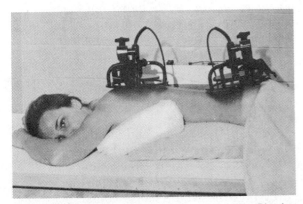

Figure 44–5. Diathermy. (From Downer, A. H.: *Physical Therapy Procedures,* 2nd ed. Springfield, Illinois, Charles C Thomas Co., 1974, p. 53.)

the patient resubmerges his limb, stir the water in the basin with a spatula to guarantee even distribution of temperature.

If the water in the basin has had medication added to it, *do not* remove some of the cooled solution and replace with warmer water as this would dilute the solution and decrease its therapeutic action. In this case, the original solution is kept in the basin for the full 20 minutes of the treatment.

Prevent patient fatigue during the treatment by positioning the patient so good body alignment is maintained; support limbs by placing small pillows under them as needed.

Dry the body surface thoroughly at the end of the treatment to enhance comfort and prevent skin breakdown from the moisture.

COMPRESSES

Compresses are dressings used in applications of either heat or cold. Hot compresses may be either sterile or nonsterile.

Sterile compresses are applied to surgical incisions, to eyes or any area where the body's defensive protection is not intact. The presence of a skin incision is evidence of penetration of the skin's protective barrier, therefore the patient's defense against pathogens is compromised. Nonsterile compresses, on the other hand, are used when the skin is intact and the area is not vulnerable. Less expensive material such as towels, sheeting or flannel is used for nonsterile compresses. Nonsterile hot wet compresses have been submerged in either water or a solution at a temperature of 55°C. (131°F.). Before the compresses are applied they are wrung out so that excess solution does not drip from the compress. If too hot, lift momentarily from the skin and reapply.

Procedure 34 details the application of sterile moist hot compresses using a bedside sterilizer. Procedure 33 in Chapter 42 presented the technique of applying a *wet sterile dressing*. A hot-water bottle can be used to provide heat. In some settings the premoistened sterile dressings are heated under an ultraviolet light in the medication room, treatment room or patient's room, then taken to the patient's bedside for application. With this method, moist 4×4 gauze dressings are packaged in a sterile foil wrap (premoistened) and placed under the ultraviolet light and left there for 10 minutes. Since the procedure is sterile the nurse opens the packages, puts on sterile gloves or uses sterile forceps to take the sterile gauze out of the package and places the dressing on the patient.

34. APPLYING STERILE MOIST HOT COMPRESSES USING BEDSIDE STERILIZER

Definition and Purpose.   *One method for applying sterile moist hot compresses by the nurse.* Used to promote healing, relieve pain, promote drainage. Sterile compresses are used for areas vulnerable to infection, e.g., open wounds or boils that are expected to open.

Contraindications and Cautions.   See Table 44–5. The application should cover an area no larger than necessary, to avoid increasing congestion.

Patient and Family Teaching Points.   Provide the patient and family with the following information as appropriate: (a) explain the procedure to the patient; (b) explain the purpose of the application; (c) explain the safety precautions the nurse has taken to minimize the chance of burns; (d) instruct the patient not to touch the sterilizer (he might get burned) or the dressings (he would cause contamination); (e) describe to the patient what he should feel from the application and instruct him to report any divergence from that sensation immediately to you; (f) explain that adaptation of the thermal receptors leads to the hot moist compress not feeling "hot enough" several minutes after it is applied. Assure the patient that compresses will be changed every few minutes to provide desired heat.

PRE-PROCEDURE ACTIVITIES

PRELIMINARY ASSESSMENT

Includes determination of:
- type of application to be used
- body part to receive treatment
- duration of treatment
- frequency of treatment
- presence of disorders that contraindicate use of heat (clarify with physician if contraindications are present)

PREPARATION OF PATIENT

- Identify patient by name and name bracelet
- Provide privacy, e.g., draw curtains
- Expose body part to receive heat application
- Provide warmth; cover all nontreatment areas with flannel blanket or bed covers
- Place waterproof sheet covered with a sheet under body part to be treated
- Have patient in good body alignment and comfortable, e.g., support limbs as needed

EQUIPMENT

- Sterile cotton swabs
- Sterile petrolatum (petroleum jelly)
- Sterile 4 × 4 gauze dressings or sterile 4 × 8 gauze dressings (number and size depend on size of area to be treated)
- Waterproof sheet
- Flannel bath blanket
- Sterile waterproof dressing
- Dressing sterilizer
- Two sterile transfer forceps
- Tie tapes or binder with pins
- Dry clean towel
- Sterile treatment (or candy) thermometer
- Waterproof bag for disposal of dressings

PREPARATION OF COMPRESSES

- Gather equipment
- Wash hands thoroughly
- Explain procedure to patient
- Wet dressings with tap water and wring out excess water so there is no water dripping from dressings
- Fluff up three dressings and put them in a fourth, which is opened up
- Put all four dressings into bedside sterilizer
- Place lid on sterilizer
- Set sterilizer at 135°C. (275°F.) for 15 minutes

PROCEDURE

SUGGESTED STEPS

1. Use sterile applicators to spread light coat of sterile petrolatum over skin surface to be treated.

2. If wound present, do *not* put petrolatum directly on wound but around area. Do not use petrolatum for eye compresses.

RATIONALE/DISCUSSION

1. Petrolatum slows down penetration of moist heat and lessens chance of burns.

2. Petrolatum may delay wound healing.

Procedure continued on the following page

SUGGESTED STEPS	RATIONALE/DISCUSSION
3. Remove the lid from the sterilizer. Remove one sterile dressing from the sterilizer by grasping the dressing with sterile transfer forceps. Hold dressing above your waist and within your sight. Replace the lid on sterilizer to keep remaining dressings hot.	3. The hand should not go over the dressing; avoid contamination.
4. Use transfer forceps to wring excess water from dressing.	4. Presence of water increases occurrence of burns.
5. Allow steam to escape from the dressing while transferring dressing from sterilizer to patient.	5. Presence of steam increases temperatures of dressing and occurrence of burns.
6. Place dressing in sterile bowl. Holding the nonregistering end of the sterile thermometer, place the registering end of the thermometer directly onto the sterile moist compress. Allow time for dressings to cool to a safe temperature. An application temperature of 55°C. (131°F.) [43°C. (110°F.) for eye compresses] is recommended unless patient is under 2 years old, is elderly, or has a vascular disorder. Then compress temperature should be 40.5°C. (105°F.).	6. Measure temperature to avoid burns. Extremes in age and certain patient conditions increase likelihood of complications from heat application.
7. Work quickly.	7. Dressings quickly lose their heat in environmental air.
8. Apply first dressing lightly and cover with other layers of 4 × 4's snugly. After a few seconds, lift dressing at edges with forceps and observe skin for signs of complications, e.g., pallor, extreme redness, red blotches, blisters, puffiness or maceration. Also, ask patient if he is experiencing pain or discomfort.	8. Initial and ongoing assessment is mandatory for prevention of complications. If dressings are not placed snugly, presence of air within and under dressings reduces heat conduction, making treatment less effective.

> *If any signs of complications appear, remove compress immediately; report verbally to doctor and charge nurse; record the occurrence in the patient's chart.*

9. Cover wet dressings with a waterproof sterile cover.	9. Cover insulates wet dressings and provides constant temperature for duration of treatment. Also, protects bedclothes from getting wet.
10. Secure dressings with tie tapes or binders depending on shape of body part.	10. Prevents dressings from falling off patient and ensures insulation.

SUGGESTED STEPS	RATIONALE/DISCUSSION
11. Change hot dressings every five minutes. Discard soiled dressings in waterproof bag.	
12. After 20 minutes remove final dressings with forceps and discard them.	12. Prolonged exposure to moisture increases skin's susceptibility to maceration and breakdown, reducing protection of intact skin.
13. Dry body part gently with sterile towel or sterile gauze dressing.	13. Moisture left on skin facilitates skin breakdown and causes cooling sensations due to moisture evaporation.
Cover area with sterile dressing.	Maintains sterile environment.
14. If continuous compresses are ordered, allow for "recovery time" and reapply.	14. Without "recovery time," heat's secondary effects appear (see p. 1148).
15. Wash hands.	

Post-Procedure Activities. Leave patient in comfortable, safe position in proper body alignment.

Patient Assessment. Observe patient's local skin reaction and systemic reaction if application was applied to large body area. Report verbally at once to the doctor and charge nurse indications of cutaneous or systemic complications. Record with exacting detail the manifestations of complications in the patient's chart. Assess treatment effectiveness in light of purpose of treatment, evaluating if the treatment goal was met, e.g., whether compress reduced pain, improved circulation, induced suppuration.

Aftercare of Equipment. Return equipment to Central Service for cleaning and reprocessing. If sterilizer is to be reused by same patient, store sterilizer in clean, tidy area of patient unit. Never place sterilizer on the floor unless the floor has been covered (newspapers) to guard against contamination.

Chart/Report. Time, kind and duration of treatment; body part treated; patient's tolerance of treatment; and condition of skin before, during and after application; results of treatment.

Hot Sterile Compresses in the Home. Moist sterile compresses can be applied at home by using 4 × 4 gauze dressings purchased at any drug store. Place gauze squares in a pan, along with two tweezers or forceps in a strainer; add water to submerge instruments and gauze and cover pan with lid. Allow the water to boil vigorously for 10 minutes, thereby destroying pathogens. At the end of the 10 minute period, lift strainer out of the water, holding until instruments dry and cool. Pick up the handle part of the tweezers or forceps, use one to pick up a corner of the moist compress, use second instrument to hold opposite corner. Wring out

1166 IX—ADVANCED CLINICAL CONSIDERATIONS

excess moisture by twisting compress between instruments. Open compress while holding in space. Apply the compress to the body part, making sure you touch nothing accidentally with the compress or forceps. If you inadvertently do touch something nonsterile, set aside the compress for reprocessing. Hold the forceps point down while transferring the sterile moist compress to the patient. Work quickly but carefully, since the compresses cool off rapidly in environmental air. Place the compress on the body part and wrap the compress with a waterproof material, e.g., Saran Wrap, to hold the compress on the body and to maintain the heat of the compress longer. Cover with towel or flannel to insulate. Leave on for 15 to 20 minutes, then remove the application and dry the body part with a sterile dry 4 × 4 gauze dressing. Discard gauze in trash.

Eye Compresses. Compresses for the eye are *sterile* because the conjunctiva (mucous membranes which line the eyelids) are very susceptible to infection.

The procedure for warm compresses is very similar to applying a wet sterile dressing (Procedure 33) with the following exceptions. A sterile basin is filled with enough sterile solution to cover compresses and is placed on a hotplate to heat. The temperature of the compresses should be 40.5°C. (105°F.)—lukewarm. Test the temperature of the solution with a sterile thermometer before wringing out excess solution.

Position the patient with his head tilted slightly back and to the side with the affected eye, so that the solution cannot run into the unaffected eye. If both eyes are being treated, use separate equipment for each eye.

Two sterile forceps or sterile gloved hands are used to wring out a sterile compress. The first compress is used to cleanse the eye by gently wiping the affected eye with one continuous movement from the inner canthus (inside angle of the eye next to the bridge of the nose) to the outer canthus (outside angle of eye approaching the temple) to remove any discharge. Avoid contamination of fingers or sterile gloves. Discard the first compress in a waterproof bag. The second compress will be applied directly on the eyelid of the closed eye and left there approximately 2 minutes. The compresses will need to be changed every 2 minutes since their retention of heat is limited. Apply the compresses for the duration ordered. Each compress is used only once, then discarded.

Nonsterile Moist Hot Packs. Nonsterile moist hot packs may be used in many situations where local heat is required. The main consideration in choosing between nonsterile applications and sterile applications is that the nonsterile can only be used when the patient's protective barriers (skin) have not been penetrated or compromised. The safe nurse practices clean technique when applying a nonsterile moist hot pack.

The hot water method for preparing nonsterile moist packs is the procedure most frequently used. Here the woolen flannel or towel packs are moistened under hot, 55°C. (130°F.) tap water, wrung out, shaken free of steam, then applied to the patient. Woolen material absorbs moisture slowly but holds moisture longer and cools off less quickly than other materials.

The nurse must assess the patient's toleration of the temperature of the packs (lift off temporarily if it feels too hot), watch carefully for complications and complete the necessary patient charting.

HIP OR SITZ BATH

Hip or sitz baths may be used to cleanse a wound, relieve pain, increase circulation, stimulate voiding or promote relaxation. For cleansing purposes the recommended temperature is 38 to 40°C. (100 to 104°F.); for increase in circulation, 43° to 46°C. (110 to 115°F.). The duration of the treatment for either purpose is usually 20 minutes. Hip or sitz baths are contraindicated if the patient is pregnant or has renal or cardiac pathology, because of the generalized systemic effect.

There are a number of appliances that can be used in providing this treatment at home or in the hospital setting. Whether the patient uses a sitz plumbing fixture, a disposable plastic model (Fig. 44–6), or a portable reusable metal model, the effects of the sitz or hip bath are obtained when the perineum is submerged in warm water.

A bathtub is sometimes used, but the sitz or hip bath is preferred to a regular tub bath for perineal soaking because there is less likelihood of marked vasodilation of the perineum and the lower extremities. The patient should bend his knees to keep his legs out of the water in a bathtub.

The disposable plastic sitz bath is used more frequently in settings outside the hospital than other methods because individual use decreases the possibility of cross contamination. The most commonly found model of sitz or hip baths in the hospital is the portable reusable metal unit. Here the patient sits in a chair-like, small, semicircular tub, submerging only his perineal area.

The nurse fills the sitz bath with the desired temperature (depending on the purpose of the treatment) warm tap water (two thirds full). The water valve located at the bottom of the sitz basin must be turned to the "closed" position before the water is poured in. Pad the metal slats which support the patient with a folded clean towel so that the patient does not come into direct contact with the metal supports; and place a bath blanket over the metal back. If the unit is a portable one, lock the wheels before the patient sits down into the tub. Assist the patient as he lowers himself, since the sitz bath level is quite low. Use the flannel bath blanket as a shawl over the shoulders. Place a second bath blanket over the legs. This cover provides warmth and privacy. (Make sure the blankets and gown do not get wet.) Check to see that the edge of the sitz bath does not put pressure on the back of the knees (this pressure is most likely to occur with shorter patients). If there is pressure behind the knees, provide a foot stool for the patient. The patient's call light should be within easy reach.

When adding warm water to re-establish the correct temperature of the sitz bath, pour away from the patient. Stir the water to facilitate its mixture with the cooler water.

With the hip or sitz bath there is sometimes the problem of "perineal pooling." The patient complains of weakness and faintness due to the shift in blood supply. When this occurs, the patient should be assisted out of the bath, dried off and assisted into bed to lie flat until normal circulation is re-established. The physician should be notified.

The heat from the sitz bath has a sedating effect; therefore, the patient may fall asleep. Take appropriate safety measures, e.g., seat belt, observation, as needed.

The patient's gown may get wet since the water usually comes up to the umbilicus. Provide a dry clean gown when the procedure is completed. After the procedure, the patient is dried thoroughly and is assisted back to bed where he can keep warm and his circulation can return to normal. The hip or sitz bath, if a reusable model, should be disinfected between each use.

CONTRAST BATHS

This procedure consists of the alternate immersion of a body part in basins of hot and cold water. Always start with a hot immersion; also end with a hot one, to prevent the patient from getting chilled. The body part is put into 40°C. (104°F.) hot water for 2 minutes, then 15°C. (59°F.) cool water for 1 minute. While the patient's body part is in the cool water basin, fill the warm water basin with more hot water to maintain the water temperature. Add more cool

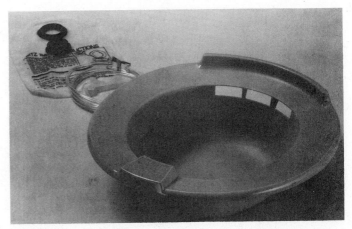

Figure 44–6. Disposable plastic sitz bath. (From Will Ross, Inc., Milwaukee, Wisconsin.)

water to that basin, while the patient's body part is in the warm water. Stir the water in the basin (after adding hot or cold water) to ensure even distribution of temperature. Contrast baths stimulate peripheral circulation in limbs without vascular impairment.[11a]

PARAFFIN BATH

The paraffin bath is most commonly used for painful hands, especially for patients with rheumatoid arthritis. The mixture for this treatment consists of wax and mineral oil. The ratio of mineral oil to paraffin is ½ to 1 ounce of oil to one pound of paraffin.[3]

Patients receiving this treatment must be able to sense the warmth and perspire. If a patient is unable to sweat (which occurs in some neurological conditions), the vessels will not dilate rapidly enough and a burn may occur. The nurse can assess the patient to see if he can sense warmth and is capable of sweating by holding a hot washcloth very close to the body part to be treated with paraffin. The patient should be able to tell the nurse he is experiencing the sensation of warmth, and the nurse must see moisture (perspiration) on the skin's surface adjacent to the hot washcloth before she proceeds with the application of paraffin. Most frequently physical therapists administer this treatment to the patient. Skin breakdown of any kind is a contraindication to the use of the paraffin bath. Remove watches and rings to prevent damage to them.

The body part (usually the hands) is submerged in the 47.7 to 52.2°C. (188 to 126°F.)

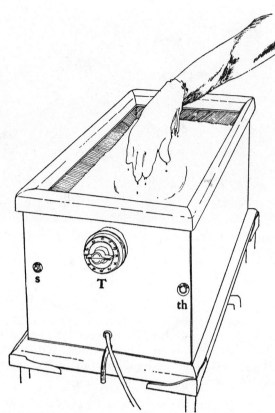

Figure 44–7. Paraffin bath. (From Millard, J. B.: *Conductive heating. In* Licht, S. (ed.): *Therapeutic Heat and Cold* (Physical Medicine Library: Vol. 2). Baltimore, Williams & Wilkins Co., 1965, p. 246.)

liquid (Fig. 44–7). If both hands are to receive the treatment, dip one hand at a time into the paraffin. Once the part is covered with paraffin, it is removed from the liquid. After the first layer has been applied, the patient must not move the part, as cracks may open that will allow the paraffin to seep in on subsequent dips, causing hot spots. Six to seven dippings are usual.

Paraffin is very flammable—caution the patient to keep the paraffin away from an open flame and to use a double boiler if he plans to do this treatment at home. A candy thermometer can serve to measure the temperature of the liquid at home. The treatment usually lasts 20 to 30 minutes; then the wax is peeled off. It can be reused if the patient is doing the procedure at home; this is not the practice in the hospital setting since usually more than one patient uses the paraffin bath.

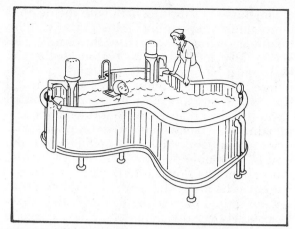

Figure 44–8. Whirlpool bath (Hubbard tank). (From Wood, L. A.: *Nursing Skills for Allied Health Services, Vol. 3.* Philadelphia, W. B. Saunders Co., 1975, p. 231.)

WHIRLPOOL BATH AND HUBBARD TANK

Full immersion baths are helpful in promoting sedation, relieving pain and encouraging débridement of widespread surface burns. Air and/or water is forced into the pool or tank to produce a bubbling effect. The agitation of the water facilitates the débridement.

When immersed in water, the body becomes buoyant and exercises are therefore performed with less effort.

The baths or tanks are usually housed in the physical therapy department (Fig. 44–8). Home models include the Jacuzzi or Vibrabath. The temperature of the water is 32 to 38°C. (90 to 100°F.).

The first treatment is usually restricted to 10 minutes, but later treatments can be as long as 30 minutes.

Watch the patient for exhaustion; he may not be able to tolerate the cardiac stimulation produced by agitation of the water. After the treatment the body may be cooled with a shower, or the heating effect may be prolonged by wrapping the patient in a warm flannel bath blanket for 30 minutes.

Application of Dry Cold

ICE PACK, BAG OR COLLAR

Appliances available for the application of local cold are used most commonly after sprains, head injuries and dental surgeries. Match the size of the area being treated with an appropriate sized bag or collar. Fill the bag or collar with cold water to check for leaks. Empty this water, then fill the appliance one half to two thirds full of crushed ice. Expel all excess air from the bag or collar since its presence in-

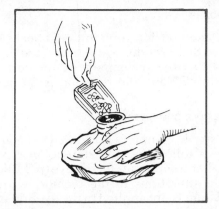

Figure 44–9.   Ice bag. (From Wood, L. A., and Rambo, B. J.: *Nursing Skills for Allied Health Services, Vol. 2,* 2nd ed. Philadelphia, W. B. Saunders Co., 1977, p. 588.)

terferes with thermal conductivity. Screw the cap on snugly. Wipe bag of any excess water. Place the bag or collar into a flannel cover or pillow case (Fig. 44–9).

Since the ice bag is colder than the patient's skin, the ice takes up heat that comes from the body, thereby reducing the local body temperature. Condensation collects on the outer surface of the ice bag or collar because it is colder than the atmosphere. The flannel absorbs this moisture and diminishes the effect of the cold. The bag or collar is applied to the area for one half hour and left off for 1 hour to allow for recovery time. Close assessment of the patient and his skin would include the patient's complaints of a burning sensation or numbness or the appearance of blisters, mottling, skin maceration, redness, extreme paleness or gray discoloration. If any of these occur, discontinue the treatment at once and immediately report to the doctor. Refill ice bag or collar and change the cover, as needed. Chart as appropriate.

CHEMICAL COLD PACKS

Similar to the chemical hot packs, a cold pack is a prefilled plastic package with two separate compartments. The nurse strikes, kneads or squeezes (depending on the manufacturer's directions) the pack to mix one chemical compound with the other and provide a controlled temperature of 10 to 26.1°C. (50 to 80°F.) (Fig. 44–10). Although the cold pack might last longer than 30 minutes before losing its coldness, the nurse must remember to provide the recovery time needed after a 30 minute application. If this time (usually 1 hour) is not provided, secondary effects could occur.

If the outer surface of a chemical cold pack is not covered with a special material, a flannel cover or pillow case must be provided before the pack is applied. The covering is used to

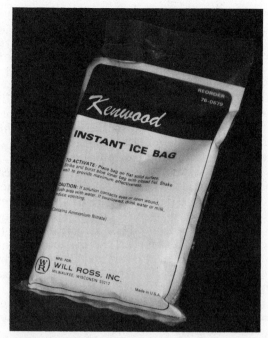

Figure 44–10.   Chemical cold pack. (Courtesy Will Ross, Inc. Milwaukee, Wisconsin.)

collect the condensation which will form on the ice pack.

This appliance is designed for "one-time" use—freezing the package for another treatment does not attain the desired temperature.

Subjective data from the patient that would indicate his tolerance of the treatment include complaints of a burning sensation or a numb feeling. Objective data would include the appearance of blisters, mottling, redness, grayness or skin maceration. Discontinue treatment promptly if your assessment reveals indications of these complications. Complete patient charting as required.

Applications of Moist Cold

COLD PACKS

The procedure for applying moist cold packs is similar to the application of moist hot packs. The pack could be a washcloth, small towel, flannel, or gauze depending on the size of the body part receiving the application. A basin of cold water is prepared and the packs are immersed into it. (The water basin can be placed into a basin of ice.) When cooled, the excess water is wrung out of the packs, and the pack applied to the body area. Replace packs as necessary to maintain coolness. The duration of treatment with moist cold packs should not exceed 20 minutes.

The patient may be able to replace his own cold packs, depending on his physical condition. Caution the patient not to put ice cubes directly on his skin because the *exposure to this extreme in cold* increases the occurrence of secondary effects and can produce burns.

The complaints of the patient and the clinical changes in his skin that indicate the occurrence of complications are the same as those given under application of chemical packs and likewise warrant immediate discontinuance of the treatment. Remember, the generalized effect is increased in relation to the size of the area. If the area is too large, treat small areas separately.

Upon terminating the treatment, dry the area gently and provide the patient with a dry gown and bed clothing as needed.

COLD SOAKS

The method for applying cold soaks is the same as that used for warm soaks (see p. 1161), except that the recommended temperature is 15°C. (59°F.) and the duration is 20 minutes.

STERILE COLD COMPRESSES

If a sterile compress is ordered to be applied to an eye, follow the same steps as discussed for sterile hot compresses for the eye (p. 1166). The notable alterations in the technique are that petrolatum is not applied to the eyelids and the large basin is two thirds full of cold water and ice chips. The smaller sterile bowl still contains the sterile water and the sterile gauze dressings. After being wrung out with the use of the sterile forceps, the compress is applied to the eye and replaced as it warms.

Procedure Summary

Table 44–7 summarizes the common methods of applying heat and cold locally for therapeutic purposes. Recommended temperatures are presented for each appliance and duration of time for the treatment is shown. The

TABLE 44–7.   MODES OF THERAPEUTIC USE OF HEAT AND COLD

APPLIANCE	TEMPERATURE	DURATION (MINUTES)
Hot-water bottle		
Infants to 2 years; aged persons	40.5 to 46°C. (105 to 115°F.)	
Adults	46 to 52°C. (115 to 125°F.)	20 to 30
Chemical heating bottles		
Infants to 2 years; aged persons	40.5 to 46°C. (105 to 115°F.)	
Adults	46 to 52°C. (115 to 125°F.)	20 to 30
Infrared, ultraviolet	18 to 24 inches from the part depending on the wattage of the heating element	20 to 30
Gooseneck lamp	25 watts; 14 inches from area	20 to 30
	40 watts; 18 inches from area	
	60 watts; 24 to 30 inches from area	
Heat cradle (Baker)	25 watts; 38° to 40.5°C. (100 to 105°F.)	Continuous or 20 to 30
Electrical heating pads	(same as hot-water bottle)	20 to 30
Aqua K pad or module	Cold: 15°C. (59°F.)	20 to 30
	Hot: 40.5°C. (105°F.)	20 to 30
Hot compresses, packs	55°C. (131°F.)	15 to 20
Hot soaks	40.5 to 43°C. (105 to 110°F.)	20
Hip or sitz bath	38°C. to 46°C. (100 to 115°F.)	20
Contrast bath	Hot: 40°C. (104°F.)	2
	Cold: 15°C. (59°F.)	1
Paraffin bath	47.7 to 52.2°C. (118 to 126°F.)	Seven immersions and settings
Whirlpool bath, Hubbard tank	32 to 38°C. (90 to 100°F.)	10 to 30
Ice bag	10 to 26.6°C. (50 to 80°F.)	30
Chemical cold packs	10 to 26.6°C. (50 to 80°F.)	30
Cold compresses, packs	15°C. (59°F.)	15 to 20
Cold soaks	15°C. (59°F.)	20

reader is reminded that these temperatures might not be tolerated by all patients. A person's reaction to different forms of heat and cold can be very individual.

THE EXPRESSIVE ROLE OF THE NURSE

We have presented technical and scientific information about the therapeutic use of heat and cold. Such information, along with expert supervision, will enable the nurse to carry out the instrumental tasks related to the application of heat and cold well. With practice, the nurse can become very skilled and may consider such procedures uncomplicated and routine. The patient, however, probably will not regard them so.

The nurse does well to anticipate that almost all patients will be experiencing some degree of anxiety. This is especially true when the patient is undergoing unfamiliar, potentially dangerous treatments. It is a nursing task to identify the sources of such anxieties and to use an expressive role to promote comfort and relative freedom from fear (see Chapter 3 for a discussion of expressive role).

There are certain factors about the application of heat and cold that commonly produce anxiety for patients. A patient may be concerned that:

▶ the medical and nursing personnel do not really understand the use of heat and cold and are prescribing it inappropriately, e.g., a patient may think heat to be more appropriate when he has been prescribed cold.

▶ the nurse does not really know how to use the equipment and may hurt him or do him no good.

▶ he will experience pain during the procedure.

▶ temperatures may be too hot or too cold and will hurt him.

▶ applications will be left on too long and hurt his skin.

▶ temperature may not be hot or cold enough to be effective.

▶ applications have not been left on long enough to be effective.

▶ moist applications may leak and his clothing and/or bed linens will become wet and uncomfortable.

These concerns may be reduced if the nurse:

▶ really understands the nature and reasons for the treatment and is skilled in the procedures. Such competence will be communicated to the patient and help him gain confidence and trust.

▶ takes time to explain the procedure quietly and clearly both before and during procedure activities.

▶ encourages the patient to ask questions and answers them clearly, making sure the patient is satisfied with the answers each time.

▶ makes certain the patient can get attention at any time during the procedure, e.g., has call bell available and feels comfortable in using it.

▶ responds to a call signal promptly.

Of course, a patient may be concerned about something quite different from any of the things identified here. A nurse *should never assume* that she knows what a patient is concerned about until she has listened carefully to what he is saying—both verbally and nonverbally. Most people require some encouragement to be able to identify and express fears and anxieties. The excellent nurse is able to provide such encouragement with the use of genuineness, accurate empathy and nonpossessive warmth as described in Chapter 3. Accurate, empathic understanding is probably the most essential element in promoting comfort during unfamiliar and fear-producing procedures. If the nurse uses this expressive skill well she will be able to:

▶ Identify the patient's fears accurately.

▶ Communicate appropriate, reassuring information at the right time and at the right level of sophistication.

▶ Assess the extent her reassurance has allayed anxieties and whether she must seek further means of promoting psychological comfort for the patient.

BIBLIOGRAPHY

1. Auld, M.: Body-temperature status. *In* Mitchell, P. H. (ed.): *Concepts Basic to Nursing.* New York, McGraw-Hill Book Co., Inc., 1973.
2. Dison, N.: *Clinical Nursing Techniques,* 3rd ed. St. Louis, C. V. Mosby Co., 1975.
3. Downer, A. H.: *Physical Therapy Procedures,* 2nd ed. Springfield, IL, Charles C Thomas, 1974.
4. DuGas, B. W.: *Introduction to Patient Care,* 3rd ed. Philadelphia, W. B. Saunders Co., 1977.

5. Feurst, E. V., Wolff, L. V., and Weitzel, M. H.: *Fundamentals of Nursing,* 5th ed. Philadelphia, J. B. Lippincott Co., 1974.

6. Glor, B. A. K., and Estes, Z. E.: Moist soaks: A survey of clinical practices. *Nursing Research, 19*:5, Sep.–Oct., 1970.

7. Goodman, L. S., and Gilman, A. (eds.): *A Pharmacological Basis of Therapeutics,* 5th ed. New York, The Macmillan Co., 1975.

8. Gragg, S. G., and Reese, O. M.: *Scientific Principles in Nursing,* 7th ed. St. Louis, C. V. Mosby Co., 1974.

9. Guyton, A. C.: *Textbook of Medical Physiology,* 5th ed. Philadelphia, W. B. Saunders Co., 1976.

10. Halsell, M.: Moist heat for relief of postoperative pain. *American Journal of Nursing, 67*:767–770, April 1967.

11. Hardy, J. D.: Thermal radiation, pain and injury. *In* Licht, S. (ed.): *Therapeutic Heat and Cold* (Physical Medicine Library: Vol. 2). Baltimore, Williams & Wilkins Co., 1965.

11a. Krusen, F. H., Kottke, F. J., and Ellwood, P. M., Jr. (eds.): *Handbook of Physical Medicine and Rehabilitation,* 2nd ed. Philadelphia, W. B. Saunders Co., 1971.

12. Leake, M. J.: *A Manual of Simple Nursing Procedures,* 5th ed. Philadelphia, W. B. Saunders Co., 1971.

13. Levine, M. E.: *Introduction to Clinical Nursing,* 2nd ed. Philadelphia, F. A. Davis Co., 1973.

14. Millard, J. B.: Conductive heat. *In* Licht, S. (ed.): *Therapeutic Heat and Cold* (Physical Medicine Library: Vol. 2). Baltimore, Williams & Wilkins Co., 1965.

14a. Miller, B. F., and Keane, C. B.: *Encyclopedia and Dictionary of Medicine, Nursing, and Allied Health,* 2nd ed. Philadelphia, W. B. Saunders Co., 1978, p. 866.

15. Moore, J., and Weinberg, M.: The case of the warm moist compress. *Canadian Nurse, 71*:625–632, March 1975.

16. Murray, M.: *Fundamentals of Nursing.* Englewood Cliffs, NJ, Prentice-Hall, Inc., 1976.

16a. O'Dell, A. J.: Hot packs for morning stiffness. *American Journal of Nursing, 75*:986–987, June 1975.

17. Petrello, J.: Temperature maintenance of hot moist compresses. *American Journal of Nursing, 6*:1050–1051, June 1973.

18. Rapier, D. H.: Hot and cold applications. *In* Rapier, D. H., et al. (eds.): *Practical Nursing,* 4th ed. St. Louis, C. V. Mosby Co., 1970.

19. Rowell, L. B.: The cutaneous circulation. *In* Ruch, T. C., et al. (eds.): *Physiology and Biophysics,* Vol. 2, 20th ed. Philadelphia, W. B. Saunders Co., 1973.

20. Scott, B.: Short wave diathermy. *In* Licht, S. (ed.): *Therapeutic Heat and Cold* (Physical Medicine Library: Vol. 2). Baltimore, Williams & Wilkins Co., 1965.

21. Sherwood, C.: Nursing procedures: you'd be amazed at what they cost. *Nursing '74, 4*:54–58, May 1974.

22. Stoner, E.: Luminous and infrared heating. *In* Licht, S. (ed.): *Therapeutic Heat and Cold* (Physical Medicine Library: Vol. 2). Baltimore, Williams & Wilkins Co., 1965.

23. Taber, C. W.: *Taber's Cyclopedic Medical Dictionary,* 12th ed. Philadelphia, F. A. Davis Co., 1973.

24. Thompson, E. M., et al.: Nursing treatments. *In* Thompson, E. M., and Rosedahl, C. B.: *Textbook of Basic Nursing,* 2nd ed. Philadelphia, J. B. Lippincott Co., 1973.

25. Wise, C. S.: Heat and cold. *In* Biermanand, W., and Licht, S. (eds.): *Physical Medicine in General Practice,* 3rd ed. New York, Hoeber, 1955.

26. Wood, L. A.: *Nursing Skills for Allied Health Services,* Vol. 2, 2nd ed. Philadelphia, W. B. Saunders Co., 1977.

27. Wood, L. A.: *Nursing Skills for Allied Health Services.* Vol. 3. Philadelphia, W. B. Saunders Co., 1975.

UNIT
X
CARING FOR PERSONS WITH SPECIAL NEEDS

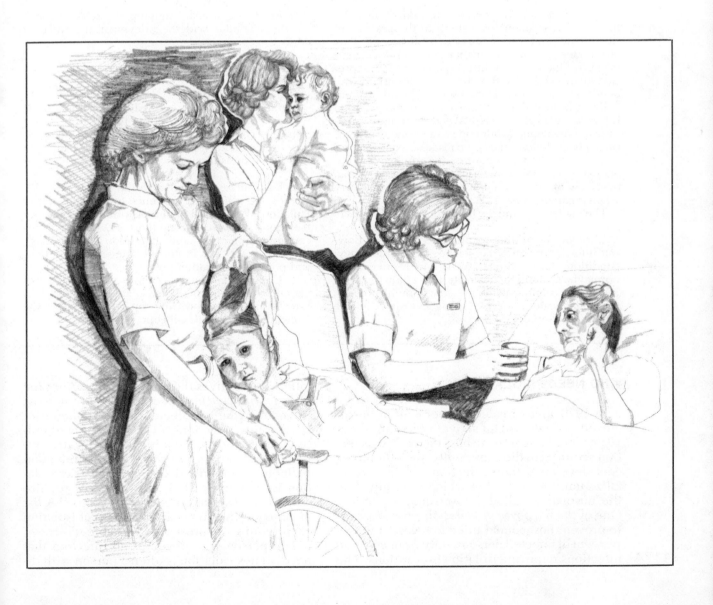

CHAPTER 45

CARING FOR PERSONS REQUIRING ISOLATION

By Joyce Zerwekh, R.N., M.A.

OVERVIEW AND STUDY GUIDE

General measures to *prevent* cross-infection in the hospital environment are central to the practice of safe nursing and were discussed in Chapter 25. This chapter focuses on those specific measures designed to *control* the spread of infection, i.e., isolation precautions. Specifically, this chapter: (a) identifies who needs isolation and how infection is spread; (b) considers a historical and international perspective on infection; (c) explores hospital and community nursing roles in relation to infection control measures; (d) presents technical and psychosocial concepts related to isolation procedures; (e) summarizes the standard isolation categories; and (f) presents an overview of common nursing procedures that vary when a patient is isolated.

The reader may find the following guide helpful to study:

1. Before beginning reading, review the following information from the science of microbiology: conditions for bacteria growth and reproduction, normal body flora, the characteristics of pathogenic organisms, common pathogens, the immune process, the inflammatory process, phagocytosis, and the definition of epidemiology.

2. After you fiinish studying this chapter, you should be familiar with the following terms and concepts:

nosocomial infection	vehicle
pathogen	vector
source	portal of entrance
portal of exit	clean and contaminated
direct contact	double bagging
droplet contact	concurrent disinfection
indirect contact	terminal disinfection.
airborne transmission	

3. Familiarize yourself with the following terms as they are used with reference to isolation: Strict Isolation, Wound and Skin Precautions, Respiratory Isolation, Enteric Precautions, Discharge Precautions (Secretion and Excretion Precautions), Blood Precautions, Protective (Reverse) Isolation, and protective isolation units.

4. Consider (a) the experiences of sensory deprivation and loneliness in the isolated patient and (b) how being viewed as "unclean" might affect the isolated patient's self-concept

WHO NEEDS ISOLATION?

In 1970 approximately 16 per cent of hospitalized patients had an active infection. About 10 per cent came into the hospital with an infection acquired in the community; the other 6 per cent developed their infections during hospitalization.[14] An infection which is acquired in the hospital is called a *nosocomial infection.* One of *the purposes of isolation procedures* is to prevent nosocomial infection. Out of the 16 per cent of infected persons, only 2 per cent had infections requiring isolation precautions. The

following list gives the *common indications for isolation precautions* beginning with the most frequent: wounds infected with *Staphylococcus aureus,* infections awaiting results of culture, tuberculosis, hepatitis, gram negative infections, staphylococcal pneumonia, infection with beta hemolytic streptococcus. Strict isolation is seldom needed; most patients require wound and skin or enteric precautions.[14] A list of common infections and the type of isolation each requires is presented in Table 45–1.

The person who develops an infection that necessitates isolation is often a person with di-

TABLE 45–1.   HOW COMMON INFECTIONS ARE ISOLATED

DISEASE	ORGANISM	TYPE OF ISOLATION PRECAUTIONS
Acute diarrhea	Multiple possibilities	Enteric precautions
Chickenpox	Varicella-zoster virus	Strict
Conjunctivitis	Bacterial/viral	Secretion precautions
Diphtheria	*Corynebacterium diphtheriae*	Strict
Food poisoning	*Clostridium perfringens*	Enteric
	Salmonella species	
	Staphylococcus aureus	
Gas gangrene	*Clostridium perfringens*	Wound and skin
Gastroenteritis	*Escherichia coli*	Enteric precautions
	Salmonella species	
	Shigella species	
German measles (rubella)	Rubella virus	Respiratory
Gonorrhea	*Neisseria gonorrhoeae*	Secretion
Hepatitis (type A and B)	Virus	Enteric and blood
Herpes simplex (local)	Virus	Secretion
Herpes zoster (local)	Virus	Wound and skin
Infectious mononucleosis	Epstein-Barr virus	Secretion precautions
Measles (rubeola)	Rubeola virus	Respiratory
Meningitis	*Neisseria meningitidis*	Respiratory
Mumps	Virus	Respiratory
Pharyngitis (strep sore throat)	*Streptococcus pyogenes*	Secretion
Pneumonia	*Staphylococcus aureus*	Strict
	Streptococcus pyogenes	Strict
	Viral	Secretion
Poliomyelitis	Polio virus	Excretion
Tuberculosis	*Mycobacterium tuberculosis*	Respiratory
Urinary tract infections	Multiple possibilities	Handwashing
Viral diseases	Viruses	Discharge precautions
Wound infections:		
Staphylococcal		
When very small wound		Secretion
When covered with dressings		Wound
When dressings cannot contain drainage		Strict
Streptococcal		
When very small wound		Secretion
When covered with dressings		Wound
When dressings cannot contain drainage		Strict
Other		Wound and skin
If very small		Secretion

(Modified from: U.S. Department of Health, Education and Welfare: Isolation Techniques for Use in Hospitals, 1975.)

minished resistance to infection, whose immediate environment is conducive to development of an infection. A community or hospital environment contributes to the spread of infection if infected persons and persons with poor resistance are existing together, so that physical contact or airborne spread may occur. Crowding makes it easier for organisms to move from person to person. Unclean food handling, unclean utensils and equipment, and especially unclean nurses' hands are common examples of methods of the spread of infection among a population. Lack of appropriate use of handwashing in either hospital or community will increase the incidence of infection spread by unclean hands. It is vital that the nurse clearly understand the scope of the infection cycle.

THE SPREAD OF INFECTION

The infection chain includes all the links in the growth, reproduction, and spread of organisms. Whenever one link is broken in the chain, the life cycle of the organism is interrupted. We systematically discuss the following six links in the infection chain:* (1) the infectious organism; (2) the source or reservoir of infection; (3) the way the organism escapes (portal of exit); (4) means of transmission of the organism; (5) the way the organism enters the host (portal of entrance); and (6) the susceptibility of the host. As you study the components of the infection chain, remember:

> *The spread of infection can be controlled only by breaking a link in the infection chain. Nursing activities are directed at breaking the infection chain.*

The Infectious Organism

An infection simply cannot occur unless infectious microorganisms are present. Microorganisms that infect human tissues, causing tissue damage and consequent disease, are called *pathogens*. Some pathogens possess various powerful characteristics which enable them to overcome body defenses and gain a foothold for producing disease. For instance, to avoid being engulfed by phagocytes, which would ingest them, pathogens may be surrounded by protective capsules, or the pathogens may secrete a substance (leukocidin) that destroys the phagocytes. Leukocidin breaks down phagocytes into pus; organisms that form pus are called pyogenic. Some pathogens secrete enzymes which destroy the body's connective tissue; others destroy fibrin clots formed by the blood in an attempt to wall off the infection.

Once body tissues are invaded, pathogens cause tissue damage primarily through the secretion of toxins. Gram-positive pathogens secrete exotoxins, while endotoxins are released from the disintegrated cell walls of gram-negative organisms. Fever, for instance, is one symptom caused by the circulation of endotoxins.

The term *virulence* is used to describe the relative ability of a pathogen to cause infection. Virulence is determined by two factors: the ability to invade body tissue and the power of toxins secreted.

The likelihood of infection increases in proportion to the actual number of pathogens

*Also frequently called "infection cycle" (see also Chap. 25).

(pathogenic organisms) to which the susceptible individual is exposed.

Antibiotics interfere with pathogens by molecular binding to vital cell components. For instance, they may inhibit cell membrane synthesis or synthesis of necessary structural proteins of the pathogens. Exposure to antibiotics causes some pathogens to change genetically into forms that are resistant to antibiotic action. Such drug resistant forms are much harder to eradicate; higher doses or more toxic drugs may be needed.

The Source of Infection

Once present, pathogens can grow and reproduce in various environments, also called *reservoirs*. Human tissues, animal tissues, or inanimate environments may all serve as reservoirs. Human reservoirs include: persons overtly ill with infectious diseases, persons with early or unrecognized illness, and persons who are pathogen "carriers." Carriers themselves show no symptoms of the disease, but their secretions or mucous membranes are found to harbor pathogens. In the developing world, insects and rodents remain significant sources of infection. Occasionally, in developed countries, pets or rodents may be reservoirs of human infection. Inanimate sources of infection are numerous and include food, water, drugs, feces, clothing, dishes, toilet articles, and medical supplies that have come in contact with pathogens.

It is also quite possible for organisms which already reside in one part of a host to become a source of infection at another site in the host's body. One common example of such a reservoir is the human intestine, teeming with organisms that are potential invaders of a vulnerable lung, bladder, or open wound.

The Portal of Exit

Organisms escape from human reservoirs through respiratory secretions, emesis or feces, urine, genital secretions, blood, or drainage from wounds and lesions. Portal of exit also includes other means by which organisms leave the reservoir, e.g., mosquitoes.

The Means of Transmission

Pathogens are transmitted (1) by contact, (2) through the air, or (3) by means of vehicles or vectors. There are three kinds of *contact transmission*. "Direct contact" occurs when a susceptible person touches an infected person. "Indirect contact" occurs when a susceptible person touches contaminated inanimate articles. "Droplet contact" occurs when coughing, sneezing, or talking by an infected person expels pathogens, which are carried on coarse droplets in the air. A person within 3 feet of the infected person may inhale droplets.[27]

Airborne transmission means that the air can carry contaminated dust particles or droplet nuclei that may be inhaled by a susceptible person at distances greater than 3 feet from the infected person. Droplet nuclei are dried clusters of organic matter and microorganisms suspended in the air.

Vehicles that may transmit pathogens include contaminated water, food, drugs, or blood. *Vectors* are living agents—animals such as mosquitoes or rats—that may transmit pathogens.

The Portal of Entrance

Pathogens can enter a potential host through natural or abnormal body orifices: mouth, nose, ears, eyes, anus, urethra, vagina, open wounds and lesions such as animal bites.

The Susceptibility of the Host

Multiple factors protect a potential host from infection. First, there are natural barriers: unbroken skin, protective secretions of the mucous membrane, and ciliary action in the respiratory tract. A pathogen cannot penetrate skin that is intact. The secretions of mucous membranes in the respiratory tract trap foreign particles as they are inhaled. The cilia are hairlike processes that clear the air passages by beating foreign particles out of the lungs towards the pharynx.

If natural barriers fail to provide protection and invasion by pathogens occurs, a host resists infection by (a) production of phagocytes to consume the organisms, (b) production of antibodies specific to the infecting organism and (c) establishment of an active, inflammatory response, which increases circulation of blood to the infected area. Host susceptibility to infection is known to be increased by elevated stress levels, fatigue, malnutrition, and general debilitation.

Breaking the Links

Control measures to break the links of the infection cycle most commonly focus on the use of *antimicrobial drugs* to diminish the human reservoirs of infection; placing *barriers at the portal of exit*, such as dressings over an infected wound or a tissue over the mouth when coughing; *covering the portal of entrance* when the tissue is known to be vulnerable, such as placing a dressing over a surgical incision; and protecting susceptible individuals by measures such as *immunization*.

Isolation precautions are specifically designed to interfere with the means of transmission of specific pathogens.

For instance, if an organism is known to be transmitted by direct contact, gloves are worn by the health worker when touching the infected person. If indirect contact spread is a known means of transmission, gloves are worn when handling all objects indirectly contaminated by the patient's pathogens. If a patient is known to be infected with pathogens that are transmitted by infected droplets in the air, the health worker wears a mask in the patient's presence.

The details of the systematic precautions derived from a knowledge of transmission are discussed later in this chapter.

HISTORICAL AND INTERNATIONAL PERSPECTIVE

Incidence of Infectious Disease

The worldwide picture of infectious diseases is undergoing constant change. In those lands where food and water supplies are plentiful and uncontaminated, where environmental sanitation is maintained, and where immunization programs are effective, the incidence of communicable disease has been dramatically diminished in recent decades. Nevertheless, communicable disease continues to be the major cause of mortality and morbidity in underdeveloped countries. Smallpox and cholera once ravaged the whole world. In contrast, in 1975 smallpox could be found only in Ethiopia, India, and Bangladesh. Cholera is once again on the rampage, moving eastward into the Mideast, Africa, and Eastern Europe, after being confined primarily to Asia during the early 1900's. Malaria continues to attack inhabitants of the tropics and subtropics, sometimes in epidemic proportions, in which the number of cases suddenly explodes out of control.

Currently the most common reportable contagious diseases in the United States are gonorrhea, chickenpox, measles, tuberculosis, hepatitis, and mumps.[24] Generally, these infections do not require hospitalization, and their control is based upon community health measures such as early case finding. screening of food handlers, safe sewage disposal.

Isolation precautions are instituted in the hospital for individuals who are admitted with infections or possible infections; or have acquired infection in the hospital (nosocomial infection). While many communicable diseases can now be controlled with medications (e.g., tuberculosis), the incidence of nosocomial infections from gram-negative bacilli and *Staphylococcus aureus* has increased sharply since the early twentieth century. Generally these infections do not appear in the healthy population, but in the already-ill person who has diminished resistance. One or two others might be isolated at the same time in a general hospital. This is in contrast to the isolation wards and contagious disease hospitals of the recent past, necessitated by fears grounded in incorrect assumptions about disease transmission.

Absent from modern advanced societies are the once numerous tuberculosis sanitoriums, replaced today by highly effective chemotherapy managed in the community environment. Gone also is the stigma that accompanied being quarantined in a colony of "unclean spirits," and gone the tribute of bravery to those nurses courageous enough to work among patients condemned to confinement and often death from contagious diseases, whose means of spread so long remained a mystery. Today knowledge has reduced the overwhelming dangers accompanying ignorance.[29] For most infections, we understand enough about transmission to be able to set up barriers effectively to protect health workers and the community from the disease.

Changing Control Measures

Infectious disease control measures have changed greatly over time, yet certain ancient methods have withstood tests of time and science and remain with us. Traditional practices were based on fear of becoming infected, religious ritual, and trial-and-error experience.

In Old Testament times, priests pronounced diagnosis of contagious disease and prescribed rigid quarantine measures and ritual cleansing as methods of control. In Leviticus chapter 15, verses 3–8, specific isolation precautions are described that compare closely with contemporary wound and skin isolation precautions:

And this is the law of uncleanness for a discharge. . . . Every bed on which he who has the discharge lies shall be unclean; and everything on which he sits shall be unclean. Anyone who touches his bed shall wash his clothes, and bathe himself in water. . . . And whoever sits on anything on which he who has the discharge has sat shall wash his clothes, and bathe himself. . . . And whoever touches the body of him who has the discharge shall wash his clothes and bathe himself in water. . . .

Control measures used to contain the plague prevalent in Europe in the 1700's included: isolating infected persons in an open field until they either recovered or died, isolating those who cared for the sick before the care-givers could re-enter society, and the wearing of elaborate protective garb by physicians as protection from the "bad air" believed to be the cause of the disease (Fig. 45–1).[13]

When bacteria were first accepted as the actual causal agents of infectious diseases, chemical disinfection and general sanitation were trusted as general infection control measures. It has taken a long time for control measures to be designed that are based upon understandings of the specific method in which each infectious microorganism is spread. Isolation techniques have long varied from institution to institution and have at times been inconsistent within the same institution. It is vital that uniform prac-

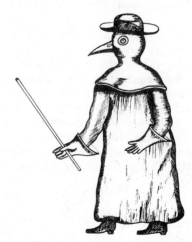

Figure 45–1. Eighteenth-century isolation garments. The foul air was filtered through aromatic herbs in the beak. (From Dubay, E., and Grubb, R.: *Infection: Prevention and Control.* St. Louis, C. V. Mosby Co., 1973, p. 11.)

tices become universally adopted and that all practices be consistent with the most current knowledge of disease spread.

In the United States, the best authority on the nature and transmission of communicable diseases is the National Center for Disease Control in Atlanta, Georgia. The manual written by this center, *Isolation Techniques for Use in Hospitals, 1975*, is the primary source for isolation guidelines discussed in this chapter and is published by the U.S. Government Printing Office.[27]

NURSING ROLES TO PREVENT AND CONTROL INFECTION

Nursing has been traditionally responsible for maintaining a therapeutic environment.* Infection control is critical to this responsibility, and nursing assumes a variety of roles to minimize the risk of spread of infection. Hospital nurses assess all patients to: (a) determine the presence and status of infection, (b) initiate and maintain appropriate isolation precautions based on the most recent knowledge about disease transmission, (c) analyze the infection chain of specific infections and implement plans to break identified links and (d) provide ongoing patient-family and staff education directed at knowledgeable use of infection control techniques. "Infection control nurses" are specialists who assume major responsibility for the implementation of infection control policies within a given institution. In the community, public health nurses also assume major responsibility for infection control. Whatever their roles, all nurses are accountable for maintaining a high level of personal practices to prevent infection and combat spread of infection in their patient care activities.

Nursing Assessment

As mentioned, nurses determine the presence and status of infection. By performing thorough, systematic assessments on all patients, nurses recognize the pattern of data that may indicate that infection is developing. Purulent drainage from body cavities or wounds and cough with purulent sputum are common indicators that infection is present. The *classical signs of inflammation* (redness, warmth, swelling, and pain) must be actively analyzed in the light of associated data; infection *could* be the cause. Fever and leukocytosis (elevated white

blood cell count) are nonspecific indications of the presence of infection. As such, they are warning signs that must be heeded. Specimens of body drainage, urine, sputum, or blood will be cultured in the clinical laboratory to determine the specific site of the infection and the virulence of the organism. Traditionally, initiating a "culture" has necessitated a physician's order, although many times it has been suggested by nursing personnel. Increasingly, nursing is assuming accountability for culturing all questionable materials when infection is suspected. Nurses need a basic understanding of culture results. They need to recognize when organisms are pathogenic in contrast to normal flora. For instance, a laboratory report that non-hemolytic streptococci are present in a patient's nasopharynx is no cause for concern, since they are known to be normal residents. In contrast, the discovery of large numbers of beta hemolytic streptococci in a patient's nasopharynx requires an immediate report to the physician so that therapy can be initiated.

In addition to determining whether infection is present, nurses constantly assess an infected person for signs and symptoms that indicate the progress or regression of known infection. For this purpose, it is vital to record accurate and complete baseline data so that all ensuing observations can be compared to that baseline. For instance, the appearance of the wound edges and character of drainage should be recorded upon admission of a patient with leg ulcers infected with *Staphylococcus aureus*. Periodic analysis of the data, together with evaluation of body temperature and blood count, will indicate the status of the infection. Since the infected patient is usually being treated with antibiotics, assessment includes determination of the medication's therapeutic effects as well as potential side effects. Thus, if the patient with infected leg ulcers were receiving intravenous Keflin as antibiotic therapy, he would need to be observed frequently for indications of thrombophlebitis at the intravenous site, impaired renal function, and/or allergic reactions.[1]

Initiating and Maintaining Isolation Precautions

Infection cannot be controlled effectively if the nurse waits for physician's orders as the only indicator of the need for isolation pre-

---

*Maintaining a therapeutic environment is discussed in Chap. 25.

cautions or unthinkingly adheres to isolation manual regulations. The competent, professional nurse does not simply rely on rules and make standardized decisions. Instead, such a nurse's decision-making process also includes making independent judgments based upon her own systematic, knowledgeable analysis of data.

> *It is vital that patients with known infections or patients manifesting symptoms indicating possible infection be promptly isolated from others. This is done to prevent spread of infection to noninfected persons.*

Some hospitals have a list of standing orders prescribing when isolation precautions are to be initiated. Other institutions delegate the authority to begin isolation precautions to their infection control nurse.[3] However, it is really the responsibility of *all* professional nurses to initiate promptly barriers against cross-infection as soon as they suspect that the condition of one patient may pose an infection threat to others, or, vice versa, that one patient is unusually susceptible to infection from others. In the first instance, the patient with a suspected infection should be isolated. In the second instance, the patient requiring protection from potential infection should be isolated. In some hospitals it is established policy for the nurse to initiate isolation precautions when the need is indicated and the physician has not yet acted.[21] However, the responsibility remains primarily the physician's to recognize when isolation is needed and to order appropriate isolation precautions.

Dubay and Grubb recommend an "alert" isolation category to be used when infection is suspected but not yet confirmed. They state that the following conditions indicate the need for an *isolation alert:* undiagnosed diarrhea, fever of undetermined origin, purulent draining wounds, suspicion of hepatitis, possible tuberculosis, possible meningitis, and suspicious skin rashes.[12]

It is vital that the professional nurse apply isolation precautions at the bedside using an ongoing problem-solving approach, rather than basing his/her actions on an attempt to memorize standardized procedures. An understanding of the underlying rationale for each precaution facilitates practice in which each action makes sense and can be modified as appropriate for individual circumstances. A large portion of this chapter is therefore devoted to helping the nurse understand the rationale behind each isolation procedure and thereby to facilitate a choice of nursing actions based upon a clear understanding of how infection is transmitted.

Discontinuing Isolation Precautions

The standardized guidelines for determining when isolation is no longer necessary are different for every disease. For instance, patients with wounds infected with *Staphylococcus aureus* must be isolated for the duration of their illness; patients with tuberculosis are isolated until 3 weeks after effective therapy has begun; patients with diphtheria are isolated until two cultures are negative.[27] Obviously, no generalizations can be made. The physician is responsible for discontinuing isolation precautions, and the nurse is responsible for working with him to be sure that isolation is not continued longer than absolutely necessary.

Analyzing the Infection Chain

Whenever nosocomial infection appears, the nurse must become a detective to analyze how the infection might have spread.[16] The nurse's investigation includes: examination of the hospital environment to identify possible sources of infection, questioning the possible route of infection, considering whether the resistance of the infected host may be impaired, and considering whether a threat to other patients remains. It is inexcusable simply to accept the emergence of a new infection without investigating its origins.

Patient-Family and Staff Education

The nurse is responsible for teaching infection control measures to patients, family, and visitors, as well as to all persons who assume responsibility for direct patient care. Details of patient-family teaching functions concerning infection control are emphasized throughout this chapter. While formal instruction for nursing team members is the official responsibility of in-service nursing educators, the staff nurse is responsible for reinforcing knowledge, functioning as a role model, and checking on team members' knowledge and performance to determine that safe levels of practice are maintained.

All persons providing bedside care for isolated patients should know: basic aseptic principles, isolation precaution procedures, disinfection procedures, the identity of common pathogens, methods of infection spread, and care measures necessary for the infected patient.[25]

Infection Control Nurse Specialists

The *hospital infection control nurse* and sometimes an additional person called a *nurse epidemiologist* are key elements in each hospital's infection control program. In order to be accredited by the American Hospital Association and the Joint Commission on Accreditation of Hospitals, each hospital must have an infection control committee to guide its infection control program.[12] This interdisciplinary committee meets regularly to determine and implement: (a) policies related to isolation and aseptic technique and (b) methods for surveillance (gathering data) of nosocomial infection.[28] The infection control specialists are responsible for applying control policies established by the committee. They also supervise isolation precautions used in the hospital and gather data about nosocomial infections. Nosocomial infections are analyzed with emphasis on investigating the route of infection spread and implementing control measures to eliminate the threat of outbreak.[2]

Control of Infection in the Community

In the previous section we looked at nurses working in hospital settings to prevent and control infections. Let us now look at infection control measures used by nurses working in the community outside the hospital. The *community health nurse:* (a) intervenes to control infection through patient-family teaching, (b) participates in case finding, and (c) is active in follow-up on identified infections.

Patient-family teaching includes several dimensions. Preventive measures such as child immunizations and household sanitation are high priorities. Patient and family need clear, accurate understanding of how the infections to which they are prone may be spread and what the signs and symptoms are which indicate they may have a disease. For example, a sexually active person requires information about the transmission of gonorrhea and how he or she can recognize the presence of gonorrheal infection.

Patient-family teaching also includes simple, realistic explanations of those control measures necessary to protect noninfected persons living in the household of an infected person. Barrier techniques needed to prevent spread of infec-

tion should be demonstrated by the health worker; return demonstration by the patient or family is essential.[18] For example, in a household where streptococcal sore throat is being passed from child to child, the health worker would teach handwashing and techniques for bagging and burning tissues soiled with exudate. It would also be appropriate to emphasize the importance of keeping separate the dishes and silverware used by the ill children and of washing their eating utensils in hot sudsy water.

The community health nurse is always involved in *case finding*. She recognizes symptom patterns indicative of those infectious diseases common to her client population. She identifies those neighborhoods or households with high incidence of disease and then works in those settings to break the infection chain. Some community nurses are involved in epidemiological investigations of the source and patterns of spread of diseases such as infectious hepatitis or tuberculosis.[18]

Finally, the community health nurse *follows patients with infections after their discharge from the hospital* into the community. For example, patients with tuberculosis or hepatitis may be only briefly hospitalized for initial therapy. The gradual home convalescence of these persons requires ongoing physical and psychosocial assessment by the nurse in addition to assessment of the patients' consistent compliance with the therapeutic plan. The community nurse implements an ongoing plan of care based on needs as they develop.

Protection for the Nurse

A nurse must maintain optimum personal resistance against infection. This includes taking responsibility for keeping immunizations current and having periodic physical examinations. The nurse's personal health program should include appropriate skin tests for tuberculosis and screening for those infectious diseases to which she is exposed. A staff health service program within health agencies offers these services to protect the nurse from infected patients and to protect patients from infection by the nurse.

The nurse also protects herself against infection by practicing good general hygiene and sound isolation technique at work. Necessary hygiene measures to diminish spread of infection include frequent appropriate handwashing, keeping hands away from hair and face, wearing a clean uniform. The remainder of this chapter focuses on sound isolation technique.

All nurses need to examine their own lifestyle for factors designed to maximize health and resistance to infection. Personal patterns concerning diet, rest, activity, smoking, use of drugs, and other life habits are all subject to scrutiny.

> *A nurse must guard against being a vehicle of infection!*

The ill nurse should not be in contact with patients. Diseases characterized by profuse sneezing, coughing, or frequent diarrhea mean that the nurse must stay home to care for herself rather than going to work and spreading her infection to patients and co-workers.

TECHNICAL CONCEPTS VITAL TO ISOLATION

Definitions of "Clean" and "Contaminated"

All isolation precautions are based on considering some areas to be free from pathogens, i.e., "clean," and other areas to be "contaminated" with pathogens. An area is designated as contaminated only on the basis of a clear understanding of how the infecting organism is transmitted. Definitions of "contaminated" have changed as our knowledge of disease spread has sharpened. An excellent example is tuberculosis. For many years the TB patient was subjected to elaborate isolation precautions. It was assumed that the organism was present in the surrounding air and on all surfaces of the patient's room. All of these areas therefore were labeled "contaminated" and barriers were placed between them and the clean person entering the tuberculosis patient's room. We now know that the TB organism is spread only through airborne droplet nuclei. Therefore, only the air is labeled as contaminated, i.e., considered to be contaminated and reacted to as contaminated. Particles that settle on the surfaces of objects in the patient's environment are known to be killed

quickly by drying, heat, and light. Such objects are not labeled as contaminated and no special barriers are needed to protect "clean" people from contacting such items.[29]

> *Any time something "clean" contacts an area defined as "contaminated," the previously clean object is immediately assumed to be contaminated and anything it subsequently touches also becomes contaminated. To avoid this "snowballing" effect, barrier techniques are used in caring for a patient requiring isolation.*

The most commonly used barriers include: handwashing; confining ("isolating") the patient in a private room; use of gown, mask, and/or gloves; and "double bagging" all contaminated materials. Each of these techniques is described in following sections. However, prior to discussing these specific barrier techniques, the major categories of isolation precautions will be presented.

All information on isolation precautions is derived directly from the 1975 recommendations of the National Center for Disease Control. These recommendations are revised continually as new knowledge develops regarding disease spread and the actual effectiveness of barrier techniques. Isolation categories are summarized in Table 45–2.

Categories of Isolation when the Patient Is Infected

The barrier techniques used for each category are determined by understanding what is contaminated. Figure 45–2 contrasts areas considered contaminated in three categories: *strict, respiratory,* and *wound and skin.*

Strict Isolation. The airborne and contact spread of highly communicable diseases necessitates the use of elaborate precautions in maintaining "Strict Isolation." This comprehensive type of isolation was until recently utilized for all types of infectious disease, regardless of the known method of spread. Strict isolation demands more time and materials than any other form of isolation precautions, and in 1970 it had come to be used least frequently of all the isolation categories, according to a Center for Disease Control study.[14] Table 45–2 summarizes the techniques required for strict isolation. Figure 45–2C illustrates strict isolation.

Wound and Skin Precautions. Infection spread by direct and indirect contact with puru-

TABLE 45–2. SUMMARY OF ISOLATION PRECAUTIONS

	Strict Isolation	Respiratory Isolation	Wound and Skin Precautions	Discharge Precautions—Secretion and Excretion	Enteric Precautions	Blood Precautions
Indications	Smallpox, staph or strep pneumonia, diphtheria, chickenpox, wound infections with staph or strep when dressings will not contain drainage	TB, meningococcal meningitis, measles, mumps, pertussis	Staph or strep wound infections without profuse drainage; other wound infections that are draining profusely	Viral diseases, minor skin infections, mononucleosis, venereal diseases, strep sore throat	Any infectious diarrhea, hepatitis	Hepatitis, malaria
Defined as Contaminated	Air, all equipment, supplies, furniture and exposed surfaces of room	Air only	Dressings, linens and patient clothing	Dressings and paper tissues and equipment	Fecal material	Blood
Room	Private essential, with door closed	Private essential, with door closed	Private desirable	Private unnecessary	Private for children, private not necessary for cooperative adults	Private unnecessary
Gown	Wear when entering	No	Wear for direct contact	No	Wear for direct contact	No
Mask	Wear when entering	Wear when entering	Wear for dressing changes	No	No	No
Gloves	Wear when entering	No	Wear for direct contact	No	Wear to touch bedpans, toilet, urinal	No
Equipment	Double bag	No special care	No special care unless purulent contaminations	Double bag contaminated	No special care, unless fecal contamination	Disposable syringes in one container; needles (unbent) in another; double bag reusable needles and syringes
Linen	Double bag	No special care	Double bag	No special care	Double bag	No special care
Dishes	Use disposable or double bag	No special care	No special care	No special care	Double bag or dispose in trash	No special care
Dressings and Tissues	Double bag	Double bag	Double bag	Double bag	Double bag	No special care
Urine and Feces	Flush down toilet immediately	No special care	No special care	Sanitary disposal	Flush down toilet immediately	No special care unless hepatitis wherein they should be double bagged and incinerated

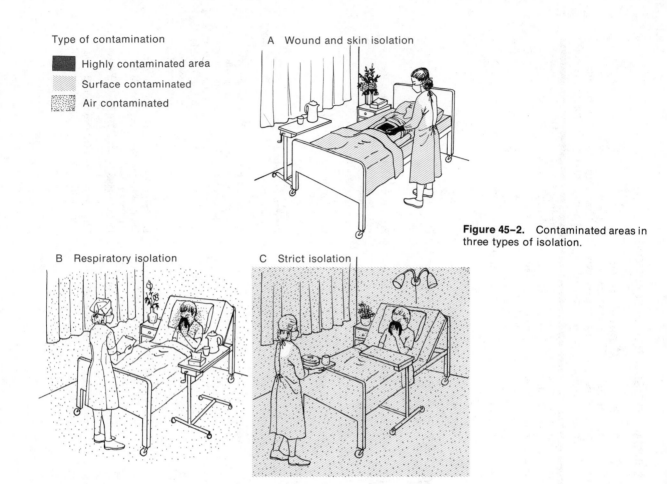

Type of contamination

▓ Highly contaminated area

▨ Surface contaminated

░ Air contaminated

A Wound and skin isolation

B Respiratory isolation

C Strict isolation

Figure 45–2. Contaminated areas in three types of isolation.

lent drainage necessitates the use of these precautions. "Wound and Skin Precautions" is the most commonly needed isolation category.[14] Table 45–2 summarizes the techniques required for wound and skin precautions, and Procedure 35 discusses this category in depth. Figure 45–2A illustrates wound and skin precautions.

35. WOUND AND SKIN PRECAUTIONS

Definition and Purposes. *Precautions used to prevent infection of other patients, visitors and staff with organisms known to be transmitted only by direct contact with wound drainage or with articles heavily contaminated by drainage.* The following conditions are indications for this type of isolation: *all* wounds or lesions with purulent drainage that can be covered with dressings that remain dry on outer surface; all profusely draining wounds that are not adequately covered by dressings, *except* beta hemolytic streptococcal infections and coagulase positive staphylococcal infections, localized herpes zoster, and gas gangrene; and extensive skin infections, e.g., impetigo with uncontrolled drainage. These latter exceptions are so contagious that *Strict Isolation* is required.

Contraindications and Cautions.   If an infected wound is very small, *Secretion Precautions* are used (p. 1183). It it becomes apparent that drainage from a staphylococcal or streptococcal infection is too profuse to be contained by dry dressings, *Strict Isolation* must be ordered (p. 1183). Never leave the patient's room with a contaminated gown on. Either remove the gown and handwash or get another staff member's assistance to bring or remove articles. Avoid vigorous movements of contaminated materials; such movements make organisms airborne. A nurse caring for a patient requiring Wound and Skin Precautions should not be assigned to a patient with lowered resistance to infection.

Patient-Family Teaching Points.   Provide the patient and family with the following information as appropriate: (a) explain clearly and simply how patient's organisms are spread by direct contact; (b) clarify what materials are considered contaminated and the special precautions needed in handling these materials; (c) for family and friends, provide step-by-step demonstrations until they master safe handwashing and gowning techniques; (d) teach the patient to wash hands whenever he comes in contact with drainage; (e) explain that procedure will be used only until drainage is no longer purulent and cultures are negative; (f) explain expected response to antibiotic therapy being used; and (g) acknowledge presence of negative feelings about isolation; encourage and accept expression of these feelings.

PRE-PROCEDURE ACTIVITIES

PRELIMINARY PATIENT ENVIRONMENT ASSESSMENT

► Determine status of infectious process from chart, e.g., temperature, leukocytosis, appearance of drainage and wound area, cultures
► Assess amount of contact will be having with patient, e.g., can enter room without gowning if not planning direct patient contact
► Determine supplies needed to take into patient's room
► Gather subjective data from patient, e.g., observations of verbal/nonverbal behaviors concerning symptoms and feelings about isolation
► Gown and glove for thorough physical assessment and/or patient care activities
► Mask for dressing change

PRELIMINARY PLANNING

► Carefully preplan to obtain supplies prior to each visit to avoid needless trips necessitating re-gowning and -gloving
► Remove rings
► Arrange for assistant to help double bag soiled linens and waste

EQUIPMENT

► Private room desirable
► Isolation label and instructions on door
► Sink, antimicrobial soap, paper towels
► Cabinet outside room with isolation gowns, (paper or cloth) masks, clean gloves, linen or plastic laundry bags and plastic trash bags, isolation labels, ties or tape, marking pen
► Moisture-proof mattress and pillow covers and furniture that is easily washable

PREPARATION OF PATIENT

► Explain why he has been placed on Wound and Skin Precautions
► Explain that he must stay in his room, but can have his door open
► Explain that individuals who have contact with him or his bed linen will wear gowns and gloves and that masks will be worn during dressing change

Procedure continued on the following page

PROCEDURE

SUGGESTED STEPS	RATIONALE/DISCUSSION

Before Entering Room

1. When *not planning contact* with patient or drainage, no special precautions are needed. But ordinary medical asepsis is observed.

1. Organisms are considered present only in drainage. Hands are washed appropriately.

2. When *planning direct contact* with patient or with materials soiled by drainage:

    a. Assemble equipment and supplies for care and dressing change.

    a. Prevents unnecessary trips in and out of patient's room.

    b. Wash hands.

    b. Soap, water and friction protect patient from additional infections.

    c. Put on isolation gown.

    c. Protects worker's uniform from possible contamination by patient's drainage.

    d. Place mask and extra gloves in bag or between layers of clean linen.

    d. Prevents contamination of mask and gloves before use.

    e. Put on clean gloves.

    e. Barrier protects nurse's hands and fingernails from massive exposure to highly concentrated organisms.

During Patient Care

1. Give hygiene care as needed.

1. Gown and gloves protect worker during direct contact with patient and his linen.

2. Use following sequence: to *change dressings:*

    a. Remove gloves and wash hands.

    a. Prevents contamination of mask and clean gloves by organisms inside moist gloves.

    b. Put on mask.

    b. Barrier protects nurse from inhaling airborne organisms when handling contaminated materials.

    c. Put on *clean gloves* to remove soiled dressings.

    c. Clean barrier protects nurse's hands since gloves used to give care may not be intact. Protects wound from other organisms.

    d. Discard soiled dressings in waterproof bag, being careful not to contaminate outside of bag. Close bag securely; put bag into wastebasket.

    d. Bag acts as barrier which immediately seals off organisms, thus reducing environmental contamination.

SUGGESTED STEPS	RATIONALE/DISCUSSION

During Patient Care (Continued)

e. Discard gloves and put on *sterile gloves.* Use sterile supplies to treat and dress wound. (See Procedures 22 and 23 and Chap. 37.)

e. Sterile barrier protects open wound from additional infectious organisms.

f. Examine wound and drainage to determine status of infection.

f. Assess the following: presence of inflammatory changes; color, consistency, and quantity of drainage; appearance of granulation tissue. (See also Chap. 42.)

g. After dressing wound, remove gloves, wash hands and remove mask.

g. Clean hands prevent contamination of helper's hair while removing mask.

2. Consider the following when *changing linens:*

a. Change gloves after handling soiled linens, whether or not linen is grossly contaminated with drainage.

a. Clean barrier protects nurse's hands and environment when highly concentrated organisms present on linens.

b. Avoid shaking linens or creating excessive air movement.

b. Shaking linens spreads organisms into air.

c. Discard soiled linens in laundry bag in patient's room, taking care not to contaminate outside of bag.

c. Linens and patient's clothing are assumed to be contaminated with drainage.

Before Leaving Patient's Room

1. Double bag linen bag with assistant when bag is two thirds full. Leave it for next worker if not sufficient soiled linen.

2. Double bag paper waste if wastebasket two thirds full.

3. Double bag accumulated equipment if contaminated by purulent material.

1. Double bagging (p. 1196) keeps outer bag completely clean and prevents cross-infection outside patient's room. Use waterproof outer bags for wet or moist trash. Use bags that can be autoclaved for instruments; discard outer bag if wet (organisms penetrate wet surface). Full linen and trash bags are difficult to handle: heavy and/or do not fit into second bag.

4. At the doorway, remove gown, and mask and gloves if worn. Discard gown in laundry; disposable gown, mask and gloves in wastebasket.

4. Wearing contaminated clothing outside patient's room would spread infection.

5. Be sure to wash hands thoroughly. Remember: sink handles are contaminated; handle them only with dry paper towel after washing.

> *Clean hands are the best means of preventing cross-infection to other patients and workers.*

Procedure continued on the following page

SUGGESTED STEPS	RATIONALE/DISCUSSION

When the Patient Leaves His Room

1. Apply fresh dressings just prior to transport of patient. Apply sufficient dressings to absorb drainage, so that outer surface of dressings will remain dry.	1. Fresh, abundant dressings control drainage, preventing spread of organisms to environment.
2. Patient can be transported in wheelchair or stretcher. Cover wheelchair or stretcher with clean sheet, assist patient to vehicle and wrap him in sheet. Cover with another clean sheet if needed to cover entire body.	2. Prevent direct contact of patient or his contaminated clothing.

Post-Procedure Activities. Hands should be thoroughly washed one final time before returning to general environment or caring for another patient. When the patient is discharged, the entire room is terminally disinfected (p. 1198).

Final Patient Assessment. Before leaving patient's room *thoroughly assess* patient's comfort and need for additional care or supplies. Thorough assessment at this time can prevent unnecessary re-donning of protective garb.

Chart/Report. Appropriate observations of: (a) patient's infectious condition (such as wound appearance) and (b) patient's psychosocial condition (reactions to his illness and his isolation).

Respiratory Isolation. Infection spread by airborne droplets necessitates the use of this isolation category. Table 45–2 summarizes the techniques required. Precautions used for tuberculosis are modified to exclude the need to wear a mask as long as the patient can control his cough or secretions; tissues are carefully disposed of. Room ventilation must be controlled to move air outside the building. Some authorities require ultraviolet lighting to be on at all times. The door is closed and the patient is masked when he leaves his room. Figure 45–2B illustrates Respiratory Isolation.

Enteric Precautions. Highly contagious infection spread by oral ingestion of fecal material necessitates the use of this category. See Table 45–2 for details. In the case of hepatitis, Blood Precautions are also required. An example of the way in which fecal material may be ingested is if a person handles food with hands that are unwashed after touching fecal matter or fecal contaminated objects, e.g., bed pans.

Discharge Precautions. This category includes three subdivisions: (1) *Secretion precautions for lesions,* used with less contagious infections that are spread by direct and indirect contact with wound drainage, (2) *Secretion precautions for oral secretions,* used for less contagious diseases spread by direct and indirect contact with nasotracheal discharges, (3) Excretion precautions, used with less contagious infections spread by ingestion of *fecal* material. Table 45–2 summarizes the techniques required. Handwashing is the critical barrier technique with this category; special garments are not indicated.

Blood Precautions. Infection spread by the parenteral injection of infected blood or serum necessitates precautions in this category. The emphasis is on safe disposal of contaminated needles and syringes. Table 45–2 summarizes the required techniques.

Isolation to Protect a Person with Diminished Resistance

Protective Isolation. This category of isolation is also called "Reverse Isolation" because it is just the opposite of caring for an infected patient. With protective isolation, the environment is considered to be the source of potential infection threatening a patient with diminished defenses. The environment and all persons except the patient are considered to be contaminated, and the patient and his area are maintained as clean. Procedure 36 discusses the rationale and procedures for Reverse Isolation.

36. PROTECTIVE ISOLATION (REVERSE ISOLATION)

Definition and Purposes. *Precautions used to prevent infection of a patient who is unusually susceptible to infection owing to his impaired defense mechanism.* Such patients are vulnerable to infection by organisms not normally considered to be "pathogenic." Three kinds of mechanisms underlie diminished resistance to infection: (1) massive destruction of skin as first line of defense; (2) impaired production of white blood cells, with consequent reduced phagocytosis and/or antibody production and (3) suppression of the normal inflammatory response. Protective isolation is used for the following conditions: (a) presence of burns; extensive dermatitis; leukemia (malignancy of leukocytes); leukopenia (profound drop in number of leukocytes); agranulocytosis (profound drop in number of leukocytes made in the marrow) and (b) administration of radiation therapy, massive doses of adrenal corticosteroids (e.g., hydrocortisone) or high doses of anti-neoplastic drugs. Protective isolation techniques are designed to protect the patient from potentially pathogenic organisms present in the environment outside the patient's room and carried by persons entering the patient's room. These techniques are directed at eliminating transmission of pathogens by direct contact and/or droplet spread.

Cautions. Protective isolation should be instituted as soon as impaired resistance to infection is suspected. Protective precautions must be meticulously followed, since exposure to potential pathogens may be life-threatening for the patient. Health workers known to have infections should *never* care for patients requiring protective isolation. Workers caring for patients in protective isolation should never be assigned to simultaneously care for a patient with an infection.

Patient-Family Teaching Points. Provide the patient-family with the following information as appropriate: (a) explain why patient is in protective isolation and how long precautions will be necessary, e.g., until white blood cell levels return to predetermined safe level; (b) explain clearly and simply how potentially hazardous organisms can be spread to the patient by direct contact and/or airborne routes; (c) explain rationale for each precaution; (d) for family and friends, provide step-by-step

Procedure continued on the following page

demonstration and have them give return demonstrations until they master safe handwashing, gowning, and masking techniques; (e) teach patient to conscientiously handwash, especially after elimination, to avoid cross-infection from one part of his body to another; (f) explain why visitors are minimized and why persons with known infections are not permitted in room; and (g) acknowledge patient's anxieties and fears about his disorder and his isolation (e.g., fears of succumbing to infection), and encourage and accept expression of these feelings.

PRE-PROCEDURE ACTIVITIES

PRELIMINARY PATIENT ASSESSMENT

▶ Make initial rapid check of room supplies and patient needs while standing in doorway briefly.
▶ To *thoroughly* assess room supplies and patient, handwash, gown, glove and mask *before* entering patient room.
▶ Determine patient's status of immunity and indications of infection from chart, e.g., check white blood cell counts, temperature, character of body secretions.

PRELIMINARY PLANNING

▶ Carefully pre-plan to obtain supplies prior to each visit to avoid needless trips necessitating regowning, gloving, and masking.
▶ Remove rings (organisms can grow under them; they may injure patient or tear gloves).

PREPARATION OF PATIENT

▶ Explain why he has been placed in protective isolation; explain that he must stay in his room with the door closed.
▶ Explain that all individuals who enter his room must wear gowns, masks, gloves, etc., to protect him.
▶ Explain that there are always staff members on the unit and that his requests will be handled as soon as possible. Show him how to signal the staff.

EQUIPMENT

▶ Private room vital
▶ Isolation label and instruction on door
▶ Sink, antimicrobial soap, paper towels
▶ Cabinet outside room with clean isolation gowns, masks, gloves
▶ For burn cases, cabinet also may contain sterile linens and sterile patient gowns
▶ Moisture-proof mattress and pillow cover and furniture that is easily washable
▶ Make certain all materials to be brought into room are clean
▶ Whenever possible keep equipment, like blood pressure cuffs, in the patient's room for his individual reuse; otherwise scrub equipment with germicide first
▶ Occasionally, caps and booties may be worn by worker.

PROCEDURE

SUGGESTED STEPS	RATIONALE/DISCUSSION

Before Entering Room (for any reason)

1. Wash hands.

1. Soap, water and friction help protect patient from potential pathogens carried by hands.

SUGGESTED STEPS	RATIONALE/DISCUSSION

Before Entering Room (Continued)

2. Put on a clean isolation gown.	2. Worker's uniform is considered to be contaminated with potential pathogens and must be covered with a clean barrier. Sterile gowns are occasionally used to protect burn wounds.
3. Put on a mask.	3. Droplets from worker's respiratory tract can contain potential pathogens.
4. Enter room and close door.	4. Door remains closed at all times; air currents may carry pathogens into room.

During Patient Care

1. Put on clean gloves for direct patient contact.	1. Since handwashing cannot eliminate all hand and nail organisms, gloves provide additional protective barrier.
2. Change mask if touched or becomes wet and every 20 minutes.	2. Masks become a source of droplet spread.
3. Put on *sterile* gloves to care for open wounds; use meticulous sterile technique. (See Procedure 23.)	3. Absolutely no pathogens should be introduced; open wound is unprotected portal of entry to body.
4. Use sterile linens and sterile gown for patients with massive skin destruction, e.g., burns.	4. Unsterile linens and gowns carry organisms which could infect patient.
5. Continually assess patient for indications of developing infection.	5. Despite protective precautions, *the patient environment* is not sterile. Chances of cross-infection are diminished but not eliminated. Patient may also be infected by his *own resident organisms.*

> *Worker must* constantly *assess and* immediately *report* early *indications of:* pulmonary infections, urinary tract infections, wound and skin infections, hepatitis, inflammations at the IV site, septicemia and septic shock.

Worker should *immediately* have cultured body discharges which appear abnormal, e.g., potentially infected, purulent.

After Leaving Patient's Room

1. Close the door.	1. Closed door provides barrier to airborne spread of infection.

Procedure continued on the following page

SUGGESTED STEPS	RATIONALE/DISCUSSION

After Leaving Patient's Room (Continued)

2. Remove and discard gown in laundry, discard mask and gloves in trash.	2. Barriers are no longer needed.
3. Wash hands.	3. Protects other patients and workers from possible cross-infection.

When the Patient Leaves His Room

1. Transport patient from his room only when absolutely essential.	1. Patient's survival is severely jeopardized by any contact with pathogens.
2. If transport is necessary, have patient put on clean isolation gown, mask and gloves before leaving his room. Cover patient completely (except face) in clean (sterile) sheet if on stretcher or in wheelchair. Have patient thoroughly handwash upon return to his room.	2. Protects patient's clothing, hands, and respiratory tract. With exposed burns, a sterile gown is donned. Handwashing further diminishes organisms transmitted by contact.

Post-Procedure Activities. When laboratory reports or clinical signs indicate that the patient no longer is unusually susceptible to infection, protective isolation is discontinued. Room, supplies and equipment are cleaned and handled as with terminal cleaning for any noninfectious patient.

Final Patient Assessment. Before leaving patient's room thoroughly assess his comfort and need for additional care or supplies. Thorough assessment at this time can prevent unnecessary re-donning of protective garb.

Chart/Report. Appropriate observations indicating (a) any signs of developing infection and (b) patient's psychosocial condition (reactions to his illness and isolation).

Special Protected Environments. Portable plastic units or tents, like the famous "Life Island," have been designed to completely enclose a patient and his bed and provide an impermeable barrier to microorganisms in the environment. The patient is cared for by gloves attached to armports, and sterilized equipment is passed through portholes. No gowning or gloving is required since staff members do not directly contact the patient. The patient is not visually isolated from others, but mobility is restricted.[10] These patient isolator units are found in experimental settings where aggressive therapy is being tried for patients with grave bone marrow depression. Levine found in 1973 that "[leukemic] patients treated within a protected environment and given an extensive prophylactic antimicrobial regimen have approximately one half as many severe infections and one fourth as many life-threatening infections as patients treated conventionally."[19] The Center for Disease Control notes in 1975 that protective isolator units may be useful for very high risk patients "who have

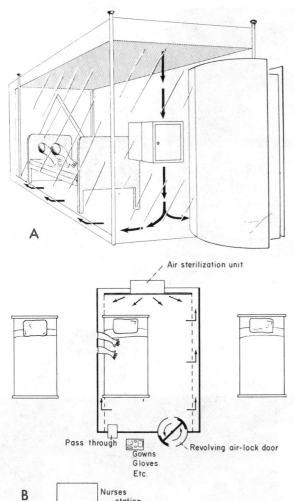

Air sterilization unit

Pass through

Gowns
Gloves
Etc.

Revolving air-lock door

Nurses
station

B

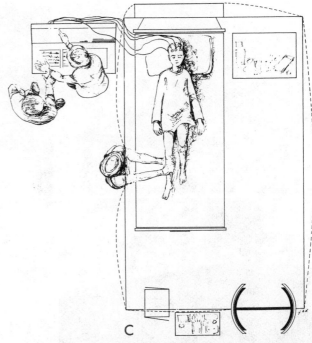

C

Figure 45–3. *A,* Bacteria-free nursing unit. Arrows indicate direction of airflow in the room and in the return ducts. Walls are of clear, flexible, plastic sheet perforated at armports, pass-throughs, and equipment taps. Revolving door at the front of the unit permits access in case of emergency. *B,* Bacteria-free nursing unit set up on an open ward. *C,* Bacteria-free nursing unit in use. Nurse is dressing an infected burn on the patient's leg while an electroencephalogram is being obtained by technicians. Note that no protective clothing or equipment is needed. (From Burke, J.: Bacteria-free nursing unit—a new approach to isolation procedures. *Hospitals, 43*:87, Jan. 1969.)

a predictable temporary period of high susceptibility." They are not needed for most patients. Such a unit is illustrated in Figure 45–3.

Handwashing

Washing of hands is "the single most important means of preventing the spread of infection."[27] The actual technique of handwashing is discussed in Chapter 25, Procedure 6. Hands are the greatest source of cross-infection from all organisms that are spread by the contact route.

Certain elements of handwashing require emphasis when you are caring for an infected person in isolation. Hands should always be washed before providing care and when leaving the room. Always wash hands after contact with any body discharges, to avoid transferring them to a new body site. Faucet handles are considered to be grossly contaminated. It is thus essential to turn off the faucet handles with a paper towel held in the hand rather than with the bare hand. Meticulous cleansing of hands and nails with at least 15 seconds of friction is vital. Rings and watches should not be worn when caring for an infected person in isolation.

The Private Room

A single room is essential for patients requiring Strict Isolation, Respiratory Isolation, and Protective Isolation. It is considered to be desirable for maintaining Enteric and Wound and

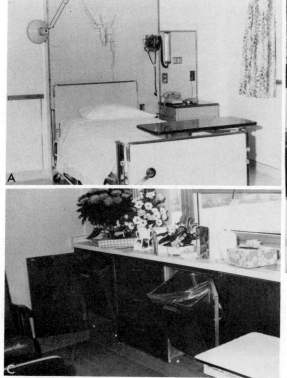

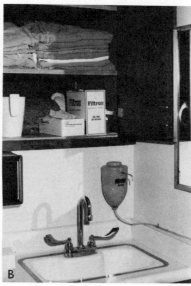

Figure 45–4. Isolation rooms. *A*, Private room with or without anteroom. *B*, Anteroom with supply cupboard and sink. *C*, Private room with anteroom having linen and waste bins opening to outside of building for removal of waste and linen. (From Dubay, E., and Grubb, R.: *Infection Prevention and Control.* St. Louis, C. V. Mosby, 1973.)

Figure 45–5. Isolation cart used when private room has no anteroom. (From Dubay, E., and Grubb, R.: *Infection Prevention and Control.*)

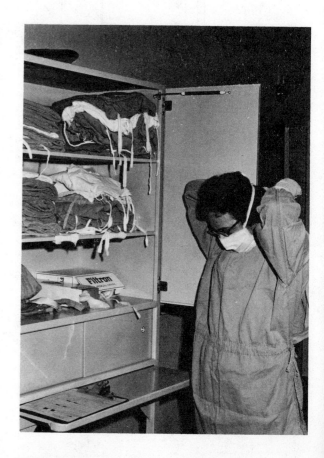

Skin Isolation. A single room is unnecessary for Discharge Precautions and Blood Precautions.[27]

A private isolation room should include washing and toilet facilities and should have its own ventilation system. An anteroom, a small chamber between the hallway and the patient's room, diminishes the exchange of airborne organisms into the corridor from the isolation room or from the corridor into the isolation room. An anteroom also provides storage space for items such as gowns, masks, gloves, paper sacks, laundry bags, plastic isolation bags, labels. When an anteroom is not present, a storage cart is placed just outside the room in the corridor. On the door of the isolation room a color-coded label is placed to identify the type of isolation required and the main precautions necessary for that isolation. Figures 45–4 and 45–5 show the isolation room and cart.

Gown, Mask, and Gloves

The Isolation Gown. The gown is freshly laundered or is disposable. It is made with long sleeves, a long skirt, and a high neck to completely cover the clothing of the wearer. When worn by the nurse caring for a person whose infection is known to be spread by indirect contact, the gown protects the nurse's clean uniform from contamination by the patient's pathogen. When worn by the infected person as he is transported outside his room, the gown prevents the patient's contaminated clothing from touching clean areas. When worn by the nurse caring for a person whose resistance to infection is diminished, the gown prevents the patient from contact with any organisms that could be on the nurse's uniform.

> *Isolation gowns should be used only once and then discarded. They are also discarded if wet.*

The older practice of reusing gowns by allowing them to hang in the patient's room between wearing is no longer recommended. An adequate supply of gowns is stored just outside the patient area. For strict isolation, watches and rings are removed before the isolation gown is donned. The gown is tied securely at the neck and overlapped at the back before tying the waist strings. The gown is removed by first untying the contaminated waist strings, washing hands, then untying the uncontaminated neck strings and pulling the gown down from the shoulders, turning it inside out as it is removed from the arms. The gown is held away

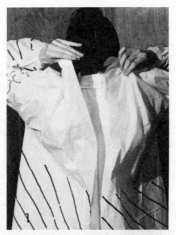

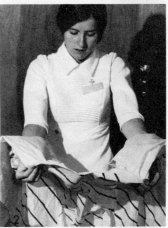

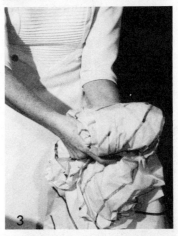

Figure 45–6. Steps in removing isolation gown. 1, With clean hands, untie the strings of your gown. 2, Grasp the top of the gown at the shoulders and pull the gown down over the arms and inside out. Draw each hand out separately. 3, Fold the gown with the contaminated portion inside and discard. (Reprinted with permission from the May 1975 issue of Nursing '75, © by Intermed Communications, Inc., 132 Welsh Rd., Horsham, PA 19044. Further reproduction in whole or part expressly prohibited by law.)

from the uniform, rolled up and discarded (Fig. 45–6).

The Mask. Whenever an infection is spread by airborne droplets or particles, the isolation mask should be worn securely over the nose and mouth. Masks are available in a variety of materials and styles. Mask materials range from gauze fiber to glass and synthetic fiber, designed to filter out airborne organisms.[15] The effectiveness of a wet mask is impaired; in fact, a wet mask is considered a hazard to the wearer and patient. Thus a new mask should be donned whenever the mask being worn becomes wet, e.g., from moisture of breathing, or when it has been worn for 20 minutes. When change of mask is anticipated, extra masks are taken into the unit. These masks must be protected in a plastic bag or between layers of clean linen. If the working part of the mask is touched by the wearer, it is considered contaminated and must be changed.

Isolation masks should be discarded after each use. Do not wear a mask longer than 20 minutes.

An adequate supply of masks is stored just outside the patient area. Masks are fitted securely over the nose and mouth and tied in a manner that prevents slipping. The mask is removed by first washing hands and then touching only the uncontaminated ties to untie and discard it.

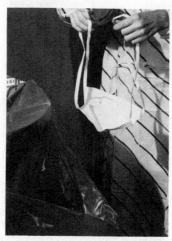

Figure 45–7. Proper disposal of masks. After untying the mask, grasp it only by the strings to discard. (Reprinted with permission from the May 1975 issue of Nursing '75, © 1975 by Intermed Communications, Inc., 132 Welsh Rd., Horsham, PA 19044. Further reproduction in whole or part expressly prohibited by law.)

The front of the mask should not be touched, since it is assumed to be contaminated by airborne pathogens. Figure 45–7 illustrates proper disposal of masks.

The Gloves. Single use (i.e., disposable) nonsterile gloves are worn in isolation: (a) whenever the helper's hands come into contact with highly contaminated areas or (b) to protect the person with poor resistance from the organisms on the helper's hands. Gloves are used in addition to thorough handwashing because of the risk of organisms remaining under fingernails. Also helper's hands which are exposed to larger numbers of pathogens soon have these pathogens as resident flora on their hands. An adequate supply of gloves is stored just outside the patient area. Gloves are changed after each contact with bodily discharges, to avoid cross-infecting the patient with his own organisms. For example, gloves used while cleansing the perineum should not be used in feeding the patient. Gloves must be changed between the two activities. The helper's hands should always be washed thoroughly after gloves are removed because pathogens on the normal skin multiply rapidly in the dark, moist environment of the gloves.

Sterile gloves are worn in isolation to care for any open wound. Even if that wound is already infected, additional organisms may be brought to the area unless meticulous attention is given to sterile technique. Sterile gloves would also, of course, be worn to perform any procedure requiring sterile technique, e.g., catheterization (see Chap. 37).

Double Bagging

All contaminated materials are "double bagged," i.e., placed in two bags, one inside the other. Both bags must be completely intact. Waterproof bags are used when possible. Paper bags are used for *dry* instruments or equipment; if paper bags become wet, they are considered contaminated.

The inner bag is considered contaminated and is handled only by contaminated hands or gloved hands. The outer bag is considered clean and is safely handled by a helper outside the contaminated unit and placed in an uncontaminated environment.

The outer bag must be tightly closed, sealed, and labeled before being sent to laundry, central supply, or the incinerator.

The procedure of "double bagging" takes some practice. An assistant stands outside the

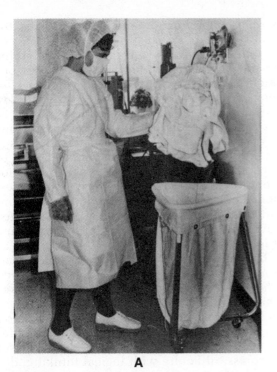

A

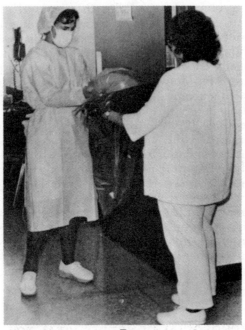

B

Figure 45–8. Double bagging technique. *A,* Placing contaminated linen into bag within the unit. *B,* Transferring bag to plastic container at door of unit. (From Elhart, Dorothy; Firsich, Sharon Cannell; Gragg, Shirley Hawke; and Rees, Olive M.: Scientific Principles in Nursing, ed. 8, St. Louis, 1978, The C. V. Mosby Co.)

door of the patient's unit, cuffs the outer bag, which is a clean plastic or paper sack or laundry bag, over her hands and holds the bag widely open. Careful not to touch the assistant, the "contaminated" helper places the closed or sealed inner bag of contaminated laundry, trash, or equipment into the outer clean bag. The "contaminated" helper may touch the *inside* of the outer bag to widen the opening. Then the assistant proceeds to close the outer bag with slow smooth movements that do not eject pathogens into the air or into her face. She does not touch the inside of the bag and holds everything away from herself. The outer bag is closed, and the completed double bag is then labeled with a sticker or marked clearly "isolation."

> Caution: *Do not refer to personnel as "contaminated," "dirty" or "clean," as this intensifies patient's feeling of being soiled, dirty or untouchable.*

Double bagged isolation linen is placed with regular soiled linen. Double bagged isolation waste is placed with other hospital waste to be incinerated. Double bagged isolation equipment is labeled with type of isolation and a list

of all equipment enclosed and placed where it can be picked up by central service. Equipment that must be autoclaved before handling must be packaged in material that can be autoclaved.

Caps and Booties

The Center for Disease Control does not recommend the covering of the nurse's head and her shoes except when observing smallpox precautions and occasionally for protecting the person with extremely poor resistance. However, hair should be pinned up so that it does not touch the collar.

Concurrent and Terminal Disinfection

Concurrent Disinfection. Isolated patient areas should be carefully cleaned once daily; in particular, the floor and sinks are highly contaminated and must be disinfected with germicidal detergent and scouring powder by housekeeping personnel. Germicidal detergents used on smooth hard surfaces include quaternary ammonium, iodophor, phenolic solution, and sodium hypochlorite. Concurrent disinfection also includes the removal of all wastes, soiled linens, and dirty equipment in double bags as discussed above. This task is performed at regular intervals as a joint responsibility of nursing and housekeeping personnel. Protective Isolation requires meticulous concurrent disinfection with a clean mop and cleaning equipment.

Terminal Disinfection. Following the discharge, transfer, or death of the infected patient, the isolation room is thoroughly cleansed by housekeeping personnel. All equipment is either discarded, returned to central supply in double bags, or washed with a germicidal detergent. Furniture, mattress and pillow covers and waterproof draw sheet are washed with germicidal detergents. Floors are wet vacuumed or mopped with a germicidal detergent. Curtains and shades or blinds are washed.

PSYCHOSOCIAL CONCEPTS VITAL TO ISOLATION

The Impact of Confinement

As indicated before, isolation precautions often demand that the patient remain alone in a private room. Patients in Strict Isolation or Protective Isolation must be confined in a single room with the door closed at all times. All human contacts must be masked and gowned. Transportation to other departments is discouraged, and if unavoidable, demands that the patient be enclosed in protective garments. Respiratory Isolation requires a private room and masking of all who enter. The patient must wear a mask when being transported elsewhere. A private room is highly desirable to prevent cross-infection with Wound and Skin Isolation and Enteric precautions. A child with diarrhea must be confined alone.

Confinement causes reduced sensory input and reduced human interaction. The isolated patient experiences these reductions and requires nursing care directed at minimizing these aspects of isolation.

Reduced Sensory Input. When a person's world is contracted to a single small hospital room, both the quantity and quality of stimuli are diminished. Consider how monotonous it would be to stay alone in a small, uninteresting room 24 hours a day, day after day. What would you look at? There would be walls, floor,

perhaps a picture on the wall, perhaps the hands of the clock. If you were fortunate, you might have a window with a view of something besides a brick wall, and hopefully your bed might provide a view out of a window. How long would you be entertained by the window view and a television? Sounds would be restricted to those from television or radio and perhaps outside traffic noises and some hospital corridor noises. Human contacts would be severely reduced, and many types of isolation would demand that all people appear faceless beneath a mask and all shrouded in the same uni-color, uni-sex long-sleeved, long-skirted gown. All of this sounds frightfully boring, and it is.

Disturbing psychosocial effects may come from the prolonged sensory deprivation necessitated by isolation precautions. Resultant *emotional changes* may range from anxiety, to mood swings, irritability and anger, and depression. *Cognitive changes* resulting from deprivation of meaningful stimuli can include decreased alertness, difficulty with logical thinking, distorted ideas, and distorted perceptions.[7] Inadequate "external" stimuli may lead the patient to direct increased attention "inward" to his bodily sensations, and the patient may complain more about discomfort than he would under more normal circumstances. He also may be more easily aggravated by mildly unpleasant stimuli, such as the crying of a confused patient down the hall or the noise of nurses' chatting; if such stimuli are among the few the patient experiences, they may come to dominate his consciousness.

Nursing care to diminish problems resulting from reduced sensory input in an isolation room begins with assessment of the environment and of the patient's behavior. Analyze the auditory and visual inputs in the environment for variety and the meaning that they may have for the individual. How much change is there in the sights and sounds of the patient's daily experience? Is outward stimulus so uninteresting that the person can be expected to turn inward? Can the patient relate to the environment, or is it totally alien, without familiar objects and people? The more restricted the sensory environment, the more predictable are deviant changes in behavior. Without planned orientation, the person whose eyes are both patched after eye surgery often becomes extremely confused and agitated. A major source of sensory input has been suddenly removed. Critically examine behavior patterns during activities of daily living, general conversation, verbalization to staff and visitors, sleep patterns. The causes of cognitive and emotional changes from normal become more difficult to assess as the patient's illness is more severe. This is because variables appear such as fever, drug toxicity, acidosis and hypoxia, which impair functioning of the brain and produce consequent abnormal behavior. Never assume that a patient's behavior is caused by a single factor, such as sensory deprivation, without careful validation of that assumption.

Nursing intervention to minimize the effects of reduced sensory input focuses on two goals: (1) to increase the quality and quantity of environmental stimuli and (2) to diminish behavioral problems. Very often if the first goal is met, the second will also be.

Approaches to meet the first goal are determined by environmental assessment, as just discussed. Consider creative ways to enrich the patient's environment visually and with sound in ways that would be most pleasant for and interesting to the individual. Examples include placing in the room pictures from home or drawings of the patient's children or playing favorite records or tapes. News of the outside world should be emphasized and discussed if the patient is able to carry on conversation. Magazines and newspapers help provide such news. Telephone contact with significant others should be encouraged. A clock and calendar help in time orientation. An occupational therapy consultant is most helpful in finding meaningful recreational activities.

Traditionally, isolation rooms have remained barren of aesthetic or personal things because it was assumed that such things would have to be burned or autoclaved afterward to prevent cross-infection. The National Center for Disease Control now notes that only those articles *visibly* contaminated with infected material need to be destroyed or disinfected.[27] As will be further discussed below, meaningful human contacts significantly decrease sensory deprivation.

The second goal of diminishing behavioral problems focuses directly on assessment of the patient's behavior. Possible approaches are highly varied and should be individualized. It is vital to provide the alert patient with an opportunity: (a) to explore emotional or thinking disturbances that he has noticed and that have troubled him, (b) to learn that the causes of such disturbances are environmental and (c) to plan together for relief. Approaches for the less alert or less cooperative patient will include the ongoing use of reorientation techniques and repeated explanation. Uncooperative and belligerent behavior should be understood as possible consequences of confinement. In addition to increasing stimuli, techniques directed at reducing such behaviors range from behavioral modification to use of restraints (as a last resort). (Restraints are discussed in Chapter 43.)

Reduced Human Interaction. The decrease in quality and number of human contacts is really the most profound deprivation experienced by the isolated patient. All the emotional and cognitive changes catalogued under "reduced sensory input" are certainly relevant. For instance, a patient might become irritable or depressed; his thinking may be distorted, with increased focus on self. In addition, forced isolation from human companionship is often a tremendously lonely experience. The isolated patient is denied the physical presence of those who have always sustained him, at a time when he is desperately in need of support. The person who has always surrounded himself with others may be alone with himself for the first time. A child's vivid encounter with loneliness is quoted by Clark Moustakas:

Empty, that's how it feels to be lonely. A sense of being in a deep dark pit, with nothing in sight, and no way out. It feels like a dark rainy day. Just there, just sitting there lonely. It's like a blue, a dark blue almost a black, but then it's a light blue washed out and dingy. It's a deep empty pit in your stomach.

Loneliness brings thinking. When lonely I feel like thinking. Not anything special, just thinking—

Loneliness leaves some after effects. Mostly just a tired feeling. Not wanting to talk to anyone, not wanting to do anything. But, most of them can be remedied by just starting to do something. Something that you like to do.[23]

The manifestations of loneliness are subtle and highly variable; they may be recognized as a strong, ongoing nurse-patient relationship develops. An insightful patient may discuss the loneliness directly; other people may use a variety of coping mechanisms to deal with the consequent anxiety. An isolated child's preoccupations and need for withdrawal are quite normal, though often painful, responses.

Nursing intervention for an isolated patient should focus on diminishing the pain of loneliness. Nursing plans include maintaining quality interactions between the patient and staff members and encouraging visits by friends and family. Of course, all visitors must be taught meticulous observance of isolation precautions. All staff members who go into the room should introduce themselves to the patient. Greeting the patient briefly from the doorway before putting on a mask is one way to minimize the patient's feelings of being subjected to a group of faceless healers. In spite of all of these efforts, confinement in an isolation room and the associated crisis of illness will result in a certain inevitable degree of loneliness for the patient. The enforced opportunity for reflection and encounter with oneself may bring new insights to the patient about his life. A nursing relationship that facilitates dialogue may also facilitate exploration of these developing thoughts with the nurse. (Therapeutic nurse-patient relationship is discussed in Chapter 3.)

Labelling a Patient as "Infected" and "Contaminated"

The experience of being separated from other persons because the illness one has poses a "danger" to others can be very troubling for a patient. In addition to feeling he is "dangerous" or "threatening," the isolated patient is also constantly reminded that he is "dirty" because others wear protective garments when they come near him. The necessity for others to wear gloves implies to the patient that he is "untouchable." The rituals involved when others enter the patient's room may make a patient feel that it is inconvenient to care for him and that he is "burdensome." Some infectious diseases still carry with them a negative social stigma which lowers a patient's self-esteem; this is especially true of venereal diseases, hepatitis, and tuberculosis. Many people, including unfortunately many health professionals, will label such patients as "unworthy and socially unacceptable"; the patients may see themselves in the same light.[6] For whatever reason, the contaminated label will impair self-image and will cause the isolated person to feel varying degrees of shame and guilt.

In caring for isolated patients the skillful nurse is attentive to manifestations of shame and guilt that the persons may feel. Shame and guilt may be manifested through body language indicating withdrawal, speech difficulties, and nervous gestures.[17] Nursing intervention focuses on acknowledging the feelings, encouraging expression of distress and exploring causes, and doing everything possible to affirm the person's dignity and sense of worth as an individual. The isolated person should always be called by name and be actively involved in decision making about his care. Physical appearance should be enhanced to maintain the patient's self-image.

Special Problems of Children in Isolation

The isolation experience is especially traumatic for a child. Because he is so dependent on family to meet basic needs, abandonment is an overwhelming threat. To minimize emotional trauma, the nurse should welcome parental visiting. Isolation precautions need not preclude the parents rooming-in with the child, if they are conscientiously taught to master the necessary precautionary techniques.

A *baby* confined in isolation is in great need of the mother's ongoing care, since his identity is not yet separate from the mother. Mobiles, toys, and music help enrich the environment of a baby's isolation room.

Developmentally, *preschool* children are acquiring a sense of autonomy and independence. They need clear, simple explanations of procedures. It is important that these children be offered as many realistic opportunities as possible to make decisions about care activities and be as independent as possible with activities of daily living.[26] The mother's supportive presence is vital.

School age children also need to receive such maternal support and to take an active part in their own care. Peer relationships are growing in importance at this age and continued contact with peers through telephone and written messages can be helpful. Developmentally the school age child is growing toward a sense of industry and struggling to overcome feelings of inferiority. Unfortunately, a child's sense of inferiority is reinforced by isolation procedures which give the child a sense of being dirty and untouchable. Invasion by germs may be difficult and frightening for the child to understand.[26] Time must be spent visiting with, explaining, and listening to the child in isolation so that he understands the situation and feels himself acceptable.

When Staff Members Avoid the Isolated Patient

Patients requiring isolation precautions are not easy to care for. The most simple nursing measures are complicated by the awkwardness of barriers like gowning, masking, or wearing gloves; by handwashing at a frequency likely to be tedious; and by the inconvenience of finding an assistant and double bagging every time materials must be removed from the patient area. The nurse caring for a person requiring isolation precautions is thus prone to be a bit busier and more tired than her colleagues! At times, staff members may tend to visit the isolated person less frequently than the other patients because of the inconvenience of techniques.

In addition to the inconveniences of isolation precautions, the nurse caring for patients in isolation must face her own feelings as she copes with the impact of her own confinement and the implication of the disease itself as she perceives it. Some nurses may find themselves feeling isolated while alone providing care for an isolated patient! All nurses must deal with their conscious and unconscious fears of contracting infection; these fears may be accentuated when caring for a person with a socially condemned illness, such as gonorrhea. The fearful nurse may tend to avoid or greatly minimize contact with the isolated patient. Whatever their own feelings, nurses caring for isolated persons need to be resourceful in dealing with the patient's behavior deviations that may develop as a result of isolation. Repeated visits to a lonely, unreasonable, or demanding isolation patient will necessitate barrier precautions each time. This can be a time-consuming responsibility.

The most effective ways to prevent avoidance of the isolation patient include increasing staff knowledge and deliberately planning time with the patient. Accurate knowledge of exactly how disease is spread should be combined with a clear understanding of human behavior in response to infection and isolation. The nurse is then more able to deal therapeutically with the emotional response to isolation experienced by herself and the patient. It is important that the complexities and inconvenience of isolation precautions be openly acknowledged by staff members and that the responsibilities of caring for isolated patients be assumed equally by the entire team. Though primary relationships are important, some visiting and caring roles may be divided among nursing team members to assure attentive care.

When Staff Members Disregard Precautions

There is nothing more frustrating and disillusioning than to have just completed a period of time-consuming nursing care meticulously following the prescribed isolation precautions, and then observe another nurse or a physician break the necessary isolation technique, e.g., barge into the room with bare face and without isolation gown, examine or treat the patient, and then leave, perhaps without even washing his or her hands! Tragically, inconsistencies in isolation technique occur far too often. Why do health professionals sometimes disregard isola-

tion precautions, and what can be done to ensure more consistent technique?

There are many different reasons for disregarding isolation precautions; these are seldom openly acknowledged by the people involved. Many health professionals actually remain ignorant about how infection is spread. Others may view isolation procedures as unnecessary rituals or as unsupported authoritarian regulations. In truth, if the institution is using the 1975 National Center for Disease Control guidelines, the isolation procedures are directly derived from the most current scientific investigation of the means of cross-infection. Some nurses or doctors possess perfectly accurate knowledge of infectious disease, but they disregard isolation precautions simply because of the inconvenience of these measures. Faced with the pressures of time and responsibilities, these persons "can't be bothered" with the isolation precautions. They do not think of them as a necessary priority.

> *The staff member who breaks isolation technique may jeopardize not only his health and that of his team members but also the safety of other patients and his own family.*

Disregarding isolation procedures is unacceptable practice. Risking the life and health of other patients is inexcusable. Florence Nightingale established the nurse as the guardian of the patient's environment; she systematically eliminated factors which rendered the environment unclean and unsafe. The responsible nurse of today must assume an equally assertive role to insist that isolation procedures be taken seriously. It is not justifiable to ignore the problem in the name of "professional courtesy" to colleagues. Our first loyalty is the protection of health and the prevention of avoidable disease.

GUIDELINES FOR ALTERING COMMON NURSING PROCEDURES

The Patient and His Visitors

Admitting the Patient. The admission procedure for a patient requiring isolation varies from standard depending on the isolation category ordered. Obviously, the patient's unit should be provided with needed supplies and should have unnecessary items removed *before* the patient arrives. Patient and family require thorough explanations about the needed precautions. The patient's room, identification bracelet, and chart should be labeled with the isolation category indicated. In the cases of Strict Isolation, Wound and Skin Precautions, and Enteric Precautions, all contaminated clothing should be double bagged and returned home. The chart is not taken into the Strict Isolation or Protective Isolation room.

Advising Visitors. Visitors are often limited because of the potential danger of cross-infection. This policy must be examined in the light of the psychosocial effects of isolation. If time is taken to explain to them clearly how infection is spread and how the required precautions prevent spread, visitors should be able to come safely to the bedside.

> *All visitors must be taught to master safe handwashing techniques, and gowning, masking, and/or gloving as indicated.*

Only those visitors who are cooperative and who understand the precautions should be permitted to visit. No more than two should be at the bedside at one time. No one can be allowed to visit unless he has first checked with a nurse and received appropriate teaching.

Transporting the Patient. To diminish the threat of cross-infection, isolated patients should leave the unit as little as possible. The department to which the patient is sent must be fully informed as to his isolation status and the barriers needed to protect other patients and staff. Transportation of the patient in Strict Isolation or Wound and Skin Precautions requires that the patient wear an isolation gown and be totally enshrouded in a blanket, with only his face exposed. The patient in Strict Isolation and the person moving the patient should wear masks. Respiratory Isolation requires only that the patient wear a mask. Discharge Precautions require that the patient's drainage be completely contained by fresh dressings. Clean pajamas and linens should be worn by the patient who needs Enteric Precautions and is continent. Extra precautions are needed for the incontinent patient, e.g., adequate numbers of disposable incontinence pads and extra protective linens beneath the patient's buttocks.

Managing Personal Possessions. Only Strict Isolation Wound and Skin Precautions, and Enteric Precautions demand special care for these items. Clothing of patients in these categories should be double bagged and returned home. There, the empty bags should be burned or placed in a clean plastic bag and discarded in the garbage. The patient's clothing and linens can be washed in a home washing machine with one cup household bleach or one cup Lysol per load.[27] Hands must be washed thoroughly after handling soiled laundry.

Books, magazines, money, toys, and letters can move freely into and out of the isolation area, as long as they are not visibly soiled with infected discharges. Soiled items must be disinfected or destroyed.

Special Nursing Techniques

Taking Vital Signs. Only Strict Isolation necessitates keeping stethoscope and sphygmomanometer in the room or discarding cloth wrap of sphygmomanometer in isolated laundry and disinfection of the remainder of the equipment after discharge. With Wound and Skin Precautions and Enteric Precautions, these items should be washed with a germicidal detergent if soiled with contaminated discharges. The glass thermometer of patients in Strict Isolation, Wound and Skin Precautions, and Enteric Precautions is kept in a disinfectant, which is changed every 3 days. Upon the patient's discharge, the thermometer is double bagged and sent to central supply, where thermometers of patients with viral disease are destroyed. Use of disposable thermometers or thermometer covers is desirable when possible (see Chap. 28).

The actual process of taking vital signs requires adaptation with Strict Isolation, Wound and Skin Precautions, and Enteric Precautions. Gowning, masking, and gloving are required for the patient in Strict Isolation. To avoid contamination, the watch must be placed on a clean paper towel or in a transparent plastic sack since all surfaces are assumed dirty. Gowning and gloving are necessary with Enteric Precautions and Wound and Skin Precautions if it is not possible to take the vital signs without direct contact; otherwise, only gloves may be worn. Meticulous handwashing afterward is essential with all categories.

Managing Dishes, Food, and Water. Only Strict Isolation and Enteric Precautions require special care for dishes and food. Disposable dishes and utensils are preferred; those that are reusable must be double bagged before being sent to the kitchen. Leftover food is discarded in wastebaskets, and leftover fluids are poured into patient's sink or toilet. To avoid cross-infection from indirect contact, water pitchers used for patients in Strict Isolation, Enteric, or Wound and Skin Precautions should not be passed and exchanged in a routine manner. It is best that the same pitcher remain at the bedside, be cleansed in the unit daily and as necessary, and be filled with ice and water without contaminating the serving vehicle. The pitcher of the patient must be filled at the door with a contaminated person holding it and an assistant filling it.

Administering Medications. The nurse must be gowned, masked, and gloved to come into the Strict Isolation room to administer medications. If direct patient contact is anticipated— for example, with all parenteral medication and whenever the patient requires assistance in swallowing oral medication—gowns and gloves are required with Enteric and Wound and Skin Precautions.

Managing Linens and Equipment. All forms of isolation precautions require double bagging of equipment known to be contaminated with infected discharges. In Strict Isolation, all equipment in the room is considered contaminated and must be either double bagged or scrubbed with germicidal detergent before being removed from the room. Strict Isolation, Wound and Skin Precautions, and Enteric Precautions require double bagging of linen before removal from the room.

Disposing of Discharges and Waste. All forms of isolation require special care with infected discharges and contaminated waste. Urine and stool are immediately flushed down the toilet in Strict Isolation and Enteric Precautions. Collections of infected drainage from body cavities are managed in the same manner. Dressings and disposable tissues soiled with infected material are double bagged in Strict Isolation, Respiratory Isolation, Enteric Precautions, Wound and Skin Precautions, and Discharge Precautions.

Collecting Specimens. If the person is in Strict Isolation, all specimens of any body discharge should be collected in containers, labeled contaminated, and double bagged in a transparent bag before being sent to the laboratory. With Enteric Precautions, specimens of urine and stool (and blood in hepatitis cases) should be handled in the same manner. Cultures from patients in Wound and Skin Precautions, Discharge Precautions, and Blood Precautions, and sputum from patients in Respiratory Isolation should be placed in a sterile container without contaminating the outside; the Center for Disease Control does not recommend double bagging for these four types of precautions and isolation.

Changing Dressings. Infected wounds must be managed with sterile technique to prevent invasion from new varieties of organisms. Standard dressing technique is used for all wounds where infections require Secretion Precautions. This procedure includes handwashing before and after, meticulous sterile technique with instruments used to handle dressings, and double bagging for soiled dressings and contaminated equipment. Special Dressing Technique is required for all infected draining wounds isolated in either Strict or Wound and Skin Precautions. In addition to the standard procedure, this technique requires gown, mask, nonsterile gloves to remove old dressings, and sterile gloves when applying sterile new dressings. Sterile gloves are considered grossly contaminated after the dressing change. They are removed, hands are washed and clean gloves are worn for continued patient care.

BIBLIOGRAPHY

a. A new way to stymie staph. *Emergency Medicine,* 9:119–121, April 1977.
1. American Medical Association, Department of Drugs: *AMA Drug Evaluations.* Acton, Mass., Publishing Sciences Group, 1973.
2. American Nurses' Association, Division on Medical-Surgical Nursing Practice: Draft, The Nurse and Infection Control, 1976.
3. Anderson, L., and Himmelsbach, C.: The nurse: first line of defense against infections. *Journal of the American Hospital Association, 41*:7, Oct. 1967.
4. Baranowski, K., and Greene, H.: Viral hepatitis: how to reduce its threat to the patient and others. *Nursing '76,* 6:31, May 1976.
5. Benenson, A.: *Control of Communicable Diseases in Man.* Washington, D.C., American Public Health Association, 1975.
6. Blackwell, B.: Stigma. *In* Carlson, C.: *Behavioral Concepts and Nursing Intervention.* Philadelphia, J. B. Lippincott Co., 1970.
7. Bolin, R.: Sensory deprivation: an overview. *Nursing Forum,* 13:241, Summer 1974.
8. Broadribb, B.: *Foundations of Pediatric Nursing.* Philadelphia, J. B. Lippincott Co., 1973.
9. Bullough, B.: Where should isolation stop? *American Journal of Nursing,* 72:733, April 1972.
10. Burke, J.: Bacteria free nursing unit—a new approach to isolation procedures. *Hospitals,* 43:86, Jan. 1969.
11. Castle, M.: Isolation: precise procedures for better protection. *Nursing '75,* 5:50, May 1975.
11a. Chavigny, K. H.: Nurse epidemiologist in the hospital. *American Journal of Nursing,* 75:638–642, April 1975.
11b. Donabedian, D.: Computer-taught epidemiology. *Nursing Outlook,* 24:749–751, Dec. 1976.
12. Dubay, E., and Grubb, R.: *Infection Prevention and Control.* St. Louis, C. V. Mosby, 1973.

13. Fuerst, E., Wolff, L., and Weitzel, M. H.: *Fundamentals of Nursing*, 5th ed. Philadelphia, J. B. Lippincott Co., 1974.

14. Garner, J., and Kaiser, A.: How often is isolation needed? *American Journal of Nursing*, 72:733, April 1972.

15. Guyton, H., and Decker, H.: Respiratory protection provided by five new contagion masks. *Applied Microbiology*, 11, 1963.

16. Hamil, E.: The role of the nurse in the control of staphylococcal infections in hospitals. *California's Health*, 17, July 1959.

17. Lange, S.: Shame. *In* Carlson, C.: *Behavioral Concepts and Nursing Intervention*. Philadelphia, J. B. Lippincott Co., 1970.

18. Lentz, J.: The nurse's role in extending infection control to the community. *Nursing Clinics of North America*, 5:165, March 1970.

19. Levine, A., et al.: Protected environments and prophylactic antibiotics. *New England Journal of Medicine*, 288:477, March 1973.

20. Lewis, L. W.: *Fundamental Skills in Patient Care*. Philadelphia, J. B. Lippincott Co., 1976.

21. Massachusetts General Hospital, Department of Nursing: *Massachusetts General Hospital Manual of Nursing Procedures*. Boston, Little, Brown & Co., 1975.

22. McInnes, B.: *Controlling the Spread of Infection*. St. Louis, C. V. Mosby, 1973.

23. Moustakas, C.: *Loneliness*. Englewood Cliffs, NJ, Prentice-Hall, 1961.

23a. Osborn, P. H.: Developing and maintaining an infection control program. *Supervisor Nurse*, 8:16–18, Dec. 1977.

24. National Center for Disease Control, summary of statistics available through July, 1978. Personal communication, September 12, 1978.

25. Parisi, J.: *Personnel Education for Infections Control*. Atlanta, Georgia, Center for Disease Control (undated USPHS reprint).

25a. Strep till the day you dye. *Emergency Medicine*, 9:108, March 1977.

25b. Turner, J. G.: The nurse epidemiologist: Selection and preparation. *Supervisor Nurse*, 9:33–41, April 1978.

26. Spicher, C.: Nursing care of children hospitalized with infections. *Nursing Clinics of North America*, 5:123, March 1970.

27. U.S. Department of Health, Education, and Welfare: *Isolation Techniques for Use in Hospitals*. Atlanta, Georgia, National Center for Disease Control (printed by U.S. Government Printing Office), 1975.

28. U.S. Department of Health, Education, and Welfare: *Outline for Surveillance and Control of Nosocomial Infections*. Atlanta, Georgia, National Center for Disease Control, 1974.

29. Weg, J.: Tuberculosis and the generation gap. *American Journal of Nursing*, 71:495, March 1971.

CHAPTER 46

CARING FOR ILL CHILDREN

By Linda A. Kent, R.N., M.N.

INTRODUCTION AND STUDY GUIDE

The pediatric nurse must develop unique and special skills to assess, plan for, and care for the child. These skills are of particular importance because children express their needs, feelings, and understandings differently than do adults, depending on multiple factors, including their stage of development, whether their illness is acute or chronic, their previous experience with illness and hospitalization, and their socioeconomic and cultural backgrounds. The nurse's ability to evaluate the physiologic and emotional changes occurring because of the effects of illness and hospitalization and hence to plan effective nursing interventions will depend on her knowledge of the unique characteristics of the child at each stage of the developmental process.

This chapter will discuss factors influencing children; an overview of childhood illness; psychophysiologic and environmental considerations in caring for children; the interaction between the parent, the child, and the nurse; and the child who is dying.

Prior to reading, consider your responses to the following questions. At the end of your reading, change or add to your responses based on what you have learned.

1. How does the level of physical, emotional, and cognitive development of the child influence (a) the nursing assessment of the child, (b) the child's response to illness and (c) the child's response to hospitalization?

2. In what ways is the child influenced by (a) his interaction with significant others in his environment, (b) his state of physical and mental health and (c) his economic and cultural background?

3. What kinds of health problems are likely to be encountered in children that are not seen in adults?

4. What should the child and parents be told before they come to the hospital?

5. In what ways can the nurse support family integrity when a child is hospitalized?

6. How and why should parents participate in caring for their child? What problems can you anticipate with this? How can they be managed?

7. What are some primary causes of anxiety in children related to hospitalization?

8. What are some specific ways in which a child's developmental needs can be met during illness and hospitalization? Include physiologic, emotional, social, and intellectual needs.

9. Why is play necessary to the well-being of the child? How can it be utilized as a tool in the hospital environment?

10. List important consideration in preparation of a child and his parents for a surgical procedure.

DEFINITION OF CHILDHOOD

"Childhood" generally refers to the several stages of growth and development occurring between birth and 11 or 13 years of age, or until the time of puberty. It includes the physical, social, sexual, psychologic, and intellectual changes and their interactions that occur with predictable sequence during this period of time. The stages composing childhood are generally considered to be: newborn, birth to 1 month; infant, 1 month to 1 year; toddler, 1 to 3 years; preschool, 3 to 6 years, and school age, 6 to 11 or 13 years.

NORMAL GROWTH AND DEVELOPMENT OF CHILDREN

An understanding of the unique characteristics of the various stages of growth, the intellectual and emotional aspects of behavior at each stage of development, and their interactions is essential to the nurse's assessment of the child and his response to illness and hospitalization. The child undergoes a variety of growth and developmental changes in the process of maturation. The changes occur in part as the result of the child's inherent, genetically acquired traits, and in part as the result of the child's interactions with the environment surrounding him. Such environmental influences include the child's interaction with important people in his environment, the quality and amount of sensory stimulation he receives and the food and nutrition available. The child, as well, will influence his surroundings, as the social interactions between himself and others will be partly based on his own individual traits. The interactions between the child and the child's environment become increasingly more complex as the child develops increased capacity to perceive and regulate himself and his environment. This occurs in a number of ways.

The child's physical growth alone represents a major change in himself to which he must accommodate. He will increase more than three times in length and more than 20 times in weight between birth and adolescence. The normal neurologic reflex patterns of infancy will change, and the crude, purposeless movements of the 4 month child, will change to the crawling of the 6 to 8 month child, to the walking of the 10 to 14 month child. Central nervous system maturation will continue to develop from the motor skills required of skipping and jumping to the very finely tuned neuromotor skills required for such skills as tying shoes and writing. This muscular and central nervous system maturation is a major influence on the child's ability to interact with and control his surroundings. Other physiologic systems mature as the child grows, and will influence nursing judgments. The respiratory system, gastrointestinal system, endocrine system, musculoskeletal system, the skin, renal system, circulatory system, and immunologic system all mature and change as the child grows older, and must be taken into ac-

count during assessment and in planning nursing care.

Psychosocial development represents another major aspect of the child's development. Erik Erikson[17] has identified eight stages of the life cycle of man, described as core problems or crises, four of which constitute childhood. Overcoming the negative component of each core problem prepares the child to move on to the next stage. A positive outcome at each level of development is influenced by the family, especially during the beginning stages, and then by others in the community.

The child's ability to perceive and interact with his environment will be heavily influenced by his cognitive and language development. A sequence of stages as described by Piaget[43] flows from the early undifferentiation between the infant's self and the world around him, to learning that certain actions have a specific effect on the environment, and to a beginning of symbolic activity. By 2 years, egocentric thinking predominates; i.e., the child considers himself the cause of outside events. Between 3 and 7 years of age, thought is intuitive and magical. The child this age lacks a concept of reversibility, and observations in the familiar world are often used for explaining the unfamiliar. He is unable to take another's view, refers every event to himself, and tends to center his attention on one aspect of an event. Development continues between 7 and 12 years of age, when the child develops a rational conceptual framework and a foundation of logical thinking that can be used for interpretation of the world.

FACTORS INFLUENCING CHILDREN

The Child's Interactions with Significant Others and the Environment

Patterns of the child's interaction with her family, significant others, and the environment begins before and at the time of birth, and continues to deeply influence the child's patterns of social relationships, psychologic growth, cognitive development, and physical and neurologic development throughout child-

TABLE 46–1.   STAGES IN THE LIFE OF CHILDREN

PERIOD OF LIFE	CORE PROBLEM OR CRISIS
1. Infancy: Birth to 1 year	Trust vs. Mistrust
2. Early Childhood: 1 to 3 years	Autonomy vs. Shame and Doubt
3. Play Age: 3 to 6 years	Initiative vs. Guilt
4. School Age: 6 to 13 years	Industry vs. Inferiority

(Adapted from Erikson, E. H.: *Childhood and Society.* New York, W. W. Norton & Company, Inc., 1963.)

hood. Factors in the child's family environment such as degree of involvement with the child, the emotional climate, degree of restriction or punishment, and amount of social, cognitive, and emotional support will affect the child's emotional and verbal responsiveness, the way in which she perceives herself, and the way she perceives and interacts with her world.

The child's physical environment, too, will affect cognitive, physical, and psychologic growth. Especially important is the quality, timing, and quantity of auditory, visual, and kinesthetic stimulation; opportunities for variety in the daily environment; opportunity for a variety of experiences; and the provision of appropriate play materials.[12] As the child grows older, relationships with peer groups, the school environment, and the community assume a major influence on the child.

A familiarity with Caldwell's *Home Observation for Measurement of the Environment*[12] will assist the nurse in assessing the child's home environment, in evaluating the parent-child relationship in the hospital, in teaching the parents, and in developing a hospital environment that meets a child's developmental needs.

The Child's State of Physical and Mental Health

The state of physical and mental health is a major factor influencing the long-term development of the child toward an integrated and productive adulthood. Her state of health will influence her self-image and body image. It will influence the way others, particularly the parents, react to and interact with the child, and therefore will influence the social and psychologic environment in which the child develops. The state of health may also form physical barriers to the child's ability to interact with her environment and may, therefore, limit the variety of experiences available to her. The state of health will greatly influence the ability of the child to complete the important developmental steps of autonomy and mastery. Illness, both chronic and acute, may impose dependency. The particular effect that the illness has on the development will depend on the type of illness or handicap, whether it is acute or chronic, and the adaptational techniques used by the parents and the child.

The Parents' and Child's Economic and Cultural Background

Culture represents patterns of interactions, values, attitudes, knowledge, belief systems, patterns of perceiving the world, and goals. It directly affects children through child-rearing practices and life-style. The child's reaction to and ability to utilize experiences will be directly affected by her cultural background. Culture especially influences language and the thought patterns that result from language.

Values that may be influenced by culture include individualism vs. group orientation, future vs. present or past time orientation, control of nature vs. being controlled by nature, planning and achievement vs. spontaneity, and the perfectibility of man vs. the unchanging nature of man. These patterns will directly influence the behavior of the child when she is stressed by illness and hospitalization and will influence the parents' and the child's overall view of illness and their participation in health care.

Poverty can also be viewed as a culture, with all of the above traits and considerations. In addition, it will directly influence the development and potential of the child by determining the availability of adequate nutrition, access to health care and other sources of help, access to education and recreation, living quarters, and social acceptability and interaction. Poverty often affects the outlook on life and results in a feeling of powerlessness and insecurity. This can be demonstrated in the way in which families of poverty participate in the health care system as well as in other aspects of life.

The Child's Level of Development

The child's level of development is a particularly important consideration during periods of illness and hospitalization. The level of development will influence the child's understanding of what he experiences in the hospital, how he is able to express his feelings related to these experiences, and how he is able to cope with the stress caused by the hospital experience. Language development will influence how the child will ask for help and how well he will be able to verbalize his questions and anxieties. His level of social and emotional development will greatly influence the kind of interaction and support needed during illness or hospitalization.

The level of development will influence how well the nurse is able to evaluate physiologic needs and respond to them. Vital signs, laboratory values, medication dosages, response to medication, nutritional needs, and fluid requirements will all depend on the size and physiologic maturity of the child. The physical maturity of the child will influence, too, the kind of disease present, and the body's physiologic response to the disease and its treatment.

The nurse can play a significant role in casefinding. Children experiencing developmental delays may not be found until they are admitted to the hospital. Percentile growth charts should be completed on every hospitalized child.[15] The Denver Developmental Screening Test[23] is one widely utilized tool that the nurse can easily learn to use and carry out in the hospital setting. Other tools, such as the Brazelton Neonatal Behavioral Assessment Scale,[17] require more in-depth learning and skill, but can give valuable information in providing guidance to families.

TYPES OF CHILDHOOD ILLNESS: AN OVERVIEW

It is generally possible for children to have almost any illness an adult has. However, the degenerative, neoplastic and metabolic disorders are much less common in children. Other disorders are much more common, have unique characteristics, or are unique in children.

Congenital anomalies exist in a wide spectrum, from the trivial to those incompatible with life. Anomalies of the heart, nervous system, skeletal system, digestive system, urinary tract, and lungs all require special treatment, often meaning multiple hospitalizations for the child for surgical repair or complications. Special disorders of the newborn—respiratory distress syndrome, erythroblastosis fetalis, hyperbilirubinemia, or prematurity—represent problems unique to pediatrics.

Nutritional abnormalities are much more common in children than in adults because of the high demands for the nutrients caused by rapid growth. "Failure to thrive" is one type of unique childhood problem that may be environmentally, genetically, or emotionally caused.

Infectious disease is more common in children than in adults and is an important cause of mortality as well as morbidity. Some diseases, suffered only once because of the ensuing immunity, are usually experienced in childhood. Other diseases may be more acute in infants and small children because of the labile temperature-regulating mechanism, the ease with which the fluid balance can be jeopardized and the small size of the airway.

Childhood accidents and *poisoning* represent a major cause of childhood illness and death. Developing eagerness to explore with newly found neuromuscular abilities, curiosity, a propensity for grabbing objects from above, a propensity for putting fingers into holes and for putting objects into any body orifices all make the toddler particularly prone to poisoning and accidents.

Neoplasms are not as common in children as in adults, but have distinctive features. Leukemia, tumors of the brain, Wilms' tumor, neuroblastoma of the adrenal, and metastatic bone tumors are the types most commonly seen in children. *Disorders requiring surgical correction* are usually related to congenital anomalies, but some disorders requiring surgery are unique in children, such as intussusception and pyloric stenosis.

Disturbances in the parent/child relationship represent an important consideration in pediatric care. Failure to thrive may be one result. The battered child is another. Various other outcomes may be behavior disorders, anxiety states, and psychosomatic illnesses.

Severe psychologic disorders are not as common in children as in adults, and psychosis is unusual. Other, more mild, psychologic disorders are sometimes seen and may relate to problems in development, may be genetically determined, or may be an outcome of an acute or chronic physical disability.

PREPARATIONS FOR HOSPITALIZATION

Preparation of the Parents

Preparation of the parents is an essential first step in the preparation of the child for hospitalization. The feeling of calm or anxiety related to the upcoming hospital experience will be sensed by the child and will be reflected in their own attitudes and feelings. Knowledgeable parents are more likely to be comfortable in preparing the child for hospitalization, and they are less likely to be threatened or upset by their child's questions.

It is essential that the parents understand the important part they play in the child's hospitalization and understand the importance of persons most significant in the child's life staying with the child when at all possible. Parents should have information about what physical arrangements they can expect, such as facilities for personal hygiene. They may need help in planning their stay in order to make arrangements with their employers, for other children, and to consider how they can best maintain family continuity during the child's hospitalization. Parents should plan to bring objects familiar to the child, such as toys or a favorite blanket, and familiar sounds, such as a music box or records, from home. They should also be prepared to bring the child's own clothing, marked with his name, if allowed by the hospital.

Parents also need to be forewarned about changes in behavior that sometimes occur in children as a reaction to the hospitalization and that the changes will be dependent on the child's age, the seriousness of the illness, the length of the hospital stay, how the child usually reacts to new situations, and how well prepared he is. They should know that behavior during and after hospitalization may sometimes be increasingly demanding, clinging, fearful, or uncooperative.

It is essential that parents understand the importance of telling the truth to the child and of not making promises that they are unable to keep. A particular example is the desire of some parents to avoid tears when they must leave the hospital; they wait until the child is preoccupied or asleep and then leave without telling the child. Parents must understand that, although good-bys may be tearful, the nursing staff is aware of the child's needs at this time and is ready to assist and that evasive answers or leaving without telling the child leads to increased anxiety in the child and increased mistrust of everyone.

Preparation of the Child

It is essential to tell the child why he is to be hospitalized and what is likely to happen during hospitalization. Some parents may be reluctant or unwilling to tell the child of the upcoming hospitalization. They may believe that the child does not have the capacity to understand, or they may not know how to go about explaining to the child. Others may not be able to deal with the child's reactions to the explanation, fearing upset in the child or questions they may not be able to answer. Parents should know that whenever an explanation concerning treatment or illness is not given or is unclear, children characteristically form their own explanation or conclusion. These conclusions, given the child's active imagination, are likely to be much more fearsome and worrisome than reality. Children, too, may interpret an unexplained hospitalization as punishment for some misdeed.

When to Tell the Child. Children over 7 years of age should be told 2 to 3 weeks in advance of the date of admission in order to provide ample opportunity for questions and to allow them to participate in the preparation. Children 4 to 7 years of age should be told 4 to 7 days in advance so that they have enough time to think about it and to ask questions, but not a long enough time to form fantasies about what will be happening to them. Children 2 to 3 years old should be told 2 to 3 days prior to admission and on the day of admission.

What to Tell the Child. The child should be told why the hospitalization is necessary and what will happen while he is there. Generally, he should know what he will feel and see, that other children will be there also, that he may wear a hospital gown, what the sleeping arrangements are, who will stay with him, what the eating arrangements are like, and equipment that he will see. He should also be told what he will feel and see that might be related to the particular reason he is hospitalized, such as x-ray equipment, anesthesia, or bandages. If he is having surgery, he should know that no other part will be operated on except what he is told. The child should know what he can do for himself while in the hospital.

How to Tell the Child. The child needs to know what will happen from his own point of view, and in ways that he can visualize and relate to past experiences. He should know what he will see and feel, but not in frightening terms. Overwhelming detail should be avoided. To make it easier for the parents to explain to the child, the nurse can help with specific words and phrases that are appropriate for the level of development of the child. The parents should be alerted to ask simple questions of the child to see what the child has retained, and to reinforce what they have taught. Ideas for explanation of specific procedures are helpful to parents if given in written form. Also the nurse can provide ideas such as doll play, specific books[2, 47, 59] or body outlines[42] that may be helpful.

Many hospitals have a special program planned to prepare the child for the hospital before the day of admission, such as a puppet show. Such preparation should take place in the presence of the trusted adult so that questions can be asked and reinforcement can take place and so that the program can be related specifically to what will be happening to that individual child.

THE CHILD, THE PARENTS, AND THE NURSE

The nurse in pediatrics thinks of the child and his parents as one unit and considers both the child and the parents in every step of the nursing process. The parent is the most important influence on the child's emotional and social well-being and will influence to a great extent the degree to which the child adjusts positively toward the hospital experience, his health problem, and the treatment needed. In most instances, the adjustment that the parent exhibits to the child's illness and the hospital experience will be reflected in the child's ability to deal with the stress of hospitalization.

Caring for the child and parent together requires a great deal of the nurse working in pediatrics. Not only must she have skills in communicating with children in a variety of developmental stages, but she must be able to communicate effectively with the adult parent. Not only will she need skills in assessment of the child at each stage of development, but she must be able to assess the parent and how the child and the parents interact. She will need skills in evaluating the effect the stress of the child's hospitalization has on the parent as well as on the child. She will need to plan for parent education as well as patient education. And she will need the knowledge and skill to analyze the interaction between parent and child in order to *support the parent in supporting the child.*

The Relationship Between the Parents and the Nurse

The relationship established by the nurse with the parents is of vital importance. The nurse involved in the care of children must carefully explore her beliefs and attitudes about the relationship between the hospitalized child, the parents, and herself. Her philosophy and attitude will be felt by the parents in the very beginning stages of the relationship and will be reflected in the success with which the relationship is established. The following understandings and attitudes will enhance a productive nurse and parent relationship.

▶ The nurse must recognize that the parents do not give up the role and responsibility of parenting to the hospital staff when the child enters the hospital. Their maintenance of the parent role in the hospital will serve as a support to the child. The nurse must communicate to the parents the expectation that they continue their parenting in the hospital and that she will support them in their parenting during a time of increased stress to the entire family.

▶ The nurse must recognize that the parents may feel, consciously or unconsciously, that health care professionals interpret the illness in their child as the result of poor parenting. They may feel that health care workers are critical and that the nurse has more knowledge about child care than they do. These feelings can lead to defensiveness and uncertainty on the part of the parents and may be a real barrier to communication.

▶ Though the nurse may at times assess problems in the parent-child relationship and parenting, she must recognize the knowledge and experience that the parent has had with this particular and unique child. She can communicate to the parents her respect for their parenting skills and experiences, beginning with the admission interview, and the parent can be a real resource to the nurse in determining what is normal and abnormal behavior for this child. The parents, before anyone else, will be able to see subtle changes in their child's condition and behavior. The wise nurse will view with respect parents' observations, concern, or warnings, for often they will signal a change or problem that is significant to the child's condition.

▶ Access to information concerning the child's hospitalization, illness, and progress is not a privilege of a parent, but a right. Knowledge of the hospital policies and their child's illness is paramount to their beginning to cope.

The nurse can work toward an open and honest hospital atmosphere and can promote parental understanding through ongoing assessment of areas of misunderstanding, lack of information, or inaccurate interpretations. She can provide information in her area of professional expertise and can see that physicians or other health professionals provide the information needed for understanding and informed decision-making. The nurse must maintain an awareness of the parents' understanding of the child's condition, nursing goals, and medical goals, and she must reinforce teaching, correct misconceptions, or call on other health team members when necessary to meet the family's need for information.

Providing for family continuity during the period of hospitalization is of utmost importance—to the child, to the parents, and to other children in the family. Research findings have demonstrated conclusively the damaging effects of separation of young children from their mothers.[6, 20] Other research is beginning to establish the periods of time (birth to 4 months) in which the interaction of the parent and child determine the whole course of the interactional and developmental processes of the child.[1] Providing opportunities for parents to stay with the child during hospitalization is most important to prevent the consequences of separation. The nurse has a vital role in assuring that the parent-child interaction is not only continued but supported during the period of hospitalization in order that the damaging effects of separation are avoided, and in order that the course of developmental process of the child and parent/child interaction is not impaired.

It is essential that the nurse caring for the child and family make available rooming-in, unrestricted visiting hours, and sibling visits. In many instances the chief obstacle is outdated and arbitrary regulations and inadequate physical facilities. The nurse will need to utilize her problem-solving skills in negotiation, communication, implementation of change, and administration to ensure that the needs of the patient are being met. She will often need ingenuity to overcome inadequate facilities and ensure that parents have a place to sleep and a way to meet their personal needs.

The nurse can promote family continuity in several other ways. She can provide the opportunity for family members to express their feelings—often including anger, resentment, guilt, and fear—about the child, the child's illness, and the hospitalization experience. The nurse can help the family members to become aware of each other's needs, attitudes, and feelings in relation to the child's illness by encouraging open and honest communication among the family members. The nurse can help the family maintain a reasonable balance between the needs of the hospitalized child and other family members. She can avoid arousal of guilt when parents are already anxious over the care of their children. As a result of these interventions, the nurse should observe a family that is able to communicate mutual concern, feelings, and support to one another, and therefore is able to deal in a positive way with the hospitalized child and the particular stresses created by the child, the illness, and the hospital experience.

The nurse also can promote family continuity by seeing that they have the community resources necessary to cope with financial, family, and emotional stresses related to the hospitalization of a child. She can be instrumental in assessing the need for social services and community agencies, and she can see that these are contacted and utilized.

Mutual Goal-Setting and Planning

The nurse will utilize information gained from evaluation of the family, their interaction, expectations, and knowledge, to plan how she will work with them as a part of the team in providing for the needs of their child. She will include the family in the development of a plan of nursing care for the child, will provide them with the opportunity to assist in physical care of the child, and will continue to solicit questions and input from the patient and family regarding the nursing care plan throughout the child's hospital stay. As a result, the child and family will understand and share in mutual goals and plans, and will participate in the plan as agreed upon by all involved.

Family Involvement in Care

The degree to which parents will participate in the care will vary with each individual, and will depend on their concept of the role of the nurse, their comfort in the hospital setting, the amount of time they are able to spend with the child, and their general desire to participate. The types of activities with which the staff would welcome involvement should be made clear, such as bathing, feeding, dressing, or accompanying the child to diagnostic procedures. They will need to know that regardless of their presence or absence, the staff will continue to meet the child's physical and emotional needs and that observations and procedures will be carried out on a 24-hour basis. Parents should not be viewed as a timesaver for routine tasks. Parents can quickly get a feeling of being exploited and fear to leave, believing children would not be cared for in their absence. The nurse may utilize the opportunity of having the parents with the child for observation of the parents and child interacting with one another and for teaching.

An important part of the role of the nurse in caring for the child and the family is to assist the parents in understanding and dealing appropriately with the unique reaction that the child in each age level will exhibit toward the hospital experience. Parents may be concerned about unusual behavior patterns and fail to understand the normal reaction of the child to the stresses he is experiencing. They may also be fearful of setting limits on unacceptable behavior of the child. The nurse can stress the importance of maintaining patterns of interaction and discipline similar to the home environment, and she can help the parents understand that behavior on their part that is consistent with what the child is used to will enhance his feelings of security in the strange situation.

The Role of the Nurse as Teacher

An important advantage of close family involvement in the care of the child is that the nurse may help them to realistically understand the child's condition, his needs, and the care that may be required when he goes home. The nurse can serve as a role model in the attitude she displays toward the child. She can explain her activities in caring for the child and can help the parents to participate in the child's care. As a result of these activities, the parents should have a positive attitude toward the child, demonstrate knowledge and comfort in caring for the child, and have a realistic plan for meeting the needs of the child at home.

The hospitalization of the child will also provide the nurse with the unique opportunity to share with the parents positive health practices that relate to the normal growth and development of the child. Her knowledge of normal development and of activities that will promote development will enable her to assess the parents' knowledge and provide teaching and counseling related to the child's development and health promotion.

When Parents Are Critical

The hospital must be prepared to deal with the inevitable conflict that the high number of interactions between staff members and parents—all under stress—will bring. Parents will be influenced in how well they deal with stress by their past experiences, their ego resources, their styles of coping, and their individual beliefs and values. They may react with flight from the situation, may concentrate on insignificant issues or problems, or may blame or become overly critical of the nursing or medical staff. They may experience guilt, resentment, fear, and pain over the pain being inflicted on their child. Honest discussion with parents, mutual support among staff, and one-to-one relationships with a primary nurse all will help. Staff acknowledgment of angry feelings of parents is particularly important, as are multidisciplinary conferences to assure consistency of planning and approach.

PSYCHOPHYSIOLOGIC CONSIDERATIONS IN CARING FOR HOSPITALIZED CHILDREN

Psychologic Considerations

Children are particularly vulnerable to the anxiety and stress caused by illness and hospitalization. It may force them into a dependency position just at the time they are gaining control and mastery over their bodily functions and their environment. They may be separated from their major source of security, comfort, and nurturing. They may experience pain and the frightening sensations of nausea or dizziness for the first time. And, they are thrust into a strange environment with different routines, people, and expectations. Because of their particular stage of development, some children may feel that hospitalization is a punishment for some thought or past misdeed. Preschool children especially have fears of body mutilation that are intensified by diagnostic or operative procedures. The fantasies and misinterpretations of reality, normal to earlier stages of cognitive development, may intensify the fear and anxiety concerning hospital routines and procedures. As a result, children frequently react strongly to procedures, especially those involving bodily intrusion, such as temperature taking, enemas, or injections, far out of proportion to the pain involved. And when children have a lack of or only partial information, their fantasy may lead to frightening interpretations of what to expect in the future. A child's interpretation of time also varies with age and intensifies the anxieties surrounding illness and hospitalization. The toddler's egocentricity and "now" orientation may prevent him from understanding that painful procedures *now* will help his *future* condition and may keep him from accepting the fact that when his parents leave *now*, they will return later.

The harmful effects of hospitalization on the child have been well documented.[6, 20, 45] The optimum approach to their prevention is to avoid hospitalization whenever possible and to explore outpatient or home care alternatives. If hospitalization is necessary, the most effective means of minimizing the trauma of the hospital experience and the potential long-term effects is through providing for and encouraging the presence and participation of those people most significant to the child.

Maintaining Developmental Level. The pediatric nurse, as a major goal, will strive to maintain the level of development the child was experiencing prior to hospitalization, and if the hospitalization is long term, to enhance growth in mastering new skills. She will assess the level of development and create a plan of care that maintains the child's level of independence, physically and emotionally. Though at times there may be forced dependency, and the child may exhibit regression, the nurse must do whatever possible to assist the child to regain his independence and mastery. She can do this by providing the opportunity for the child to exercise control over his environment by enlisting the child's help in decision-making, as with the daily schedule, injection site, or menu. And if the child has mastered a particular step in development at home, such as toilet training or a cup, the nurse can avoid those activities that would encourage regression, such as putting a diaper on the child or providing a bottle when none is used at home.

Promoting Communication and Understanding. The stage of cognitive development[43] will influence the child's understanding of and his reaction to what he experiences in the hospital, how he is able to express his feelings related to these experiences, and therefore how he is able to cope with the stress caused by the hospital experience. The nurse's understanding of the conceptual level within which the child is functioning will enable her to provide explanations that are effective in providing reassurance and understanding. For example, the child's understanding of the content and function of his body will change as the level of cognitive development changes.[25]

It is of vital importance for the nurse to assess the child's language ability, for it may give important clues about how the child will ask for help, how well he will be able to explain how he feels, how well he will be able to verbalize his questions and anxieties, and how the child views and interprets the experiences related to hospitalization. His parents will be important resources in determining how he usually communicates his needs, for example, the words or gestures used for toileting, and for food or drink.

Because of a desire of concerned adults to shield a child from frightening or upsetting information, or because of a feeling that the child will not understand, facts concerning the reason for illness or hospitalization or of upcoming events are often not shared with the child. Yet, because of the child's active fantasy, because of the child's sensitivity to anxiety and fear in those around him, and because he will undoubtedly hear bits of information related to his illness, it is important for the health professional to assure that the child understands what is happening to him. This is of vital importance in giving the child the means to deal with the situation in which he finds himself, and in preventing a situation where the child fears the unknown and anxiety is created by active fantasies, but where no one will discuss honestly and openly his expressed concerns. Michael Rothenberg[49] suggests that the health professional must "talk to the child" and in so doing provide the answers for the following six questions, always present, but seldom explicitly stated:

1. What do I have?
2. How did I get it?
3. Why did I get it?
4. Will I get well?
5. When will I get well?
6. Why did my parents leave me in the hospital?

Providing a Secure Environment. A world lacking in behavioral limits is frightening and anxiety-provoking to the child, and the anxiety is intensified when those he meets in the strange hospital environment react to his actions in a variety of ways. One of the important functions of the nurses on a pediatric unit is to provide a consistent social milieu where the child will be able to predict the outcomes of his behavior and the behaviors of others in his environment. She can do this by expecting that age-appropriate behavior will continue during hospitalization, by setting limits when necessary, and by providing acceptable ways in which anger and aggressiveness can be expressed. It is important that each nurse caring for the child manage a particular behavior problem in the same way and that agreements made with the child are followed through. Parents will need support in understanding the reasons for behavior changes during hospitalization and in providing consistency of discipline during this stressful time. Communication with the parents and among nurses, then, is important, and the approach decided upon should be recorded in the care plan.

The nurse can also provide a secure environment by protecting the child from overhearing discussions which may arouse fear and by shielding him from disturbing sights and sounds. If such incidents do occur, misinterpretations should be watched for, and the child should be encouraged to discuss the meaning of these incidents for him.

The pediatric unit should have areas that are "off limits" for painful procedures, such as the playroom and the child's room. Painful tests and procedures should be restricted to specific areas, such as a treatment room. The child, then, will have the security of knowing that the unexpected will not occur in these "safe" places. The child must also have the security of knowing that he will be informed, prior to a procedure, what the nurse or other health professional is going to do, what he can anticipate, and what will be expected of him.

Play.   Play, for the child, is a necessary way of learning about himself and his world. It is one of the child's most effective means of managing stress. Play can be the means by which the crisis of illness and hospitalization is broken into manageable segments, When a child is unable to verbalize feelings and questions, anxieties and fears are often intensified, but through play the child is able to clarify reality and to express feelings he is not able to articulate. Play can provide for the child mastery over an overwhelming situation and can move him from a passive to an active position in relating to the experiences imposed by the illness and hospitalization. Play can be a useful tool in helping a child to understand intrusive and surgical procedures and can be an important motivator for mobility and activity after surgery. Observation of play activities may also serve as a useful diagnostic tool, in which level of development, social interactions, and success of coping mechanisms can be assessed. Play, then, is an essential part of the child's hospital environment and of the nursing care planning.

An adequate play environment includes adults who permit noise, activity, and some messiness. It includes space. It includes play equipment for big muscle activity, such as tricycles, wagons, and carts. It includes materials for release of anger, such as clay, pounding boards, paints, and puppets. It includes materials for playing hospital, such as beds, dolls,

bandages, plastic syringes and thermometers, IV tubing, stethoscope, and tongue blades; it includes materials for playing nurse and doctor, such as hats, kits, and dolls. Most important, it includes a sensitivity by health care professionals to the needs of children for play, and a flexibility and ingenuity in providing ongoing opportunity for play as a natural part of the child's daily activities.

Maintaining   Intellectual   Growth: School.   School is a most influential factor in the school-age child's social and intellectual growth. The child's illness and hospitalization may have major consequences on the child's ability to progress satisfactorily in school. In order to promote this important part of development, the nurse must determine the effect the child's illness has had on past school accomplishment, the resources available from the child's school in terms of materials and/or teacher time, resources available in the hospital, and the degree to which the child might be able to continue study while in the hospital. Though physical needs often will take precedence over school in the initial stages of admission, every opportunity should be taken to include school in the daily planning for the child. This will require flexibility and planning but will give the child the message of "wellness" and "returning to home environment" important to hospitalized children, and it will ensure that they may return to the important social and intellectual environment of the school without the hospitalization having caused a major setback. As an important social influence on the child, contact with the child's own school is important, both during and after hospitalization, to reassure the child of his continuing school belongingness, to assure maintenance of his academic levels, and to effectively reintegrate the child into the school community.

Maintaining   Social   and   Emotional Growth.   The child experiences social and emotional needs unique to each stage of development that must be included in nursing care planning. Most important, the nurse must see that the child's need for affection and emotional support is met, especially in the absence of parents. She can do this by providing physical closeness for the child through activities such as rocking or reading, by staying with the child when the parents leave, and by comforting and staying with the child through painful and frightening procedures.

Also important to maintaining social and emotional growth is a physical environment that provides sensory stimulation appropriate to the developmental level of the child. Providing visual and auditory stimulation in the crib of infants, talking and playing with the infants and children, providing a variety of age-appropriate toys, and providing variety in the daily environment of the child are all examples of activities the nurse can carry out to assure that the child will continue to develop appropriate communication and social adaptive skills.

The nurse must be particularly sensitive to the effect that the illness or health problem, whether long term and chronic, or acute, has on the child's overall emotional and social development. Chronic illness and congenital malformations in particular can affect the child's self-image, the relationship between the child and his parents, the child's social relationships with other children, and the opportunity to interact in a normal way with the physical environment. The nurse is in a strategic position to evaluate the effect of the illness on the overall social and emotional development of the child and to see that appropriate counseling and long-term community support are made available.

The mobility of the child is particularly important to his development. With a new-found ability to walk, the child can explore and control his environment. He can explore space relationships, build his perception of form and movement, and experience control of a situation by moving toward or away from it. It is a way in which a child can express aggression and a way in which he can choose to relate with other people and objects. When immobilized through restraint, a cast, or having to remain in bed, generally the child will demonstrate an increased expression of aggressive feelings, increased verbal aggression, and increased restlessness and irritability. Special devices to provide self-directed mobility for the spina bifida child, wagons, and even 24-hour urine collection systems on a wheelchair for a child who has not been potty trained are all examples of possible methods to assure that the important mobility is maintained.

The restriction of mobility, restriction of variety of social experiences available to the child, and the lessened interaction with other children or siblings that result from illness and hospitalization are all factors that need to be taken into consideration by the nurse in planning care. Planning for group mealtimes, encouragement of group play activities, moving beds into the hallway to increase social accessibility of children who must remain in bed, assuring sibling visits, enlisting the help of children in some of the "jobs" on the unit, and encouraging ongoing relationships between mutually supporting children are all ways in which the nurse can assure that social growth continues during the hospital experience.

Physiologic Considerations

Physiologic Assessment of the Child. The physiologic assessment of the child must be interpreted based on a knowledge of normal ranges for children of various weights and ages. The normal range of pulse, respiration, and blood pressure will vary depending on the age and weight of the child.[15] Normal blood chemistry values will also change as the infant and child matures, particularly during the first year of life.[15]

With assessment of physiologic status of the child, care must be used in selecting the tools and criteria appropriate to the age, size, and developmental level of the child. The nurse must select both an approach to the child consistent with his developmental level, and the tools, such as the proper sized blood pressure cuff and the right type of thermometer, that will provide her with accurate and reliable information.

Considerations in Meeting Nutritional and Fluid Needs. Promoting adequate nutrition in children is one of the challenges of a pediatric nurse. It will require a knowledge of the caloric needs at various stages and an understanding of the unique interaction of the psychosocial stage of development, physical growth, the effect of the illness on the child, and the effect of hospitalization on the child. As well, the nurse must have a working knowledge of various formulas and foods available for children to enable a selection of a diet that is

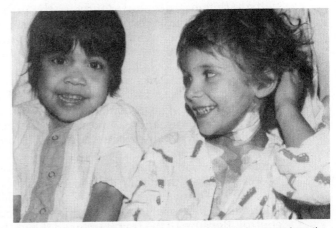

Figure 46–1. Maintaining children's social development is an important part of the nurse's role. (Photograph by Ronald C. McDonald.)

both nutritionally balanced and acceptable to the infant or child.

The child's nutritional and fluid requirements will change as the child grows older. An infant, for example, will require approximately 110 calories per kilogram per day, and 150 ml./kg./day of fluids. These requirements will gradually decrease to 70 cal./kg./day and 75 ml./kg./day for the 10 year old. The average daily excretion of urine will also change as the child grows older. The nurse must become familiar with normal requirements in order for her to assess the adequacy of a child's diet and fluid intake, to assess the influence of the illness on the nutritional and fluid and electrolyte status, and to plan and evaluate appropriate nursing interventions.

Illness places both nutritional status and fluid and electrolyte balance in jeopardy. The younger the child, the greater are the proportional needs for water, and the less are the fluid reserves. The fever, vomiting, diarrhea, and increased metabolic rate frequently accompanying illness, coupled with an inability or unwillingness to take in fluids, can cause life-threatening dehydration and electrolyte imbalances in young children. Likewise, the demand for calories for the normal growth of the child is intensified by the increased metabolism of illness at the same time the nutritional intake is likely to be decreased. Careful recording of fluid intake and output, especially with vomiting or diarrhea, is essential in children where the illness may lead to fluid and electrolyte imbalances. Fluid imbalances and dehydration may develop rapidly, so the nurse must be particularly concerned with the signs of weight loss, decreased urine, dry skin, sunken orbits, or rapid respirations, as shock may shortly follow.

A nurse can play an important role in assuring adequate fluid and caloric intake by skillful encouragement of oral intake. If intravenous fluid replacement and maintenance are required, the nurse must assure accuracy in administration. Too great a volume of fluid too quickly can be deleterious and must be guarded against through frequent observation and use of "mini drips," Buretrols, or similar equipment for careful fluid monitoring and control. Because of the trauma caused the child in starting the IV and the difficulty of starting the IV in small veins, care must be used to stabilize and maintain an IV once it is started.

Initiating intravenous infusion will be painful and frightening to the child, and the nurse must use her knowledge of development in preparing the child prior to the procedures, and supporting and comforting the child during the procedure.

Administration of Medications. Several physiologic factors must be considered in the administration of drugs to children. The effects of physiologic immaturity will increase as the child's age decreases. In infants particularly, organ immaturity is an important consideration in the degradation and excretion of drugs; slow detoxification and excretion result in enhanced toxicity and prolonged effects of some drugs. In addition, drugs are usually used when an infant is already sick, when water requirements and losses rise together with a decreased fluid intake, further decreasing the excretion of drugs.

Another physiologic factor to consider is the inefficient blood/brain barrier that exists in infants. This will mean enhanced neurologic effects of some drugs, such as morphine. In addition, the nurse must be aware of the possibility that some drugs, particularly steroids, will affect the child's growth when given over prolonged periods of time.

An added consideration in administration of drugs to children is the difficulty in the administration itself. The nurse must use her knowledge of growth and development and of the child to administer the medication in a manner least traumatic to the child while still assuring that the child receives the dose prescribed.

Observation for side effects of drugs is particularly important in children since often they are unable to communicate their response. Side effects to some drugs may be the same as with adults. With others, the side effects may be enhanced because of organ immaturity, and some drugs will have unique side effects in children, such as a change in behavior. The nurse must be aware of the possible side effects of the drugs she administers, specific to the pediatric population she is working with.

Dosages with drugs for children are usually prescribed according to the weight of the child and sometimes according to the body surface area. Because of the small size of children, an error in prescription or in administration can have serious, even fatal, results. The nurse must use extreme caution to assure that both the dosage ordered and the dosage administered are appropriate for the size of the child for which ordered. The nurse should continue to double-check dosages calculated by the physician until she is familiar with normal doses for children. She should question the physician if she has any doubt that the dosage ordered is appropriate. Because of the serious consequences of error, all doses and calculations of narcotics and digoxin should be checked with another nurse.

The ease with which a child accepts medications and the resulting long-term fears or lack of fear associated with them will depend in part on the skill of the nurse giving them. Whether or not the child receives the prescribed dose will also depend on her skill.

Oral medications may be given to infants in several ways, such as on the tip of a spoon, in a medicine dropper with a rubber tip, a syringe, nipple, or small cup. Whichever way is chosen, careful consideration should be given to safety. Infants have not yet learned to keep liquid from rolling out of their mouth and can easily choke. To assure that the infant gets the prescribed dose and to prevent choking, small amounts of the medication should be given slowly enough for the infant to swallow. For the same reason, it is preferable to give the medication when the infant is sitting or to at least elevate the infant's head. Though other methods are preferable, if one must use a syringe to administer oral medications, it should be directed to the side, not the back of the mouth. The method of medication administration will depend partly on the taste of the medication. Oral medications may be made more palatable to the infant by mixing with syrup or honey.

Injections for infants are usually given with a 25-gauge, ⅝ inch needle and are given in the mid-anterior thigh (quadriceps) or mid-lateral thigh (vastus lateralis). The gluteal area is small and poorly developed and should not be used at least until the child is walking, and preferably not until 5 to 6 years because of the potential damage to the sciatic nerve. The deltoid area should also be avoided because of the potential danger to the radial nerve. To ensure safety of administration, the nurse may wish to use a mummy restraint, leaving one leg exposed, or she may require the help of another nurse in giving the injection. The infant probably will not cry in anticipation of the injection, but he should be picked up and comforted by the nurse or by a parent after the injection.

Special consideration must be given to the developmental needs of toddlers and preschoolers when administering medications. They are in the stages of autonomy and mastery. This means that they wish for control, that often they are egocentric and unable to put themselves in another's place, and often their favorite word is *no*. At the same time they have a wish to please, so that they may feel this conflict in any situation, sometimes resulting in dawdling. By the time they are preschool age, they have acquired an interest in rituals and routines.

These characteristics hold several implications for the nurse administering medication to toddlers and preschoolers. She can be aware that a reaction to her approach with medication to be taken orally may be "no" and a tightly closed mouth, and she can understand this as a normal result of the developmental stage of the child. The nurse can avoid phrasing questions so the child can say "no," but can give the opportunity for a choice when it is realistic. Force should be avoided, but if you must resort to it, the basis for mastery later can be developed by telling the child that even though you know he does not like the medicine, someday he will be able to take it himself. Putting medication in food that a child needs nutritionally or attempting to disguise the medication must be avoided. If the medication is mixed with something else, like jelly or syrups, the child should be told.

Injections are particularly difficult for this age group. There is a universal fear among hospitalized children, well documented, surrounding injections. Preschoolers, especially, have increased fears and imagination. It is important that you tell them what you are going to do, so that they have the security of knowing that they will always be told before receiving an injection. The nurse can promote mastery by allowing the child to help, such as by cleaning the injection site or choosing the area where the injection will be given. The nurse should remain with the child until he has reestablished his equilibrium, and play materials should be provided to assist him to "work out" the particular feelings related to injections.

Nursing Procedures Unique to Children. The nurse will be required to carry out several procedures in caring for the child that are unique to the pediatric population. She will need to be familiar with a wide variety of urine collection techniques, for example, or may be confronted with unique methods of administration of oxygen, such as the croupette or "dog house." She may care for infants requiring Isolettes, and she will need to learn to use infant scales. Though use of restraints should be avoided if possible, there are times when they are necessary for the successful outcome of a procedure, and the nurse will need to learn a variety of approaches to restraining the child. Procedures such as gavage feeding are commonplace, and the approach to cardiopulmonary resuscitation is unique in the child. These represent only a few of the skills that are unique to pediatrics, and the pediatric nurse must be comfortable in carrying them out, so that she can concentrate on meeting the child's developmental and emotional needs.

ENVIRONMENTAL CONSIDERATIONS IN CARING FOR CHILDREN

The Emotional Environment

The emotional climate on a pediatric unit is far more important than the building or decor. A quality pediatric environment is welcoming, unthreatening, nurturing, supporting, consistent, and flexible to meet the needs of children and their families. Staff and volunteers are carefully selected for their sensitivity to the needs of children and their warmth. Nursing staff are well prepared in child development, child care, and counseling. The environment fosters open communication and human relationships among staff and patients. It invites, welcomes, and accommodates parents in the hospital, and encourages involvement of children and families in decisions related to their care. It is responsive to a variety of developmental, emotional, social and cultural needs and provides the educational and social activities, toys, equipment, and books to meet these needs. Children have the opportunity for self-expression, especially concerning their stress, anger, and fears, through talk with staff who are open, receptive, and sensitive to childhood concerns; and through easy availability of materials such as clay, paper and paints, or beanbags. It is an environment that emphasizes optimum use of potential of each child through promotion of a "wellness" atmosphere. This occurs when children dress in their own clothes during the day, when children are encouraged to be out of bed whenever possible, and when children eat and play together as a normal happening on the unit. And, it is an environment that encourages the maintenance of the relationship between the child, the family, and his home environment through unlimited visiting and rooming-in for those most important to the child.

The Safety Environment

Because their developmental immaturity makes children particularly susceptible to ac-cidents, safety is a significant consideration in caring for children. Children should be placed in a bed that resembles that which they are used to at home. A child in a crib whose mother gives a history of falls from the crib at home should have a protective "bubble" or other device placed over the crib. Siderails on cribs should be securely latched. The nurse must be aware of the rapidity with which a child, even an infant, can roll over or change positions; she must use extreme care to see that a child does not fall off a scale or out of a crib when the siderail is down. If she must look away for a moment, she should keep a hand on the child. Nothing should be left within reach of a crib or bed that the child might put into his mouth, swallow, or choke on, such as pins, medication, or syringe tops. All medication, cleaning agents, and chemicals or solutions must be out of the reach of children. A child in a highchair should be restrained, to prevent him from falling out. When restraints are used, they should be applied carefully so as not to impair circulation and in such a way that the child cannot manipulate himself into a position where he will be choked or strangled. Toys should be checked for sharp edges or small breakable or removable parts that could be swallowed or aspirated.

Bottles must never be propped, nor feedings or medications forced because of the danger of aspiration. Children's skin, particularly infants', is sensitive to heat and will burn easily. For this reason, hot-water bottles are never placed directly against the skin without wrapping, and they are filled with water no hotter than 46°C. (115°F.). Plastic sheets or pads should not be used in the beds of infants because of the danger of suffocation. Windows, staircases, electrical outlets, and fans must be made safe. Glass thermometers should be used with supervision because of the danger of breakage. When children cannot hold still for injections or treatments, help should be obtained so that the procedure can be conducted safely. Children must always wear identification bands.

PREPARATION OF THE PARENTS AND CHILD FOR SURGICAL AND DIAGNOSTIC PROCEDURES

Preparation of children and their families for surgical or diagnostic procedures is an important part of the role of the nurse caring for children. It is essential that every child be properly prepared before any surgical or other type of procedure. A study by Madelon A. Visintainer and John A. Wolfer has shown that systematic preparation for procedures, together with support from a consistent person, would "increase children's cooperation, decrease their upset behavior and problems in posthospital adjustment, and result in less anxiety, better information, and more satisfaction with care by parents."[57] These findings generally support other similar studies.[36] Preparation will help the child to marshal her resources to master new experiences, and even to utilize them in a positive way in her developmental process. It will replace the anxiety and fear of the unknown with trust and the knowledge that those around her will be truthful and will help her to manage the difficult experience. The outcome will be that the child will recover more quickly, without the long-term outcomes seen when children are not adequately prepared: general anxiety and regression, separation anxiety, anxiety about sleep, eating disturbances, mistrust and resistance of authority, apathy, and withdrawal.

It is a nursing responsibility to guarantee that children and parents have the information they need in order to cope with the experiences of surgery and procedures. Children generally learn best when they can be active participants in the process rather than passive listeners. They will want to know what they actually will experience—sounds, feelings, smells, sights—and will need to know what will be expected of them and what they can do to help. If the procedure is a treatment, children should be given a choice as to approach whenever possible and should be allowed to perform as much as possible themselves. Any preparation should be broken into segments that are manageable for the child, considering her anxiety level, attention span, age, time needed for assimilation, and previous understanding.

Any preparation must begin with an assessment of the child's and the parents' understanding. The nurse can review the teaching that the parents did, finding out what terms were used, what symptoms the child exhibited, and how they were related to the child's condition. Other sources of prior preparation can be considered, such as their physician, Public Health Nurse, clinic visits, or previous hospitalization. The child's understanding must be assessed: What has her illness meant to her? What is her understanding of why she came to the hospital? If she was hospitalized before, what kind of experience did she have? Based on conversations with parents, it must be decided if they should be involved in the teaching, and if so, whether they will teach the child with the nurse present, or the nurse will teach the child with the parents present. The nurse then must gather as much information as possible about what actually will happen—time of surgery; kind of anesthetic and preoperative medication; and

the procedure itself, such as where the incision will be, what kinds of tubes and monitors or other equipment the child will experience.

Next, an appropriate explanation and approach to the child must be decided upon. Words must be chosen based on the child's understanding, and an approach selected based on cognitive level. Care must be used to avoid so much detail that the child becomes frightened. Neutral words, such as open, drain, and ooze, should be chosen rather than words such as "cut" and "bleed." Still, enough information must be given in order that the child can anticipate and prepare for some of the more unpleasant aspects, such as the preoperative injection, or that postoperatively she will experience pain, a sore throat, or will need to cough and walk even though it hurts.

Two to three year olds will respond best to a multisensory approach by which they can actually explore equipment they will experience and see, such as surgical masks, tubings, stethoscopes, and dolls with appropriate appearance for a particular procedure. A child this age will be most concerned about separation and will want to know that she will see her parents after the procedure is over. Preschoolers may respond best to a rehearsal or dramatization of events they will experience, the nurse playing one role and the child another. Then the roles are reversed so that the nurse can assess the child's understanding. Dolls, animals, and puppets can be used to encourage participation in this kind of preparation. Children this age are capable of understanding the inside of the body, so a simple explanation of anatomy and physiology may be given on a body outline. Children this age fear separation but also are concerned with punishment and bodily mutilation. They need to know the procedure is not a punishment and that no other part of their body will be operated on. School-age children may respond to a more scientific approach, using pictures, books, and body outlines. The nurse can take advantage of the more mature concept of time and reason a child of this age has.

Anesthesia is often a frightening aspect for the child, and some have a fear of not awakening. They need an opportunity to handle and experiment with an anesthesia mask and should know that anesthesia is only a temporary sleep until the operation is over. Children will need to know the operative site and their postoperative appearance, such as surgical dressings, incision line, sutures, IV's, and monitors. If the child is to be in an intensive care unit, a visit there with the parents and a nurse can be helpful in "inoculation"[27] of the child to the sights and sounds she will be exposed to while there. Postoperative expectations—suctioning, coughing, and turning—must be explained and practiced. Children need a realistic understanding of pain but should know that they can receive medication to help decrease it. Closer to the actual time of surgery, such events as fasting after bedtime and in the morning, the starting of an IV, the pHisoHex bath, transportation to the OR, and who will be with him need explanation. An evaluation should be made of the anxiety caused by injections. If highly anxiety provoking, it may be wise to wait until the morning of surgery to explain this aspect. Children should have the opportunity to review and repeat what has been learned and to ask questions. The nurse must use care to ask the child simple questions throughout the preparation period to assess understanding.

Parents will want to know when the child will go to the operating room, how long it will take, how far they may accompany the child, where they should wait, whether they can leave during the surgery, when they will see the doctor, and when they will be able to see their child postoperatively. They should be prepared for what their child will look like—his restlessness, crying, possible slurred speech, very flushed or very pale skin, or occasional nausea and vomiting. Parents should know that their child will react to and reflect their own attitudes and emotions. Whenever possible, they should have the opportunity to see their child in the recovery room or intensive care unit before he is awake so that they may react to the child's appearance and ask questions. In doing so, they have the opportunity to regain their composure before their child awakens. Parents should know what resources will be available to them during the time they are waiting for the surgery to be over and immediately postoperatively. Nursing staff familiar with the child, for example, can visit them during the waiting period to see that their needs are being met and to answer questions.

After surgery, a return to normal habits should be encouraged as rapidly as possible, such as visiting, eating, playing, and moving about. Opportunities for dramatic play with equipment they have experienced should be encouraged. If they are verbal, they should be encouraged to talk about their experiences. Communication with friends by phone or letter should be encouraged. They may use colors, paint, and drawings to tell a story, or they may make a scrapbook or keep a diary. All of these activities will help them in understanding, integrating, and controlling what has happened to them.

DEATH: THE CHILD, THE FAMILY, AND THE NURSE

Though the role that the pediatric nurse plays in promoting wellness in the child is important, one of the greatest needs of the child and family will be for her sensitive, available, and integrated support during the time surrounding anticipated death and death. The nurse can play an invaluable role in assuring the child a peaceful and dignified death and in supporting the child's significant others. (See also Chapters 48 and 49.)

The child's perception of death changes and grows with his change in time perspective, logic, and reasoning ability. Under 3 years of age a child's greatest fear is separation from comforting adults and loss of love. Between 3 and 6 years, the child is concerned with punishment, and may view death as reversible. There are reports of children of 4 years who have questions about their own survival. Between 6 and 10 years, the child begins to fear death itself, the changed perception being consistent with a general broadening of thinking and more realistic ideas. His greatest fears may be unexpected pain, mutilation, and the mystery surrounding death. From 9 years of age on, children can comprehend the permanence of death and its universality.

The nurse may assume that a child who is oriented to the future wonders why he has not gotten well. Research by Waechter[58] on children 6 to 10 years of age showed that children with fatal illness, even though not directly informed as to the nature of their illness, demonstrated significantly greater anxiety related to death than did other groups. They showed considerable preoccupation with death in fantasy and demonstrated feelings of loneliness and isolation and a sense of loss of control. One of the significant findings was that children who had the opportunity to discuss their illness and prognosis expressed less anxiety than did the children with fatal illness who did not have the same opportunity.

Death is the ultimate loneliness and isolation for the child when there is no opportunity for discussion of his fear and when there is a feeling of not being understood. Because of society's attitude toward death and the taboo in talking about death, the child may feel inhibited in expressing his concerns. Children are extremely perceptive of emotional climate, evasiveness, or false cheerfulness. Often they may have knowledge or fears of their impending death, have overheard whispered discussions, but have no one they feel they can discuss it with. They may, as well, have a knowledge of their condition, but wish to shield their family from the pain surrounding it.

Parents will go through the phases of shock, denial and disbelief, anger, and guilt before acceptance. When the death of a child can be anticipated, anticipatory grief is almost universal. Parents may be preoccupied with thoughts concerning the impending death and have periods of depression and crying. Often somatic symptoms such as apathy and weakness are a part of the grieving. They may feel guilt for previous omissions in raising their child, and their anger may be displaced to medical and nursing personnel. Some parents derive comfort from being able to provide physical care to their child. Others will need to escape from the situation.

The nurse may experience increased difficulty in working with the dying child. Often there is a greater sense of loss than with adults because the child has not yet experienced life. The pain of close contact with the child is difficult, and often the defenses of isolation or "professional behavior" make it easier to avoid forming a relationship with the dying child and are common attempts to deal with the helplessness and ambivalence felt by the nurse. But she is in the key position to provide support to the child and family during this difficult time, and avoidance can result in extreme loneliness at the very time the child needs closeness and comfort. It takes courage and maturity to undergo the experience of a child's death with his family and retain openness and compassion as a human being. The nurse must explore her own feelings, resources, and mechanisms of support. Often, staff conferences or discussion with individual resource persons will be helpful to the nurse in dealing with her feelings about the child and family, feelings about death, and her own sadness and grieving. Only through a continuing self-assessment and seeking of resources to meet her own needs can a nurse retain sensitivity to the child's and family's needs and her effectiveness in providing them needed guidance and support.

It is important that the team of health care professionals decide together on the approach to the dying child and the family. They need to determine the family's usual coping mechan-

isms, how much support is needed, and what family or community support is available to them. Parents should be consulted concerning their attitudes, how much they are comfortable in telling the child themselves, and how much they want imparted by the staff. Information is needed on how much the child knows, as well. When to tell the child that he will not recover requires careful consideration. Too early disclosure may inhibit normal relationships, but dealing with the fact too late may leave the child to deal with his knowledge in isolation. An atmosphere of openness should be promoted, and if children ask questions, they deserve to be answered. Parents may need help in understanding the importance of honesty with the child and in understanding that their attempts to shield the child from painful knowledge will promote anxiety, loneliness, and isolation in the child at the time when he most needs the closeness and support of his family. Parents can be helped to tell the child the truth with specific words and phrases. Staff and parents should be prepared to accept that honesty concerning death will involve feelings of sadness and helplessness and be prepared to deal with these feelings. Both the parents and the child should be allowed hope, and a feeling of active coping should be promoted.

It is always a surprise to adults, who have a romantic view of childhood, that children have the capacity for a "making the best of it" attitude and are in some ways inventive and practical about their afflictions. However, their inventiveness and play of mind to develop new solutions depends on keeping their anxiety at a minimum.[42]

The usual activities and normal relationships with family and friends should be maintained as long as possible. Whenever possible, the child should be encouraged to dress in play clothes, stay out of bed and play and eat with other children. Placement on the nursing unit is significant and is important in decreasing feelings of isolation. Expressions of anger and hostility must be accepted.

The child's mother particularly may feel a need to be physically close to the child in order to cope with the impending separation and guilt. The nurse can support the parents in providing physical care and emotional support to the child, emphasizing their value as parents despite the helplessness of the situation. If, on the other hand, the parents feel a need to escape the situation, the nurse can recognize this as a normal reaction and can help them in establishing a closer relationship with the child during this difficult period.

The topic of how the parents plan to tell the child's siblings should be approached. Siblings often react to the emotional changes parents are experiencing, to a concern that they may die of the same disease their brother or sister has, or to a feeling of parental neglect or abandonment. Helping parents to deal appropriately with the siblings of the dying child may do much to prevent the school failures, depression, hyperactivity, and feelings of parental neglect or abandonment that siblings often experience.

At the actual time of death, parents need consideration, empathy, and emotional support. They will need privacy and respect for the social and cultural customs related to grieving. If at all possible, the health care professional, whether nurse, physician, or social worker, who has worked most closely with the family in dealing with the death of the child should be present to provide support. It is natural that the nurse too will feel grief at this time, and it can be shared with the parents. This is a time, however, when it will be important to not allow her own grief to supersede a supporting relationship with the family.

Other children on the unit may have questions about the empty room of the child. Their questions should be answered truthfully, and they should be allowed the opportunity of exploring the meaning of the event for them. Hiding the truth can promote increased fantasy and anxiety.

Routine follow-up care is important to the family of the child who has died. Ideally, bereaved families are sought out 1 to 3 months after the child's death. The health professional responsible for this activity must assess how effectively the family is dealing with the loss of their child, recognize signs of maladaptive coping if present, and help them toward a healthy resolution of their loss.

SUMMARY

Children are influenced by a variety of factors, especially their interaction with their family and environment and their particular level of development. These factors must be considered in evaluating the effects of illness and hospitalization on the child and in planning nursing interventions. This chapter has provided a broad overview of the nursing role in caring for children experiencing illness and should serve as a basis for further in-depth study.

BIBLIOGRAPHY

1. Barnard, K., and Erres, S. S. (eds.): *Nursing Child Assessment Contract, Results of the First Twelve Months of Life.* Final report submitted to Division of Nursing, Bureau of Health Resources Development, USPHS, HEW, Contract NOI-NU-14174, May 1977 (unpublished manuscript).
2. Bemelmans, L.: *Madeline.* New York, Viking Press, Inc., 1969.
3. Blake, F. G.: *Open Heart Surgery in Children.* Washington, D.C., U.S. Government Printing Office, U.S. Department of Health, Education, and Welfare, Public Health Service Publication No. 2075, 1964.
4. Blake, F. G.: *The Child, His Parents and the Nurse.* Philadelphia, J. B. Lippincott Co., 1954.
5. Blake, F. G., Wright, F. H., and Waechter, E. H.: *Nursing Care of Children.* Philadelphia, J. B. Lippincott Co., 1970.
6. Bowlby, J., et al.: *Maternal Care and Mental Health; Deprivation of Maternal Care: A Reassessment of Its Effects.* New York, Schocken Books, 1966.
7. Bowlby, J.: *Attachment and Loss: Vol. 1. Attachment.* New York, Basic Books, 1969.
8. Brazelton, T. B.: *Infants and Mothers.* New York, Dell Publishing Co., Inc., 1969.
9. Brazelton, T. B.: *The Neonatal Behavioral Assessment Scale.* Philadelphia, J. B. Lippincott Co., 1973.
10. Brooks, M. M.: Why play in the hospital? *Nursing Clinics of North America,* 5:431, Sep. 1970.
11. Butler, A., Chapman, J., and Stuible, M.: Child's play is therapy. *The Canadian Nurse,* 71:35, Dec. 1975.
12. Caldwell, B. M.: *Instruction Manual Inventory for Infants (Home Observation for Measurement of the Environment).* Little Rock, Ark., University of Arkansas, 1970.
12a. Chadwick, B. J., Pflederer, D., and Ray, M. A.: Maintaining the hospitalized child's home ties. *American Journal of Nursing,* 78:1360–1362, Aug. 1978.
13. Chenevert, M.: Taking the hurt out of the hospital. *Family Health,* 2:30, Feb. 1970.
14. Chilman, C. S.: *Growing Up Poor.* Washington, D.C., U.S. Government Printing Office, SRS Publication No. 109, 1966.
15. Chinn, P. L.: *Child Health Maintenance.* St. Louis, C. V. Mosby Co., 1974.
16. Chinn, P. L., and Leitch, C. J.: *Handbook for Nursing Assessment of the Child.* Salt Lake City, University of Utah Printing Service, 1973.
16a. Christophersen, E. R.: Behavioral pediatrics. *American Family Physician,* 17:134–139, March 1978.
17. Erikson, E. H.: *Childhood and Society.* New York, W. W. Norton & Company, Inc., 1963.
18. Erickson, F.: The toddler during illness. *Hospital Topics,* 42:95, Sep. 1964.
19. Erickson, M. L.: *Assessment and Management of Developmental Changes in Children.* St. Louis, C. V. Mosby Co., 1976.
19a. Everson, S.: Sibling counseling. *American Journal of Nursing,* 77:644–646, April 1977.
20. Fagin, C. M.: *The Effects of Maternal Attendance During Hospitalization on the Post-Hospital Behavior of Young Children: A Comparative Survey.* Philadelphia, F. A. Davis, 1966, pp. 61–65.
21. Farrell, S. E., and Kiernan, B. S.: A positive approach to nutrition for hospitalized children. *Maternal Child Nursing,* 2:113, March/April 1977.

22. Fond, K. I.: Dealing with death and dying through family-centered care. *Nursing Clinics of North America*, 7:53, March 1972.

23. Frankenburg, W. K., Dodds, J. B., and Fendal, A. W.: *The Denver Developmental Screening Test.* Denver, University of Colorado Medical Center, 1970.

24. Galligan, A. C.: Books for hospitalized children. *American Journal of Nursing*, 75:2164, Dec. 1975.

25. Gellert, E.: Children's conceptions of the content and functions of the human body. *In Genetic Psychology Monographs*, 65:297, May 1962.

26. Gesell, A., Ilg, F. L., and Ames, L. B.: *Infant and Child in the Culture of Today.* New York, Harper & Row, 1974.

27. Hardgrove, C.: Emotional inoculation: the 3 R's of preparation. *Journal of the Association for the Care of Children in Hospitals*, 5:17, Spring 1977.

28. Hardgrove, C. B., and Dawson, R. B.: Ideas, A to Z, for personalizing pediatric units. *Nursing '76*, 6:57, April 1976.

29. Haynes, U.: *A Developmental Approach to Casefinding.* Washington, D.C., U.S. Government Printing Office, Children's Bureau Publication No. 449, 1967.

30. Holt, J. L.: Discussion of the method and clinical implications from the study "Children's recall of a preschool age hospital experience after an interval of five years." *In* Batey, M. V. (ed.): *Communicating Nursing Research; The Research Critique.* Boulder, Colo., Western Interstate Commission for Higher Education, 1:56, 1968.

31. Irelan, L. M. (ed.): *Low Income Life Styles.* Washington, D.C., U.S. Government Printing Office, Welfare Administration Publication No. 14, 1967.

31a. Isler, C.: The fine art of handling a hospitalized child. *RN*, 41:41–45, March 1978.

32. Klaus, M. H., and Kennell, J. H.: *Maternal-Infant Bonding.* C. V. Mosby Co., St. Louis, 1976.

33. Kunzman, L.: Some factors influencing a young child's mastery of hospitalization. *Nursing Clinics of North America*, 7:13, March 1972.

34. Lawson, B. A.: Chronic illness in the school-aged child: effects on the total family. *The American Journal of Maternal Child Nursing*, 2:49, Jan./Feb. 1977.

35. Lichtenberg, P., and Norton, D. G.: *Cognitive and Mental Development in the First Five Years of Life.* Washington, D.C., U.S. Government Printing Office, DHEW Publication No. (HSM) 72–9102, 1970.

36. Mahaffy, P. R.: The effects of hospitalization on children admitted for tonsillectomy and adenoidectomy. *Nursing Research*, 14:12, Winter 1965.

37. Mahaffy, P. R.: Nurse-parent relationships in living-in situations. *Nursing Forum*, 3:53, Feb. 1964.

38. Mattsson, A.: Long-term illness in childhood: a challenge to psychosocial adaptation. *Pediatrics*, 50:801, Nov. 1972.

38a. Miller, C.: Working with parents of high-risk infants. *American Journal of Nursing*, 78:1228–1230, July 1978.

39. Morrissey, J. R.: Death anxiety in children with a fatal illness. *In* Parad, H. J. (ed.): *Crisis Intervention: Selected Readings.* New York, Family Service Association of America, 1965.

40. Murray, R., and Zentner, J.: *Nursing Assessment and Health Promotion through the Life Span.* Englewood Cliffs, N. J., Prentice-Hall, Inc., 1975.

41. Petrillo, M.: Preventing hospital trauma in pediatric patients, *American Journal of Nursing*, 68:1469, July 1968.

42. Petrillo, M., and Sanger, S.: *Emotional Care of Hospitalized Children.* Philadelphia, J. B. Lippincott Co., 1972.

43. Phillips, J. L.: *The Origins of Intellect: Piaget's Theory.* San Francisco, W. H. Freeman and Co., 1969.

44. Piper, W. (ed.): *Little Engine that Could.* Bronx, N.Y., Platt & Munk Publishers, 1976.

45. Prugh, D. G., et al.: A study of the emotional reactions of children and families to hospitalization and illness. *American Journal of Orthopsychiatry*, 23:70, 1953.

46. Redl, F.: *When We Deal With Children.* New York, Free Press, 1966.

47. Rey, M., and Rey, H. A., *Curious George Goes to the Hospital.* New York, Houghton Mifflin Co., 1966.

48. Robertson, J.: *Young Children in Hospitals.* London, Tavistock Publications, 1968, pp. 20–23.

49. Rothenberg, M. B.: Reactions of children to illness and hospitalization. *In* Smith, D. W., and Marshall, R. E. (eds.): *Introduction to Clinical Pediatrics.* Philadelphia, W. B. Saunders Co., 1972.

49a. Schleicher, I. M.: Teaching parents to cope with behavior problems. *American Journal of Nursing*, 78:838–839, May 1978.

49b. Shufer, S.: Communicating with children: teaching via the play-discussion group. *American Journal of Nursing*, 77:1960–1962, Dec. 1977.

50. Simon, J. I.: Emotional aspects of physical disability. *The American Journal of Occupational Therapy*, 25:408, Nov.–Dec. 1971.

51. Slattery, J. S.: Nutrition for the normal healthy infant. *Maternal Child Nursing*, 2:105, March/April, 1977.

51a. Smith, E. C.: Are you really communicating? *American Journal of Nursing*, 77:1966–1968, Dec. 1977.

51b. Smith, E. C., et al.: Reestablishing a child's body image. *American Journal of Nursing*, 77:445–447, March 1977.

52. Snell, B., and McLellan, C.: Whetting hospitalized preschoolers' appetites. *American Journal of Nursing*, 76:413, March 1976.

53. Spock, B.: *Baby and Child Care.* New York, Pocket Books, Inc., 1976.

54. Turtle, W. J.: *Dr. Turtle's Babies.* New York, Popular Library, Inc., 1974.

55. Vaughan, V. C., McKay, R. J., and Nelson, W. E.: *Nelson Textbook of Pediatrics*, 10th ed. Philadelphia, W. B. Saunders Co., 1975.

56. Vernick, J., and Karon, M.: Who's afraid of death on a leukemia ward? *American Journal of Diseases of Children*, 109:393, May 1965.

57. Visintainer, M. A., and Wolfer, J. A.: Psychological preparation for surgical pediatric patients: the effect on childrens' and parents' stress responses and adjustment. *Pediatrics*, 56:187, Aug. 1975.

58. Waechter, E. H.: Death anxiety in children with fatal illness. *Nursing Research Conference (ANA)*, 5:83, March 1969.

59. Weizenbach, J. F., and Cline, N.: *Wendy Well and Billy Better Say Hello Hospital.* Chicago, R. R. Donnelley Sons Co., 1970.

60. Weizenbach, J. F., and Cline, N.: *Wendy Well and Billy Better Ask a "Mill-Yun" Hospital Questions.* Chicago, R. R. Donnelley Sons Co., 1970.

61. Weizenbach, J. F., and Cline, N.: *Wendy Well and Billy Better and the Hospital See-through Machines.* Chicago, R. R. Donnelley Sons Co., 1970.

62. Weizenbach, J. F., and Cline, N.: *Wendy Well and Billy Better Meet the Hospital Sandman.* Chicago, R. R. Donnelley Sons Co., 1970.

63. Wolff, S.: *Children Under Stress.* Middlesex, England, Penguin Books Ltd., 1973.

64. Young, R. K.: Chronic sorrow: parents' response to the birth of a child with a defect. *The American Journal of Maternal Child Nursing*, 2:38, Jan./Feb. 1977.

CHAPTER 47

CARING FOR ILL ELDERLY PERSONS

By Alma Miller Ware, R.N., M.N.

The task of analyzing the physiology and behavior of those requiring nursing care is enormously complex in any case, and it is especially so with the ill elderly. Everyone involved with this care bears a major responsibility and needs to be continually reminded why their particular functions are being performed. The nursing person, in particular, needs to remember that her primary responsibility is concerned with the person's daily living activities which have been disrupted by either the development of a disease process or consequences of normal aging changes.

INTRODUCTION AND STUDY GUIDE

It is more and more evident that people are living longer than they used to. As one examines the predictions of demographers the actual number of individuals alive is also increasing. At the turn of the century only 4 per cent of Americans were over 65; at present 10 per cent are. By the middle of the next century, this group will exceed 25 per cent of our population. Accompanying this rise in number is an increase in the number of persons experiencing pathologies that may interfere with positive self-regard and self-esteem during the senior years.

One implication of these facts is that those persons now living have few role models to pattern their senescence after.[30] The hope is that this absence of role models will change as the longevity of present and future populations continues.

Certainly we think we know what aging is. We have been counting birthdays as far back as we can remember. We probably recognize, too, that chronologic age is not the only way of defining where we are on the time scale. In fact, chronologic age can be completely misleading if we use it as the sole basis for decisions of any kind, especially health care. Effective nursing action requires us to recognize the distinction between what is meant by chronologic aging and what is meant by functional aging. Functional aging presents itself in wide variations in individuals and is experienced as a creeping loss of vitality. It is determined by how one performs rather than how many years one has lived. If it is clear to most of us that no two adolescents are the same, it should be even more apparent that persons who have lived a long period of time will show even greater evidence of individual variations. Those persons who deal with the ill elderly must recognize and clearly identify both the positive and negative functions in the individuals they are working with.

One's physiology determines the parameters within which one functions. In order to deal with abnormalities, such as disease, the nursing student must understand what is normal for the long-lived person. It is the nurse who, by tradition and at times by default, has inherited the crucial responsibility of caring for many of the nation's long-lived ill elderly. One only needs to scan the needs of residents in any long-term care facility to appreciate nursing's responsibility. Indeed, the care of the person who has lived a long time offers one of the most challenging opportunities to the nursing process. The effectiveness with which nursing meets the challenge depends upon an understanding of both physiology and behavioral science of normal aging. Generally, long-lived persons do not seek direct nursing care until they are ill. For this reason, understandably, the nursing student may begin by focusing on the pathology present. Thus the knowledge and understanding base of the whole person is limited. This constricted focus may become one of the prime reasons for the ineffective nursing care of the ill elderly.

The Learner

Persons working with the ill elderly will need to recognize what their own experiences, expectations, and attitudes are.[2] Where do our attitudes come from? They come from our personal experiences and from what society has taught us about aging. How can a beginning nursing student assess her own attitudes? Start by examining your contacts with long-lived persons, think about the attitudes you have developed from exposure to television, newspapers, magazines, comics, jokes, songs (for example *Old Man Take A Look at Me* and *MacArthur Park*)—even school texts. Did the students around you even note the nursing home scandals of 1975 and, if so, were they as concerned about them as they were about Watergate? Did they see films such as *Harry and Tonto* or that classic, *Harold and Maude*? What kind of feelings for the aging process do these films produce?

Has your own direct contact with the elderly been limited or do you really *know* an old person—someone you've had long talks with, someone who has shared his view of life with you? Has your contact included awareness of the joys of long-term living as well as the problems? Can you imagine what it is like to be 70 years old? Have you thought about your own development from one age to another (e.g., from early childhood to adolescence and from adolescence into early adulthood)? What have you observed about your parents' and grandparents' aging transitions?

Answers to these questions will most likely reveal gaps in knowledge about the aging process. One misconception is that growing old is synonymous with being ill. This attitude is understandable since, until the 1950's, most of the emphasis and study of older people focused on their diseases or the aftermath of illnesses. During the last decade more interest has been directed to looking at the positive side of long-term living.[36] *Learning to Grow Old* by Paul Tournier, a well-known Swiss psychiatrist in his mid-seventies, was published in 1972 and reflects this change in attitude.[41]

The purposes of this chapter include:

1. To enable those who have nursing responsibilities in the care of the ill elderly to effectively assist in, direct, and provide realistic nursing programs

2. To provide a workable base for expanding and developing new approaches to the needs of the ill elderly

3. To promote understanding of the unique factors facilitating the assessment process for care of the aged

4. To relate these assessment findings with the student's increased knowledge and understanding

As one becomes more familiar with the literature from this field an understanding of the vocabulary is necessary. Familiarity with the following words and concepts will facilitate the learner's appreciation of the literature and research:

chronological age	life space
cohort	life span
cross-sectional	lipofuscin
life review	long-term care
demography	longevity
developmental tasks	longitudinal
functional age	nursing homes
geriatric	senility
gerontology	senescence
identity crisis	significant others

After completion of this chapter, the student should be able to discuss the following:

1. How does the chronologic age, the perspective, and attitude of the health care worker influence scope and implementation of the established care plan?

2. How do energy levels of the long-lived person differ throughout the aging process?

3. How do energy levels affect functioning ability?

4. In interpreting blood chemistry reports, what other factors must be taken into consideration for adequate assessment of the report?

5. What sensory changes occur with normal aging?

6. How might these sensory changes determine the specificity of nursing care orders?

7. What are the unique responsibilities for the nurse involved in geriatric/gerontological practice?

8. What factors determine effective assessments of the long-lived person?

IMPACT OF AGING

Age-related changes manifest themselves variously, and the changes which do occur are gradual in their development. All of us grow and develop in our own unique ways. Listing possible or probable changes in aging is to grossly oversimplify the myriad variations with which these changes reveal themselves in each human being. Comprehensive reviews of the alterations resulting from normal age changes are available.[7, 9, 22, 47] To be clinically competent, the student needs to be able not only to recognize the changes but also to understand the basis for the identified changes.

The fact that the care of the ill elderly is first and foremost an interactional process between the patient and the nurse practitioner cannot be overemphasized. The reciprocal relationship between the physiologic and psychosocial processes of human beings is also well recognized.[40] However, the general approach to and knowledge base of clinical practice have tended to be psychosocial, with the physiologic consequences of normal aging often being overlooked. An exception to this psychosocial emphasis has been in understanding physiologic specifics of diseases.[22a]

Physiologic Changes

Declining reserve physiologic support impairs the older person's recuperative power, in that homeostatic readjustments become slower as we age.[38, 40] There is a difference in the ability of cells and tissues to reproduce themselves during the life span. Skin, gut lining, liver and bone marrow cells retain their ability to reproduce themselves throughout the life span with adequate physiological support. Neurons, muscle and kidney cells of the older person, however, do not have this regenerative ability; these cells lose this ability either shortly before or shortly after birth.

Decrease of physiologic reserves is affected by any change, but particularly by stress imposed by an illness, and places the aged in an even more vulnerable situation. Almost every organ of the body loses some function with aging, but the degree and rate of loss will depend on the person's genetic makeup, life experiences, and past and current environments. Changes may occur in any of all body systems, but three systems are probably of core importance in the aging process: the cardiovascular, the central nervous, and the endocrine. The nerve cells' need for adequate blood supply is acute, while the body's primary control mechanisms, i.e., temperature and blood pressure regulation, operate either through the endocrine or nervous systems. The failure of these systems probably accounts for the major illnesses and significant decrements in the functioning of aging people. This inability of the body's systems to function effectively leads to many of the conditions causing the elderly to be ill or unable to function optimally without the assistance of nursing care.

The Cardiovascular System. The cardiovascular system is in a central position because the decrease in the heart's effectiveness leads to many of the pathologies seen in the long-lived person. The specific effects of age itself on the heart are not clear. Generally it is considered that the age changes are due to decreased vascular elasticity of blood and heart vessels. Separation of the role of coronary arteriosclerosis from the intrinsic changes within the myocardial fibers is difficult. Also, the importance of changes in cardiac output itself is unclear. There is a fall in stroke volume, and

TABLE 47–1.   CARDIOVASCULAR SYSTEM: SELECTED CHANGES OF NORMAL AGING

ORGAN, FUNCTION, OR REPORT	CHANGES COMMON IN THE LONG-LIVED PERSON
1. Arterial blood pressure	Rate of systolic increase is greater than rate of diastolic increase
2. Baroreceptor sensitivity	Decreases
3. Circulation time	Increases
4. Heart	As a pump, functions well under ordinary circumstances Loses physiologic reserve Difficulty in responding normally to stress situations (blood loss, excess parenteral infusions)
a. Contractility	Decreases Time is prolonged; therefore increasing O_2 requirement
b. Stroke volume	Decreases
c. Cardiac output	Decreases
d. Electrocardiogram (EKG)	Usually shows no change with age
e. Atrial gallop	Commonly heard even in the absence of disease
5. Organ perfusion	Decreases
6. Peripheral vascular resistance	Increases
7. Postural hypotension	Occurs fairly frequently Increases with febrile disease
8. Pulse pressure	Individual's range widens

contractibility is slower, which narrows the range of optimal heart rate.

Resting cardiac output decreases 30 to 40 per cent between the ages of 25 and 65. Regional perfusion decreases during this same age span: coronary flow decreases slightly less than 30 per cent; cerebral flow decreases 14 per cent; and a 40 to 45 per cent decrease occurs in both the liver visceral flow and the flow within the kidney. Two important symptoms of cardiac disease which are modified by the aging process are cardiac pain and dyspnea. Edema, when it is present in the elderly, may be due to cardiac disease or it may arise as a result of other physiological imbalances; i.e., kidney failure, hormonal imbalances, immobility.

Despite these changes, however, the changes in the aging heart are such that the ability of the heart to function as a pump under ordinary circumstances remains. Table 47–1 outlines other known changes of the cardiovascular system.

Central Nervous System. The central nervous system coordinates and integrates the body's muscular, neuronal, glandular and circulatory systems; this system organizes the overall behavior and regulates vital autonomic functions. Specific changes due to aging have yet to be fully clarified.[22] The cell changes presently known to be more often correlated with nervous tissue are: lipofuscin deposits, neurofibrillary tangles, and amyloid plaques. Our knowledge of the neurobiology of aging is truly in its very early stage.

Prior to 1960 the consequences of aging to the central nervous system were assumed to be insurmountable. We now know that the morphological changes occur very slowly. Effective therapeutic programs presently are being explored to intervene with the changes before aging consequences are clinically irreversible.

In long-lived persons, interdependence of the central nervous system physiology and emotional stability becomes significantly increased.[44] Cognitive decline can be one of the earliest indications of central nervous system changes. Additional data are necessary before conclusions can be made, but available evidence supports a more optimistic view of central nervous system aging consequences.

Sensory losses are particularly significant, since any such impairment affects the individual's ability to interact satisfactorily with his external or internal environment. Sensory systems are the means used for "getting the message to the C.N.S." Because of alterations due to aging, the long-lived individual often loses control over what is perceived; Table 47–2 lists some of the sensory impairments that commonly occur.

TABLE 47–2. SENSORY SYSTEM: SELECTED CHANGES OF NORMAL AGING

Sensory Systems in General
  a. Decreased efficiency
  b. General decline of awareness of environmental stimuli
  c. After 75 years, three out of five persons have some sensory deficits.

Hearing (Audition)[10]
  a. Auditory threshold decreases with aging
  b. Greater loss of higher frequency sounds
  c. Ability to discriminate speech declines
  d. Long-time exposure to noise pollution increases loss
  e. For some, "feeling of paranoia" occurs

Proprioception (perception of position and relationship in and to space)
  a. Impaired
  b. Balance and coordination are affected

Smell
  a. Research findings conflicting
  b. Some decline usually present

Taste
  a. Changes studied with conflicting results
  b. Increased complaints about food
  c. Older persons may prefer tart beverages

Touch Sensation
  a. Declines
  b. Adaptation to environment is affected

Vibration
  a. Sense loss is greater in lower than in upper extremities
  b. Begins at about 50 years
  c. Greater amplitude of change required[12]

Vision[10]
1. Accommodation
  a. Rate diminishes
  b. Decreases, but generally after age 60 there is no further decrease
  c. Adaptation to darkness declines
  d. Affected by glare
2. Pupil size and reactivity
  a. Reduction of both is commonly observed
3. Acuity
  a. Decreases
  b. Decrease progressively greater for females than males
4. Color perception
  a. Transmission of colors from green to violet decreases
  b. Sensitivity to blue and possibly red also decreases
5. Critical flicker fusion
  a. Decreases
  b. Linked to a general decline in central nervous system efficiency
6. Depth perception
  a. Less accurate

Endocrine System. The stability of the human body results from the coordinated functions and interrelationships of the endocrine and autonomic nervous system. At one time it was

TABLE 47–3.   CHANGES OF PLASMA HORMONES DURING AGING

	HORMONE CONCENTRATION IN BLOOD	RESPONSE TO PHYSIOLOGIC OR PHARMACOLOGIC STIMULATION	METABOLISM (DISPOSAL RATE)	END-ORGAN SENSITIVITY
Growth Hormone	↔	↓		↓
Gonadotropins	↑*			
Thyrotropin (TSH)	↔	↓		↔
Thyroxine (T4)	↔	↔	↓	↑
Triiodothyronine (T3)	↓			
Parathyroid Hormone	↓			↑
Cortisol	↔	↔	↓	
Adrenal Androgens	↓	↓		
Aldosterone	↓		↓	
Insulin	↔	↓	↔	↔
Glucagon	↔	↔		
Testosterone	↓		↓	
Estrogens	↓		↓	

(From Williams, R. H.: *Textbook of Endocrinology*, 5th ed. Philadelphia, W. B. Saunders Co., 1974.)
Symbols: ↑, increase; ↓, decrease; ↔, no change; *, postmenopausal.

believed that deficiencies resulting from failure of the endocrine glands to secrete their hormones lead to aging. This thinking is now known to be much too simple. The age-related endocrine changes which do occur vary.[24] Table 47–3 indicates the known hormonal changes of the system.

Psychosocial Changes

Since conventional thinking already places so much emphasis on understanding psychosocial behaviors of the elderly, this topic can be treated more briefly here. However, these behaviors do occur, accumulate, and compound the normal physiologic losses.[40]

In a society whose values are founded on being young, the psychosocial damage suffered by many of the aging is often overwhelming.[26] The negative stereotypes of the elderly are entrenched and widespread, particularly in modern industrial societies. Some cultures and ethnic groups affirm the unique and special qualities of the aged—maturity, wisdom, compassion, spirituality and self-acceptance.[27]

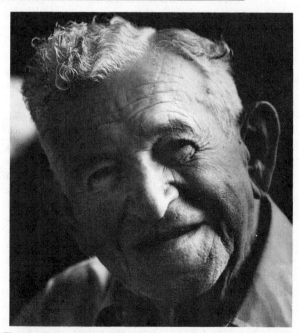

Figure 47–1. Modern industrial society places little value on the special qualities of the aged—maturity, wisdom, compassion, spirituality and self-acceptance. (Photograph by Josef Scaylea, courtesy Kline Galland Home, Seattle, Washington.)

However, these values tend not to be recognized in technologically oriented groups.

Consequently, in our culture few people really prepare to grow old, and when they find themselves suddenly classified as elderly, they may be swamped with problems. One of the most difficult of these is the feeling that they are no longer needed by others. This is not necessarily true, but it is an idea presently inculcated

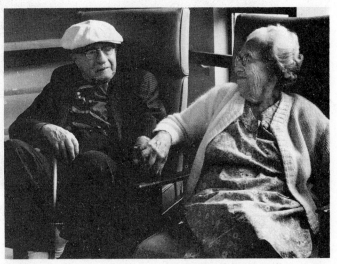

Figure 47-2. The need for closeness with others continues throughout life. (Photograph by Josef Scaylea, courtesy Kline Galland Home, Seattle, Washington.)

TABLE 47-4.   AREAS OF PSYCHOSOCIAL CONCERN: SELECTED EXPECTED CHANGES FOR THE LONG-LIVED PERSON

1. Confidence in cognitive function
   a. Decreases.

2. Cosmetic appearance
   a. Societal values impose a negative appreciation.

3. Familiar environments
   a. Lack of control over number of changes.
   b. Imposed limitations by others increases.
   c. Need for change of residence increases.[25]
   d. Need for transportation facilities increases.

4. Financial
   a. Income decreases.
   b. Amount available is usually fixed.
   c. Inflation adjustments difficult.

5. Future expectations
   a. Zest for new experiences decreases.
   b. Lowered energy reserves interfere with planning for future.
   c. Sustaining anticipation difficult.

6. Importance to others
   a. Decreases.
   b. Value of cohort relationships increases.

7. Intimacy
   a. Availability decreases.
   b. Need often misunderstood.

8. Legal rights
   a. Retained.

9. Political participation
   a. Tends to increase.

10. Reminiscence
    a. Increases.
    b. Source of pleasure.
    c. Focus on past rather than present uncertainties.
    d. Not a function of memory disturbance.[14]

11. Sexuality[15]
    a. Overall ability remains.
    b. Orgasmic capacity slows and decreases.
    c. Slower erection.
    d. Decreased pressure to ejaculate.
    e. At times, lower abdominal pain experienced by females during orgasm.
    f. Increased time for nipple erection.
    g. Increased time for clitoral engorgement.
    h. Higher proportion of females to males.
    i. Societal taboo against sexual involvement between elderly persons. May be used by some as an excuse for not engaging in sexual activity.

12. Social functioning
    a. Closely related to personal satisfaction.
    b. At times, may be voluntarily curtailed.

by American culture. Usually, those who have depended on the long-lived person or provided support in the past are gone or not readily available. This absence of significant others, either through death or increased mobility of family members and friends, leaves the elderly with a feeling there is no one to share the day-to-day events with. Emotional readjustments, which are always difficult, are especially so for the elderly. Younger people often fail to comprehend that the need for closeness with others continues throughout life.

The aging person also fears the loss—real or not—of his cognitive functions, i.e., problem solving and learning skills. Although some progress has been made in breaking the myth that "only the young can learn," many elderly persons are concerned that their faculties are deteriorating with age.[45] They wonder if they are still capable of learning.

Another great worry for many is decreased financial security. Not only are the elderly forced to live on a more limited income, but they must make that fixed amount cover ever-increasing prices. The eroding effects of inflation hit the elderly more severely than any other cohort group. The high cost of health care also particularly affects the ill elderly; this frequently inhibits their seeking health care until a crisis occurs. Additional psychosocial areas are indicated on Table 47–4.

One concept among people in the field of gerontology is that there are three essentials for

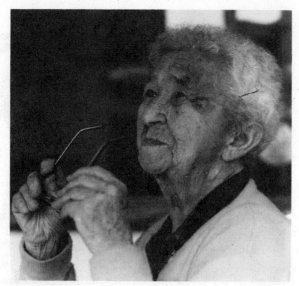

Figure 47–3. The changes and stress of illness compound the normal changes of aging. (Photograph by Josef Scaylea, courtesy of Kline Galland Home, Seattle, Washington.)

the successful experience of aging: friends, health, and money. If a person continues to have any two of the three, adaptation to normal aging is more comfortable. For example, if one has a sufficient number of friends and the money to deal with an illness, one's loss of health may not have as great an impact.

ASSESSMENT

In assessing nursing care needs of the ill elderly we must guard against compartmentalizing our observations. The information gathered from the assessment will be inadequate if limited to pathological findings. It is the person in his entirety who is experiencing the effects of long-term living, compounded by the aftermath of illness. Obviously, with the older individual there is a great deal of information to be obtained.

Recognizing that the changes normal to aging are difficult to separate from the changes resulting from a pathology (also, the long-lived person seldom has only *one* pathology) is basic to effective assessment. Detailed assessment areas and procedures are beyond the scope of this chapter. The OARS Methodology, developed at a well-known center for the study of aging, is a comprehensive tool for gauging assessment needs.[34]

As with any assessment, the evaluation of the older person is facilitated by early recognition of the presenting situation. The ease and potential for the individual's adjustment to the existing situation is linked to an early assessment. Certain points must be remembered about assessment of the long-lived person who is ill:

1. The reliability of the data base is influenced by the scope and depth of the information gathered. Thus, the data base for the long-lived person should include a longitudinal review of the person's life events as well as health history.

2. Knowledge of the family's health history provides some information of the genetic background. For example, did the person's parents or siblings die of natural causes? At what age? How were they functioning at the time of death? Was the death due to the occurrence of an acute or chronic pathology for which therapy had not been developed at the time?

3. Careful monitoring of the person's energy level at the time of the assessment is necessary to determine whether the informant's responses to the questions are reliable and whether the function being evaluated is at a representative level. The energy level can also determine the values of blood chemistry. Results from blood drawn at a time when the person was well rested can differ from results at a time of low energy level, e.g., after physical exertion.

4. Understanding the purpose of the assessment improves the older person's attitude and cooperation. The person may have already responded to the same questions or experienced the same assessment procedure before. Repetition may well be necessary, but if you take time to be sure the older person knows why it is necessary, a trusting relationship can be facilitated.

5. Usually there is already information available from other health professionals. This should be reviewed and considered for data relevant to nursing care goals.

6. Direct observation of the individual's functional abilities related to activities of daily living, i.e., dressing, bathing, mobility, sleeping patterns, continency, can provide valuable information without requiring extra assessment time.

Other baseline information that should be readily available for comparison with findings as changes occur includes:

1. Condition of skin.
2. Weight.
3. Urinary output and frequency.
4. Characteristics of blood pressure, cardiac output, respiration, and digestion.
5. Mental acuity.

6. Descriptions of vision, hearing and speech.

ACUTE AND LONG-TERM CARE SETTINGS

The difference between health care in the acute care setting and health care in the long-term care setting is that the acute care situation is designed and staffed for identification and evaluation of diseases plus establishment and stabilization of therapy related to a specific illness. In a long-term care setting, however, activities are usually directed towards rehabilitative and maintenance services for persons who are experiencing chronic physiologic and/or psychosocial disabilities.

A 1975 study of long-term care facilities disclosed that 4 of 5 persons in those settings had some chronic condition, resulting either from negative developments in aging or a pathology occurring in aging or—most likely—a combination of both.[42] This study established the median age of residents to be 82 years; within these nursing homes there were twice as many 84-year-old residents as 65-year-old people. Thirty per cent of the residents in long-term care situations had major activity limitations, and at least 15 per cent were unable to carry on any major activity without assistance. Approximately two thirds of the residents were admitted from an acute care situation, with another 20 per cent being admitted directly from their homes. Finally, 13 per cent of the residents were admitted as transfers from other long-care facilities.

Hospitalization in acute care setting occurs three times as often for persons over 75, and the average stay for the ill elderly is twice as long as for younger persons.

NURSING CARE CONCERNS

The processes of aging must be a basic consideration for clinical practice. These processes are also manifested in the variety of clinical problems associated with aging. These manifestations usually present themselves as disruptions in the established patterns of daily living and are most apparent when the long-lived person is experiencing stress and/or change.[38] Variations and rates of these alterations may be as different as the individuals experiencing the imposed change.

When the various individual consequences of normal aging are compounded by the additional alterations that illness produces, the elderly person is placed in double jeopardy. The changes experienced from both processes (aging and illness) compound each other. The presenting signs and symptoms may lack the clarity present in younger persons. Table 47–5 indicates selected clinical concerns and the expected alterations. The beginning student must realize that this list is only the barest outline and must not form an oversimplified impression of clinical nursing concerns.

It is important to keep in mind that the least alike cohort group is composed of those who have experienced a long life. The nurse's skill in separating aging effects from pathology facilitates development of therapies specially suitable for the individual older person.

CONCLUSIONS

Nurses are professionals unique in having developed the philosophy, commitment, and personal resources for providing care for persons who have lived a long time.[3, 4, 17] These elderly usually need services because of the effects of normal aging, compounded by pathology. One way to facilitate the beginning student's understanding of the nursing role in the care of the ill elderly is to ensure that these students learn basic concepts of normal age-related changes.

Because of their longevity, the elderly have highly complex backgrounds. Thus, assessment in these cases requires astute observational skills. Both the strengths and weaknesses of the aged person must be identified and considered by those who determine the nursing care plan. Also necessary is a firm sense of accountability to the individuals who receive nursing care, as well as to their significant others. This responsibility extends to keeping others who are concerned with the care of the ill elderly person informed of nursing observations and goals.

Care of the long-lived person is rewarding. Understanding of the older person's experiences can become a stimulating nursing care challenge. Even though problems of the ill elderly may seem alien to you at the beginning of your nursing studies, you can develop an understanding of the elderly by reviewing your own experiences with them and reexamining your approach to nursing care of the long-lived person in light of what you learn about the aging developmental processes. From this in-

Cognition[6, 10]
   a. Effects "felt" from decreased cardiopulmonary support increase.
   b. Information overload increases "neural noise."
   c. Need for activities with meaningful outcomes increases.
   d. Decline may be related to nearness of death.
   e. Dividing attention increasingly penalizes the older person.
1. Reaction time to external stimuli
   a. Change is small but a slowing does occur.
2. Psycho-motor functions
   a. Nature of decline, if present, is not fully understood.
   b. Differences cannot be explained on the basis of education.
   c. Motivation effects.
   d. Not always affected by practice.
   e. Appear to be correlated with slower electroencephalogram (EEG) waves.

Drug Therapy[22a]
   a. Most dynamic effects are frequently accomplished not in giving drugs but in the withdrawal.[39]
   b. Age related changes may greatly affect rate of absorption, distribution, metabolism and excretion.[1]
   c. Increased vulnerability to adverse effects.
   d. Problems related to intravenous fluid therapy increase.

Elimination
   a. Disturbances usually due to diet and/or fluid intake change.
1. Constipation
   a. Usually due to decrease of bulk in diet.
   b. Decreased fluid intake.
   c. Poor dentition influences.
2. Diarrhea
   a. If present, usually due to laxative abuse.
   b. Incidence in women is higher than in males.
3. Urinary
   a. Increased kidney sensitivity to sudden acid/base balance changes.
   b. Nocturia increases.
   c. Significance of adequate fluid intake increases.
   d. Lack of control increases social isolation.
   e. Prostatic enlargement increases frequency.

Nutritional state
   a. Adversely affected by poor income.
   b. Loneliness can interfere with.
   c. Degree of physical activity a major consideration.
   d. Condition of mouth is a factor.
1. Vitamin deficiency
   a. Not common.
2. Absorption of nutrients
   a. No valid evidence of change.
3. Basal metabolism rate.
   a. Decreases.

Pain
   a. Sensitivity changes have been both asserted and disputed.
   b. Indications exist that threshold is more dependent upon physiological changes.
   c. Tolerance is more related to psychological factors.
   d. Tolerance to deep pain decreases.
   e. Tolerance to subcutaneous pain increases.[46]
   f. Death can be welcomed.

Physical Body Care
   a. Increased vulnerability to abrasions.
   b. Significance of routine attention increases.
1. Skin[41a]
   a. Appears dry and brittle, looks fragile.
   b. Increased wrinkling due to loss of subcutaneous fat.
   c. Decreased turgor.
   d. Loses ability to keep properly hydrated.
   e. Collagen content greatly increases.
   f. Sexual and cultural differences are manifested.
   g. Sweat gland support decreases.
   h. Pigmentation spots increase.
   i. Decreased number of capillary loops and other blood vessels.
2. Nails
   a. Slight slowing of growth.
   b. Detrophies are usually due to circulatory impairments.
3. Hair
   a. Loss occurs but varies in the sexes.
   b. Grays.
   c. Axillary hair often disappears.
   d. Overall body and pubic hair decreases.
4. Mouth
   a. Dentures increase.
   b. Increase in periodontal disease.
   c. Diminished secretions.
   d. Increased attention to hygiene necessary.[35]

Physical Exercise and Mobility[23]
1. Muscle support
   a. Size diminishes.
   b. Tone decreases.
   c. Strength decreases, maximum peak between 20 and 30 years.
   d. Loss may be secondary to decreased activity.
   e. Grip strength one of the earliest indications of change.
   f. Potassium content declines.
2. Bone mass
   a. Widespread decrease.
   b. Fractures occur more frequently in weight-bearing areas.
   c. May have slight loss of stature due to intravertebral disc changes.

Safety
   a. Ambiguous environments increase confusion.
   b. Need for specific environmental clues increases (for example, hand rails on walls, large-size room numbers).
   c. Need for appropriately designed equipment and personal furnishings increases.
   d. Slick and uneven walking surfaces predispose to falling.

Sleep
   a. General pattern frequently changes to shorter periods.
   b. Spontaneous interruptions increase.
   c. Proportion of REM and non-REM remains fairly constant till about 60 years.
   d. Reduction in slow wave sleep.
   e. Deep sleep (Stage 4) often absent.
   f. Concern and anxiety for pattern changes increases.

Time Perception
   a. Tendency to underestimate.
   b. Persons with current life satisfactions are less likely to underestimate.
   c. Need for structure and adherence to time schedules is increased.

creased understanding and from actual clinical experience in caring for the elderly can come questions that will quicken interest in the literature on the subject. The uniqueness of geriatric/gerontological nursing derives from the understanding of the physiological and psychosocial changes that occur during the entire life span; from the appreciation of life's later stages of development—the positive, as well as the negative; and finally, from the necessity for dealing with the ever-increasing imminence of death.

BIBLIOGRAPHY

1. Aagaard, G. W.: Drug therapy in the aged. *Postgraduate Medicine, 52*:115, Aug. 1972.
2. Aldridge, J. W.: *In the Country of the Young.* New York, Harper Magazine Press, 1969.
3. American Nurses' Association, Committee on Skilled Nursing Care: *Nursing and Long-term Care for the Aging.* Kansas City, MO, 1975.
4. American Nurses' Association, Executive Committee, Division on Gerontological Nursing Practice: *Standards for Gerontological Nursing Practice.* Kansas City, MO, 1976.
5. Andrus Gerontology Center: *Drugs and the Elderly.* Los Angeles, University of Southern California, 1973.
6. Baltes, P. B., and Schaie, K. W.: The myth of the twilight years. *Psychology Today, 7*:35, March 1974.
7. Binstock, R. H., and Shanas, E. (eds.): *Handbook of Aging and the Social Sciences.* New York, Van Nostrand Reinhold Co., 1976.
8. Birchenall, J., and Streight, M. E.: *Care of the Older Adult.* Philadelphia, J. B. Lippincott Co., 1973.
9. Birren, J. E., and Schaie, K. W. (eds.): *Handbook of the Psychology of Aging.* New York, Van Nostrand Reinhold Co., 1977.
10. Botwinick, J.: *Aging and Behavior.* New York, Springer Publishing Co., Inc., 1973.
10a. Bowers, J. E.: Caring for the elderly. *Nursing '78, 8*:42–47, Jan. 1978.
11. Boyle, E., Jr., et al.: Auditory and visual memory loss in aging populations. *Journal of the American Geriatrics Society, 23*:284, June 1975.
11a. Brock, A. M., and Madison, A. S.: The challenge in gerontological nursing. *Nursing Forum, XVI*:95–105, No. 1, 1977.
12. Burnside, I. M.: *Nursing and the Aged.* New York, McGraw-Hill Book Co., 1976.
13. Burnside, I.: Touching is talking. *American Journal of Nursing, 73*(12):2060, Dec. 1973.
14. Butler, R. N.: Successful aging and the role of the life review. *Journal of the American Geriatrics Society, 22*(12):529, Dec. 1974.
15. Butler, R. N.: Sex after sixty. *In* Brown, L., and Ellis, E. (eds.): *The Later Years.* Acton, MA, Publishing Sciences, 1975.
16. Caird, F. I., and Judge, T. G.: *Assessment of the Elderly Patient.* Kent, England, Pitman Medical, 1974.
17. Campbell, M. E.: Study of attitudes of nursing personnel toward the geriatric patient. *Nursing Research, 20*(2):147, March–April 1971.
17a. Combs, K. L.: Preventive care in the elderly. *American Journal of Nursing, 78*:1339, Aug. 1978.
18. Davis. B. A.: Gerontological nursing comes of age. *Journal of Gerontological Nursing, 1*:6, March–April 1975.

19. de Vries, H. A.: *Vigor Regained.* Englewood Cliffs, NJ, Prentice-Hall, 1974.
20. Eisdorfer, C., et al.: Improvement of learning in the aged by modification of autonomic nervous system activity. *Science, 170*:1327, 1970.
21. Eisdorfer, C., and Jann, W. E. (eds.): *Psychopharmacology and Aging.* New York, Plenum Press, 1973.
22. Finch, C. E., and Hayflicks, L. (eds.): *Handbook of the Biology of Aging.* New York, Van Nostrand Reinhold Co., 1976.
22a. Friedman, S. A., and Steinheber, F. U. (eds.): Symposium on geriatric medicine. *Medical Clinics of North America.* Vol. 60, Nov. 1976.
22b. Gotz, B. E., and Gotz, V. P.: Drugs and the elderly. *American Journal of Nursing, 78*:1347, Aug. 1978.
23. Greenberg, B.: Reaction time in the elderly. *American Journal of Nursing, 73*(12):2056, Dec. 1973.
24. Gregerman, R. I., and Bierman, E. L.: Aging and hormones. *In* Williams, R. H.: *Textbook of Endocrinology,* 5th ed. Philadelphia, W. B. Saunders Co., 1974.
24a. Hanan, Z. I.: Geriatric medications: How the aged are hurt by drugs meant to help. *RN, 41*:57, Jan. 1978.
24b. Hogstel, M. O.: How do the elderly view their world? *American Journal of Nursing, 78*:1335, Aug. 1978.
25. Huttman, E. D.: *Housing and Social Services for the Elderly.* New York, Praeger Publishers, 1977.
26. The Institute of Gerontology: *No Longer Young: The Older Woman in America.* Detroit, University of Michigan, 1975.
27. Kalish, R. A.: A gerontological look at ethnicity, human capacities, and individual adjustments. *The Gerontologist, 11*:78, Jan. 1971.
28. Kimmel, D. C.: *Adulthood and Aging.* New York, John Wiley and Sons, Inc., 1974.
28a. King, G., and Vaughn, S.: You may be the aged's only advocate. *RN, 41*:48, May 1978.
29. Knowles, L.: Putting geriatric nursing standards into practice. *The Nursing Clinics of North America. 7*(2):201, June 1972.
30. Leaf, A.: Getting old. *Scientific American, 229*(3):44, Sep. 1973.
30a. McGreehan, D. M., and Warburton, S. W.: How to help families cope with caring for elderly members. *Geriatrics, 33*:99, June 1978.
31. Moore, J.: Situational factors affecting minority aging. *The Gerontologist, 11*:88, Jan. 1971.
32. Palmore, E. (ed.): *Normal Aging.* Durham, NC, Duke University Press, 1970.
33. Palmore, E. (ed.): *Normal Aging II.* Durham, NC, Duke University Press, 1974.
34. Pfeiffer, E. (ed.): *Multidimensional Functional Assessment: The OARS Methodology.* Durham, NC, Center for the Study of Aging and Human Development, 1975.
35. Pope, W., Reitz, M., and Patrick, M.: A study of oral hygiene in the geriatric patient. *International Journal of Nursing Studies, 12*:65–92, 1975.
36. Rosenfeld, A.: *Prolongevity.* New York, Alfred A. Knopf, Inc., 1976.
37. Schwab, Sr. M.: Caring for the aged. *American Journal of Nursing, 73*:2049–2053, Dec. 1973.
38. Selye, H. A.: Stress and aging. *Journal of American Geriatrics Society, 18*(9):699, 1970.
39. Shields, E. M.: Introduction to drug therapy. *Journal of Gerontological Nursing, 1*:6, March–April 1975.

40. Timiras, P. S.: Nature of aging processes. *In* Timiras, P. S. (ed.): *Developmental Physiology and Aging.* New York, The Macmillan Company, 1972.

41. Tournier, P.: *Learning to Grow Old.* New York, Harper and Row, 1972.

41a. Uhler, D. M.: Common skin changes in the elderly. *American Journal of Nursing,* 78:1342, Aug. 1978.

42. U.S. Department of Health, Education and Welfare, Office of Nursing Home Affairs: *Long Term Care Facility Improvement Study* (Interim Report). Rockville, MD, Public Health Service, March 1975.

43. U.S. Department of Health, Education and Welfare, Office of Nursing Home Affairs, Ad Hoc Nurse–Physician Advisory Group: *Assessing Health Care Needs in Skilled Nursing Facilities: Health Professional Perspectives.* Washington, D.C., March 1976.

44. Walker, J., and Hertzog, C.: Brain function and behavior. *In* Woodruff, D. S., and Birren, J. E. (eds.): *Aging: Scientific Perspectives and Social Issues.* New York, D. Van Nostrand Co., 1975.

45. Wilkie, F., and Eisdorfer, C.: Intelligence and blood pressure in the aged. *Science, 172*:959, May 1971.

46. Woodrow, R. M., et al.: Pain tolerance: differences according to age, sex, and race. *Psychosomatic Medicine, 34*(6):548, 1972.

47. Woodruff, D. S., and Birren, J. E. (eds.): *Aging: Scientific Perspectives and Social Issues.* New York, D. Van Nostrand Co., 1975.

CHAPTER 48

CARING FOR GRIEVING PERSONS

By Margaret Helen Parkinson, R.N., R.M.N., Dip.N., B.Soc.Sc., M.N.

INTRODUCTION AND STUDY GUIDE

This chapter is written to help you develop the understandings and skills that will enable you to identify grief reactions and to plan and implement appropriate nursing care for grieving persons.

As you work to develop a functional understanding of the concept of loss, you will find yourself becoming involved in both cognitive and affective learning. You will gain knowledge about: (a) the kinds of losses people commonly experience; (b) the signs and symptoms of the grieving process; (c) the specific experience of bereavement (i.e., loss through death of a significant other) and (d) appropriate interventions to assist a grieving person with grief work. This is the *cognitive learning.*

Also, it is likely that your own reactions to loss will become clearer to you. You may be reminded of losses you have experienced in your own life; losses that still hold pain for you. You will be encouraged to examine your own feelings and how you handle them when you are in a close therapeutic relationship with a grieving person. These are examples of *affective learning.* Both cognitive and affective learning are important to your development as a professional nurse.

To help you with the task of developing a functional understanding of the concept of loss you may find it helpful to follow suggestions included in the study guide below. As you read this chapter:

1. Write, in your own words, the meanings of the terms loss, grief, grief work, mourning, bereavement, anticipatory grief and unresolved grief.

2. Learn carefully the symptoms of grief described by Lindemann and the stages of grief and mourning described by Engel.

3. Identify the special elements involved in grieving for a life partner, a child, a parent, a peer.

4. Identify the differential signs of "normal" and "pathological" grief.

You may also find it useful to keep a journal during the time you are studying this material. Journal writing is often a very useful way to identify and clarify feelings. In your journal you could record:

1. Your feelings and reactions while reading the material in this chapter.

2. Your experiences with grieving people. Include the objective behavioral signs you observe in a grieving person; the things such a person tells you; and your feelings and reactions while interacting with a grieving person. Try to include people who have experienced a variety of losses, not only losses related to death but also other losses such as the loss of a body part or a body function.

3. The thoughts and feelings that arise as you reflect on your own past losses and as you consider present losses and future anticipated losses.

You may also find it useful to:

1. Make process recordings of your conversation with grieving people. Discuss these recordings with your instructor to try to identify the places you functioned well and the places where alternate responses on your part may have been more useful to the grieving person.

2. Develop nursing care plans for grieving people. Discuss your plans with your instructor to try to identify the nursing interventions that would be appropriate and those that would be inappropriate in the nursing care of a grieving person. Such nursing care plans would probably be of most use to you if they related to a real person rather than a hypothetical patient.

You may find that material presented in this chapter has very personal meanings to you. If this occurs, you may experience some significant emotional reactions. It is important that you do not keep such reactions bottled up inside yourself where you cannot work to resolve them. Share your emerging feelings with someone you trust. A useful experience may be to share your reactions with a group of nursing students who are having the same experiences. You may ask your instructor to join such a group as facilitator.

Our *objectives* for this chapter are that by studying this material you will:

1. Identify the kinds of losses most commonly experienced by people throughout life

2. Understand that bereavement is only one kind of loss and differs only in severity from other losses

3. Know the signs and symptoms most often seen in grieving people

4. Know the stages of grieving through which most people pass during a loss experience

5. Become aware of your own reactions to loss and appreciate how these may influence the kind of nursing care you can offer

6. Develop skills appropriate to helpful therapeutic relationships with grieving persons

LOSS IS EXPERIENCED THROUGHOUT LIFE

The concept of loss is an important one for nurses. In their professional practice nurses come in contact with many people who have lost or are anticipating losing something of importance to them. Such people are said to be *grieving.* It is helpful for the reader to know that the terms "loss," "grief," and "mourning" are used in overlapping ways to describe what happens when a person has to do without something or someone upon which he had come to depend. The term "grief work" is sometimes used synonymously with the term "mourning." These terms are defined in appropriate places in the chapter.

Engel defines *grief* as: "... typical reaction to the loss of a source of psychological gratification. ..."[15] Carlson describes grief as: "... the series of emotional responses that follow the perception, or anticipation, of a loss of one or more valued or significant objects. These responses often include helplessness, loneliness, hopelessness, sadness, guilt, anger and the like."[13]

Health professionals, including nurses, are often inclined to think of a grieving person as someone who has experienced a death in some way. This is not altogether true. People grieve for other losses as well as those associated with death. Benoliel states that:[5]

The process of grieving . . . is not reserved for those in the terminal stages of living nor for families undergoing bereavement associated with death. It occurs whenever there is a loss that carries psychosocial significance either for an individual or a group of individuals or both.

The exact nature of a loss varies among individuals. Each person places different value on various lost objects, experiences and persons. Examples of situations which may produce grief include the loss of:

▷ A sentimentally valued object, e.g., memento, piece of jewelry, ornament or book

▶ An economically valued object, e.g., diamond ring, stolen car or quantity of cash

▶ An indispensably useful object, e.g., crutches for a crippled person, pair of glasses, appointment calendar, patient's record, craftsman's tools, passport

▶ A social role, e.g., occupational position upon retirement or dismissal from a job or social group

▶ Social or personal relationships, e.g., a circle of friends disrupted by a move from one city to another, the ending of a friendship or some other significant relationship such as by divorce

▶ A pet such as a loved cat or dog which strays away or dies

▶ A significant other person through death

Loss and change are closely connected.

Grieving may result from changes such as:

▶ A change in social role, e.g., when a parent feels "less needed," as when a child begins a first job and leaves home

▷ A change in environment, e.g., when a person leaves a house or leaves a city or a school that was enjoyable and satisfying

Pause in your reading for a few minutes and try to extend these lists by adding other situations you think could create a gap in the life of an individual and therefore be an experience of loss.

Maybe you extended the lists to include some *losses specific to people experiencing illness* and others specific to people *during hospitalization.* These may have included:

▶ *Physical losses,* e.g., loss of vision, loss of hearing, loss of a limb (amputation), loss of a body organ

▶ Loss of "normal" *body image,* e.g., with surgical removal of breast, excessive scarring, colostomy, amputations, paralysis

▶ Loss of *social role* that may occur when a person enters hospital as a patient or takes on the "sick role" outside a hospital

▶ Loss of *control over one's day-to-day living* that may occur when a person enters a hospital as a patient or takes on the "sick role" outside a hospital

▶ Loss of *control over one's body* when a body part is lost or functionally altered, e.g., loss of bowel or bladder control, paralysis of limbs

▶ *Anticipated loss of life* that occurs with a serious diagnosis, e.g., cancer, heart attack

> *Whatever the specific circumstances, losses of any kind cause some degree of psychologic pain and demand some functional readjustment.*

Identification of people experiencing loss is important in nursing for three major reasons:
1. So that avoidable losses can be eliminated or reduced
2. So that a person can be comforted and supported while grieving over unavoidable losses
3. Because loss itself predisposes to further illness

Holmes[27] illustrates this last point with his social readjustment rating scale. Holmes has identified 43 common life changes and has evaluated each according to the amount of life readjustment required for each specific life change. Holmes has shown that the greater the readjustment required by a person over a period of 2 years the greater is his susceptibility to illness. The majority of items on Holmes' Social Readjustment Rating Scale imply some degree of loss.

Benoliel[5] describes three forms of significant loss that would be accompanied by a grief reaction: *personal loss, group loss* and *multiple loss.*

We most commonly think of grief reactions in terms of personal loss. Certainly, significant loss produces intense psychologic pain that requires serious functional readjustment for the individual. Benoliel points out, however, that personal loss very often exists simultaneously with group loss.

Whenever a group member, e.g., a member of a family or some other social group, is lost by death or some other cause, a social readjustment must take place to accommodate the ab-

sence of a member. The social readjustment required may be seen as a grief reaction. Benoliel points out that the effects of a group loss may be seen in hospitals and clinics when patients die.

Losses do not always occur one at a time. Individuals, families and other social groups sometimes experience several losses at the same time. Elderly people are often in a position of experiencing a combination of physical and relationship losses. Whenever several losses occur at the same time (multiple losses), grief reactions are compounded.

A NURSE'S DIFFICULTY IN COPING WITH LOSS

It is sometimes very difficult for nurses to acknowledge and respond appropriately to the kinds of losses they see people experiencing within a medical setting. This difficulty may be based in part on the fact that it is tempting to equate "success" with "cure." When a patient is not completely cured, a nurse may experience a sense of partial or complete failure. None of us likes to fail. Thus we are likely to avoid, either physically or psychologically, situations where failure may become inevitable. Dying persons and grieving persons may therefore tend to be avoided, leaving them lonely and isolated.

If nurses can see "care" as important as "cure," they are less likely to engage in such untherapeutic, avoiding practices. Nurses can gain a sense of satisfaction in comforting and supporting individuals or groups through loss experiences whether or not cures are likely outcomes.

> *A nurse does well to remember that her primary function is to* care for *an individual, whether or not a* cure *is possible.*

SIGNS AND SYMPTOMS OF LOSS

It is important that nurses be familiar with the signs and symptoms of grief so that they can: (a) *recognize* grief reactions present in patients and their social groups and (b) *anticipate* reactions that are likely to occur for grieving people with the passage of time.

No doubt you have experienced many of the

symptoms of grief. Pause in your reading for a few minutes and try to remember how it was for you when you experienced a significant loss. To help you with this recapitulation, follow the fantasies described below and write down your responses where indicated. Take your time over this exercise and try to really "get into" your feelings.

▶ Think back to a time when you lost an object (not a person) that was especially valuable to you.

▶ Recall that special object for a few minutes. Remember what it looked like, what it felt like, what it smelt like. Remember what you did with it. Remember how you liked it.

▶ Write down a series of adjectives that describe the value of that special object to you.

▶ Now recall the *first moment* you realized that you did not have that object any more. What did you say? What did you do? What did you feel?

▶ Write down your responses to the above questions, relative to the first time you realized you had lost your special object.

▶ Next remember back to a *few days or a week or two after the loss* of your special object. You did not find it. What did you do? What did you think? What did you feel?

▶ Write down your responses to the questions listed immediately above.

▶ Think about that special lost object again and try to identify the feelings you have about it *now*. What are the things you remember about it now? How do you feel about it now? Has any other object replaced it in any way?

▶ Write down your responses to the questions listed immediately above.

It may be helpful for you to share your responses to the above fantasy with others who have undergone the same exercise. You may be surprised to find that others respond in similar ways.

We now suggest that you repeat the exercise described above two more times. First, replace the "special object" with memories of a time when you were separated from someone you loved and with whom you had a very special relationship. The third time you go through this exercise, recall a time when someone very important to you died. Each time you go through the exercise, follow the same process and write down your responses. When you finish the exercise it would be helpful to you to share your experience with others who have completed the same exercise.

As you undertake the above exercises, it is likely that you will find that your reactions were similar to those of others. It is also likely that you will find that the kinds of reactions you experienced were similar in each of the exercises. Any differences would likely be in the intensity or quality of your responses rather than in the nature of the responses themselves. Possibly you felt grief much more intensely when you lost your friend than when you lost your special object. Was this so?

It is likely that your responses to the preceding fantasy exercises were similar to the descriptions Lindemann[39] has made of the symptoms of grieving. He interviewed over 100 people who had experienced losses and identified a number of somatic, psychologic and social reactions.

The somatic symptoms associated with grieving tend to center around the respiratory and gastrointestinal systems and tend to occur in "waves," lasting 20 to 60 minutes. These somatic symptoms include:

1. A tightness in the throat
2. A sense of choking and shortness of breath
3. Excessive sighing
4. An empty feeling in the abdomen
5. Loss of appetite, nausea
6. Tenseness and inability to relax
7. Loss of strength—lethargy

The psychologic symptoms commonly experienced with grieving are:

1. A sense of unreality
2. An increased emotional distance from people
3. Preoccupation with images of the "lost object"
4. Preoccupation with feelings of guilt
5. Repeated questioning as to why the loss had occurred
6. A fear of loss of mental stability ("I felt as if I was going out of my mind.")

The social and behavioral symptoms commonly experienced with grieving are:

1. Loss of warmth toward others
2. Relationships with others characterized by irritability, anger and the "desire not to be bothered." If the bereaved person is aware of tension in relationships with others, formal and stiff interactions may occur as an overcompensation.
3. Restlessness and aimlessness in movements

4. Inability to maintain organized daily patterns or, conversely, a rigid adherence to a daily routine

5. Nervous speech

6. Limited concentration and disoriented béhavior

A person's response to loss almost always includes some or all of the symptoms described above. However, symptom patterns tend to be very individualized, varying from person to person.

Grieving is a very personal although common human behavior. Many people feel that their grief experiences are different from anyone else's. There are common grieving patterns, however, and knowledge of these patterns helps a nurse communicate accurate empathetic understanding with grieving persons.

In addition, if a nurse is well acquainted with the symptoms of loss, she can identify a loss reaction in a person from his behavioral signs and his verbal descriptions of symptoms. This is important, as the specific cause of a loss reaction is not always obvious even to the person himself.

PROCESS OF RECOVERY FROM LOSS

Mourning is the way that people slowly recover from significant losses in their lives. It is an inevitable process and follows certain fairly predictable patterns. Carlson defines *mourning* as:

. . . The psychological processes that follow a loss of a significant or valued object, or that follow the realization that such a loss may occur. These processes usually lead to giving up the lost object. Mourning, therefore, includes the processes that are necessary to overcome the subjective state of grief.[13]

Engel[15] equates the healing process of mourning to the healing process of a physical wound. Just as there is a progressive pattern with wound healing, *there is a progressive pattern to grieving.* Engel describes this grieving pattern as occurring over three stages: (1) shock and disbelief, (2) developing awareness and (3) restitution.

Shock and Disbelief

The first responses to a severe loss are usually feelings of "shock" and "disbelief." The person is likely to say "No! It can't be true!" or make similar comments. Sometimes a person will appear to have accepted the loss and will proceed with necessary activities in a calm manner. This is usually only an intellectual acceptance, however. Such people are usually shielding themselves from acute pain by blocking out intense emotional responses. The pain comes a little later.

During this initial state the person is often numbed and dazed. Such an individual appears to be functioning automatically and to be out of contact with himself, his environment or what is happening.

The main function at this stage appears to be protection from overwhelming distress. The individual who has suffered a severe loss may need such a period of denial in order to be able to survive the intense initial stress. This stage of shock and disbelief may last only a few minutes or it may go on longer, e.g., several days.

Developing Awareness

As the grieving person moves from the stage of shock and disbelief into the second stage of developing awareness, the reality of the loss becomes very clear. The person feels acute psychologic pain and experiences the symptoms described previously. Everything seems empty and pointless because the "valued object" (or lost person) is missing.

At this time the person may experience *anger.* This anger may be directed toward others or toward the self. It is very important for a nurse to understand this grieving phenomenon as she may, at times, become the recipient of anger from a person experiencing loss. It is important at such times that the nurse respond to this expression of anger with understanding rather than defensiveness.

Crying also commonly occurs during this period of developing awareness. The shedding of tears may be very helpful for a person experiencing the acute pain of recent loss. The amount of crying done by a grieving person is variable, depending in part upon the general acceptance of tears within this individual's cultural and social environment. The Anglo-Saxon culture tends generally to discourage tears. Sometimes in this cultural group the gentle reassurance of another person (e.g., saying "it's OK to cry") may give the grieving individual "permission" to use this form of emotional release.

Some people find they are quite unable to shed tears. The absence of tears does not necessarily mean the absence of grief. The grieving person who cannot cry may be experiencing the acute distress of loss intensely and may, in fact, say he is suffering and "crying inside."

Restitution

The third stage of recovery from loss is the stage of restitution. This begins the sometimes long process of *grief work,* during which the person gradually resolves the loss and is able to make the adjustments necessary to function again in a satisfying way. Restitution is complete when a person is able once more to allow himself some pleasure in life. Much intrapsychic work must be done, however, before this can occur. Such work may take up to a year to complete following a severe loss such as the death of a significant other.

When death is the cause of a loss, the various cultural rituals associated with funerals can help with the recovery process of the grieving person. A funeral or memorial service allows the grieving person to say "good-bye" to the lost person in an institutionalized manner. Additionally, such a service provides the support of the social group, which gathers together at times of bereavement. It is important that excessive use of tranquilizing drugs be avoided at this time. A bereaved person who is heavily tranquilized may be denied this important phase of recovery.

During the restitution stage of recovery from loss, the grieving person may become very aware of himself. He may experience somatic (physical) sensations and discomfort. If the loss is a death, the grieving person may experience the same kinds of symptoms that were previously experienced by the dead person. The appearance of such symptoms is normally brief, however.

The grieving person is commonly preoccupied with thoughts of the lost object during the restitution stage, and he has a need to talk about it over and over again. The most helpful person to the griever at this time is someone who will listen understandingly and patiently to stories that are often repeated. A grieving person can sometimes get very tired of talking repeatedly about his loss, yet he continues to have this need.

The phenomenon of idealization of the lost object occurs at this time, i.e., the grieving person represses all the negative aspects of the lost object. For example, if the loss is a death, the griever perceives the deceased person as altogether good and perfect. Feelings of *guilt* also may be present, e.g., "I didn't give him enough attention."

Gradually these preoccupations with the lost object lessen, and the grieving person is able to gain an increasing sense of independence. Over a period of time, the lost object is remembered more realistically and the griever begins to take pleasure from such memories. Also, he can begin to reinvest himself in other valued objects.

Pause in your reading for a few moments and recall the fantasy exercise you were encouraged to do earlier in this chapter. Re-examine your responses to remembered losses: (a) at the time of the loss, (b) a few days or weeks after the loss and (c) a long time after the loss. It is likely you will find your responses consistent with the stages of grieving just discussed, described by Engel.[15] There may be some variation, of course, depending largely on the value of the lost object to you. As mentioned earlier, the loss of a "special object" is less likely to cause as severe a response pattern as the loss of a significant other through death. On the whole, however, the processes of recovery from loss are similar for whatever kind of loss occurs.

HOW A NURSE CAN HELP A GRIEVING PERSON

It has already been pointed out that a nurse needs to be very familiar with the symptoms, behavioral signs and processes of grieving so that she can recognize such patterns in patients she cares for. What is actually lost may not be clear to either the nurse or the person concerned. If a nurse suspects a grief reaction, she may need to talk at length with the person, encouraging him to share with her some of his recent life experiences. During such sharing the helpful nurse listens very carefully and empathetically in order to be able to identify circumstances that may have precipitated feelings of loss in the client. The nurse must remember that almost any loss can produce a grief reaction—anything that was of value and is now no longer present. Premature interpretations of the client's situation or guesses about the basis of the feeings of loss are not appropriate.

Once a nurse is *reasonably sure* that her client is grieving, the following three general principles can guide her nursing intervention:

1. Acknowledge the loss to the client
2. Facilitate the expression of feelings by the client
3. Support the client as he moves through the stages of grieving

In *acknowledging the loss* the nurse lets the client know she understands that something that was of great value is now no longer available to him.

Suppose, for example, that nursing student Ms. Smith is caring for Mr. Thompson (admitted to the hospital for investigation of recurring abdominal pain). Ms. Smith notices that Mr. Thompson picks at his food, is very agitated and does not seem to be able to sit still. During visiting time, Ms. Smith notices that Mr. Thompson's visitors talk to each other and do not really involve Mr. Thompson in their conversations. Ms. Smith takes the time to sit down and talk with Mr. Thompson, using the skills of therapeutic communication (see Chap. 3). She gradually learns some things about Mr. Thompson's recent life experiences that suggest he may be having a grief reaction to a significant change in his social role.

Mr. Thompson has just turned 65 years of age. He had worked for 35 years in a large insurance firm. Mr. Thompson enjoyed his job and commonly spent a lot of extra hours at his work. The firm he worked for has a policy of compulsory employee retirement at age 65. Consequently, Mr. Thompson was recently given his "golden handshake" and asked to leave. Now he is at home all the time and at a loss concerning how to spend his time. Mr. Thompson is not a man of varied interests. Over the years he allowed his work to take up most of his energies. His mate has long established daily patterns that do not really include her husband. So much changed so quickly.

After hearing Mr. Thompson talk about his recent life changes, Ms. Smith acknowledges her perception of his loss by saying warmly to him: "You have had a very big change in your life lately. Are you missing your life as a businessman very much? It sounds rather like you might be grieving for your job in a way." Mr. Thompson may then be able to think about that and see if he does in fact feel that he is experiencing grief over the loss of his job.

To take this example a little further, Ms. Smith could continue to *facilitate expression of feeling* for Mr. Thompson by having further conversations with him. During these conversations she could help him to talk about his job, what it meant to him, and his feelings and thoughts since he is no longer going to work each day. Ms. Smith would do this most successfully by showing genuine caring, nonpossessive warmth and accurate empathy and by using the listening and communication skills of attending, reflecting, paraphrasing and summarizing described in Chapter 3. If Mr. Thompson is indeed grieving over his change in social role, he may be greatly helped by conversations of this nature.

Through conversations such as those described above, a therapeutic nurse-patient relationship may develop that gives Mr. Thompson *support as he moves through the stages of grieving*. Ms. Smith may notice that Mr. Thompson needs to talk a lot about his job— how good it was, how good he was at it, how pleased the executives were with his work. He may also express anger at his enforced retirement or he may think that maybe he didn't work hard enough while he had the job (ex-

pression of guilt). Mr. Thompson may also begin to realize that his abdominal pains did not occur until after he had left his job.

As his grief begins to be resolved, Mr. Thompson may begin to think more positively about the future and begin to consider what new possibilities for using his time appeal to him. This may all take some time, however, and Mr. Thompson may be discharged from the hospital before the process is completed. Ms. Smith would therefore do well to include Mrs. Thompson in the discussions so that she, too, could better understand what Mr. Thompson is experiencing. It is to be hoped that the two of them could support each other as they adjust to this major life change.

In the example above, Ms. Smith uses: (a) her knowledge of the symptoms, behavioral signs and process of grieving and (b) her skills in therapeutic interaction to plan nursing interventions that help a family adjust to the loss of a social role. Such knowledge and skills could be used similarly for persons experiencing other kinds of losses.

BEREAVEMENT: THE MOST SEVERE EXPERIENCE OF LOSS

We have considered the concept of loss as applying to the removal of any valued object, person or experience from the life space of an individual or group. We will now consider *death,* the ultimate of losses, more specifically.

The Dying Person

The psychosocial adjustments that must be faced by a person experiencing terminal illness are discussed in Chapter 49. It is important to remember, however, that the *dying person is also grieving*. In fact, it could be said that the dying person has more to grieve for than the bereaved persons who survive him.

> *The person who is dying must say good-bye to every one, everything and every experience he has ever loved or valued. He must separate from his whole earthly life—past, present and future.*

The person anticipating death will experience *preparatory grief* for all that he values. It is not surprising then that the stages of dying described by Kübler-Ross,[33] i.e., Denial, Anger, Bargaining, Depression, and Acceptance (see Chap. 49), are rather similar to the stages of grieving described by Engel. A difference is that the dying person is often a few steps ahead of his significant others in the grief process. This fact can precipitate tension between a dying patient and his loved ones. Imagine, for example, if the patient were at the stage of "acceptance" and the family were still at "anger," the family might incorrectly interpret the patient's detachment as rejection of themselves. A nurse can help relieve such tensions by listening to the feelings of the family and explaining the kind of grieving the patient himself is going through. He has to say good-bye to so much, he must inevitably become detached as he does it.[33]

The Significant Others of a Dying Person

John Donne's famous line "No man is an island" is worth remembering in any nursing situation. This is certainly true in relation to the care of a dying person. Few people die as isolates. There is usually someone or frequently many people whose lives have been so entwined with the dying person's that they experience a loss when death does actually occur. Such people are commonly the patient's family members, but they may also include friends. A nurse needs to carefully identify the social network surrounding a patient so that she is able to offer support to those who need it. In some settings other patients may become involved to such an extent that they too will experience a grief reaction when another patient dies, e.g., in long-term care facilities.

Whoever they are, the nurse has as much responsibility to care for the significant others of a dying person as she does to care for the patient himself. The nurse does well to get to know these people, if it is possible, before the patient's death is imminent. This means that a helpful relationship may already be established between the significant others and the nurse before the time of greatest stress comes.

Give Attention and Listen.   Family and friends can often feel that their loved one has been removed from them when the terminal stages of illness occur. This is especially true if a dying patient is admitted to a hospital. A patient's significant others should be permitted to remain connected with the patient and his life even during the final days, if they wish to maintain such connections. A nurse can help a dying patient's significant others to maintain contact with the patient by:

▶ Welcoming them to the hospital

▶ Acknowledging them by name

▶ Giving them information about the patient's condition and comfort

▶ Providing private time with the patient as appropriate

▶ Orienting them to the hospital and the facilities available to them, e.g., cafeteria, telephones, a private place to sit

▶ Arranging for interviews with the patient's doctors

▶ Explaining medical and nursing procedures and equipment being used

▶ Discussing the nursing care plan with them

▶ Permitting them to do caring things for the patient, such as feeding him, washing his face or rubbing his back

▶ Demonstrating that the patient is being carefully and thoughtfully cared for

▶ Encouraging them to talk and share feelings with the patient—even if he appears unresponsive

▶ Showing concern for the family and friends themselves, e.g., noticing their kindness and worry

▶ Listening to and encouraging their expression of feelings

Listening to the expression of feelings may be the most therapeutic thing a nurse can do for people about to be bereaved.

The grieving process begins before the loved one actually dies. The more *anticipatory grief* a person can experience, the "easier" the process is after the death has occurred. A nurse can help with anticipatory grief by empathetic, warm and genuine listening.

When death is imminent, every effort should be made to inform the significant others in time for them to be with the patient when he dies. Needless to say, news of the patient's imminent death should be given gently. It is better to give the news of death or impending death to a group of significant others rather than to an individual. A nurse may have been able to identify the "strongest" member of the group beforehand so that she can encourage his/her presence to support those who will need it. The nurse may assist with summoning religious counselors or other persons according to the wishes of the patient and other significant persons.

When death has occurred the patient's significant others need to be:

▶ Given time alone with their deceased loved one so they can say "good-bye" in their own way.

▶ Given a private place where they can express themselves during this stage of shock, away from public scrutiny.

▶ Accepted and understood. Much of their behavior is a consequence of shock and they must not be judged for it.

▶ Given the opportunity to carry out cultural or religious practices that are of significance to them.

As has been pointed out, grieving takes a long time and may continue for a year or more after the death of a significant other. The grieving person needs the support of others throughout this time while they work through the various processes involved in readjustment to life without the loved person.

The Death of a Life Partner. Particular attention should be paid to the person who has lost a life partner through death. Such a person has to restructure a life that may have been built around the relationship with the deceased person. A life that was cooperative is now singular.

While the husband-wife dyad is the usual life commitment relationship in our society, it is not the only one that exists. Couples of the same sex may also enter into lifetime commitments to each other that should be recognized. These persons can experience intense feelings of loneliness and abandonment at times of bereavement when it is not recognized that they have, in effect, lost a "spouse." Holmes and Rahe[27] rate the death of a spouse as the life change that requires the greatest amount of social readjustment.

The Death of a Child. It is particularly difficult to accept the death of a child. There seems to be a sense of "wrong timing" about it, especially for a parent. Parents do not normally expect to survive their children. So the grief of parents may be especially painful and poignant. It is of prime importance that parents be allowed to care for their dying child if this is what they wish to do. Guilt is often experienced sharply after the death of a child. Ways in which parents can feel that they have been useful and attentive to the child will help them and the dying child. (Ill children are discussed in Chap. 46.)

Grief in the Elderly Person. "Bereavement-pain is one of the commonest pains an elderly person endures."[9] The older a person gets, the more likely he is to experience multiple loss through deaths of longstanding friends, acquaintances and family. Gramlich[22] suggests that elderly people may show a pattern of grief which he calls "chronic grief." He suggests that elderly people may not experience grief intensely at a conscious level, but may be more inclined to suppress grieving feelings and then exhibit them as somatic symptoms. In other words, an elderly grieving person may hurt physically rather than psychologically. Such a person needs a lot of love, attention and encouragement to express feelings more directly. (See also Chap. 47.)

The Religious Needs of the Bereaved. Some people obtain comfort from religious practices, others do not. The most important thing for a nurse to remember in this regard is to make it possible for patients and significant others to receive spiritual help, guidance and comfort in ways and at times that *they* want. Nurses or anyone else, for that matter, should never impose their values and beliefs upon other persons.

DIFFERENTIATING "NORMAL" FROM PATHOLOGIC GRIEF

Grief is a "normal" process. It is universal (i.e., happens to everyone) and it is self-limiting. As stated before, grief is usually resolved in about a year, especially if appropriate support is given to the grieving person. Note that when we say grief is resolved, we do not mean that the griever is never again lonely for the deceased.

Occasionally a person experiences a pathologic (abnormal) reaction to loss that requires professional treatment, e.g., skilled counseling. Such *unresolved grief* may take several forms:[16]

▶ *Prolonged denial* of the loss. This is really a psychotic response that is an exaggeration of the denial that normally occurs in the beginning phases of grief. The person rejects reality and continues to behave as if the loss had not occurred.

▶ *Denial of the significance of the loss* can be a pathological response. Here the person does not allow himself to feel the depth of pain that the loss brings. Psychotic depression or a manic reaction can result from this.

▶ Attempts to substitute another mourner in the role of the deceased person (as a "vicarious object") may occur in pathologic grieving. Sometimes a person can expect another mourner to take on the role of the deceased person. In this way such a person is made a vicarious object. If such a role is not accepted, a severe depression may result.[16]

If a nurse suspects any of the above pathologic reactions, a psychiatric referral should be made so that professional evaluation and treatment can be undertaken as appropriate.

A NURSE NEEDS SUPPORT TOO

It is always important to remember that *nurses are people too*. Caring for grieving people is very difficult, and nurses often experience the despair and hopelessness that patients in their care express.

> *Nurses need to have opportunities to share their feelings and concerns with others in the nursing and health team.*

It is impossible to be continually caring for others unless a nurse experiences caring and concern that is directed toward herself. It is sometimes hard to find such support within institutional nursing, but it can be created if it is considered important enough.

CONCLUSION

Loss is an experience that comes to all of us over and over again in the course of life. It is not the losses themselves that are harmful, painful as they are. It is the failure to grieve satisfacto-

rily that is potentially dangerous. As Ujhely observes:[62]

The danger of grief does not lie in what one feels, but rather in one's inability to tolerate one's experience, one's thinking one should feel differently, one's blocking or repressing one's feeling state, one's consciously forbidding oneself to feel the way one does because one thinks it is not befitting to oneself or to the lost one.

BIBLIOGRAPHY

1. Armstrong, M. E.: Dying and death—and life experiences of loss and gain. A proposed theory. *Nursing Forum, 14*:95–104, No. 1, 1975.
2. Averill, J. R.: Grief: its nature and significance. *Psychological Bulletin, 70*(6):721–748, 1968.
3. Beachy, W.: Assisting the family in time of grief. *In* Montgomery, D. W. (ed.): *Healing and Wholeness.* Richmond, WA, John Knox Press, 1971.
4. Bendiksen, R., and Fulton, R.: Death and the child: an anterospective test of the childhood bereavement and later behavior disorder hypothesis. *Omega, 6*(1):45–59, 1975.
5. Benoliel, J. Q.: Assessments of loss and grief. *Journal of Thanatology, 1*:182–194, May–June 1971.
6. Benoliel, J. Q.: Talking to patients about death. *Nursing Forum, 9*:254–268, No. 3, 1970.
7. Benoliel, J. Q.: The concept of care for a child with leukemia. *Nursing Forum, 11*:194–204, No. 2, 1972.
8. Binger, C. M., et al.: Childhood leukemia—emotional impact on patient and family. *New England Journal of Medicine, 280*:415–416, Feb. 1969.
8a. Breu, C., and Dracup, K.: Helping the spouses of critically ill patients. *American Journal of Nursing, 78*:50–53, Jan. 1978.
8b. Bunch, B., and Zahra, D.: Dealing with death: The unlearned role. *American Journal of Nursing, 76*: 1486–1488, Sep. 1976.
9. Burnside, I. M.: Grief work in the aged patient. *Nursing Forum, 8*:416–427, No. 4, 1969.
10. Caine, L.: *Widow.* New York, William Morrow, 1974.
11. Caplan, L. M., and Hackett, T. P.: Emotional effects of lower limb amputation in the aged. *New England Journal of Medicine, 269*(22):1166–1171, 1963.
12. Carr, A. C., and Schoenberg, B.: Object-loss and somatic symptom formation. *In* Schoenberg, B. (ed.): *Loss and Grief: Psychological Management in Medical Practice.* New York, Columbia University Press, 1970, pp. 36–48.
13. Carlson, C.: Grief and mourning. *In* Carlson, C. (ed.): *Behavioral Concepts and Nursing Intervention.* Philadelphia, J. B. Lippincott Co., 1970, pp. 95–116.
14. Clayton, P.: The effect of living alone on bereavement symptoms. *American Journal of Psychiatry, 132*(2): 133–137, Feb. 1975.
14a. Encounters with grief (collection of articles). *American Journal of Nursing, 78*:414–425, March 1978.
15. Engel, G. L.: Grief and grieving. *American Journal of Nursing, 64*:93–98, Sep. 1964.
16. Engel, G. L.: Is grief a disease? A challenge for medical research. *Psychosomatic Medicine, 23*(1):18–22, 1961.
17. Engel, G. L.: *Psychological Development in Health and Disease.* Philadelphia, W. B. Saunders Co., 1962.

18. Friedman, S. B.: After sudden death. *Emergency Medicine,* 6:52–60, Sep. 1974.
19. Fulton, R.: *Death and Identity.* New York, John Wiley & Sons, Inc., 1965.
20. Glick, I. O., Weiss, R. S., and Parkes, C. M.: *The First Year of Bereavement.* New York, John Wiley & Sons Inc., 1974.
21. Gorer, G.: *Death, Grief and Mourning.* Garden City, NY, Doubleday Books, 1965.
22. Gramlich, E.: Recognition and management of grief in elderly patients. *Geriatrics,* 23:87–92, July 1968.
23. Gray, V. R.: Grief. *Nursing '74,* 4:25–27, Jan. 1974.
24. Gut, E.: Some aspects of adult mourning. *Omega,* 5(4):323–342, Winter 1974.
25. Hampe, S. O.: Needs of the grieving spouse in a hospital setting. *Nursing Research, 24*:113–120, March–April 1975.
26. Hinton, J.: *Dying.* Harmondsworth, England, Penguin Books, 1967.
27. Holmes, T. H., and Rahe, R. H.: The social readjustment rating scale. *Journal of Psychosomatic Research, 11*:213–218, 1967.
28. Kalish, R.: The effects of death upon the family. *In* Pearson, L. (ed.): *Death and Dying.* Cleveland, The Press of the Case Western Reserve University, 1969.
29. Kastenbaum, A. H. (ed.): *Death and Bereavement.* Springfield, IL, Charles C Thomas, 1969.
30. Keith, R.: *Acute Grief and the Funeral.* New York, Columbia University Press, 1974.
31. Krant, M. J.: *Dying and Dignity.* Springfield, IL, Charles C Thomas, 1974.
32. Krupp, G. R., and Kligfeld, B.: The bereavement reaction: a cross cultural evaluation. *Journal of Religion and Health, 1*:222–246, April 1962.
33. Kübler-Ross, E.: *Death: The Final Stage of Growth.* Englewood Cliffs, NJ, Prentice-Hall, Inc., 1975.
34. Kübler-Ross, E.: *On Death and Dying.* New York, Macmillan Publishing Co., Inc., 1969.
35. Kübler-Ross, E.: *Questions and Answers on Death and Dying.* New York, Macmillan Publishing Co., Inc., 1974.
36. Kutsher, A. (ed.): *Death and Bereavement.* Springfield, IL, Charles C Thomas, 1969.
37. Levin, S.: Depression and the aged. *In* Berezin, M. A., and Cath, S. H. (ed.): *Geriatric Psychiatry: Grief, Loss and Emotional Disorders in the Aging Process.* New York, International Universities Press, Inc., 1965, p. 210.
38. Lewis, C. S.: *A Grief Observed.* London, Faber and Faber, 1964.
39. Lindemann, E.: Symptomatology and management of acute grief. *In* Fulton, R. (ed.): *Death and Identity.* New York, John Wiley & Sons, Inc., 1965.
40. Lopata, H. Z.: *Widowhood in an American City.* Cambridge, Schenkman Publishing Company, Inc., 1973.
40a. McCawley, A.: Help patients cope with grief. *Consultant, 17*:64, Nov. 1977.
41. Maddison, D., and Raphael, B.: The family of the dying patient. *In* Schoenberg, B. (ed.): *Psychosocial Aspects of Terminal Care.* New York, Columbia University Press, 1972.
42. Mandelbaum, D. G.: Social uses of funeral rites. *In* Fulton, R. (ed.): *Death and Identity.* New York, John Wiley & Sons, Inc., 1965.
42a. Marks, M. J. B.: The grieving patient and family. *American Journal of Nursing,* 76:1488–1490, Sep. 1976.
42b. Mercer, R. T.: Crisis: A baby is born with a defect. *Nursing '77,* 7:45–47, Nov. 1977.
43. Miles, H. S., and Hays, D. R.: Widowhood. *American Journal of Nursing,* 75:280–282, Feb. 1975.
44. Morris, S.: *Grief and How to Live with It.* New York, Grosset and Dunlap, 1972.
45. Neels, R. J.: The experience of dying and death. *New Zealand Medical Journal,* 82:233–236, April 1976.
46. Parkes, C. M.: Bereavement and mental illness (Parts 1 and 2). *British Journal of Medical Psychology,* 38:1–26, March 1966.
47. Parkes, C. M.: *Bereavement: Studies of Grief in Adult Life.* New York, International Universities Press, Inc., 1972.
48. Parkes, C. M.: "Seeking" and "finding" a lost object: evidence from recent studies of reaction to bereavement. *Social Science and Medicine, 4*:187–201, 1970.
49. Pevetz, D.: Development, object-relationships and loss. *In* Schoenberg, B. (ed.): *Loss and Grief: Psychological Management in Medical Practice.* New York, Columbia University Press, 1970, pp. 3–19.
50. Pevetz, D.: Reaction to loss. *In* Schoenberg, B. (ed.): *Loss and Grief: Psychological Management in Medical Practice.* New York, Columbia University Press, 1970, pp. 20–35.
51. Pincus, L.: *Death and the Family: The Importance of Mourning.* New York, Random House, 1974.
52. Prattes, D. R.: Helping the family face an impending death. *Nursing '73,* 3:17–20, Feb. 1973.
53. Quint, J.: *The Nurse and the Dying Patient.* New York, Macmillan Publishing Co., Inc., 1967.
54. Quint, J.: The threat of death: some consequences for patients and nurses. *Nursing Forum,* 8:286–300, No. 3, 1969.
55. Rinear, E. E.: Helping the survivors of expected death. *Nursing '75,* 5:60–65, March 1975.
56. Rinear, E. E.: The nurse's challenge when death is unexpected. *R.N.,* 38:50–55, Dec. 1975.
57. Schmale, A. H., Jr.: *Bereavement: Its Psychosocial Aspects.* New York, Columbia University Press, 1975.
58. Schoenberg, B., et al. (ed.): *Loss and Grief: Psychological Management in Medical Practice.* New York, Columbia University Press, 1970.
59. Shneidman, E. S. (ed.): *Death: Current Perspectives.* Palo Alto, CA, Jason Aronson, Inc., 1976.
59a. Sonstegard, L., et al.: The grieving nurse. *American Journal of Nursing,* 76:1490, Sep. 1976.
60. Switzer, D. K.: *The Dynamics of Grief, Its Source, Pain and Healing.* Nashville, Abingdon, 1970.
61. Thaler, O. R.: Grief and depression. *Nursing Forum,* 5:9–22, No. 2, 1966.
62. Ujhely, G. B.: Grief and depression: implications for prevention and therapeutic nursing care. *Nursing Forum,* 5:23–25, No. 2, 1966.
63. Volkart, E., and Michael, S. T.: Bereavement and mental health. *In* Fulton, R. (ed.): *Death and Identity.* New York, John Wiley & Sons, 1965.
63a. Wachowiak, K. D.: Sudden infant death syndrome: What you can do to help the family. *RN,* 41:46–49, Feb. 1978.
64. Weisman, A. D.: Coping with untimely death. *Psychiatry,* 36:366–378, Nov. 1973.
65. Westhoff, M. E.: Listening to relieve the fear of death. *Supervisor Nurse,* 3:80–87, March 1972.

CHAPTER 49*

CARING FOR DYING PERSONS

When death confronts us, life always seems like a downward flow or like a clock that has been wound up and whose eventual "running down" is taken for granted. We are never more convinced of this "running down" than when a human life comes to its end before our eyes, and the question of the meaning and worth of life never becomes more urgent or more agonizing than when we see the final breath leave a body which a moment before was living.[70]

CARL JUNG, "THE SOUL AND DEATH"

INTRODUCTION AND STUDY GUIDE

The care of the dying involves far more than merely passively watching the sands of time run out; caring for the dying need not be an experience of helplessness for the nurse. While the ultimate fact of death is out of the nurse's control, there is much that she *can* control and much that she *can* do. The same is frequently true for the dying person.

Providing care for a dying person is both a challenge and an opportunity for the nurse. The nurse is challenged to use many of her special skills in "caring for" and "comforting" the dying person psychologically and physically, i.e., caring for the total person. Also, the nurse is often given the opportunity to help the dying patient to both live well and die well.

The nursing role of "caring" is uniquely primary in working with terminally ill persons. Emphasis on "curing" the patient is replaced with a total effort to preserve and meet the rights (we could say "needs") of the dying person. The Dying Person's Bill of Rights is presented below. A review of these rights demonstrates that they are best met by the activities of nurses (whose primary role is to "care") rather than by physicians (whose primary role is to "cure"). A review of the rights of the dying person also shows that most of them can best be met through effective, sensitive interactions. (See also Chapters 3 and 4. Refer to Figure 4–2 [p. 53] for clarification of care-cure models.)

For some nurses the care of persons who are dying is one of the most uncomfortable situations in their

nursing practice. Other nurses find it very satisfying to care for patients as they pass through this inevitable experience. Patients in this ultimate situation are greatly in need of the compassionate understanding and skills that they believe nurses should possess. It is indeed unfortunate when nurses feel they are not meeting their own expectations or those of the dying patient and his significant others.

Interaction with a dying person and the physical care given through terminal illness do *not* need to be sources of discomfort for nurses. The care of the dying involves learned skills that mature with increments of thoughtful practice. Interaction patterns and attitudes are learned, and they are amenable to change through peer-support, introspection, education and practice. The administration of comfort measures and other aspects of physical care are also learned. With the development of skills and understandings, confidence emerges—and with these essential attributes the novice nurse moves from *self*-doubt and *self*-concern to a professional ability to care for and about *others*. Thus, in addition to "self-awareness" the nurse gains "patient-awareness" and awareness of the needs of the patient's significant others.

Like any other nursing activity, the care of the dying can become a source of pride for the nurse who achieves skill in this area and who obtains a sense of satisfaction in helping others through perhaps the most anxiety-laden period of their lives. One nurse expresses her satisfaction in caring for terminally ill persons as follows:

Many people have said to me, "How depressing it must be knowing that in spite of all your efforts they will not get

---

*Our thanks to Margaret Helen Parkinson, R.N., R.M.N., Dip.N., B.Soc.Sc., M.N., for her critical review of this chapter.

(From Donovan, M. I., and Pierce, S. G.:
Cancer Care Nursing. New York, Appleton-
Century-Crofts, 1976, p. 33.)

The Dying Person's Bill of Rights*

I have the right to be treated as a living human being until I die.

I have the right to maintain a sense of hopefulness however changing its focus may be.

I have the right to be cared for by those who can maintain a sense of hopefulness, however changing this might be.

I have the right to express my feelings and emotions about my approaching death in my own way.

I have the right to participate in decisions concerning my care.

I have the right to expect continuing medical and nursing attention even though "cure" goals must be changed to "comfort" goals.

I have the right not to die alone.

I have the right to be free from pain.

I have the right to have my questions answered honestly.

I have the right not to be deceived.

I have the right to have help from and for my family in accepting my death.

I have the right to die in peace and dignity.

I have the right to retain my individuality and not be judged for my decisions which may be contrary to beliefs of others.

I have the right to discuss and enlarge my religious and/or spiritual experiences, whatever these may mean to others.

I have the right to expect that the sanctity of the human body will be respected after death.

I have the right to be cared for by caring, sensitive, knowledgeable people who will attempt to understand my needs and will be able to gain some satisfaction in helping me face my death.

This Bill of Rights was created at a workshop on "The Terminally Ill Patient and the Helping Person," in Lansing, Mich., sponsored by the Southwestern Michigan Inservice Education Council and conducted by Amelia J. Barbus, associate professor of nursing, Wayne State University, Detroit.

---

better." I suppose that it would be if one measured achievement in that way, but I believe that there is an entirely different way to look at this work. Surely, to provide the support and care and attention that practically every human being will need in his turn, is worthy of all the skill and thought and experience that nursing can provide.[46]

A nurse's position in the care of a dying person is frequently central and exceptional. Commonly a patient's last home is a hospital ward or convalescent center, and his last contact with the living is with a nurse. Often, too, a nurse is the first professional person to meet with the friends and relatives of a deceased person. The nurse frequently has the daily care of a terminally ill patient and spends the final moments with him and his significant others. The patient and his significant others all look to the nurse for empathy, comfort and direction. The character of a nurse's actions as she participates in the intimate experience of another person's dying can not only lend support but may also help impart meaning to the process.

The life of a dying person is influenced powerfully by those who are with him and take care of him. Since nurses are often the persons with whom dying patients spend most of their time, the nurses' views of a dying person and of that person's remaining life-time are thus extremely important. Quint comments:

Perhaps from time to time we need to remind ourselves that patients who are dying are not just dying. They are also living. Whether or not they have the opportunity to live this final human experience to the fullest—each in his own way—is influenced in great measure by us who take care of them.[124]

Quint believes that the behavior of the dying patient is a product of his interactions with significant persons around him. The dying person can gain the

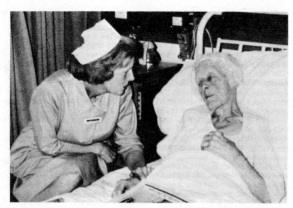

Figure 49–1. The nurse supports a dying patient. (From Saunders, C.: Living with dying. *Man and Medicine.* *1*(3):241, Spring 1976.)

added psychological strength he needs to face death's approach if these interactions are such that he is enabled to *live* each moment as it comes.

> *The terminally ill person who is cared for successfully can die feeling that he is a person of worth. Such a patient can know that others feel that his remaining life and his death are important to them.*

His worth will be proved to him by the facts that others are staying with him, listening to him, talking with him about whatever he wishes to discuss, and helping him to master and pass through difficult times. The dying person can come to recognize his strengths and his worth through others—just as we all do each day. Even in the process of dying away from home in a care facility, it is still possible to form meaningful relationships with others, and it is possible to continually grow, master and control. A dying person can be helped to feel that death is not just an event imposed upon him, leaving him totally out of control and helpless. *He* can determine the character of his response to the knowledge of death; he can determine the quality of his present time—just as he has always done.

The nurse who works effectively with dying patients and their significant others is aware that her attitudes affect the experiences of those in her care and of her coworkers. She, thus, carefully and frequently evaluates her philosophies about living and dying. She also thoughtfully assesses her professional interactions and the other ways in which she actualizes her philosophies.

The needs of the dying are many, complex, individualized and often debatable. Some controversial issues related to death which are commonly discussed in nursing include: suicide, abortion,

whether or not a patient should be told that his illness appears fatal, whether or not a dying person should be cared for at home or in a care facility, and euthanasia.

Euthanasia (derived from the Greek meaning a good death, dying well or an easy, peaceful death) refers to painlessly inducing death in patients who appear to be incurable. Euthanasia may be practiced actively or passively. *Active* euthanasia (also called positive euthanasia) is presently illegal in treating humans. However, it is commonly practiced in veterinary medicine, e.g., by injecting an overdose of an anesthetic agent. *Passive* euthanasia (also called negative euthanasia) is advisedly practiced in the care of human beings, e.g., when a decision is made not to use extraordinary life-sustaining measures or when a patient is removed from life-support systems such as respirators and intravenous nourishment.

The philosophic, moral and ethical facets of the controversial issues involved in caring for dying persons are not discussed here. These are issues, however, to which every nurse should address her attention.

In 1963 one of the authors of this book published, with Joan Baker, one of the first articles on death to appear in nursing literature. Only in recent years has the taboo on discussing dying been weakened. Currently, literature on death and dying is abundant; seminars are commonly given on these subjects, and the study of death *(thanatology)* has emerged. The care of terminally ill persons is now the chosen specialty of some nurses, and special settings *(hospices)* are emerging devoted entirely to providing care for dying persons. Our society is making some progress toward being less death-denying and more death-accepting. Still, in actual practice we have a long way to go.

Much of the credit for the important progress that has been made goes to Dr. Elisabeth Kübler-Ross (psychiatrist), whose chosen area of interest has become identifying ways of helping dying persons. Other significant contributions have been made by Dr. Cicely Saunders (social worker–nurse–physician), founder and medical director of the first hospice, and Dr. Jeanne Quint Benoliel (nurse–sociologist), investigator and teacher in the areas of death and dying.

As you proceed to study this chapter the following study guide may prove helpful. (Many topics are suitable for group discussion.)

1. First, identify what your personal attitudes are toward death. Consider natural death, traumatic death, expected death, sudden unexpected death, and death in various age groups. Reflect on your personal experiences in these areas. Identify attitudes of your significant others toward death, and cultural attitudes about death which may have influenced your development of attitudes.

2. Identify your reactions to losses. (Review as necessary Chapters 3, 5 and 48.)

3. Carefully study the Kübler-Ross stages of dying and appropriate care.

4. Identify your personal attitudes toward: suicide, abortion, whether or not a patient should be told that his illness appears fatal, whether or not a dying person should be cared for at home or in a care

facility, and euthanasia. As you consider your attitudes toward each topic, think about whether your attitudes differ between what you would think best for *another person* in each situation and what you would think best for *you* as the subject in each situation. Consider the origins of your opinions about each topic. Also, in addition to reflecting on your attitudes and opinions relative to each subject, try to become aware of how each topic causes you to "feel" (mentally and physically) as you think about it. Recall your experiences in each of these areas.

5. Clarify your philosophy of nursing, e.g., its relationships to the medical "cure" model and the nursing "care" model. (Refer to Chap. 4.)

6. Consider how all of the above can influence *your* nursing practice.

7. Summarize factors of importance in giving nursing care to persons who are terminally ill and in the process of dying.

8. Finally, pause and think carefully about how you will want others to be with you when you are dying.

ATTITUDES TOWARD DEATH

Patients and nurses each bring to the experience of dying their own unique feelings and attitudes about death. Everything one has seen, heard, read, dreamed, felt or otherwise experienced about death influences how the experience of death is ultimately viewed. Numerous events and attitudes are prevalent in our society that tend to make us uncomfortable in thinking about death and may make it difficult for us to be with dying or dead persons or creatures. As mentioned earlier, if a nurse hopes to help others accept death, she herself needs to (a) reach acceptable philosophic conclusions about death, (b) recognize that cultural and religious beliefs vary concerning death and (c) understand that each individual's personal experiences with the dying and dead markedly affect his perspective of death. The more completely a nurse can understand and accept various individual's perspectives about death, the less inclined she will feel to force her own viewpoint upon others.

Factors Influencing Attitudes Toward Death

Summarized below are some of the factors that cause us all to have our particular attitudes about death. We begin with some statements about how children become aware of death and progress to look at society in general.

▶ Anxiety about death is first experienced in childhood, and a certain amount of this anxiety is normal. A fellow human being or a pet dies; perhaps a dead bug is found . . . all of these kinds of experiences create concern in the child. The child may feel responsible for the death that has occurred.

▶ Childhood experiences with death influence later adult responses. Some children lose loved ones through death; others

do not. Because no two people have the same experiences in growing up, each person reacts differently from others in adult life.

▶ Children's reactions to the knowledge of death and to the dying are influenced by the ways in which adults around them behave. Attitudes about death are thus learned responses to a large degree. Children also learn from adults ways in which they can reduce their anxieties about death. (Some of these are discussed in a following section.)

▶ Children may be markedly influenced by "symbolic representations" of death or of the dead, e.g., the grim reaper carrying a scythe, ghosts, skulls and crossbones, spooks, goblins, coffins, graves.

▶ Children are often lied to about the dead, e.g., "He is sleeping," and thus reality is confused for them. Some children's questions about death may be brushed aside ("We'll talk about it later. Don't worry yourself about it now") or children may feel too uncomfortable to even express their questions.

▶ Children are rarely exposed to dying persons because the dying are commonly moved out of the home and placed in care facilities to die. The dying are isolated from their homes and communities.

▶ Children are often excluded from the places where the dying are placed; also they are commonly excluded from mourning activities and from seeing dead persons, e.g., at funeral homes. The process of dying and the dead thus become frightening "unknowns" in their minds . . . topics and experiences which are left open, for speculation and imagination to fill.

▶ Families are frequently mobile today and family members are scattered. Consequently children and adults may be less likely to be with a dying relative, because they do not live in the same geographic area. Exposure to the dying is thus reduced, and adults lack helpful experiences that would enable them to serve as useful role models for children.

▶ Our society emphasizes youth and health; thus death and illness often become rejected as meaningful life experiences and are denied as realities.

▶ Discussing death is often considered to be "in poor taste," morbid or gruesome. We frequently can't talk with others comfortably about death because of our lack of experience in discussing this topic. Because we do not talk with very many people about death, we lack exposure to the variety of differing philosophies about it . . . we lack enlightenment and education upon which we can formulate our own philosophies. Some persons are raised with exposure to only one viewpoint about death and also with the idea that other views are "strange," "silly" or "nonsense."

▶ Our society consists of persons with a variety of ethnic and religious backgrounds. Because of this, wide varieties of conflicting views about death occur, and conflicts may arise in individuals attempting to formulate their personal philosophy of death.

▶ Because our society is composed of persons from various cultures, we lack clear broad societal "guidelines" which indicate how one should behave when: (a) with the dying, (b) dying himself or (c) mourning the dead. For example, once one is aware of impending death a dilemma arises: should the fact that death is approaching be faced and dealt with, or should death's presence be denied or ignored—encouraging us to be uncomfortable and dishonest with ourselves and others?

▶ Emphasis in health professions has been on saving life ("curing"), and so the loss of life may be viewed as failure and may produce feelings of anger and disappointment in the therapist, patient and others.

▶ Finally, because none of us has ever died, we have no experience with death upon which we can base our thoughts. We also cannot talk with anyone who has experienced death. This situation is unique, un-like any other aspect of life. Typically we have personal experiences or the experiences of others to guide us; we can share our experiences with others and learn from theirs, e.g., experiences with illness, surgery, business matters, pleasurable experiences. In dealing with death, familiar problem-solving methods cannot be used.

Broad Cultural Attitudes

It has been noted that three broad cultural attitudes toward death can be identified: death-accepting, death-defying, and death-denying. The *death-accepting* attitude views death as not merely inevitable, but necessary to give a meaningful coherence to the cycle of life and to existence as a whole. A *death-defying* attitude has been that of traditional Western civilization, with its Judeo-Christian heritage. In this century, however, with a lack of traditional values and a decline in religious values, there has been a shift rapidly toward a *death-denying* attitude, particularly in America. "So modern medicine is devoted to the preservation of life, and death is viewed as an intrusion into a scientific quest for eternal existence."[116]

Nurses cannot handle death by running from it, defying it, denying it or trying to conceal it from themselves or others. They have *chosen* to accept professional responsibilities which *require* them to be death-accepting and thus to examine personal feelings, possibly fears, that they may have harbored for years. *If nurses cannot become death-accepting—they will become patient-rejecting!*

Ultimately the experience of death is one which cannot be prevented. One *must* die; it is inescapable. And, in many nursing situations, one must care for the dying.

To be aware of the separateness of self is to be aware of one's insignificance and helplessness, and this entails the knowledge that one will die . . . death remains. Eventually nothing avails against it, for it is not a misfortune but an inevitability.[160]

Accepting death may require a long, difficult process that consists of interactions between thinking, experiencing and consulting with others. However, persons who have gone through this process feel that it has been most worthwhile.

VIEWS OF DEATH

Death is conceived of in many ways. A Japanese court poem expresses one person's view.

I now must set
"Out of darkness on yet a darker path"
O blest moon
Hovering upon the mountain rim,
Shine clearly on the way I take ahead.

IZUMI SHIKIBU[16]

The path of science ends with death, for death is the province of speculation, faith and doubt. Because there is no absolute proof of what happens after death, it is not surprising that a variety of beliefs have evolved. For some people death is not an incomprehensible mystery, because they have assigned certain beliefs and values to it. Other people feel that they do not understand the mystery of death at all and that they cannot predict anything about what the unknown will be like.

People who arrive at definite conclusions about death may either believe that there is no afterlife or that there is a life after death.

Those who view death as the real *beginning of life* believe that following death man enters into timeless eternity where he will live forever. Some believe that the physical self will be present in the afterlife; others think that only the spiritual self transcends. Many believe that this life is a preparation for the next and that, while this life is often incomprehensible ("Why should man suffer?"), the next life is clearly defined and will explain life on earth.

Persons who believe in an afterlife, in our society, often believe that the afterlife will be pleasant for those who have lived a life relatively free of sin but will be a time of punishment for sinners. Persons with this belief may fear that their own sins in life will be punished when they die and thus may be afraid when dying.

Death may be viewed as a punishment and, thus, the dying may feel as if they are being killed by an outside force. Kübler-Ross comments:

Death will always be distasteful to man. It is inconceivable to imagine an ending to our own life here on Earth. And if our life has to end, the ending is always attributed to a malicious intervention from the outside. In our unconscious mind we can only be killed. It is inconceivable to die of a natural cause, or of old age. Therefore, death is associated with a bad act, a frightening happening, something that calls for retribution and punishment.[81]

People who believe in an afterlife believe in *immortality*. This belief is not uncommon in our society or in others. Let us briefly look more closely at immortality.

Regardless of the kinds of experiences children have with death, they all individually come to realize that there is an end to life as they know it. Also, they come to think of death in relation to themselves. When the idea of death first comes into association with the idea of self, a normal, critical anxiety is likely to develop. This anxiety tends to be reduced by the development of a belief, in one form or another, in *immortality*. Each person has a certain feeling, much of the time, that he will be immortal: *he* will be invulnerable to death. While others may die and their lives will end forever, he will remain alive. This feeling is in part a necessity for life. If the consciousness of inevitable death were everpresent in one's mind its reality would be immobilizing and crushing: "Neither the sun nor death can be looked at steadily" (La Rochefoucauld).

Another view of death is the belief in *reincarnation* (from Latin, meaning "taking on flesh again"). This belief holds that after death the soul occupies a new body. Beliefs vary as to whether or not a period of time of disembodiment occurs before the soul enters the new body, and whether or not the soul is consistently reincarnated in the same species.

Those persons who view death as the *end of life* believe that human beings are not immortal. Experience after death may be looked upon, by these persons, as similar to experience prior to birth; namely, there is no awareness. Death begins a blank void and existence becomes nonexistence; life is "being" and death is "nonbeing."

Consider the following view of death: It is a fundamental aspect of the inorganic thermodynamic process that living organisms are never in actual environmental equilibrium with the inorganic world, and that this lack of equilibrium with the inorganic world is the result of homeostasis. In other words, the process of homeostasis in the living "organic" organisms keeps us from going into equilibrium and becoming part of the "inorganic" environment: homeostatic mechanisms in life keep us alive and organic. When homeostatic failure occurs, the organism dies and goes into thermodynamic equilibrium with the environment, or, to state it in another manner, it becomes one with its inorganic environment. With death, then, the living organism is reduced to an inorganic system and reacts like other inorganic systems. When viewed in this context, death appears almost as a relaxation of the energetic homeostatic attempts to keep the body infused with life and pulled away from the inorganic environment during its life span.

*The eclipse is decreasing. The man gets together
with elements with which he has a natural affinity.*

I CHING

Age and Views of Death

Each age group tends to view death uniquely. Dying *children* may experience fears of pain, separation, punishment and mutilation. Children who have been told that death is "going to sleep" may be afraid to go to sleep. Those who are told that God selects people he loves to come to live with him may experience anger with God for taking them or loved ones away. And then they feel guilty about their anger. Children may personify death, i.e., endow death with human qualities. For example, a child may think of death as "a man who comes and takes you."

Adolescents tend to view death more in terms of an extremely remote possibility that is really not likely to happen to them. These strong feelings of being invulnerable to death, typical of adolescents, may prompt them to be reckless, e.g., to perform death-defying acts or go into battle feeling secure that they will survive.

The *adult* often experiences a major feeling of loss (see Chap. 48). The *losses* include loss of activity, work, play; loss of identity, body, self-image, importance; loss of people, friends, colleagues, loved ones, pets; loss of place, home, life on earth, nature; and loss of respect, responsibilities, and self-control. In addition to fearing these losses, the dying adult may have other *fears* such as fear of the unknown, pain and suffering, regression, and loneliness. These fears and feelings of losses may be intermingled with concerns about the welfare of those who will be left behind and thoughts about the meaning, history and consequences of one's life.

Older people tend to think more personally about death because they view themselves as closer to it. Also, they have usually become more familiar with death than younger persons because they have experienced more losses through the deaths of loved ones and acquaintances.

We have presented several divergent views of death and attitudes toward death. Over a period of time the practicing nurse may care for dying persons who hold these various beliefs.

One patient may be death-accepting, anticipating death comfortably and looking ahead to a pleasant afterlife with reunions with loved ones or looking ahead to reincarnation. Another may hold no belief in an afterlife yet also be death-accepting . . . ready to pass on into the apparent state of thermodynamic equilibrium. Still another dying person may be fearful of death, viewing it as mysterious, dark and incomprehensible. The excellent nurse will not be judgmental in giving care.

COPING WITH ANXIETIES ABOUT DEATH

"Death is the one reality in which most men cannot believe."[105] Psychologic adaptive mechanisms are commonly used for protection against this reality. Some adaptive mechanisms which help to reduce the fear of death are: belief in immortality (previously discussed), denial, displaced feelings, and intellectualization. These may become so interwoven that they are difficult to distinguish at times.

One of the strongest adaptive mechanisms, or basic adjustive techniques, used against knowledge of death is *denial* that one will die. Even the dying may deny that they are going to die. Most people, however, can deny the reality of death for only so long. Sooner or later most people realize that they will die and that death must be faced.

*Though formerly I heard
About the road that all must travel
At the inevitable end,
I never thought, or felt, today
Would bring that far tomorrow.*

ARIWARA NARIHIRA[16]

Denial has been described as a buffer after shocking news, allowing the patient to collect himself and, with time, mobilize other defenses that are less radical. In the dying, denial often tends to be temporary and may be replaced by partial acceptance and feelings of anger, hostility, resentment and envy.

The above feelings may be *displaced* in various directions, e.g., toward nurse and loved ones. Often, displaced feelings are more difficult to cope with than denial, because they are directed at someone, while denial is more inner-directed. It helps if those persons who are the targets of displaced feelings can try to put themselves in the patient's situation and attempt to accept the patient's feelings without retaliation. Below are some examples of displaced feelings:

▶ Dying is experienced with overwhelming feelings of helplessness at times. There is nothing the individual (nurse or patient) can do to prevent it. All of science, all of man's history of conquest and cleverness leave him powerless against death. Feelings of personal inadequacy create feelings of frustration, which are expressed as *anger, rage, envy,* and *resentment.* The dying may feel inadequate to cope with the dying process and experience bewilderment, unspecified fear, anxiety, and confusion.

▶ Death taboos in our society, e.g., reluctance to discuss death, add to the burden of the dying by contributing to feelings of isolation. The dying are made to feel they should not discuss, or at times even acknowledge, their death because they will make others feel uncomfortable. The dying may, therefore, feel *angry* that they must keep others comfortable though they themselves are despairing, in need of solace and wanting to talk with someone about their dying.

▶ Feelings of *anger* and *hostility* may be present in both the terminal patient and in those providing care. Those who are well may feel uncomfortable that they are healthy and will probably be living after the dying person is dead. The well persons may feel guilty over their survival and health. Those dying, who want to live, may *resent* their situation, *envying* those who are well. The dying may feel a marked separation between "we the dying" and "you the living."

▶ The person who knows he is going to die may unconsciously want to *punish* those who will survive. This is one reason why a nurse may respond to the dying person with a feeling of *hostility.* Unconsciously the nurse senses the anger that the dying individual feels because he is dying and the nurse, and others, will live longer.

Finally, *intellectualization* about death may occur in an attempt to reduce fear. In this situation death is acknowledged intellectually, however it is not acknowledged emotionally. The emotional self does not confront reality and remains sheltered.

IMPENDING DEATH: THE NURSE'S REACTIONS

Dying people often evoke fears and anxieties in those around them, for the dying are a reminder that we will each, in our turn, die. It is natural for frightened, anxious persons to employ defense mechanisms (basic adjustive techniques) of various kinds in an attempt to protect themselves from awareness of their own vulnerabilities. Nurses are no exceptions to this natural occurrence of events. However, because a nurse is a professional person, she recognizes that her defensive behaviors can impede her therapeutic effectiveness and even increase the distress of persons in her care. The excellent nurse thus strives to gain awareness of her defensive feelings and how they are causing her to act toward others. This process of self-examination is not as easy as it might seem. Therefore, the nurse may enlist the assistance of valued colleagues, requesting their help (and giving hers in return) in a process of peer assessment.

As the reader will note, defenses express themselves in a wide range of behaviors. Presented below are some examples of protective defenses that nurses may use when they are uncomfortable in working with terminally ill persons.

▶ Unconsciously the nurse may wish to *punish* a dying person by viewing his dying as an act which is hostile on his part. The "punishment" may be expressed in numerous ways, e.g., delaying care, roughness in handling the patient, rudeness.

▶ A nurse may feel *angry* with a patient who talks about death, responding as if he is deliberately trying to make her uncomfortable. At times a nurse may actually feel angry at a patient for dying while she was responsible for his care . . . as if he could control the time of his death. Such anger is apparent when a nurse says, "Why did he have to die on my shift?" Becoming angry with a patient for dying is actually a *displacement* of the nurse's feelings about her own coming death. If she cannot keep a patient alive, she realizes that the time will come when she cannot be kept alive. Also, the nurse may experience a feeling of *guilt* that she didn't say the "right" things to the patient in talking of death, or that she could have done something more to keep the patient alive.

▶ Because talking about death makes her feel uncomfortable, the nurse may try in various ways to get the patient to *stop talking* about it, "Aw . . . come on . . . don't talk that way." Or she may make the patient feel guilty for bringing the subject of death up, "You shouldn't talk this way." or "It's wrong to talk like that!" Perhaps she minimizes his concerns, "You don't need to worry about that." Or, she may give false reassurance, "I just know that everything is going to be O.K." When the patient speaks of death the nurse may simply ignore what he is saying, change the subject, use social chit-chat (talk of the weather or television) to avoid talking about death. Other ways of *controlling conversation* are to use obscure or technical professional language which the patient cannot understand, or to use "hospital rules" and the doctor's authority to completely put off talking about the patient's concerns. Other ways of ignoring conversation about death are to busy oneself with objects and manual tasks while with the patient or to keep the patient so sedated that he doesn't talk about anything.

▶ *Flight* and *avoidance* are other defenses. The nurse may *rationalize* her behavior and say to herself, "I really would like to sit down and talk with him about his dying, but I simply don't have the time." Or, "I should answer his call light, but I think it's more important if I do. . . . Someone else can go to him." The nurse in a room with a patient close to death, who appears comatose, may want to leave the room and rationalizes her behavior by thinking, "I'm not really leaving him alone. He's unconscious and doesn't know what's going on or whether I'm here or not." It is wise to remember, nevertheless, that people who have recovered from comas sometimes have remembered what was going on during that time. While they appeared unaware of everything, they were actually able to hear what was being said or were aware of the presence of others, but they were unable to respond. A dying patient may never be able to tell the nurse that he was comforted by her presence and by the way she talked to him, kept him clean, changed his position, smoothed his hair, sponged his face. And yet, he may well be aware of her actions and may be perceiving them with heartfelt gratitude.

▶ Viewing the patient in a *depersonalized* manner is another defense. An increasingly complex, mechanized approach to the care of the dying may result in depersonalized care, which is protective to staff members. Defensively they may blame the machines for failing to keep the patient alive. Or, they may focus only on the "case," the patient's

physiology, and attempt to defensively ignore his "self" (soul, personality, consciousness, psychic existence).

As a nurse comes to understand and accept death—and as she gains experience in caring for the dying in a supportive environment—she is able to recognize and discard her protective defenses more easily. As the nurse works to reduce her defensive behaviors, it may be helpful for her to recall that her defenses are natural and to realize that those which interfere with patient care can be altered through conscious efforts on her part.

We emphasize that recognizing and reducing one's defenses concerning dying does not mean becoming void of feelings or "hardened" toward death.

Our task is analogous to that of the harp player. The harp player develops a callus on the tip of each finger so that his finger won't bleed when he plays the harp and plucks the strings. Yet, if he is a good harp player, through these calluses he preserves an amazing sensitivity. Those calluses do not prevent him from being a good harp player; they make him a good harp player. . . . Courage is not the absence of fear, it is the ability to function effectively in the presence of fear.[157]

Several situations have been identified which make death particularly stressful for nurses.[42] For example, a patient's death may be especially stressful if the patient was not considered to be in critical condition but suddenly developed an irreversible complication that caused death. Also, death may be highly stressful if the patient who died (a) was someone the nurse felt especially fond of, (b) was someone to whom the nurse had devoted considerable time and attention or (c) was in an age group in which death is usually unlikely, e.g., child or young person. A patient's death may also be stressful for a nurse when she is the one who will inform the patient's significant others and will perform the postmortem (after-death) care. The nurse may experience feelings of remorse for not having done more for the patient while he was alive. She may wonder if she really did everything possible to keep the patient alive or if she was, in some way, responsible for his death.

As mentioned, the nurse who works with dying persons is herself in need of support. This intense work, involving in part the nurse's own grief work, is draining and demanding when done well. A team approach is helpful to the nurse. She needs understanding people to turn to for support and guidance. If the nurse is unable to share her experiences and express her grief with colleagues, she will take these personal emotions into the nurse-patient, nurse-family relationships in ways which may be untherapeutic. Additionally, it is helpful for the nurse who works frequently with dying persons to have pleasant personal experiences confirming *life*.

It should be acknowledged that "while it is true that a nurse is committed to care for the sick without discrimination, it is realistic to remember that terminal care may not be within the competency of every nurse."[53]

Let us reemphasize a point made earlier. If a nurse is highly "cure" oriented, she will tend to consider dying persons as "failures," and with this view she may withdraw her interest in providing supportive care.

IMPENDING DEATH: THE PATIENT'S REACTIONS

. . . dying . . . is a highly individualistic human experience which defies precise identification or principles and guidelines. It is as if each person, in his dying, forever and irrevocably declares his uniqueness as an individual and vigorously disputes society's designation of him as "mass man."[156]

Dying *is* an individual experience and generalizations about such experiences must always be tentative. Nevertheless it has been possible to obtain some insight into divergent ways of approaching death by talking with large numbers of people as they were dying and those who were close to dying but recovered.

Dr. Elisabeth Kübler-Ross, pioneer in studying people's reactions to knowledge of impending death, has interviewed hundreds of dying patients. On the basis of these interviews Kübler-Ross[80, 83, 84] identified *five psychologic stages* that dying patients typically pass through:

1. Denial
2. Anger
3. Bargaining
4. Depression
5. Acceptance.

These stages, which may occur in reaction to any loss, are described in Table 49–1, along with some suggested nursing actions for each stage. Stages 2 and 4 are commonly the most difficult to experience and work with.

We do not here discuss in detail the various stages of dying and helpful responses. The reader is strongly encouraged to study Kübler-Ross's publications, in which she provides skilled guidance and numerous examples (see bibliography).

It is helpful for the nurse to work toward gaining awareness, acceptance and understanding of each stage so she can eventually be comfortable with it. In talking with dying and grieving persons (as in talking with anyone), be genuine in your responses. Refer to Chapter 3 in this text for discussions of genuineness and use of accurate empathy. Patients do not always use the words "death" and "dying" when talking about these topics. Instead they may use various disguised, individualized terms. Listen carefully for these.

It is important to realize that *all dying persons do not move in an orderly progression through these stages;* however, at least one stage is usually experienced. Some stages may be missed; others may be returned to (a process called "regression") after moving ahead to more advanced stages. All dying persons, for example, may not die in a state of acceptance. Likewise, bargaining may periodically reoccur. A dying person may move from a state of acceptance back into anger and depression. This latter situation may occur when a patient is ready to accept death; however, his loved ones cannot accept his death and let him peace-

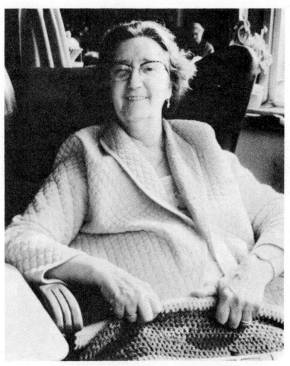

Figure 49–2. The cheerful smile can mask deep anxiety or denial. Here Mrs. L's hands are more revealing than her face. (From Saunders, C.: Living with dying. *Man and Medicine, 1* (3):240, Spring 1976.)

TABLE 49–1. STAGES OF DYING (LOSS) IDENTIFIED BY KÜBLER-ROSS AND SOME SUGGESTED NURSING ACTIONS

STAGE OF DYING	SUGGESTED NURSING ACTIONS
Stage 1: Denial. Characterized by the comment, "No, not me! It can't be true!" Denial is a coping period, usually of brief duration. Most patients do not need denial long for themselves, but may use it to try to protect others, e.g., loved ones, nurses. Almost all patients use denial briefly in the first stage of terminal illness. It may then be used intermittently and is gradually given up. An occasional patient needs to sustain denial until he dies.	**Stage 1: Denial** *In all stages: Do not strip the patient of his defense; however, do not lie to him either. Let the patient tell you what he knows about his condition. Try to use his own words when talking with him (e.g., "the long journey"). Maintain a genuine, honest attitude of interest. Listen carefully. Be warm, supportive and understanding. Use accurate empathy (see Chap. 3). Sustain an appropriate feeling of hope. Coordinate your approach to the patient with those of other health team members, e.g., find out what the doctor has told the patient about his condition. If the patient asks if he is dying it may be best to say he is seriously ill. Let the patient know you are ready to discuss his concerns and feelings whenever he is ready. Be present for the patient and let him know he will not be abandoned. Help the patient's significant others as they experience these stages and also assist them to understand why the patient is behaving as he does.*
Stage 2: Anger. "Why me?" As denial resolves, it is replaced with questioning and feelings of anger, rage, resentment and envy. These feelings are projected onto others, e.g., nurse, family. The patient blames, complains and finds fault easily. This is a very difficult period for the patient's significant others and staff to handle well as they tend to want to retaliate against the patient, thus increasing his distress and frustration.	**Stage 2: Anger.** View the anger as a healthy, adjusting response which is helpful to the patient. Try not to take the "attacks" personally. Remember the anger is not actually with you, but rather arises from the patient's feelings of fear and helplessness and the knowledge that he is dying. *Try to not retaliate with your own expressions of anger or avoidance.* Acknowledge how the patient appears to feel. Don't tell the patient he "shouldn't act this way" or "shouldn't say that." Let the patient express his anger and "pour out his feelings." When observing the patient's anger, it may help to comment, "I'd be angry too. Get it off your chest!" Try to remain with the patient

when appropriate so he won't feel his anger has driven you away. Do not feel you must answer those questions which are philosophic, e.g., "Why is God doing this to me?"

Stage 3: Bargaining. A temporary truce occurs as the "Why me?" stage is replaced by, "Yes, it's me *but. . .*" or, "Why now?" In an attempt to obtain a prolongation of life, the patient tries to bargain with God or fate. "If I can just live until. . . I promise I will. . ." This stage, helpful to the patient, may be intermittent or brief.

Stage 3: Bargaining. You may not notice this stage as the patient may do his bargaining privately. However, if you do see it, understand that this stage is helpful to the patient and that he is trying to postpone his fate by being cooperative and good.

Stage 4: Depression. Now the bargaining period is past. Progression toward death is obvious to the patient and he simply acknowledges, "Yes, . . . me." Markedly depressed, deeply saddened, the patient experiences the intense psychologic pain of grieving. He may cry and express other indications of grief (see Chap. 48). He may withdraw, ask to see certain people for the final time, then want just one loved one to remain nearby. Depression may be long term. The stage of depression has two phases: (1) *Reactive grief* or depression related to what he has already lost, e.g., body part removed surgically, symbolic losses of self-esteem, etc.; and (2) *Preparatory grief* or depression in anticipation of losing all his love objects and life itself.

Stage 4: Depression. Allow the patient to mourn, cry and talk about his losses. (See also Chaps. 15 and 48.) Recognize that patients may try to cover up their depressions. (See Fig. 49–2.) Also, understand that it may be more difficult for men (socialized to "be strong and act like a *man*") to express grief and mourn than it is for women. Realize that depression and grieving are *normal* for a dying person and that he needs to be allowed to freely express these feelings.

Stage 5: Acceptance. It is desirable for the patient to be able to move out of depression and into the stage of acceptance. (Acceptance is not resignation, i.e., is not the bitter "giving up," seen when a person has no reason to live.) The patient feels he has taken care of all his unfinished business with others, his work is done, he is ready to accept death. Fears, anxieties and most pain are gone.

Stage 5: Acceptance. Allow the patient to be calm, quiet and detached. Don't force interaction. Continue to be present and appropriately supportive.

fully die. This is indeed tragic, and brings up other important points for discussion here.

The stages identified by Kübler-Ross *are commonly passed through not only by the patient, but also by the dying person's significant others and often by members of the health team.* All of these people do not pass through the stages at the same rate of speed or in the same sequence. It is therefore possible, for example, for the dying person to be in the stage of acceptance while his spouse in still in the stage of denial—or vice versa. Or, perhaps the nurse is angry and the patient is depressed. These variances, when unrecognized and improperly handled, can create serious disturbances that increase the burdens and suffering of all involved.

There is nothing you can do to hurry people through the stages to reach the stage of acceptance. You can, however, facilitate and support their progression. Remain present for them and communicate understanding and warmth. Also, try to maintain the patient's *hope.* "If we can elicit the patient's hope and support *his* hope, then we can help him the most."[84] The nature of his hope may change. Listen closely to identify what he is hoping for and support that. You can ask the patient who has accepted your invitation to talk about dying, what kinds of things you can do now to help make the remaining time more meaningful and more bearable.

In sum, reactions to knowledge of impending death vary markedly, depending on many factors. Some of these factors are: philosophy of life, happiness with living, presence or absence of loved ones, religion, personality and cultural background. A patient's dying causes reactions not only within the patient, but also in his significant others, staff and other patients.

The skilled nurse realizes that patients react *individually* to the fact that they are dying, and she assesses each patient carefully in an attempt to identify each patient's unique situation. While one person may easily reach a comfortable stage of acceptance and actually feel ready to die, another may rage and resist the knowledge that he is dying until the end. The poet Dylan Thomas wrote: "Do not go gentle into that good night. Rage, rage against the dying of the light."*

The Poems of Dylan Thomas. New York, New Direction, 1971.

Whether a dying person denies, accepts, rages or resigns himself to his fate, each is within his right to view death and approach it in his unique manner.

As pointed out, dying patients may gradually become more drowsy, tired, weak, withdrawn, eventually reaching a time when they seem ready to stop struggling for life and wanting to live. They come to accept death and quietly enter a void of feeling and are ready to die. ". . . a patient reaches a point when death comes as a great relief, and . . . [they can] die easier if . . . allowed to detach themselves slowly from all the meaningful relationships in their life."[81]

Some among the dying may wish they had lived differently and may realize that there is no longer time to do all that was "wished for" or "put off." Now there won't be time to smooth over animosities, to travel, to relax, to read those unread books. There isn't going to be time to watch the children grow or possibly to see the next change of season. One can see that many hopes will never be realized. The "tomorrow" that could always be counted on will no longer appear. Time assumes new meaning for many as they are dying.

> *"Lament on the Instability of Human Life"*
>
> How I yearn to be
> Unalterably what I once was,
> Immovable as a rock,
> But because I belong to this world,
> There is no stop to time.
>
> OKURA[16]

Kübler-Ross comments frequently that dying people can teach us an extremely valuable lesson: *How to live!* To enjoy the simple joys of everyday life. To enjoy today without waiting for tomorrow. To use our time well and enjoy it fully.

IMPENDING DEATH: PROVIDING PSYCHOLOGIC SUPPORT

It is crucially important to look beyond the physical symptoms and complaints to see the human being in profound psychological suffering. The patient may be dying but his capacity to experience fear, despair and grief is very much alive. Very often, the psychological management of the patient by the medical staff and the family will determine not only whether he is a cooperative patient or not, but whether he will be able to face death with dignity.[53]

For some persons, the mental preparations for death are more difficult than the physical act of dying. Anxieties and fears need to be coped with and meanings assigned to death. Unresolved conflicts and other "unfinished business" (emotional and practical) are often revived and are in need of being resolved. *Grieving* (i.e., normal, healthy yet painful reactions to loss) must be experienced and *grief work* (i.e., remorse and pain over unfinished business) needs to be completed. An enormous amount of psychologic "work" is commonly performed by dying persons. All of this may come at a time when the person is feeling ill and low on energies, is experiencing overwhelming emotions, and is perhaps facing long-suppressed fears. Clearly, the dying person is in need of the strong, yet sensitive psychologic support which can be given by a professional nurse.

DISCLOSING THE DIAGNOSIS

A question of central importance appears: *Should the patient be told he is dying?* Some believe that persons who have illnesses that will probably be fatal should not be told they are "dying," but that most should be told that they are "seriously ill." Kübler-Ross has observed that frequently persons who are near death comment that they wish they had been told about their situation sooner than they were. These persons stated they needed the valuable "missed time" to prepare themselves and their significant others.

We have learned that our patients all know when they are dying, and I think that's consoling for us to know. Half of them have never been told that they have a serious illness. We are often asked what or whether a patient should be told that he is dying. He will tell *you* that when you dare to listen, when you are able to hear it.

But patients should, I think, with very few exceptions, be told when they have a serious illness. Our patients say that they would like to be told this under two conditions: one is that the person telling them allows for some hope, and the second is that "you are going to stick it out with me—not desert me—not leave me alone." If we can, indeed "stick it out" with them, then I think we can help them the most.[84]

Psychiatrists tend to favor telling patients the diagnosis and the possible fatal outcome of their illness. Supporting an "honest relationship" with patients, they often feel that the question of concern should not be whether or not to tell the patient but rather, how to *best* share with the patient a realization of his life situation.

Physicians practicing medicine in fields other than psychiatry may not agree that a patient should be told if he has an illness that is possibly irreversible. Thus, many surgeons and medical practitioners may tell relatives that a patient's illness appears to be of a terminal nature, but they will not tell the patient. And obviously, not all patients feel the same way; some want to be told, others do not.

Because there are considerations pro and con as to whether or not persons should be informed of an illness which might be fatal, nurses need to discuss with physicians: (a) whether or not a given patient and his significant others have been informed and (b) exactly what information was given. The nurse needs to recognize that the practices of physicians vary and the wishes of individual patients also vary. The nurse will want to be extremely sensitive to the apparent wishes of each patient. Does he appear to be wanting to talk about his concerns about death? Does he seem to be avoiding any mention of his condition and wish to deny the reality of his situation? Am *I* wanting to avoid discussion of his condition? Patients should not be forced to discuss impending death. However, they must not be made to feel that they must bear in silence the loneliness of one who is about to leave the only reality he has ever known.

> *Although terminally ill persons should not be forced to talk about their dying, they should know that you are available to talk with them about their concerns whenever they are ready.*

Some Benefits From Honesty

It is possible to simply and privately help a patient realize that he has a serious illness without removing all hope of recovery. Summarized below are some of the *benefits* of an honest and reasonable discussion:

▶ Patients, their significant others and staff may all feel more comfortable in an atmosphere free of suspicion and deception. If patients learn the truth about their illness from persons other than those taking care of them, they may lose their faith and trust in those caring for them.

▶ Honesty may provide greater mental ease for patients and their significant others during their final time of life together. Patients often do come to know the truth about their situation even if they are not told. If they have not been told, they may feel uncomfortable in bringing up the subject. They may believe that they were not told because no one wanted to talk with them about their situation and that they are expected to play the game of "Everything Is Just Fine" even though they are dying. Such impressions contribute to the feelings of many dying persons that they are isolated and that they make others uncomfortable.

▶ Terminally ill persons may be able to better accept the course of their illnesses if they understand the illness. The uncertainty of the unknown and the realm of imagination are reduced somewhat by realizing what is happening to them, e.g., why they continue to feel ill.

▶ Finally, the patient can take some control and decide how he may choose to spend his remaining time. He can take care of unfinished business, clear up relationships with others that need "tending," and deal with the realistic matters of getting his will in order, discussing burial wishes, transferring business obligations, attending to religious concerns, and so on.

Once the dying person begins to talk about his impending death the nurse may be able to help him identify unfinished business and attend to this business. Also, she may help the patient to live his remaining life more fully by identifying his needs and hopes and then finding appropriate persons to help meet them.

> *It should be* expected *that upon realizing that he may die from his illness a patient may react defensively, e.g., with denial and/or feelings of anger, resentment or envy directed at persons around him. The patient should be assisted to feel comfortable in expressing his feelings and discussing them. Carefully assess both verbal and nonverbal behaviors.*

Where to Die?

Should a person die at home or in a care facility? When a person is dying this question becomes real and must be answered individually. The nurse has her own ideas on this matter. However, her role is to *nonjudgmentally* help the patient and his significant others decide what will be done, rather than to pass her own opinions about "what is right." Many factors must be considered, e.g., the patient's wishes, the wishes of those who will care for him if he remains at home, the patient's condition (his strengths, impairments, potential complications, probable course), the home environment and availability of helpers there, financial matters, where the patient will be most comfortable, etc. Some persons require admission to a care facility; others do not.

Increasingly, persons about to die are brought to hospitals or nursing homes. This is a change from the pattern of not too many years ago, when it was accepted in our society that dying persons should remain at home. Today, many people say *they* want to die at home, however they do not want *others* to die at home. The basis of such a statement may be honorable, "I don't think we could give him the best care if he stayed here at home," and the decision may also be partially based in deep rooted fears about the dying and lack of experience in being with people as their lives end.

Sometimes one will hear family members say, "We would like to keep him at home to die, but the children shouldn't be exposed to it." Kübler-Ross discusses the desirability of dying at home and the influence on children of having a dying person in the home as follows:

If a patient is allowed to terminate his life in a familiar and beloved environment it requires less adjustment for him. His own family knows him well enough to replace a sedative with a glass of his favorite wine; or the smell of a homecooked soup may give him the appetite to sip a few spoons of fluid which is still more enjoyable than an infusion.

The fact that children were allowed to stay home where a fatality has struck, and are included in the talk and fears, gives them the feeling that they are not alone in the grief. It gives them the comfort of shared responsibility and shared mourning. It helps them view death as part of life, an experience which may help them grow and mature.[81]

When a patient prefers to die at home and his loved ones intend to provide most of the care, the nurse may function in various supportive ways, e.g., counseling, teaching, administering part-time care. For example, a spouse may be taught how to administer injectable medications; equipment for home care (e.g., wheelchair) may be rented; and a nurse may visit on a regular (or on-call) basis to assist with some of the more difficult aspects of care and to provide counseling-teaching services.

In some areas there are now special settings devoted entirely to the care of persons with terminal illness. These settings are called *hospices*. Some are separate agencies not affiliated with hospitals; others are special units (hospice units) based in hospitals. The original idea of a hospice was introduced by Dr. Cicely Saunders when she founded St. Christopher's Hospice in London in 1967. Hospices may have both in-patient and out-patient services. The home-care (out-patient) concept is extremely important since one goal in the successful care of dying persons is to prevent their isolation from home and significant others. Some hospices have round-the-clock "on call" teams which help people to die at home. Persons admitted to a hospice may find they can have unlimited visiting hours which allow visits by children and pets, in addition to adult visitors. Also, in a hospice the patient's significant others may participate along with the staff in caring for him.

Facilitating Interaction About Death

As already indicated, awareness of impending death raises many doubts, concerns and questions. *Often there is a great need for the dying (and their significant others) to talk about what they are experiencing.*

When we have concerns, usually we seek out others to talk with us, or, sometimes, to just *be* with us. Yet, when faced with one of life's most stressful and most meaningful experiences, one often finds that the door to communication with others is closed. When friends can't help with concerns, one often turns to professional persons for guidance or, at least, support and understanding. A patient typically turns to "his" nurse.

The nurse can help by first providing an atmosphere of acceptance, in which the patient feels comfortable and can talk openly. Acceptance is an important quality that a patient expects to find in a professional person. If a patient is to be helped to talk about death, he must be allowed to express his feelings freely, without censure. Thus, the nurse tries to show the patient that she is not going to impose her beliefs about death on him or judge his beliefs or his behavior.

The following information may be helpful in providing care that is directed at facilitating interaction about death.

▶ Recognize that patients may be at their *peak of mental distress* when they are first coming to realize that their disorder is probably terminal. Stages 2 (anger) and 4 (depression) described by Kübler-Ross (see Table 49–1) are especially difficult to experience. In facing death an individual's anxiety typically mounts to a peak and then falls. At the peak point the person either mobilizes his coping mechanisms to deal with the anxiety or else he capitulates to it and experiences disorganization. Regardless of the solution the peak of acute anxiety is commonly reached prior to death, and a state of diminishing anxiety usually occurs as the individual approaches death. Thus, the later stages of a terminal illness may not be as stressful psychologically to the patient. (This may

well not be true for the patient's significant others or the nurse.) *Early* supportive psychologic care may help the patient to adapt to his situation and contribute to making his remaining life more mentally peaceful.

▶ Attempt to determine what the *meaning of death* is for the patient rather than assuming that death has the same meaning for him that it may have for you. Plan care according to the patient's view of death. For example, as discussed earlier, while some individuals do not hold a belief in an afterlife, others do. The latter may not consider the end of physical life as "death," but rather view it as the "birth" of a soul.

▶ Realize that awareness of coming death may awaken problems from a person's near or distant past. *Unresolved conflicts and fears* resurface, e.g., problems of identity, inadequacy, dependency, passivity, independence, or fears of pain, isolation, loneliness, humiliation, loss of privacy, invasion of one's body. These problems contribute to the stress which the dying are trying to cope with. The nurse strives to identify the patient's individual conflicts and fears and then to plan (with the patient when possible) ways of resolving conflicts and reducing fears.

▶ Attempt to identify those *adaptive mechanisms (basic adjustive techniques)* employed by a specific dying person, and plan care accordingly. For example, denial may be a protective shelter for some persons and they may not wish to discuss their deaths. Respect such wishes. (See Table 49–1.) When a person who has been denying death, or who has otherwise found it difficult to discuss, seems ready to talk about his situation— don't put off the discussion. Interact immediately, even if you can do so only briefly. When ending the discussion always leave the door open for further communication, e.g., "We can talk about this more again . . . whenever you wish." Recognize, also, when the person shows signs of being ready to terminate discussion of death.

Nurses (and others) are often troubled about "what to say" to persons who wish to talk about death. Often *what* is said is not nearly as important as *how* it is said. While much of a nurse's education prepares her to "know the answers," those questions pertaining to death are often rhetorical and the nurse cannot realistically expect that she should be able to answer them. Often a person talking about death actually simply wants a chance to think out loud, rather than to hear about someone else's conclusions. He is trying to formulate his own answers. (Role playing can be very useful in developing interaction skills. Why not practice talking about death with a peer? Take turns being the dying person and the helper.)

When patients ask questions about the possibility of their conditions being fatal, try to decide *why* you think the question is being asked. Is an answer expected? Is this a way of letting the nurse know of fear and of the desire to discuss this fear? Or, is the question being asked to test you and see if your answer is the same as that of others? You might begin by asking the patient to tell you what he thinks about the nature of his condition. This may encourage him to express more clearly the basis of his original question, and often the original question may not require a specific answer.

Familiarization with the basic beliefs and practices of major faiths will help you talk with persons about death and to understand and facilitate specific requests for contact with priests, rabbis and ministers.

Even persons with deep religious faith, however, may be fearful of death or may express anger with God because they are dying. As with others, they should not be intimidated for their concerns or feelings. And they should not be made to feel that their faith is not "strong enough."

Many people are not accustomed to talking seriously about death and dying. They may joke about these subjects or refer to them in slang terms, e.g., "Who croaked?" You will want to recognize that jokes, teasing and slang often indicate underlying anxiety, e.g., "I think I'll die laughing." "You wouldn't let me die, would you?" (said while smiling or with mild laughter). "I guess I'll just kick the bucket." Recognizing that such expressions may come from lack of experience in talking about death and anxiety over what is happening, try to not act offended or amused by what the patient says. Avoid joking in return and express what you believe the patient's feelings might be, e.g., "Are you feeling concerned about the seriousness of your condition?" Quips, jokes, changing the subject, making "Pollyanna" remarks ("Everything will be all right, don't worry.") are not helpful to troubled people.

Summarized below are some helpful guidelines. In interacting about dying with patients attempt to:

▶ be supportive without being invasive

▶ express concern, not curiosity

▶ use accurate empathy and understanding

▶ give control and identify strengths

▶ continue to "be present"; do not withdraw

▶ listen carefully

▶ use the patient's own language with reference to death

▶ identify and reduce specific fears and concerns

▶ facilitate grieving

▶ identify and sustain the patient's hopes, at whatever level they may be; early in illness he may "hope" for recovery, later he may "hope" for a peaceful death and an afterlife

Reducing Specific Fears and Concerns

Dying people harbor many fears and concerns. They can obtain a great deal of relief through the expression of these fears and concerns and from measures undertaken to reduce these individualized psychologic discomforts. "Once fears have been voiced, they are easier to dispel; even as they are expressed, they lose much of their power to disturb."[134]

> Help the dying person to identify his specific fears and concerns about dying. Then plan and implement appropriate measures to reduce these worries.

Kübler-Ross observes that dying children are easier to work with than adults, because children are less afraid. "Grownups make such a nightmare out of death, but very young children are not afraid of death. They pick up this fear as they get older."[85]

Some common fears expressed by dying persons include fear of: isolation, abandonment, loneliness, pain, loss of control, loss of privacy, invasion of one's body. A person's specific fears can be voiced and discussed, one by one, in a supportive environment. Plans can then be made of ways to reduce these fears.

A common concern of the dying is over the welfare of their significant others. This concern can also be discussed and a course of action can be planned to help meet it.

This entire process can begin by a nurse helping a dying person to identify his particular fears and concerns. The patient should be allowed to name them, rather than the nurse stating what she thinks they might be. The latter course may only serve to introduce new, previously unthought of worries. For example, a patient says, "I'm afraid to die." One appropriate response might be, "Have you thought about what it is that you are particularly afraid of?" After he has talked about one of his fears or concerns you might say, "I'm wondering if there are other worries you might talk with me about."

An almost universal need of the dying was expressed quite simply by Dr. Charles W. Mayo, "I hope that when I die, it will be quick. But if there is some delay, I hope I'll have somebody I love with me—somebody to hold my hand."[148]

Many people fear dying *alone* in a care facility, out of contact with loved ones and perhaps without any other human being present. In some intensive care settings the patient may be denied much of the important contact he needs with loved ones. In some settings only "immediate family" is admitted. This is unfair in instances where patients have no immediate family and in those instances where relatives are not the most significant persons in a patient's life. *We should never assume that we know who is most significant for another person, but rather we should let him identify who is most important for him and closest to him.*

If patients fear dying alone or out of contact with loved ones, this needs to be discussed and appropriate plans implemented. Let the patient state who he would like to have with him if possible and make plans to contact that person. In all instances assure the patient that he will not die alone, and then make every effort to see that this does not happen. It helps if the nurse makes a point of stopping in to see a terminally ill person at times when he has not specifically summoned her. This gives confidence to the patient that he is indeed being thought of and looked out for.

Some patients fear *dying with strangers looking after them.* It may help terminally ill patients with this fear if they are assigned to the same nurses instead of a rotating staff. While an assignment to one nurse may be more comfortable for the patient, the increased intensity of the relationship may make it difficult for the individual nurse. Obviously patient and nurse need to be compatible, and this is an important consideration in planning staff assignments. Assignment to the same nurse on each shift can help reduce feelings of strangeness and depersonalization in a care facility. Thus, the patient's security may increase as he comes to have significant others on the staff.

In some care facilities terminally ill persons are *isolated* in private rooms. Often the rooms occupied by the dying tend to be avoided. Studies[75] have noted that nurses tend to unconsciously express their aversion to death by being slow to answer the calls of patients near death. Recognizing this natural tendency, nurses assigned to terminally ill persons must *consciously* try to increase their responsiveness to these patients.

A dying patient who is experiencing *pain* or *discomfort* can be made more comfortable psychologically if he knows that the nurse will work with him and make every effort to keep him as comfortable as possible. The patient gains some feeling of *control* if he knows his statements about pain or discomfort are not merely dismissed as "complaints," but rather are heard and understood and responded to by staff members. Interaction is thus important in this area of care; merely carrying out physical aspects of care is not enough. Examples of some statements which may be helpful are: "I can tell that you are uncomfortable: what do you think might help?" "Tell me exactly how you are feeling and together we will try to find out what might be helpful." "Now that we have changed your position are you still uncomfortable anywhere?" "Let me try something new and will you tell me if it helps?" "How are you feeling since having your pain medication?"

Loneliness is often the companion of the dying. In an attempt to reduce loneliness, the thoughtful nurse *sits down* beside her patient periodically rather than standing and looking down at him all of the time. She might plan specific times to sit with the patient and may tell him in advance so he can look forward to her coming. Visits from volunteers and other patients may be helpful for some persons. In long-term care facilities, patients commonly support one another, often becoming quite close. (An important point to remember: when a patient dies in a long-term care facility, other patients may grieve and be in need of support.)

Companionship can reduce loneliness and fear. The companions need not always talk. The mere physical presence of another human being can be comforting.

The needs of the dying were summed up for us for all times in the simple words "Watch with Me." This did not mean "take away"; it could not have meant "understand"; and it did nothing to explain or to seek an explanation. Its simple command was "Be there." If we are ready to "be there" as another person, as well as to "be there" as a skilled and understanding professional, we will experience something of the human spirit and what it can achieve. As we see them "living with dying," I think we are led to believe that we are seeing glimpses of another dimension in which both living and dying are fulfilled beyond time.[134]

One must also consider respecting the need for *privacy* in the dying. Privacy, without loneliness, is essential. Too often the dying are shut off and avoided in the guise of "providing privacy." Patients' needs for privacy with loved ones and privacy from observation by strangers need to be respected and provided for.

Some dying persons express fears about how their bodies will be dealt with after death. A patient may fear *invasion of his body* after death and may request that he not be embalmed or that autopsy not be performed. Another patient may not want *cremation* or may not want the opposite, to be *buried*. All of these concerns can be minimized by planning with the patient to meet his expressed wishes.

It is to be expected that many dying persons are deeply concerned about the *welfare of their significant others*. Some persons will want to tend to legal matters before they die, e.g., matters concerning estates, wills, etc. It may be comforting for the patient and his life partner to discuss and plan together some future actions, such as children's education, investments, where the surviving member will be living, management of income. The dying person may also want to review what he would like done with his possessions. All of these matters may provide opportunity for the nurse to be helpful when appropriate. Referrals may be made for a visiting nurse at home so the patient will feel less burdensome to his family in some aspects of his care or a referral may be made to a social worker. The nurse may talk with the patient about his planning and may contact religious advisors if requested. These are but a few examples of ways in which the nurse can help a dying patient handle his concerns about his significant others.

Assisting with Grieving

It is common practice to assist with the grieving of the loved ones of a person who has died or is dying. However, it has been only in recent years that recognition has been given to the fact that the dying person is himself experiencing a grieving process which may be even more profound.

However it is expressed, the major crisis *appears* to be not so much a fear of death, per se, but the intense pain of separation from everyone and everything one has ever loved. Hence, to speak of the "fear of death" may prove to be a misnomer, it is not so much a fear of life ending, but the pain which comes from breaking love bonds and commitments which causes intense suffering for the dying patient. . . . In the single act of dying he loses not just a person he loves, he loses everything . . . and he loses his life![53]

As previously discussed (see Table 49–1), the nurse assists the dying person as he moves psychologically through the various stages of dying identified by Kübler-Ross. The nurse also helps the patient's significant others move through these stages and she recognizes that she is herself experiencing many of the feelings related to the various stages. Just as the nurse helps the patient and his loved ones, so, in turn, must she be helped and supported. Commonly the patient's significant others and the nurse are *slower* to move through the stages than the patient; they lag behind his psychologic state. The skillful nurse recognizes what is occurring. She is familiar with the various stages and how they might be behaviorally expressed. She also recognizes her powerful position to facilitate or hinder the movement of others (including the patient) through the difficult stages. Thus the skilled nurse is not only familiar with helpful responses, but she also recognizes those responses that impede progression. It is essential that the nurse realize that the behaviors expressed in the various stages are *not* abnormal, e.g., a psychiatric referral need not be made merely because the dying patient is angry and depressed. (See also Chap. 48.)

Unfortunately, it is not uncommon to observe dying persons who are "psychologically disinherited" by significant others and staff, long before death occurs. Let us strive to remember the essential fact that the dying are *living* until they die—and should be treated accordingly. We need to show respect for a person's life regardless of its time limit. Present time should not be devalued merely because there is little expectation for a long-range future.

IMPENDING DEATH: PROVIDING PHYSICAL CARE

While a nurse cannot control the inevitability of death, there is much that she *can* control in attempting to make the final stages of life as satisfying as possible for the terminal patient. In previous sections of this chapter we have discussed many aspects of providing psychologic care for the dying person and his significant others. Here our emphasis is primarily on physical care. Of course, in practice, both aspects are interrelated.

Cautiously, and with sensitivity, try constantly to discern what the dying person is physically capable of doing: when he needs to be dependent and when it is best to encourage or allow independence. The skillful nurse helps terminally ill persons to be independent and in control for as long as possible; they will *need* to be dependent soon enough. When dependency is necessary, it is handled in ways that preserve the patient's self-respect and dignity and that do not call undue attention to his need to be dependent.

Help to maintain the dying patient's physical appearance, bodily functions and activities of daily living for as long as feasible. Tub baths, showers, exercises, getting up and dressed, shampoos, shaves, and hair sets—*all* should be continued as long as appropriate without unduly fatiguing the patient.

By focusing on the *present*, the nurse can help to make the dying patient's life as natural as possible. Actually we all live only in the present; although we may recall the past or try to think ahead to the future, we really only *live* in each present moment. The dying person is no different in that respect. (We do not mean that he is to be forced to live in the present and denied opportunities to discuss the future as he wishes.)

We all want to be physically more comfortable, and we are typically more or less in constant motion in an effort to attain comfort. We change our position, comb our hair, brush our teeth, take a bath, and so on, to attain physical comfort. Much can be done to help the dying patient stay physically comfortable when he can no longer help himself, if you try to anticipate what he needs and what would be helpful. Remember to do the "minor" activities that we all do frequently throughout the day to feel physically refreshed, e.g., wash hands. (Basic patient hygiene is discussed in Chap. 27.)

A summary of some changes that may occur with approaching death and with death are presented in Table 49–2. Appropriate care is discussed below.

Nursing Actions in the Care of the Terminally Ill*

Facial Appearance and Sight, Speech, and Hearing. Remove *dentures* if they obstruct breathing, contribute to nausea, or do not fit prop-

---

*Chap. 33 discusses minimizing the hazards of immobility. Refer to Chap. 21 for discussions of biomechanics, positioning and moving patients.

erly. Lubricate the patient's lips. Close the patient's mouth if it is open following death; place a rolled towel under his chin to keep his mouth closed. As *vision* fails, communicate more with speech and touch. Tell the patient what you are doing. Keep the room comfortably illuminated; prevent bright lights from shining in the patient's face. If the patient's eyes are open during terminal stage, protect them with normal saline pads or protective ophthalmic ointment.

TABLE 49–2.   CHANGES THAT OCCUR WITH APPROACHING DEATH AND AFTER DEATH

A. Facial Appearance, and Sight, Speech, and Hearing: Facial muscles relax; cheeks become flaccid, moving in and out with each breath. Facial structure may change so dentures cannot be worn. With dentures removed, mouth structure may collapse, lips pucker and sink in. Loss of muscle tone and anemia cause *facies hippocratica:* prominent cheeks and chin; pinched sharp nose; pale ashy skin; and sunken, glazed eyes. Sides of nose draw in with each inspiration. *Sight* gradually fails. Patient instinctively turns toward light; eyes may remain half open and glazed. With death, pupil fixes and does not react to light. *Speech* becomes increasingly difficult, confused, or unintelligible, and finally impossible. *Hearing* is believed to be the sense retained longest.

B. Skin and Muscular-Skeletal System: Muscles relax gradually, lose their irritability, and patient is increasingly less able to move. Lips first lose reflexes, sensation and ability to move. Following death, muscles become fixated. *Rigor mortis* occurs: stiffening of body, beginning a few hours following death, starting with jaw and progressing successively down body. Immediately following death, body movement of muscles may occur. With death's approach, *skin* may become pale, cool, covered with profuse perspiration, and extremities mottled; all owing to peripheral circulatory failure. Following death, body cools rapidly initially, then gradually reaches environmental temperature.

C. Respiratory System: As respiratory system progressively fails, respirations become: irregular, Cheyne-Stokes; rapid and shallow, or very slow. Respirations may be noisy (stertorous) if patient unable to handle respiratory secretions. Patient may become unable to swallow; gag reflex disappears. Oxygen lack (due to circulatory and respiratory failure) is ultimate cause of death.

D. Central Nervous System: Mental status varies from mental clarity to coma. Reflexes and pain (if present due to pathology) are gradually lost. Restlessness may occur owing to need for oxygen and sensation of heat experienced although body surface is cooling. Consciousness is lost with death; reflexes are absent.

E. Circulatory System: Circulatory changes cause alterations in temperature, pulse, and respiration as circulatory system gradually fails. Rapid, irregular pulse may precede death. Radial pulse gradually fails; once it stops, apical heart rate may continue briefly. Usually heart beats a while following cessation of respirations. Following death, blood may settle, causing *postmortem hypostasis:* bruise-like red or blue discolorations.

F. Gastrointestinal and Genitourinary Systems: Hiccoughs, nausea, vomiting, and weight loss may occur. Impaction, urine retention, distention, and bladder and bowel incontinence may be present. Decreasing peristalsis prevents stomach from emptying its contents into intestine; stomach thus distends with whatever is swallowed. Impaction may occur because of lack of energy needed to evacuate bowels. Incontinence is due to relaxation of anal and bladder sphincters.

After death, close the patient's eyes by gently pushing down on his eyelids. Keep a flashlight and ophthalmoscope at bedside for use in determining death. As *speech* fails, anticipate needs that the patient cannot express; continue to talk to him although he cannot reply. Since *hearing* remains longer than might seem obvious, speak to the patient as you approach his bed and say only what is appropriate for the patient to hear when in his presence. Speak clearly, close to the patient when making statements directed to him. Avoid whispering. Continue to comfort the patient by telling him when you are about to do something, even though he appears unable to hear you.

Skin and Muscular-Skeletal System. Patients in terminal stages of illness may be markedly "wasted" physically and lack sufficient adipose tissue to cushion bony prominences. Careful, frequent *skin inspection* and *care* are essential over all bony prominences. Pad the bedpan for emaciated patients. Weakened patients who cannot turn themselves should be placed on alternating pressure mattresses. Pad bony prominences. Make every effort to *prevent* decubitus ulcers; they are physically and mentally distressing, contributing to body image changes and a sense of despair about dying.

Patients greatly appreciate being comfortably *positioned and frequently turned.* Movements should be accomplished as smoothly and effortlessly as possible so that the patient's increasing dependency is not emphasized. A patient having terminal cancer should be turned by two persons, even though he may not weigh much. Painful metastasis to the bone is common, and therefore smooth, gentle handling is important. Proper positioning can greatly lessen pain. Even though it may be initially painful for a patient to be moved, he may feel markedly better a few minutes after turning than he did before he was turned. It is essential to use ample pillows, pads, towels, trochanter rolls, and so forth, to position patients correctly. Remember to use proper biomechanics as you handle patients who are physically dependent. Doing so will not only reduce your fatigue but may also prevent injury to you or the patient.

Continue *range-of-motion* exercises as long as the doctor believes it is advisable. Although the patient may see little purpose in this, such exercises may prevent discomforts of inactivity, e.g., aching, contractures, and so on. Exercises are carried out with the goal of maintaining

present comfort in this situation, rather than enabling future function.

Keep the patient with *diaphoresis* dry, also his gown and bed. Following death, place the patient in good body alignment as much as possible.

Respiratory System. It is distressing to feel *short of breath.* Thus, the terminally ill patient who is alert, apprehensive, restless, and short of breath may be given inhalation therapy to ease his discomfort. However, this would not be given to prolong the life of a comatose patient expected to die. Elevation of the patient's head and shoulders may make breathing easier. Keep room air as fresh as possible with comfortable circulation.

In the final stages of life the patient may be unable to move his secretions by coughing, swallowing, and turning in bed. As a result, his respirations become noisy (stertorous), and periodic suctioning is required. Keep suctioning equipment available and suction gently, as necessary, to keep the patient comfortable. Avoid letting the patient remain too long in one position because this encourages pooling of secretions; keep him positioned on his sides rather than flat on his back. (Chap. 36 discusses support of respiratory function.)

Carefully observe the patient's respirations. Morphine may be given in an attempt to slow rapid respirations and prevent regurgitation and coughing. When respirations are very shallow, a mirror held up to the patient's nose and mouth may indicate if he is breathing; the clouding of the mirror with moisture indicates that he continues to breathe. Ultimately, respirations cease. (Monitoring respiration is discussed in Chap. 29.)

Central Nervous System. Some patients are alert and mentally clear until the moment of death; others may be confused, delirious, or only partially conscious; still others are comatose and unresponsive to external stimuli. Continuously evaluate the patient's mental status; plan care accordingly. For example, protect the restless patient with side rails and provide supervision.

If the patient is conscious, assess the necessity for blankets according to what he says is comfortable. Even though his skin may feel cool to you, the patient may feel quite warm. Too many covers can increase restlessness. Avoid exposing the patient; see that he is covered at least with a sheet.

Circulatory System. Follow the progression of the patient's circulatory vital signs. Have a stethoscope and sphygmomanometer at the bedside. Check both apical and radial pulse; when the radial pulse ceases, continue to listen to the apical. Following death, elevate the patient's head and shoulders to prevent discoloration of the face due to *postmortem hypostasis*. (Pulse and blood pressure are discussed in Chap. 29.)

Gastrointestinal and Genitourinary Systems. Often the terminally ill are nauseated and perhaps vomiting. They may ultimately be unable to tolerate food or oral liquids and may be placed on intravenous therapy. Give oral liquids cautiously, checking first for the presence of the gag reflex if in doubt about the patient's ability to swallow. This can be done as unobtrusively as possible while giving mouth care. The patient may drown from oral liquids if the gag reflex is absent and he cannot swallow. Terminal patients may be very thirsty because of diaphoresis. Some patients receive IV therapy to relieve thirst at the time of terminal care. Carry out IV therapy as ordered and monitor it carefully. A restless patient may dislodge the IV needle, causing painful infiltration. (See Chaps. 24, 38 and 39.)

Give frequent oral hygiene. If the patient is conscious and able to handle secretions, mouthwash may be used. Glycerin and lemon juice swabs are useful for persons who are semiconscious or unconscious. (Oral hygiene is discussed in Chap. 27.)

Terminal patients may require assistance with drinking and eating. It may be helpful to give liquids from a teaspoon with the patient turned slightly onto one side. One of the most common causes of death in chronic illness is starvation. Attractive food service with foods served at their proper temperatures, small amounts of alcoholic beverages, medications, and mouth care are all activities that can help to stimulate the appetite. Moreover, the patient should ideally receive food when it is best for *him* rather than when it is most convenient for the staff. The patient's food preferences should be observed and if he is hungry for some special food item it should be prepared for him if possible. Intake, output, and weight should be recorded and subjected to careful evaluation. (See Unit VII.)

Change of position and medications may help to control nausea and vomiting. Antiemetics may be given 30 to 45 minutes before meals. Other activities that may help to reduce nausea are to keep 7-Up, ginger ale, crackers, and ice chips at the bedside and to order small but frequent servings of food. Avoid jarring the patient, as this can upset a nauseated patient to the point of provoking vomiting.

Elimination can cause severe distress for the weakened, terminally ill. Common problems are: constipation, impaction, urine retention, distention, and bladder and bowel incontinence. Analgesics may cause constipation and the patient may lack the energy to evacuate his bowels. Palpate the bladder to detect urine re-

tention; check for abdominal distention; observe for signs of fecal impaction. Each of these problems should receive appropriate treatment; each should be *prevented* if possible. The incontinent patient requires frequent and thorough skin, perineal, and catheter care. Every effort should be made to reduce both the physical and mental distress that incontinence can cause. (See Chap. 30, Maintaining Bowel and Kidney Functions, and Chap. 40 for discussion of patients with urethral catheters).

General Care. Hospital routines may need modifications for the terminal patient. The skillful nurse makes every attempt to modify her care to maintain a patient's welfare rather than for purposes of nursing convenience. For example, the patient who is restless from pain and bed rest should not be awakened for early morning care; his hours of pain and discomfort are long enough and he should be allowed to wait to be washed and have his linens changed when he awakens. Moreover, it might be that the patient sleeps poorly at night and is in need of sleep. (See Chap. 26, Promoting Rest and Sleep, and Chap. 34, Providing Pain Relief.)

Rest periods need to be planned with the patient. A sign posted on the door when a patient is resting may spare him unnecessary interruptions or noises, e.g.: "Mr. Johnson is resting from 1 to 2 this afternoon. Please do not disturb him." However, he should not feel ignored or forgotten. It is possible to greatly relieve a patient's apprehensions by letting him know that you are "keeping in touch with him." For example, drop in and visit at times when the patient hasn't called you so he won't feel he must call each time he needs help. He may feel relieved to know that you are watching out for him in the event tht he should be unable to call you. Often it is reassuring for the patient to know that you are periodically stopping by his bed, even though he is sleeping. For example you might say, "I came in to see how you were several times while you were resting. Now that you are awake is there anything you would like?"

Because the terminally ill person may tire easily, the nurse may need to limit visitors and to space procedures to prevent undue fatigue. The patient is kept physically clean, but a "total bath" may not be necessary, and may be too painful or fatiguing. Limiting visitors must be done thoughtfully, bearing in mind the patient's wishes and remembering that he and his loved ones must soon be permanently separated in this life.

Dressings are changed as frequently as necessary, and the atmosphere around the patient is kept fresh, without draft, comfortably lit, and quiet. Even though every effort is made to keep the patient and the environment clean, there may be situations in which distressing odors are present and pleasant air sprays may be helpful. These should be used as discreetly as possible to lessen the patient's feeling that he is offensive. (See Chap. 25, Providing a Safe and Therapeutic Environment.)

All unnecessary or soiled equipment should be removed from the room. Perhaps the patient will enjoy having some familiar objects in his room, and these should be permitted as much as possible.

In managing the pain, nausea, and other problems of the terminally ill, the nurse will have opportunity to ease patients' discomforts by skillfully administering medications so that they will be most effective. Her consultations with physicians regarding the effectiveness of medications will help to keep orders current with patients' changing needs.

Pain of increasing intractability and severity will be a source of great distress for some patients. Pain control should be as intensive as possible; that is to say, the nurse should employ all her nursing skills to control it, and not rely just on medications.

A question that has long concerned people is whether or not the act of dying is itself painful.

An expert on pain, Dr. W. K. Livingston, has discussed this question in the following way in a classic article:

I am convinced that neither a dying man nor a person undergoing anesthesia feels any pain, though their groans and body movements, those physical manifestations which we so naturally associate with pain, may seem to support the contrary view.

With these convictions I can tell the man who fears death will be painful that dying is merely the closing event in a sequential loss of function which accompanies brain depression. . . . A dying man may welcome death because it offers his exhausted body rest. Before all his senses fail, before he loses all power of speech and movement, before his heart stops beating, long before his nerves lose their capacity to transmit pain signals, the ability of the brain to translate these signals into pain perception has been lost. For pain is a product of consciousness in which the essential element is awareness.[95]

THE MOMENT OF DEATH

Is he then dead?
What, dead at last, quite, quite forever dead?

WILLIAM CONGREVE—The Mourning Bride

The fear of premature pronouncement of death has always worried man and indeed this has occasionally happened. Thus, pronouncement of the moment of death must be a procedure which follows established guidelines, policies and a thorough examination for signs of death. Likewise, most of us are concerned about what will be done with our bodies after death. After-death care of the body is thus also subject to protective procedures and regula-

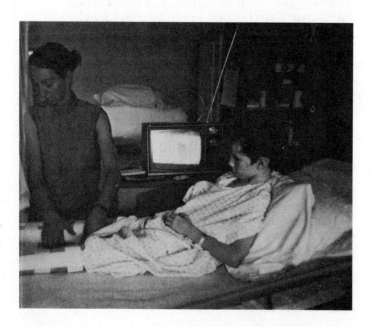

Figure 49–3. It is important for parents to be informed and involved in the care of children who have life-threatening illnesses. In some settings all medical records are open to parents, meetings are held with parents, parents may live in the hospital, and patients, parents and staff all share the ward day room. (From Shuman, R.: *Day by Day.* San Francisco, Scrimshaw Press, 1977.)

tions. The reader is directed to observe those policies established in her place of practice.

There are certain situations in which it is particularly difficult to decide whether or not a person is actually dead, i.e., whether or not the "moment of death" has been reached. Some of these situations are: (a) when the patient's vital functions are being maintained by artificial means, (b) in patients in cataleptic, hypnotic, hypothermic or drugged states, (c) in infants striving to survive birth, (d) in patients with animation suspended following electric shock, and (e) in persons so ill that signs of life may barely flicker.

While "death" has been defined as the *final* cessation of the vital functions, the problem of determining the moment of death has become increasingly difficult in care centers due to the use of artificial and mechanical means to maintain vital functions, e.g., respirators, pacemakers, defibrillators. Moreover, at times the problem of determining the moment of death is compounded by the need to obtain suitable tissues or organs (for grafting or transplant purposes) from persons who have just died. These tissues must be rapidly obtained following death before degenerative changes can set in.

There are situations where a patient's tissues are maintained temporarily in a living state and his vital functions are mechanically assumed for purposes of treatment or in the hope that these functions will recover sufficiently for necessary surgery to be performed. Our abilities to scientifically prolong life create problems in determining when such prolongation actually becomes inhumane and unreasonable.

A crucial question is: *When patients are being kept alive by artificial means, when and how is it determined to stop the machines and let them die?* An equally important question is: *When and how is it decided to not use "heroic" measures even initially to prolong life?*

These critical decisions are ideally best made by the patient in consultation with his physician; however this ideal state is often not possible. It is extremely helpful to care-givers and the patient's significant others when the patient's wishes on this matter are known. Some persons, concerned that their dying may be prolonged, sign *living wills* (see Fig. 49–4) and give copies of these to their physician and significant others. These may be obtained free from the Euthanasia Education Council, 250 W. 57th St., New York, NY 10019.

In the absence of a statement from the patient, the physician makes individual judgments about when it is not in a patient's best interests to keep him alive. The patient's questionable, faint hold on life is then released as gently and comfortably as possible. For example, persons with evidence of severe brain damage following cardiac arrest are usually not kept alive by mechanical means; the machines are disconnected and the patient is allowed to die. And cardiopulmonary resuscitation is typically not employed with persons expected to die, for whom there is no expectation of recovery (see also Chap. 35).

The only certain criterion for determining death is failure to spontaneously respond to resuscitation and, ultimately, production of a still electrocardiogram and electroencephalogram. Obviously it is not possible to run an electrocardiogram and electroencephalogram on every person to determine death. However, these procedures should be carried out in a hospital when death is doubtful, or when they are the established procedure. Out-patients in doubtful states of death may be given resuscitation and admitted to a hospital for tests by electrical detectors. In cases of hypothermia or profound drug coma, for example, a weak heart beat may be imperceptible for several hours by means of a stethoscope; however, life may still be present.

In more usual situations, when death is expected, the nurse remains with the patient and monitors his vital signs as she provides care. The physician may have left word whether or not he wants to be called concerning the vital sign changes as they occur. A stethoscope, sphygmomanometer, flashlight, and ophthalmoscope are usually placed at the bedside of the patient near death for use in assessing vital signs and determining moment of death. It is usually established procedure that a physician pronounce a patient dead. In a care facility when a patient's vital signs cease, the time is charted, the patient is screened (if this has not already been done), the physician is notified and someone is left in attendance with the body.

The *classic signs of death* are: absence of pulse, heartbeat and respirations; red blood cells rolling to a stop or forming rouleaux in the retinal vessels (as observed via ophthalmoscope); and pupils of the eye becoming fixed and nonreactive to light shined into them (flashlight). While the absence of reflexes is another sign of death, it should be realized that reflexes may be elicited long after death.

Examination of the patient for signs of death should be carried out in a quiet place since it is necessary to continue listening for some minutes with a stethoscope. *All* of the signs should

TO MY FAMILY, MY PHYSICIAN, MY LAWYER, MY CLERGYMAN
TO ANY MEDICAL FACILITY IN WHOSE CARE I HAPPEN TO BE
TO ANY INDIVIDUAL WHO MAY BECOME RESPONSIBLE FOR MY HEALTH, WELFARE OR
AFFAIRS

Death is as much a reality as birth, growth, maturity and old age—it is the one certainty of life. If the time comes when I, _____ can no longer take part in decisions for my own future, let this statement stand as an expression of my wishes, while I am still of sound mind.

If the situation should arise in which there is no reasonable expectation of my recovery from physical or mental disability, I request that I be allowed to die and not be kept alive by artificial means or "heroic measures". I do not fear death itself as much as the indignities of deterioration, dependence and hopeless pain. I, therefore, ask that medication be mercifully administered to me to alleviate suffering even though this may hasten the moment of death.

This request is made after careful consideration. I hope you who care for me will feel morally bound to follow its mandate. I recognize that this appears to place a heavy responsibility upon you, but it is with the intention of relieving you of such responsibility and of placing it upon myself in accordance with my strong convictions, that this statement is made.

Signed _____

Date _____

Witness _____

Witness _____

Copies of this request have been given to _____

_____

_____

_____

Figure 49–4. This form is called a "Living Will." It expresses formally the signer's wish to not have "heroic" life-prolonging measures used in the event of an irreversible illness. (Reprinted with permission from the Euthanasia Educational Council, New York, NY.)

be carefully assessed by the physician, since they may be difficult to discern. For example, the pulse may be so faint it is difficult to be certain whether it is present or absent; the heartbeat may also be difficult to detect if weak and may be intermittent or suspended; pupil reactions may be fixed by fear, drugs or injury. A mirror may be held close to the patient's nose and mouth in an attempt to discern if he is breathing (if so the mirror may become clouded and moist); however, this may be difficult to determine.

Because the examination is a difficult one to conduct, for the reasons just mentioned, and because it is such an important one, the nurse may assist by keeping the room as quiet as possible, preventing interruptions and having the necessary equipment available. Of course, the examination for death and the after-death care should be carried out with respect for the patient's dignity. Following the examination, the patient's significant others are notified if this has not already been done. They may be with the patient, or if they are not, they may want to come to be with the patient at the care facility before the body is transferred to a funeral home or morgue. Both physician and nurse complete necessary paper work for the patient's record, and the physician signs a death certificate.

Many authorities on grieving state that it is helpful to survivors if they can view the body of the deceased. If possible before the patient's significant others view him, it is desirable to remove equipment, tubes, etc. (not dressings), and straighten up the room and bed environments. The visible body parts are washed if necessary, the hair combed, and one pillow placed beneath the head. Follow institutional policies concerning aftercare of the body, e.g., concerning insertion of dentures and preparation of the body for transfer.

In talking about the sudden deaths of children Kübler-Ross comments:

After sudden death, it's especially important that the family be allowed to see the corpse. Otherwise peope can have prolonged, pathological grief. . . . If the body is mutilated, bandage the mutilated parts. Even if the whole face is bandaged, it's OK. As long as the family see a familiar scar, or something that they can identify, or if they can touch the person and know it is truly their daughter or son, they can face the reality of death.[85]

When a patient dies in a care facility, the patient's significant others can be asked if they would like to spend some time with the deceased and if so, whether they would like someone to accompany them into the room. Often a dimly lit room is most appropriate.

Survivors frequently find it comforting to learn some details about the patient's final moments. These details are, of course, personalized. While your remarks are based on the truth, it is unnecessary to provide detail about situations of discomfort. Depending on the circumstances, you might make remarks such as: "He died quite peacefully, holding my hand." "A calm look came into his eyes." "He spoke your name." "He said. . . ." "Everything possible was done by everyone who was here." "He wasn't left alone for a minute all evening until he died." "He was a strong man, but it was finally time for him to go." What you say to the patient's loved ones at this time can be a source of great comfort to them and can be a final privileged service which you can provide for the patient.

I would give *anything* to stand in your place. I would give anything to look at her face. To hold her, to comfort her—to take her home! Will one of you help? Will you? Can I count on you . . . strangers all . . . will just one of you comfort her? She's tiny, she's small. Or, must she turn from this bed where I now lie dead, and face the final insult . . . the pain that is too much . . . alone? Will she feel your indifference as you hand her the plastic bag with my clothes? If it is there, she *will* know it. For, she is sensitive you see. That's one of the qualities I love about her. And now, that sensitivity will cause her to hurt. She's bent now, and broken with grief . . . but, remember she's not blinded. I would give *anything* to put my arms around her, to lead her gently from this room of death. Oh, . . . won't you . . .?

CARING FOR THE PATIENT'S SIGNIFICANT OTHERS

At least, my dear,
You did not have to live to see me die . . .
The most I ever did for you was to outlive you
But that is much.

EDNA ST. VINCENT MILLAY*

It is the ultimate gift of love when one can shepherd another through dying and to a peaceful death. To do so requires releasing the dying person from earthly life. Often, however, a surviving person is unable to accept the impending loss of the dying person and as death approaches she tries to tighten even more firmly her grip on his fading life. With gentleness and skill a nurse can help to separate familiar hand from familiar hand, supporting each person so each can embark with relative strength, dignity and peace on their separate journeys. The survivor requires support to "survive"; the dying person needs a reliable companion to keep the pace with him as he approaches death. The nurse can help both in their separate tasks. Also, perhaps most importantly, she can help them to recognize that they are not abandoning one another. But rather, they are moving together through this final life process, the course of which neither has the power to change . . . and, they are doing it quite well.

As previously mentioned, the nurse finds out from the dying person who his "important people" (significant others) are. It is particularly important to do this when the patient is an adult who is unmarried. Once identified, the nurse may find that both the dying person and his loved ones want her to act as "mediator"

---

*Collected Poems of Edna St. Vincent Millay, Harper & Row, 1956.

and "facilitator" between them during their time of mutual grief.

Often realization of the separation which death will bring is stunning, and there may be an inability for patient and his loved ones to communicate for a while. Realizing that they will soon be forced apart, they may find it initially unbearable to be together. The nurse talks with both the patient and his significant others. She ascertains how they are viewing the impending death and what their specific concerns are. Then she works to find ways of helping to reduce the identified concerns. Often merely having the chance to talk with a nurse reduces the tensions enough that the dying person and his loved ones are able to begin to talk with one another about the crisis in their situation. It may be helpful for a dying person and his loved ones to realize that the love which is present between them need not die merely because they will no longer be physically present for one another.

When *young children* will be surviving a parent, the considerate nurse talks with the surviving parent about how he or she is managing at home and how the children seem to be reacting. The nurse may help the parent to recognize and understand how the children may be thinking about the loss of their mother or father. The nurse also helps the surviving parent to think about ways in which the children's lives may be changed by the death of one parent. A child who strongly resembles the dying parent may be smothered with affection by the surviving parent. Or, it may be that because of his or her intense grieving the surviving parent rejects the children, wishing only that the dying husband or wife could live.

Young children may feel that the death of a parent is a loss which they somehow precipitated. They may think they were "left" (abandoned) because their parent did not love them or that because they were "bad" they drove the dying parent away. Surviving young children may believe that their own anger at their deceased parent (which all children experience in growing up, as parents tell them how to behave) "killed" the parent, e.g., that their *wishes* that the parent "were dead" actually killed the parent. Such magical thinking is common and can make a child feel guilty about the death of the parent and responsible for it. When appropriate, the nurse may work directly with the children in assisting them with their grieving.

As Kübler-Ross's observations point out (see Table 49–1), often the dying gradually withdraw and no longer feel the need to remain with the living. They prepare to face the final step of death alone . . . as they must ultimately.

The nurse recognizes, as she helps the patient's significant others through their individual stages of grieving, that *they will probably move through the stages more slowly than the patient*. Thus, the patient may have reached a stage of acceptance and be ready to die, while his spouse may still be in a stage of denial, anger, bargaining or depression. The dying person may feel greatly distressed and "pulled" between living and dying if his loved ones cannot accept his death. For example, loved ones may want a dying patient to keep undergoing additional procedures which might keep him alive for a while longer, e.g., surgery, chemotherapy. Or, loved ones may make remarks to the patient such as, "You simply *must* stay alive, I can't make it without you!"

When the dying patient has reached the stage in preparatory grief of acceptance, and he is more withdrawn than he has been and is not really in need of much interaction, remember to continue to give attention and support to his significant others. Help them to understand that the patient's detachment does not mean rejection of them, but rather is an indication that he is beginning to accept his death. "His outer detachment matches his inner renouncement of what once mattered to him. . . Hence, he needs much less contact with family and friends."[48]

The patient's wishes should be respected concerning whom he wants to see during his remaining time. The nurse may need to help those persons the patient feels he has terminated with (and, hence, does not want to see) to understand that he is not rejecting what they have had in life together. Rather, he is dying now and in need of the privacy he has chosen.

At times during the final stages of illness, when death is imminent, loved ones may be hesitant or uncomfortable in entering the patient's room alone. They may also fear being left alone with the patient. If this appears to be the situation, the nurse may offer to enter the room with the visitor and demonstrate how she may be summoned if needed, e.g., call bell, intercom. Or, she might offer to remain in the room.

The nurse can frequently assist the patient's close survivors in carrying out his religious desires or in managing after-death details. In the terminal stages of his illness if the patient's loved ones seem to want to do something for the patient (e.g., participate in his care), the nurse provides direction and suggestion concerning ways in which they might help make him more comfortable. For example, "He seems more peaceful when you hold his hand. Would you like to sit in a chair close by his bed?" "He seems very warm, perhaps you would like to sponge his face and hands a bit." "He is wanting sips of water. Perhaps you can help him with that."

Above all, the dying patient's loved ones should not be made to feel that they are an intrusion. Their "complaints" need to be examined closely and understood as expressions of frustration and helplessness when that is the case. The dying person is not "owned" by the staff who cares for him, yet he is sometimes treated as if he were. Consideration needs to be given to the important bonds formed in his pre-illness life.

The dying patient's significant others are in frequent need of the direction and concern of the nurse. Small acts of kindness and thoughtfulness are often appreciated. "You have been here a long time. Could I direct you to the cafeteria?" "I'm concerned about you. Would you like to sit down in the lounge for a few moments and talk?" "Are you familiar with the hospital? Do you know where the telephones, rest rooms, lounges and cafeteria are?" "You seem tired; would you like some coffee?" "How can I help?" Remarks such as these are comforting and helpful. Helping *doesn't* take a lot of time.

The nurse who shows consideration of a patient's significant others is often indirectly providing additional comfort to the patient. Seeing the concern of others for his loved ones may provide some solace to the patient who finds himself helpless to ease their anguish.

Let us remember to take advantage of opportunities to compliment dying patients and their significant others on their strengths and uniqueness. We all are helped by hearing from others about what we do well or about what other people enjoy in us. In appropriate ways we can thank the people we professionally give care to for what they give us of themselves and for what they teach us. Patients and visitors are too often the only ones to say "Thank-you" in their interactions with nurses.

Kübler-Ross comments:

It's most difficult for people whose loved ones die suddenly. They can't finish unfinished business. They can't tell their lost one, "I love you." What I try to teach people is to live in such a way that you say those things while the other person can still hear it. What do you think dying people teach you? They teach you how to live. That's all. I mean, if I die today after having told my family "I love you," I've said it. If I got home and found that a loved one had died, I'd say, "Thank heavens I've said all those things I've always wanted to say."[85]

CONCLUSION

As the reader will observe, much of the nurse's assistance to the dying individual involves recognition of the fact that man is, as we said in the beginning of this text, a "dream animal." That is, he has the gift of an intellect which allows him to wonder about things. He can think ahead in time and image himself and others in a variety of situations . . . and thus he appears to differ from other creatures and has excelled over them.

However, in contemplating his death, the intellect of man may not be uplifting to him at times, but rather may pull him down into states of despair, fear and disillusionment. He can recognize the existential dilemma of life (although he may not do so in those actual terms): a man finds himself in a life that he did not choose to enter and that he can leave only by dying and he knows he will die.

Death is puzzling to the "dream animal." As a scientific man, he feels uncomfortable in his lack of knowledge. As an intellectual man he is baffled, for he likes to be able to understand his life and maintain control. As a loving man, he finds himself bereft by the death of loved ones. Death has distressed and hurt him in his life. In dying and approaching his own death he needs to be helped with his feelings as well as helped physically.

While man can foresee his own death, he is often not helpless in dying in the way that other animals are. He has some powers to control his dying and some choices to make about it. For example, he can take his own life; or he can use his ability to philosophize or use his religious faith to spiritually and intellectually face death. Also, a man need not die alone and without the help of others if it is known that he is dying. Thus, in dying he can help himself and be helped.

A summary of care of the dying has been expressed as follows:

1. Sharing the responsibility for the crisis of dying with the patient so that he has help in dealing with the first impact of anxiety and bewilderment.
2. Clarifying and defining the realities of the day-to-day existence which can be dealt with by the patient. These are the realities of his daily life.
3. Making continued contact available and rewarding.
4. Assisting in the separation from and grief over the realistic losses of family, body-image and self-control, while retaining communication and meaningful relationships with those who will be lost.
5. Assuming necessary body and ego functions for the person without incurring shame or depreciation,

maintaining respect for the person, and helping him maintain his self-respect.

6. Encouraging the person to work out an acceptance of his life situation with dignity and integrity so that gradual regression may occur without conflict or guilt.[116]

Providing the kind of complete care described in this chapter for a dying person and his significant others "may pose a burden to the nurse's time and even her psyche, but this is also her challenge as a professional committed to the highest standards of nursing."[53]

It is not easy to care for the dying—to give them the nursing care and support that they are entitled to have and need. Patients who die may not make us "feel good" as nurses, as do those who recover and bolster our feelings of healing omnipotence. Other people's deaths influence us and we feel their loss. John Donne wrote, "Any man's death diminishes me because I am involved in Mankind." Such losses hurt. Nevertheless, it would not be possible to feel losses from terminally ill persons if we had not experienced gains from those same individuals.

There comes a time to die. It is as natural to die as it is to be born and to breathe. The acts of life are all interrelated, and in many ways there is a natural progression toward death throughout life.

The dying person begins to return to a state of being at one with the world where there is a helplessness and timeless existence, where I (the ego) and you (outer world) no longer are differentiated. At this point, one is rapidly approaching the state of surrender to the process of renunciation of life and return to union with the earth out of which we have sprung. Indeed, psychic death is now acceptable, desirable, and now at hand.[116]

BIBLIOGRAPHY

1. Annas, G. J.: Rights of the terminally ill patient. *Journal of Nursing Administration*, 4:40–44, March–April, 1974.
2. Anonymous: Notes of a dying professor. *Nursing Outlook*, 20:502–506, Aug. 1972.
3. Aries, P.: *Western Attitudes Toward Death*. Baltimore, The Johns Hopkins University Press, 1974.
4. Armstrong, M. E.: Dying and death—and life experiences of loss and gain: a proposed theory. *Nursing Forum*, 14:95–104, No. 1, 1975.
4a. Autonomy, authenticity, ethics and death. *Emergency Medicine*. 10:148–151, Feb. 1978.
5. Bahra, R. J.: The Potential for Suicide. *American Journal of Nursing*, 75:1782, Oct. 1975.

6. Baker, J., and Sorensen, K.: A patient's concern with death. *American Journal of Nursing*, 63:90, July 1963.
7. Barbus, A. J.: The dying person's bill of rights. *American Journal of Nursing*, 75:99, Jan. 1975.
8. Bassett, S. D.: Death, dying, and grief: a personal view. *Texas Reports on Biology and Medicine*, 32:347–350, Spring 1974.
9. Beauchamp, J. M.: Euthanasia and the nurse practitioner. *Nursing Forum*, 14:56–73, No. 1, 1975.
10. Beaumont, E., and Wiley, L. (eds.): Innovations in nursing: what should hospitals do with the dying? *Nursing '73*, 3:45, July 1973.
11. Benoliel, J. Q.: Talking to patients about death. *Nursing Forum*, 9:254–268, No. 3, 1970.
12. Benoliel, J. Q.: The concept of care for a child with leukemia. *Nursing Forum*, 11:194, No. 2, 1972.
12a. Berg, D. L., and Isler, C.: The right to die dilemma: Where do you fit in? *RN*, 40:48–54, Aug. 1977.
13. Black, P. M. L.: Criteria of brain death: review and comparison. *Postgraduate Medicine*, 57:69–74, Feb. 1975.
14. Blewett, L. J.: To die at home. *American Journal of Nursing*, 70:2602, Dec. 1970.
15. Bliss, V. J.: Sharing another's death. *Nursing '76*, 6:30, April 1976.
15a. Brimigion, J.: Living with dying. *Nursing '78*, 8:76–79, Sep. 1978.
16. Brower, R. H., and Miner, E.: *Japanese Court Poetry*. Stanford, CA, Stanford University Press, 1961.
17. Browning, M. H., and Lewis, E. P. (comp.): *The Dying Patient: A Nursing Perspective*. New York, The American Journal of Nursing Company, 1972.
18. Bunch, B., and Zahra, D.: Dealing with death: The unlearned role. *American Journal of Nursing*, 76:1486, Sep. 1976.
19. Burgess, K. E.: The Influence of Will on Life and Death. *Nursing Forum*, 15:238–258, No. 3, 1976.
20. Burkhalter, P. K.: Fostering staff sensitivity to the dying patient. *Supervisor Nurse*, 6:54–59, April 1975.
21. Calderaro, P.: A time to die. *American Journal of Nursing*, 77:861, May 1977.
22. Campbell, M. A.: On dying. *American Journal of Nursing*, 75:796, May 1975.
23. Cawley, M.: Euthanasia: should it be a choice? *American Journal of Nursing*, 77:859, May 1977.
24. Craig, D. B.: The good days of life—and the last. *RN*, 39:51–56, April 1976.
25. Craven, J., and Wald, F. S.: Hospice care for dying patients. *American Journal of Nursing*, 75:1816, Oct. 1975.
26. Creighton, H.: Brain death. *Supervisor Nurse*, 7:47, March 1976.
27. Creighton, H.: Choose life or let die? *Supervisor Nurse*, 6:12–14, Aug. 1975.
28. Cutter, F.: *Coming to Terms With Death*. Chicago, Nelson-Hall Co., 1974.
29. Daniels, J.: The victory. *Nursing '76*, 6:39, May 1976.
30. *Dealing with death and dying*. (Nursing '77 Skillbook Series). Jenkintown, PA, Intermed Communications, 1977.
31. de Beauvoir, S.: *A Very Easy Death*. New York, Warner Communications Co., 1973.
32. Delbridge, P. M.: Identifying the suicidal person in the community. *The Canadian Nurse*, 70:14–17, Nov. 1974.
33. Denton, J. A., and Wisenbaker, V. B., Jr.: Death experience and death anxiety among nurses and nursing students. *Nursing Research*, 26:61–64, Jan.–Feb. 1977.
34. Des Pres, T.: *The Survivor: An Anatomy of Life in the Death Camps*. New York, Oxford University Press, 1976.

35. Diran, M. O. K.: You can prevent suicide. *Nursing '76,* 6:60–64, Jan. 1976.
36. Donovan, M. I., and Pierce, S. G.: *Cancer Care Nursing.* New York, Appleton-Century-Crofts, 1976 (Chap. 3, Dying).
37. Edwards, J.: The nursing challenges of OB: when the baby is stillborn. *RN,* 34:44, Nov. 1971.
38. Fallon, B.: "And certain thoughts go through my head." *American Journal of Nursing,* 72:1257, July 1972.
39. Feifel, H., and Branscomb, A. B.: Who's afraid of death? *Journal of Abnormal Psychology,* 81:282, June 1973.
40. Fischer, H. K., and Olin, B. M.: Psychogenic determination of time of illness or death by anniversary reactions and emotional deadlines. *Psychosomatics,* 13:170, May–June 1972.
41. Fletcher, J.: Ethics and euthanasia. *American Journal of Nursing,* 73:670, April 1973.
42. Fox, D., et al.: *Satisfying and Stressful Situations.* In *Basic Programs in Nursing Education.* New York, Bureau of Publications, Teachers College, Columbia University, 1964.
43. Fox, N. L.: A good birth, a good life, why not a good death? *The Journal of Practical Nursing,* 24:19, Oct. 1974.
44. French, J., and Schwartz, D. R.: Home care of the dying in two cultures. *American Journal of Nursing,* 73:502, March 1973.
45. Friedman, S. B.: After sudden death. *Emergency Medicine,* 6:53, Sep. 1974.
46. Garland, D.: The care of the dying. *Nursing Times,* 64:355, March 1968.
47. Gelein, J. L.: Needs of the terminally ill aged. *In ANA Clinical Sessions, 1972, Detroit.* New York, Appleton-Century-Crofts, 1973.
48. Goleman, D.: We are breaking the silence about death. *Psychology Today,* 10:44, Sep. 1976.
49. Gottheil, E. W., McGurn, C., and Pollak, O.: Truth and/or hope for the dying patient. *Nursing Digest,* 4:12, March–April 1976.
50. Griffin, J. J.: Family decision: a crucial factor in terminating life. *American Journal of Nursing,* 75:794, May 1975.
51. Grollman, E. A. (ed.): *Concerning Death: A Practical Guide for the Living.* Boston, Beacon Press, 1974.
52. Guimond, J.: We knew our child was dying. *American Journal of Nursing,* 74:248, Feb. 1974.
53. Gullo, S. V.: Thanatology: the study of death and the care of the dying. *Bedside Nurse,* 5:11–14, 1972.
54. Hirsh, H. L.: Brain death. *In Medical Trial Technique Quarterly 1975 Annual.* Chicago, Callaghan & Company, 1975.
55. Halacki, S.: A lesson you won't learn in lectures. *RN,* 39:46, May 1976.
56. Hancock, S.: A death in the family: a lay view. *British Medical Journal,* 1:29–30, Jan. 1973.
57. Hardgrove, C., and Warrick, L. H.: How shall we tell the children? *American Journal of Nursing,* 74:448, March 1974.
58. Hendrickson, S.: A philosophy of death made personal. *American Journal of Nursing,* 76:90, Jan. 1976.
59. Heusinkveld, K. B.: Cues to communication with the terminal cancer patient. *Nursing Forum,* 11:105, No. 1., 1972.
60. Hinton, J.: Assessing the views of the dying. *Social Science & Medicine,* 5:37, Feb. 1971.
61. His own executioner. *Emergency Medicine,* 6:24, Jan. 1974.
62. Hiscoe, S.: The awesome decision. *American Journal of Nursing,* 73:291, Feb. 1973.
63. Hobbins, W. B.: What is a day of life worth? *RN,* 38:33, April 1975 (includes 4 parts; four distinctive views of the dying patient).
64. Isler, C.: Breaking down the barriers to total cancer nursing: approaching the final days. *RN,* 41:63–65, April 1978.
65. Jackson, P. L.: The child's developing concept of death: implications for nursing care of the terminally ill child. *Nursing Forum,* 14:204–215, No. 2, 1975.
66. Janzen, E.: Relief of pain: prerequisite to the care and comfort of the dying. *Nursing Forum,* 13:48–51, No. 1, 1974.
67. Johnson, P.: Just what is life? *Nursing '76,* 6:28–29, June 1976.
68. Johnson, P.: The long, hard dying of Joe Rodriguez. *American Journal of Nursing,* 77:54, Jan. 1977.
69. Jourard, S. M.: Suicide: an invitation to die. *American Journal of Nursing,* 70:269–275, Feb. 1970.
70. Jung, C.: The soul and death. *In* Feifel, H. (ed.): *The Meaning of Death.* New York: McGraw-Hill Book Co., 1959.
71. Kastenbaum, R.: On death and dying: should we have mixed feelings about our ambivalence toward the aged? *Journal of Geriatric Psychiatry,* 7:94–107, No. 1, 1974.
72. Kavanaugh, R. E.: Dealing naturally with dying. *Nursing '76,* 6:21–29, Oct. 1976.
73. Kavanaugh, R. E.: Helping patients who are facing death. *Nursing '74,* 4:35–42, May 1974.
74. Kittleson, J. A.: Nursing experience: in spite of everything Tommy died in peace. *RN,* 41:97, Feb. 1978.
75. Kneisl, C. R.: Dying patients and their families: how staff members can give support. *Hospital Topics,* 45:37, Nov. 1967.
76. Kneisl, C. R.: Thoughtful care for the dying. *American Journal of Nursing,* 68:550–553, March 1968.
77. Kobrzycki, P.: Dying with dignity at home. *American Journal of Nursing,* 75:1312, Aug. 1975.
78. Krant, M. J.: *Dying and Dignity.* Springfield, IL, Charles C Thomas, Publishers, 1974.
79. Kübler-Ross, E.: *Death: The Final Stage of Growth.* Englewood Cliffs, NJ, Prentice-Hall, Inc., 1975.
80. Kübler-Ross, E.: Dying with dignity. *The Canadian Nurse,* 67:31–35, Oct. 1971.
81. Kübler-Ross, E.: How to face death. *Seattle Post-Intelligencer, Northwest Today,* June 8, 1969; June 15, 1969, June 22, 1969.
82. Kübler-Ross, E.: Letter to a nurse about death and dying. *Nursing '73,* 3:11–13, Oct. 1973.
83. Kübler-Ross, E.: *On Death and Dying.* New York, The Macmillan Co., 1969.
84. Kübler-Ross, E.: What is it like to be dying? *American Journal of Nursing,* 71:54, Jan. 1971.
85. Kübler-Ross, E., and Goleman, D.: "The child will always be there, real love doesn't die." *Psychology Today,* 10:48–52, Sep. 1976.
86. Lacasse, C. M.: A dying adolescent. *American Journal of Nursing,* 75:433, March 1975.
87. Lande, S.: A gift of hope. *American Journal of Nursing,* 77:639, April 1977.
88. Larsen, K. S., et al.: Attitudes toward death: a desensitization hypothesis. *Psychological Reports,* 35:687–690, Oct. 1974.
88a. Lee, A.: The Lazarus syndrome: Caring for patients who've 'returned form the dead'. *RN,* 41:53–64, June 1978.
89. LeRoux, R. S.: Communicating with the dying person. *Nursing Forum,* 16:144–155, No. 2, 1977.
90. LeShan, L., and LeShan, E.: Psychotherapy and the patient with a limited life span. *Psychiatry,* 24:318, 1961.

91. Lester, D., Getty, C., and Kneisl, C. R.: Attitudes of nursing students and nursing faculty toward death. *Nursing Research, 23*:50–53, Jan.–Feb. 1974.

92. Levine, C. W.: The dying patient: can you help when you care too much? *Nursing '77, 7*:40, March 1977.

93. Lewis, F. M.: A time to live and a time to die: an instructional drama. *Nursing Outlook, 25*:762, Dec. 1977.

94. Lifton, R. J., and Olson, E.: *Living and Dying.* New York, Praeger Publishers, 1974.

95. Livingston, W. K.: What is pain? *Scientific American Reprint,* March 1953.

96. Marino, E. B.: Vinnie was dying. But he wasn't the problem. I was. *Nursing '74, 4*:46–47, Feb. 1974.

97. Martin, L. B., and Collier, P. A.: Attitudes toward death: a survey of nursing students. *Journal of Nursing Education, 14*:28–35, Jan. 1975.

98. Martinson, I. M., et al.: Home care for the dying child. *American Journal of Nursing, 77*:1816, Nov. 1977.

99. Martinson, I. M.: Why don't we let them die at home? *RN, 39*:58, Jan. 1976.

100. Maxey, D.: In the presence of death, a determined fight for life. *Psychology Today, 10*:57–61, Sep. 1976.

101. Maxwell, S. M. B.: A terminally ill adolescent and her family. *American Journal of Nursing, 72*:925, May 1972.

102. McCorkle, R.: The advanced cancer patient: how he will live—and die. *Nursing '76, 6*:46–49, Oct. 1976.

103. McGuire, M. A.: Have you ever let a patient die by default? *RN, 40*:56, Nov. 1977.

104. Miya, T. M.: The child's perception of death. *Nursing Forum, 11*:214–220, No. 2., 1972.

105. Montagu, A.: *Immortality.* New York, Grove Press, 1955.

106. Moody, R. A., Jr.: *Life After Life.* New York, Bantam Books, 1975.

107. Muslin, H. L., Levine, S. P., and Levine, H.: Partners in dying. *American Journal of Psychiatry, 131*:308–310, March 1974.

108. Northrup, F. C.: The dying child. *American Journal of Nursing, 74*:1066, June 1974.

109. Notes and quotes: Bar Association suggests change in legal definition of death. *RN, 38*:29–30, May 1975.

110. Noyes, R., Jr.: The art of dying. *Perspectives in Biology and Medicine, 14*:432–447, Spring 1971.

111. Nursing '74 Questionnaire: Probe: death & dying: how do you really feel about it? *Nursing '74, 4*:58–63, Nov. 1974.

112. Oraftik, N.: Only time to touch. *Nursing Forum, 11*:205–213, No. 2, 1972.

113. O'Sullivan, D. D.: Post-mortem investigation of death. *In Medical Trial Technique Quarterly 1974 Annual.* Chicago, Callaghan & Company, 1974.

114. Owens, N. F.: The patient's right to live: critical aspects of nurse intervention in radical treatment. *In ANA Clinical Sessions,* 1972, pp. 149–156.

115. Paige, R. L., and Looney, J. F.: Hospice care for the adult. *American Journal of Nursing, 77*:1812, Nov. 1977.

116. Pattison, M.: The experience of dying. Paper presented at Institute, *Death: Children and Adults,* University of Washington, School of Nursing, May 12–13, 1966.

116a. Pennington, E. A.: Postmortem care: More than ritual. *American Journal of Nursing, 78*:846–847, May 1978.

117. Popoff, D., and Nursing '75: What are your feelings about death and dying? Part 1. *Nursing '75, 5*:15–24, Aug. 1975.

118. Popoff, D., and Nursing '75: What are your feelings about death and dying? Part 2. *Nursing '75, 5*:55–62, Sep. 1975.

119. Popoff, D., and Nursing '75: What are your feelings about death and dying? Part 3. *Nursing '75, 5*:39–50, Oct. 1975.

120. Prattes, O. R.: Helping the family face an impending death. *Nursing '73, 3*:17–20, Feb. 1973.

121. Preston, C. E.: Behavior modification: a therapeutic approach to aging and dying. *Postgraduate Medicine, 54*:64–68, Dec. 1973.

122. Proulx, J. R.: Ministering to the dying: a joint pastoral and nursing effort. *Hospital Progress, 56*:62–63, March 1975.

123. Pruitt, R. D.: Death as an expression of functional disease. *Mayo Clinic Proceedings, 49*:627–634, Sep. 1974.

124. Quint, J. C.: Obstacles to helping the dying. *American Journal of Nursing, 66*:1568, July 1966.

125. Quint, J. C.: *The Nurse and the Dying Patient.* New York, The Macmillan Co., 1967.

126. Rachels, J.: Active and passive euthanasia. *New England Journal of Medicine, 292*:78, 1975.

127. Raft, D.: How to help the patient who is dying. *American Family Physician, 7*:112–115, April 1973.

128. Reynolds, D. K., and Kalish, R. A.: The social ecology of dying: observations of wards for the terminally ill. *Hospital and Community Psychiatry, 25*:147–152, March 1974.

129. Rinear, E. E.: The nurse's challenge when death is unexpected. *RN, 38*:50–55, Dec. 1975.

130. Robinson, L.: *Liaison Nursing: Psychological Approach to Patient Care.* Philadelphia, F. A. Davis Co., 1974 (Chap. 12, The Dying Patient).

131. Robinson, L.: "We have no dying patients." *Nursing Outlook, 22*:651–653, Oct. 1974.

132. Rosenthal, T.: *How Could I Not Be Among You?* New York, George Braziller, 1973.

133. Russell, R.: The choice. *Nursing '75, 5*:19, July 1975.

134. Saunders, C.: Living with dying. *Man and Medicine, 1*:227–242, Spring 1976.

135. Saunders, C.: The last stages of life. *American Journal of Nursing, 65*:70–75, March 1965.

136. Schroeder, O. C., Jr. (ed.): Suicide: a dilemma for medicine, law and society. *Postgraduate Medicine, 53*:55–57, Jan. 1973.

137. Schulz, R., and Aderman, D.: Clinical research and the stages of dying. *Omega, 5*:137–143, No. 2, 1974.

138. Schwartz, R. S.: On sudden, unexpected death. *In Lane, F. (ed.): Medical Trial Technique Quarterly 1975 Annual.* Chicago, Callaghan & Company, 1975.

139. Seldon, E.: . . . Even the elderly, *RN, 39*:66–70, Jan. 1976.

140. Shneidman, E. S. (ed.): *Death: Current Perspectives.* Palo Alto, CA, Jason Aronson, Inc., 1976.

141. Shusterman, L. R.: Death and dying: a critical review of the literature. *Nursing Outlook, 21*:465–471, July 1973.

142. Shusterman, L. R., and Sechrest, L.: Attitudes of registered nurses toward death in a general hospital. *Psychiatry in Medicine, 4*:411–426, Fall 1973.

143. Sobel, D. E.: Death and dying. *American Journal of Nursing, 74*:98, Jan. 1974.

144. Sorensen, K., and Baker, J.: Curriculum implications for student-patient verbal interaction about death. *In* Pesznecker, B. L., and Hewitt, H. E. (eds.): *Psychiatric Content in the Nursing Curriculum.* Seattle, University of Washington Press, 1963.

145. Stolorow, R. D.: A note on death anxiety as a developmental achievement. *American Journal of Psychoanalysis,* 34:351–353, Winter 1974.

146. Storlie, F.: Gloria. *American Journal of Nursing,* 75:118, July 1975.

147. Sumner, F., and Gwozdz, T.: A nurse for suicidal patients. *American Journal of Nursing,* 76:1792, Nov. 1976.

148. Thanatology, death and modern man. *Time,* November 20, 1964.

149. Timmons, A. L.: Is it so awful? *American Journal of Nursing,* 75:988, June 1975.

150. Toole, J. F.: The neurologist and the concept of brain death. *Perspectives in Biology and Medicine,* 14:599–607, Summer 1971.

151. Ufema, J. K.: Dare to care for the dying. *American Journal of Nursing,* 76:88, Jan. 1976.

152. Ufema, J.: Do you have what it takes to be a nurse-thanatologist? *Nursing '77,* 7:96–99, May 1977.

153. Vaillot, M. C., Sr.: Living—hope: the restoration of being. *American Journal of Nursing,* 70:268–273, Feb. 1970.

154. Vollen, K. H., and Watson, C. G.: Suicide in relation to time of day and day of week. *American Journal of Nursing,* 75:263, Feb. 1975.

155. Waechter, E. H.: Children's awareness of fatal illness. *American Journal of Nursing,* 71:1168, June 1971.

156. Wagner, B. M.: Teaching students to work with the dying. *American Journal of Nursing,* 64:128, Nov. 1964.

157. Wahl, C. W.: Death. Lecture presented to nursing students, University of California at Los Angeles, 1957.

158. Walker, M.: The last hour before death. *American Journal of Nursing,* 73:1592, Sep. 1973.

159. Weber, L. J.: Ethics and euthanasia—another view. *American Journal of Nursing,* 73:1228, July 1973.

160. Weelis, A.: *The Quest for Identity.* New York, W. W. Norton and Company, Inc., 1958.

161. Weisman, A. D.: Coping with untimely death. *Psychiatry,* 36:366–378, Nov. 1973.

162. Weisman, A. D.: On death and dying. Does old age make sense? Decisions and destiny in growing older. *Journal of Geriatric Psychiatry,* 7:84–93, No. 1, 1974.

163. Weisman, A. D.: *On Dying and Denying: A Psychiatric Study of Terminality.* New York, Behavioral Publications, Inc., 1972.

164. Wentzel, K. B.: The dying are the living. *American Journal of Nursing,* 76:956, June 1976.

165. Westercamp, T. M.: Suicide. *American Journal of Nursing,* 75:260, Feb. 1975.

166. Westhoff, M. E.: Listening to relieve the fear of death. *Supervisor Nurse,* 3:80–87, March 1972.

167. Whitman, H. H., and Lukes, S. J.: Behavior modification for terminally ill patients. *American Journal of Nursing,* 75:98, Jan. 1975.

168. Wiley, L. (ed.): Salvaging an unwilling life. *Nursing '76,* 6:54–57, Feb. 1976.

169. Williams, R. H.: The end—of life in the elderly. *Postgraduate Medicine,* 54:55–59, Dec. 1973.

170. Wise, D. J.: Learning about dying. *Nursing Outlook,* 22:42–44, Jan. 1974.

APPENDIX
TABLES OF NORMAL VALUES*

ABBREVIATIONS USED IN APPENDIX

< = less than
> = greater than

kg = kilogram
gm = gram
cg = centigram
mg = milligram
µg = microgram
ng = nanogram
pg = picogram

L = liter
dl = deciliter
ml = milliliter
µl = microliter
nl = nanoliter
pl = picoliter

km = kilometer
m = meter
cm = centimeter
mm = millimeter

mEq = milliequivalent
IU = International Unit
mIU = milliInternational Unit
µIU = microInternational Unit
U = Unit
mOsm = milliosmole
M = mole
mM = millimole
µM = micromole

sec = second
msec = millisecond
min = minute
hr = hour

Conversions:
1 kg = 2.2 pounds (lb)
1 kg = 35.27 ounces (oz)
1 liter = 1.06 quarts (qt)
1 liter = 33.81 ounces
1 kilometer = 5/8 mile
1 meter = 39.37 inches
1 inch = 2.54 centimeters

*Adapted from Halstead, J. A.: *The Laboratory in Clinical Medicine: Interpretation and Application.* Philadelphia, W. B. Saunders Co., 1976, p. 792.

Hematologic Values (Adults)

Red blood cell count		Men: 4.6–6.2 million/ml
		Women: 4.2–5.4 million/ml
		Pregnancy: >3.6 million/ml
White blood cell count		4500–11,000/ml

Differential white blood cell count	Range in per cent	Range of absolute counts
Segmented neutrophils	55–75	1800–7000/ml
Bands	0–5	0–700/ml
Lymphocytes	25–45	1000–4000/ml
Monocytes	2–6	100–900/ml
Eosinophils	0.5–4	50–450/ml
Basophils	0.3	0–200/ml

Platelet count	150,000–400,000/ml
Hemoglobin	Men: 14.0–16.5 gm/100 ml
	Women: 12.6–14.2 gm/100 ml
	Pregnancy: >10.6 gm/100 ml
Hematocrit (packed cell volume, PCV)	Men: 42–52%
	Women: 37–47%
	Pregnancy: >34%
Reticulocyte count	0.2–2.0%

Red blood cell indices
Mean corpuscular volume (MCV)	82–92 cu μ
Mean corpuscular hemoglobin (MCH)	27–31 pg
Mean corpuscular hemoglobin concentration (MCHC)	32–36%

Blood volume (7–8% of body weight in kg)	Men: 69 ml/kg
	Women: 65 ml/kg
Plasma volume	Men: 44 ml/kg
	Women: 40 ml/kg
Red blood cell volume	Men: 26 ml/kg
	Women: 21 ml/kg
Erythrocyte sedimentation rate (ESR) (Westergren)	Men: 5–15 mm/hr
	Women: 10–25 mm/hr
Leukocyte alkaline phosphatase index	13–130 units

Osmotic fragility
Beginning hemolysis at	0.45–0.39 gm NaCl/100 ml
Complete hemolysis at	0.33–0.30 gm NaCl/100 ml

Haptoglobin	30–200 mg/100 ml (as hemoglobin binding)
Viscosity	1.4–1.8 times water

Normal differential count of bone marrow; 0.2 ml
  aspirated

Hemoglobin F	<2%
Hemoglobin A_2	1.5–3.5%

Coagulation tests
Bleeding time (Ivy)	1–6 min
Clotting time (Lee-White)	3–15 min
Clotting time (Silicone)	15–42 min
One-stage prothrombin time (to be compared with control)	12–14 sec
Kaolin—cephalin clotting time (activated partial thromboplastin time, PTT)	45–65 sec

Urine Measurements

Test	Type of Specimen	Normal Value	Comment
Acetone	Random	Negative	
Addis count	12-hr collection	WBC and epithelial cells: 1,800,000/12 hr RBC: 500,000/12 hr Hyaline casts: 0–5000/12 hr	Rinse bottle with some neutral formalin; discard excess
Albumin, qualitative quantitative	Random 24 hr	Negative 10–100 mg/24 hr	
Aldosterone	24 hr	2–26 μg/24 hr	Keep refrigerated
Amylase	24 hr	800–4200 Somogyi units per 24 hr	
Bence Jones protein	Random	Negative	
Bilirubin, qualitative	Random	Negative	
Blood, occult	Random	Negative	
Calcium, qualitative (Sulkowitch) Quantitative	Random 24 hr	1 + turbidity Average diet: 100–250 mg/24 hr Low calcium diet: <150 mg/24 hr High calcium diet: 250–300 mg/24 hr	Compare with standard
Catecholamines, total norepinephrine epinephrine	24 hr 24 hr 24 hr	<100 μg/24 hr <80 μg/24 hr <20 μg/24 hr	
Chloride	24 hr	110–250 mEq/24 hr	
Coproporphyrin	24 hr	34–234 μg/24 hr	Use fresh specimen and do not expose to direct light; preserve 24-hr urine with 5 gm Na_2CO_3
Creatine	24 hr	Male: 0–40 mg/24 hr Female: 0–100 mg/24 hr Higher in children and during pregnancy	
Creatinine	24 hr	Male: 20–26 mg/kg/24 hr 1.0–2.0 gm/24 hr Female: 14–22 mg/kg/24 hr 0.8–1.8 gm/24 hr	
Glucose, qualitative	Random	Negative	Not detectable by ordinary clinical qualitative techniques
Gonadotropins, pituitary (FSH and LH)	24 hr	10–50 mouse units/24 hr	
17-Hydroxycorticosteroids (Porter-Silber)	24 hr	2–12 mg/24 hr After 25 USP units ACTH, IM, a 2- to 4-fold increase	Keep refrigerated
5-Hydroxyindoleacetic acid (5-HIAA), qualitative	Random	Negative	Some muscle relaxants and tranquilizers interfere with test
Ketone bodies	Random	Negative	Fresh, keep cool
17-Ketosteroids	24 hr	Male: 8–23 mg/24 hr Female: 5–15 mg/24 hr Children: 12–15 yr, 5–12 mg/24 hr; <8 yr, <2 mg/24 hr After 25 USP units ACTH, IM: 50–100% increase	Keep refrigerated; tranquilizers interfere with test

Table continued on the following page

Urine Measurements — *Continued*

Test	Type of Specimen	Normal Value	Comment
Lead	24 hr	$<100~\mu g/24$ hr	
Osmolality	Random	500–800 mOsm/L	May be lower or higher, depending on state of hydration
pH	Random	4.6–8.0	
Phenolsulfonphthalein (PSP)	Urine, timed after 6 mg PSP IV		As screening procedure, the 15-min specimen alone is sufficient
	15 min	28–50% dye excreted	
	30 min	16–24% dye excreted	
	60 min	9–17% dye excreted	
	120 min	3–10% dye excreted	
Phenylpyruvic acid, qualitative	Random	Negative	
Phosphorus	Random	0.9–1.3 gm/24 hr	Varies with intake
Porphyrins, quantitative	24 hr		
Coproporphyrin		34–234 $\mu g/24$ hr	
Uroporphyrin		14–56 $\mu g/24$ hr	
Porphobilinogen		0–2.0 mg/24 hr	
Potassium	24 hr	40–80 mEq/24 hr	Varies with diet
Pregnancy tests	Concentrated morning specimen	Positive in normal pregnancies or with tumors producing chorionic gonadotropin	
Pregnanediol	24 hr	Male: 0–1 mg/24 hr Female: 1–8 mg/24 hr Peak: 1 week after ovulation Pregnancy: 60–100 mg/24 hr Children: Negative	Keep refrigerated
Pregnanetriol	24 hr	Male: 1.0–2.0 mg/24 hr Female: 0.2–3.5 mg/24 hr Children: <0.5 mg/24 hr	Keep refrigerated
Protein, qualitative	Random	Negative	
quantitative	24 hr	10–100 mg/24 hr	
Reducing substances, total	24 hr	0.5–1.5 mg/24 hr	
Sodium	24 hr	80–180 mEq/24 hr	Varies with dietary ingestion of salt
Specific gravity	Random	1.016–1.022 (normal fluid intake) 1.001–1.035 (range)	
Sugars (excluding glucose)	Random	Negative	
Titratable acidity	24 hr	20–50 mEq/24 hr	Collect with toluene
Urea nitrogen	24 hr	6–17 gm/24 hr	
Uric acid	24 hr	250–750 mg/24 hr	Varies with diet
Urobilinogen	2 hr 24 hr	0.3–1.0 Ehrlich units 0.05–2.5 mg/24 hr or 0.5–4.0 Ehrlich units/24 hr	
Vanillylmandelic acid (VMA)	24 hr	1.5–7.0 mg/24 hr	
Volume, total	24 hr	600–1600 ml/24 hr	
Zinc	24 hr	0.20–0.75 mg/24 hr	

Examination of Cerebrospinal Fluid

Opening pressure	Less than 200 mm H_2O
Color	Clear
Lumbar fluid	
Cells, adults	Less than 5 per cu mm, all lymphocytes
newborn	Less than 15 per cu mm, may be up to 60% polymorphonuclear cells
Protein	15 to 45 mg/100 ml
Gamma globulin	Less than 13% of the total protein (valid only when total protein between 20 mg/100 and 80 mg/100)
Qualitative test for globulins (Pandy test)	Negative
Colloidal gold	No figure greater than 2 in any tube
Glucose	Above 40 mg/100 ml (two-thirds of a concomitant fasting blood glucose if below 200 mg/100 ml)
Chloride	120–130 mEq/L
pH	7.31
Creatine phosphokinase*	Less than 5.5
Lactic dehydrogenase*	Less than 65
Glutamic oxaloacetic transaminase*	Less than 26

*Culebras-Fernándes, A., and Richards, N. G.: Cleveland Clin. Q., 38:113, 1971.

INDEX